Veterinary Parasitology

Professor Domenico Otranto
Professor of Parasitology and Parasitic Diseases of Animals
University of Bari, Italy

Distinguished Visiting Professor
Department of Veterinary Clinical Sciences
City University of Hong Kong

Professor Richard Wall
Professor of Zoology
University of Bristol, UK

Fifth Edition

WILEY Blackwell

This edition first published 2024
© 2024 John Wiley & Sons Ltd

Edition History
Longman Scientific and Technical (1e, 1987)
Blackwell Scientific Ltd (2e, 1996)
John Wiley & Sons Ltd (3e, 2007), (4e, 2016)

Registered Offices
John Wiley & Sons, Inc., 111 River Street, Hoboken, NJ 07030, USA
John Wiley & Sons Ltd, The Atrium, Southern Gate, Chichester, West Sussex, PO19 8SQ, UK

For details of our global editorial offices, customer services, and more information about Wiley products visit us at www.wiley.com.

Wiley also publishes its books in a variety of electronic formats and by print-on-demand. Some content that appears in standard print versions of this book may not be available in other formats.

Library of Congress Cataloging-in-Publication Data

Names: Otranto, Domenico, author. | Wall, Richard (Richard), author. |
   Veterinary parasitology.
Title: Veterinary parasitology / Professor Domenico Otranto, Professor
   Richard Wall.
Description: Fifth edition. | Hoboken, NJ : Wiley-Blackwell, 2024. |
   Preceded by Veterinary parasitology / M.A. Taylor, R.L. Coop, R.L. Wall.
   2016. | Includes bibliographical references and index.
Identifiers: LCCN 2024000397 (print) | LCCN 2024000398 (ebook) | ISBN
   9781394176342 (cloth) | ISBN 9781394176366 (adobe pdf) | ISBN
   9781394176359 (epub)
Subjects: MESH: Animals, Domestic–parasitology | Parasitic Diseases,
   Animal
Classification: LCC SF810.A3 (print) | LCC SF810.A3 (ebook) | NLM SF
   810.A3 | DDC 636.089/696–dc23/eng/20240124
LC record available at https://lccn.loc.gov/2024000397
LC ebook record available at https://lccn.loc.gov/2024000398

Cover Design: Wiley
Cover Images: Courtesy of Riccardo Paolo Lia, Domenico Otranto, and Richard L. Wall

Set in 9/11pt MinionPro by Straive, Pondicherry, India

Printed and bound in Great Britan by Bell & Bain Ltd, Glasgow

Contents

Preface to the fifth edition

This is a textbook for students, teachers and researchers in universities and institutes, veterinarians in practice and in government service, and others involved in any aspects of parasitic disease. The first edition was published in 1987 as a much slimmer volume, written by Professor G.M. Urquhart and others. Subsequently it has gone through a number of changes, with new editions published at approximately seven-year intervals. Each new edition has attempted to update developments in classification, diagnostics and treatment, while swelling in size as each attempted to become more comprehensive than the previous one and simultaneously address the requirements of its diverse readership. The latter creates an inherent tension in the book structure, associated with the fact that some readers are primarily interested in the biology of the parasites while others are more concerned with the pathological consequences of infestation and treatment of resultant disease. The first and second editions were structured entirely taxonomically; the third and fourth editions, led by Professor Mike Taylor, added a host and organ/system-based structure in addition to taxon-based chapters, while striving to be definitively comprehensive. However, this structure proved problematic for some readers.

In this fifth edition, therefore, we have attempted to reduce repetition, clarify, by removing some of the less important parasites, and divide the material more clearly into two parts. The first is a taxon-based overview of the biology of key parasites of veterinary importance, their life cycles, morphology, diagnosis and identification, along with the general principles of treatment and epidemiology. The second contains specific clinical details of the pathogenesis, epidemiology, control and treatment of individual parasite species, still structured by host and organ system. The result, we hope, is an edition that is easier for readers to navigate.

The classification of parasites has been updated to reflect many of the systematic changes. This is a rapidly developing field given the insights being provided by molecular genetics. As a result, throughout, synonyms have been provided and changes in classification are explained and matched with older nomenclature. However, ultimately, where various classification issues remain unsettled, the overriding principle to the nomenclature provided is to ensure clarity and consistency. This fifth edition also contains updated information, particularly relating to treatment and emerging parasites that have become more prevalent over the last decade. A novelty of this fifth edition is represented by new life-cycle figures, and the most exciting development is the addition of video-based practical guides that can be accessed by QR codes embedded in the text.

In considering treatment of parasitic infections, we have used the generic names of drugs to avoid listing the wide range of products currently marketed in different countries. Dose rates of drugs are not always stated as many vary from country to country, being influenced by the relevant regulatory authorities. In all cases, readers are advised to consult the manufacturer's data sheets for current information and local regulations.

Overall, while working on this fifth edition, we realised that one of the most important messages for readers is that parasitology is a science in constant evolution as it reflects the world where parasites and hosts live together.

This new edition combines the expertise of two of the leading international veterinary parasitologists.

Professor Domenico Otranto DVM, PhD, Diplomate European Veterinary Parasitology College (EVPC) is Professor of Animal Parasitic Diseases at the University of Bari and Distinguished Visiting Professor at the Department of Veterinary Clinical Sciences, City University of Hong Kong. He has been closely involved in promoting parasitology in various capacities, being also President of both the European Veterinary Parasitology College and the World Association for the Advancement of Veterinary Parasitology. His research focuses on the study of arthropods and arthropod-borne diseases in various countries of the world, from Brazil to China passing through the Mediterranean Basin and Middle East. He currently works on different aspects of canine and feline vector-borne diseases of zoonotic concern with both basic and applied approaches. In recent years, his activities have focused on research and education projects in low- and middle-income countries, as he has been part of many international boards to promote the One Health approach.

Professor Richard Wall graduated in zoology from the University of Durham followed by a PhD in insect population ecology at the University of Liverpool. He is Professor of Zoology at the University of Bristol. He specialises in the biology of arthropod ectoparasites and vectors, and has worked extensively on agents of myiasis, mange mites, lice and ticks. His research ranges widely from fundamental studies of arthropod taxonomy and physiology, through to field population ecology and farm-level investigations of the application of sustainable control technologies. He has taught extensively: entomology to biologists and parasitology to veterinary students. He has been closely involved in the work of the World Association for the Advancement of Veterinary Parasitology, in various capacities, for many years.

Acknowledgements

The authors were greatly assisted by many people, in particular:

Laura Rinaldi (University of Naples, Italy) added material on diagnostics to Chapter 4, building on the extensive contribution of Philip Skuse in the fourth edition. Emanuele Brianti (University of Messina, Italy) and Frédéric Beugnet (Boehringer Ingelheim Animal Health) added material on treatment for Chapter 5. Filipe Dantas-Torres (Aggeu Magalhaes Institute, Fiocruz, Brazil) checked the taxonomy and biological life cycles. Jairo Alfonso Mendoza Roldan (University of Bari, Italy) prepared the biological life cycle drawings and Nicole Szafranski assisted in the preparation of the biological life cycle text. Cinzia Cantacessi (University of Cambridge, UK) reviewed the biological life cycles and glossary. Giovanni Sgroi (Istituto Zooprofilattico Sperimentale del Mezzogiorno), Marielisa Carbonara, Iniobong Chukwuebuka Ugochukwu, Renata Fagundes Moreira, Viviane Noll Louzada Flores, Livia Perles, Rossella Samarelli, Pedro Paulo de Abreu Teles (University of Bari, Italy) and Emilia Rumsey (University of Bristol, UK) assisted in the edition of chapters. Grazia Greco (University of Bari, Italy) and Marialetizia Fioravanti (University of Bologna, Italy) advised on taxonomy.

We thank Antonio Varcasia, Francesca Nonnis and Claudia Tamponi (University of Sassari, Italy) oversaw the preparation of the videos. Ranju Manoj (Cornell University, USA), Hira Muqaddas (Women University Multan, Pakistan), Alicia Rojas (University of Costa Rica), Jairo Alfonso Mendoza Roldan (University of Bari, Italy) and Nicole Szafranski (University of Tennessee, USA) for their participation on the tutorial videos.

The whole collaborative work was supervised and coordinated by Marcos Antonio Bezerra Santos (University of Bari, Italy).

Finally, the authors are grateful to Elanco, Boehringer Ingelheim and Merck Sharp and Dohme for financial support for editorial assistance, figures and the creation of the videos.

August 2023

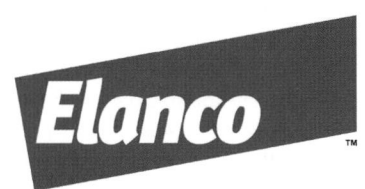 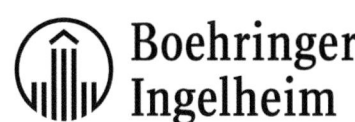 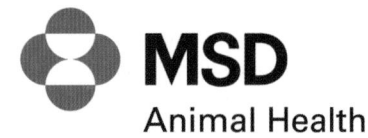

Introduction

In the context of this book, parasites are considered as organisms which live for a considerable portion of their lives in (endoparasites) or on (ectoparasites) another organism, the **host**. During this association, parasites are dependent on the host and benefit at the host's expense. They derive nutrition from the host and may also gain other benefits such as a protected habitat in which to grow and reproduce. This book also includes the arthropods that act as vectors of the pathogens that may cause disease.

The activity of parasites on or in their host results in direct harm to the host. If no harm ensues, the relationship is described as commensal. However, the harm that parasites cause their host is not always easy to demonstrate as an individual parasite may cause little or no measurable damage. Disease is frequently a population phenomenon, with small numbers of parasites having little discernible impact but large numbers causing effects ranging from subclinical damage to debilitating fatal disease. Relationships can also change from commensal to parasitic as a function of density. This change and resultant damage to the host may also result from the host's defence mechanisms reacting to the presence of parasites.

Many parasites are entirely dependent upon a specific host or hosts in order to complete their life cycle and survive, and these organisms are known as **obligate parasites** of that particular host. Where an organism can either act as a parasite or can survive or complete its life cycle independently from a host, then it is called a facultative parasite. There are instances where for various reasons parasites become established in hosts other than their definitive host and in which they cannot complete their normal life cycle. These hosts are termed **accidental hosts** and in the case of some zoonotic parasites of veterinary importance, humans are an example.

Every parasite must have at least one host in its life cycle and many species have several hosts. The host in which the parasite is best adapted and in which it develops to an adult or sexually mature stage and reproduces is known as the **definitive, primary** or **final** host. If there is only a single host in the life cycle, then transmission is said to be direct and the parasite to have a direct life cycle. Many parasites have more complex life cycles with additional hosts in which essential development to a new parasite stage occurs. These stages either do not reproduce or if they do, then it is by asexual multiplication. These hosts are known as **intermediate** or **transitional** hosts. Some of these hosts can also be vectors (such as ticks, mosquitoes), which carry and spread disease-causing parasites from one host to another. These life cycles with more than one host are known as **indirect** or **complex** life cycles.

There are some parasites that use additional hosts to overcome adverse environmental conditions or to increase the likelihood that the parasite will be transmitted to the definitive host. There is no further development of the parasite in these hosts. They are known as **paratenic** or **transport** hosts.

Part 1: Parasites and infection

1 VETERINARY HELMINTHOLOGY

Kingdom Animalia

Phylum	Class	Order (Suborder)	Superfamily	Family	Genus
Nematoda	**Chromadorea**	**Rhabditida (Rhabditina)**	**Trichostrongyloidea**	Trichostrongylidae	*Trichostrongylus*
					Marshallagia
					Hyostrongylus
					Mecistocirrus
					Graphidium
					Obeliscoides
					Libyostrongylus
					Graphinema
					Impalaia
					Ostertagia
					Teladorsagia
					Spiculopteragia
					Apteragia
					Camelostrongylus
					Haemonchus
				Cooperidae	*Cooperia*
				Amidostomidae	*Amidostomum*
					Epomidiostomum
				Molineidae	*Nematodirus*
					Nematodirella
					Lamanema
					Molineus
					Ollulanus
					Tupaiostrongylus
				Helligmoneillidae	*Nippostrongylus*
					Nematospiroides
				Ornithostrongylidae	*Ornithostrongylus*
				Dictyocaulidae	*Dictyocaulus*
			Strongyloidea	Strongylidae	*Codiostomum*
					Craterostomum
					Oesophagodontus
					Oesophagostomum
					Poteriostomum
					Strongylus
					Triodontophorus
					Cyathostomum
					Cylicocyclus
					Cylicodontophorus
					Cylicostephanus
				Chabertidae	*Agriostomum*
					Chabertia
				Syngamidae	*Cyathostoma*
					Mammomonogamus
					Syngamus
					Stephanurus
				Deletrocephalidae	*Deletrocephalus*
					Paradeletrocephalus
			Ancylostomatoidea	Ancylostomatidae	*Ancylostoma*
					Bunostomum
					Gaigeria
					Globocephalus
					Necator
					Uncinaria

	Diaphanocephaloidea	Diaphanocephalidae	*Kalicephalus*
	Metastrongyloidea	Metastrongylidae	*Metastrongylus*
		Protostrongylidae	*Cystocaulus*
			Elaphostrongylus
			Muellerius
			Neostrongylus
			Parelaphostrongylus
			Protostrongylus
			Spiculocaulus
			Varestrongylus
		Filaroididae	*Filaroides*
			Oslerus
		Angiostrongylidae	*Aelurostrongylus*
			Angiostrongylus
		Crenosomatidae	*Crenosoma*
			Troglostrongylus
	Rhabditoidea	Panagrolaimidae	*Halicephalobus*
		Rhabditidae	*Rhabditis*
		Rhabdiasidae	*Rhabdias*
	Strongyloidoidea	Strongyloididae	*Strongyloides*
Ascaridida	**Ascaridoidea**	Ascarididae	*Angusticaecum*
			Ascaris
			Baylisascaris
			Parascaris
			Polydelphus
			Porrocaecum
			Ophidascaris
			Toxascaris
			Toxocara
		Ascaridiidae	*Ascaridia*
		Heterakiidae	*Heterakis*
		Anisakidae	*Anisakis*
			Contracaecum
			Pseudoterranova
			Sulcascaris
		Raphidascarididae	*Hysterothylacium*
		Aspidoderidae	*Paraspidodera*
	Subuluroidea	Subuluridae	*Subulura*
Oxyurida	**Oxyuroidea**	Oxyuridae	*Aspiculuris*
			Dermatoxys
			Enterobius
			Oxyuris
			Passalurus
			Skrjabinema
			Syphacia
		Kathlaniidae	*Probstmayria*
		Pharyngodonidae	*Tachygonetria*
Spirurida	**Spiruroidea**	Spirocercidae	*Ascarops*
			Physocephalus
			Simondsia
			Spirocerca
			Streptoparagus
		Habronematidae	*Habronema*
			Draschia
			Parabronema
			Histiocephalus
		Gongylonematidae	*Gongylonema*
		Thelaziidae	*Oxyspirura*
			Thelazia

(Continued)

Kingdom Animalia *Continued*

Phylum	Class	Order (Suborder)	Superfamily	Family	Genus
				Gnathostomatidae	*Gnathostoma*
				Spiruridae	*Odontospirura*
					Protospirura
					Spirura
				Tetrameridae	*Tetrameres*
				Hartertiidae	*Hartertia*
				Pneumospiridae	*Metathelazia*
					Vogeloides
			Physalopteroidea	Physalopteridae	*Physaloptera*
			Dracunculoidea	Dracunculidae	*Avioserpens*
					Dracunculus
			Acuarioidea	Acuaridae	*Cheilospirura*
					Dispharynx
					Echinuria
					Streptocara
			Filarioidea	Filariidae	*Loa*
					Parafilaria
					Suifilaria
					Stephanofilaria
				Onchocercidae	*Acanthocheilonema*
					Brugia
					Cercopithifilaria
					Chandlerella
					Dirofilaria
					Dipetalonema
					Elaeophora
					Mansonella
					Onchocerca
					Paronchocerca
					Pelecitus
					Setaria
					Splendidofilaria
					Wuchereria
	Enoplea	Enoplida	**Trichuroidea**	Trichuridae	*Anatrichosoma*
					Trichosomoides
					Trichuris
				Capillariidae	*Capillaria*
					Eucoleus
			Trichinelloidea	Trichinellidae	*Trichinella*
			Dioctophymatoidea	Dioctophymatidae	*Dioctophyma*
					Eustrongyloides
					Hystrichis
Acanthocephala	**Archiacanthocephala**	**Oligacanthorhynchida**		Oligacanthorhynchidae	*Macracanthorhynchus*
					Oncicola
				Polymorphidae	*Polymorphus*
					Filicollis
Platyhelminthes	**Trematoda**	**Plagiorchiida**		Fasciolidae	*Fasciola*
					Fascioloides
					Fasciolopsis
				Paramphistomatidae	*Bothriophoron*
					Calicophoron
					Cotylophoron
					Gigantocotyle
					Paramphistomum
					Pseudodiscus
					Orthocoelium
				Gastrodiscidae	*Gastrodiscus*
					Homalogaster

		Gastrothylacidae	*Carmyerius*
			Fischoederius
			Gastrothylax
		Echinostomatidae	*Echinochasmus*
			Echinoparyphium
			Echinostoma
			Euparyphium
			Hypoderaeum
			Isthmiophora
		Philophthalmidae	*Philophthalmus*
		Cyclocoelidae	*Hyptiasmus*
			Typhlocoelum
		Notocotylidae	*Catatropis*
			Cymbiforma
			Notocotylus
			Paramonostomum
			Ogmocotyle
		Dicrocoeliidae	*Dicrocoelium*
			Eurytrema
			Platynosomum
		Paragonimidae	*Paragonimus*
		Nanophyetidae	*Nanophyetus*
		Collyriclidae	*Collyriclum*
		Prosthogonimidae	*Prosthogonimus*
		Plagiorchiidae	*Plagiorchis*
		Lecithodendriidae	*Novetrema*
			Odeningotrema
			Phaneropsolus
			Primatotrema
		Opisthorchiidae	*Apophallus*
			Clonorchis
			Cryptocotyle
			Opisthorchis
			Metorchis
			Parametorchis
			Pseudamphistomum
	Strigeidida	Brachylaemidae	*Brachylaemus*
			Postharmostomum
			Skrjabinotrema
		Heterophyidae	*Haplorchis*
			Heterophyes
			Metagonimus
			Pygidiopsys
		Schistosomatidae	*Austrobilharzia*
			Bilharziella
			Heterobilharzia
			Orientobilharzia
			Ornithobilharzia
			Schistosoma
			Trichobilharzia
		Diplostomatidae	*Alaria*
			Diplostomum
		Strigeidae	*Apatemon*
			Cotylurus
			Parastrigea
Cestoda	**Cyclophyllidea**	Taeniidae	*Taenia*
			Echinococcus

(Continued)

Kingdom Animalia *Continued*

Phylum	Class	Order (Suborder)	Superfamily	Family	Genus
				Anoplocephalidae	*Anoplocephala*
					Avitellina
					Cittotaenia
					Moniezia
					Paranoplocephala
					Stilesia
					Thysanosoma
					Thysaniezia
				Dipylidiidae	*Dipylidium*
					Diplopylidium
					Joyeuxiella
				Dilepididae	*Amoebotaenia*
					Choanotaenia
				Paruterinidae	*Metroliasthes*
				Davaineidae	*Cotugnia*
					Davainea
					Houttuynia
					Raillietina
				Hymenolepididae	*Fimbriaria*
					Hymenolepis
				Mesocestoididae	*Mesocestoides*
		Diphyllobothriidea		Diphyllobothriidae	*Diphyllobothrium*
					Spirometra

2 VETERINARY PROTOZOOLOGY

Kingdom Protozoa

Phylum	Class	Order	Family	Genus
Amoebozoa	**Archamoebea**	**Entamoebida**	Entamoebidae	*Endolimax* *Entamoeba* *Iodamoeba*
	Discosea	**Centramoebida**	Acanthamoebidae	*Acanthamoeba*
Percolozoa	**Heterolobosea**	**Schizopyrenida**	Vahlkampfiidae	*Naegleria*
Euglenozoa	**Kinetoplastea**	**Trypanosomatida**	Trypanosomatidae	*Leishmania* *Trypanosoma*
Metamonada	**Trichomonadea**	**Trichomonadida**	Trichomonadidae	*Tritrichomonas* *Trichomonas* *Tetratrichomonas* *Trichomitus* *Pentatrichomonas* *Cochlosoma*
			Dientamoebidae	*Histomonas* *Dientamoeba*
			Monocercomonadidae	*Monocercomonas* *Chilomitus*
			Hexamastigidae	*Hexamastix*
			Proteromonadidae	*Proteromonas*
	Trepomonadea	**Retortamonadida**	Retortamonadidae	*Retortamonas* *Chilomastix*
		Diplomonadida	Spironucleidae	*Spironucleus*
			Caviomonadidae	*Caviomonas*
			Enteromonadidae	*Enteromonas*
			Giardiidae	*Giardia*
	Anaeromonadea	**Oxymonadida**	Polymastigidae	*Monocercomonoides*
Apicomplexa	**Conoidasida**	**Eucoccidiorida**	Eimeriidae	*Caryospora* *Cyclospora* *Eimeria* *Hoarella* *Isospora* *Tyzzeria* *Wenyonella*
			Sarcocystidae	*Besnoitia* *Cystoisospora* *Hammondia* *Neospora* *Frenkelia* *Sarcocystis* *Toxoplasma*
			Lankesterellidae	*Lankesterella* *Schellakia*
			Klossiellidae	*Klossiella*
			Hepatozoidae	*Hepatozoon*
			Haemogregarinidae	*Haemogregarina*
		Cryptogregarinorida	Cryptosporidiidae	*Cryptosporidium*
	Aconoidasida	**Haemosporida**	Plasmodiidae	*Haemoproteus* *Hepatocystis* *Leucocytozoon* *Plasmodium*
		Piroplasmida	Babesiidae	*Babesia*
			Theileriidae	*Theileria* *Cytauxzoon*
Ciliophora	**Litostomatea**	**Vestibuliferida**	Balantidiidae	*Balantioides*
			Pycnotrichidae	*Buxtonella*
			Nyctotheridae	*Nyctotherus*

3 VETERINARY ENTOMOLOGY

Kingdom	Phylum	Class	Order	Suborder	Family	Genus
Animalia	Arthropoda	Insecta	Diptera	Nematocera	Ceratopogonidae	*Culicoides*
					Simuliidae	*Simulium*
					Psychodidae	*Phlebotomus* *Lutzomyia*
					Culicidae	*Aedes* *Anopheles* *Culex*
				Brachycera	Tabanidae	*Chrysops* *Haematopota* *Tabanus*
					Muscidae	*Musca* *Hydrotaea* *Stomoxys* *Haematobia*
					Fanniidae	*Fannia*
					Hippoboscidae	*Hippobosca* *Melophagus* *Lipoptena* *Pseudolynchia*
					Glossinidae	*Glossina*
					Calliphoridae	*Lucilia* *Calliphora* *Protophormia* *Phormia* *Cochliomyia* *Chrysomya* *Cordylobia*
					Sarcophagidae	*Sarcophaga* *Wohlfahrtia*
					Oestridae	*Oestrus* *Rhinoestrus* *Gedoelstia* *Cephenemyia* *Cephalopina* *Oedemagena* *Pharyngomyia* *Gasterophilus* *Hypoderma* *Przhevalskiana* *Cuterebra* *Dermatobia*
			Psocodea	Anoplura	Haematopinidae	*Haematopinus*
					Linognathidae	*Linognathus* *Solenopotes*
					Microthoraciidae	*Microthoracius*
					Polyplacidae	*Polyplax*
					Pedicinidae	*Pedicinus*
					Pediculidae	*Pediculus*
					Pthiridae	*Pthirus*
				Amblycera	Menoponidae	*Menacanthus* *Menopon* *Holomenopon* *Ciconiphilus* *Trinoton* *Amyrsidea*
					Boopidae	*Heterodoxus*
					Gyropidae	*Gyropus* *Gliricola* *Aotiella*
					Trimenoponidae	*Trimenopon*

		Ischnocera	Philopteridae	*Cuclotogaster*
				Lipeurus
				Goniodes
				Goniocotes
				Columbicola
				Struthiolipeurus
				Meinertzhageniella
				Dahlemhornia
				Tricholipeurus
				Anaticola
				Acidoproctus
				Anatoecus
				Ornithobius
				Lagopoecus
				Trichophilopterus
			Trichodectidae	*Felicola*
				Trichodectes
				Eutrichophilus
				Cebidicola
			Bovicolidae	*Bovicola*
	Siphonaptera		Ceratophyllidae	*Ceratophyllus*
				Nosopsyllus
			Pulicidae	*Ctenocephalides*
				Spilopsyllus
				Echidnophaga
				Pulex
				Xenopsylla
				Archaeopsylla
			Tungidae	*Tunga*
			Leptopsyllidae	*Leptopsylla*
	Hemiptera	**Heteroptera**	Cimicidae	*Cimex*
	Hemiptera	**Heteroptera**	Reduviidae	*Triatoma*
				Rhodnius
				Panstrongylus
Arachnida	**Sarcoptiformes**	**Astigmata**	Sarcoptidae	*Sarcoptes*
				Notoedres
				Trixacarus
			Psoroptidae	*Psoroptes*
				Chorioptes
				Otodectes
			Knemidocoptidae	*Knemidocoptes*
			Listrophoridae	*Leporacarus*
			Myocoptidae	*Myocoptes*
			Cytoditidae	*Cytodites*
			Laminosioptidae	*Laminosioptes*
			Analgidae	*Megninia*
			Atopomelidae	*Chirodiscoides*
				Listrocarpus
			Dermoglyphidae	*Dermoglyphus*
			Freyanidae	*Freyana*
			Epidermoptidae	*Epidermoptes*
				Rivoltasia
				Microlichus
				Promyialges
				Lynxacarus
			Pterolichidae	*Pterolichus*
				Sideroferus
			Gabuciniidae	*Gabucinia*
			Hypoderatidae	*Hypodectes*
	Trombidiformes	**Prostigmata**	Demodicidae	*Demodex*
			Cheyletidae	*Cheyletiella*
			Trombiculidae	*Trombicula*
				Neotrombicula
				Eutrombicula
				Leptotrombidium
				Neoschongastia
			Psorergatidae	*Psorobia*
			Pyemotidae	*Pyemotes*

(Continued)

Continued

Kingdom	Phylum	Class	Order	Suborder	Family	Genus
					Myobiidae	*Myobia*
						Radfordia
					Syringophilidae	*Syringophilus*
					Cloacaridae	*Cloacarus*
					Pterygosomatidae	*Geckobiella*
						Pimeliaphilus
						Hirstiella
						Ixodiderma
						Scapothrix
						Zonurobia
			Mesostigmata		Macronyssidae	*Ornithonyssus*
						Ophionyssus
					Dermanyssidae	*Dermanyssus*
						Liponyssoides
					Halarachnidae	*Pneumonyssoides*
						Pneumonyssus
						Rhinophaga
						Raillietia
					Entonyssidae	*Entonyssus*
						Entophionyssus
					Rhinonyssidae	*Sternosoma*
					Haemogamasidae	*Haemogamasus*
					Laelapidae	*Laelaps*
						Androlaelaps
			Ixodida		Ixodidae	*Ixodes*
						Dermacentor
						Haemaphysalis
						Rhipicephalus
						Amblyomma
						Hyalomma
					Argasidae	*Argas*
						Otobius
						Ornithodoros
		Crustacea (Pentostomida)	**Porocephalida**		Linguatulidae	*Linguatula*
					Armilliferidae	*Armillifer*
					Porocephalidae	*Porocephalus*

4 KINGDOM BACTERIA

Phylum	Class	Order	Family	Genus
Proteobacteria	Alphaproteobacteria	**Rickettsiales**	Rickettsiaceae	*Rickettsia*
			Anaplasmataceae	*Anaplasma*
				Ehrlichia
				Neorickettsia
				Aegyptianella
		Hyphomicrobiales	Bartonellaceae	*Bartonella*
		Legionellales	Coxiellaceae	*Coxiella*
Firmicutes	Mollicutes	**Mycoplasmatales**	Mycoplasmataceae	*Mycoplasma* (haemominutum group)
				Mycoplasma (haemofelis group)

5 KINGDOM FUNGI

Phylum	Class	Order	Family	Genus
Microsporidia	Microsporea	Microspororida	Unikaryonidae	*Encephalitozoon*
		Enterocytozoonida	Enterocytozoonidae	*Enterocytozoon*
Ascomycota	Pneumocystidomycetes	Pneumocystidales	Pneumocystidaceae	*Pneumocystis*

6 KINGDOM CHROMALVEOLATA

Phylum	Class	Order	Family	Genus
Opalinata	Blastocystae	Blastocystida	Blastocystidae	*Blastocystis*

CHAPTER 1

Veterinary helminthology

PRINCIPLES OF CLASSIFICATION

When examined, living organisms can be seen to form natural groups with features in common. These similarities may be morphological, but increasingly may be based on DNA analysis. Groups of organisms are combined into biologically meaningful groups, usually attempting to represent evolutionary pathways. A group of this sort is called a **taxon** and the study of this aspect of biology is called **taxonomy**. The study of the complex systems of interrelationship between living organisms is called **systematics**. The taxa into which organisms may be placed are recognised by international agreement; the primary ones are **kingdom**, **phylum**, **class**, **order**, **family**, **genus** and **species**. The intervals between these are large, and some organisms cannot be allocated to them precisely, so intermediate taxa, prefixed appropriately, have been formed; examples of these are the **suborder** and the **superfamily**. As an example, the taxonomic status of one of the common abomasal parasites of ruminants may be expressed as shown below.

Kingdom	Animalia
Phylum	Nematoda
Class	Chromadorea
Order	Rhabditida
Suborder	Rhabditina
Superfamily	Trichostrongyloidea
Family	Trichostrongylidae
Subfamily	Haemonchinae
Genus	*Haemonchus*
Species	*contortus*

The names of taxa must follow a set of internationally agreed rules, but it is permissible to anglicise the endings, so that members of the superfamily Trichostrongyloidea in the example above may also be termed trichostrongiloids. The names of the genus and species are expressed in Latin form, the generic name having a capital letter, and they must be in grammatical agreement. It is customary to print Latin names in italics. Accents are not permitted. If an organism is named after a person, amendment may be necessary; the name of Müller, for example, has been altered in the genus *Muellerius*.

HELMINTHOLOGY

Parasitic helminths can affect humans, animals and plants, with estimated numbers of between 75 000 and 300 000 species. The higher taxa containing helminths of veterinary importance are as follows.

Major
- Nematoda (roundworms)
- Platyhelminthes (flatworms)
  - Trematoda (flukes)
  - Cestoda (tapeworms)

Minor
- Acanthocephala (thorny-headed worms)

PHYLUM NEMATODA

The nematodes (Nematoda) are commonly called **Roundworms** from their appearance in cross-section, and are parasitic or free-living. In the majority of nematodes the sexes are separate.

CLASSES CHROMADOREA AND ENOPLEA

The system of classification of nematodes of veterinary importance, which is based on current taxonomic literature, is given in taxonomic tables. In this system, nematode genera and species are divided in the classes Chromadorea and Enoplea, which are grouped into several **superfamilies**. The superfamilies can be conveniently divided into **bursate** and **non-bursate** groups, the most typical features of which are summarised in Table 1.1.

STRUCTURE AND FUNCTION

Most nematodes have a cylindrical unsegmented form, tapering at either end, and the body is covered by a colourless, somewhat translucent, layer: the cuticle. The tough **cuticle** is secreted by the underlying **hypodermis**, which projects into the body cavity forming two **lateral cords,** which carry the excretory canals, and a dorsal and ventral cord carrying the **nerves** (Fig. 1.1). The muscle cells, arranged longitudinally, lie between the hypodermis and the body cavity. The latter contains fluid at a high pressure, which maintains the turgidity and shape of the body (pseudocoelom). Locomotion is effected by undulating waves of muscle contraction and relaxation that alternate on the dorsal and ventral aspects of the worm. A circular muscle layer is absent in nematodes. Most of the internal organs are filamentous and suspended in the fluid-filled body cavity (Fig. 1.1). The **digestive system** is tubular (Fig. 1.2a). The mouth, or stoma, of many nematodes is a simple opening, which may be

Veterinary Parasitology, Fifth Edition. Domenico Otranto and Richard Wall.
© 2024 John Wiley & Sons Ltd. Published 2024 by John Wiley & Sons Ltd.

Table 1.1 Characteristic features of parasitic nematodes of veterinary importance.

Superfamily	Typical features
Bursate nematodes	
Trichostrongyloidea *Trichostrongylus, Ostertagia, Dictyocaulus, Haemonchus,* etc.	Buccal capsule small. Life cycle **direct**; infection by L_3
Strongyloidea *Strongylus, Syngamus,* etc.	Buccal capsule well developed; leaf crowns and teeth usually present. Life cycle **direct**; infection by L_3
Ancylostomatoidea *Ancylostoma, Uncinaria,* etc.	
Metastrongyloidea *Metastrongylus, Muellerius, Protostrongylus,* etc.	Buccal capsule small. Life cycle **indirect**; infection by L_3 in intermediate host
Non-bursate nematodes	
Rhabditoidea *Strongyloides, Rhabditis,* etc.	Very small worms; buccal capsule small. Free-living and parasitic generations. Life cycle **direct**; infection by L_3
Ascaridoidea *Ascaris, Toxocara, Parascaris,* etc.	Large white worms. Life cycle **direct**; infection by L_2 in egg
Dioctophymatoidea *Dioctophyma,* etc.	Very large worms. Life cycle **indirect**; infection by L_3 in aquatic annelids
Oxyuroidea *Oxyuris, Skrjabinema,* etc.	Female has long pointed tail. Life cycle **direct**; infection by L_3 in egg
Spiruroidea *Spirocerca, Habronema, Thelazia,* etc.	Spiral tail in male. Life cycle **indirect**; infection by L_3 from insects
Filarioidea *Dirofilaria, Onchocerca, Parafilaria,* etc.	Long thin worms. Life cycle **indirect**; infection by L_3 from insects
Trichuroidea *Trichuris, Capillaria*	Whip-like or hair-like worms. Life cycle **direct** or **indirect**; infection by L_1
Trichinelloidea *Trichinella,* etc.	

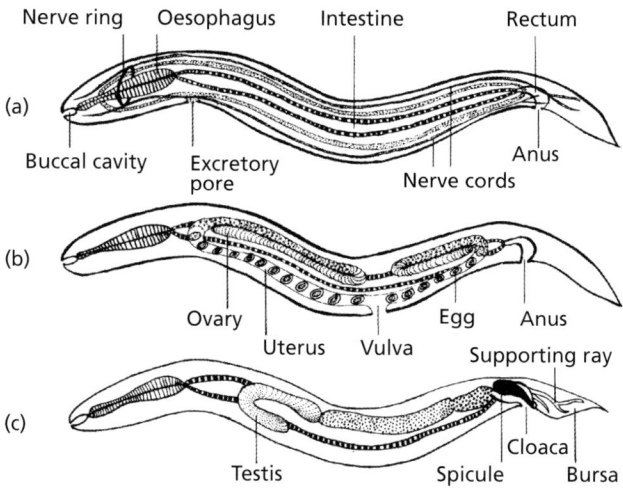

Fig. 1.2 Longitudinal sections of a generalised nematode. (a) Digestive, excretory and nervous system. (b) Reproductive system of a female nematode. (c) Reproductive system of a male nematode.

surrounded by two or three lips, and leads directly into the oesophagus. Where the mouth opening is large and well developed it is often surrounded by a leaf crown. In others, such as the strongyloids, it is large, and opens into a **buccal capsule**, which may contain blades or teeth. Such parasites, when feeding, draw a plug of mucosa into the buccal capsule, where it is broken down by the action of enzymes, which are secreted into the capsule from adjacent glands. Some of these worms may also secrete anticoagulant, and small vessels, ruptured in the digestion of the mucosal plug, may continue to bleed for some minutes after the worm has moved to a fresh site.

Those nematodes with very small buccal capsules, like the trichostrongyloids, or simple oral openings, like the ascaridoids, generally feed on mucosal fluid, products of host digestion and cell debris, while others, such as the oxyuroids, appear to scavenge on

the contents of the lower gut. Worms living in the bloodstream or tissue spaces, such as the filarioids, feed exclusively on body fluids. The **oesophagus** is usually muscular and pumps food into the intestine. It is of variable form (Fig. 1.3) and is a useful preliminary identification character for groups of worms. It may be **filariform**, simple and slightly thickened posteriorly, as in the bursate nematodes; **bulb shaped**, with a large posterior swelling, as in the ascaridoids; or **double bulb shaped**, as in the oxyuroids. In some

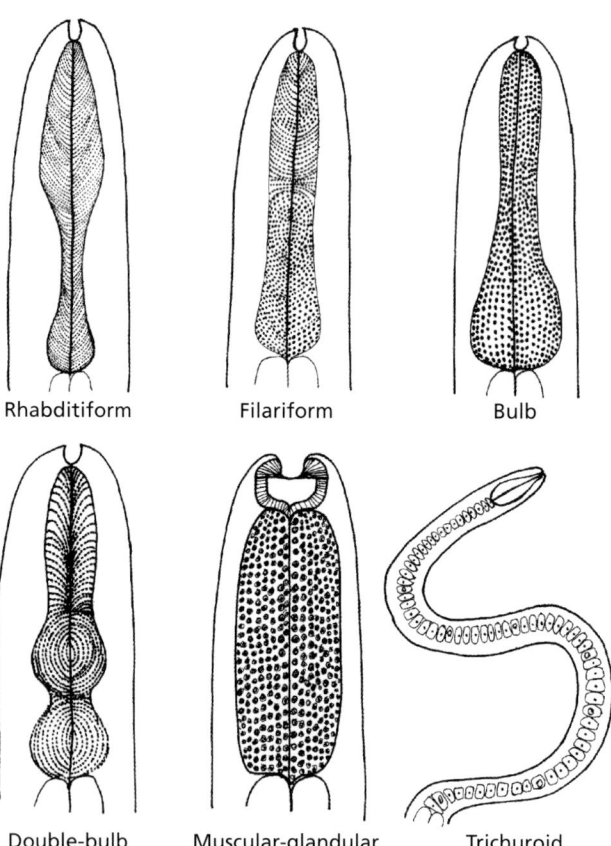

Fig. 1.3 The basic forms of oesophagus found in nematodes.

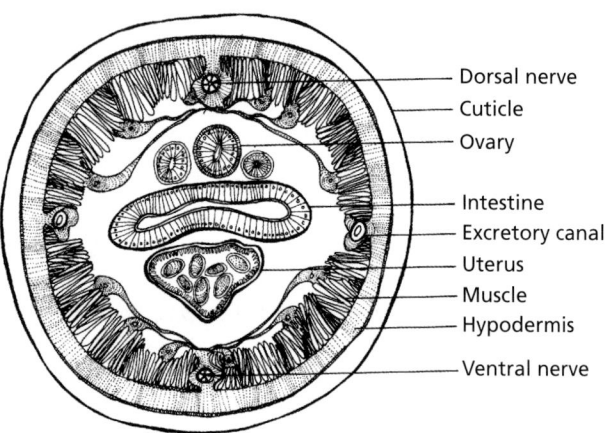

Fig. 1.1 Transverse section of a generalised female nematode.

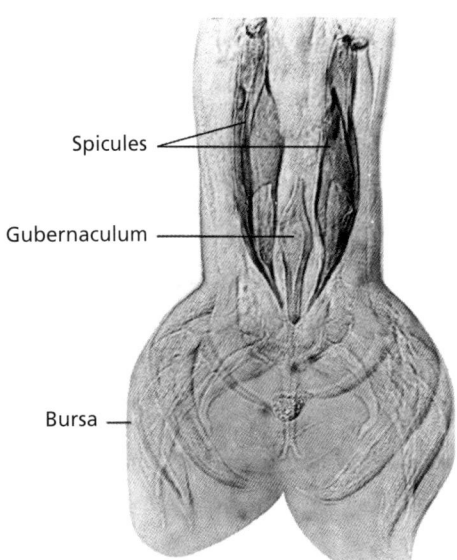

Spicules

Gubernaculum

Bursa

Fig. 1.4 Male trichostrongiloid nematode bursa showing spicules and bursa.

groups this wholly muscular form does not occur: the filarioids and spiruroids have a **muscular–glandular** oesophagus which is muscular anteriorly, the posterior part being glandular; the **trichuroid** oesophagus has a capillary form, passing through a single column of cells, the whole being known as a stichosome. A **rhabditiform** oesophagus, with slight anterior and posterior swellings, is present in the preparasitic larvae of many nematodes, and in adult free-living nematodes.

The **intestine** is a simple tube descending from the oesophagus whose lumen is enclosed by a single layer of epithelial cells or by a syncytium. The luminal surfaces possess microvilli, which increase the absorptive capacity of the cells. In female worms the intestine terminates in an anus, while in males there is a cloaca which functions as an anus, into which opens the vas deferens and through which the copulatory spicules may be extruded.

The so-called 'excretory system' is very primitive, consisting of a canal within each lateral cord joining at the excretory pore in the oesophageal region. The **reproductive systems** consist of filamentous tubes, which float in the body cavity. The **female organs** comprise ovary, oviduct and uterus, which may be paired (didelphic) or sometimes single (monodelphic), ending in a common short vagina, which opens at the vulva (Fig. 1.2b). The location of the vulva can be a useful aid in diagnosis, being at the anterior end (opisthodelphic), middle (amphidelphic) or posterior end (prodelphic). At the junction of uterus and vagina in some species, there is a short muscular organ, the ovejector, which regulates and assists in egg laying. A vulval flap may also be present. Nematodes can be oviparous, ovoviviparous or viviparous. The **male organs** consist of a single continuous testis and a vas deferens terminating in a muscular ejaculatory duct into the cloaca (Fig. 1.2c). Accessory male organs are sometimes important in identification, especially of the trichostrongyloids, the two most important being the spicules and gubernaculum (Fig. 1.4). The **spicules** are chitinous organs, usually paired, which are inserted in the female genital opening during copulation. In some species they are absent (e.g. *Trichinella*) or only one spicule is present (e.g. *Trichuris*). The **gubernaculum**, also chitinous, is a small structure located in the dorsal wall, which acts as a guide for the spicules. When the guide is located in the ventral

wall it is referred to as a **telamon**. With the two sexes in close apposition, the amoeboid sperm are transferred from the cloaca of the male into the uterus of the female. The **cuticle** may be modified to form various structures (Fig. 1.5), the more important of which include the following.

- **Leaf crowns** consisting of rows of papillae occurring as fringes round the rim of the buccal capsule (external leaf crowns) or just inside the rim (internal leaf crowns). They are especially prominent in certain nematodes of horses. Their function is not known, but it is suggested that they may be used to pin a patch of mucosa in position during feeding, or that they may prevent the entry of foreign matter into the buccal capsule when the worm has detached from the mucosa.
- **Cervical papillae** occur anteriorly in the oesophageal region, and **caudal papillae** posteriorly at the tail. They are spine-like or finger-like processes, and are usually diametrically placed. Their function may be sensory or supportive.
- **Cervical** and **caudal alae** are flattened wing-like expansions of the cuticle in the oesophageal and tail regions respectively.

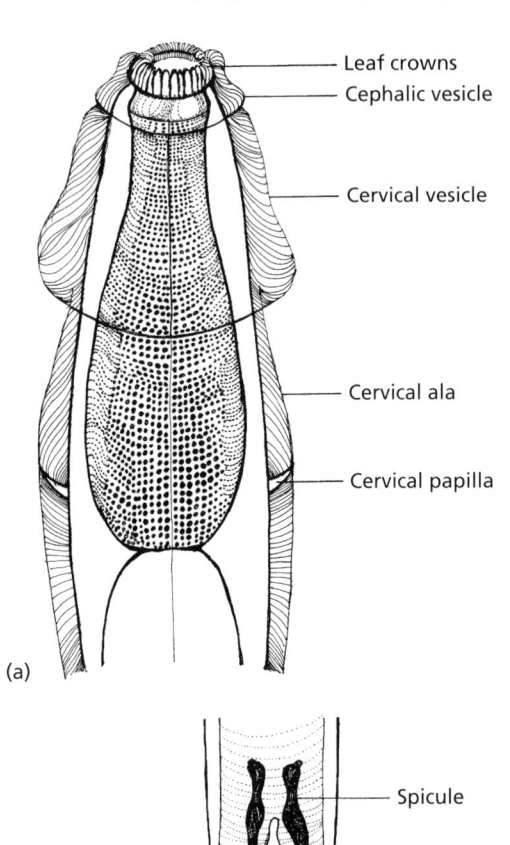

Leaf crowns
Cephalic vesicle
Cervical vesicle
Cervical ala
Cervical papilla

(a)

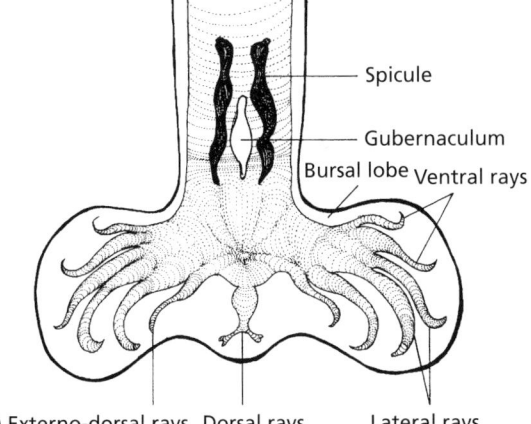

Spicule
Gubernaculum
Bursal lobe Ventral rays

(b) Externo-dorsal rays Dorsal rays Lateral rays

Fig. 1.5 Cuticular modifications of a generalised nematode: (a) anterior region; (b) posterior region of a male.

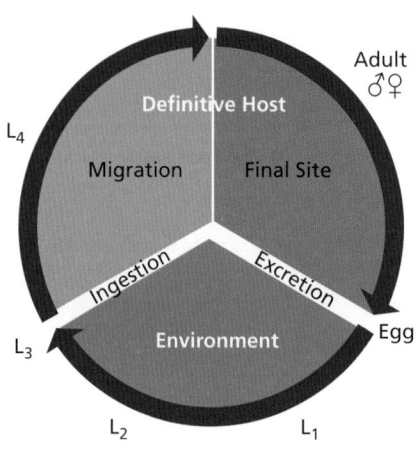
(a) Direct life cycle

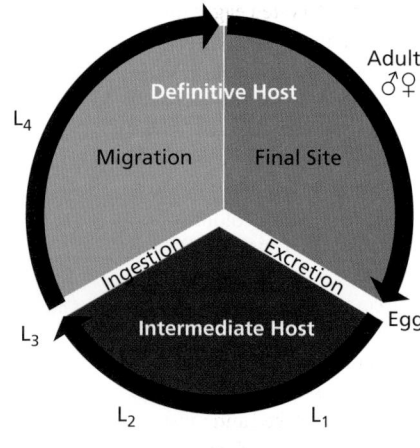
(b) Indirect life cycle

Fig. 1.6 Generalised nematode life cycles: (a) direct; (b) indirect.

- **Cephalic** and **cervical vesicles** are inflations of the cuticle around the mouth opening and in the oesophageal region.
- The **copulatory bursa**, which embraces the female during copulation, is important in the identification of certain male nematodes and is derived from much expanded caudal alae, which are supported by elongated caudal papillae called **bursal rays**. It consists of two lateral lobes and a single small dorsal lobe. It is particularly well developed in the strongylids.
- **Plaques** and **cordons** are plate-like and cord-like ornamentations present on the cuticle of many nematodes of the superfamily Spiruroidea.

BASIC NEMATODE LIFE CYCLE

In the Nematoda, the sexes are separate and the males are generally smaller than the females, which lay eggs or larvae. During development, a nematode moults at intervals, shedding its cuticle. In the complete life cycle there are four moults, the successive larval stages being designated L_1, L_2, L_3, L_4 and finally L_5, which is the immature adult.

One feature of the basic nematode life cycle is that immediate transfer of infection from one **final host** to another rarely occurs. Some development usually takes place either in the faecal pat or in a different species of animal, the **intermediate host**, before infection can take place.

In the common form of **direct** life cycle (Fig. 1.6a), the free-living larvae undergo two moults after hatching and infection is by ingestion of the free L_3 stage. There are some important exceptions, however, infection sometimes being by larval penetration of the skin or by ingestion of the egg containing a larva. In **indirect** life cycles (Fig. 1.6b), the first two moults usually take place in an intermediate host and infection of the final host is either by ingestion of the intermediate host or by inoculation of the L_3 when the intermediate host, such as a blood-sucking insect, feeds.

After infection, two further moults take place to produce the L_5 or immature adult parasite.

Following copulation, a further life cycle is initiated. In the case of gastrointestinal parasites, development may take place entirely in the gut lumen or with only limited movement into the mucosa. However, in many species, the larvae travel considerable distances

through the body before settling in their final (predilection) site and this is the migratory form of life cycle. One of the most common routes is the **hepatic–tracheal**. This takes developing stages from the **gut** via the portal system to the **liver** then via the hepatic vein and posterior vena cava to the **heart** and from there via the pulmonary artery to the **lungs**. Larvae then travel via the bronchi, trachea and oesophagus to the **gut**. It should be emphasised that the above is a basic description of nematode life cycles and that there are many variations.

DEVELOPMENT OF THE PARASITE

Egg

Nematode eggs differ greatly in size and shape, and the shell is of variable thickness, usually consisting of three layers. The inner membrane, which is thin, has lipid characteristics and is impermeable. A middle layer, which is tough and chitinous, gives rigidity and, when thick, imparts a yellowish colour to the egg. In many species this layer is interrupted at one or both ends with an operculum (lid) or plug. The third outer layer consists of protein, which is very thick and sticky in the ascaridoids and is important in the epidemiology of this superfamily. In contrast, in some species the eggshell is very thin and may be merely present as a sheath around the larva. The survival potential of the egg outside the body varies, but appears to be connected with the thickness of the shell, which protects the larva from desiccation. Thus parasites whose infective form is the larvated egg usually have very thick-shelled eggs which can survive for years on the ground.

Hatching

Depending on the species, eggs may hatch outside the body or after ingestion. Outside the body, hatching is controlled partly by factors such as temperature and moisture and partly by the larva itself. In the process of hatching, the inner impermeable shell membrane is broken down by enzymes secreted by the larva and by its own movement. The larva is then able to take up water from the environment and enlarges to rupture the remaining layers and escape.

When the larvated egg is the infective form, the host initiates hatching after ingestion by providing stimuli for the larva, which then completes the process. It is important for each nematode species that hatching should occur in appropriate regions of the gut and hence the stimuli will differ, although it appears that dissolved carbon dioxide is a constant essential.

Larval development and survival

Three of the important superfamilies, the trichostrongyloids, the strongyloids and the rhabditoids, have a completely free-living preparasitic phase. The first two larval stages usually feed on bacteria but the L_3, sealed off from the environment by the retained cuticle of the L_2, cannot feed and must survive on the stored nutrients acquired in the early stages. Growth of the larva is interrupted during moulting by periods of lethargus in which it neither feeds nor moves.

The cuticle of the L_2 is retained as a sheath around the L_3; this is important in larval survival with a protective role analogous to that of the eggshell in egg-infective groups. The two most important components of the external environment are temperature and humidity. The optimal temperature for the development of the maximum number of larvae in the shortest feasible time is generally in the range 18–26 °C. At higher temperatures, development is faster and the larvae are hyperactive, thus depleting their lipid reserves. The mortality rate then rises, so that few will survive to L_3. As the temperature falls, the process slows and below 10 °C, the development from egg to L_3 usually cannot take place. Below 5 °C movement metabolism of L_3 is minimal, which in many species favours survival.

The optimal humidity is 100%, although some development can occur down to 80% relative humidity. It should be noted that even in dry weather where the ambient humidity is low, the microclimate in faeces or at the soil surface may be sufficiently humid to permit continuing larval development.

In the trichostrongyloids and strongyloids, the embryonated egg and the ensheathed L_3 are best equipped to survive in adverse conditions such as freezing or desiccation; in contrast, the L_1 and L_2 are particularly vulnerable. Although desiccation is generally considered to be the most lethal influence in larval survival, there is increasing evidence that by entering a state of anhydrobiosis, certain larvae can survive severe desiccation.

On the ground most larvae are active, although they require a film of water for movement and are stimulated by light and temperature. It is now thought that larval movement is mostly random and encounter with grass blades accidental.

Infection

As noted previously, infection may be by ingestion of the free-living L_3, and this occurs in the majority of trichostrongyloid and strongyloid nematodes. In these, the L_3 sheds the retained sheath of the L_2 within the alimentary tract of the host, the stimulus for exsheathment being provided by the host in a manner similar to the hatching stimulus required by egg-infective nematodes. In response to this stimulus the larva releases its own exsheathing fluid, containing an enzyme, leucine aminopeptidase, which dissolves the sheath from within, either at a narrow collar anteriorly, so that a cap detaches, or by splitting the sheath longitudinally. The larva can then wriggle free of the sheath.

As in the preparasitic stage, growth of the larva during parasitic development is interrupted by two moults, each of these occurring during a short period of lethargus. The time taken for development from infection until mature adult parasites are producing eggs or larvae is known as the **prepatent period** and this is of known duration for each nematode species.

METABOLISM

The main food reserve of preparasitic nematode larvae, whether inside the eggshell or free-living, is lipid, which may be seen as droplets in the lumen of the intestine. The infectivity of these stages is often related to the amount of lipid present; larvae which have depleted their reserves are not as infective as those which still retain quantities of lipid.

Apart from these reserves, the free-living first- and second-stage larvae of most nematodes feed on bacteria. However, once they reach the infective third stage, they are sealed in the retained cuticle of the second stage, cannot feed and are completely dependent on their stored reserves.

In contrast, the adult parasite stores its energy as glycogen, mainly in the lateral cords and muscles, and this may constitute 20% of the dry weight of the worm.

Free-living and developing stages of nematodes usually have an aerobic metabolism, whereas adult nematodes can metabolise carbohydrate by both glycolysis (anaerobic) and oxidative decarboxylation (aerobic). However, in the latter, pathways may operate which are not present in the host and it is at this level that some antiparasitic drugs operate.

The oxidation of carbohydrates requires the presence of an electron transport system, which in most nematodes can operate aerobically down to oxygen tensions of 5 mmHg or less. Since the oxygen tension at the mucosal surface of the intestine is around 20 mmHg, nematodes in close proximity to the mucosa normally have sufficient oxygen for aerobic metabolism. Otherwise, if the nematode is temporarily or permanently some distance from the mucosal surface, energy metabolism is probably largely anaerobic.

As well as the conventional cytochrome and flavoprotein electron transport system, many nematodes have 'haemoglobin' in their body fluids which gives them a red pigmentation. This nematode haemoglobin is chemically similar to myoglobin and has the highest affinity for oxygen of any known animal haemoglobin. The main function of nematode haemoglobin is thought to be to transport oxygen, acquired by diffusion through the cuticle or gut, into the tissues; blood-sucking worms presumably ingest a considerable amount of oxygenated nutrients in their diet.

The end products of the metabolism of carbohydrates, fats or proteins are excreted through the anus or cloaca, or by diffusion through the body wall. Ammonia, the terminal product of protein metabolism, must be excreted rapidly and diluted to non-toxic levels in the surrounding fluids. During periods of anaerobic carbohydrate metabolism, the worms may also excrete pyruvic acid rather than retaining it for future oxidation when aerobic metabolism is possible.

The 'excretory system' terminating in the excretory pore is almost certainly not concerned with excretion, but rather with osmoregulation and salt balance.

Two phenomena which affect the normal parasitic life cycle of nematodes and which are of considerable biological and epidemiological importance are arrested larval development and the periparturient rise in faecal egg counts.

ARRESTED LARVAL DEVELOPMENT

(Synonyms: inhibited larval development, hypobiosis)
This phenomenon may be defined as the temporary cessation in development of a nematode at a precise point in its parasitic development. It is usually a facultative characteristic and affects only a proportion of the worm population. Some strains of nematodes have a high propensity for arrested development while in others this is low. The stage at which larvae become arrested varies between species of nematodes; for example, L_3 stage in *Trichostrongylus*, Cyathostominae and *Ancylostoma*, L_4 stage in *Ostertagia*, *Teladorsagia*, *Haemonchus* and *Obeliscoides*, or immature adults as in *Dictyocaulus*.

Conclusive evidence for the occurrence of arrested larval development can only be obtained by examination of the worm population in the host. It is usually recognised by the presence of large numbers of larvae at the same stage of development in animals withheld from infection for a period longer than that required to reach that particular larval stage.

The nature of the stimulus for arrested development and for the subsequent maturation of the larvae is still a matter of debate. Although there are apparently different circumstances which initiate arrested larval development, most commonly the stimulus is an environmental one received by the free-living infective stages prior to ingestion by the host. It may be seen as a ruse by the parasite to avoid adverse climatic conditions for its progeny by remaining sexually immature in the host until more favourable conditions return. The name commonly applied to this seasonal arrestment is **hypobiosis**. Thus, the accumulation of arrested larvae often coincides with the onset of cold autumn/winter conditions in the northern hemisphere or very dry conditions in the subtropics or tropics. In contrast, the maturation of these larvae coincides with the return of environmental conditions suitable to their free-living development, although it is not clear what triggers the signal to mature and how it is transmitted.

The degree of adaptation to these seasonal stimuli and therefore the proportion of larvae which do become arrested seem to be heritable traits and are affected by various factors, including grazing systems and the degree of adversity in the environment. For example, in Canada where the winters are severe, most trichostrongyloid larvae ingested in late autumn or winter become arrested, whereas in southern Britain with moderate winters, about 50–60% are arrested. In the humid tropics where free-living larval development is possible all the year round, relatively few larvae become arrested.

However, arrested development may also occur as a result of both acquired and age immunity in the host and although the proportions of larvae arrested are not usually so high as in hypobiosis, they can play an important part in the epidemiology of nematode infections. Maturation of these arrested larvae seems to be linked with the breeding cycle of the host and occurs at or around parturition.

The epidemiological importance of arrested larval development from whatever cause is that, first, it ensures the survival of the nematode during periods of adversity and, second, the subsequent maturation of arrested larvae increases the contamination of the environment and can sometimes result in clinical disease.

PERIPARTURIENT RISE IN FAECAL EGG COUNTS

(Synonyms: postparturient rise, spring rise)
Periparturient rise (PPR) refers to an increase in the numbers of nematode eggs in the faeces of animals around parturition. This phenomenon is most marked in ewes, goats and sows and recent data support the hypothesis that there is competition for nutrients between the immune system, the rapidly growing fetus in late pregnancy and the udder during lactation, particularly metabolisable protein. This relaxation of immunity can be largely restored by supplementation with rumen-undegradable protein and is also influenced by the body protein status of the ewe.

The source of the PPR is threefold.
1 Maturation of larvae arrested due to host immunity.
2 An increased establishment of infections acquired from the pastures and a reduced turnover of existing adult infections.
3 An increased fecundity of existing adult worm populations.

Contemporaneously, but not associated with the relaxation of host immunity, the PPR may be augmented by the maturation of hypobiotic larvae.

The importance of the PPR is that it occurs at a time when the numbers of new susceptible hosts are increasing and so ensures the survival and propagation of the worm species. Depending on the magnitude of infection, it may also cause a loss of production in lactating animals and, by contamination of the environment, lead to clinical disease in susceptible young stock.

NEMATODE SUPERFAMILIES

SUPERFAMILY TRICHOSTRONGYLOIDEA

In some recent taxonomic classification, this superfamily is included within the superfamily Strongyloidea. The trichostrongyloids are small, often hair-like, worms in the bursate group, which, with the exception of the lungworm *Dictyocaulus*, parasitise the alimentary tract of animals and birds. Structurally, they have few cuticular appendages and the buccal capsule is vestigial and possesses no leaf crowns. Teeth are usually absent. The males have a well-developed bursa with large lateral lobes and two spicules, the configuration of which is used for species differentiation. The life cycle is direct and usually non-migratory and the ensheathed L_3 is the infective stage. The trichostrongiloids are responsible for considerable mortality and widespread morbidity, especially in ruminants.

The most important alimentary genera are *Ostertagia*, *Haemonchus*, *Trichostrongylus*, *Cooperia*, *Nematodirus*, *Hyostrongylus*, *Marshallagia* and *Mecistocirrus*. *Dictyocaulus* is an important genus affecting the respiratory tract of ruminants and horses. Other genera of lesser importance are *Graphidium*, *Obeliscoides*, *Ollulanus*, *Libyostrongylus*, *Graphinema*, *Impalaia*, *Ornithostrongylus*, *Amidostomum*, *Epomidiostomum*, *Nematodirella*, *Lamanema*, *Nippostrongylus* and *Nematospiroides*.

FAMILY TRICHOSTRONGYLIDAE

Trichostrongylus

Adult worms are small, slightly reddish/brown in colour, slender and hair-like, usually less than 7 mm long (Fig. 1.7) and difficult to see with the naked eye. The worms have no obvious buccal capsule and cephalic inflations are absent. A most useful generic character is the distinct excretory notch in the oesophageal region (Fig. 1.8). The male bursa has long lateral lobes, while the dorsal lobe is not well defined with a slender dorsal ray, which is cleft near its tip into two branches. The ventro-ventral ray is well separated from the other rays. The spicules are thick and unbranched and a gubernaculum is present. Species identification is based on the shape and size of the spicules (Tables 1.2 and 1.3). In the female,

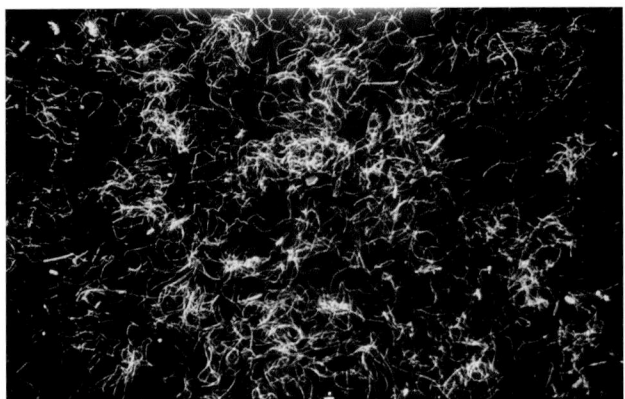

Fig. 1.7 Adult *Trichostrongylus* worms.

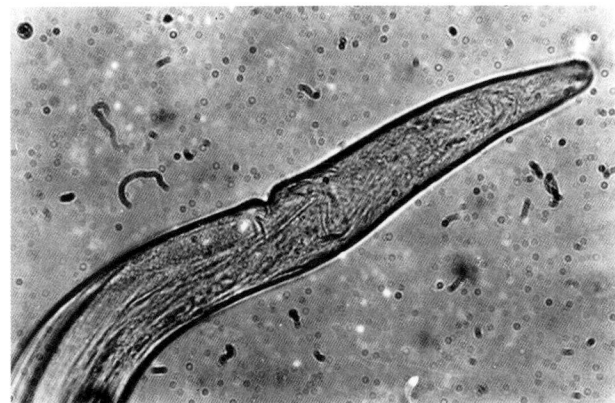

Fig. 1.8 Characteristic excretory notch in the oesophageal region of *Trichostrongylus*.

the tail is bluntly tapered (Fig. 1.9) and there is no vulval flap and the vulva opens a short distance from the middle of the body. The females possess double ovejectors.

Life cycle: This is direct and the preparasitic phase is typically trichostrongyloid, eggs developing to the infective L_3 in about 7–10 days under optimal conditions. Following ingestion and exsheathment, larvae penetrate the mucosa of the small intestine (Fig. 1.10) and after two moults the fifth-stage worms are present under the intestinal epithelium around two weeks after initial infection. The prepatent period is generally 2–3 weeks.

Table 1.2 Identification of *Trichostrongylus* spp. based on male spicule morphology.

Species	Spicules: description	Spicules: morphology
Trichostrongylus axei	Spicules are dissimilar and unequal in length (the right being shorter than the left)	(a)
Trichostrongylus colubriformis	Thick, brown, unbranched, of equal length and terminate in a barb-like tip	(b)
Trichostrongylus vitrinus	Thick, unbranched, of equal length and end in a point	(c)
Trichostrongylus longispicularis	The spicules are stout, brown, unbranched, slightly unequal in length and terminate in a tapering blunt tip that has a small semi-transparent protrusion	(d)
Trichostrongylus rugatus	Spicules are unequal and dissimilar, bearing transverse ridges near the tip	(e)
Trichostrongylus falculatus	Spicules subequal – 100 µm long	(f)
Trichostrongylus capricola	Spicules are equal in length. Thinner distally than anteriorly and terminate in a rounded tip	(g)
Trichostrongylus retortaeformis	Spicules are stout, unequal in length and terminate in a barb-like tip	(h)

Table 1.3 *Trichostrongylus* species.

Species	Hosts	Site
Trichostrongylus axei (syn. *Trichostrongylus extenuatus*)	Cattle, sheep, goats, deer, horses, pigs	Abomasum or stomach
Trichostrongylus colubriformis	Cattle, sheep, goats, camels, rabbits, pigs, dogs, humans	Duodenum, anterior small intestine
Trichostrongylus vitrinus	Sheep, goats, camels, deer, rabbits	Duodenum, small intestine
Trichostrongylus capricola	Sheep, goats	Small intestine
Trichostrongylus falculatus	Sheep, goats, antelopes	Small intestine
Trichostrongylus longispicularis	Sheep, cattle, goats, camels, deer, llamas	Small intestine
Trichostrongylus probolurus	Sheep, goats, camels, occasionally humans	Stomach, small intestine
Trichostrongylus rugatus	Sheep, goats	Small intestine
Trichostrongylus retortaeformis	Rabbits, hares	Small intestine
Trichostrongylus calcaratus	Rabbits, hares	Small intestine
Trichostrongylus affinus	Rabbits, sheep, occasionally humans	Small intestine
Trichostrongylus tenuis	Gamebirds (grouse, partridges, pheasants), chickens, ducks, geese, turkeys, emus	Small intestine, caecae

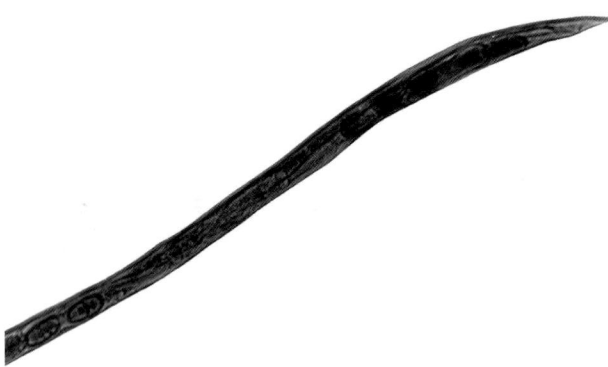

Fig. 1.9 Tail of adult female *Trichostrongylus*.

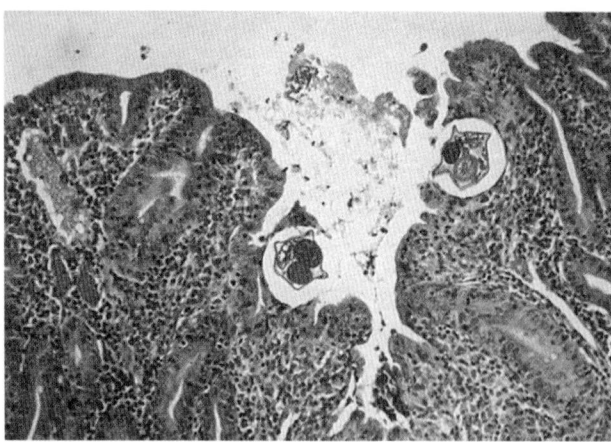

Fig. 1.10 Developing *Trichostrongylus vitrinus* in the small intestinal mucosa.

Trichostrongylus axei

Synonym: *Trichostrongylus extenuatus*

Common name: Stomach hairworm

Description, gross: The adults are small, hair-like, light brownish-red and difficult to see with the naked eye. Males measure around 3–6 mm and females 4–8 mm in length. There is no buccal capsule and the anterior of the worm and the vulval area lack any accessory cuticular structures. The bursa is simple in form and the ventro-ventral ray is positioned well apart from the other rays. The male spicules are dissimilar and unequal in length, the right being shorter than the left (Fig. 1.11; Table 1.2a). The female has double ovejectors. The eggs are medium-sized, an irregular ellipse and measure about 70–106 by 30–45 μm. The poles are dissimilar, one being more rounded, and are not very wide (see Fig. 4.4).

Trichostrongylus colubriformis

Synonym: *Trichostrongylus instabilis*

Common name: Black scour or bankrupt worm

Description: Males measure around 4–5.5 mm and females 5.5–7.5 mm in length. There is no buccal capsule and the anterior of the worm and the vulval area lack any accessory cuticular structures. The bursa is simple in form and the ventro-ventral ray is positioned well apart from the other rays. The spicules are thick, brown, unbranched, of equal length and terminate in a barb-like tip (Fig. 1.12; Table 1.2b). The female has double ovejectors. The thin-shelled eggs are medium-sized, an irregular ellipse and measure about 79–101 by 38–50 μm. The poles are dissimilar, one being more rounded, and are not very wide. The eggs are segmenting when laid.

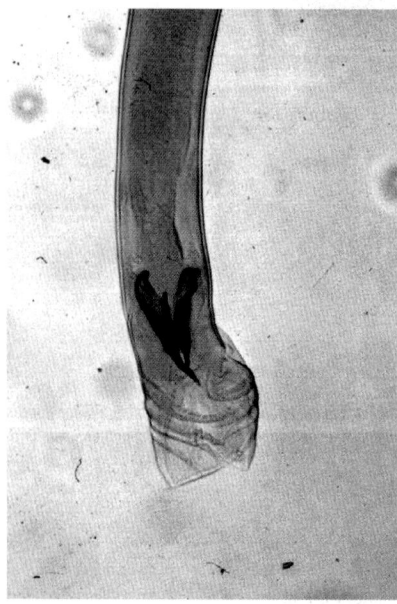

Fig. 1.11 Copulatory bursa and spicule of *Trichostrongylus axei*.

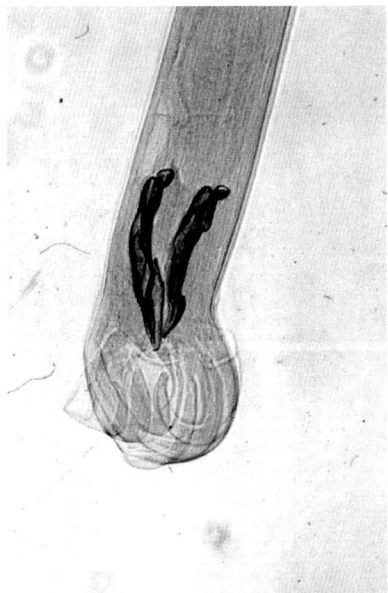

Fig. 1.12 Copulatory bursa and spicule of *Trichostrongylus colubriformis*.

Trichostrongylus vitrinus

Common name: Black scour worm

Description: Males measure around 4–6 mm and females 5–8 mm in length. The spicules are thick, unbranched, of equal length and end in a point (Fig. 1.13; Table 1.2c). Eggs are slightly 'brazil nut'-shaped and measure 93–118 by 41–52 µm.

Trichostrongylus capricola

Description: Males measure around 4–5 mm and females 6–7 mm in length. The male spicules are of equal length, thicker anteriorly than distally and end in a rounded tip (Table 1.2g).

Trichostrongylus falculatus

Description: Males measure around 4.5–5.5 mm. The spicules are thick, brown, of almost equal length with a sickle-shaped offshoot (Table 1.2f). The gubernaculum is bent anteriorly at right angles.

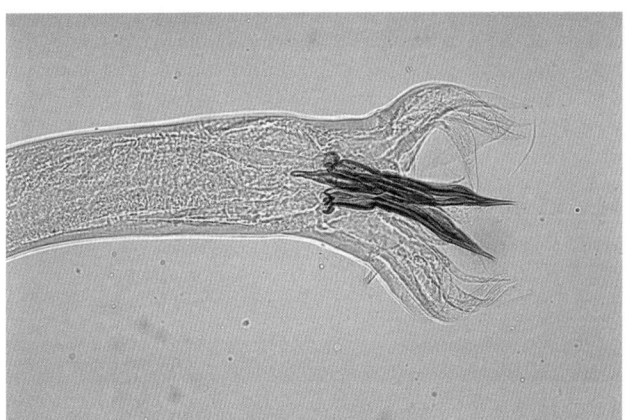

Fig. 1.13 Copulatory bursa and spicule of *Trichostrongylus vitrinus*. (Courtesy of Aránzazu Meana).

Trichostrongylus longispicularis

Description: Males are around 5.5 mm in length. The spicules are stout, brown, unbranched, and slightly unequal in length terminating in a tapering blunt tip that has a small semi-transparent membranous protrusion (Table 1.2d).

Trichostrongylus probolurus

Description: Males are 4.5–6.5 mm and females 6–7.5 mm in length. The spicules are large and of equal size with two triangular projections.

Trichostrongylus rugatus

Description: Males are 4.5–5.5 mm and females 4.5–7 mm in length. The spicules differ in size and dimensions and have a complex form with transverse ridges near the tip of the spicule (Table 1.2e).

Trichostrongylus retortaeformis

Description: The adults are small, white and hair-like, usually less than 7 mm long and difficult to see with the naked eye. In the male, the ventro-ventral ray tends to be disparate from the other rays and spicules are stout, unequal in length and terminate in a barb-like tip (Table 1.2h). The females possess double ovejectors. The medium-sized eggs are an irregular ellipse with dissimilar poles. One of the side walls may be slightly flattened (see Fig. 4.9). Eggs measure about 85–91 by 46–56 µm. The thin chitinous shell has a smooth surface and contains 16–32 blastomeres.

Trichostrongylus calcaratus

Description: The adults are small, white and hair-like, usually less than 7 mm long. Male worms have an asymmetrical dorsal ray and two short, nearly equal spicules.

Trichostrongylus affinus

Description: Males measure 5–7.5 mm and females 8.5–9 mm in length. The male spicules are short, broad and equal in length, bent ventrally and taper distally into two blunt hooks.

Trichostrongylus tenuis

Description: Males measure around 5–6.5 mm and females 7–9 mm in length. The spicules are curved distally and possess an auricular offshoot anteriorly. The worms have no buccal capsule. A useful generic character is the distinct excretory notch in the oesophageal region. The medium-sized eggs are long and ovoid with dissimilar poles and parallel side walls and are pale coloured with an almost colourless shell (see Fig. 4.8). They have a thin shell with a smooth surface and measure about 65–75 by 35–42 µm.

Life cycle: The prepatent period is short (7–10 days).

Marshallagia

Similar to *Ostertagia* spp. and can be differentiated by its greater length (males 10–13 mm; females 15–20 mm).

Life cycle: The life cycle is similar to *Ostertagia* except that L$_2$ can hatch from the egg. Following ingestion, larvae burrow into the abomasal mucosa and form small greyish white nodules, which may contain several developing parasites. The young L$_5$ emerge from the nodules around day 16 post infection and egg laying is usually apparent by three weeks. Arrested development of larvae can occur. The main species is *Marshallagia marshalli* which infects the abomasum of sheep, goats, deer and camels.

Marshallagia marshalli

Synonyms: *Ostertagia tricuspis, Ostertagia marshalli*

Description: Males have a long thin dorsal ray, which bifurcates near the posterior extremity (Fig. 1.14). The end of the spicule is divided into three small processes (Fig. 1.15), surrounded by a transparent membrane. The ellipsoidal eggs are much larger than those of *Ostertagia* spp., measuring 160–200 by 75–100 µm, and resemble those of *Nematodirus battus*. The thick-shelled eggs have almost parallel sides and contain a morula in an advanced stage of development when passed in the faeces (see Fig. 4.4). The eggs can be differentiated from those of *Nematodirus* as the morula is more developed and the geographical distribution of the worms is different.

Hyostrongylus

Slender reddish worms when fresh, with males measuring around 5–7 mm and females 6–10 mm in length (Fig. 1.16). The body cuticle is both transversely and longitudinally striated with 40–45 longitudinal striations.

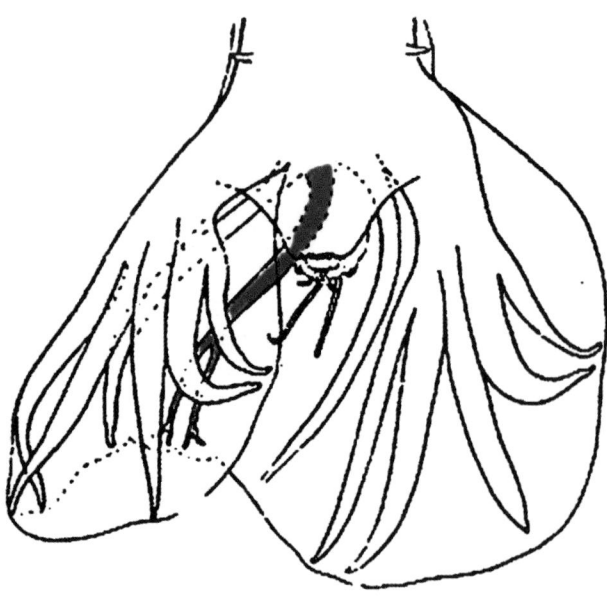

Fig. 1.14 Copulatory bursa of *Marshallagia marshalli* highlighting long thin bifurcating dorsal ray. (Adapted from Ransom, 1907.)

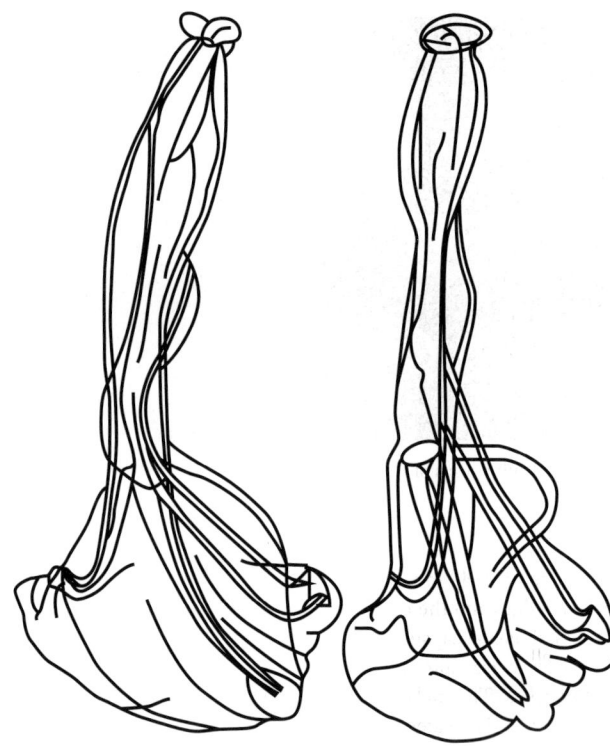

Fig. 1.15 Spicules of *Marshallagia marshalli*. (Adapted from Ransom, 1907.)

Life cycle: The free-living and parasitic stages are similar to those of *Ostertagia* in cattle; infection is through oral ingestion of L$_3$. The prepatent period is about three weeks. Hypobiosis of L$_4$ may occur following repeated infection, or be induced by seasonal changes, and is often seen in older animals. In sows, these hypobiotic larvae may resume their development during the periparturient relaxation of immunity and/or early lactation, leading to an increase in the faecal egg count. The main species is *Hyostrongylus rubidus* which infects the stomach of pigs.

Hyostrongylus rubidus

Description: Slender reddish worms when fresh, males measuring around 5–7 mm and females 6–10 mm in length (see Fig. 1.16). The body cuticle is both transversely and longitudinally striated with 40–45 longitudinal striations. A small cephalic vesicle is present and the spicules resemble *Ostertagia* in ruminants, but have only two distal branches. The bursa of the male is well developed and the dorsal lobe small. There is a well-developed telamen and short spicules. The vulva of the female opens in the posterior third of the body. Eggs are medium-sized, 71–78 by 35–42 µm, strongyle type and often difficult to differentiate from those of *Oesophagostomum*. They are ovoid with almost similar rounded poles and slightly barrel-shaped side walls. The eggshell is colourless with a thin wall and in fresh faeces contains a minimum of 32 blastomeres.

Mecistocirrus

Worms of this genus are similar in appearance to *Haemonchus contortus*, except that in the female the slit-shaped flapless vulva is located close to the anus. The males measure up to around 30 mm

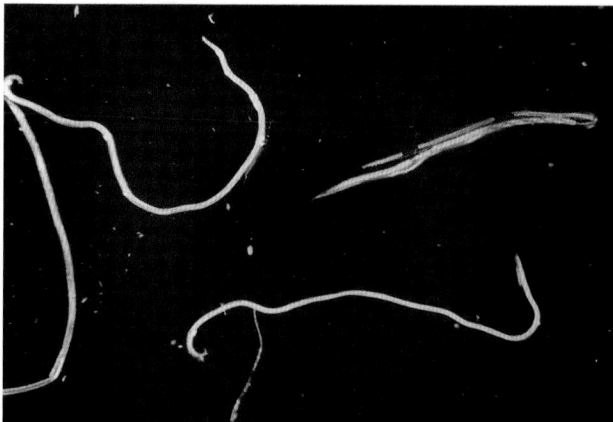

Fig. 1.16 Adult worms of *Hyostrongylus rubidus*.

and the females 42 mm in length. The cuticle contains many longitudinal ridges and the paired cervical papillae are readily apparent. The small buccal capsule is armed with a small lancet. In the female the ovaries are spirally coiled round the intestine, similar to *Haemonchus*. The male spicules are thin and long and in the bursa the dorsal ray is located symmetrically.

Life cycle: This is direct and similar to that of *Haemonchus*. The prepatent period is longer than in *Haemonchus*, being 60–80 days, partly the result of the longer duration of the fourth stage in the abomasal mucosa. The main species is *Mecistocirrus digitatus* which infects the abomasum of cattle, buffalos, sheep, goats and pigs.

Mecistocirrus digitatus

Description: To the naked eye, the worm is indistinguishable from *Haemonchus contortus*, although it is closely related to *Nematodirus*. The white ovary is wrapped around the red blood-filled intestine, giving it a 'barber's pole' appearance. The males measure up to around 30 mm and the females 42 mm in length. The male is distinguishable from *Haemonchus* by the presence of long narrow spicules that are fused together for the majority of their length and the tips are enclosed in a spindle-shaped appendage (in *Haemonchus* the spicules are thicker, separate and barbed at the tips). The dorsal ray is symmetrically located in the bursa, whereas in *Haemonchus* the dorsal ray is asymmetrical. The female differs from *Haemonchus* in that the slit-shaped vulva is positioned nearer to the tip of the tail and there is no vulval flap. The cuticle contains many longitudinal ridges and the cervical papillae are readily apparent. The small buccal capsule is armed with a lancet. The eggs are large and, unlike *Nematodirus*, typically strongylate and measure around 100 μm in length.

Graphidium

Stomach worms of lagomorphs found throughout Europe.

Life cycle: The life cycle is direct. Infection is by ingestion of infective larvae, which develop to the adult stage in the stomach in about 12 days. The main species is *Graphidium strigosum* which infects the stomach and small intestine of rabbits and hares.

Graphidium strigosum

Description: The adults are reddish worms when fresh, with 40–60 longitudinal lines and fine transverse striations. The male is 8–16 mm and female 11–20 mm long. The male bursa has large lateral lobes and a small dorsal lobe. Spicules are long, slender and each ends distally in several points. The medium-sized eggs are typically trichostrongyle, ovoid and measure 98–106 by 50–58 μm (see Fig. 4.9). The egg contains a large number of blastomeres or may contain an L_1 larva. The eggs are larger than those of *Trichostrongylus*.

Obeliscoides

This genus contains several species of worms found in a number of rabbit species in the USA.

Life cycle: The life cycle is direct. Infection is by ingestion of infective larvae, which develop to the adult stage in the stomach in about 19 days. The main species is *Obeliscoides cuniculi* which infects the stomach of rabbits, hares and occasionaly white-tailed deer.

Obeliscoides cuniculi

Description: Adults are red-brownish in colour and males measure 10–16 mm and the females 15–18 mm in length. The brown spicules are bifurcated at their distal tips and terminate in a hook. The female worm tapers in the distal 20% of the body. The male spicules are brown and bifurcated at the distal end. The body of the female is tapered over the posterior 20% of its length. Eggs are typically trichostrongyle, ovoid and measure 76–86 by 44–45 μm (see Fig. 4.9).

Libyostrongylus

Libyostrongylus douglassi and *Libyostrongylus dentatus* are parasites of ratites (ostrich) commonly referred to as 'Wireworms' found in the proventriculus and gizzard.

Life cycle: The life cycle is typically strongyle. Following ingestion, infective larvae burrow into the proventricular glands and under the kaolin layer of both the proventriculus and gizzard where they develop into adult worms 4–5 weeks later. Eggs which contain fully developed larvae are very resistant to desiccation and can survive a couple of years.

Libyostrongylus douglassi

Description: Small yellowish-red nematodes, males 4–6 mm and females 5–6 mm in length. The male bursa is well developed; the dorsal ray is long and split in its distal half forming three small branches either side. The spicules each end in a large and small spine. Eggs measure 59–74 by 36–44 μm. Third-stage larvae are characterised by a small knob at the tip of the tail and measure around 745 μm in length (Fig. 1.17).

Libyostrongylus dentatus

Description: Males are 6–8 mm and females 10–12 mm in length. There is a prominent dorsal, oesophageal tooth. The male has a large bursa; the dorsal ray is long and bifurcated, extending into a

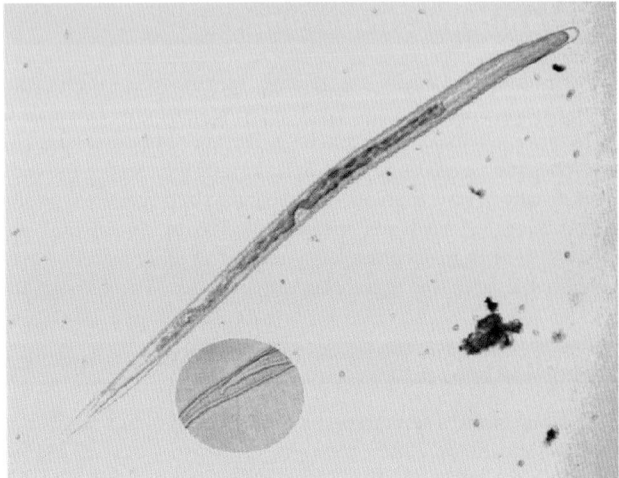

Fig. 1.17 *Libyostrongylus douglassi* L$_3$. Inset shows magnified larval tail tip within the third cuticle.

Table 1.4 *Ostertagia* species.

Species	Hosts	Site
Ostertagia ostertagi *Ostertagia* (syn. *Skrjabinagia*) *lyrata*	Cattle, deer, rarely goats	Abomasum
Ostertagia leptospicularis (syn. *Ostertagia crimensis*) *Skrjabinagia* (*Ostertagia*) *kolchida* (syn. *Grosspiculagia podjapolskyi*)	Deer, cattle, sheep and goats	Abomasum
Teladorsagia circumcincta *Ostertagia trifurcata* *Teladorsagia davtiani*	Sheep, goats, deer, camels, llamas	Abomasum
Spiculopteragia spiculoptera (syn. *Apteragia spiculoptera*, *Rinadia spiculoptera*, *Mazamostrongylus spiculoptera*)	Deer (red deer, fallow deer, roe deer), cattle, sheep, goats	Abomasum
Spiculopteragia asymmetrica (syn. *Ostertagia asymmetrica*, *Apteragia asymmetrica*, *Rinadia asymmetrica*, *Mazamostrongylus asymmetrica*)	Deer (roe deer, sika deer, fallow deer)	Abomasum
Apteragia quadrispiculata	Deer (roe deer, sika deer, fallow deer)	Abomasum
Spiculopteragia (*Apteragia*) *bohmi* *Spiculopteragia* (*Rinadia*) *mathevossiani*	Mouflons, deer (fallow deer, roe deer)	Abomasum
Spiculopteragia peruvianus	Llamas, vicunas	Abomasum

rounded lobe of the bursal membrane. The spicules have a dorsal process arising two-thirds from the anterior and the main shaft ending in a rounded point capped by a hyaline sheath.

Graphinema

Graphinema aucheniae

Description: Male worms measure 5.5–8 mm and females 9–12 mm in length. These worms have a small buccal capsule, a claviform oesophagus and cervical papillae. The male bursa has a small anteroventral ray and a widely divergent posteroventral ray. The dorsal ray bifurcates near the distal tip, with each branch dividing distally. The spicules are long and pointed.

Life cycle: Similar to that of other trichostrongyles. The main species is *Graphinema aucheniae* which infects the abomasum of llamas and vicunas.

Impalaia

Impalaia tuberculata and *Impalaia nudicollis* are parasites of the abomasum of camels, very similar in dimensions (i.e. males are 7–9 mm and females 14–18 mm long). *Impalaia tuberculata* has the cervical cuticle studded with papillae and spicules are equal in length, slender and with a fine pointed end, whereas *Impalaia nudicollis* males have long spicules and a long gubernaculum.

SUBFAMILY OSTERTAGINAE

Species within the subfamily Ostertaginae are considered together as they form a large and complex group, the taxonomy of which has not been fully elucidated. Some species names are considered synonymous and species polymorphism is commonly reported (Table 1.4).

The adults are slender reddish-brown worms up to 1 cm long, occurring on the surface of the abomasal mucosa and are only visible on close inspection (Fig. 1.18). They possess a short buccal cavity and a very small pair of cervical papillae. The short spicules are brown in colour and terminate in two or three processes, depending on the species. In the female, the vulva can be covered with a flap or this may be absent and the tip of the tail is annulated.

The larval stages occur in the gastric glands and can only be seen microscopically following processing of the gastric mucosa. Species differentiation is generally based on the structure of the male spicules. These worms occur in cattle, sheep and other ruminants.

Life cycle: Eggs are passed in the faeces and, under optimal conditions, develop within the faecal pat to the infective third stage within two weeks. When moist conditions prevail, the L$_3$ migrate from the faeces on to the herbage. After ingestion, the L$_3$ exsheaths in the rumen and further development takes place in the lumen of an abomasal gland. Two parasitic moults occur before the L$_5$ emerges from the gland around 18 days after infection to become sexually mature on the mucosal surface. The entire parasitic life cycle usually takes tyree weeks, but under certain circumstances many of the ingested L$_3$ become arrested in development at the early fourth larval stage (EL$_4$) for periods of up to six months (also referred to as hypobiosis). See **life cycle 1**.

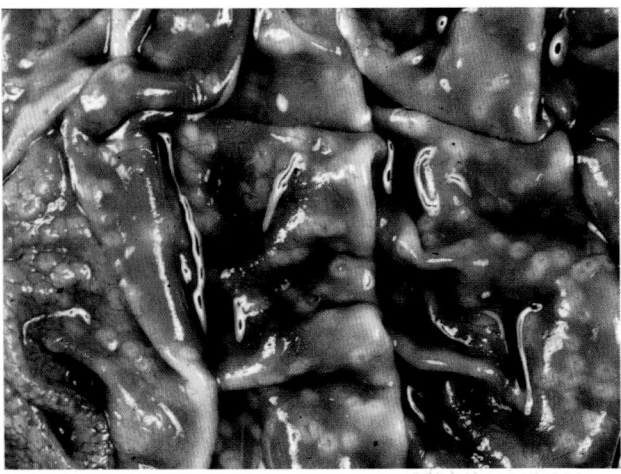

Fig. 1.18 *Ostertagia ostertagi* on the abomasal mucosa.

LIFE CYCLE 1. LIFE CYCLE OF *OSTERTAGIA* SPP.

Adults of *Ostertagia* spp. live on the surface of the abomasum (1) of cattle and small ruminants. Worms are thin and whitish in colour, with a vestigial buccal capsule. Males are ~7 mm long and characterised by a well-developed copulatory bursa and distinct spicules, whose morphology is useful for species identification (2). Females are ~11 mm long, and in some species the vulva is covered by a cuticular expansion known as a 'vulvar flap' (3). The eggs are elliptical in shape, thin-walled and transparent (80–100 × 50 μm), with 16–32 blastomeres (4); eggs are eliminated into the environment with the faeces. Under optimal conditions of temperature and humidity, eggs hatch into L_1 (5) which, after two moults, develop into second-stage (6) and infective third-stage larvae (L_3) (7). Once ingested by grazing ruminants (8), the larvae lose their external sheath in the rumen and travel to the abomasum, where they penetrate the gastric glands (9) and continue their development. Here, the L_3 moult to L_4 and grow from 1.3 mm to 8 mm in length, thus forming nodules ~1–2 mm in diameter with a characteristic central hole; the glandular mucosa appears hyperplasic and undergoes functional changes that lead to a significant reduction in the production of gastric pepsin. During winter, the larvae can undergo hypobiosis (reduced metabolism and developmental arrest). The larvae develop to L_5 (10) and emerge in the lumen of the abomasum. The prepatent period, from ingestion of infective larvae to development of sexually mature adults, takes ~3 weeks. The life cycle of other Trichostrongylidae is similar to that of *Ostertagia* spp., except for *Nematodirus* spp. whose infective L_3 develop inside the eggs, prior to hatching in the environment.

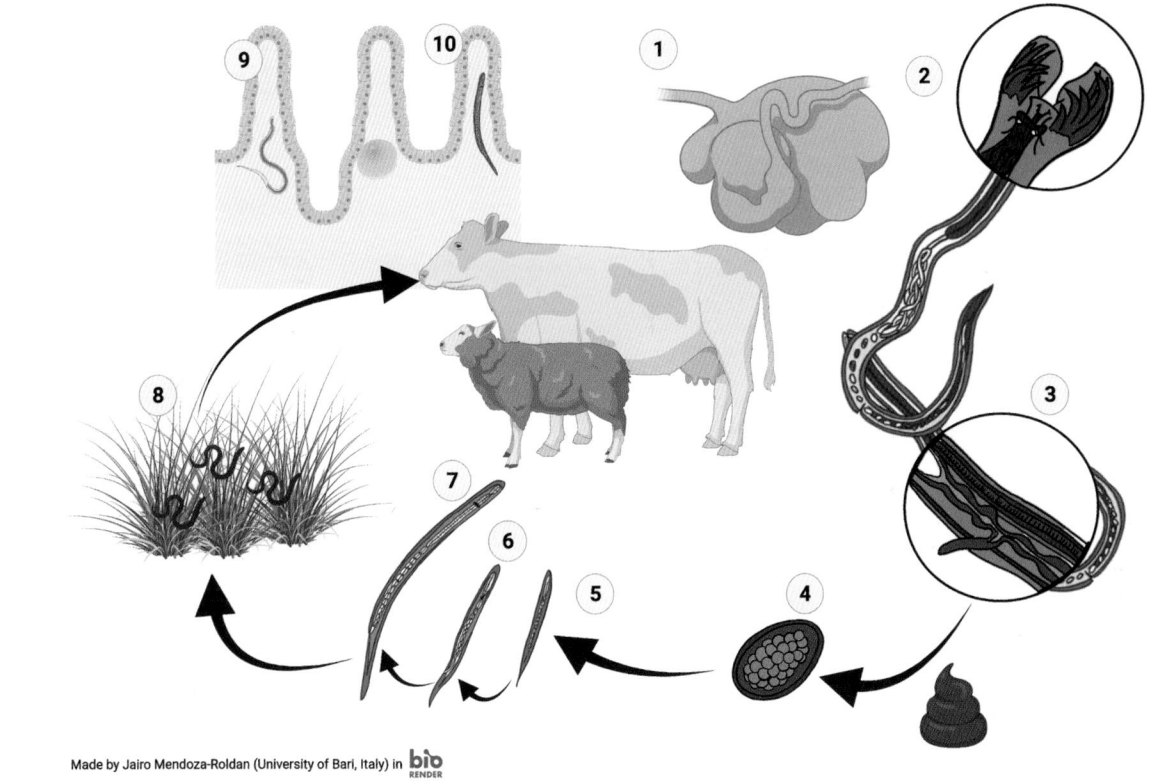

Made by Jairo Mendoza-Roldan (University of Bari, Italy) in bioRENDER

Ostertagia ostertagi

Morph species: *Ostertagia* (syn. *Skrjabinagia*) *lyrata*

Description: Adults are small, slender reddish-brown worms with a short buccal cavity. Males measure 6–8 mm and females 8–11 mm in length. The cuticle in the anterior region is striated transversely whereas the rest of the body is unstriated and bears around 30 longitudinal ridges.

- *Ostertagia ostertagi*: The spicules are divided in the posterior region where two thin lateral branches arise from the main stem (Table 1.5a). The bursa is small and the accessory bursal membrane is supported by two divergent rays (Fig. 1.19). In the female, the vulva is sited about 1.5 mm from the posterior and is covered with a flap (Fig. 1.20).

- *Ostertagia lyrata*: The spicules are stout and divided into three branches posteriorly. The main branch is solid and ends in a shoe-like expansion. One lateral branch is thick and massive, terminating in a hat-like expansion; the other is small and pointed (Table 1.5b and Fig. 1.21). The gubernaculum is spindle-shaped.

Ostertagia leptospicularis

Synonym: *Ostertagia crimensis*

Morph species: *Skrjabinagia* (*Ostertagia*) *kolchida* (syn. *Grosspiculagia podjapolskyi*)

Description: Adults are slender reddish-brown worms with a short buccal cavity. Males measure 6–8 mm and females 8–9 mm in length.

Table 1.5 Identification of Ostertaginae based on male spicule morphology.

Species	Spicules: description	Spicules: morphology
Ostertagia ostertagi	The spicules are of equal length and shape, tapering towards the distal end into three processes	(a)
Ostertagia lyrata	The spicules are stout and divided into three branches posteriorly. The main branch is solid and ends in a shoe-like expansion. One lateral branch is thick and massive, terminating in a hat-like expansion; the other is small and pointed	(b)
Ostertagia leptospicularis	The spicules are slender, of equal length and shape, tapering towards the distal end into three processes, with the two lateral branches extremely fine and pointed	(c)
Skrjabinagia kolchida	The spicules are of equal length and shape, tapering towards the distal end into three branches terminating in an 'ice-skate'-like structure. The medial branch is the shortest and truncated	(d)
Teladorsagia circumcincta	Spicules are variable in length but normally long and thin. The posterior end is split into two branches of equal length. A third short offshoot, not readily seen, arises in front of the bifurcation	(e)
Ostertagia trifurcata	Spicules are short and broad; the posterior end is divided into three processes, one long and thick with a truncated end, and two short slender branches each tapering to a point	(f)
Spiculopteragia spiculoptera	The spicules are of equal length, bifurcating distally where they contain a cavity and distally ending in a fan-shaped expansion	(g)
Spiculopteragia bohmi	Spicules of equal size but asymmetrical. The right spicule divides into three branches and the left spicule into two branches	(h)

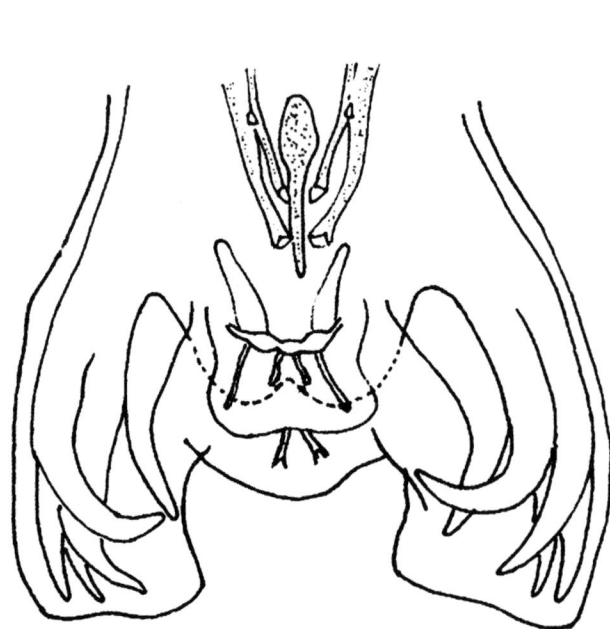

Fig. 1.19 Male bursa and spicules of *Ostertagia ostertagi*.

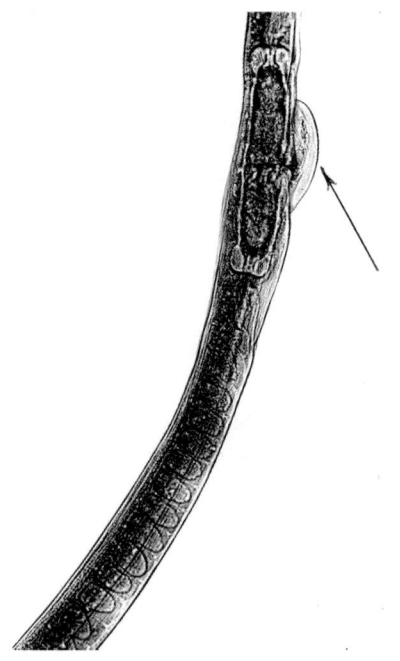

Fig. 1.20 Female vulva and flap (arrowed) of *Ostertagia ostertagi*.

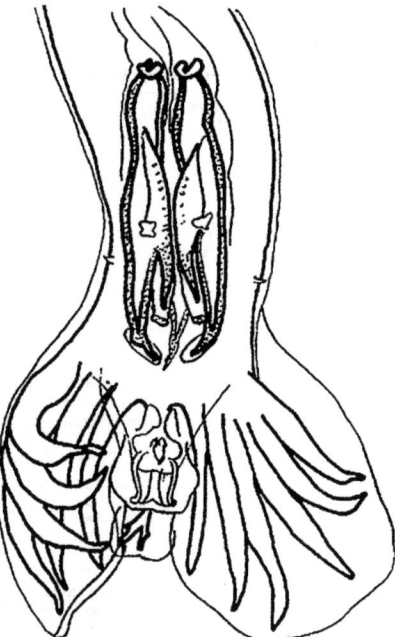

Fig. 1.21 Male bursa and spicules of *Ostertagia lyrata*.

Distinguished from other ostertagian species by the length of the oesophagus, which is longer (0.7 mm compared with approximately 0.6 mm in other species). In cattle, the worms are thinner than *O. ostertagi* and male worms are differentiated on spicule morphology.

- *Ostertagia leptospicularis*: The spicules are of equal length and shape, tapering towards the distal end into three processes (Table 1.5c and Fig. 1.22). The gubernaculum is racket-shaped.
- *Skrjabinagia kolchida*: The spicules are of equal length and shape, tapering towards the distal end into three branches terminating in a shoe-like structure (Table 1.5d and Fig. 1.23). The medial branch is the shortest and truncated. The gubernaculum is longer than in *O. leptospicularis* and twisted.

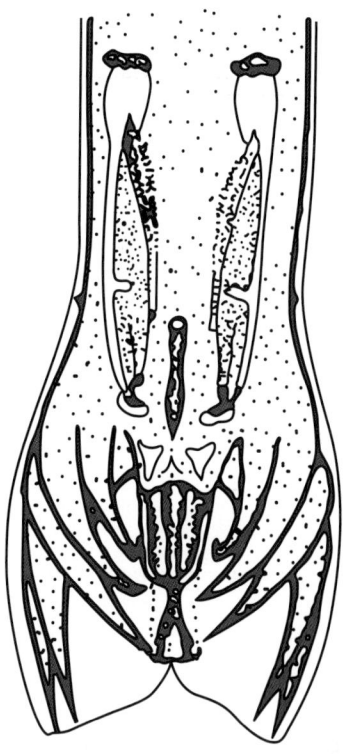

Fig. 1.23 Male bursa and spicules of *Skrjabinagia kolchida*.

Teladorsagia circumcincta

Synonym: *Ostertagia circumcincta*

Morph species: *Ostertagia trifurcata, Teladorsagia davtiani*

Description: Adults are slender reddish-brown worms with a short buccal cavity. Males measure 6–8 mm and females 8–10 mm.

- *Teladorsagia circumcincta*: The lateral lobes of the bursa are well developed but the dorsal lobe is small; a telamon is present in the genital cone; the accessory bursal membrane is small and supported by two divergent rays (Fig. 1.24). Spicules are variable in length but

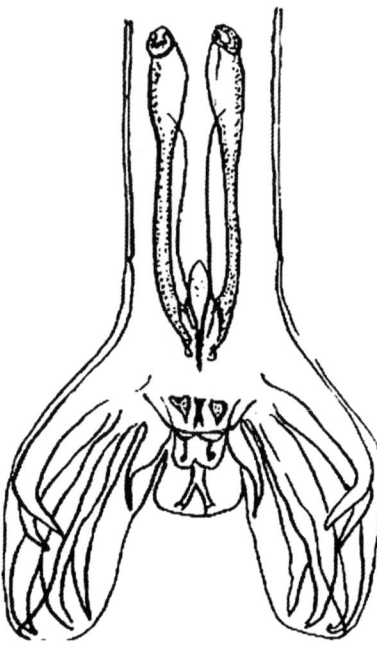

Fig. 1.22 Male bursa and spicules of *Ostertagia leptospicularis*.

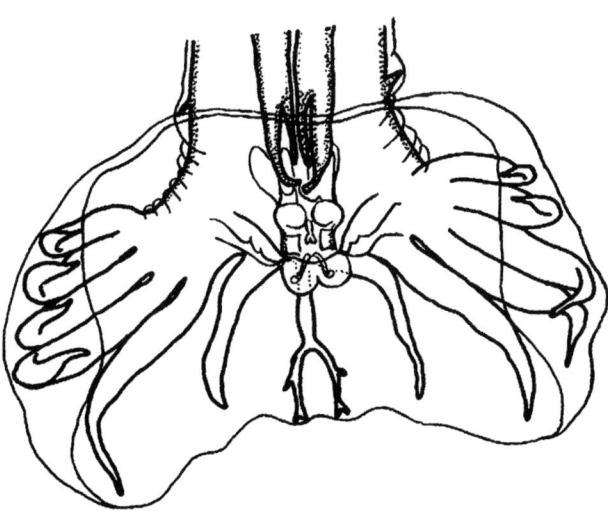

Fig. 1.24 Male bursa and spicules of *Teladorsagia circumcincta*.

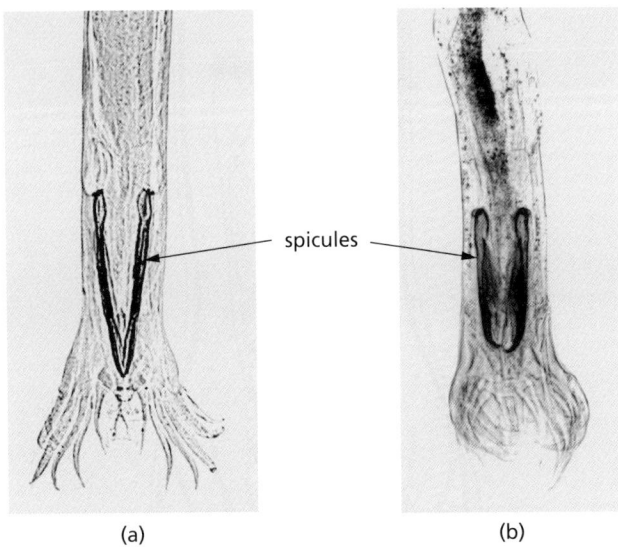

spicules

(a)   (b)

Fig. 1.25 Comparison of spicules of (a) *Teladorsagia circumcincta* and (b) *Ostertagia trifurcata*. Those of *T. circumcincta* are long and thin whereas *O. trifurcata* spicules are short and broad.

normally long and thin (Table 1.5e and Fig. 1.25a). The posterior end is split into two branches of equal length. A third short offshoot, not readily seen, arises in front of the bifurcation. The gubernaculum is racket-shaped. In the female, the vulva is usually covered with a large flap and opens near the posterior of the body.

- *Ostertagia trifurcata*: The bursa is longer than in *T. circumcincta*. The lateral lobes of the bursa are well developed and the dorsal lobe is small (Fig. 1.26). A well-developed telamon is present in the genital cone. The accessory bursal membrane is modified to form Sjoberg's organ supported by two rays. The spicules are short and broad (Table 1.5f and Figs 1.25b and 1.26) with the posterior ends divided into three processes, one long and thick with a truncated end and two short slender branches each tapering to a point. The gubernaculum is somewhat spindle-shaped.
- *Teladorsagia davtiani*: This morph species is similar in appearance to *O. trifurcata*. The accessory bursal membrane is modified to form Sjoberg's organ and resembles a pair of sessile papillae on the posterior extremity of the genital cone (Fig. 1.27).

Spiculopteragia spiculoptera

Synonyms: *Apteragia spiculoptera, Rinadia spiculoptera, Mazamostrongylus spiculoptera*

Description: The spicules are of equal length, bifurcating distally where they contain a cavity, and distally ending in a fan-shaped expansion (Table 1.5g). The gubernaculum is absent.

Spiculopteragia asymmetrica

Synonyms: *Ostertagia asymmetrica, Apteragia asymmetrica, Rinadia asymmetrica, Mazamostrongylus asymmetrica*

Description: Males measure 4.5–6 mm. Spicules are distally asymmetrical and pointed, with a T-shaped offshoot near the distal end of the right spicule. The gubernaculum is small and boat-shaped.

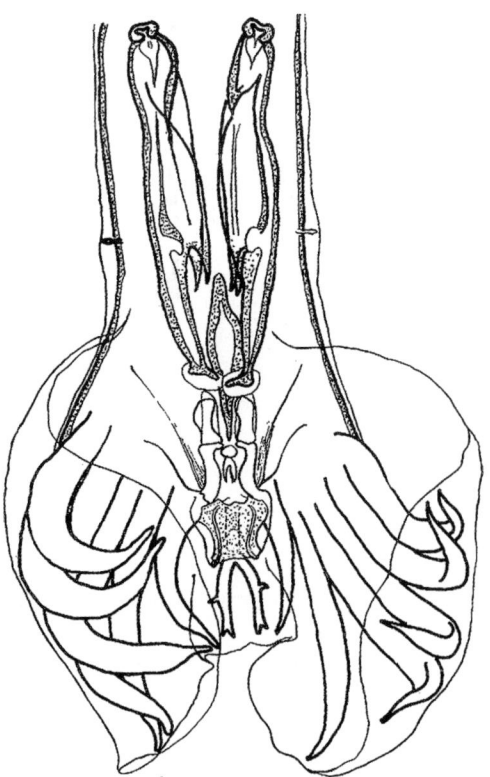

Fig. 1.26 Male bursa and spicules of *Ostertagia trifurcata*.

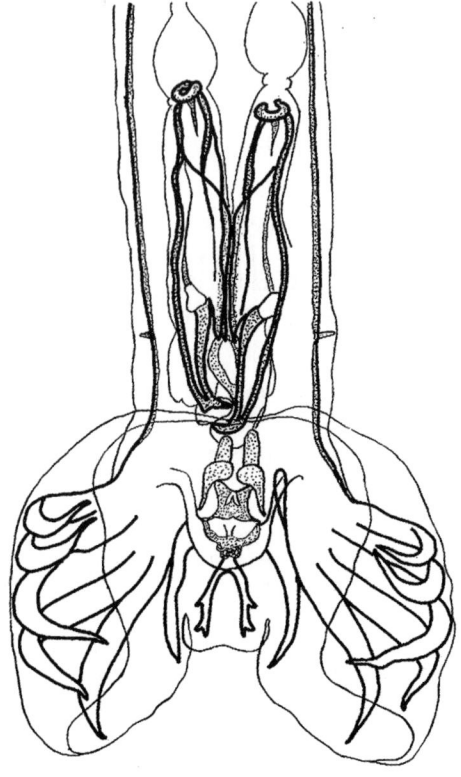

Fig. 1.27 Male bursa and spicules of *Teladorsagia davtiani*.

Apteragia quadrispiculata

Description: Males measure 6–8.5 mm. Spicules possess four branches distally.

Spiculopteragia bohmi

Synonyms: *Apteragia bohmi, Rinadia bohmi, Mazamostrongylus bohmi, Ostertagia bohmi*

Morph species: *Spiculopteragia (Rinadia) mathevossiani*

Description: Considered to be a polymorphic species with two male morphs, *Spiculoptergia bohmi* and *Spiculoptergia mathevossiani*. Males measure 6–7 mm.

- *Spiculopteragia bohmi*: Spicules of equal size but asymmetrical. The right spicule divides into three branches and the left spicule into two branches (Table 1.5h). The gubernaculum is absent.
- *Spiculopteragia mathevossiani*: The spicules have asymmetrical distal thirds each ending in three branches. The gubernaculum is absent.

Spiculopteragia peruvianus

Description: Males measure 6.5–8 mm and females 8.5–10 mm in length.

Camelostrongylus

The main species is *Camelostrongylus mentulatus* which infects the abomasum and small intestine of camels, sheep and goats.

Camelostrongylus mentulatus

Synonym: *Ostertagia mentulatus*

Description: *Camelostrongylus mentulatus* is similar in size to *Ostertagia ostertagi*. Males are 6.5–7.5 mm and females 8–10 mm long. The bursa possesses two large lateral lobes and the spicules are narrow, long, denticulated and of equal length (Fig. 1.28). Eggs measure about 75–85 by 40–50 μm.

SUBFAMILY HAEMONCHINAE

Haemonchus

The adult *Haemonchus* spp. (Table 1.6) are easily identified because of their specific location in the abomasum and their large size (2–3 cm). In fresh female specimens, the white ovaries winding spirally around the blood-filled intestine produce a 'barber's pole' appearance (Fig. 1.29). The buccal cavity is small and contains a small lancet-like tooth. The anterior body possesses prominent cervical papillae. The vulva is usually protected by a cuticular flap which can have a range of shapes. In the male, the lateral lobes of the bursa are large, whereas the dorsal ray is small and asymmetrical.

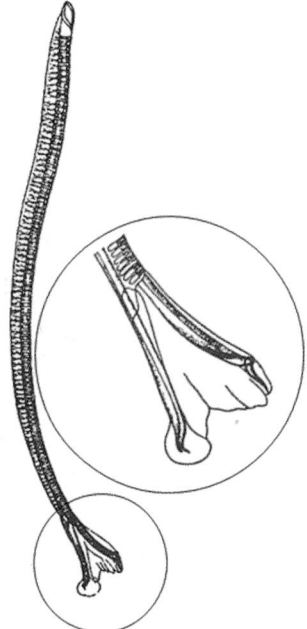

Fig. 1.28 Male bursa and spicule of *Camelostrongylus mentulatus*. (Adapted from Skrjabin *et al.*, 1954.)

Table 1.6 *Haemonchus* species.

Species	Hosts	Site
Haemonchus contortus (syn. *Haemonchus placei*)	Sheep, goats, cattle, deer, camels, llamas	Abomasum
Haemonchus similis	Cattle, deer	Abomasum
Haemonchus longistipes	Camels, sheep	Abomasum

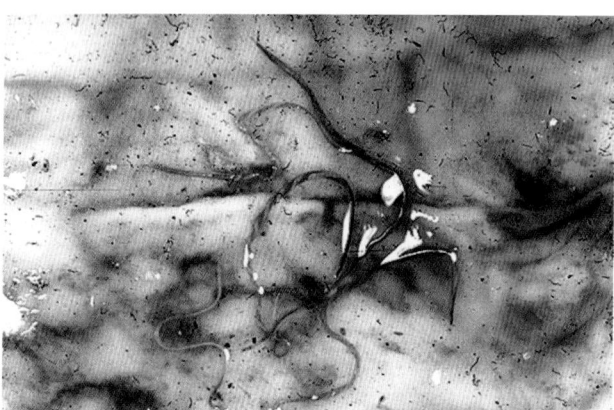

Fig. 1.29 Adult male and female worms of *Haemonchus contortus* on the abomasal mucosa.

Life cycle: This is direct and the preparasitic phase is typically trichostrongyloid. The females are prolific egg layers. The eggs hatch to L_1 on the pasture and may develop to L_3 in as little as five days but development may be delayed for weeks or months under cool conditions. After ingestion and exsheathment in the rumen, the larvae moult twice in close apposition to the gastric glands. Just before the final moult, they develop the piercing lancet which enables them to obtain blood from the mucosal vessels. As adults, they move freely on the surface of the mucosa. The prepatent period is 2–3 weeks in sheep and four weeks in cattle.

Haemonchus contortus

Synonym: *Haemonchus placei*

Description: Males are about 10–22 mm and females 20–30 mm in length. The male has an asymmetrical dorsal lobe and barbed spicules (Fig. 1.30a). The vulva is situated at the beginning of the posterior third of the body. This is a useful feature for distinguishing *Haemonchus* from *Mecistocirrus*, in which the vulva is positioned near the tip of the tail. In both sexes there are cervical papillae (Fig. 1.30b) and a tiny lancet inside the buccal capsule. Infective larvae have 16 gut cells, the head is narrow and rounded and the tail of the sheath is offset. The egg is medium-sized (64–95 × 40–50 μm) and is a regular broad ellipse with barrel-shaped side walls and flattened wide poles (see Fig. 4.4). The chitinous shell is thin, slightly light-yellowish in colour and smooth, and the egg contains numerous blastomeres which nearly fill the entire volume. The blastomeres are not readily distinguished. Infective larvae measure around 690 μm (see Fig. 4.15).

Notes: Until recently, the sheep species was *H. contortus* and the cattle species *H. placei*. However, there is now increasing evidence that these are the single species *H. contortus* with only strain adaptations for cattle and sheep.

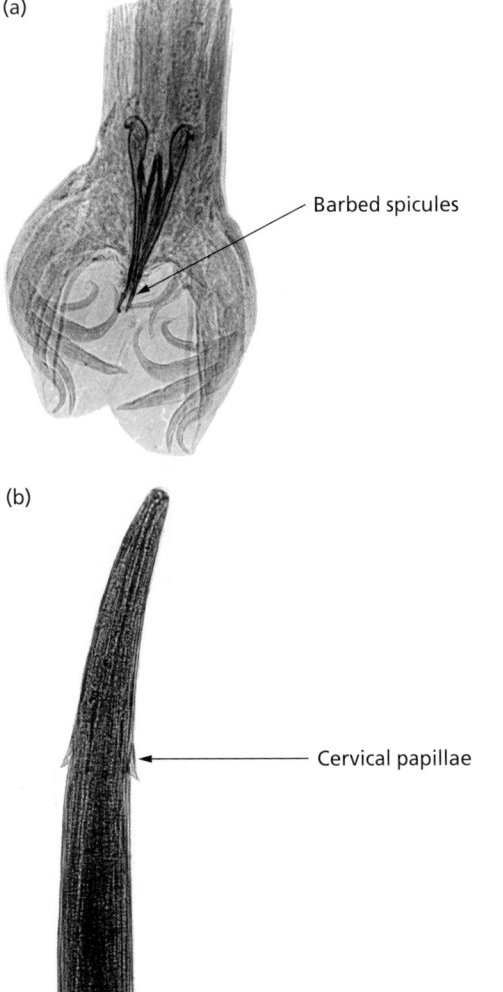

(a)

Barbed spicules

(b)

Cervical papillae

Fig. 1.30 (a) Barbed spicules and bursa of a mature *Haemonchus contortus* male worm. (b) Anterior of *H. contortus* showing the position of the cervical papillae.

Haemonchus similis

Description: The adults are 2–3 cm and reddish in colour. The male has an asymmetrical dorsal lobe and barbed spicules, differing from *H. contortus* in that the terminal processes of the dorsal ray are longer and the spicules shorter.

Haemonchus longistipes

Description: Relatively small worms; males are 10–20 mm and females 18–30 mm long. Females have a reduced knob-like vulval flap (cf. *H. contortus* which has a well-developed linguiform vulvar flap).

FAMILY COOPERIDAE

Cooperia

Cooperia spp. (Table 1.7) are relatively small worms (usually less than 9 mm long), which appear pinkish-white when fresh. The main generic features are the small cephalic vesicle and the marked transverse cuticular striations in the oesophageal region (Fig. 1.31). The body possesses longitudinal ridges. The male bursa is relatively

Table 1.7 *Cooperia* species.

Species	Hosts	Site
Cooperia oncophora	Cattle, sheep, goats, deer, camels	Small intestine
Cooperia curticei	Sheep, goats, deer (red deer, fallow deer)	Small intestine
Cooperia punctata	Cattle, deer, rarely sheep	Small intestine
Cooperia pectinata	Cattle, deer, rarely sheep	Small intestine
Cooperia surnabada (syn. *Cooperia mcmasteri*)	Cattle, sheep, goats, camels	Small intestine

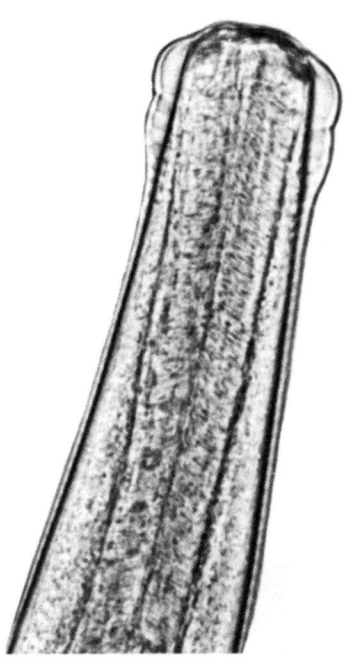

Fig. 1.31 Anterior of *Cooperia* spp. showing the cephalic vesicle and cuticular striations.

large compared to the size of the body. It has a small dorsal lobe, and the brown-coloured spicules are short and stout with distinct wing-like expansions in the middle region, which often bear transverse ridged striations (except in *C. surnabada*) (Table 1.8). There is no gubernaculum. The females have a long tapering tail and the vulva may be covered by a vulval flap and is located posterior to the middle of the body. The egg contains many blastomeres that are not easily distinguished. The small poles are very similar and the side walls are parallel. This feature allows the eggs to be differentiated from those of *Ostertagia* which have wider poles and more spherical walls.

Life cycle: The life cycle is direct and typical of the superfamily. Ingested L_3 exsheath, migrate into the intestinal crypts for two moults and then the adults develop on the surface of the intestinal mucosa. The prepatent period is 2–3 weeks. The bionomic requirements of the free-living stages are similar to those of *Teladorsagia*.

Cooperia oncophora

Description: In size, *C. oncophora* is similar to *Ostertagia* but with a large bursa. Males measure around 5.5–9 mm and females 6–8 mm in length. Spicules have a longitudinal line pattern with the distal end rounded and bearing cuticular formations (Table 1.8a).

Cooperia curticei

Description: *Cooperia curticei* is moderately small with a large bursa with fleshy supporting rays. The most notable feature is the 'watch spring'-like posture. Males measure around 4.5–6 mm and females 6–8 mm in length. When fresh, they appear pinkish white. The main generic features are the very small cephalic vesicle and the transverse cuticular striations in the oesophageal region. The body possesses longitudinal ridges. Spicules are equal in length and have a central protuberance with a transverse striation and end in a rounded disc-like structure (Table 1.8b). The females have a long tapering tail. Eggs are oval with nearly similar poles and parallel side walls (see Fig. 4.4). They are thin-shelled with a smooth surface and contain many blastomeres which are hard to distinguish. Infective larvae measure around 780 μm (see Fig. 4.15).

Cooperia surnabada

Synonym: *Cooperia mcmasteri*

Description: The males measure around 7 mm and the females 8 mm in length. The appearance is very similar to *C. oncophora*, although the bursa is larger and the bursal rays tend to be thinner. The spicules are thinner with a posterior bifurcation into an external branch with a small conical appendage and an internal branch that is shorter and pointed (Table 1.8c).

Cooperia punctata

Description: Males measure around 4.5–6 mm and females 6–8 mm in length. Spicules are short and bear a large protuberance at the distal half, tapering to a slightly blunted point (Table 1.8d).

Table 1.8 Identification of *Cooperia* spp. based on male spicule morphology.

Species	Spicules: description	Spicules: morphology
Cooperia oncophora	Spicules are 240–300 μm long and have a longitudinal line pattern with the distal end rounded and bearing cuticular formations	(a)
Cooperia curticei	Spicules are equal in length (135–145 μm) and have a central protuberance with a transverse striation and end in a rounded 'disc-like' structure	(b)
Cooperia surnabada	The spicules are 270 μm long and thin with a posterior bifurcation into an external branch with small conical appendage and an internal branch that is shorter and pointed	(c)
Cooperia punctata	Spicules are short (120–150 μm) and bear a large protuberance at the distal half, tapering to a slightly blunted point	(d)
Cooperia pectinata	Spicules are 240–280 μm long with a large protuberance centrally, and are bent ventrally, with a wrinkled inner surface	(e)

Cooperia pectinata

Description: Males measure around 7–8 mm and females 7.5–10 mm in length. Spicules bear a protuberance centrally and are bent ventrally, with a wrinkled inner surface (Table 1.8e).

FAMILY ORNITHOSTRONGYLIDAE

Ornithostrongylus

The adult worms, which measure up to 2.5 cm, are bloodsuckers, have a reddish colour and can be seen by the naked eye. The life cycle is direct and typically trichostrongyle. The main species is *Ornithostrongylus quadriradiatus* which infects the crop, proventriculus and small intestine of pigeons and doves.

Ornithostrongylus quadriradiatus

Description: Males measure 9–12 mm and females 18–24 mm in length. The cuticle of the head is slightly inflated and the body bears longitudinal cuticular ridges. The anterior of the worm has a long, slightly inflated vesicle, which is present from the cephalic area to the cervical region. The tail of the female worm is blunt with a small spine. In the male bursa, the ventral rays are close together and the dorsal ray is short. The telamon is shaped like a small bar with two arms and covers the tips of the spicules. Spicules end in three pointed processes. Eggs are ovoid and measure 70–75 by 38–40 μm.

FAMILY AMIDOSTOMIDAE

Amidostomum

The slender adult worms, bright red in colour when fresh and up to 2.5 cm in length, are easily recognised at necropsy where they predominate in the horny lining of the gizzard (Fig. 1.32). These worms have a shallow buccal cavity and do not possess leaf crowns. Three longitudinal ridges/plates line the oesophagus.

Life cycle: Direct and similar to other strongyles. Infection is via ingestion of L_3 or through skin penetration. Eggs passed in the faeces are already embryonated and develop to L_3 in the egg. Ingested larvae penetrate the submucosa of the gizzard. Patency is around 2–3 weeks in geese.

Amidostomum anseris

Synonym: *Amidostomum nodulosum*

Description: The slender adult worms, bright red in colour when fresh and up to 2.5 cm in length, are easily recognised at necropsy where they predominate in the horny lining of the gizzard. Males measure about 10–17 mm and females 15–25 mm. Characterised by a shallow buccal capsule with three pointed teeth, the middle one being the largest. The male spicules are of equal length and are divided into two branches at the posterior. The medium-sized eggs are thin-shelled with a smooth surface, ellipsoidal and measure around 90–110 by 50–80 µm and contain a large number of blastomeres or a segmented embryo when laid (see Fig. 4.8). The egg hatches when the L_3 larva is present.

Amidostomum acutum

Synonym: *Amidostomum skrjabini*

Description: Characterised by a shallow buccal capsule with one pointed tooth. The spicules have 2–3 branches at the distal end.

Epomidiostomum

These worms are similar to *Amidostomum* but smaller.

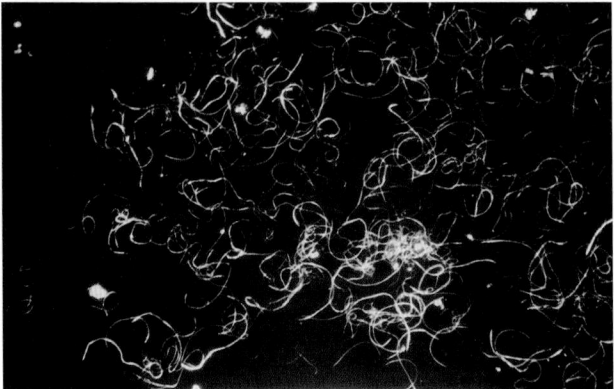

Fig. 1.32 Adult worms of *Amidostomum anseris*.

Epomidiostomum uncinatum

Synonyms: *Epomidiostomum anatinum*, *Strongylus uncinatus*, *Amidostomum anatinum*

Description: Males measure about 10 mm and females 15 mm in length. Teeth are absent from the rudimentary buccal capsule. The cuticle bears distinct thickenings, 'epaulettes', at the anterior end and tooth-like projections form a fringe around the mouth. The posterior of the female is rounded and has a small button-shaped tip. Three branches occur on each spicule.

Epomidiostomum orispinum

Synonyms: *Strongylus anseris*, *Strongylus orispinum*
Description: Males measure around 11 mm and females 16 mm in length. The anterior of the worm possesses four posteriorly pointing offshoots and lateral festoons bearing a pair of papillae. Spicules are equal with three shafts pointing distally. The body of the female tapers abruptly, towards the digitate tail.

Epomidiostomum skrjabini

Description: The size of the males and females is similar to that of *E. orispinum*. The head of the worm possesses a cuticular prominence which is armed with four symmetrical, lateral-pointing spines. There are also two epaulette formations. The mouth is surrounded by four small spines. The bursa has three lobes, the central lobe being poorly developed. Spicules are equal and the posterior ends are split into three sharp-tipped branches. The anterior ends are blunt. The female tail terminates in a finger-like appendage, which is bent ventrally.

FAMILY MOLINEIDAE

Nematodirus

Nematodirus spp. adult worms (Table 1.9) are whitish, slender and relatively long, with the anterior thinner than the posterior region. They may appear slightly coiled. Adult males are 10–15 mm and females 15–24 mm in length. A small but distinct cephalic vesicle is present (Fig. 1.33) and the cuticle possesses about 14–18 longitudinal ridges. The male bursa has elongated lateral lobes and the spicules are long and slender; the tips of the spicules are fused together and terminate in a small expansion, which varies in shape and is a useful feature for species differentiation (Table 1.10). The ventral

Table 1.9 *Nematodirus* species.

Species	Hosts	Site
Nematodirus battus	Sheep, goats, occasionally cattle	Small intestine
Nematodirus filicollis	Sheep, goats, occasionally deer	Small intestine
Nematodirus spathiger	Sheep, goats, cattle	Small intestine
Nematodirus helvetianus	Cattle, occasionally sheep, goats	Small intestine
Nematodirus abnormalis	Camels, sheep, goats	Small intestine
Nematodirus mauritanicus	Camels	Small intestine
Nematodirus lamae	Llamas, alpacas, vicunas	Small intestine
Nematodirus leporis	Rabbits	Small intestine

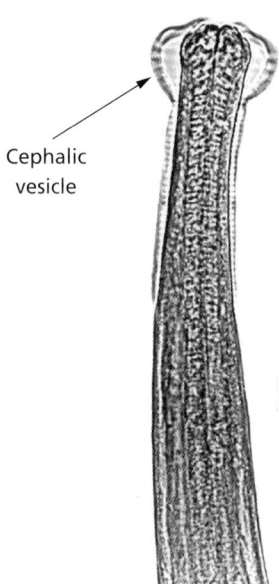

Cephalic
vesicle

Fig. 1.33 Anterior of *Nematodirus battus* illustrating the small cephalic vesicle.

Table 1.10 Identification of *Nematodirus* species based on male spicule morphology.

Species	Spicules: description	Spicules: morphology
Nematodirus battus	The spicules are long and slender and the tips are fused into a small, flattened oval-shaped projection	(a)
Nematodirus filicollis	The spicules are long and slender with fused tips and terminate in a narrow pointed swelling	(b)
Nematodirus spathiger	The spicules are long and slender with fused tips and terminate in a spoon-shaped tip	(c)
Nematodirus helvetianus	The long slender spicules terminate in a fused point with the surrounding membrane being lanceolate	(d)
Nematodirus abnormalis	The spicules are asymmetrical with the distal ends bent to form an asymmetrical lancet	(e)

rays are parallel and are situated close together. The female worm has a short tail with a slender terminal appendage. The eggs are large and readily distinguishable from other trichostrongiloid species.

Life cycle: The preparasitic phase is almost unique in the trichostrongyloids in that development to the L_3 stage takes place within the eggshell. Species differences occur regarding the critical hatching requirements.

Nematodirus battus

Description: The adults are long and slender, the males measuring around 11–16 mm and females 15–25 mm in length. The anterior of the worm is thinner than the posterior region and the cuticle

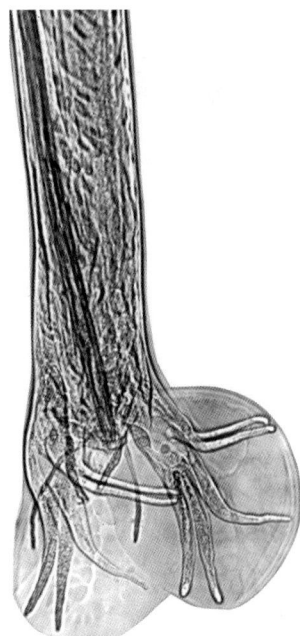

Fig. 1.34 Male bursa and spicules of *Nematodirus battus* with single sets of parallel rays in the dorsal lobes.

possesses longitudinal ridges. The body is usually twisted or coiled so that the worms tend to tangle together. A small but distinct cephalic vesicle is present (see Fig 1.33). Males are characterised by having only one set of divergent rays in each bursal lobe (Fig. 1.34) and the tips of the spicules are fused into a small, flattened, oval-shaped projection (Table 1.10a). The female worm has a long pointed tail. The large egg is brownish with parallel sides and measures around 150–180 by 67–80 μm (see Fig. 4.4). The chitinous eggshell is thin-walled, smooth and contains 4–8 darkly stained blastomeres when passed in faeces.

Life cycle: Development to the L_3 takes place within the eggshell. Hatching of most eggs requires a prolonged period of chill followed by a mean day/night temperature of more than 10 °C, conditions which occur in late spring in the northern hemisphere. Hence most of the eggs from one season's grazing remain unhatched on the ground during the winter and usually only one generation is possible each year for the bulk of this species. However, some *N. battus* eggs deposited in the spring are capable of hatching in the autumn of the same year, resulting in significant numbers of L_3 on the pasture at this time. The ingested L_3 penetrate the mucosa of the small intestine and moult to the L_4 stage around the fourth day. After moulting to the L_5, the parasites inhabit the lumen, sometimes superficially coiled around villi. The prepatent period is 14–16 days.

Nematodirus filicollis

Description: The adults are long slender worms, males measuring 10–15 mm and females 15–24 mm in length. A small but distinct cephalic vesicle is present. The male has two sets of parallel rays in each of the main bursal lobes (Fig. 1.35). The spicules are long and slender with fused tips and terminate in a narrow pointed swelling (Table 1.10b). The female has a truncate blunt tail with a small spine (similar to *N. spathiger*), and the egg is

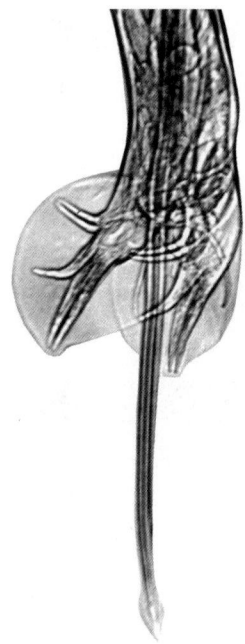

Fig. 1.35 Male bursa and spicules of *Nematodirus filicollis* with two sets of parallel rays in the dorsal lobes.

large, ovoid (130–200 × 70–90 µm), thin-shelled and colourless and twice the size of the typical trichostrongyle egg (see Fig. 4.4).

Life cycle: Development to the L₃ takes place within the eggshell. *Nematodirus filicollis* does not have the same critical hatching requirements as *N. battus*. Hatching occurs over a more prolonged period and so larvae often appear on the pasture within 2–3 months of the eggs being excreted in the faeces. The parasitic phase within the host is similar to that of *N. battus*. The prepatent period is 2–3 weeks.

Nematodirus spathiger

Description: The adults are slender worms, males measuring around 10–15 mm and females 15–25 mm in length. A small but distinct cephalic vesicle is present. The male has two sets of parallel rays in each of the main bursal lobes. The spicules are long and slender with fused tips and terminate in a spoon-shaped tip (Table 1.10c). The female has a truncate blunt tail with a small spine (similar to *N. filicollis*), and the egg is large, ovoid, thin-shelled and colourless and twice the size of the typical trichostrongyle egg. The egg measures 175–260 by 106–110 µm and usually contains an embryo of eight cells when passed in the faeces. Infective larvae measure around 1100 µm and have eight gut cells (see Fig. 4.15).

Life cycle: As for *N. fillicollis*.

Nematodirus helvetianus

Description: Adult males measure around 11–16 mm and females 17–24 mm in length. The male has two sets of parallel rays in each of the main bursal lobes and the dorsal lobe is not

separated from the lateral lobe. The long slender spicules terminate in a fused point, with the surrounding membrane being lanceolate (Table 1.10d). The female has a truncate tail with a small spine. The egg is large (160–233 by 87–121 µm), ovoid with slightly sharp poles and clear, and twice the size of the typical trichostrongyle egg. The chitinous eggshell is thin with a smooth surface and contains 2–8 large dark blastomeres, which are separated from the yolk membrane by quite a large fluid-filled cavity.

Life cycle: *Nematodirus helvetianus* does not have the same critical hatching requirements as *N. battus* and so the larvae often appear on the pasture within 2–3 weeks of the eggs being excreted in the faeces. More than one annual generation is therefore possible. The parasitic phase within the host is similar to that of *N. battus*. The prepatent period is around three weeks.

Nematodirus abnormalis

Description: Adult males measure around 11–17 mm and females 18–25 mm. The spicules are asymmetrical with the distal ends bent to form an asymmetrical lancet (Table 1.10e).

Nematodirus mauritanicus

Description: Adult females are 21–24 mm and males 13–15 mm long. Male spicules are joined for part of their length with the tips enclosed in a thin lanceolate membrane.

Nematodirus lamae

Description: These are small worms, females 14–20 mm, males 10–13 mm long. Male worms have a deeply emarginated dorsal lobe with two distinct lobules and long spicules, with the distal end enlarged and terminating in two distinct bifurcated medioventral processes.

Nematodirus leporis

Description: Male worms are 8–15 mm and female worms 16–20 mm in length. The bursa has rounded lobes with parallel posterolateral and mediolateral bursal rays and the spicules are long. The eggs are large (250 × 100 µm).

Nematodirella

Nematodirella spp. (Table 1.11) are narrow worms and are similar to *Nematodirus*. Male spicules are extremely long and thin.

Nematodirella dromedarii

Description: Males are 10–15 mm and females 10–30 mm in size. The very long spicules can measure up to half the body length and are equal in size (Fig. 1.36). Eggs are large, measuring about 250 by 125 µm.

Table 1.11 *Nematodirella* species.

Species	Hosts	Site
Nematodirella dromedarii	Camels (dromedaries)	Small intestine
Nematodirella cameli	Camels (Bactrians), elk, reindeer	Small intestine
Nematodirella alcides (syn. *Nematodirus longispiculata*, *Nematodirella longissimespiculata*)	Elk	Small intestine

Life cycle: This is thought to be similar to that of *Nematodirus* spp. (not *N. battus*).

Nematodirella cameli

Description: Males are 16–17 mm and females 21–25 mm in size. In the males, the spicules are asymmetrical, thin and extremely long, adjoining each other closely over their entire length, forming rounded swellings distally from which branch off spine-shaped distal extremities.

Nematodirella alcides

Synonyms: *Nematodirus longispiculata*, *Nematodirella longissimespiculata*

Description: Males are 15–17 mm and females 23–25 mm in size. The spicules are long, thin and filiform with a spear-like tip.

Lamanema

The main species is *Lamanema chavezi* which infects the small intestine of alpacas and vicunas.

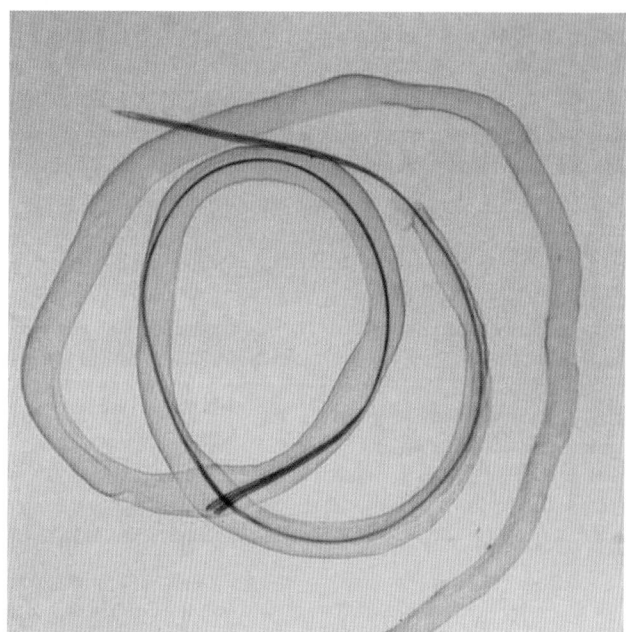

Fig. 1.36 *Nematodirella dromedarii* showing the very long male spicules.

Lamanema chavezi

Description: Small worms, females measuring 14–18 mm and males 9–11 mm long. There is a shallow buccal capsule with dorsal tooth and two small lateroventral teeth at the base. In the male, the lateral lobes are large, the dorsal lobe is small and there are short spicules and a large gubernaculum.

Life cycle: Ingested infective larvae penetrate the intestinal mucosa and migrate to the liver and lungs. Maturation is completed by migration of the worms back to the intestine via the trachea.

Ollulanus

These are very minute worms. Males are 0.7–0.8 mm and females 0.8–1 mm long. The buccal cavity is small. Microscopic identification is by the presence of the spiral coil of the head.

Life cycle: The worms are viviparous, the larvae developing to the L_3 stage in the uterus of the females. Autoinfection can occur, the shed L_3 developing into adult worms on the gastric mucosa in around 4–5 weeks. The whole life cycle may be completed endogenously and transmission, at least in the cat, is thought to be via ingestion of vomit containing the L_3. The worms live under a layer of mucus in the stomach wall and the anterior end of the worm is often located within the gastric crypts. The main species is *Ollulanus tricuspis* which infects the stomach of cats, wild felids, pigs, dogs and foxes.

Ollulanus tricuspis

Description: It is identified microscopically by the spiral coil of the head. The male bursa is well developed and the spicules are stout and each is split into two for a considerable portion of its length. The female has a tail, which terminates in three or four short cusps. The vulva is in the posterior part of the body and there is only one uterus and ovary.

FAMILY HELLIGMONELLIDAE
Nippostrongylus

The main species is *Nippostrongylus brasiliensis* (syn. *Nippostrongylus muris*, *Heligmosomum muris*) which infects the small intestine of rats, mice, hamsters, gerbils, rabbits and chinchillas.

Nippostrongylus brasiliensis

Synonyms: *Nippostrongylus muris*, *Heligmosomum muris*

Description: Adults are filiform and reddish in colour; males measure 2.1–4.5 mm and females 2.5–6 mm in length. They usually appear as a tight coil. The medium-sized eggs are ellipsoidal, thin-shelled with a smooth surface and measure about 52–63 by 28–35 μm. They contain a morula.

Life cycle: The life cycle is direct and typically trichostrongyloid. Infection is usually percutaneous and larvae migrate via the lungs.

Worms are adult by around five days post infection and are usually short-lived. The prepatent period is 5–6 days.

Nematospiroides

The main species is *Nematospiroides dubius* (syn. *Heligmosomoides polygyrus*) which infects the small intestine of rats and mice.

Nematospiroides dubius

Description: Adults are long red worms measuring 0.6–1.3 cm in length, with a coiled tail and a cephalic vesicle. The medium-sized eggs are ovoid with a thin smooth shell, measure around 68 by 43 μm and contain a morula.

Life cycle: Typically trichostrongyloid with infection via the L_3. The prepatent period is nine days and patency may last for up to eight months.

FAMILY DICTYOCAULIDAE

Dictyocaulus

Adults of *Dictyocaulus* spp. (Table 1.12) are slender thread-like worms, white/light grey in colour and up to 8–10 cm in length. Their location in the trachea and bronchi and their size are diagnostic. The buccal capsule and the bursa are small. The brown spicules are short and often have a slightly granular appearance. There is some debate over the species taxonomy in deer.

Life cycle: The female worms are ovoviviparous, producing eggs containing fully developed larvae, which hatch almost immediately. The L_1 migrate up the trachea, are swallowed and pass out in the faeces. The larvae are unique in that they are present in fresh faeces, are characteristically sluggish, and their intestinal cells are filled with dark-brown food granules (Fig. 1.37). In consequence, the preparasitic stages do not need to feed. Under optimal conditions, the L_3 stage is reached within five days but usually takes longer in the field. The L_3 leave the faecal pat to reach the herbage either by their own motility or through the agency of the ubiquitous fungus *Pilobolus*. After ingestion, the L_3 penetrate the intestinal mucosa and pass to the mesenteric lymph nodes where they moult. The L_4 then travel via the lymph and blood to the lungs, and break out of

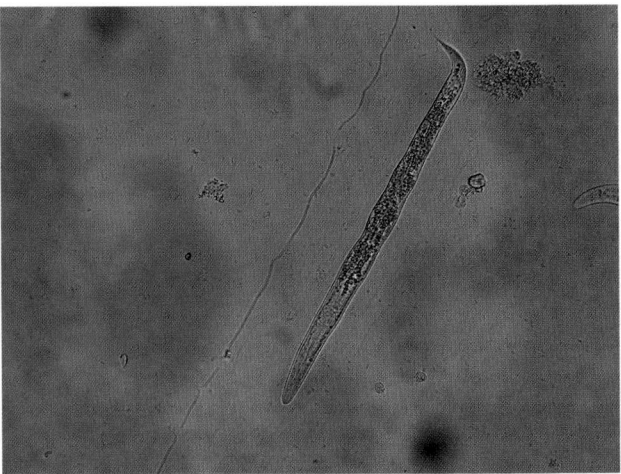

Fig. 1.37 First-stage larvae of *Dictyocaulus viviparus*. (Courtesy of Laura Rinaldi).

the capillaries into the alveoli about one week after infection. The final moult occurs in the bronchioles a few days later and the young adults then move up the bronchi and mature. See **life cycle 2**.

Dictyocaulus viviparus

Description: The adults are slender thread-like worms; males measure around 4–5.5 cm and females 6–8 cm in length. The buccal ring is triangular in shape. They are very similar to *D. filaria* but the posterolateral and mediolateral rays are entirely fused together. First-stage larvae present in fresh faeces are about 300–450 μm in length and 25 μm in width, the intestinal cells containing numerous brownish chromatin granules (see Fig. 1.37). The head is rounded, there being no protruding anterior knob (cf. *D. filaria* in sheep and goats). The oesophagus is simple strongyloid and the tail terminates in a blunt point.

Life cycle: The prepatent period is around 3–4 weeks in cattle. The prepatent period in red deer is 20–24 days.

Dictyocaulus filaria

Description: The worms are white with the intestine visible as a dark band. Males measure around 4–8 cm and females 6–10 cm in length. In the bursa, the posterolateral and mediolateral rays are fused together, except at their extremities. The dark-brown spicules are stout and shaped like a boot. The vulva is located just posterior to the middle of the worm. The eggs measure 112–138 by 69–90 μm and contain fully formed first-stage larvae when laid. The L_1 resembles that of *D. viviparus* but has a characteristic small protruding cuticular knob at the anterior extremity (see Fig. 4.13b). The larva measures 550–580 μm in length, has a blunt tail (see Fig. 1.59a) and its intestinal cells contain numerous dark food granules.

Life cycle: The prepatent period is about 4–5 weeks.

Table 1.12 *Dictyocaulus* species.

Species	Hosts	Site
Dictyocaulus viviparus	Cattle, buffalo, deer, camels	Trachea, lungs
Dictyocaulus filaria	Sheep, goats, camelids	Trachea, lungs
Dictyocaulus arnfieldi	Horses, donkeys, zebras	Trachea, lungs
Dictyocaulus eckerti (syn. *Dictyocaulus noerneri*)	Deer (roe deer, fallow deer, red deer), cattle	Trachea, lungs
Dictyocaulus capreolus	Deer (roe deer, moose)	Trachea, lungs

LIFE CYCLE 2. LIFE CYCLE OF *DICTYOCAULUS VIVIPARUS*

Dictyocaulus viviparus causes bronchopulmonary disease in cattle. Adult parasites live in the trachea and large bronchi (1) and induce productive bronchitis with severe cellular infiltration (mainly eosinophils, neutrophils and macrophages) that may obstruct the alveolar lumen. The surface of infected lungs displays extended emphysematous areas, oedema and atelectasis. Adult females are ovoviviparous, and release eggs containing the L_1 (2) that, in most cases, hatch in the bronchi (3). The larvae migrate up the trachea and, once swallowed, are excreted with the faeces (4). In the environment, larvae develop into infective L_3 (5) within

five days; these are poorly motile and in order to exit the faecal pat, they climb up the sporangium of *Pilobolus* fungi (6). When the sporangium discharges, the larvae are also discharged on the surrounding vegetation (7). Once ingested by the grazing hosts, the larvae penetrate the intestinal mucosa (8) and, via the lymphatic circulation, travel to the mesenteric lymph nodes (9) where they moult to L_4. The latter travel via the lymphatics and blood vessels (10) to the lungs (11) where they penetrate the alveoli. From here, within ~7 days, the immature adults reach the bronchi where they develop into sexually mature adults.

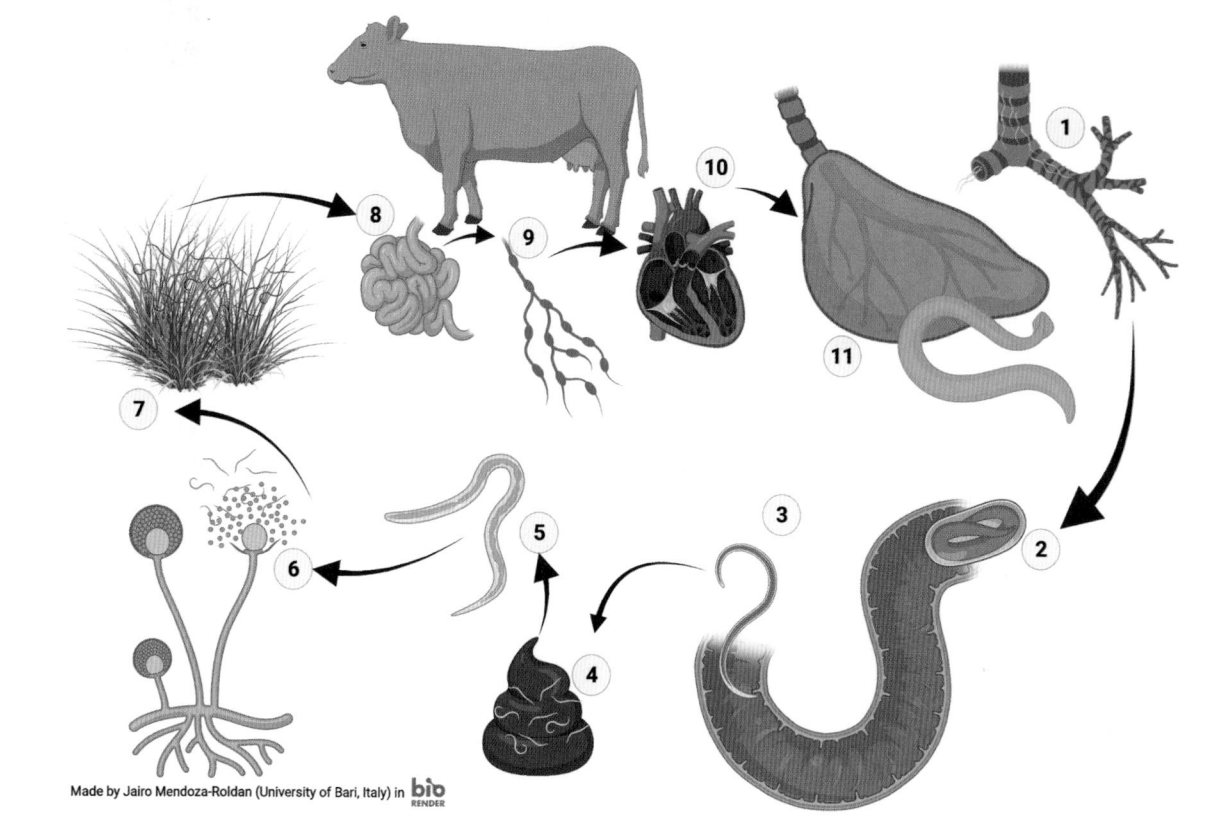

Made by Jairo Mendoza-Roldan (University of Bari, Italy) in **bio**RENDER

Dictyocaulus arnfieldi

Description: The adults are slender, thread-like and whitish in colour, the adult males measuring around 3.5 cm and the females 6.5 cm in length. Male worms have a small non-lobulated bursa with short rays, with the mediolateral and posterolateral rays fused for half their length. The spicules are short, of equal length and slightly curved. The medium-sized, ellipsoidal, thin-walled eggs measure 80–100 by 50–60 µm and are embryonated. First-stage larvae emerge from the egg very early and measure 290–480 µm, with a posterior transparent protuberance (Fig. 1.38). The contents are granular in appearance.

Life cycle: The detailed life cycle is not fully known, but is considered to be similar to that of the bovine lungworm, *D. viviparus*, except in the following respects. The adult worms are most often found in the small bronchi and their thin-shelled eggs, containing the first-stage larvae, are coughed up before they are swallowed, passed in the faeces and then hatch soon after being deposited. The prepatent period is around 2–3 months. Patent infections are common in donkeys of all ages, but in horses generally only occur in foals and yearlings. In older horses, the adult lungworms rarely attain sexual maturity.

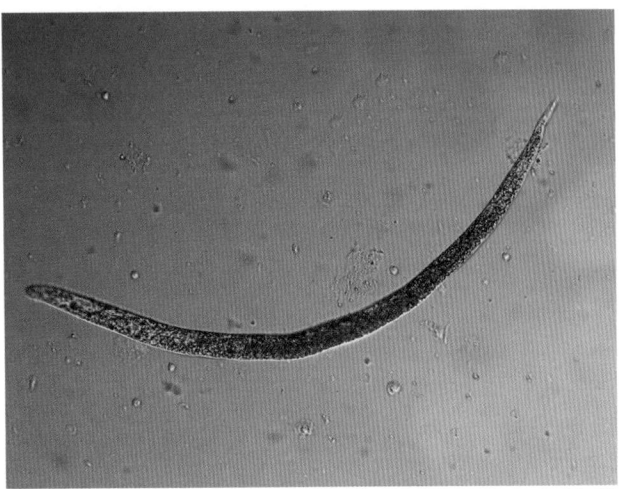

Fig. 1.38 *Dictyocaulus arnfieldi* first-stage larva showing the terminal protuberance.

Dictyocaulus eckerti

Synonym: *Dictyocaulus noerneri*

Description: Similar to *D. viviparus* but the mouth opening is elongate and the buccal ring is kidney-shaped.

Dictyocaulus capreolus

Description: Distinguished from *D. eckerti* on the basis of the morphology of the buccal capsule and the bursa.

SUPERFAMILY STRONGYLOIDEA

There are several important parasites of domestic mammals and birds in this superfamily of bursate nematodes. Most are characterised by a large buccal capsule, which often contains teeth or cutting plates, and in some there are prominent leaf crowns surrounding the mouth opening. The bursa of males is well developed and a gubernaculum or telamon is usually present. The spicules are usually of equal length. The adults occur on mucosal surfaces of the gastrointestinal and respiratory tracts and feeding is generally by the ingestion of plugs of mucosa.

With the exception of three genera, *Syngamus*, *Mammomonogamus* and *Cyathostoma*, which are parasitic in the trachea and major bronchi, and *Stephanurus* found in the perirenal area, all other genera of veterinary importance in this superfamily are found in the intestine and can be conveniently divided into two groups, the strongyles and hookworms.

The strongyles are parasitic in the large intestine and the important genera are *Strongylus*, *Triodontophorus* ('large strongyles' of horses), *Chabertia* and *Oesophagostomum*. Also in this group of

small strongyles are the genera *Poteriostomum*, *Craterostomum* and *Oesophagodontus*.

The cyathostomins (cyathostomes or trichonemes) or 'small strongyles' of horses (subfamily Cyathostominae) include the genera *Cyathostomum*, *Cylicocyclus*, *Cylicodontophorus* and *Cylicostephanus* (formerly the single genus *Trichonema*).

Syngamus and *Cyathostoma* are important parasites of the respiratory tract of birds. *Mammomonogamus* are parasites of the respiratory tract of cattle, sheep and goats.

FAMILY STRONGYLIDAE

SUBFAMILY STRONGYLINAE

Strongylus

Members of this genus (Table 1.13) live in the large intestine of horses and donkeys. These are robust dark-red worms which are easily seen against the intestinal mucosa (Fig. 1.39). The well-developed deep buccal capsule of the adult parasite is prominent, as is the bursa of the male. The anterior margin of the buccal capsule usually bears leaf-like cuticular structures (leaf crowns or corona radiata). Species differentiation is based on size and the presence and shape of the teeth in the base of the buccal capsule. See **life cycle 3**.

Table 1.13 *Strongylus* species.

Species	Hosts	Site
Strongylus edentatus (syn. *Alfortia edentatus*)	Horses, donkeys	Large intestine
Strongylus equinus	Horses, donkeys	Large intestine
Strongylus vulgaris (syn. *Delafondia vulgaris*)	Horses, donkeys	Large intestine

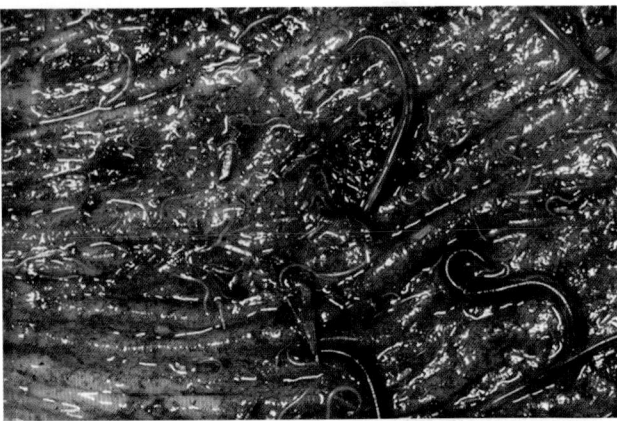

Fig. 1.39 *Strongylus* spp. adult worms (large strongyles) on the intestinal mucosa with smaller cyathostomins (small strongyles) also present.

LIFE CYCLE 3. LIFE CYCLE OF *STRONGYLUS* SPP. (LARGE STRONGYLES OF EQUINES)

Adults of *Strongylus vulgaris*, *Strongylus edentatus* and *Strongylus equinus*, known as large strongyles, live in the lumen of the caecum and colon, where they attach to the mucosa with their buccal capsule. The infected horse sheds elliptical, unembryonated eggs in the faeces (1) into the environment (2). The rhabditiform first-stage larva hatches from the egg (3) and moults to second- (4) and third-stage larva (5), becoming infective within two weeks. Horses acquire the infection by ingesting infective L_3 contaminating the environment (6). After ingestion, depending on species, the larvae undergo different somatic migrations before establishing in the final site of infection.

Larvae of *S. vulgaris* (7a) penetrate the intestinal wall and, after a week, moult in the submucosa and penetrate the small arteries to reach the main branches of the cranial mesenteric artery and the ileo-caeco-colic system. Here, the larvae persist for many months and after a further moult, return to the intestinal wall via the blood vessels. As the larvae grow, nodules form within the

caecal and colonic walls. These eventually rupture and release the immature adults in the intestinal lumen. Here, the worms reach sexual maturity and reproduce, thus completing the life cycle.

Larvae of *S. edentatus* (7b) penetrate the intestinal wall and travel to the liver parenchyma, where they moult to become fourth-stage larvae and migrate to the subserosa, in proximity to the hepatorenal ligament and parietal peritoneum, where they form haemorrhagic nodules. Here, the larvae moult to become pre-adults and return to the intestine, where they form purulent nodules containing the immature adults. The latter are subsequently released from the nodules and develop to sexually mature adults, completing the life cycle.

Larvae of *S. equinus* (7c) penetrate the caecal and colonic wall, where they form nodules within the muscular and subserosal layers. After moulting, the larvae migrate to the liver parenchyma, and subsequently to the pancreas and intestinal lumen, where the parasites complete development to sexually mature adults.

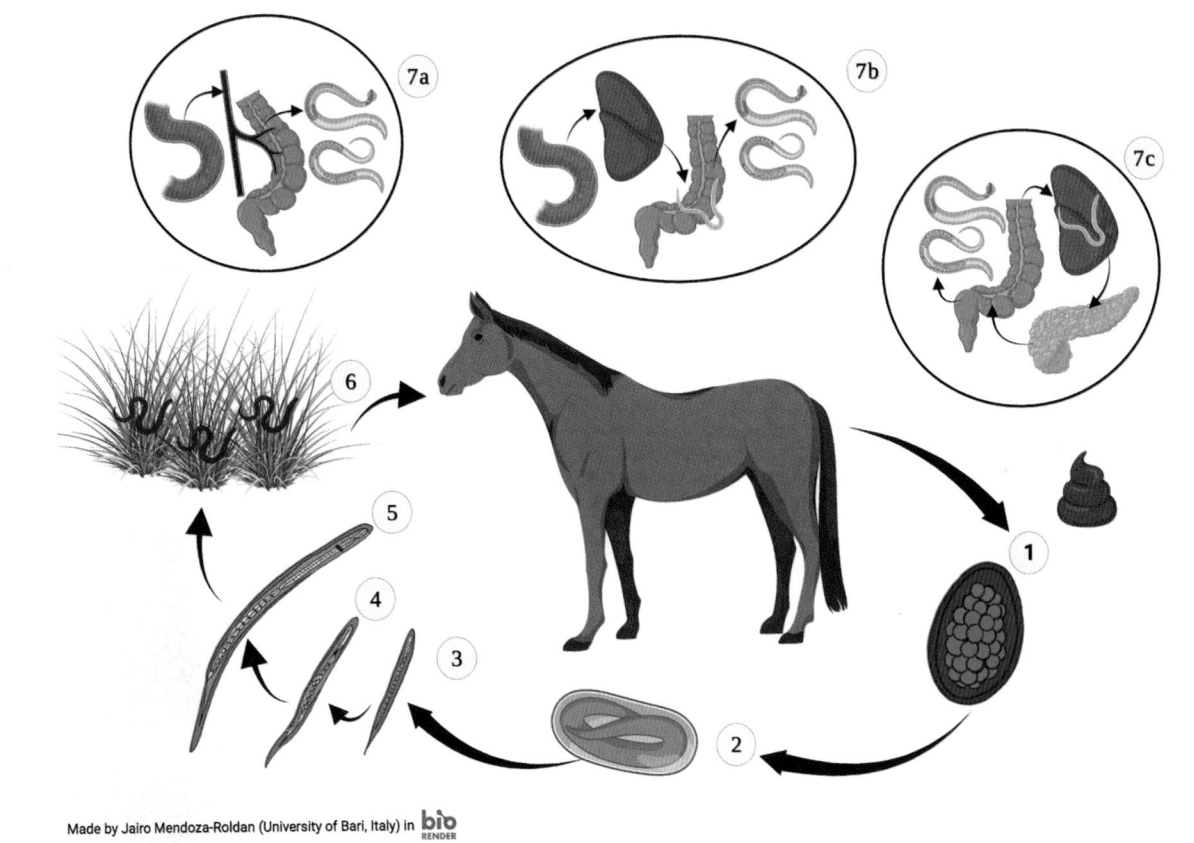

Made by Jairo Mendoza-Roldan (University of Bari, Italy) in **bio**RENDER

Strongylus edentatus

Description: Robust dark-red worms that are easily seen against the intestinal mucosa (Fig. 1.40). The well-developed buccal capsule of the adult parasite is prominent, as is the bursa of the male. Male are 2.3–2.8 cm and females 3.3–4.4 cm. The head end is wider than the rest of the body. Species differentiation is based on size and the presence and

shape of the teeth in the base of the buccal capsule. The buccal capsule is wider anteriorly than at the middle and contains no teeth (Fig. 1.41a). The medium-sized eggs have almost similar poles and barrel-shaped side walls. They have a smooth thin shell, measure 78–88 by 48–52 µm and contain a morula with several large blastomeres.

Life cycle: Eggs, which resemble those of the trichostrongyles, are passed in the faeces and development from egg to the L_3 under

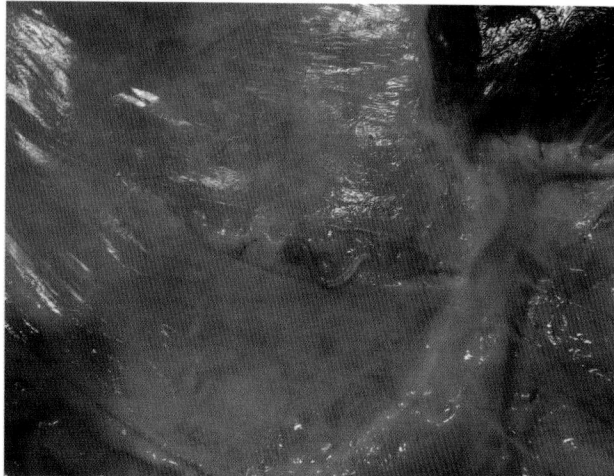

Fig. 1.40 *Strongylus edentatus* feeding on the mucosa of the large intestine. (Courtesy of Aránzazu Meana).

summer conditions in temperate climates requires approximately two weeks. Infection is by ingestion of the L_3. Subsequently, parasitic larval development of the three species of *Strongylus* differs and will be dealt with separately.

After penetration of the intestinal mucosa, L_3 travel via the portal system and reach the liver parenchyma within a few days. About two weeks later, the moult to L_4 takes place; further migration then occurs in the liver and by 6–8 weeks post infection, larvae can be found subperitoneally around the hepatorenal ligament. The larvae then travel under the peritoneum to many sites, with a predilection for the flanks and hepatic ligaments. The final moult occurs after four months and each L_5 then migrates, still subperitoneally, to the wall of the large intestine where a large purulent nodule is formed, which subsequently ruptures with release of the young

adult parasite into the lumen. The prepatent period is usually about 10–12 months and is the longest of the strongyles.

Strongylus equinus

Description: Robust dark-red worms that are easily seen against the intestinal mucosa. The well-developed buccal capsule of the adult parasite is prominent, as is the bursa of the male. Males are 2.6–3.5 cm and females 3.8–4.7 cm. The head end is not marked off from the rest of the body. Species differentiation is based on size and the presence and shape of the teeth in the base of the buccal capsule. The buccal capsule is oval in outline and there are external and internal leaf crowns. At the base of the buccal capsule is a large dorsal tooth with a bifid tip and two smaller subventral teeth (Fig. 1.41b). The dorsal oesophageal gland opens into the buccal capsule through a number of pores situated in a thickened ridge, the dorsal gutter, formed by the wall of the buccal capsule. The male has two simple slender spicules. In the female, the vulva lies 12–14 mm from the posterior extremity. The eggs are similar to those of *S. edentatus* and measure 75–92 by 41–54 µm.

Life cycle: The adult parasites live in the caecum and colon. The free-living phase is as described for *S. edentatus*. Of the three *Strongylus* species, least is known of the larval migration of *S. equinus*. It appears that the L_3 lose their sheaths while penetrating the wall of the caecum and ventral colon and within one week provoke the formation of nodules in the muscular and subserosal layers of the intestine. The moult to L_4 occurs within these nodules and the larvae then travel across the peritoneal cavity to the liver where they migrate within the parenchyma for six weeks or more. After this time, L_4 and L_5 have been found in and around the pancreas before their appearance in the large intestinal lumen. The prepatent period is 8–9 months.

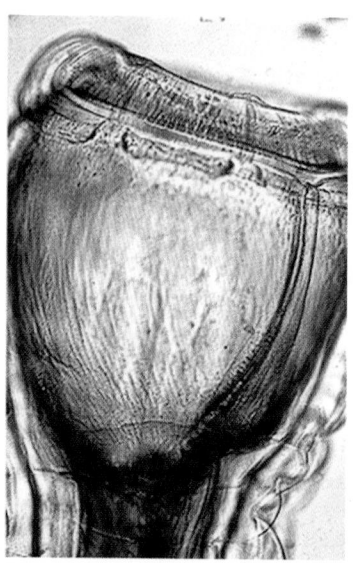
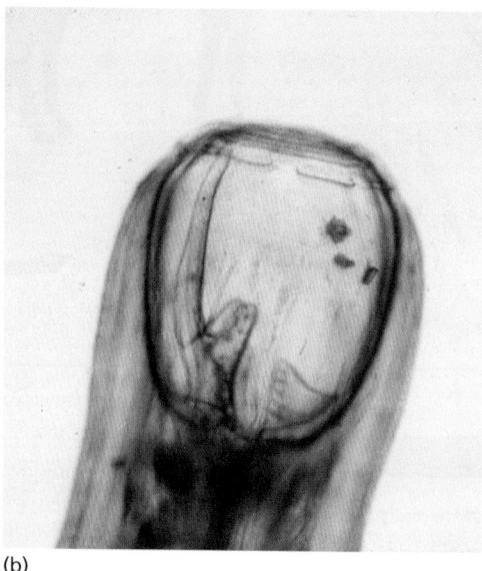
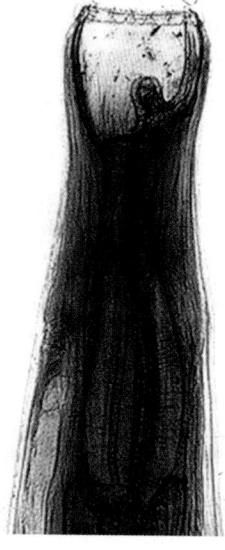

(a)   (b)   (c)

Fig. 1.41 (a) Anterior of *Strongylus edentatus* showing the cup-shaped buccal capsule, which is devoid of teeth. (b) Anterior of *Strongylus equinus* showing oval buccal capsule with a large dorsal tooth and smaller subventral conical teeth. (c) Anterior of *Strongylus vulgaris* showing ear-shaped rounded teeth at the base of the buccal capsule.

Strongylus vulgaris

Description: Adults of this species are shorter and thinner than the other two *Strongylus* species. Robust dark-red worms that are easily seen against the intestinal mucosa. The well-developed buccal capsule of the adult parasite is prominent, as is the bursa of the male. Males are 14–16 mm and females 20–24 mm. The head end is not marked off from the rest of the body. Species differentiation is based on size and the presence and shape of the teeth in the base of the buccal capsule. The buccal capsule is oval in outline and contains two ear-shaped teeth at its base (Fig. 1.41c). The elements of the leaf crowns are fringed at their distal extremities. The dorsal oesophageal gland opens into the buccal capsule through a number of pores situated in a thickened ridge, the dorsal gutter, formed by the wall of the buccal capsule. The thin-shelled eggs are similar to those of *S. edentatus* and measure 83–93 by 48–52 μm.

Life cycle: The free-living phase is as described for the other two species. Following ingestion, the L$_3$ penetrate the intestinal mucosa and moult to L$_4$ in the submucosa of the caecum and ventral colon seven days later. These then enter small arteries and arterioles and migrate on the endothelium to their predilection site in the cranial mesenteric artery and its main branches. After a period of development of several months, the larvae moult to L$_5$ and return to the intestinal wall via the arterial lumina. Nodules are formed around the larvae mainly in the wall of the caecum and colon when, due to their size, they can travel no further within the arteries, and subsequent rupture of these nodules releases the young adult parasites into the lumen of the intestine. The prepatent period is 6–7 months.

Triodontophorus

Members of the genus *Triodontophorus* (Table 1.14) are non-migratory, large strongyles frequently found in large numbers in the colon of horses and donkeys. They are reddish worms 1–2.5 cm in length, readily visible on the colonic mucosa. The buccal capsule is subglobular and thick-walled with three pairs of large oesophageal teeth, each composed of two plates, the anterior rim of which is thickened and surrounded by six plate-like structures (Fig. 1.42). The dorsal gutter is prominent. The spicules of the male terminate in small hooks.

Life cycle: Little information is available on the developmental cycle of this genus, but it is thought to be similar to that of cyathostomes.

Triodontophorus brevicauda

Description: Medium-sized worms, varying in size from around 9 to 25 mm. The buccal capsule is subglobular and thick-walled with three large oesophageal teeth composed of two plates which are

Table 1.14 *Triodontophorus* species.

Species	Hosts	Site
Triodontophorus brevicauda	Horses, donkeys	Large intestine
Triodontophorus minor	Horses, donkeys	Large intestine
Triodontophorus nipponicus	Horses, donkeys	Large intestine
Triodontophorus serratus	Horses, donkeys	Large intestine
Triodontophorus tenuicollis	Horses, donkeys	Large intestine

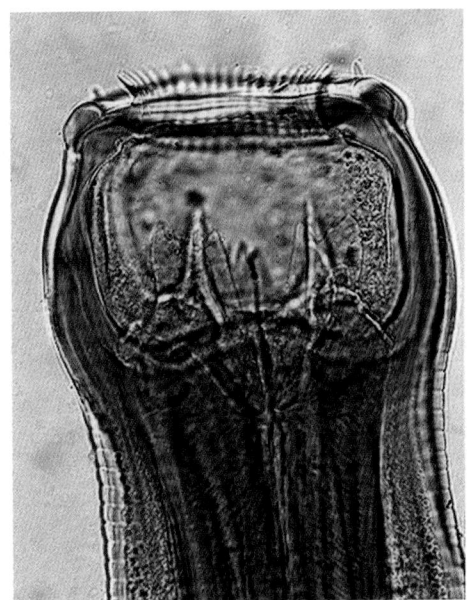

Fig. 1.42 Head of *Triodontophorus* spp. showing the location of teeth at the base of the buccal capsule.

smooth except for three elevations on each and protrude into the buccal capsule. The anterior rim of the buccal capsule is thickened anteriorly and surrounded by six plate-like structures. The submedian papillae are short, broad and conical. The external leaf crown consists of numerous slender elements protruding from the buccal collar, with an equal number of inner leaf crown elements. In the female, the vulva is close to the anus and the tail is very short. The large smooth egg is ovoid with almost similar poles and barrel-shaped side walls and contains a morula with very dark blastomeres. It measures 130–140 by 55–65 μm.

Triodontophorus minor

Description: Medium-sized worms, varying in length from around 9 to 15 mm. The buccal capsule is subglobular and thick-walled with three large oesophageal teeth composed of two plates which are strongly denticulated and protrude into the buccal capsule. The anterior rim of the buccal capsule is thickened anteriorly and surrounded by six plate-like structures. The cuticle is strongly serrated in the cervical region. The external leaf crown consists of 44–50 slender elements protruding from the buccal collar, with an equal number of inner leaf crown elements. In the female, the vulva is close to the anus and the tail is short. The eggs are similar to those of *T. brevicauda*.

Triodontophorus nipponicus

Description: Medium-sized worms, varying in size from about 9 to 15 mm. The buccal capsule is subglobular and thick-walled with three large oesophageal teeth composed of two plates which are strongly denticulated, with three large denticulations, and protrude into the buccal capsule. The anterior rim of the buccal capsule is thickened anteriorly and surrounded by six plate-like structures. The cuticle is strongly serrated in the cervical region. The external leaf crown consists of 56–69 slender elements protruding from the buccal collar, with an equal number of inner leaf crown elements. In the female, the vulva is close to the anus and the tail is short. The eggs are similar to those of *T. brevicauda*.

Triodontophorus serratus

Description: This is the largest species of the genus. Males measure 18–20 mm and females 20–26 mm in length. The buccal capsule is subglobular and thick-walled with three large oesophageal teeth composed of two plates that protrude into the buccal capsule. The anterior rim of the buccal capsule is thickened anteriorly and surrounded by six plate-like structures. The mouth collar appears as an inflated round tube around the mouth. The external leaf crown consists of numerous slender elements protruding from the buccal collar, with an equal number of inner leaf crown elements. In the female, the vulva is close to the anus and the tail is long. The eggs are similar to those of *T. brevicauda*.

Triodontophorus tenuicollis

Description: Males are around 17 mm and females 22 mm long. The buccal capsule is subglobular and thick-walled with three large oesophageal teeth composed of two plates which are finely denticulated and protrude into the buccal capsule. The anterior rim of the buccal capsule is thickened anteriorly and surrounded by six plate-like structures. The cuticle is strongly serrated in the cervical region; the dorsal lobe of the bursa is short and teeth are finely denticulated. The external leaf crown consists of numerous slender elements protruding from the buccal collar, with an equal number of inner leaf crown elements. In the female, the vulva is close to the anus. The eggs are similar to those of *T. brevicauda*.

Oesophagostomum

Worms of this genus (Table 1.15) are stout and whitish with a narrow cylindrical buccal capsule and measure 1–2 cm in length (Fig. 1.43). The body is often slightly curved. A ventral cervical groove is located near the anterior end of the worm and the anterior cuticle is dilated to form a cervical vesicle. Leaf crowns are present.

Life cycle: The preparasitic phase is typically strongyloid. The egg hatches on the ground, releasing the first-stage larva which moults to the second stage, and then to the infective third stage. Infection is by ingestion of L_3. There is no migration stage in the body, although there is limited evidence that skin penetration is possible. The larvae moult again and the fourth-stage larvae attach to, or enter, the wall of the intestine. These L_4 then emerge on to the mucosal surface, migrate to the colon and develop to the adult stage. The prepatent period is 5–7 weeks. On reinfection, the larvae may remain arrested as L_4 in nodules for up to one year.

Oesophagostomum columbianum

Description: Male worms are 12–17 mm and females 15–22 mm with large cervical alae, which induce a dorsal curvature of the anterior part of the body. The cuticle forms a high mouth collar

Table 1.15 *Oesophagostomum* species.

Species	Hosts	Site
Oesophagostomum columbianum	Sheep, goats, camels, wild ruminants	Large intestine
Oesophagostomum venulosum (syn. *Oesophagostomum virginimembrum*)	Sheep, goats, deer, camels	Large intestine
Oesophagostomum asperum	Sheep, goats	Large intestine
Oesophagostomum multifoliatum	Sheep, goats	Large intestine
Oesophagostomum radiatum	Cattle, water buffalo	Large intestine
Oesophagostomum dentatum	Pigs	Large intestine
Oesophagostomum brevicaudum	Pigs	Large intestine
Oesophagostomum longicaudatum	Pigs	Large intestine
Oesophagostomum quadrispinulatum	Pigs	Large intestine
Oesophagostomum georgianum	Pigs	Large intestine
Oesophagostomum granatensis	Pigs	Large intestine
Oesophagostomum apiostomum	Primates	Large intestine
Oesophagostomum bifurcum	Primates	Large intestine
Oesophagostomum aculeatum	Primates	Large intestine
Oesophagostomum stephanostomum	Primates	Large intestine

shaped like a truncate cone. This is separated from the remainder of the body by a constriction. The cephalic vesicle is anterior to a cervical groove, behind which arise the cervical alae pierced by cervical papillae. External leaf crowns consist of 20–24 elements and the internal ones have two small elements to each external element. The male bursa is well developed with two alate spicules of equal length. The smooth, colourless, thin-shelled egg is a medium-sized (70–89 × 36–45 μm), regular broad ellipse with barrel-shaped walls and round wide poles, and contains 8–16 blastomeres when passed in the faeces (see Fig. 4.4). The L_3 have long filamentous tails, 32 gut cells and a rounded head and measure around 790 μm.

Life cycle: The prepatent period is about 45 days.

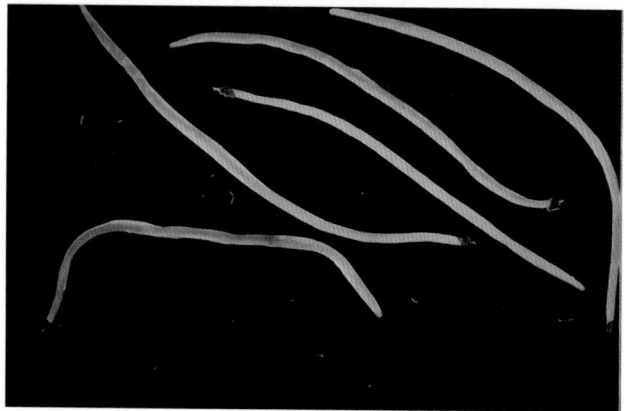

Fig. 1.43 Adult worms of *Oesophagostomum venulosum*.

Oesophagostomum venulosum

Synonym: *Oesophagostomum virginimembrum*

Description, gross: Males worms are 11–16 mm and females 13–24 mm long. Around the anterior oesophagus there is an inflated cuticular cephalic vesicle (Fig. 1.44). This terminates in a cervical groove, which is followed in some species by broad cervical alae. In the male the bursa is well developed. The head has a shallow buccal capsule with an external leaf crown of 18 elements. The external crown is compressed and so there is only a narrow opening into the buccal capsule. There are no lateral cervical alae and the worms are therefore not curved anteriorly. The cervical papillae are posterior to the oesophagus. The smooth, colourless, thin-shelled egg is a medium-sized (85–120 × 45–60 μm), regular broad ellipse with barrel-shaped walls, and contains 16–32 blastomeres when passed in the faeces. The L_3 have long filamentous tails, 32 gut cells and a rounded head.

Life cycle: The prepatent period is about 5–7 weeks.

Oesophagostomum multifolium

Description: Males measure 12–14 mm and females 14–17 mm in length.

Oesophagostomum radiatum

Description: Adult male worms are 12–17 mm and females 16–22 mm long. The cuticle forms a rounded mouth collar and large cephalic vesicle, constricted around the middle by a shallow annular groove (Fig. 1.45). External leaf crowns are missing and the internal ring consists of 38–40 small triangular denticles. Cervical papillae are present, just posterior to the cervical groove. The male bursa is well developed. The egg is a medium-sized (75–98 × 46–54 μm), regular,

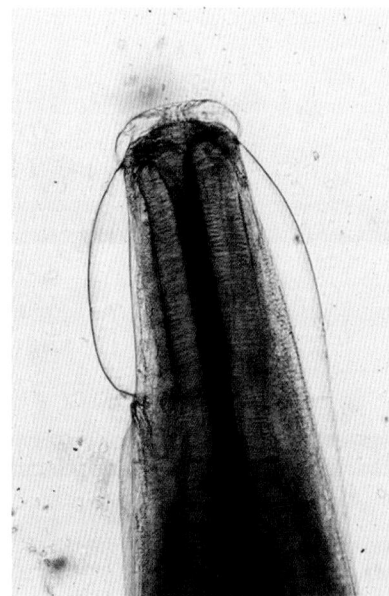

Fig. 1.45 Anterior of *Oesophagostomum radiatum* showing the large cephalic vesicle.

broad ellipse with barrel-shaped side walls and rounded poles, and contains 16–32 blastomeres when passed in the faeces. The colourless chitinous shell is thin with a smooth surface. Infective larvae (L_3) have long filamentous tails, 32 gut cells and a rounded head.

Life cycle: The prepatent period is about 40 days.

Oesophagostomum dentatum

Description: Adult males are 8–10 mm and females 11–14 mm in length (Fig. 1.46). The cephalic vesicle is prominent but cervical alae are virtually absent. The nine elements of the leaf crown project forward and the internal leaf crown has 18 elements. The buccal capsule is shallow with parallel sides and the oesophagus is club-shaped with a narrow anterior end. In the female, the tail is

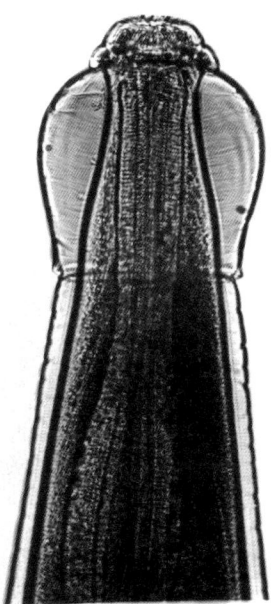

Fig. 1.44 Anterior of *Oesophagostomum venulosum* showing the large inflated cephalic vesicle.

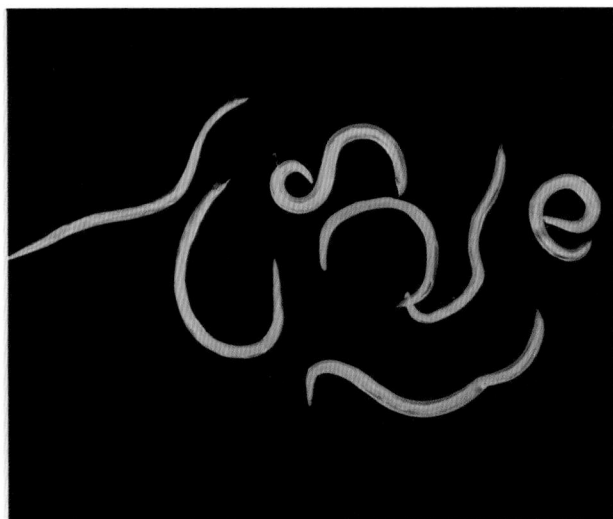

Fig. 1.46 *Oesophagostomum dentatum* adult worms.

relatively short. Eggs are ovoid, smooth with almost similar rounded poles and strongly barrel-shaped side walls. The shell is thin and colourless. They measure around 60–80 by 35–45 µm and contain 8–16 blastomeres in fresh faeces. L_3 are less than 600 µm with a tail less than 60 µm.

Oesophagostomum brevicaudum

Description: Males measure 6–7 mm and females 6.5–8.5 mm in length. There are 28–32 elements and 14–16 elements in the internal and external leaf crowns respectively. In the female, the tail is bent dorsally.

Oesophagostomum quadrispinulatum

Description: This worm is similar to *O. dentatum*, although the oesophagus is slightly more slender and the tail of the female is almost twice as long.

Poteriostomum

These worms (Table 1.16) measure about 9–21 mm in length. This genus is closely related to the genus *Cylicodontophorus*. The two genera are easily separated based on characteristics of the buccal capsule, especially the point of insertion of the internal leaf crowns, and on the character of the dorsal rays. The externodorsal ray and the dorsal ray of the bursa in this genus arise from a common trunk and the dorsal ray gives off, almost at 90°, two lateral branches near the origin of the externodorsal rays and the dorsal ray is cleft only to about half its length.

Poteriostomum imparidentatum

Description: Males are 9–14 mm and females 13–21 mm. This genus is closely related to the genus *Cylicodontophorus*. The two genera are easily separated based on characteristics of the buccal capsule, especially the point of insertion of the internal leaf crown and the character of the dorsal ray. In *P. imparidentatum* six elements of the internal leaf crown are markedly longer than the others.

Poteriostomum ratzii

Description: Males are 9–14 mm and females 13–21 mm. This genus is closely related to the genus *Cylicodontophorus*. The two genera are easily separated based on characteristics of the buccal

Table 1.16 *Poteriostomum* species.

Species	Hosts	Site
Poteriostomum imparidentatum	Horses, donkeys	Large intestine
Poteriostomum ratzii	Horses, donkeys	Large intestine
Poteriostomum skrjabini	Horses, donkeys	Large intestine

capsule, especially the point of insertion of the internal leaf crown and the character of the dorsal ray. In *P. ratzii*, all elements of the internal leaf crown are of equal length.

Poteriostomum skrjabini

Description: Distinguished by a poorly defined dorsal gutter.

Craterostomum

These are relatively small worms, 6–11 mm long, and in general are similar to *Triodontophorus* (apart from the lack of protruding teeth and also the female vulva is located more anteriorly). The buccal capsule is of greatest diameter in the middle, with the wall thickened behind the anterior edge. The dorsal gutter is strongly developed. There is a shallow oesophageal funnel with three small triangular teeth that do not project into the buccal cavity. Elements of the external leaf crown are large and transparent and less numerous than the short broad elements of the inner leaf crown that ring the anterior ridge of the buccal capsule. Submedian papillae extend beyond the depressed mouth collar. In the female, the tail is long and pointed and the vulva is relatively far from the anus.

Craterostomum acuticaudatum

Description: The males measure about 6–10 mm and the females 7–11 mm in length. The internal leaf crown has 22–26 short elements and the external leaf crown bears 6–8 petal-shaped elements. The bottom of the buccal capsule is funnel-shaped and possesses a row of papillae which appear like a leaf crown. Teeth are absent from the buccal cavity. The buccal capsule is of greatest diameter in the middle, the wall being thickened behind the anterior edge. The dorsal gutter is strongly developed. The shallow oesophageal funnel has three small triangular teeth that do not project into the buccal cavity. Elements of the external leaf crown are large and transparent and less numerous than the short broad elements of the inner leaf crown that ring the anterior ridge of the buccal capsule. Submedian papillae extend beyond the depressed mouth collar. In the female, the tail is long and pointed and the vulva is relatively far from the anus.

Craterostomum tenuicauda

Description: Small worms, 6–10 mm long. The buccal capsule is of greatest diameter in the middle, the wall being thickened behind the anterior edge. The dorsal gutter is strongly developed. The shallow oesophageal funnel has three small triangular teeth that do not project into the buccal cavity. The elements of the external leaf crown (nine) are large and transparent and less numerous than the short broad elements of the inner leaf crown (18) that ring the anterior ridge of the buccal capsule. Submedian papillae are unnotched and extend beyond the depressed mouth collar. In the female, the tail is short and pointed and the vulva is relatively far from the anus.

Oesophagodontus

There is only one species in the genus. Male worms are 15–18 mm and females 19–24 mm in size. There is a slight constriction between the anterior region and the remainder of the body. The main species is *Oesophagodontus robustus* which infects the large intestine of horses and donkeys.

Oesophagodontus robustus

Description: Male worms are 15–18 mm and females 19–24 mm. There is a slight constriction between the anterior end and the rest of the body. The buccal capsule is shaped like a funnel with a thickened ring encircling its posterior margin. The oesophageal funnel has three lancet-like teeth that do not project into the buccal capsule. There is no dorsal gutter.

Codiostomum

The main species is *Codiostomum struthionis* which infects the large intestine and caecum of ostriches and rheas.

Codiostomum struthionis

Description: Adult worms are 13–17 mm in length. The large buccal capsule is subglobular with external and internal leaf crowns, but no teeth. The male bursa has a large projecting dorsal lobe. The third-stage larva has a rounded cephalic region and an acute termination of the tail, beyond which is a long filamentous sheath tail.

Life cycle: The life cycle is unknown but is considered to be direct.

SUBFAMILY CYATHOSTOMINAE

The 'small strongyles' include over 50 species, popularly known as trichonemes, cyathostomes or cyathostomins. For many years there has been a great deal of confusion in the classification of this group of parasites and in a new revision it has been proposed that the genus *Trichonema* be discarded and replaced by four main genera, namely *Cyathostomum*, *Cylicocyclus*, *Cylicodontophorus* and *Cylicostephanus*, these being collectively referred to as cyathostomes or, more recently, cyathostomins.

Small strongyles are small (5–12 mm long) bursate nematodes ranging in colour from white to dark red, the majority being visible on close inspection of the large intestinal mucosa or contents (Fig. 1.47). The well-developed short buccal capsule is cylindrical, without teeth, and species differentiation is based on characteristics of the buccal capsule and the internal and external leaf crowns.

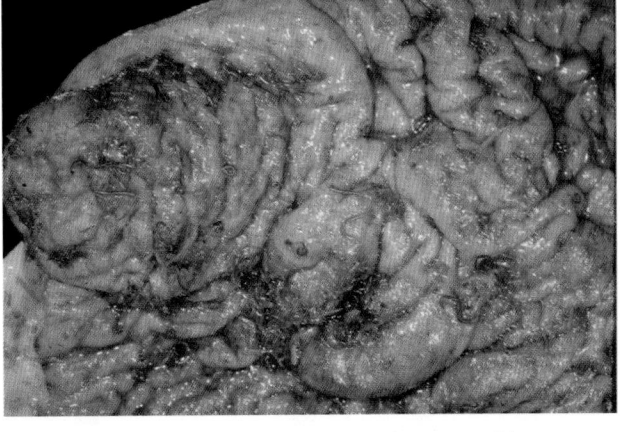

Fig. 1.47 Small strongyles (cyathostomins) on the mucosa of the ventral colon.

Life cycle: Hatching of eggs and development to L_3 are complete within two weeks during the summer in temperate areas, after which the larvae migrate from the faeces on to the surrounding herbage. After ingestion, the L_3 exsheath and invade the wall of the ileum and large intestine where they develop to L_4 before emerging into the gut lumen and moulting to become young adult worms. The prepatent periods of members of this genus are generally between two and three months, although this may be extended due to hypobiosis in some species. See **life cycle 4**.

Cyathostomum

Cyathostomum spp. (Table 1.17) are small (5–12 mm in length) bursate nematodes ranging in colour from white to dark red, the majority being visible on close inspection of the large intestinal mucosa or contents. These parasites have a moderately high mouth collar, with cephalic papillae not very prominent. The well-developed short buccal capsule is cylindrical, without teeth, and species differentiation is based on characteristics of the buccal capsule and the internal and external leaf crowns. The buccal capsule is broader than deep and has no dorsal gutter. Elements of the external leaf crown are larger, broader and fewer than elements of the internal leaf crown. The inner leaf crown is deep in the buccal capsule and has sclerotised extrachitinous supports at or near the anterior edge of the buccal capsule (Fig. 1.48a). The dorsal ray of the male bursa is split to the origin of the externodorsal rays and the spicules are filiform, equal in length with 'pick'-shaped tips. In the female, the vulva is close to the anus. The tail may be straight or bent dorsally with a ventral bulge, anterior to the vulva. The eggs are medium-sized, a long ellipse, measuring about 100–110 by 40–45 μm. The shells are smooth and thin with almost similar poles and parallel side walls and contain a morula with several large blastomeres. It is not possible to distinguish between the eggs of the different species of cyathostomes.

LIFE CYCLE 4. LIFE CYCLE OF CYATHOSTOMINAE (SMALL STRONGYLES OF EQUINES)

Adult stages of small strongyles live in the lumen of the large intestine of the horse (1) that sheds unembryonated eggs with the faeces (2). After embryonation and first-stage larva formation (3) in the external environment, the egg hatches, releasing the first-stage larva, which moults twice to become an infective, third-stage larva (4) in about one week. The horse acquires the infection by ingesting infective larvae while grazing (5) or drinking contaminated water. After ingestion, the larvae migrate to the ileal, caecal and colonic glands (depending on genera and species of Cyathostominae), where they become encysted, thus forming nodules within the intestinal and submucosal wall (6). Within the nodules, the larvae continue their development and subsequently emerge within the intestinal lumen where they become adults. Adult males are characterised by a copulatory bursa with chitinous rays (7), whilst in females the location of the vulva and the morphology of the caudal end differ depending on genera (8). The morphology of the buccal capsule, with its external and internal chitinous crowns, is also taxonomically important and differs depending on species (9).

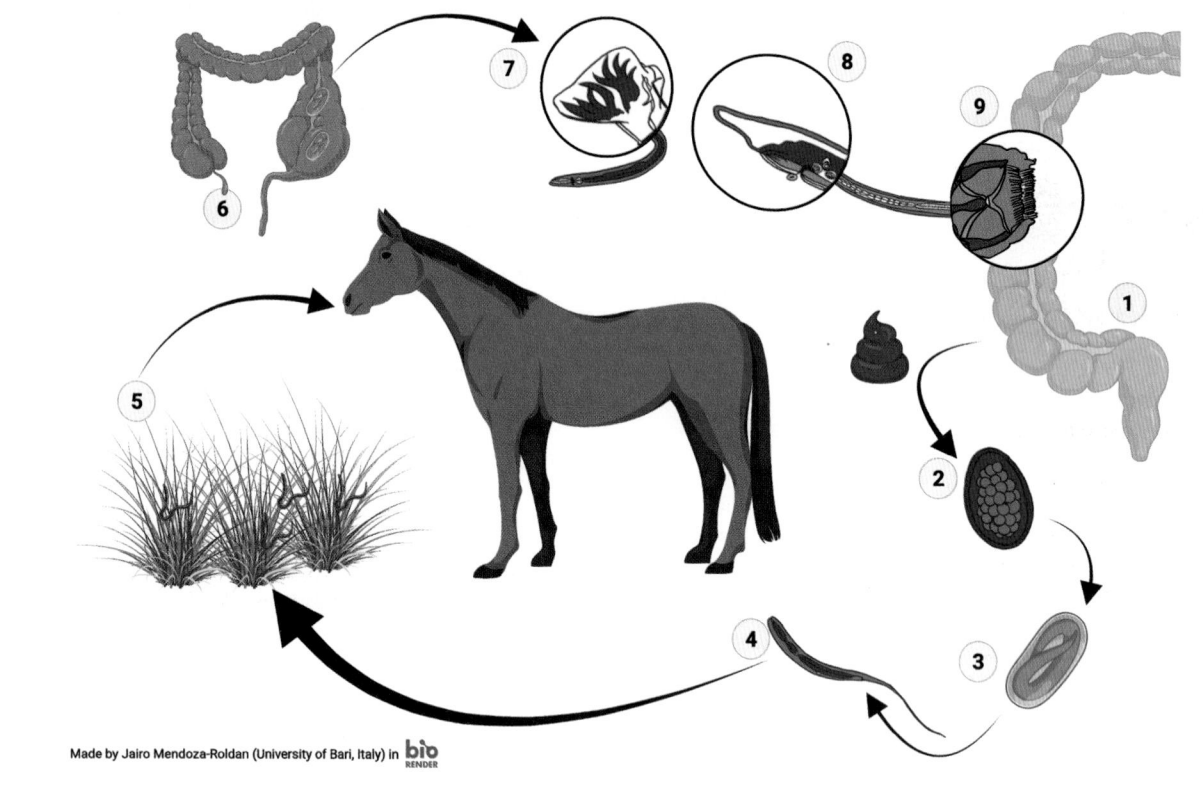

Made by Jairo Mendoza-Roldan (University of Bari, Italy) in bio RENDER

Table 1.17 *Cyathostomum* species.

Species	Hosts	Site
Cyathostomum alveatum (syn. *Cylichnostomum alveatum, Cylicostomum alveatum, Trichonema alveatum, Cylicocercus alveatus*)	Horses, donkeys	Large intestine
Cyathostomum catinatum (syn. *Cylichnostomum catinatum, Cylicostomum catinatum, Trichonema catinatum, Cylicocercus catinatum*)	Horses, donkeys	Large intestine
Cyathostomum coronatum (syn. *Cylichnostomum coronatum, Cylicostomum coronatum, Trichonema coronatum, Cylicostomias coronatum*)	Horses, donkeys	Large intestine
Cyathostomum labiatum (syn. *Cyathostomum labratum, Cylichnostomum labiatum, Cylicostomum labiatum, Trichonema labiatum, Cylicostomias labiatum*)	Horses, donkeys	Large intestine
Cyathostomum labratum (syn. *Cylichnostomum labratum, Cylicostomum labratum, Trichonema labratum, Cylicostomias labratum*)	Horses, donkeys	Large intestine
Cyathostomum montgomeryi (syn. *Cylicostomum montgomeryi, Trichonema labratum, Cylicotoichus montgomeryi*)	Horses, donkeys	Large intestine
Cyathostomum pateratum (syn. *Cylicodontophorus pateratum, Cylicostomum pateratum, Trichonema pateratum, Cylicostocercus pateratum*)	Horses, donkeys	Large intestine
Cyathostomum saginatum (syn. *Cylicostomum sagittatum, Trichonema sagittatum, Cylicostomias sagittatum, Cylicodontophorus sagittatum*)	Horses, donkeys	Large intestine
Cyathostomum tetracanthum (syn. *Strongylus tetracanthus, Sclerostomum tetracanthum, Cylichnostomum tetracanthum, Cylicostomum tetracanthum, Trichonema tetracanthum, Trichonema arcuata, Trichonema aegypticum, Cylicostomum aegypticum*)	Horses, donkeys	Large intestine

lef crowns. Chitinous supports are spindle-shaped. The excretory pore is sited near the junction of the mid to posterior third of the oesophagus.

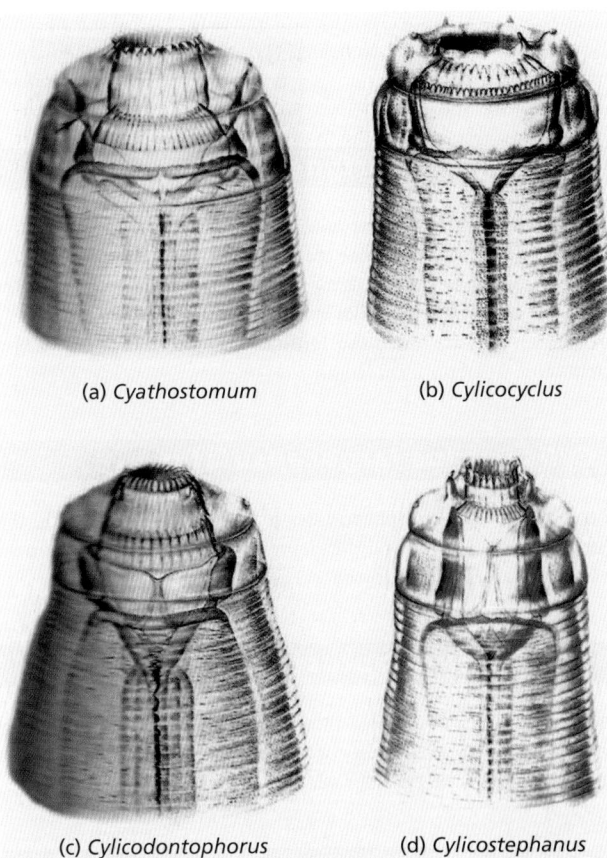

(a) Cyathostomum   **(b) Cylicocyclus**

(c) Cylicodontophorus   **(d) Cylicostephanus**

Fig. 1.48 Cystostomins showing characteristic features of the heads and buccal capsules used in generic and species identification: (a) *Cyathostomum*; (b) *Cylicocyclus*; (c) *Cylicodontophorus*; (d) *Cylicostephanus*. (Redrawn from Lichtenfels, 1975. Reproduced with permission from the Helminthological Society of Washington.)

Cyathostomum alveatum

Description: The walls of the buccal capsule have a uniform thickness posterior to the inner leaf crown, which is about one-third the depth of the buccal capsule.

Cyathostomum catinatum

Description: The inner leaf crown is more anterior on the lateral sides of the buccal capsule compared with the dorsal and ventral sides, but not in a sinuous line.

Cyathostomum coronatum

Description: Extrachitinous supports are prominent and the inner leaf crown forms an even line around the buccal cavity, which is as deep as it is broad and with walls that are thick and bent inwards.

Cyathostomum labiatum

Description: The mouth collar is notched and forms four distinct lips; the inner leaf crown elements are half the length of the external

Cyathostomum labratum

Description: The mouth collar is not notched; the inner leaf crown elements are greater than half the length of the external leaf crowns. Chitinous supports are pyriform-shaped and the excretory pore is located near the middle of the oesophagus.

Cyathostomum montgomeryi

Description: Similar to *C. labiatum* but without well-defined lips. The wall of the buccal capsule is longer in dorsoventral view.

Cyathostomum pateratum

Description: The inner leaf crown is in a sinuous line deep in the buccal cavity (seen in lateral view).

Cyathostomum saginatum

Description: Similar to *C. coranatum* but the buccal capsule is shallow.

Cyathostomum tetracanthum

Description: The extrachitinous supports are nearly as large as the wall of the buccal capsule and appear as extensions of the buccal capsule wall.

Cylicocyclus

These parasites (Table 1.18) are small to medium-sized (10–25 mm in length) bursate nematodes ranging in colour from white to dark red, the majority being visible on close inspection of the large intestinal mucosa or contents. The well-developed short buccal capsule is cylindrical, without teeth, and species differentiation is based on characteristics of the buccal capsule and the internal and external leaf crowns. *Cylicocyclus* have a high mouth collar with broad lateral papillae. Elements of the external leaf crown are larger, fewer and broader than those of the inner leaf crown, the latter being short, with thin rods at or near the anterior edge of the buccal capsule. The buccal capsule is short, broader than deep, with thin walls tapering anteriorly, with a hoop-shaped thickening around the posterior margin. A dorsal gutter is usually absent from the buccal capsule (Fig. 1.48b). In the male the dorsal ray is split to the origin of the externodorsal rays and the spicules are filiform, of equal length with pick-shaped tails. In females, the vulva is near the anus and the tail is usually straight but may be bent slightly dorsally.

Table 1.18 *Cylicocyclus* species.

Species	Hosts	Site
Cylicocyclus adersi (syn. *Cylicostomum adersi, Trichonema adersi*)	Horses, donkeys	Large intestine
Cylicocyclus auriculatus (syn. *Cylichnostomum auriculatum, Cylicostomum auriculatum, Trichonema auriculatum, Cyathostomum auriculatum*)	Horses, donkeys	Large intestine
Cylicocyclus brevicapsulatus (syn. *Cylicostomum brevispiculatum, Cylichobrachytus brevispiculatum, Trichonema brevispiculatum*)	Horses, donkeys	Large intestine
Cylicocyclus elongatus (syn. *Cyathostomum elongatum, Cylichnostomum elongatum, Trichonema elongatum, Cylicoostomum elongatum*)	Horses, donkeys	Large intestine
Cylicocyclus insigne (syn. *Cylichnostomum insigne, Cylicostomum insdigne, Cylicostomum zebra, Trichonema insigne*)	Horses, donkeys	Large intestine
Cylicocyclus largocapsulatus (syn. *Trichonema largocapsulatus*)	Horses, donkeys	Large intestine
Cylicocyclus leptostomus (syn. *Cylichnostomum leptostomum, Trichonema leptostomum, Schultzitrichonema leptostomum, Cylicotetrapedon leptostomum*)	Horses, donkeys	Large intestine
Cylicocyclus maturmurai (syn. *Trichonema maturmurai*)	Horses, donkeys	Large intestine
Cylicocyclus nassatus (syn. *Cyathostomum nassatum, Cylichnostomum nassatum, Cylicostomum nassatum, Trichonema nassatum, Cylicocyclus bulbiferus*)	Horses, donkeys	Large intestine
Cylicocyclus radiatus (syn. *Cyathostomum radiatum, Cylichnostomum radiatum, Trichonema radiatum, Cylicostomum prionodes*)	Horses, donkeys	Large intestine
Cyliocyclus triramosus (syn. *Cylicostomum triramosum, Trichonema triramosum*)	Horses, donkeys	Large intestine
Cylicocyclus ultrajectinus (syn. *Cylicostomum ultrajectinum, Trichonema ultrajectinum*)	Horses, donkeys	Large intestine

Cylicocyclus adersi

Description: Buccal capsule is not shallow and the walls are of uniform thickness. The dorsal gutter is short but well developed. The inner leaf crown elements are few and wider than the external leaf crown elements and are of uniform length.

Cylicocyclus auriculatus

Description: The buccal capsule is not shallow and the dorsal gutter is absent. Lateral papillae are long ear-like or horn-like extending much higher than the mouth collar. The excretory pore and cervical papillae are located behind the oesophago-intestinal junction.

Cylicocyclus brevicapsulatus

Description: The buccal capsule is extremely shallow with delicate inconspicuous walls.

Cylicocyclus elongatus

Description: The buccal capsule is not shallow, the dorsal gutter is absent and the lateral papillae are not long. The excretory pore and cervical papillae are anterior to the oesophago-intestinal junction.

The oesophageal funnel is nearly as large as the buccal capsule, and the oesophagus is greatly elongated with the posterior half enlarged and cylindrical.

Cylicocyclus insigne

Description: The buccal capsule is not shallow, the dorsal gutter is absent and the lateral papillae are not long. The excretory pore and the cervical papillae are anterior to the oesophago-intestinal junction. The external leaf crown elements are narrow; the inner leaf crown elements are much shorter than the external leaf crown elements and are of uniform length.

Cylicocyclus largocapsulatus

Description: The oesophago-intestinal valve is not elongate, the buccal capsule is large and the elements of the external leaf crown are about half as long as the buccal capsule is deep.

Cylicocyclus leptostomus

Description: The oesophago-intestinal valve is elongate, the buccal capsule is small and elements of the external leaf crown are almost as long as the buccal capsule is deep.

Cylicocyclus maturmurai

Description: The buccal capsule is not shallow and the walls are of uniform thickness. The inner leaf crown elements outnumber the external leaf crown elements and are of uniform length.

Cylicocyclus nassatus

Description: The buccal capsule is not shallow, with both lateral papillae and external leaf crown extending beyond the mouth collar. A dorsal gutter is present extending half of the depth of the buccal capsule. Submedian papillae are long and extend beyond the mouth collar. The external leaf crown has 20 elements. The buccal capsule has an internal shelf-like cuticular projection.

Cylicocyclus radiatus

Description: The oesophago-intestinal valve is not elongate, the buccal capsule is large and the elements of the external leaf crown are almost about one-third as long as the buccal capsule is deep.

Cyliococyclus triramosus

Description: The buccal capsule is not shallow, with both lateral papillae and the external leaf crown extending beyond the mouth collar. The dorsal gutter is short and button-like. The submedian papillae are short and do not extend beyond the mouth collar. The external leaf crown has 30 elements. The buccal capsule is without an internal projection.

Cylicocyclus ultrajectinus

Description: The buccal capsule is not shallow, the dorsal gutter is absent and the lateral papillae are not long. The excretory pore and cervical papillae are located near the oesophago-intestinal junction. The external leaf crown elements are broad; the inner leaf crown elements are as long, or longer, than the external leaf crown elements.

Cylicodontophorus

Small (7–14 mm in length) bursate nematodes (Table 1.19) ranging in colour from white to dark red, the majority being visible on close inspection of the large intestinal mucosa or contents. The well-developed short buccal capsule is cylindrical, without teeth, and species differentiation is based on characteristics of the buccal capsule and the internal and external leaf crowns. *Cylicodontophorus* have a high mouth collar, with inconspicuous lateral papillae and short and conical submedian papillae. The buccal capsule is short, thick-walled, of nearly uniform thickness and broader than deep. Inner leaf crown elements are longer, broader and less numerous than the external leaf crown elements, and are inserted near the anterior edge of the buccal capsule (Fig. 1.48c). The dorsal ray of the male bursa is split only to the proximal branch, and the spicules are filiform, equal in length with 'hook'-shaped tips. In the female, the tail is short with a sharp tip, and a prominent ventral bulge may be present anterior to the vulva.

Cylicodontophorus bicoronatus

Description: The dorsal gutter is well developed. The elements of the external and internal leaf crowns are nearly equal in size.

Cylicodontophorus euproctus

Description: The dorsal gutter is absent. The elements of the internal leaf crowns are twice as long as the elements of the external leaf crown. The oesophageal funnel is not well developed.

Cylicodontophorus mettami

Description: The dorsal gutter is absent. The elements of the internal leaf crowns are less than twice as long as the elements of the external leaf crown. The oesophageal funnel is well developed.

Table 1.19 *Cylicodontophorus* species.

Species	Hosts	Site
Cylicodontophorus bicoronatus (syn. Cyathostomum bicoranatum, Cylichnostomum bicoronatum, Cylicostomum bicoranatum, Trichonema bicoranatum)	Horses, donkeys	Large intestine
Cylicodontophorus euproctus (syn. Cylichnostomum euproctus, Cylicostomum euproctus, Trichonema euproctus)	Horses, donkeys	Large intestine
Cylicodontophorus mettami (syn. Cylicostoma mettami, Cylicostomum mettami, Trichonema mettami, Cylicocercus mettami, Cylicostomum ihlei)	Horses, donkeys	Large intestine

Cylicostephanus

These are small (4–10 mm in length) bursate nematodes (Table 1.20) ranging in colour from white to dark red, the majority being visible on close inspection of the large intestinal mucosa or contents. The well-developed short buccal capsule is cylindrical, without teeth, and species differentiation is based on characteristics of the buccal capsule and the internal and external leaf crowns. *Cylicostephanus* have a depressed mouth collar, with inconspicuous lateral papillae and prominent submedian papillae. The buccal capsule is slightly narrow anteriorly, with a wall of varying thickness and with a dorsal gutter. External leaf crown elements are longer, broader and less numerous than the internal leaf crown elements, which are short thin rods inserted near the anterior edge of the buccal capsule (Fig. 1.48d). The dorsal ray of the male bursa is split only to the proximal branch, and the spicules are filiform, equal in length with pick-shaped tips. In the female, the vulva is near the anus and the tail is usually straight.

Cylicostephanus asymetricus

Description: The walls of the buccal capsule are markedly thicker anteriorly, the elements of the external leaf crown are as broad as long, and the dorsal gutter extends almost to the base of the inner

Table 1.20 *Cylicostephanus* species.

Species	Hosts	Site
Cylicostephanus asymetricus (syn. Cylicostomum asymetricum, Cylicotrapedon asymetricum, Schulzitrichonema asymetricum)	Horses, donkeys	Large intestine
Cylicostephanus bidentatus (syn. Cylicostomum bidentatum, Cylicotrapedon bidentatum, Trichonema bidentatum, Schulzitrichonema bidentatum)	Horses, donkeys	Large intestine
Cylicostephanus calicatus (syn. Cyathostomum calicatum, Cylichnostomum calicatum, Cylicostomum calicatum, Trichonema calicatum, Cylicostomum barbatum, Trichonema tsengi)	Horses, donkeys	Large intestine
Cylicostephanus goldi (syn. Cylichnostomum goldi, Cylicostomum goldi, Trichonema goldi, Schulzitrichonema goldi, Cylicostomum tridentatum)	Horses, donkeys	Large intestine
Cylicostephanus hybridus (syn. Cylicostomum hybridus, Trichonema hybridum, Schulzitrichonema hybridum, Trichonema parvibursatus)	Horses, donkeys	Large intestine
Cylicostephanus longibursatus (syn. Cylicostomum longibursatum, Trichonema longibursatum, Cylicostomum nanum, Cylicostomum calicatiforme)	Horses, donkeys	Large intestine
Cylicostephanus minutus (syn. Cylicostomum minutum, Trichonema minutum)	Horses, donkeys	Large intestine
Cylicostephanus ornatus (syn. Cylicostomum ornatum, Trichonema ornatum, Cylicostomias ornatum, Cyathostomum ornatum, Cylicodontophorus ornatum)	Horses, donkeys	Large intestine
Cylicostephanus poculatus (syn. Cyathostomum poculatum, Cylichnostomum poculatum, Cylicostomum poculatum, Trichonema poculatum, Petrovina poculatum)	Horses, donkeys	Large intestine
Cylicostephanus skrjabini (syn. Trichonema skrjabini, Petrovinema skrjabini)	Horses, donkeys	Large intestine

leaf crown. The buccal capsule is asymmetrical in lateral view and the walls of the capsule are concave. The teeth in the oesophageal funnel are not prominent.

Cylicocyclus bidentatus

Description: The walls of the buccal capsule are markedly thicker anteriorly, the elements of the external leaf crown are as broad as long, and the dorsal gutter extends almost to the base of the inner leaf crown. The buccal capsule is asymmetrical in lateral view and the walls of the capsule are concave. The teeth in the oesophageal funnel are not prominent.

Cylicostephanus calicatus

Description: The buccal capsule is as broad as deep and the wall is of uniform thickness. The external leaf crowns are composed of 8–18 triangular elements and the submedian papillae are notched near their tips.

Cylicostephanus goldi

Description: The walls of the buccal capsule are of uniform thickness, the elements of the external leaf crown are twice as numerous as the elements of the inner leaf crown, and the dorsal gutter is button-like. The walls of the buccal capsule have a slight compound curve, being slightly thicker posteriorly. The female tail is bent dorsally. There are no prominent teeth in the oesophageal funnel.

Cylicostephanus hybridus

Description: The walls of the buccal capsule are of uniform thickness, the elements of the external leaf crown are twice as long as broad, and the dorsal gutter extends halfway to the base of the inner leaf crown. The walls of the buccal capsule are straight, slightly thicker posteriorly in dorsal view.

Cylicostephanus longibursatus

Description: The walls of the buccal capsule are of uniform thickness, the elements of the external leaf crown are twice as long as broad, and the dorsal gutter is button-like. The walls of the buccal capsule have a slight compound curve and are slightly thicker posteriorly.

Cylicostephanus minutus

Description: The buccal capsule is as broad as deep and the walls are of uniform thickness. The external leaf crowns are composed of 8–18 triangular elements and the submedian papillae are notched midway.

Cylicostephanus ornatus

Description: The walls of the buccal capsule are markedly thicker anteriorly, the elements of the external leaf crown are as broad as

long, and the dorsal gutter extends almost to the base of the inner leaf crown. The buccal capsule is asymmetrical in lateral view and the walls of the capsule are concave. The teeth in the oesophageal funnel are not prominent.

Cylicostephanus poculatus

Description: The buccal capsule is deeper than broader in lateral view and the walls are much thicker posteriorly. The external leaf crown is composed of approximately 36 elements.

Cylicostephanus skrjabini

Description: The buccal capsule is deeper than broader in lateral view and the walls are much thicker posteriorly. The external leaf crown is composed of approximately 36 elements. It lacks a lateral projection on the inner wall of the buccal capsule and has a rim of dentiform processes at the bottom of the buccal capsule.

FAMILY CHABERTIDAE

Chabertia

Worms of this genus are usually found in low numbers in the majority of sheep and goats. The adults are 1.5–2 cm in length and are the largest nematodes found in the colon of ruminants. They are white with a markedly truncated and enlarged anterior end due to the presence of the very large buccal capsule. The anterior is curved slightly ventrally (Fig. 1.49).

Life cycle: The life cycle is direct. Eggs are passed in the faeces and hatch on the ground, releasing the first-stage larva which moults to the second stage, and then to the infective third stage. The host is infected by ingestion of the larva with the herbage. In the parasitic phase, the L_3 enter the mucosa of the small intestine and occasionally that of the caecum and colon; after a week they moult, the L_4 emerge on to the mucosal surface and migrate to congregate in the caecum where development to the L_5 is completed about 25 days

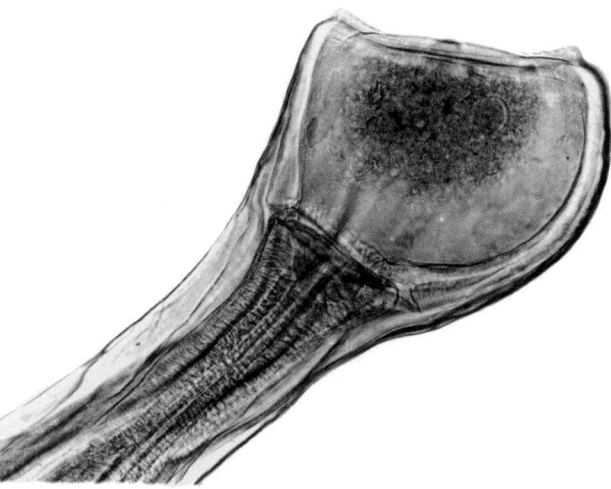

Fig. 1.49 Head of *Chabertia ovina* illustrating the large bell-shaped buccal capsule.

after infection. The young adults then travel to the colon. There is no migration stage in the body. The prepatent period is about 6–7 weeks. The main species is *Chabertia ovina* which infects the large intestine of sheep, goats and occasionally cattle.

Chabertia ovina

Description: The adults range from about 1.3 to 2 cm in length and are the largest nematodes found in the colon of ruminants. They are white and stout with a markedly truncated and enlarged anterior end due to the presence of the very large buccal capsule (Fig. 1.49). The huge buccal capsule, which is bell-shaped, has a double row of small papillae around the rim. There are no teeth. There is a shallow ventral cervical groove and anterior to it a slightly inflated cephalic vesicle. In the male, the bursa is well developed and the spicules are 1.3–1.7 mm long, with a gubernaculum. In the female, the vulva opens about 0.4 mm from the posterior extremity. The egg is a thin-shelled, smooth, medium-sized (90–100 × 45–55 μm), regular broad ellipse with wide slightly flattened poles (see Fig. 4.4). It contains 16–32 blastomeres. Infective larvae have a rounded head, 32 gut cells and a long filamentous tail and measure around 730 μm.

Agriostomum

Worms are stout and greyish-white in colour. Males are around 9–11 mm and females 13–16 mm in length. The main species is *Agriostomum vryburgi* which infects the small intestine of cattle, buffalo, oxen and zebu.

Agriostomum vryburgi

Description: The shallow buccal capsule opens anterodorsally and contains four pairs of large teeth on its margin and has a rudimentary leaf crown. The large wide oesophageal opening at the base of the buccal capsule houses two small subventral lancets. The bursa is well developed and the ventral rays are close together and parallel. A gubernaculum is present and the spicules are equal in length. Eggs measure about 130–190 by 60–90 μm.

FAMILY SYNGAMIDAE

Syngamus

The large reddish female and the small whitish male are permanently *in copula* forming a 'Y' shape (Fig. 1.50). They are the only parasites found in the trachea of domestic birds. Males possess two spicules.

Life cycle: Eggs escape under the bursa of the male and are carried up the trachea in the excess mucus produced in response to infection; they are then swallowed and passed in the faeces. Unlike other strongyloids, the L$_3$ develops within the egg. Infection may occur by one of three ways: first by ingestion of the L$_3$ in the egg, second by ingestion of the hatched L$_3$, or third by ingestion of a transport (paratenic) host containing the L$_3$. The most common paratenic host is the common earthworm, but a variety of other invertebrates including slugs, snails, beetles and some flies may act as transport hosts. After penetrating the intestine of the final host, the L$_3$ travel,

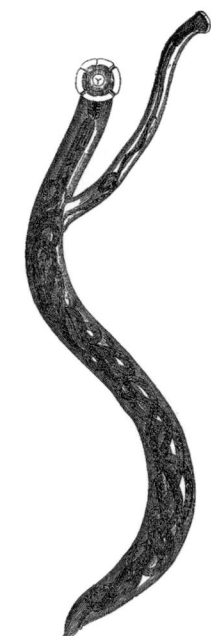

Fig. 1.50 *Syngamus trachea* male and female worms *in copula*. (Redrawn from Neumann, trans. Fleming, 1892).

via the liver, to the lungs, probably in the blood since they are found in the alveoli 4–6 hours after experimental infection. The two parasitic moults take place in the lungs within five days, by which time the parasites are 1–2 mm long. Copulation occurs around day 7 in the trachea or bronchi, after which the female grows rapidly. The prepatent period is 16–20 days. Longevity is around nine months. The main species is *Syngamus trachea* which infects the trachea of chickens, turkeys, gamebirds (pheasants, partridges, guinea fowl), pigeons and various wild birds.

Syngamus trachea

Synonyms: *Syngamus parvis*, *Syngamus gracilis*

Description: The large reddish female (around 1–3 cm) and the small whitish male (up to 0.5 cm) are permanently *in copula* forming a 'Y' shape (Fig. 1.50); they are the only parasites found in the trachea of domestic birds (Fig. 1.51). The worms have large, shallow, cup-shaped buccal capsules that have up to 10 teeth at their base.

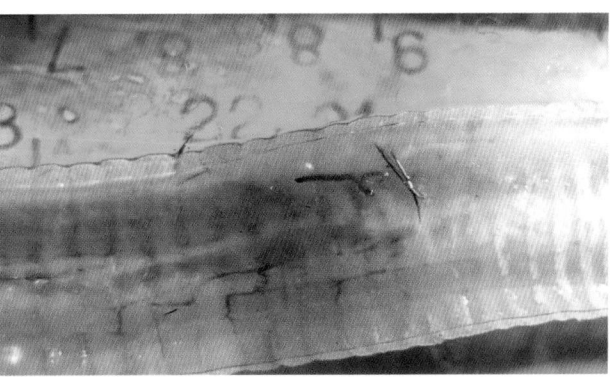

Fig. 1.51 *Syngamus trachea*: adult *in situ* (arrow). (Courtesy of Călin Mircea GHERMAN).

There are no leaf crowns. The bursal rays are short and thick and the two spicules are long and of simple form. The ellipsoidal thin-shelled eggs are 70–100 by 43–46 µm with a thick operculum at both ends. They are in the 16-cell stage when ejected.

Cyathostoma

The male bursa is well developed but worms in this species are not permanently *in copula*, as observed in *Syngamus*.

Life cycle: The life cycle is thought to be similar to that of *Syngamus*.

Cyathostoma bronchialis

Synonym: *Syngamus bronchialis*

Description: The worms are reddish in colour when fresh. Adult male worms are 4–6 mm and females much larger at 15–30 mm in length. The buccal capsule is large, deep and cup-shaped with 6–7 teeth at its base. The male bursa is well developed but worms in this species are not permanently *in copula*, as seen in *Syngamus trachea*. The medium-sized, lightly coloured eggs are ovoid with a smooth shell and possess a hardly perceptible operculum at one pole. They measure about 74–89 by 47–62 µm and the morula contains eight blastomeres.

Cyathostoma variegatum

Description: Adult worms are 0.4–3 cm long; males are 4–6 mm and females 16–31 mm. The buccal capsule is cup-shaped with 6–7 teeth at its base. The male bursa is well developed but worms in this species are not permanently *in copula*, which contrasts with the situation in *Syngamus trachea*. Eggs are 74–83 by 49–62 µm.

Mammomonogamus

These nematodes (Table 1.21) are similar to *Syngamus*. The worms are reddish in appearance and about 0.6–2 cm long. The females and males are found in permanent copulation. The large buccal capsule lacks a cuticular crown. There is a cervical papilla. Species of *Mammomonogamus* found in cats may be synonyms of the species found in ruminants.

Life cycle: The life cycle is direct but the mode of transmission is unknown.

Table 1.21 *Mammomonogamus* species.

Species	Hosts	Site
Mammomonogamus nasicola (syn. *Syngamus nasicola, Syngamus kingi*)	Sheep, goats, cattle, deer	Nasal cavities
Mammomonogamus laryngeus (syn. *Syngamus laryngeus*)	Cattle, buffalo, goats, sheep, deer, rarely humans	Larynx
Mammomonogamus auris (syn. *Syngamus auris*)	Cats	Ear canals
Mammomonogamus ierei (syn. *Syngamus ierei*)	Cats	Nasal cavities
Mammomonogamus mcgaughei (syn. *Syngamus mcgaughei*)	Cats	Nasal sinuses, pharynx

Mammomonogamus nasicola

Synonyms: *Syngamus nasicola, Syngamus kingi*

Description: The worms are reddish in appearance and about 1–2 cm long. Males are 4–6 mm and females 11–23 mm long and found in permanent copulation. The buccal capsule lacks a cuticular crown. Eggs are ellipsoid, 54–98 µm, with no operculum at either end.

Mammomonogamus laryngeus

Synonym: *Syngamus laryngeus*

Description: The worms are reddish in appearance and about 1–2 cm long. The females and males are found in permanent copulation. The buccal capsule lacks a cuticular crown. Eggs are ellipsoid, 42–45 by 75–85 µm, with no operculum at either end.

Mammomonogamus ierei

Synonym: *Syngamus ierei*

Description: Female worms are about 20 mm long, while male worms are 5–6.9 mm long and rather stocky in appearance. The worms are found with the bursa of the male attached at the level of the vulva of the female. There is a large buccal capsule that has eight large teeth at its base.

Stephanurus

Large worms found in the kidneys and perirenal tissues.

Life cycle: Preparasitic development from egg to L_3 is typically strongyloid, though earthworms may intervene as transport hosts. There are three modes of infection: by ingestion of the free L_3, ingestion of earthworms carrying the L_3, and percutaneously. After entering the body, there is an immediate moult and the L_4 travel to the liver in the bloodstream, either from the intestine by the portal stream or from the skin by the lungs and systemic circulation. In the liver, the final moult takes place and the young adults wander in the parenchyma for three months or more before piercing the capsule and migrating in the peritoneal cavity to the perirenal region. There they are enclosed in a cyst by the host reaction, and complete their development. The cyst communicates with the ureter either directly or, if it is more distant, by a fine connecting canal, allowing the worm eggs to be excreted in the urine. The prepatent period is 6–19 months and the worms have a longevity of about 2–3 years. The main species is *Stephanurus dentatus* which infects the kidney of pigs.

Stephanurus dentatus

Description: A large stout worm up to 4.5 cm long, with a prominent buccal capsule and transparent cuticle through which the internal organs may be seen. Males are 2–3 cm and females 3–4.5 cm long. The colour is usually pinkish. The size and site are diagnostic. The buccal capsule is cup-shaped with small leaf crowns and six external cuticular thickenings (epaulettes), of which the ventral and dorsal are most prominent, and six cusped teeth at the base. The male bursa is short and the two spicules of either equal or unequal length. The medium-sized eggs are a broad ellipse with a thin transparent shell and appear only in the urine. They measure about 90–120 by 53–70 μm and contain numerous blastomeres (32–64).

FAMILY DELETROCEPHALIDAE

Deletrocephalus

The main species is *Deletrocephalus dimidiatus* which infects the small intestine of rheas.

Deletrocephalus dimidiatus

Description: Adult worms are stout and robust with a well-developed buccal capsule. Male worms are 9–11 mm and females 14–16 mm long. Males are bursate with long thin spicules. The eggs are 160 by 70 μm (Fig. 1.52). Third-stage larvae are approximately 720 μm long, with a rounded head, 28–31 intestinal cells and a short to medium tail.

Paradeletrocephalus

The main species is *Paradeletrocephalus minor* which infects the small intestine of rheas.

Paradeletrocephalus minor

Description: Adult worms are similar in size and appearance to *Deletrocephalus* spp. The buccal capsule has vertical ridges and there are no external, or internal, coronary rings.

SUPERFAMILY ANCYLOSTOMATOIDEA

Hookworms are parasites of the small intestine and the genera of veterinary importance are *Ancylostoma*, *Uncinaria*, *Bunostomum* and, to a lesser extent, *Gaigeria* and *Globocephalus*. In humans important hookworm genera are *Ancylostoma* and *Necator*.

FAMILY ANCYLOSTOMATIDAE

Ancylostoma

Ancylostoma spp. (Table 1.22) are reddish-grey worms, the colour depending on whether the worm has fed, and are readily recognised on the basis of size. The anterior extremity is usually bent dorsally. The worms have a well-developed buccal capsule, which is devoid of leaf crowns but is armed with teeth or chitinous cutting plates on its ventral edge.

Ancylostoma caninum

Description: The worms are reddish-grey in colour, depending on whether the worm has fed, and are readily recognised on the basis of size and by their characteristic hook-like posture (Fig. 1.53). Males are about 12 mm and females 15–20 mm in length (much smaller than the common ascarid nematodes, which are also found in the small intestine). The anterior end is bent dorsal and the oral aperture is directed anterodorsally. The buccal capsule is large with three pairs of sharp marginal teeth and a pair of ventrolateral teeth and possesses a dorsal gutter (Fig. 1.54). The male bursa is well developed. Eggs are typically 'strongylate' with slightly dissimilar bluntly rounded poles, barrel-shaped side walls and a thin smooth shell (see Fig. 4.7). They measure about 56–75 by 34–47 μm and contain 2–8 blastomeres when passed in faeces.

Life cycle: The life cycle is direct and, given optimal conditions, the eggs may hatch and develop to L_3 in as little as five days. Infection is

Table 1.22 *Ancylostoma* species.

Species	Hosts	Site
Ancylostoma braziliense	Dogs, foxes, cats, wild canids	Small intestine
Ancylostoma caninum	Dogs, foxes, wild canids, occasionally humans	Small intestine
Ancylostoma ceylanicum	Dogs, cats, wild felids, occasionally humans	Small intestine
Ancylostoma tubaeforme (syn. *Strongylus tubaeforme*)	Cats	Small intestine
Ancylostoma duodenale	Humans, primates	Small intestine

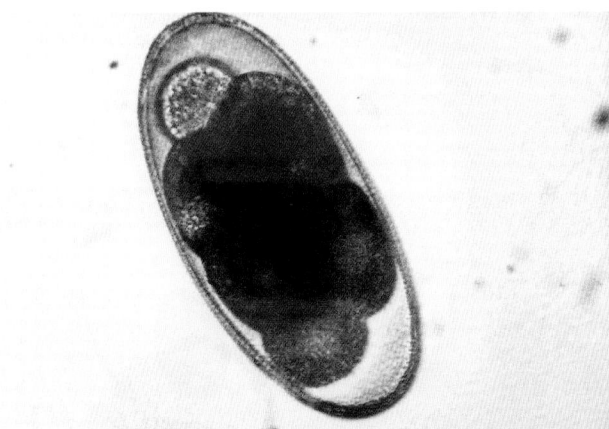

Fig. 1.52 *Deletrocephalus dimidiatus* egg.

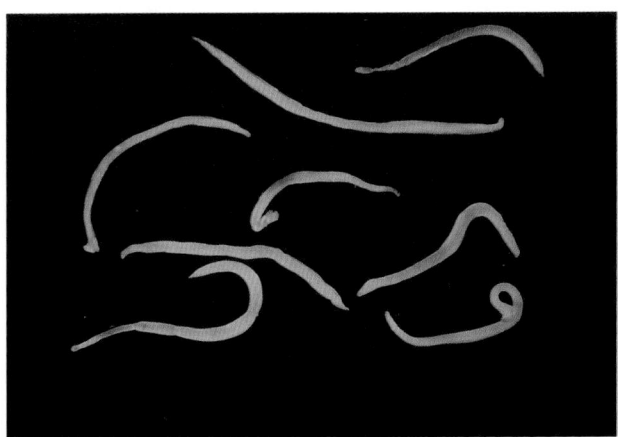

Fig. 1.53 *Ancylostoma caninum* adult worms.

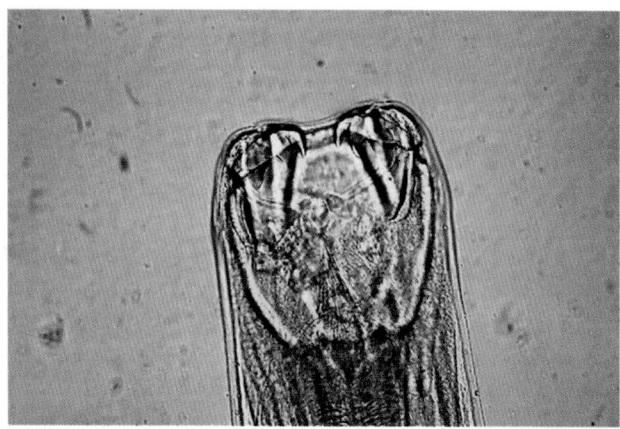

Fig. 1.54 Head of *Ancylostoma caninum* showing the large buccal capsule containing pairs of teeth.

by skin penetration or ingestion, both methods being equally successful. Paratenic hosts can also be important. In percutaneous infection, larvae migrate via the bloodstream to the lungs where they moult to L$_4$ in the bronchi and trachea, and are then swallowed and pass to the small intestine where the final moult occurs. If infection is by ingestion, the larvae may either penetrate the buccal mucosa and undergo the pulmonary migration or pass directly to the intestine where the adult worms burrow their buccal capsules into the mucosa. Whichever route is taken, the prepatent period is 14–21 days. The worms are prolific egg layers and an infected dog may pass millions of eggs daily for several weeks. An important feature of *A. caninum* infection is that, in susceptible bitches, a proportion of the L$_3$ that reach the lungs migrate to the skeletal muscles where they remain dormant until the bitch is pregnant. They are then reactivated and, still as L$_3$, are passed in the milk of the bitch for a period of about three weeks after whelping. Transplacental transmission does not occur. See **life cycle 5**.

LIFE CYCLE 5. LIFE CYCLE OF *ANCYLOSTOMA CANINUM*

Adults of *Ancylostoma caninum* live in the lumen of the small intestine of the dog, that acts as definitive host (1). After mating, adult females release elliptical eggs, that contain 4–8 blastomeres (2). Once excreted in the environment with the host faeces, the egg develops (3) and after 24–48 hours, contains a rhabditoid first-stage larva (4). After hatching, within ~5 days, the larva moults to second- (5) and infective third-stage larva (L$_3$) (6). Infection occurs predominantly via percutaneous penetration or ingestion of the infective larvae. The larvae that penetrate the skin (7) migrate via the circulation to the lungs, where they moult and travel up the respiratory system (8), where they are coughed up and swallowed. Once swallowed, the larvae reach the small intestine and develop

into adults (9). In infections that occur via ingestion of L$_3$ (directly or via paratenic hosts, that harbour infective larvae in their somatic tissues), these may reach the intestine immediately, there developing into adults, or penetrate the buccal mucosa and travel to the lungs and the upper respiratory system, where they are swallowed to reach the small intestine. A proportion of L$_3$ travel from the lungs to the skeletal muscles via the circulatory system; in the muscles, these larvae encyst to then become mobilised during pregnancy. These larvae are then excreted via the colostrum and milk and transmitted to the litter via the transmammary route (10) over the first three weeks from parturition. In humans, L$_3$ can penetrate the skin and cause cutaneous *larva migrans*.

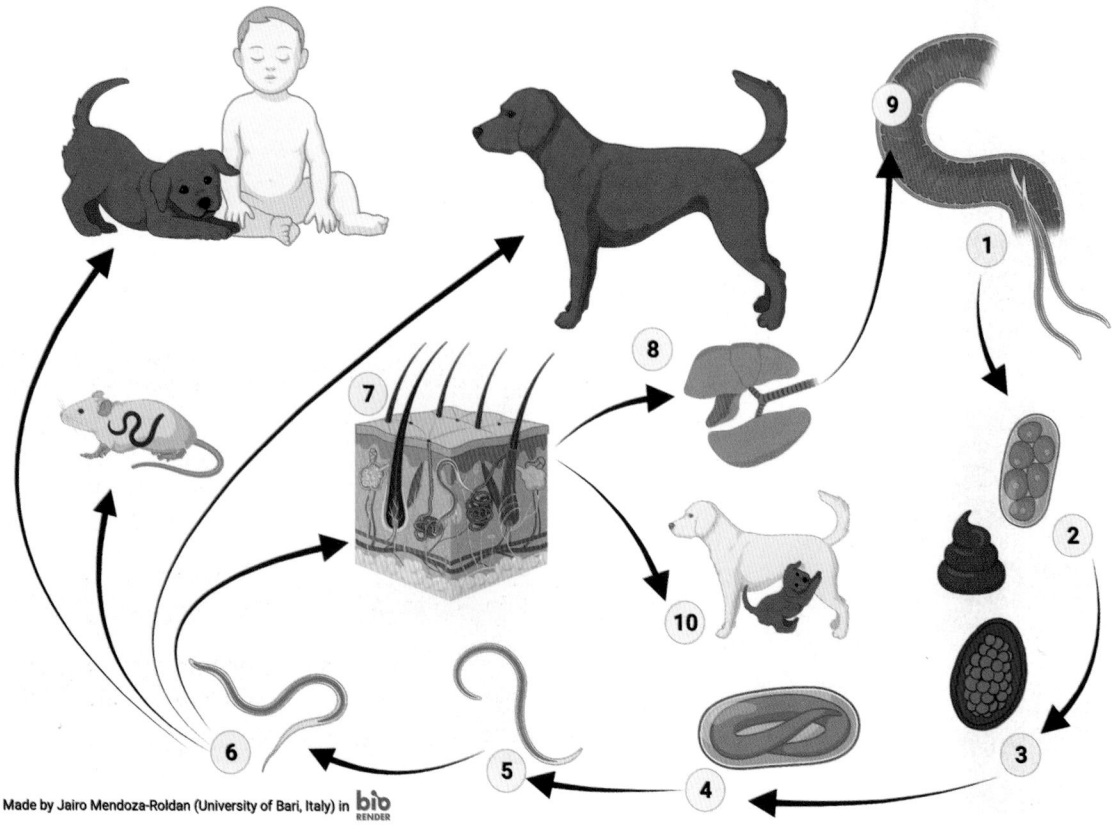

Made by Jairo Mendoza-Roldan (University of Bari, Italy) in **bio**RENDER

Ancylostoma braziliense

Description: As for *A. caninum* except it is smaller than either *A. caninum* or *A. tubaeforme*. In the dog, males measure around 7.5 mm and females 9–10 mm in length. The buccal capsule is deep with two pairs of large dorsal and very small ventral teeth. Eggs are similar to those of *A. caninum*, measuring around 75–95 by 41–45 μm.

Life cycle: Similar in many respects to *A. caninum*, with both oral and percutaneous routes of infection, but transmammary transmission has not been demonstrated. Rodents can act as paratenic hosts. The prepatent period is about two weeks in the dog and cat.

Ancylostoma ceylanicum

Description: Almost identical to *A. braziliense*. The cuticular striations are wider than in *A. braziliense* and the inner pair of ventral teeth in the buccal capsule are larger.

Life cycle: Similar to *A. braziliense*. The prepatent period is about two weeks in the dog.

Ancylostoma tubaeforme

Synonym: *Strongylus tubaeforme*

Description: Almost identical to *A. caninum* but slightly smaller, the males measuring around 10 mm and the females 12–15 mm. The buccal capsule is deep with the dorsal gutter ending in a deep notch on the dorsal margin of the buccal capsule, the ventral margin of which bears three teeth on each side. The cuticle is thicker and the deep 'oesophageal' teeth are slightly larger than in *A. caninum*. The male bursa is well developed and the spicules are about 50% longer than in *A. caninum*. Eggs are similar to those of *A. caninum* and measure about 56–75 by 34–47 μm.

Life cycle: As for *A. braziliense*. The prepatent period is about three weeks.

Ancylostoma duodenale

Description: A small cylindrical worm, greyish-white in colour. There are two ventral plates on the anterior margin of the buccal capsule, each with two large teeth that are fused at their bases. A pair of small teeth is present in the depths of the buccal capsule. Males are 8–11 mm long with a copulatory bursa at the posterior end. Females are 10–13 mm long, with the vulva located at the posterior end. Eggs are typically 'strongylate' with slightly dissimilar bluntly rounded poles, barrel-shaped side walls and a thin smooth shell (Fig. 1.55).

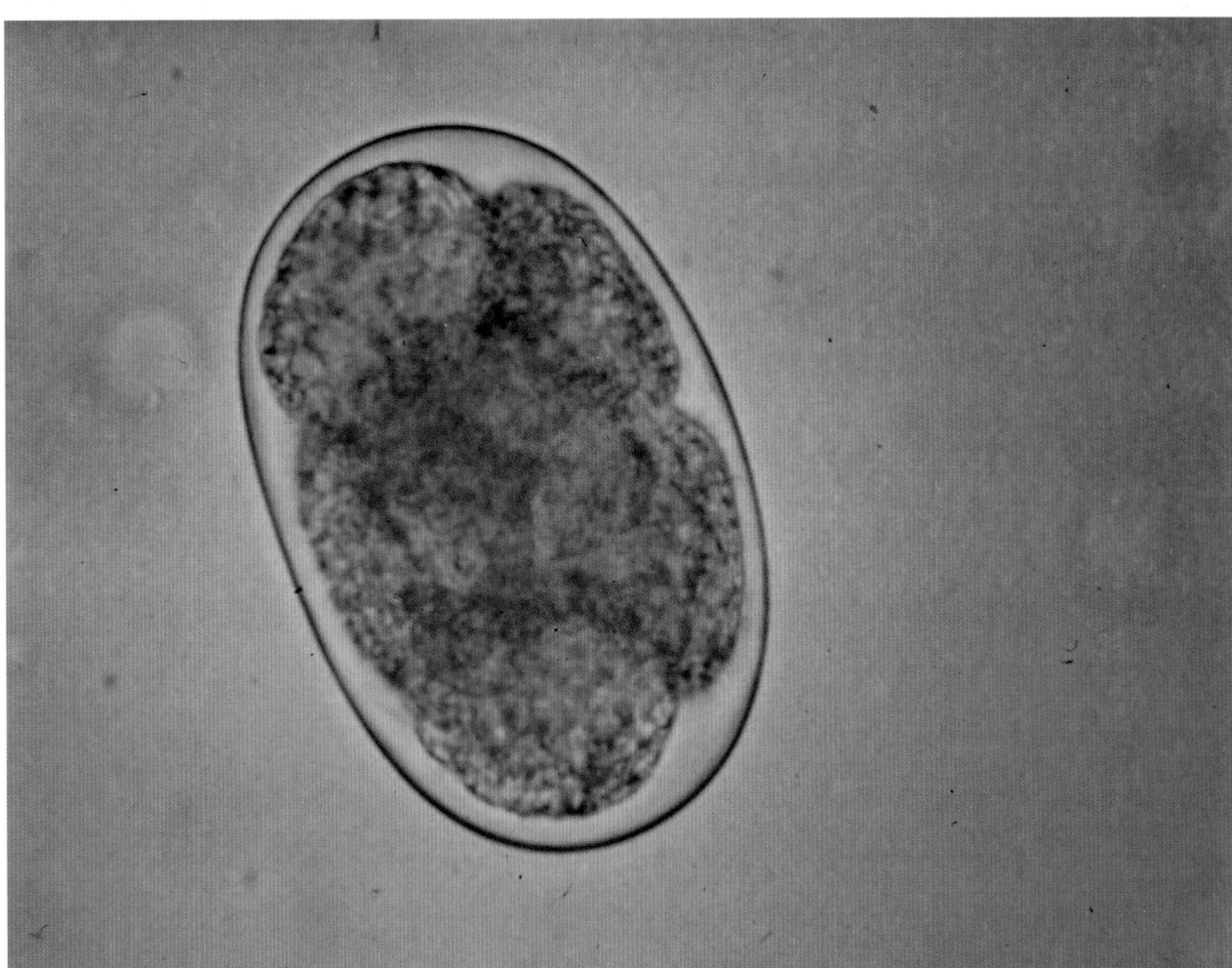

Fig. 1.55 Hookworm egg.

Life cycle: Similar to *A. caninum*. The prepatent period is about five weeks in the dog.

Uncinaria

The genus consists of a single species. The worms are small, up to about 1 cm long; males are 5–8.5 mm and females 7–12 mm long.

Life cycle: Infection with infective L₃ by oral infection, without pulmonary migration, is the usual route. Although the infective larvae can penetrate the skin, the infection rarely matures and there is no evidence as yet of transmammary or intrauterine transmission. Carnivores may become infected via the consumption of paratenic hosts, such as infected mice. The prepatent period is about 15 days. The main species is *Uncinaria stenocephala* which infects the small intestine of dogs, cats, foxes, other wild canids and felids.

Uncinaria stenocephala

Description: A small worm, up to about 1 cm long; males are 5–8.5 mm and females 7–12 mm. The adult worms have a large funnel-shaped buccal capsule, which has a pair of chitinous plates, lacks dorsal teeth, but has a pair of subventral teeth at the base (Fig. 1.56). The dorsal cone does not project into the buccal capsule. The male worm has a well-developed bursa with a short dorsal lobe and two large and separate lateral lobes and slender spicules. The eggs resemble those of *Ancylostoma caninum* but are slightly longer and wider and have a thicker shell. They are ovoidal with dissimilar poles and the thin smooth side walls are almost parallel. Eggs measure 65–80 by 40–50 μm and contain large blastomeres.

Necator

Male worms are usually 7–9 mm long and females about 9–11 mm in length. The main species is *Necator americanum* which infects the small intestine of humans, primates, dogs, cats and pigs.

Necator americanus

Description: Males are 7–9 mm and females about 9–11 mm long. The buccal capsule has two dorsal and two ventral cutting plates around the anterior margin. There is also a pair of subdorsal and a pair of subventral teeth located close to the rear of the buccal capsule.

Bunostomum

Bunostomum is one of the larger nematodes of the small intestine of ruminants (Fig. 1.57), being 1–3 cm long, stout, greyish-white and characteristically hooked at the anterior end, with the buccal capsule opening anterodorsally (Fig. 1.58). In the buccal capsule area there are cuticular festoons.

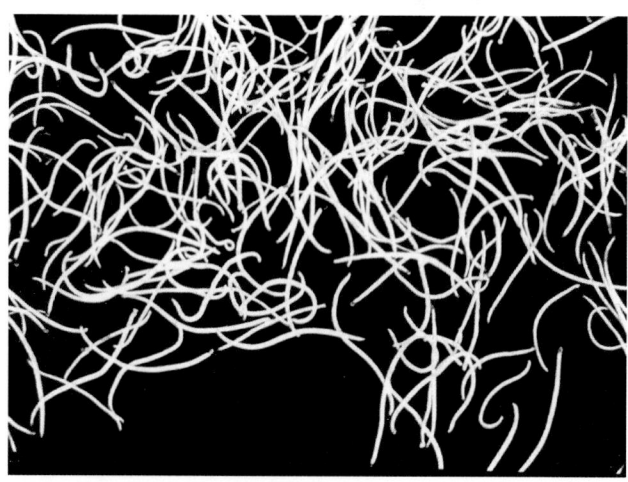

Fig. 1.57 Adult *Bunostomum phlebotomum*.

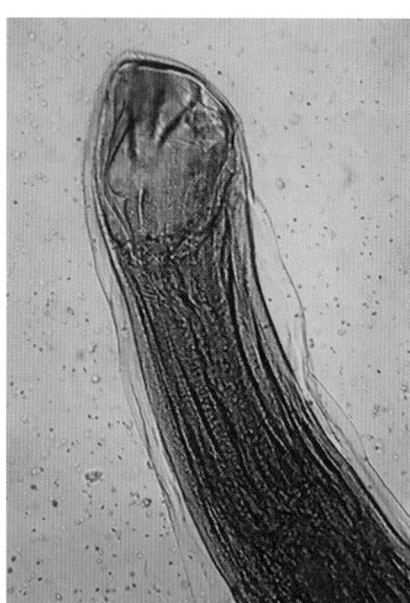

Fig. 1.56 Head of *Uncinaria stenocephala* showing the funnel-shaped buccal capsule and the pair of chitinous plates.

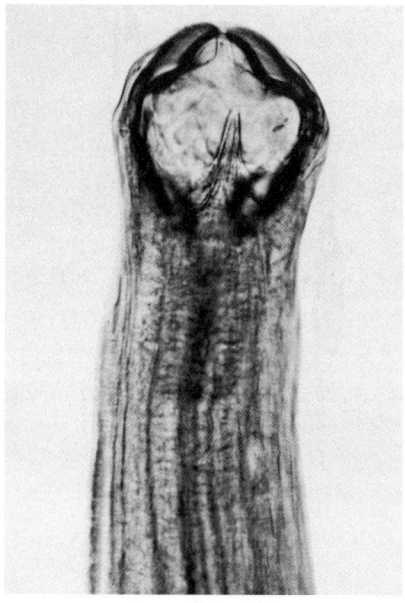

Fig. 1.58 Head of *Bunostomum phlebotomum* showing the large buccal capsule and cutting plates.

Life cycle: Infection with the L$_3$ may be percutaneous or oral. After skin penetration, the larvae travel to the lungs and moult to fourth-stage larvae before re-entering the gastrointestinal tract after approximately 11 days. Ingested larvae usually develop without a migration. Further development continues in the gut.

Bunostomum phlebotomum

Description: Male worms are 10–18 mm and female worms 24–28 mm in length. This species is very similar to *B. trigonocephalum* in sheep, but the dorsal cone is shorter and there are two pairs of small subventral lancets at its base. The large buccal capsule opens antero-dorsally and bears on the ventral margin a pair of chitinous cutting plates and internally a large dorsal cone. Dorsal teeth are absent from the buccal capsule but there are two pairs of small subventral lancets at its base. In the male the bursa is well developed and has an asymmetrical dorsal lobe. The right externodorsal ray arises higher up on the dorsal stem and is longer than the left. It arises near the bifurcation of the dorsal ray, which divides into two tridigitate branches. The spicules are very long and slender. In the female the vulva opens a short distance in front of the middle of the body. The infective larva is small with 16 gut cells and a short filamentous tail. The egg is a medium-sized (97–106 by 45–55 µm), thin-shelled, irregular broad ellipse with blunt ends and dissimilar side walls, one being flattened. It contains four to eight darkly pigmented blastomeres.

Life cycle: The prepatent period is about 6 weeks after skin penetration, and 7–10 weeks after ingestion.

Bunostomum trigonocephalum

Synonym: *Monodontus trigonocephalum*

Description: Male worms are 12–17 mm and females 19–26 mm. The large buccal capsule opens anterodorsally and bears on the ventral margin a pair of chitinous cutting plates and internally a large dorsal cone. Dorsal teeth are absent from the buccal capsule but there are a pair of small subventral lancets at its base. In the male the bursa is well developed and the dorsal lobe is asymmetrical. The right externodorsal ray emerges higher up on the dorsal stem and is longer than the left. The left externodorsal ray arises near the bifurcation of the dorsal ray, which divides into two tridigitate branches. The spicules are slender, twisted and relatively short. In the female the vulva opens a short distance in front of the middle of the body. The infective larva is small with 16 gut cells and a short filamentous tail. The egg is medium-sized (75–104 × 45–57 µm), an irregular broad ellipse in shape, with similar wide poles and dissimilar side walls, one being flattened. The thin-shelled egg contains 4–8 darkly stained blastomeres.

Life cycle: The prepatent period is 4–8 weeks.

Gaigeria

The single species of this genus is a hookworm that occurs mainly in the duodenum of small ruminants.

Life cycle: The life cycle is thought to be direct; the main route of infection is percutaneous. Infective L$_3$ larvae resemble those of *Bunostomum trigonocephalum* and are susceptible to desiccation. The main species is *Gaigeria pachyscelis* which infects the duodenum and small intestine of sheep, goats and wild ruminants.

Gaigeria pachyscelis

Description: The worms are very similar in shape and size to *Bunostomum trigonocephalatum*. Adult male worms measure up to 2 cm and females up to 3 cm long. The buccal capsule contains a large dorsal cone and a pair of subventral lancets, which have several cusps each. There is no dorsal tooth. The male bursa has a large dorsal lobe and small lateral lobes, which are joined together ventrally. The anterolateral ray is short and rounded and is separated quite widely from the other lateral rays. The externo-dorsal rays arise from the main stem of the dorsal ray. The dorsal ray is split for about one-quarter of its length, and the two short branches terminate in three minute digitations. The spicules are short and stout and terminate with recurved unbarbed ends. The eggs measure 105–129 by 50–55 µm and their poles are bluntly rounded.

Globocephalus

Several species of this genus parasitise the small intestine of pigs. The worms are stout and whitish, and approximately 4–8 mm in length. The mouth opens subdorsally and the buccal capsule is globular in shape but with an absence of chitinous structures in the buccal capsule. There are no leaf crowns. The male bursa is well developed and possesses a gubernaculum and the spicules are slender.

Life cycle: The life cycle is direct, either by oral ingestion of L$_3$ larvae or by percutaneous penetration. Larval migration through the heart, lungs, trachea, oesophagus and stomach occurs. The main species is *Globocephalus urosubulatus* (syn. *Globocephalus longemucronatus*, *Globocephalus samoensis*) which infects the small intestine of pigs and wild boards.

Globocephalus urosubulatus

Synonyms: *Globocephalus longemucronatus*, *Globocephalus samoensis*

Description: A very small, stout, whitish worm. Males measure 4–7 mm and females 6–9 mm in length. The mouth opens subdorsally and the buccal capsule is globular. There are two raised cuticular rings near the opening of the mouth. There are small triangular chitinous plates in the buccal capsule. Leaf crowns are absent. The male bursa is well developed and the spicules are slender. Eggs are medium-sized, ovoid, smooth, with a thin colourless shell. They measure 50–60 by 26–35 µm and only have 6–8 blastomeres.

SUPERFAMILY DIAPHANOCEPHALOIDEA

FAMILY DIAPHANOCEPHALIDAE

Nematodes of the genus *Kalicephalus* are hookworms of snakes. The life cycle is direct with a prepatent period of 2–4 months.

SUPERFAMILY METASTRONGYLOIDEA

Most worms in this superfamily inhabit the lungs or the blood vessels adjacent to the lungs. The typical life cycle is indirect and the intermediate host is usually a mollusc. They may be conveniently divided into four groups according to host: those occurring in **pigs** (Metastrongylidae: *Metastrongylus*); in **sheep** and **goats** (Protostrongylidae: *Muellerius, Protostrongylus, Cystocaulus, Spiculocaulus, Neostrongylus* and *Varestrongylus*); in **deer** (*Elaphostrongylus, Parelaphostrongylus*); and in the domestic and wild **carnivores** (Filaroididae: *Oslerus, Filaroides*, Angostrongylidae: *Angiostrongylus, Aelurostrongylus*; and Crenosomatidae: *Crenosoma, Troglostrongylus*).

FAMILY METASTRONGYLIDAE

Metastrongylus

Members of this genus (Table 1.23) are slender white worms, up to 6 cm in length, found in pigs. The site and long slender form are sufficient for generic identification. These worms have two lateral trilobed lips. Individual species are differentiated on the size and shape of the male spicules. The dorsal ray of the bursa is small. The life cycle involves an earthworm intermediate host. The ellipsoid eggs have rough thick shells, are 45–57 by 38–41 µm in size and are larvated when laid.

Life cycle: In cold temperatures the eggs are very resistant and can survive for over a year in soil. Normally, however, they hatch almost immediately, the intermediate host ingesting the L_1. In the earthworm, development to L_3 takes about 10 days at optimal temperatures of 22–26 °C. The longevity of the L_3 in the earthworm is similar to that of the intermediate host itself and may be up to seven years. The pig is infected by ingestion of earthworms and the L_3, released by digestion, travel to the mesenteric lymph nodes and moult. The L_4 then reach the lungs by the lymphatic–vascular route, the final moult occurring after arrival in the air passages.

Metastrongylus apri

Synonym: *Metastrongylus elongatus*

Description: The slender white adult male worms measure up to 25 mm and the females up to 58 mm in length. There are six small papillae located around the oral opening. The male bursa is relatively small and the dorsal rays are reduced. The spicules are filiform, around 4 mm long, and each terminates in a single hook. The vulva of the female is near the anus and both are covered in cuticu-

Table 1.23 *Metastrongylus* species.

Species	Hosts	Site	Intermediate hosts
Metastrongylus apri (syn. *Metastrongylus elongatus*)	Pigs, wild boar	Lung	Earthworms (*Lumbricus, Dendrobaena, Eisena, Helodrilus* spp.)
Metastrongylus pudendotectus (syn. *Metastrongylus brevivaginatus*)	Pigs, wild boar	Lung	Earthworms (*Lumbricus, Dendrobaena, Eisena, Helodrilus* spp.)
Metastrongylus salmi	Pigs, wild boar	Lung	Earthworms (*Lumbricus, Dendrobaena, Eisena, Helodrilus* spp.)

lar swellings. Eggs measure around 50–63 by 33–42 µm and contain a fully developed first-stage larva when laid.

Life cycle: The prepatent period is about 24 days.

Metastrongylus pudendotectus

Synonym: *Metastrongylus brevivaginatus*

Description: Differs from *M. apri* in having a larger bursa and smaller spicules (<1.5 mm long) with double hooks in the male. Males are about 16–18 mm and females 20–37 mm in length. The female possesses a straight tail. Eggs measure about 57–63 by 39–42 µm.

Life cycle: The prepatent period is about four weeks.

Metastrongylus salmi

Description: Similar to *M. pudendotectus* but with longer spicules, which are approximately 2 mm in length.

FAMILY PROTOSTRONGYLIDAE

See **life cycle 6**.

Muellerius

These are grey-reddish, slender hair-like worms about 1–4 cm long, which, although large, are often difficult to discern with the naked eye as they are embedded in lung tissue.

Life cycle: The life cycle is indirect and involves a molluscan intermediate host. The worms are ovoviviparous, the L_1 being passed in the faeces; these penetrate the foot of the molluscan intermediate host and develop to L_3 in a minimum period of 2–3 weeks. The sheep or goat is infected by ingesting the mollusc. The L_3, freed by digestion, travel to the lungs by the lymphatic–vascular route, the parasitic moults occurring in the mesenteric lymph nodes and lungs. The prepatent period of *Muellerius* is 6–10 weeks. The period of patency is very long, exceeding two years. The main species is *Muellerius capillaris* which infects the lung of sheep, goats, deer and wild ruminants. This parasite has slugs (*Limax, Agrolima* spp.) and snails (*Helix, Succinea* spp.) as intermediate hosts.

Muellerius capillaris

Description: Males are 12–24 mm and females 19–25 mm long. The posterior end of adult male *Muellerius* is spirally coiled and the bursa is very small and folded inwards. The spicules consist of a proximal alate region and two distal serrated arms. Two sclerotised rods represent the gubernaculum. Eggs measure about 100 by 20 µm and are unsegmented when laid and develop in the lungs before being passed as L_1 larvae in the faeces. The first-stage larva

LIFE CYCLE 6. LIFE CYCLE OF BRONCHOPULMONARY PROTOSTRONGILIDAE IN SHEEP AND GOATS

The four most common species of bronchopulmonary protostrongylids, also known as small bronchopulmonary strongylids of small ruminants, can be differentiated based on size, location in the lung of the host and morphology of the caudal end of the first-stage larvae (L_1) (A – *Protostrongylus rufescens*, B – *Muellerius capillaris*, C – *Cystocaulus ocreatus*, D – *Neostrongylus linearis*).

In definitive hosts, adult protostrongylids live in the lungs (1). After mating, the females release eggs (2) that hatch into L_1; these are excreted in the external environment through the expectorate and nasal mucus (3) and, more frequently, via the faeces (4) after having been swallowed enveloped in bronchial catarrh. In order to become infective, the larvae require passage

through pulmonate gastropods, that act as intermediate hosts (5); larvae penetrate the foot of these hosts and moult from L_1 to L_2 and L_3. Small ruminants acquire the infection by ingesting infected intermediate hosts (6). Once ingested, the L_3 penetrate the intestinal submucosa (7) and, via the circulatory system, travel to the mesenteric lymph nodes where they moult to fourth-stage larvae (L_4). The latter travel to the lung capillaries via the thoracic duct, vena cava and right heart (8). Once in the capillaries, the larvae penetrate the lung parenchyma and develop into adult worms in the secondary branches of the bronchi, in the alveoli or underneath the pleura (9), depending on species.

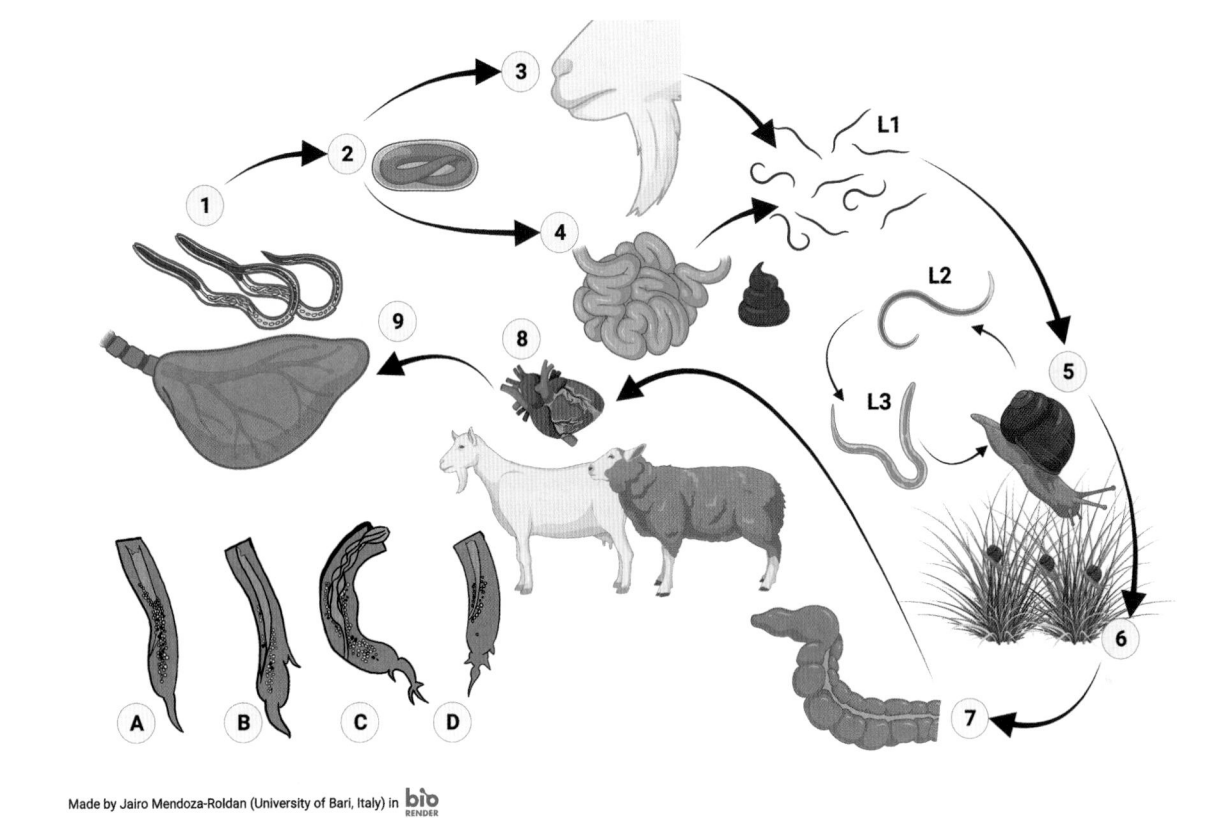

Made by Jairo Mendoza-Roldan (University of Bari, Italy) in bio RENDER

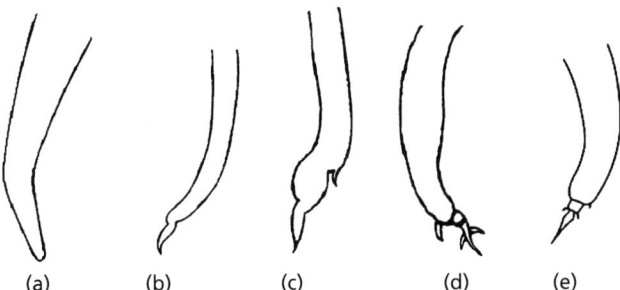

Fig. 1.59 Comparison of the posterior region of the first-stage larvae of (a) *Dictyocaulus filaria*, (b) *Protostrongylus rufescens*, (c) *Muellerius capillaris*, (d) *Cystocaulus ocreatus* and (e) *Neostrongylus linearis*.

has an S-shaped wavy tail (see Fig. 4.13c) and a small dorsal spine adjacent to the tip (Fig. 1.59c). It measures 300–320 μm and contains fine granules.

Protostrongylus

Adult worms are slender, hair-like, reddish worms found in the small bronchioles of the lung (Table 1.24).

Life cycle: The worms are ovoviviparous, the L_1 being passed in the faeces; these penetrate the foot of the molluscan intermediate host and develop to L_3 in a minimum period of 2–3 weeks. The final host is infected by ingesting the mollusc. The L_3, freed by digestion,

Table 1.24 *Protostrongylus* species.

Species	Hosts	Site	Intermediate hosts
Protostrongylus rufescens	Sheep, goats, deer, wild ruminants	Lung	Snails (*Helicella, Theba, Abida, Zebrina* spp.)
Protostrongylus brevispiculum	Sheep	Lung	Snails
Protostrongylus stilesi	Sheep	Lung	Snails
Protostrongylus skrjabini	Sheep	Lung	Snails
Protostrongylus rushi	Sheep	Lung	Snails
Protostrongylus davtiani	Sheep	Lung	Snails

travel to the lungs by the lymphatic–vascular route, the parasitic moults occurring in the mesenteric lymph nodes and lungs. The prepatent period of *Protostrongylus* is 5–6 weeks. The period of patency is very long, exceeding two years.

Protostrongylus rufescens

Description: Adult worms are slender and reddish; males measure up to 4.5 cm and females up to 6.5 cm. In the male, the bursa is well developed but small. The dorsal ray is globular in shape with six papillae on the ventral side. The spicules are almost straight; the distal ends bear two membraneous alae. The male worms can be differentiated from *D. filaria* by these long comb-like spicules. The gubernaculum has two boot-shaped prolongations bearing several knobs posteriorly. In the female, the vulva is close to the anus and the conoid tail. Both horns of the uterus extend anteriorly (prodelphic). This differs from *D. filaria* where the vulva is situated near the middle of the body and where the two horns of the uterus extend in opposite directions (amphidelphic). The eggs measure around 75–120 by 45–82 μm and are unsegmented when laid. The first-stage larva has a wavy outline with a pointed tail but is devoid of a dorsal spine (Fig. 1.59b). It measures 320–400 μm and contains fine granules.

Protostrongylus brevispiculum

Description: The adult worms are small and hair-like. In the male, the dorsal ray is small and rounded and the externodorsal rays are elongate. The spicules are much shorter than in *P. rufescens* and the gubernaculum consists of two parts that are smooth and pointed and curve medially and ventrally. The telamon is well developed.

Cystocaulus

Adult worms are slender, thread-like, dark-brown worms found in the small bronchioles of the lung.

Life cycle: Similar to *Muellerius*. The prepatent period is 5–6 weeks.

Cystocaulus ocreatus

Description: Male worms are up to 4–5 cm and females up to 9 cm long. In the male, the bursa is small; the spicules consist of a proximal cylindrical region joined distinctly to a distal lance-shaped region. The gubernaculum has a complex structure, with the posterior part

consisting of two pointed boot-shaped structures. In the female, the vulva is protected by a bell-shaped expansion of the cuticle. The first-stage larva has a kinked tail and dorsal and ventral spine (Fig. 1.59d).

Spiculocaulus

The main species is *Spiculocaulus austriacus* which infects the lung of sheep and goats. This parasite has snails as intermediate hosts.

Neostrongylus

Small worms found in the lungs.

Life cycle: Similar to the other metastrongylid lungworms. The prepatent period in sheep is around 8–10 weeks. The main species is *Neostrongylus linearis* which infects the lung of sheep and goats. This parasite has snails as intermediate hosts.

Neostrongylus linearis

Description: Adult worms are small; the males are 5–8 mm and females 13–15 mm long. In the male, the spicules are unequal in size. The first-stage larva has a straight tail with a small dorsal and two small lateral spines (Fig. 1.59e).

Varestrongylus

Thread-like worms found in the lung parenchyma and bronchioles of sheep and goats (i.e. *Varestrongylus schulzi*), and of red deer and fallow deer (i.e. *V. sagittatus, V. capreoli*).

Life cycle: Ingested third-stage larvae present within the intermediate host migrate through the intestinal wall to the lymph nodes, migrating via the lymph and blood to the lungs. They then form 'breeding clusters' in which they grow to sexual maturity. Female worms are ovoviviparous with first-stage larvae coughed up and swallowed. When ingested by a molluscan intermediate host, the larvae develop to infective L_3 in 3–4 weeks.

Elaphostrongylus

The main species is *Elaphastrongylus cervi* (syn. *Elaphostrongylus rangiferi*) which infects the connective tissue and CNS of deer (red, roe, sika, reindeer). This parasite has slugs and snails as intermediate hosts.

Elaphostrongylus cervi

Synonym: *Elaphostrongylus rangiferi*

Description: The mature worms are long and slender. Males are up to 40 mm and females up to 60 mm long. First-stage larvae have a dorsal spine on the tail and measure 395–440 μm in length.

Life cycle: Female worms lay eggs that either hatch *in situ* or are carried to the lungs via the bloodstream and then hatch.

Larvae migrate through the lungs to the airways and are then swallowed and pass out in the faeces. The larvae may survive in the environment for up to two years before infecting a molluscan intermediate host. The parasites develop through the second-stage to the infective third-stage larvae in the mollusc within 27–50 days and can retain their infectivity for up to another two years. Deer become infected when they ingest snails containing infective larvae. After ingestion, the larvae burrow through the gut wall and migrate to the final tissue site, at the same time developing into adult worms. The prepatent period is about 112 days.

Parelaphostrongylus

The main species is *Parelaphostrongylus tenuis* (syn. *Odocoileostrongylus tenuis*, *Elaphostrongylus tenuis*) which infects the cranial meninges and CNS of white-tailed deer, moose, wapiti and others. This parasite has slugs and snails as intermediate hosts.

Parelaphostrongylus tenuis

Synonyms: *Odocoileostrongylus tenuis, Elaphostrongylus tenuis*

Description: The mature worms are long and thread-like; males are up to 40 mm and females up to about 90 mm long. First-stage larvae have a dorsal spine on the tail and measure about 350 μm.

Life cycle: Unembryonated eggs are released into the bloodstream and travel to the lungs where they lodge in the capillaries and complete their development to L_1 before moving to the alveoli, from where they are coughed up and swallowed and passed in the faeces. To develop further, they must penetrate or be eaten by a slug or snail. In the foot of the snail, the larvae develop through the second-stage to the infective third-stage larvae. Deer become infected when they accidentally ingest slugs or snails containing infective larvae. After ingestion, the larvae burrow through the gut wall and migrate to the CNS via the spinal nerves and spinal cord, at the same time developing into adult worms. The prepatent period is about 82–137 days.

FAMILY FILAROIDIDAE

Oslerus

This genus was part of the larger genus *Filaroides*, but has now been separated on morphological grounds from the other members. Though distinction has been made on morphology, it is also useful from the veterinary standpoint, for it separates the single harmful species, *Oslerus osleri*, living in the upper air passages, from the relatively harmless species which are retained in the genus *Filaroides* and which live in the lung parenchyma. *Oslerus*, and its closely related genus *Filaroides*, are exceptional in the superfamily Metastrongyloidea in having direct life cycles.

Life cycle: The females are ovoviviparous and most eggs hatch in the trachea. Many larvae are coughed up and swallowed and passed in the faeces and infection may occur by ingestion of these; more commonly, transmission occurs when an infected bitch licks the pup and transfers the newly hatched L_1, which are present in her sputum. After ingestion, the first moult occurs in the small intestine

and the L_2 travel to the lungs by the lymphatic–vascular route. Development through to L_5 takes place in the alveoli and bronchi, and the adults migrate to their predilection site, the tracheal bifurcation. The prepatent period varies from 10 to 18 weeks.

Oslerus osleri

Description: The worms, which are embedded in fibrous nodules in the trachea in the region of the bifurcation and in the adjacent bronchi, are small, pale and slender; males are 5 mm and females 9–15 mm long and slightly thicker. The tail of the male is rounded without obvious bursal lobes and bears a few papillae. The short spicules are slightly unequal. In the female the vulva is located close to the anus. The larva has a short S-shaped tail and measures 232–266 μm in length. The medium-sized eggs have thin shells, measure around 80 by 50 μm and contain a larva.

Oslerus rostratus

Synonyms: *Anafilaroides rostratus, Filaroides rostratus*

Description: The adult males are about 28–37 mm long and the adult females 48–64 mm long. The vulva in the female is located just anterior to the anus.

Filaroides

The worms (Table 1.25) are very small (0.5–1 cm long), slender, hair-like and greyish, and are not only difficult to see with the naked eye in the lung parenchyma but are also unlikely to be recovered intact from the tissue. These lungworms have a direct life cycle.

Filaroides hirthi

Description: The worms are very small (0.5–1 cm long), slender, hair-like and greyish, and are not only difficult to see with the naked eye in the lung parenchyma but are unlikely to be recovered intact from the tissue. *Filaroides hirthi* is smaller than *F. milksi* (see next section). The L_1, present in the faeces and sputum, are coiled and the tail has a notch, followed by a constriction, and has a terminal lance-like point. Larvae measure about 240–290 μm.

Life cycle: The life cycle is direct. The worms are ovoviviparous and the hatched L_1 are passed in faeces or expelled in sputum. Though infection may be acquired by ingestion of faecal larvae, the important route, as in *Oslerus* infection, is thought to be by transfer of L_1 in the bitch's saliva when the pup is licked. The prepatent period of *F. hirthi* is around five weeks.

Table 1.25 *Filaroides* species.

Species	Hosts	Site
Filaroides hirthi	Dogs	Lung
Filaroides milksi (syn. *Andersonstrongylus milksi*)	Dogs	Lung
Filaroides bronchialis (syn. *Filaroides martis*)	Mink, polecats, other Mustelidae	Lung

Filaroides milksi

Description: As for *F. hirthi*. *Filaroides milksi* is larger than *F. hirthi*.

FAMILY ANGIOSTRONGYLIDAE

Angiostrongylus

Three main species are reported within this genus (Table 1.26).

Angiostrongylus vasorum

Description: These are small reddish worms. The slender males measure 14–18 mm and the stouter females 18–25 mm in length. Males have a small bursa and females have a 'barber's pole' appearance with the white ovaries coiled round the red intestine, similar to that in *Haemonchus*. The ventral rays are fused for most of their length and the dorsal ray is stout with stout terminal branches. In the female, the white ovaries are coiled round the red intestine (Fig. 1.60) with the vulva in the posterior half of the body. Eggs are

Table 1.26 *Angiostrongylus* species.

Species	Hosts	Site	Intermediate hosts
Angiostrongylus vasorum	Dogs, foxes	Heart, pulmonary vessels	Slugs and snails
Angiostrongylus cantonensis	Rats, humans	Pulmonary artery (rats), meninges (humans)	Slugs and snails
Angiostrongylus costaricensis	Rats, humans	Ileocaecal arteries (rats), intestines (humans)	Slugs and snails

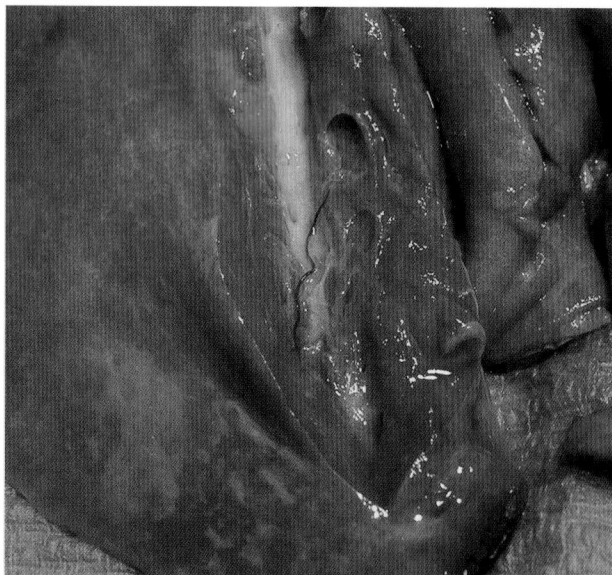

Fig. 1.60 Female *Angiostrongylus vasorum* in the pulmonary artery.

unsegmented when laid in the lung and measure about 70–80 by 40–50 μm. First-stage larvae are 330–360 μm in length and have a small cephalic button and a wavy tail with a subterminal notch (see Fig. 4.13e).

Life cycle: The genus is ovoviviparous. The adult worms in the larger pulmonary vessels lay eggs, which are carried to the capillaries, where they hatch. The L_1 break into the alveoli, migrate to the trachea and thence to the alimentary tract to be passed in the faeces. Further development takes place after entry into the intermediate host, the infective third stage being reached in 17 days. After the mollusc has been ingested by the dog, the infective L_3, freed by digestion, travel to the lymph nodes adjacent to the alimentary tract, where both parasitic moults take place, and then to the vascular predilection site. L_5 have also been found in the liver. The prepatent period is around seven weeks, and the worms can live in the dog for more than two years.

Angiostrongylus cantonensis

Description: The body is filariform and tapered at both ends. Males measure about 18 mm and females 23 mm in length. Fresh female worms have a 'barber's pole' appearance as the white uterine tubules spiral round the blood-filled intestine. The slender spicules are of equal length and are striated. A gubernaculum is present. The ovoid eggs laid in the pulmonary arteries are thin-shelled, transparent and unembryonated.

Life cycle: Infection is acquired through ingestion of a mollusc containing L_3 larvae. The larvae are released in the digestive tract and migrate via the hepatic portal system and lungs to the central nervous system where they undergo two moults. The young worms eventually migrate via the cerebral vein to the pulmonary arteries. The adult worms mate and lay eggs that pass to the capillaries; these eggs embryonate and hatch and L_1 larvae enter the alveoli and eventually are coughed up, swallowed and pass out in the faeces. These larvae are about 270–300 μm long. The L_1 are ingested by, or penetrate, the intermediate host. The prepatent period is around six weeks.

Angiostrongylus costaricensis

Description: The worms are tapered at both ends and are filiform in shape. Males measure about 20 mm and females 30–40 mm in length. The spicules are equal in length, slender and striated. The cephalic ends of the spicules are blunt and the caudal tips are pointed. A gubernaculum is present. The ovoid eggs laid in the mesenteric arterioles are thin-shelled, transparent and unembryonated. The embryonated eggs shed in faeces measure around 90 μm.

Life cycle: Larvae are shed in the faeces of the rodent and are ingested by a mollusc in which development to the L_3 stage takes place. Following ingestion of the mollusc by rats, or ingestion of vegetation contaminated with infective mucous trails, the L_3 migrate via the lymphatics. After two moults, the worms migrate to the ileocaecal arteries where they mature, reproduce and lay eggs, which are then carried to the intestinal wall. Eggs embryonate and hatch to L_1 larvae which migrate to the lumen of the intestine and pass out in the faeces. The prepatent period is around 3–4 weeks.

Aelurostrongylus

The genus consists of one species, *Aelurostrongylus abstrusus*, which is common in the lungs of the domestic cat.

Life cycle: The life cycle is indirect. The worms are ovoviviparous, and the L_1 are passed in the faeces. These penetrate the foot of the molluscan intermediate host and develop to the infective L_3 and during this phase paratenic hosts, such as birds and rodents, may eat the mollusc. The cat is usually infected by ingestion of these paratenic hosts and less frequently by ingestion of the intermediate hosts. The L_3 released in the alimentary tract travel to the lungs by the lymphatics or bloodstream. After the final moult, the adults are located in the alveolar ducts and the terminal bronchioles. The prepatent period is between four and six weeks, and the duration of patency is about four months, though some worms may survive in the lungs for several years despite the absence of larvae in the faeces. This parasite has slugs and snails as intermediate hosts. See **life cycle 7**.

LIFE CYCLE 7. LIFE CYCLE OF *AELUROSTRONGYLUS ABSTRUSUS*

Adults of *Aelurostrongylus abstrusus* live in the bronchioles and alveolar ducts of cats (1), that act as definitive hosts. After mating, the females release elliptical eggs (2) containing larvae (L_1) that, after hatching, travel up the respiratory system and are either eliminated with the expectorate or, more frequently, swallowed and excreted with the faeces (3). In the external environment (4), the larvae penetrate terrestrial molluscs that act as intermediate hosts (5); inside these hosts, the larvae moult twice to reach the infective, third-larval stage (6). The intermediate hosts may be ingested by parastenic hosts, e.g. reptiles, amphibians, rodents and birds (7). Cats acquire the infection by ingesting infected intermediate or paratenic hosts. Following infection, the larvae migrate via the circulatory system through several organs (8, 9) before reaching the respiratory tract (10), where they develop into sexually mature adult nematodes within four weeks.

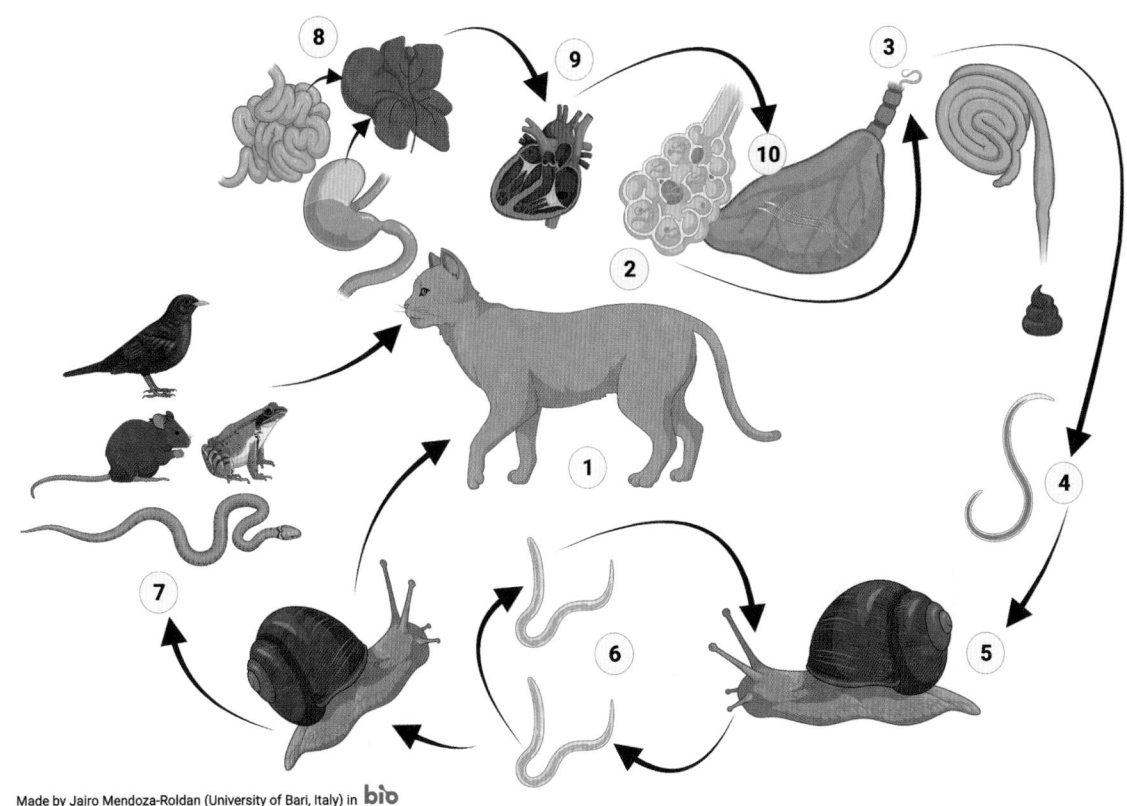

Made by Jairo Mendoza-Roldan (University of Bari, Italy) in bio RENDER

Aelurostrongylus abstrusus

Description: Aggregations of worms, eggs and larvae are present throughout the lung tissue. The worms, about 1 cm long, are very slender and delicate, and are difficult to recover intact for examination; a squeeze preparation from a cut surface of the lung will show the worm material including the characteristic L_1, which bear a subterminal spine on their S-shaped tail (Fig. 1.61). The male bursa is short and the lobes are indistinct. The spicules are stout. Eggs have a thin shell, measure around 70–80 by 50–75 μm and embryonate in the lung. L_1 in faeces are short and thick with a conical anterior they are about 360–400 μm long with granular contents.

FAMILY CRENOSOMATIDAE

This family includes several species that infect trachea, bronchi, bronchioles of many animal species. In particular, *Crenosoma vulpis* infects dogs, foxes and wolves, and *Troglostrongylus brevior* domestic and wild felids.

Life cycle: Adult females deposit thin-shelled eggs containing first-stage larvae (L_1), which ascend the trachea and pass into the intestinal tract and out in the faeces. These larvae penetrate the foot of the intermediate molluscan host and are present as infective third-stage larvae (L_3) in about three weeks. After ingestion of the molluscan host by the final host, the L_3 are released by digestion and travel to the lungs, via the lymphatic glands and hepatic circulation, where both parasitic moults take place. The prepatent period is around three weeks. The transmammary transmission of *Troglostrongylus brevior* has been demonstrated being this parasite infection of major concern in kittens.

Crenosoma vulpis

Description: Slender white worms, up to 1.5 cm long. Males are 4–8 mm with well-developed bursae with a large dorsal ray. Females are 12–16 mm. The two horns of the uterus extend in opposite directions (amphidelphic). The ovejector sphincter is prominent. The host and site are usually sufficient for generic diagnosis. Microscopic confirmation is based on the presence of annular

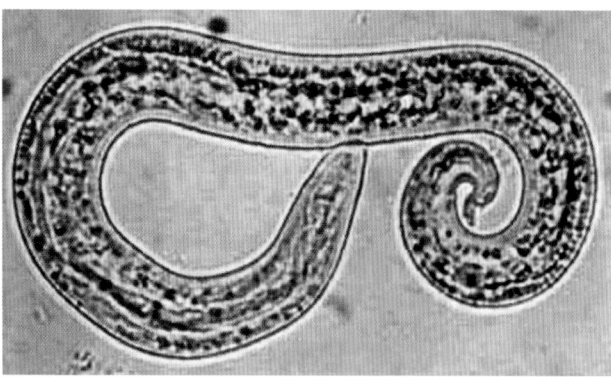

Fig. 1.61 *Aelurostrongylus abstrusus* L_1: S-shaped tail bears a subterminal spine.

crenated folds of the cuticle, which bear small backwardly directed spines on their margins. Larvae are about 265–330 μm in length and have a straight pointed tail.

Troglostrongylus brevior

Description: Adults are slender worms located in the frontal sinuses and bronchi of the definitive hosts. The female worms are up 1.3 cm long (longer than *A. abstrusus*) with a cuticle finely striated with transverse striations and inflated at the apical and caudal ends where it throws into folds. In the male, the bursa is small in comparison with the total body size and is supported by short rays. The dorsal ray of *T. brevior* is elongated with two pairs of papillae and externodorsal and anterolaterals rays arising independently while postero- and mediolaterals are partially fused. Spicules of *T. brevior* are 510–631 μm long, each terminating with a thin and long appendage and four small digitiform projections.

Considering the strong similarities between the first-stage larvae (L_1) and those of the better known *Aelurostrongylus abstrusus*, their identification is often challenging and the actual impact of these lungworm infestations has yet to be fully appreciated. First-stage larvae of *T. brevior* are 300–357 μm long and present a pointed anterior extremity and a subterminal (dorsal) oral opening (in *A. abstrusus* the oral opening is terminal).

SUPERFAMILY RHABDITOIDEA

This is a primitive group of nematodes which are mostly free-living, or parasitic in lower vertebrates and invertebrates. *Rhabdias* are respiratory parasites in reptiles. A few normally free-living genera such as *Halicephalobus* (*Micronema*) and *Rhabditis* occasionally cause problems in animals.

FAMILY PANAGROLAIMIDAE
Halicephalobus (syn. Micronema)

Occasional cases of infection of horses with the saprophytic free-living nematode *Halicephalobus deletrix* (syn. *Halicephalobus gingivalis*, *Micronema deletrix*) have been described from various parts of the world. In affected animals the very small worms, less than 0.5 mm in length, have been found in nasal and maxillary granulomas and in the brain and kidney.

FAMILY RHABDITIDAE
Rhabditis

Several members of this free-living genus of nematodes may become casual parasites, the larvae invading the skin and causing an intense pruritus. The larvae do not migrate but die and so adults are not present in animals. Cases have been most frequently reported in dogs housed in kennels with damp hay or straw bedding and the lesions, usually confined to areas of the body in contact with the ground, show hair loss, erythema and pustule formation if infected with bacteria. The very small worms (1–2.8 mm in length) with a rhabditiform oesophagus may be recovered from skin scrapings. Treatment is symptomatic and the condition can be prevented by housing animals on clean dry bedding. *Rhabditis* infection has also been associated with otitis externa in cattle in the tropics. The main species is *Rhabditis strongyloides* (syn. *Pelodera strongyloides*) which infects the subcutaneous tissue and skin of dogs, cattle and horses.

FAMILY RHABDIASIDAE

Lungworms of the genus *Rhabdias* are common parasites of amphibians and reptiles, with about 60 species reported worldwide.

Life cycle: Only females are parasitic and these produce larvated, oval, thin-shelled eggs. After hatching, larvae may develop through four larval stages into free-living adult male and female worms and this can be followed by a succession of free-living generations. Infection is usually via the oral route (but percutaneous infection is also possible) and larvae penetrate the oesophageal tissue and then pass via the body cavity and primarily reside near the lower lung as ungravid adults. These adults then penetrate the lungs and feed on blood, becoming gravid and passing embryonated eggs in the faeces. Usually no intermediate hosts are involved. However, transport hosts such as physid snails, earthworms or frogs can be involved for some *Rhabdias* species.

SUPERFAMILY STRONGYLOIDIDEA

FAMILY STRONGYLOIDIDAE

Strongyloides

Members of this genus are common parasites of the small intestine in very young animals and although generally of little pathogenic significance, under certain circumstances may give rise to severe enteritis.

These worms (Table 1.27) are slender, hair-like, colourless worms generally less than 10 mm long and only the female worms are parasitic. The long cylindrical oesophagus (typically rhabditiform in shape) may occupy up to one-third of the body length and the filamentous uterus is intertwined with the intestine, giving the appearance of contorted twisted thread (Fig. 1.62). Unlike other intestinal parasites of similar size, the tail has a blunt point. Species identification is generally based on identification of the characteristic female worms, or eggs, in the host species.

Life cycle: *Strongyloides* is unique among the nematodes of veterinary importance, being capable of both parasitic and free-living reproductive cycles. The parasitic phase is composed entirely of female worms in the small intestine and these produce larvated eggs by parthenogenesis, i.e. development from an unfertilised egg. In herbivores, it is the larvated egg which is passed out in the faeces, but in other animals it is the hatched L_1. After hatching, larvae may develop through four larval stages into free-living adult male and female worms and this can be followed by a succession of free-living generations. However, under certain conditions, possibly related to temperature and moisture, the L_3 can become parasitic, infecting the host by skin penetration or ingestion and migrating via the venous system, the lungs and trachea to develop into adult female worms in the small intestine. Young animals may acquire

Table 1.27 *Strongyloides* species.

Species	Hosts	Site
Strongyloides papillosus	Sheep, cattle, goats, wild ruminants, rabbits	Small intestine
Strongyloides westeri	Horses, donkeys, zebras, rarely pigs	Small intestine
Strongyloides ransomi	Pigs	Small intestine
Strongyloides avium	Chickens, turkeys, geese, wild birds	Small intestine, caecae
Strongyloides stercoralis (syn. *Strongyloides canis, Strongyloides intestinalis, Anguillula stercoralis*)	Dogs, foxes, cats, humans, Old World monkeys, apes	Small intestine
Strongyloides planiceps	Cats	Small intestine
Strongyloides felis (syn. *Strongyloides cati*)	Cats	Small intestine
Strongyloides tumefaciens	Cats	Large intestine
Strongyloides ratti	Rats	Small intestine
Strongyloides cebus	New World monkeys	Small intestine
Strongyloides fulleborni	Old World monkeys, apes	Small intestine

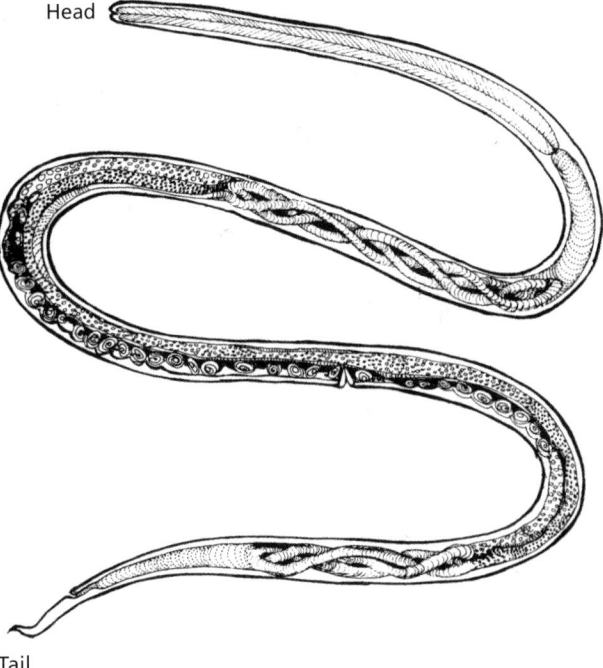

Head

Tail

Fig. 1.62 *Strongyloides* spp. adult female.

infection immediately after birth from the mobilisation of arrested larvae in the tissues of the ventral abdominal wall of the dam, which are subsequently excreted in the milk. In addition, prenatal infection has been demonstrated experimentally in cattle. The prepatent period in most species is 8–14 days.

LIFE CYCLE 8. LIFE CYCLE OF *STRONGYLOIDES* SPP.

Strongyloides infects several animal species (e.g. ruminants, equids, carnivores, pigs, birds), including humans (1). Adult females are the only parasitic life cycle stage; these are <1 cm long and characterised by a well-developed oesophagus (spanning one-third of the whole-body length) and uterus coiled around the intestine (2). Adult females live in the small intestine, where they reproduce by parthenogenesis, releasing larvated eggs (3). The eggs (35 × 45 μm) are oval in shape and with a thin outer membrane (4). They are excreted in the faeces of herbivore hosts while, in other hosts, they hatch in the intestine, thus releasing the L_1. The eggs are characterised by different chromosome numbers (n). Eggs 1n and 2n hatch L_1 (5) that, following moults to L_2 (6) and L_3 (7), develop into free-living males (8) and heterogametic females (9), respectively. The 3n type egg develops directly via L_1–L_3 into the homogonic female; this may occur via free L_3 on soil or inside the host's intestine (internal autoinfection cycle). Mating results in eggs (10) that may give rise to new free-living generations (8, 9) or develop via L_3 into parthenogenic females upon penetration into the vertebrate host (11). L_3, hatched from 3n eggs, penetrate the skin of the host (11) and, through the haemolymphatic circulation (12), travel to the lungs (13), where they may cause microhaemorrhages. After travelling up the trachea, larvae are swallowed and reach the intestine, where they develop into adult females that release larvated eggs by parthenogenesis.

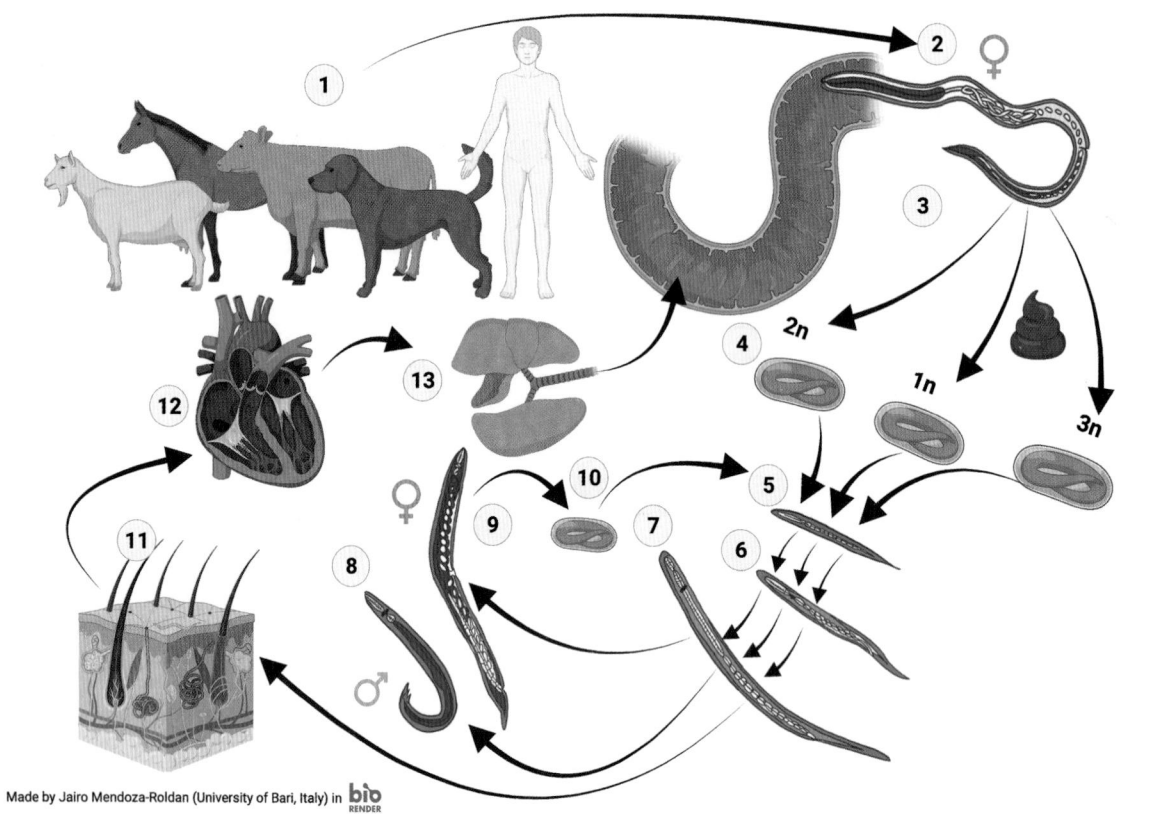

Made by Jairo Mendoza-Roldan (University of Bari, Italy) in **bio** RENDER

Strongyloides papillosus

Description: Adult female worms are 3.5–6 mm long with an oesophagus 0.6–0.8 mm in length. *Strongyloides* eggs are oval with blunt poles and slightly barrel-shaped side walls, thin-shelled and small, being half the size of typical strongyle eggs. These colourless eggs have a smooth shell and measure about 43–60 by 20–25 μm and contain an L_1 larva. Infective larvae measure about 600 μm.

Strongyloides westeri

Description: Adult female worms are up to 9 mm long with an oesophagus measuring 1.2–1.5 mm in length. The long oesophagus may occupy up to one-third of the body length and the uterus is intertwined with the intestine, giving the appearance of twisted thread. Unlike other intestinal parasites of similar size, the tail has a blunt point. *Strongyloides* eggs are oval, thin-shelled, smooth and small (40–52 × 32–40 μm), being half the size of typical strongyle eggs (see Fig. 4.5). The side walls are symmetrical and the poles are wide and the egg contains a short thick larva. The hatched L_1 is passed out in the faeces.

Strongyloides ransomi

Description: Slender hair-like worms 3.4–4.5 mm long (Fig. 1.62). Only females are parasitic. The long oesophagus may occupy up to one-third of the body length and the uterus is intertwined with the intestine, giving the appearance of twisted thread. Unlike other intestinal parasites of similar size, the tail has a blunt point.

Strongyloides eggs are oval, thin-shelled and small, 45–55 by 26–35 μm. They have a very fine wall and always contain a thick, short, first-stage larva (see Fig. 4.6).

Life cycle: The prepatent period is 6–9 days.

Strongyloides avium

Description: Adult female worms are approximately 2 mm long with an oesophagus 0.7 mm in length. The long oesophagus may occupy up to one-third of the body length and the uterus is intertwined with the intestine, giving the appearance of twisted thread (Fig. 1.62). Unlike other intestinal parasites of similar size, the tail has a blunt point. *Strongyloides* eggs are oval, thin-shelled and small, 52–56 by 36–40 μm, being half the size of typical strongyle eggs. The larvated egg is usually passed in the faeces.

Strongyloides stercoralis

Synonyms: *Strongyloides canis, Strongyloides intestinalis, Anguillula stercoralis*

Description: Slender hair-like worms around 2 mm long. Only females are parasitic. The long oesophagus may occupy up to one-third of the body length and the uterus is intertwined with the intestine, giving the appearance of twisted thread. Unlike other intestinal parasites of similar size, the tail has a blunt point. *Strongyloides* eggs are oval, thin-shelled and small, 50–58 by 30–34 μm. The hatched L$_1$ is passed out in the faeces.

Strongyloides planiceps

Description: Parasitic females are 2.4–3.3 mm long (mean 2.8 mm). The tail of the parasitic female narrows abruptly to a blunt tip, and the worms have ovaries with a spiral appearance.

Strongyloides felis

Synonym: *Strongyloides cati*

Description: Similar to *S. planiceps*. Parasitic females of *S. felis* have a long tail narrowing slowly to the tip. Ovaries are straight.

Strongyloides tumefaciens

Description: The parasitic females are 5 mm long and found in tumours of the large intestine.

SUPERFAMILY ASCARIDOIDEA

The ascaridoids are among the largest nematodes and occur in most domestic animals, both larval and adult stages being of veterinary importance. While the adults in the intestine may cause unthriftiness in young animals, and occasional obstruction, an important feature of the group is the pathological consequences of the migratory behaviour of the larval stages.

With a few exceptions, the genera have the following characteristics in common. They are large, white or cream, opaque worms that inhabit the small intestine. There is no buccal capsule, the mouth consisting simply of a small opening surrounded by three large conspicuous lips. A posterior bulb is usually absent from the oesophagus. The males possess two spicules but do not have a bursa. The common mode of infection is by ingestion of the thick-shelled egg containing the L$_2$. However, the cycle may involve transport and paratenic hosts.

Genera of veterinary interest include *Ascaris, Toxocara, Toxascaris, Parascaris, Ascaridia, Heterakis, Porrocaecum, Bayliascaris, Paraspidodera* and to a lesser extent the anisakids (Anisakidae: *Anisakis, Contracaecum, Hysterothylacium, Pseudoterranova*). Other acaridoids occur in reptiles and include *Ophidascaris* and *Polydelphus* found in snakes and *Angusticaecum* and *Sulcascaris* found in chelonia.

FAMILY ASCARIDIDAE

Ascaris

The genus includes large, stout, white worms, around 15–40 cm in length, infecting the small intestine of pigs (*Ascaris suum*) and humans (*Ascaris lumbricoides*).

Ascaris suum

Description: *Ascaris suum* is by far the largest nematode of the pig; the white/cream-coloured rigid females are up to 40 cm long and the males up to 25 cm in length (Fig. 1.63), and could only be confused with *Macracanthorhynchus* where this occurs. The dorsal lip possesses two double papillae, and each ventrolateral lip has one double papilla and a small lateral papilla. These lips have a row of very small denticles on their interior surface. The oesophagus is about 6.5 mm long and simple in shape. The male spicules are stout and the males tend to be slightly curved posteriorly. The eggs are ovoid and yellowish-brown, with a thick shell, the outer layer of which is irregularly mamillated (see Fig. 4.6). They measure 50–75 by 40–55 μm and the contents consist of granules and unsegmented cells. The egg is larvated when passed in the faeces and the thick multilayered eggshell enables the egg to survive desiccation and

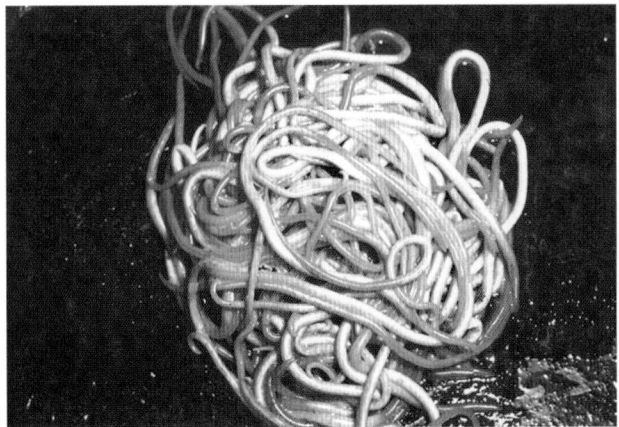
Fig. 1.63 *Ascaris suum* adult worms.

freezing in the environment for several years. Occasionally, the population of worms will comprise only females and unfertilised eggs can appear in the faeces. Where an outer albuminous layer is present, it is thinner than that of a fertilised egg.

Life cycle: The life cycle is direct. Though the preparasitic moults occur by about three weeks after the egg is passed, a period of maturation is necessary and the egg is not usually infective until a minimum of four weeks after being passed, even in the optimal temperature range of 22–26°C. The egg is very resistant to temperature extremes, and is viable for more than four years. After ingestion, the larvated egg hatches in the small intestine, the L_3 larva penetrates the intestinal mucosa and then travels to the liver. The larva then passes in the bloodstream to the lungs and thence to the small intestine via the bronchi, trachea and pharynx. In the intestine, the final moult occurs and the young adult worms inhabit the lumen of the small intestine. If the eggs are ingested by an earthworm or dung beetle, they will hatch and the L_3 travel to the tissues of these paratenic hosts, where they can remain, fully infective for pigs, for a long period. The prepatent period is 7–9 weeks, and each female worm is capable of producing more than 200 000 eggs per day. Longevity is around 6–9 months.

Ascaris lumbricoides

Description: Male worms are 15–31 cm long and the posterior end is curved ventrally and has a bluntly pointed tail. Female worms are 20–49 cm long with the vulva located in the anterior end, which

accounts for about one-third of its body length. The egg is ovoid and yellowish-brown, with a thick shell, the outer layer of which is irregularly mamillated (Fig. 1.64).

Toxocara

Nematodes in this genus (Table 1.28) are large white/cream-coloured worms, with females up to 18 cm and males up to 10 cm in length. There are no interlabia or intestinal caeca.

Toxocara canis

Description: Adult male worms measure up to 10 cm and females 18 cm in length, although the size can vary considerably (Fig. 1.65). The adult head is elliptical due to the presence of a pair of large

Table 1.28 *Toxocara* species.

Species	Hosts	Site
Toxocara canis	Dogs, foxes	Small intestine
Toxocara mystax (syn. *Toxocara cati*)	Cats	Small intestine
Toxocara malayiensis	Cats	Small intestine
Toxocara vitulorum (syn. *Neoascaris vitulorum*)	Buffalo, cattle	Small intestine

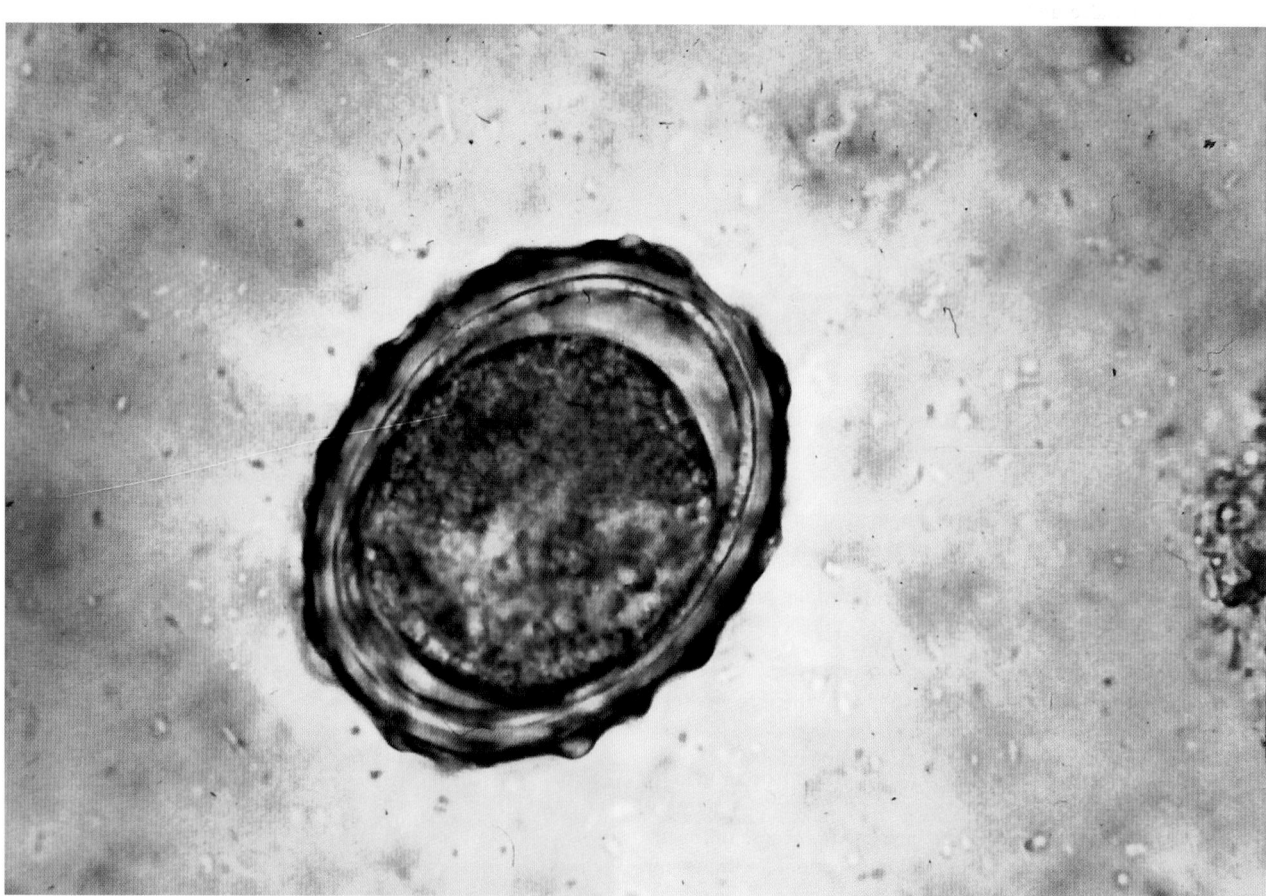

Fig. 1.64 *Ascaris* egg.

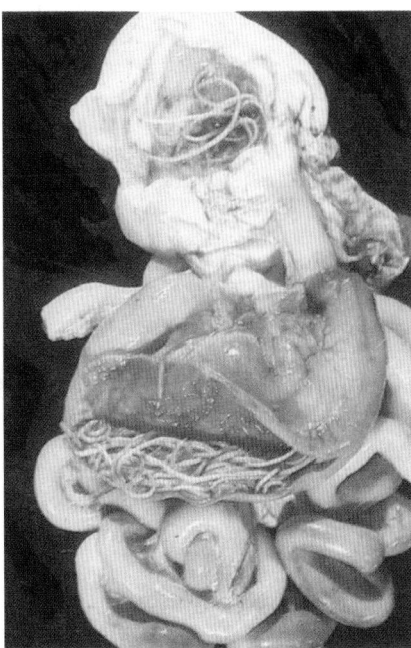

Fig. 1.65 Heavy *Toxocara canis* infection in the small intestine of a pup.

lanceolate cervical alae and the anterior body is curved ventrally. The mouth is surrounded by three large lips. There is no buccal capsule and the oesophagus lacks a posterior bulb. The tail of the male has caudal alae and a narrow terminal appendage. Female genital organs extend both anteriorly and posteriorly to the vulval area. The medium-sized egg is dark brown and subglobular, with a thick rough pitted shell. The granular unsegmented contents are very dark and normally fill the whole volume of the shell. Eggs measure 90 by 75 μm. The egg is very similar to that of *Parascaris*.

Life cycle: This species has the most complex life cycle in the superfamily, with four possible modes of infection. The basic form is typically ascaridoid, the egg containing the L₃ being infective, at optimal temperatures, four weeks after being passed. After ingestion, and hatching in the small intestine, the larvae travel by the bloodstream via the liver to the lungs, where the second moult occurs. The larvae then return via the trachea to the intestine where the final two moults take place. This form of ascaridoid migration occurs regularly only in dogs of up to about 2–3 months old.

In dogs over three months of age, hepatic–tracheal migration occurs less frequently and at around 4–6 months, it has almost ceased and is replaced by somatic migration, followed by hypobiosis. However, some dogs will support hepatic–tracheal migration as adults. Instead of hepatic–tracheal migration, the L₃ travel to a wide range of tissues including the liver, lungs, brain, heart and skeletal muscle, and the walls of the alimentary tract.

In the pregnant bitch, prenatal infection occurs, larvae becoming mobilised at about three weeks prior to parturition and migrating to the lungs of the fetus where they moult just before birth. In the newborn pup, the cycle is completed when the larvae travel to the intestine via the trachea, and the final moults occur. A bitch, once infected, will usually harbour sufficient larvae to infect all her subsequent litters, even if she never again encounters the infection. A few of these mobilised larvae, instead of going to the uterus, complete the normal migration in the bitch, and the resulting adult worms produce a transient but marked increase in faecal *Toxocara* egg output in the weeks following parturition.

The suckling pup may also be infected by ingestion of L₃ in the milk during the first three weeks of lactation. There is no migration in the pup following infection by this route. Paratenic intermediate hosts such as rodents, sheep, pigs or birds may ingest the infective eggs and the L₃ travel to their tissues where they remain until eaten by a dog, when subsequent development is apparently confined to the gastrointestinal tract.

A final complication is recent evidence that bitches may be reinfected during late pregnancy or lactation, leading directly to transmammary infection of the suckling pups and, once patency is established in the bitch, to contamination of the environment with eggs. The bitch may be reinfected via the ingestion of larval stages from the fresh faeces of puppies through her coprophagic activities. See **life cycle 9**.

The known minimum prepatent periods are as follows.
- Direct infection following ingestion of eggs or larvae in a paratenic host: 4–5 weeks.
- Prenatal infection: 2–3 weeks.

Toxocara mystax

Synonym: *Toxocara cati*

Description: Typical of the superfamily, *Toxocara mystax* is a large white/cream-coloured worm (up to 10 cm in length), often occurring as a mixed infection with the other ascarids of cats, such as *Toxascaris leonina*. Males are 3–6 cm and females 4–10 cm in length. The tail of the male has a terminal narrow appendage. Differentiation is readily made between *Toxocara mystax* and *Toxascaris leonina* on gross examination or with a hand lens, when the cervical alae of the former are seen to have an arrowhead form, with the posterior margins almost at a right angle to the body, whereas those of *Toxascaris* taper gradually into the body (Fig. 1.66a). The male, like that of *Toxocara canis*, has a small finger-like process at the tip of the tail. The egg is subglobular with

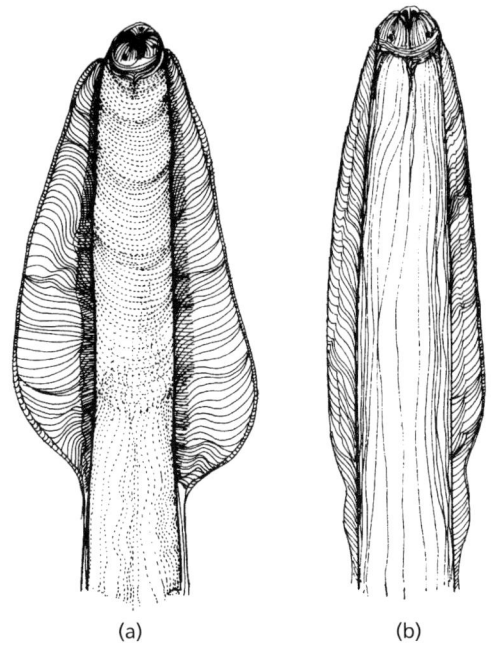

(a)   (b)

Fig. 1.66 Comparison of the anterior region of (a) *Toxocara mystax* and (b) *Toxascaris leonina*. The cervical alae of *Toxocara mystax* are arrow-shaped whereas those of *Toxascaris leonina* are more slender and less protrusive.

LIFE CYCLE 9. LIFE CYCLE OF *TOXOCARA CANIS*

Toxocara canis lives in the intestine of the dog (1), which acts as definitive host and sheds the nematode eggs with the faeces (2); these are spherical and characterised by a beehive-like outer shell encased in albuminous material. The egg contains a single undifferentiated embryo that, once in the external environment, matures (3) into an infective second-stage larva (4). The dog becomes infected by ingesting the larvated egg or paratenic hosts harbouring larvae in somatic tissues (5). Following ingestion of a larvated egg by a dog <3 months in age, an entero-hepatic-pneumo-tracheo-enteric migration occurs (6). In particular, the eggs hatch in the gastrointestinal tract (7) and, via the circulation, the larvae travel to the liver. Here, the larvae moult and, via the suprahepatic veins, reach the lungs (8), migrate up to the larynx and pharynx (9), and are swallowed to reach the intestine, where they mature to adult nematodes (10).

In dogs >3 months of age, this migration is gradually replaced by a visceral or somatic migration (11) whereby, following ingestion of larvated eggs, larvae migrate via the haemolymphatic circulation to several organs and tissues (e.g. liver, lung, heart, kidneys and skeletal muscles, 12) where they become latent. In male dogs, this phase marks the end of the life cycle; conversely, in pregnant bitches, the larvae become mobilised and migrate transplacentally to the livers of the fetuses (13). After birth, the larvae migrate to the lungs, moult, travel up the respiratory system and are swallowed, thus reaching the intestine where they develop into adult nematodes. Puppies can also acquire the infection via transmammary transmission (14), as mobilised larvae of *T. canis* are also excreted in the colostrum and milk. In humans (15), accidental ingestion of larvated eggs results in entero-pneumo-somatic migration of larvae (16), that cause visceral *larva migrans* (17), encephalic *larva migrans* (18) or ocular *larva migrans* (19), depending on where migration occurs.

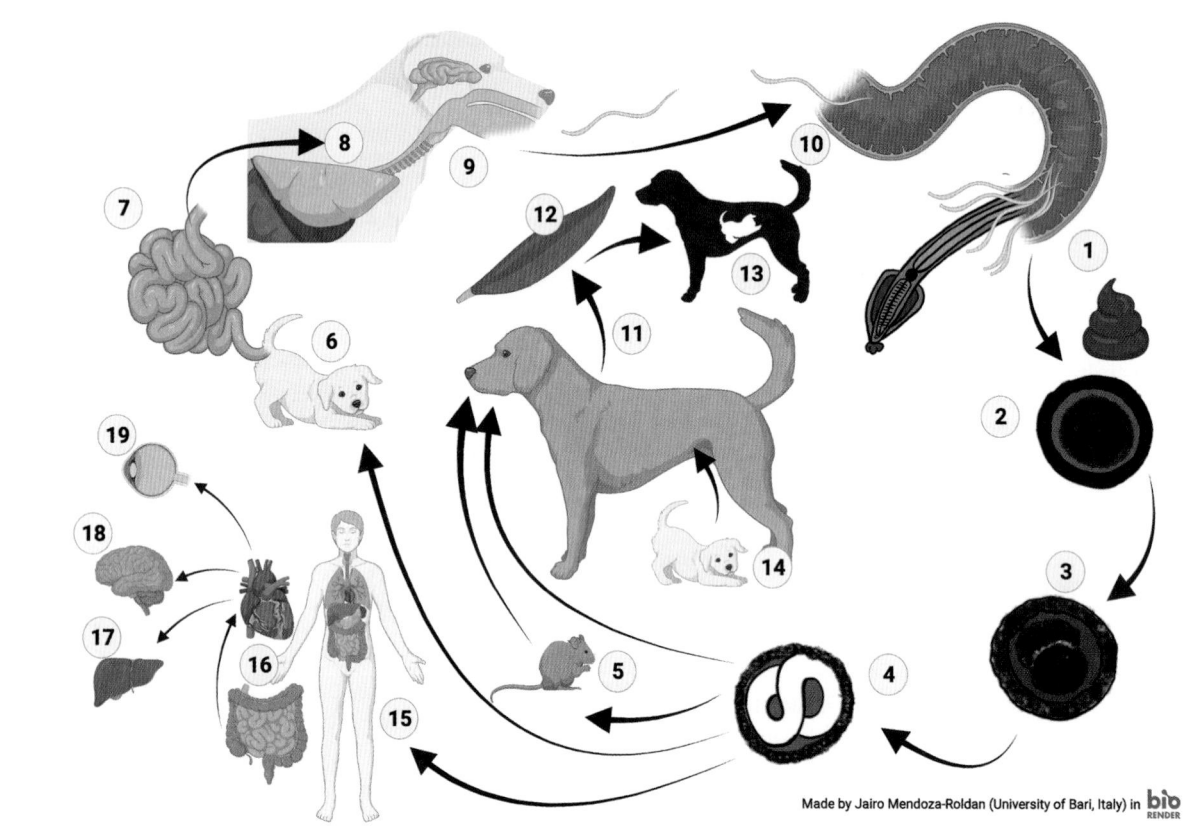

Made by Jairo Mendoza-Roldan (University of Bari, Italy) in **bio** RENDER

a thick, rough, pitted shell. The granular unsegmented contents are dark brown to black in colour and usually occupy the whole volume of the shell. Eggs measure 65 by 75 μm and are characteristic in cat faeces.

Life cycle: The life cycle of *T. mystax* is migratory when infection occurs by ingestion of the L_2 in the egg, and non-migratory after transmammary infection with L_3 or after ingestion of a paratenic host. Following ingestion of eggs containing an infective second-stage larva, the larvae enter the stomach wall and then migrate via the liver, lungs and trachea back to the stomach and moult to L_3, while L_4 occur in the stomach contents, the intestinal wall and bowel contents. Rodent infections also play an important part in the life cycle. In these, larvae remain as second-stage forms but when an infected mouse is eaten by a cat, the larvae, liberated by digestion, enter the stomach wall of the cat and develop to L_3. As well as mice acting as 'intermediate hosts', L_2 may be found in the tissues of earthworms, cockroaches, chickens, sheep and other animals fed infective eggs. Transmammary infection is common throughout lactation, particularly in acutely infected cats, and the lactogenic route of transmission is the most important. Prenatal infection through the placenta does not occur, which is dissimilar to *T. canis*. The prepatent period from egg infection is about eight weeks.

Toxocara malayiensis

Description: *Toxocara malayiensis* is a large white worm, typically 3 to 15 cm in length. It is morphologically similar to *T. canis* in dogs. There are three well-defined lips, each with a deep median notch lined with denticles: a dorsal lip with two large outer papillae, and two subventral lips each with one outer papilla. Cervical alae arise immediately behind the lips, gradually increasing in width to mid-length, then tapering gradually posteriorly.

Life cycle: The life cycle has not been fully described.

Toxocara vitulorum

Description: This is a very large whitish nematode. The adult male is up to 25 cm and the female up to 30 cm in length. The cuticle is less thick than other ascarids and somewhat soft and translucent.

There are three lips, broad at the base and narrowing anteriorly. The oesophagus is 3–4.5 mm long and has a posterior granular ventriculus. The tail of the male usually forms a small spike-like appendage. There are about five pairs of postcloacal papillae; the anterior pair is large and double. Precloacal papillae are variable in number. The vulva is situated about one-eighth of the body length from the anterior end. The medium-sized egg of *T. vitulorum* is subglobular, with a thick, finely pitted albuminous shell, is almost colourless and measures 75–95 by 60–74 µm. The egg is unsegmented and the granular contents frequently only occupy part of the internal volume.

Life cycle: The most important source of infection is the milk of the dam, in which larvae are present for up to 3–4 weeks after parturition. There is no tissue migration in the calf following milk-borne infection and the prepatent period is 3–4 weeks. The ingestion of larvated eggs by calves over six months of age seldom results in patency, the larvae migrating to various tissues where they remain dormant; in female animals, resumption of development in late pregnancy allows further transmammary transmission. See **life cycle 10**.

LIFE CYCLE 10. LIFE CYCLE OF *TOXOCARA VITULORUM*

Adults of *Toxocara vitulorum* live in the small intestine of cattle (1) and excrete the parasite eggs via the faeces; the eggs are spherical and characterised by a granular outer shell (2). In the environment, the eggs embryonate (3) and become infective, containing the third-stage larva (4). Once ingested by the bovine host, the larva is released from the egg in the forestomach (5); subsequent development depends on the animal's age (adult cattle or calves). In adult cattle (black arrows), the larvae undergo somatic or visceral migration, thus reaching several organs and tissues, e.g. liver (6), heart (7), lungs (8), skeletal muscles (9) and udder (10), where they become latent. In pregnant cattle, the latent larvae become mobi-lised and migrate through the circulation and the placenta to the liver of the fetus (11). After the birth of the calves (dashed green arrows), the larvae migrate from the liver (6) to the heart (7) and lungs (8), where they moult to fourth-stage larvae and, via the trachea, travel up the respiratory system where they are swallowed and reach the intestine. Here they develop to adult nematodes (1). Calves can acquire the infection through their mother's colostrum and milk, as somatic larvae that become mobilised during pregnancy can be excreted via the udder (10, 12). In the case of trans-mammary infection, larval migration does not occur and the parasites develop into adults in the intestine within 20–23 days.

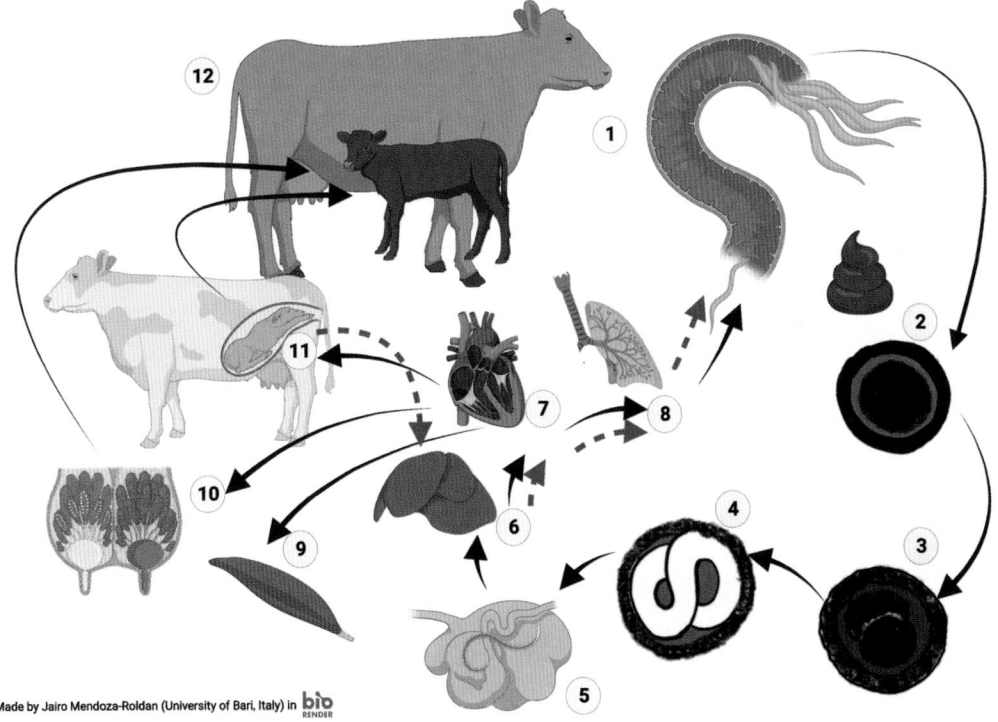

Made by Jairo Mendoza-Roldan (University of Bari, Italy) in **bio** RENDER

Toxascaris

Large worms grossly very similar to *Toxocara canis* with cervical alae present. A posterior bulb is absent from the oesophagus. The tail of the male does not possess a narrow terminal appendage as is the case for *T. canis* and *T. mystax*. The main species is *Toxascaris leonina* (syn. *Toxascaris limbata*) which infects the small intestine of dogs, cats, foxes, wild canids and felids.

Toxascaris leonina

Synonym: *Toxascaris limbata*

Description: Males measure up to 7 cm and females up to 10 cm long. Adults have an elliptical head due to the presence of cervical alae, which are slender and arrow-like, and taper posteriorly (Fig. 1.66b). Three large lips surround the mouth, there is no buccal capsule and the oesophagus lacks a bulb. The tail of the male is simple. The female genital organs lie behind the level of the vulva. The egg is slightly ovoid, with a smooth, thick, almost colourless shell. The yellowish-brown granular unsegmented contents fill only part of the shell. Eggs measure about 75–85 by 60–70 μm and are characteristic in dog and cat faeces.

Life cycle: The infective stage is the egg containing a second-stage larva or the third-stage larvae present in a mouse intermediate host. The eggs develop rapidly to the infective stage (about one week) compared with that for *Toxocara* species (around four weeks). Following ingestion and hatching, larvae enter the wall of the small intestine and remain for about two weeks. No migration of larvae occurs, as with other ascarid species. Third-stage larvae appear after about 11 days and moult to L_4 about 3–5 weeks post infection. Adult stages appear from about six weeks post infection and lie in the lumen of the intestine. The prepatent period is 10–11 weeks.

Parascaris

This very large, rigid, stout, whitish nematode, up to 40 cm in length, is found in the small intestine of equids (Fig. 1.67).

Life cycle: The life cycle is direct and migratory, involving a hepatopulmonary route. Eggs produced by the adult female worms are passed in the faeces and can reach the infective stage containing the L_2 in as

little as 10–14 days, although development may be delayed at low temperatures. After ingestion and hatching, the larvae penetrate the intestinal wall and within 48 hours have reached the liver. By two weeks, they have arrived in the lungs where they migrate up the bronchi and trachea, are swallowed and return to the small intestine. The site of occurrence and timing of the parasitic larval moults of *P. equorum* are not precisely known, but it would appear that the moult from L_2 to L_3 occurs between the intestinal mucosa and the liver and the two subsequent moults occur in the small intestine. The minimum prepatent period of *P. equorum* is 10 weeks; longevity is up to two years. There is no evidence of prenatal infection. The main species is *Parascaris equorum* (syn. *Ascaris equorum*, *Ascaris megacephala*) which infects the small intestine of horses, donkeys and zebras.

Parascaris equorum

Description: This very large, rigid, stout, whitish nematode cannot be confused with any other intestinal parasite of equines. Males measure 15–25 cm and females up to 40–50 cm in length. The adult parasites have a simple mouth opening surrounded by three large lips, and in the male the tail has small caudal alae. The dorsal lip has two double papillae and each ventrolateral lip has one double subventral and a small lateral papilla. Spicules are long and stout. The medium-sized egg of *P. equorum* is almost spherical (85–100 × 80–90 μm), brownish and thick-shelled with an outer pitted albuminous coat.

Porrocaecum

Species of this genus are parasites of a range of birds and various fish-eating mammals.

Life cycle: Similar to other ascarid species. The main species is *Porrocaecum crassum* which infects the small intestine of ducks. This parasite has earthworms as intermediate hosts.

Porrocaecum crassum

Description: The worms are reddish-white in colour, males measuring 12–30 mm and females 40–55 mm in length. Caudal alae are absent. The tail of the male is conical.

Bayliascaris

Species of the genus *Bayliascaris* are found in a wide range of mammal hosts. *Bayliascaris procyonis*, whose definitive host is the raccoon, is of veterinary importance because it has the ability to infect a wide range of wild and domestic animals and occasionally humans, causing visceral *larva migrans*.

Life cycle: The definitive hosts for this parasite are mammals such as skunks and raccoons, in which the nematode localises in the small intestine, eliminating eggs out in the faeces. These eggs can remain viable in the environment for several years. When ingested by paratenic hosts (e.g. dogs, cats, rodents, lagomorphs, gallinaceous birds, ostriches and occasionally humans), the larvae develop and penetrate into the circulation and eventually enter the brain and spinal cord.

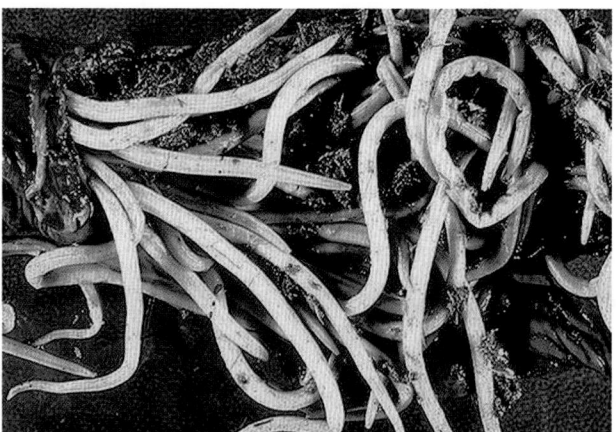

Fig. 1.67 *Parascaris equorum* adult worms in the small intestine.

Bayliascaris procyonis

Description: Adult worms in the definitive host are whitish in colour, and measure 15–20 cm in length and 1 cm in width.

FAMILY ASCARIDIIDAE

Ascaridia

The worms (Table 1.29) are stout and densely white; male worms are 50–75 mm and female worms 70–120 mm long (Fig. 1.68). *Ascaridia* is by far the largest nematode of poultry.

Life cycle: The egg becomes infective at optimal temperatures in a minimum of three weeks and the parasitic phase is non-migratory, consisting of a transient histotrophic phase in the intestinal mucosa after which the adult parasites inhabit the lumen of the intestine. The egg is sometimes ingested by earthworms, which may act as transport hosts. Eggs can remain viable for several months under moist cool conditions but are killed by a dry hot environment. The prepatent period ranges from 4–6 weeks in chicks to eight weeks or more in adult birds. The worms live for about one year.

Ascaridia galli

Synonyms: *Ascardia lineata*, *Ascaridia perspicillum*

Description: Male worms are 50–75 mm and female worms 70–120 mm long. The anterior end is characterised by a prominent mouth, which is surrounded by three large trilobed lips. The edges

Table 1.29 *Ascaridia* species.

Species	Hosts	Site
Ascaridia galli (syn. *Ascaridia lineata*, *Ascaridia perspicillum*)	Chickens, turkeys, geese, ducks, guinea fowl and a number of wild galliform birds	Small intestine
Ascaridia dissimilis	Turkeys	Small intestine
Ascaridia columbae (syn. *Ascaridia maculosa*)	Pigeons	Small intestine

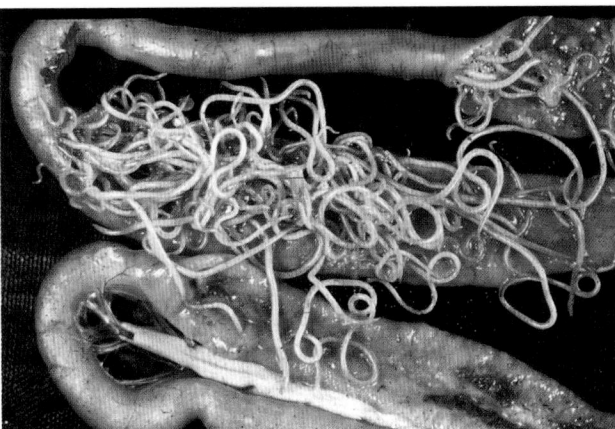

Fig. 1.68 *Ascaridia galli* adult worms in the small intestine.

of the lips bear teeth-like denticles. A posterior bulb is absent from the oesophagus. The tail of the male possesses small alae and also bears 10 pairs of papillae. Spicules are almost equal in length. In the male, there is a circular precloacal sucker, which has a thick cuticular rim. The medium-sized pale-brown egg is distinctly oval, with barrel-shaped side walls, and they are unsegmented when laid (see Fig. 4.8). They measure about 75–80 by 45–50 μm. The smooth thick shell has three layers, the middle one being more prominent. Eggs cannot easily be distinguished from those of the other common poultry ascaridoid, *Heterakis*.

Ascaridia dissimilis

Description: The worms are stout and densely white. Males measure 35–50 mm and females 50–75 mm in length. The males of this species and those of *A. galli* are separated by differences in the position of the first and fourth pairs of ventral caudal papillae, and by the form of the spicules. The egg is distinctly oval, with a smooth shell, and is 80–95 μm in size.

Ascaridia columbae

Synonym: *Ascardia maculosa*

Description: The worms are stout and densely white; males are 16–70 mm and females 20–95 mm in length. The egg is distinctly oval, with a smooth shell, and measures 80–90 by 40–50 μm.

FAMILY HETERAKIIDAE

Heterakis

These are small to medium whitish worms up to 1.5 cm long, with elongated pointed tails (Table 1.30). Gross examination readily indicates the genus but for specific identification, microscopic examination is necessary to determine the shape of the oesophagus (in *Heterakis* the oesophagus has a large posterior bulb) and the size and shape of spicules. A buccal capsule is absent. Generic identity may be confirmed by the presence of a large, chitinous, circular precloacal sucker in the male and prominent caudal alae supported by 12 pairs of caudal papillae (Fig. 1.69). The precloacal sucker is much less prominent in *Ascaridia*.

Life cycle: The direct life cycle is similar to that of *Ascaridia* spp. The egg is infective on the ground in about two weeks at optimal temperatures. Eggs may remain viable in the soil for several months. Earthworms may be transport hosts, the eggs simply passing through

Table 1.30 *Heterakis* species.

Species	Hosts	Site
Heterakis gallinarum (syn. *Heterakis papillosa*, *Heterakis gallinae*, *Heterakis vesicularis*)	Chickens, turkeys, pigeons, pheasants, partridges, grouse, quails, guinea fowl, ducks, geese and a number of wild galliform birds	Caeca
Heterakis isolonche	Pheasants, grouse, quails, ducks, chickens	Caeca
Heterakis dispar	Ducks, geese, chickens	Caeca
Heterakis brevispeculum	Ducks, geese, guinea fowl, chickens	Caeca

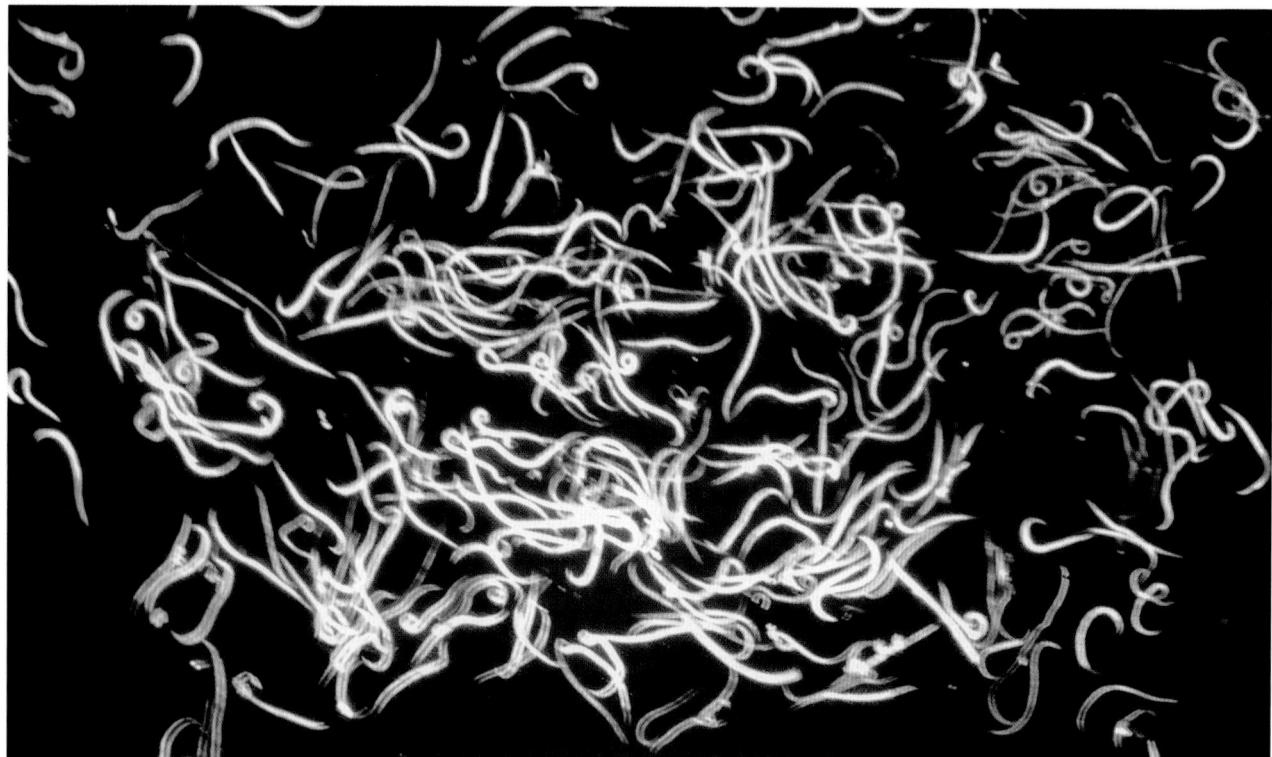

Fig. 1.69 Adult *Heterakis gallinarum* worms.

the gut, or paratenic hosts in which the egg hatches and the L$_3$ travel to the tissues to await ingestion by the fowl. The prepatent period of the genus is about four weeks. Longevity is about 12 months.

Heterakis gallinarum

Description: The male is 7–13 mm long and the female 10–15 mm (Fig. 1.70). Gross examination readily indicates the genus but for specific identification, microscopic examination is necessary to determine the shape of the oesophagus and the size and shape of spicules. The oesophagus has a large posterior bulb. Generic identity may be confirmed by the presence of a large circular pre-cloacal sucker in the male and prominent caudal alae supported by 12 pairs of caudal papillae (Fig. 1.70). The spicules are unequal in length, the left (about 0.7 mm) has broad alae and the right is slender (about 2 mm). The egg is ovoid, thick and smooth-shelled with almost parallel side walls (see Fig. 4.8). Eggs measure 65–80 by 35–46 μm and are unsegmented when laid. *Heterakis* eggs are sometimes difficult to distinguish from those of *Ascaridia*, although in the latter species the eggs are larger and have slightly barrel-shaped side walls.

Heterakis isolonche

Description: Male worms measure about 7–13 mm and females 10–15 mm in length. The spicules are long and of equal length.

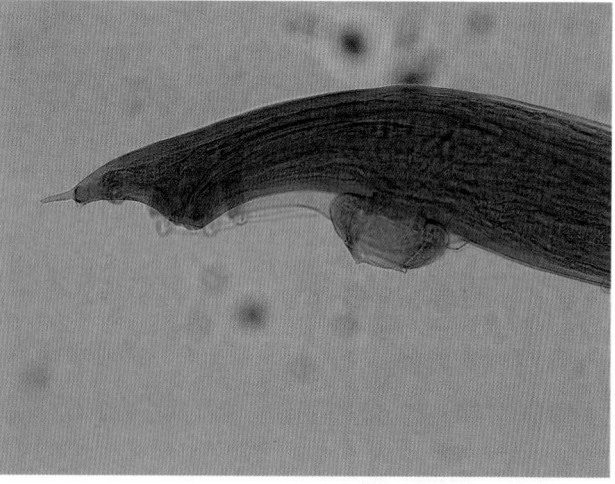

Fig. 1.70 Tail of male *Heterakis gallinarum* showing prominent caudal alae supported by 12 pairs of caudal papillae. (Courtesy of Georgiana Deak).

The spicules are asymmetrical and generic identity may be confirmed by the presence of a large circular precloacal sucker in the male and prominent caudal alae supported by large caudal papillae. The egg is ovoid, thick and smooth-shelled, about 65–75 by 38–45 μm. More details of the eggs are given under *H. gallinarum*.

Heterakis dispar

Description: Worms are larger than the other species, with males measuring 11–18 mm and females 16–23 mm in length. The spicules are short and equal in length (40–50 µm).

Heterakis brevispeculum

Description: The spicules are of equal length (about 0.5 mm) and possess a barb near the tip.

Other ascarids (Table 1.31) found in reptiles are briefly mentioned and covered in Chapter 16. Members of the genera *Ophidascaris* and *Polydelphus* are mainly parasites of snakes and lizards, occasionally of amphibians. *Angusticaecum* spp. are ascarids of tortoises.

Table 1.31 Reptilian ascarid species.

Species	Hosts	Site
Ophidascaris spp.	Snakes, lizards	Intestine
Polydelphus spp.	Snakes	Intestine
Angusticaecum holopterum	Reptiles (chelonia)	Intestine

FAMILY ANISAKIDAE

Members of the Anisakidae (Table 1.32) have life cycles involving marine mammals and fish and are of importance mainly in human medicine as some species can cause disease through the ingestion of raw or uncooked fish. Detailed descriptions are not within the scope of this book. See **life cycle 11**.

Table 1.32 Anisakidae species.

Species	Final hosts	Site	Intermediate hosts
Anisakis simplex	Whales, dolphins, seals	Stomach and intestine	Crustaceans, fishes
Contracaecum spiculigerum	Ducks, geese, swans, waterfowl	Small intestine	Invertebrates (copepods, crustaceans, insects, etc.) Damselflies, fishes, tadpoles
Contracaecum spp.	Whales, dolphins, seals	Stomach and intestine	Copepods, fishes
Pseudoterranova decipiens (syn. *Phocanema decipiens*)	Seals	Stomach	Crustaceans, fishes
Sulcascaris spp.	Reptiles (turtles)	Intestine	Molluscs

LIFE CYCLE 11. LIFE CYCLE OF *ANISAKIS* SPP.

Anisakis spp. are nematode parasites of several animal species, including humans. Adult *Anisakis* live in the intestine of fishes and sea mammals. The unembryonated eggs (2) reach the marine environment via the host faeces. Following embryonation (3), formation of first- (L_1) (4) and second-stage larvae (L_2) (5) occurs inside the egg, which subsequently hatches, releasing the L_2 (6). The L_2 are ingested by small marine crustaceans (7) and invade the host haemocoel where they moult to third-stage larvae (L_3). Once infected crustaceans are eaten by cephalopods (8) or predatory fish (9), the larvae migrate from the intestinal tract of the new host to the coelomatic cavity, where they encapsulate on the surface of organs and skeletal muscles (particularly following the death of the host). Predatory fish (9) represent a key element of the life cycle, as these hosts accumulate and transmit larvae ingested by infected fish, crustaceans and cephalopods. The definitive host acquires the infection via ingestion of infected fish or cephalopods. In humans, the larvae present in raw or undercooked fish may migrate through the intestinal mucosa or other tissues.

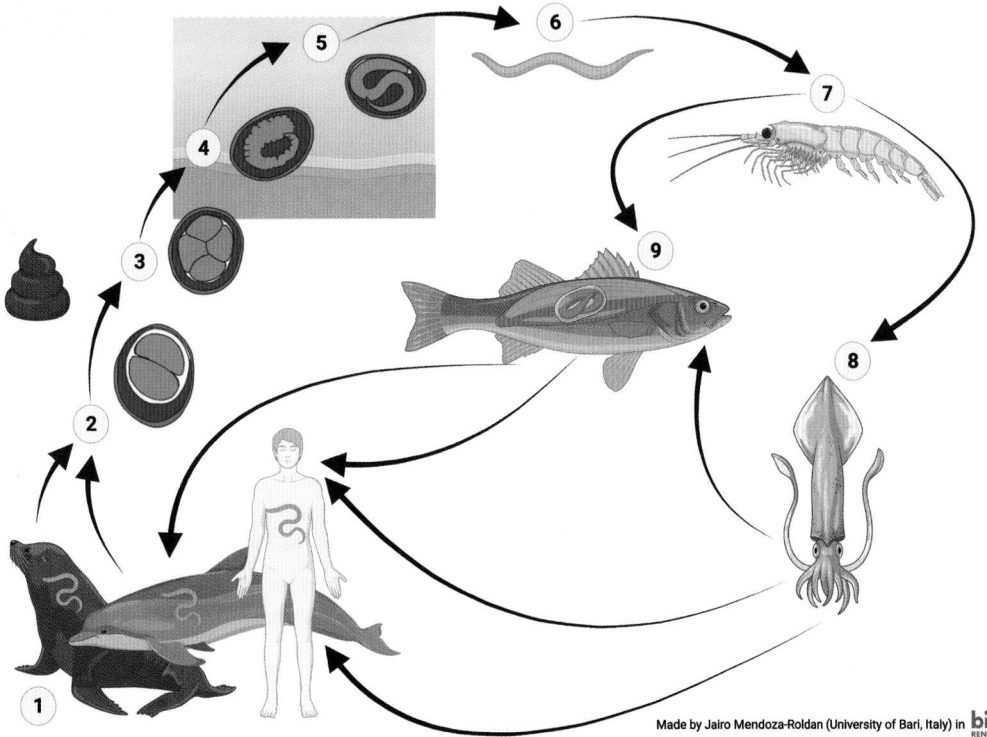

Made by Jairo Mendoza-Roldan (University of Bari, Italy) in **bio** RENDER

FAMILY ASPIDODERIDAE

Paraspidodera

The main species is *Paraspidodera uncinata* which infects the large intestine of guinea pigs.

Paraspidodera uncinata

Description: Male worms are 16–17 mm and females 18–21 mm in length. Both sexes have a large bulb-shaped oesophagus. Caudal alae are absent. The male spicules are of equal length. The male has a precloacal sucker. The egg is small, ellipsoidal and measures about 43 by 31 μm. The shell is thick with a smooth surface and the contents are unsegmented.

SUPERFAMILY SUBULUROIDEA

Members of this superfamily are parasites mainly of rodents and are characterised by weakly developed lips with sensilla and a thick-walled stoma that is armed with three teeth. The only genus of veterinary importance is *Subulura*, species of which are parasites of poultry.

FAMILY SUBULIRIDAE

Subulura

Species of this genus, found in birds, are small worms located in the caecae. They are similar to *Heterakis*, although the tail is not as pointed. The males measure around 8–10 mm and the females up to 14–18 mm in length.

Life cycle: Eggs passed in faeces are ingested by the intermediate host where they develop to the infective L_3 stage after about two weeks. Following ingestion by the final host, the larvae migrate to the lumen of the caeca. The prepatent period is 6–8 weeks. The main species is *Subulura suctoria* (syn. *Subulura brumpti*, *Subulura differens*, *Allodapa suctoria*) which infects the caeca of chickens, turkeys, guinea fowl, quails, grouse, pheasants and ducks. This parasite has beetles and cockroaches as intermediate hosts.

Subulura suctoria

Synonyms: *Subulura brumpti*, *Subulura differens*, *Allodapa suctoria*

Description: The buccal capsule is small and possesses three teeth at its base. The oesophagus is dilated posteriorly, followed by a bulb. The tail of the male has large lateral alae and is curved ventrally. Two long thin curved spicules are present. A slit-like precloacal sucker is present, surrounded by radiating muscle fibres. In the female, the vulva is situated just anterior to the middle of the body.

ORDER OXYURIDA

SUPERFAMILY OXYUROIDEA

Adult oxyuroids of animals inhabit the large intestine and are commonly called 'Pinworms' because of the long pointed tail of the female parasite. The ventrolateral papillae are often absent and where present are very much reduced. The number of spicules can vary in the males from zero, one or two depending on the species. They have a double bulb oesophagus, the posterior bulb being well developed. The life cycle is direct. The genera of veterinary interest are *Oxyuris* and *Probstmayria*, both parasitic in the horse; *Skrjabinema*, which are parasites of ruminants; *Syphacia* and *Aspiculuris* found in rodents; *Passalurus* and *Dermatoxys* found in rabbits and hares; and *Tachygonetria* found in reptiles. Oxyurids also include the common human pinworm, *Enterobius*.

FAMILY OXYURIDAE

Oxyuris

The adult female worms, which may reach 10–15 cm in length, are found in the lumen of the caecum and large colon of equids. The much smaller males are difficult to observe in digesta. The main species is *Oxyuris equi* and infects the caecum, colon and rectum of horses and donkeys.

Life cycle: The life cycle is direct. The adult worms are found in the lumen of the caecum and the small and large colon. After fertilisation, the gravid female migrates to the anus, extrudes her anterior end and lays her eggs in clumps (up to 50 000 eggs per female), seen grossly as yellowish-white gelatinous streaks on the perineal skin or perianal region. Development is rapid and within 4–5 days the egg contains the infective L_3. Eggs are rubbed off and contaminate the environment. Infection is by ingestion of embryonated eggs on fodder, grass, bedding, etc. The larvae are released in the small intestine, move into the large intestine and migrate into the mucosal crypts of the caecum and colon where development to L_4 takes place within 10 days. The L_4 then emerge and feed on the mucosa before maturing to adult stages that inhabit the lumen and feed on intestinal contents. The prepatent period of *O. equi* is about five months. Longevity of female worms is around six months.

Oxyuris equi

Description: The mature females are large, greyish-white, opaque worms with very long tapering tails that may reach 10–15 cm in length, whereas the mature males are generally less than 1.2 cm long (Fig. 1.71). *Oxyuris equi* L_4 are 5–10 mm in length, have long tapering tails and are often attached orally to the intestinal mucosa. There is a double oesophageal bulb (Fig. 1.72; see also Fig. 1.3) and the tiny males have caudal alae and a single pin-shaped spicule. In the female the vulva is situated anteriorly. *Oxyuris equi* eggs are ovoid, yellowish, thick-shelled, smooth and slightly flattened on one side with a transparent mucoid operculate plug at one end (see Fig. 4.5). Eggs measure 80–95 by 40–45 μm and contain a late-stage morula or a first larval stage when shed in faeces.

Skrjabinema

Skrjabinema are small non-pathogenic pinworms in the caecum of domestic and wild ruminants (Table 1.33).

Life cycle: The life cycle is direct. Embryonated eggs are deposited on the perineal skin by the adult female worms. Infection is by ingestion of the embryonated egg.

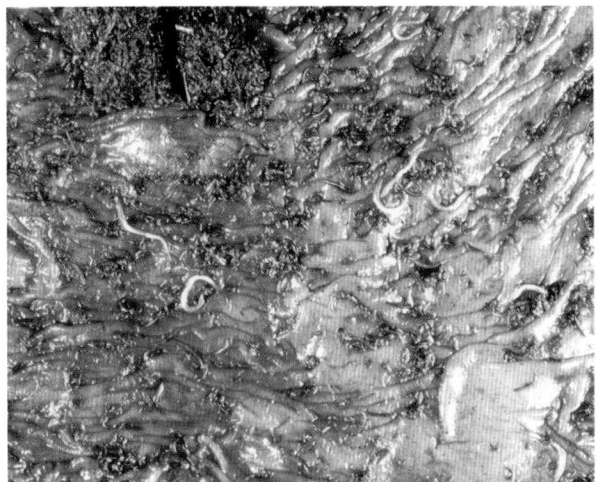

Fig. 1.71 Mixed infection of *Oxyuris equi* adults (white) and small strongyles in the colon.

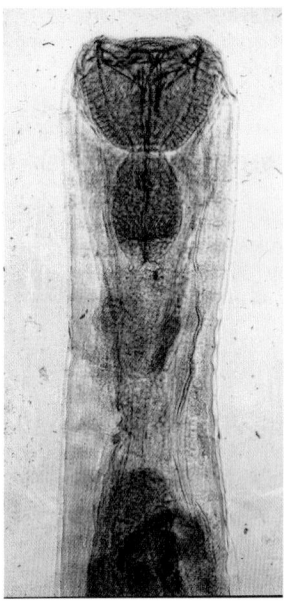

Fig. 1.72 Head of *Oxyuris equi* with double oesophageal bulb.

Table 1.33 *Skrjabinema* species.

Species	Hosts	Site
Skrjabinema ovis (syn. *Oxyuris ovis*)	Goats, sheep	Caecum, colon
Skrjabinema alata	Sheep	Caecum, colon
Skrjabinema caprae	Goats	Caecum, colon
Skrjabinema parva	Deer (white-tailed)	Caecum, colon

Skrjabinema ovis

Description: Small worms, up to 7 mm in size; male are around 3 mm and females 6–7 mm in length. There are three large intricate lips and three small intermediate lips. The oesophagus is cylindrical in cross-section and ends in a large spherical bulb. The male worm has a single spicule and the tail is rounded with a cuticular expansion supported by two pairs of processes. Eggs are asymmetrically flattened, larvated and measure 55–60 by 32–35 μm.

Life cycle: The prepatent period for this species is about 25 days.

Aspicularis

These are small pinworms of rodents. Males are 2–4 mm and females 3–4 mm long.

Life cycle: The life cycle is direct. Females deposit embryonated eggs on the perineal skin. Infection occurs in three ways:

1 directly by ingestion of embryonated eggs from the perineum
2 indirectly with food
3 by retro-infection when eggs hatch in the perineal region and migrate back via the anus.

The main species is *Aspicularis tetraptera* which infects the caecum and colon of mice and rats.

Aspicularis tetraptera

Description: The oesophageal bulb is oval, the oesophagus is club-shaped and the mouth has three lips. The cervical alae are broad and their posterior margin ends abruptly. There is no spicule or gubernaculum in the male.

Syphacia

These are small whitish worms, up to 6 mm in size, localised in the caecum and colon of mice and rats. Males measure 1–1.5 mm and females 3.4–6 mm. The mouth has three distinct lips without a buccal capsule. The oesophagus has a prebulbular swelling and a posterior globular bulb. Small cervical alae, with rounded posterior margins, are present. The males have a single long slender spicule.

Syphacia obvelata

Description: The adult male is 1.1–1.6 mm long and 125 μm wide with the tail length about equal to its body width. Female worms measure 3.4–5 mm in length.

Syphacia muris

Description: The adult male is 1.2–1.3 mm long and 100 μm wide and the tail length is about twice the body width. The females measure 2.8–3.4 mm in length. The vulva of *S. muris* is further posterior, in relation to the oesophageal bulb, than that of *S. obvelata*.

Passalurus

Species of *Passalurus* are common pinworms localised in the caecum and colon of rabbits and hares.

Life cycle: Development is direct and infection occurs through the ingestion of infective eggs. Immature stages are found in the mucosa of the small intestine and caecum.

Passalurus ambiguus

Description: Adult worms are 4–11 mm in size and semi-transparent; males are 4–5 mm and females 9–11 mm. The oesophagus has the typical oxyurid oesophageal bulb. The distal extremity of the female tail possesses around 40 circular striations. The male spicule is simple in appearance and the tail has an appendix shaped like a whip. Eggs are thin-walled, with slightly flattened walls on one side and measure 95–103 by 43 μm.

Dermatoxys

Species of *Dermatoxys* are common pinworms of rabbits and hares.

Life cycle: Details of the life cycle are not known. It is probably direct and similar to other pinworms. The main species is *Dermatoxys veligera* which infects the caecum and colon of rabbits and hares.

Dermatoxys veligera

Description: Female worms are 16–17 mm and males 8–11 mm long. Males have small spicules. Females have a vulva located in the cranial half of their body.

Enterobius

This genus includes the human pinworm, *Enterobius vermicularis*, which is also found in apes, and *Enterobius anthropopitheci* of chimpazees. Both are found in the caecum and colon.

Life cycle: Gravid female worms in the caecum and colon migrate to the rectum and deposit eggs on the perineum. Eggs become infective within a few days and infection is via the embyonated egg. The prepatent period is about eight weeks.

Enterobius vermicularis

Description: Adults are slender cream-coloured worms with long tails. Males measure 2–5 mm and females 8–13 mm in length.

FAMILY KATHLANIIDAE

Probstmayria

Small, slender, viviparous nematodes that are perpetual parasites, living from generation to generation in the equine large intestine. The main species is *Probstmayria vivipara* which infects the colon of horses.

Probstmayria vivipara

Description: Adult worms are 2–3 mm long with long filamentous tails. The mouth has six small lips and the buccal capsule is cylindrical and long. The oesophagus has an expanded posterior bulb. A large sucker-like excretory pore is present. The tail of the male is curved into a hook shape.

Life cycle: *Probstmayria vivipara* is unusual in that it is a perpetual parasite and lives from generation to generation in the equine caecum and colon. The females are viviparous and give birth to larvae almost as large as the adults. Both adults and larvae may be passed in the faeces.

FAMILY PHARYNGODONIDAE

The Pharyngodonidae includes a number of genera that are pinworms of reptiles. The genus *Tachygonetria* is commonly found in Mediterranean tortoises (*Testudo* spp.).

ORDER SPIRURIDA

SUPERFAMILY SPIRUROIDEA

The precise classification of a number of genera currently assigned to this superfamily is controversial, but there are some of significance in veterinary medicine: *Spirocerca*, *Habronema*, *Draschia*, *Parabronema*, *Thelazia*, *Gnathostoma*, *Gongylonema* and to a lesser extent *Ascarops*, *Physocephalus*, *Simondsia*, *Physaloptera*, *Spirura*, *Odontospirura*, *Tetrameres*, *Histiocephalus*, *Hartertia*, *Oxyspirura*, *Metathalazia* and *Vogeloides*. A major characteristic of this group is the tight, spirally coiled tail of the male. The life cycles are indirect, involving arthropod intermediate hosts.

Members of the genus *Thelazia* are principally found in or around the eyes of animals and can be responsible for keratitis. Unlike most spiruroids, the L_1 stage is not ingested from the faeces but by flies feeding on ocular secretions.

The genus *Gongylonema* is unusual among the spiruroids in having a very wide final host range, which includes all the domesticated animals, though it is most prevalent in ruminants. Like most spiruroids, the favoured location of the adults is the upper alimentary tract, the oesophagus and the forestomachs and stomach of mammals and the crop of birds. Species belonging to the genera *Cheilospirura*, *Echinuria*, *Dispharynx* and *Streptocara* are now considered to be members of the superfamily Acuarioidea.

FAMILY SPIROCERCIDAE

Spirocerca

These are stout, reddish, spirally coiled worms, 3–8 cm long, are found in tumour-like granulomas in the wall of the oesophagus and stomach.

Life cycle: The thick-shelled elongate egg containing a larva is passed in the faeces or vomit, and does not hatch until ingested by a dung beetle. In this, the intermediate host, the larva develops to the L_3 and encysts. Paratenic hosts may also be involved if the dung beetle, in turn, is ingested by any of a variety of other animals including the domestic chicken, wild birds and lizards. In these, the L_3 become encysted in the viscera. On ingestion of the intermediate or paratenic host by the final host, the L_3 are liberated, penetrate the stomach wall and migrate via the coeliac artery to the thoracic aorta. About three months later, the majority of larvae cross to the adjacent oesophagus where they provoke the development of granulomas as they develop to the adult stage in a further three months. Adults are usually located in cystic nodules which communicate with the lumen of the stomach or oesophagus through fistulae. The prepatent period is therefore about 5–6 months. Eggs, however, may not be found in the faeces of a proportion of animals with adult infections where the granulomas have no openings into the oesophageal lumen. The main species is *Spirocera lupi* which infects the oesophagus, stomach and aorta of dogs, foxes, wild canids, occasionally cats and wild felids. This parasite has coprophagous beetles as intermediate hosts. See **life cycle 12**.

LIFE CYCLE 12. LIFE CYCLE OF *SPIROCERCA LUPI*

Adults of *Spirocerca lupi* (1) live in nodules that develop within the wall of the thoracic section of the oesophagus of dogs and other canids, which act as definitive hosts. Adult females release larvated eggs (2) that reach the oesophageal lumen through a round opening of the nodule (nipple-like) and are excreted in the environment with the faeces or emesis. The life cycle continues when eggs are ingested by free-living biological vectors (coprophagous Coleoptera) (3) that act as intermediate hosts; within these hosts, the parasites develop into infective third-stage larvae. Other animals, such as amphibians, reptiles and birds, may act as paratenic hosts (4), harbouring live infective larvae. The dog acquires the infection by ingesting intermediate or paratenic hosts harbouring infective larvae of *S. lupi*. After ingestion, the larvae penetrate the gastric wall and, via the coeliac artery, migrate to the thoracic aorta and subsequently to the oesophageal wall (5, 6) where they moult and develop into sexually mature adults ~6 months after initial infection.

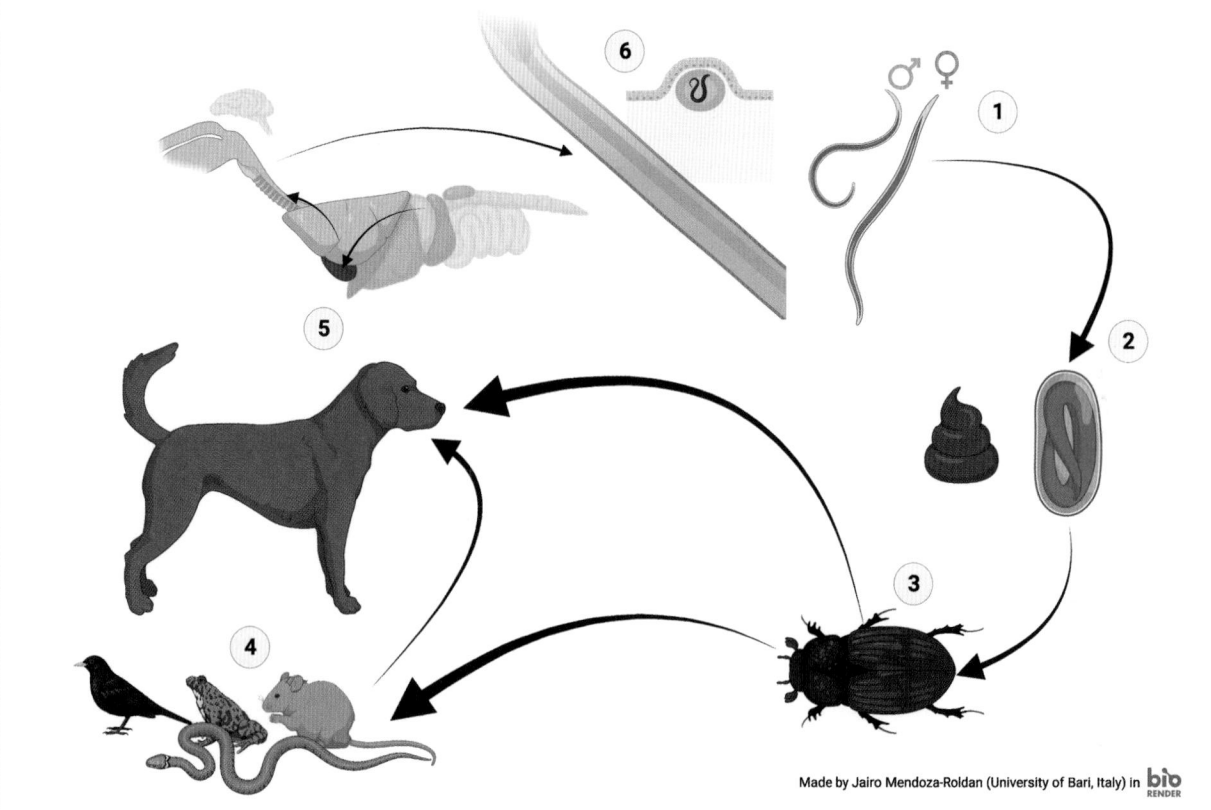

Made by Jairo Mendoza-Roldan (University of Bari, Italy) in **bio**RENDER

Spirocerca lupi

Description: Adult worms are spirally coiled and have a blood-red colour; males are around 30–55 mm and females 55–80 mm. The lips are trilobed and the pharynx is short. The male tail bears lateral alae (four pairs and one unpaired), median precloacal papillae and two pairs of postcloacal papillae, with a group of minute papillae near the tail tip. The very small eggs have smooth thick shells and are elongate with parallel side walls. They measure about 30–37 by 11–15 μm and are larvated when passed in faeces.

Ascarops

Worms of this genus, and of the genera *Physocephalus* and *Simondsia*, live on the stomach wall of pigs and wild boar under a layer of mucus, and occasionally in the small intestine.

Life cycle: The life cycle is typically spiruroid. Eggs passed in the faeces of the infected host develop into infective larvae, if ingested by coprophagous beetles. The life cycle is completed when pigs ingest the beetles. The prepatent period is about four weeks.

Ascarops strongylina

Synonym: *Arduenna strongylina*

Description: Small slender filiform worms, the males measuring up to 15 mm and the reddish females about 22 mm long. A cervical ala is located only on the left side of the body. The wall of the pharynx contains several spiral supports and a small tooth is present on each of the two lips. The right caudal alae in the male are much larger than the left and there are four pairs of asymmetrical precloacal papillae and one pair of caudal papillae. The left spicule is about 4–5 times longer than the right spicule. Eggs are small, thick-shelled, 34–39 by 20–22 μm, and are embryonated when passed.

Ascarops dentata

Synonym: *Arduenna dentata*

Description: Similar to *A. strongylina* but much bigger; male worms are 35 mm and female worms are 55 mm long. The buccal capsule has two teeth anteriorly.

Physocephalus

Small slender worms found on the surface of the stomach wall.

Life cycle: The life cycle is typically spiruroid. Eggs passed in the faeces of the infected host develop into infective larvae, if ingested by coprophagous beetles. The prepatent period is about six weeks. The main species is *Physocephalus sexalatus* which infects the stomach of pigs and camels, rarely rabbits and hares. This parasite has coprophagous beetles as intermediate hosts.

Physocephalus sexalatus

Description: Small slender filiform worms which are reddish when fresh, the males measuring about 10–12 mm and the females up to 22 mm long. The anterior of the body is thinner than the posterior region and just posterior to the vestibule is a cuticular swelling. There are three cervical alae on either side and the cervical papillae are asymmetrically located. The wall of the pharynx contains a single spiral support. In the male worm, the caudal alae are narrow and symmetrical and there are four pairs of precloacal papillae. The left spicule is about 6–7 times longer than the right spicule. Eggs are small, an elongated ellipse, thick-shelled, measure around 34–39 by 15–17 μm and are embryonated when passed.

Simondsia

Male worms live on the surface of the gastric mucosa, but the females are found in small cysts in the mucosal crypts with their anterior ends protruding.

Life cycle: The life cycle is indirect. Eggs are passed in the faeces and ingested by beetles in which they hatch and develop to infective larvae. The parasites continue development when the intermediate host is ingested by a pig. The main species is *Simondsia paradoxa* (syn. *Spiroptera cesticillus*) which infects the stomach of pigs, rarely rabbits and hares. This parasite has coprophagous beetles as intermediate hosts.

Simondsia paradoxa

Synonym: *Spiroptera cesticillus*

Description: The males are small slender worms measuring about 12–15 mm in length and possess a spirally coiled tail. Female worms measure up to about 15–20 mm in length. They have large lateral alae and a large ventral and dorsal tooth. The gravid female has a characteristic form, the posterior end of the body being a rounded sac filled with eggs and the anterior end is slender. The small eggs are oval or ellipsoid, 20–29 μm, and are embryonated when laid.

Table 1.34 *Streptopharagus* species.

Species	Hosts	Site	Intermediate hosts
Streptopharagus armatus	Rhesus monkeys, cynomolgus monkeys, Japanese macaques, guenons, baboons, gibbons	Stomach	Coprophagous beetles
Streptopharagus pigmenatus	Rhesus monkeys, cynomolgus monkeys, Japanese macaques, guenons, baboons, gibbons	Stomach	Coprophagous beetles

Streptopharagus

Worms of this genus are found in the stomachs of Old World monkeys and apes (Table 1.34).

FAMILY HABRONEMATIDAE

Habronema

Members of the genus *Habronema* are small, slender, white translucent worms 1.5–2.5 cm long (Fig. 1.73). The male has wide caudal alae and the tail has a spiral twist. Together with the closely related genus *Draschia*, they are parasitic in the stomach of the horse. *Habronema* inhabits the mucus layer of the gastric mucosa and may cause a catarrhal gastritis, but is not considered an important pathogen. The chief importance of these parasites is as a cause of cutaneous habronematidosis or 'summer sores' in warm countries.

Life cycle: The life cycle is similar for all species. Eggs or L_1 are passed in the faeces and the L_1 are ingested by the larval stages of various muscid flies of the genera *Musca*, *Stomoxys* and *Haematobia* (*Lyperosia*), that are often present in faeces. Development to L_3 occurs synchronously with the development to maturity of the fly intermediate host. When the fly feeds around the mouth, lips, ocular conjunctiva and nostrils of the horse, the larvae pass from its mouthparts onto the skin and are swallowed. Alternatively, infected flies may be swallowed whole in feed and drinking water. Development to adult takes place in the stomach where the larvae burrow into the glandular area of the mucosa and induce the formation of nodules. The worms develop to mature adults within the nodules in about eight weeks. When the larvae are deposited on a skin wound or around the eyes, they can invade the tissues; they do not complete their development but may cause granulomatous skin lesions. See **life cycle 13**.

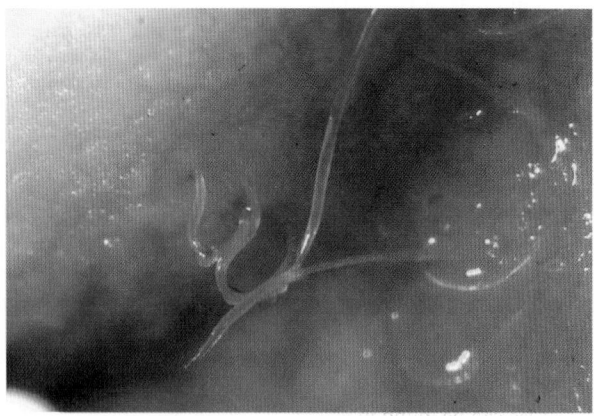

Fig. 1.73 Adult *Habronema* worms.

LIFE CYCLE 13. LIFE CYCLE OF *HABRONEMA MUSCAE*, *HABRONEMA MICROSTOMA* AND *DRASCHIA MEGASTOMA*

The adults of *Habronema muscae*, *Habronema microstoma* and *Draschia megastoma* live in the stomach (1) and, after mating, the females release larvated eggs, a proportion of which hatch during transit through the gastrointestinal tract, thus freeing the L_1, with the remainder excreted with the faeces and hatching in the external environment (2). The life cycle requires larval stages of flies that act as intermediate hosts. Briefly, fly larvae hatching from the eggs deposited on the host faecal pat (3) ingest the nematode larvae (4), and the development of the fly larvae occurs simultaneously to that of the nematodes (5), with adult flies harbouring infective third-stage larvae (L_3) (6). Infected flies, attracted by host secretions, land on the latter and release larvae of *Habronema* and *Draschia* (7). The larvae deposited near the lips and perilabial area (8) are swallowed, thus reaching the stomach (9) and developing to sexually mature adults within two months, completing the life cycle. Definitive hosts may also acquire the infection via ingestion of water and feedstuffs contaminated by infected flies (10). The larvae deposited on the skin (11), particularly on wounds and abrasions, cause cutaneous habronemiasis (12), while those deposited on the nasal mucosa can migrate to the lungs and establish in the bronchioles and alveoli, causing pulmonary habronemiasis (13).

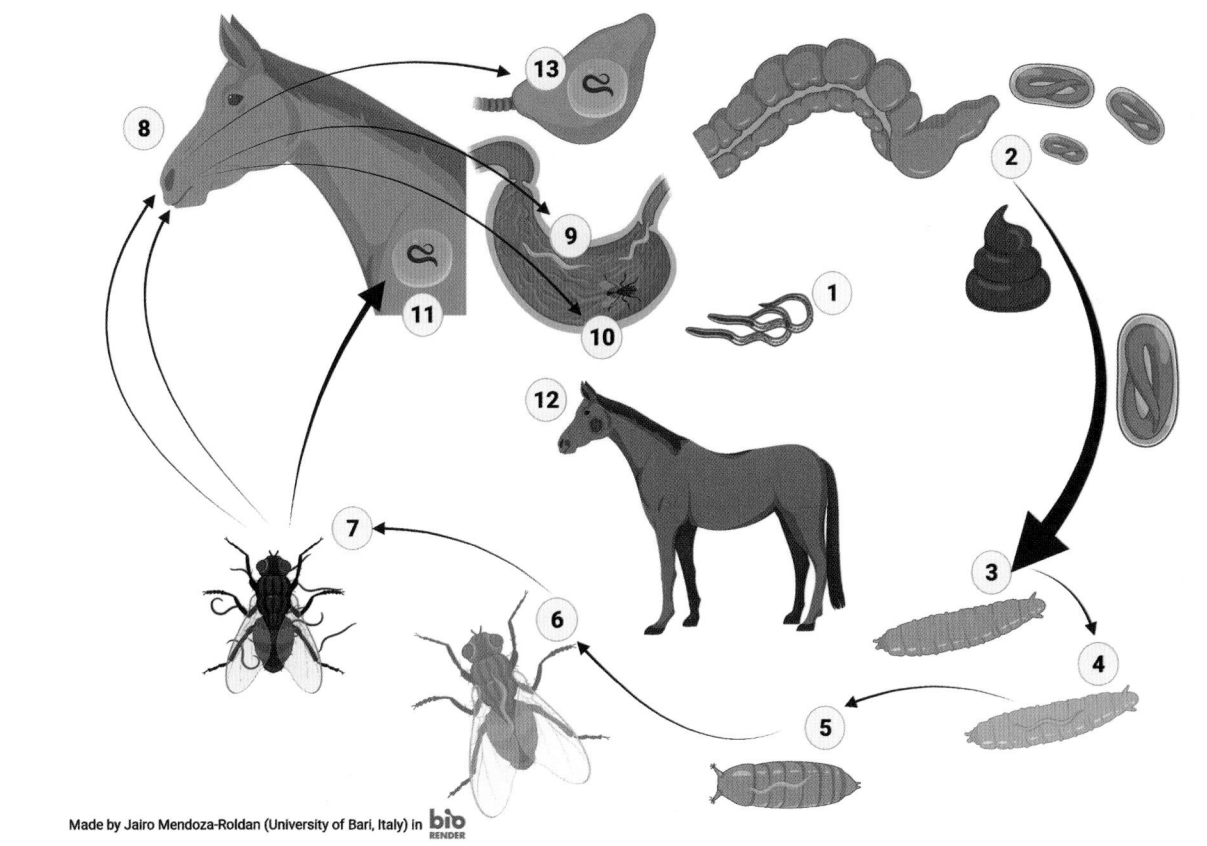

Made by Jairo Mendoza-Roldan (University of Bari, Italy) in bio RENDER

Habronema microstoma

Description: Adult males are 16–22 mm and females 15–25 mm long. The anterior region of the cylindrical pharynx contains a small dorsal and ventral tooth in its anterior region. Four pairs of precloacal papillae are present in the male worm. Spicules are uneven in length, with the left spicule (0.8 mm) being about twice as long as the right (0.4 mm). The buccal cavity is cylindrical in shape and the pharynx contains a dorsal and ventral tooth in its anterior part. The male has four pairs of precloacal papillae. Spicules are uneven in length, with the slender left one longer than the right. The very elongated, ellipsoidal, small eggs are thin-shelled, about 45–59 by 10–16 µm, and larvated when shed in faeces. Both eggs and larvae can be found in faeces. Eggs resemble those of *Draschia* but are slightly larger.

Habronema muscae

Description: Slender white translucent worms, 1–2.5 cm long; adult males are 8–14 mm and females 13–25 mm. The male has wide caudal alae and the tail has a spiral twist. It is unlikely to be confused with other nematodes in the stomach since *Draschia* is associated with characteristic lesions and *Trichostrongylus axei* is less than 1 cm in length. There are two lateral trilobed lips; the pharynx is cylindrical and has a thick cuticular lining. There are four pairs of precloacal papillae and one or two papillae behind the cloaca. The cloacal region is covered with small cuticlar ridges. Spicules are uneven in length, with the slender left one about five times longer than the right. The vulva is situated near the middle of the body and opens dorsolaterally. The elongated, oval, small eggs are thin-shelled, 40–50 by 10–12 µm, and larvated when shed in faeces. Eggs or larvae may be observed in the faeces.

Draschia

These worms are very similar to *Habronema* but smaller with a distinct collar in the anterior region. *Draschia* parasitises the fundic region of the stomach wall and provokes the formation of large fibrous nodules that are occasionally significant. The female worms are ovoviviparous. The main species is *Draschia megastoma* (syn. *Habronema megastoma*) which infects the stomach of horses and other equids. This parasite has dipteran flies, *Musca*, *Stomoxys* and *Haematobia* (*Lyperosia*) as intermediate hosts.

Draschia megastoma

Description: Slender white translucent worms 7–13 mm long; adult males are 7–10 mm and females 10–13 mm. The worms are recognised by their heads, which are slightly constricted from the main body by a deep groove which circles the body just posteriorly to the oral region (Fig. 1.74). The pharynx is funnel-shaped. Male worms have four pairs of precloacal papillae. The spicules are short and uneven in length with the left (0.5 mm) longer than the right (0.25 mm). The eggs are thin-shelled and elongate and measure around 35 by 8 μm and hatch in the stomach.

Parabronema

Parabronema are found in the abomasum of ruminants. The genus is readily distinguished from the other abomasal worms by the presence of large cuticular shields and cordons in the cephalic region.

Life cycle: Eggs or L_1 are passed in the faeces and the L_1 are ingested by the larval stages of various muscid flies that are often present in faeces. Development to L_3 occurs synchronously with the develop-

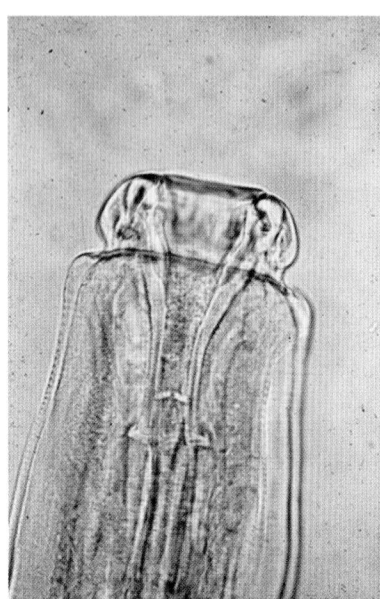

Fig. 1.74 Head of *Drachsia megastoma*.

ment to maturity of the fly intermediate host. When the fly feeds around the mouth, lips and nostrils of the host, the larvae pass from its mouthparts onto the skin and are swallowed. Alternatively, infected flies may be swallowed whole in feed and drinking water. Development to adult takes place in the glandular area of the abomasum. The main species is *Parabronema skrjabini* which infects the abomasum of sheep, goats, cattle and camels. This parasite has muscid flies of the genera *Stomoxys*, *Lyperosia* and *Haematobia* as intermediate hosts.

Parabronema skrjabini

Description: The white slender adult worms (up to 3.6 cm long) resemble *Haemonchus* spp. somewhat in gross form and size, but without the red spiral coloration, while the younger worms are closer to *Ostertagia* in appearance. Males measure 15–18 mm with one spicule. The genus is readily distinguished from the other abomasal worms by the presence of large cuticular shields and cordons in the cephalic region. The tail of the male is spiral with four pairs of preanal papillae.

Histiocephalus

The main species is *Histiocephalus laticaudatus* which infects the gizzard of chickens and ducks. The intermediate host of this parasite is unknown.

Histiocephalus laticaudatus

Description: Males measure around 7–7.5 mm and females 13–16 mm in length. The mouth is surrounded by four lips and the pseudolips are indented, forming 10 finger-like expansions, each with two or three points. Adult worms have ornate leaf-like structures and a cervical collar. The buccal cavity is cylindrical. Males have two large alae and four pairs of precloacal papillae and two pairs of postcloacal papillae. Spicules are long and of equal length. A gubernaculum is absent. The vulva in the female is situated anteriorly.

Life cycle: Little is known of the life cycle.

FAMILY THELAZIDAE

Thelazia

Members of this genus are parasites of the conjunctival sac and lacrimal duct and because of their location are also known as 'eye-worms' (Table 1.35). Worms have a large vestibule and lips are absent in this genus. Prominent striations are present on the anterior cuticle. Caudal alae are absent in the male worms.

Life cycle: The worms are viviparous. The L_1 passed by the female worm into the lacrimal secretion are ingested by the fly intermediate host as it feeds. Development from L_1 to L_3 occurs in the ovarian follicles of the fly in 15–30 days during the summer months. L_3 migrate to the mouthparts of the fly and are transferred to the final host when the fly feeds. Development in the eye takes place without further migration. See **life cycle 14**.

Table 1.35 *Thelazia* species.

Species	Hosts	Site	Intermediate hosts
Thelazia rhodesi	Cattle, buffalo, occasionally sheep, goats, camels	Eye, conjunctival sac, lacrimal duct	Muscid flies, particularly *Fannia* spp.
Thelazia gulosa (syn. *Thelazia alfortensis*)	Cattle, sheep, wild ruminants	Eye, conjunctival sac, lacrimal duct	Muscid flies (*Musca* spp.)
Thelazia skrjabini	Cattle, sheep, wild ruminants	Eye, conjunctival sac, lacrimal duct	Muscid flies (*Musca* spp.)
Thelazia callipaeda	Dogs, cats, humans, primates, rabbits, foxes, bears, wolves, badgers	Eye, conjunctival sac, lacrimal duct	Muscid flies, fruit flies
Thelazia californiensis	Dogs, cats, sheep, deer, humans	Eye, conjunctival sac, lacrimal duct	Muscid flies
Thelazia lacrymalis	Horses, cattle	Eye, conjunctival sac, lacrimal duct	Face flies (*Musca* spp.)
Thelazia leesi	Camels	Conjunctival sac	Muscid flies

LIFE CYCLE 14. LIFE CYCLE OF *THELAZIA CALLIPAEDA*

Thelazia spp. are spirurid nematodes that infect the eye (1) of several mammals, including dogs, cats, rabbits, foxes, wolves and humans. The adult nematodes live under the eyelids and nictitating membrane of the hosts (1), and are sexually dimorphic. After mating, the females (viviparous) release large numbers of first-stage larvae (2) in the lacrimal secretions. The latter, free on the cornea, are ingested by sucking insects (*Phortica variegata*) that feed on eye secretions (3). *Phortica variegata* is active in Mediterranean regions between April and October when it actively seeks to feed on lacrimal secretions, thus acting as intermediate host of *T. callipaeda*. Within the insect, the L_1 remain encapsulated and develop to second- and third-stage larvae (4). The latter migrate from the coelomatic cavity of the intermediate host to the thorax and the buccal apparatus within 21 days. When the intermediate host feeds on a new susceptible host, the larvae are released from the proboscis and deposited onto the ocular mucosa (5), where they develop into sexually mature adults within four weeks, depending on the season. The other species of *Thelazia* are characterised by a similar life cycle, except for their intermediate hosts, belonging to flies of the family Muscidae.

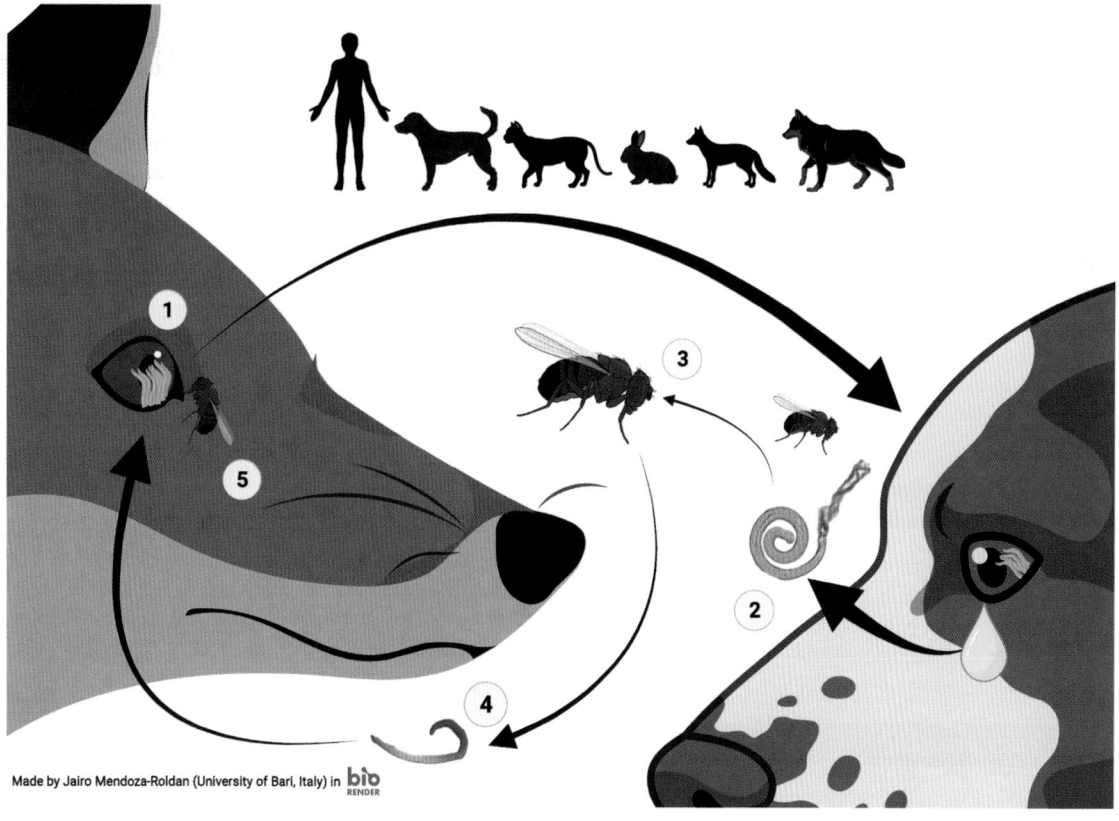

Made by Jairo Mendoza-Roldan (University of Bari, Italy) in **bio** RENDER

Thelazia rhodesi

Description: Small, thin, yellowish-white worms 1–2 cm long. Males are 8–12 mm and females are 12–20 mm in length. A mouth capsule is present and the cuticle has prominent striations at the anterior end. The male worms have about 14 pairs of precloacal and three pairs of postcloacal papillae.

Life cycle: The prepatent period is 20–25 days.

Thelazia gulosa

Synonym: *Thelazia alfortensis*

Description: *Thelazia gulosa* are milky-white worms, with thin transverse cuticular striations (less evident in rear part of the body), and a large, deep, cup-shaped buccal cavity. Males are 4.8–10.9 mm long and have a variable number of precloacal papillae (from 8 to 33 pairs) and three pairs of postcloacal papillae. There are two asymmetrical spicules. The females are 4.8–18.8 mm long with a tapered caudal extremity.

Thelazia skrjabini

Description: Adult worms are whitish in colour, with transverse fine cuticular striations. The buccal cavity is small and shallow. Males are 5–11.5 mm long and curved posteriorly, with 16–32 pairs of precloacal and three pairs of postcloacal papillae. The spicules are unequal in length. The females are 7.5–21 mm long with a truncated caudal extremity.

Thelazia callipaeda

Description: Small thin white worms 1–1.7 cm long; males are 7–11.5 mm and females 7–17 mm in length. The cuticle bears fine transverse striations. The male has one single and five pairs of precloacal papillae and two pairs of postcloacal papillae. The left spicule is much longer (about 10 times) than the right. In the female, the vulva is in the oesophageal region. When laid, the eggs contain fully developed larvae.

Thelazia californiensis

Description: Small thin white worms 1–1.5 cm long. A mouth capsule is present and the cuticle has prominent striations at the anterior end. The male has 10 pairs of caudal papillae. The left spicule is long and slender and the right spicule short and stout.

Thelazia lacrymalis

Description: Small thin yellowish-white worms 1–2 cm long. Males are 8–12 mm and females 14–18 mm. A mouth capsule is present and the cuticle has prominent striations at the anterior end. In the male, the tail is blunt and recurved with caudal alae.

Life cycle: The prepatent period is about 3–6 weeks.

Oxyspirura

Eyeworms of birds found on the conjunctiva, under the nictitating membrane or in the nasal–lacrimal ducts.

Life cycle: The life cycle is indirect. Eggs pass through the lacrimal duct, are swallowed and shed in the faeces. These are ingested by an intermediate host and development to the infective stage occurs. Following consumption of the intermediate host by the definitive host, the larvae migrate from the oesophagus and pharynx to the eye via the lacrimal duct. The main species is *Oxyspirura mansoni* (syn. *Oxyspirura parvorum*) which infects the eye, conjunctiva and lacrimal ducts of chickens, turkeys and guinea fowl. This parasite has cockroaches and mayflies (Ephemeroptera) as intermediate hosts.

Oxyspirura mansoni

Synonym: *Oxyspirura parvorum*

Description: These are slender worms with a smooth cuticle and a globular-shaped pharynx; in the female, the vulva is near the tail. The males measure around 10–15 mm and the females 14–20 mm. The tail of the male is curved ventrally and alae are absent. Spicules are uneven, the right being short and stubby, the left long (about 15 times the length of the right spicule) and slender. In the female worm, the vulva is near the tail. The medium-sized ovoid egg is embryonated when laid and measures on average about 65 by 45 µm.

FAMILY GNATHOSTOMATIDAE

Gnathostoma

These are parasites of the stomach of carnivores (Table 1.36). The presence of the worms in gastric nodules is sufficient for generic diagnosis.

Gnathostoma spinigerum

Description: Thick-bodied worms, reddish at the front and greyish posteriorly. The males are 1–2.5 cm and the females up to 3 cm long. The presence of the worms in gastric nodules is sufficient for generic diagnosis. Confirmation is easily made with a hand lens when the swollen anterior head bulb covered with transverse rows of 6–11 small hooks will be seen. The head contains four submedian cavities that each communicate with a cervical sac. The anterior of the body is covered with flat cuticular spines and the ventral caudal region of the male bears small spines and four pairs of large

Table 1.36 *Gnathostoma* species.

Species	Hosts	Site	Intermediate hosts
Gnathostoma spinigerum	Cats, dogs, humans, mink, polecats and several wild carnivores	Stomach	Freshwater crustaceans, copepods
Gnathostoma hispidum	Pigs, rarely humans	Stomach	Freshwater crustaceans, *Cyclops* spp.
Gnathostoma doloresi	Pigs, wild boar	Stomach	Freshwater crustaceans

pedunculate papillae as well as several smaller sessile ones. The left spicule is longer than the right. The medium-sized eggs are oval, with a greenish shell which possesses fine granulations, and they have a thin cap at one pole. Eggs measure 69 by 37 μm and contain one cell or a morula when passed in faeces.

Life cycle: The adult worms live in tunnels in the gastric nodules, and the eggs pass from there into the lumen and are dropped into the water in the faeces where they hatch after several days. The crustaceans (first intermediate hosts) ingest L_1 and development to L_2 takes place. The crustaceans are themselves ingested by vertebrates (second intermediate hosts), such as fish, frogs and reptiles, and development to L_3 occurs and the larvae become encysted. The L_3 can also encyst in many mammals such as mice, rats and dogs. The final host is infected by ingestion of the vertebrate vector and further development occurs in the stomach wall, where the worms provoke the growth of fibrous lesions.

Gnathostoma hispidum

Description: Thick-bodied worms; the males are 1.5–2.5 cm and the females 2–4.5 cm long. Spiny scales cover the whole body of the worm. The left spicule is about three times longer than the right spicule. Eggs are oval, 72–74 by 39–42 μm, with a thin cap at one pole (Fig. 1.75).

Life cycle: The young worms migrate in the abdominal organs of the host, particularly the liver. Adult worms live in tunnels in the gastric nodules, and the eggs pass from there into the lumen and are dropped into the water in the faeces where they develop to L_2 before hatching after several days. Crustaceans ingest L_2 and development to L_3 takes place within about 10 days. The final host is infected by ingestion of the crustacean intermediate host and further development occurs in the stomach wall, where the deeply embedded worms provoke the growth of fibrous lesions. A second intermediate host is not required with *G. hispidum*.

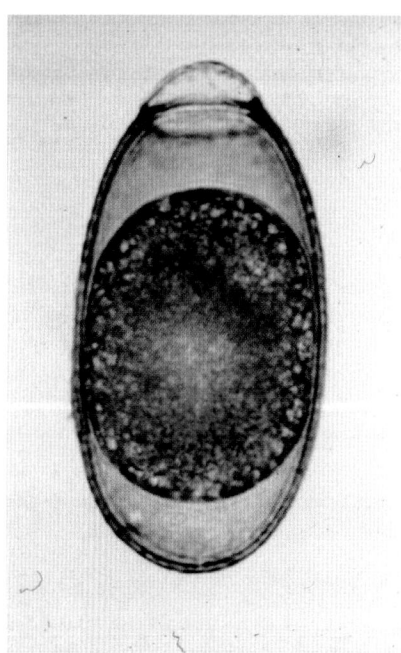

Fig. 1.75 *Gnathostoma hispidum* egg.

Gnathostoma doloresi

Description: Adult male worms are 2.6–2.8 cm long and female worms 3–4 cm long. The entire body surface has numerous transverse rows of backwardly directed cuticular spines. Anteriorly, the spines are broad and short, with several unequal teeth, becoming gradually smaller, with single-pointed spines posteriorly. The spicules are unequal, stout and curved, tapering evenly from root to tip.

Life cycle: As for *G. hispidum*.

FAMILY GONGYLONEMATIDAE

Gongylonema

Thread-like parasitic worms of mammals and birds often referred to as 'gullet worms', with over 30 species described (Table 1.37). Both sexes have cervical alae and the males possess caudal alae which are often asymmetrical.

Life cycle: The life cycle is typically spiruroid. Eggs are passed in faeces and when eaten by an intermediate host, they hatch and develop to the infective stage within about four weeks. Infection of the definitive host is through the ingestion of infected coprophagous beetles or cockroaches. The adult worms live spirally (in a zipper fashion) embedded in the mucosa or submucosa with their anterior and/or posterior ends protruding into the lumen. The prepatent period is about eight weeks.

Gongylonema ingluvicola

Description: These are long slender worms. The female worm is about 32–55 mm and the males around 18 mm long. The anterior end of the body has a number of longitudinal rows of round or oval, wart-like cuticular plaques. The eggs measure approximately 58 by 35 μm.

Table 1.37 *Gongylonema* species.

Species	Hosts	Site	Intermediate hosts
Gongylonema ingluvicola	Chickens, turkeys, partridges, pheasants, quails	Crop, oesophagus	Coprophagous beetles, cockroaches
Gongylonema monnigi	Sheep, goats	Rumen	Coprophagous beetles, cockroaches
Gongylonema pulchrum (syn. *Gongylonema scutatum*)	Sheep, goats, cattle, pigs, zebus, buffalo, horses, donkeys, deer, camels, humans, primates	Oesophagus, rumen	Coprophagous beetles, cockroaches
Gongylonema verrucosum	Cattle, sheep, goats, deer, zebus	Rumen, reticulum, omasum	Coprophagous beetles, cockroaches
Gongylonema macrogubernaculum	Old and New World Monkeys	Oesophagus, tongue, buccal cavity	Coprophagous beetles, cockroaches

Gongylonema monnigi

Description: A long, slender, whitish worm, the males being about 4 cm and the females up to about 11 cm in length. Similar to G. verrucosum except the cervical ala is not festooned and the shape of the gubernaculum differs.

Gongylonema pulchrum

Synonym: *Gongylonema scutatum*

Description: A long, slender, whitish worm, the males being about 5 cm and the females up to about 14 cm in length. Worms are easily distinguished microscopically by the presence of longitudinal rows of cuticular bosses in the anterior region of the body. Asymmetrical cervical alae are prominent. The tail of the male has asymmetrical alae with 10 pairs of papillae. The left spicule is long and slender whereas the right spicule is short and stout. The male has a gubernaculum. The egg is thick-shelled and possesses two opercula. It measures 50–70 by 25–37 μm and contains an L_1 when passed in faeces.

Gongylonema verrucosum

Description: Long slender worms, reddish when fresh. The males are about 3.5 cm and the females 7–9.5 cm in length. The adult worms have a festooned cervical ala and cuticular bosses only on the left side of the body. The males' spicules are unequal in length with the left spicule considerably longer than the right.

Gongylonema macrogubernaculum

Description: These are long thin whitish worms, the males measuring about 5 cm and the females around 14 cm in length. Worms are characterised by the presence of longitudinal rows of cuticular bosses in the anterior region of the body.

FAMILY SPIRURIDAE

Nematodes of the family Spiruridae are found in the upper digestive tract of mammals and birds (Table 1.38).

Spirura/Odontospirura

Life cycle: The life cycle is typically spiruroid. Eggs develop into infective larvae within an intermediate host. Larvae may be ingested by paratenic hosts, such as rodents and lizards, in which they

Table 1.38 *Spirura* species.

Species	Hosts	Site	Intermediate hosts
Spirura ritypleurites	Cats, rarely dogs, foxes	Stomach	Beetles, cockroaches
Spirura uncinipenis (syn. Sicarius uncinipenis)	Rheas	Proventriculus	Beetles, cockroaches
Spirura zschokkei (syn. Vaznema zschokkei)	Rheas	Proventriculus	Beetles, cockroaches
Odontospirura cetiopenis	Rheas	Proventriculus, gizzard	Beetles, cockroaches

become encapsulated. The final host becomes infected by ingesting the insects or their transport hosts.

Spirura ritypleurites

Description: Thick, short, white worms with the posterior region thicker than the anterior and twisted in a spiral. Male worms measure up to 26 mm and females can be 30 mm in length. The anterior area of the cuticle is inflated on the underside and the transverse striations are prominent. The eggs have a thick shell and are embryonated when passed and measure up to 52 by 36 μm.

Spirura uncinipenis

Synonym: *Sicarius uncinipenis*

Description: Males measure 15–20 mm and females 16–26 mm. The spicules are short and unequal in length.

Spirura zschokkei

Synonym: *Vaznema zschokkei*

Description: Male worms measure 16–17 mm and females 17–25 mm in length. The spicules are long and filiform.

Odontospirura cetiopenis

Description: The body is spirally coiled, with male worms measuring 15–17 mm and females 20–23 mm. Four pairs of cephalic papillae are present at the base of the lips. Males have caudal alae and long spicules of equal length.

FAMILY TETRAMERIDAE

Tetrameres

Parasites of this genus show sexual dimorphism. The male worms are pale white, small and slender and lie in the lumen of the proventriculus of birds (Table 1.39). The females are bright red and almost spherical, and lie embedded in the proventricular glands. Cordons are absent.

Life cycle: Eggs are shed with the faeces and hatch when eaten by an intermediate host. The final host becomes infected following ingestion of the intermediate host and the males and females locate in the glands of the proventriculus. Males inhabit the mucosal surface and upper regions of the glands but after mating they leave the glands and die. The females are embedded deep in the mucosal glands.

Tetrameres americana

Synonym: *Tropisurus americana*

Description: The adults show sexual dimorphism. The males are pale, white, slender and only about 5–6 mm long. The females are bright red and almost spherical, with a diameter of about

Table 1.39 *Tetrameres* species.

Species	Hosts	Site	Intermediate hosts
Tetrameres americana (syn. *Tropisurus americana*)	Chickens, turkeys, ducks, geese, grouse, quails, pigeons	Proventriculus	Cockroaches, grasshoppers, beetles
Tetrameres fissispina (syn. *Tropisurus fissispina*)	Ducks, geese, chickens, turkeys, pigeons and wild aquatic birds	Proventriculus	Crustaceans (*Daphnia* and *Gammarus*), grasshoppers, earthworms
Tetrameres crami	Domestic and wild ducks	Proventriculus	Crustaceans (*Gammarus* and *Hyalella*)
Tetrameres confusa	Chickens	Proventriculus	?
Tetrameres mohtedai	Chickens	Proventriculus	?
Tetrameres pattersoni	Quails	Proventriculus	?

3.5–4.5 mm (Fig. 1.76). Males have spiny cuticles and no cordons; females have four longitudinal deep furrows on the surface. Eggs are oval, thick-shelled, 42–60 by 24–45 µm and embryonated when passed. They are transparent in appearance and have thickened poles (see Fig. 4.8).

Tetrameres fissispina

Synonym: *Tropisurus fissispina*

Description: See *T. americana*. Males are pale, white, slender and 5–6 mm long. The females are bright red, ovoid/spherical, with a diameter varying from around 2.5 to 6 mm. Males have four longitudinal rows of spines along the median and lateral lines and no cordons; females have four longitudinal deep furrows on the surface. Eggs are essentially similar to those of *T. americana* and measure 48–56 by 26–30 µm.

Tetrameres crami

Description: Males are white, slender and about 4 mm long. The red ovoid/spherical females measure around 2 mm by 1.5 mm.

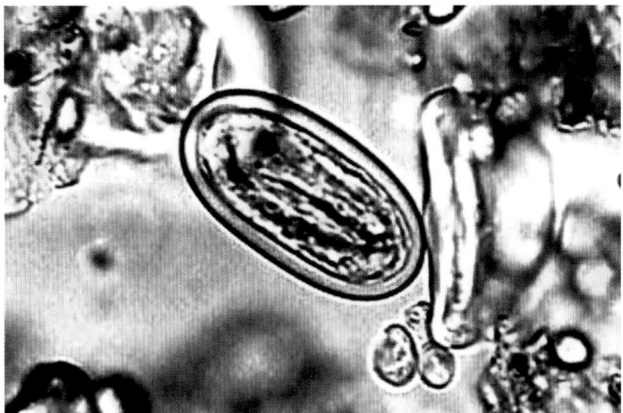

Fig. 1.76 Adult female *Tetrameres americana*.

FAMILY HARTERTIIDAE

Hartertia

The main species is *Hartertia gallinarum* which infects the small intestine of chickens and bustards. This parasite has termites as intermediate hosts.

Hartertia gallinarum

Description: Slender worms and exceptionally long for a spiruroid. The males measure up to around 40 mm and the females up to 110 mm in length. The gross appearance of the worms closely resembles that of *Ascaridia galli* and they have two lateral lips, each divided medially into three lobes. The posterior of the male has lateral alae, ventral cuticular bosses and four pairs of precloacal and two pairs of postcloacal papillae. The left spicule has a barbed expansion at its tip and is about four times larger than the blunt-ended right spicule. Eggs are thick-shelled, 45–53 by 27–33 µm, and are embryonated when passed.

Life cycle: Eggs are passed in faeces and, when ingested by a termite, develop to the infective stage in the body cavity. Following ingestion of an infected intermediate host, the larvae develop to maturity in the final host in about three weeks.

FAMILY PNEUMOSPIRIDAE

Members of this family are lungworms of wild felids and include species within the genera *Metathelazia* and *Vogeloides*.

SUPERFAMILY PHYSALOPTEROIDEA

FAMILY PHYSALOPTERIDAE

Physaloptera

The genus *Physaloptera* includes a number of species that are parasites of the stomach of mammals and other vertebrates. In particular, *Physaloptera praeputialis* infects cats, wild felids and rarely dogs, whereas *Physaloptera rara* infects cats and dogs.

Life cycle: The life cycle is typically spiruroid. Eggs passed in the faeces of the infected host develop into infective larvae if ingested by coprophagous beetles, crickets and other insects. The life cycle is completed when cats ingest the intermediate hosts. Various cold-blooded transport hosts may also be involved in transmission of infection. The prepatent period is around 8–10 weeks.

Physaloptera praeputialis

Description: Adult worms are white or pinkish in colour and larger than most spiruroids, being stout and resembling ascarids. Males measure 1–45 mm and females 2–60 mm. The cuticle in both sexes extends posteriorly as a sheath (pseudolabia) beyond the end of the body and the mouth is surrounded by a cuticular collar. The lips are simple and bear a set of three flattened internal teeth and a single conical external tooth. The male bears lateral alae, joined anteriorly

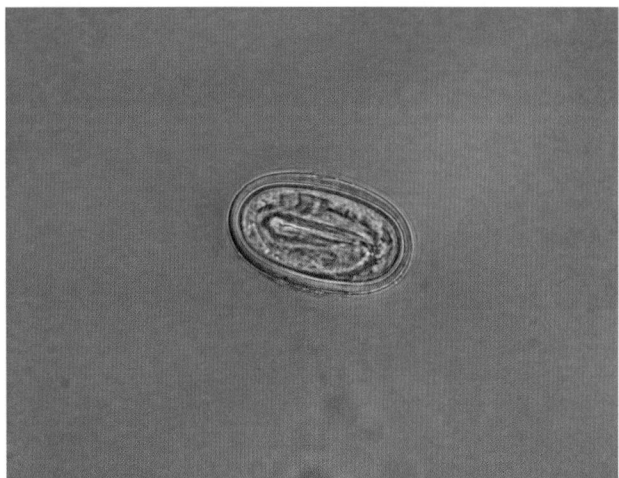

Fig. 1.77 *Physaloptera* egg. (Courtesy of Jana Bulantová).

across the ventral surface. In the female, the vulva is slightly anterior to the mid-body. The larvated eggs have a thick clear shell and measure 45–58 by 30–36 μm (Fig. 1.77).

Physaloptera rara

Description: Adult male worms are 2.5–3 cm and females 3–6 cm long. This species differs from *P. praeputialis* in that there is no sheath over the posterior portion of the body in both sexes. The female vulva is anterior to the middle of the body. Eggs are thick-shelled and ellipsoid, 42–53 by 29–35 μm.

SUPERFAMILY DRACUNCULOIDEA

Members of this superfamily are parasites of the subcutaneous tissues. The two genera of veterinary significance are *Dracunculus* and *Avioserpens*. The life cycle involves development in a species of *Cyclops* before becoming infective to the final host.

FAMILY DRACUNCULIDAE

Dracunculus

This genus includes the 'guinea worm', an important parasite affecting humans, and the North American guinea worm found in carnivores. The male worms are very much smaller than the females and the latter are one of the longest of the common nematodes in human and animals.

Life cycle: This is indirect. Adult worms mature in deep connective tissue and then migrate to peripheral subcutaneous tissue about nine months after initial infection. A cutaneous blister develops around the head end of the worm and when this makes contact with water, the uterus of the worm ruptures and liberates large numbers of L_1 larvae. Release of larvae can continue over several weeks if the lesion is repeatedly immersed in water. These larvae develop to the infective stage in a species of *Cyclops*. Infection of the final host is through ingestion of infected copepods with drinking water or within paratenic hosts.

Dracunculus medinensis

Description: Males measure about 2–3 cm; females are much larger, being around 100 cm long and 1.5–2 mm in width, but they can reach up to 300 cm in length. The anterior of the worms possess a 'helmet'. Females have no vulva.

Life cycle: Infection is caused by drinking water containing copepods, which are infected with larvae of *D. medinensis*. Following ingestion by the hosts (e.g. human; occasionally cattle, horse, dog, cat and other mammals), the copepods die and release the larvae, which penetrate the host stomach and intestinal wall and enter the abdominal cavity. After maturation into adults and copulation, the male worms die and the females migrate in the subcutaneous tissues near the skin surface, where the female worm induces a blister on the skin that ruptures. When this lesion comes into contact with water, the female worm emerges and releases larvae, which if ingested by a copepod develop into infective larvae after about two weeks. The prepatent period is around 12 months.

Dracunculus insignis

Description: Adults are white cylindrical worms 17.6–23 cm in length and 3–4 mm at maximum width. The females are much larger than the males and are filled with first-stage larvae. This species can be differentiated from *D. medinensis* by the number of preanal papillae and also the length of the gubernaculum.

Life cycle: Similar to *D. medinensis*. Development in the copepod is around three weeks. Hosts are mink, raccoon, otter, wild carnivores; occasionally dog and cat. Frogs can also act as paratenic intermediate hosts.

Avioserpens

Avioserpens are parasites of ducks and are found in subcutaneous swellings.

Life cycle: Larvae are released into water and infective stages have been shown to occur in *Cyclops*. Infection of the final host occurs through ingestion of the intermediate host.

Avioserpens taiwana

Synonyms: *Filaria taiwana*, *Oshimaia taiwana*, *Avioserpens denticulophasma*, *Petroviprocta vigissi*

Description: The female measures up to about 25 cm in length by 0.8 mm in width. The anterior end is blunt and a chitinous rim, carrying two prominent lateral papillae, surrounds the mouth. Four smaller papillae are found further back on the head. The large uterus contains larvae. The anus, vagina and vulva are atrophied. A conical papilla is sited at the termination of the tail. The male worm is unknown.

SUPERFAMILY ACUARIOIDEA

Members of the Acuarioidea (formerly Spiruroidea) are small to medium-sized nematodes inhabiting the upper alimentary tract of birds. The species are characterised by the presence of peculiar cuticular cephalic structures (cordons) extending posteriorly, and sometimes recur forwards.

FAMILY ACURIDAE

Echinuria

The main species is *Echinuria uncinata* (syn. *Acuaria uncinata*) which infects the oesophagus, proventriculusand gizzard of ducks, geese, swans and various aquatic birds. This parasite has *Daphnia* and *Gammarus* as intermediate hosts.

Echinuria uncinata

Synonym: *Acuaria uncinata*

Description: These are small whitish worms with a slender body. Males measure 8–10 mm and females 12–18.5 mm long. The cuticle is ornamented with four wavy cordons that are non-recurrent and they anastomose in pairs and do not extend beyond the oesophagus section. Four rows of longitudinal spines are present on the cuticle. In the male, there are four pairs of precloacal papillae in two groups of two either side, and four pairs of postcloacal papillae. The left spicule is about 3–4 times longer than the right spicule. The small ellipsoidal eggs are thick-shelled with a smooth surface. They measure on average 37 by 20 μm and are embryonated when passed (see Fig. 4.8).

Life cycle: Eggs are passed in the faeces and ingested by water fleas in which they hatch and develop to infective larvae. The parasites continue development when the intermediate host is ingested by an aquatic bird.

Dispharynx

The main species is *Dispharynx nasuta* (syn. *Dispharynx spiralis, Acuaria spiralis, Acuaria nasuta*) which infects the oesophagus and proventriculus of chickens, turkeys, pigeons, guinea fowl, grouses pheasants and other birds. This parasite has isopods, including sowbugs (*Porcellio*) and pillbugs (*Armadillidium*), as intermediate hosts.

Dispharynx nasuta

Synonyms: *Dispharynx spiralis, Acuaria spiralis, Acuaria nasuta*

Description: The body is slender and coiled, particularly the posterior of the male. Males measure up to around 8 mm and the females 10–12 mm long. The cuticle is ornamented with four wavy cordons that recurve anteriorly and do not fuse. The male has four pairs of precloacal and five pairs of postcloacal papillae. The left spicule is slender and the right spicule shorter and oval-shaped. The eggs are thick-shelled, 33–40 by 18–25 μm, and embryonated when passed.

Life cycle: The intermediate host ingests embryonated eggs and development to L_3 takes place in the body cavity. When the isopod is consumed by the final host, the worms develop to the final stage in the proventriculus or oesophagus.

Cheilospirura

The main species is *Cheilospirura hamulosa* (syn. *Acuaria hamulosa*) which infects the gizzard of chickens and turkeys. This parasite has grasshoppers (*Melanoplus*), weevils and beetles as intermediate hosts.

Cheilospirura hamulosa

Synonym: *Acuaria hamulosa*

Description: The worms have four, double-wavy, irregular, cuticular ridged cordons that extend to more than half the length of the body. These cordons do not anastomose or recur anteriorly. Male worms measure up to 15 mm and females 30 mm. The males have four pairs of precloacal and six pairs of postcloacal papillae, a short flattened spicule on the right and a longer slender spicule on the left side. The oval eggs measure about 40–45 by 24–47 μm and are embryonated when passed. The egg is very similar in size and appearance to that of *Dispharynx*.

Life cycle: Eggs shed in the faeces are ingested by the intermediate host where they develop to the infective stage in about three weeks. The final host becomes infected after consuming this intermediate host and the prepatent period is about three weeks.

Streptocara

These worms are of minor importance in domestic livestock. The main species is *Streptocara crassicauda* which infects the gizzard of ducks and chickens. This parasite has crustacea (*Gammarus*) as intermediate hosts.

Streptocara crassicauda

Description: Males are about 5 mm and females up to 10 mm in length. The cervical alae are well developed and possess small teeth on the posterior margin.

Life cycle: Little is known of the life cycle.

SUPERFAMILY FILARIOIDEA

This superfamily is closely related to the Spiruroidea and, as in the latter, all its genera have indirect life cycles. None of them inhabits the alimentary tract, and they depend on insect vectors for transmission.

Within the superfamily, differences in biological behaviour are seen, the more primitive forms laying eggs, which are available to the vectors in dermal exudates, and the more highly evolved forms laying larvae, termed microfilariae. The latter, which may be enclosed in a flexible sheath-like 'eggshell', are taken up by parasitic insects feeding on blood and tissue fluids. In some species, the microfilariae only appear in the peripheral blood and tissues at regular intervals, some appearing in the daytime and others at night; this behaviour is termed diurnal or nocturnal periodicity.

Genera of interest in veterinary medicine include the Filariidae: *Parafilaria, Stephanofilaria, Suifilaria*; and the Onchocercidae: *Onchocerca, Dirofilaria, Acanthocheilonema, Pelecitus, Chandlerella, Setaria, Elaeophora, Splendidofilaria* and *Paronchocerca*.

FAMILY FILARIIDAE

Parafilaria

Adults of this genus of primitive filarioids live under the skin of cattle and buffalo (i.e. *Parafilaria bovicola*), horse, donkey and other equids (*Parafilaria multipapillosa*), where they produce inflammatory lesions or nodules.

Parafilaria bovicola

Description: Small slender white worms about 3–6 cm in length. Males are 2–3 cm and females 4–6 cm long. Anteriorly, there are numerous papillae and circular ridges in the cuticle. The rest of the cuticle is striated transversely. In the female, the vulva is situated anteriorly near the simple mouth opening and the tail is blunt with no papillae. The tail of the male is blunt and short. The caudal alae are supported by precloacal and postcloacal papillae. Small embryonated eggs, 45 by 30 μm, that have a thin flexible shell are laid on the skin surface where they hatch to release the microfilariae or L_1, which are about 200 μm in length.

Life cycle: Eggs or free L_1 present in exudates from bleeding points in the skin surface are ingested by muscid flies (e.g. *Musca autumnalis* in Europe, *M. lusoria* and *M. xanthomelas* in Africa) in which they develop to L_3 within several weeks to months, depending on air temperature. Transmission occurs when infected flies feed on lacrimal secretions or skin wounds in other cattle and the L_3 deposited then migrate in the subcutaneous tissue and develop to the adult stage under the skin in 5–7 months. Bleeding points develop 7–9 months after infection, which is about the same duration as patency.

Parafilaria multipapillosa

Synonym: *Filaria haemorrhagica*

Description: Slender white worms 3–7 cm in length. Adult males are 28 mm and females 40–70 mm in length. The anterior end of the worm bears a large number of papilliform thickenings. The small embryonated eggs (around 55 × 30 μm) have a thin flexible shell and are laid on the skin surface where they hatch to release the microfilariae or L_1; these are about 200 μm in length and have a rounded posterior extremity.

Life cycle: Eggs or free L_1 larvae present in exudates from bleeding points in the skin surface are ingested by horn flies (*Haematobia*), in which they develop to L_3 within several weeks to months, depending on air temperature. Transmission occurs when infected flies feed on lacrimal secretions or skin wounds in other horses and the L_3 deposited then migrate in the subcutaneous tissue and develop to the adult stage under the skin in 9–12 months.

Stephanofilaria

Worms of this genus inhabit the dermis and cause chronic dermatitis in cattle, buffalo, rhinoceros and elephants in the tropics and subtropics (Table 1.40). The genus is readily recognised because the worms are small, and the oral opening is surrounded by numerous spines.

Life cycle: The fly vectors are attracted to the open lesions in the skin caused by the adult parasites, and ingest the microfilariae in the exudate. Development to L_3 takes about three weeks, and the final host is infected when the flies deposit larvae on normal skin.

Stephanofilaria dedoesi

Description: Small nematodes; males are 2.3–3.2 mm and females 6.1–8.5 mm in length. A protruding cuticular rim, with a denticulate edge, surrounds the oral aperture. The anterior of the worms has a circular thickening, which possesses a number of small cuticular

Table 1.40 *Stephanofilaria* species.

Species	Hosts	Site	Intermediate hosts
Stephanofilaria assamensis	Cattle, goats, buffalo	Skin, back	Muscid flies
Stephanofilaria kaeli	Cattle	Skin, head, legs, teats	Muscid flies
Stephanofilaria dedoesi	Cattle	Skin, head, legs, teats	Muscid flies
Stephanofilaria okinawaensis	Cattle	Skin, face and teats	Muscid flies
Stephanofilaria stilesi	Cattle	Skin, lower abdomen	Horn flies (*Haematobia* spp.)
Stephanofilaria zaheeri	Buffalo, cattle	Skin, ears, legs, teats	Muscid flies

spines. An anus is absent in female worms. The male spicules are of unequal length.

Stephanofilaria stilesi

Description: Small nematodes; males are 2.6–3.7 mm and females 3.7–6.9 mm in length. There are 4–5 cephalic spines and 18–19 peribuccal spines. The male spicules are unequal and the female worms have no anus. The thin-shelled eggs are 58–72 by 42–55 μm in size. Microfilariae are 45–60 μm in length and are characterised by a peribuccal elevation with a single spine and a short and rounded tail.

Stephanofilaria okinawaensis

Description: The parasites are small, rounded, whitish and slender bodied. Females are 7–8.5 mm and males 2.7–3.5 mm in length.

Suifilaria

These worms can be associated with dermal abscesses but are generally of little veterinary significance.

Life cycle: Not known. The females appear to lay their eggs in the skin of the pig. The main species is *Suifilaria suis* which infects the subcutaneous connective tissue of pigs. The intermediate host is not known.

Suifilaria suis

Description: These are slender worms. Male are 17–25 mm and females 34–40 mm in length. The male only has one caudal ala and this is on the left. The hind end of the male is spirally coiled and the spicules are unequal, with the left shorter than the right. The tail of the female bears a number of small tubercles on its tip, which ends abruptly. Small embryonated eggs, 51–61 by 28–32 μm, have a thin flexible shell and are laid on the skin surface where they hatch to release the microfilariae or L_1, which are about 200 μm in length.

FAMILY ONCHOCERCIDAE

Dirofilaria

Of the two species occurring in domestic carnivores, *Dirofilaria immitis* is by far the more important since adults are found in the right side of the heart and adjacent blood vessels of dogs, being responsible for canine heartworm disease. Adults of *Dirofilaria repens* are localised in the subcutaneous tissues. Both species infect dog, fox, wild canids, occasionally cat and rarely human and primates.

Dirofilaria immitis

Description: Long slender white/grey worms measuring 15–30 cm in length with a tough cuticle. Adult females measure 25–30 cm, with the males about half as long. Many worms are usually found together in a tangled mass. The size and site are diagnostic for *D. immitis*. The male tail has the typical loose spiral common to the filarioids (Fig. 1.78), and the tail bears small lateral alae. There are 4–6 pairs of ovoid papillae. The left spicule is long and pointed; the right spicule is smaller and ends bluntly. In the female, the vulva is situated just behind the end of the oesophagus. The microfilariae in the blood are not ensheathed and are 307–332 μm in length by 6.8 μm wide. They have a tapered anterior end and blunt posterior end.

Life cycle: The adults live in the heart and adjacent blood vessels and the females release microfilariae directly into the bloodstream. These microfilariae can live for several months in the visceral blood vessels. Microfilariae are ingested by female mosquitoes during feeding. Development to infective L_3 in the malpighian tubules of

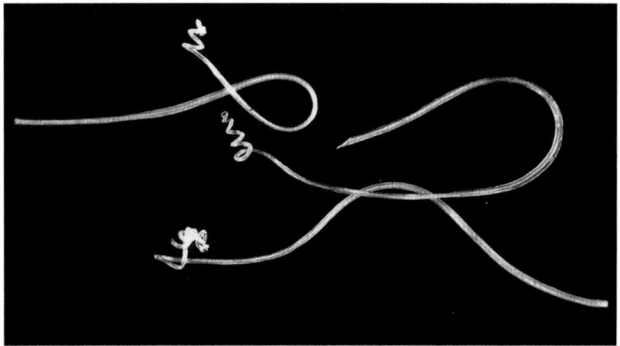

Fig. 1.78 Adult *Dirofilaria immitis* heartworms.

the mosquito takes about two weeks. The infective L_3 then migrate to the mouthparts and the final host is infected when the mosquito takes a further blood meal. In the dog, the L_3 migrate to the subcutaneous or subserosal tissues in the thorax or abdomen and undergo two moults over the next few months; only after the final moult do the young *D. immitis* pass to the heart via the venous circulation. The minimum prepatent period is about six months. The adult worms survive for several years and patency has been recorded for over five years. See **life cycle 15**.

LIFE CYCLE 15. LIFE CYCLE OF *DIROFILARIA IMMITIS*

Adults of *Dirofilaria immitis* live in the right side of the heart, and in the pulmonary artery and its branches of dogs and cats, that act as definitive hosts (1). After mating, the females release first-stage larvae (microfilariae, 2) directly into the circulatory system. When intermediate hosts (mosquitoes of the genera *Culex*, *Aedes* and *Anopheles*) feed on an infected host, they ingest the microfilariae; these pass through the midgut into the haemocoel and eventually, in the malpighian tubules, they moult within 2–4 weeks to second-stage larvae ('sausage-like', 3) and subse-

quently to infective third-stage larvae (long and thin) (4). The larvae then migrate to the labium of the mosquito mouthparts (5); from here, they can be inoculated into the circulation of a susceptible host during the insect's next blood meal (6). The larvae then begin migrating toward the final site of infection; the first preadult forms in the pulmonary artery and right ventricle at 70–85 days post infection and reaches sexual maturity at 120 days post infection (1). Microfilariae start to be produced 6–9 months post infection and can be detected in blood vessels.

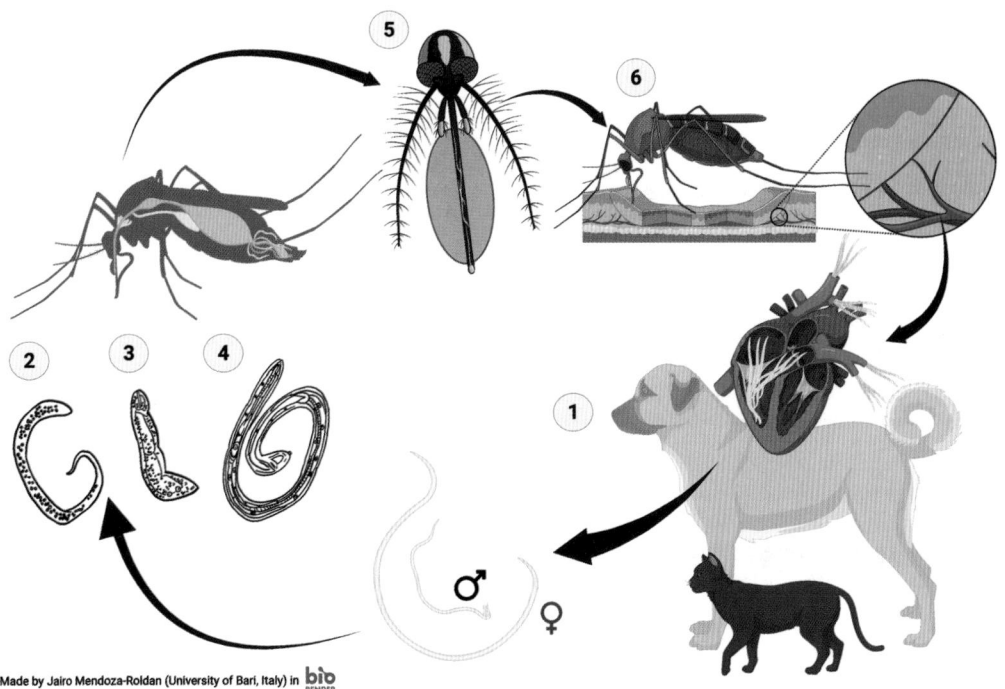

Made by Jairo Mendoza-Roldan (University of Bari, Italy) in **bio**RENDER

Dirofilaria repens

Synonym: *Nochtiella repens*

Description: The adults are long slender worms measuring from around 5 cm up to 17 cm in length. Males are 5–7 cm and females 13–17 cm. Microfilariae measure 360 by 12 μm.

Life cycle: The adults live in subcutaneous nodules and the females release microfilariae, which migrate to the blood and are ingested by female mosquitoes during feeding. Development to L_3 takes place in the mosquito and the final host is infected when the mosquito takes a further blood meal. In the dog, the L_3 migrate to the subcutaneous or subserosal tissues and undergo two moults over the next few months. The prepatent period is 27–34 weeks.

Acanthocheilonema

Several species of *Acanthocheilonema* (formerly *Dipetalonema*), transmitted mainly by fleas, lice and mosquitoes, occur in the subcutis of dogs and various canids in tropical and subtropical zones. While *A. reconditum* is mainly present in the subcutaneous tissues, *A. dracunculoides* is found in the peritoneum and kidney, being transmitted by louse flies.

Acanthocheilonema reconditum

Synonym: *Dipetalonema reconditum*

Description: The slender male worms measure on average 1.5 cm and females about 2.5 cm. The male spicules are unequal. The unsheathed microfilariae are less than 300 μm in length and have a blunt head and hooked posterior end with button-hook tails.

Life cycle: Following ingestion of a blood meal, the microfilariae develop to the infective third stage in about 7–14 days and then migrate to the head. Larvae pass to the host when the intermediate host next feeds. The prepatent period in the dog is 8–10 weeks. *Acanthocheilonema reconditum* shows a diurnal periodicity.

Acanthocheilonema dracunculoides

Synonym: *Dipetalonema dracunculoides*

Description: The adult worms are small; male worms are 2.4–3 cm, females 3.2–6 cm in length. Males have broad unequal spicules.

Cercopithifilaria

Cercopithifilaria bainae

Description: Skin microfilariae are unsheathed and the cephalic end is rounded with a slight protuberance bearing a tiny cephalic hook. The body is short (mean length of 183.1 ± 7.8), flattened dorsoventrally and constant along its length, except for the posterior conical end (Fig. 1.79). The body cuticle is thick bearing transverse striations.

Life cycle: The life cycle occurs in *Rhipicephalus sanguineus* sensu lato in which microfilariae develop to infective larvae in about four weeks under experimental conditions. Larvae pass to dogs when the intermediate host next feeds on another individual.

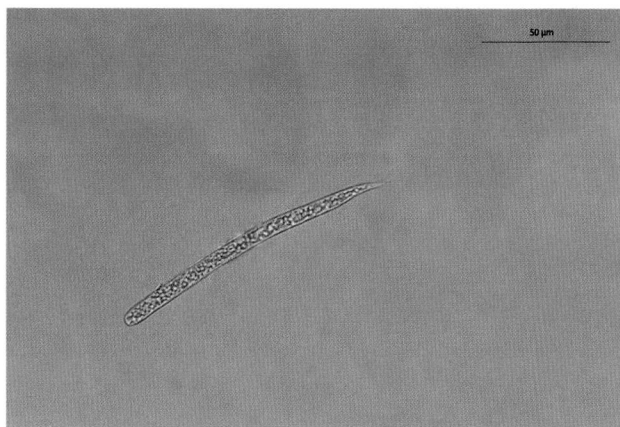

Fig. 1.79 Microfilaria of *Cercopithifilaria bainae*.

Cercopithifilaria grassii

Synonym: *Dipetalonema grassii, Acanthocheilonema grassii*

Description: The adult worms are small, the females measuring about 2.5 cm in length. Microfilariae are large, up to 800 μm in length, with a hook-shaped tail.

Life cycle: The life cycle has not been described in detail. Following ingestion of a blood meal, the microfilariae develop to infective larvae in the intermediate hosts, which are ticks. Larvae pass to the host when the intermediate host next feeds off blood on a dog.

Dipetalonema

Several species of *Dipetalonema*, transmitted mainly by mosquitoes, occur in the subcutis, peritoneum, pleura or blood vessels of mammals in tropical and subtropical zones. The main species is *Dipetalonema evansi* (syn. *Deraiophoronema evansi*) which infects the heart, arteries and veins, pulmonary arteries, spermatic arteries and lymph nodes of camels. This parasite has mosquitoes of the genus *Aedes* as intermediate hosts.

Dipetalonema evansi

Synonym: *Deraiophoronema evansi*

Description: These are fairly large filarial worms; adult male worms are 8–11 cm, adult females 14.5–18.5 cm. Microfilariae are ensheathed, 200–315 μm in length and found in the peripheral blood.

Life cycle: The life cycle has not been described in detail but *Aedes* mosquitoes are thought to act as intermediate hosts. Following ingestion of a blood meal, the microfilariae develop to infective larvae in the intermediate host. Larvae pass to the host when the intermediate host next feeds.

Onchocerca

Though onchocercosis is an important filarial infection in human medicine (*Onchocerca volvulus* causing river blindness), most species in domestic animals are relatively harmless (Table 1.41).

Table 1.41 *Onchocerca* species.

Species	Hosts	Site	Intermediate hosts
Onchocerca gutturosa (syn. Onchocerca lienalis)	Cattle, camels	Connective tissue, ligamentum nuchae, gastrosplenic ligament	Blackflies (Simulium)
Onchocerca gibsoni	Cattle	Connective tissue	Midges (Culicoides)
Onchocerca ochengi (syn. Onchocerca dermata)	Cattle	Connective tissue, scrotum and udder	Unknown
Onchocerca armillata	Cattle, buffalo, sheep, goats, occasionally camels	Thoracic aorta	Midges (Culicoides), blackflies (Simulium)
Onchocerca dukei	Cattle	Abdomen, thorax, thighs	Unknown but probably blackflies
Onchocerca cebei (syn. Onchocerca sweetae)	Buffalo	Abdomen, thorax, thighs	Midges (Culicoides)
Onchocerca cervicalis	Horses	Cervical ligament	Midges (Culicoides)
Onchocerca fasciata	Camels	Connective tissue, ligamentum nuchae	Unknown
Onchocerca lupi	Dogs, cats, humans, wolves	Eyeball, conjunctiva, sclera, spinal channel	Unknown
Onchocerca tarsicola	Deer	Legs	Blackflies (Simulium)
Onchocerca reticulata	Horses, donkeys	Connective tissue, flexor tendons	Midges (Culicoides)
Onchocerca volvulus	Humans	Dermis, eye	Blackflies (Simulium)

Life cycle: The life cycle of *Onchocerca* is typically filarioid, with the exception that the microfilariae occur in the tissue spaces of the skin rather than in the peripheral bloodstream. Microfilariae migrate in subdermal connective tissue in the skin of the back, sometimes ears and neck, where biting flies, feeding in this area, ingest microfilariae, which then develop to the infective stage in around three weeks. When these infected insects feed on another animal, host transmission of L$_3$ occurs.

Onchocerca gutturosa

Synonym: *Onchocerca lienalis*

Description: Slender whitish worms; males range from 2 to 6 cm, while females are up to 60 cm in length or longer and are coiled in fibrous tissues. The cuticle possesses spiral thickenings to aid attachment. Microfilariae are 250–265 µm long and unsheathed.

Onchocerca gibsoni

Description: The slender worms range from 2 cm to over 20 cm in length and lie tightly coiled in tissue nodules. Males are 3–5 cm and females 14–20 cm although there have been reports of worms up to 50 cm in length. The tail of the male is ventrally curved and bears lateral alae and 6–9 papillae at either side. The spicules are unequal in size. Microfilariae are not sheathed and are 240–280 µm long and found mainly in the brisket area. The cuticle possesses transverse striations.

Onchocerca lupi

After its first description in a Caucasian wolf from Georgia, *Onchocerca lupi* remained almost unknown for decades until being reported in dogs from southern Europe (Greece, Portugal) and Germany, Israel, Hungary, Romania and Switzerland, and cats from the south of Iran, Portugal and Romania. In the western United States, cases of canine and feline onchocercosis are also reported. Since 2011, when the first report of human ocular infestation was described in Turkey, other human cases of *O. lupi* have been identified in patients from Germany, Turkey, Tunisia, Iran and the US.

Description: Adults of *O. lupi* are white and slender with rounded anterior ends and a multilayer tick cuticle with characteristic annular ridges 2–3 µm high and wide and evenly spaced at 25–30 µm intervals. Males are 4.3–5 cm long with two unequal spicules and the females longer (up to 16.5 cm) containing two uteri. However, their exact length is currently unknown due to the difficulty in removing complete adult females from the subcutaneous nodules where males and females copulate. The females develop microfilariae inside their uteri, which are released to subcutaneous tissues. Microfilariae are unsheathed, straight (81–115 µm in length) and have a bluntly rounded anterior end and a bent tail posterior end (Fig. 1.80).

Life cycle: The life cycle of *O. lupi* involves canids as definitive hosts and unknown arthropod species as intermediate hosts. Many aspects of the biology and ecology of *O. lupi* remain unknown. In the definitive hosts, male and female adult stages usually develop in the connective tissue of the subconjunctiva, conjunctiva, eyelids and nictitating membrane sitting on top of the sclera until reaching sexual maturity. Aberrant migration to the laryngeal soft tissue in dogs and spinal cord in humans has also been reported. The lifespan of adult worms in dogs has been estimated to be 3–8 years.

Onchocerca armillata

Description: Slender whitish worms. Male worms are about 7 cm and female worms up to 70 cm long. Microfilariae are unsheathed and measure 346–382 µm.

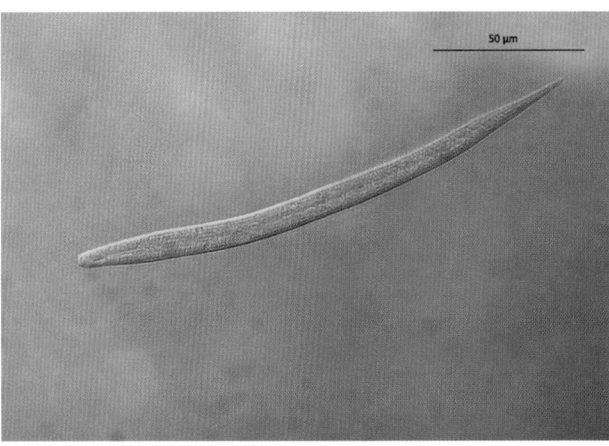

Fig. 1.80 Microfilaria of *Onchocerca lupi*.

Onchocerca cervicalis

Description: The male is 6–7 cm in length and the female up to 30 cm long.

Onchocerca reticulata

Description: Slender whitish worms; males are 15–20 cm and females over 50 cm long. Microfilariae are 330–370 μm and possess a long whiplash tail.

Life cycle: The prepatent period is around 12–16 months.

Pelecitus

The members of this genus are filarioid worms of birds and mammals (Table 1.42).

Pelecitus clavus

Synonym: *Eulimdana clava*

Description: Small to medium-sized worms which have helical turns. Male worms are 6–7 mm and female worms 17–20 mm long. The male spicules are unequal in length, the left being larger than the right.

Life cycle: Microfilariae are present in the blood or subcutaneous space of infected birds and are ingested by biting ectoparasite vectors when they feed.

Pelecitus scapiceps

Synonyms: *Dirofilaria scapiceps, Loaina scapiceps*

Description: Male worms are 11–16 mm in length with spicules of unequal length. Female worms are 25–30 mm long.

Life cycle: Microfilariae circulate in the blood of infected lagomorph hosts (there is no circadian periodicity). Microfilariae ingested by a mosquito develop into infective third-stage larvae and these are then injected into the definitive host during feeding. These larvae migrate in the subcutaneous tissue to a maturation site, such as the main body, and develop to the early fifth stage before migrating to the hocks where they develop into mature adult worms. The prepatent period can vary around 130–220 days.

Table 1.42 *Pelecitus* species.

Species	Hosts	Site	Intermediate hosts
Pelecitus clavus (syn. *Eulimdana clava*)	Pigeons, wild birds and occasionally humans	Subcutaneous, connective tissue	Unknown
Pelecitus mazzanti	Pigeons	Subcutaneous, connective tissue	Unknown
Pelecitus scapiceps (syn. *Dirofilaria scapiceps, Loaina scapiceps*)	Rabbits, hares	Synovial sheaths of the feet	Species of mosquitoes

Chandlerella

Members of this genus are filarioid worms of birds. The main species is *Chandlerella quiscali* which infects the brain of emus and wild birds. This parasite has midges (*Culicoides* spp.) as intermediate hosts.

Chandlerella quiscali

Description: Slender worms, with males 8–15 mm and female worms 17–24 mm in length. In the male, the spicules are thick and equal in length and there are 3–4 pairs of postanal papillae.

Setaria

The members of this genus are usually harmless inhabitants of the peritoneal and pleural cavities (Table 1.43). The worms are slender and whitish, up to 12 cm long, and the posterior end is spirally coiled. The mouth is surrounded by a cuticular ring with dorsal, ventral and frequently lateral prominences, which give the worms a characteristic appearance. The tail of the male has four pairs of precloacal and usually four pairs of postcloacal papillae. The spicules are dissimilar and unequal in length. The tail of female worms usually has spines of several large conical projections. The site and gross appearance are sufficient for generic identification (Fig. 1.81).

Table 1.43 *Setaria* species.

Species	Hosts	Site	Intermediate hosts
Setaria congolensis (syn. *Setaria bernardi*)	Pigs	Peritoneum, pleural cavity	Mosquitoes
Setaria equina	Horses, donkeys, other equids	Peritoneum, pleural cavity	Mosquitoes
Setaria labiato-papillosa (syn. *Setaria digitata, Setaria altaica, Setaria cervi*)	Cattle, buffalo, bison, yaks, deer, antelopes, rarely sheep	Peritoneum, pleural cavity	Mosquitoes
Setaria digitatus	Cattle, buffalo	Peritoneum, pleural cavity	Mosquitoes

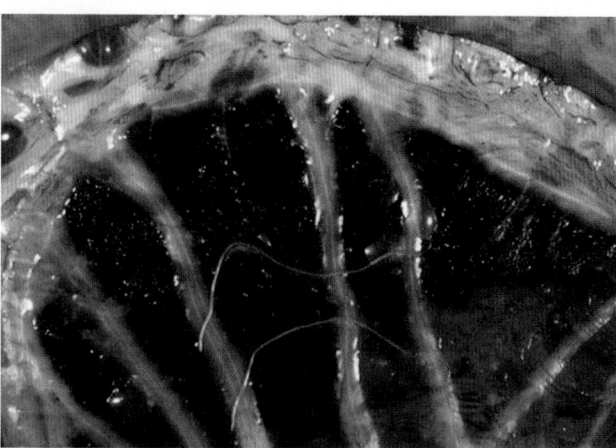

Fig. 1.81 *Setaria labiato-papillosa* in bovine mesentery.

Setaria congolensis

Synonym: *Setaria bernardi*

Description: Male worms are 8 cm and female worms 11–14 cm in length. The male worm has three pairs of small precloacal papillae and four pairs of large postcloacal papillae. The right spicule is spiny and the left spicule is comparatively long with a flagellated end.

Setaria equina

Description: The adults are long and slender with cephalic papillae. Males measure 8–10 cm and females 13–15 cm in length. Worms have an elevated chitinous peribuccal ring. The spiral tail of the female terminates in a point. Male spicules are unequal, the left being about three times longer than the right. The microfilariae present in the blood are sheathed and measure about 190–256 μm in length.

Life cycle: Larvae produced by adult worms in the body cavity circulate in the blood and are taken up by culicine mosquitoes, including *Aedes* and *Culex* species. Infective larvae develop in the mosquito muscles in two weeks and are reinjected into horses when the mosquitoes feed. The prepatent period is 8–10 months.

Setaria labiato-papillosa

Synonyms: *Setaria digitata*, *Setaria altaica*, *Setaria cervi*

Description: Males are 40–60 mm and females 60–120 mm in length. The dorsal and ventral prominences and the peribuccal ring are clearly perceptible. The tail of the female ends in a marked button, which is divided into a number of papillae. The male spicules are of unequal length, the left being around 2.5 times longer than the right. Microfilariae are sheathed and measure 240–260 μm.

Life cycle: Larvae produced by adult worms in the body cavity circulate in the blood and are taken up by culicine mosquitoes, including *Aedes* and *Culex* species. Infective larvae develop in the mosquito muscles in 12–16 days, and are reinjected into the final host when the mosquitoes feed. The prepatent period is 8–10 months.

Elaeophora

These long slender worms inhabit large blood vessels but are generally of local importance, leading to filarial dermatosis caused by circulating microfilariae (Table 1.44).

Table 1.44 *Elaeophora* species.

Species	Hosts	Site	Intermediate hosts
Elaeophora poeli	Cattle, buffalo, zebus	Aorta	Unknown
Elaeophora schneideri	Deer, sheep, goats	Blood vessels	Tabanid flies
Elaeophora bohmi	Horses	Blood vessels	Unknown

Elaeophora poeli

Description: Slender worms, males measuring around 4–7 cm and females up to 30 cm in length. The oesophagus is very long and lips are absent. The tail of the male possesses 5–7 pairs of papillae, of which two pairs are precloacal. Spicules are short and robust. Microfilariae are 340–360 μm.

Life cycle: The life cycle is indirect. The microfilariae are ingested by the intermediate host and the L$_3$, when developed, are released into the wound made when the insect next feeds. The male occurs in nodules in the wall of the aorta, while the female is fixed in nodules by its anterior extremity with the rest of the body free in the lumen of the aorta. Microfilariae occur in the blood and in subcutaneous connective tissue.

Elaeophora schneideri

Description: Slender worms; males are around 5–8 cm and females up to 12 cm long with a very long oesophagus. The tail of the male is coiled and the spicules are long, slender and unequal. Microfilariae are 270 μm, bluntly rounded anteriorly and tapering posteriorly.

Life cycle: Similar to *E. poeli*. Early development in the host appears to be in the meningeal arteries, then the worms migrate to the carotid arteries and are mature and producing microfilariae about 4.5 months after infection. The adult worms are embedded in the arterial intima of the carotid, mesenteric and iliac arteries; occasionally they are found in the digital and tibial arteries with only the anterior part of the female free in the lumen. The prepatent period is around 4–5 months.

Elaeophora bohmi

Description: These are slender worms, the males measuring 4.5–6 cm and females 4–20 cm in length. Microfilariae are 230–290 μm with a long tail.

Life cycle: The microfilariae are ingested by the intermediate host (tabanid flies) when blood feeding and the L$_3$, when developed, are released into the wound made when the insect next feeds. Microfilariae occur in the blood and in subcutaneous connective tissue.

Splendidofilaria

Parasites of birds, characterised by a relatively long tail and subequal spicules. The main species is *Splendidofilaria fallisensis* (syn. *Ornithofilaria fallisensis*) which infects the subcutaneous tissue of ducks. This parasite has slugs and blackflies (*Simulium*) as intermediate hosts.

Splendidofilaria fallisensis

Synonym: *Ornithofilaria fallisensis*

Description: These are delicate transparent nematodes, with male worms measuring 9–15 mm and female worms 24–40 mm in length.

Paronchocerca

This genus of filarial heartworms is of little veterinary importance. *Paronchocerca struthionis* has been reported in ostriches and rheas; *Paronchocerca ciconarum* has been reported to cause myocardial degeneration in storks. Intermediate hosts are unknown.

Paronchocerca struthionis

Description: Long abursate nematodes, 3–5 cm in length with bluntly rounded extremities. Male spicules are dissimilar in length; a gubernaculum is absent.

Filariosis in humans

Filarioid worms are probably the most important group of helminth infections in humans, but are of only marginal concern to the veterinarian since domestic animals are of little significance in their epidemiology. Of greatest importance in human medicine are the genera *Onchocerca*, *Brugia*, *Loa*, *Wuchereria* and *Mansonella*.

1 *Onchocerca volvulus*: Human onchocerciasis, due to *O. volvulus*, occurs around the world in the equatorial zone and is transmitted by *Simulium* spp. (blackflies). The adult worms live in subcutaneous nodules, and almost the entire pathogenic effect is caused by the microfilariae; dermatitis and elephantiasis are common, but the most important effect is ocular onchocerciasis ('river blindness'), so called because of its distribution along the habitats of *Simulium* spp. Dying microfilariae cause a sclerosing keratitis in the cornea that leads to corneal opacification and retinochoroiditis. It has been estimated that in Africa, about 20 million people are affected by onchocerciasis. The only other animals to which it is transmissible are the higher primates, chimpanzee and gorilla. Ivermectin is effective in reducing skin microfilarial counts in *O. volvulus* infection and repeated treatment should help reduce transmission. The onchocerciasis-associated pathology in the eye and skin has also been shown to be reduced with ivermectin treatment.
2 *Brugia* spp. are carried by many species of mosquito and occur in Southeast Asia, notably in Malaysia, causing elephantiasis. The most important species, *B. malayi*, is also infective for monkeys and domestic and wild carnivores, and has been transmitted experimentally to the cat and dog. The lesser species occurring in human, *B. pahangi*, has a reservoir in many species of domestic and wild animals, including the dog and cat. Adult parasites inhabit lymph nodes and afferent lymphatic vessels.
3 *Wuchereria bancrofti* is also mosquito borne and affects the lymphatic system, causing elephantiasis in Africa, Asia and South America. It is exclusive to humans. As with *Brugia* spp., the main pathogenic effects are associated with adult worms rather than with microfilariae.
4 *Loa loa* is transmitted by *Chrysops* spp. (tabanid flies), and occurs in West, Central and East Africa, where it causes the transient subcutaneous enlargements known as 'Calabar swellings'. It is confined to humans, apes and monkeys. Longevity can be up to 20 years.
5 *Mansonella ozzardi*, carried by *Culicoides* and *Simulium* spp., occurs in the Caribbean and Central and South America. It lives in the fat and on the mesentery or pleural cavity, and is usually considered to be non-pathogenic, though recently it has been associated with allergic signs. The prevalence is extremely high in endemic areas, where parasites closely resembling *M. ozzardi* are commonly found in monkeys, horses and cattle. However, there is reluctance to presume that these animals may be reservoir hosts until positive identification is made.

CLASS ENOPLEA

ORDER ENOPLIDA

SUPERFAMILY TRICHUROIDEA

The members of this superfamily are found in a wide variety of domestic animals. A common morphological feature is the 'stichosome' oesophagus that is composed of a capillary-like tube surrounded by a single column of cells. The male has only one spicule within a sheath, or it may be completely absent (e.g. *Trichinella*). There are several genera of veterinary interest in the family Trichuridae. The Trichuridae include species of *Trichuris*, which are found in the caecum and colon of mammals; *Capillaria* (*Eucoleus*) species are most commonly present in the alimentary or respiratory tract of mammals or birds. Both lay eggs with plugs at both poles. *Trichosomoides* species are bladder worms found in rodents and are of minor interest. *Anatrichosoma* are parasites of primates, occasionally reported in humans, and are found in the skin and nasal passages.

FAMILY TRICHURIDAE

Trichuris

Worms belonging to this genus are commonly known as 'Whipworms' because the thick broad posterior end tapers rapidly to a long filamentous anterior end (about twice as long as the posterior region) that is characteristically embedded in the mucosa (Fig. 1.82; Table 1.45). The anterior of the worm bears a small point. The male tail is tightly coiled and possesses a single spicule in a protrusible sheath.

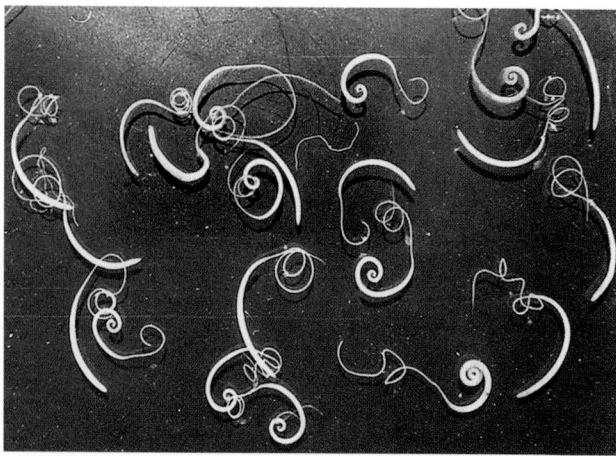

Fig. 1.82 *Trichuris suis* adult worms.

Table 1.45 *Trichuris* species.

Species	Hosts	Site
Trichuris campanula	Cats	Large intestine
Trichuris capreoli	Deer	Large intestine
Trichuris discolor	Cattle, buffalo, occasionally sheep, goats	Large intestine
Trichuris globulosa	Cattle, occasionally sheep, goats, camels, other ruminants	Large intestine
Trichuris leporis	Rabbits, hares, coypus	Large intestine
Trichuris muris	Rats, mice	Large intestine
Trichuris ovis	Sheep, goat, occasionally cattle and other ruminants	Large intestine
Trichuris serrata	Cats	Large intestine
Trichuris skrjabini	Sheep, goats, camels	Large intestine
Trichuris suis	Pigs, wild boar	Large intestine
Trichuris trichiura	Humans, primates	Large intestine
Trichuris vulpis	Dogs, foxes, cats	Large intestine
Trichuris cameli	Camels	Large intestine
Trichuris tenuis	Llamas, alpacas	Large intestine

Trichuris trichiura, the whipworm of human and simian primates, is morphologically indistinguishable from *T. suis*. However, it is generally considered that these two parasites are strictly host specific. Worldwide, the number of cases in humans is several hundred million, with around 10 000 deaths per year attributed to trichuriosis. It is more common in children. The taxonomic status of *Trichuris* species is very confused because many described species may be synonymous, reflecting the fact that an accepted species has been found in a different host and determined as a new species.

Life cycle: The infective stage is the L_1 within the egg, which develops within 1–2 months of being passed in the faeces, depending on the temperature. Under optimal conditions, these larvated eggs may subsequently survive and remain viable for several years. After ingestion, the plugs are digested and the released L_1 penetrate the mucosal glands of the distal ileum, caecum and colon. Subsequently, all four moults occur within these glands, the adults emerging to lie on the mucosal surface with their anterior ends embedded in the mucosa. The prepatent period is about 7–10 weeks. See **life cycle 16**.

LIFE CYCLE 16. LIFE CYCLE OF *TRICHURIS VULPIS*

Adults of *Trichuris vulpis* (1) live in the caecum and colon of the dog. After mating, the females release elliptical eggs, characteristically lemon-shaped, defined by the presence of 'polar plugs' at each end (2). The eggs are non-segmented and are eliminated in the external environment with the faeces, where they mature (3) until an infective first-stage larva (L_1)

forms inside each egg (4). The dog acquires the infection by ingesting larvated eggs. After hatching in the intestinal lumen, the larvae begin migrating through the mucosa. After 8–10 days, the larvae return to the intestinal lumen (5), attach to the mucosa with their cephalic end and develop into sexually mature adults (1).

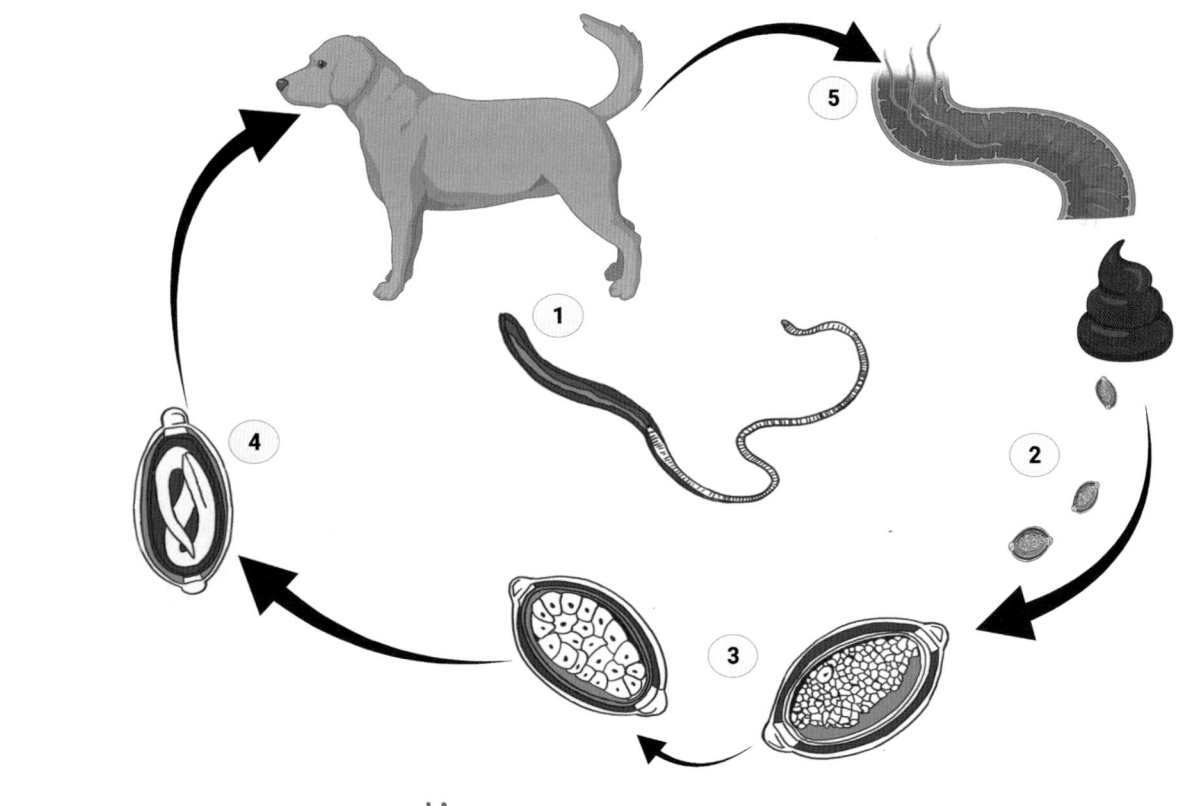

Made by Jairo Mendoza-Roldan (University of Bari, Italy) in **bio** RENDER

Trichuris discolor

Description: Worms are similar to *T. globulosa* but the females are yellow-orange in colour. Eggs measure about 65 by 30 µm.

Trichuris globulosa

Description: The adults are long white worms, with males measuring 4–7 cm and females 4–6 cm in length. The single spicule sheath bears a terminal spherical expansion, on which are spines larger than on the rest of the sheath. The male tail is coiled and possesses a single spicule in a protrusible sheath. The sheath is covered with minute spines and bears a spherical appendage; the female tail is merely curved. The characteristic medium-sized eggs are lemon-shaped, 70–80 by 30–40 µm, with a thick smooth shell and a conspicuous protruding transparent polar plug (operculum) at both ends. The content of the egg is granular, there being no blastomeres. In the faeces these eggs appear yellowish or brown in colour.

Trichuris leporis

Description: Adult males measure 1.9–2.1 cm and adult females 1.7–2.1 cm in length.

Trichuris ovis

Description: The adults are long white worms, the males measuring 5–8 cm and the females 3.5–7 cm in length with a thick broad posterior end tapering rapidly to a long filamentous anterior end that is characteristically embedded in the mucosa. The male tail is coiled and possesses a single spicule in a protrusible sheath. The sheath bears an oblong swelling a short distance from its distal extremity and is covered with minute spines, which decrease in size towards the distal end. The female tail is merely curved. The characteristic eggs are lemon-shaped, with a thick smooth shell and a conspicuous protruding transparent polar plug (operculum) at both ends (see Fig. 4.4). In the faeces these eggs appear yellow or brown in colour. They measure around 70–80 by 30–42 µm and when laid, they contain an unsegmented embryo.

Trichuris skrjabini

Description: Males of *T. skrjabini* have one short spicule (0.82 mm) with a rounded tip that is always fully covered by the spicule sheath and large conical caudal papillae.

Trichuris suis

Description: The adults are whitish and about 3–5 cm long with a thick broad posterior end tapering rapidly to a long filamentous anterior end that is characteristically embedded in the mucosa (Fig. 1.83). The male tail is coiled and possesses a single spicule in a protrusible sheath. The sheath is variable in shape and in the extent of its spinous armature. The female tail is curved. The characteristic eggs are lemon-shaped, 50–68 by 21–31 µm, with a thick smooth shell and a conspicuous transparent protruding polar plug at both

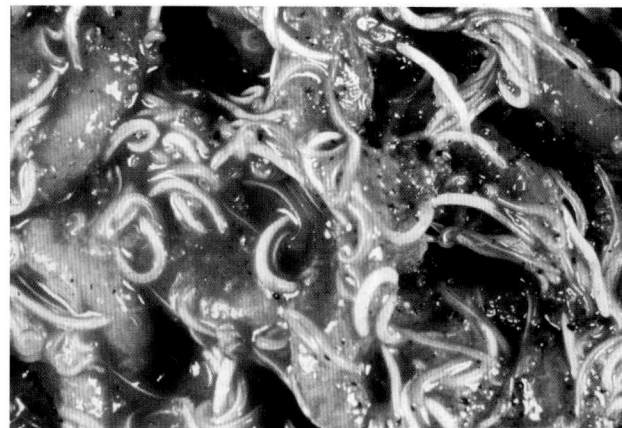
Fig. 1.83 *Trichuris suis* on the surface of the large intestine.

ends; in the faeces these eggs appear yellow or brown in colour. The contents are granular, unsegmented and brownish.

Trichuris trichiura

Description: Females are slightly larger than male worms (approximately 3.5–5 cm compared to 3–4.5 cm). The females have a bluntly round posterior compared to their male counterparts with a coiled posterior end.

Trichuris vulpis

Description: The adults are whitish and about 4.5–7.5 cm long with a thick broad posterior end tapering rapidly to a long filamentous anterior end that is characteristically embedded in the mucosa (Fig. 1.84). The male tail is coiled and possesses a single spicule in a protrusible sheath. The sheath bears small spines only on its anterior portion. The characteristic eggs are lemon-shaped, with a thick smooth shell, slightly barrel-shaped side walls and conspicuous protruding transparent polar plugs at both ends. They measure 80–90 by 36–42 µm and in the faeces these eggs appear yellow or brown in colour with granular unsegmented contents (see Fig. 4.7).

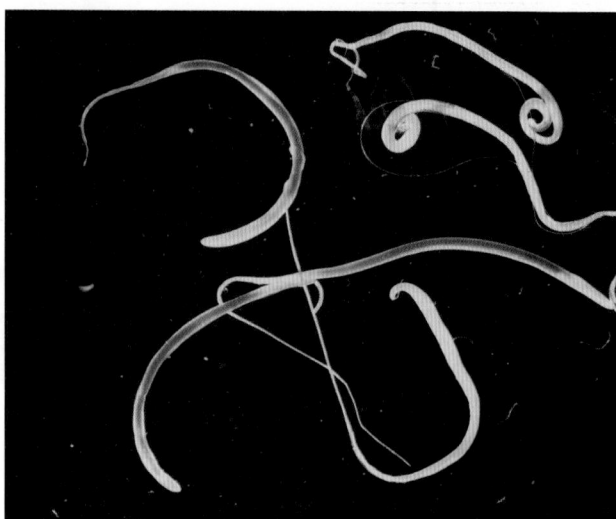
Fig. 1.84 *Trichuris vulpis* adults recovered from an infected intestine.

Trichosomoides

These are permanent hyperparasites that inhabit the urinary bladder of rats.

Life cycle: Infection is by ingestion of embryonated eggs voided in the urine. Eggs hatch in the stomach, penetrate the stomach wall and are carried in the blood to the lungs and other parts of the body. Only those larvae that reach the kidneys or urinary bladder survive. The life cycle takes 8–9 weeks and the prepatent period is 8–12 weeks. The main species is *Trichosomoides crassicauda* which infects the bladder of rats.

Trichosomoides crassicauda

Description: The female is 10–19 mm long; the male measures 1.5–3.5 mm and is a permanent hyperparasite living within the reproductive tract of the female. The medium-sized egg is lemon-shaped with protruding transparent polar plugs and measures about 60–70 by 30–36 µm. The shell is thick and brown in colour, and contains either a morula or an L_1 larva. Eggs are only found in the urine.

Anatrichosoma

Members of this genus have been reported from the skin and nasal mucosa of primates and the skin and mucosa of wild rodents and marsupials. There have been some reports of infections with species of these parasites in dogs, cats and humans.

FAMILY CAPILLARIIDAE

Capillaria

Worms belonging to this genus, commonly known as 'Hairworms' or 'Threadworms', are very fine whitish filamentous worms, the narrow stichosome oesophagus occupying about one-third to half the body length (Table 1.46). There is a simple mouth and a buccal capsule is absent. The males have a long thin colourless single spicule and often possess a primitive bursa-like structure. The small eggs are slightly lemon-shaped (similar to *Trichuris*) but the side walls are almost parallel. They measure 45–50 by 22–25 µm, are colourless and have thick shells that are slightly striated with two protruding transparent bipolar plugs. The contents are granular with no blastomeres.

Life cycle: The life cycles are generally direct but some species found in birds have indirect life cycles, with earthworms acting as intermediate hosts. The infective L_1 develops within the egg in about 3–4 weeks. Infection of the final host is through ingestion of this embryonated infective stage and development to adult worms occurs usually without a migration phase. The taxonomy and systematics of these parasites have been changed many times because of a difficulty in designation of particular species' features and there are many synonyms in this group. Some species of *Capillaria* are now listed under the generic name *Eucoleus*, although they may universally still be referred to as *Capillaria*.

Capillaria anatis

Synonyms: *Capillaria brevicollis, Capillaria collaris, Capillaria mergi, Thornix anatis*

Table 1.46 *Capillaria/Eucoleus* species.

Species	Hosts	Site
Capillaria anatis (syn. Capillaria brevicollis, Capillaria collaris, Capillaria mergi, Thornix anatis)	Chickens, turkeys, gallinaceous birds (pheasants, partridges), pigeons, ducks, geese	Caeca
Capillaria anseris (syn. Baruscapillaria anseris)	Geese, ducks	Small intestine
Capillaria bovis (syn. Capillaria brevipes)	Cattle	Small intestine
Capillaria bilobata	Zebus	Abomasum
Capillaria bursata	Chickens, turkeys, pheasants, ducks and wild birds. Intermediate hosts: earthworms	Small intestine
Capillaria caudinflata (syn. Aonchotheca caudinflata)	Chickens, turkeys, geese, pigeons and wild birds. Intermediate hosts: earthworms	Small intestine
Capillaria feliscati (syn. Pearsonema feliscati)	Cats	Bladder
Capillaria hepatica (syn. Callodium hepatica, Hepaticola hepatica)	Rats, mice, squirrels, rabbits and farmed mustelids; occasionally dogs, cats, humans, primates	Liver
Capillaria longipes	Sheep, goat, cattle	Small intestine
Capillaria obsignata (syn. Baruscapillaria obsignata, Capillaria columbae)	Pigeons, chickens, turkeys, pheasants and wild birds	Small intestine
Capillaria phasianina (syn. Thornix phasianina)	Pheasants, grey partridges	Small intestine, caecae
Capillaria philippinensis	Humans	Small intestine
Capillaria plica (syn. Pearsonema plica)	Dogs, cats, foxes, wolves	Bladder
Capillaria putorii (syn. Aonchotheca putorii)	Cats, dogs, mustelids, hedgehogs, bears, raccoons	Stomach, small intestine
Capillaria uropapillata	Pheasants	Oesophagus, crop
Eucoleus aerophila (syn. Capillaria aerophila)	Foxes, mustelids, occasionally dogs, coyotes, cats and humans	Trachea, bronchi
Eucoleus boehmi (syn. Capillaria boehmi)	Foxes, dogs	Nasal, frontal and maxillary sinuses
Eucoleus annulata (syn. Capillaria annulata)	Chickens, turkeys, ducks and wild birds. Intermediate hosts: earthworms	Oesophagus, crop
Eucoleus contorta (syn. Capillaria contorta)	Chickens, turkeys, pheasants, ducks and wild birds. Intermediate hosts: earthworms	Oesophagus, crop
Eucoleus perforans (syn. Capillaria perforans)	Pheasants, guinea fowls	Oesophagus, crop

Description: Males measure around 16–24 mm and females 28–38 mm in length. The males have a long thin single spicule and often possess a primitive bursa-like structure. The eggs are slightly barrel-shaped, light brown and with protruding transparent polar plugs (see Fig. 4.8). They measure around 48–65 by 23–35 μm and the outer shell is thick, striated and rugose. More details of the eggs are given under *Capillaria contorta*.

Life cycle: The life cycle is direct. The infective L_1 develops within the egg in about 3–4 weeks. Infection of the final host is through ingestion of this embryonated infective stage, and development to adult worms occurs without a migration phase. The prepatent period is 3–4 weeks.

Capillaria bursata

Description: Males measure around 6–12 mm and females up to 25 mm.

Life cycle: The life cycle of this species is indirect.

Capillaria bovis

Synonym: *Capillaria brevipes*

Description: Males measure around 8–9 mm and females up to 12 mm.

Capillaria caudinflata

Synonym: *Aonchotheca caudinflata*

Description: See *Eucoleus annulata*. Males measure around 6–12 mm and females up to 25 mm. Females have a characteristic projecting vulval appendage. The medium-sized eggs measure 43–69 by 20–27 μm and have a finely sculptured thick shell; their other characteristics are more fully described under *Eucoleus contorta*.

Life cycle: The life cycle of this species is indirect.

Capillaria hepatica

Synonyms: *Callodium hepatica, Hepaticola hepatica*

Description: These are very fine filamentous worms generally measuring 10–50 mm in length. The males have a long thin single spicule and often possess a primitive bursa-like structure. The medium-sized eggs are barrel-shaped and almost colourless. They have thick shells that are slightly striated with minute pores and the bipolar plugs protrude. Eggs measure about 48–62 by 29–37 μm and contain a morula.

Life cycle: The life cycle is direct and differs from that of other *Capillaria* species. Adult *C. hepatica* worms reproduce in the liver and females lay groups of eggs in the parenchyma where they become encapsulated by the host's reaction. These eggs are therefore not released directly from the host. Infection is acquired by ingestion of either the liver, following predation, cannibalism or carrion feeding, or eggs on the ground, which have been freed by decomposition of the host. Eggs in the soil will embryonate and be infective in about four weeks. When infective eggs are ingested by the host, they hatch

in the intestine and the larvae penetrate the intestinal wall and are carried to the liver via the lymphatics and the bloodstream.

Capillaria longipes

Description: These are very fine filamentous worms, the narrow stichosome oesophagus occupying about one-third to half the body length. Males measure around 10–13 mm and females up to 20 mm. The males have a long thin single spicule, 1.2 mm long, and often possess a primitive bursa-like structure. The females contain eggs that resemble those of *Trichuris* in possessing bipolar plugs. The eggs are only slightly barrel-shaped, the midregions of the shell wall being parallel. They measure 45–50 by 22–25 μm and are colourless, and have thick shells that are slightly striated with slightly projecting transparent bipolar plugs (see Fig. 4.4).

Life cycle: The prepatent period is 3–4 weeks.

Capillaria obsignata

Synonyms: *Baruscapillaria obsignata, Capillaria columbae*

Description: See *Eucoleus annulata*. Males measure around 10–12 mm and females up to 15 mm in length. The tail of the female worm tapers posteriorly. The medium-sized eggs are barrel-shaped with slightly striated bipolar plugs and possess a shell with a reticulate pattern. They measure around 50–62 by 20–25 μm; their other characteristics are more fully described under *Eucoleus contorta*.

Life cycle: This species has a direct life cycle. The infective L_1 develops within the egg in about 7–10 days. Infection of the final host is through ingestion of this embryonated infective stage, and development to adult worms occurs without a migration phase. The prepatent period is around three weeks.

Capillaria plica

Synonym: *Pearsonema plica*

Description: Fine, whitish, filamentous worms 1–6 cm long; males measure 13–30 mm and females 30–60 mm. The males have a long thin single spicule and often possess a primitive bursa-like structure. The medium-sized ovoid eggs are barrel-shaped, and have thick yellowish shells that are slightly striated with protruding transparent flattened bipolar plugs. They measure 63–68 by 24–27 μm and the almost colourless contents are granular and unsegmented. The egg is only observed in urine.

Life cycle: This parasite requires an earthworm intermediate host, ingested eggs developing to the infective L_3 within 30 days. The prepatent period is around eight weeks.

Capillaria feliscati

Synonym: *Pearsonema feliscati*

Description: Adult worms are small thread-like parasites; adult females measure 30–60 mm, males 13–30 mm long. Eggs are oval and colourless with a thick capsule and typical bipolar plugs, and measure 50–68 by 22–32 μm.

Capillaria putorii

Synonym: *Aonchotheca putorii*

Description: Thin filamentous worms, about 10 mm long; males are 5–8 mm and females 9–15 mm. The medium-sized, oval, elongate eggs have broad flat poles with two protruding semi-transparent polar plugs. They measure around 60 by 30 µm and contain granular unsegmented contents.

Eucoleus aerophila

Synonym: *Capillaria aerophila*

Description: These are very fine, whitish, filamentous worms, the narrow stichosome oesophagus occupying about one-third to half the body length. Males measure around 24 mm and females 32 mm. The males have a long thin single spicule and often possess a primitive bursa-like structure. The females contain eggs that resemble those of *Trichuris* in possessing bipolar plugs. The elongate, oval, medium-sized eggs are barrel-shaped and possess a thick, granular, slightly striated shell. The poles of each egg have a protruding transparent plug. Eggs measure about 59–80 by 30–40 µm and have a greenish to yellowish-brown colour and contain granular unsegmented contents. These eggs can be differentiated from those of *Trichuris vulpis*, which are larger and possess a smooth shell, and from those of *Capillaria plica*, which are almost colourless and are passed in the urine.

Eucoleus boehmi

Synonym: *Capillaria boehmi*

Description: These are fine, whitish, filamentous worms with adults measuring 15–40 mm long. The males have a long thin single spicule. The females contain eggs that macroscopically resemble those of *E. aerophila* in possessing bipolar plugs. Microscopically, the eggs can be differentiated: the surface of *E. boehmi* eggs are pitted whereas those of *E. aerophila* are covered with a network of branching ridges.

Eucoleus annulata

Synonym: *Capillaria annulata*

Description: These are very fine filamentous worms, the narrow stichosome oesophagus occupying about one-third to half the body length. Males measure around 15–25 mm and females 37–80 mm. The males have a long thin single spicule, with a spiny spicule sheath, and often possess a primitive bursa-like structure. This species has a cuticular swelling at the back of the head. The females contain eggs that resemble those of *Trichuris* in possessing bipolar plugs. The medium-sized eggs are barrel-shaped and colourless to pale brown, 60–65 by 25–28 µm, and have thick shells that are slightly striated with bipolar plugs.

Life cycle: The life cycle is indirect. Eggs passed in faeces are ingested by earthworms and develop to the infective stage in 2–3 weeks. The prepatent period is about 3–4 weeks in the final host.

Eucoleus contorta

Synonym: *Capillaria contorta*

Description: General description as for other *Eucoleus/Capillaria* species. Males measure around 12–17 mm and females 27–38 mm. The medium-sized lemon-shaped eggs measure about 48–60 by 21–28 µm. They have slightly barrel-shaped asymmetrical side walls with protruding transparent polar plugs. Eggs have a thick brown shell with a smooth surface and their granular contents are unsegmented.

Life cycle: *Eucoleus contorta* appears to be able to develop both directly and indirectly. In the direct life cycle, the infective L_1 develops within the egg in about 3–4 weeks. Infection of the final host is through ingestion of this embryonated infective stage, and development to adult worms occurs without a migration phase. In the indirect life cycle, the egg needs to be ingested by an earthworm in which it hatches, the final host being infected by ingestion of the earthworm. The prepatent period is about 3–4 weeks in the final host.

Capillariosis in humans

Three species of *Capillaria*, *C. philippinensis*, *C. hepatica* and *Eucoleus* (*Capillaria*) *aerophila*, can infect humans. Humans acquire *C. hepatica* infection through ingestion of soil containing embryonated eggs or by consuming contaminated food or water. Heavy infections in human induce similar hepatic lesions to those seen in other mammalian hosts and hepatic capillariosis is usually fatal.

Capillaria philippinensis infects the small intestine and causes a severe enteropathy that can be fatal. It occurs mainly in the Philippines and Thailand, with sporadic outbreaks in other parts of Southeast Asia, India, the Middle East and southern Europe. Eggs shed into water embryonate and are ingested by freshwater or brackish-water fish and develop to the infective stage in the intestinal mucosa. Infection is acquired through the consumption of raw or undercooked fish. Large infections can accumulate through autoinfection. Fish-eating birds are thought to be the reservoir host. Clinical signs include intermittent diarrhoea, followed by anorexia, abdominal distension and weight loss. There is a protein-losing enteropathy. Human capillariosis resulting from *E. aerophila* is very rare.

SUPERFAMILY TRICHINELLOIDEA

FAMILY TRICHINELLIDAE

Trichinella are found in the small intestine of mammals and produce larvae that immediately invade the tissues of the same host.

Trichinella

The taxonomy of the genus has been controversial until very recently. It is composed of several sibling species that cannot be differentiated morphologically but molecular typing, and other criteria, have now identified eight species of *Trichinella* (Table 1.47).

Table 1.47 *Trichinella* species.

Species	Distribution	Principal hosts	Resistance to freezing
Capsule forming			
Trichinella spiralis	Cosmopolitan	Pigs, rats, horses, wide range of mammals, humans	No
Trichinella nativa	Arctic and subarctic zones: North America, Finland, Sweden	Wild carnivores, seals, polar bears, walruses	High
Trichinella nelsoni	Tropical Africa	Wild carnivores and omnivores	No
Trichinella britovi	Temperate zone of Palaearctic region	Wild carnivores, foxes, wild boar, horses, humans	Low
Trichinella murrelli	North America	Wildlife, horses, humans	No
Non-capsule forming			
Trichinella pseudospiralis	Cosmopolitan	Mammals, birds	No
Trichinella papuae	Papua New Guinea	Wild pigs, humans	No
Trichinella zimbabwensis	Zimbabwe	Crocodiles	No

Description: Because of their short lifespan, the adult worms are rarely found in natural infections. The male is about 1.5 mm and the female 3.5–4 mm long. The oesophagus is at least one-third of the total body length, and the tail in the male has two small knob-shaped conical cloacal flaps but no copulatory spicule nor a spicule sheath. In the female, the uterus contains developing larvae. The vulva is sited in the midoesophageal region of the worm. *Trichinella* infection is most easily identified by the presence of coiled larvae in striated muscle (Fig. 1.85). These larvae measure about 800–1000 µm in length. The cysts are lemon-shaped, 0.3–0.8 by 0.2–0.4 mm in size and often transparent. Adult worms are unlikely to be encountered during gross examination of intestinal digesta.

Life cycle: The life cycle is indirect. The adult parasites and infective larvae (muscle trichinae) are unusual in being present within a single host (i.e. development from larva to adult to larva in a single host). *Trichinella* does not have a free-living stage. The very small developing adults lie between the villi of the small intestine. After fertilisation, the males die while the females burrow deeper into the intestinal mucosa. About a week later, they produce L_1 which enter the lymphatic vessels and travel via the bloodstream to the skeletal muscles. There, still as L_1, they penetrate striated muscle cells where they are encapsulated by the host, grow and assume a characteristic coiled position; the parasitised muscle cell is transformed by microvascularisation into a 'nurse cell'. This process is complete within about 3–4 weeks, by which time the larvae are infective and may remain so for many years. Development is resumed when muscle, containing the encysted trichinae, is ingested by another host, usually as a result of predation or carrion feeding. The L_1 is liberated in the stomach and in the intestine undergoes four moults to become sexually mature within about a week. Patent infections persist for only a few weeks at the most. See **life cycle 17**.

SUPERFAMILY DIOCTOPHYMATOIDEA

This group contains three genera: *Dioctophyma*, found in the kidney of carnivores, and *Hystrichis* and *Eustrongyloides*, which occur in aquatic fowl. The alimentary canal is attached to the abdominal wall by four longitudinal muscles and the tail of the male has a terminal cup-shaped bursa which lacks bursal rays. A single spicule is present.

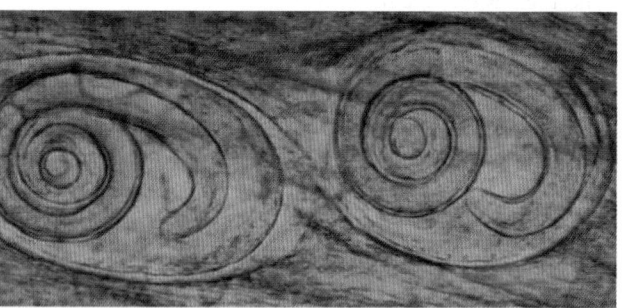

Fig. 1.85 Coiled infective larvae of *Trichinella spiralis* in striated muscle.

FAMILY DIOCTOPHYMATIDAE

Dioctophyma

Dioctophyma renale (syn. *Dictophyme renale*, *Eustrongylus gigas*), 'kidney worm', is the largest parasitic nematode known in domestic animals and is found in the abdominal cavity and kidneys of dogs, foxes, mink, ferrets, otters, pine martens, polecats and seals, occasionally in cats, pigs, horses and humans. This parasite has aquatic oligochaetes (annelids) as intermediate hosts.

Dioctophyma renale

Synonym: *Dictophyme renale*, *Eustrongylus gigas*

Description: Female worms usually measure more than 60 cm in length, with a diameter of around 1 cm but can occasionally be as long as 100 cm. The male is about 35–40 cm long with a bell-shaped bursa which is lined with papillae and a supporting ray is absent (Fig. 1.86). A single brown spicule is present. The worms are deep red–purple in colour. Their size and predilection site are sufficient for identification. Male worms have only one spicule and possess a bell-shaped copulatory bursa. The eggs are lemon-shaped, yellowish-brown, with a thick pitted shell and slightly protruding bipolar plugs. They measure about 71–84 by 46–52 µm and the granular contents are unsegmented when passed. The eggs are observed in the urine.

LIFE CYCLE 17. LIFE CYCLE OF *TRICHINELLA* SPP.

Trichinella spp. is the only genus of nematodes that completes its whole life cycle within a single host. These parasites infect the vast majority of mammalian species, including humans, and also birds and reptiles. Trichinellosis is regarded as a severe zoonosis, with an incidence varying widely between different countries. *Trichinella* spp. are common in wildlife, and infections have been reported in boars, foxes, bears, wolves, coyotes, badgers, lynx and small rodents, as well as pigs, horses and domestic carnivores. Thus, trichinellosis is an infection mostly occurring in sylvatic environments, and transmission to humans occurs via the ingestion of raw or undercooked game meat, or pig and horse meat from infected animals (1). Adult parasites live among the villi of the small intestine (2) and are rarely detected during natural infections as they are short-lived (six weeks at most). Males are $1.5 \times 40 \, \mu m$, with a well-developed oesophagus (over one-third of the whole-body length), without spicules but with a cloaca featuring two small 'flaps' (3). Females ($3-4 \, mm \times 60 \, \mu m$) are viviparous (4). After mating, the males die, whilst the females travel deeper through the villi and, within 3–5 days, begin releasing L_1

(5). Within 4–16 weeks, females release up to 2000 larvae that penetrate the lymphatic system and, via the circulation, travel to the skeletal muscles, especially the diaphragm, masseter, tongue, extraocular, laryngeal and intercostal muscles. The larvae (6) ($100 \times 8 \, \mu m$) feature a rounded tail, long oesophagus and an apical stiletto; on penetrating the muscular fibres (7), the larvae induce transformation of the latter into 'mother cells' (also known as 'nurse cells', 8). The L_1 grow and, without moulting, begin to coil ~18 days later. Due to the onset of reactive processes, a thin connective capsule forms around the cysts of some *Trichinella* species, with each larva encased in a structure resembling a lemon with groups of adipocytes deposited at each pole. Inside these cysts, the parasite remains alive and infective for long periods of time. Nevertheless, after ~6 months, a calcification process may begin around the cysts. Ingestion of infected meat by a new host allows the larvae to exit the cysts thanks to the activity of gastric juices (9), and to travel to the duodenum. Here, the L_1 undergo three moults (from L_1 to L_4, 10), and subsequent sexual development.

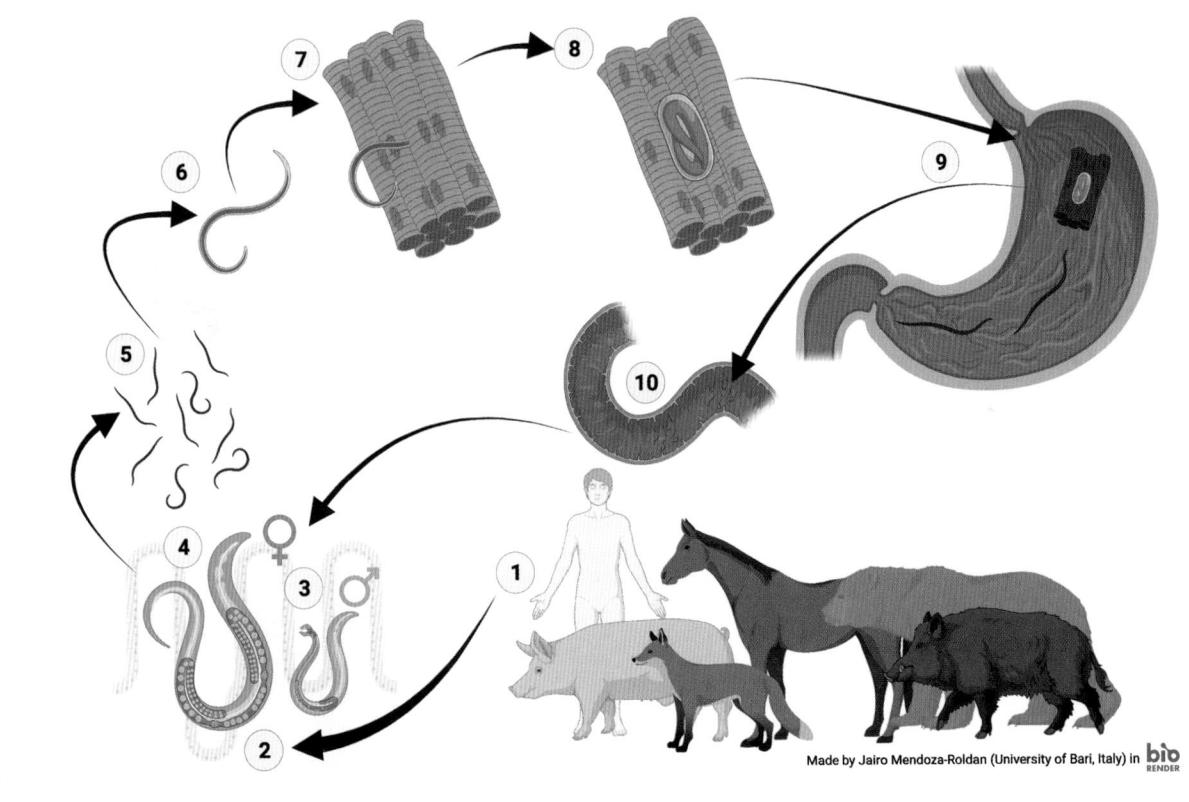

Made by Jairo Mendoza-Roldan (University of Bari, Italy) in **bio** RENDER

Life cycle: The worms are oviparous. The eggs, in the single-cell stage, are passed in the urine in clumps or chains and are ingested by the annelid intermediate host, in which the two preparasitic moults occur. The development phase in the annelid is about 2–4 months. The final host is infected by swallowing the annelid with the drinking water, or by the ingestion of a paratenic host, such as a frog or fish, which has itself eaten the infected annelid. In the final host, the infective larvae penetrate the intestinal wall, enter the peritoneal cavity and eventually penetrate the kidney.

The prepatent period is about six months but has been observed to be as long as two years.

Hystrichis

The main species is *Hystrichis tricolor* which infects the proventriculus oesophagus of domestic and wild ducks and anatid birds. This parasite has aquatic oligochaetes (annelids) as intermediate hosts.

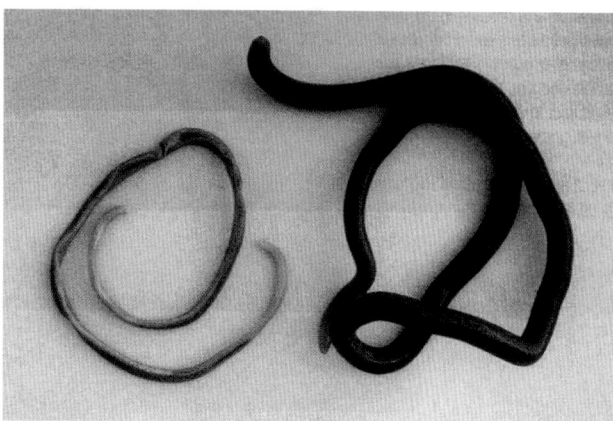

Fig. 1.86 Male and female worms of the kidney worm *Dioctophyma renale*.

Hystrichis tricolor

Description: Adult female worms are up to about 4 cm and males 2.5 cm in length. The cephalic area is expanded, and possesses many regularly positioned spines. The eggs are thick-shelled, coated with tubercles and have truncated poles. They measure about 85–88 by 36–40 μm and only develop slowly in water, taking around 8–9 weeks to reach the embryonated stage.

Life cycle: This is indirect. Fowl and other birds become parasitised through ingestion of infected oligochaetes. The adult worms are deeply embedded in the mucosa, with their caudal and cephalic regions lying within the lumen of the tract. The prepatent period is around two weeks.

Eustrongyloides

Parasites of waterfowl found in the oesophagus and proventriculus (Table 1.48).

Life cycle: The life cycles of *Eustrongyloides* species are not fully known but oligochaetes are likely to be involved as intermediate hosts and various fish as paratenic hosts.

Eustrongyloides papillosus

Description: Females measure about 3 cm in length. The male has a bursal cup with a fringed margin.

Eustrongyloides tubifex

Description: Males measure around 3–3.5 cm and females 3.5–4.5 cm in length. This worm has a small mouth and the head lacks spines. The cuticle is annulated. The male bursal cup is shaped like a trumpet and the spicule is slender and long.

Table 1.48 *Eustrongyloides* species.

Species	Hosts	Site	Intermediate hosts
Eustrongyloides papillosus	Ducks, geese	Proventriculus, oesophagus	Aquatic oligochaetes Fishes
Eustrongyloides tubifex (syn. *Strongylus tubifex, Eustrongylus tubifex, Hystrichis tubifex*)	Waterfowl	Proventriculus, oesophagus	Aquatic oligochaetes Fishes

PHYLUM ACANTHOCEPHALA

This is a separate phylum, closely related to the Nematoda, that contains a few genera of veterinary importance. They are generally referred to as 'thorny-headed worms' due to the presence of a hook-covered proboscis anteriorly (Fig. 1.87), and most are parasites of the alimentary tract of vertebrates. The body is usually cylindrical, although some are flattened. The hollow proboscis armed with recurved hooks, which aid in attachment, is retractable and lies in a sac. There is no alimentary canal, with absorption taking place through the thick cuticle, which is often folded and invaginated to increase the absorptive surface. The sexes are separate, males being much smaller than females. Posteriorly, the male has a muscular bursa and penis. After copulation, eggs, discharged by ovaries into the body cavity of the female, are fertilised and taken up by a complex structure called the uterine bell, which only allows mature eggs to pass out. These are spindle-shaped, thick-shelled and contain a larva which has an anterior circlet of hooks and spines on its surface and is called an **acanthor**.

Life cycle: The life cycle is indirect, involving either an aquatic or terrestrial arthropod intermediate host. On ingestion by the intermediate host, the egg hatches and the acanthor migrates to the haemocoel of the arthropod where it develops to become a **cystacanth** after 1–3 months. The definitive host is infected by ingestion of the arthropod intermediate host, and the cystacanth, which is really a young adult, attaches and grows to maturity in the alimentary canal. The prepatent period varies from five to 12 weeks.

FAMILY OLIGACANTHORHYNCHIDAE

The major genera of veterinary significance are *Macracanthorhynchus*, which is found in pigs, *Oncicola* found in dogs and other canids, and *Prosthenorchis* (*Oncicola*) which is found in primates.

Macracanthorhynchus

The main species is *Macracanthorhynchus hirudinaceus* which infects the small intestine of pigs and wild boar. This parasite has various dung beetles and water beetles as intermediate hosts.

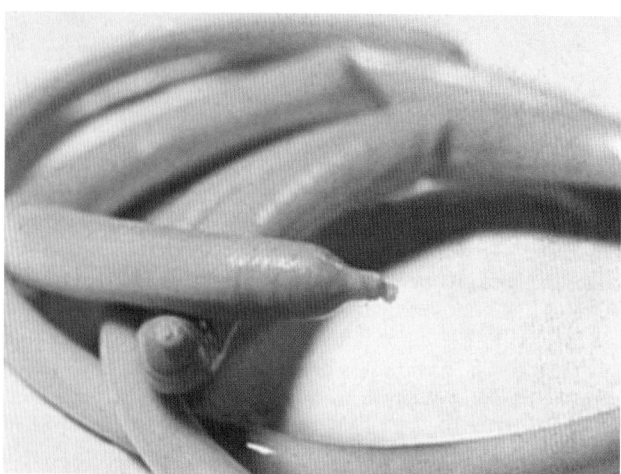

Fig. 1.87 Head of *Macracanthorhynchus hirudinaceus* showing the retractible proboscis.

Macracanthorhynchus hirudinaceus

Description: Adults resemble *Ascaris suum*, but taper posteriorly. The anterior of the worm possesses a retractable proboscis, which is covered with recurved hooks (Fig. 1.87). Male worms are up to 10 cm long and the females around 40–60 cm in length and are slightly curved and white/pinkish in colour when fresh. The worms are thick (5–10 mm in width) and flattened and the cuticle is transversely wrinkled. This pseudo-segmentation can sometimes cause misidentification as a tapeworm. There is no alimentary canal. The anterior of the worm possesses a small retractable proboscis, which is covered with about six transverse rows of recurved hooks. The size of the hooks decreases posteriorly. The larva has a small circle of minute hooks at the anterior. The eggs are ovoid, yellowish-brown in colour, with a thick shell, the outer layer of which is irregularly mamillated (see Fig. 4.6) and measure 50–75 by 40–55 μm.

Life cycle: The prepatent period is 2–3 months and longevity can be around one year.

Oncicola

The main species is *Oncicola canis* which infects the small intestine of dogs, coyotes and occasionally cats. This parasite has beetles as intermediate hosts.

Oncicola canis

Description: These are thick worms (around 2–4 mm in width). Males are 6–13 mm and females 7–14 mm in length. The body is conical, tapering backwards, and is dark grey in colour. The proboscis bears six transverse rows, each with six hooks. The shapes of the hooks are taenioid in the anterior region and more like a rose thorn in the posterior section.

FAMILY POLYMORPHIDAE

A few genera are parasites of rodents (*Moniliformis*), aquatic birds (*Polymorphus*, *Filicollis*) and fishes (*Echinorhynchus*, *Acanthocephalus*). These are frequently small worms with a cylindrical body, although *Moniliformis* species can be very large, up to 30 cm in length.

Life cycle: The definitive host is infected following ingestion of an intermediate host that contains an infective cystacanth. The adult worm establishes in the posterior small intestine. The prepatent period is 3–4 weeks.

Polymorphus

The main species is *Polymorphus boschadis* (syn. *Polymorphus minutus*, *Echinorhynchus polymorphus*) which infects the small intestine of ducks, geese, chickens, swans and various wild aquatic birds. This parasite has crustaceans, including *Gammarus pulex*, freshwater shrimp and sometimes the crayfish *Potamobius astacus*, as intermediate hosts.

Polymorphus boschadis

Synonyms: *Polymorphus minutus*, *Echinorhynchus polymorphus*

Description: Males measure around 3 mm and females up to 10 mm in length and are orange-coloured when fresh. The anterior region possesses small spines and the cylindrical body has a constriction along its length, about one-third from the head. The proboscis has 16 rows of small hooks, their size increasing anteriorly. The spindle-shaped eggs have a thick middle shell, which is irregularly constricted towards the poles, and a thin outer shell, the embryo being slightly orange in colour. Eggs measure around 110 by 20 μm.

Filicollis

The main species is *Filicollis anatis* which infects the small intestine of ducks, geese, swans and various wild aquatic birds. This parasite has crustaceans, isopods such as *Asellus aquaticus*, as intermediate hosts.

Filicollis anatis

Description: The whitish male is about 7 mm in length and the anterior region possesses many small spines. The ovoid proboscis is armed with 18 longitudinal rows of small hooks. The neck of the female worm is elongate, slender and bears a globular-shaped proboscis, the crown of which is armed with 18 rows of minute hooks in a star-shaped pattern. The oval eggs measure approximately 62–67 by 19–23 μm. The eggs are smaller than those of *Polymorphus* and are oval rather than spindle-shaped.

PHYLUM PLATYHELMINTHES

This phylum contains the two classes of parasitic flatworms, the **Trematoda** and the **Cestoda**. A third class, the **Turbellaria** (planarians), which are mainly free-living carnivorous flatworms, are of no veterinary significance.

CLASS TREMATODA

Parasites of the class Trematoda (commonly called 'Flukes') include species of veterinary importance, which occur primarily in the bile ducts, alimentary tract and vascular system. Most flukes are flattened dorsoventrally, have a blind alimentary tract, suckers for attachment and are hermaphrodite (except Schistosomatidae where the sexes are separate). Depending on the predilection site, the eggs pass out of the final host, usually in faeces or urine, and the larval stages develop in a molluscan intermediate host. For a few species, a second intermediate host is involved, but the mollusc is essential for all members of the group.

There are many families in this class, and those which contain parasites of major veterinary importance include the Fasciolidae, Dicrocoeliidae, Paramphistomatidae and Schistosomatidae. Of lesser importance are the Echinostomatidae, Gastrodiscidae, Cyclocoeliidae, Opisthorchiidae, Brachylaemidae, Heterophyidae, Diplostomatidae, Strigeidae and Lecithodendriidae. The most important family by far is the Fasciolidae and our discussion of structure, function and life cycle is largely oriented towards this group.

STRUCTURE AND FUNCTION OF TREMATODES

The adult is usually flat and leaf-like and possesses two muscular suckers for attachment. The oral sucker at the anterior end surrounds the mouth and the ventral sucker (called the acetabulum), as the name indicates, is on that surface. The body surface is a tegument, which is absorptive and is often covered with spines or scales. The muscles lie immediately below the tegument. There is no body cavity and the organs are packed in a parenchyma (Fig. 1.88).

The digestive system is simple, the oral opening leading into a pharynx, oesophagus and a pair of branched intestinal caeca, which end blindly. Undigested material is presumably regurgitated as flukes lack an anus. The excretory system consists of a large number of ciliated flame cells, which impel waste metabolic products along a system of tubules that ultimately join and open to the exterior, or to an excretory bladder. The nervous system is simple, consisting of a pair of longitudinal trunks connecting anteriorly with two ganglia.

The trematodes are usually hermaphrodite and both cross- and self-fertilisation may occur. The male reproductive system consists of a pair of testes, simple or branched, each leading into a vas deferens; these join to enter the cirrus sac containing a seminal vesicle and the cirrus, a primitive penis which terminates at the common genital opening (Fig. 1.88). In some flukes there is a cirrus sac surrounding these terminal organs. The female system has a single ovary leading into an oviduct (where eggs are fertilised), which is expanded distally to form the ootype. There the ovum acquires a yolk from the secretion of the vitelline glands and ultimately a shell. As the egg passes along the uterus, the shell becomes hardened and toughened and is finally extruded through the genital opening adjacent to the ventral sucker. The mature egg is usually yellow because of the tanned protein shell and most species have an operculum. The eggs of many species of fluke develop in the uterus and are therefore able to hatch once they are expelled. Food, generally blood or tissue debris, is ingested and passed into the caeca where it is digested and absorbed. Metabolism appears to be primarily anaerobic.

LIFE CYCLE OF TREMATODES

There is wide variation in the complex digenean life cycle. In general, the life cycle may have two or more obligate hosts, sometimes with transport or paratenic hosts. In most species, the first intermediate host is a mollusc in which futher development of hatched larvae takes place. The essential point of the life cycle is that whereas one nematode egg can develop into only one adult, one trematode egg may eventually develop into hundreds of adults. This is due to the phenomenon of asexual multiplication, **parthenogony**, in the molluscan intermediate host, i.e. the production of new individuals by single larval forms.

The adult flukes are always oviparous and lay eggs with an operculum or lid at one pole. In the egg, the embryo develops into a pyriform (pear-shaped) ciliated larva called a **miracidium** (Fig. 1.89). The eggs of some digenean flukes may be passively eaten by snails, in which they hatch. In many species of digenean flukes (e.g. *Fasciola hepatica*), the egg hatches in water and under the stimulus of light and temperature, the miracidium releases an enzyme that attacks the proteinaceous cement holding the operculum in place. The latter springs open like a hinged lid and the miracidium emerges within a few minutes.

The miracidium, propelled through the water by its cilia, does not feed and must, for its further development, find a suitable snail within a few hours before it exhausts its energy reserves. It is believed to use chemotactic responses to 'home in' on the snail and, on contact, it adheres by suction to the snail and penetrates its soft tissues using its conical papilla and aided by a cytolytic enzyme. The entire process of penetration takes about 30 minutes, after which the cilia are lost and the miracidium develops into an elongated sac, the **sporocyst**, containing a number of undifferentiated germinal cells. These cells develop into **rediae**, which migrate to the hepatopancreas of the snail; rediae are also larval forms possessing an oral sucker, some flame cells and a simple gut. From the germinal cells of the rediae arise the final stages, the **cercariae** (Fig. 1.90), although if environmental conditions for the snail are unsuitable, a second or daughter generation of rediae is often produced instead.

The cercariae, in essence young flukes with long tails, emerge actively from the snail, usually in considerable numbers. The actual stimulus for emergence depends on the species but is most commonly a change in temperature or light intensity. Once a snail is infected, cercariae continue to be produced indefinitely, although

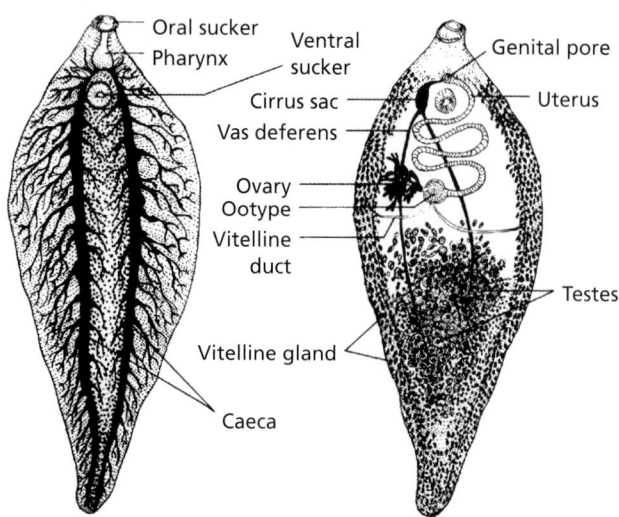

Fig. 1.88 Internal structure of a generalised digenetic trematode.

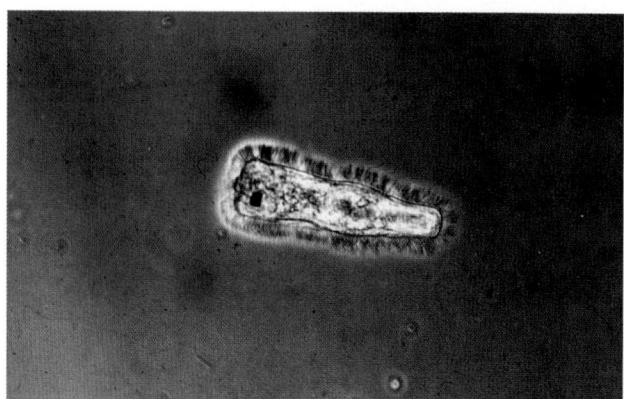

Fig. 1.89 Miracidium of *Fasciola hepatica*.

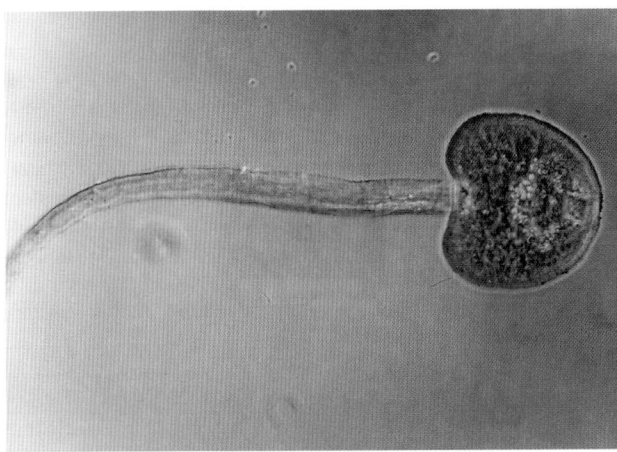

Fig. 1.90 Cercaria of *Fasciola hepatica*.

the majority of infected snails die prematurely from gross destruction of the hepato-pancreas.

Typically, the cercariae swim for some time, utilising a film of water, and within an hour or so attach themselves to vegetation, shed their tails and encyst. This stage is called a **metacercaria** (Fig. 1.91), which is the infective stage for grazing animals. Encysted metacercariae have great potential for survival extending to months. Once ingested, the outer cyst wall is removed mechanically during mastication. Rupture of the inner cyst occurs in the intestine and depends on a hatching mechanism, enzymatic in origin, triggered by a suitable oxidation–reduction potential and a carbon dioxide system provided by the intestinal environment. The emergent juvenile fluke, often called a marita, then penetrates the intestine and migrates to the predilection site where it becomes adult after several weeks and starts to lay eggs, thus completing the cycle.

The location of the metacercariae varies between different flukes but in general they have a pattern. Those from fasciolids and paramphistomatids encyst on herbage. The metacercariae from troglotrematids, opisthorchiids and heterophyids encyst in fish, crab or crayfish intermediate hosts, whereas those from diplostomatids prefer amphibian or other vertebrate paratenic hosts. Schistosomatids do not have a metacercarial stage; the cercariae are able to penetrate the definitive host percutaneously.

ORDER PLAGIORCHIIDA

FAMILY FASCIOLIDAE

These are large, flat leaf-shaped flukes. The anterior end is usually elongated into the shape of a cone and the anterior sucker is located at the end of the cone. The ventral sucker is placed at the level of the 'shoulders' of the fluke. The internal organs are branched while the cuticle is covered in spines. There are three important genera: *Fasciola*, *Fascioloides* and *Fasciolopsis*.

Fasciola

The members of this genus are commonly known as Liver flukes. They are responsible for widespread morbidity and mortality in sheep and cattle. The two most important species are *Fasciola hepatica* and *F. gigantica*. *F. hepatica* is found in the liver of sheep, cattle, goats, horses, deer, rabbits, humans and other mammals of temperate areas and in cooler areas of high altitude in the tropics and subtropics. *F. gigantica* predominates in tropical areas and is localised in the liver of cattle, buffalo, sheep, goats, pigs, camels, deer and humans (Fig. 1.92). Both species have lymnaeid snails as intermediate hosts.

Fasciola hepatica

Description: The young fluke at the time of entry into the liver is 1–2 mm in length and lancet-like (Fig. 1.92a). Adult flukes are leaf-shaped (being broader anteriorly than posteriorly), grey-brown in colour and around 2.5–3.5 cm in length and 1 cm in width (Fig. 1.93). The anterior end is conical and marked off by distinct shoulders from the body. The tegument is covered with backwardly

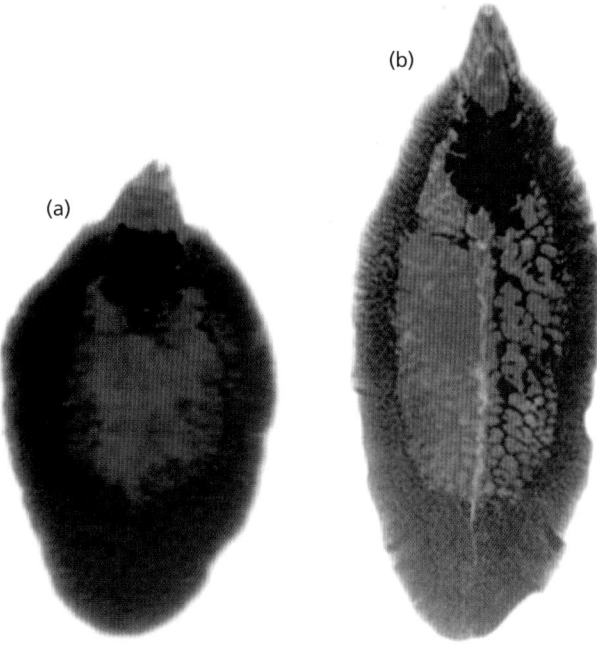

(a) (b)

Fig. **1.92** Outline of (a) *Fasciola hepatica* and (b) *F. gigantica*. The former has broader shoulders and is shorter in length.

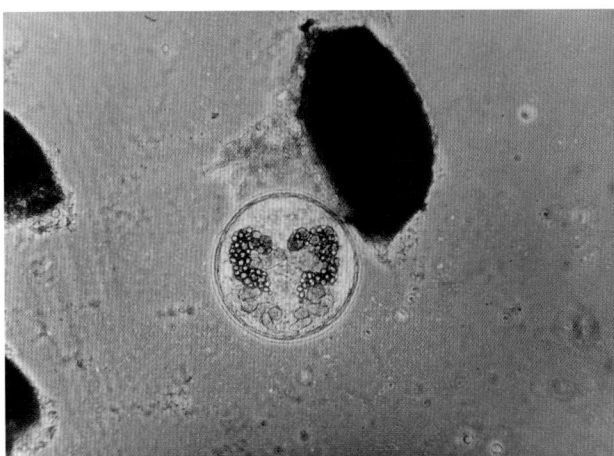

Fig. **1.91** Metacercariae of *Fasciola hepatica*.

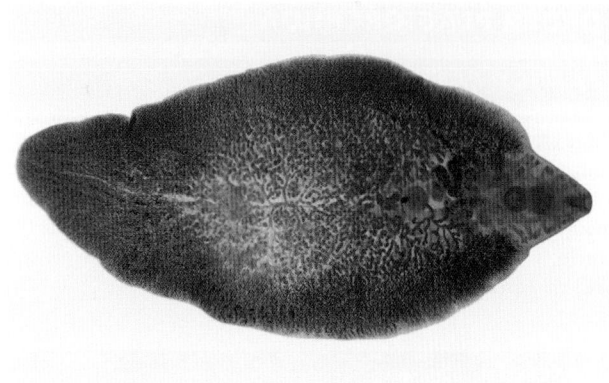

Fig. 1.93 Adult *Fasciola hepatica* fluke. (Courtesy of Jana Bulantova).

projecting spines. An oral and ventral sucker, situated at the level of the shoulders, may be readily seen. The intestinal caeca have many branches and extend a considerable distance posteriorly. The testes and ovary are multibranched. The uterus is positioned anterior to the testes. The cirrus is well developed. Immature flukes at the time of entry into the liver are 1–2 mm in length and lancet-like. The egg is thin-shelled, oval with symmetrical barrel-shaped side walls, operculate, browny-yellow and large (130–150 × 65–90 μm), and about twice the size of a trichostrongyle egg (Fig. 1.94; see also Fig. 4.3). The granular contents fill the whole of the egg.

Life cycle: Adult flukes in the bile ducts shed eggs into the bile and these enter the intestine. Eggs passed in the faeces of the mammalian host develop and hatch, releasing motile ciliated miracidia. This takes 9–10 days at optimal temperatures of 22–26 °C and little development occurs below 10 °C. The liberated miracidium has a short lifespan and must locate a suitable snail within about three hours if successful penetration of the latter is to occur. In infected snails, development proceeds through the sporocyst and redial stages to the final stage in the intermediate host, the cercaria; these are shed from the snail as motile forms, which attach themselves to firm surfaces, such as grass blades, and encyst there to form the infective metacercariae. It takes a minimum of 6–7 weeks for completion of development from miracidium to metacercaria, although under unfavourable circumstances a period of several months is required.

Infection of a snail with one miracidium can produce over 600 metacercariae. Metacercariae ingested by the final host excyst in the small intestine, migrate through the gut wall, cross the peritoneum and penetrate the liver capsule. The young flukes tunnel through the liver parenchyma for 6–8 weeks and then enter the small bile ducts where they migrate to the larger ducts and occasionally the gallbladder and reach sexual maturity. The prepatent period is 10–12 weeks. The minimal period for completion of one entire life cycle of *F. hepatica* is therefore 17–18 weeks. The longevity of *F. hepatica* in untreated sheep may be years; in cattle it is usually less than one year. See **life cycle 18**.

Fasciola gigantica

Description: The adult fluke is larger than *F. hepatica*, reaching 7.5 cm in length and 1.5 cm in breadth, and the body is more transparent. The shape is more leaf-like, the conical anterior end is very short and the shoulders, characteristic of *F. hepatica*, are barely perceptible (Fig. 1.92b). The gut caeca are more highly branched than in *F. hepatica*. The eggs are larger than those of *F. hepatica*, measuring 170–190 by 90–100 μm.

Life cycle: This is similar to *F. hepatica*, the main differences being in the time scale of the cycle. The immature stages migrate through the liver parenchyma, the adults reaching the bile ducts about 12 weeks after infection. Most parasitic phases are longer and the prepatent period is 13–16 weeks.

Fascioloides

The genus comprises a single species, *Fascioloides magna*, also known as the giant liver fluke, large American liver fluke or deer fluke. It is one of the largest of the trematodes and is easily identified.

Life cycle: The life cycle is similar to that of *F. hepatica*. The eggs hatch to miracidia after four weeks or longer. Development in the snail takes 7–8 weeks. The prepatent period in deer is around 30 weeks. The main species is *Fascioloides magna* which infects the liver and occasionally bile duct of deer, cattle, sheep, goats, pigs, horses and llamas. This parasite has lymnaeid snails (*Fossaria* spp., *Lymnaea* spp., *Stagnicola* spp.) as intermediate hosts.

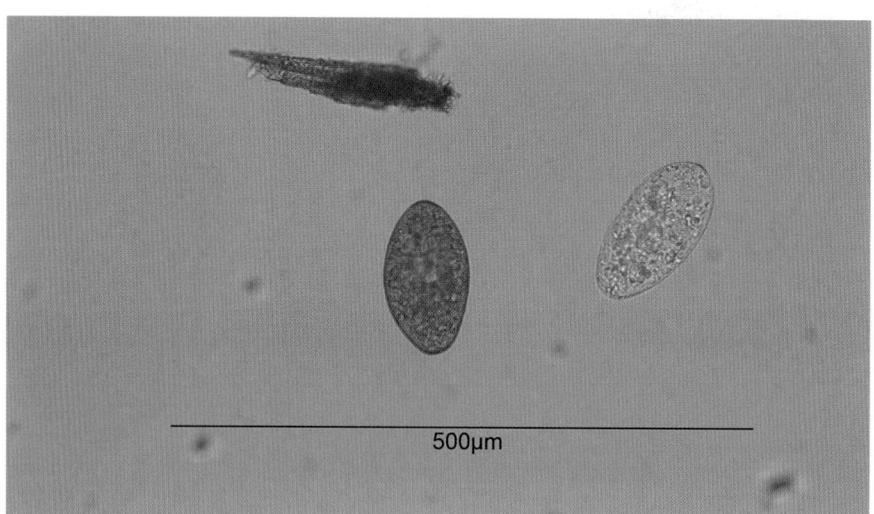

500μm

Fig. 1.94 Rumen fluke eggs (Paramphistomatidae) with yellow-brown egg of *Fasciola hepatica* (left). (Courtesy of Anja Joachim).

LIFE CYCLE 18. LIFE CYCLE OF *FASCIOLA HEPATICA*

Fasciola hepatica is a trematode parasite of the biliary ducts (1) of small and large ruminants, which excrete the parasite eggs with the faeces (2). Upon contact with water, miracidia (larvae with vibrating cilia, 3) hatch from the egg and actively swim to seek out a suitable intermediate host, freshwater snails of the family Lymnaeidae (4). The miracidium enters the foot of the snail and travels to the hepatopancreas where it develops into a sporocyst (5). Subsequently, the sporocyst generates rediae (6), that localise in the respiratory tract, and then several cercariae (7). The latter stage is highly motile, and actively leaves the intermediate host to become encysted as metacercaria (8) on aquatic plants, such as watercress (9). Once ingested by suitable definitive hosts (including humans) (10), the metacercaria hatches and begins migrating as a juvenile form (adolescaria) from the intestine through the peritoneum to the parenchyma of the liver and finally to the biliary ducts, where it develops into a sexually mature adult trematode.

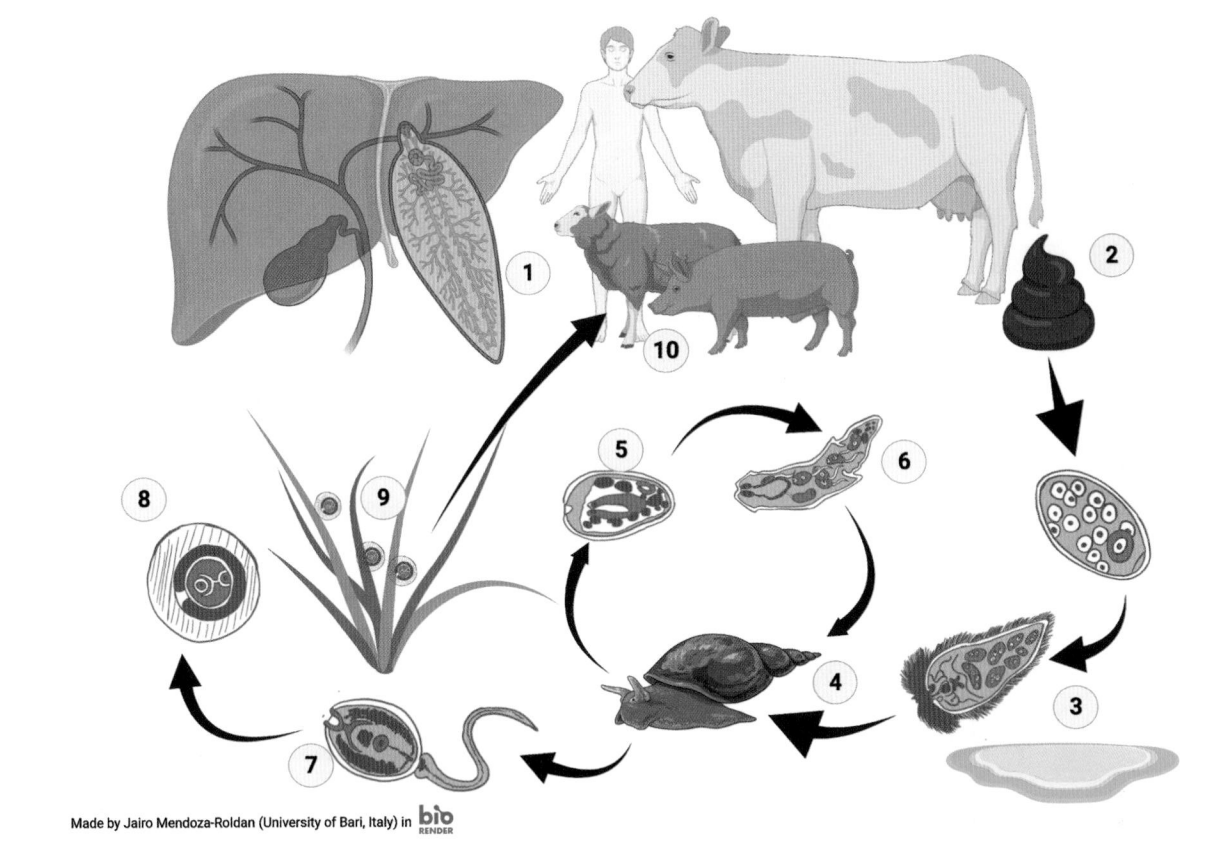

Made by Jairo Mendoza-Roldan (University of Bari, Italy) in **bio** RENDER

Fascioloides magna

Description: Flukes are large and thick and measure up to 10 cm long by 2.5 cm broad and around 3–4 mm in depth. The flukes are oval, with a rounded posterior end. They possess no anterior cone projection and when fresh are flesh-coloured (Fig. 1.95). In deer, adult *F. magna* occur in cysts which communicate with the bile ducts. Eggs are large, operculate, measure 109–168 by 75–96 μm and have a protoplasmic appendage at the pole opposite the operculum.

Fasciolopsis

The single species of this genus is primarily a parasite of humans in India, Pakistan, Southeast Asia and China, but can occur in the pig which may act as a reservoir host.

Life cycle: The life cycle is similar to that of *F. hepatica*. The final host is infected through ingestion of metacercariae that encyst on aquatic plants. The prepatent period is 9–13 weeks. The main species is *Fasciolopsis buski* which infects the small intestine of humans, pigs and occasionally dogs. This parasite has freshwater snails (*Planorbis*, *Segmentina*, *Hippeutis*) as intermediate hosts.

Fasciolopsis buski

Description: Large, thick, elongate–oval, fleshy pink flukes without shoulders, broader posteriorly, and variable in size but usually measuring 30–75 mm long by 8–20 mm wide. The ventral sucker is located near the anterior extremity and is much larger than the oral sucker. The cuticle is covered in spines that are frequently lost as adults. The intestinal caeca are unbranched and extend to near the posterior of the fluke. The testes are branched and tandem; the ovary is also branched. Eggs are oval, yellowish-brown, thin-shelled with an operculum, and measure 125–140 by 70–90 μm (Fig. 1.96). They resemble those of *Fasciola*.

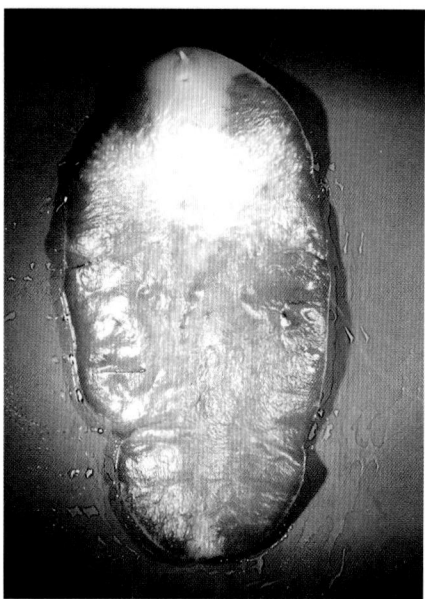

Fig. 1.95 *Fascioloides magna.*

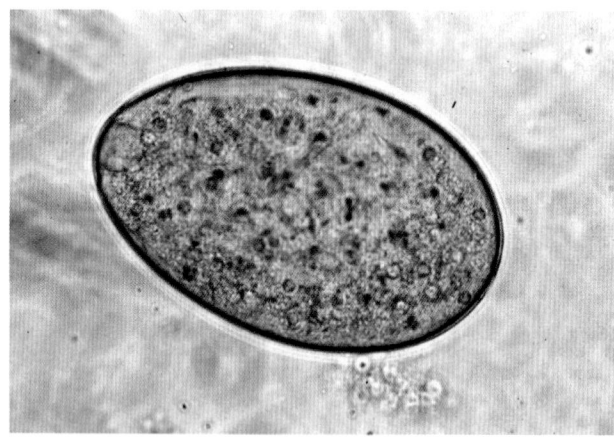

Fig. 1.96 Egg of *Fasciolopsis buski.*

FAMILY PARAMPHISTOMATIDAE

Adult paramphistomes (amphistomes) are mainly parasitic in the forestomachs of ruminants, although *Gigantocotyle* is found in the liver and duodenum. Their shape is not typical of the trematodes, being conical and thick and fleshy rather than flat. All require a water snail as an intermediate host. There are several genera: *Paramphistomum*, *Cotylophoron*, *Bothriophoron*, *Orthocoelium* and *Gigantocotyle*, of which *Paramphistomum* is the most common and widespread in ruminants. The taxonomy of the paramphistomes is complex and unresolved and many of the species described may be synonymous, being differentiated mainly on size and shape of the suckers.

Paramphistomum

Members of this genus (rumen fluke) are found in the rumen and reticulum of ruminants (Table 1.49). The adults are small, conical (pear-shaped), maggot-like flukes about 1 cm long and 3–5 mm wide and light red in colour when fresh. Unlike other flukes, the large ventral sucker is located at the posterior extremity of the body and is well developed.

Life cycle: Eggs shed in the faeces are undeveloped. In an aquatic environment, miracidia develop and hatch to penetrate water snails in which they develop to cercaria, following sporocyst and redial stages. The cercariae encyst (metacercariae) on vegetation in, or bordering, watercourses and ponds. Development in the snail intermediate host is similar to that of *Fasciola* and under favourable conditions (26–30 °C) can be completed in four weeks. Following ingestion by a definitive host, the metacercariae excyst in the duodenum, where the young flukes attach and feed for about six weeks, before migrating forward to the forestomachs where they mature. The prepatent period is between seven and 10 weeks.

Paramphistomum cervi

Synonym: *Paramphistomum explanatum*

Description: Adult flukes measure about 6–13 mm by 3–5 mm. The adults are small, conical (pear-shaped), maggot-like flukes

Table 1.49 *Paramphistomum (Calicophoron, Cotylophoron, Bothriophoron)* species.

Species	Hosts	Site	Intermediate hosts
Paramphistomum cervi (syn. *Paramphistomum explanatum*)	Cattle, sheep, goats, deer, buffalo, antelopes	Rumen	Freshwater snails (*Bulinus* spp., *Planorbis* spp.)
Calicophoron daubneyi (syn. *Paramphistomum daubnei, Paramphistomum daubneyi*)	Cattle, goats	Rumen	Freshwater snails (*Omphiscola* spp.)
Paramphistomum microbothrium	Cattle, sheep, goats, deer, buffalo, antelopes	Rumen	Freshwater snails (*Fossaria* spp., *Bulinus* spp.)
Paramphistomum ichikawa	Sheep, cattle	Rumen	Planorbid snails (*Gyraulus, Helicorbis, Segnetilia*)
Cotylophoron cotylophorum (syn. *Paramphistomum cotylophorum*)	Sheep, goats, cattle and wild ruminants	Rumen, reticulum	Freshwater snails (*Bulinus* spp.)
Paramphistomum bothriophoron (syn. *Bothriophoron bothriophoron*)	Zebus	Rumen	Freshwater snails (*Bulinus* spp., *Planorbis* spp.)
Paramphistomum streptocoelium (syn. *Ceylonocotyle streptocoelium, Orthocoelium streptocoelium*)	Cattle, sheep, goats and wild ruminants	Rumen	Freshwater snails (*Glyptanisus* spp.)
Calicophoron calicophorum (syn. *Paramphistomum calicophorum*)	Cattle, sheep, other ruminants	Rumen, reticulum	Water snails

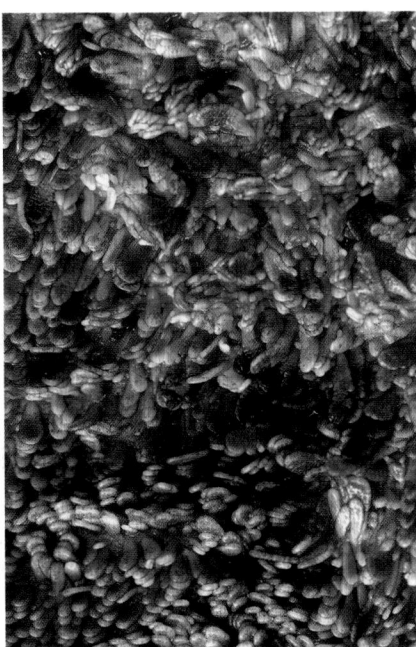

Fig. 1.97 Adult flukes of *Paramphistomum*. (Courtesy of Andrei Mihalca).

about 1 cm long and light red in colour when fresh (Fig. 1.97). One sucker is visible at the tip of the cone and the other well-developed sucker is at the base. The tegument has no spines. The larval stages are less than 5 mm, fresh specimens having a pink colour. The egg resembles that of *Fasciola hepatica*, being large (about 115–175 by 75–100 µm) and operculate, but is transparent or slightly greenish rather than yellowish-brown and slightly smaller than eggs of *F. hepatica* (see Fig. 1.94). In the early stages of segmentation, the egg contains 4–8 blastomeres surrounded by yolk cells.

Cotylophoron cotylophorum

Synonym: *Paramphistomum cotylophoron*

Description: The fluke is very similar to *Paramphistomum cervi* but the genital pore is surrounded by a genital sucker. The egg measures 125–135 by 60–68 µm.

Gigantocotyle

Gigantoctyle is found in the liver and duodenum of cattle and other ruminants. The life cycle is similar to that of *F. hepatica* and requires snails of the genus *Galba* as intermediate hosts. The main species is *Gigantocotyle explanatum* (syn. *Explanatum explanatum*, *Paramphistomum explanatum*) which infects the liver, bile ducts, gallbladder and duodenum of cattle, buffalo and other ruminants. This parasite has freshwater snails as intermediate hosts.

Gigantocotyle explanatum

Synonyms: *Paramphistomum explanatum, Paramphistomum fraturnum, Explanatum explanatum*

Description: These are conical pinkish flukes when fresh. Adult fluke are 8–10 mm long and 4.7–5.7 mm wide. The body tapers anteriorly and is curved ventrally with no tegumental papillae.

The acetabulum is very large and the genital pore is bifurcal. The oval eggs measure 180–200 by 110–130 µm, are colourless and have an operculum.

Pseudodiscus

Adult flukes have a conical anterior end widening gradually to an oval leaf-like shape. The main species is *Pseudodiscus collinsi* which infects the caecum and colon of horses. This parasite has freshwater snails (*Indoplanorbis* spp.) as intermediate hosts.

Pseudodiscus collinsi

Description: Adult flukes are 6–12 mm by 3–7 mm in size. The conical body has conspicuous serrations along the anterior lateral margins. There is a ventral sucker and the oral sucker has paired pouch-like diverticula.

FAMILY GASTRODISCIDAE

Gastrodiscus spp. are found in the large intestines of horses and pigs. *Homalogaster* is found in the large intestine of cattle and buffalo.

Gastrodiscus

Intestinal flukes with a short conical anterior end and a large posterior discoid body covered ventrally with large papillae (Table 1.50).

Life cycle: The life cycle of the different species is generally similar. Eggs are passed in the faeces and, following development, release miracidia into water where they enter a species of water snail. Development in the snail proceeds through sporocyst and redial stages leading to the release of cercariae, which encyst to form metacercariae. Infection of the final host is by ingestion of metacercariae with herbage. Excystation occurs in the intestine where the immature paramphistomes develop to reach maturity.

Gastrodiscus aegyptiacus

Description: Adult flukes are reddish-pink in colour when fresh and measure 9–17 mm by 8–11 mm. The anterior region measures up to 4 mm by 2.5 mm and is cylindrical, while the remainder of the body is saucer-shaped, with the margins curved inwards (Fig. 1.98). The ventral surface is covered by a large number of regularly arranged papillae. The oral sucker has two posterolateral pouches;

Table 1.50 *Gastrodiscus* species.

Species	Hosts	Site	Intermediate hosts
Gastrodiscus aegyptiacus	Horses, donkeys, pigs, warthogs	Large and small intestine	Freshwater snails (*Bulinus* spp., *Cleopatra* spp.)
Gastrodiscus hominis (syn. *Gastrodiscoides hominis*)	Pigs, humans	Caecum, colon	Planorbid snails (*Helicorbis* spp.)
Gastrodiscus secundus	Horses, elephants	Large intestine	Freshwater snails (*Bulinus* spp.)

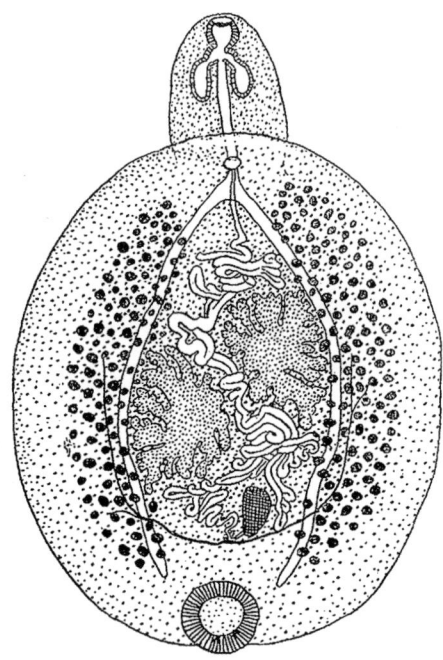

Fig. 1.98 *Gastrodiscus aegyptiacus.* (Adapted from Mönnig, 1934).

the posterior sucker is small and subterminal. Eggs are oval and measure 131–139 by 78–90 μm.

Gastrodiscus hominis

Synonym: *Gastrodiscoides hominis*

Description: Adult flukes are pink in colour when fresh and measure 8–14 mm by 5–8 mm, with a conical anterior body and a large discoidal posterior body lacking tegumental papillae.

Gastrodiscus secundus

Description: Identical to *G. aegyptiacus* but the genital pore is located posterior to the level of the caecal origin and the vitelline glands are distributed all over the discoid posterior body.

Homalogaster

These are intestinal flukes in which the body is divided into two, with a large anterior region and a small cylindrical posterior region.

Life cycle: The life cycle is presumed to be similar to other paramphistomes of the rumen. The main species is *Homalogaster paloniae* which infects the large intestine of cattle and buffalo. This parasite has freshwater snails (*Hippeutis* spp., *Polypylis* spp.) as intermediate hosts.

Homalogaster paloniae

Description: Adult flukes are 8–15 mm long and 4.5–7.5 mm wide. The anterior body is large, flat, ellipsoidal and bluntly pointed anteriorly with large numbers of papillae present on the ventral tegument. The posterior body is small and spherical.

FAMILY GASTROTHYLACIDAE

Pouched amphistomes are similar in appearance to the paramphistomes, with a number of species belonging to the genera *Gastrothylax*, *Fischoederius* and *Carmyerius* parasitic in ruminants throughout Africa and Asia. These flukes differ in having an extremely large ventral pouch that opens anteriorly and which covers the ventral surface of the fluke as far as the large ventral sucker.

Gastrothylax

The main species is *Gastrothylax crumenifer* which infects the rumen and reticulum of cattle, buffalo, zebu, sheep and other ruminants. This parasite has freshwater snails as intermediate hosts.

Gastrothylax crumenifer

Description: This is an elongated fluke, being circular in transverse section and reddish in colour when fresh. The body is 10–16 mm long and 5–8 mm wide. This fluke differs in having an extremely large ventral pouch that opens anteriorly and which covers the ventral surface of the fluke as far as the large ventral sucker. The ventral pouch is normally triangular in cross-section with a dorsally directed apex. The terminal genitalium opens into the ventral pouch about halfway between the intestinal bifurcation and the pharynx. The terminal oval sucker is small. Eggs are 115–135 by 66–70 μm.

Fischoederius

Fischoederius spp. complete their biological life cycle in freshwater snails, and are localised in the rumen and duodenum of cattle, buffalo, zebu, sheep and other ruminants. *Fischoederius elongatus* may rarely infect humans.

Fischoederius elongatus

Description: The flukes are reddish when fresh. The body is 10–20 mm long and 3–5 mm wide. The terminal genitalium is within the ventral pouch. The uterus is situated along the midline. The testes are lobed and one is sited dorsally to the other. Eggs measure 125–150 by 65–75 μm.

Fischoederius cobboldi

Description: The flukes are reddish in colour when fresh. The body measures 8–10 mm in length. Eggs measure 110–120 by 60–75 μm.

Carmyerius

Carmyerius spp. complete their biological life cycle in freshwater snails, and are localised in the rumen of cattle, buffalo and antelopes.

Carmyerius spatiosus

Synonym: *Gastrothylax spatiosus*

Description: Flukes measure 8.5–12 mm in length and 2.5–3 mm in width. The posterior sucker is quite small and is spherical. The intestinal caeca extend down into the last quarter of the body. The ventral pouch is either circular or slightly triangular with blunt angles and the terminal genitalium lies within the pouch. The testes lie horizontally, one on each side of the median line, which differs from the position in *Fischoederius*. Eggs measure 115–125 by 60–65 μm.

Carmyerius gregarius

Description: The flukes are 7–10 mm in length. The intestinal caeca extend only a short distance below the middle of the body.

FAMILY ECHINOSTOMATIDAE

The family Echinostomatidae includes the genera *Echinostoma*, *Echinoparyphium* and *Hypoderaeum*, which are parasites of birds, and *Echinochasmus*, *Isthmiophora* and *Euparyphium*, which are parasites of fish-eating mammals.

Life cycle: The life cycle involves two intermediate hosts, namely freshwater snails and fish or frogs. Eggs passed in the faeces of infected birds hatch to produce a miracidium, which infects the first intermediate snail host. Subsequently, cercariae encyst within the snail or are shed and migrate to infect other snails. Cercariae can also encyst in the kidneys of tadpoles and adult frogs. The definitive host is infected through eating the second intermediate host containing encysted metacercariae (mesocercariae). The prepatent period is 1–2 weeks.

Echinostoma

Echinostoma revolutum are localised in the rumen, caecum, cloaca and rectum of ducks, geese, fowl, partridges and pigeons (*Echinostoma revolutum*), and occasionally humans. *Echinostoma paraulum* are localised in the small intestine of ducks, pigeons and humans. Both species complete their biological life cycle in snails and frogs.

Echinostoma revolutum

Description: The fluke is about 10–20 mm long and up to 2 mm in width. The head-collar is armed with around 37 spines, some forming groups of 'corner' spines. The anterior of the cuticle is covered in spines. The ovary is anterior to the tandem testes.

Echinostoma paraulum

Synonym: *Echinoparyphium paraulum*

Description: The fluke measures 6–10.5 mm in length by 0.8–1.5 mm in width. The tegument is usually almost completely covered in spines, but in some instances these can be absent. The head-collar is armed with 37 spines, some forming a double dorsolateral row. The tandem testes are located in the third quarter of the body.

Echinoparyphium

The main species is *Echinoparyphium recurvatum* which infects the small intestine of ducks, geese, chickens, pigeons, wild birds and humans. This parasite has snails, fish, shellfish and tadpoles as intermediate hosts.

Echinoparyphium recurvatum

Description: The fluke is about 4 mm long by 0.7 mm wide and curved ventrally. Spines are present anterior to the ventral sucker and the head-crown is armed with spines. Eggs measure about 110 by 82 μm.

Hypoderaeum

The main species is *Hypoderaeum conoideum* which infects the small intestine of chickens, turkey, ducks, geese, pigeons and other aquatic birds. This parasite has snails, fish, shellfish and tadpoles as intermediate hosts.

Hypoderaeum conoideum

Description: Adult flukes have an elongate body 5–12 mm long and tapering posteriorly. The anterior body is armed with about 50 small spines and bears a large ventral sucker. The testes are elongate and slightly lobed, and situated just beyond the midline.

Echinochasmus

The main species is *Echinochasmus perfoliatus* which infects the small intestine of dogs, cats, foxes and pigs. This parasite has snails and fish as intermediate hosts.

Echinochasmus perfoliatus

Description: Adult flukes are 2–4 mm long with a head-crown bearing 24 spines arranged in a single row. The testes are large and situated just beyond the midline, with the ovaries to the right and anterior to the testes.

Euparyphium

Euparyphium spp. complete their biological life cycle in snails and amphibian tadpoles, and are localised in the small intestine of cats, foxes, polecats, mink, badgers, otters, hedgehogs (*Euparyphium melis*), humans, dogs and rats (*Euparyphium ilocanum*).

Euparyphium melis

Description: Adult flukes have an elongate body 3.5–12 mm long that bears a large ventral sucker and a dorsal head-collar with 27 spines. The whole ventral surface is covered with small spines. The testes are situated midline, with one lying posterior to the other. The ovary lies anterior to the testes and to the right of the midline.

FAMILY PHILOPHTHALMIDAE

Philophthalmus are eye flukes of birds.

Life cycle: Embryonated eggs are shed from the eyes, mouth and nostrils, and hatch immediately on contact with water. After penetrating a snail intermediate host, a single redia is released. The mother redia penetrates the heart of the snail, releasing daughter rediae that migrate to the digestive glands and after about 95 days produce cercariae, which are released from the snail and encyst on aquatic vegetation. Following ingestion, metacercariae excyst in the mouth or crop and young flukes may be found in the oesophagus, nasal passages, orbit and lacrimal gland within a few hours following ingestion.

Philophthalmus

The main species is *Philophthalmus gralli* (the Oriental avian eye fluke) which infects the conjunctival sac of ostriches, chickens and wild birds. This parasite has freshwater snails as intermediate hosts.

Philophthalmus gralli

Description: Adult flukes are very small (2–3 mm) and fusiform shaped. The body surface is covered by small spines and the two suckers are orally and subterminally located. The pharynx is located immediately posterior to the oral sucker.

FAMILY CYCLOCOELIDAE

These are medium-sized to large slightly flattened flukes, parasites of aquatic birds in the body cavity, air sacs or nasal cavities. They do not possess an oral sucker and often the ventral sucker is absent. The intestinal caeca are joined together posteriorly and their structure is simple or branched. The lateral vitellaria similarly meet posteriorly. Genera include *Typhlocoelum* in the respiratory tract of ducks and *Hyptiasmus* in the nasal and orbital sinuses of ducks and geese.

Typhlocoelum

Life cycle: Eggs are coughed up and swallowed in the faeces of ducks. A miracidium, containing a single redia, hatches from the egg. The redia, not the miracidium, enters a snail and after 11 days produces small numbers of cercariae. There is no sporocyst stage. The cercariae are retained within the snail and encyst. Birds are infected by eating infected snails of the genera *Helisoma* and *Planorbis*. The larval fluke reaches the bronchi via the bloodstream.

Typhlocoelum cucumerinum

Synonyms: *Distoma cucumerinum*, *Typhloceolum obovlae*

Description: Adult flukes are 6–12 mm long by 2–5 mm broad. The body is oval and blunter anteriorly than posteriorly. The testes are deeply lobed and lie diagonally one behind the other with the unlobed ovary situated in front of the posterior testis.

Typhlocoelum cymbium

Synonym: *Tracheophilus sisowi*

Description: Adult flukes are 6–11.5 mm long by 3 mm broad. The body has rounded ends and is wide in the middle. The testes are rounded, not lobed, and lie in a diagonal position in the posterior part of the body with the unlobed ovary situated in front of the anterior testis. Eggs measure about 122 by 63 µm.

Hyptiasmus

The main species is *Hyptiasmus tumidus* (syn. *Hyptiasmus arcuatus*, *Cyclocoelum arcuatum*) and infects the nasal and orbital sinuses of ducks and geese. This parasite has water snails as intermediate hosts.

Hyptiasmus tumidus

Synonyms: *Hyptiasmus arcuatus*, *Cyclocoelum arcuatum*

Description: Adult flukes are 7–20 mm long by 2–5 mm wide. The body is pyriform and more rounded posteriorly. The gonads are arranged in a straight line.

FAMILY NOTOCOTYLIDAE

The family Notocotylidae includes the genera *Notocotylus*, *Paramonostomum* and *Catatropis*, which are parasites of birds, and *Cymbiforma*, which occur in sheep, goats and cattle. The small eggs are characterised by long filaments at the poles. The intermediate hosts are water snails.

Notocotylus

The main species is *Notocotylus attenuatus* which infects the caecum and rectum of chickens, ducks, geese and wild aquatic birds. This parasite has snails as intermediate hosts.

Notocotylus attenuatus

Description: The adult flukes are 2–5 mm long by 0.7–1.5 mm wide, narrow anteriorly and have no ventral sucker. The testes are situated posteriorly and the ovary lies between them. The uterus forms regular transverse coils extending from the posterior ovary to the elongate cirrus sac, situated anteriorly.

Catatropis

The main species is *Catatropis verrucosa* which infects the caeca of chickens, ducks, geese and other aquatic birds. This parasite has snails as intermediate hosts.

Catatropis verrucosa

Description: The fluke is 2–6 mm long and rounded anteriorly and posteriorly and has no ventral sucker. The testes are situated posteriorly and the ovary lies between them.

Cymbiforma

The main species is *Cymbiforma indica* (syn. *Ogmocotyle indica*) which infects the small intestine of sheep, goats and cattle. This parasite has snails as intermediate hosts.

Cymbiforma indica

Synonym: *Ogmocotyle indica*

Description: Adult flukes are pear-shaped, concave ventrally and measure 0.8–2.7 cm in length and 0.3–0.9 mm in width. There is no ventral sucker and the cuticle is armed with fine spines ventrally and anteriorly. The ovary has four demarcated lobes. The fluke lacks a pharynx and the oesophagus is short. The genital opening is sited just anterior to the middle of the body and to the left of the midline. Eggs bear long filaments at both poles and measure 18–27 by 11–13 µm.

FAMILY DICROCOELIIDAE

These trematodes are small lancet-like flukes occurring in the biliary and pancreatic ducts of vertebrates. Miracidia are present in the eggs when they are passed in the faeces; there is no redial stage during development in the snail and 2–3 intermediate hosts may be involved in the life cycle. Members of this family are found in ruminants (*Dicrocoelium*, *Eurytrema*), cats and birds (*Platynosomum*).

Dicrocoelium

The single species of this genus is found in the bile ducts of the liver of ruminants. There is no possibility of confusion with other flukes in the bile ducts of ruminants due to their small size and distinct lanceolate shape.

Life cycle: The egg does not hatch until ingested by the first intermediate host, a terrestrial snail, in which two generations of sporocysts develop which then produce cercariae. The latter are extruded in masses cemented together by slime and adhere to vegetation. This phase of development takes at least three months. The slime balls of cercariae are ingested by ants in which they develop to metacercariae, mainly in the body cavity and occasionally the brain. The presence of a brain lesion in the ant, induced by metacercariae, impels the ant to climb up and remain on the tips of the herbage, thus increasing the chance of ingestion by the final host. This phase in the ant is completed in just over one month in summer temperatures. Infection of the final host is by passive ingestion of ants containing metacercariae. The metacercariae hatch in the small intestine and the young flukes migrate up the main bile duct and thence to the smaller ducts in the liver. There is no parenchymal migration and the prepatent period is 10–12 weeks. The total life cycle takes approximately six months. The flukes are long-lived and can survive in the final host for several years. See **life cycle 19**.

Dicrocoelium dendriticum

Synonym: *Dicrocoelium lanceolatum*

Description: Adult flukes are 6–12 mm long and 1.5–2.5 mm wide, distinctly lanceolate and semi-transparent/translucent allowing the internal organs to be readily seen (Fig. 1.99). They are almost symmetrical in shape and the cuticle is smooth. The oral sucker is smaller than the ventral sucker and is located in close proximity. The gut is simple, consisting of two branches resembling a tuning fork. Behind the ventral sucker, the lobed testes lie in tandem with the ovary immediately posterior. The uterus is usually dark brown and convoluted, filling the space behind the genital gland. The cirrus is small. There are no spines on the cuticle (cf. *Fasciola*). The thick-shelled egg is small, 35–45 µm in length by 22–30 µm in width, dark brown with small round poles and slightly barrel-shaped walls and operculate, usually with a flattened side. The operculum is often difficult to see. It contains a miracidium that completely fills the egg when passed in the faeces.

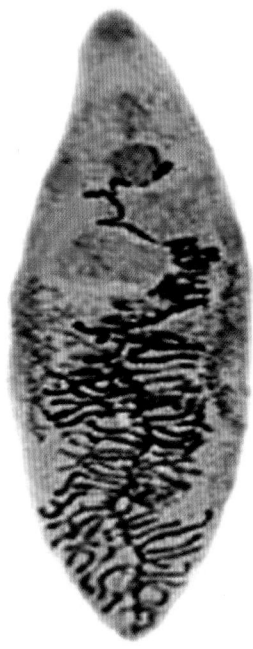

Fig. 1.99 *Dicrocoelium dendriticum.*

LIFE CYCLE 19. LIFE CYCLE OF *DICROCOELIUM DENDRITICUM*

Adult *Dicrocoelium dendriticum* live in the biliary ducts and gall-bladder of cattle and other grazing animals, which are definitive hosts; humans can be accidental definitive hosts (1). These excrete parasite eggs with the faeces (2). In the environment, a miracidium develops inside the egg (3). Once eggs containing the miracidia are ingested by terrestrial gastropods (first intermediate hosts, 4), the miracidia hatch (5) and migrate to the snail hepatopancreas, where they form first- and second-generation sporocysts (6); these generate tailed cercariae (7) that leave the intermediate hosts via mucus secretions (slime balls, 8) and are ingested by the second intermedi-

ate hosts (9), i.e. ants (e.g. *Formica fusca* and *Formica rufibarbis*). Once ingested, the cercariae encyst in the body of the ant, thus becoming metacercariae (9), with one or two localising to the pharyngeal ganglion (10); during the cooler evening hours of the day, the latter enlarge, causing infected ants to undergo spastic paralysis (11). Thus, infected ants cling to the tips of grass blades, facilitating their ingestion by suitable definitive hosts. Once in the intestine of the definitive host, the metacercariae begin migrating to the liver via the common bile duct, and mature into adult trematodes within 70–85 days (1).

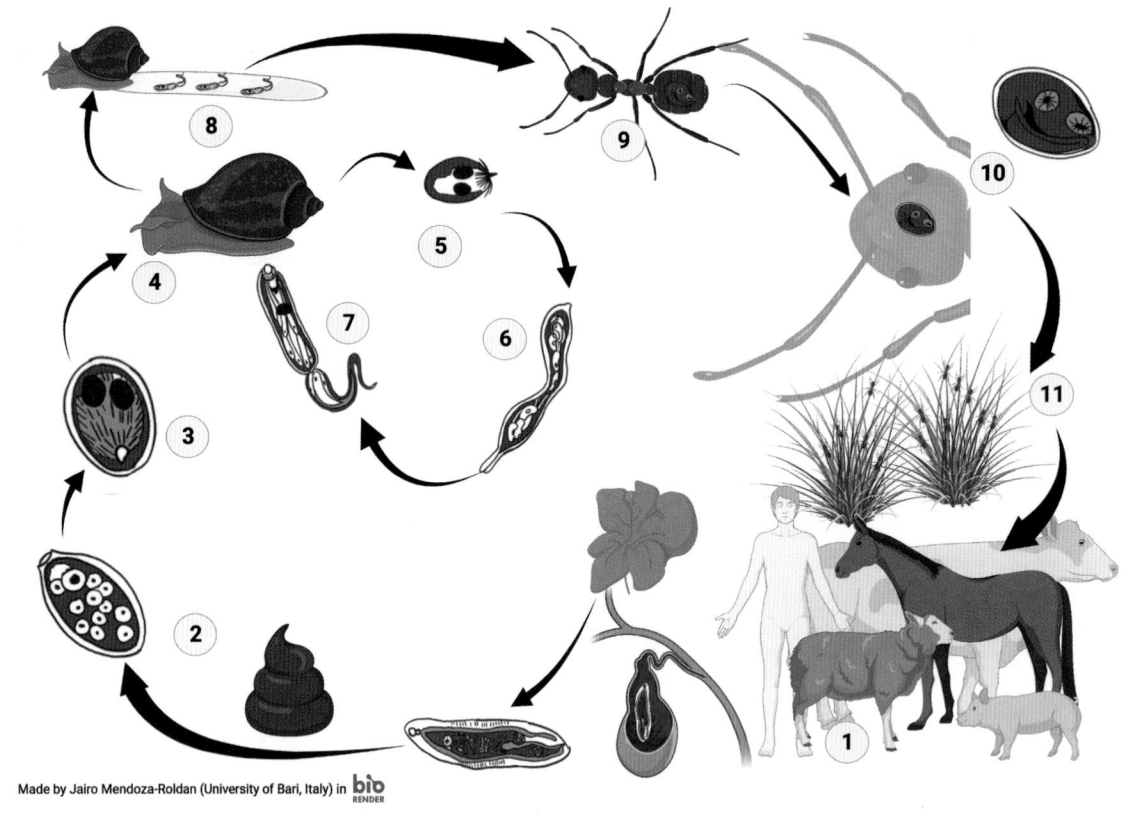

Made by Jairo Mendoza-Roldan (University of Bari, Italy) in **bio** RENDER

Dicrocoelium hospes

Description: Details are essentially similar to *D. dendriticum* and the flukes are usually found in the liver and gallbladder of cattle, oxen and occasionally sheep and goats in parts of Africa.

Eurytrema

This genus inhabits the pancreatic ducts and sometimes the bile ducts of ruminants (Table 1.51).

Eurytrema pancreaticum

Synonyms: *Distoma pancreaticum, Eurytrema ovis*

Description: Oval, leaf-shaped, reddish-brown flukes measuring around 8–16 mm long by 5–8.5 mm wide (Fig. 1.100). The body is

thick and the juvenile flukes are armed with spines which are often absent by the adult stage. The oral sucker is larger than the ventral sucker and the pharynx and oesophagus are short. The testes are

Table 1.51 *Eurytrema* species.

Species	Hosts	Site	Intermediate hosts
Eurytrema pancreaticum (syn. *Distoma pancreaticum, Eurytrema ovis*)	Cattle, buffalo, sheep, goats, pigs, camels, humans, primates	Pancreas; rarely bile ducts Perirenal fat	Land snails, particularly of the genus *Bradybaena* Grasshoppers of the genus *Conocephalus* or tree crickets (*Oecanthus*)
Eurytrema coelomaticum (syn. *Distoma coelomaticum*)	Cattle, sheep	Pancreas; rarely bile ducts	Land snails, particularly of the genus *Bradybaena* Grasshoppers of the genus *Conocephalus* or tree crickets (*Oecanthus*)
Eurytrema procyonis	Cats, foxes, raccoons	Pancreas	Snails of the genus *Mesodon* Grasshoppers

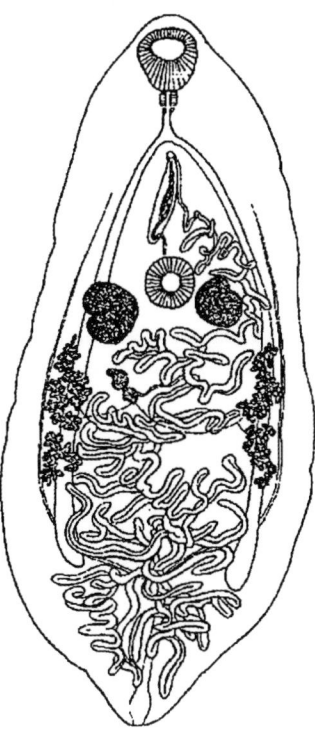

Fig. 1.100 *Eurytrema pancreaticum.* (Soulsby, 1971. Reproduced with permission from Lord Soulsby of Swaffham Prior.)

positioned horizontally just behind the ventral sucker. A tubular cirrus sac is present. The uterus completely occupies the posterior body. Eggs measure around 40–50 by 25–35 μm and are similar to those of *Dicrocoelium*.

Life cycle: Eggs passed in faeces are ingested by a snail where two generations of sporocysts occur. Cercariae are released onto the herbage about five months after initial infection and these are ingested by grasshoppers. Infective metacercariae are produced in about three weeks. The final host becomes infected by accidentally eating the second intermediate host. Metacercariae encyst in the duodenum and migrate to the pancreas via the pancreatic duct and reside in the small ducts of the pancreas. The prepatent period in cattle is 3–4 months.

Eurytrema coelomaticum

Synonym: *Distoma coelomaticum*

Description: A leaf-shaped reddish brown fluke with adults measuring around 8–12 by 6–7 mm.

Eurytrema procyonis

Description: The adult measures about 2.9 mm long by 1.2 mm wide. The oral sucker is subterminal with a dorsal lip-like projection. The eggs are small, 45 by 35 μm, asymmetrical, dark brown with an operculum and a miracidium.

Life cycle: The life cycle is unknown but is thought to involve snail intermediate hosts of the genus *Mesodon*. Animals are likely to become infected by ingestion of the snail intermediate host.

Table 1.52 *Platynosomum* species.

Species	Hosts	Site	Intermediate hosts
Platynosomum fastosum (syn. *Eurytrema fastosum*)	Cats	Bile and pancreatic ducts	Land snails (*Sublima*) and woodlice Lizards are obligate paratenic hosts
Platynosomum concinnum	Cats	Bile and pancreatic ducts	Land snails (*Sublima*) and woodlice Lizards are obligate paratenic hosts
Platynosomum illiciens	Cats	Bile and pancreatic ducts	Land snails (*Sublima*) and woodlice Lizards are obligate paratenic hosts

Platynosomum

Flukes of this genus are found in wild birds, but some species are also found in the liver of cats (Table 1.52).

Platynosomum fastosum

Description: The adult fluke is lanceolate and measures 4–8 mm by 1.5–2.5 mm in size. The testes lie obliquely horizontal. The eggs are brown, oval, thick-shelled and operculate and measure about 34–50 by 23–35 μm. They are embryonated when laid.

Life cycle: Eggs passed in the faeces develop in a land snail (*Sublima*) and a crustacean (woodlouse). Cercariae encyst when a lizard, gecko, skink or toad eats the woodlouse. The cat is infected by ingesting a lizard or other host containing metacercariae, which acts as an obligate paratenic host. The prepatent period is around 2–3 months.

FAMILY PARAGONIMIDAE

Trematodes in this family mainly have a flattened fleshy body and a tegument covered with spines. The oral sucker is subterminal and the ventral sucker is located around the middle of the body. The genital pore is situated just below the ventral sucker. Several genera are of local veterinary interest. *Paragonimus*, commonly referred to as the 'Lung fluke', is found in cats, dogs and other carnivores and in humans in North America and Asia. Pulmonary signs are comparatively rare in cats or dogs and the veterinary interest is in the potential reservoir of infection for humans.

Life cycle: The life cycle involves an amphibious or water snail, and a crayfish or freshwater crab. Snails of the genera *Melania*, *Ampullaria* or *Pomatiopsis* are infected by miracidia in which further development through sporocyst, redia and cerceria takes place. After escaping the snail, the cercariae swim about and, on contact with a freshwater crab or crayfish, penetrate it and encyst. Crabs and crayfish can also eat cercaria-infected snails. Infection of the final host occurs by ingestion of the metacercariae in the liver or muscles of the crustacean. Infection can also be acquired through consumption of paratenic hosts which have eaten infected crabs or crayfish. The young flukes migrate to the lungs where they are encapsulated by fibrous cysts connected by fistulae to the bronchioles to facilitate egg excretion. Eggs pass up from the lung in the sputum, which the animal usually swallows such that eggs are passed in the faeces. The prepatent period is 5–6 weeks.

Paragonimus

Parasites of this genus are localised in the lungs of several vertebrate hosts (Table 1.53).

Paragonimus westermani

Description: The parasite is rounded (lemon-shaped) and thick (7.5–16 mm by 4–8 mm), reddish-brown in colour and covered in very small scale-like spines. The oral and ventral suckers are similar in size, with the ventral sucker situated slightly anterior to the middle of the fluke (Fig. 1.101). The testes are located in the posterior half of the body. Species differentiation is based on the shape of the spines. Those in *P. westermani* are large and have bifid points. Eggs are yellowish-brown in colour, operculate, 75–118 by 42–67 µm, and the shell is thickened at the opposite end to the operculum (Fig. 1.102).

Table 1.53 *Paragonimus* species.

Species	Hosts	Site	Intermediate hosts
Paragonimus westermani	Dogs, cats, pigs, goats, cattle, foxes, other carnivores, humans and primates	Lung	Snails of the genera *Melania, Ampullaria, Pomatiopsis* Crabs and crayfish
Paragonimus kellicotti	Cats, pigs, dogs	Lung	Snails of the genera *Melania, Ampullaria, Pomatiopsis* Crabs and crayfish

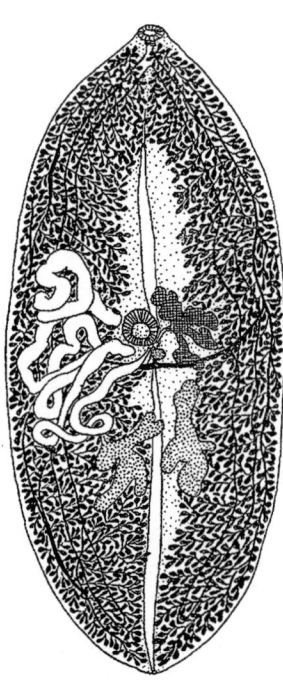

Fig. 1.101 *Paragonimus westermani.* (Adapted from Mönnig, 1934.)

Paragonimus kellicotti

Description: Adult flukes are usually located in pairs in cysts in the lungs of the final host. The parasite is rounded, reddish-brown in colour, 7.5–16 by 4–8 mm and covered in scale-like spines. The ventral sucker is situated slightly anterior to the middle of the fluke. Species differentiation is based on the shape of the spines. Those in *P. kellicotti* are very large and have a number of points. Eggs are golden-brown in colour, 80–118 by 48–60 µm, and have a partly flattened operculum.

FAMILY NANOPHYETIDAE

The genus *Nanophyetus* is a fluke found mainly in the small intestine of dogs, mink and other fish-eating mammals. It occurs in the northwest USA and parts of Siberia and is of importance because the flukes are vectors of the rickettsial organism *Neorickettsia helminthoeca*, which causes severe haemorrhagic enteritis of dogs, so-called 'salmon poisoning'. This name is derived from the cycle of the fluke, which involves a water snail and a fish that is often one of the salmonid type.

Life cycle: Undeveloped eggs are passed in the faeces of the host and after hatching, which takes about three months, infect the snail first intermediate host where cercariae develop in rediae. The liberated cercariae swim for a while before penetrating a fish and encysting in the kidneys, muscles and other organs. Infection of the final host occurs when the fish is eaten. The prepatent period is as short as five days in the dog.

Nanophyetus

The main species is *Nanophyetus salmincola* (syn. *Troglotrema salmincola*) which infects the small intestine of dogs, foxes, cats, raccoons, mink, bears, lynxes, other fish-eating mammals and, rarely, humans. This parasite has snails (*Oxytrema, Goniobasis, Semisulcospira* spp.), salmonid fishes, other fish and salamanders as intermediate hosts.

Nanophyetus salmincola

Synonym: *Troglotrema salmincola*

Description: These trematodes are generally very small, oval or elongate, and white or cream in colour. Adult flukes measure about 1–2.5 mm long by 0.3 mm wide. The oral sucker is well developed and is located terminally and the ventral sucker is usually found in the mid-third of the body. The large testes are oval and situated side by side in the posterior third of the segment. The spherical ovary is situated behind the ventral sucker and to its right. The genital pore is just to the posterior of the ventral sucker and the cirrus sac is large. The vitellaria consist of large follicles. Eggs are yellowish-brown in colour, unembryonated and measure about 64–80 by 34–50 µm. They have an indistinct operculum and a small rounded abopercular knob at the opposite pole.

FAMILY COLLYRICLIDAE

Parasites of the genus *Collyriclum* occur within subcutaneous cysts in chickens, turkeys and wild birds. Intermediate hosts are snails and dragonflies.

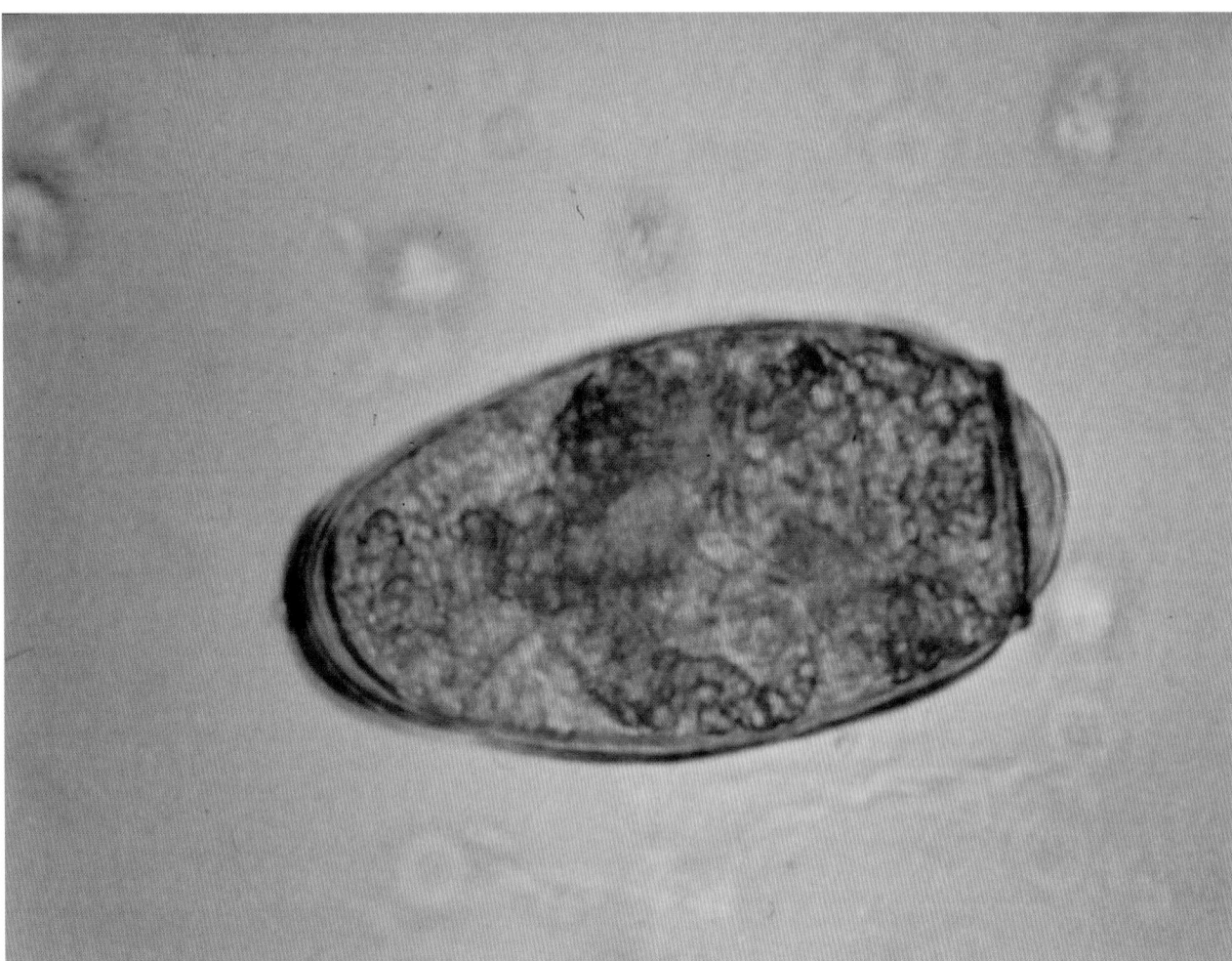

Fig. 1.102 *Paragonimus westermani* egg.

Life cycle: Cysts in the subcutaneous tissues usually contain a pair of flukes. Eggs are passed through an opening in the wall of the cyst and hatch in the environment to produce a miracidium, which penetrates a snail. These directly produce cercariae, there being no redial development, and the cercariae are shed from the snail and will enter dragonfly larvae, where they encyst to the metacercaria stage. Infection of the final host occurs through ingestion of the infected dragonfly. The immature trematodes then migrate to the subcutaneous tissues.

Collyriclum

The main species is *Collyriclum faba* (syn. *Monostoma faba*) which infects the skin and subcutaneous tissues of chickens, turkeys and wild birds. This parasite has snails and dragonfly nymphs as intermediate hosts.

Collyriclum faba

Synonym: *Monostoma faba*

Description: The flukes occur in pairs in a tissue cyst. The fluke has a spiny tegument, is dorsally convex and venterally flattened, and measures about 4 by 5 mm. There is no ventral sucker and the oral

sucker is small. The ovary is multilobular and the vitellaria are located in the anterior half of the body. Eggs are very small, measuring about 19–21 by 9–11 μm.

FAMILY PROSTHOGONIMIDAE

Prosthogonimus are parasites found in the cloaca and reproductive tract of birds.

Life cycle: Eggs passed in faeces hatch to produce a miracidium, which penetrates a snail to form a mother sporocyst, which produces daughter sporocysts. These directly produce cercariae, there being no redial development, and the cercariae are shed from the snail and will enter dragonfly larvae via the rectal respiratory chamber where they eventually encyst as the metacercaria stage in the haemocoel. Infection of the final host occurs through ingestion of the infected nymphal stage or the adult dragonfly. The immature trematodes then migrate to the cloaca and bursa of Fabricius or enter the oviduct. The fluke is mature after about a week.

Prosthogonimus

Parasites of this genus infect several bird species (Table 1.54)

Table 1.54 *Prosthogonimus* species.

Species	Hosts	Site	Intermediate hosts
Prosthogonimus pellucidus (syn. *Prosthogonimus intercalandus, Prosthogonimus cuneatus*)	Chickens, turkeys, other fowl, geese, ducks	Cloaca, oviduct, bursa of Fabricius	Water snails (*Bithynia*) Dragonfly nymphs
Prosthogonimus macrorchis	Chickens, turkeys, other fowl, ducks	Lower gut, cloaca, oviduct, bursa of Fabricius	Water snails (*Bithynia*) Dragonfly nymphs
Prosthogonimus ovatus	Chickens, turkeys, other fowl, geese	Cloaca, oviduct, bursa of Fabricius	Water snails (*Bithynia*) Dragonfly nymphs

Prosthogonimus pellucidus

Synonyms: *Prosthogonimus intercalandus, Prosthogonimus cuneatus*

Description: Adult flukes are pear-shaped, semi-transparent, pale orange when fresh and measure around 9–12 mm in length, being broader towards the posterior. The fluke has a spiny cuticle and two suckers are present. The posterior width of the fluke increases from the middle region. The ovoid eggs are around 26–32 by 10–15 μm in size, dark brown and have a small spine at the opposite pole to the operculum.

Prosthogonimus macrorchis

Description: These flukes are very similar to *P. pellucidus* but possess larger testes.

Prosthogonimus ovatus

Description: Adult flukes are smaller than the other two species, measuring 3–6 mm. The testes are slightly elongate and lie side by side in the midline.

FAMILY PLAGIORCHIIDAE

Plagiorchis are parasites of birds and are mainly located in the gut. One species, *P. arcuatus*, has a similar pathogenesis to *Prosthogonimus*, affecting the bursa of Fabricius in young birds and the oviduct in older birds.

Life cycle: The life cycle involves two intermediate hosts, namely freshwater snails and larvae of dragonflies. The definitive host is infected through eating the dragonflies or their nymphs containing encysted metacercariae.

Plagiorchis

The main species is *Plagiorchis arcuatus* which infects the oviduct and bursa of Fabricius of chickens and other poultry. This parasite has snails, crustacea and insects as intermediate hosts.

Plagiorchis arcuatus

Description: The fluke is oval, about 4–5 mm in length and 1.5 mm in breadth, and tapers to a point at both ends. The cuticle possesses small spines, which are more numerous in the anterior region. The testes are rounded or oval and lie obliquely behind each other. The ovary is rounded, situated near the end of the cirrus sac, and to the right of the ventral sucker.

FAMILY LECITHODENDRIIDAE

The Lecithodendriidae include the genera *Novetrema*, *Odeningotrema*, *Phaneropsolus* and *Primatotrema*, which are intestinal flukes of primates.

FAMILY OPISTHORCHIIDAE

The members of this family require two intermediate hosts, the first being water snails and the second a wide variety of fish, in which the metacercariae are encysted. The final hosts are fish-eating mammals in which they inhabit the bile ducts. These oval or fusiform flukes are of medium size and possess suckers which are small and weak and located fairly close together. The ovary and uterus are anterior to the testes. This feature avoids confusion with the similarly sized and shaped dicrocoeliid flukes where they are positioned posteriorly to the testis. *Clonorchis* is by far the most important genus, with *Apophallus*, *Cryptocotyle*, *Opisthorchis*, *Metorchis*, *Parametorchis* and *Pseudamphistomum* being of lesser importance.

Apophallus

Parasites of this genus are localised in the small intestine of gulls, cormorants, dogs, cats, foxes and seals. Fishes are the intermediate hosts.

Apophallus muhlingi

Synonym: *Cotylophallus muhlingi*

Description: Adult flukes are small and measure 1.2–1.6 mm by 0.2 mm. The cuticle is covered in fine spines. The suckers are small, equal in size and located in the midbody. The testes are rounded and lie diagonally one behind the other. The ovary is rounded and is opposite the anterior testis.

Apophallus donicum

Synonym: *Rossicotrema donicum*

Description: Flukes are small, measuring 0.5–1.15 mm by 0.2–0.4 mm. The cuticle is covered in spines and the testes are round and large and located in the posterior section of the body.

Cryptocotyle

The main species is *Cryptocotyle lingua* which infects the small intestine of gulls, terns, kittiwakes, seals, mink, dogs, cats and humans. This parasite has shellfish, snails and fish as intermediate hosts.

Cryptocotyle lingua

Description: Spatula-shaped body, 0.5–2 mm long by 0.2–0.9 mm wide. The cuticle is armed with spines and the suckers are small, with the anterior larger than the ventral sucker. The testes are slightly lobed and lie side by side or diagonally at the posterior end of the body. The ovary is trilobed and lies in front of the testes.

Clonorchis

The main species is *Clonorchis sinensis* (syn. *Opisthorchis sinensis*) which infects the bile ducts, pancreatic ducts and occasionally small intestine of humans, dogs, cats, pigs, mink, weasels and badgers. This parasite has operculated snails (*Parafossalurus*, *Bulimus* spp., *Bithynia*, *Melania* and *Vivipara*) and cyprinid fishes as intermediate hosts.

Clonorchis sinensis

Synonym: *Opisthorchis sinensis*

Description: The adult fluke is flat, transparent–pinkish, wide posteriorly and tapering anteriorly, and may reach a size of 25 mm long by 5 mm wide (Fig. 1.103). The cuticle is spiny in the young fluke but smooth in the adult. The testes are multibranched and posterior to the ovary and uterus. A cirrus sac is absent. Eggs have a thick, light yellowish-brown wall and measure 27–35 by 12–20 μm; they contain a miracidium when they are laid, the internal structure of

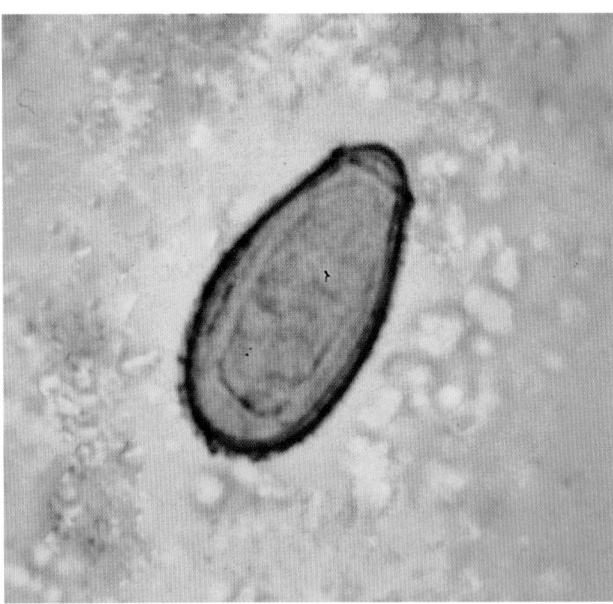

Fig. **1.104** *Clonorchis sinensis* egg.

which is asymmetrical. The convex operculum of the egg slots into a prominent rim of the shell (Fig. 1.104). A small hook-like structure is frequently present on the opposite pole.

Life cycle: The eggs normally hatch only after they have been swallowed by the snail first intermediate host. In the snails, the miracidium develops into a sporocyst, which produces rediae and these in turn produce cercariae, which have fairly long tails and elongate bodies with pigmented eye-spots. After breaking out of the snail, the cercaria swims about and on meeting a suitable fish, it penetrates partly or completely into the tissues of the fish and, losing its tail, becomes encysted in the fish. Infection of the final host occurs through eating raw infected fish. The metacercariae are liberated in the duodenum of the final host and reach the liver by way of the bile duct. The prepatent period is 16 days.

Opisthorchis

The main species is *Opisthorchis felineus* (syn. *Opisthorchis tenuicollis*, *Opisthorchis viverrini*) which infects the liver, bile ducts and occasionally pancreatic ducts of cats, dogs, foxes, pigs, humans and cetaceans. This parasite has freshwater snails (*Bithynia* spp.) and freshwater fish as intermediate hosts.

Opisthorchis felineus

Synonyms: *Opisthorchis tenuicollis*, *Opisthorchis viverrini*

Description: Adult flukes are reddish in colour, with a smooth cuticle and measure 7–12 by 1.5–2.5 mm (Fig. 1.105). The testes are lobed and not branched. Eggs are about 26–30 by 11–15 μm in size, and contain a miracidium when they are laid, the internal structure of which is asymmetrical. The operculum of the egg fits into a prominent rim of the shell and may have a tubercular appendage (Fig. 1.106).

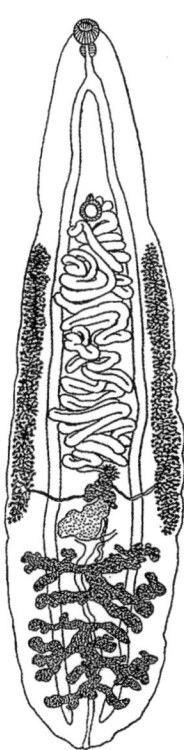

Fig. **1.103** *Clonorchis sinensis*. (Soulsby, 1971. Reproduced with permission from Lord Soulsby of Swaffham Prior.)

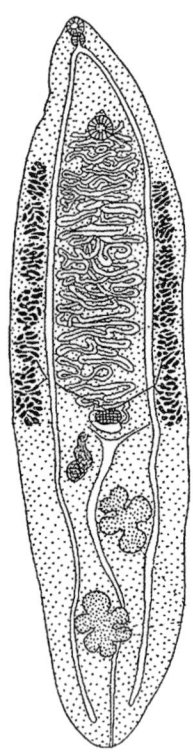

Fig. 1.105 *Opisthorchis felineus*. (Adapted from Mönnig, 1934.)

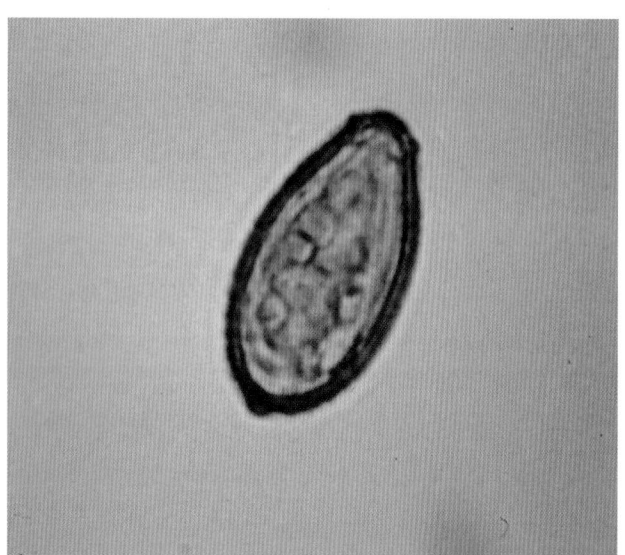

Fig. 1.106 *Opisthorchis felineus* egg.

Life cycle: The prepatent period is 2–3 weeks and deposited eggs are ingested by a snail in which cercariae develop in rediae. The cercariae encyst in fish as metacercariae and infect the definitive host when ingested. See **life cycle 20**.

Metorchis

Parasites of this genus are localised in the liver, bile ducts and gall-bladder of dogs, cats, foxes, seals, some poultry, mink, raccoons and occasionally humans (*Metorchis albidus*).

Metorchis albidus

Synonyms: *Distoma albicum, Opisthorchis albidus*

Description: The fluke is spatulate, pointed anteriorly, rounded and flat posteriorly, 2.5–6.5 mm long by 1–1.6 mm broad with a spinous cuticle in the young fluke. The genital pore is in front of the ventral sucker. The testes are located diagonally in the posterior region of the body and they are lobed. The ovary is fairly circular and lies just in front of the anterior testis. The operculate eggs are small, 24–30 by 13–16 μm.

Metorchis conjunctus

Description: Adults measure 1–6.5 mm long by 0.6–2.6 mm broad. The suckers are equal in diameter. The genital pore lies at the anterior margin of the acetabulum. The cuticle of the young fluke possesses spines.

Parametorchis

The main species is *Parametorchis complexus* which infects the liver and bile ducts of cats and dogs. The intermediate hosts of this parasite are not known, but probably are freshwater snails.

Parametorchis complexus

Description: The fluke is 5–10 mm long by 1.5–2 mm broad. The uterus forms a rosette around the ventral sucker. The testes are lobed and lie together in the posterior part of the body. The vitelline glands are restricted to the anterior third of the fluke.

Pseudamphistomum

The main species is *Pseudamphistomum truncatum* which infects the liver and bile ducts of dogs, cats, foxes and rarely humans. This parasite has snails and fish as intermediate hosts.

Pseudamphistomum truncatum

Description: Adult flukes are small, measuring 2–2.5 mm, with a spiny body that is truncate posteriorly. The testes are spherical and lie horizontally at the posterior end of the body (Fig. 1.107).

LIFE CYCLE 20. LIFE CYCLE OF *OPISTHORCHIS FELINEUS*

The parasite lives in the biliary and pancreatic ducts (1) and occasionally in the small intestinal lumen of the definitive host, which includes fish-eating mammals such as dogs, cats, foxes, seals, lions, wolverines, martens, polecats and humans, but also pigs and rabbits. The eggs (2) are excreted with the faeces, and are ingested by aquatic snails (3) that act as first intermediate hosts. In the snail, the egg hatches to release a miracidium (4), that subsequently becomes a sporocyst (5), rediae (6) and then cercariae (7). The latter are highly motile and actively leave the first intermediate host to seek out a freshwater fish, the second intermediate host (8). On penetrating the fish skin, the cercariae lose their tails and become encysted in muscular tissues as metacercariae (9). When a susceptible definitive host ingests raw or undercooked fish containing the metacercariae (10), these hatch in the duodenum (11) and migrate to the liver via the biliary ducts (12), where the parasites mature to adult trematodes (1). The prepatent period is ~16 days.

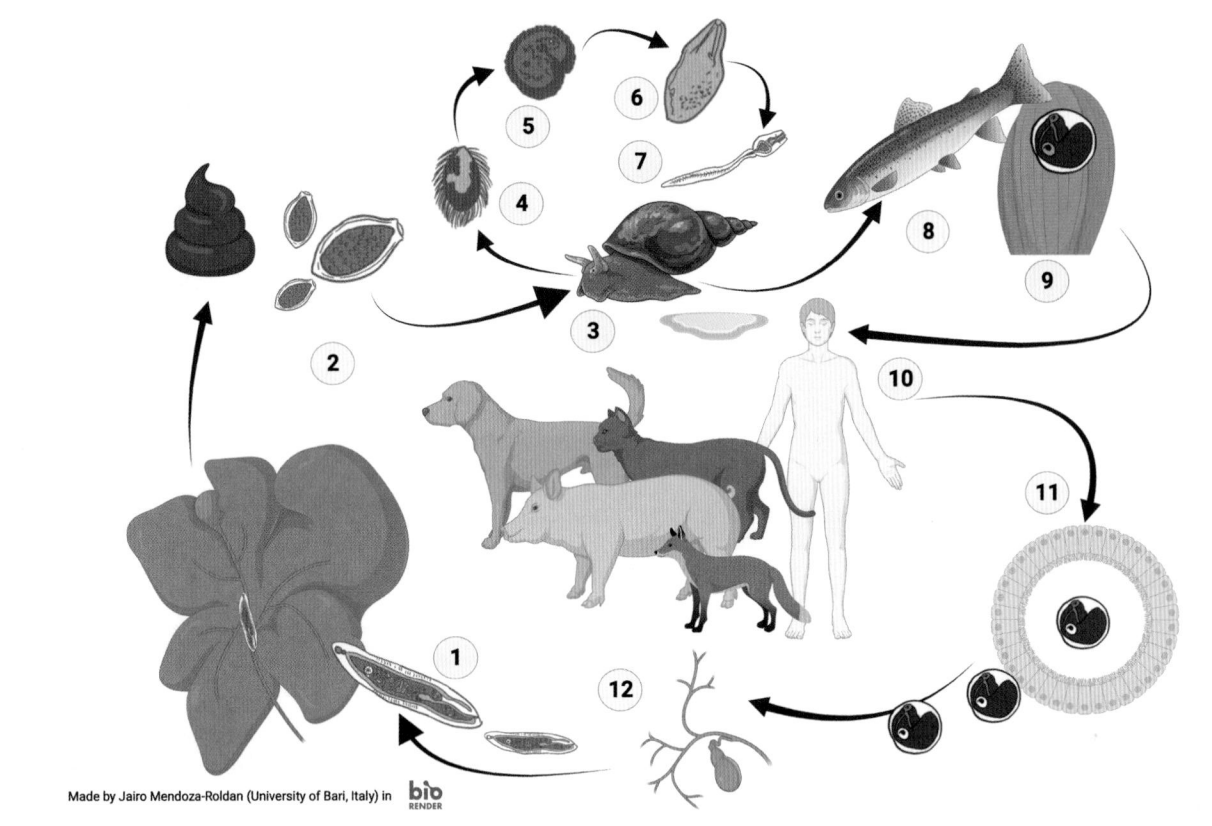

Made by Jairo Mendoza-Roldan (University of Bari, Italy) in BioRender

ORDER STRIGEIDIDA

FAMILY BRACHYLAEMIDAE

Members of this family are parasites of birds (*Brachylaemus*), sheep (*Skrjabinotrema*) and pigs (*Postharmostomum*). The intermediate hosts are snails. They are of only minor veterinary importance.

Skrjabinotrema

The main species is *Skrjabinotrema ovis* which infects the small intestine of sheep. This parasite has snails as intermediate hosts.

Skrjabinotrema ovis

Description: Adult flukes are small with smooth bodies and measure about 1 mm long by 0.3–0.7 mm wide. Eggs measure 24–32 by 16–20 µm and are slightly flattened on one side with a large operculum at one end and a small appendage at the other.

Postharmostomum

The main species is *Postharmostomum suis* which infects the small intestine of pigs. This parasite has snails as intermediate hosts.

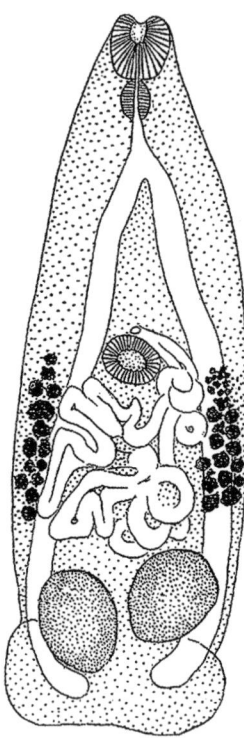

Postharmostomum suis

Description: The body is smooth, elongate and around 4–8 mm in length.

FAMILY HETEROPHYIDAE

These are small trematodes found in the intestines of mammals and birds. The genital pore and ventral sucker are located in a ventro-genital sac. More than 10 species of the family Heterophyidae have been reported in humans and fish-eating mammals. The life cycle generally involves two intermediate hosts, namely freshwater snails and fishes or frogs. Genera of veterinary interest are *Heterophyes* found in dogs, cats, foxes and humans; *Metagonimus* in the small intestines of dogs, cats, pigs and humans; *Cryptocotyle* of seabirds, reported in dogs and cats; and *Apophallus* (*Rossicotrema*) normally found in seabirds or seals but also reported in cats, dogs and foxes.

Heterophyes

Parasites of this genus are localised in the small intestine of dogs, cats, foxes and humans. Snails of the genus *Pirenella* and *Cerithida*, and fish are intermediate hosts.

Heterophyes heterophyes

Description: This is a small pear-shaped fluke that is wider posteriorly than anteriorly, measuring 1–1.7 mm by 0.3–0.7 mm. The ventral sucker is anterior to the middle of the body and the genital sucker lies immediately behind it and to one side and bears an incomplete circle of 70–80 small rods. The testes are located horizontally and are oval in shape (Fig. 1.108).

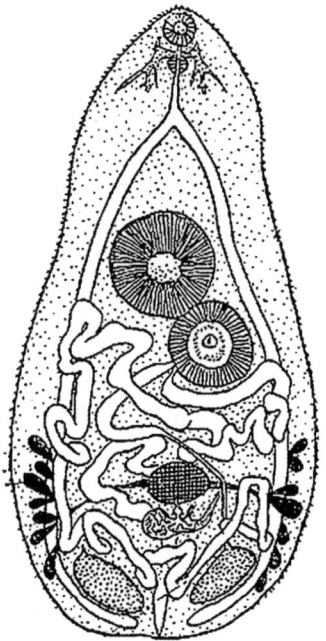

Fig. 1.108 *Heterophyes heterophyes*. (Neveu-Lemaire, 1936. Reproduced with permission from Editions Vigot.)

Heterophyes nocens

Description: Small ovoid fluke measuring 0.8–1 mm in length by 0.5–0.6 mm in width. The genital sucker is armed with 50–60 small rods and is located close to the ventral sucker.

Metagonimus

The main species is *Metagonimus yokagawai* which infects the small intestine of dogs, cats, pigs and humans. This parasite has snails (*Semisulcospira* spp.), cyprinid fish, mullet and trout as intermediate hosts.

Metagonimus yokagawai

Description: Small flukes that are wider posteriorly than anteriorly, measuring 1–2.5 mm by 0.4–0.7 mm. The cuticle bears spines over its whole surface. The ventral sucker is right of the median line and close to the genital pore, which opens anteriorly. The testes are slightly oblique and the ovary is median in position.

FAMILY SCHISTOSOMATIDAE

This family is primarily parasitic in the blood vessels of the alimentary tract and bladder. In humans, schistosomes are often responsible for severe and debilitating disease and veterinary interest lies in the fact that they can cause a similar disease in animals, some of which may act as reservoirs of infection for humans. The schistosomes differ from other flukes in that the sexes are separate, the small adult female lying permanently in a longitudinal groove, the gynaecophoric canal, in the body of the male (Fig. 1.109). The most important genus is *Schistosoma*, with *Bilharziella*, *Trichobilharzia*, *Orientobilharzia*, *Ornithobilharzia*, *Heterobilharzia* and *Austrobilharzia* other genera of lesser importance.

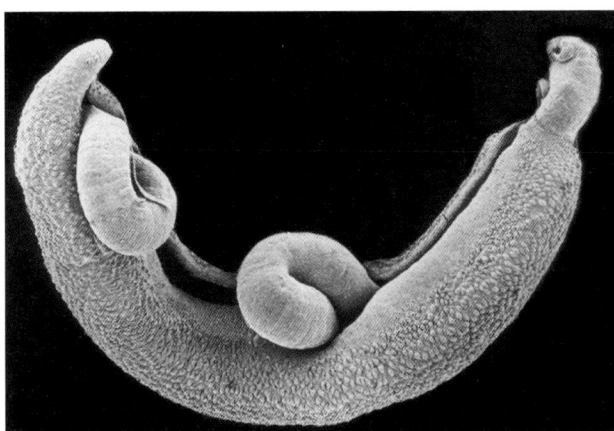

Fig. 1.109 Male and female *Schistosoma* in copula.

Schistosoma

The sexes are separate, with the male, which is broad and flat and about 2 cm long, carrying the slender female in the hollow of its inwardly curved body. This characteristic and the vascular predilection site are sufficient for generic identification. Suckers are either absent or weak and there is no pharynx. The genus, as currently defined, is paraphyletic so revisions are likely. The genus has been divided into four groups: *haematobium*, *indicum*, *mansoni* and *japonicum*. Species found in Africa are divided into two groups: those with a lateral spine on the egg (*mansoni* group) and those with a terminal spine (*haematobium* group) (Fig. 1.110; Table 1.55).

Schistosoma bovis

Description: The male is 9–22 mm long and 1–2 mm wide, and the female 12–28 mm long. In the male, the suckers and the tegument behind the suckers are armed with minute spines, while the dorsal surface of the tegument bears small cuticular tubercles. The slender female worm lies permanently in a ventral groove in the broad flat body of the male. The eggs are usually spindle-shaped, but smaller eggs may be oval and have a mean measurement of 187 by 65 μm when passed in the faeces. There is no operculum.

Life cycle: The ovigerous female penetrates deeply into the small vessels of the mucosa or submucosa of the intestine and inserts her tail into a small venule. Since the genital pore is terminal, the eggs are deposited, or even pushed, into the venule. There, aided by their spines and by proteolytic enzymes secreted by the unhatched miracidia, they penetrate the endothelium to enter the intestinal submucosa and ultimately the gut lumen; they are then passed out in the

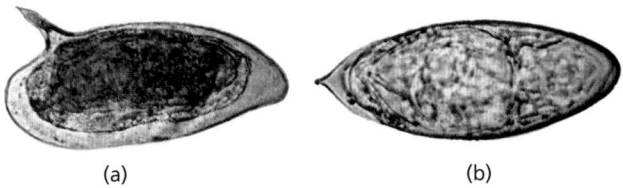

(a)   (b)

Fig. 1.110 *Schistosoma* egg morphology: (a) *mansoni* group; (b) *haematobium* group.

Table 1.55 *Schistosoma* species.

Species	Hosts	Site	Intermediate hosts
Haematobium *group*			
Schistosoma bovis	Cattle, sheep, goats, camels	Portal, mesenteric and urogenital veins	Snails (*Bulinus* spp., *Physopsis* spp.)
Schistosoma haematobium	Humans, primates	Bladder veins and urethra	Snails (*Bulinus* spp.)
Schistosoma mattheei	Cattle, sheep, goats, camels, humans, primates	Portal, mesenteric and bladder veins	Snails (*Physopsis* spp.)
Schistosoma leiperi	Cattle, antelopes	Mesenteric veins	Snails (*Bulinus* spp.)
Indicum *group*			
Schistosoma indicum	Cattle, buffalo, sheep, goats, horses, donkeys, camels	Portal, pancreatic, hepatic and mesenteric veins	Snails (*Indoplanorbis*)
Schistosoma nasale (syn. *Schistosoma nasalis*)	Cattle, goats, sheep, buffalo, horses	Nasal mucosa veins	Snails (*Lymnaea* spp., *Indoplanorbis* spp.)
Schistosoma spindale	Cattle, buffalo, horses, pigs and rarely dogs	Mesenteric veins	Snails (*Planorbis* spp., *Indoplanorbis* spp., *Lymnaea* spp.)
Mansoni *group*			
Schistosoma mansoni	Humans, primates, wild animals	Mesenteric veins	Snails (*Biomphalaria* spp.)
Japonicum *group*			
Schistosoma japonicum	Cattle, horses, sheep, goats, dogs, cats, rabbits, rodents, pigs, humans	Portal and mesenteric veins	Snails (*Oncomelania* spp.)
Others			
Schistosoma incognitum (syn. *Schistosoma suis*)	Pigs, dogs	Mesenteric veins	Snails (*Radix* spp.)
Schistosoma turkestanica (syn. *Orientobilharzia turkestanicum*)	Cattle, buffalo, sheep, goats, camels, horses, donkeys, cats	Mesenteric veins and small veins of the pancreas and liver	Snails (*Lymnaea* spp.)

faeces. Worms present in the vesical veins penetrate the endothelial lining of the bladder where eggs may be passed in the urine. Some eggs are carried away in the bloodstream and locate in other organs such as the liver. The eggs hatch in water and the miracidia penetrate appropriate snails. Cercariae develop from daughter sporocysts, which replace the redia stage, and there is no metacercarial phase; penetration of the final host by the motile cercariae occurs via the skin or by ingestion in drinking water. After penetration or ingestion, the cercariae lose their forked tails, transform to schistosomula or young flukes, and travel via the bloodstream through the heart and lungs to the systemic circulation. In the liver, they locate in the portal veins and become sexually mature before migrating to their final site, the mesenteric veins. The prepatent period is 6–7 weeks.

Schistosoma mattheei

Description: The male flukes measure around 9–22 mm in length and about 1–2 mm wide. Females range from 12 to 28 mm in length. The body of the male behind the suckers is armed with very long spines, as are the suckers. The dorsal surface possesses small cuticular tubercles. The eggs passed in faeces are usually spindle-shaped, but smaller ones may be oval. They measure 170–280 by 72–84 μm. There is no operculum.

Schistosoma indicum

Description: The sexes are separate; the males are 5–19 mm and the females 6–22 mm in length. The eggs are oval with a terminal spine and measure 57–140 by 18–72 μm.

Schistosoma spindale

Description: The male measures 5–16 mm and the female 7.2–16.2 mm long. The sexes are separate, with the male, which is broad and flat and up to about 1.5 cm in length, carrying the female in the hollow of its inwardly curved body. The eggs are spindle-shaped, measure 200–300 by 70–90 μm and have a lateral or terminal spine. There is no operculum.

Schistosoma nasale

Synonym: *Schistosoma nasalis*

Description: The sexes are separate. The male, which is broad and flat and about 0.6–1 cm long, carries the female in the hollow of its inwardly curved body. The flukes closely resemble those of *S. spindale*. The eggs measure 350–380 by 50–80 μm and are boomerang-shaped, with a terminal spine.

Life cycle: Details of the life cycle are not completely known. The female in the veins of the nasal mucosa lays her eggs, which presumably enter the nasal sinuses and are sneezed out. The eggs hatch in minutes in water and the miracidia penetrate appropriate snails. Development to the cercarial stage occurs without a redial form and there is no metacercarial phase. After penetration or ingestion, the cercariae transform to schistosomula, or young flukes, and travel to their final site, the nasal veins.

Schistosoma mansoni

Description: The adult male is up to 10 mm in length and possesses a longitudinal groove, the gynaecophoric canal, that enfolds the female, which is longer (12–16 mm) and thinner. The tegument of the male has tubercles on the dorsal surface, whereas the tegument of the female is smooth. The male has 6–9 testes, and the male genital pore opens ventrally, immediately posterior to the ventral sucker. The female possesses a single ovary located in the anterior portion of the body.

Schistosoma japonicum

Description: The male is broad and flat and 9.5–20 mm long, carrying the female (12–26 mm long) in the hollow of the inwardly curved body. The suckers lie close together near the anterior end. The cuticle is spiny on the suckers and in the gynaecophoric canal. This characteristic and the vascular predilection site are sufficient for generic identification. The eggs are short, oval, measuring

70–100 by 50–80 μm, and may have a small lateral subterminal spine. There is no operculum.

Life cycle: This is similar to that of *S. bovis*. Development to the cercarial stage occurs through two generations of sporocyst without a redial form and there is no metacercarial phase, penetration of the final host by the motile cercariae occurring via the skin. The developmental period in the snail can be as short as five weeks. Schistosomula, or young flukes, that reach the abdominal vessels and pass to the portal veins become sexually mature in about four weeks.

Schistosoma turkestanica

Synonym: *Orientobilharzia turkstanicum*

Description: This is a small species; the male is 4.2–8 mm and the female 3.4–8 mm in length. The spirally coiled ovary is positioned in the anterior part of the body. In the male there are around 70–80 testes. The female uterus is short and contains only one egg at a time, which measures 72–77 by 16–26 μm with a terminal spine and a short appendage at the opposite end.

OTHER SCHISTOSOMES

The main species is *Bilharziella polonica* which infects the mesenteric and pelvic veins of ducks. This parasite has snails of the genus *Planorbis* as intermediate hosts.

Bilharziella polonica

Description: The body is lancet-shaped posteriorly and the sexes are separate. Males are about 4 mm and females 2 mm in size. The female genital pore is just behind the ventral sucker and the short uterus contains one egg at a time. The eggs have a long, narrow and elongate anterior end and a swollen posterior end with a terminal spine, and measure 400 by 100 μm.

Life cycle: Eggs are laid in the small vessels of the intestinal wall through which they penetrate and are passed out in the faeces. Development takes place in the snail intermediate host and leads to the release of cercariae, which infect the intermediate host either percutaneously or following ingestion.

FAMILY DIPLOSTOMATIDAE

The family Diplostomatidae includes the genera *Alaria* and *Diplostomum*, which are flukes of mammals and birds. Only the former genus is of veterinary significance. The life cycle involves two intermediate hosts, namely freshwater snails and frogs. The definitive host is infected through eating frogs containing encysted metacercariae (mesocercariae).

Alaria

Alaria are found in the small intestine of dogs, cats, foxes and mink (Table 1.56). The anterior forebody of the fluke is flattened or spoon-shaped, and the posterior hindbody is conical and contains

Table **1.56** *Alaria* species.

Species	Hosts	Site	Intermediate hosts
Alaria alata	Dogs, cats, foxes, mink, wild carnivores and rarely humans	Small intestine	Snails (*Planorbis* spp.), frogs, toads Paratenic: snakes, rodents
Alaria americana	Dogs, foxes and other canids	Small intestine	Snails (*Planorbis* spp.), frogs, toads
Alaria canis	Dogs, foxes	Small intestine	Snails (*Heliosoma* spp.), frogs, toads
Alaria marcianae	Cats, raccoons	Small intestine	Snails (*Heliosoma* spp.), frogs, toads Paratenic: snakes, rodents
Alaria michiganensis	Dogs, foxes, coyotes	Small intestine	Snails (*Planorbis* spp.), frogs, toads

the reproductive organs. The oral and ventral suckers are located in the forebody. The life cycle involves freshwater snails as first intermediate hosts, and amphibians or reptiles as second intermediate hosts.

Life cycle: Unembryonated eggs are passed in the faeces from which miracidia eventually hatch and enter freshwater snails (*Planorbis*). Sporocysts produce cercariae with bifurcated tails. These leave the snail and infect tadpoles or frogs where the cercariae encyst in the muscles, forming mesocercariae. If a frog, snake or mouse eats the tadpole, the mesocercariae become encysted, these animals acting as paratenic hosts. Dogs and foxes may be infected by eating rodents infected with mesocercariae. Once infected, the mesocercariae migrate extensively, including passage through the lungs and diaphragm, becoming metacercariae before returning to the small intestine and maturing into flukes. The prepatent period is 2–4 weeks.

Alaria alata

Description: Adult flukes are 2–6 mm in length and the flat, spoon-shaped, expanded anterior part is much longer than the posterior cylindrical hindbody which contains the reproductive organs. At the anterior lateral corners of the anterior part, there are two tentacle-like processes (Fig. 1.111). The suckers are very small and the adhesive organ consists of two long folds with distinct lateral margins. The yellowish-brown eggs are large, 98–134 by 62–68 µm, operculate and unembryonated (Fig. 1.112).

Alaria americana

Description: Adult flukes range from 2.5 to 4 mm in length. The genital pore is located posteriorly on the mid-hindbody. This species is additionally characterised by the presence of pointed processes flanking the oral sucker.

Alaria canis

Description: Adult flukes are 2.5–4.2 mm long. There is a conical tentacle-like appendage on each side of the oral sucker. There is an oval holdfast organ with a longitudinal median depression

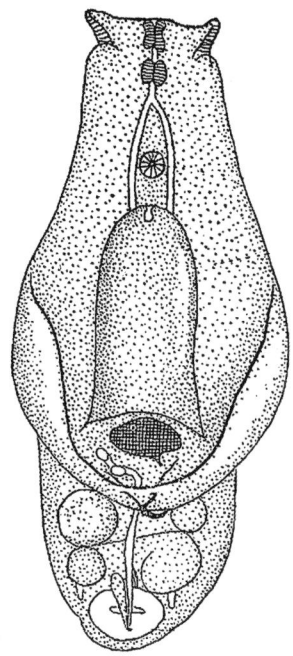

Fig. 1.111 *Alaria alata.* (Adapted from Baylis, 1929.)

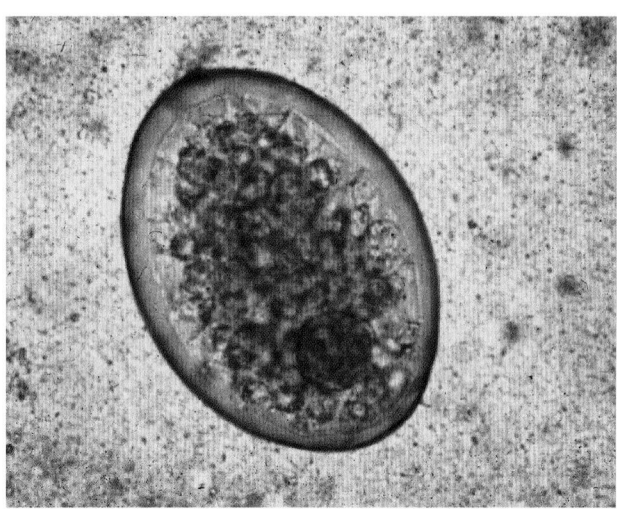

Fig. 1.112 *Alaria* egg.

extending from the ventral sucker to the constriction between the anterior and posterior parts of the body. Testes are lobed, with the posterior one much larger.

FAMILY STRIGEIDAE

These flukes are characterised by a constriction dividing the body into an anterior flattened adhesive organ and a posterior cylindrical or oval part, which contains the reproductive system. A cup-shaped adhesive organ is present in the anterior region. They are parasites of the alimentary tract of birds. The life cycle involves two intermediate hosts: freshwater snails of many genera and a second host that may be a fish or leech. Genera include *Apatemon* and *Cotylurus* in the intestine of pigeons and ducks, and *Parastrigea* in ducks.

Apatemon

The main species is *Apatemon gracilis* which infects the intestine of ducks, pigeons and wild birds. This parasite has snails and leeches as intermediate hosts.

Apatemon gracilis

Description: Adult flukes have a cup-like anterior region, containing an adhesive organ, and a posterior cylindrical region and measure 1.5–2.5 mm by 0.4 mm. The suckers are fairly well developed and the testes and ovary are arranged one behind the other with the ovary foremost. Vitellaria are limited to the posterior region of the body.

Parastrigea

The main species is *Parastrigea robusta* which infects the intestine of ducks. The intermediate host of this parasite is unknown.

Parastrigea robusta

Description: The flukes are 2–2.5 mm long and broader in the anterior region (1.5 mm) than the posterior region (1 mm). The genital papilla is large and oviform and the testes are compact and only slightly lobed. The vitellaria are mainly located in the adhesive organ and the lateral expansions, although some extend into the posterior part of the body.

Cotylurus

The main species is *Cotylurus cornutus* which infects the intestine of ducks, pigeons and wild birds. This parasite has snails as intermediate hosts.

Cotylurus cornutus

Description: The adult flukes are around 1.2–1.5 mm long and 0.5 mm wide with a rounded anterior region and an ovoid posterior region. The oral sucker is smaller than the ventral sucker and the testes and ovary are arranged one behind the other. They are similar to *Apatemon* species but a strong copulatory organ is located in the bursa.

CLASS CESTODA

This class differs from the Trematoda in having a tape-like body with no body cavity or alimentary canal. There is a wide variation in length, ranging from a few millimetres to several metres. The body is segmented, each segment containing one and sometimes two sets of male and female reproductive organs. Almost all the tapeworms of veterinary importance are in the order Cyclophyllidea, the two exceptions being in the order Pseudophyllidea.

ORDER CYCLOPHYLLIDEA

STRUCTURE AND FUNCTION

The adult cestode (Fig. 1.113) consists of a globular head or **scolex** bearing attachment organs, a short unsegmented neck and a chain of segments. The chain is known as a **strobila** and each segment as a **proglottid**. The organs of attachment are four suckers on the sides of the scolex and these may bear hooks. The scolex usually bears anteriorly a mobile protrusible cone or rostellum and in some species this may be armed with one or more concentric rows of hooks, which aid in attachment.

The proglottids are continuously budded from the neck region and become sexually mature as they pass down the strobila to the distal end of the tapeworm. Each proglottid is hermaphrodite with one or two sets of reproductive organs, the genital pores usually opening on the lateral margin or margins of the segment (Fig. 1.114); both self-fertilisation and cross-fertilisation between proglottids may occur. The structure of the genital system is generally similar to that of the trematodes. As the segment matures, its internal structure largely disappears and the fully ripe or gravid proglottid eventually contains only remnants of the branched uterus packed with eggs. The gravid segments are usually shed intact from the strobila and pass out with the faeces, either singly or occasionally in chains. Outside the body, the eggs are liberated by disintegration of the segment or are shed through the genital pore.

The fully embryonated egg consists of:
1 the hexacanth (six-hooked) embryo or **oncosphere**
2 a thick, dark, radially striated 'shell' called the **embryophore** (in the Mesocestoididae it is apparent as a thin cellular membrane)
3 a true shell, which is a delicate membrane and is often lost while still in the uterus.

The tegument of the adult tapeworm is highly absorptive, the worm deriving all its nourishment through this structure. Below the tegument are muscle cells and the parenchyma, the latter a syncytium of cells, which fills the space between the organs. The nervous system consists of ganglia in the scolex from which nerves run posteriorly

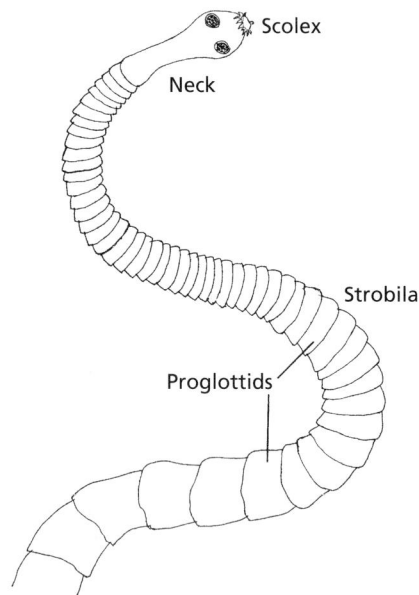

Fig. 1.113 Structure of a typical cyclophyllidean cestode.

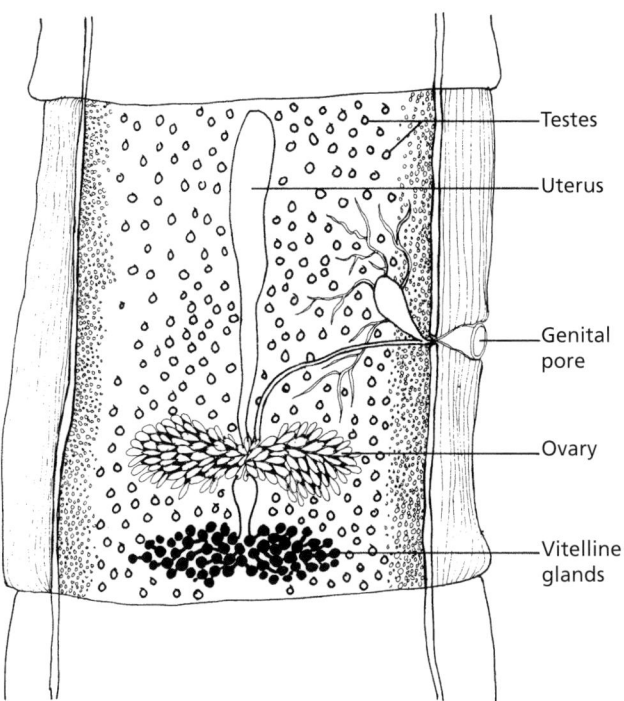

Fig. 1.114 Mature segment illustrating the reproductive organs.

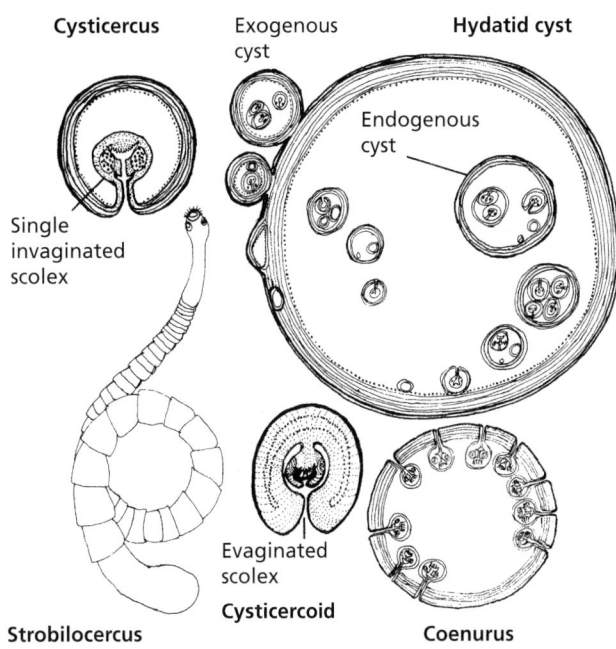

Fig. 1.115 Larval stages of cyclophyllidean cestodes.

and enter the strobila. The excretory system, as in the Trematoda, is composed of flame cells leading to efferent canals that run through the strobila to discharge at the terminal segment.

LIFE CYCLE

The typical life cycle of these cestodes is indirect with one or more intermediate hosts. With few exceptions, the adult tapeworm is found in the small intestine of the final host, the segments and eggs reaching the exterior in the faeces. When the egg is ingested by the intermediate host, the gastric and intestinal secretions digest the embryophore and activate the oncosphere. Using its hooks, it tears through the mucosa to reach the blood or lymph stream or, in the case of invertebrates, the body cavity. Once in its predilection site, the oncosphere loses its hooks and develops, depending on the species, into one of the following larval stages, often known as **metacestodes** (Fig. 1.115).

- **Cysticercus**: Single fluid-filled cyst or bladder containing an attached single invaginated scolex, sometimes called a protoscolex.
- **Coenurus**: This large cyst is similar to a cysticercus, but with numerous invaginated scolices attatched to the cyst wall.
- **Strobilocercus**: The scolex is evaginated and is connected to the cyst by a chain of segmented asexual proglottids. The latter are digested away after ingestion by the final host, leaving only the scolex.
- **Hydatid**: This is a large, fluid-filled, complex cyst lined with germinal epithelium from which are produced invaginated scolices which lie free or in bunches, surrounded by germinal epithelium (brood capsules). The contents of the cysts other than the fluid (i.e. scolices and brood capsules) are frequently described as 'hydatid sand'. Occasionally also, daughter cysts complete with cuticle and germinal layer are formed endogenously or, if the cyst wall ruptures, exogenously.

- **Cysticercoid**: A single evaginated scolex embedded in a small solid cyst. Typically found in very small intermediate hosts such as arthropods.
- **Tetrathyridium**: Worm-like, flattened and elongate larva with an invaginated acetabular scolex; found only in Mesocestoididae.

When the metacestode is ingested by the final host, the scolex attaches to the mucosa, the remainder of the structure is digested off and a chain of proglottids begins to grow from the base of the scolex.

The seven main families of veterinary interest in the order Cyclophyllidea are the Taeniidae, Anoplocephalidae, Dilepididae, Davaineidae, Hymenolepididae, Mesocestoididae and Paruterinidae.

FAMILY TAENIIDAE

The adults are, in most cases, large tapeworms and are found in domestic carnivores and humans in the small intestine. Genera of importance are *Taenia* (syn. *Multiceps*) and *Echinococcus*. The scolex has an armed rostellum with a concentric double row of hooks (the important exception is *Taenia saginata* whose scolex is unarmed). The gravid segments are longer than they are wide. The intermediate stage is a cysticercus, strobilocercus, coenurus or hydatid cyst and these occur only in mammals. Historically, the intermediate stage has been named according to the type of metacestode stage present in the intermediate host. Thus, *Cysticercus tenuicollis* found in the ruminant host is the metacestode stage of *Taenia hydatigena* in the dog. The correct nomenclature now is for the intermediate host stage to be referred to as the 'metacestode stage' of the adult *Taenia* species.

Taenia

Members of the genus *Taenia* are large tapeworms comprising a number of species (Table 1.57). Differentiation is usually based on the size of the scolex, the size of the rostellum and number of hooks, and on the morphology of the genital system within the mature proglottids.

Table 1.57 *Taenia* species.

Species	Final hosts	Intermediate hosts (larval stage)	Site
Taenia asiatica (syn. *Taenia saginata asiatica*)	Humans	Cattle	Muscle
Taenia crassiceps	Foxes, coyotes	Rodents	Abdominal cavity, various tissues
Taenia hydatigena (syn. *Taenia marginata*)	Dogs, foxes, wild canids, mustelids	Cattle, sheep, goats, pigs (*Cysticercus tenuicollis*)	Abdominal cavity, liver
Taenia multiceps (syn. *Multiceps multiceps*)	Dogs, foxes, wild canids	Sheep, cattle, goats, pigs, horses, deer, camels, humans (*Coenurus cerebralis*)	Brain, spinal cord
Taenia skrjabini		Sheep (*Coenurus skrjabini*)	Muscle, subcutaneous tissue
Taenia (Multiceps) gaigeri		Goat (*Coenurus gaigeri*)	
Taenia ovis (syn. *Taenia cervi, Taenia krabbei, Taenia hyaenae*)	Dogs, foxes, wild canids	Sheep, goats (*Cysticercus ovis*) Deer (*Cysticercus cervi*) Reindeer (*Cysticercus tarandi*) Camels (*Cysticercus dromedarii, Cysticercus cameli*)	Muscle
Taenia pisiformis	Dogs, foxes, wild canids	Rabbits, hares (*Cysticercus pisiformis*)	Peritoneum, liver
Taenia saginata (syn. *Taeniarhynchus saginata*)	Humans	Cattle, occasionally other ruminants (*Cysticercus bovis*)	Muscle
Taenia serialis (syn. *Multiceps serialis*)	Dogs	Rabbits, hares (*Coenurus serialis*)	Connective tissue
Taenia solium	Humans	Pigs, wild boar (*Cysticercus cellulosae*)	Muscle
Taenia taeniaeformis (syn. *Hydatigera taeniaeformis, Taenia crassicollis*)	Cats, wild felids	Small rodents (*Strobilocercus fasciolaris*; syn. *Strobilocercus crassicollis*)	Liver

The adults of *Taenia* are usually of minor importance in domesticated animals, and it is the larval stages which are of veterinary interest.

Taenia asiatica

Synonym: *Taenia saginata asiatica*

Description: Similar to *T. saginata*. The adult tapeworm is about 3.5 m long with a scolex bearing four simple suckers and the rostellum is usually surrounded by two rows of rudimentary hooklets. It is unique in having posterior protuberances in the gravid proglottid (which are absent in other taeniids, including *T. saginata*) and it presents 11–32 uterine buds. The metacestode differs morphologically from that of *T. saginata* in having wart-like formations on the external surface of the bladder wall.

Taenia hydatigena

Synonyms: *Taenia marginata*

Description: *Taenia hydatigena* is a large tapeworm measuring up to 5 m in length. The scolex is large and has two rows of 26 and 46 rostellar hooks. Four suckers are present. Gravid proglottids measure 12 by 6 mm and the uterus has 5–10 lateral branches. The mature metacestode (*Cysticercus tenuicollis*) is about 5–7 cm in diameter (see Fig. 9.26) and contains a watery fluid and invaginated scolex with a long neck. Eggs are subspherical or slightly elliptical and measure 36–39 by 31–35 μm. They have a smooth thick shell with a radially striated embryophore and contain a hexacanth embryo.

Life cycle: Dogs and wild canids are infested by consuming the cysticercus in the intermediate host. The intermediate host is infected through the ingestion of tapeworm eggs that hatch in the intestine. The oncospheres, infective to sheep, goats, cattle and pigs, are carried in the blood to the liver in which they migrate for about four weeks before they emerge on the surface of this organ and attach to the peritoneum. Within a further four weeks, each develops into the characteristically large metacestode, *Cysticercus tenuicollis*. The complete life cycle of this tapeworm is around 7–8 months. See **life cycle 21**.

Taenia multiceps

Synonyms: *Multiceps multiceps, Coenurus cerebralis, Taenia skrjabini, Coenurus skrjabini, Taenia (Multiceps) gaigeri, Coenurus gaigeri*

Description: Adult tapeworms are 40–100 cm in length and have a small head about 0.8 mm in diameter with four suckers (Fig. 1.116). There is a double ring of 22–32 rostellar hooks (Fig. 1.117). The gravid segments measure 8–12 mm by 3–4 mm and the uterus has 18–26 lateral branches which contain taeniid eggs. Eggs are approximately 29–37 μm in diameter and have thick smooth shells with a radially striated embryophore. They contain a hexacanth embryo. The metacestode larval stage (*Coenurus cerebralis*) is readily recognised when mature as a large fluid-filled cyst up to 5 cm or more in diameter bearing random clusters of invaginated scolices, sometimes up to several hundred, on its internal wall (Fig. 1.118). The coenurus bears clusters of several hundred protoscolices on its internal wall.

Life cycle: The intermediate host is infected through the ingestion of *T. multiceps* eggs. Each egg contains an oncosphere that hatches and is activated in the small intestine. The oncosphere then penetrates the intestinal mucosa and is carried via the blood to the brain or spinal cord where each oncosphere develops into the metacestode larval stage (*Coenurus cerebralis*). In goats, the cysts can also

LIFE CYCLE 21. LIFE CYCLE OF *TAENIA HYDATIGENA*

Taenia hydatigena is a hooked cestode that, at the adult stage, lives in the small intestine of dogs, which act as definitive hosts (1). Eggs are released from the proglottids shed with the host faeces (2); following ingestion of the eggs by suitable intermediate hosts (i.e. cattle, sheep, pigs), the hexacanth larvae are released in the small intestine (3). From here, the larvae migrate via the circulation to the parenchyma of the liver (4). In the latter, the larva, known as '*Cysticercus tenuicollis*', grows into an immature vesicle (5) containing the invaginated protoscolex immersed in clear fluid. The cysticercus actively traverses the hepatic serosa and, once in the peritoneum (final site), adheres to the peritoneal serosa and completes development into a pear-shaped vesicle (up to 8 cm) with a thin and long neck; the protoscolex occurs at the neck's extremity (6). Dogs become infected by ingesting raw or undercooked offal from infected sheep or sheep carcasses abandoned on pasture. Once ingested, the protoscolices evaginate in the small intestine and develop to adult tapeworms within two months (1).

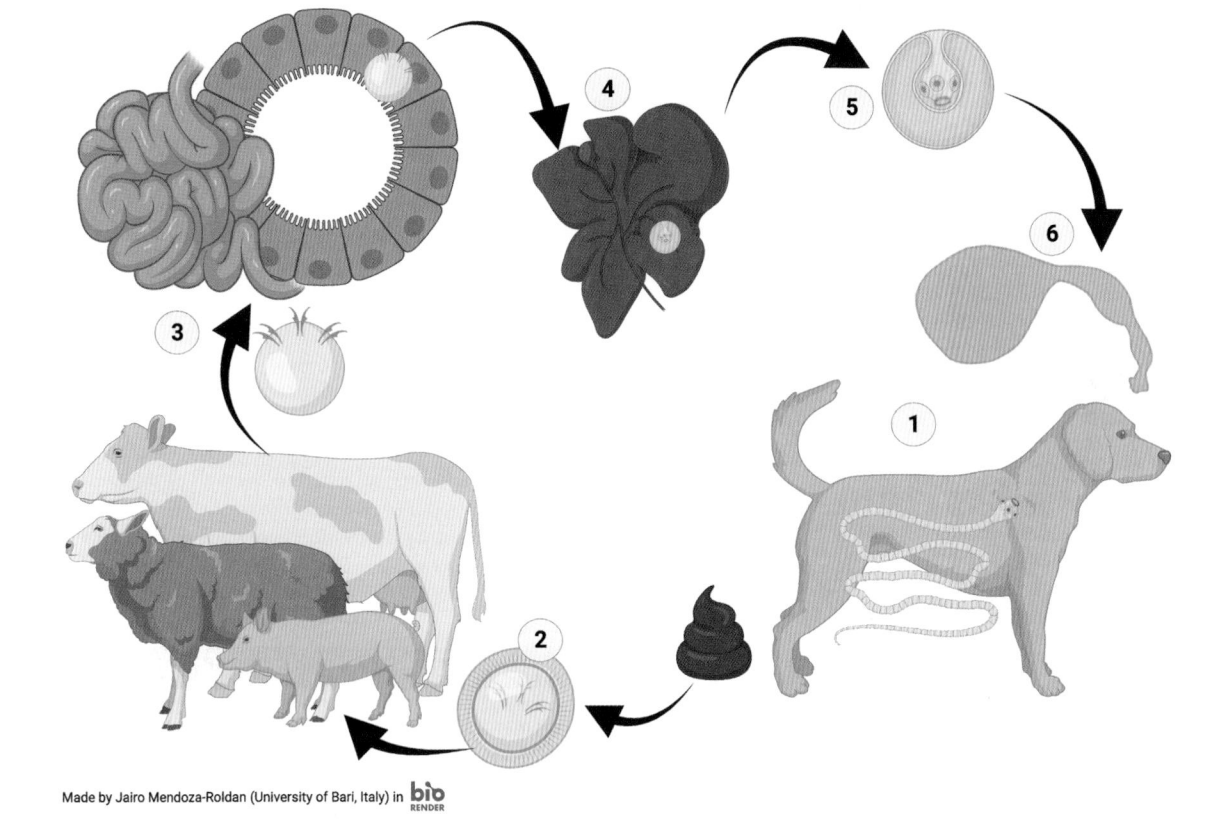

Made by Jairo Mendoza-Roldan (University of Bari, Italy) in **bio**RENDER

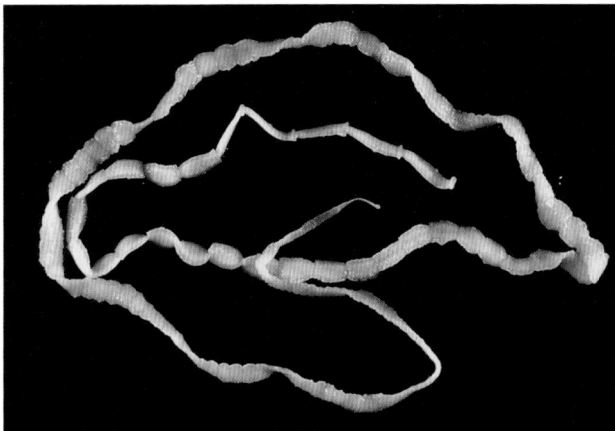

Fig. 1.116 Mature tapeworm, *Taenia multiceps.*

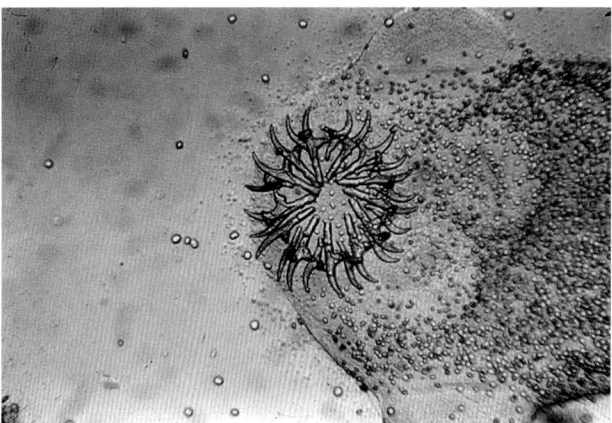

Fig. 1.117 Rostellar hooks of *Taenia* (*Multiceps*) *multiceps.*

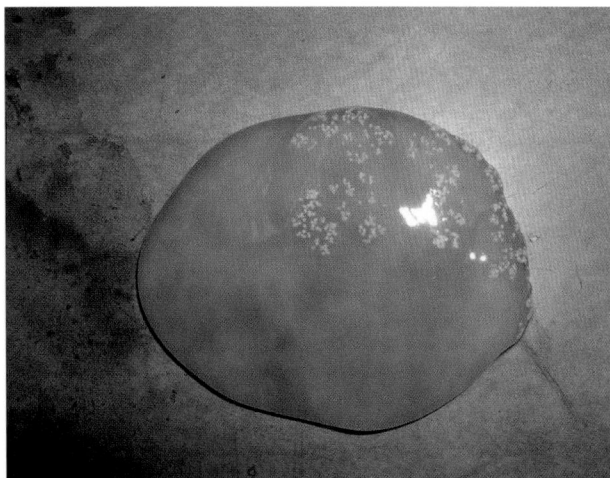

Fig. 1.118 *Coenurus cerebralis* metacestode stage of *Taenia multiceps*. (Courtesy of Andrei Mihalca).

mature in subcutaneous and intramuscular sites. The cysts in sheep and goats often persist throughout the life of the animal. The life cycle is completed when the final host, dog or wild canid, eats an infected sheep brain or spinal cord.

Taenia ovis

Synonyms: *Cysticercus ovis, Taenia cervi (Cysticercus cervi), Taenia krabbei (Cysticercus tarandi), Taenia hyaenae (Cysticercus dromedarii, Cysticercus cameli)*

Description: The adult tapeworm is large, measuring 0.5–1.5 m in length. The rostellum bears 24–36 hooks. The strobila has a scalloped edge and is often coiled into a spiral. The mature proglottids have a vaginal sphincter and the ovary and vagina cross each other. The uterus of the gravid proglottids has 20–25 lateral branches on either side. The oval egg measures 34 by 24–28 µm. Mature cysticerci are ovoid, white and around 3.5–10 mm and contain a single protoscolex, which is invaginated and armed with hooks and a rostellum (Fig. 1.119). In the intermediate host, each cysticercus occurs within a small cyst measuring about 4 mm or less in length.

Life cycle: Dogs and wild canids are infested by consuming the cysticercus in the intermediate host. The intermediate host is infected through the ingestion of tapeworm eggs that hatch in the intestine. The metacestode stage (*Cysticercus ovis*) infects the musculature and cysts are usually located in the skeletal muscle, heart, diaphragm and intermuscular connective tissue. The cyst becomes infective around 2–3 months after infection of the host. The prepatent period in dogs is around 6–9 weeks.

Taenia pisiformis

Synonym: *Cysticercus pisiformis*

Description: The adult tapeworm can measure up to 2 m in length. It has a large scolex with narrow strobila and the rostellum has 34–48 hooks in two rows (Fig. 1.120). Gravid segments have a uterus with 8–14 lateral branches on either side. The cysticercus is a small pea-like transparent cyst and usually occurs in bunches. Eggs are oval or elliptical, approximately 48 by 46 µm in size, and have thick smooth shells with a radially striated embryophore. They contain a hexacanth embryo.

Life cycle: Infection of the intermediate host is through ingestion of tapeworm eggs shed by dogs. Ingested eggs hatch in the small intestine of the intermediate host and penetrate the intestinal wall and pass via the portal system to the liver. Juvenile stages migrate through the liver parenchyma and locate in the abdominal cavity after 2–4 weeks, where they develop into cysts (*Cysticercus pisiformis*) attached to the wall of the mesentery and omentum. Cysts can survive the life of the host. The final host is infected by ingesting the cysticercus. The prepatent period in the dog is around 6–8 weeks.

Taenia saginata

Synonyms: *Taeniarhynchus saginata, Cysticercus bovis*

Description: The adult tapeworm is usually 5–8 m long, rarely up to 15 m. The scolex has neither a rostellum nor hooks. Gravid segments are 16–20 mm long by 4–7 mm wide and the uterus has

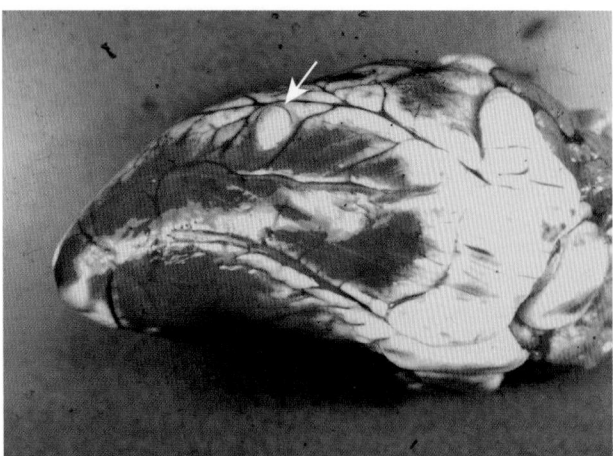

Fig. 1.119 *Cysticercus ovis* metacestode stage of *Taenia ovis* in sheep heart (arrowed).

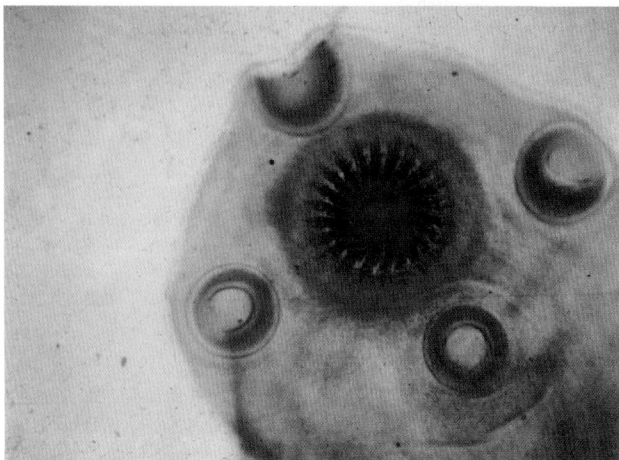

Fig. 1.120 Scolex of *Taenia pisiformis* showing the four suckers and armed rostellum.

15–35 lateral branches on either side. In cattle, the mature cysticercus, *C. bovis*, is greyish-white, oval, about 0.5–1 by 0.5 cm long, and filled with fluid in which the scolex is usually clearly visible. As in the adult tapeworm, it has neither rostellum nor hooks.

Life cycle: An infected human may pass millions of eggs daily, either free in the faeces or as intact segments each containing about 250 000 eggs, and these can survive on pasture for several months. After ingestion by a susceptible bovine, the oncosphere travels via the blood to striated muscle. It is first grossly visible about two weeks later as a pale semi-transparent spot about 1 mm in diameter, but is not infective to humans until about 12 weeks later when it has reached its full size of around 1 cm. By then, it is enclosed by the host in a thin fibrous capsule but despite this the scolex can usually still be seen. The longevity of the cysts ranges from weeks to years. When they die, they are usually replaced by a caseous crumbly mass, which may become calcified. Both living and dead cysts are frequently present in the same carcass. Humans become infected by ingesting raw or inadequately cooked meat. Development to patency takes 2–3 months. See **life cycle 22**.

Taenia serialis

Synonyms: *Multiceps serialis*, *Coenurus serialis*

Description: The adult tapeworm is of medium length, around 0.5–0.7 m long. The scolex is armed with two rows of 26–32 hooks (Fig. 1.121). The metacestode cysts may be 4–6 cm in size and the scolices are distributed in packed rows within the cyst. The numerous scolices in the coenurus are arranged in lines or strands, as the name '*serialis*' implies. The gravid uterus has 10–18 lateral branches and the vaginal sphincter is well developed. The slightly elliptical eggs measure 31–34 by 29–30 μm and have thick smooth shells with a radially striated embryophore. They contain a hexacanth embryo.

Life cycle: Infection of the intermediate host is through ingestion of tapeworm eggs shed by dogs. The intermediate stage, *Coenurus serialis*, is found in the rabbit, usually subcutaneously or in the intermuscular connective tissue. The final host is infected by ingesting the metacestode stage.

LIFE CYCLE 22. LIFE CYCLE OF *TAENIA SAGINATA*

Taenia saginata is a harmless 8–12 meter-long cestode, found in the small intestine of humans, which act as definitive hosts (1). Each gravid proglottid features several uterus branches (15–30) and may contain up to 80 000 eggs (2). The egg contains a hexacanth larva that features three pairs of hooks (3). Cattle, which act as intermediate hosts (4), acquire the infection by ingesting eggs or gravid proglottids shed in the faeces of the human definitive hosts. In the bovine intestine, eggs hatch the oncospheres (5) that migrate via the circulation to the masseter muscle, heart, diaphragm and tongue. In these sites, the larva, known as '*Cysticercus bovis*', grows, forming a vesicle containing the invaginated protoscolex immersed in citrine fluid (6). The fully developed vesicle is elongated and measures 5 × 10 mm. Humans become infected by ingesting raw or undercooked bovine meat containing the cysticerci (7); in the intestine of the definitive host, the protoscolices evaginate and develop to adult tapeworms within 2–3 months (8).

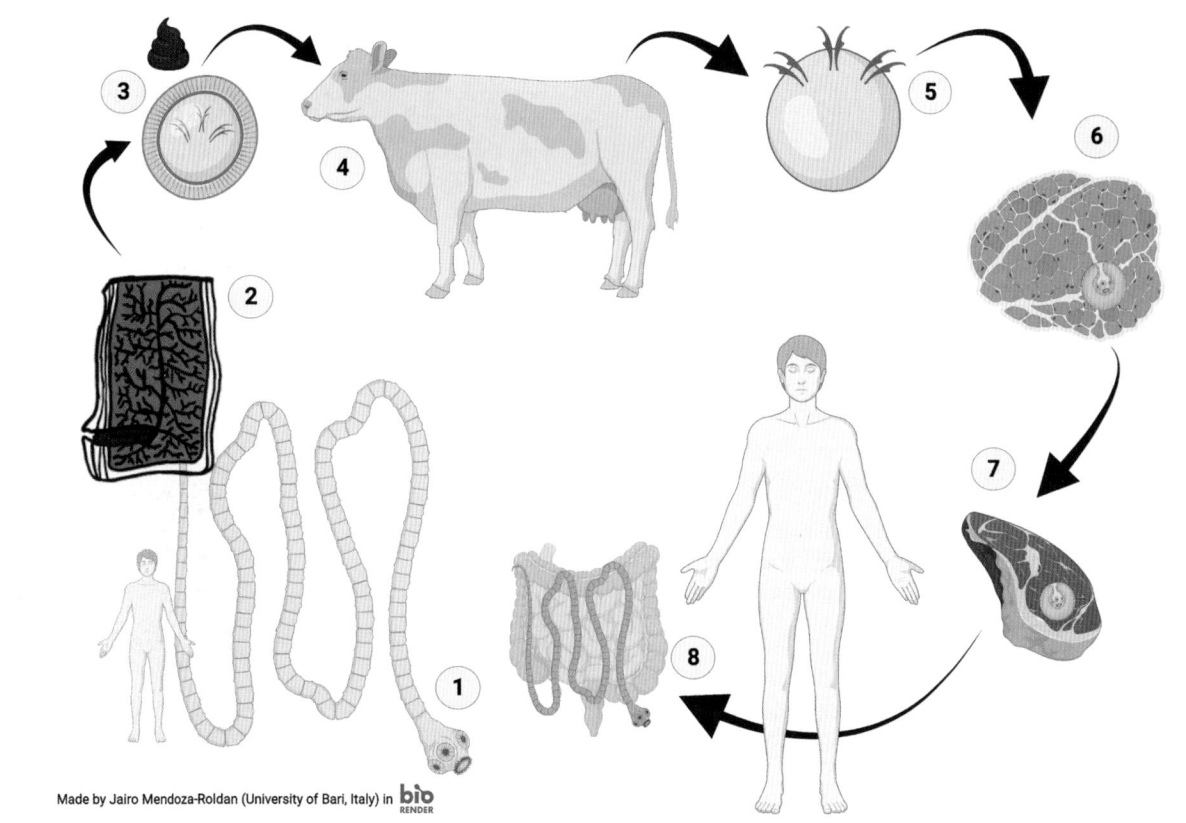

Made by Jairo Mendoza-Roldan (University of Bari, Italy) in **bio**RENDER

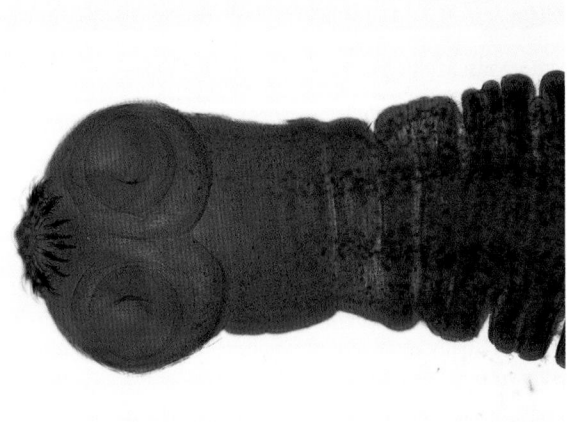

Fig. 1.121 Scolex of *Taenia serialis*.

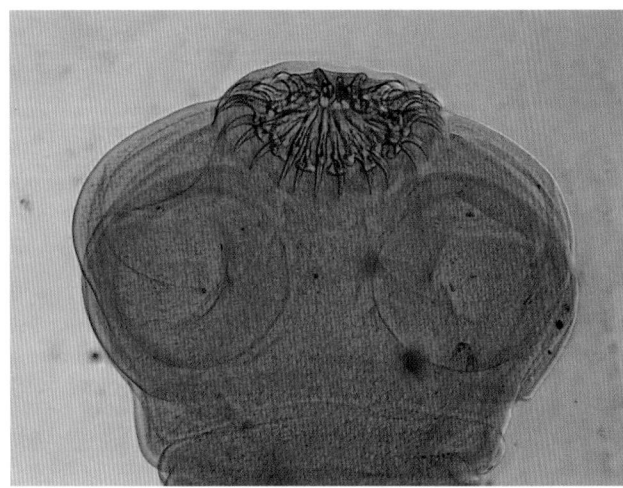

Fig. 1.122 Scolex of *Taenia solium*. (Courtesy of Libor Mikeš).

Taenia solium

Synonym: *Cysticercus solium*

Description: The adult tapeworm is 3–5 m long, rarely up to 8 m. The rostellum has four radially arranged suckers and bears four suckers and 22–32 hooks in two rows (Fig. 1.122), one row of large hooks measuring 0.14–0.18 mm and one row of smaller hooks measuring 0.11–0.14 mm. Gravid segments are 10–12 mm long and 5–6 mm wide. The ovary is in the posterior third of the proglottid and has two lobes with an accessory third lobe. The uterus has 7–12 lateral branches on either side. Adults can survive in humans for many years. Cysts are milky white and have a scolex bearing a rostellum and hooks similar to the adult. The small egg is slightly ellipsoidal with a smooth shell with a radially striated embryophore. They are yellowish-brown and measure about 35–40 by 30–35 μm and contain a hexacanth embryo. Eggs are released when the shed gravid proglottid disintegrates. The cysticerci have morphologically distinct types. The most common is the 'cellulose' cysticercus which has a fluid-filled bladder that is 0.5–1.5 cm in length with an invaginated scolex. The 'racemose' form has no evident scolex, but is larger and up to 20 cm in length.

Life cycle: Gravid segments passed in the faeces, frequently in chains, each contain around 40 000 eggs and because they are non-motile they tend to be concentrated over a small area. Eggs can also resist destruction for a relatively long period. After ingestion by a susceptible pig, the oncosphere travels via the blood to striated muscle. The principal location is the striated muscles but cysticerci may also develop in other organs, such as the lungs, liver, kidney and brain. Humans become infected by ingesting raw or inadequately cooked pork containing viable cysticerci. The human final host may also act as an intermediate host and become infected with cysticerci. This is most likely to occur from the accidental ingestion of *T. solium* eggs via unwashed hands or contaminated food. There is also, apparently, a minor route of autoinfection in a person with an adult tapeworm, from the liberation of oncospheres after the digestion of a gravid segment that has entered the stomach from the duodenum by reverse peristalsis. The prepatent period is 2–3 months. See **life cycle 23**.

Taenia taeniaeformis

Synonyms: *Hydatigera taeniaeformis, Taenia crassicollis, Strobilocercus fasciolaris, Strobilocercus crassicollis*

Description: The adult tapeworm is of medium size, up to 70 cm in length. The scolex is large with a double row of rostellar hooks and there is no neck region (Fig. 1.123). The uterus has 5–9 lateral branches and the posterior proglottids are bell-shaped. The metacestode stage is a strobilocercus (*Strobilocercus fasciolaris*), which is a small cyst connected with an evaginated scolex by a segmented juvenile strobila. The subspherical eggs measure on average about 31–37 μm and have thick smooth shells with a radially striated embryophore. They contain a hexacanth embryo.

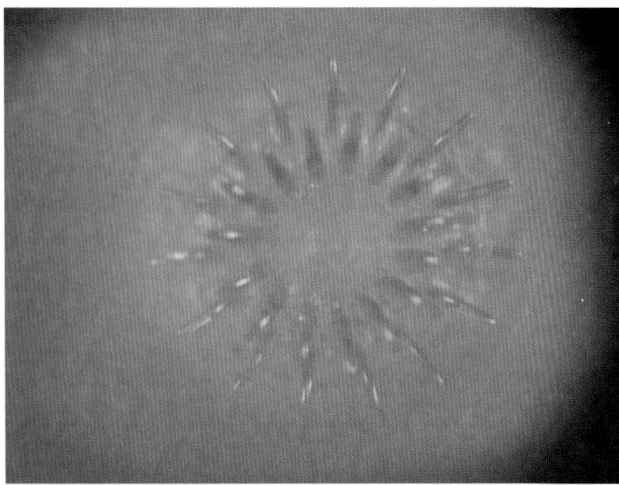

Fig. 1.123 Scolex of *Taenia taeniaeformis*. (Courtesy of Andrei Mihalca).

LIFE CYCLE 23. LIFE CYCLE OF *TAENIA SOLIUM*

Taenia solium is a 2–8 meter-long hooked cestode that, at the adult stage, is found in the small intestine of humans, which act as definitive hosts (1). The parasite's gravid proglottids are eliminated with the host faeces (2); each of these proglottids features 7–13 uterus branches and contains up to 40 000 eggs. Each egg contains a hexacanth larva, that features three pairs of hooks (3). Pigs act as intermediate hosts, which become infected by ingesting eggs or proglottids shed by infected humans (4). In the small intestine of the pig host, the eggs hatch and the oncospheres traverse the duodenal wall to invade the circulation and migrate to the skeletal muscles, particularly the masseter, tongue, heart and diaphragm (5). In these sites, the larval stage, known as 'Cysticercus

cellulosae', grow to form a whitish vesicle (20 × 10 mm) that contains the invaginated protoscolex immersed in a clear fluid (5). Humans acquire the infection by ingesting raw or undercooked pork meat containing the cysticerci (6). Once in the intestine of the definitive host, the protoscolices evaginate, attach to the intestinal mucosa (7) via the hooks and develop to adult tapeworms.

Humans can also act as accidental dead-end intermediate hosts by ingesting parasite eggs (3) or via autoinfection. If this occurs, the eggs (8) hatch in the intestine and the parasites migrate through the liver (9) and the circulatory system (10) to several organs and tissues, including skeletal muscles, eyes and central nervous system.

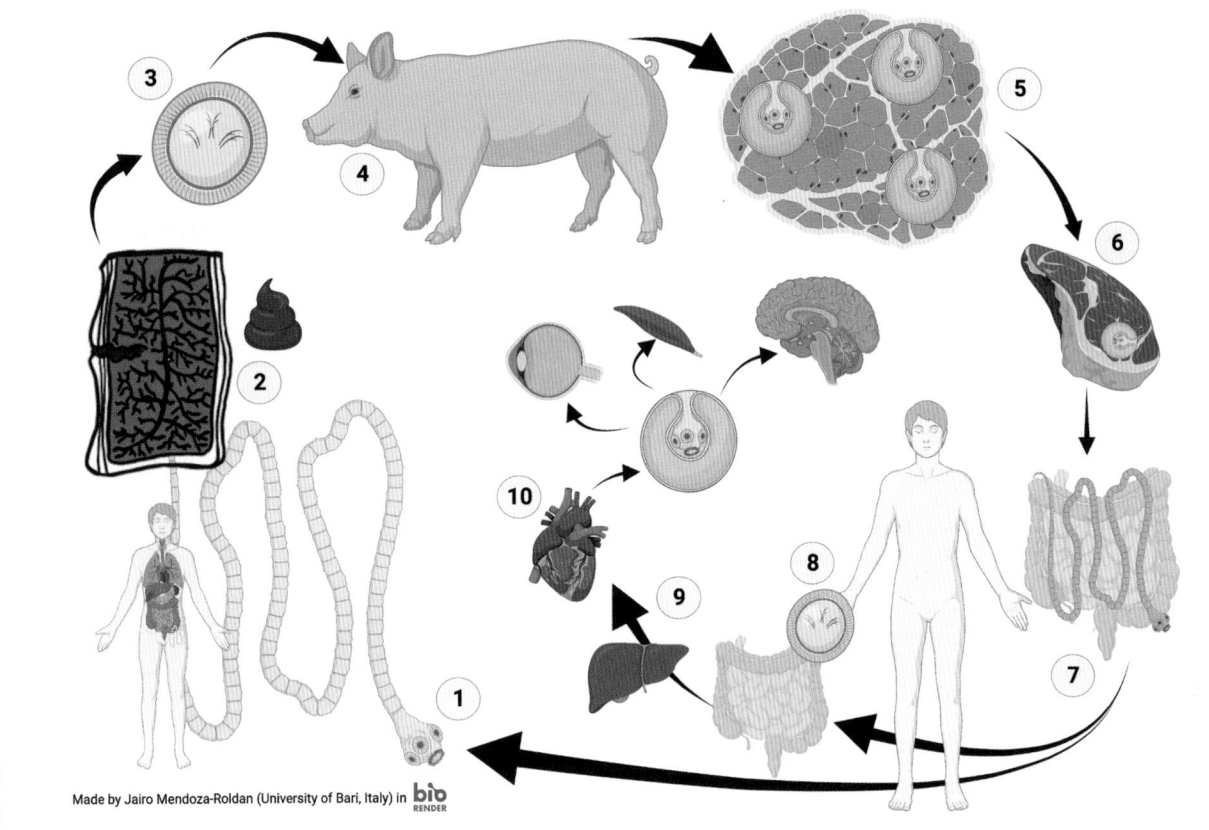

Made by Jairo Mendoza-Roldan (University of Bari, Italy) in **bio** RENDER

Life cycle: The metacestode (*Cysticercus fasciolaris*) develops in the liver of rodents and is infective to cats after about nine weeks. When a cat ingests the metacestode, the scolex attaches to the wall of the intestine. Tapeworms in cats become patent around six weeks and eggs are ingested by the intermediate host. Cats can remain infected for up to about two years.

Echinococcus

The genus *Echinococcus* is composed of several species that exploit predator–prey systems between carnivores (mainly canids) as principal hosts and intermediate hosts that range from rodents to

livestock depending on the species (Table 1.58). Six species are currently recognised in the genus *Echinococcus*, with a seventh, *Echinococcus shiquicus*, recently described. Considerable phenotypic and genetic variability has been observed within the species *E. granulosus* and several strains have been identified based on molecular genotyping.

New data demonstrate that '*E. granulosus*' is an assembly of several rather diverse strains and genotypes (designated G1–G10) that show fundamental differences, not only in their epidemiology but also in their pathogenicity to humans. *Echinococcus equinus* was formerly known as the horse strain (G4) of *E. granulosus*. *Echinococcus ortleppi*, the former cattle strain (G5), is adapted to transmission by cattle. *Echinococcus oligarthus* and *E. vogeli* exist in

Table 1.58 *Echinococcus* species.

Species	Hosts	Intermediate hosts	Site
Echinococcus granulosus	Dogs, foxes, wild canids	Sheep, cattle, camels, pigs, buffalo, deer, humans	Liver, lungs
Echinococcus equinus (G4)	Dogs	Horses, donkeys	Liver
Echinococcus orteleppi (G5)	Dogs	Cattle	Liver
Echinococcus multilocularis	Dogs, foxes, cats, wild canids, humans	Rodents, pigs	Liver
Echinococcus vogeli	Wild canids	Rodents	Liver
Echinococcus oligarthus	Wild felids	Rodents	Liver

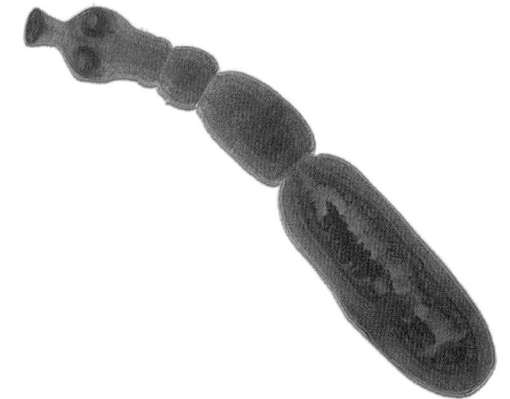

Fig. 1.124 *Echinococcus granulosus* showing the scolices and the large gravid posterior proglottids. (Courtesy of Aránzazu Meana).

wildlife cycles and are morphologically similar to *E. multilocularis* and cause polycystic echinococcosis in humans.

Echinococcus granulosus (Echinococcus equinus, Echinococcus orteleppi)

Description: The entire cestode is only about 6 mm long, and is therefore difficult to find in the freshly opened intestine. It consists of a scolex and usually three or four segments, the terminal gravid one occupying about half the length of the complete tapeworm (Fig. 1.124). The scolex is typically taeniid and the rostellum has two rows of hooks, varying in number from 30 to 60. Each segment has a single genital opening, with the penultimate segment sexually mature and the last segment gravid. The genital pores alternate irregularly. The gravid proglottid normally disintegrates in the alimentary tract and only eggs are expelled in faeces. The small, almost spherical eggs have a smooth thick shell and are typically 'taeniid'. They measure 32–36 by 25–30 µm and the lamellar embryophore is radially striated with a six-hooked oncosphere. Hydatid cysts are large fluid-filled vesicles, 5–10 cm in diameter, with a thick concentrically laminated cuticle and an internal germinal layer. The germinal layer produces numerous small vesicles or brood capsules each containing up to 40 scolices, invaginated into their neck portions and attached to the wall by stalks. Brood capsules may become detached from the wall of the vesicle and float freely in the vesicular fluid and form 'hydatid sand'.

Life cycle: The prepatent period in the final host is around 40–50 days, after which only one gravid segment is shed per week. The oncospheres are capable of prolonged survival outside the host, being viable on the ground for about two years. After ingestion by the intermediate host, the oncosphere penetrates the gut wall and travels in the blood to the liver or in the lymph to the lungs. These are the two most common sites for larval development, but occasionally oncospheres escape into the general systemic circulation and develop in other organs and tissues. Growth of the hydatid is slow, maturity being reached in 6–12 months. In the liver and lungs, the cyst may have a diameter of up 20 cm, but in the rarer sites, such as the abdominal cavity, where unrestricted growth is possible, it may be very large and contain several litres of fluid. The cyst capsule consists of an outer membrane and an inner germinal epithelium from which, when cyst growth is almost complete, brood capsules each containing a number of scolices are budded off. Many

of these brood capsules become detached and exist free in the hydatid fluid; collectively, these and the scolices are often referred to as 'hydatid sand'. Sometimes, complete daughter cysts are formed either inside the mother cyst or externally; in the latter case, they may be carried to other parts of the body to form new hydatids. See **life cycle 24**.

Echinococcus multilocularis

Description: *Echinococcus multilocularis* is a very small tapeworm (2–4 mm) and is generally similar to *E. granulosus*, but usually with 3–5 segments, the terminal one measuring less than half the length of the whole worm (Fig. 1.125). The scolex has four suckers and possesses a double row of large and small hooks (about 14–34). The third segment of the adult tapeworm is sexually mature and the genital pores are in front of the middle of each segment. The uterus is sac-like with no lateral sacculations in the terminal proglottid. Gravid segments contain around 200–300 spherical eggs. Eggs that are shed have a diameter of about 30–40 µm. The structure of the metacestode consists of a germinative gelatinous matrix forming a cystic structure with internal brood capsules and protoscolices

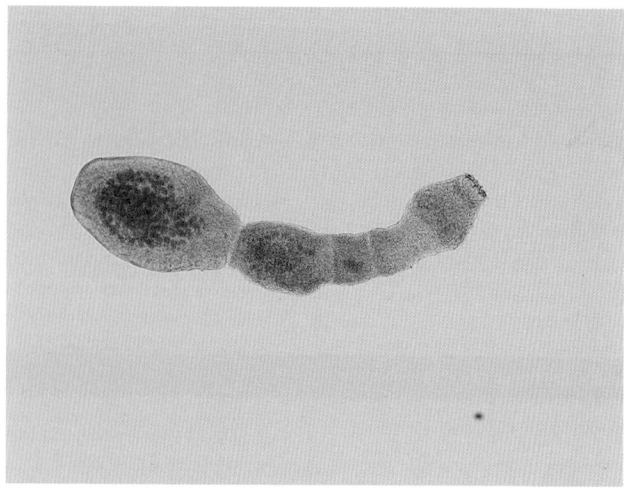

Fig. 1.125 *Echinococcus multilocularis*. (Courtesy of Libor Mikeš).

LIFE CYCLE 24. LIFE CYCLE OF *ECHINOCOCCUS GRANULOSUS*

Adult stages of *Echinococcus granulosus* (~6 mm in length) live in the small intestine of the dog, which acts as definitive host (1). The dog sheds the last proglottid of the adult tapeworm with the faeces (2); in the environment, the proglottid releases several eggs (3) that contaminate the surroundings. Depending on the genotype of *Echinococcus*, several animal species may act as intermediate hosts. The main intermediate host is the sheep (4), that acquires the infection by ingesting eggs contaminating the environment. In the sheep intestine, the eggs hatch, releasing hexacanth larvae that, via the circulation, travel to the liver (5) (where the vast majority of them establish), lungs and other organs and tissues. In these sites, the hexacanth embryos develop slowly to form cysts; these are characterised by an external capsule, a middle layer and an internal membrane, known as the 'germinative membrane'. The cysts are known as 'hydatids' and represent the larval form of the parasite (metacestode), that are also named 'Echinococcus polymorphus' (syn. Echinococcus granulosus). The hydatids contain a clear fluid and several daughter and grand-daughter cysts, each of which contains protoscolices (6). The life cycle is complete when a definitive host (dog) ingests infected sheep offal (7) containing the hydatids. In the small intestine of the dog, the protoscolices evaginate and, after attaching to the intestinal mucosa, develop into adult tapeworms. Humans acquire the infection by ingesting food (particularly poorly washed fruit and vegetables) contaminated with tapeworm eggs. In such an occurrence, humans act as intermediate hosts, with the parasite undergoing an identical cycle to that described for the sheep, with hydatid cysts forming in several organs and tissues, particularly liver and lungs (8).

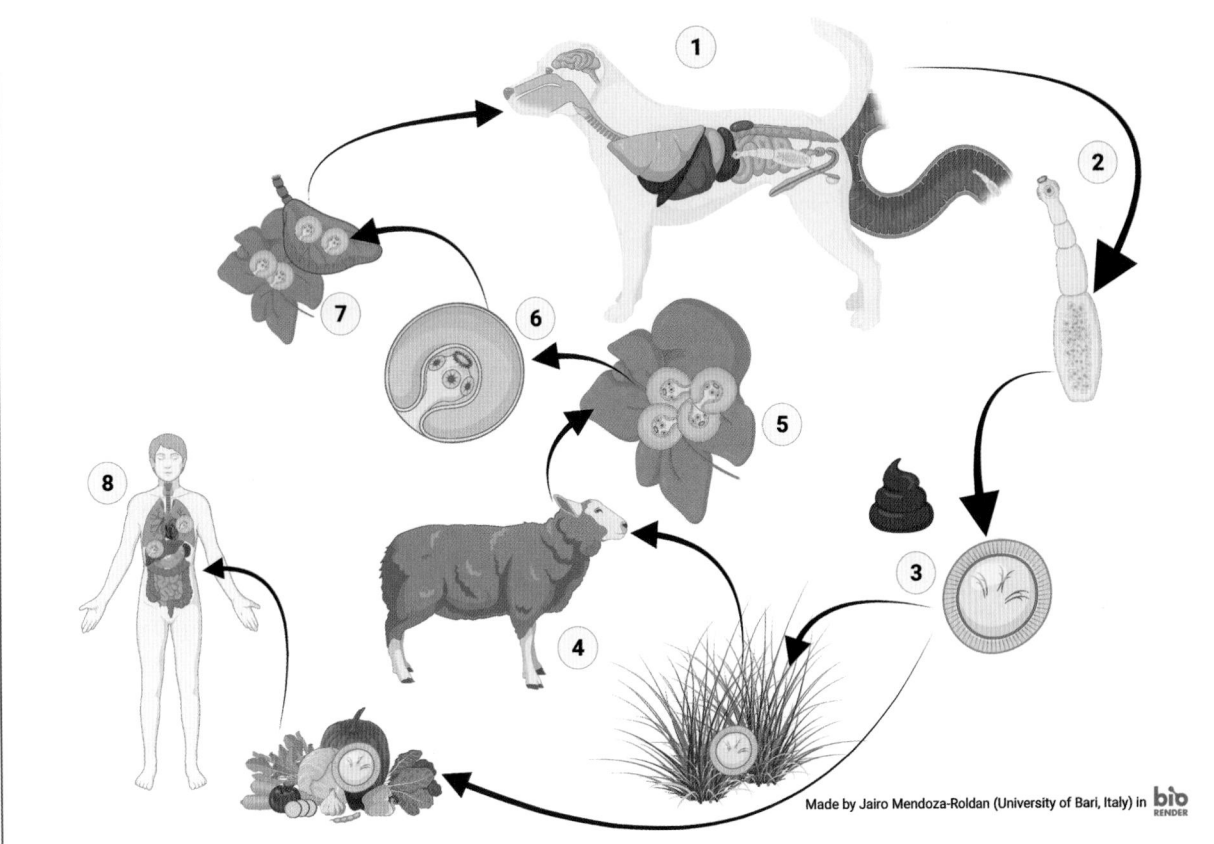

Made by Jairo Mendoza-Roldan (University of Bari, Italy) in bio RENDER

which form racemose proliferative masses of metacestodes within infected livers of the intermediate hosts.

Life cycle: *Echinococcus multilocularis* is typically maintained in a sylvatic (wildlife) cycle, although in some rural communities a synanthropic cycle occurs with the domestic dog acting as definitive host. The intermediate host is infected by ingestion of the oncosphere and subsequent passage, via the circulatory system, to the liver where it develops into a multilocular or alveolar cyst (metacestode stage). The cycle is completed when the definitive host consumes an infected intermediate host, the mature tapeworm developing in about five weeks. Adult tapeworms are relatively short-lived, about six months.

Echinococcus vogeli

Description: *Echinococcus vogeli* is a very small tapeworm (4–6 mm) and usually has three segments, the terminal gravid segment being very long in comparison to the rest of the tapeworm. The uterus is sac-like, long and tubular in shape. The metacestode has a polycystic structure.

Echinococcus oligarthus

Description: *Echinococcus oligarthus* is an extremely small tapeworm (2.5–3 mm) and usually has three segments. The uterus is sac-like, long and tubular in shape. The metacestode has a polycystic structure.

FAMILY ANOPLOCEPHALIDAE

These are essentially tapeworms of horses (*Anoplocephala*, *Paranoplocephala*) and ruminants (*Moniezia*, *Stilesia*, *Thysanosoma*, *Thysaniezia* and *Avitellina*) (Table 1.59). Species of *Cittotaenia* are found in lagomorphs. The scolex has neither rostellum nor hooks and the gravid segments are wider than they are long. The intermediate stage is a cysticercoid present in forage mites of the family Oribatidae.

Life cycle: Mature segments are passed in the faeces and disintegrate, releasing the eggs. These are ingested by forage mites in which they develop to the cysticercoid stage in 2–4 months. The adult tapeworms are found in the intestine of horses 1–2 months after the ingestion of infected mites in the herbage.

Anoplocephala

Cestodes of this genus infect the gut of horses, donkeys and other equids, and are transmitted by Oribatidae mites.

Anoplocephala perfoliata

Description: Adult tapeworms measure 4–8 cm in length and 1.2 cm in width. There is a small rounded scolex, 2–3 mm in diameter, with a pair of 'lappets' just behind the four suckers, but there is neither rostellum nor hooks. It has a very short neck and the strobila widens rapidly, individual proglottids being much wider than they are long and containing only a single set of reproductive organs. The large gravid uterus is lobed and shaped like a sac. Eggs are irregularly spherical or triangular, 65–80 μm in diameter, and contain a hexacanth embryo. They have a thin smooth multilayered shell. The oncosphere is supported by a pair of chitinous projections, the pyriform apparatus. Gravid proglottids release the eggs as they disintegrate. Oncospheres can survive for 6–9 months in the environment unless they are frozen.

Anoplocephala magna

Description: *Anoplocephala magna* is similar morphologically to *A. perfoliata* but much longer, up to 80 cm long by 2.5 cm wide, and is similar to a broad ribbon. The scolex is large, 4–6 mm wide, with suckers opening anteriorly, and there are no lappets on the scolex. The neck is short, as are the segments. The genital organs are single and the pores are unilateral. Eggs are similar to those of *A. perfoliata* but slightly smaller and rounder, measuring 50–60 μm.

Paranoplocephala

Cestodes of this genus infect the small intestine of horses and donkeys (*Paranoplocephala mamillana*), and rabbits (*Paranoplocephala cunniculi*), and are transmitted by Oribatidae mites.

Table 1.59 Tapeworms of ruminants.

Tapeworm	Description
Moniezia	Long, wide tapeworms up to 600 cm long. Segments broader than long with two sets of genital organs
M. expansa	Row of interproglottid glands along whole breadth of posterior border
M. benedeni	Interproglottid glands confined to short row close to the middle of the posterior margin
Thysanosoma actinoides	Short tapeworms up to 30 cm long. Segments short and fringed posteriorly containing two sets of genital organs
Thysaniezia ovilla	Long tapeworms up to 200 cm long. Segments wider than long with single genital pore alternating irregularly
Stilesia globipunctata	Short thin tapeworms up to 60 cm long. Single genital pore alternating irregularly. Two distinct set of testes present
Avitellina centripunctata	Long thin tapeworms up to 300 cm in length. Segments wider than long and indistinct except for last few. Single genital pore alternating irregularly

Source: Drawings reproduced from Ransom (1911) and Soulsby (1971). Reproduced with permission from Lord Soulsby of Swaffham Prior.

Paranoplocephala mamillana

Synonym: *Anoplocephaloides mamillana*

Description: *Paranoplocephala mamillana* is only 10–50 mm long by 4–6 mm wide and is often referred to as the Equine 'dwarf tapeworm'. There are no lappets on the narrow scolex and the suckers are slit-like and located ventrally and dorsally. The scolex is large and without rostellum and hooks. The gravid segments are wider than they are long. Eggs are irregularly spherical or triangular and measure 51 by 37 μm in diameter.

Life cycle: Mature proglottids or eggs are passed in the faeces and on to pasture where the oncospheres are ingested by forage mites. The oncospheres are only infective for mites for about three months. The embryos migrate into the body cavity of the mite where they develop to cysticercoids in 1–4 months and infection of the final host is by ingestion of infected mites during grazing. The prepatent period is approximately six weeks but the adult worms appear to be short-lived, patent infections persisting for only about three months.

Moniezia

Cestodes of this genus infect the small intestine of sheep, goats, cattle and buffalo, and are transmitted by Oribatidae mites.

Moniezia expansa

Description: These are long tapeworms, up to 2 m or more, which possess unarmed scolices and have four prominent suckers (Fig. 1.126). Segments are broader than they are long (up to 1.5 cm wide) and contain two sets of genital organs grossly visible along the lateral margin of each segment (Fig. 1.127; see also Table 1.59). There is a row of interproglottid glands extending along the whole breadth of the posterior border of each segment, which may be used in species differentiation. In *M. expansa* they extend along the full breadth of the segment; in *Moniezia benedeni* they occupy only the midzone of the segment. The irregularly triangular-shaped eggs have a well-defined pyriform apparatus and vary from about 50 to 67 μm in diameter (see Fig. 4.4). See **life cycle 25**.

Moniezia benedeni

Description: Grossly similar to *M. expansa*. Segments are broader than they are long (up to 2.5 cm wide). There is a row of interproglottid glands at the posterior border of each segment, which may be used in species differentiation; in *M. benedeni* they are confined to a short row close to the middle of the segment (see Table 1.59). The medium-sized irregularly quadrangular eggs have a well-defined pyriform apparatus and vary from 80 to 90 μm in diameter. The egg has a thick smooth shell and contains an embryo.

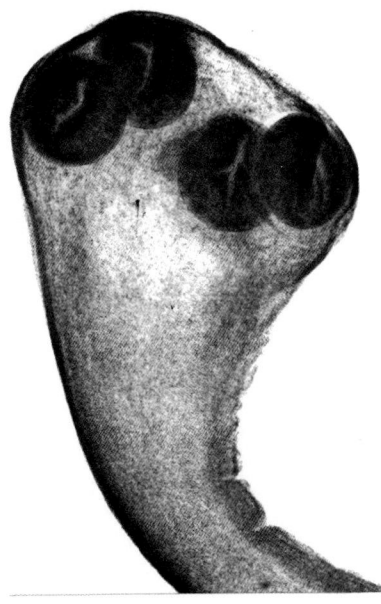

Fig. 1.126 Scolex of *Moniezia expansa* with four prominent suckers.

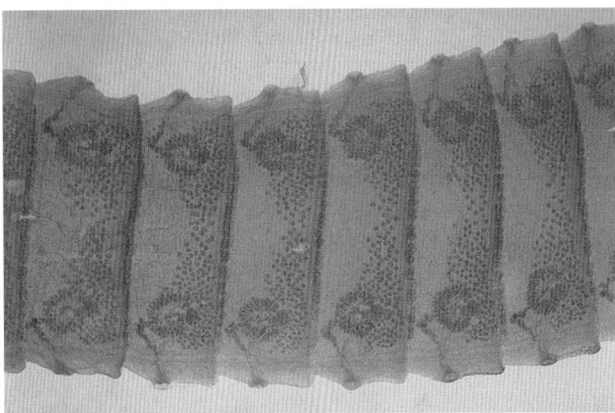

Fig. 1.127 Proglottids of *Moniezia expansa* containing two sets of genital organs. (Courtesy of Aránzazu Meana).

Thysanosoma

The main species is *Thysanosoma actinoides* which infects the small intestine, bile and pancreatic ducts of sheep, cattle and deer. This parasite has oribatid mites (*Galuma*, *Scheloribates*) and psocids (bark lice, dust lice) as intermediate hosts.

Thysanosoma actinoides

Description: The adult 'fringed' tapeworms measure 15–30 cm in length by 8 mm in width. The scolex is up to 1.5 mm in breadth; segments are short and fringed posteriorly. In the distal regions of the tapeworm, the 'fringes' are as long as the proglottid (Fig. 1.128; see also Table 1.59). Each proglottid contains two sets of genital organs with the testes lying medially. Several parauterine organs are present in each proglottid and the oval eggs (measuring about 27 × 18 μm) have no pyriform apparatus.

Life cycle: Mature segments are passed in the faeces of the infected host onto pasture, where forage mites ingest the oncospheres. Cysticercoids develop within the oribatid intermediate hosts and infection of the final host is by ingestion of infected mites during grazing.

Thysaniezia

The main species is *Thysaniezia ovilla* (syn. *Thysaniezia giardia*, *Helictometra giardi*) which infects the small intestine of cattle, sheep, goats, camels, wild ruminants and occasionally pigs. This parasite has oribatid mites (*Galuma*, *Scheloribates*) and psocids (bark lice, dust lice) as intermediate hosts.

Thysaniezia ovilla

Synonyms: *Thysaniezia giardia*, *Helictometra giardi*

Description: Adults reach 200 cm in length, varying in width up to 12 mm. The scolex is small, measuring up to 1 mm in diameter. Segments are short, bulge outwards, giving the margin of the worm an irregular appearance, and contain a single set of genital organs, rarely two, with genital pores alternating irregularly (see Table 1.59).

LIFE CYCLE 25. LIFE CYCLE OF *MONIEZIA EXPANSA* AND *MONIEZIA BENEDENI*

Moniezia parasites live in the intestine of ruminants (1) and gravid proglottids are eliminated with the faeces. *Moniezia expansa* is characterised by groups of interproglottid glands that localise along the entire posterior length of each proglottid (2). The egg of *M. expansa* is hexagonal in shape, and the oncosphere is enclosed within a pear-shaped apparatus (3). In *Moniezia benedeni*, the interproglottid glands localise to the centre of the posterior side of each proglottid (4) and the eggs are rhomboid in shape (5). In the external environment, the oncospheres resume their development once ingested by oribatid mites (intermediate hosts) (6). Inside these hosts, within 1-4 months, the oncospheres develop into cysticercoid larvae (7). The life cycle is complete when infected mites are ingested by ruminant hosts (8). In these hosts, the cysticercoids develop into adult tapeworms (1) after ~6 weeks.

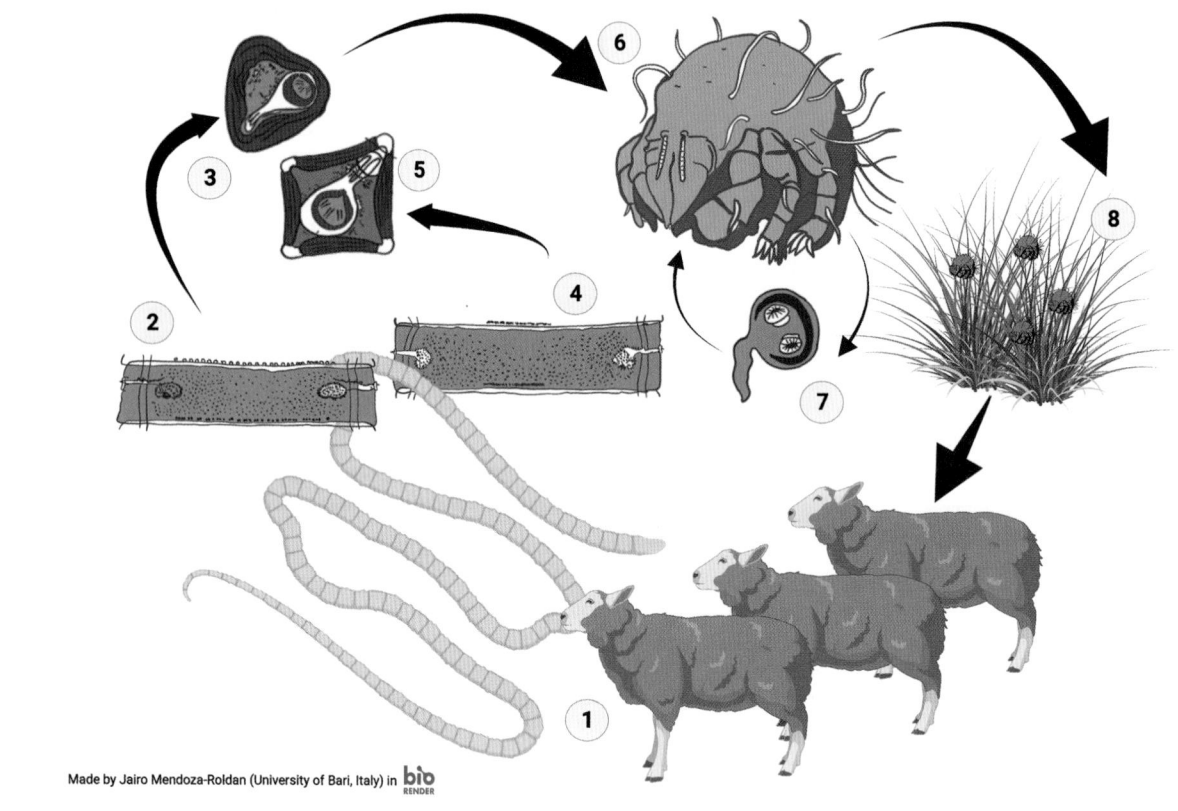

Made by Jairo Mendoza-Roldan (University of Bari, Italy) in **bio**RENDER

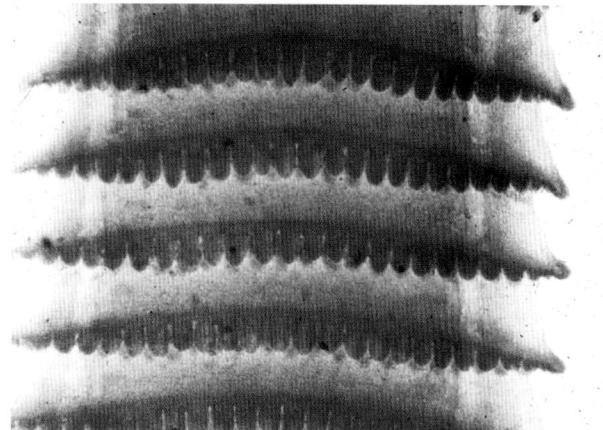

Fig. 1.128 *Thysanosoma actinoides* showing 'fringed' proglottids.

The oval eggs (measuring up to 27 by 19 μm) have no pyriform apparatus and have a thick grey shell and a protuberance at one end. They are found in groups of 10–15 in the numerous elongated parauterine organs (100 μm long) in each proglottid.

Life cycle: Mature segments are passed in the faeces of the infected host onto pasture, where forage mites ingest the oncospheres. Cysticercoids develop within the oribatid intermediate hosts and infection of the final host is by ingestion of infected mites during grazing.

Stilesia

Cestodes of this genus infect the guts and liver of several ruminants (Table 1.60).

Table 1.60 *Stilesia* species.

Species	Hosts	Site	Intermediate hosts
Stilesia globipunctata	Sheep, goats, cattle, other ruminants	Small intestine	Oribatid mites and psocid lice
Stilesia hepatica	Sheep, goats, cattle, wild ruminants	Liver, bile ducts	Oribatid mites?
Stilesia vittata	Camels	Small intestine	Oribatid mites?

Stilesia globipunctata

Description: Adults measure 45–60 cm in length by 3–4 mm in width. The narrow scolex has four large suckers but no hooks. Strobila is broader than long. A single set of genital organs is present and genital pores alternate irregularly (see Table 1.59). Two distinct sets of testes are present in each segment, one on each side, but no testes in the median line. Eggs lack a pyriform apparatus and measure around 27 by 15 µm. See **life cycle 26.**

Stilesia hepatica

Description: The adult tapeworm measures 20–50 cm in length and 2–3 mm in width. The neck is narrow and the scolex is large with prominent suckers. The genital organs are single and the opening pores alternate irregularly. There are 10–12 testes on either side lying dorsal to the ventral canal. The proglottids are short. The oval eggs lack a pyriform apparatus and measure about 26–30 by 16–19 µm.

Life cycle: The life cycle is not known but probably involves oribatid mites.

Stilesia vittata

Description: Adults are 18–23 cm long. Mature proglottids contain 5–7 testes lying lateral to the ventral canal.

Avitellina

Species of this genus occur in the small intestine of ruminants in parts of Africa, Europe and India (Table 1.61).

Life cycle: The life cycle is similar to that of *Moniezia.*

Avitellina centripunctata

Synonym: *Avitellina woodlandi*

LIFE CYCLE 26. LIFE CYCLE OF *STILESIA HEPATICA* AND *STILESIA GLOBIPUNCTATA*

Stilesia globipunctata and *Stilesia hepatica* are harmless cestodes (up to 50 cm in length) that, in the adult stage (1), live in the small intestine (2) and the biliary ducts (3), respectively, of small ruminants (definitive hosts). The proglottids are wider than long and feature irregularly distributed genital pores. The ovoid-shaped eggs contain an oncosphere with a pear-shaped apparatus (4). Once excreted into the environment with the host's faeces, the eggs are ingested by coprophagic oribatid mites (*Scheloribates* spp., 5), which act as intermediate hosts. Inside the mite, the oncosphere develops into a cysticercoid (6). Small ruminants become infected while grazing on pastures contaminated with mites containing the cysticercoids (7); once in the small intestine of the definitive host (8), the cysticercoids evaginate and develop to adult tapeworms (1).

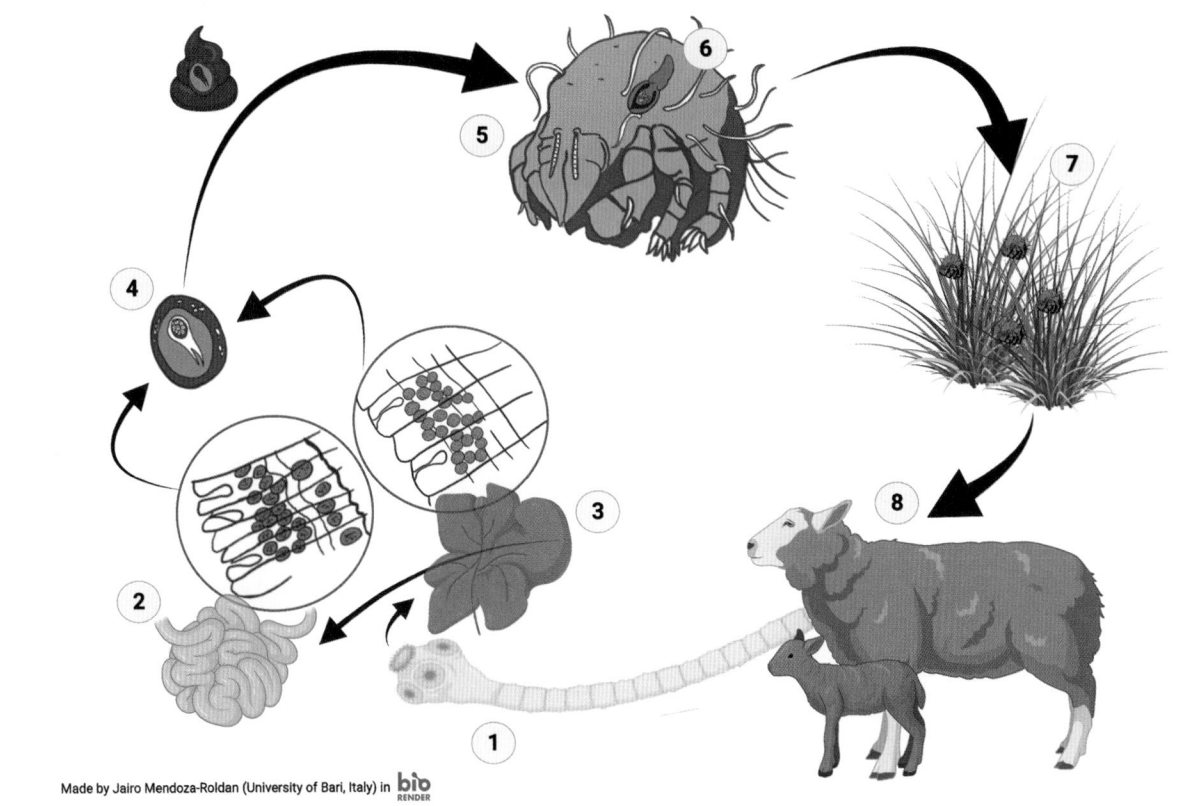

Made by Jairo Mendoza-Roldan (University of Bari, Italy) in bio RENDER

Table 1.61 *Avitellina* species.

Species	Hosts	Site	Intermediate hosts
Avitellina centripunctata (syn. *Avitellina woodlandi*)	Sheep, goats, camels and other ruminants	Small intestine	Oribatid mites or psocid lice
Avitellina goughi	Sheep	Small intestine	Oribatid mites or psocid lice
Avitellina chalmersi	Sheep	Small intestine	Oribatid mites or psocid lice
Avitellina tatia	Goats	Small intestine	Oribatid mites or psocid lice

Description: This tapeworm resembles *Moniezia* on gross inspection except that the segmentation is so poorly marked that it appears somewhat ribbon-like. It can reach 3 m in length and about 3–4 mm in width and the posterior end is almost cylindrical in appearance. Proglottids are short with indistinct segmentation and single genitalia present with the pores alternating irregularly (see Table 1.59). Eggs lack a pyriform apparatus and measure around 20–45 μm. They are contained in capsules in a single parauterine organ in each proglottid.

Cittotaenia

Parasites of this genus are found in rabbits and hares (Table 1.62).

Life cycle: Mature proglottids or eggs are passed in the faeces and onto pasture where the oncospheres are ingested by forage mites. The embryos migrate into the body cavity of the mite where they develop to cysticercoids. Infection of the final host is by ingestion of infected mites during grazing.

Cittotaenia ctenoides

Description: Mature tapeworms grow up to 80 cm long and 1 cm wide. The scolex is about 0.5 mm wide and bears a short neck. The proglottids are much wider than they are long and each contains two sets of genital organs containing 60–80 testes behind an ovary on each side.

Cittotaenia denticulata

Description: Differs from *C. ctenoides* by having a wider scolex (0.8 mm) and no neck.

Cittotaenia pectinata

Description: Very similar to *C. ctenoides* but with a smaller scolex (0.25 mm) but also bears a short neck.

Table 1.62 *Cittotaenia* species.

Species	Hosts	Site	Intermediate hosts
Cittotaenia ctenoides	Rabbits	Small intestine	Oribatid mites
Cittotaenia denticulata	Rabbits	Small intestine	Oribatid mites
Cittotaenia pectinata	Rabbits, hares	Small intestine	Oribatid mites

FAMILY DIPYLIDIIDAE

These are small to medium-sized tapeworms of the dog and cat (*Dipylidium, Diplopylidium, Joyeuxiella*). The scolex usually has an armed rostellum with several rows of hooks. The suckers may also possess fine hooks. The gravid uterus is retained as a transverse sac. The intermediate stage is a cysticercoid.

Dipylidium

This is the most common tapeworm genus of the domestic dog and cat. *Dipylidium* is a much shorter tapeworm than *Taenia*, the maximum length being about 50 cm.

Life cycle: The newly passed segments are active, and can crawl about on the tail region of the animal. The oncospheres are contained in egg packets or capsules, each with about 20 eggs, and these are either expelled by the active segment or released by its disintegration. After ingestion by the intermediate host, the oncospheres travel to the abdominal cavity where they develop into cysticercoids. All stages of the biting louse can ingest oncospheres but the adult flea, with its mouthparts adapted for piercing, cannot do so and infection is only acquired during the larval stage, which has chewing mouthparts. Development in the louse, which is permanently parasitic and therefore enjoys a warm habitat, takes about 30 days but in the flea larva and the developing adult in the cocoon, both of which are on the ground, development may extend over several months. The final host is infected by ingestion of the flea or louse containing the cysticercoids, usually while grooming. Development to patency, when the first gravid segments are shed, takes about three weeks. The main species is *Dipylidium caninum* which infects the small intestine of dogs, foxes, cats and rarely humans. This parasite has fleas (*Ctenocephalides* spp., *Pulex irritans*) and lice (*Trichodectes canis*) as intermediate hosts. See **life cycle 27**.

Dipylidium caninum

Description: *Dipylidium* is a much shorter tapeworm than *Taenia*, the maximum length being about 50 cm. The scolex has four suckers and a protrusible retractable rostellum, which is armed with four or five rows of small rose thorn-shaped hooks (Fig. 1.129). The proglottid is easily recognised, being elongate, like a large rice grain or cucumber seed, and has two sets of genital organs, with a pore opening on each margin (Fig. 1.130). Eggs are yellowish-brown in colour and almost spherical. They contain a hexacanth embryo and measure about 25–50 μm and are contained in an egg capsule (about 120–200 μm), which may hold up to 30 eggs (Fig. 1.131; see also Fig. 4.7).

Amoebotaenia

Small tapeworms found in the duodenum of chickens, with earthworms as intermediate hosts.

Life cycle: See *Raillietina cesticillus*. The prepatent period is around 4–5 weeks. The main species is *Amoebotaenia sphenoides* (syn. *Amoebotaenia cuneata*) which infects the small intestine of chickens. This parasite has earthworms as intermediate hosts.

LIFE CYCLE 27. LIFE CYCLE OF *DIPYLIDIUM CANINUM*

Dipylidium caninum is a hooked cestode (1), up to 90 cm in length, that lives in the small intestine of companion animals (dogs and cats) (2), which act as definitive hosts. The gravid proglottids containing egg capsules detach from the strobila (3) and are eliminated with the faeces. Once in the environment, the external wall of the proglottid disintegrates, thus releasing eggs (4) contained in egg capsules (5); these are ingested by flea larvae (6), in which development of cysticercoids takes place. The development of the cysticercoids (7,

8) occurs simultaneously to that of the flea, and terminates once the flea has reached the adult stage. The definitive hosts become infected by ingesting fleas containing the cysticercoids (9); in the small intestine of these hosts, the cysticercoids mature to adult tapeworms that attach to the intestinal mucosa via the rostellum and suckers (1). Some species of lice can also act as intermediate hosts. Humans, and children in particular, may acquire the infection by ingesting fleas or lice containing the cysticercoids.

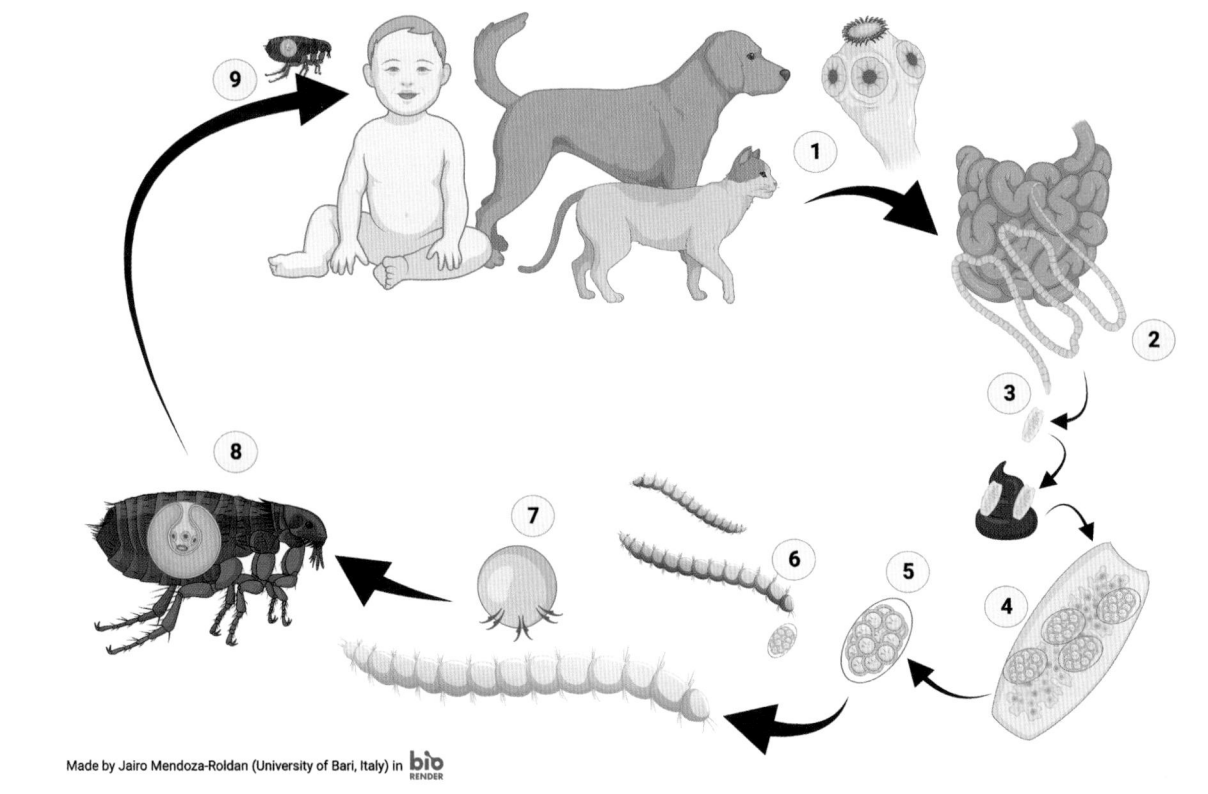

Made by Jairo Mendoza-Roldan (University of Bari, Italy) in **bio** RENDER

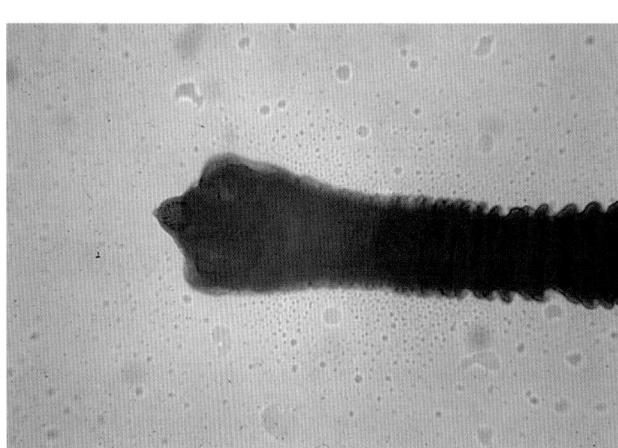

Fig. 1.129 Scolex of *Dipylidium caninum* with four suckers and protrusible rostellum.

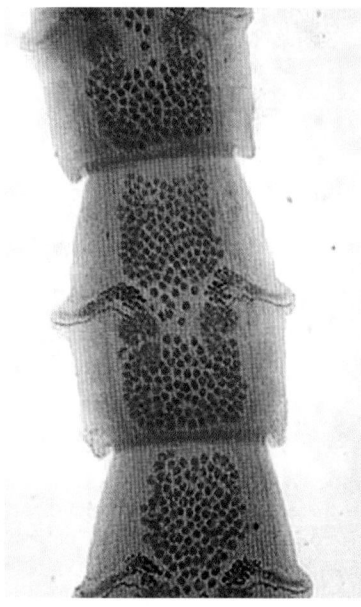

Fig. 1.130 Proglottids of *Dipylidium caninum* with two sets of genital organs.

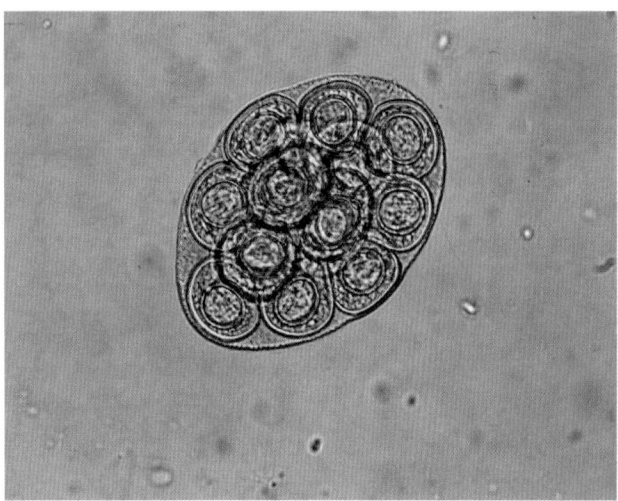

Fig. 1.131 *Dipylidium caninum* egg packet.

FAMILY DILEPIDIDAE

Amoebotaenia sphenoides

Synonym: *Amoebotaenia cuneata*

Description: A very small tapeworm, up to about 4 mm long by 1 mm wide, with up to 20 proglottids, each wider than long. These proglottids are approximately triangular in shape, although the last few segments decrease in size. Its overall appearance is slightly fluke-like. The rostellum bears a single circular row of 12–14 hooks. In the single reproductive organ, the genital pores alternate regularly.

Choanotaenia

These are large robust tapeworms, up to 20 cm in length, found in chickens, turkeys and other gallinaceous birds. The main species is *Choanotaenia infundibulum* which infects the small intestine of chickens, turkeys and gamebirds. This parasite has house fly (*Musca domestica*), beetles (*Aphodius, Calathus, Geotrupes, Tribolium*) and grasshoppers as intermediate hosts.

Choanotaenia infundibulum

Description: A relatively large tapeworm up to 20 cm in length and 1.5–3 mm in width. Each segment is wider posteriorly, giving the margin of the tapeworm a 'saw-edge' appearance. The scolex is triangular, pointed anteriorly with a distinctive rostellum, ringed with about 18 slender hooks. A single set of reproductive organs is present in each proglottid and the genital pores alternate regularly.

Joyeuxiella and Diplopylidium

These two genera contain a couple of species of restricted veterinary importance. In these tapeworms, the genital apertures are sited anterior to the middle of the proglottid. Each egg capsule contains only one egg. *Joyeuxiella pasquale* has been found in the cat and the dog in Africa, the Middle East and Australia. It is very similar to

Dipylidium. It requires two intermediate hosts: first, various beetles and second, a lizard or small mammals. *Diplopylidium nolleri* and *D. trinchesi* occur in the cat and dog in the Middle East. Two intermediate hosts are involved: first, various beetles and second, a reptile or small mammal.

FAMILY PARUTERINIDAE

Members of this family, which are parasites of birds, are closely related to the Dilepididae but possess a parauterine organ.

Metroliasthes

The main species is *Metroliasthes lucida* (syn. *Hexaparuterins lucida*) which infects the small intestine of turkeys and chickens. This parasite has grasshoppers (*Chorthippus, Paroxya, Melanopus*) as intermediate hosts.

Metroliasthes lucida

Synonym: *Hexaparuterins lucida*

Description: The tapeworm is about 20 cm long and 1.5–2 mm wide. The scolex has no rostellum or hooks and the suckers are devoid of spines. The single genital pores are irregularly alternating and can be prominent. Each gravid proglottid possesses a single parauterine organ containing one egg.

FAMILY DAVAINEIDAE

These are mainly parasites of birds (*Davainea, Raillietina, Cotugnia, Houttuynia*). These tapeworms usually have rows of hooks on both rostellum and suckers. Egg capsules replace the uterus in this family. The intermediate stage is a cysticercoid.

Davainea

This genus contains *Davainea proglottina*, the most pathogenic cestode of poultry.

Life cycle: Gravid proglottids are shed in faeces and eggs are ingested by various gastropod molluscs, in which they develop to the cysticercoid stage after about three weeks. Following ingestion of the mollusc by the final host, the cysticercoids develop into adult tapeworms in about two weeks. The main species is *Davainea proglottina* which infects the small intestine of turkeys, chickens, pigeons and other gallinaceous birds. This parasite has slugs (*Agriolimax, Arion, Cepaea* and *Limax*) and land snails as intermediate hosts.

Davainea proglottina

Description: *Davainea proglottina* is an extremely small cestode up to 1–4 mm long, and usually possesses only 4–9 segments (Fig. 1.132). The rostellum bears 80–94 hooks, arranged in a double

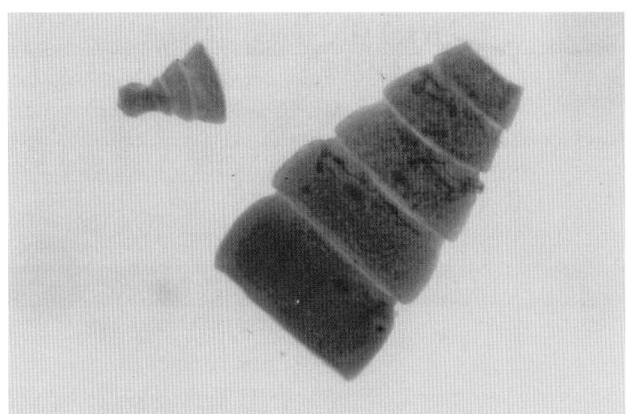

Fig. 1.132 *Davainea proglottina*: scolex and proglottids.

row, and the suckers bear a few rows of small hooks. Each segment contains a single set of reproductive organs. The genital pores alternate regularly. Eggs are spherical and measure about 30–40 µm and are found singly within the parenchymatous capsules in the gravid segment.

Raillietina

Species of this genus are found in the small intestine of chickens and turkeys and other fowl with the cysticercoid intermediate stage, depending on the species, in ants or beetles (Table 1.63).

Life cycle: Gravid proglottids are passed in faeces and eggs are ingested by various intermediate hosts. The embryo hatches from the egg in the intestine and then changes into a cysticercoid in the body cavity. Following ingestion by the final host, the activated cysticercoid attaches to the mucosa of the anterior or mid small intestine. The prepatent period is around 2–3 weeks.

Raillietina cesticillus

Description: A small tapeworm that can reach around 10–14 cm in length, but is often much shorter at about 4–5 cm long. The broad scolex is large and the rostellum wide. The unarmed suckers are not prominent and the rostellum is armed with several hundred small hammer-shaped hooks arranged in a double row. The gravid proglottids contain several thin-walled egg capsules, each housing a

Table 1.63 *Raillietina* species.

Species	Hosts	Site	Intermediate hosts
Raillietina cesticillus (syn. *Skrjabinia cesticillus*)	Chickens, turkeys, guinea fowl	Small intestine	Various genera of beetles, cockroaches, *Musca domestica*
Raillietina echinobothrida	Chickens, turkeys	Small intestine	Ants of the genera *Pheidole* and *Tetramorium*
Raillietina tetragona	Chickens, guinea fowl, peafowl and pigeons	Small intestine	Houseflies (*Musca domestica*) and ants of the genera *Pheidole*, *Tetramorium* and *Onthophagus*
Raillietina georgiensis	Turkeys	Small intestine	Ants of the genera *Pheidole* and *Tetramorium*

single egg. Eggs are spherical to slightly ellipsoidal and measure approximately 75 by 90 µm. They have a thick smooth shell and contain a hexacanth embryo (see Fig. 4.8). Eggs are shed only after the gravid proglottid or the egg capsule disintegrates.

Raillietina echinobothrida

Description: *Raillietina echinobothrida*, which may be up to 25 cm in length, is similar in shape to *R. tetragona*. The suckers are circular and armed with several rows of small hooklets and the rostellum is well endowed with two rows of around 200 hooks (these features distinguish it from *R. tetragona*). A 'neck' is absent behind the scolex. The gravid proglottids contain multiple fibrous-walled egg capsules, each housing several eggs (around 6–12). Eggs are identical to those of *R. cesticillus* and measure approximately 75 by 95 µm.

Raillietina tetragona

Description: Often the largest tapeworm of fowl, reaching around 20–25 cm in length. The scolex is smaller than that of *R. echinobothrida* and the 'neck' is quite prominent. The oval suckers are lightly armed with several rows of fine hooklets and the rostellum bears one or sometimes two rows of around 100 hooks. The gravid proglottids contain multiple fibrous-walled egg capsules, each housing many eggs (about 8–14). Eggs measure approximately 50 by 25 µm. *Raillietina tetragona* has a larger number of egg capsules in the gravid proglottid than either *R. cesticillus* or *R. echinobothrida*.

Raillietina georgiensis

Description: The length of this tapeworm is around 15–35 cm. The rostellum is covered with about 100 hooks.

Cotugnia

Parasites of this genus infect the small intestine of birds (Table 1.64).

Cotugnia digonopora

Description: The tapeworm is up to 10 cm long. The head is large with a small rudimentary retractile rostellum, which is armed with two rows of small hooklets. The suckers are large and unarmed and the proglottids are wider than long. Segments possess a double set of genital organs.

Life cycle: The life cycle is unknown but is thought to involve ants or beetles.

Table 1.64 *Cotugnia* species.

Species	Hosts	Site	Intermediate hosts
Cotugnia digonopora	Chickens	Small intestine	Ants, beetles?
Cotugnia fastigata	Ducks, geese	Small intestine	Unknown
Cotugnia cuneata	Pigeons	Small intestine	Unknown

Houttuynia

The main species is *Houttuynia struthionis* which infects the small intestine of ostriches and rheas. The intermediate hosts of this parasite are unknown.

Houttuynia struthionis

Description: These are large, long, flat, white segmented tapeworms (60–120 cm long by 9 mm wide). The scolex is 1–2 mm wide and bears a double row of about 160 large and small hooks. The eggs are contained within parenchymatous capsules in the gravid proglottid. There are around 15–25 eggs in each capsule. Genital pores are unilateral.

Life cycle: The life cycle is unknown.

FAMILY HYMENOLEPIDIDAE

These small to medium-sized parasites are of minor veterinary importance. Members of this family, which have a characteristically slender strobila with a conical rostellum, infect birds, humans and rodents (*Hymenolepis*, *Rodentolepis*, *Fimbriaria*). The intermediate stage is a cysticercoid present in an arthropod host.

Hymenolepis

This genus contains a large number of species that are usually narrow and thread-like in appearance with three testes in each segment (Table 1.65).

Hymenolepis cantaniana

Synonym: *Stephylepis cantaniana*

Description: A slender tapeworm, reaching a length of up to 2 cm. The rostellum is rudimentary and the suckers are unarmed.

Table 1.65 *Hymenolepis* species.

Species	Hosts	Site	Intermediate hosts
Hymenolepis cantaniana (syn. *Stephylepis cantaniana*)	Chickens, turkeys, pheasants, quails and other fowl	Small intestine	Beetles (Scarabeidae)
Hymenolepis carioca (syn. *Echinolepis carioca*) Small intestine	Chickens, turkeys and other fowl	Small intestine	Dung and flour beetles; occasionally *Stomoxys* spp.
Hymenolepis lanceolata (syn. *Drepanidotaenia lanceolatum*)	Ducks, geese	Small intestine	Freshwater crustaceans (copepods)
Hymenolepis nana (syn. *Rodentolepis nana*, *Rodentolepis fraterna*, *Vampirolepis nana*)	Rats, mice, humans	Small intestine	Flour beetles (*Tenebrio*) or fleas
Hymenolepis diminuta (syn. *Rodentolepis diminuta*)	Rats, mice, humans	Small intestine	Moths, cockroaches, fleas, beetles, millipedes

Hymenolepis carioca

Synonym: *Echinolepis carioca*

Description: This is a slender thread-like tapeworm reaching a length of up to 8 cm. The scolex is unarmed. The proglottids number 500–1100 and are broader than they are long.

Hymenolepis lanceolata

Synonym: *Drepanidotaenia lanceolatum*

Description: A slender tapeworm reaching up to 15–20 cm in length. The proglottids are much wider than they are long.

Hymenolepis nana

Synonyms: *Rodentolepis nana*, *Rodentolepis fraterna*, *Vampirolepis nana*

Description: The tapeworm is small, 2.5–4 cm in length, and has a characteristically slender strobila with about 200 segments. The scolex has four suckers and is armed with a retractable rostellum bearing a single row of 20–30 hooks. The genitalia are single and the segments are wider than they are long. Eggs are small, round or oval in shape and measure 44–62 by 30–55 µm. They are colourless with a smooth shell and contain a lemon-shaped embryophore with protruding polar plugs that bear long fine undulated filaments. The embryo has three pairs of small hooks.

Life cycle: The life cycle can be direct, the cysticercoids developing in the villi of the small intestine of the final host and then emerging to develop to the adult tapeworm in the intestinal lumen. Otherwise, flour beetles or fleas can serve as intermediate hosts.

Hymenolepis diminuta

Synonym: *Rodentolepis diminuta*

Description: A small tapeworm, about 20–60 mm in length. The rostellum does not possess hooks. The eggs are larger than those of *R. nana*, measuring about 60 µm, and the outer membrane is darker and may be striated.

Fimbriaria

The main species is *Fimbriaria fasciolaris* which infects the small intestine of chickens, ducks, geese and wild anseriform birds. This parasite has copepods (*Cyclops* spp. and *Diaptomus* spp.) as intermediate hosts.

Fimbriaria fasciolaris

Description: This is not a common cestode. The adult tapeworms vary in length from 2.5 cm up to about 40 cm. The scolex is small with 10 hooks but the anterior part of the body possesses a 'pseudoscolex' (a folded body expansion) for attachment to the host. The presence of this expansion aids diagnosis. The uterus is a continuous tube which separates into small tubules in the posterior of the worm. These tubules contain eggs which retain the outer spindle-shaped shell and they contain the oval embryophores. The genital pores are unilateral with three testes to each set of genital organs.

FAMILY MESOCESTOIDIDAE

Also of minor veterinary importance, these cestodes of carnivorous animals and birds have two metacestode stages. The first is a cysticercoid in an insect or mite, and the second a solid larval form, a tetrathyridium, in a vertebrate. Genera include *Mesocestoides* found in dogs, cats and wild mammals, and *Dithyridium* in chickens, turkeys and wild birds.

Mesocestoides

Adult tapeworms are found in the small intestine of dogs, cats and wild carnivores. The second intermediate stages (tetrathyridia) occur in the peritoneal and pleural cavities or subcutaneous tissue of a wide variety of vertebrate hosts (*Dithyridium*, *Tetrathyridium*).

Life cycle: The life cycle requires two intermediate hosts. A cysticercoid is produced in the first intermediate host which, when eaten by the second intermediate host, forms a tetrathyridium; this may remain as an encapsulated form for some time. The tetrathyridium is located in the peritoneal cavity in reptiles and mammals and in the lungs in birds. Dogs and cats can start to shed tapeworm segments in faeces as early as three weeks after infection. The main species is *Mesocestoides lineatus* which infects the small intestine of dogs, cats, foxes, mink, wild carnivores and occasionally humans. This parasite has oribatid mites (cysticercoid), coprophagus beetles, birds, amphibians, reptiles and mammals (tetrathyridium) as intermediate hosts.

Mesocestoides lineatus

Synonyms: *Dithyridium variable*, *Tetrathyridium bailetti*, *Tetrathyridium elongatum*

Description: The adult tapeworm ranges from 30 to 250 cm in length and up to 3 mm wide. The scolex is large, unarmed and without a rostellum, and the four suckers are elongate and oval. The strobila is thin and narrow, up to 1.5 cm in length. Mature segments are longer than wide and each contains a single set of central reproductive organs, the central genital pore opening on the dorsal surface (Fig. 1.133). The ovary and vitelline glands are bilobed and there are numerous testes. Oncospheres in gravid segments progress from the uterus into a parauterine organ. Eggs accumulate in the parauterine organ as the segments mature. The eggs are oval and measure 40–60 by 35–43 μm.

ORDER DIPHYLLOBOTHRIIDEA

The morphology of the Diphyllobothriidea is generally similar to that of the Cyclophyllidea, but there are three distinct features. First, the unarmed scolex has no suckers and instead has two

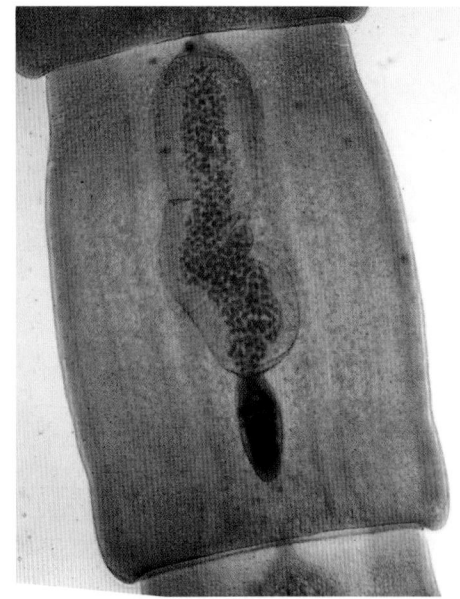

Fig. 1.133 Proglottid of *Mesocestoides lineatus* with a single set of central genital organs opening dorsally.

weakly muscular, shallow longitudinal grooves or **bothria**, which become flattened to form organs of attachment. Second, the proglottids possess a uterine pore that enables eggs to be discharged from a large length of the strobila. The terminal proglottids are not gravid and usually are exhausted and may become detatched in short chains. Third, the eggshell is thick, brownish-yellow and operculate, and the **coracidium**, which emerges after hatching, is an oncosphere with an embryophore which is ciliated for mobility in water.

The pseudophyllidean life cycle utilises two intermediate hosts. The coracidium must first be ingested by a crustacean in whose body cavity a larval procercoid develops. Subsequently, if the crustacean is eaten by a freshwater fish, amphibian or reptile, the procercoid is liberated and in the muscles of the new host develops into a second larval stage, a plerocercoid, which possesses the characteristic scolex; it is only this stage which is infective to the final host.

This order contains only two genera of veterinary importance: *Diphyllobothrium* and *Spirometra*.

FAMILY DIPHYLLOBOTHRIIDAE

Parasites of cetaceans, fish-eating mammals and other vertebrates with well-developed bothria.

Diphyllobothrium

The genus *Diphyllobothrium* is an important cestode of humans and fish-eating mammals, such as dogs, cats, pigs and polar bears. They are long tapeworms with an unarmed scolex, with two muscular bothria.

Life cycle: Eggs are continuously discharged from the genital pores of the attached gravid segments of the strobila and pass to the exterior in the faeces. They resemble *F. hepatica* eggs, being

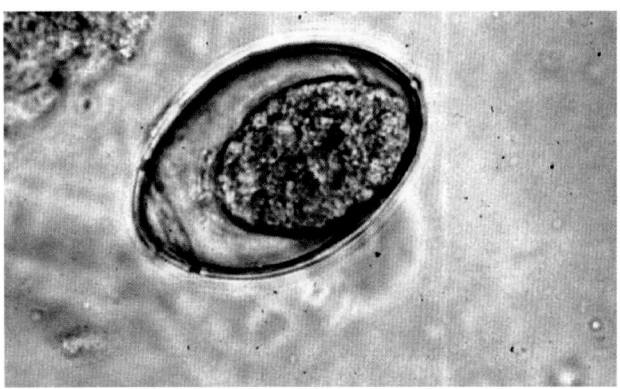

Fig. 1.134 Egg of *Diphyllobothrium latum*.

yellow and operculate, but are approximately half the size (Fig. 1.134). The eggs must develop in water and within a few weeks, each hatches to liberate a motile ciliated coracidium which, if ingested by a copepod, develops into the first parasitic larval stage, a worm-like procercoid. When the copepod is ingested by a freshwater fish, the procercoid migrates to the muscles or viscera to form the second larval stage, the plerocercoid; this solid larval metacestode is about 5 mm long and possesses the characteristic scolex. The life cycle is completed when the infected fish is eaten raw, or insufficiently cooked, by the final host. Development to patency is rapid, occurring within 3–4 weeks of ingestion of the plerocercoid. However, if the infected fish is eaten by a larger fish, the plerocercoid has the ability to establish itself in its new host. See **life cycle 28**.

LIFE CYCLE 28. LIFE CYCLE OF *DIPHYLLOBOTRIUM LATUM*

Adult parasites live in the small intestine of the definitive host (mainly humans and other fish-eating mammals) (1). This long cestode (that may grow to up to 25 m in length) features a chain of large proglottids, each with a central uterus and a lateral opening (tocostoma) from which eggs are released (2). The operculated, non-embryonated eggs are continuously eliminated by the proglottids (3). Once they reach an aquatic environment within the host faeces, the eggs mature and hatch into motile coracidia (4) that, upon ingestion by aquatic copepods (first intermediate hosts, 5) develop and moult (6) to become procercoids (7). When an infected copepod is ingested by freshwater fish (second intermediate host, 8), the procercoids migrate to the muscles or viscera and become plerocercoids (9). The life cycle is complete when raw or undercooked infected fish is ingested by a suitable definitive host (10). In this host, the plerocercoids, already provided with a scolex, develop into adult cestodes. If the second intermediate host (freshwater fish) is ingested by another predatory fish (11), the plerocercoids remain infective in the muscles of the latter, thus allowing completion of the life cycle if this is ingested by a suitable definitive host (1).

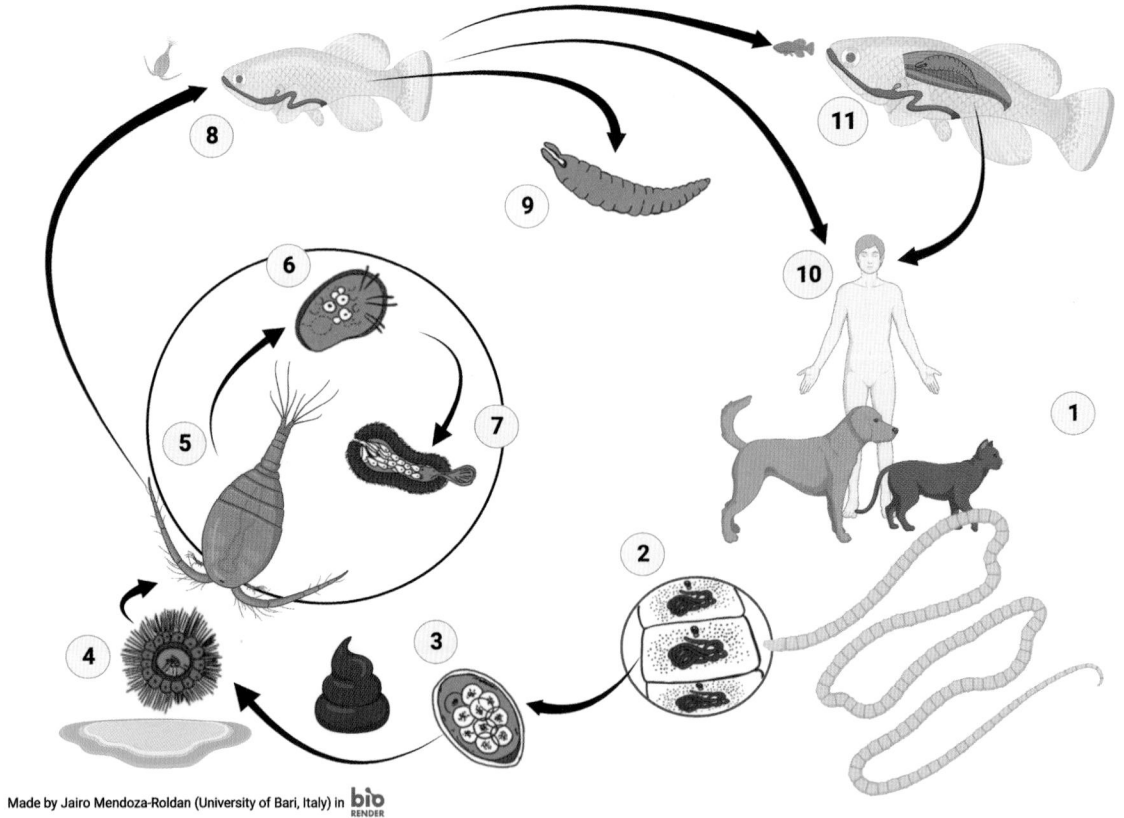

Made by Jairo Mendoza-Roldan (University of Bari, Italy) in **bio**RENDER

Diphyllobothrium latum

Synonym: *Dibothriocephalus latus*

Description: A very long, ivory-coloured tapeworm measuring up to 10–15 m in length or longer, with several hundred, or in some cases a few thousand, proglottids. The scolex is unarmed, with two weak muscular longitudinal grooves or bothria as organs of attachment. Anterior proglottids are broader than long while the mature and gravid segments are rectangular with a central genital pore. The uterus is situated centrally and is rosette-shaped. The mature and gravid segments are rectangular with a central genital pore, being broader than they are long. The reproductive organs are located at the centres of the segments. Eggs are yellowish-light brown, ovoid with rounded poles, operculate and measure around 66–70 by 45–50 μm (Fig. 1.134). Note that eggs of *Spirometra* spp. are very similar but have more pointed poles (Fig. 1.135).

Spirometra

Spirometra are small to medium-sized tapeworms of dogs, cats and wild carnivores and an occasional human zoonosis (sparganosis). A couple of features enable differentiation from the very similar genus *Diphyllobothrium*: the vagina and uterus exit separately onto the ventral surface of the proglottid; and the uterus has a spiral form whereas in *Diphyllobothrium* it has a rosette shape (Table 1.66).

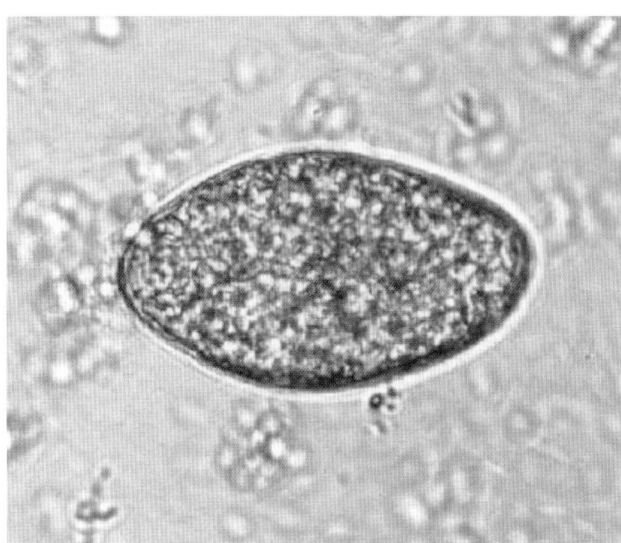

Fig. 1.135 *Spirometra* egg.

Table 1.66 *Spirometra* species.

Species	Hosts	Site	Intermediate hosts
Spirometra mansoni	Dogs, cats, wild carnivores, occasionally humans	Small intestine	Copepods: *Cyclops* spp. (**procercoid**) Amphibians, reptiles, birds (**plerocercoid**)
Spirometra mansonoides (syn. *Diphyllobothrium mansonoides*)	Cats, bobcats, raccoons, occasionally dogs	Small intestine	Crustaceans (**procercoid**) Rats, snakes, mice (**plerocercoid** or **spargana**)
Spirometra erinacei (syn. *Spirometra erinaceieuropaei*)	Cats, dogs, foxes	Small intestine	Crustaceans (**procercoid**) Frogs (**plerocercoid**)

Life cycle: The morphology and life cycle of these tapeworms are similar to those of *D. latum*, the procercoids being found in crustaceans, such as *Cyclops*, and the plerocercoids in a wide variety of hosts. These can also act as paratenic hosts. The plerocercoids can also transfer between intermediate hosts. The prepatent period is around 20–30 days.

Spirometra mansoni

Description: The adult tapeworms are very similar to *Diphyllobothrium*, the scolex being unarmed and possessing two muscular longitudinal slit-like grooves as organs of attachment. Proglottids possess both a uterine and a vaginal pore and the uterus is spiral in shape. The plerocercoids, also called spargana, are white, ribbon-like, crinkled and can measure around 300–400 mm. The operculate eggs have pointed ends and measure on average 65 by 45 μm (Fig. 1.135).

Spirometra mansonoides

Synonym: *Diphyllobothrium mansonoides*

Description: The adult worms are pinkish in color and gravid proglottids have a tightly coiled uterus full of brown eggs.

Spirometra erinacei

Synonym: *Spirometra erinaceieuropaei*

Description: Adult tapeworms can reach 1.5 m in length and possess a finger-like scolex with the bothria fading into the strobila. The proglottids contain a spiral uterus with 2–3 coils and a dumbbell-shaped ovary that is transversely long.

CHAPTER 2
Veterinary protozoology

KINGDOM PROTOZOA

Protozoa are unicellular organisms that are more primitive than animals, and no matter how complex their bodies may be, all the different structures are contained in a single cell.

Protozoa, like most organisms, are **eukaryotic**, in that their genetic information is stored in chromosomes contained in a nuclear envelope. In this way, they differ from bacteria which do not have a nucleus and whose single chromosome is coiled like a skein of wool in the cytoplasm. This primitive arrangement, found only in bacteria, rickettsia and certain algae, is called **prokaryotic** and such organisms may be regarded as neither animal nor plant, but as a separate kingdom of prokaryotic organisms, the Monera.

STRUCTURE AND FUNCTION OF PROTOZOA

Protozoa, like other eukaryotic cells, have a nucleus, an endoplasmic reticulum, mitochondria and a Golgi body and lysosomes. In addition, because they lead an independent existence, they possess a variety of other subcellular structures or organelles with distinct organisational features and functions.

Thus, locomotion in, for example, the genus *Trypanosoma* (Fig. 2.1) is facilitated by a single **flagellum**, and in some other protozoa by several flagella. A flagellum is a contractile fibre arising from a structure called a basal body, which in some species is attached to the body of the protozoan along its length, so that when the flagellum beats, the cell membrane (pellicle) is pulled up to form an **undulating membrane**. Sometimes, also, it projects beyond the protozoan body as a free flagellum. During movement, the shape of these organisms is maintained by microtubules in the pellicle.

Other protozoa, such as *Balantioides* (Fig. 2.2), move by means of **cilia** which are fine short hairs, each arising from a basal body; these cover much of the body surface and beat in unison to effect movement. In such species, a mouth or **cytostome** is present and the ciliary movement is also used to waft food towards this opening.

A third means of locomotion, used by protozoa such as *Entamoeba* (Fig. 2.3), is **pseudopodia**, which are prolongations of cytoplasm. Movement occurs as the rest of the cytoplasm flows into this prolongation. The pseudopodium also possesses a phagocytic capacity and can function as a cup, which closes, enveloping particulate food material in a vacuole.

Finally, some protozoa, such as the extracellular stages of *Eimeria*, have no obvious means of locomotion but are nevertheless capable of gliding movements.

The nutrition of parasitic protozoa usually occurs by pinocytosis or phagocytosis, depending on whether tiny droplets of fluid or small objects of macromolecular dimension are taken into the cell. In both cases, the process is the same, the cell membrane gradually enveloping the droplet or object which has become adherent to its

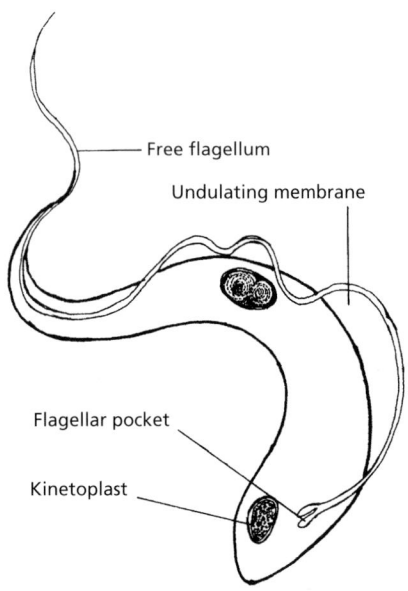

Fig. 2.1 *Trypanosoma brucei* showing the flagellum and undulating membrane.

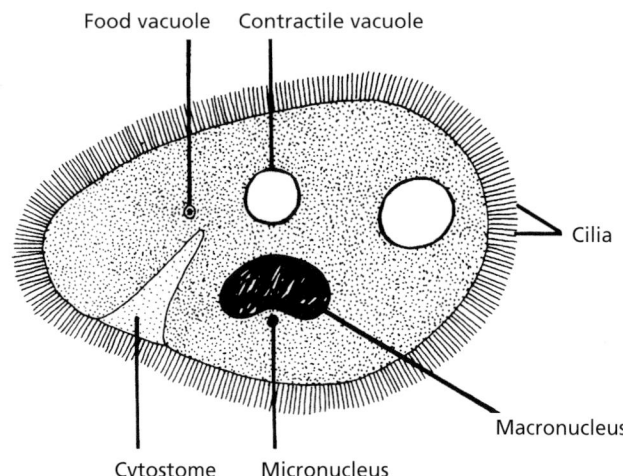

Fig. 2.2 The morphology of the intestinal protozoan *Balantioides*.

Veterinary Parasitology, Fifth Edition. Domenico Otranto and Richard Wall.
© 2024 John Wiley & Sons Ltd. Published 2024 by John Wiley & Sons Ltd.

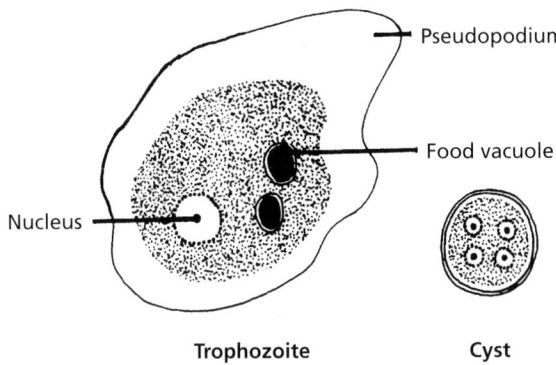

Fig. 2.3 *Entamoeba histolytica* has an amoeboid trophozoite stage and a non-motile cystic stage with four nuclei.

outer surface. When this is complete, the particle is carried into the cell where fusion with lysosomes effects digestion. Finally, undigested material is extruded from the cell. As noted above, some ciliated protozoa and also some stages of the organisms causing malaria obtain food through a cytostome. At the base of the cytostome, the food enters a vacuole for digestion within the cell. Metabolic products are excreted by diffusion through the cell membrane.

The infective stage of some protozoa is called a **sporozoite**, while the term **trophozoite** is applied to that stage of the protozoa in the host, which feeds and grows until division commences. In most protozoa, reproduction is asexual and is accomplished by binary fission or, in the case of *Babesia* within erythrocytes, by budding. Another form of asexual reproduction, which occurs in the Order Eucoccidiorida, is **merogony** (**schizogony**). In this process, the trophozoite grows to a large size while the nucleus divides repeatedly. This structure is called a **meront** (**schizont**) and, when mature, each nucleus has acquired a portion of the cytoplasm so that the meront is filled with a large number of elongated separate organisms called **merozoites**. The meront eventually ruptures, liberating the individual merozoites.

Protozoa that only divide asexually generally have a short generation time, and since they cannot exchange genetic material, rely on mutants to provide the variants necessary for natural selection. However, most Sporozoa at certain stages in their life cycle also have a sexual phase of reproduction, called **gametogony**, which may be followed by a free-living maturation phase, or **sporogony**. Sometimes, as in *Eimeria*, both asexual and sexual phases occur in the same host while in others, such as *Plasmodium*, the asexual phase occurs in the vertebrate host and the sexual phase in the arthropod vector.

Finally, it should be noted that although this section deals with pathogenic protozoa of veterinary importance, there are many other species, particularly in the rumen, which are purely commensal or even symbiotic. These protozoa assist in the digestion of cellulose, and on being passed to the abomasum act as a source of protein for the host.

CLASSIFICATION

Classification of the kingdom Protozoa is extremely complex and undergoing constant revision. The classification given below is intended to give an outline of the basic differences in the structure and life cycles of the main groups.

The most recent classification of the protozoa now recognises 13 phyla. Under the older system of classification, as described in most veterinary textbooks, there were four phyla containing parasites of veterinary interest: Sarcomastigophora (containing Sarcodina and Mastigophora), Apicomplexa, Microspora and Ciliophora. Under the new classification system, there are now nine phyla containing the genera of veterinary importance. The old phylum Microspora has been moved to the kingdom Fungi, as the phylum Microsporidia.

PHYLUM AMOEBOZOA

Members of the phylum Amoebozoa move by means of pseudopods, which are also used for feeding. Their cytoplasm is divided into endoplasm, containing food vacuoles and nucleus, and relatively clear ectoplasm. Reproduction is asexual by binary fission. Only a few species of the Sarcodina are pathogenic.

ORDER ENTAMOEBIDA

FAMILY ENTAMOEBIDAE

Members of this family are parasitic in the digestive tract of vertebrates and invertebrates. Three genera contain parasites of animals and humans (*Entamoeba*, *Iodamoeba*, *Endolimax*) but only *Entamoeba* contains pathogenic species of veterinary significance. Genera are differentiated on the basis of their nuclear structure. The only species known to be pathogenic to mammals is *Entamoeba histolytica*.

Entamoeba

Members of the genus can be divided into distinct types based on the trophozoite and cyst structures and species within the groups are differentiated on the basis of size and hosts infected (Table 2.1). Many species are probably synonymous.

Life cycle: Trophozoites divide by binary fission. Before encysting, the amoebae round up, become smaller and lay down a cyst wall. Amoebae emerge from the cysts and grow into trophozoites.

The genus *Entamoeba* found in humans and animals has been arbitrarily divided into four groups based on trophozoite and cyst structure.

1 Histolytica group (*E. histolytica*, *E. hartmanni*, *E. equi*, *E. anatis*) in which the nucleus has a small central endosome, with a few scattered chromatin granules. Cysts when mature have four nuclei.
2 Coli group (*E. coli*, *E. wenyoni*, *E. muris*, *E. caviae*, *E. cuniculi*, *E. gallinarum*) in which there is a larger and eccentric nucleus with a ring of coarse peripheral granules and scattered chromatin granules between them. Cysts have eight nuclei.
3 Bovis group (*E. bovis*, *E. ovis*, *E. suis*, *E. chattoni*) in which the endosome of the nucleus varies in size and the ring of peripheral granules is fine or coarse. Cysts have one nucleus when mature.
4 Gingivalis group (*E. gingivalis*, *E. equibuccalis*, *E. suigingivalis*) in which the nucleus has a small central endosome and a ring of small peripheral granules. There are no cysts.
5 Others (*E. dedoelsti*, *E. invadens*).

Table 2.1 *Entamoeba* species.

Species	Hosts	Site
Histolytica group		
Entamoeba histolytica (syn. Entamoeba dysenteriae, Endamoeba histolytica)	Humans, apes, monkeys, dogs, cats, pigs, rats	Large intestine, liver, lungs; rarely brain, spleen
Entamoeba hartmanni	Humans, apes, monkeys	Caecum, colon
Entamoeba equi	Horses	Caecum, colon
Entamoeba anatis	Ducks	Caeca
Coli group		
Entamoeba coli (syn. Amoeba coli, Endamoeba hominis, Entamoeba cynocephalusae)	Humans, apes, monkeys, reported in pigs and deer (white-tailed)	Caecum, colon
Entamoeba wenyoni	Goats, camels	Caecum, colon
Entamoeba muris	Rats, mice	Caecum, colon
Entamoeba caviae	Guinea pigs	Caecum
Entamoeba cuniculi	Rabbits	Caecum
Entamoeba gallinarum	Chickens, turkeys, ducks, geese, guinea fowl	Caeca
Bovis group		
Entamoeba bovis	Cattle, deer	Rumen
Entamoba ovis	Sheep, goats	Large intestine
Entamoeba suis	Pigs	Caecum, colon
Entamoeba chattoni	Monkeys, rarely humans	Caecum, colon
Gingivalis group		
Emtamoeba gingivalis (syn. Amoeba gingivalis, Amoeba buccalis, Amoeba dentalis, Entamoeba buccalis, Entamoeba maxillaris, Entamoeba canibuccalis)	Humans, chimpanzees, macaques, baboons	Mouth
Entamoeba equibuccalis	Horses	Mouth
Entamoeba suigingivalis	Pigs	Mouth, teeth
Others		
Entamoeba gedoelsti	Horses	Caecum, colon
Entamoeba invadens	Reptiles	Intestines

Entamoeba histolytica

Description: Two forms of the parasite exist. Trophozoites of the large form are 20–30 μm in diameter, those of the small form are 12–15 μm. The nucleus, when stained, has a small central endosome with a ring of small peripheral granules. The cysts of both forms are 10–12 μm in size and contain four nuclei when mature and often contain rod-like chromatin bodies with rounded ends.

Entamoeba bovis, Entamoeba ovis, Entamoeba suis

Description: Trophozoites vary in size from 5 to 25 μm in diameter. The endosome of the nucleus varies in size with a ring of peripheral granules of varying sizes around its periphery. The cysts are 4–17 μm in diameter and contain a single nucleus when mature. A large glycogen granule may or may not be present.

Entamoeba coli, Entamoeba muris, Entamoeba caviae, Entamoeba cuniculi

Description: The nucleus is large and eccentric and has a ring of coarse peripheral granules with scattered chromatin granules. The cysts have eight nuclei and splinter-like chromatin granules. Glycogen granules, when present, are fairly well defined.

Entamoeba gingivalis, Entamoeba equibuccalis, Entamoeba suigingivalis

Description: Trophozoites vary in size (10–20 μm long) and have no cysts. The nucleus has a small central endosome and a ring of small peripheral granules.

Entamoeba gedoelsti

Description: Trophozoites are 7–13 μm in diameter. The nucleus has an eccentric endosome and a row of relatively coarse chromatin granules around its periphery. Cysts have not been reported.

Entamoeba invadens

Description: Trophozoites are 11–20 μm and cysts approximately 16 μm.

Iodamoeba

A single species is recognised with a large nuclear endosome rich in chromatin surrounded by a layer of globules. The cysts each contain a large glycogen body. It infects the caecum and colon of pigs, humans, apes and monkeys.

Iodamoeba buetschlii

Description: Trophozoites are 4–20 μm with blunt pseudopods that form slowly. The nucleus is large and contains a large nuclear endosome rich in chromatin surrounded by a layer of globules. The cysts are irregular in form, ranging from 5 to 14 μm, and contain a single nucleus and a large glycogen body.

Endolimax

Small amoebae 6–15 μm in diameter with a vesicular nucleus containing a large irregular-shaped endosome composed of chromatin granules (Table 2.2). Mature cysts are generally oval and contain four nuclei.

Table 2.2 *Endolimax* species

Species	Hosts	Site
Endolimax nana (syn. Amoeba limax, Entamoeba nana, Endolimax intestinalis, Endolimax suis, Endolimax ratti)	Humans, pigs, apes, monkeys, rats	Caecum, colon
Endolimax caviae	Guinea pigs	Caecum
Endolimax gregariniformis	Chickens, turkeys, guinea fowl, pheasants, geese, ducks, wild birds	Caeca

Endolimax nana

Description: Trophozoites are 6–15 μm with granular vacuolated cytoplasm and a nucleus which contains an irregular endosome composed of chromatin granules. Mature cysts are oval, 8–10 μm long, and contain four nuclei.

FAMILY ACANTHAMOEBIDAE

Members of this family are found in soil and water and have a specific form of pseudopodia (acanthopodia) that are continuously formed and resorbed to induce locomotion. Most species are free-living, but some *Acanthamoeba* species are opportunistic pathogens in animals and humans.

PHYLUM PERCOLOZOA

Members of this phylum are free-living amoebae in soil, water and faeces and can exist in either amoeboid or flagellate forms.

ORDER SCHIZOPYRENIDA

FAMILY VAHLKAMPFIDAE

Includes the genus *Naegleria*, which is an opportunist pathogen infecting the nasal mucosa and CNS of various animal species (e.g. cattle, monkeys, reptiles), and humans.

Naegleria

Description: The trophozoites are characterised by a nucleus and a surrounding halo. They travel by pseudopodia – temporary round processes which fill with granular cytoplasm. The pseudopodia form at different points along the cell, thus allowing the trophozoite to change direction.

PHYLUM EUGLENOZOA

These are flagellate protozoa having one or more flagellae. Multiplication is mainly asexual by binary fission, with some species producing cysts.

CLASS KINETOPLASTEA

ORDER TRYPANOSOMATIDA

The haemoflagellates all belong to the family Trypanosomatidae, and include the trypanosomes and leishmanias.

FAMILY TRYPANOSOMATIDAE

Members of the genus *Trypanosoma* are found in the bloodstream and tissues of vertebrates throughout the world. However, a few species are of overwhelming importance as a serious cause of morbidity and mortality in animals and humans in tropical regions. With one exception – *T. equiperdum*, which is transmitted venereally – all have an arthropod vector. Trypanosomiasis is one of the world's most important diseases of animals and humans. Most African species are transmitted by the tsetse fly (*Glossina*).

MORPHOLOGY

Trypanosomes have a leaf-like or rounded body containing a vesicular nucleus, and a varying number of subpellicular microtubules lying beneath the outer membrane. There is a single flagellum arising from a **kinetosome** or basal granule. An undulating membrane is present in some genera and the flagellum lies on its outer border. Posterior to the kinetosome is a rod-shaped or spherical **kinetoplast** containing DNA. Members of this family were originally parasites of the intestinal tract of insects, and many are still found in insects. Others are heteroxenous, spending part of their life cycle in a vertebrate host and part in an invertebrate host.

Members of the genus *Trypanosoma* are heteroxenous and pass through amastigote, promastigote, epimastigote and trypomastigote stages in their life cycle. In some species, only trypomastigote forms are found in the vertebrate host; in others, presumably more primitive species, both amastigote and trypomastigote forms are present.

- In the **trypomastigote** form, the kinetoplast and kinetosome are near the posterior end and the flagellum forms the border of an undulating membrane that extends along the side of the body to the anterior end.
- In the **epimastigote** form, the kinetoplast and kinetosome are just posterior to the nucleus and the undulating membrane runs forward from there.
- In the **promastigote** form, the kinetoplast and kinetosome are still further anterior in the body and there is no undulating membrane.
- In the **amastigote** form, the body is rounded and the flagellum emerges from the body through a wide funnel-shaped reservoir.

TRANSMISSION OF TRYPANOSOME INFECTION IN ANIMALS

With one exception, all trypanosomes have arthropod vectors in which transmission is either cyclical or non-cyclical.

In **cyclical transmission**, the arthropod is a necessary intermediate host in which the trypanosomes multiply, undergoing a series of morphological transformations before forms infective for the next mammalian host are produced. When multiplication occurs in the digestive tract and proboscis, so that the new infection is transmitted when feeding, the process is known as **anterior station development**; the various species of trypanosomes which use this process are often considered as a group, the **Salivaria**. All are trypanosomes transmitted by tsetse flies, the main species being *Trypanosoma congolense* (subgenus *Nanomonas*), *T. vivax* (subgenus *Duttonella*) and *T. brucei* (subgenus *Trypanozoon*).

In other trypanosomes, multiplication and transformation occur in the gut and the infective forms migrate to the rectum and are passed with the faeces; this is **posterior station development** and the trypanosome species are grouped together as the **Stercoraria**. In domestic animals, these are all relatively non-pathogenic trypanosomes such as *T. theileri* and *T. melophagium* transmitted by tabanid flies and sheep keds, respectively. This is certainly not the case in humans, in which *T. cruzi*, the cause of the serious Chagas disease in South America, is transmitted in the faeces of reduviid bugs.

Non-cyclical transmission is essentially mechanical transmission in which the trypanosomes are transferred from one mammalian host to another by the interrupted feeding of biting insects, notably tabanids and *Stomoxys*. The trypanosomes, in or on the contaminated proboscis, do not multiply and die quickly so that cross-transmission is only possible for a few hours. *Trypanosoma evansi*, widely distributed in livestock in Africa and Asia, is transmitted mechanically by biting flies. However, in Central and South America, *T. evansi* is also transmitted by the bites of vampire bats in which the parasites are capable of multiplying and surviving for a long period. Strictly speaking, this is more than mere mechanical transmission since the bat is also a host, although it is certainly non-cyclical since the multiplying trypanosomes in the bat's blood do not undergo any morphological transformation before they migrate into the buccal cavity.

It is important to note that the salivarian trypanosomes, normally transmitted cyclically in tsetse flies, may on occasion be transmitted mechanically. Thus, in South America, *T. vivax* has established itself, presumably by the importation of infected cattle, and is thought to be transmitted mechanically by biting flies.

Finally, apart from classic cyclical and non-cyclical transmission, dogs, cats and wild carnivores may become infected by eating fresh carcasses or organs of animals that have died of trypanosomosis, allowing the parasites to penetrate through oral abrasions.

The important trypanosome infections of domestic animals differ considerably in many respects and are best treated separately. The African species responsible for the 'tsetse-transmitted trypanosomoses' (i.e. Salivaria) are generally considered to be the most significant.

Trypanosoma

A number of species of *Trypanosoma* (Table 2.3), found in domestic and wild animals, are all transmitted cyclically by *Glossina* in much of sub-Saharan Africa. Reproduction in the mammalian host is continuous, taking place in the trypomastigote stage. Salivarian trypanosomes are highly pathogenic for certain mammals, such that the presence of trypanosomiasis precludes the rearing of livestock in many areas, while in others, where the vectors are not so numerous, trypanosomiasis is often a serious problem, particularly in cattle. The disease, sometimes known as nagana, is characterised by lymphadenopathy and anaemia accompanied by progressive emaciation and, often, death.

Salivarian trypanosomes are elongated spindle-shaped protozoa ranging from 8 to 39 μm long and the posterior end of the body is usually blunt. All possess a flagellum, which arises at the posterior end of the trypanosome from a basal body at the foot of a flagellar pocket. The flagellum runs to the anterior end of the body and is attached along its length to the pellicle to form an undulating membrane. Thereafter, the flagellum may continue forward as a free flagellum. Within a stained specimen, a single centrally placed nucleus can be seen, and adjacent to the flagellar pocket is a small structure, the kinetoplast, which contains the DNA of the single mitochondrion.

In stercorarian trypanosomes, the free flagellum is always present in the trypomastigote and the kinetoplast is large and not terminal.

Table 2.3 *Trypanosoma* species.

Species	Subgenus	Hosts	Vector
Salivarian			
Trypanosoma vivax	Duttonella	Cattle, sheep, goats, horses, camels, wild ruminants	Tsetse flies
Trypanosoma congolense	Nannomonas	Cattle, sheep, goats, horses, camels, pigs, wild ruminants	Tsetse flies
Trypanosoma simiae	Nannomonas	Pigs, camels, sheep, goats	Tsetse flies
Trypanosoma brucei T. brucei brucei T. brucei evansi	Trypanozoon	Cattle, sheep, goats, horses, donkeys, camels, pigs, dogs, cats, wild game animals	Tsetse flies (T. b. evansi: Tabanus, Stomoxys, Haematopota, Stomoxys)
T. brucei gambiense T. brucei rhodesiense		Humans	Tsetse flies
T. equiperdum		Horses	None (coitus)
Trypanosoma suis	Pycnomonas	Pigs	Tsetse flies
Trypanosoma avium	Trypanomorpha	Birds	Biting insects, red mites
Trypanosoma gallinarum	Trypanomorpha	Chickens	Biting insects
Stercorarian			
Trypanosoma theileri	Megatrypanum	Cattle, wild ruminants	Tabanid, hippoboscid flies
Trypanosoma melophagium	Megatrypanum	Sheep	Sheep keds
Trypanosoma cervi	Megatrypanum	Deer	Tabanid, hippoboscid flies
Trypanosoma lewsii	Herpetosoma	Rats	Fleas
Trypanosoma musculi	Herpetosoma	Mice	Fleas
Trypanosma cruzi	Schizotrypanum	Humans, primates, dogs, cats	Reduvid bugs

The posterior end of the body is pointed. Multiplication in the mammalian host is discontinuous, typically taking place in the epimastigote or amastigote stages with the trypomastigotes typically not pathogenic. See **life cycle** 29.

SALIVARIAN TRYPANOSOMES

SUBGENUS *DUTTONELLA*

These are monomorphic trypanosomes with a free flagellum and large kinetoplast, which is usually terminal. Development in the tsetse fly vector occurs only in the proboscis.

Trypanosoma vivax

Description: *Trypanosoma vivax* is monomorphic, ranging in size from 20 to 27 μm. The undulating membrane is inconspicuous, the large kinetoplast is terminal and the posterior end is broad and rounded. A short free flagellum is present (Figs 2.4 and 2.5). In fresh blood smears, *T. vivax* moves rapidly across the microscope field.

LIFE CYCLE 29. LIFE CYCLE OF *TRYPANOSOMA BRUCEI, TRYPANOSOMA CONGOLENSE* AND *TRYPANOSOMA VIVAX*

Trypanosomes are transmitted to domestic and wild mammalian species by flies of the genus *Glossina* (invertebrate host, 1) as metacyclic trypomastigotes (infective form) encased in a glycoprotein sheet (2). In the vertebrate hosts, trypomastigotes undergo binary fission (3), first around the inoculation site and subsequently in the circulatory system; the latter leads to detectable parasitaemia within 1–3 weeks following infection. The glycoproteins covering the surface of trypanosomes (surface antigens) undergo cyclic variation, thus allowing the parasites to elude the host immune response. The trypomastigotes (4) are ingested by the vector (5) during blood feeding on an infected host. Inside the arthropod host, trypanosomes lose the surface glycoproteins (6) and divide by binary fission (7) either in the midgut (*T. congolense* and *T. brucei*) or in the proboscis (*T. vivax*). Then, trypanosomes travel to the salivary glands (*T. brucei*) and the proboscis (*T. congolense* and *T. vivax*) where they become epimastigotes (8). In epimastigotes, the kinetoplast localises in front of the cell nucleus. Epimastigotes replicate by binary fission and acquire surface glycoproteins, thus becoming infective metacyclic trypomastigotes. The life cycle inside the arthropod host is completed within 15–35 days.

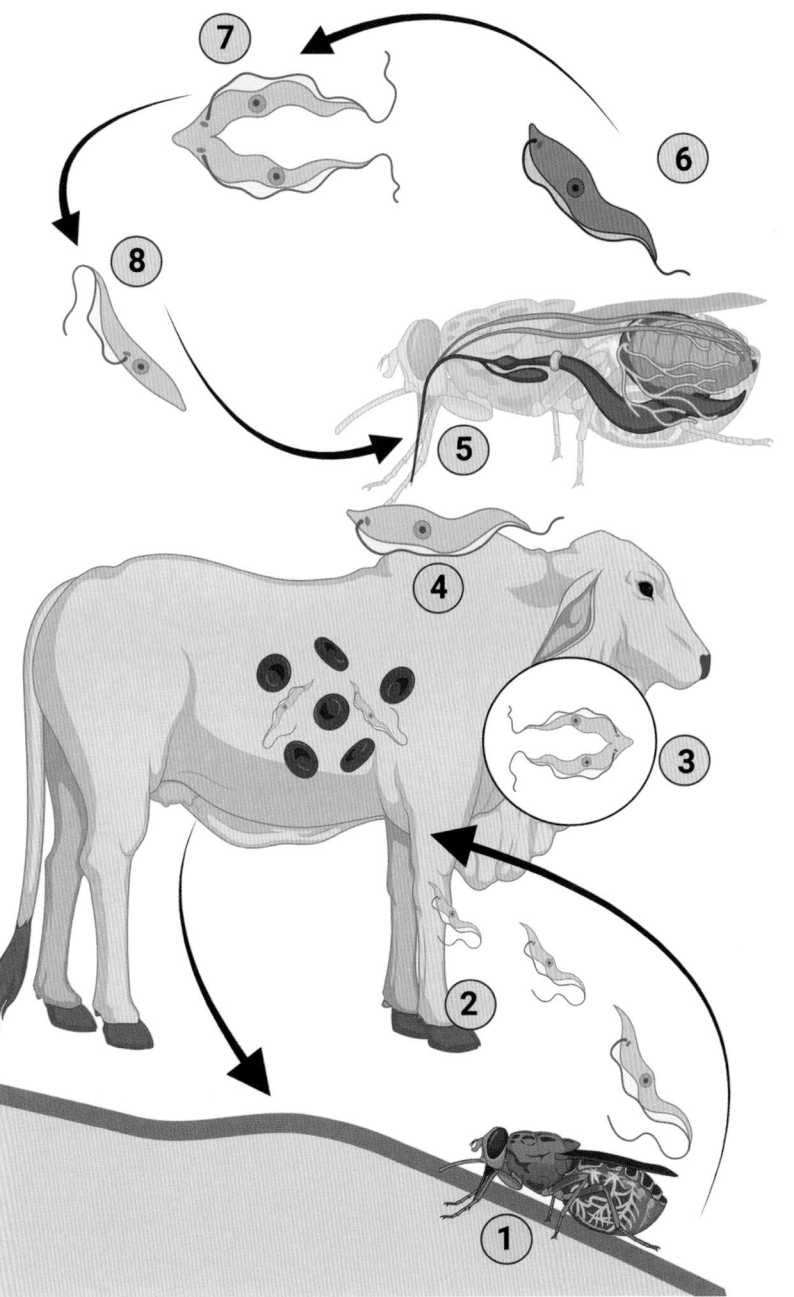

Made by Jairo Mendoza-Roldan (University of Bari, Italy) in bio render

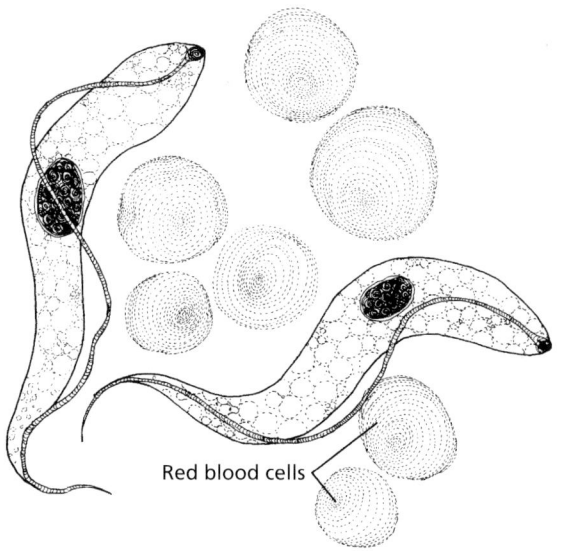

Fig. 2.4 *Trypanosoma vivax* is monomorphic and has a short flagellum and terminal kinetoplast.

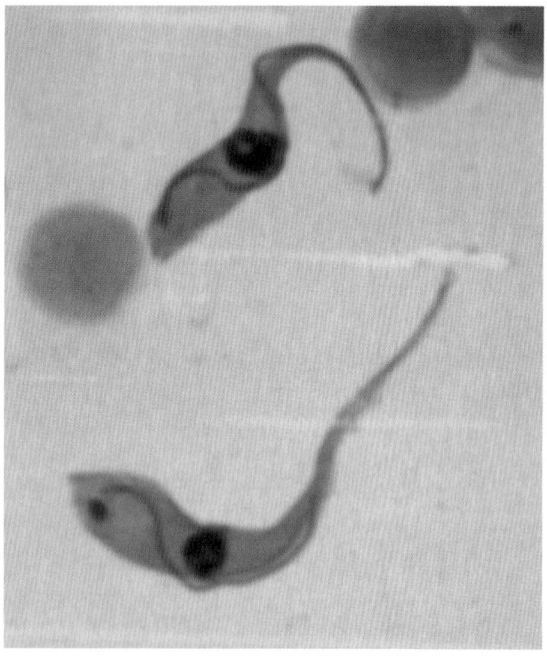

Fig. 2.5 Trypomastigotes of *Trypanosoma vivax*. (Courtesy of Marcos A. Bezerra-Santos).

Life cycle: Development in the insect vector takes place only in the proboscis. The trypanosomes turn first into the epimastigote form and then the metacyclic infective trypanosomes, which pass to the hypopharynx and infect new hosts when the tsetse flies bite and feed.

SUBGENUS *NANNOMONAS*

These are small forms usually without a free flagellum and a typically marginal medium-sized kinetoplast. Development in the tsetse fly vector occurs in the midgut and proboscis.

Trypanosoma congolense

Description: *Trypanosoma congolense* is small, monomorphic in form and 8–20 μm long. The undulating membrane is inconspicuous, the medium-sized kinetoplast is marginal and the posterior end is blunt. There is no free flagellum (Figs 2.6 and 2.7). In fresh blood smears, the organism moves sluggishly, often apparently attached to red cells.

Life cycle: The trypanosomes divide by longitudinal binary fission in the vertebrate host. After ingestion by the tsetse fly, they develop in the midgut as long trypomastigotes without a free flagellum. They attach first to the wall of the proboscis and multiply there for a time before passing to the hypopharynx where they develop into metacyclic infective trypomastigotes similar in appearance to the blood forms. These are injected into the vertebrate when the fly bites. Development to the infective stage in *Glossina* takes from 15 to well over 20 days at 23–34 °C.

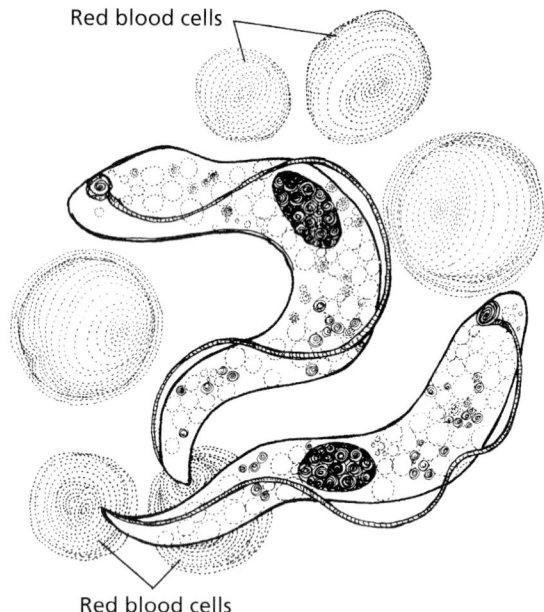

Fig. 2.6 *Trypanosoma congolense* is monomorphic and possesses a marginal kinetoplast.

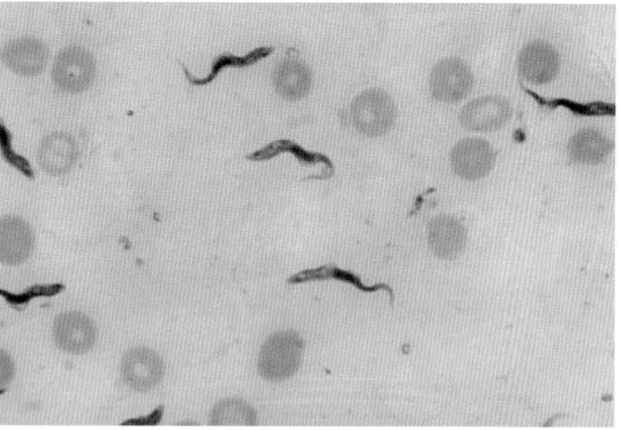

Fig. 2.7 Trypomastigotes of *Trypanosoma congolense*.

SUBGENUS *TRYPANOZOON*

These are pleomorphic (slender to stumpy) forms with or without a free flagellum and with a small subterminal kinetoplast. Development occurs in the midgut and salivary glands of the tsetse fly vector. Some forms are transmitted mechanically by tabanid vectors or by contact.

Trypanosoma brucei brucei

Description: *Trypanosoma brucei brucei* is pleomorphic in form and ranges from long and slender, up to 42 μm (average 29 μm), to short and stumpy, 12–26 μm (mean 18 μm), the two forms often being present in the same blood sample. The undulating membrane is conspicuous, the kinetoplast is small and subterminal and the posterior end is pointed. In the slender form, the kinetoplast is up to 4 μm from the posterior end, which is usually drawn out, tapering almost to a point, and has a well-developed free flagellum; in the stumpy form, the flagellum is either short or absent and the posterior end is broad and rounded with the kinetoplast almost terminal. Intermediate forms average 23 μm long and have a blunt posterior end and moderately long flagellum (Figs 2.8 and 2.9). A fourth form with a posterior nucleus may be seen in laboratory animals. In fresh unfixed blood smears, the organism moves rapidly within small areas of the microscope field.

Life cycle: Tsetse flies ingest trypanosomes in the blood or lymph while feeding on an infected host. Thereafter, the trypanosomes lose their glycoprotein surface coat and become elongated and multiply in the midgut before migrating forward to the salivary glands. There they undergo a transformation, losing their typical trypanosome, or trypomastigote, form and acquire an epimastigote form, characterised by the fact that the kinetoplast lies just in front of the nucleus. After further multiplication of the epimastigotes, they transform again into small, typically trypomastigote forms with a glycoprotein surface coat. These are the infective forms for the next host and are called **metacyclic** trypanosomes. The entire process takes at least 2–3 weeks and the metacyclic trypanosomes are inoculated into the new host when the tsetse fly feeds. At the site of inoculation, the metacyclic forms multiply locally as the typical

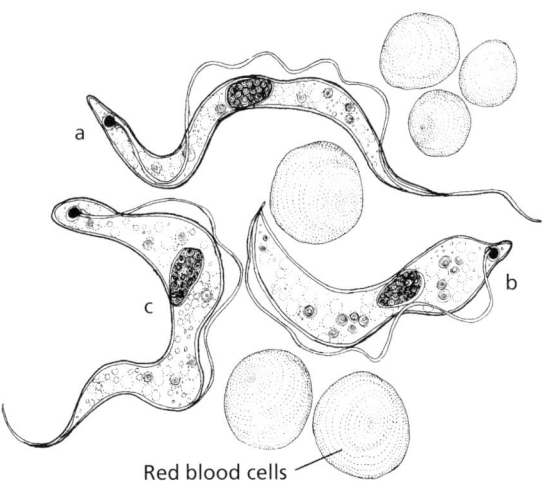

Fig. 2.8 *Trypanosoma brucei* is pleomorphic, showing (a) long slender, (b) short stumpy and (c) intermediate forms.

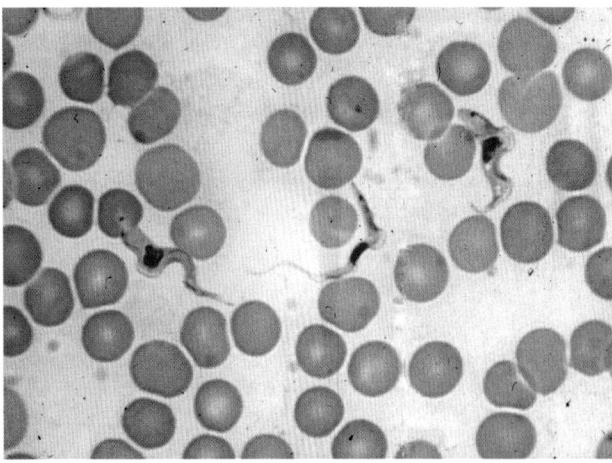

Fig. 2.9 Trypomastigotes of *Trypanosoma brucei brucei*.

blood forms, producing within a few days a raised cutaneous inflammatory swelling called a **chancre**. Thereafter, they enter the bloodstream and multiply; a parasitaemia, detectable in the peripheral blood, usually becomes apparent 1–3 weeks later. Subsequently, the parasitaemia may persist for many months, although its level may wax and wane due to the immune response of the host.

Trypanosoma brucei evansi

Description: *Trypanosoma brucei evansi* is identical to, and structurally indistinguishable in appearance from, the slender forms of *T. brucei*. The mean length varies considerably, with typical forms 15–34 μm long (mean 24 μm). Most are slender or intermediate in shape but stumpy forms occur sporadically. Strains that lack a kinetoplast, visible with the light microscope, have occasionally arisen spontaneously or can be produced by treatment with certain dyes, drugs or frozen storage.

Trypanosoma equiperdum

Description: The organism is identical to, and structurally indistinguishable in appearance from, *T. brucei evansi*. The organism is polymorphic, with slender, intermediate and stumpy forms. The mean length varies considerably, with typical forms 15–34 μm long (mean 24 μm). The undulating membrane is conspicuous and the kinetoplast small and subterminal. Strains that lack a kinetoplast, visible with the light microscope, have occasionally arisen spontaneously or can be produced by treatment with certain dyes, drugs or frozen storage.

Life cycle: The trypanosome is transmitted at coitus. The organism divides by longitudinal binary fission in various tissue fluids, particularly in subcutaneous urticarial plaques and in the reproductive system.

SUBGENUS *PYCNOMONAS*

These are stout monomorphic forms with a short free flagellum and small subterminal kinetoplast. Development in the tsetse fly vector occurs in the midgut and salivary glands.

Trypanosoma suis

Description: Trypomastigotes are monomorphic, stout, 14–19 μm long with a small marginal kinetoplast and a short free flagellum.

SUBGENUS *TRYPANOMORPHA*

These are pleomorphic, often large trypanosomes, with a long flagellum. Development occurs in biting flies.

Trypanosoma gallinarum

Description: Pleomorphic organisms, 26–29 μm long or even longer, with a free flagellum.

Life cycle: Multiplication occurs in the avian host by longitudinal binary fission of the epimastigote form in various tissues. Following ingestion by the invertebrate host, they multiply in the midgut before migrating forward to the salivary glands, forming trypomastigotes. Metacyclic trypanosomes are inoculated into the new host when the arthropod feeds.

STERCORARIAN TRYPANOSOMES

SUBGENUS *MEGATRYPANUM*

These are large mammalian trypanosomes with the kinetoplast typically situated near the nucleus and far from the posterior end of the body. Known vectors are hippoboscid or tabanid flies.

Trypanosoma theileri

Description: Large trypanosomes, 60–70 μm in length, although they may be up to 120 μm with the posterior end long and pointed (Figs 2.10 and 2.11). There is a medium-sized kinetoplast with a prominent undulating membrane and a free flagellum. Both trypomastigote and epimastigote forms may appear in the blood.

Life cycle: Multiplication occurs in the vertebrate host by longitudinal binary fission of the epimastigote form in the lymph nodes and various tissues. The trypanosomes develop into small

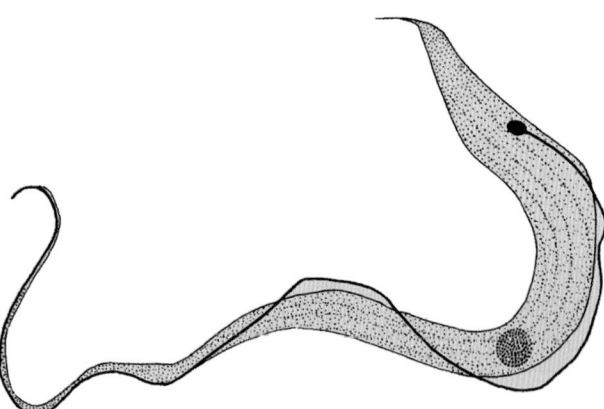

Fig. 2.10 *Trypanosoma theileri* is a large trypanosome with a prominent undulating membrane.

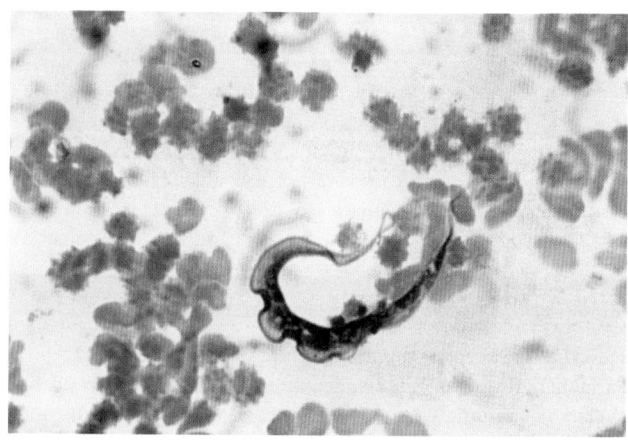

Fig. 2.11 Trypomastigotes of *Trypanosoma theileri*.

metacyclic trypomastigotes in the hindgut of tabanid flies (stercorarian development). Transmission back to the vertebrate host occurs through fly faeces, containing the parasite, deposited on mucous membranes.

SUBGENUS *HERPETOSOMA*

These trypanosomes are of medium size with a subterminal kinetoplast lying at some distance from the pointed end of the body. Reproduction in the mammalian host is in the amastigote and/or epimastigote stages. Fleas are the main vectors.

SUBGENUS *SCHIZOTRYPANUM*

These are relatively small, typically 'C'-shaped trypanosomes with a large kinetoplast close to the short, pointed posterior end of the body. Multiplication in the mammalian host is typically intracellular, primarily in the amastigote form and secondarily in the epimastigote form. Known vectors are reduviid bugs.

Trypanosoma cruzi

Description: Trypanosomes are monomorphic, 16–20 μm long, with a pointed posterior end, a curved stumpy body and a narrow undulating membrane with a trailing flagellum. The kinetoplast is large and subterminal, causing the body to bulge around it. Amastigotes are 1.5–4 μm in diameter and occur in groups.

Life cycle: Trypomastigote forms enter cells of the reticuloendothelial system, muscles and especially the heart, where they form rounded amastigotes. These multiply by binary fission, forming groups of parasites that turn into trypomastigote forms and which re-enter the blood. The vectors of *T. cruzi* are kissing bugs (Reduviidae) and, once ingested, the trypomastigotes pass to the midgut where they turn into amastigote forms. These multiply by binary fission and turn into either metacyclic trypomastigote or epimastigote forms. Epimastigote forms multiply further and extend into the rectum, where they turn into metacyclic trypomastigotes, which pass out in the faeces.

Infective trypomastigotes can actively penetrate the mucous membrane or skin of the final host.

Leishmania

Leishmania are ovoid organisms within the macrophage and possess a rod-shaped kinetoplast associated with a rudimentary flagellum. The parasites are found as the amastigote stage in cells of the vertebrate host and as the promastigote stage in the intestine of the sand fly (Table 2.4).

In the vertebrate host, *Leishmania* is found in the macrophages and other cells of the reticuloendothelial system in the skin, spleen, liver, bone marrow, lymph nodes and mucosa. It may also be found in leucocytes in the blood.

Description: *Leishmania* amastigotes are small, round or oval bodies, 1.5–3 by 2.5–6.5 µm, located within macrophages and possessing a large nucleus and rod-shaped kinetoplast associated with a rudimentary flagellum (Fig. 2.12).

Life cycle: After ingestion by a sand fly, the leishmanial, or amastigote, form transforms in the insect gut into a promastigote form in which the kinetoplast is situated at the posterior end of the body (Fig. 2.12a). These divide repeatedly by binary fission, migrate to the proboscis and are inoculated into a new host when the insect subsequently feeds. Once within a macrophage, the promastigote reverts to the amastigote form (Fig. 2.12b) and again starts to divide. See **life cycle** 30.

Leishmania occur primarily in mammals, although 10 species have been described in Old World lizards. They cause disease in humans, dogs and various rodents. *Leishmania* have a heteroxenous life cycle and are transmitted by sand flies of the genus *Phlebotomus* in the Old World and *Lutzomyia* in the New World.

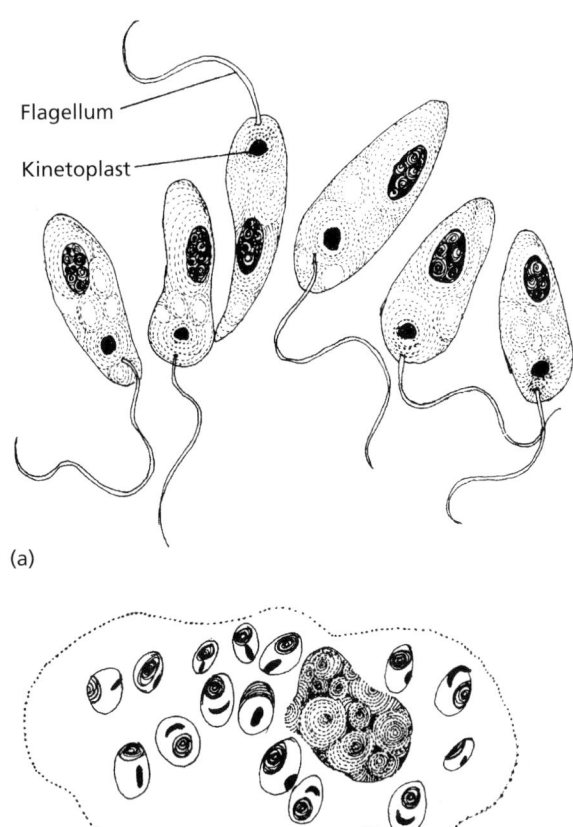

Fig. 2.12 *Leishmania*: (a) promastigote form; (b) amastigote form.

Hypopylaria are primitive species found in Old World lizards, which become infected following ingestion of sand flies. Development occurs in the sand fly hindgut.

Peripylaria develop in both the hindgut and foregut of sand flies and infect both lizards and mammals. Transmission in mammals is by bite of sand flies.

Suprapylaria develop in the sand fly midgut and foregut and occur only in mammals, with transmission by sand fly bite.

PHYLUM METAMONADA
CLASS TRICHOMONADEA
ORDER TRICHOMONADIDA

Members of the families Trichomonadidae, Dientamoebidae and Monocercomonadidae occur predominantly in the gastrointestinal tract of vertebrates. While many are considered to be commensals, some may be important causes of enteritis and diarrhoea.

FAMILY TRICHOMONADIDAE

The family Trichomonadidae ('trichomonads') includes a number of genera of medical and veterinary interest: *Tritrichomonas*, *Trichomonas*, *Tetratrichomonas*, *Trichomitus* and *Pentatrichomonas*.

Table 2.4 *Leishmania* species.

Species	Hosts	Site	Sand fly vector
Leishmania infantum (syn. *Leishmania chagasi*)	Humans, dogs, cats, rodents, rabbits, foxes, opossums, wild canids	Skin, liver, spleen, bone marrow, lymph nodes, mucoses	*Phlebotomus* spp., *Lutzomyia* spp.
Leishmania tropica (syn. *Leishmania killicki*)	Humans, dogs, hyraxes, foxes, cats	Skin, liver, spleen, bone marrow, lymph nodes	*Phlebotomus* spp.
Leishmania major	Humans, dogs, cats, rodents, gerbils, jirds	Skin	*Phlebotomus* spp.
Leishmania aethiopica	Humans, hyraxes	Skin, mucoses	*Phlebotomus* spp.
Leishmania donovani sensu stricto	Humans, dogs, rodents	Skin, liver, spleen, bone marrow, lymph nodes, mucoses	*Phlebotomus* spp.
Leishmania peruviana	Humans, dogs	Skin, mucoses	*Lutzomyia* spp.
Leishmania braziliensis	Humans, dogs, rodents, horses	Skin, mucoses	*Lutzomyia* spp.
Leishmania martinquensis (syn. *Leishmania siamensis*)	Horses, cows, humans	Skin, liver, spleen, bone marrow, lymph nodes	Unknown (probably *Culicoides* spp.)
Leishmania tarentolae	Reptiles	Erythropoietic organs	*Sargentomyia* spp.

LIFE CYCLE 30. LIFE CYCLE OF *LEISHMANIA INFANTUM*

Infection by *Leishmania infantum* occurs via inoculation of the metacyclic promastigote form during blood feeding by the haematophagous arthropod vector, phlebotomine sand flies (invertebrate host, 1) on vertebrate hosts (2). Promastigotes enter the cytoplasm of monocytes and macrophages (3), lose the flagellum and become amastigotes (4). Inside the cytoplasm of monocytes and macrophages, the parasites replicate several times by binary fission, thus causing cell membrane rupture and subsequent release of free amastigotes (5) that thus can penetrate other macrophages (5). In dogs, this process causes systemic reticuloendotheliosis that leads to severe disease, characterised by weight loss, enlarged lymph nodes, onychogryphosis, epistaxis and cutaneous ulcers (6). The arthropod host acquires amastigotes while blood feeding on an infected host, whether symptomatic or asymptomatic (7). In the abdominal midgut, the blood meal is encased by peritrophic matrix (PM), and amastigotes transform to small and slow procyclic promastigotes (with a short flagellum) which soon begin to multiply (8). Procyclic promastigotes evolve into nectomonad promastigotes (9), larger and slimmer in shape, which migrate to the thoracic portion of the midgut where they develop into leptomonad promastigotes (10). This form is shorter and undergoes a second cycle of multiplication inside the insect (5–7 days after infection). Finally, the parasites develop into metacyclic promastigotes within 4–20 days, depending on the species of *Leishmania* and sand fly vector. Metacyclic promastigotes, with a small cell body, an elongated flagellum and lively movements, are the infective forms of the protozoan (11) and travel through the insect pharynx to be injected into the host's skin during the subsequent blood meal of the vector arthropod.

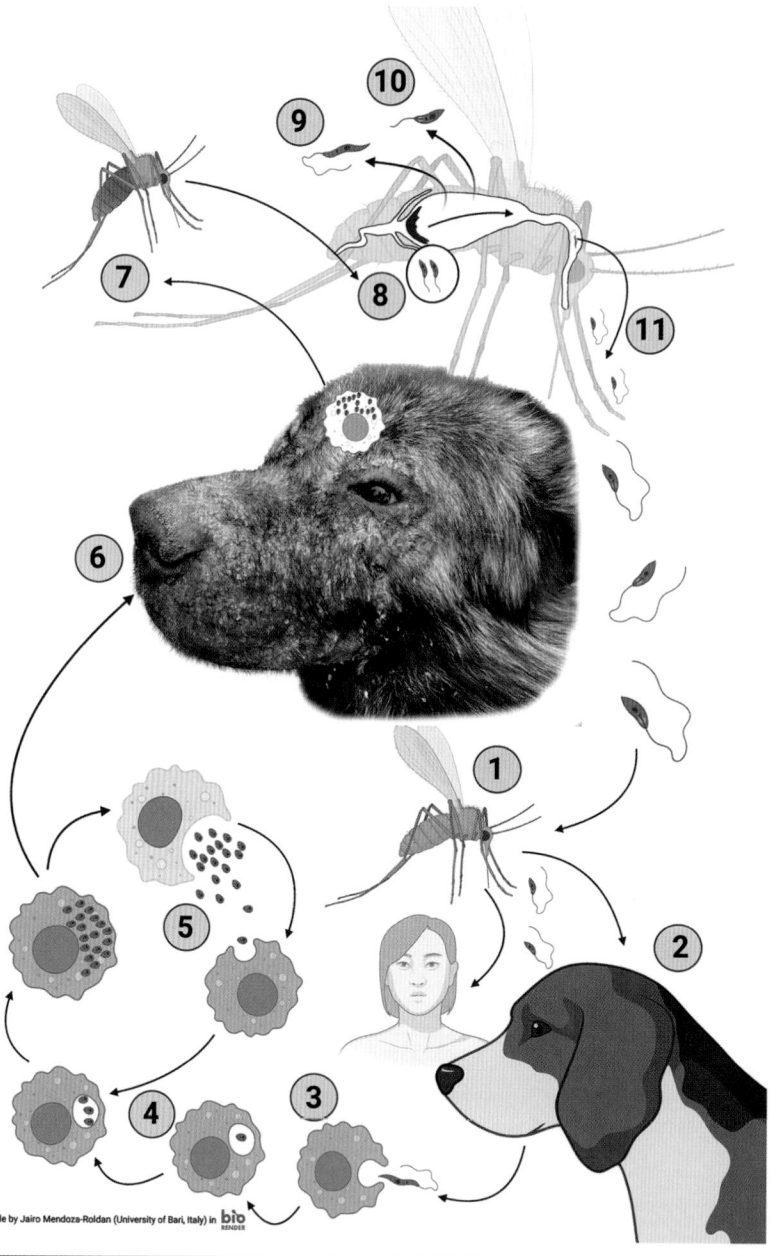

Made by Jairo Mendoza-Roldan (University of Bari, Italy) in bioRENDER

Trichomonads have 3–5 flagella, of which one is usually recurrent and attached to an undulating membrane, and have been found in the caecum and colon of virtually all species of mammals and birds, and also in reptiles, amphibians, fish and invertebrates. Specific identification and host–parasite relationships of many species remain unclear and several species are thought to be synonymous.

Tritrichomonas in cattle is an important venereal disease causing infertility and abortion.

Tritrichomonas

Members of this genus have three anterior flagella and a posterior flagellum, and lack a pelta (Table 2.5).

Life cycle: The trichomonads reproduce by longitudinal binary fission. No sexual stages are known and there are no cysts.

Tritrichomonas eberthi

Description: The body is elongate, 8–14 by 4–7 μm, with vacuolated cytoplasm and three anterior flagella. The undulating membrane is prominent and extends the full length of the body. The posterior flagellum extends about half the length of the body beyond the undulating membrane (Fig. 2.13). An accessory filament is present. The blepharoplast is composed of four granules; the axostyle is massive and hyaline, and its anterior end is broadened to form a capitulum and a ring of chromatin granules is present at the point where the axostyle emerges from the body. The parabasal body is shaped like a flattened rod and is of variable length.

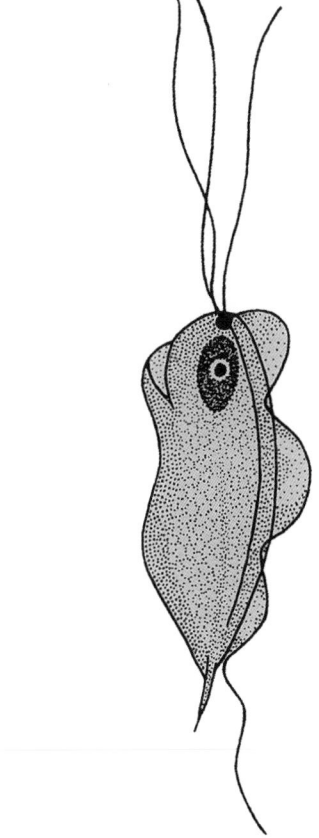

Fig. 2.13 *Tritrichomonas eberthi.*

Tritrichomonas foetus

Description: The organisms found in cats are morphologically indistinguishable from those seen in cattle. Trophozoites is pear-shaped, approximately 10–25 μm long and 3–15 μm wide and has a single nucleus and four flagella, each arising from a basal body situated at the anterior rounded end (Fig. 2.14). Three of the flagella are free anteriorly, while the fourth extends backwards to form an

Table 2.5 *Tritrichomonas* species.

Species	Hosts	Site
Tritrichomonas eberthi (syn. *Trichomonas eberthi*)	Chickens, turkeys	Caeca
Tritrichomonas foetus (syn. *Trichomonas foetus*)	Cattle / Cats	Prepuce, uterus / Small intestine
Tritrichomonas muris (syn. *Trichomonas criceti*)	Mice, rats, voles	Large intestine
Tritrichomonas suis (syn. *Trichomonas suis*) (considered synonymous with *T. foetus*)	Pigs	Nasal passages, stomach, caecum, colon
Tritrichomonas enteris (syn. *Trichomonas enteris*)	Cattle, zebu	Caecum, colon
Tritrichomonas minuta	Rats, mice, hamsters	Large intestine
Tritrichomonas wenyoni (syn. *Trichomitus wenyoni*)	Rats, mice, hamsters, monkeys	Large intestine
Tritrichomonas caviae	Guinea pigs	Caecum

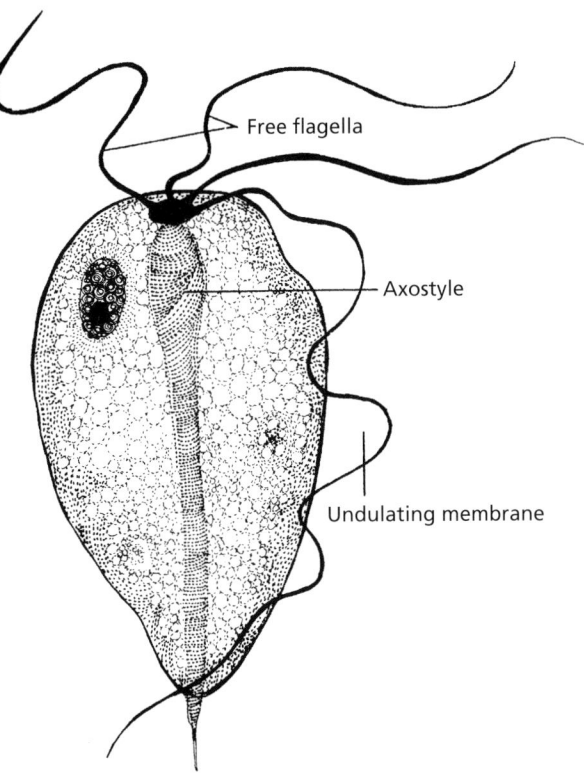

Free flagella

Axostyle

Undulating membrane

Fig. 2.14 *Tritrichomonas foetus.*

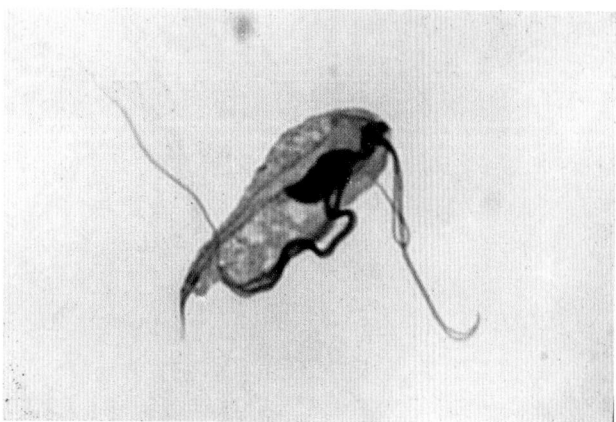

Fig. 2.15 *Tritrichomonas foetus* showing three anterior flagella and trailing posterior flagellum.

undulating membrane along the length of the organism and then continues posteriorly as a free flagellum (Fig. 2.15). The axostyle, a hyaline rod with a skeletal function, extends the length of the cell and usually projects posteriorly. The costa is prominent but there is no pelta. In fresh preparations, the organism is motile and progresses by rolling jerky movements, the flickering flagella and the movements of the undulating membrane being readily seen. Occasionally, rounded immobile forms are observed and these are possibly effete.

Tritrichomonas muris

Description: The body is pyriform, 12–20 μm long, and there are three anterior flagella which arise from a conspicuous blepharoplast. The undulating membrane is prominent and extends the length of the body in ribbon-like folds bounded by a thick marginal filament, which extends beyond the body as a free trailing flagellum. The costa is well developed and the axostyle is present as a thick tubular structure and has a short posterior extension.

Tritrichomonas suis

Description: The body is characteristically elongate or spindle-shaped, but may occasionally be pyriform or rotund, 9–16 by 2–6 μm (mean 11 × 3 μm), with three anterior flagella which are approximately equal in length and each ending in a round or spatulate knob. The undulating membrane runs the full length of the body and has 4–6 folds and its marginal filament continues as a posterior free flagellum (Fig. 2.16). An accessory filament is present. The costa runs the full length of the body and fine subcostal granules are present. The axostyle is a hyaline rod with a bulbous capitulum and extends beyond the body as a cone-shaped projection narrowing abruptly to a short tip. There is a chromatic ring around its point of exit. The parabasal body is usually a single, slender, tube-like structure, and the nucleus is ovoid or elongated and has a large conspicuous endosome surrounded by a relatively clear halo.

Tritrichomonas enteris

Description: The body measures 6–12 by 5–6 μm and there are three anterior flagella of equal length, which arise from a single blepharoplast. The flagellum at the edge of the undulating

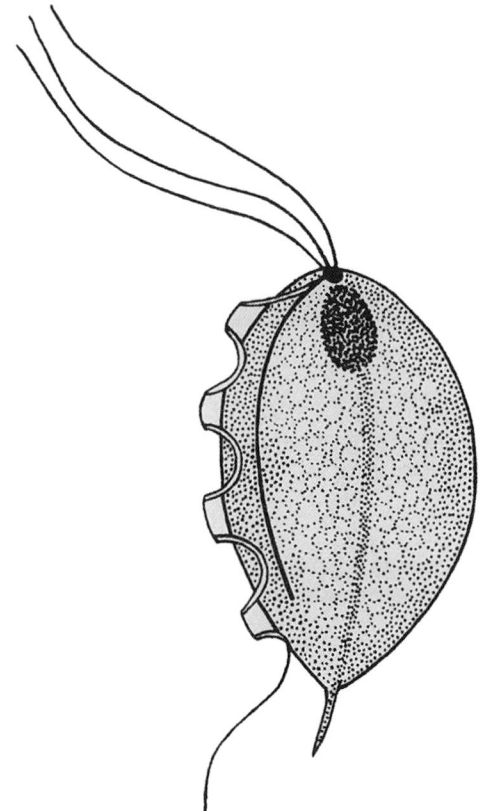

Fig. 2.16 *Tritrichomonas suis.*

membrane is single and lacks an accessory filament. The undulating membrane extends three-quarters of the body length and a free flagellum extends beyond the undulating membrane. The axostyle is straight and slender, bending around the nucleus to give a spoon shape and extending most one-quarter of the body length beyond the body.

Tritrichomonas minuta

Description: The body measures 4–9 μm long and there are three anterior flagella. The undulating membrane extends almost the length of the body and there is a trailing posterior flagellum.

Tritrichomonas wenyoni

Description: The body measures 4–16 μm long and there are three anterior flagella. The undulating membrane extends the length of the body and has a long trailing posterior flagellum. The axostyle is broad and hyaline.

Tritrichomonas caviae

Description: The body is 10–22 μm long with a flat cylindrical nucleus, three anterior flagella and a prominent undulating membrane extending the length of the body (Fig. 2.17). The axostyle is well defined with a prominent costa.

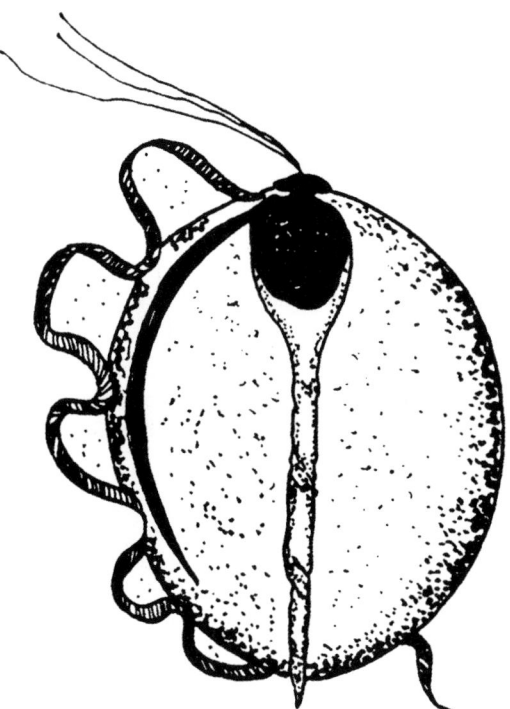

Fig. 2.17 *Tritrichomonas caviae.*

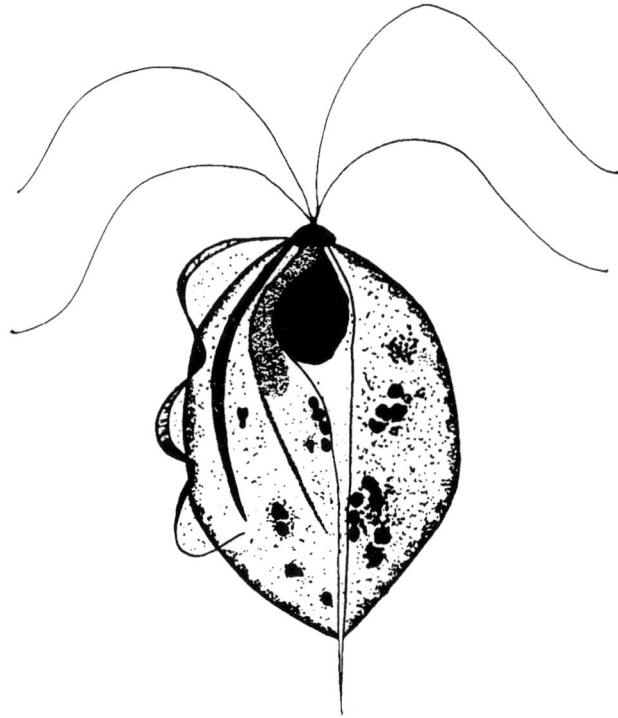

Fig. 2.18 *Trichomonas gallinae.*

Trichomonas

Trichomonas gallinae has four anterior flagella, an undulating membrane but no trailing flagellum. It infects the pharynx, oesophagus, crop and proventriculus of pigeons, turkeys and raptors (hawks, falcons, eagles).

Trichomonas gallinae

Description: The body is elongate, ellipsoid or pyriform, 5–19 by 2–9 μm, with four anterior flagella that arise from the blepharoplast. The undulating membrane does not reach the posterior end of the body and a free posterior flagellum is absent (Fig. 2.18). An accessory filament is present. The axostyle is narrow, protrudes 2–8 μm from the body and its anterior portion is flattened into a spatulate capitulum. There is a crescent-shaped pelta anterior to the axostyle and there is no chromatic ring at its point of emergence. The parabasal body is hook-shaped and has a parabasal filament and the costa is a very fine rod running three-quarters the length of the body.

Tetratrichomonas

Members of this genus have four flagella, a posterior (trailing) flagellum, an undulating membrane and a pelta (Table 2.6).

Life cycle: Reproduction is by longitudinal binary fission. No sexual stages are known and there are no cysts.

Tetratrichomonas anatis

Description: The body is broadly beet-shaped, 13–27 by 8–18 μm, with four anterior flagella and an undulating membrane that

Table 2.6 *Tetratrichomonas* species.

Species	Hosts	Site
Tetratrichomonas anatis (syn. *Trichomonas anatis*)	Ducks	Small and large intestine
Tetratrichomonas anseris (syn. *Trichomonas anseris*)	Geese	Caeca
Tetratrichomonas buttreyi (syn. *Trichomonas buttreyi*)	Cattle, pigs	Caecum, colon
Tetratrichomonas canistomae	Dogs	Mouth
Tetratrichomonas felistomae	Cats	Mouth
Tetratrichomonas gallinarum (syn. *Trichomonas gallinarum*, *Trichomonas pullorum*)	Chickens, turkeys, guinea fowl, quails, pheasants	Caeca
Tetratrichomonas microti (syn. *Trichomonas microti*)	Rats, mice, hamsters, voles	Large intestine
Tetratrichomonas ovis (syn. *Trichomonas ovis*, *Ditrichomonas ovis*)	Sheep	Caecum, rumen
Tetratrichomonas pavlovi (syn. *Trichomonas pavlovi*, *Trichomonas bovis*)	Cattle	Large intestine

extends most of the length of the body and terminates in a free posterior flagellum. There is a costa and a slender fibrillar axostyle.

Tetratrichomonas anseris

Description: The body is elongate, 8–14 by 4–7 μm, with vacuolated cytoplasm and three anterior flagella. The undulating membrane is prominent and extends the full length of the body. The posterior flagellum extends about half the length of the body beyond the undulating membrane. An accessory filament is present. The blepharoplast is composed of four granules; the axostyle is massive and hyaline, and its anterior end is broadened to form a capitulum. A ring of chromatin granules is present at the point where the axostyle emerges from the body. The parabasal body is shaped like a flattened rod and is of variable length.

Tetratrichomonas buttreyi

Description: The body is ovoid or ellipsoid, and 4–7 by 2–5 μm (mean 6 × 3 μm) in size. Cytoplasmic inclusions are frequently present. There are three or four anterior flagella, which vary in length from a short stub to more than twice the length of the body, and each ends in a knob or spatulate structure. The undulating membrane runs the full length of the body and has 3–5 undulations ending in a free posterior flagellum. The accessory filament is prominent and the costa relatively delicate. The axostyle is relatively narrow, has a spatulate capitulum and extends 3–6 μm beyond the body. There is no chromatic ring at its point of exit. A pelta is present. The nucleus is frequently ovoid (2–3 × 1–2 μm) but is variable in shape and has a small endosome.

Tetratrichomonas canistomae

Description: The body is pyriform, 7–12 by 3–4 μm. The four anterior flagella are about as long as the body and arise in pairs from a large blepharoplast. The undulating membrane extends almost the length of the body and terminates in a free posterior flagellum, which is about half the length of the body (Fig. 2.19). The axostyle is thread-like and extends a considerable length

beyond the body. The costa is slender and there are no subcostal granules.

Tetratrichomonas felistomae

Description: The body is pyriform, 6–11 by 3–4 μm (mean 8 × 3 μm). There are four anterior flagella, which are longer than the body. The undulating membrane extends most of the body length and terminates in a free posterior flagellum and the axostyle extends a considerable distance beyond the body.

Tetratrichomonas gallinarum

Description: The body is pyriform and is 7–15 by 3–9 μm. There are four anterior flagella and a posterior flagellum that runs along the undulating membrane and extends beyond it. An accessory filament is present. The axostyle is long, pointed and slender, and lacks a chromatic ring at its point of emergence. Supracostal granules are present but there are no subcostal or endoaxostylar granules. The pelta is elaborate and terminates in a short ventral extension which is more or less free from the ventral edge of the axostyle. The parabasal body usually consists of a ring of variously spaced granules plus one or two fibrils or rami.

Tetratrichomonas microti

Description: The body is 4–9 μm long and there are four anterior flagella. The undulating membrane extends almost the length of the body and there is a trailing posterior flagellum (Fig. 2.20). The axostyle is slender.

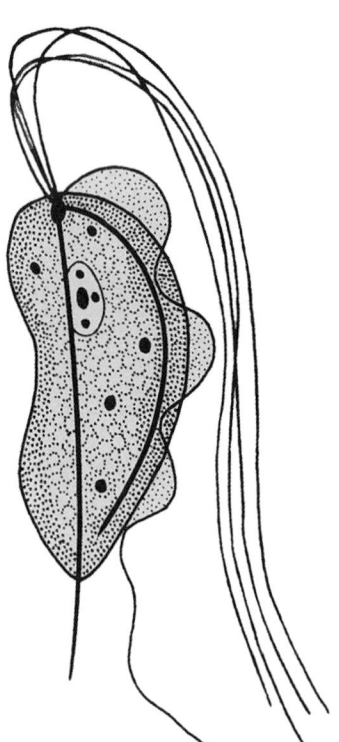

Fig. 2.19 *Tetratrichomonas canistomae.*

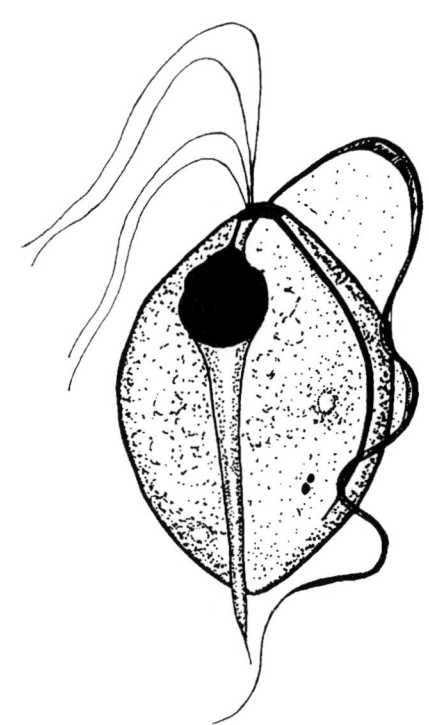

Fig. 2.20 *Tetratrichomonas microti.*

Tetratrichomonas ovis

Description: The body is pyriform, 6–9 by 4–8 μm (mean 7 × 6 μm) and the four anterior flagella are of unequal length. There is a slender hyaline axostyle which extends approximately 5 μm beyond the body and gradually tapers to a point. There is no chromatic ring at the point where the axostyle leaves the body. There is an anterior nucleus and a prominent pelta at the anterior end. There is a prominent undulating membrane which extends 75–100% the length of the body, and which continues as a free posterior flagellum. The costa is prominent and there are several irregular rows of paracostal granules, an ovoid or club-shaped parabasal body containing an intensely chromophilic body, and a parabasal filament.

Tetratrichomonas pavlovi

Description: The body is pyriform and is usually 11–12 by 6–7 μm. It has four anterior flagella, which are about the same length as the body. The undulating membrane is well developed and has 2–4 waves that extend almost to the posterior end of the body. There is a free posterior flagellum, an accessory filament and a costa. The nucleus is round or ovoid. The axostyle is slender, broadening to form a capitulum at the anterior end.

Trichomitus

Members of this genus have three anterior flagella, an undulating membrane, a pelta and posterior (trailing) flagellum.

Trichomitus rotunda

This species infects the caecum and colon of pigs.

Description: The body is typically broadly pyriform, but may occasionally be ovoid or ellipsoid. It measures 7–11 by 5–7 μm (mean 9 × 6 μm). Cytoplasmic inclusions are frequently present. The three anterior flagella are approximately equal in length and each terminates in a knob or spatulate structure. The blepharoplast appears to consist of a single granule. The undulating membrane together with the costa extends about 50–75% the length of the body. The free posterior flagellum is generally shorter than the body. The axostyle is a narrow, straight, non-hyaline rod with a crescent or sickle-shaped capitulum extending about 4 μm beyond the body. The nucleus is practically spherical, 2–3 μm in diameter, with an endosome surrounded by a clear halo. The parabasal body is 2–3 by 0.4–1.3 μm and is composed of two rami forming a 'V'. Each ramus has a parabasal filament.

Pentatrichomonas

Members of this genus have five anterior flagella, an undulating membrane, a pelta and a sixth trailing flagellum (Table 2.7).

Life cycle: The trichomonads reproduce by longitudinal binary fission. No sexual stages are known and there are no cysts.

Table 2.7 *Pentatrichomonas* species.

Species	Hosts	Site
Pentatrichomonas hominis (syn. *Pentatrichomonas felis, Cercomonas hominis, Monocercomonas hominis, Trichomonas intestinalis, Trichomonas felis*)	Humans, monkeys, dogs, cats, rats, mice, hamsters, guinea pigs	Large intestine
Pentatrichomonas gallinarum	Chickens, turkeys, guinea fowl	Caeca, liver

Pentatrichomonas hominis

Synonyms: *Pentatrichomonas felis, Cercomonas hominis, Monocercomonas hominis, Trichomonas intestinalis, Trichomonas felis*

Description: The body is pyriform, 8 by 20 μm, and there are usually five anterior flagella. Four of the anterior flagella are grouped together and the fifth is separate and directed posteriorly. A sixth flagellum runs along the undulating membrane and extends beyond the body as a free trailing flagellum. The undulating membrane extends the length of the body. The axostyle is thick and hyaline with a sharply pointed tip. The pelta is crescent-shaped.

Pentatrichomonas gallinarum

Description: The body is usually spherical, measuring 7 by 5 μm with five anterior flagella, and an undulating membrane extends the length of the body with a free flagellum at its end. The axostyle is slender, projecting from the posterior end (Fig. 2.21).

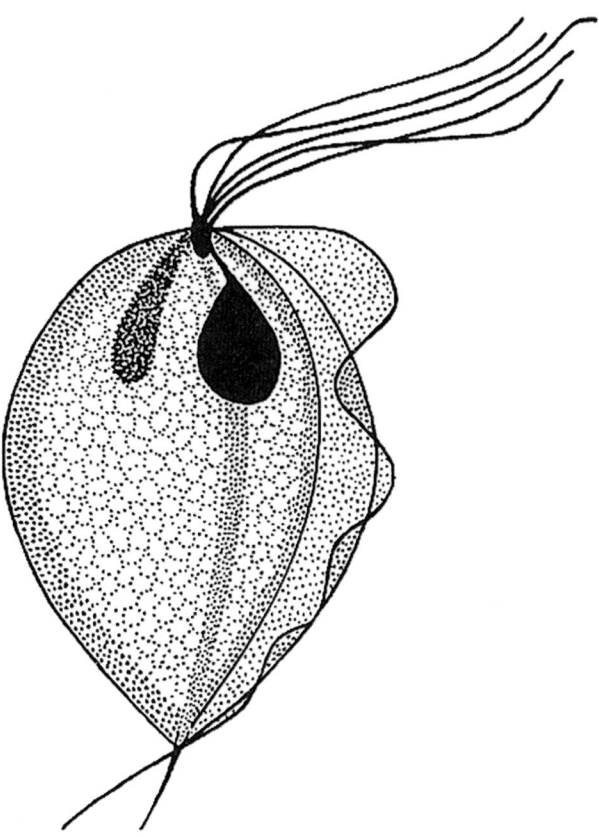

Fig. 2.21 *Pentatrichomonas gallinarum.*

Cochlosoma

Cochlosoma anatis

Synonym: *Cochlosoma rostratum*

This species infects the large intestine, cloaca and caeca of ducks.

Description: The body is beet-shaped, 6–12 by 4–7 μm, with a nucleus in the middle of the body. There are six flagella of unequal length arising from a blepharoplast at the anterior end, and two trailing flagella lying in a longitudinal groove. A sucker covers one-third to half of the body length.

FAMILY DIENTAMOEBIDAE

Histomonas

A single species, *Histomonas meleagridis*, is recognised to infect the caeca and liver of turkeys, pheasants, partridges and chickens. The body is actively amoeboid with a single flagellum arising from a basal granule close to the nucleus.

Life cycle: Birds become infected by ingestion of the embryonated egg of the caecal worm, *Heterakis gallinarum*, the flagellate being carried in the unhatched larva. When the egg hatches, the histomonads are released from the larva and enter the caecal mucosa where they cause ulceration and necrosis. They reach the liver in the portal stream and colonise the liver parenchyma, producing circular necrotic foci which increase in size as the parasites multiply in the periphery of the lesion. The next phase of the life cycle is not clear, but it is presumed that the *Heterakis* worms become infected with the caecal histomonads, possibly by ingestion, and that these subsequently reach the ovary of the worm. It is certainly established that the histomonads become incorporated in a proportion of the *Heterakis* eggs, and thus reach the exterior. Infection of birds may also result from the ingestion of earthworms, which are transport hosts for *Heterakis* eggs and larvae.

Histomonas meleagridis

Description: A pleomorphic organism, with its morphology depending on organ location and stage of disease. In the caecum, the organism is round or oval, amoeboid, with clear ectoplasm and granular endoplasm, 6–20 μm in diameter, and bears a single flagellum (Fig. 2.22), although this appears to be lost when in the mucosal tissue or the liver. The nucleus is vesicular and a flagellum arises from a small blepharoplast near the nucleus. In the caecal mucosa and liver, the organism is found singly or in clusters and is amoeboid, 8–15 μm in diameter, with no flagellum. Both luminal and tissue stages exhibit pseudopodial movement.

Dientamoeba

There is a single species, *D. fragilis*, which occurs in the caecum and colon of humans and some species of monkeys. Only trophozoites have been described, and these are 3–22 μm in diameter and contain one or two vesicular nuclei connected by a filament or desmose.

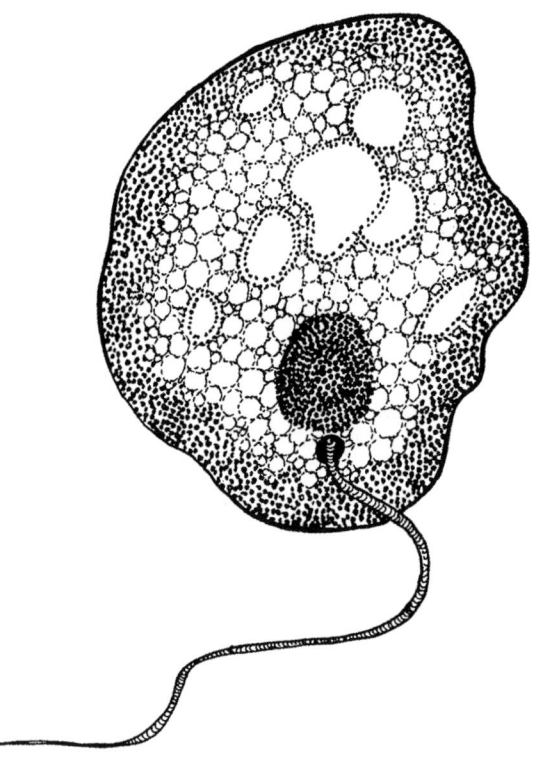

Fig. 2.22 *Histomonas meleagridis.*

FAMILY MONOCERCOMONADIDAE

These are similar in appearance to the trichomonads except there is no undulating membrane. The genus *Histomonas* is of veterinary importance, causing major losses in turkeys and gamebirds. *Monocercomonas* occurs in a wide range of mammals, birds, reptiles, amphibians and fish and is generally considered non-pathogenic. Organisms in the single species of the genus *Dientamoeba* were originally thought to be amoebae but are now classed as trichomonads.

Monocercomonas

Members of this genus have three anterior flagella, a trailing flagellum with no undulating membrane and the axostyle usually projects beyond the posterior end of the body (Table 2.8).

Life cycle: The life cycle is simple, with trophozoites dividing by binary fission. No sexual stages are known and there are no cysts.

Monocercomonas ruminantium

Synonyms: *Trichomonas ruminantium, Tritrichomonas ruminantium*

Table 2.8 *Monocercomonas* species.

Species	Hosts	Site
Monocercomonas ruminantium (syn. *Trichomonas ruminantium, Tritrichomonas ruminantium*)	Cattle, sheep	Rumen
Monocercomonas cuniculi (syn. *Trichomastix cuniculi*)	Rabbits	Caecum

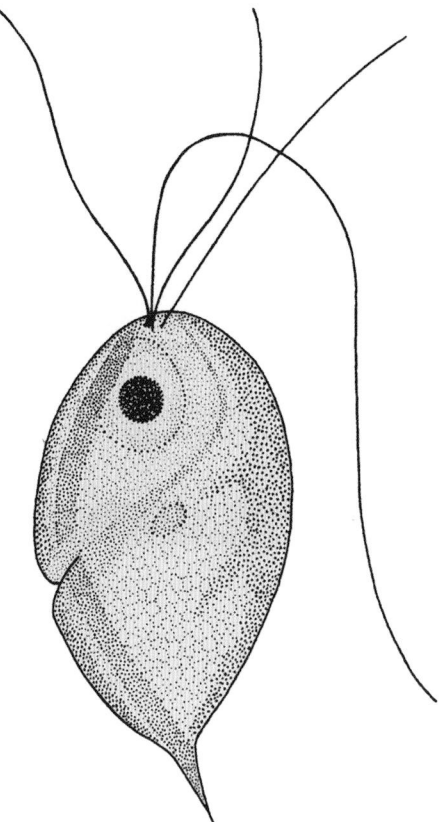

Fig. 2.23 *Monocercomonas ruminantium* trophozoite.

Description: The trophozoite is subspherical (3–8 × 3–7 μm) with a rounded anterior end. The axostyle is curved and may or may not extend beyond the body. A pelta and parabasal body are present. The cytostome and anterior nucleus are anterior. There are three anterior flagella and a trailing flagellum (Fig. 2.23).

Monocercomonas cuniculi

Synonym: *Trichomastix cuniculi*

Description: The body is pyriform, 5–14 μm long, with a slender hyaline axostyle projecting from the body.

Chilomitus

Trophozoites have an elongate body, an anterior nucleus, a rudimentary axostyle and a cup-like cytostome at the anterior end from which arise four flagella. Species of this genus infect the caecum of guinea pigs.

Chilomitus caviae

Description: Trophozoites are 6–14 μm long and 3–5 μm wide.

Chilomitus conexus

Description: Trophozoites are 4–7 μm long by 1–2 μm wide.

FAMILY HEXAMASTIGIDAE

Hexamastix

Hexamastix has a pyriform body with an anterior nucleus and cytostome, a pelta, a conspicuous, axostyle and five anterior flagella, and a trailing flagellum (Table 2.9).

Hexamastix caviae

Synonym: *Pentatrichomastix caviae*

Description: Trophozoites are 4–10 μm long by 3–5 μm wide.

Hexamastix robustus

Synonym: *Pentatrichomastix robustus*

Description: Trophozoites are 7–14 μm long by 3–8 μm wide.

Hexamastix muris

Synonym: *Pentatrichomastix robustus*

Description: Trophozoites are 5–12 μm long.

FAMILY PROTEROMONADIDAE

Proteromonas

Trophozoites are spindle-shaped with an anterior and free trailing posterior flagellum. The nucleus is anterior to the body and lies next to a paranuclear body of similar size.

Proteromonas brevifilia

This species infects the caecum of guinea pigs.

Description: Trophozoites are 4–9 μm long by 2–4 μm wide.

CLASS TREPOMONADEA

ORDER RETORTAMONADIDA

FAMILY RETORTAMONADIDAE

These protozoa are predominantly inhabitants of stagnant water but occur in a wide range of mammals, birds, reptiles and insects, and are generally considered non-pathogenic. Species of *Retortamonas* and *Chilomastix* are found in humans, monkeys, cattle, sheep, rabbits, guinea pigs, amphibians, reptiles and insects.

Table 2.9 *Hexamastix* species

Species	Hosts	Site
Hexamastix caviae (syn. *Pentatrichomastix caviae*)	Guinea pigs	Caecum
Hexamastix robustus (syn. *Pentatrichomastix robustus*)	Guinea pigs	Caecum
Hexamastix muris (syn. *Pentatrichomastix muris*)	Rats	Caecum

Table 2.10 *Retortamonas* species.

Species	Hosts	Site
Retortamonas ovis (syn. *Embadomonas ovis*, *Embadomonas ruminantium*)	Sheep, cattle	Caecum
Retortamonas cuniculi (syn. *Embadomonas cuniculi*)	Rabbits	Caecum
Retortamonas caviae	Guinea pigs	Caecum
Retortamonas intestinalis (syn. *Embadomonas intestinalis*, *Waskia intestinalis*)	Humans, chimpanzees, monkeys	Caecum

Table 2.11 *Chilomastix* species.

Species	Hosts	Site
Chilomastix mesnili (syn. *Chilomastix suis*, *Chilomastix hominis*, *Macrostoma mesnili*)	Humans, apes, monkeys, pigs	Caecum, colon
Chilomastix gallinarum	Chickens, turkeys	Caeca
Chilomastix equi	Horses	Intestine
Chilomastix caprae	Goats	Rumen
Chilomastix cuniculi	Rabbits	Caecum
Chilomastix intestinalis	Guinea pigs	Caecum
Chilomastix wenrichi	Guinea pigs	Caecum
Chilomastix bettencourti	Rats, mice, hamsters	Caecum

Retortamonas

Retortamonas has a pyriform body with large cytostome and two flagella (Table 2.10).

Retortamonas ovis

Synonyms: *Embadomonas ovis, Embadomonas ruminantium*

Description: Trophozoites are pyriform and average 5.2 by 3.4 μm. There is a large cytostome near the anterior end containing a cytostomal fibril that extends across the anterior end and posteriorly along each side. An anterior flagellum and a posterior trailing flagellum emerge from the cytostomal groove. Cysts are pyriform and ovoid, containing one or two nuclei, and retain the cytostomal fibril.

Retortamonas cuniculi

Synonyms: *Embadomonas cuniculi*

Description: Trophozoites are ovoid, 7–13 by 5–10 μm, with an anterior flagellum and a posterior trailing flagellum emerging from the cytostomal groove. Cysts are pyriform or ovoid, 5–7 by 3–4 μm.

Retortamonas caviae

Description: Trophozoites are 4–8 μm long by 4 μm wide with cysts 4–6 μm by 3–4 μm wide.

Retortamonas intestinalis

Synonyms: *Embadomonas intestinalis, Waskia intestinalis*

Description: The trophozoite is small, measuring 4–9 μm long by 4–7 μm wide, with two anterior flagella and a prominent cytostome. It has a relatively large nucleus at the anterior end with a small compact karyosome.

Chilomastix

Trophozoites are pyriform with a large cytostomal groove near the anterior end. There are three anterior flagella and a short fourth flagellum within the cytostomal cleft. Species of this genus are found in mammals, birds, reptiles, amphibians, fish and insects and are considered to be non-pathogenic (Table 2.11).

Chilomastix mesnili

Synonyms: *Chilomastix suis, Chilomastix hominis, Macrostoma mesnili*

Description: Trophozoites are pear-shaped, 6–24 by 3–10 μm, with a spiral groove crossing the middle half of the body and three anterior flagella. A slit-like cytostome, enclosing a fourth flagellum, is located in the anterior portion of the body. The lemon-shaped cysts are 6–10 μm in diameter and contain a single nucleus and cytostome (Fig. 2.24).

Chilomastix gallinarum

Description: The body is pear-shaped, 11–20 by 5–12 μm, with a nucleus at the anterior end of the body. There are three anterior flagella and a short fourth flagellum that undulates within a cytostomal cleft that is shaped like a figure 8, which is located on the ventral body spiralling to the left and extending half to two-thirds of the body length (Fig. 2.25). Cysts are lemon-shaped (7–9 × 4–6 μm) with a single nucleus.

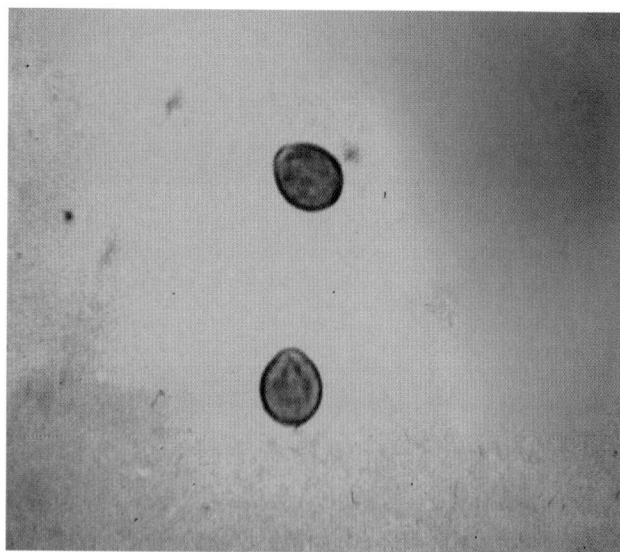

Fig. 2.24 Cysts of *Chilomastix mesnili*.

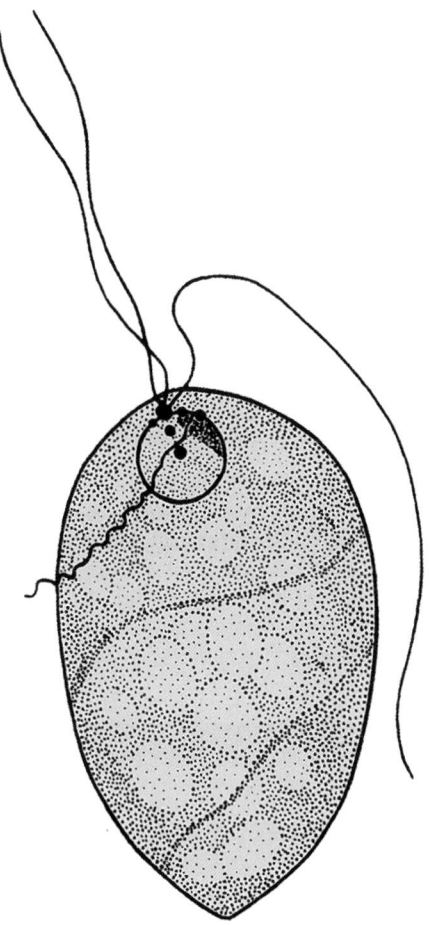

Fig. 2.25 *Chilomastix gallinarum.*

Chilomastix equi

Description: Trophozoites are pyriform, 16–32 by 6–16 μm with a posterior spike.

Chilomastix caprae

Description: Trophozoites are pear-shaped, 8–10 by 4–6 μm.

Chilomastix cuniculi

Description: Trophozoites are pyriform, 10–15 μm long.

Chilomastix intestinalis

Description: Trophozoites are pyriform and 9–28 μm long by 7–11 μm wide. Cysts are 9–11 by 7–10 μm.

Chilomastix wenrichi

Description: Trophozoites are pyriform and 7.5–12 μm long.

Chilomastix bettencourti

Description: Trophozoites are pyriform and 6–24 by 3–10 μm.

ORDER DIPLOMONADIDA

FAMILY SPIRONUCLEIDAE

The family Spironucleidae contains one main genus of veterinary interest, *Spironucleus*, and a few minor genera considered to be non-pathogenic in animals. *Spironucleus* (*Hexamita*) is a cause of enteritis and diarrhoea in birds (particularly poultry, gamebirds and pigeons) and rodents.

Spironucleus

Trophozoites are bilaterally symmetrical, possessing two nuclei, two sets of three anterior flagella and two flagella which pass through the body to emerge posteriorly (Table 2.12). These parasites used to be referred to as *Hexamita*, but members of the latter genus are usually free-living.

Spironucelus columbae

Synonyms: *Hexamita columbae, Octomitus columbae*

Description: Trophozoites are small, measuring 5–9 by 2.5–7 μm.

Spironucleus meleagridis

Synonyms: *Hexamita meleagridis*

Description: Trophozoites are bilaterally symmetrical, 6–12 by 2–5 μm, and possess two nuclei, two sets of three anterior flagella and two flagella that pass through the body to emerge posteriorly (Fig. 2.26).

Spironucleus muris

Synonyms: *Hexamita muris, Octomitus muris, Syndyomita muris*

Description: The body is pyriform, 7–9 by 2–3 μm, with two nuclei near the anterior end and six anterior and two posterior flagella. There is no cytostome.

Table 2.12 *Spironucleus* species.

Species	Hosts	Site
Spironucleus columbae (syn. Hexamita columbae, Octomitus columbae)	Pigeons	Small intestine
Spironucleus meleagridis (syn. Hexamita meleagridis)	Turkeys, gamebirds (pheasants, quails, partridges)	Small intestine, caeca
Spironucleus muris (syn. Hexamita muris, Octomitus muris, Syndyomita muris)	Mice, rats, hamsters	Small intestine, caecum
Spironucleus pitheci	Monkeys	Large intestine

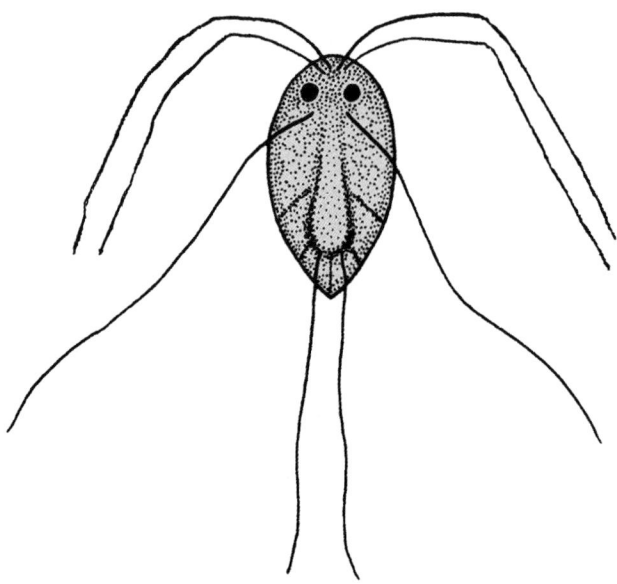

Fig. 2.26 *Spironucleus meleagridis.*

FAMILY CAVIOMONADIDAE

Members of the family include *Caviomonas* which are found in the caecum of guinea pigs.

Caviomonas

Trophozoites have a single flagellum and no cytostome.

Caviomonas mobilis

This species infects the caecum of guinea pigs and hamsters.

Description: Trophozoites have an ovoid to carrot-shaped body, 2–7 μm long by 2–3 μm wide, with a pointed posterior end. A single flagellum arises from the nucleus at the anterior end and extends posteriorly along the periphery of the body surface.

FAMILY ENTEROMONADIDAE

Enteromonas

Trophozoites are spherical or pyriform and possess an anterior nucleus, a strand-like funis, three short anterior flagella and a long fourth flagellum extending posteriorly beyond the body (Table 2.13).

Table 2.13 *Enteromonas* species.

Species	Hosts	Site
Enteromonas caviae	Guinea pigs	Caecum
Enteromonas hominis (syn. *Octomitus hominis*, *Tricercomonas intestinalis*, *Enteromonas bengalensis*)	Rats, hamsters, humans, primates (chimpanzees, macaques)	Caecum

Enteromonas caviae

Description: Trophozoites are 3–5 μm long and 2–4 μm wide.

Enteromonas hominis

Synonyms: *Octomitus hominis, Tricercomonas intestinalis, Enteromonas bengalensis*

Description: Trophozoites are 4–10 μm long and 3–6 μm wide and contain numerous food vacuoles.

FAMILY GIARDIIDAE

Giardia is a common cause of chronic diarrhoea in humans and infection also occurs in wild and domestic animals (Table 2.14). The organism is bilaterally symmetrical and possesses eight flagella, six of which emerge as free flagella at intervals around the body. It is unique in possessing a large adhesive disc on the flat ventral surface of the body, which facilitates attachment to the epithelial cells of the intestinal mucosa.

Giardia

Trophozoites of *Giardia* have a pyriform to ellipsoid, bilaterally symmetrical body, 12–15 μm long by 5–9 μm wide. The dorsal side is convex and there is a large sucking disc on the ventral side (Fig. 2.27). There are two anterior nuclei, two slender axostyles, eight flagella in four pairs and a pair of darkly staining median bodies (Fig. 2.28). The median bodies are curved bars resembling the claws of a hammer. Cysts are ovoid, 8–12 by 7–10 μm, and contain four nuclei (Fig. 2.29).

At least 10 species have been distinguished on the basis of light microscopic characteristics (shape of trophozoite and median body) and more recently using molecular methods, which group the species into assemblages, a system which is still evolving.

Table 2.14 *Giardia* species.

Species	Assemblages	Hosts	Site
Giardia intestinalis (syn. *Giardia duodenalis*)	A	Humans, primates, dogs, cats, livestock, rodents, wild mammals	Small intestine
Giardia enterica	B	Humans, primates, dogs, cats, some wild mammals	Small intestine
Giardia canis	C, D	Dogs, other canids	Small intestine
Giardia bovis	E	Cattle, other ungulates	Small intestine
Giardia cati	F	Cats	Small intestine
Giardia simondi	G	Rats	Small intestine
Giardia spp.	H	Pinnipeds	Small intestine
Giardia muris		Rodents	Small intestine
Giardia microti		Rodents	Small intestine
Giardia psittaci		Birds	Small intestine
Giardia ardeae		Birds	Small intestine

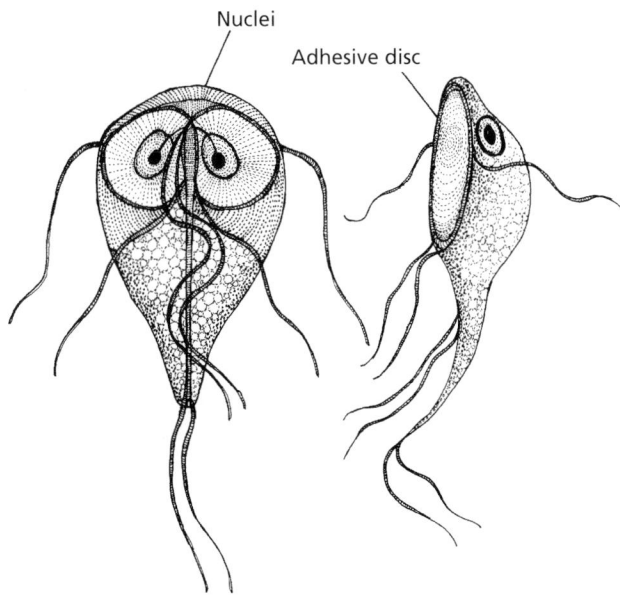

Nuclei

Adhesive disc

Fig. 2.27 Trophozoite of *Giardia intestinalis*.

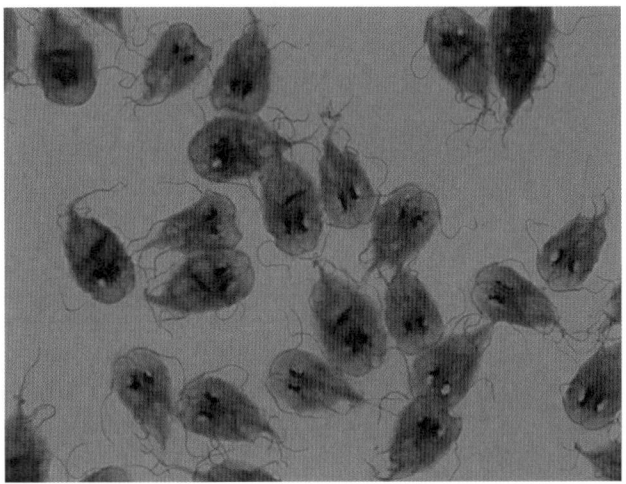

Fig. 2.28 *Giardia intestinalis* trophozoite. (Courtesy of Andrei Mihalca).

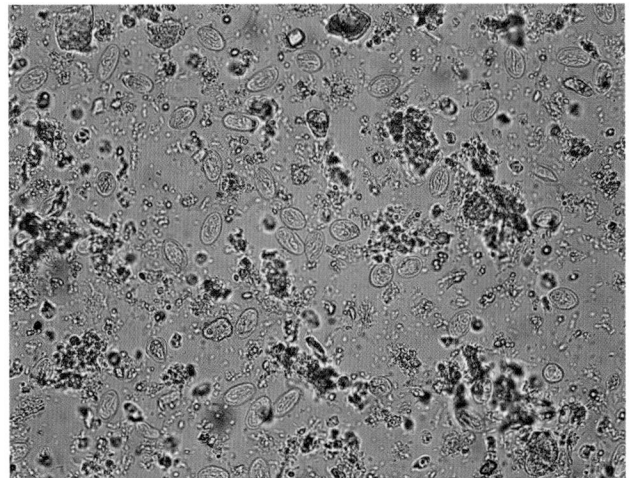

Fig. 2.29 *Giardia* cysts. (Courtesy of Walter Basso).

Life cycle: The life cycle is simple and direct, the trophozoite stage dividing by binary fission to produce further trophozoites. Intermittently, trophozoites encyst, forming resistant cyst stages that pass out of the host in the faeces. See **life cycle** 31.

CLASS ANAERONONADEA

ORDER OXYMONADIDA

FAMILY POLYMASTIGIDAE

Monocercomonoides

Species of this genus have an anterior nucleus, two pairs of anterior flagella, a pelta and a filamentous axostyle. There are 1–4 costa-like structures (funises) extending backwards beneath the body surface. Members of this genus occur in mammals, amphibian, reptiles and insects and are considered non-pathogenic (Table 2.15).

Monocercomonoides caviae

Description: Trophozoites are ovoid, 4–8 µm long by 3–7 µm wide and have three funises.

Monocercomonoides wenrichi

Description: Trophozoites are 3–12 µm long by 3–8 µm wide and have a thick, single, sinuous funis.

Monocercomonoides quadrifunilis

Description: Trophozoites are 3–13 µm long by 3–11 µm wide and have four funises.

Monocercomonoides exilis

Description: Trophozoites are 4–9 µm long by 3–6 µm wide and have a single short funis.

Monocercomonoides caprae

Synonyms: *Monocercomonas caprae, Monocercomonoides sayeedi*

Description: Trophozoites are ovoid, 6–12 µm long by 4–8 µm wide.

PHYLUM APICOMPLEXA

Protozoa within the phylum Apicomplexa (Sporozoa) are characterised by their intracellular lifestyle and possession of an apical complex at some stage of their development. The trophozoites have no cilia or flagella. Reproduction involves both asexual (merogony or schizogony) and sexual (gametogony) phases.

LIFE CYCLE 31. LIFE CYCLE OF *GIARDIA INTESTINALIS*

Giardia intestinalis is a flagellate protozoan intestinal parasite with an oro-faecal life cycle, infecting several animal species (e.g. canids, felids, ruminants), including humans (1). Hosts acquire the infection through the ingestion of cysts excreted with the faeces (2). Following ingestion, and once in the intestinal tract, the outer wall of the cysts ruptures, thus freeing trophozoites (3). Each pear-shaped trophozoite (10 × 15 µm) is binucleate and provided with four pairs of flagella; the trophozoite is also equipped with a ventral disc that adheres to the surface of enteric cells (4). Trophozoites replicate in the colon by binary fission (5) and eventually generate mature cysts (6). The cysts are oval in shape (8 × 10 µm) and characterised by a double outer wall, posterior tail, four nuclei and corresponding parabasal bodies (6). The cysts, excreted via the host faeces, contaminate water and feedstuffs, and can thus be ingested by and infect new susceptible hosts (1).

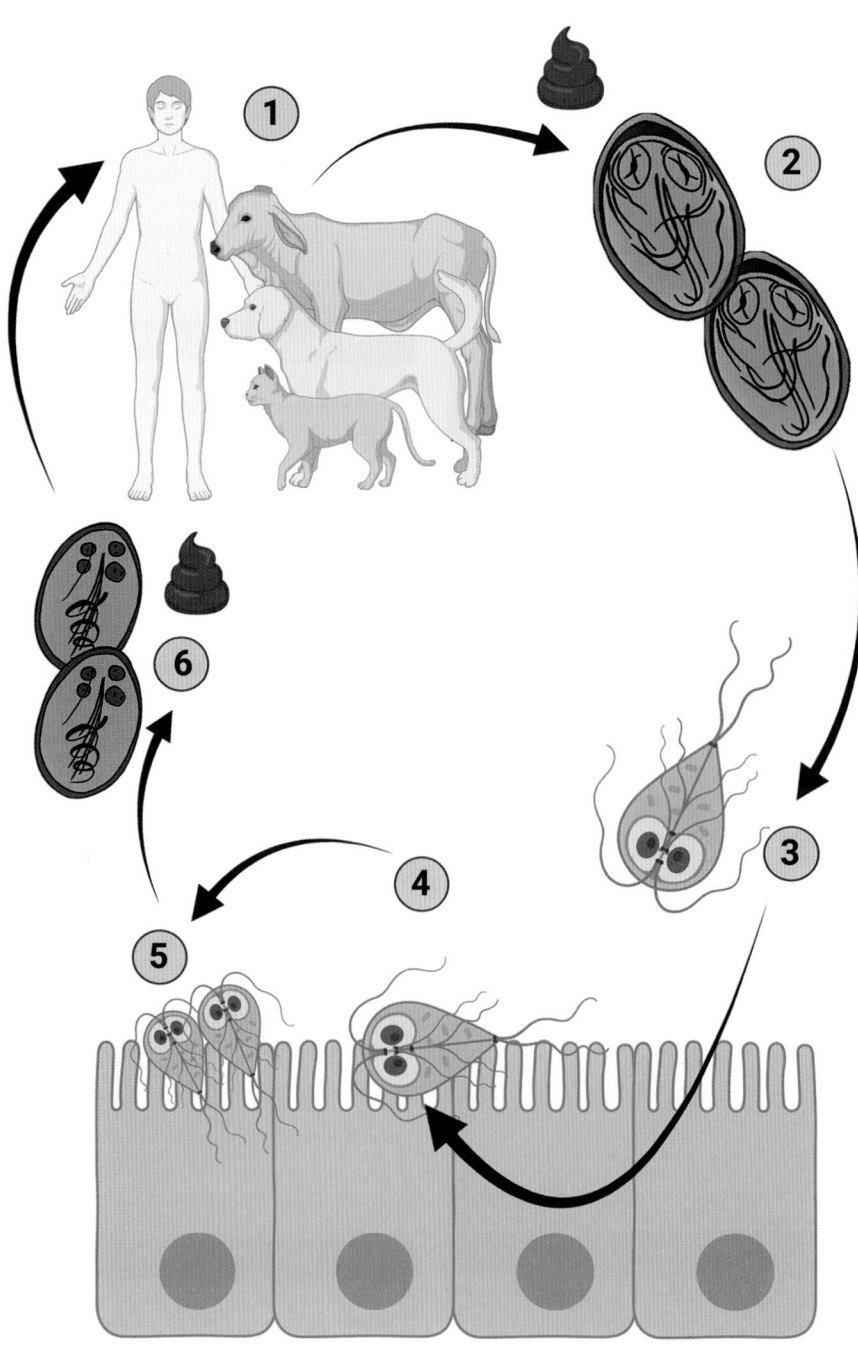

Table 2.15 *Monocercomonoides* species.

Species	Hosts	Site
Monocercomonoides caviae	Guinea pigs	Caecum
Monocercomonoides wenrichi	Guinea pigs	Caecum
Monocercomonoides quadrifunilis	Guinea pigs	Caecum
Monocercomonoides exilis	Guinea pigs	Caecum
Monocercomonoides caprae (syn. *Monocercomonas caprae, Monocercomonoides sayeedi*)	Goats	Rumen

Following gametogony, a zygote is formed which divides to produce spores (sporogony).

Within the class Conoidasida there is one order of veterinary significance, the Eucoccidiorida, which are intestinal sporozoa. In the class Aconoidasida, there are two genera of veterinary interest, the Haemospororida and Piroplasmorida, which are blood sporozoa.

ORDER EUCOCCIDIORIDA

SUBORDER EIMERIORINA

The Eimeriorina contains parasites which occur mainly in vertebrates. Those of major veterinary importance fall into two families, the Eimeriidae and Sarcocystidae. Other families of lesser significance include the Lankesterellidae, Klossiellidae and Hepatozoidae.

GENERALISED LIFE CYCLE

The life cycle is divided into three phases: sporulation, infection and merogony (schizogony), and finally gametogony and oocyst formation, as represented by the life cycle of the genus *Eimeria*. For differences in life cycles of *Eimeria* spp. see host chapters.

Sporulation

Unsporulated oocysts, consisting of a nucleated mass of protoplasm enclosed by a resistant wall, are passed to the exterior in the faeces. Under suitable conditions of oxygenation, high humidity and optimal temperatures of around 27 °C, the nucleus divides twice and the protoplasmic mass forms four conical bodies radiating from a central mass. Each of these nucleated cones becomes rounded to form a **sporoblast**, while in some species the remaining protoplasm forms the oocyst residual body. Each sporoblast secretes a wall of refractile material and becomes known as a **sporocyst**, while the protoplasm within divides into two banana-shaped **sporozoites**. In some species, the remaining protoplasm within the sporocyst forms a sporocyst residual body and the sporocyst may have a knob at one end, the **Stieda body**. The time taken for these changes varies according to temperature but under optimal conditions usually requires 2–4 days. The oocyst, now consisting of an outer wall enclosing **sporocysts** each containing **sporozoites**, is referred to as a **sporulated oocyst** and is the infective stage.

Infection and merogony (asexual reproduction)

The host becomes infected by ingesting the sporulated oocyst. The sporocysts are then liberated either mechanically or by carbon dioxide, and the sporozoites, activated by trypsin and bile, leave the sporocyst. In most species, each sporozoite penetrates an epithelial cell, rounds up and is then known as a **trophozoite**. After a few days, each trophozoite has divided by multiple fission to form a **meront** (schizont), a structure consisting of a large number of elongated nucleated organisms known as **merozoites**. When division is complete and the meront is mature, the host cell and the meront rupture and the merozoites escape to invade neighbouring cells. Merogony may be repeated, the number of meront generations depending on the species.

Gametogony and oocyst formation (sexual reproduction)

Merogony terminates when the merozoites give rise to male and female gametocytes. The factors responsible for this switch to gametogony are not fully known. The **macrogametocytes** are female and remain unicellular, but increase in size to fill the parasitised cell. They may be distinguished from trophozoites or developing meronts by the fact that they have a single large nucleus. The male **microgametocytes** each undergo repeated division to form a large number of flagellated uninucleate organisms, the **microgametes**. It is only during this brief phase that coccidia have organs of locomotion. The microgametes are freed by rupture of the host cell, one penetrates a macrogamete, and fusion of the microgamete and macrogamete nuclei then takes place. A cyst wall forms around the resulting **zygote**, now known as an oocyst, and no further development usually takes place until this **unsporulated oocyst** is liberated from the body in the faeces.

FAMILY EIMERIIDAE

This family contains 16 genera and some 1340 named species, of which the most important are *Eimeria* and *Isospora*, and infections with these genera are often referred to as 'coccidiosis'. The genera are differentiated on the basis of the number of sporocysts in each oocyst and the number of sporozoites in each sporocyst (Table 2.16). Members of this family are intracellular parasites and most undergo merogony in the intestinal cells of their hosts. The life cycle is usually homoxenous (occurring within one host) and the majority of species are highly host specific. See **life cycle** 32.

Eimeria is the largest genus in the family, containing well over 1000 named species, with a number of important species affecting domestic mammals and birds. Oocysts contain four sporocysts, each with two sporozoites. Oocysts are unsporulated when passed in the faeces and require a period of development before becoming

Table 2.16 Generic identification of coccidian parasites.

Genus	Sporocysts per oocyst	Sporozoites per sporocyst	Total sporozoites per oocyst
Eimeria	4	2	8
Isospora	2	4	8
Caryospora	1	8	8
Cyclospora	2	2	4
Hoarella	16	2	32
Octosporella	8	2	16
Pythonella	16	4	64
Wenyonella	4	4	16
Dorisiella	2	8	16
Tyzzeria	0	8	8

LIFE CYCLE 32. LIFE CYCLE OF *EIMERIA* SPP. IN POULTRY

The main species of *Eimeria* infecting poultry live in the small intestine (*Eimeria necatrix* and *Eimeria acervulina*), the caecum (*Eimeria tenella*) and the large intestine (*Eimeria brunetti*). Chicks ingest sporulated oocysts from the contaminated environment; oocysts are characterised by the presence of four sporocysts, each containing two sporozoites (1). In the intestine, the outer wall of the oocyst and sporocyst ruptures, thus releasing the banana-shaped sporozoites (2); the sporozoites penetrate the enterocytes (3), where they grow in size and become trophozoites (4). A process of nuclear fission occurs inside the infected enterocytes (schizogony), culminating in the formation of a schizont (5). Following a series of cytoplasmic divisions, the enterocyte ruptures, thus freeing several merozoites (6). The merozoites invade other enterocytes and repeat the process of schizogony (asexual replication) for 2–3 additional cycles. Following schizogony, some merozoites become telomerozoites (7), which begin sexual reproduction (gametogony).

Some telomerozoites become microgametocytes (8), while others become macrogametocytes (9). Microgametocytes are motile and characterised by the presence of a flagellum (10), while macrogametocytes are static and characterised by a large nucleus (11). Microgametocytes fertilise the macrogametocytes, thus producing a zygote (12). The zygote is characterised by a double outer wall and represents the precursor of a non-sporulated oocyst (13) which contains the sporont (unorganised genetic material, 14). Once excreted in the environment with the host faeces, the oocyst undergoes sporulation (sporogony), i.e. the process by which the sporont initially forms four conical bodies (sporoblasts, 15) that, in turn, progressively differentiate into four elliptical sporocysts, each containing two sporozoites with a residual body (16). Following sporogony, the mature oocysts (infective stage) contain eight sporozoites, each characterised by a central residual body (17) and an apical micropyle (18).

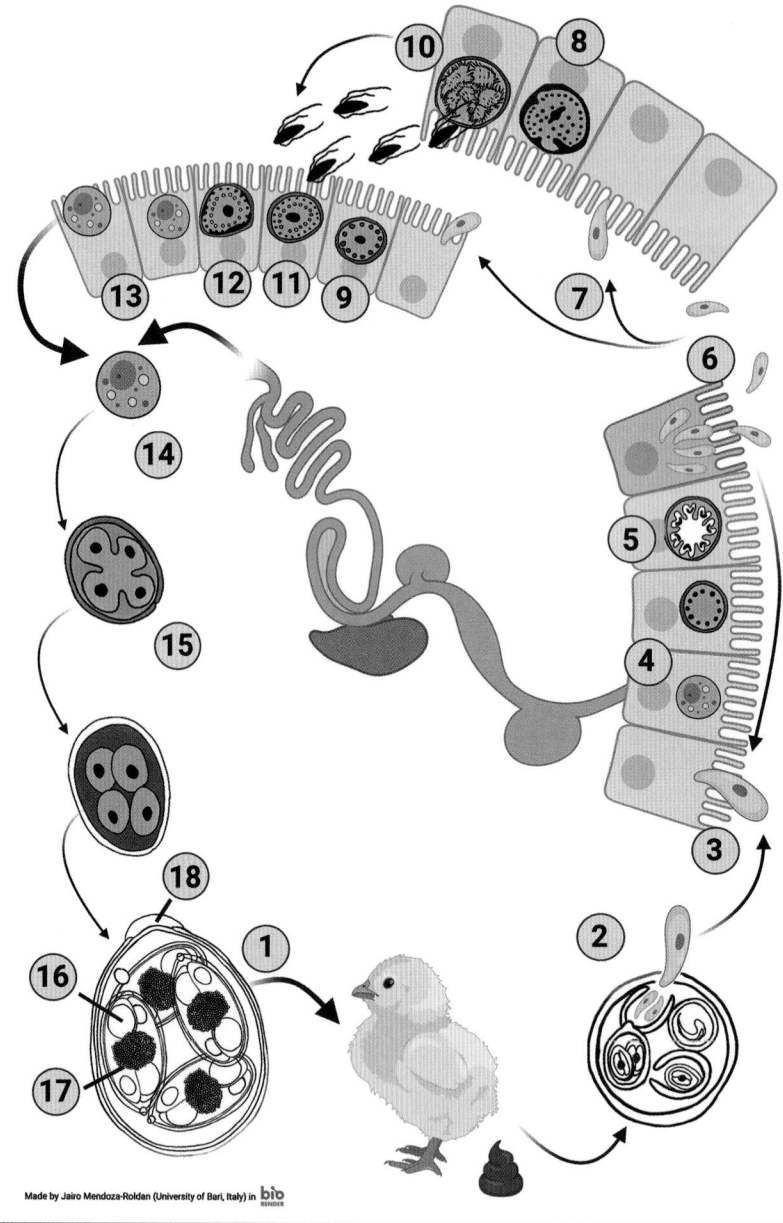

infective. Species of *Eimeria* are capable of causing significant morbidity and mortality and are discussed in detail under their respective hosts. *Isospora* can cause disease in cage birds.

Cyclospora has been reported in monkeys, reptiles and insectivores and has been reported as a cause of gastrointestinal food-borne disease in humans. Oocysts consist of two sporocysts each with two sporozoites.

Caryospora are found primarily in birds and snakes and have a two-host life cycle in which the hosts manifest a predator–prey relationship. Oocysts consist of a single sporocyst with eight sporozoites.

The genus *Isospora* occurs in birds, with about 17 named species. Transmission is by ingestion of sporulated oocysts.

Other genera in this family include *Tyzzeria* and *Wenyonella* in birds and *Hoarella*, *Octosporella*, *Pythonella* and *Dorisiella* in reptiles.

Eimeria

In this genus (Table 2.17), the oocysts contain four sporocysts each with four sporozoites (Fig. 2.30). Both structural and biological characteristics are used to differentiate species of *Eimeria*. Since the endogenous stages of many coccidia are unknown, identification is generally based on oocyst size, morphology and knowledge of the host animal.

Because of the large number of species and host specificity of *Eimeria* species, descriptions of the oocysts by host are detailed in Tables 2.18–2.37. More detailed descriptions, including life cycle stages, are provided within the respective host chapters.

Table 2.17 *Eimeria* species.

Species	Hosts	Site
Eimeria acervulina	Chickens	Duodenum
Eimeria adenoides	Turkeys	Lower small intestine, caeca
Eimeria ahsata	Sheep	Small intestine
Eimeria alabamensis	Cattle, buffalo	Small and large intestine
Eimeria alijevi	Goats	Small and large intestine
Eimeria alpacae	Alpacas	Unknown
Eimeria anatis	Ducks	Small intestine
Eimeria anseris	Geese	Small and large intestine
Eimeria ankarensis	Buffalo	Unknown
Eimeria arctica	Reindeer	Unknown
Eimeria arloingi	Goats	Small intestine
Eimeria asymmetrica	Deer (red deer)	Unknown
Eimeria aspheronica	Goats	Unknown
Eimeria auburnensis	Cattle, buffaloes	Small intestine
Eimeria austriaca	Deer (red deer)	Unknown
Eimeria bactriani (syn. *E. nolleri*)	Camels	Small intestine
Eimeria bakuensis	Sheep	Small intestine
Eimeria bateri	Quails (Japanese, Cortunix)	Unknown
Eimeria bareillyi	Buffalo	Small intestine
Eimeria bovis	Cattle, buffalo	Small and large intestine
Eimeria brasiliensis	Cattle, buffalo	Unknown
Eimeria brunetti	Chickens	Lower small intestine, caeca, rectum
Eimeria bukidnonensis	Cattle, buffalo	Unknown
Eimeria cameli	Camels	Small and large intestine

Table 2.17 *Continued*

Species	Hosts	Site
Eimeria canadensis	Cattle, buffalo	Unknown
Eimeria capralis	Goats	Unknown
Eimeria capreoli	Deer (roe deer)	Unknown
Eimeria caprina	Goats	Small and large intestine
Eimeria caprovina	Goats	Unknown
Eimeria catubrina	Deer (roe deer)	Unknown
Eimeria caucasica	Partridges (rock)	Unknown
Eimeria caviae	Guinea pigs	Large intestine
Eimeria cervi	Deer (red deer)	Unknown
Eimeria charlestoni	Goats	Unknown
Eimeria christenseni	Goats	Small intestine
Eimeria coecicola	Rabbits	Small intestine
Eimeria colchici	Pheasants	Caeca
Eimeria colini	Quails (*Colinus*)	Unknown
Eimeria columbae	Pigeons	Unknown
Eimeria coturnicus	Quails (*Cortunix*)	Unknown
Eimeria crandallis	Sheep	Small and large intestine
Eimeria cylindrica	Cattle	Unknown
Eimeria debliecki	Pigs	Small intestine
Eimeria dispersa	Turkeys	Duodenum
Eimeria dromedarii	Camels	Small intestine
Eimeria duodenalis	Pheasants	Small intestine
Eimeria elaphi	Deer (red deer)	Unknown
Eimeria ellipsoidalis	Cattle, buffalo	Small intestine
Eimeria exigua	Rabbits	Small intestine
Eimeria falciformis	Mice	Small and large intestine
Eimeria faurei	Sheep	Small and large intestine
Eimeria ferruginea	Primates (prosimians)	Unknown
Eimeria flavescens	Rabbits	Small and large intestine
Eimeria galago	Primates (prosimians)	Unknown
Eimeria gokaki	Buffalo	Unknown
Eimeria gallapovonis	Turkeys	Ileum, caeca, rectum
Eimeria gilruthi	Sheep, goats	Abomasum
Eimeria granulosa	Sheep	Unknown
Eimeria grenieri	Guinea fowl	Small intestine
Eimeria hasei	Rats	Unknown
Eimeria hindlei	Mice	Unknown
Eimeria hirci	Goats	Unknown
Eimeria innocua	Turkeys	Small intestine
Eimeria intestinalis	Rabbits	Small intestine
Eimeria intricata	Sheep	Small and large intestine
Eimeria irresidua	Rabbits	Small intestine
Eimeria ivitaensis	Alpacas	Unknown
Eimeria jolchijevi	Goats	Unknown
Eimeria keilini	Mice	Unknown
Eimeria koifoidi	Partridges (grey, chukar, rock)	Small intestine
Eimeria krijgsmanni	Mice	Unknown
Eimeria labbaena (syn. *E. peifferi, E. columbarum*)	Pigeons, doves (rock, collared)	Small intestine
Eimeria lamae	Alpacas	Unknown
Eimeria legionensis	Partridges (red, rock)	Small intestine
Eimeria lemuris	Primates (prosimians)	Unknown
Eimeria leuckarti (syn. *Globidium leuckarti*)	Horses, donkeys	Small intestine
Eimeria macusaniensis	Alpacas	Unknown
Eimeria magna	Rabbits	Small intestine
Eimeria marsica	Sheep	Unknown
Eimeria masseyensis	Goats	Unknown

Continued

Table 2.17 *Continued*

Species	Hosts	Site
Eimeria maxima	Chickens	Mid small intestine
Eimeria mayeri	Reindeer	Unknown
Eimeria media	Rabbits	Small intestine
Eimeria megalostoma	Pheasants	Unknown
Eimeria meleagridis	Turkeys	Caeca
Eimeria meleagrimitis	Turkeys	Duodenum
Eimeria mitis	Chickens	Small and large intestine
Eimeria modesta	Primates (prosimians)	Unknown
Eimeria musculi	Mice	Unknown
Eimeria necatrix	Chickens	Small intestine
Eimeria neodebliecki	Pigs	Unknown
Eimeria nieschulzi	Rats	Small intestine
Eimeria ninakohlyakimovae	Goats	Small and large intestine
Eimeria nocens	Geese	Small intestine
Eimeria nochti	Rats	Unknown
Eimeria numidae	Guinea fowl	Small and large intestine
Eimeria otolicni	Primates (prosimians)	Unknown
Eimeria ovinoidalis	Sheep	Small and large intestine
Eimeria ovoidalis	Buffalo	Unknown
Eimeria pachylepyron	Primates (prosimians)	Unknown
Eimeria pacifica	Pheasants	Small intestine, caeca
Eimeria pallida	Sheep, goats	Unknown
Eimeria panda	Deer (roe deer)	Unknown
Eimeria parva	Sheep	Small and large intestine
Eimeria patavina	Deer (roe deer)	Unknown
Eimeria pellerdyi	Camels	Unknown
Eimeria pellita	Cattle	Unknown
Eimeria perforans	Rabbits	Small intestine
Eimeria perminuta	Pigs	Unknown
Eimeria peruviana	Llamas, alpacas	Unknown
Eimeria phasiani	Pheasants	Small and large intestine
Eimeria pyriformis	Rabbits	Colon
Eimeria polita	Pigs	Small intestine
Eimeria ponderosa	Deer (roe deer)	Unknown
Eimeria porci	Pigs	Small intestine
Eimeria praecox	Chickens	Small intestine
Eimeria procera	Partridges (grey)	Unknown
Eimeria punctata	Sheep, occasionally goats (?)	Unknown
Eimeria punonensis	Alpacas	Unknown
Eimeria rajasthani	Camels	Unknown
Eimeria ratti	Rats	Unknown
Eimeria robusta	Deer (red deer)	Unknown
Eimeria rotunda	Deer (roe deer)	Unknown
Eimeria scabra	Pigs	Small and large intestine
Eimeria scheuffneri	Mice	Unknown
Eimeria separata	Rats	Large intestine
Eimeria solipedum	Horses, donkeys	Small intestine
Eimeria sordida	Deer (red deer)	Unknown
Eimeria spinosa	Pigs	Small intestine
Eimeria stiedai	Rabbits	Liver, bile ducts
Eimeria subrotunda	Turkeys	Small intestine
Eimeria subspherica	Cattle	Unknown
Eimeria suis	Pigs	Unknown
Eimeria superba	Deer (roe deer)	Unknown
Eimeria taldykurganica	Quails (Japanese, Cortunix)	Unknown
Eimeria tarandi	Reindeer	Unknown

Table 2.17 *Continued*

Species	Hosts	Site
Eimeria tenella	Chickens	Small intestine
Eimeria thianethi	Buffalo	Unknown
Eimeria truncata	Geese	Kidney
Eimeria tsunodai	Quails (Japanese)	Caeca
Eimeria tupaiae	Primates (prosimians)	Unknown
Eimeria uniungulata	Horses, donkeys	Small intestine
Eimeria uzura	Quails (Japanese)	Unknown
Eimeria vejdovsyi	Rabbits	Small intestine
Eimeria weybridgensis	Sheep	Small intestine
Eimeria wapiti	Deer (wapiti)	Unknown
Eimeria wyomingensis	Cattle, buffalo	Unknown
Eimeria zuernii	Cattle, buffalo	Small and large intestine

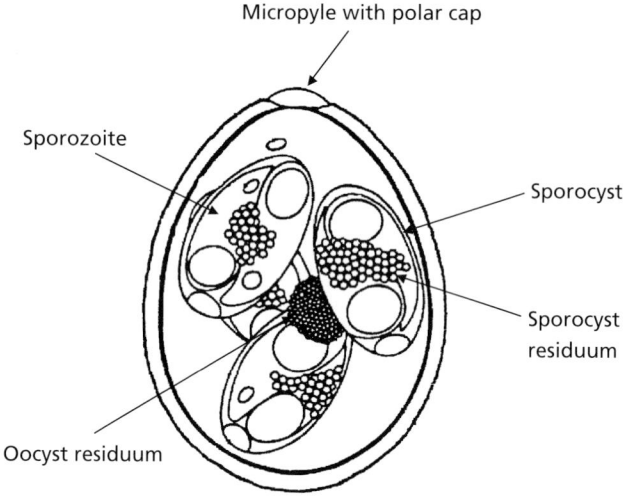

Fig. 2.30 Sporulated oocyst of *Eimeria* with four sporocysts each containing two sporozoites.

Tyzzeria

Parasites of birds; the oocysts contain eight sporozoites and no sporocysts. Species of this genus infect the small intestine of ducks (*Tyzzeria perniciosa*) and geese (*Tyzzeria anseris*).

Tyzzeria perniciosa

Description: Oocysts are ellipsoid, colourless, 10–13 by 9–11 μm (mean 12 × 10 μm), without a micropyle and with a residuum. Sporulated oocysts have no sporocysts and contain eight free-sporozoites (see Table 2.16). First-generation meronts are 12 by 8 μm and contain only a few merozoites. Further meront generations are 15–16 by 14–15 μm and contain more and larger merozoites.

Tyzzeria anseris

Description: Oocysts are ellipsoid, colourless, 10–16 by 9–14 μm, without a micropyle or residuum, with eight free sporozoites.

Table 2.18 *Eimeria* species (cattle).

Species	Description
Eimeria bovis	Oocysts are ovoid or subspherical, colourless, 23–34 by 17–23 μm (mean 27.7 × 20.3 μm) and have a smooth wall with an inconspicuous micropyle, no polar granule or oocyst residuum (Fig. 2.31). Sporocysts are elongate ovoid, 13–18 by 5–8 μm, and have an inconspicuous Stieda body and a sporocyst residuum. The sporozoites are elongate and lie lengthwise head to tail in the sporocysts and usually have a clear globule at each end.
Eimeria zuernii	Oocysts are subspherical, colourless, 15–22 by 13–18 μm (mean 17.8 × 15.6 μm), with no micropyle or oocyst residuum (Fig. 2.32). Sporocysts are ovoid, 7–14 by 4–8 μm, each with a tiny Stieda body, and a sporocyst residuum is usually absent. The sporozoites are elongate and lie head to tail in the sporocysts; each has a clear globule at the large end.
Eimeria alabamensis	Oocysts are usually ovoid, 13–24 by 11–16 μm (mean 18.9 by 13.4 μm) with a smooth colourless wall with no micropyle, polar body or residuum. Sporocysts are ellipsoid, 10–16 by 4–6 μm with a tiny Stieda body and a sporocyst residuum. The sporozoites lie lengthwise head to tail in the sporocysts and have 1–3 clear globules. First-generation meronts are usually ovoid, 7–9 by 5.5–8 μm, containing 8–16 merozoites. Second-generation meronts are 9–12 by 6–9 μm, ovoid or ellipsoid in shape and contain 18–26 merozoites.
Eimeria auburnensis	Elongated, ovoid, yellowish-brown, with smooth or heavily granulated wall with a micropyle and polar granule, but no oocyst residuum (mean 38 by 23 μm).
Eimeria brasiliensis	Ellipsoid, yellowish-brown, with a micropyle covered by a distinct polar cap. Polar granules may also be present but there is no oocyst residuum (mean 37 by 27 μm).
Eimeria bukidnonensis	Pear-shaped or oval, tapering at one pole, yellowish-brown, with a thick, radially striated wall and micropyle. A polar granule may be present but there is no oocyst residuum (mean 49 by 35 μm).
Eimeria canadensis	Ovoid or ellipsoid, colourless or pale yellow, with an inconspicuous micropyle, one or more polar granules and an oocyst residuum (mean 33 by 23 μm).
Eimeria cylindrica	Elongated, cylindrical, with a colourless smooth wall, no micropyle and no oocyst residuum (mean 23 by 12 μm).
Eimeria ellipsoidalis	Ellipsoid to slightly ovoid, colourless, with no discernible micropyle, polar granule or oocyst residuum (mean 23 by 16 μm).
Eimeria pellita	Egg-shaped, very thick brown wall with evenly distributed protuberances, with a micropyle and polar granule consisting of several rod-like bodies but no oocyst residuum (mean 40 by 28 μm).
Eimeria subspherica	Round or subspherical, colourless, with no micropyle, polar granule or oocyst residuum (mean 11 by 10 μm).
Eimeria wyomingensis	Ovoid, yellowish brown, with a thick wall, a wide micropyle but no polar granule or oocyst residuum (mean 40 by 28 μm).
Eimeria ankarensis	Oocysts are ovoid, with a micropyle and thick yellowish-brown wall (mean 37.5 by 27 μm). Sporocysts are elongate, almost ellipsoid, with a Stieda body and residuum, with sporozoites that are elongate and comma-shaped with two clear globules. Sporulation time is 3–4 days.
Eimeria bareillyi	Oocysts are pyriform, with a micropyle and residuum and a smooth brown wall (mean 29.5 by 20 μm). Sporocysts are lemon-shaped, with a Stieda body and residuum, and with sporozoites that are banana-shaped with a clear globule at the large end and sometimes 1–2 smaller ones.
Eimeria gokaki	Oocysts are ovoid, with an orange wall and micropyle but without a residuum (mean 26.5 by 21.5 μm). Sporocysts are elongate.
Eimeria ovoidalis	Oocysts are ovoid, with a pinkish-orange wall and micropyle but without a residuum (mean 36 by 24 μm). Sporocysts are ovoid with a Stieda body and residuum. The sporulation time is 4–5 days.
Eimeria thianethi	Oocysts are ovoid, with a greyish-yellow wall and distinct micropyle but without a residuum (mean 44 by 26 μm). Sporocysts are lemon-shaped with a pointed end and residuum.

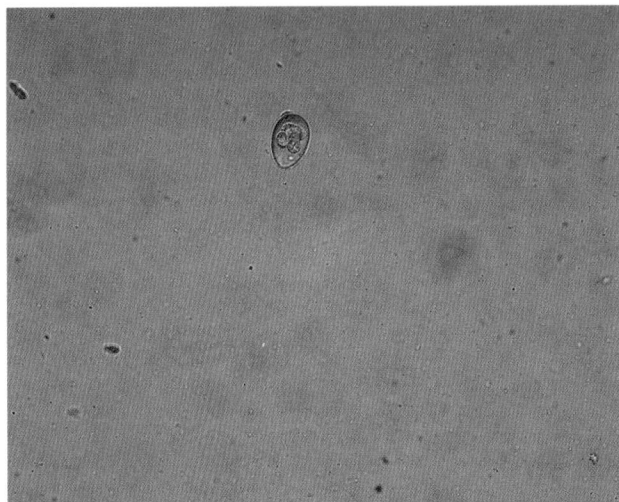

Fig. 2.31 Oocysts of *Eimeria bovis*. (Courtesy of Laura Rinaldi).

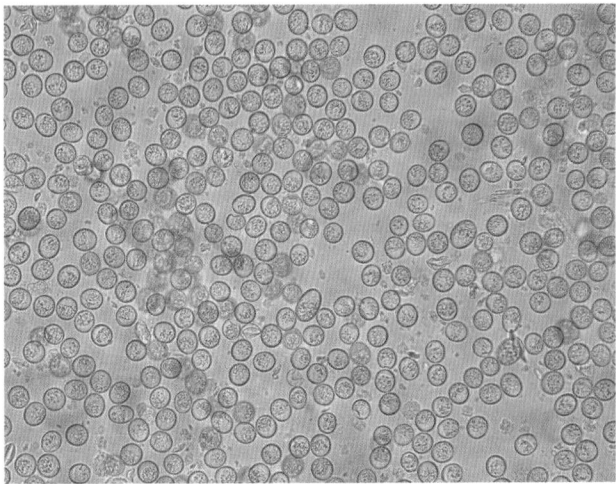

Fig. 2.32 Oocysts of *Eimeria zuernii*. (Courtesy of Anja Joachim).

Table 2.19 *Eimeria* species (sheep).

Species	Description
Eimeria crandallis	Oocysts are subspherical to broadly ellipsoid, 17–23 by 17–22 µm (mean 21.9 × 19.4 µm), with a micropyle, which may be distinct or indistinct, and a micropylar cap (Fig. 2.33; see also Fig. 4.37). One or more polar granules may be present and there is no residuum. The sporocysts are broadly ovoid, 8–13 by 6–9 µm. There is no Stieda body but a residuum may be present. The sporozoites lie transversely at the ends of the sporocysts and have 1– clear globules. Mature first-generation meronts are 250 µm in diameter and are visible to the naked eye as pin-point white spots, occurring most frequently in the lower jejunum. They contain an average of 253 000 first-generation merozoites measuring 10 by 1.7 µm.
Eimeria ovinoidalis	Oocysts are ellipsoid, colourless or pale-yellow, 17–30 by 14–19 µm (mean 19 × 13 µm). There is an inconspicuous micropyle without a micropylar cap (Fig. 2.34; see also Fig. 4.37). Two or more polar granules are present and there is no residuum. Sporocysts are elongate ovoid, 10–14 by 4–8 µm. Each has a Stieda body and a residuum. The sporozoites are elongate, 11–14 by 2–4 µm, and lie lengthwise head to tail in the sporocysts. Each has one large and one small globule. First-generation meronts, at 10 days, average 290 µm in diameter and contain many thousands of merozoites (Fig. 2.35). Second-generation meronts mature at about 10–11 days and have a mean diameter of 12 µm, each containing an average of 24 merozoites. The mature microgamonts average 15 by 12 µm and contain many microgametes arranged peripherally around a central residuum, while mature macrogamonts average 16 by 12 µm.
Eimeria ahsata	The oocysts are ellipsoid to ovoid, yellowish-brown, 29–37 by 17–28 µm (mean 33.4 × 22.6 µm) with a micropyle and a micropylar cap and have one or occasionally more polar granules, without a residuum (Fig. 2.36; see also Fig. 4.37). Sporocysts are 12–22 by 6–10 µm without a Stieda body and with a residuum. The sporozoites are elongate, and lie lengthways head to tail in the sporocysts, and have 1–3 clear globules each. First-generation meronts average 184 by 165 µm and may reach 265 by 162 µm by 15 days post infection and contain several thousand merozoites. Second-generation meronts measure 52 by 39 µm and contain approximately 50 merozoites. Intranuclear stages have been observed in small intestinal epithelial cells 15, 18 and 19 days after experimental infection. The developing parasites are 1.6–5 µm in size and are mostly localised within a tiny cavity of the nucleus. Each intranuclear parasite is surrounded by a halo, and most contain 2–4 dark-staining and probably dividing nuclei and appear to be second-generation merozoites. The macrogamonts are 35–45 µm in diameter and the microgamonts are 6.5 by 26 µm.
Eimeria bakuensis	Oocysts are ellipsoid, pale yellowish-brown, and measure 23–36 by 15–24 µm. There is a micropyle and micropylar cap, one or more polar granules and no residuum (Fig. 2.37; see also Fig. 4.37). The sporocysts are elongate ovoid, 11–17 by 6–9 µm, and contain a residuum and sometimes an inconspicuous Stieda body. Sporozoites are elongate and lie lengthwise head to tail in the sporocysts and have a large clear globule at the broad end and a smaller one at the narrow end. Meronts when mature are 122–146 µm in diameter and contain hundreds of thousands of merozoites (9 × 2 µm).
Eimeria faurei	Ovoid, pale yellowish-brown, without oocyst residuum or sporocyst residuum (mean 32 by 23 µm) (Fig. 2.38).
Eimeria granulosa	Urn-shaped with large micropolar cap at broad end, yellowish-brown, without oocyst residuum (mean 29 by 21 µm) (Fig. 2.39).
Eimeria intricata	Ellipsoid, thick and striated wall, brown, no oocyst residuum (mean 48 by 44 µm) (Fig. 2.40).
Eimeria marsica	Ellipsoid, with inconspicuous micropyle, colourless or pale yellow, without oocyst or sporocyst residuum (mean 19 by 13 µm) (Fig. 2.41).
Eimeria pallida	Ellipsoid, thin-walled, colourless to pale yellow, without oocyst residuum but with sporocyst residuum (mean 14 by 10 µm) (Fig. 2.42).
Eimeria parva	Spherical to subspherical, colourless, no oocyst residuum, sporocyst residuum composed of few granules (mean 17 by 14 µm) (Fig. 2.43).
Eimeria weybridgensis	Broadly ellipsoid or subspherical, micropyle with or without polar cap, without oocyst or sporocyst residuum (mean 24 by 17 µm) (Fig. 2.44).
Eimeria punctata	Oocysts are ellipsoid to ovoid, micropyle with or without polar cap, with oocyst residuum; sporocyst elongate ovoid with residuum (mean 24 by 18 µm).

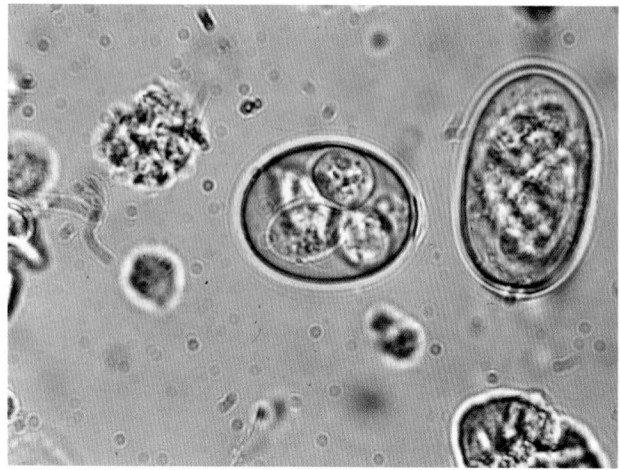

Fig. 2.33 Oocysts of *Eimeria crandallis*.

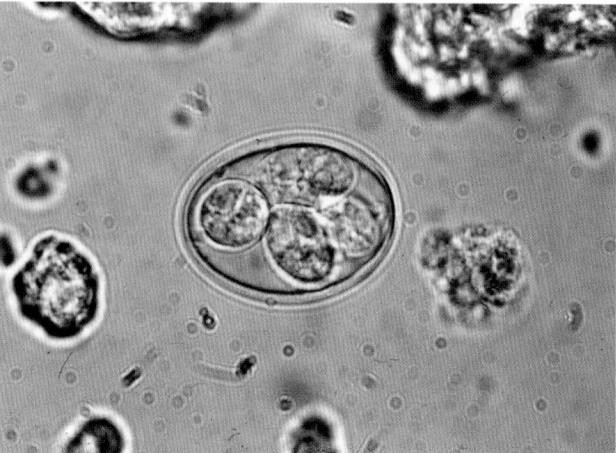

Fig. 2.34 Oocyst of *Eimeria ovinoidalis*.

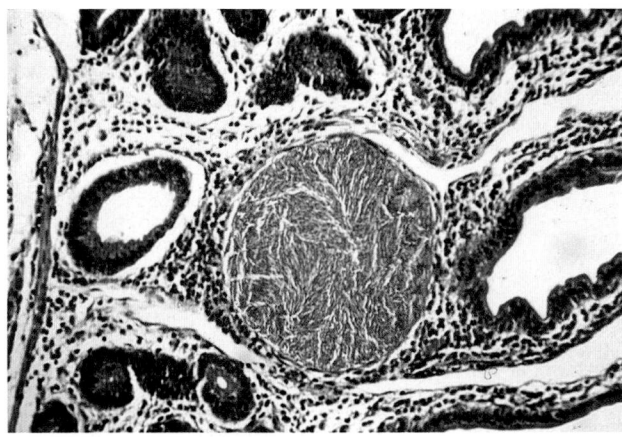

Fig. 2.35 First-generation ('giant') meront of *Eimeria ovinoidalis*. Each meront contains thousands of merozoites.

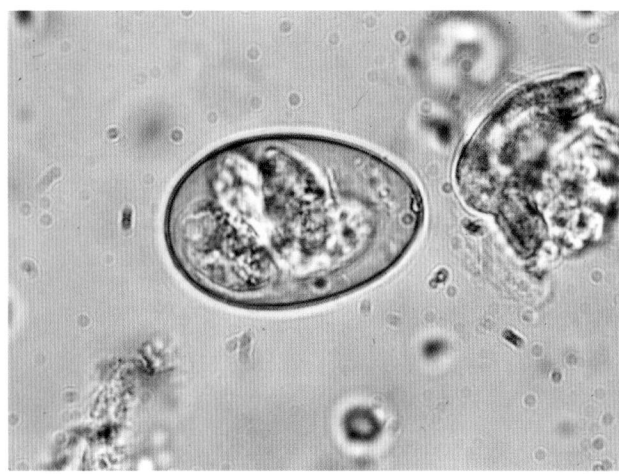

Fig. 2.38 Oocyst of *Eimeria faurei*.

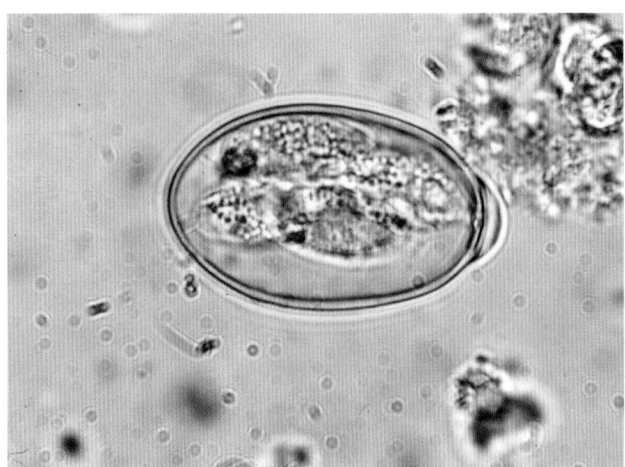

Fig. 2.36 Oocyst of *Eimeria ahsata*.

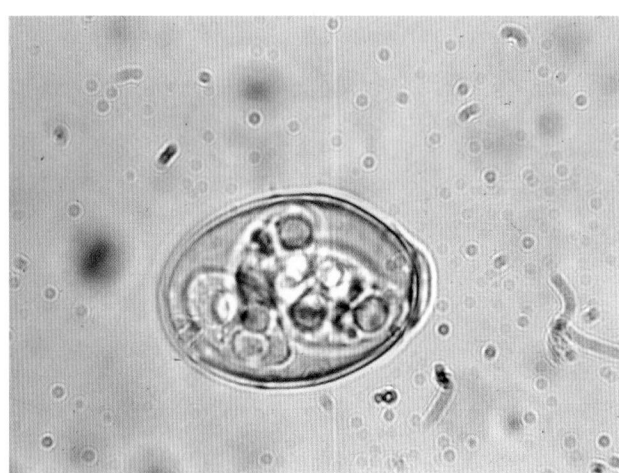

Fig. 2.39 Oocyst of *Eimeria granulosa*.

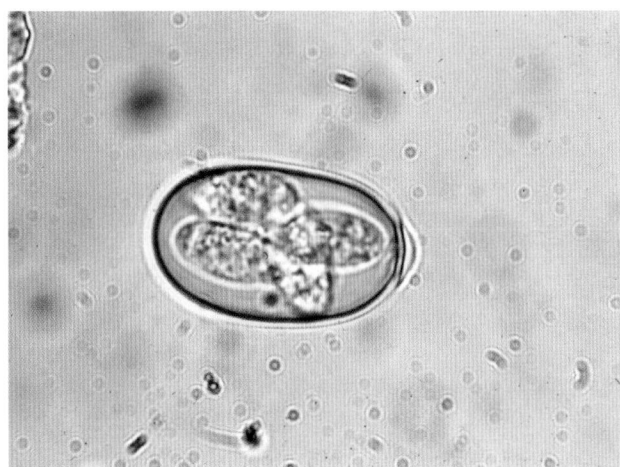

Fig. 2.37 Oocyst of *Eimeria bakuensis*.

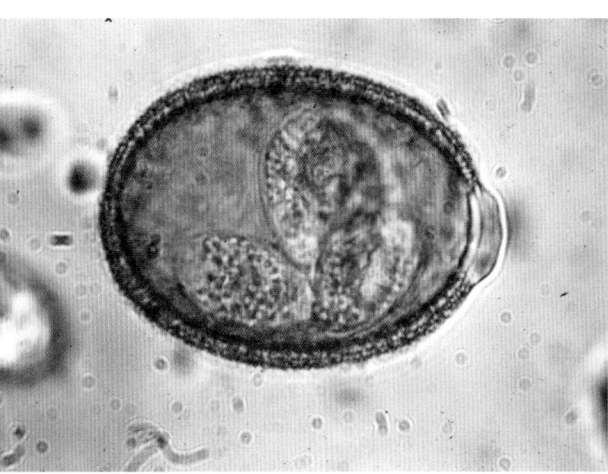

Fig. 2.40 Oocyst of *Eimeria intricata*.

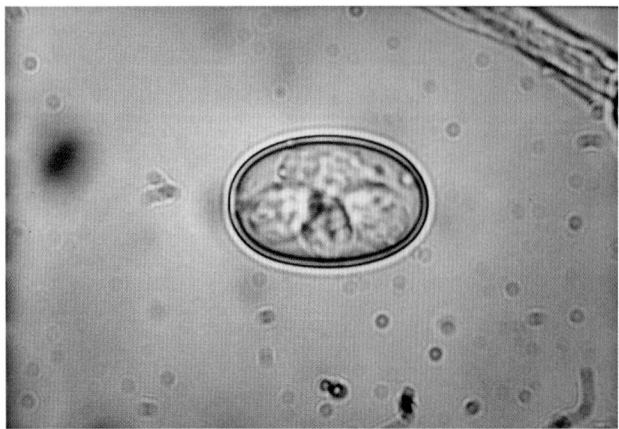

Fig. 2.41 Oocyst of *Eimeria marsica*.

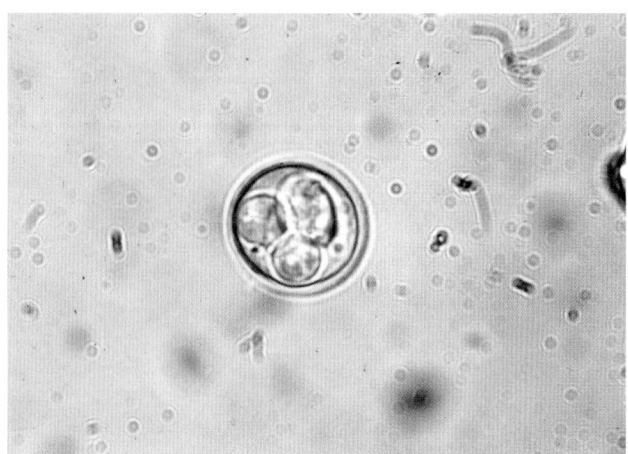

Fig. 2.43 Oocyst of *Eimeria parva*.

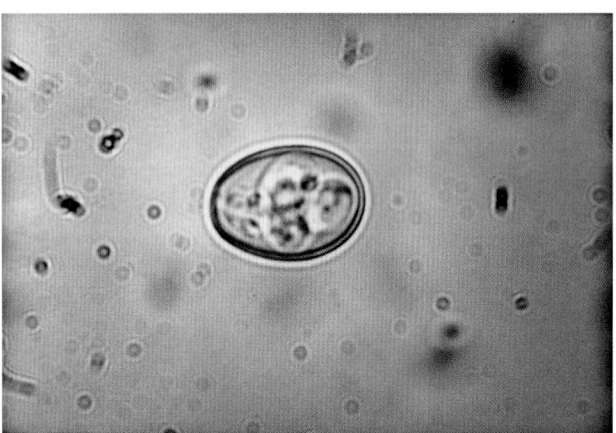

Fig. 2.42 Oocyst of *Eimeria pallida*.

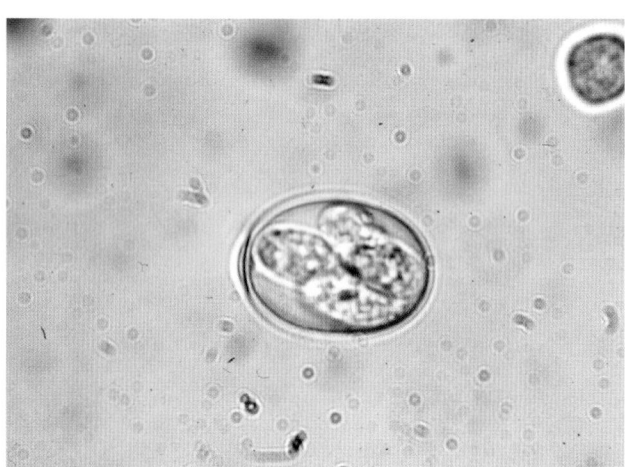

Fig. 2.44 Oocyst of *Eimeria weybridgensis*.

Table 2.20 *Eimeria* species (goats).

Species	Description
Eimeria caprina	Oocysts are ellipsoid or slightly ovoid, dark brown to brownish-yellow in colour, 27–40 by 19–26 µm with a smooth wall. There is a micropyle but no micropylar cap or oocyst residuum (Fig. 2.45; see also Fig. 4.37). One or more polar granules are present. Sporocysts are elongate ovoid, 13–17 by 7–10 µm, with a small Stieda body and a residuum. The sporozoites are elongate, lie lengthwise head to tail in the sporocysts and usually have a large clear globule at the large end and a smaller one at the small end.
Eimeria ninakohlyakimovae	Ellipsoid, thin-walled, colourless, micropyle absent or indistinct, without oocyst residuum but with sporocyst residuum (mean 21 by 15 µm) (Fig. 2.46).
Eimeria christenseni	The oocysts are ovoid or ellipsoid, 27–44 by 17–31 µm (mean 38 × 25 µm), colourless to pale yellow, with a micropyle and micropylar cap (Fig. 2.47; see also Fig. 4.37). One or more polar granules are present but there is no oocyst residuum. Sporocysts are broadly ovoid, 12–18 by 8–11 µm. Each has a residuum and the Stieda body is either vestigial or absent. The sporozoites are elongate and lie lengthwise head to tail in the sporocysts. Each has one or more clear globules. First-generation meronts when mature are ellipsoid, 100–277 by 81–130 µm and contain thousands of straight merozoites about 6–8 by 1–2 µm. Second-generation meronts are 9–20 by 8–12 µm and contain 8–24 merozoites and sometimes a residuum. Mature macrogametes are 19–35 by 13–25 µm and mature microgamonts are 19–50 by 12–40 µm and contain hundreds of comma-shaped microgametes (3 × 0.5 µm) and a residuum.
Eimeria hirci	Oocysts are ellipsoid to subspherical, light brown to brownish-yellow, 18–23 by 14–19 µm (mean 20.7 × 16.2 µm), with a micropyle and micropylar cap, one or more polar granules but no oocyst residuum (Fig. 2.48; see also Fig. 4.37). Sporocysts are ovoid, 8–14 by 4–9 µm with a tiny Stieda body and a residuum. The sporozoites lie lengthwise, at an angle, or even at the ends of the sporocysts and have 1–2 clear globules.
Eimeria alijevi	Oocysts are ovoid or ellipsoid, pale yellowish to colourless, 15–23 by 12–22 µm (mean 17 × 15 µm), with an inconspicuous micropyle without a micropylar cap or residuum, and one polar granule (Fig. 2.49; see also Fig. 4.37). Sporocysts are elongate to ovoid, 7–13 by 4–9 µm, with or without a Stieda body and with a sporocyst residuum. The sporozoites are elongate and lie at an angle or lengthwise head to tail in the sporocysts and usually have 1–2 clear globules. First-generation meronts are 260 by 180 µm and can be seen grossly as whitish bodies. Second-generation meronts are 15–18 by 9–12 µm. The macrogamonts are 14–18 by 9–14 µm, and the microgamonts 22–25 by 15–20 µm.

Table 2.20 *Continued*

Species	Description
Eimeria arloingi	Oocysts are ellipsoid or slightly ovoid, 17–42 by 14–19 µm (mean 27 × 18 µm), with a thick wall and a micropyle and micropylar cap present (Fig. 2.50; see also Fig. 4.37). There are one or more polar granules but no oocyst residuum. Sporocysts are ovoid, 10–17 by 5–10 µm with a sporocyst residuum, but the Stieda body is either vestigial or not present. The sporozoites are elongate and lie lengthwise head to tail in the sporocysts and usually have a large clear globule at the large end and a small one at the small end. First-generation meronts are 130–350 by 65–240 µm and contain many thousands of merozoites 9–12 by 1–2 µm. Second-generation meronts are 11–44 by 9–20 µm and contain 8–24 merozoites, which are 4–10 µm long. The microgamonts are 19–34 by 13–29 µm and contain a large residuum and several hundred microgametes. The macrogametes are similarly sited and are 19–28 by 14–20 µm.
Eimeria aspheronica	Ovoid, greenish to yellow-brown, with micropyle, without oocyst residuum but with sporocyst residuum (mean 31 by 32 µm) (Fig. 2.51).
Eimeria caprovina	Oocysts are ellipsoid to subspherical, 26–36 by 21–28 µm (mean 30 × 24 µm), colourless, with a micropyle but without a micropylar cap (Fig. 2.52; see also Fig. 4.37). One or more polar granules are present. There is no oocyst residuum. Sporocysts are elongate ovoid, 13–17 by 8–9 µm, and each has a Stieda body and a residuum. The sporozoites are elongate, lie lengthwise head to tail in the sporocysts and have a large clear globule at each end.
Eimeria jolchijevi	Oocysts are ellipsoid or ovoid, pale yellow, 26–37 by 18–26 µm (mean 31 × 22 µm), with a micropyle at the broad end and a prominent micropylar cap (Fig. 2.53; see also Fig. 4.37). There is no oocyst residuum. Sporocysts are ovoid, 12–18 by 6–10 µm, with a small Stieda body and a residuum. The sporozoites are elongate and lie lengthwise head to tail in the sporocysts and have one or more large clear globules.
Eimeria capralis	Ellipsoid with a distinct micropylar cap, with Stieda body and sporocyst residuum (mean 29 by 20 µm) (Fig. 2.54).
Eimeria masseyensis	Ellipsoid to ovoid, with Stieda body and distinct micropylar cap (mean 22 by 17 µm) (Fig. 2.55).
Eimeria charlestoni	Ellipsoid with no micropylar cap. Distinctive elongate sporocysts containing prominent refractile bodies (mean 23 by 17 µm) (Fig. 2.56).

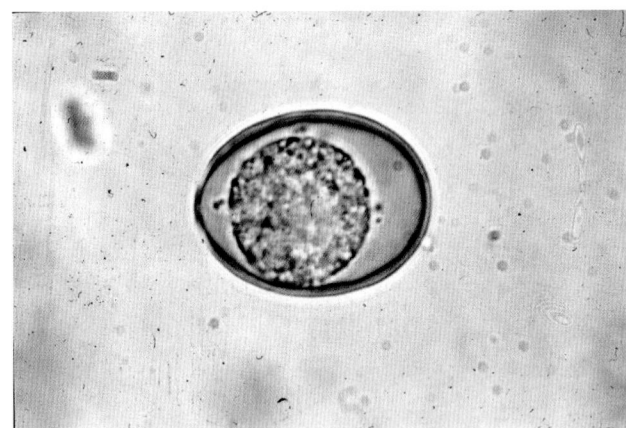

Fig. 2.45 Oocyst of *Eimeria caprina.*

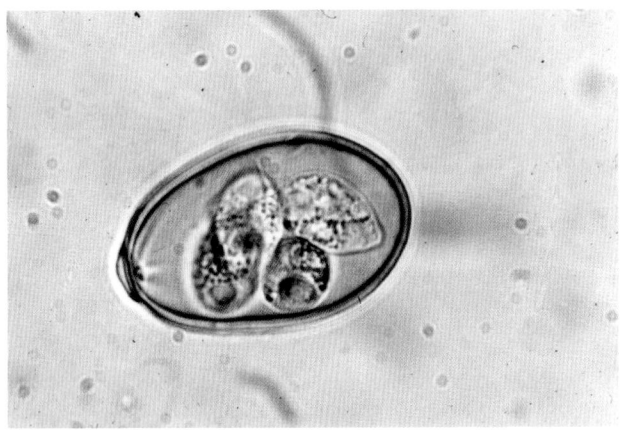

Fig. 2.47 Oocyst of *Eimeria christenseni.*

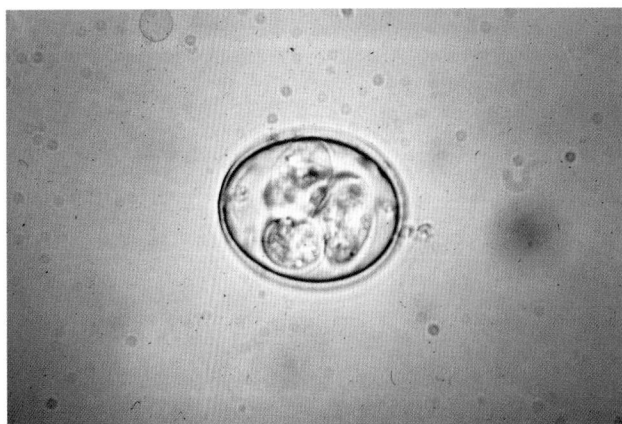

Fig. 2.46 Oocyst of *Eimeria ninakohlyakimovae.*

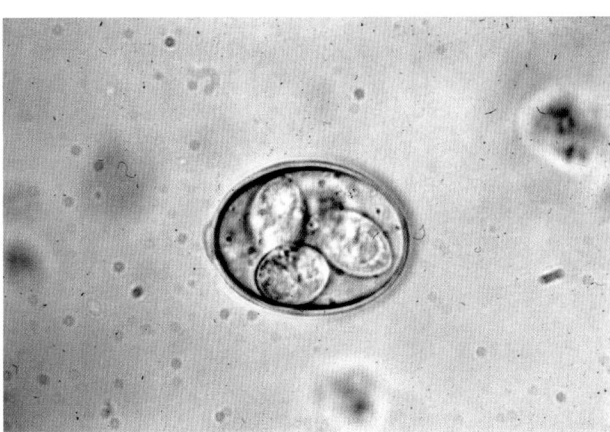

Fig. 2.48 Oocyst of *Eimeria hirci.*

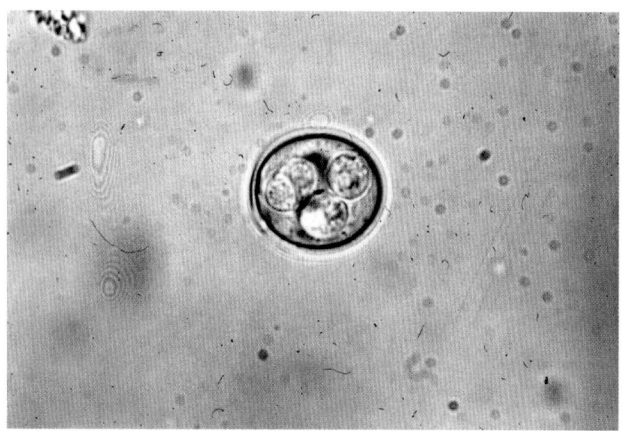

Fig. 2.49 Oocyst of *Eimeria alijevi*.

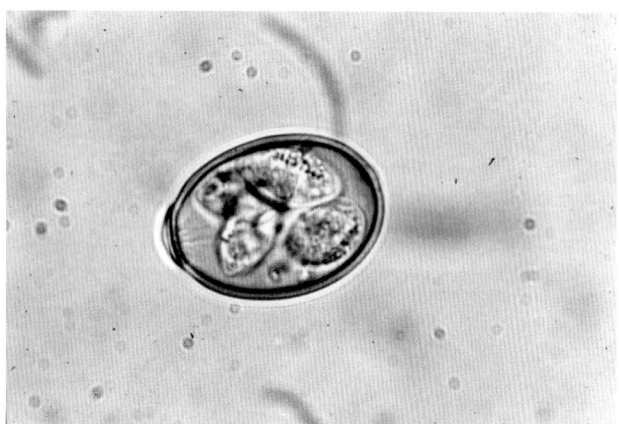

Fig. 2.50 Oocyst of *Eimeria arlongi*.

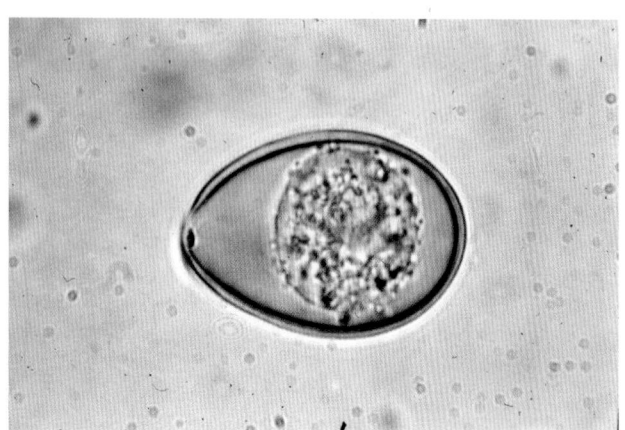

Fig. 2.51 Oocyst of *Eimeria aspheronica*.

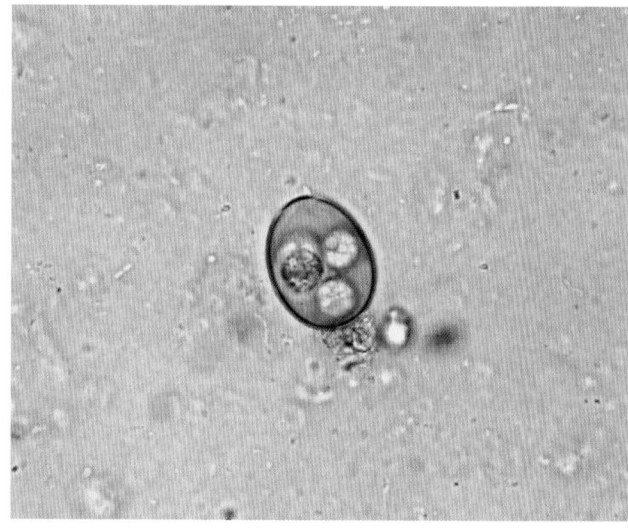

Fig. 2.52 Oocyst of *Eimeria caprovina*. (Courtesy of Antonio Ruiz Reyes).

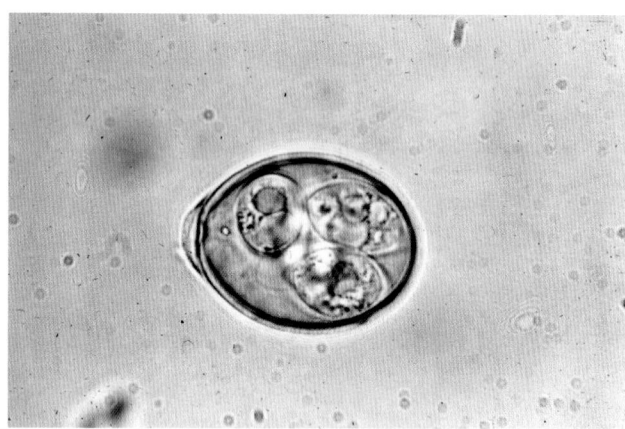

Fig. 2.53 Oocyst of *Eimeria jolchijevi*.

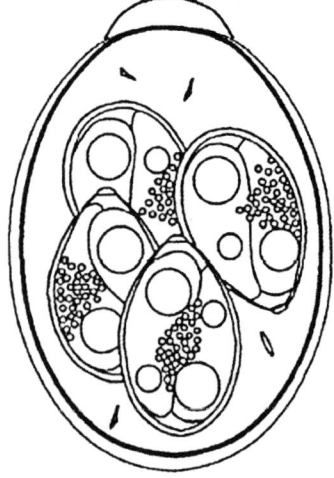

Fig. 2.54 Oocyst of *Eimeria capralis*. (From Soe and Pomroy, 1992. Reproduced with permission from Springer Science and Business Media.)

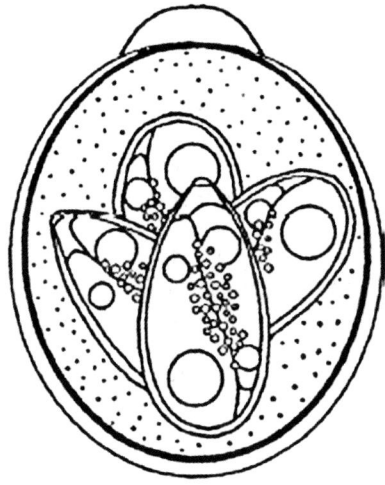

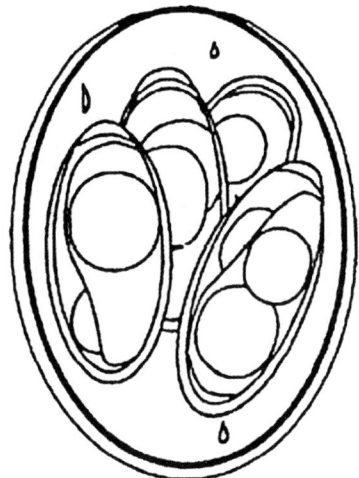

Fig. 2.55 Oocyst of *Eimeria masseyensis*. (From Soe and Pomroy, 1992. Reproduced with permission from Springer Science and Business Media.)

Fig. 2.56 Oocyst of *Eimeria charlestoni*. (From Soe and Pomroy, 1992. Reproduced with permission from Springer Science and Business Media.)

Table 2.21 *Eimeria* species (horses).

Species	Description
Eimeria leuckarti	Oocysts are ovoid or pyriform, flattened at the small end and very large, measuring 70–90 by 49–69 μm (mean 80 × 60 μm), with a thick dark shell and distinct micropyle. Sporocysts are elongate, 30–43 by 12–15 μm, with a Stieda body and residuum. The sporozoites are up to 35 μm long, lie lengthwise head to tail in the sporocysts and have a clear globule at the broad end.
Eimeria solipedum	Oocysts are spherical, orange to yellowish-brown, 15–28 μm in diameter, without an oocyst residuum or micropyle. Sporocysts are ellipsoid to oval, 5 by 3 μm.
Eimeria uniungulata	Oocysts are oval or ellipsoid, light orange, without an oocyst residuum or micropyle (mean 20 by 15 μm).

Table 2.22 *Eimeria* species (pigs).

Species	Description
Eimeria perminuta	Oocysts are ovoid to subspherical, 12–15 by 10–13 μm (mean 13.3 × 11.7 μm), yellow in colour, and the wall has a rough surface. A polar granule is present but no micropyle or oocyst residuum (see Fig. 4.38). Sporocysts are ellipsoid to broadly ovoid, 6–8 by 4–6 μm, each with a Stieda body and residuum. Sporozoites are elongate with two clear globules and lie lengthwise head to tail in the sporocysts.
Eimeria suis	Oocysts are ellipsoid, 15–23 by 12–18 μm (mean 18.2 × 14 μm), with a smooth and colourless wall. There is a polar granule but no micropyle or oocyst residuum (see Fig. 4.38). Sporocysts are elongate ovoid, 8–12 by 4–6 μm, each with a prominent Stieda body and a sporocyst residuum. The sporozoites are elongate and lie lengthwise head to tail in the sporocysts and each has a clear globule at the broad end.
Eimeria spinosa	Oocysts are ovoid, 17–24 by 12–19 μm (mean 20.6 × 16.2 μm), with a thick, rough, brown wall with long spines. There is a polar granule but no micropyle or oocyst residuum (see Fig. 4.38). Sporocysts are elongate ovoid, 10–14 by 5–7 μm, each with a prominent Stieda body and residuum. The sporozoites are elongate, and lie lengthwise head to tail in the sporocysts and each has a clear globule at the large end.
Eimeria neodebliecki	Oocysts are ellipsoid, 17–26 by 13–20 μm (mean 21.2 × 15.8 μm), and the wall is smooth and colourless; there is no micropyle or oocyst residuum but there is a polar granule (see Fig. 4.38). Sporocysts are elongate or broadly ovoid (9–14 by 5–8 μm); each has a Stieda body and a sporocyst residuum. The sporozoites are vermiform and lie lengthwise head to tail in the sporocysts and each has two clear globules.
Eimeria debliecki	Oocysts are ellipsoid or ovoid, 15–23 by 11–18 μm (mean 18.8 × 14.3 μm), with a smooth and colourless wall (see Fig. 4.38). There is a polar granule but no micropyle or oocyst residuum. Sporocysts are elongate ovoid, 13–20 by 5–7 μm, with a large Stieda body and a large sporocyst residuum. The sporozoites are vermiform, and each contains two large clear globules.
Eimeria polita	Oocysts are ellipsoid or broad ovoid, 20–33 by 14–22 μm (mean 25.9 × 18.1 μm), with a slightly rough yellowish-brown wall (see Fig. 4.38). There is no micropyle or oocyst residuum, although a polar granule may be present. Sporocysts are ellipsoid to ovoid, 13–19 by 5–9 μm, and each has a Stieda body and a residuum. The sporozoites are elongate with one or two clear globules, and lie lengthwise head to tail in the sporocysts. The mature meronts are about 14–24 by 11–23 μm and contain 15–30 merozoites. Macrogametes are 16–29 by 15–25 μm and microgamonts 16–29 by 13–29 μm and possess a residuum.
Eimeria porci	Oocysts are ovoid, 18–27 by 13–18 μm (mean 21.6 × 15.5 μm), colourless to yellowish-brown, with an indistinct micropyle, a polar granule but no oocyst residuum (see Fig. 4.38). Sporocysts are ovoid, 8–12 by 6–8 μm. Each has a Stieda body and a sporocyst residuum. The sporozoites are elongate and lie at either end of the sporocysts, or lie lengthwise head to tail. Each has an indistinct clear globule.
Eimeria scabra	Oocysts are ovoid or ellipsoid, 24–42 by 20–24 μm (mean 31.9 × 22.5 μm), with a thick rough striated wall, yellow–brown in colour (see Fig. 4.38). There is a micropyle and polar granule, but no oocyst residuum. Sporocysts are ovoid, 14–18 by 7–9 μm, each with a prominent Stieda body and sporocyst residuum. The sporozoites are elongate with two clear globules and lie lengthwise head to tail in the sporocysts. First-generation meronts are 16 by 13 μm in size at three days post infection and contain 16–24 merozoites. Second-generation meronts are 16 by 12 μm (five days), containing 14–22 merozoites; third-generation meronts are 21 by 16 μm in size (seven days) and contain 14–28 merozoites. The macrogametes are 18 by 12 μm and the microgamonts 17 by 13 μm.

Table 2.23 *Eimeria* species (camels).

Species	Description
Eimeria bactriani	The oocysts are spherical to ellipsoid, pale yellow–brown, smooth, 21–34 by 20–28 µm, with a micropyle but without micropylar cap and oocyst residuum. Sporocysts are spherical or elongate, 8–9 by 6–9 µm with a residuum. Meronts in the small intestine are 16 by 10 µm and contain 20–24 merozoites; mature microgamonts are 25 by 20 µm.
Eimeria cameli	The oocysts are large, pyriform, 80–100 by 55–94 µm, have a rough brown wall, with a micropyle, with or without a micropylar cap, and without an oocyst residuum. Sporocysts are elongate or ellipsoid, pointed at both ends, 30–50 by 14–20 µm without a Stieda body but with a residuum. Sporozoites are comma-shaped, lie lengthwise head to tail in the sporocyst, and have a clear globule at the large end. Giant meronts in the small intestine are up to 350 µm and contain many merozoites.
Eimeria dromedarii	The oocysts are ovoid, 23–33 by 20–25 mm, have a brown wall, with a micropylar cap, but without a polar granule or oocyst residuum (Fig. 2.57). Sporocysts are ovoid or spherical, 8–11 by 6–9 µm, without a Stieda body or residuum. Sporozoites are comma-shaped, with one to two clear globules.
Eimeria pellerdyi	The oocysts are ovoid or ellipsoid, smooth, colourless, 22–24 by 12–14 µm, without a micropyle, polar granule or oocyst residuum. Sporocysts are ovoid, 9–11 by 4–6 µm, with a small Stieda body and a residuum. Sporozoites are club-shaped, 8–10 by 1–3 µm, with a clear globule at the large end.
Eimeria rajasthani	The oocysts are ellipsoid, light yellowish-green, 34–39 by 25–27 µm, with a micropylar cap, but without a polar granule or oocyst residuum. Sporocysts are ovoid, 14–15 by 8–11 µm, with a Stieda body and a residuum. Sporozoites are elongate, 10–14 by 3–4 µm, with two or more clear globules.

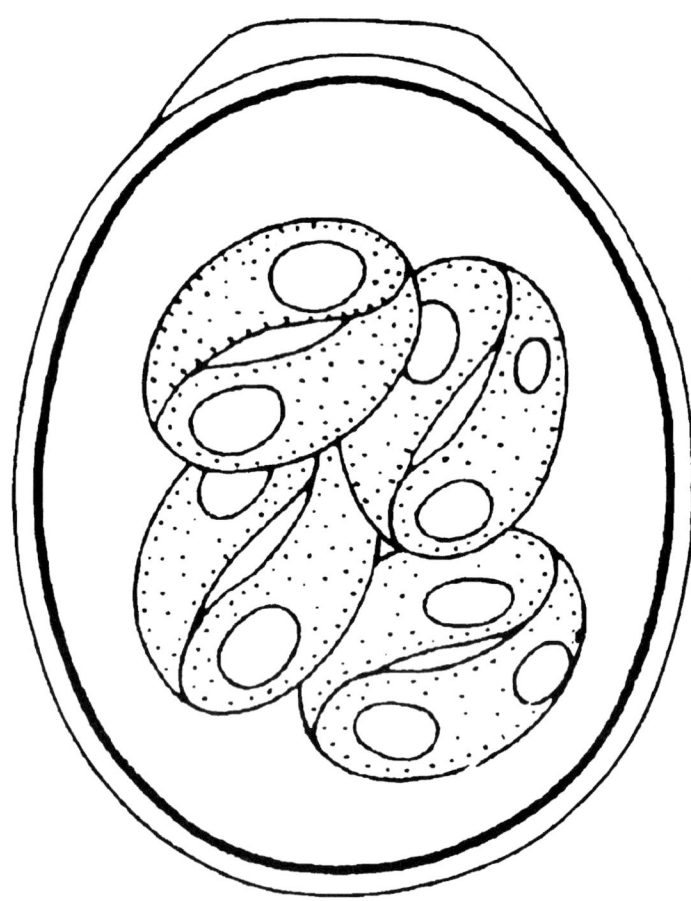

Fig. 2.57 Oocyst of *Eimeria dromedarii*.

Table 2.24 *Eimeria* species (camelids).

Species	Description
Eimeria lamae	The oocysts are ellipsoid to ovoid, smooth, bluish to greenish yellow, 30–40 by 21–30 µm, with a micropyle and micropylar cap, with or without a polar granule, but without an oocyst residuum (Fig. 2.58). Sporocysts are elongate ovoid, 13–16 by 8–10 µm, with a Stieda body and a residuum. Sporozoites are elongate, with one to three clear globules.
Eimeria alpacae	The oocysts are ellipsoid, rarely ovoid, pale green-blue, smooth, 22–26 by 18–21 µm, with a micropyle and micropylar cap, with or without polar granules and without an oocyst residuum. Sporocysts are ovoid, 10–13 by 7–8 µm, with a faint Stieda body and a residuum. Sporozoites are elongate and lie lengthwise head to tail in the sporocyst with one to three clear granules.
Eimeria punonensis	Oocysts are ellipsoid, smooth, 17–22 by 14–19 µm (mean 19.9 × 16.4 µm), with a micropyle, micropylar cap and polar granules. Sporocysts are elongate, 9.2 by 6.1 µm, with a faint Stieda body and a sporocyst residuum.
Eimeria macusaniensis	The oocysts are ovoid, sometimes pyriform, brown with a thick wall, 81–107 by 61–80 µm, with a micropyle and micropylar cap, but without a polar granule or oocyst residuum. Sporocysts are elongate ovoid, 33–40 by 16–20 µm, with a faint Stieda body and a residuum. Sporozoites are elongate, with a clear globule at the large end and a small one at the small end.
Eimeria ivitaensis	The oocysts are dark brown in colour and ellipsoid in shape (mean 89 by 52 µm) with a micropyle. The sporozoites are elongate with a residuum with a clear globule at the large end and a small globule at the smaller end
Eimeria peruviana	Oocysts are ovoid and lack a micropyle (mean 32 by 19 µm).

Table 2.25 *Eimeria* species (rabbits).

Species	Oocyst description
Eimeria coecicola	Oocysts are smooth-walled, ellipsoid, 34 by 20 μm (range 27–40 × 15–22 μm), light yellow to light brown in colour, with a distinct micropyle having a slight collar-like protrusion, and with oocyst residuum but no polar granule (Fig. 2.59; see also Fig. 4.39).
Eimeria exigua	Spherical or subspherical, colourless, with no micropyle, polar granule or oocyst residuum (mean 15 by 14 μm).
Eimeria flavescens	Oocysts are ovoid, 30 by 21 μm (range 25–35 × 16–21 μm), yellowish in colour, with a prominent micropyle at the broad end. There is no polar granule or oocyst residuum (Fig. 2.60; see also Fig. 4.39).
Eimeria intestinalis	Oocysts are pyriform, 27 by 19 μm (range 22–30 × 16–21 μm), yellowish-brown in colour, with a micropyle at the narrow end and a large oocyst residuum but no polar granule (Fig. 2.61; see also Fig. 4.39).
Eimeria irresidua	Oocysts are ovoid and smooth, barrel-shaped, yellowish in colour, with a wide micropyle, a residuum may be present but there are no polar granules, and measure 39 by 23 mm (range 31–44 × 20–27 mm) (Fig. 2.62; see also Fig. 4.39).
Eimeria magna	Oocysts are ovoid, 36 by 24 μm (range 31–42 × 20–28 μm), dark yellow in colour, and truncated at the micropylar end with a marked collar-like thickening around the micropyle. There is a very large oocyst residuum but no polar granules (Fig. 2.63; see also Fig. 4.39).
Eimeria media	Oocysts are ovoid or ellipsoid, 31 by 17 μm (range 25–35 × 15–20 μm), smooth and 'pinkish' with a micropyle with a pyramidal-shaped protuberance. There is a medium to large oocyst residuum and no polar granule (see Fig. 4.39).
Eimeria perforans	Oocysts are ellipsoid to subrectangular, 22 by 14 μm (range 15–27 × 11–17 μm), smooth and colourless with a uniformly thin wall. There is an inconspicuous micropyle and an oocyst residuum but no polar granule (see Fig. 4.39).
Eimeria pyriformis	Oocysts are pyriform, often asymmetrical, 30 by 18 μm (range 25–33 × 16–21 μm), yellowish-brown in colour, with a prominent micropyle but no polar granule or oocyst residuum (see Fig. 4.39).
Eimeria stiedai	Slightly ellipsoid, colourless or pinkish orange, with an inapparent micropyle and no oocyst residuum (mean 37 by 20 μm).
Eimeria vejdovsyi	Oocysts are elongate or ovoid, 32 by 19 μm (range 25–38 × 16–22 μm), a micropyle is present without collar-like protrusion and there is a medium-sized oocyst residuum.

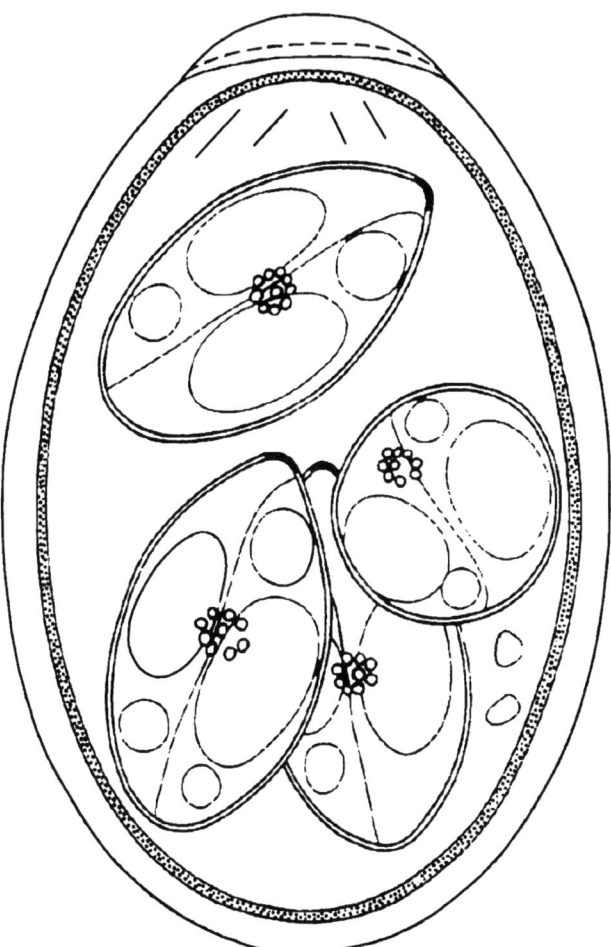

Fig. 2.58 Oocyst of *Eimeria lamae*.

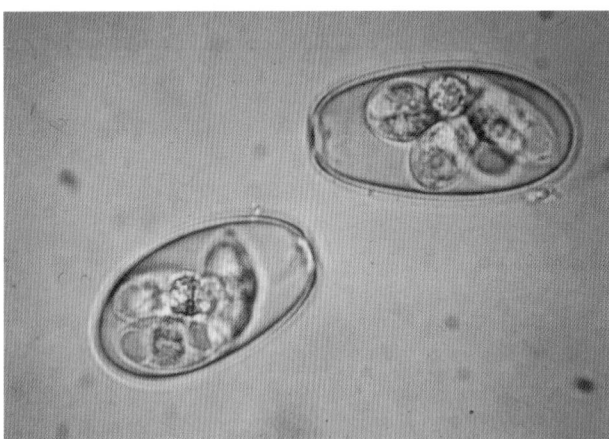

Fig. 2.59 Oocysts of *Eimeria coecicola*.

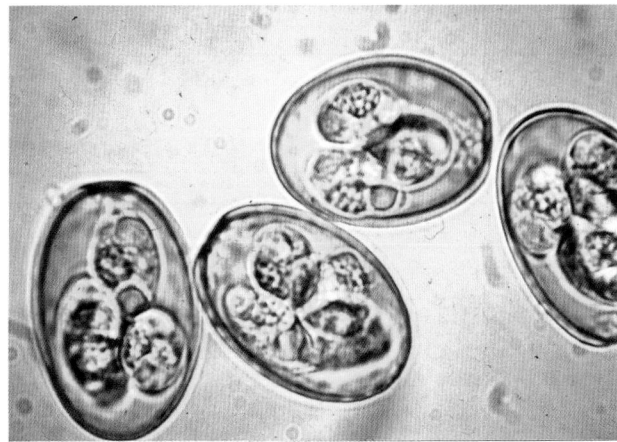

Fig. 2.60 Oocysts of *Eimeria flavescens*.

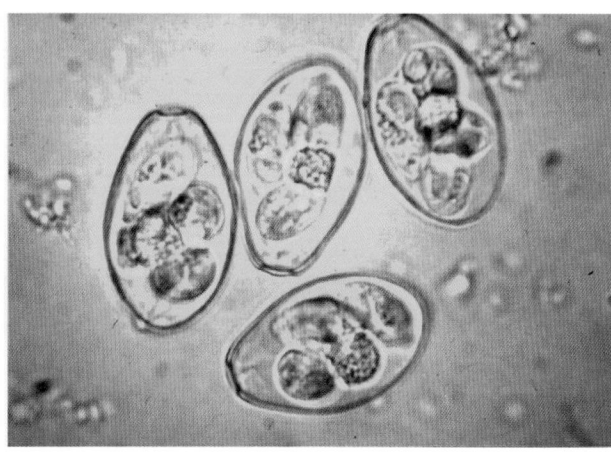

Fig. 2.61 Oocysts of *Eimeria intestinalis*.

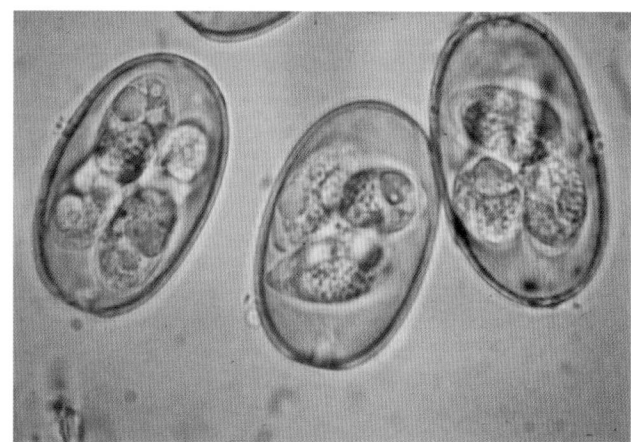

Fig. 2.62 Oocysts of *Eimeria irresidua*.

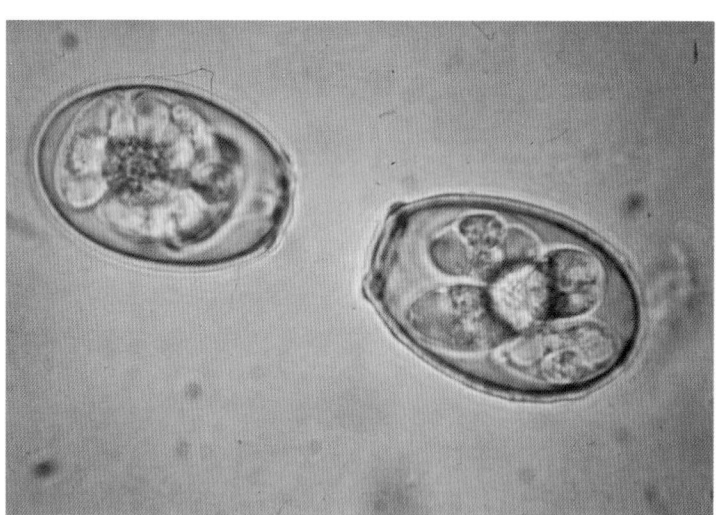

Fig. 2.63 Oocysts of *Eimeria magna*.

Table 2.26 *Eimeria* species (guinea pigs).

Species	Oocyst description
Eimeria caviae	Oocysts are ellipsoid or ovoid, smooth, brown, 13–26 by 12–23 μm, without a micropyle or polar granule but with a residuum.

Table 2.27 *Eimeria* species (mice).

Species	Oocyst description	Mean size (μm)
Eimeria falciformis	Oocysts are broadly ellipsoid, smooth, colourless, 14–26 by 13–24 μm, without a micropyle or oocyst residuum. Sporocysts are elongate and have a Stieda body and residuum. Sporozoites lie longitudinally within the sporocyst (Fig. 2.64).	20 × 19
Eimeria musculi	Oocysts spherical, smooth, greenish, without a micropyle, or oocyst residuum.	23 × 23
Eimeria scheuffneri	Oocysts ellipsoid, smooth, colourless or yellowish, without a micropyle or oocyst residuum.	21 × 15
Eimeria krijgsmani	Oocysts cylindrical, smooth, colourless without a micropyle or oocyst residuum.	22 × 16
Eimeria keilini	Oocysts ellipsoid, smooth, yellowish, without a micropyle or oocyst residuum.	28 × 20
Eimeria hindlei	Oocysts ovoid, smooth, greenish, without a micropyle or oocyst residuum.	25 × 20

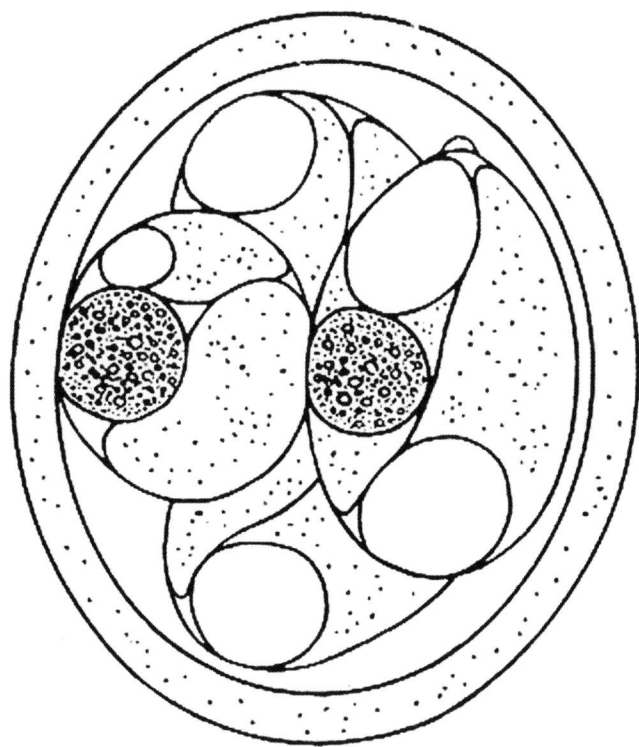

Fig. 2.64 Oocyst of *Eimeria falciformis*. (Adapted from Schneider, 1875.)

Table 2.28 *Eimeria* species (rats).

Species	Oocyst description	Mean size (μm)
Eimeria nieschulzi	Oocysts are ellipsoid or ovoid, smooth, colourless or yellowish, 16–26 by 13–21 μm, without a micropyle or oocyst residuum but with a polar granule. Sporocysts are elongate, ovoid and have a small Stieda body and residuum. Sporozoites contain a central nucleus with an eosinophilic globule at each end (Fig. 2.65).	21 × 17
Eimeria hasei	Oocysts ellipsoid or ovoid, without a micropyle, or oocyst residuum but with a polar granule.	18 × 14
Eimeria nochti	Oocysts are ovoid, without a micropyle, oocyst residuum or polar granule.	18 × 17
Eimeria ratti	Oocysts are cylindrical to ovoid, without a micropyle, oocyst residuum but with a polar granule.	22 × 16
Eimeria separata	Oocysts are ellipsoid or ovoid, smooth, colourless or yellowish, without a micropyle or oocyst residuum, but with 1–3 polar granules. Sporocysts are ellipsoid and have a small Stieda body and residuum (Fig. 2.66).	10–19

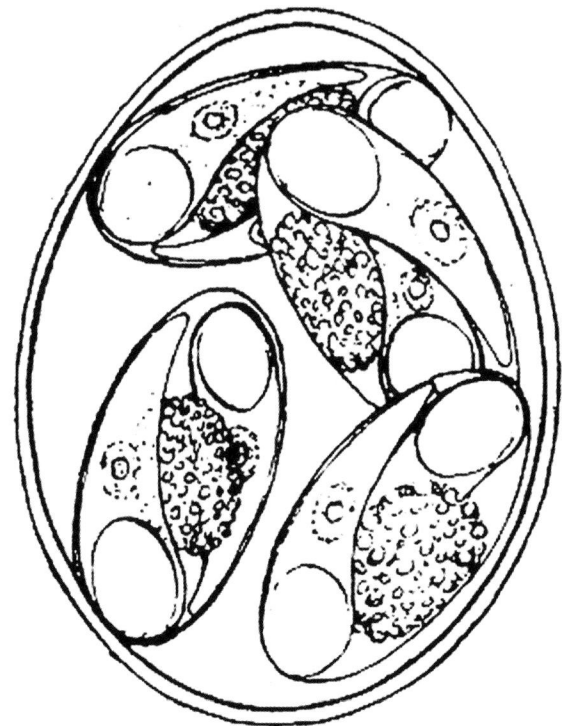

Fig. 2.65 Oocyst of *Eimeria nieschulzi*. (Adapted from Pérard, 1926.)

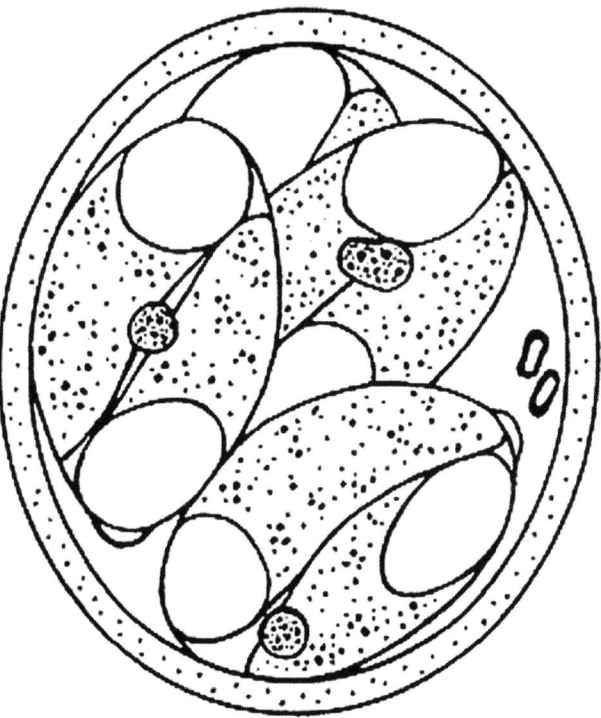

Fig. 2.66 Oocyst of *Eimeria separata*.

Table 2.29 *Eimeria* species (chickens).

Species	Description
Eimeria acervulina	Oocysts are ovoid, smooth, 12–23 by 9–17 μm (mean 18 × 14 μm), without a micropyle or residuum but with a polar granule (Fig. 2.67). The sporocysts are ovoid, with a Stieda body and without a residuum. First-generation meronts are 9–11 μm long and mature in 36–48 hours to produce 8–16 merozoites with a small residuum. Second-generation meronts mature in 41–56 hours to produce 16 merozoites with no residuum; third-generation meronts mature 56–72 hours after inoculation to produce eight merozoites with a residuum; and fourth-generation meronts mature 80–96 hours after inoculation and produce 32 merozoites with a large residuum. The macrogamonts are 14.5–19 μm in diameter and the microgamonts 7–8 μm. The latter produce many triflagellate microgametes 2–3 μm long.
Eimeria brunetti	Oocysts are ovoid, smooth, 14–34 by 12–26 μm (mean 26 × 22 μm), without a micropyle or residuum but with a polar granule. The sporocysts are ovoid (13 × 7.5 μm), with a Stieda body and a sporocyst residuum. First-generation meronts are 28 by 21 μm long and contain 318 merozoites. Second-generation meronts are smaller than first-generation meronts and contain 15–120 merozoites. The microgamonts contain several centres of microgamete development and are larger than the macrogamonts, which are 25 by 22 μm.
Eimeria maxima	Oocysts are ovoid, yellowish and smooth, 21–42 by 16–30 μm (mean 30 × 20 μm), without a micropyle or residuum but with a polar granule (Fig. 2.68). Sporocysts are ovoid, 15–19 by 8–9 μm, with a Stieda body and without a residuum. The sporozoites are 19 by 4 μm and each has a conspicuous clear globule.
Eimeria mitis	Oocysts are subspherical, smooth, 10–21 by 9–18 μm (mean 16 × 15 μm), without a micropyle or residuum but with a polar granule. The sporocysts are ovoid, 10–16 μm, with a Stieda body and without a residuum. Merogony stages have not been described. The microgamonts are 9–14 μm in diameter, and the microgamonts somewhat larger.
Eimeria necatrix	Oocysts are ovoid, smooth, colourless, 12–29 by 11–24 μm (mean 20 × 17 μm), without a micropyle or residuum but with a polar granule. The sporocysts are ovoid, with a Stieda body and without a residuum.
Eimeria praecox	Oocysts are ovoid, smooth, colourless, 20–25 by 16–20 μm (mean 21 × 17 μm), without a micropyle or residuum but with a polar granule. The sporocysts are ovoid, with a Stieda body and without a residuum.
Eimeria tenella	Oocysts are ovoid, smooth, colourless, 14–31 by 9–25 μm (mean 25 × 19 μm), without a micropyle or residuum but with a polar granule (Fig. 2.69). The sporocysts are ovoid, with a Stieda body and without a residuum.

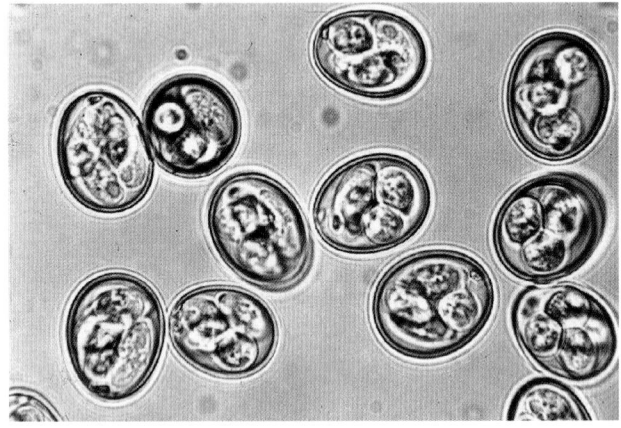

Fig. 2.67 Oocysts of *Eimeria acervulina*.

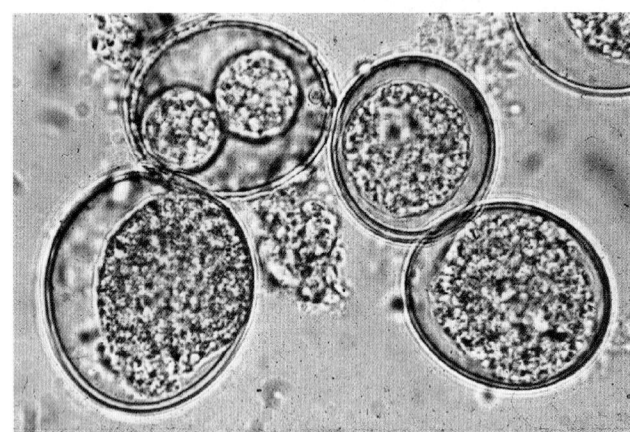

Fig. 2.68 Oocysts of *Eimeria maxima*.

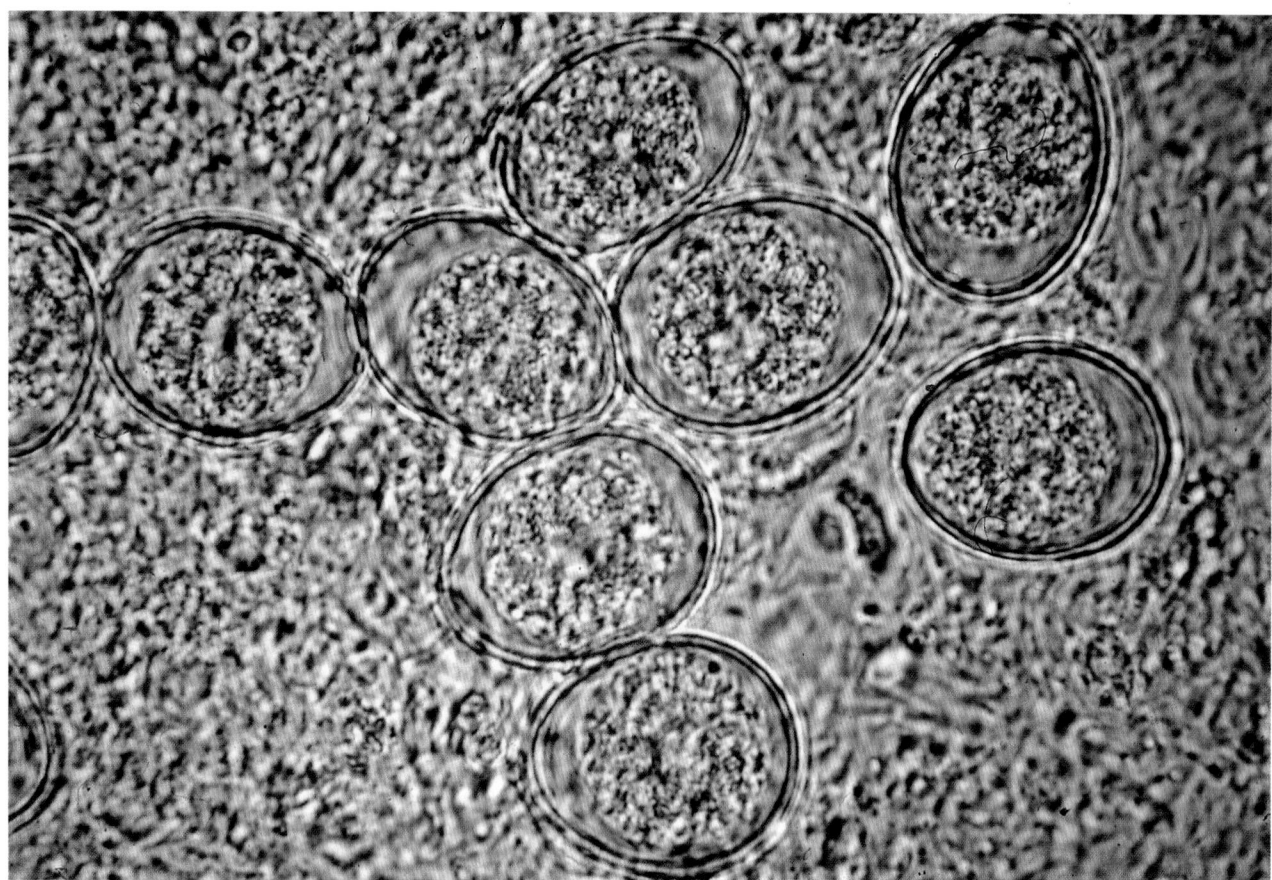

Fig. 2.69 Oocysts of *Eimeria tenella*.

Table 2.30 *Eimeria* species (turkeys).

Species	Description
Eimeria adenoides	Oocysts are ellipsoid or ovoid, smooth, colourless, 19–31 by 13–21 µm (mean 26 × 17 µm), with a micropyle, 1–3 polar granules but with no oocyst residuum. The sporocysts are elongate, with a Stieda body and a residuum, and contain a clear globule at the large end. First-generation meronts are 30 by 18 µm when mature (after 30 hours) and contain approximately 700 merozoites, 4–7 by 1.5 µm, with a central nucleus. Second-generation meronts are 10 by 10 µm and produce 12–24 merozoites, 10 by 3 µm, with the nucleus slightly nearer the rounded end. The mature macrogamonts and microgamonts are 20 by 18 µm.
Eimeria dispersa	Oocysts are ovoid, smooth, 22–31 by 18–24 µm (mean 26 × 21 µm), with no micropyle, polar granule or oocyst residuum. Sporocysts are ovoid and have a Stieda body. First-generation meronts are 14 by 13 µm and contain an average of 19 merozoites; second-generation meronts are 8 by 7 µm and contain an average of 13.5 merozoites; third-generation meronts are 9 by 9 µm and contain an average of 15 merozoites; and fourth-generation meronts are 12 by 10.5 µm and contain an average of seven merozoites. Mature macrogametes are 18–20 µm in diameter, with microgamonts slightly smaller.
Eimeria meleagridis	Oocysts are ellipsoid, smooth, 19–31 by 14–23 µm (mean 23 × 16 µm), with no micropyle and no oocyst residuum but with 1–2 polar granules. Sporocysts are ovoid with a Stieda body and a residuum. First-generation meronts are 20 by 15 µm and contain 50–100 merozoites; second-generation meronts are approximately 9 µm in diameter and contain 8–16 merozoites. Mature gamonts are 18 by 13 µm.
Eimeria meleagrimitis	Oocysts are subspherical, smooth, colourless, 16–27 by 13–22 µm (mean 19 × 16 µm), with no micropyle or oocyst residuum, but with 1–3 polar granules. The sporocysts are ovoid, with a Stieda body and a residuum and contain a clear globule at the large end. First-generation meronts are 17 by 13 µm when mature (after 48 hours) and contain approximately 80–100 merozoites, 4.5 by 1.5 µm, with a nucleus at the larger end. Second-generation meronts are 8 by 7 µm and produce 8–16 merozoites, 7 by 1.5 µm, with the nucleus slightly near the centre. Third-generation meronts are the same size as the second-generation meronts but differ in possessing a residuum and have a nucleus nearer the large end. The mature macrogamonts are 15 by 11 µm and the microgamonts contain a residuum.
Eimeria gallapovonis	Oocysts are ovoid, smooth, 22–31 by 18–24 µm (mean 26 × 21 µm), with no micropyle, polar granule or oocyst residuum. Sporocysts are ovoid and have a Stieda body. First-generation meronts are 14 by 13 µm and contain an average of 19 merozoites; second-generation meronts are 8 by 7 µm and contain an average of 13.5 merozoites; third-generation meronts are 9 by 9 µm and contain an average of 15 merozoites; and fourth-generation meronts are 12 by 10.5 µm and contain an average of seven merozoites. Mature macrogametes are 18–20 µm in diameter with microgamonts slightly smaller.
Eimeria innocua	Subspherical, smooth, without a micropyle or polar granules (mean 22 by 21 µm).
Eimeria subrotunda	Subspherical, smooth, without a micropyle or polar granules (mean 22 by 21 µm).

Table 2.31 *Eimeria* species (ducks).

Species	Description
Eimeria anatis	Oocysts are ovoid, smooth and colourless, with thickened ring around the micropyle, and without a polar granule or residuum (mean 17 by 14 μm).
Eimeria truncata	Oocysts are ovoid, smooth, with a narrow truncate small end, 14–27 by 12–22 μm, with a micropyle and micropylar cap, sometimes with a residuum. Mature meronts in the renal epithelial cells are 13 μm in diameter and contain 20–30 merozoites. Macrogametes are 12–18 by 11–15 μm and microgamonts are 15–22 by 13–18 μm.

Table 2.32 *Eimeria* species (geese).

Species	Description
Eimeria anseris	Oocysts are small and pear-shaped, with a truncated cone, smooth, colourless, 16–24 by 13–19 μm (mean 21 × 17 μm), with a micropyle and without a polar granule but with a residuum just beneath the micropyle. Sporocysts are ovoid and almost completely fill the oocysts, 8–12 by 7–9 μm, with a slightly thickened wall at the small end and with a residuum. Mature meronts are 12 by 20 μm and contain approximately 15–25 merozoites. The macrogametes are usually spherical and 12–26 by 10–15 μm. The microgamonts are 12–66 by 8–18 μm.
Eimeria nocens	Oocysts are ellipsoid or ovoid, thick-walled, brown, 25–33 by 17–24 μm (mean 29 × 20 μm), with a distinct micropyle, which is covered by the outer layer of the oocyst wall. Mature meronts are 15 by 30 μm and contain approximately 15–35 merozoites. The macrogametes are usually ellipsoid or irregularly spherical and 20–25 by 16–21 μm. The microgamonts are spherical or ellipsoid and 28–36 by 23–31 μm.

Table 2.33 *Eimeria* species (pheasants).

Species	Description
Eimeria colchici	Oocysts are elongate, ellipsoid with one side less rounded than the other, colourless, 19–33 by 11–21 μm (mean 27 × 17 μm) with an inconspicuous micropyle, a polar granule but no oocyst residuum (Fig. 2.70). Sporocysts are elongate, 11.5–15.5 by 6–7.5 μm (mean 14.6 × 6.6 μm). Sporozoites are arranged head to tail in the sporocysts and possess a single large refractive globule. First-generation meronts are 18 by 13 μm and contain 50–100 elongate merozoites; second-generation meronts are 28 by 21 μm and contain large numbers of merozoites; and third-generation meronts measure 8.5 by 7 μm and contain on average 19 merozoites.
Eimeria duodenalis	Oocysts are subspherical to broadly ellipsoid, smooth, colourless to pale yellowish-brown, 18–24 by 15.4–21.4 μm (mean 21.2 × 18.6 μm), with no micropyle and no oocyst residuum (Fig. 2.71). The ellipsoid sporocysts measure 11.6–13.6 by 6.1–6.8 μm (mean 12.6 × 6.7 μm). There is a small Stieda body and a larger sub-Stieda body. The sporocyst residuum largely obscures the sporozoites, which possess a large refractile body and occasionally a second smaller one.
Eimeria megalostoma	Oocysts are ovoid, yellowish-brown, 24 by 19 μm, with a thick oocyst wall and prominent micropyle.
Eimeria pacifica	Oocysts are ovoid, with a mammillated oocyst wall (mean 22 by 17 μm).
Eimeria phasiani	Oocysts are ellipsoid, smooth, yellowish, 20.1–30.9 by 13.4–20.5 μm (mean 25 × 17 μm), with no micropyle and no oocyst residuum, but with 1–3 polar granules. Sporocysts are elongate, pyriform, each with a prominent Stieda body, 12.9–15.9 by 5.6–7.4 μm (mean 14.3 × 6.7 μm). Sporozoites contain a single refractile body.

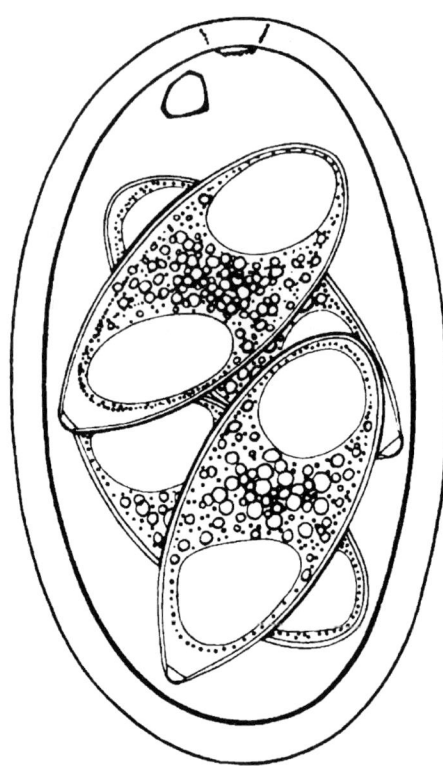

Fig. 2.70 Oocyst of *Eimeria colchici*.

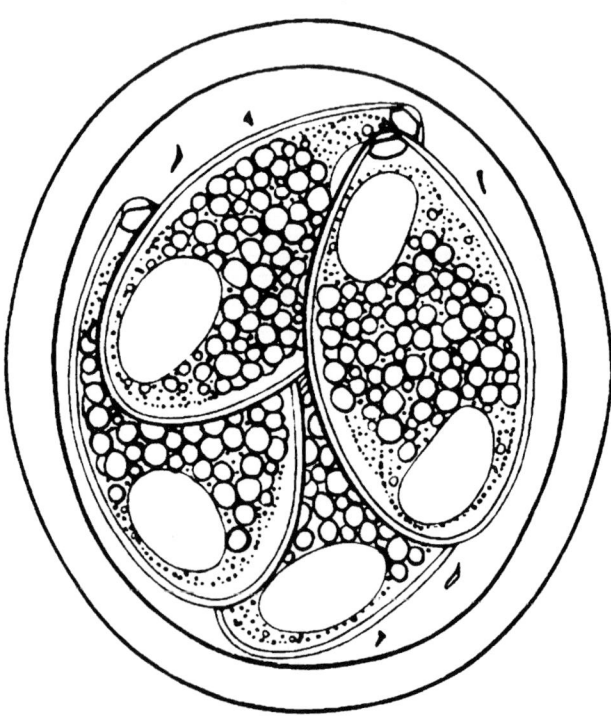

Fig. 2.71 Oocyst of *Eimeria duodenalis*.

Table 2.34 *Eimeria* species (partridges).

Species	Description
Eimeria caucasica	Oocysts elongate, rarely ovoid (mean 33 by 19 μm).
Eimeria procera	Oocysts elongate-elliptic (mean 30 by 17 μm).
Eimeria koifoidi	Oocysts ovoid (mean 20 by 18 μm).
Eimeria legionensis	Oocysts elliptic, almost symmetrical, sometimes slightly flattened, 18–24 by 12–16 μm (mean 21.3 by 14.6 μm).

Table 2.35 *Eimeria* species (quails).

Species	Description
Eimeria bateri	Oocysts ellipsoid, ovoid or infrequently round (mean 23 by 18 μm). Single refractive polar granule present, but micropyle and the residual body absent.
Eimeria colini	Oocysts broadly ellipsoid, oocysts with sporocyst residuum, Stieda body and an inconspicuous micropyle, without oocyst residuum and polar granule (mean 25 by 21 μm).
Eimeria coturnicus	Oocysts ovoid (mean 33 by 23 μm).
Eimeria taldykurganica	Oocysts ovoid (mean 24 by 13 μm), 1–2 polar granules present but micropyle and residual body absent.
Eimeria tsunodai	Oocysts ovoid (mean 19 by 18 μm).
Eimeria uzura	Oocysts broadly elliptic or ovoid (mean 22 by 16 μm), 2–5 polar granules present but micropyle and residual body absent.

Table 2.36 *Eimeria* species (guinea fowl).

Species	Description
Eimeria grenieri	Oocysts are ellipsoid, smooth, 15–27 by 12–18 μm (mean 21 × 15 μm), with a micropyle and polar granules but without a residuum. Sporocysts are ovoid, with a Stieda body and a residuum.
Eimeria numidae	Oocysts are ellipsoid, smooth (mean 18 by 15 μm), with a button-shaped micropyle and a polar granule but without a residuum.

Table 2.37 *Eimeria* species (pigeons).

Species	Description
Eimeria labbeana (syn *Eimeria columbarum*)	Oocysts are subspherical to spherical, smooth, colourless or slightly yellowish-brown, 13–24 by 12–23 μm, without a micropyle or a residuum but with a polar granule. Sporocysts are elongate ovoid, with a Stieda body and residuum. The sporozoites are slightly crescent-shaped with one end wider than the other, lie lengthwise head to tail in the sporocysts, and have a clear globule at each end.

Wenyonella

Parasites of birds; the oocysts contain four sporocysts each with four sporozoites.

Wenyonella gallinae

This species infects the caeca and rectum of chickens.

Description: Oocysts are ovoid, rough, punctate and measure 29–34 by 20–23 μm (mean 31 × 21 μm). There are four sporocysts, which are flask-shaped (19 × 8 μm), and each contains four sporozoites.

Life cycle: Details of the life cycle have not been described. The prepatent period is 7–8 days and patent period is three days. The sporulation time is 4–6 days.

Wenyonella columbae

This species infects the small intestine of pigeons.

Description: Oocysts are spherical or slightly ovoid, 21–27 by 21–26 μm, without a micropyle, polar granule or oocyst residuum.

Caryospora

The species in this genus infect birds and reptiles, with the majority of described species infecting snakes. Sporulated oocysts have one sporocyst containing eight sporozoites.

FAMILY SARCOCYSTIDAE

Seven genera (i.e. *Besnoitia*, *Hammondia*, *Sarcocystis*, *Neospora*, *Frenkelia*, *Toxoplasma* and *Cystoisospora*) are of veterinary interest. Their life cycles are similar to those of *Eimeria* and *Isospora* except that the asexual and sexual stages occur in intermediate and final hosts, respectively. Oocysts have two sporocysts each with four sporozoites. With the exception of the genus *Toxoplasma*, they are normally non-pathogenic to their final hosts and their significance is due to the cystic tissue stages in the intermediate hosts, which include ruminants, pigs, horses and humans. The tissue phase in the intermediate host is obligatory, except in *Toxoplasma* where it is facultative.

Table 2.38 *Besnoitia* species.

Species	Hosts	Intermediate hosts	Site
Besnoitia besnoiti (syn. *Sarcocystis besnioti*)	Cats, wild cats (lions, cheetahs, leopards)	Cattle, goats, wild ruminants (wildebeest, impalas, kudus)	Skin, conjunctiva
Besnoitia bennetti	Unknown	Horses, donkeys	Skin, conjunctiva
Besnoitia tarandi	Unknown	Reindeer, caribou	Skin, conjunctiva

Table 2.39 *Hammondia* species.

Species	Hosts	Intermediate hosts	Site
Hammondia hammondi (syn. *Isospora hammondi*, *Toxoplasma hammondi*)	Cats and other felids	Rodents	Skeletal muscle
Hammondia heydorni	Dogs and other canids	Cattle, sheep, goats, rodents, guinea pigs	Skeletal muscle

Besnoitia

Species of *Besnoitia* have been found in cattle, horses, deer, rodents, primates and reptiles. Cats are the definitive hosts (Table 2.38). The parasites develop in connective tissue, particularly of the skin, causing skin thickening and hair loss.

Life cycle: Members of the genus are heteroxenous, reproducing sexually, and producing unsporulated oocysts in felids and multiplying by merogony in a variety of prey animals.

Besnoitia besnoiti

Synonym: *Sarcocystis besnoiti*

Description: Oocysts in the definitive hosts are ovoid, 14–18 by 12–14 μm, unsporulated and without a micropyle when passed in the faeces of cats. After sporulation, they contain two sporocysts each with four sporozoites. The pseudocysts in the intermediate hosts are non-septate and about 100–600 μm in diameter, with a thick wall containing thousands of merozoites but no metrocytes (Fig. 2.72). The prepatent period in cats is 4–25 days and the patent period 3–15 days.

Besnoitia bennetti

Description: Oocysts have not been described. The pseudocysts in the intermediate hosts are non-septate and about 100–1000 μm in diameter.

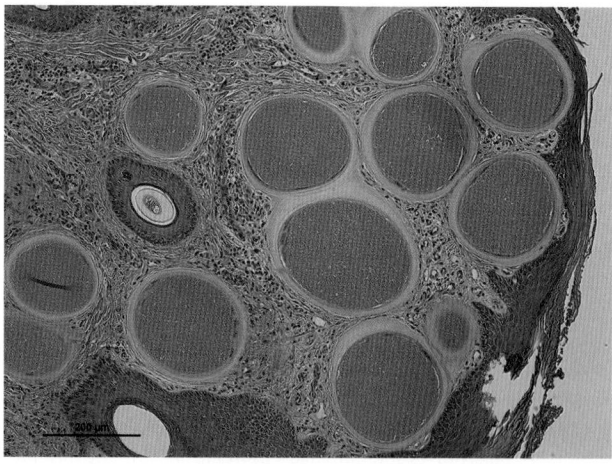

Fig. 2.72 Tissue cyst of *Besnoitia besnoiti*. (Courtesy of Walter Basso).

Hammondia

The genus is closely related to *Toxoplasma* and has a heteroxeneous life cycle with a carnivore definitive host and an intermediate (prey species) host (Table 2.39). Reproduction (gametogony) occurs in the small intestine of the final host. Cysts containing bradyzoites occur in the skeletal muscle of the prey host.

Hammondia hammondi

Synonyms: *Isospora hammondi*, *Toxoplasma hammondi*

Description: Unsporulated oocysts are colourless, spherical to subspherical, 11–13 by 10–13 μm without a micropyle or residuum; after sporulation, they are subspherical to ellipsoid, 13–14 by 10–11 μm (mean 13 × 11 μm). The sporocysts are ellipsoid, 8–11 by 6–8 μm (mean 10 × 6.5 μm) and have no Stieda body but have a residuum. The sporozoites are elongate and curved with a nucleus near the centre.

Life cycle: The cat is infected by ingesting infected rodents containing meronts. After ingestion, there is multiplication in the small intestine epithelium followed by gametogony. The prepatent period in the cat is 5–16 days and the patent period can be as long as 136 days.

Hammondia heydorni

Synonyms: *Isospora heydorni*, *Toxoplasma heydorni*

Description: Unsporulated oocysts are colourless, spherical to subspherical, 11–13 by 10–13 μm without a micropyle or residuum; after sporulation, they are subspherical to ellipsoid, 13–14 by 10–11 μm (mean 13 × 11 μm). The sporocysts are ellipsoid, 8–11 by 6–8 μm (mean 10 × 6.5 μm) and have no Stieda body but have a residuum. The sporozoites are elongate and curved with a nucleus near the centre.

Life cycle: Unsporulated oocysts are produced in the faeces and, following infection of the intermediate hosts, the multiplication of tachyzoites in the lamina propria of the intestinal wall is followed by the production of cysts containing bradyzoites in the skeletal muscle. The prepatent period is 6–7 days. Sporulation time is three days.

Sarcocystis

There are about 130 recognised species in this genus reported from the striated muscles of mammals, birds, reptiles and humans (Table 2.40). *Sarcocystis* is one of the most prevalent parasites of livestock and infects mammals, including humans, birds and lower vertebrates. The parasites derive their name from the intramuscular cyst stage (sarcocyst) present in the intermediate (prey) host (Fig. 2.73). Most *Sarcocystis* species infecting human and domestic

Table 2.40 *Sarcocystis* species.

Species	Final hosts	Intermediate hosts	Site
Sarcocystis alceslatranis	Dogs, coyotes	Deer (moose)	Muscle
Sarcocystis aucheniae (syn. *Sarcocystis tilopodi*, *Sarcocystis guanicocanis*)	Dogs	Llamas, guanacos, alpacas	Muscle
Sarcocystis bovicanis (syn. *Sarcocystis cruzi*, *Sarcocystis fusiformis*)	Dogs, foxes, wolves, coyotes	Cattle	Muscle
Sarcocystis bovifelis (syn. *Sarcocystis hirsuta*, *Sarcocystis fusiformis*)	Cats	Cattle	Muscle
Sarcocystis bovihominis (syn. *Sarcocystis hominis*)	Humans, primates	Cattle	Muscle
Sarcocystis cameli	Dogs	Camels (Bactrians, dromedaries)	Muscle
Sarcocystis capracanis	Dogs	Goats	Muscle
Sarcocystis capreolicanis	Dogs, foxes	Deer (roe deer)	Muscle
Sarcocystis cervicanis	Dogs	Deer (red deer)	Muscle
Sarcocystis cuniculi	Cats	Rabbits	Muscle
Sarcocystis equicanis (syn. *Sarcocystis bertrami*)	Dogs	Horses	Muscle
Sarcocystis fayeri	Dogs	Horses	Muscle
Sarcocystis gracilis	Dogs	Deer (roe deer)	Muscle
Sarcocystis grueneri	Dogs, foxes, coyotes	Deer (red deer, reindeer)	Muscle
Sarcocystis hircicanis	Dogs	Goats	Muscle
Sarcocystis hircifelis (syn. *Sarcocystis moulei*)	Cats	Goats	Muscle
Sarcocystis hofmani	Dogs, raccoon dogs	Deer (red deer, roe deer, fallow deer, sika deer)	Muscle
Sarcocystis hovarthi (syn. *Sarcocystis gallinarum*)	Dogs	Chickens	Muscle
Sarcocystis ippeni	Unknown	Camels (dromedaries)	Muscle
Sarcocystis jorrini	Unknown	Deer (fallow deer)	Muscle
Sarcocystis lamacenis	Unknown	Llamas	Muscle
Sarcocystis muris	Cats	Mice	Muscle
Sarcocystis neurona	Horses	Opossums	Brain, spinal cord
Sarcocystis ovicanis (syn. *Sarcocystis tenella*)	Dogs	Sheep	Muscle
Sarcocystis ovifelis (syn. *Sarcocystis tenella*, *Sarcocystis gigantea*, *Sarcocystis medusiformis*)	Cats	Sheep	Muscle
Sarcocystis porcifelis (syn. *Sarcocystis suifelis*)	Cats	Pigs	Muscle
Sarcocystis randiferi	Unknown	Deer (reindeer)	Muscle
Sarcocystis rangi	Dogs	Deer (reindeer)	Muscle
Sarcocystis sinensis	Unknown	Buffaloes	Muscle
Sarcocystis suicanis (syn. *Sarcocystis porcicanis*, *Sarcocystis miescheriana*)	Dogs	Pigs	Muscle
Sarcocystis suihominis (syn. *Sarcocystis porcihominis*)	Humans, primates	Pigs	Muscle
Sarcocystis sybillensis	Dogs	Deer (red deer, roe deer)	Muscle
Sarcocystis tarandi	Unknown	Deer (reindeer)	Muscle
Sarcocystis tarandivulpis	Dogs, foxes, raccoon dogs	Deer (reindeer)	Muscle
Sarcocystis wapiti	Dogs, coyotes	Deer (red deer, roe deer)	Muscle

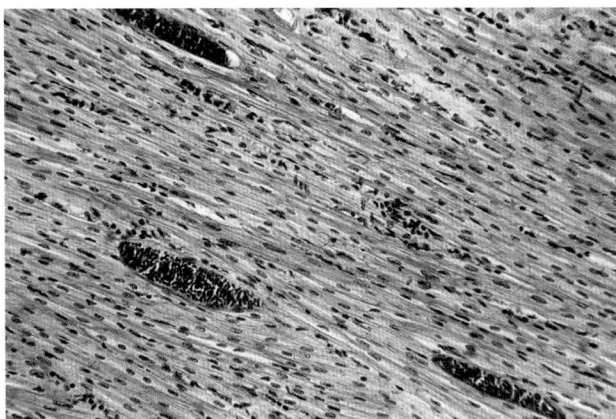

Fig. 2.73 Sarcocysts in bovine muscle.

animals are species specific for their intermediate hosts and family specific for their final hosts. *Sarcocystis* infections in the intermediate hosts are usually asymptomatic. Gastrointestinal disease is occasionally reported in humans.

Sarcocysts are found in striated and heart muscles and may be either microscopic or visible to the naked eye and contain metrocytes initially and bradyzoites when mature. Oocysts sporulate within the predator host and are passed in the faeces. Revision of the taxonomy of the genus is ongoing, and many of the currently recognised species may be synonyms of species that can infect multiple hosts.

Life cycle: The life cycle for all species is heteroxenous. Sexual stages occur in the predator and oocysts are passed in the faeces. Infection in the dog and cat is by ingestion of bradyzoite cysts in the muscles of infected intermediate hosts. The bradyzoites are liberated in the intestine and the freed zoites pass to the subepithelial lamina propria and differentiate into micro- and macrogametocytes. Following conjugation of gametes, thin-walled oocysts are formed which, unlike those of most other enteric sporozoans, sporulate within the body. Two sporocysts are formed, each containing four sporozoites. Usually the fragile oocyst wall ruptures and free sporocysts are found in the faeces. See **life cycle** 33.

Sarcocystis bovicanis

Synonyms: *Sarcocystis cruzi*, *Sarcocystis fusiformis*

Description: In cattle, the meronts found in the endothelial cells are quite small, measuring 2–8 μm in diameter. The bradyzoite cysts can be large and visible to the naked eye as whitish streaks running in the direction of the muscle fibres. They have been reported as reaching several centimetres in length, but more commonly range from 0.5 to 5 mm. The cyst wall is thin and smooth and has a small number of flattened protrusions 0.3–0.6 μm long, without fibrils.

Sporulated oocysts are fully sporulated and dumb-bell shaped if passed in the faeces, 19–21 by 15–18 μm, with a thin oocyst wall sunken between two sporocysts, without a micropyle, polar granule or oocyst residuum (Fig. 2.74). However, it is usually the sporulated sporocyst that is found free in the faeces. Sporocysts are ellipsoid, 14.3–17.4 by 8.7–13.3 μm (mean 16.3 × 10.8 μm), smooth, colourless without a Stieda body but with a residuum and each has four sporozoites.

LIFE CYCLE 33. LIFE CYCLE OF *SARCOCYSTIS*

All species of *Sarcocystis* are characterised by a heteroxenous life cycle, with sexual reproduction occurring in predatory species (definitive hosts). The oocysts sporulate in the intestinal lumen, forming two sporocysts, each containing four sporozoites (1). The outer wall of the oocyst is thin and fragile, and therefore free sporocysts are frequently observed in faeces (2). Intermediate hosts, including humans, acquire the infection by accidentally ingesting oocysts (3). In these hosts, parasites replicate several times by schizogony in endothelial cells of the blood vessels (4), thus generating free merozoites (5). The latter infect mononuclear (6) or muscular cells (7). In both cell types, merozoites replicate by endodyogeny and form muscular cysts that contain bradyzoites (8). Following ingestion of the large muscular cysts (sometimes >1 cm in size) by a predatory animal (9), the bradyzoites are released in the intestine and penetrate the lamina propria (10), where they form micro- and macrogametes (11, 12) which, after fertilisation, generate the zygote (13). The latter develops into an oocyst that sporulates in the intestine, thus becoming infective (1).

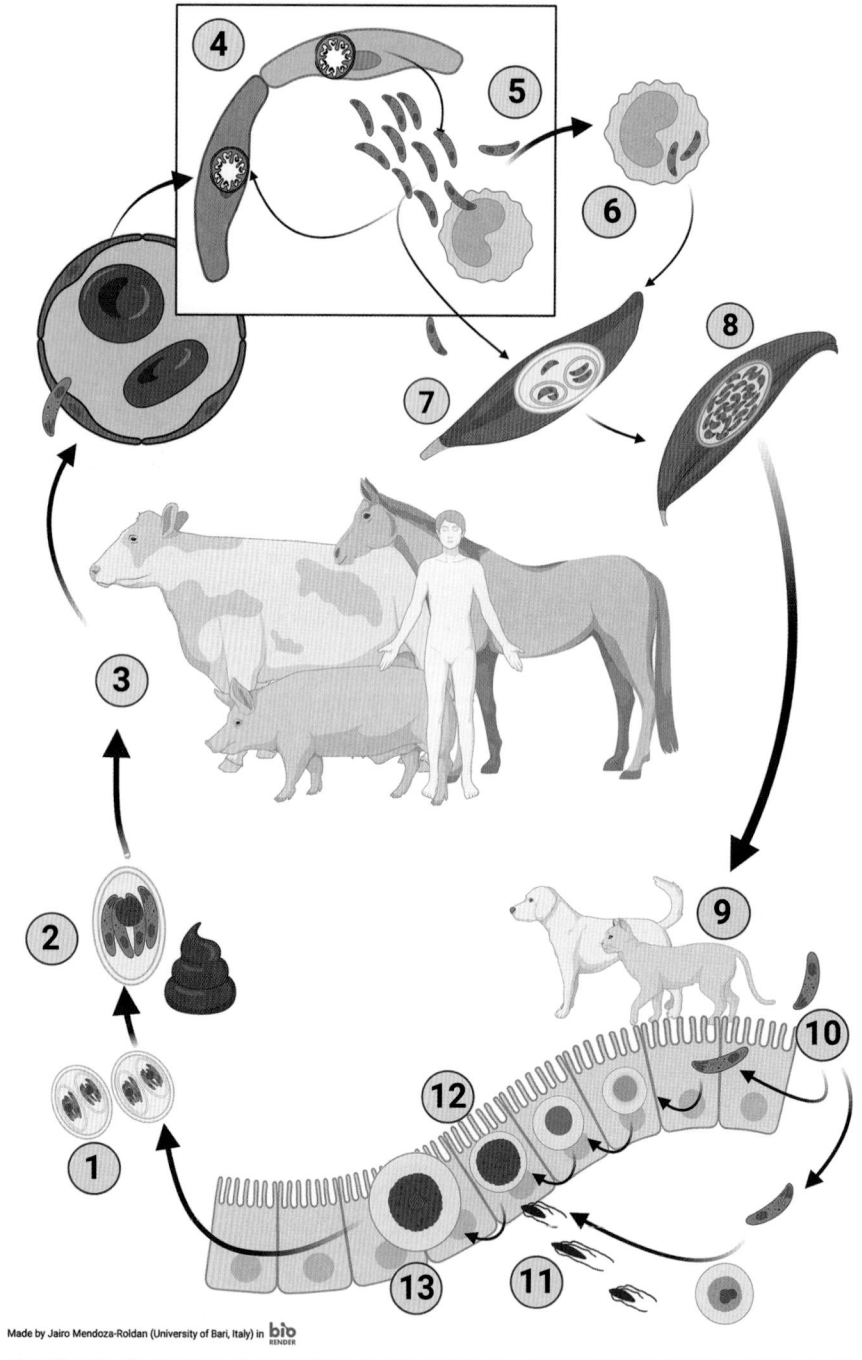

Made by Jairo Mendoza-Roldan (University of Bari, Italy) in **bio**RENDER

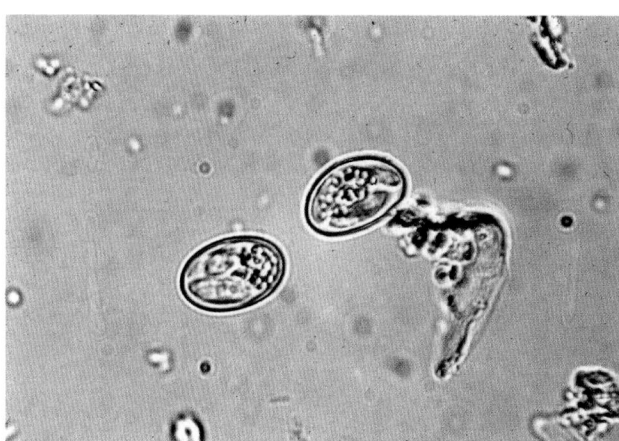

Fig. 2.74 Oocysts of *Sarcocystis bovicanis*.

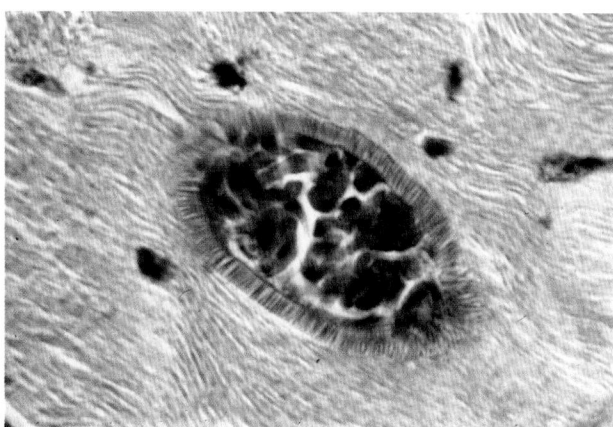

Fig. 2.75 Sarcocyst (*Sarcocystis ovicanis*) in sheep muscle.

Sarcocystis bovifelis

Synonyms: *Sarcocystis hirsuta, Sarcocystis fusiformis*

Description: The first-generation meronts measure 37 by 22 µm and contain more than 100 tachyzoites. Second-generation meronts, when mature, are 14 by 6.5 µm and contain up to 35 tachyzoites. Sarcocysts are up to 8 mm long with a striated wall, 7 µm thick, and may be visible to the naked eye.

Oocysts are smooth, colourless, 12–18 by 11–14 µm and contain two sporocysts each with four sporozoites, dumb-bell shaped in appearance, and with no micropyle, polar granule or oocyst residuum. Sporocysts are ellipsoid, 11–14 by 7–9 µm (mean 12.5 × 7.8 µm) without a Stieda body but with a residuum.

Sarcocystis bovihominis

Synonym: *Sarcocystis hominis*

Description: First-generation meronts are 37 by 22 µm and contain more than 100 tachyzoites. Second-generation meronts, when mature, are 14 by 6.5 µm and contain up to 35 tachyzoites. In the intermediate host, sarcocysts are compartmented with a radially striated wall of about 6 µm in thickness.

Sarcocystis ovicanis

Synonyms: *Sarcocystis tenella, Isospora bigemina*

Description: In the intermediate host, first-generation meronts found in the endothelial cells are 19–29 by 7.5–24 µm and contain 120–280 merozoites. Tissue cysts are microscopic in size (500 × 60–100 µm) and are found in skeletal and cardiac muscle (Fig. 2.75). The wall of the cyst appears thick (up to 2.5 µm) and radially striated with long palisade-like protrusions without fibrils visible on electron microscopy. Oocysts are sporulated when passed in the faeces and contain two sporocysts each with four sporozoites; usually the sporulated sporocyst is found free in the faeces. In *S. ovicanis*, the sporulated sporocysts measure approximately 13.1–16.1 by 8.5–10.8 µm (mean 14.8 × 9.9 µm).

Life cycle: Sheep become infected by ingesting sporocysts passed in the faeces of the dog. Once ingested, there are three asexual generations. In the first, sporozoites, released from the sporocysts, invade the intestinal wall and enter the capillaries where they locate in endothelial cells in many organs and undergo two merogony cycles. A third asexual cycle occurs in the circulating lymphocytes, the resulting merozoites penetrating muscle cells. There they encyst and then divide by a process of budding or endodyogeny, giving rise to broad banana-shaped bradyzoites contained within a cyst; this is the mature sarcocyst and is the infective stage for the dog final host.

Sarcocystis ovifelis

Synonyms: *Sarcocystis tenella, Sarcocystis gigantea, Sarcocystis medusiformis, Isospora bigemina*

Description: In the intermediate host, the meronts found in the endothelial cells are quite small, measuring 2–8 µm in diameter. Bradyzoite cysts have been reported as reaching several centimetres in length, but more commonly they range up to 1.5 cm by 0.2–5 mm. The cyst wall has numerous cauliflower-like protrusions 1–4.5 µm long, each containing numerous fibrils. The parasitised host cell is enclosed in connective tissue forming a secondary cyst wall. Sporulated sporocysts are ellipsoid and measure 10.8–13.9 by 7.7–9.3 µm (mean 12.4 × 8.1 µm).

Life cycle: Infection is by ingestion of the sporocysts and this is followed by a single asexual generation in capillaries and arterioles of the lung, kidney and brain, from which the resulting merozoites penetrate muscle cells. There they encyst and then divide by a process of budding or endodyogeny, giving rise to broad banana-shaped bradyzoites contained within the sarcocyst. Sarcocysts are found primarily in the muscles of the oesophagus, larynx, tongue and, to a lesser extent, diaphragm and skeletal muscles. Cats are the final host.

Sarcocystis capracanis

Description: Tissue cysts are microscopic in size (130–800 × 50–70 µm) and are found in skeletal and cardiac muscle. The wall of the cyst appears thick (up to 2.6 µm) and radially striated with long finger-like protrusions. The oocysts have not been described.

The sporulated sporocysts are ellipsoid and measure approximately 12–15 by 8–10 μm.

Life cycle: As described for sheep species. There are three merogony cycles.

Sarcocystis hircicanis

Description: In the intermediate hosts, tissue cysts are up to 2.5 mm in size and are found in skeletal and cardiac muscle. The wall of the cyst is thin, smooth and striated with long hair-like protrusions. The oocysts have not been described. The sporulated sporocysts are ellipsoid and measure approximately 15–17.3 by 10.5–11.3 μm.

Life cycle: As for *S. capracanis*. The number of merogony stages is unknown.

Sarcocystis hircifelis

Synonym: *Sarcocystis moulei*

Description: The sarcocysts are elongate, compartmented and up to 12 mm in length and have a thick striated wall. Sporocysts measure 12.4 by 9.1 μm.

Life cycle: As described for *S. hircicanis* except that the cat is the final host. The number of merogony stages is unknown.

Sarcocystis equicanis

Synonym: *Sarcocystis bertrami*

Description: Tissue cysts are segmented, up to 10 mm long with a smooth wall less than 1 μm thick with no radial striations. A small number of 0.4–2 μm protrusions are evident on electron microscopy. Sporulated sporocysts measure 15–16.3 by 8.8–11.3 μm (mean 15.2–10 μm).

Sarcocystis fayeri

Description: Tissue cysts are up to 900 μm long by 70 μm wide. The cyst wall is 1–2 μm thick and radially striated. Sporulated sporocysts measure 11–13 by 7–8.5 μm (mean 12 × 7.9 μm).

Sarcocystis neurona

Description: Meronts present in the cytoplasm of neural cells, leucocytes and giant cells in the grey and white matter of the brain and spinal cord measure 5–35 by 5–20 mm and contain 4–40 merozoites when mature.

Life cycle: Details of the life cycle are not completely known. The North American opossum is thought to be one definitive host with transmission to the horse via sporocysts in faeces. The life cycle may also involve opossums scavenging on bird carcasses containing an identical organism, *Sarcocystis falcatula*, a parasite of several North American bird species. In this respect, horses may be acting as an abnormal, aberrant host.

Sarcocystis suicanis

Synonyms: *Sarcocystis porcicanis*, *Sarcocystis miescheriana*

Description: Tissue cysts are compartmented up to 0.5–1.5 mm long by 15–100 μm. The cyst wall has numerous palisade-like processes with randomly arranged filaments seen on electron microscopy. Sporulated sporocysts found free in the faeces measure approximately 12.7 by 10.1 μm.

Life cycle: Infection is by ingestion of the sporocysts and this is followed by three asexual generations. In the first, sporozoites, released from the sporocysts, invade the venules of the liver where they locate in endothelial cells. The second-generation meronts are found in the endothelial cells of capillaries of all organs and the resulting merozoites penetrate muscle cells. There they encyst and then divide by a process of budding or endodyogeny, giving rise to broad banana-shaped bradyzoites contained within a cyst; this is the mature sarcocyst and is the infective stage for the carnivorous final host. Cysts are found in skeletal and cardiac muscle.

Sarcocystis porcifelis

Synonym: *Sarcocystis suifelis*

Description: The sporulated sporocysts are ellipsoid and measure 13.2–13.5 by 7.2–8 μm, without a Stieda body, but with a residuum.

Sarcocystis suihominis

Synonym: *Sarcocystis porcihominis*

Description: Mature sarcocysts are thin-walled, compartmented, up to 1.5 mm long and have protrusions up to 13 μm long, folded closely on the surface.

Life cycle: Infection is by ingestion of the sporocysts and this is followed by at least three asexual generations. In the first, sporozoites, released from the sporocysts, invade the intestinal wall and the endothelial cells of blood vessels in the liver, where they undergo two merogony cycles. Sarcocysts can be found in the striated muscles, heart and brain. At first, they contain only metrocytes but these divide rapidly to form bradyzoites contained within the thin-walled cyst; this is the mature sarcocyst and is the infective stage for the final host. The prepatent period is about 12–14 days and the patent period lasts at least 18 days.

Sarcocystis hovarthi

Synonym: *Sarcocystis gallinarum*

Description: Tissue cysts are 1–10 mm long with striated walls and are found in skeletal muscles of the breast, thigh, neck and oesophagus. The oocysts have not been described. The sporulated sporocysts are ellipsoid and measure approximately 10–13 by 7–9 μm.

Frenkelia

The closely related genus, *Frenkelia*, differs from *Sarcocystis* in that its last-generation meronts occur in the brain rather than in the muscles. The protozoa in this genus infect the gastrointestinal tract of birds of prey (definitive hosts) and the tissues of small rodents (intermediate hosts).

Neospora

The single species in this genus, *Neospora caninum*, is an important pathogen in cattle and dogs. *Neospora* is a cause of paralysis in dogs and abortion in cattle. Recent evidence indicates members of the dog family are the final hosts.

Neospora caninum

This species infects the brain, heart, liver and placenta of ruminants (intermediate hosts) and the small intestine of dogs and other canids (definitive hosts).

Description: Unsporulated oocysts in dogs are reported to measure 11.7 by 11.3 μm (10.6–12.4 × 10.6–12 μm). Tachyzoites measure 6 by 2 μm and are usually located in the cytoplasm of cells. Tissue cysts are oval, 107 μm long, and have a thick wall (up to 4 μm) and are found only in neural tissue.

Life cycle: The complete life cycle of *Neospora caninum* has only recently been elucidated. Oocysts are passed in the faeces of the definitive host 8–23 days after infection. When ingested by the intermediate hosts, such as cattle, they become permanently infected and form tissue cysts. Pregnancy activates these cysts and may cause spontaneous abortion. If the aborted fetus and placenta are eaten by the final carnivore host, they become infected and the life cycle is complete. Transplacental infection has been shown to occur in cattle, sheep, dogs and cats. Dogs and foxes can also act as intermediate hosts. See **life cycle** 34.

Toxoplasma

The genus *Toxoplasma* contains a single species. Unsporulated oocysts are passed in the faeces of cats and other felids. *Toxoplasma* shows a complete lack of species specificity in the intermediate host and is capable of infecting any warm-blooded animal, and is an important zoonosis.

    Life cycle: The final host is the cat, in which gametogony takes place. A range of mammals (and birds) act as intermediate hosts, in which the cycle is extraintestinal and results in the formation of tachyzoites and bradyzoites, which are the only forms found in non-feline hosts. Infection usually occurs through the ingestion of sporulated oocysts. The liberated sporozoites rapidly penetrate the intestinal wall and spread by the haematogenous route. This invasive and proliferative stage is called the tachyzoite and, on entering a cell, it multiplies asexually in a vacuole by a process of budding or endodyogeny, in which two individuals are formed within the mother cell, the pellicle of the latter being used by the daughter cells. When 8–16 tachyzoites have accumulated, the cell ruptures and new cells are infected. This is the acute phase of toxoplasmosis. In most instances, the host survives and antibody is produced which limits the invasiveness of the tachyzoites and results in the formation of cysts containing thousands of organisms which, because endodyogeny and growth are slow, are termed bradyzoites. The cyst containing the bradyzoites is the latent form, multiplication being held in check by the acquired immunity of the host. If this immunity wanes, the cyst may rupture, releasing the bradyzoites, which become active and resume the invasive characteristics of the tachyzoites. See **life cycle** 35.

Toxoplasma gondii

This species infects the muscles, lungs, liver, reproductive system and central nervous system of any mammal, including humans, or birds (intermediate hosts) and has cats and other felids as definitive hosts.

Description: Oocysts are round to slightly oval and measure 11–15 μm (mean 13 μm) by 8–12 μm (mean 11 μm). Sporulated oocysts contain two ellipsoid sporocysts (8.5 × 6 μm) each containing four sporozoites (Fig. 2.76). Tachyzoites are found developing in vacuoles in many cell types, for example fibroblasts, hepatocytes, reticular cells and myocardial cells. In any one cell there may be 8–16 organisms, each measuring 6–8 μm. Tissue cysts, measuring up to 100 μm in diameter, are found mainly in the muscle, liver, lung and brain and may contain several thousand lancet-shaped bradyzoites (Fig. 2.77).

Cystoisospora

The genus *Cystoisospora* contains many species that parasitise a wide range of hosts. *Cystoisospora* includes species previously classified as *Isospora* in mammals, based on the absence of Stieda bodies in their sporocysts (Table 2.41). The life cycles of *Cystoisospora* species differ from those of *Eimeria* in three respects. First, the sporulated oocyst contains two sporocysts each with four sporozoites (Fig. 2.78). Second, extraintestinal stages occurring in the spleen, liver and lymph nodes, as found in the pig for example, may reinvade the intestinal mucosa and cause clinical signs. Third, rodents may, by the ingestion of oocysts from the dog and cat, become infected with asexual stages and act as reservoirs. See **life cycle** 36.

Cystoisospora canis

Synonym: *Isospora canis*

Description: Oocysts are ellipsoid to slightly ovoid, 34–42 by 23–36 μm (mean 38 × 30 μm) with a smooth pale wall without a micropyle, polar granule or residuum, but with a tiny blob adherent to the oocyst wall at the broad end. The two sporocysts are ellipsoid (18–28 × 15–19 μm) with a smooth colourless wall and a prominent residuum and each contains four sausage-shaped sporozoites with clear subcentral globules.

Life cycle: Three merogony generations occur in the subepithelium of the lamina propria of the small intestine. Gamonts appear within the epithelial cells about seven days post infection. The prepatent period is 9–11 days and infections can remain patent for about four weeks.

LIFE CYCLE 34. LIFE CYCLE OF *NEOSPORA CANINUM*

The protozoan parasite *Neospora caninum* is amongst the primary aetiological agents of bovine abortion. Dogs act as definitive hosts (1), while several domestic and wild mammalian species act as intermediate hosts (2). Dogs release oocysts via the faeces (3) into the environment in about 8–23 days post infection. The oocysts are ovoid in shape, similar to other species of coccidia, and sporulate in the environment (4); from here, sporulated oocysts can contaminate water and feedstuffs (5). The intermediate hosts acquire the infection by accidentally ingesting oocysts (horizontal transmission) (6); following ingestion, the parasite replicates in the cytoplasm of several cell types, particularly those of the central nervous system, where it forms tissue cysts (7). The tissue cysts are very resistant and are surrounded by a thick wall. When cattle ingest oocysts during pregnancy, the oocyst outer wall ruptures in the gastrointestinal tract, releasing pear-shaped tachyzoites (8) that, through the placenta, reach the fetus (vertical transmission, 9). Depending on the stage of gestation when infection occurs, the fetus may be reabsorbed (first trimester of pregnancy), become mummified and aborted, stillborn or born weak and symptomatic (second trimester), or born asymptomatic but with persistent infection (last trimester, 10). The latter occurs most frequently, although stillbirths are also possible. Persistently infected calves may abort their own fetuses following reactivation of tachyzoites in the central nervous system. Tachyzoites present in the aborted fetuses represent the source of infection for the definitive host (11).

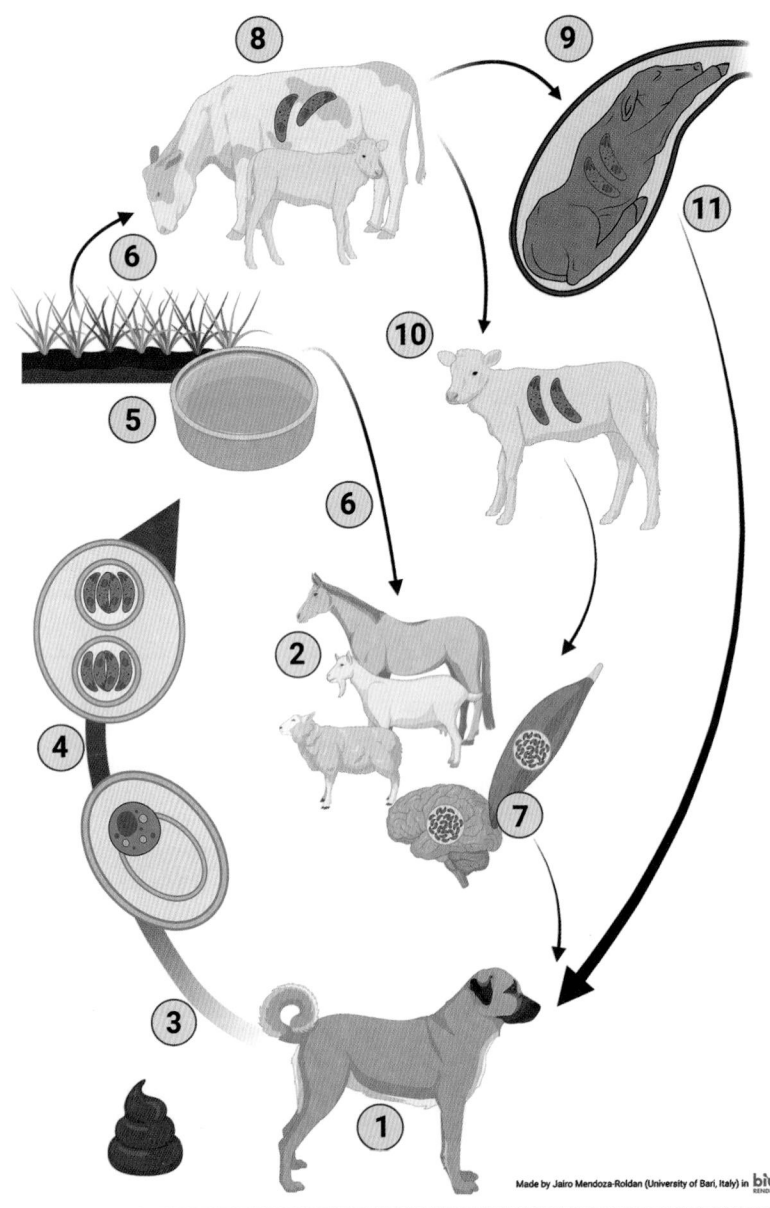

Made by Jairo Mendoza-Roldan (University of Bari, Italy) in bio RENDER

LIFE CYCLE 35. LIFE CYCLE OF *TOXOPLASMA GONDII*

Cats and some wild felids act as definitive hosts of *Toxoplasma gondii*, while several mammalian species (e.g. ruminants, pigs, equids, rodents), as well as birds, act as intermediate hosts. In the definitive host, *T. gondii* undergoes intestinal and extraintestinal cycles, while in intermediate hosts only the latter occurs. The definitive host excretes unsporulated oocysts of *T. gondii* via the faeces (1); in the environment, unsporulated oocysts undergo sporogony within 2–5 days, depending on temperature (2). Sporogony is terminated with the formation of a sporulated oocyst that contains two elliptical sporocysts, each including four sporozoites (2). Following ingestion by an intermediate host (3), the oocyst ruptures in the intestine, releasing the sporozoites that infect reticuloendothelial cells; from here, the parasite reaches several organs and tissues. Inside the reticuloendothelial cells, the sporozoites replicate by endodyogeny (i.e. daughter cells produced inside mother cells). The daughter cells (rapidly multiplying tachyzoites) continue endodyogeny (4) inside host cells (pseudocyst), leading to the formation of 8–16 tachyzoites. The pseudocyst can rupture, thus releasing the tachyzoites that invade other reticuloendothelial cells (5), eventually forming other pseudocysts (acute phase). Following activation of the host immune response, the parasite replication slows, particularly in tissues of the central nervous system and muscles, where *T. gondii* forms terminal cysts (6). In the terminal cysts, the

parasites undergo slow replication and are known as bradyzoites. Cats become infected by ingesting sporulated oocysts or pseudo- or terminal cysts infecting the tissues of intermediate hosts (e.g. rodents or birds, 7).

In the cat, ingestion of a sporulated oocyst is followed by a phase of coccidia-like replication, consisting of schizogony (8) and gametogony (9) which will produce a zygote (10) and thus an oocyst (11). Once the intestinal cycle is complete, the cat excretes non-sporulated oocysts with the faeces (1). Meanwhile, in cats an extraintestinal cycle may occur identical to that of intermediate hosts. Depending on whether cats become infected by ingesting sporulated oocysts or pseudo- or terminal cysts, the prepatent phase may be long (14–28 days) or short (4–10 days). Humans acquire the infection (12) by accidental ingestions of sporulated oocysts contaminating the environment (e.g. through contaminated vegetables, 13) or, more often, by eating raw or undercooked meat from intermediate hosts containing tissue cysts (14). Transmission through direct contact of mucosal lesions or body fluids containing the tachyzoites has been reported. In pregnant women, as well as in other intermediate hosts (e.g. sheep), the infection can be transmitted transplacentally to the unborn foetus (15), thus causing abortion, fetal malformations or central nervous system lesions, depending on the stage of gestation when infection occurs.

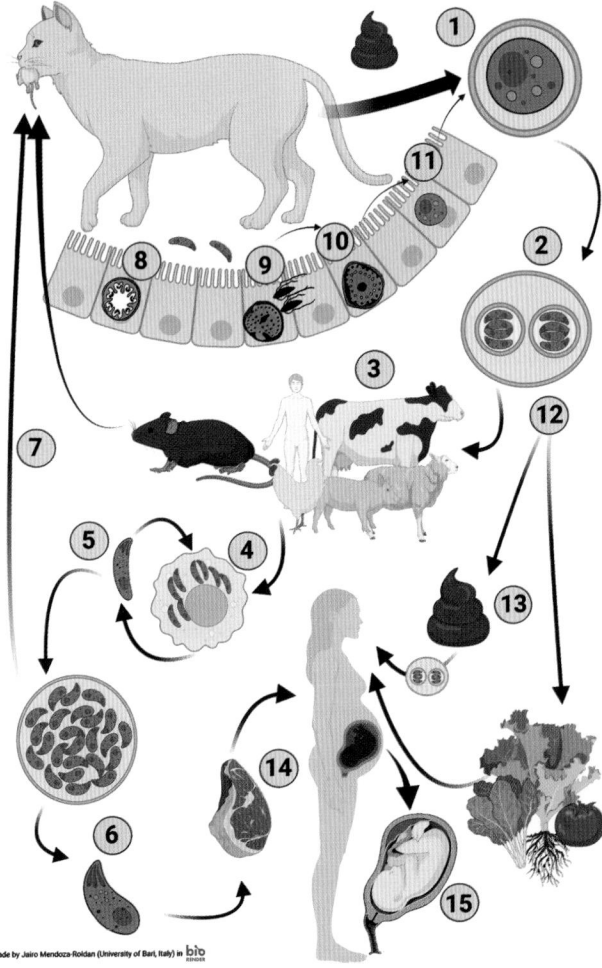

Made by Jairo Mendoza-Roldan (University of Bari, Italy) in bioRender

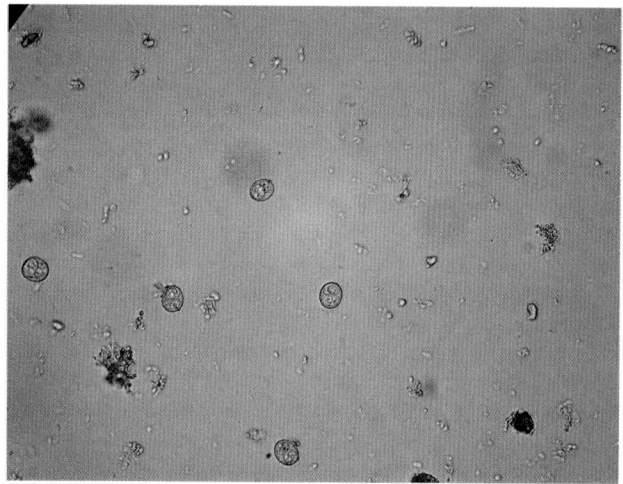

Fig. 2.76 Oocysts of *Toxoplasma gondii*. (Courtesy of Anja Joachim).

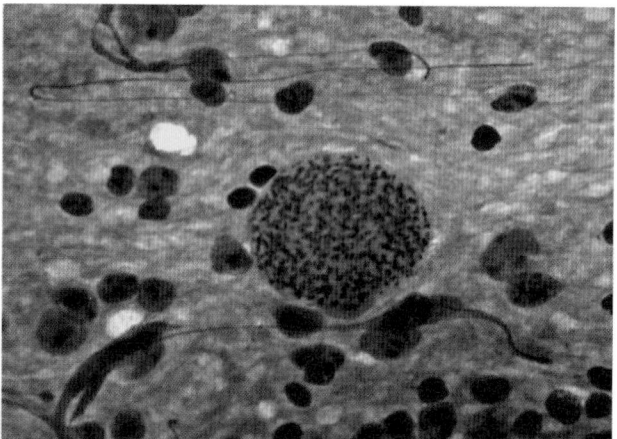

Fig. 2.77 Tissue cyst of *Toxoplasma gondii*. (Courtesy of Anja Joachim).

Table 2.41 *Cystoisospora* species.

Species	Hosts	Site
Cystoisospora canis (syn. *Isospora canis*)	Dogs	Small intestine
Cystoisospora felis (syn. *Isospora felis*)	Cats	Small intestine
Cystoisospora ohioensis (syn. *Isospora ohioensis*)	Dogs	Small intestine
Cystoisospora burrowsi (syn. *Isospora burrowsi*)	Dogs	Small intestine
Cystoisospora rivolta (syn. *Isospora rivolta*)	Cats	Small intestine
Cystoisospora suis (syn. *Isospora suis*)	Pigs	Small intestine
Cystoisospora orlovi (syn. *Isospora orlovi*)	Camels	Unknown
Cystoisospora belli (syn. *Isospora belli*)	Humans	Small intestine
Cystoisospora aectopitheci (syn. *Isospora aectopitheci*)	Primates	Small intestine
Cystoisospora callimico (syn. *Isospora callimico*)	Primates	Small intestine
Cystoisospora papionis (syn. *Isospora papionis*)	Primates	Small intestine

Cystoisospora felis

Synonym: *Isospora felis*

Description: Oocysts are ovoid, measuring 32–53 by 26–43 μm (mean 43 × 32 μm) with a smooth, yellowish to pale brown wall without a micropyle, polar granule or residuum. The two sporocysts are ellipsoid (20–27 × 17–22 μm) with a smooth colourless wall and

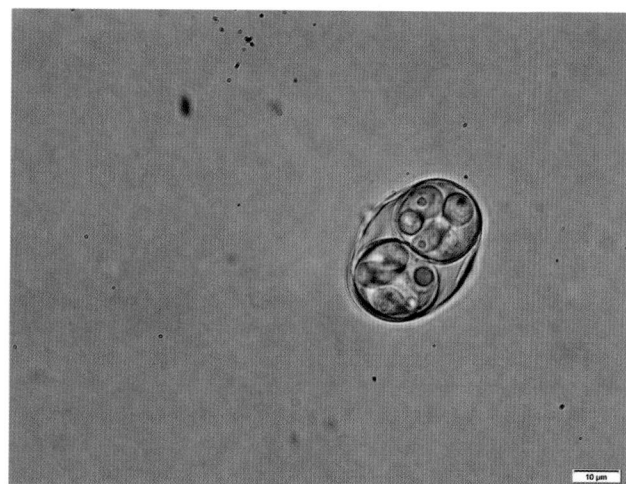

Fig. 2.78 Sporulated oocyst of *Cystoisospora* with two sporocysts each containing four sporozoites. (Courtesy of Anja Joachim).

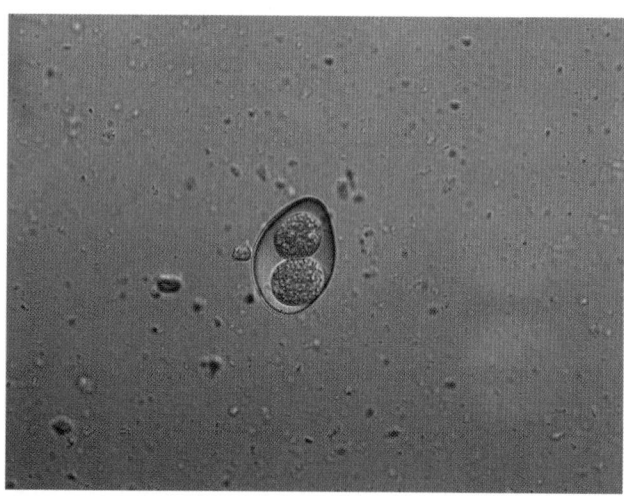

Fig. 2.79 Oocysts of *Cystoisospora felis*. (Courtesy of Riccardo Paolo Lia).

a prominent residuum and each contains four sausage-shaped sporozoites with clear subcentral globules (Fig. 2.79).

Life cycle: All stages are found above the host cell nuclei in the epithelium of the lower small intestine. Gamonts appear from six days after infection. The prepatent period is 7–10 days. Infections can remain patent for about 1–3 weeks.

Cystoisospora ohioensis

Synonym: *Isospora ohioensis*

Description: Oocysts are ellipsoid to oval, measuring 20–27 by 14–24 μm (mean 23 × 19 μm) with a smooth, colourless to pale yellow wall without a micropyle, polar granule or residuum. The two sporocysts are ellipsoid, 12–19 by 9–13 μm (mean 14.5 × 10 μm), with a residuum and four sporozoites with one or more clear globules.

Life cycle: All stages occur in the epithelium of the small intestine; gamonts can also be found in the caecum and large intestine 4–5 days post infection. The prepatent period is 4–5 days and patency is 3–5 weeks.

LIFE CYCLE 36. LIFE CYCLE OF *CYSTOISOSPORA* SPP. IN DOGS AND CATS

Species of *Cystoisospora* infect the small intestine of dogs (*Cystoisospora canis* and *Cystoisospora ohioensis*) and cats (*Cystoisospora felis* and *Cystoisospora rivolta*). Puppies and kittens become infected by ingesting sporulated oocysts contaminating the environment (1); once in the intestine, sporozoites (banana-shaped and motile) are released (2) and penetrate the enterocytes (3), thus growing in size and becoming trophozoites (4). Inside the enterocytes, the trophozoites divide by nuclear fission, eventually forming the schizont (asexual reproduction, schizogony) (5). Subsequently, enterocytes rupture, releasing several merozoites that invade other enterocytes (6), further repeating the cycle of schizogony, 2–3 times (3–5). Following schizogony, some merozoites become telomerozoites (7), which begin a phase of sexual reproduction (gametogony); some telomerozoites become microgametes (male gametes, 8), motile and possessing a flagellum (9), while others become macrogametes, which are static and characterised by a large nucleus (10). The microgametes fertilise the macrogametes, thus producing a zygote (11), characterised by a double outer wall. The zygote is the precursor to the unsporulated oocysts, which contain the sporont (unorganised genetic material, 12). Once excreted in the environment with the host faeces (13), the oocyst undergoes sporulation (sporogony), progressively differentiating into two sporoblasts (14). Subsequently, the sporoblasts differentiate into two sporocysts, each containing four banana-shaped sporozoites (1). Once sporogony is complete, the mature oocyst (infective stage) contains eight sporozoites.

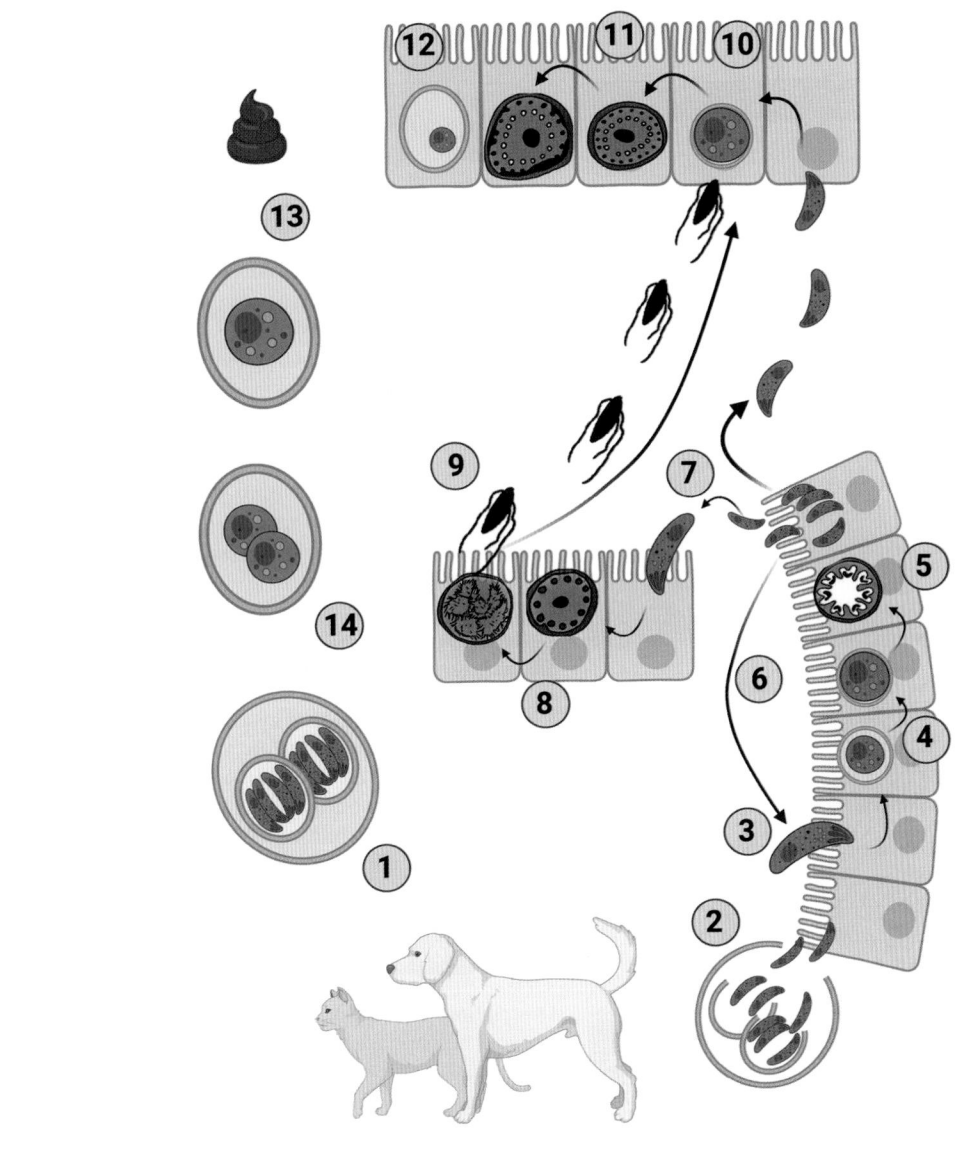

Made by Jairo Mendoza-Roldan (University of Bari, Italy) in bioRENDER

Cystoisospora orlovi

Synonym: *Isospora orlovi*

Description: Oocysts contain two sporocysts each with four sporozoites. The oocysts are ellipsoid, oval, cylindrical or shaped like a figure 8, smooth, 27–35 by 15–20 μm, without a polar granule, micropyle or residuum. Sporocysts are ellipsoid, ovoid (15–20 × 13–17 μm) or spherical (13–15 μm diameter) without a Stieda body, but with a residuum.

Cystoisospora rivolta

Synonym: *Isospora rivolta*

Description: Oocysts are ellipsoid to ovoid, measuring 21–29 by 18–26 μm (mean 25 × 21 μm) with a smooth, colourless to pale brown wall without a micropyle, polar granule or residuum. The two sporocysts are ellipsoid (14–16 × 10–13 μm) with a residuum and four sporozoites each with clear subcentral globules.

Cystoisospora suis

Synonym: *Isospora suis*

Description: Oocysts are spherical to subspherical, wall colourless and thin, measuring 17–25 by 16–22 μm (mean 20.6 × 18.1 μm) and without a micropyle or residuum. The two sporocysts are ellipsoid (13–14 × 8–11 μm) without a Stieda body but with a sporocyst residuum. The four sporozoites in each sporocyst are sausage-shaped with one pointed end.

Life cycle: Meronts are found in the epithelial cells of the villi of the small intestine, usually in the distal third and below the host cell nucleus. First-generation meronts are present 2–3 days after infection. Second-generation meronts are present four days and mature gamonts five days after infection. The prepatent period is 4–6 days and the period of patency 3–13 days.

FAMILY LANKESTERELLIDAE

Lankesterella occur in amphibians; *Schellakia* are found in reptiles. Transmission is by leeches, mites and insects.

FAMILY KLOSSIELLIDAE

Klossiella is the only genus in this family. Its members are essentially non-pathogenic, with most species occurring in the kidneys. The oocysts reside in the kidney tubules, where they contain as many as 40 sporocysts, each with 8–15 sporozoites. The sporocysts pass out in the urine and infect new hosts when they are ingested.

Klossiella

Members of the genus are homoxenous, with meronts and merozoites present in the Bowman's capsules and gamonts in the tubules of the kidney (Table 2.42).

Life cycle: The life cycle is not clearly understood. Within epithelial cells of kidney tubules, trophozoites form meronts and merozoites, which in turn form gamonts. Fertilised gametes are believed to

Table 2.42 *Klossiella* species.

Species	Hosts	Site
Klossiella equi	Horses, donkeys, zebras	Kidney
Klossiella cobayae	Guinea pigs	Kidney
Klossiella muris	Mice	Kidney
Klossiella boae	Snakes	Kidney

develop into sporonts, which bud to form sporoblasts. Each of these sporoblasts undergoes successive divisions to form sporocysts that contain sporozoites. Mature sporocysts are surrounded by a thick wall and pass from the body in the urine. When ingested by another host, the sporozoites are released from the sporocyst and move to the kidney, where they enter epithelial cells and initiate the cycle.

Klossiella equi

Description: Meronts in endothelial cells of Bowman's capsule in the kidneys are 8–12 μm in diameter with 20–30 nuclei. Second-generation meronts found in epithelial cells of the proximal convoluted tubules are 15–23 μm in diameter and contain 15–20 merozoites. Gamogony and sporogony occur in the epithelial cells of the thick limb of Henle's loop. The microgamonts form 4–10 microgametes. Sporonts, 20–23 μm in diameter, have about 40 buds on their periphery before becoming sporoblasts, 35–45 μm in diameter. Each sporoblast divides by multiple fission forming 10–15 or more nuclei, which condense and come to lie along the periphery of the sporoblast. The sporocysts each contain 10–15 sporozoites and are themselves contained in a sac formed by the host cell.

FAMILY HEPATOZOIDAE

The genus *Hepatozoon* has been reported from mammals, reptiles and birds and is of importance in dogs. Definitive hosts include ticks, mites, sand flies, tsetse flies, mosquitoes, fleas, lice, reduviid bugs and leeches.

Hepatozoon

Parasites of this genus share a basic life cycle that includes sexual development and sporogony in a haematophagous invertebrate definitive host, and merogony followed by gametogony in a vertebrate intermediate host (Table 2.43). Transmission takes place by ingestion of the definitive host, an invertebrate containing *Hepatozoon* oocysts, by the intermediate host.

Hepatozoon canis

Description: Gamonts, found in circulating neutrophils, are ellipsoid in shape, about 11 by 4 μm, and are enveloped in a thick membrane (Fig. 2.80). Meronts are usually round to oval, about 30 μm in diameter, and include elongated micromerozoites with defined nuclei, which in cross-section have a 'wheel-spoke' appearance.

Life cycle: The life cycle involves two hosts. The tick is a final host in which syngamy occurs, and the dog is an intermediate host in which asexual reproduction occurs. Nymphal ticks engorge with gamont-infected leucocytes in an infected dog. Following ingestion, the

Table 2.43 *Hepatozoon* species.

Species	Hosts	Intermediate hosts	Site
Hepatozoon canis	Ticks (*Rhipicephalus*)	Dogs, cats	Blood, liver, kidney
Hepatozoon americanum	Ticks (*Amblyomma*)	Dogs	Blood, muscle
Hepatozoon felis	Unknown	Cats and wild felids	Myocardium, skeletal muscles, lungs
Hepatozoon silvestris	Unknown	Cats and wild felids	Myocardium, skeletal muscles, intestine
Hepatozoon cuniculi	Unknown	Rabbits	Spleen
Hepatozoon muris	Spiny rat mite (*Echinolaelaps*)	Rats	Blood, liver

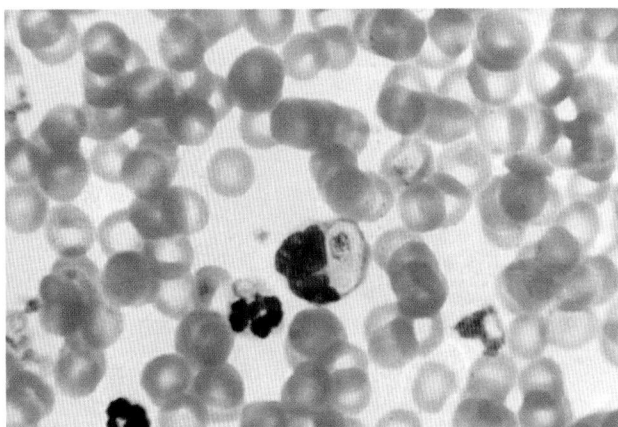

Fig. 2.80 Gamont of *Hepatozoon canis* in circulating neutrophil.

gamonts are freed from the leucocytes, associate in pairs and transform into male and female gametes, leading to the formation of zygotes and oocysts. Each mature oocyst contains numerous sporocysts, each containing 10–26 sporozoites. After the tick moults, oocysts are found in the haemocoel and each tick may carry thousands of infective sporozoites. Since the sporozoites remain in the body cavity, the dog is apparently infected by ingesting the tick. Once ingested, the sporozoites are released from the oocysts, penetrate the intestinal wall and are transported to target tissues and organs in the blood and lymph. They primarily infect the spleen, lymph nodes and bone marrow where merogony occurs in macrophages and endothelial cells. Two forms of meronts are found in infected tissues, one type containing 2–4 macromerozoites and a second type containing 20 elongated micromerozoites. When the meront matures and ruptures, merozoites are released and penetrate circulating neutrophils, in which they develop into gamonts that circulate in peripheral blood. The cycle is completed when the tick ingests infected blood. The period of development in the dog from infection to the appearance of gamonts is about 28 days. See **life cycle** 37.

Hepatozoon americanum

Description: Gamonts present within neutrophils are ellipsoid in shape, 8.8 by 3.9 μm, with a central compact nucleus and enveloped in a thick membrane. The cytoplasm stains pale blue and the nucleus dark reddish with Giemsa stain. Muscle cysts are round to oval, 250–500 μm in diameter, with the outer portion composed of concentric layers of fine, pale-staining laminar membranes that give the cyst an 'onion skin' appearance.

Life cycle: Similar to that of *H. canis*. The parasite infects skeletal and cardiac muscle, where it develops between myocytes within host cells of undetermined origin. Mucopolysaccharide layers encyst the infected cells in the muscle where the parasite undergoes merogony. At maturation, the cyst ruptures, releasing merozoites into adjacent tissue. Neutrophils and macrophages are recruited to the area and many become infected, leading to pyogranuloma formation with increased vascularisation, allowing infected leucocytes containing gamonts to enter the circulation and repeat the asexual reproductive phase at other sites. The cycle is completed when the tick ingests infected blood. The period of development in the dog from infection to the appearance of gamonts is about 32 days.

Hepatozoon felis

Description: Meronts may reach 39 μm in diameter. Gamonts in the cytoplasm of neutrophils and/or monocytes are elongated and can present basophilic staining granules. Compared with *H. canis*, *H. felis* gamonts have a rounder nucleus and a mean length of 10.5 μm.

Life cycle: Similar to that of *H. canis*. Cats become infected by ingesting ticks or other arthropod vectors. Once ingested, the sporozoites primarily infect myocardium, skeletal muscles and lungs, where merogony occurs. Merozoites released penetrate the circulating neutrophils and/or monocytes, developing into gamonts that can be found in peripheral blood. The level of parasitaemia is usually low in felid hosts, with less than 1% of the neutrophils and monocytes containing gamonts.

Hepatozoon silvestris

Description: Meronts may reach 32 μm in diameter. Gamonts in neutrophils are up to 11.2 μm length.

Life cycle: Similar to that of *H. felis*.

Hepatozoon cuniculi

Description: Merocysts may reach 4–6 mm in diameter.

Life cycle: The life cycle is unknown. Meronts are found in the spleen and gamonts within leucocytes.

Hepatozoon muris

Synonyms: *Hepatozoon perniciosum, Leucocytozoon muris, Leucocytozoon ratti*

Description: Meronts in the liver are 10–30 μm in diameter. Gamonts in the lymphocytes appear in stained blood smears as elongated oval bodies, 8–12 by 3–6 μm.

LIFE CYCLE 37. LIFE CYCLE OF *HEPATOZOON CANIS*

Hepatozoon canis is a protozoan parasite infecting the white blood cells of dogs. The life cycle of *H. canis* involves a phase of gametogony and one of sporogony in the tick vectors, and a phase of schizogony, followed by the formation of gamonts, in canine hosts. When a dog ingests a tick infected with oocysts (1), sporozoites are released in the dog's intestine (2). The sporozoites invade the intestinal epithelium and, via the circulation, travel to several organs and tissues, such as liver (3), spleen (4), bone marrow (5), lungs, lymph nodes (6) and muscles (7). In all tissues above, and in particular in the liver, spleen and bone marrow, the sporozoites undergo schizogony, thus forming schizonts (8) that subsequently differentiate into macroschizonts (9) and microschizonts (that contain several micromerozoites) (10). The macroschizonts generate macromerozoites (11) that undergo secondary schizogony, leading to the formation of new schizonts (8). The merozoites released by the microschizonts (12) invade the white blood cells (13), especially neutrophils and monocytes, and become gamonts (14). The tick vector ingests *H. canis* gamonts during the blood meal (15). In the tick's gut, the white blood cells rupture, releasing the gamonts that, following fertilisation (16), form the zygote. In turn, the zygote forms a mobile ookinete (17) that travels through the midgut epithelium to the tick's haemocoel and becomes an oocyst (18). Once mature, the oocyst contains several sporozoites (19). Since the sporozoites do not migrate to the tick's salivary glands, infection of a canine host occurs following ingestion of infected ticks.

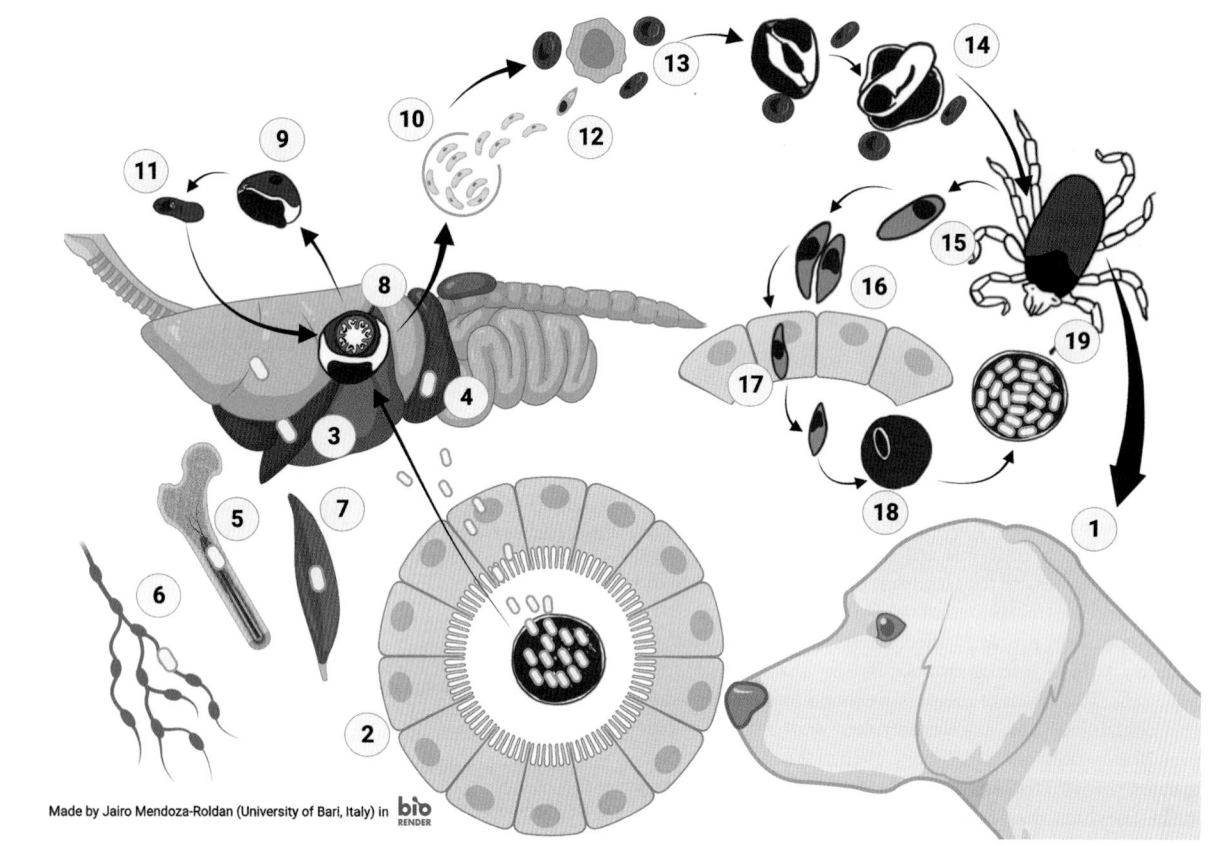

Made by Jairo Mendoza-Roldan (University of Bari, Italy) in **bio**RENDER

Life cycle: Rats become infected by ingesting the invertebrate host, the spiny rat mite *Echinolaelaps echidninus*. Sporozoites are released in the intestine, enter the hepatic portal system and are transported to the liver. Merogony takes place in the liver parenchymal cells. Merozoites enter the lymphocytes in the blood and become gamonts. Fertilisation and sporogony occur in the arthropod vector following ingestion.

FAMILY HAEMOGREGARINIDAE

Parasites of the genus *Haemogregorina* have been described from the red blood cells of chelonia and are generally considered to be non-pathogenic. The definitive hosts are leeches.

ORDER CRYPTOGREGARINORIDA

FAMILY CRYPTOSPORIDIIDAE

This family, in the order Cryptogregarinorida, contains a single genus, *Cryptosporidium*, occurring in mammals, birds, reptiles and fish. Members of this family are small parasites infecting the brush border of epithelial cells mainly in the gastrointestinal tract.

Life cycle: The life cycle is monoxenous, but some species are capable of infecting a range of vertebrate hosts. Oocysts, each with four sporozoites, are liberated in the faeces (Fig. 2.81). Development is intracellular but extracytoplasmic and oocysts lack sporocysts. Gametogony follows after 1–2 generations of meronts, leading to

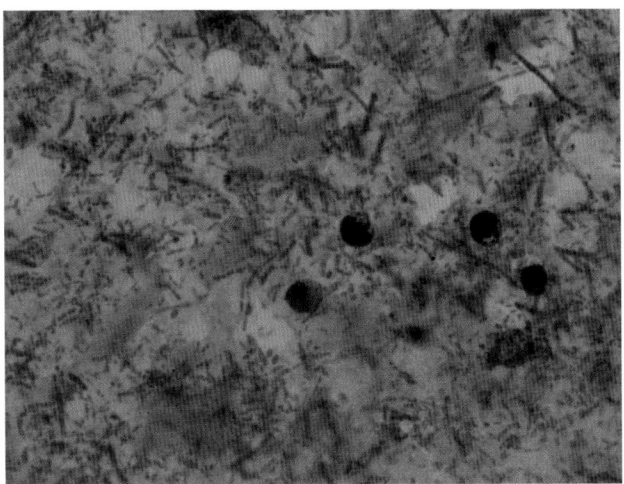

Fig. 2.81 Oocysts of *Cryptosporidium parvum* (Ziehl–Neelsen stain ×1000). (Courtesy of Georgiana Deak).

Table 2.44 *Cryptosporidium* species.

Species	Hosts	Site	Oocyst size (μm)
Cryptosporidium parvum	Cattle, sheep, goats, horses, pigs, deer, humans	Small intestine	5 × 4.5
Cryptosporidium hominis	Humans, sheep, dugongs	Small intestine	5.5 × 4.5
Cryptosporidium bovis	Cattle, sheep	Small intestine	5 × 4.5
Cryptosporidium andersoni	Cattle, camels	Abomasum	7.4 × 5.5
Cryptosporidium ryanae	Cattle, deer	Small intestine	3.2 × 3.7
Cryptosporidium muris	Rodents, humans, rock hyraxes	Stomach	6.1 × 8.4
Cryptosporidium wrairi	Guinea pigs	Small intestine	5.40 × 4.6
Cryptosporidium canis	Dogs, humans	Small intestine	4.7 × 5
Cryptosporidium fayeri	Marsupials	Small intestine	4.9 × 4.3
Cryptosporidium felis	Cats	Small intestine	4.5 × 5
Cryptosporidium suis	Pigs	Small and large intestine	5.2 × 4.1
Cryptosporidium xiaoi	Sheep, goats	Small intestine	4 × 3.4
Cryptosporidium ubiquitum	Deer, ruminants, rodents, carnivores	Small intestine	5 × 4.7
Cryptosporidium baileyi	Chickens, parrots, ducks, oysters	Bursa, conjunctiva, trachea	4.6 × 6.2
Cryptosporidium meleagridis	Turkeys, chickens, ducks and other birds, rarely dogs, humans	Small intestine	4.7 × 4.9
Cryptosporidium galli	Finches, parrots, canaries and other bird species	Proventriculus	8.3 × 6.3
Cryptosporidium serpentis	Snakes	Stomach	6.2 × 5.3
Cryptosporidium saurophilum	Lizards	Stomach and small intestine	4.7 × 5
Cryptosporidium molnari	Fishes	Stomach and intestines	4.7 × 4.5

the production of oocysts. Sporulation takes place within the host so that oocysts are immediately infective. Evidence also indicates that in some species, two types of oocysts are produced. The first, the majority, are thick-walled and passed in the faeces. The remaining oocysts are thin-walled and release their sporozoites in the intestine, causing autoinfection.

Cryptosporidium

Cryptosporidium is a phenotypically and genotypically heterogeneous assemblage of largely morphologically identical genotypes and species. Species differentiation is determined largely by molecular genotyping and subtyping (Table 2.44). See **life cycle** 38.

Cryptosporidium parvum

Description: Mature oocysts are ovoid or spheroidal, 5 by 4.5 μm (range 4.6–5.4 by 3.8–4.7 μm) and have a length/width ratio of 1.19.

Cryptosporidium andersoni

Description: Oocysts are ellipsoid, 7.4 by 5.5 μm (range 6–8.1 × 5–6 μm); length/width ratio, 1.35.

Cryptosporidium baileyi

Description: Oocysts are ellipsoid, 6.2 by 4.6 μm (range 5.6–6.3 × 4.5–4.8 μm); length/width ratio, 1.3.

Cryptosporidium meleagridis

Description: Oocysts are ellipsoid, 5.6–6.3 by 4.5–4.8 μm (mean 6.2 × 4.6 μm). length/width ratio, 1.1.

Cryptosporidium muris

Description: Oocysts are small, ovoid, 7.4 by 5.6 μm, and contain four free sporozoites (Fig. 2.82). Trophozoites attached to the surface of a gland cell consist of a small amount of cytoplasm with a nucleus, and often appear to be surrounded by a cyst wall (peritrophic membrane). The maturing first-generation meronts reach a maximum size of 7 by 6 μm and contain eight merozoites. Microgametocytes are 5 by 4 μm and contain 16 microgametes; macrogametocytes are 7 by 5 μm.

Cryptosporidium ryanae

Description: Oocysts measure 2.94–4.41 by 2.94–3.68 μm (mean 3.16 × 3.73 μm); length/width shape index, 1.18.

LIFE CYCLE 38. LIFE CYCLE OF *CRYPTOSPORIDIUM PARVUM*

Infected animals excrete small round oocysts (2–6 μm) with the faeces; each oocyst contains four infective sporozoites (1). Once ingested by susceptible hosts, the oocysts rupture, thus releasing the sporozoites (2). Each sporozoite adheres to an enterocyte (3) and is enveloped by the microvilli, thus forming the parasitophorous vacuole (4). In the latter, the sporozoite becomes trophozoite and then schizont, which contains eight merozoites (schizogony, 5) that subsequently invade other enterocytes (6); schizogony is repeated twice. Following this phase of asexual reproduction, some merozoites become gamonts (7) and then non-flagellated microgametes (8) and static macrogametes (9). The zygote forms following fertilisation of the macrogamete by the microgamete (10), and subsequently develops into an oocyst containing four sporozoites (1). The oocysts are excreted into the environment with the faeces (11), and contaminate water and pasture, thus exposing susceptible hosts to the infection. A proportion of oocysts characterised by thin outer walls may hatch in the intestine prior to excretion, thus leading to the frequent phenomenon known as 'autoinfection'.

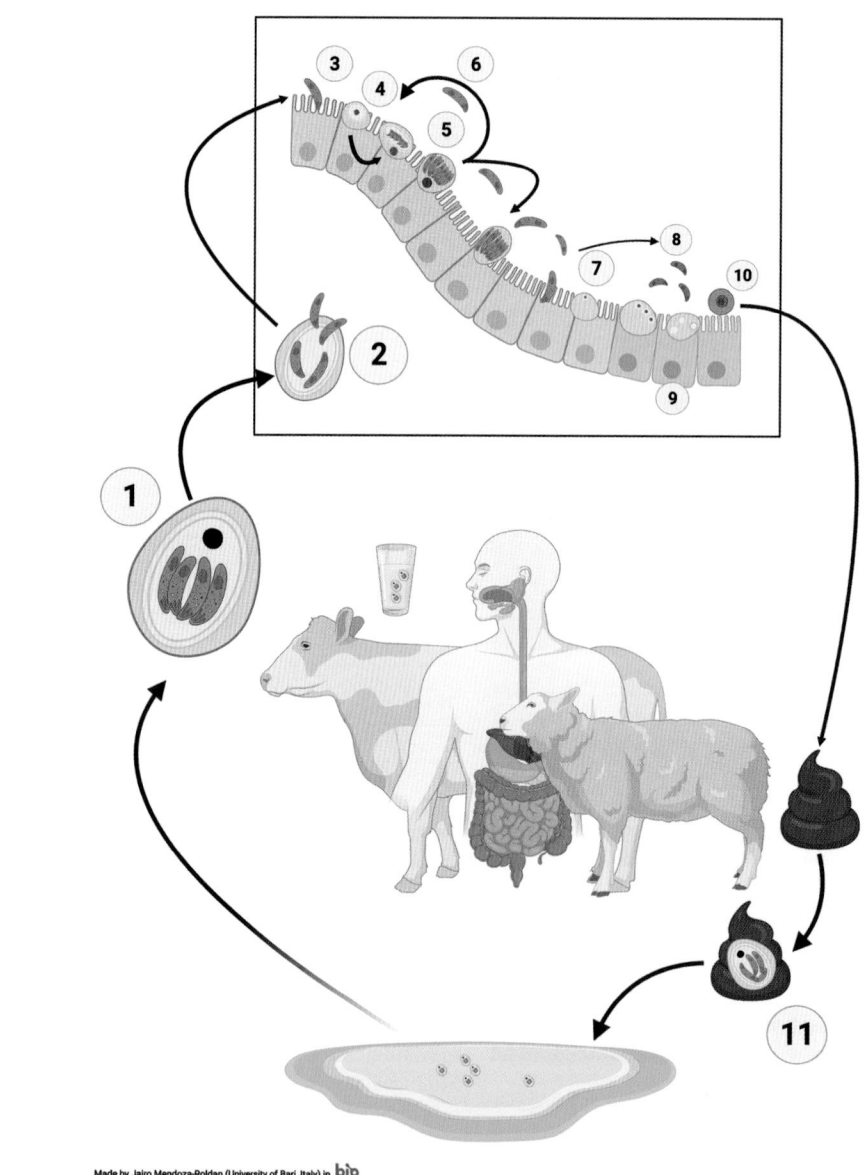

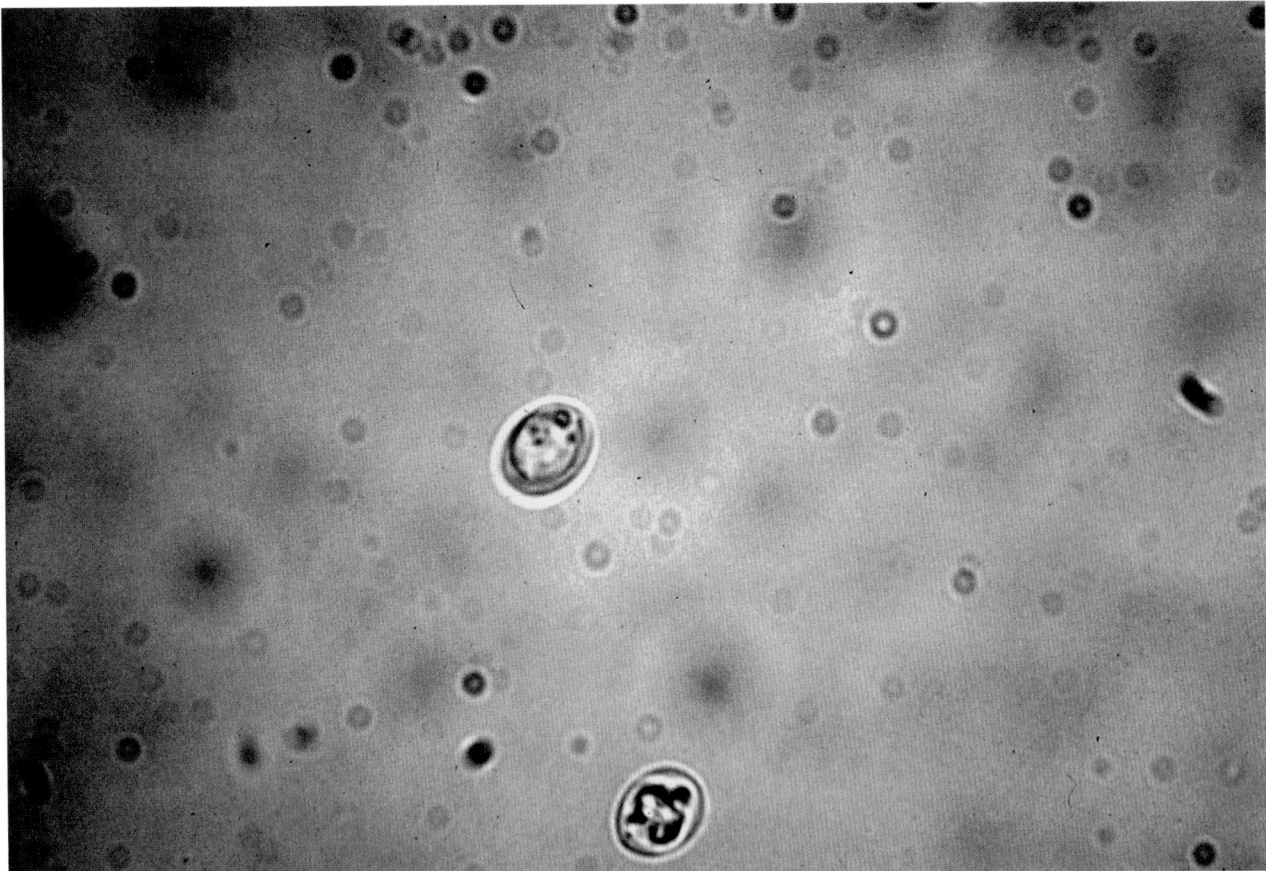

Fig. 2.82 Oocysts of *Cryptosporidium muris*.

Cryptosporidium wrairi

Description: Mature oocysts are ovoid, 4.8–5.6 by 4–5 μm (mean 5.40 × 4.6 μm); length/width ratio, 1.17. First-generation meronts are 3.4–4.4 μm when mature and contain eight merozoites; second-generation meronts contain four merozoites. Developing macrogametes are 4–7 μm in size.

Cryptosporidium fayeri

Description: Mature oocysts are ovoid and measure 4.5–5.1 by 3.8–5 μm (mean 4.9 × 4.3 μm); length/width ratio, 1.02–1.18 (mean 1.14).

Cryptosporidium xiaoi

Description: Oocysts measure 3.94 by 3.44 μm (range 2.94–4.41 × 2.94–4.41 μm); length/width shape index, 1.15.

Cryptosporidium ubiquitum

Description: Oocysts measure 5.04 by 4.66 μm (range 4.71–5.32 × 4.33–4.98 μm); length/width shape index, 1.08.

Cryptosporidium serpentis

Description: Oocysts measure 6.2 by 5.3 μm (range 5.6–6.6 × 4.8–5.6 μm); length/width shape index, 1.16.

CLASS ACONOIDASIDA

ORDER HAEMOSPORIDA

A single family, the Plasmodiidae, contains a number of genera of medical and veterinary interest. All species are heteroxenous with merogony occurring in a vertebrate host and sporogony in an invertebrate host. There are no sporocysts, with the sporozoites lying free within the oocysts.

FAMILY PLASMODIIDAE

Within the family Plasmodiidae are the species of *Plasmodium* which cause malaria in humans, one of the most prevalent diseases of humans in the world. Sporozoites are inoculated into humans by female anopheline mosquitoes. *Plasmodium falciparum* causes malignant tertian or falciparum malaria; *P. vivax* causes benign malaria; *P. malariae* causes quartan or malariae malaria; and *P. ovale* causes a type of tertian malaria. Malaria is also one of the most common haemoprotozoal parasitic diseases of primates in tropical

Table 2.45 Species of *Plasmodium* from non-human primates.

Prosimians	Old World Monkeys	New World Monkeys	Apes
Quotidian			
	Plasmodium knowlesi		
Tertian			
Plasmodium lemuris	*Plasmodium cynomolgi* *Plasmodium coatneyi* *Plasmodium fragile* *Plasmodium siminovale* *Plasmodium fieldi* *Plasmodium gonderi* *Plasmodium eylesi* *Plasmodium jefferyi* *Plasmodium youngi*	*Plasmodium simium*	*Plasmodium pitheci* *Plasmodium reichenowi* *Plasmodium schwetzi* *Plasmodium silvaticum*
Quartan			
Plasmodium girardi	*Plasmodium inui* *Plasmodium hylobati* *Plasmodium shortii*	*Plasmodium brazilianum*	*Plasmodium malariae* (syn. *Plasmodium rodhaini*)

and subtropical regions. Malaria parasites that infect the apes are different from those affecting monkeys and are homologous to the human malaria parasites and morphologically indistinguishable (Table 2.45).

Three separate genera in this family, *Plasmodium*, *Haemoproteus* and *Leucocytozoon*, are the causes of avian 'malaria' in domestic and wild birds, a disease most common in the tropics and transmitted by biting dipteran flies. The vectors differ, in that avian species of *Plasmodium* are transmitted by mosquitoes, *Haemoproteus* by midges or hippoboscid flies, and *Leucocytozoon* by *Simulium* spp.

Plasmodium

Avian malaria is a common mosquito-transmitted disease of wild birds that infects domestic fowl and cage birds when suitable vectors and wild reservoir hosts are present. There are over 30 species of *Plasmodium* affecting birds which differ widely in host range, geographical distribution, vectors and pathogenicity. Avian species of malaria fall into two groups, with either round or elongate gamonts present within the erythrocytes, and can be grouped into five subgenera (Table 2.46) according to morphological characteristics that include size and shape of the gamonts and meronts. Species that infect domestic birds occur in four of the five subgenera.

Plasmodium spp. (Table 2.47) are distinguished from the genera *Haemoproteus* and *Leucocytozoon* by the presence of merogony in circulating erythrocytes. Meronts for the majority of avian *Plasmodium* species are found within endothelial cells of the lymphoid–macrophage system. With one exception, all species of *Plasmodium* are transmitted by culicine mosquitoes. Pre-erythrocytic meronts develop in the liver and produce merozoites, which enter into the erythrocytes producing gamonts. Intraerythrocytic merogony may continue indefinitely, leading to persistent infection with frequent relapses.

Plasmodium gallinaceum

Subgenus: *Haemamoeba*

Description: The trophozoite is a small rounded form containing a large vacuole, which displaces the cytoplasm of the parasite to the periphery of the erythrocyte (Fig. 2.83). The nucleus is situated at

Table 2.46 Avian subgenera of *Plasmodium*.

Description	Subgenus
Parasites without pigment	
Gametocytes and meronts large and when mature displace host cell nucleus; present only in circulating leucocytes	*Plasmodioides*
Parasites with pigments	
Rounded gametocytes displacing host cell nucleus towards pole	*Haemamoeba*
Gametocytes elongate; no displacement of host cell nucleus; meronts in circulating erythrocyte precursors only	*Huffia*
Gametocytes elongate; no displacement of host cell nucleus; meronts in mature erythrocytes only; larger than host cell nucleus containing large amounts of cytoplasm	*Giovannolaia*
Meronts in mature erythrocytes only; smaller than host cell nucleus with little cytoplasm	*Novyella*

Table 2.47 Avian *Plasmodium* species.

Species	Subgenus	Hosts
Plasmodium gallinaceum	*Haemamoeba*	Chickens, guinea fowl
Plasmodium relictum	*Haemamoeba*	Pigeons, doves, ducks, wild birds
Plasmodium hermani	*Huffia*	Turkeys, wild birds
Plasmodium durae	*Giovannolaia*	Turkeys, peafowl
Plasmodium juxtanucleare	*Novyella*	Chickens, other gallinaceous birds
Plasmodium struthionis	?	Oysters

one of the poles, giving the young form a 'signet ring' appearance when stained by Giemsa. Both gametocytes and meronts can be round, oval or irregular in shape. The nucleus of host cells is rarely expelled during infection, but may be displaced by the parasite. Each meront produces 8–36 merozoites and on average there are 16–20 merozoites in erythrocytic meronts.

Life cycle: Following the introduction of the sporozoites from infected mosquitoes, numerous pre-erythrocytic meronts (cryptozoites) are found in the macrophages and fibroblasts of the skin near the point of entry. Merozoites from this first generation of pre-erythrocytic meronts form a second generation of pre-erythrocytic meronts, the metacryptozoites, which reach maturity at about 72 hours. Merozoites from the metacryptozoites enter erythrocytes

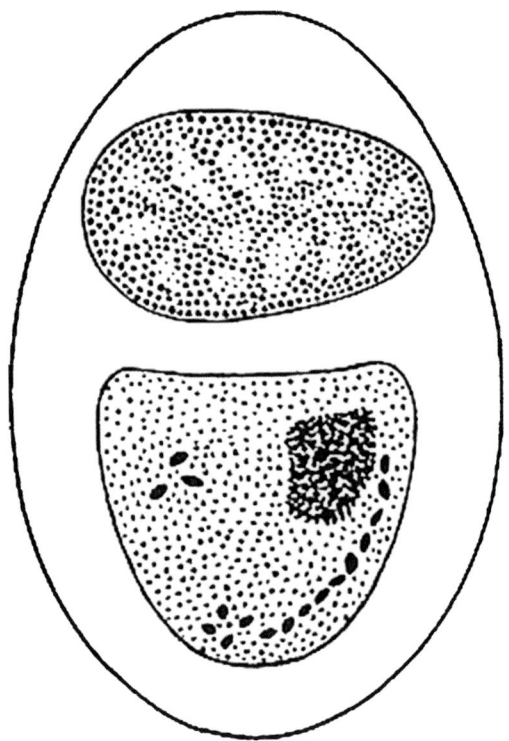

Fig. 2.83 *Plasmodium gallinaceum* macrogamont within an erythrocyte located below the cell nucleus.

and cells of the lymphoid–macrophage system in the skin, spleen, lungs and capillary endothelial cells of the major organs. In this species, the exoerythrocytic developmental stages may be added to by forms which are derived from the erythrocytic cycle. These are known as phanerozoites, being derived from the merozoites of the meronts in the erythrocytic cycle.

The erythrocytic cycle is initiated 7–10 days after infection by merozoites from metacryptozoites and at other times by merozoites from exoerythrocytic meronts located, according to species, in the endothelial or haemopoietic cells. Once within the erythrocyte, the merozoite rounds up to form a trophozoite. The early trophozoites undergo merogony to produce merozoites, which are released from the meronts synchronously. After a number of asexual generations have occurred, some merozoites undergo sexual development with the formation of microgametocytes and macrogametocytes, the latter being generally more numerous and staining more intensely blue with Giemsa than do the microgametocytes. Further development of the gametocyte stages can take place only when a suitable mosquito host ingests the blood. Development in the mosquito is rapid. Following ingestion, the nucleus of the microgametocyte divides and, through a process of exflagellation, 6–8 μm long, thin, flagella-like microgametes are extruded from the parent cell, become detached and swim away to find, and fertilise, the macrogamete. The resulting zygote (ookinete) is motile and penetrates the midgut mucosa and comes to lie on the outer surface of the stomach, forming an early oocyst about 50–60 μm in diameter. The nucleus of the oocyst divides repeatedly to produce a very large number of sporozoites. Maturation of the oocyst takes a variable period of time depending on the species of parasite, temperature and the species of mosquito, but in general it is 10–20 days. When mature, the oocyst ruptures, liberating the

sporozoites into the body cavity of the mosquito, which then migrate all over the body of the mosquito but eventually reach the salivary glands and are now infective to a new host, infection occurring when the mosquito takes a blood meal. A mosquito remains infected for its lifespan, transmitting malarial parasites every time it takes a blood meal.

Plasmodium relictum

Subgenus: *Haemamoeba*

Description: Gamonts are round or irregular, larger forms displacing or expelling the host cell nucleus. Pigment granules are relatively fine. Meronts produce 8–32 merozoites.

Plasmodium hermani

Subgenus: *Huffia*

Description: Meronts are oval or round with 6–14 merozoites and are only present in immature erythrocytes. Gamonts are elongate and present in mature erythrocytes.

Plasmodium juxtanucleare

Subgenus: *Novyella*

Description: Meronts are small, round, ovoid or irregular and usually in contact with the erythrocyte host cell nucleus and produce 2–7 (mean: four) merozoites. Gamonts are round, ovoid, irregular or elongate pyriform, leading to the host erythrocyte often being distorted.

Life cycle: Details of the pre-erythrocytic development following inoculation by a mosquito vector are not known. Extraerythrocytic meronts have been reported in lymphoid–macrophage cells of the spleen, liver, kidney, heart, lung, bone marrow, testes, pancreas and brain, being most common in the spleen. Erythrocytic cycles peak at 6–8 days, with merozoites undergoing sexual development with the formation of microgametocytes and macrogametocytes; the latter are generally more numerous and stain more intensely blue with Giemsa than do the microgametocytes. Further development of the gametocyte stages can take place only when a suitable mosquito host ingests the blood. Development in the mosquito is similar to that in other species.

Plasmodium durae

Subgenus: *Giovannolaia*

Description: Trophozoites are amoeboid in appearance. Mature meronts rarely displace the host cell nucleus and contain 6–14 (mean eight) merozoites. Gamonts are elongate, at the end or side of the host cell, and often displace the host cell nucleus, although the host cell is not usually enlarged. Pigment granules are usually large, round and black.

Life cycle: The detailed life cycle has not been described. Exoerythrocytic meronts have been found in capillary endothelial cells of lung, liver, spleen and brain tissue, but are especially numerous in the brain. In turkeys, parasitaemias peak between 15 and 25 days post infection. Within the erythrocytes, the merozoites round up to form trophozoites. The early trophozoites undergo merogony to produce merozoites, which are released from the meronts synchronously. After a number of asexual generations, some merozoites undergo sexual development with the formation of microgametocytes and macrogametocytes. Further development of the gametocyte stages can take place only when a suitable mosquito host ingests the blood. Development in the mosquito is similar to that in other species.

Hepatocystis

Hepatocystis parasitise arboreal tropical mammals such as squirrels, fruit bats and monkeys and are transmitted by midges of the genus *Culicoides* spp. (Table 2.48). *Hepatocystis* spp. are distributed throughout the Indian subcontinent and Africa south of the Sahara.

Life cycle: The life cycle resembles that of *Plasmodium*, with the major exception that schizogony takes place in the liver, producing grossly visible cysts (merocysts). Macrogamonts and microgamonts develop within erythrocytes and, following ingestion by the vector host, the microgametes are formed and fertilisation and sporogony take place.

Haemoproteus

Gamonts present within erythrocytes are usually elongate and curved (halter-shaped) around the host cell nucleus (Fig. 2.84). Merogony takes place in the endothelial cells of the blood vessels, especially in the lungs. Members of this genus are parasites of birds, reptiles and some amphibians, and are very common in domestic pigeons, ducks and turkeys (Table 2.49). Known vectors are louse flies (hippoboscids) and midges (*Culicoides*).

Table 2.48 *Hepatocystis* species.

Species	Hosts	Vectors
Hepatocystis kochi (syn. Hepatocystis simiae)	Monkeys	Midges (Culicoides)
Hepatocystis semnopitheci	Monkeys	Midges (Culicoides)
Hepatocystis taiwanensis	Monkeys	Midges (Culicoides)
Hepatocystis bouillezi	Monkeys	Midges (Culicoides)
Hepatocystis cercopitheci	Monkeys	Midges (Culicoides)
Hepatocystis foleyi	Monkeys	Midges (Culicoides)

Table 2.49 *Haemoproteus* species.

Species	Hosts	Vectors
Haemoproteus meleagridis	Turkeys	Midges or hippoboscid flies?
Haemoproteus nettionis (syn. Haemoproteus anatis, Haemoproteus anseris, Haemoproteus hermani)	Ducks, wild ducks, geese, swans	Midges or hippoboscid flies?
Haemoproteus columbae	Pigeons, doves	Hippoboscid flies
Haemoproteus sacharovi	Pigeons, doves	Hippoboscid flies?

Haemoproteus meleagridis

Description: Macrogametes and microgametes present in erythrocytes are elongate and curve around the host cell nucleus, occupying about half to three-quarters of the host cell. The nucleus of macrogametocytes is generally more compact, the cytoplasm denser and melanin granules evenly distributed compared with the polar clustering in microgametocytes.

Life cycle: Details of the life cycle are incomplete. Sporozoites in the salivary gland of the insect vector enter the circulation of the host when the insect bites. Meronts occur in the vascular epithelium of the lung, liver, kidney and spleen. Merozoites develop within the meront in clusters and when mature are released into the circulation as tiny round bodies which transform into macrogametes and microgamonts within erythrocytes.

Haemoproteus nettionis

Synonyms: *Haemoproteus anatis*, *Haemoproteus anseris*, *Haemoproteus hermani*

Description: Macrogametes and microgametes are elongate and curve around the erythrocyte cell nucleus, partially encircling the host cell nucleus and often displacing it. They contain a few to 30 or more pigment granules, which are usually coarse and round and often grouped at the ends of the cell. The host cell is not enlarged.

Life cycle: Details as for *H. meleagridis*.

Haemoproteus columbae

Description: Macrogametes and microgametes present in erythrocytes range from tiny ring forms to elongate crescent shapes that curve around the host cell nucleus in the form of a halter (Fig. 2.84). Macrogametes stain dark blue with Giemsa stains, the nucleus is red to dark purple and compact, and pigment granules are dispersed throughout the cytoplasm.

Life cycle: Sporozoites in the salivary gland of the fly enter the circulation of the host when the insect bites and penetrate endothelial cells of blood vessels, where they develop into meronts forming 15 or more cytomeres, each producing large numbers of merozoites. When merozoites are mature, they are released into the circulation as tiny round bodies which transform into macrogametes and microgamonts within erythrocytes. Further development takes place in the insect host after blood feeding. After fertilisation, a zygote forms in the insect midgut where sporogony takes place, forming sporozoites. These are liberated in the body cavity and pass to the salivary glands.

Haemoproteus sacharovi

Description: Macrogametes and microgametes completely fill the erythrocyte when mature, distorting and pushing the nucleus to one side. Pigment granules are sparse compared with other species.

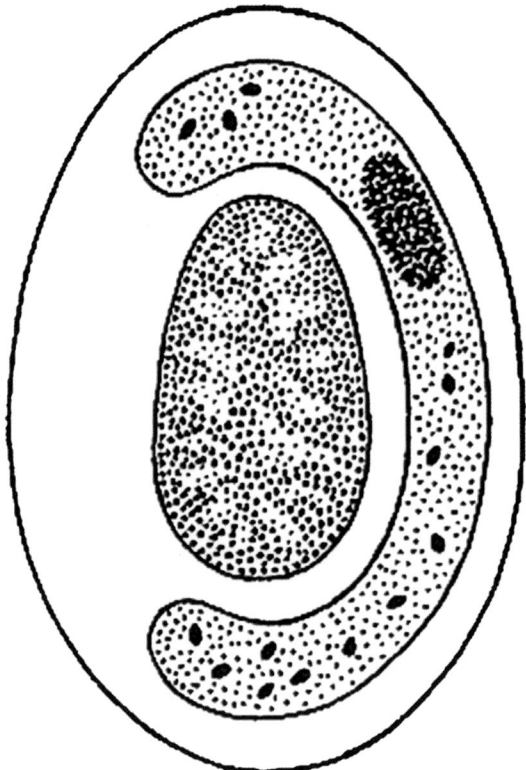

Fig. 2.84 *Haemoproteus columbae* elongate gamont surrounding the erythrocyte nucleus.

Table 2.50 *Leucocytozoon* species.

Species	Hosts	Vectors
Leucocytozoon caulleryi	Chickens, guinea fowl	Midges (*Culicoides*)
Leucocytozoon sabrezesi	Chickens, guinea fowl	Midges (*Culicoides*)
Leucocytozoon smithi (syn. *Leucocytozoon schueffneri, Leucocytozoon macleani*)	Turkeys	Blackflies (*Simulium*)
Leucocytozoon simondi	Ducks, geese	Blackflies (*Simulium*)
Leucocytozoon marchouxi (syn. *Leucocytozoon turtur*)	Pigeons, doves	Blackflies (*Simulium*)
Leucocytozoon struthionis	Oysters	Blackflies (*Simulium*)

Leucocytozoon

Leucocytozoon are parasites of birds (Table 2.50). Macrogametes and microgametes reside in the leucocytes or, with some species, occasionally in the erythrocytes. Merogony takes place in the parenchyma of the liver, heart, kidney and other organs, with meronts forming large bodies (megalomeronts) divided into cytomeres. Merogony does not occur in erythrocytes or leucocytes. Known vectors are blackflies (*Simulium*) or midges (*Culicoides*).

Leucocytozoon caulleryi

Description: Gamonts present in erythrocytes when mature are round, 15.5 by 15 μm, and distort the host cell, causing the host cell nucleus to form a narrow dark band extending about one-third

around the parasite. Megalomeronts present within tissues are 26–300 μm in diameter.

Life cycle: Sporozoites are introduced into a new host by the feeding insects. Parasites undergo merogony in the endothelial cells of the liver, heart, kidney, spleen, thymus, pancreas and other organs of the avian host. The meronts are spherical or lobed and divide at first into cytomeres which eventually fuse, forming megalomeronts, which produce a great number of merozoites. Gamonts appear in the blood about 14 days post infection and are found in erythrocytes or sometimes erythroblasts, and the infected host cells become distorted and assume a spindle shape. When mature, the parasites break out of the host cell and lie free in the plasma. When ingested during blood feeding by the vector insect, *Culicoides* spp., a zygote is formed which elongates into an ookinete about 21 μm long, which passes through the midgut wall to form subspherical oocysts on the midgut outer wall. Sporozoites are formed and pass to the salivary glands and are introduced to the new host when the midges bite them.

Leucocytozoon sabrezesi

Description: Gamonts present in erythrocytes when mature are elongate, 22–24 by 4–7 μm, and distort the host cell, which becomes spindle-shaped, 67 by 6 μm, with long cytoplasmic horns extending beyond the parasites. The host cell nucleus forms a narrow, darkly staining band along one side of the parasite.

Life cycle: As for *L. caulleryi.*

Leucocytozoon smithi

Synonyms: *Leucocytozoon schueffneri, Leucocytozoon macleani*
Description: The mature gamonts are rounded at first but later become elongate, averaging 20–22 μm in length. Their host cells are elongate, averaging 45 by 14 μm, with pale cytoplasmic horns extending out beyond the enclosed parasite. The host cell nucleus is elongate, forming a thin dark band along one side of the parasite (Fig. 2.85), often splitting to form a band on each side of the parasite. Meronts in the hepatocytes of the liver are 10–20 by 7–14 μm (mean 13.5 × 10.5 μm).

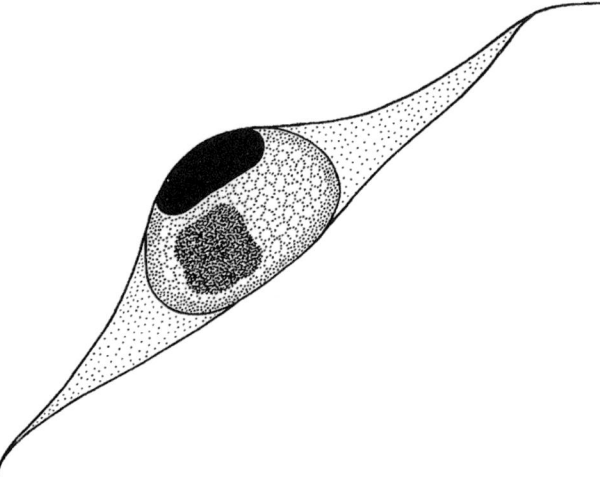

Fig. 2.85 *Leucocytozoon smithi* gamont within an elongated lymphocyte.

Life cycle: Birds become infected when bitten by a blackfly vector. The sporozoites enter the bloodstream, invade various tissue cells, round up and become meronts. Hepatic meronts occur in the liver cells, the earliest stage containing round and crescent-shaped basophilic cytomeres, which develop into masses of deeply staining merozoites that completely fill the host cell cytoplasm. Megalomeronts have not been seen but eventually merozoites enter blood cells and form gamonts. In the blackfly's midgut, microgametes are formed and develop into oocysts to produce sporozoites, which break out of the oocysts and pass to the salivary glands, where they accumulate. The prepatent period is nine days.

Leucocytozoon simondi

Description: Mature macrogametes and microgamonts are elongate, sometimes rounded, 14–22 μm long, and present within erythrocytes or leucocytes, which become elongate, up to 45–55 μm long, with their nucleus forming a long, thin, dark band along one side. Infected host cells have pale cytoplasmic horns extending out beyond the parasite and the nucleus. Hepatic meronts are 11–18 μm in diameter; megalomeronts found in various tissues of the body are 6–164 μm in diameter when mature.

Life cycle: Birds become infected when bitten by a blackfly vector. The sporozoites enter the bloodstream, invade various tissue cells, round up and become meronts. Two types of meront occur in the duck. Hepatic meronts occur in the liver cells, forming a number of cytomeres, which in turn form small merozoites by multiple fission. Megalomeronts are found in the brain, lungs, liver, heart, kidney,

gizzard, intestine and lymphoid tissues 4–6 days after exposure. They are more common than the hepatic meronts. Each megalomeront produces many thousands of bipolar merozoites. The merozoites enter blood cells and form gamonts. Merogony continues in the internal organs for an indefinite but long time, although at a much reduced rate. During this relapse phase, adult birds are not seriously affected but they are the source of infection for the new crop of ducklings. In the blackfly's midgut, 4–8 microgametes are formed by exflagellation from the microgamonts. These fertilise the macrogametes to form a motile zygote or ookinete about 33 by 5 μm. Ookinetes are present in the blackfly midgut 2–6 hours after ingestion of infected blood. They develop into oocysts both in the midgut wall and in the midgut itself and produce several slender sporozoites 5–10 μm long, with one end rounded and the other pointed. They break out of the oocysts and pass to the salivary glands, where they accumulate. Viable sporozoites can be found for at least 18 days after an infective feeding.

Leucocytozoon marchouxi

Description: Macrogametes are rounded or elliptical, stain dark blue with Giemsa and have a compact, reddish nucleus (Fig. 2.86). This species forms rounded megalomeronts in nearly all internal organs (Fig. 2.87).

Life cycle: Sporozoites are introduced into a new host by the feeding insects. Parasites undergo merogony in the endothelial cells of internal organs, forming megaloschizonts. These lead to the production of gametocytes in the blood which, after ingestion by the vector insect, form zygote and oocysts. These undergo sporogony

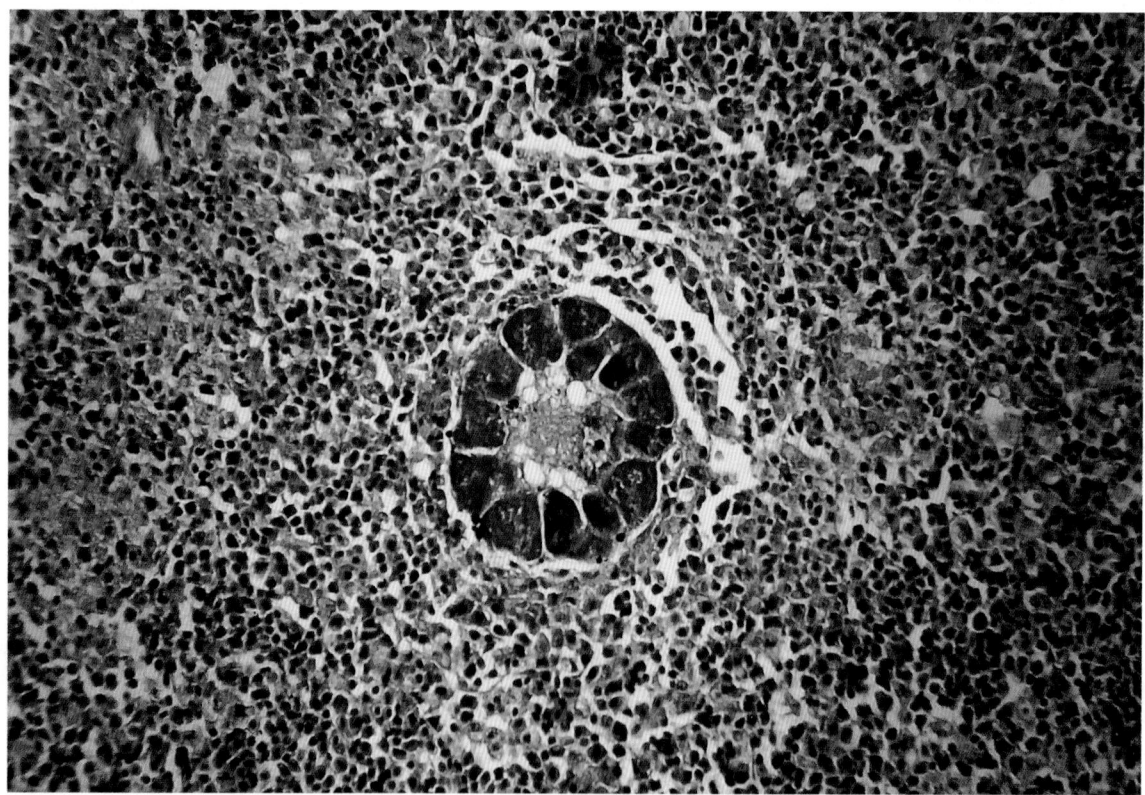

Fig. 2.86 Macrogamont of *Leucocytozoon marchouxi*.

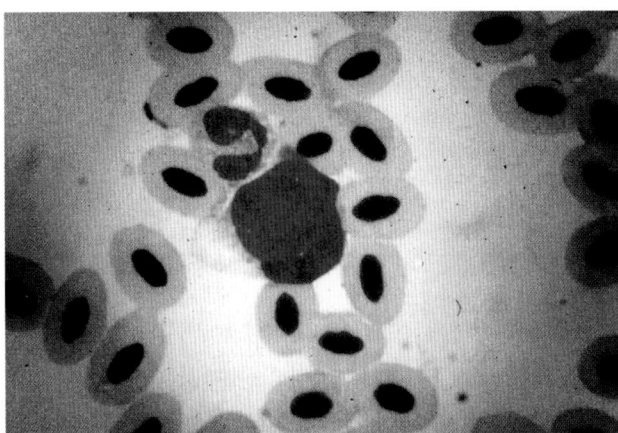

Fig. 2.87 Megalomeront of *Leucocytozoon marchouxi* in the spleen.

leading to the formation of sporozoites, which pass to the salivary glands and are introduced to the new host when the insect vectors feed.

Leucocytozoon struthionis

Description: Gamonts are round and present within erythrocytes.

Hepatocystis kochi

Description: The intraerythrocytic parasites have an unusual nucleus that, when stained with Giemsa, displays a large, oval, pink nucleoplasm that occupies one-third or more of the parasite. Within the nucleus are numerous red chromatin granules.

ORDER PIROPLASMIDA

Often referred to as 'piroplasms', these parasites are found mainly in the erythrocytes or leucocytes of vertebrates. No oocysts are formed and reproduction in the vertebrate host is asexual, with sexual reproduction occurring in the invertebrate host. The piroplasms are heteroxenous with known vectors ixodid or argasid ticks.

FAMILY BABESIIDAE

Babesia

The genus *Babesia* are intraerythrocytic parasites of domestic animals and are transmitted by ticks in which the protozoan passes transovarially, via the egg, from one tick generation to the next (Table 2.51). The disease, babesiosis, is particularly severe in naive animals introduced into endemic areas and is a considerable constraint on livestock development in many parts of the world.

Life cycle: Infective sporozoites present in the tick are injected into the host within saliva when the tick feeds. Multiplication in the vertebrate host occurs in the erythrocytes by binary fission, endodyogeny, endopolyogeny (budding) or merogony to form merozoites. The erythrocytes rupture during repeated phases of merogony, releasing merozoites that invade other erythrocytes. In

Table 2.51 *Babesia* species.

Species	Hosts	Vectors
Babesia bigemina	Cattle, buffalo	*Rhipicephalus (Boophilus) annulatus, R. (B.) microplus* and *R. (B.) decoloratus*
Babesia bovis (syn. *Babesia argentina*)	Cattle, buffalo, deer	*Rhipicephalus (Boophilus) annulatus, R. (B.) microplus*
Babesia caballi	Horses, donkeys	*Dermacentor reticulatus, D. variabilis, D. albipictus, D. silvarum, D. nitens, Hyalomma anatolicum excavatum, H. scupense, H. detritum Rhipicephalus bursa, R. sanguineus*
Babesia canis	Dogs, cats	*Dermacentor reticulatus*
Babesia rossi	Dogs	*Haemaphysalis leachi*
Babesia vogeli	Dogs, cats	*Rhipicephalus sanguineus* sensu lato
Babesia divergens	Cattle	*Ixodes ricinus*
Babesia felis (syn. *Nuttalia felis, Babesia cati*)	Cats	Unknown, possibly *Haemaphysalis leachi*
Babesia gibsoni	Dogs	*Haemaphysalis longicornis, H. bispinosa, Rhipicephalus sanguineus*
Babesia vulpes (syn. *Theileria annae, Babesia annae*)	Dogs	*Ixodes hexagonus? I. ricinus?*
Babesia major	Cattle	*Haemaphysalis punctata*
Babesia motasi	Sheep, goats	*Haemaphysalis punctata, Dermacentor silvarum, Rhipicephalus bursa*
Babesia occultans	Cattle	*Hyalomma marginatum rufipes*
Babesia orientalis	Buffalo	*Rhipicephalus haemaphysaloides*
Babesia ovata	Cattle	*Haemaphysalis longicornis*
Babesia ovis	Sheep, goats	*Rhipicephalus bursa*, possibly *Ixodes ricinus, I. persulcatus* and *Dermacentor reticulatus*
Babesia perroncitoi	Pigs	*Rhipicephalus appendiculatus, R. sanguineus, Dermacentor reticulatus*
Babesia trautmanni	Pigs	*Rhipicephalus appendiculatus, R. sanguineus, Dermacentor reticulatus, Rhipicephalus (Boophilus) decloratus*
Babesia pitheci	Monkeys	Unknown

chronic infections, parasites become sequestered within capillary networks of the spleen, liver and other organs, from where they are released periodically into the circulation. On ingestion by the tick, these forms become vermiform and enter the body cavity, then the ovary and penetrate the eggs where they round up and divide to form small round organisms. When the larval tick moults into the nymph stage, the parasites enter the salivary gland and undergo a series of binary fissions, entering the cells of the salivary gland. They multiply further until the host cells are filled with thousands of minute parasites. These become vermiform, break out of the host cell, lie in the lumen of the gland and are injected into the mammalian host when the tick feeds. See **life cycle** 39.

Babesia bigemina

Description: *Babesia bigemina* is a large pleomorphic *Babesia* but characteristically is identified by the pear-shaped bodies joined at an acute angle within the mature erythrocyte (Fig. 2.88). Round forms measure 2 μm and the pear-shaped elongated ones

LIFE CYCLE 39. LIFE CYCLE OF *BABESIA CANIS*

Babesia canis is mainly transmitted by *Dermacentor reticulatus*, which inoculate the infective sporozoites contained in the saliva during the blood meal (1). Following inoculation, the sporozoites invade the red blood cells (2), become trophozoites (3) and divide by binary fission (4), thus forming paired merozoites. Once the red blood cell ruptures (5), the free merozoites enter circulation and invade other red blood cells (6). The red blood cells containing merozoites (usually 2–4) are ingested by the tick during the course of the blood meal (7), rupture in the tick's gut and the merozoites become isogametes, which feature thin cytoplasmic extensions (8). The fusion of two gametes (gametogony, 9) marks the formation of the zygote (10). From the latter, in the tick's intestine, 'vermiform' parasites originate (vermicula) (11) that invade the arthropod's body cavities and, in particular, the salivary glands (12). Sporogony (asexual reproduction) occurs in the salivary glands (13), thus allowing the parasites to be transmitted to a susceptible host via the blood meal. The vermicula can also invade the tick's ovaries and eggs (14, 15), where they undergo sporogony. The transfer of the parasites from the infected female to her offspring is known as transovarial passage or transovarial transmission. The infection may also be transferred from an infected larva (16) to the nymphal stage (17) and from an infected nymph to the adult stage (18), a process known as trans-stadial passage or trans-stadial transmission. Therefore, all developmental stages of the tick vector may potentially transmit the infection to a receptive host during the blood meal.

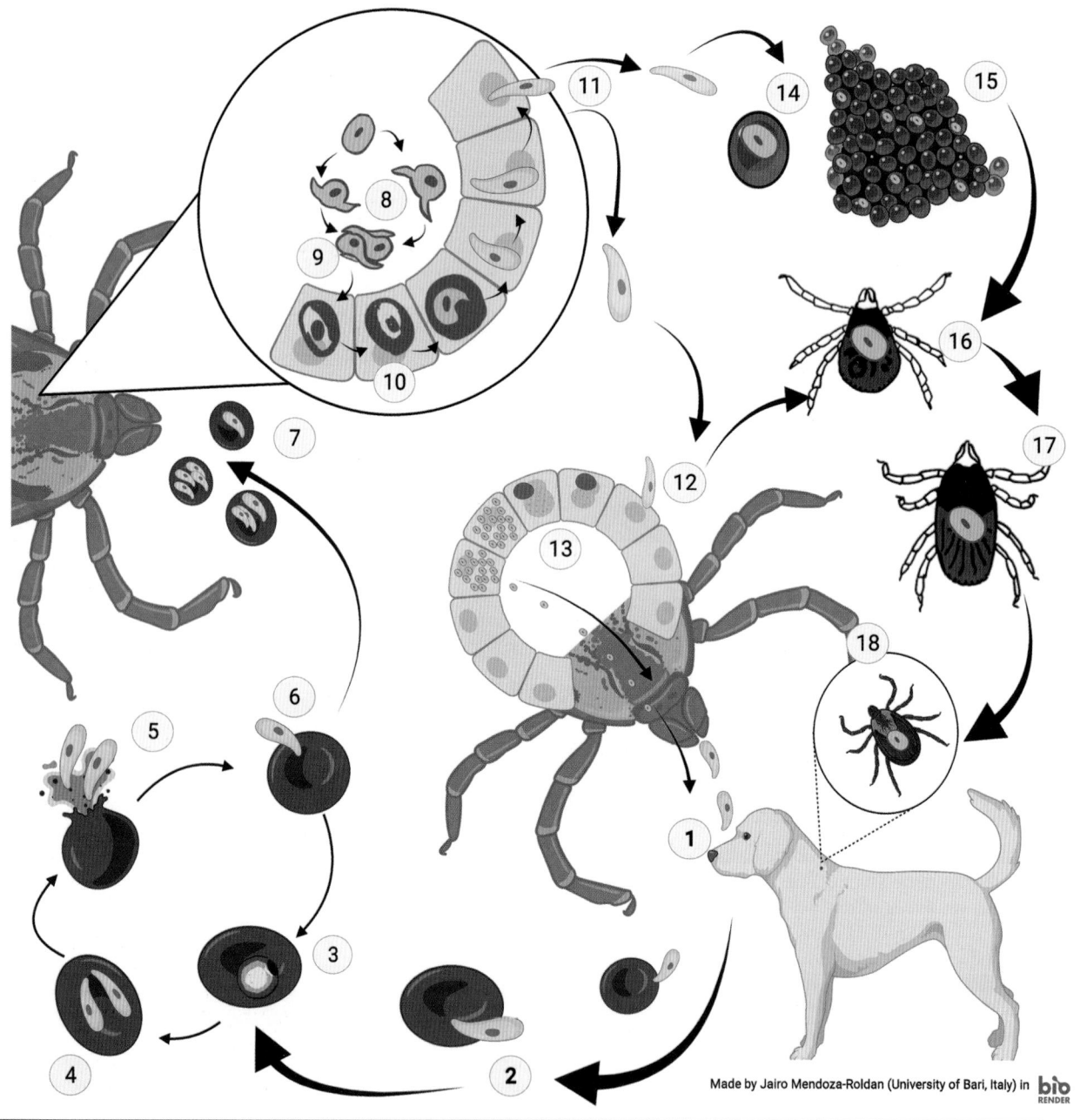

Made by Jairo Mendoza-Roldan (University of Bari, Italy) in **bio**RENDER

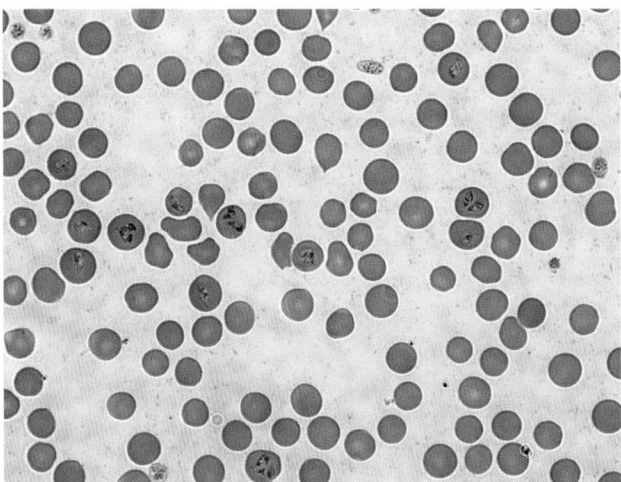

Fig. 2.88 Intraerythrocytic stages of *Babesia bigemina*. (Courtesy of Riccardo Paolo Lia).

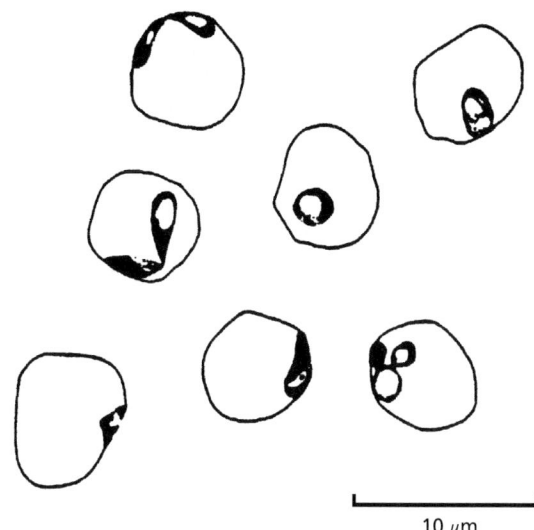

10 μm

Fig. 2.89 Diverse forms of *Babesia divergens* in bovine red cells.

are 4–5 μm. The erythrocytic stages lack a conoid, micropores and typical mitochondria, but have an anterior and posterior polar ring and typically two rhoptries.

Babesia bovis

Synonym: *Babesia argentina*

Description: *Babesia bovis* is a small pleomorphic *Babesia*, typically identified as a single body, as small round bodies or as paired pear-shaped bodies joined at an obtuse angle within the centre of the mature erythrocyte. The round forms measure 1–1.5 μm and the pear-shaped bodies 1.5 by 2.4 μm in size. Vacuolated signet ring forms are especially common.

Babesia divergens

Description: The organisms within red cells are almost always found singly or in pairs, often arranged at a characteristic angle with their narrow ends opposed. Typically, they are pyriform but may be round, elongated or cigar-shaped. *Babesia divergens* is a 'small *Babesia*' and in blood smears typically appears as paired, widely divergent organisms, 1.5 by 0.4 μm, lying near the edge of the red cell. Other forms may be present measuring 2 by 1 μm, while some are circular up 2 μm in diameter and a few may be vacuolated (Fig. 2.89).

Babesia major

Description: This is a 'large *Babesia*', with pyriform bodies 2.6 by 1.5 μm, being characteristically paired at an acute angle less than 90° and found in the centre of the erythrocyte (Fig. 2.90), although round forms about 1.8 μm diameter may also occur.

Babesia motasi

Description: *Babesia motasi* is a large species, 2.5–4 by 2 μm, and is usually pyriform. The merozoites occur singly or in pairs, and the angle between members of a pair is usually acute.

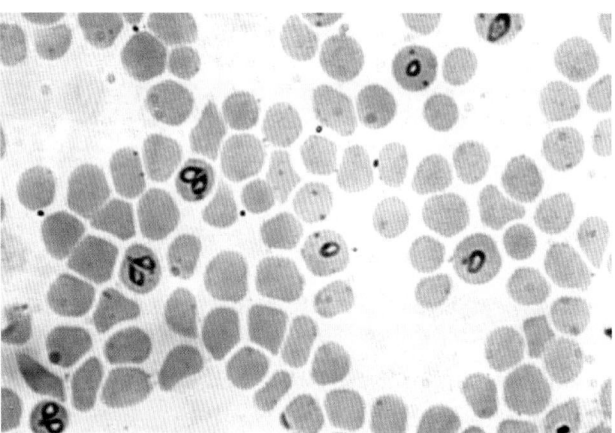

Fig. 2.90 Intraerythrocytic stages of *Babesia major*.

Babesia ovis

Description: *Babesia ovis* is a small species, 1–2.5 μm long, mostly rounded and located in the margin of the host erythrocytes, with paired pyriform trophozoites usually lying at an obtuse angle.

Babesia caballi

Description: Trophozoites within erythrocytes are pear-shaped measuring 2–5 μm in length, commonly occurring in pairs joined at the posterior ends, with the angle between the organisms acute. Round or oval forms 1.5–3 μm in diameter may also occur.

Babesia perroncitoi

Description: A 'small *Babesia*' occurring most commonly as annular forms measuring 0.7–2 μm, although oval to pyriform forms, 1–3 by 1–2 μm in size, may also occur. Merozoites usually occur singly in erythrocytes, but sometimes two or more may be present.

Babesia trautmanni

Description: A 'large *Babesia*' occurring as oval, pyriform and, less commonly, round forms. Merozoites measure 2.5–4 by 1.5–2 μm, and usually occur in pairs within erythrocytes, but sometimes four or more may be present.

Babesia canis

The large *Babesia* of dogs were referred as to three subspecies of *Babesia canis* (i.e. *Babesia canis canis*, *Babesia canis rossi*, *Babesia canis vogeli*). Nowadays, the above are considered as three different species, (i.e. *Babesia canis*, *B. rossi* and *B. vogeli*).

Subspecies: *Babesia canis canis*, *Babesia canis rossi*, *Babesia canis vogeli*

Description: Large piroplasms, pyriform in shape, 4–5 μm in length, pointed at one end and rounded at the other (Fig. 2.91). Amoeboid forms have been described that are 2–4 μm in diameter and usually contain a vacuole.

Babesia vogeli

Description: Large *Babesia* with pyriform merozoites measuring over 2.5 μm in length. Ring-shaped forms usually measure less than or equal to 2.5 μm.

Babesia rossi

Description: Large piroplasms of 2–5 μm length, varied in shape from round to oval to pyriform. Merozoites usually occur individually or in pairs; only occasionally more than three parasites can be found within one erythrocyte.

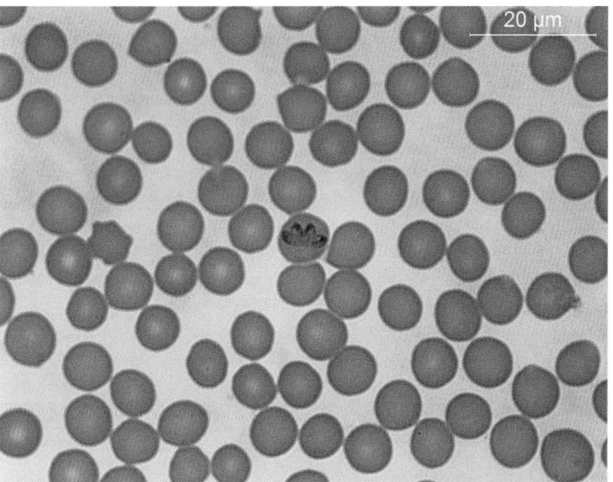
20 μm

Fig. 2.91 Intraerythrocytic stages of *Babesia canis*. (Courtesy of Riccardo Paolo Lia).

Babesia gibsoni

Description: A small piroplasm, annular or oval in shape, and no more than one-eighth the diameter of the host erythrocyte.

Babesia felis

Synonyms: *Nuttalia felis*, *Babesia cati*

Description: Small piroplasms, with the majority of merozoites present in erythrocytes, round, irregularly round and 1.5–2 μm in diameter; some are elongate 2–3 μm long and may form cruciform meronts.

Babesia vulpes

Synonyms: *Theileria annae*, *Babesia annae*, *Babesia microti*-like

Description: Merozoites are small, usually singular, 1 by 2.5 μm.

Life cycle: The life cycle has not been described but *T. annae* is thought to be transmitted by the hedgehog tick, *Ixodes hexagonus*.

Babesia pitheci

Description: The piroplasms are pyriform in shape and measure 2–6 μm long. Round, oval and lanceolate shapes have also been reported.

FAMILY THEILERIIDAE

The diseases caused by several species of *Theileria* are a serious constraint on livestock development in Africa, Asia and the Middle East. The parasites, which are transmitted by ticks, undergo repeated schizogony in the lymphocytes, ultimately releasing small merozoites which invade the red cells to become piroplasms. *Theileria* are widely distributed in cattle and sheep in Africa, Asia, Europe and Australia, have a variety of tick vectors and are associated with infections that range from clinically inapparent to rapidly fatal (Table 2.52).

Various species of *Cytauxzoon* occur as *Theileria*-like piroplasms in the red cells of wild animals. The genus differs from *Theileria* in that schizogony occurs in the reticuloendothelial cells rather than lymphocytes. *Cytauxzoon* is the cause of a fatal disease of domestic cats, characterised by fever, anaemia and icterus, in southern USA. The reservoir hosts are wild cats.

Theileria

Life cycle: The life cycle of *Theileria* spp. involves erythrocytic merozoites, which are ingested by the tick intermediate host and develop into macrogamonts and microgamonts to produce zygotes. These develop and enter the haemolymph to become kinetes and then the salivary glands to become fission bodies. In adult ticks, the primary fission bodies divide into secondary (primary sporoblasts)

Table 2.52 *Theileria* species.

Species	Hosts	Vector
Theileria annulata	Cattle, buffalo	Hyalomma detritum, H. anatolicum excavatum, H. truncatum, H. dromedarii, H. turanicum, H. marginatum
Theileria cervi (syn. Theileria tarandi)	Deer (fallow, red, sika, white-tailed, reindeer)	Unknown
Theileria camelensis	Camels	Hyalomma dromedarii
Theileria equi (syn. Babesia equi, Nuttalia equi)	Horses, donkeys	Dermacentor reticulatus, D. albipictus, D. variabilis, D. nitens, Hyalomma marginatum, H. scupense (syn. H. detritum), H. anatolicum, H. dromedarii, Rhipicephalus bursa, R. evertsi, R. sanguineus
Theileria hirci (syn. Theileria lestoquardi)	Sheep, goats	Rhipicephalus bursa, Hyalomma anatolicum
Theileria orientalis complex Theileria mutans Theileria buffeli Theileria sergenti	Cattle, buffalo	Amblyomma variegatum, A. cohaerens, A. hebraeum, Haemaphysalis bispinosa
Theileria ovis	Sheep, goats	Rhipicephalus bursa, R. evertsi
Theileria recondita	Sheep, goats, deer	Haemaphysalis punctata
Theileria separata	Sheep, goats	Rhipicephalus evertsi
Theileria parva (subsp. Theileria parva lawrencei, Theileria parva parva)	Cattle, buffalo	Rhipicephalus appendiculatus
Theileria taurotragi (syn. Cytauxzoon taurotragi)	Cattle, antelopes, particularly the eland	Rhipicephalus appendiculatus, R. pulchellus
Theileria velifera (syn. Haematoxenus veliferus)	Cattle, zebus	Amblyomma variegatum, A. lepidum, A. hebraeum

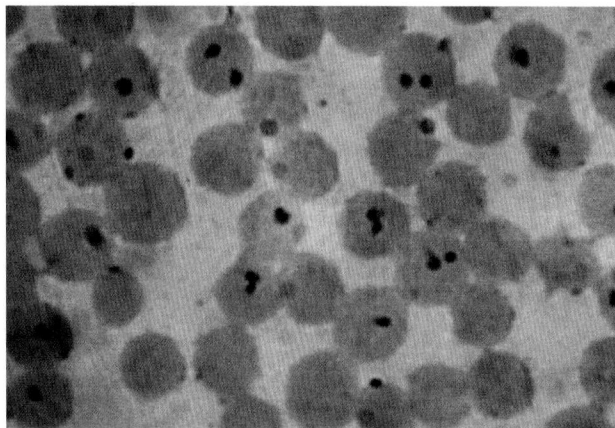

Fig. 2.92 Intraerythrocytic stages of *Theileria parva*.

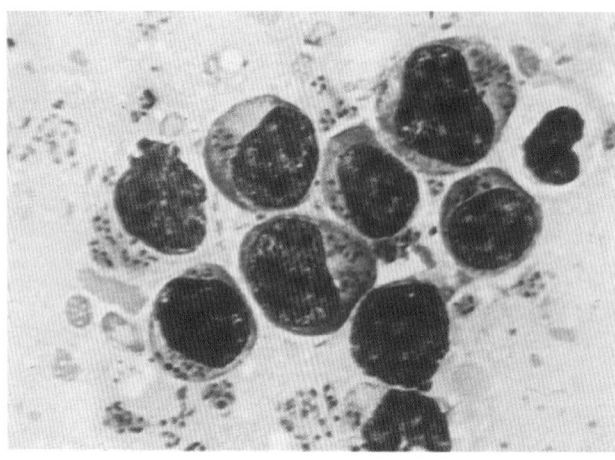

Fig. 2.93 Macroschizonts of *Theileria parva* in a smear of a lymph node.

and tertiary (secondary sporoblasts) fission bodies and produce sporozoites that are released into the saliva. Animals are infected when the ticks suck blood. Species in this genus undergo exoerythrocytic merogony in the lymphocytes, histiocytes, erythroblasts and other cells of the internal organs. Leucocytes filled with meronts (schizonts) are called Koch bodies. Both macromeronts and micromeronts occur, producing micromerozoites that invade erythrocytes, where usually another round of division occurs, producing a generation of merozoites which in turn infect new erythrocytes. Multiplication in erythrocytes results in four (rarely two) merozoites forming characteristic tetrads (the Maltese cross). Some species (*T. parva*) do not multiply in the red blood cells, and asexual division is confined only to lymphocytes. Gametogony occurs in the tick vector's intestine and sporogony in the salivary glands.

Theileria parva

Subspecies: *Theileria parva lawrencei, Theileria parva parva*

Description: Trophozoite forms in the erythrocyte are predominantly rod-shaped (1.5–2 × 0.1–1 μm), but may also be round, oval and comma-shaped (Fig. 2.92). Koch bodies are found in the lymphocytes and endothelial cells of the spleen or lymph nodes where they are very numerous and average 8 μm but can range up to 12 μm or more. Two types have been described: macroschizonts containing chromatin granules 0.4–2 μm in diameter (Fig. 2.93); these divide further to become microschizonts that contain chromatin granules 0.3–0.8 μm in diameter and produce merozoites 0.7–1 μm in diameter.

Life cycle: Erythrocytic merozoites are ingested by the tick intermediate host, *Rhipicephalus appendiculatus* (the brown ear tick), and develop into macrogamonts and microgamonts to produce zygotes. These develop and enter the haemolymph to become kinetes. These enter the salivary glands to become fission bodies. In adult ticks, the primary fission bodies divide into secondary (primary sporoblasts) and tertiary (secondary sporoblasts) fission bodies and produce sporozoites that are released into the saliva.

Cattle are infected when the ticks suck blood. The sporozoites are inoculated into cattle and quickly enter lymphocytes in an associated lymph gland, usually the parotid. The parasitised lymphocyte transforms to a lymphoblast, which divides rapidly as the macroschizont develops. This division is apparently stimulated by the parasite, which itself divides synchronously with the lymphoblast to produce two infected cells. The rate of proliferation is such that a 10-fold increase in infected cells may occur every three days. About 12 days after infection, a proportion of the macroschizonts develop into microschizonts and within a day or so these produce the micromerozoites that enter erythrocytes, which after a few binary fissions produce the varied forms present in the red cells.

For completion of the life cycle, the piroplasms have to be ingested by the larvae or nymphal stages of the three-host vector, *R. appendiculatus*. In these, the sexual phase described above occurs in the tick gut followed by the formation of sporoblasts in the salivary glands. No further development occurs until the next stage of the tick starts to feed, when the sporoblasts produce infective sporozoites from about day 4 onwards. Since female ticks feed continuously for about 10 days and males intermittently over a longer period, this allows ample time for infection of the host. Transmission is trans-stadial, i.e. by the next stage of the tick, and transovarian transmission does not occur. The incubation period following tick transmission is 8–24 days. See **life cycle** 40.

LIFE CYCLE 40. LIFE CYCLE OF *THEILERIA PARVA*

Infection by *Theileria parva* occurs when the tick vector (mainly *Rhipicephalus appendiculatus*) (1) inoculates the sporozoites into the bovine host during the blood meal. The sporozoites invade the lymphocytes (2), particularly in the lymph nodes, and undergo schizogony (3). During schizogony, infected lymphocytes become lymphoblasts, which divide rapidly into two infected cells (4). Approximately 12 days post infection, micromerozoites are released by the lymphocytes (5) and invade other lymphocytes and/or red blood cells (6), in which they divide by binary fission. Completion of the life cycle relies on ingestion of infected red blood cells by larvae or nymphs of the competent tick vector (7), in which the parasites are passed trans-stadially. Gamogony occurs in the tick's intestine and leads to the formation of micro- and macrogametes that, following fertilisation, generate the zygote (8). In the tick's haemolymph, the zygote becomes a sporokinete (9); the latter reaches the salivary glands (10), where three consecutive cycles of sporogony occur (11). Sporogony terminates with the formation of infective sporozoites (12) that are transmitted to a new susceptible host during the tick's blood meal.

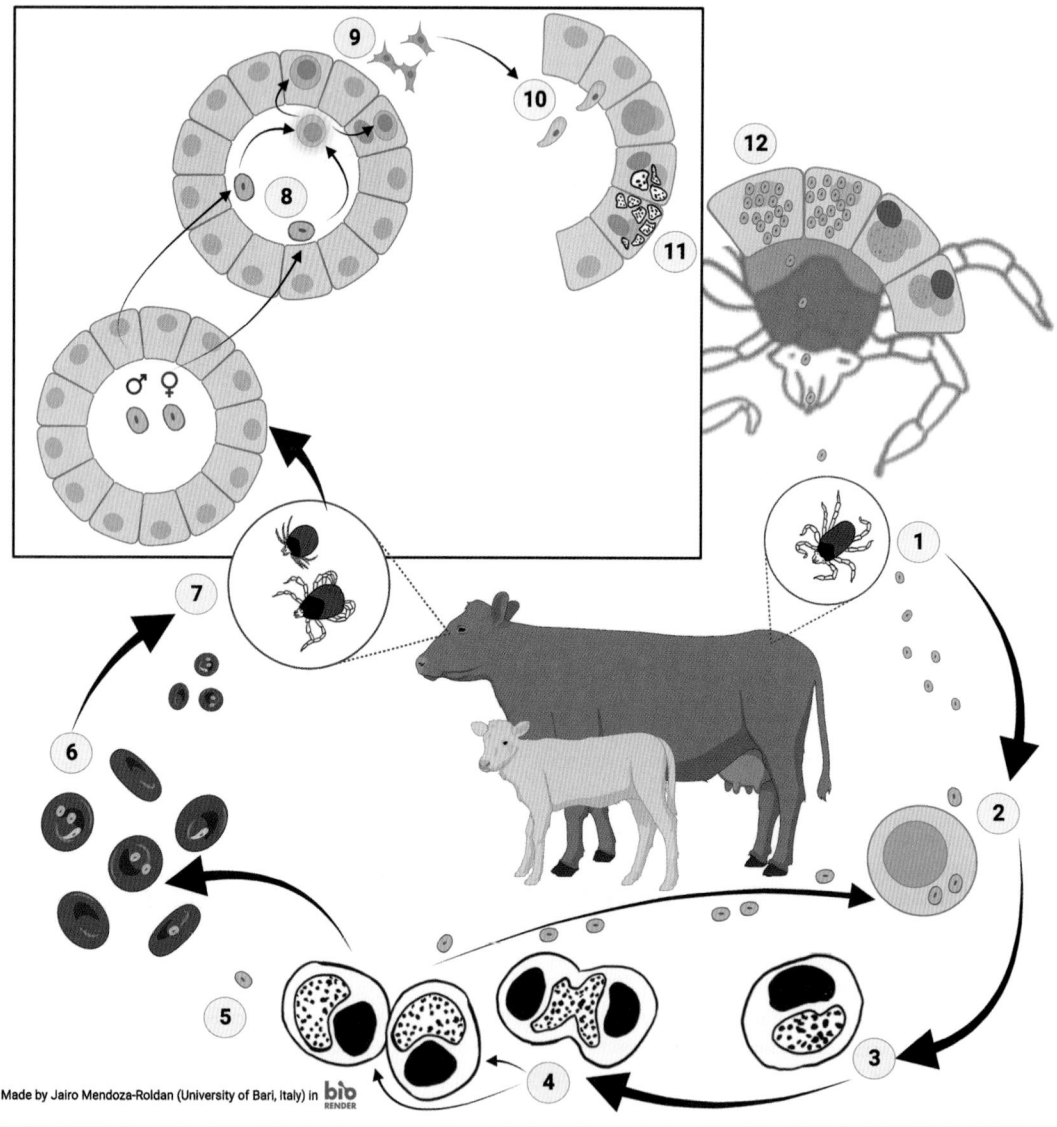

Made by Jairo Mendoza-Roldan (University of Bari, Italy) in **bio** RENDER

Theileria annulata

Description: Trophozoite forms in the erythrocyte are predominantly round (0.5–2.7 μm) to oval (2 × 0.6 μm), but may also be rod-shaped or comma-shaped (1.2 × 0.5 μm). Division by binary fission may form two or four daughter cells, the latter in the shape of a cross. Koch bodies are in the lymphocytes of the spleen or lymph nodes or even free in these organs. They average 8 μm but can be up to 27 μm. Two types have been described: macromeronts containing chromatin granules 0.4–1.9 μm in diameter; these divide further to become micromeronts that contain chromatin granules 0.3–0.8 μm in diameter and produce merozoites 0.7–1 μm in diameter.

Life cycle: Erythrocytic merozoites, ingested by the tick intermediate host, develop into macrogamonts and microgamonts to produce zygotes. These develop and enter the haemolymph to become kinetes, which then enter the salivary glands to become fission bodies. In adult ticks, the primary fission bodies divide into secondary (primary sporoblasts) and tertiary (secondary sporoblasts) fission bodies and produce sporozoites that are released into the saliva. Cattle are infected when the ticks suck blood. The sporozoites enter lymphocytes and become meronts, initially macromeronts and then micromeronts. Micromerozoites enter erythrocytes, and after a few binary fissions produce the varied forms that are taken up by other ticks. The incubation period following tick transmission is 9–25 days (mean 15 days).

Theileria equi

Description: The merozoites in the erythrocytes are relatively small, 2–3 μm, rounded, amoeboid or most often pyriform, and are readily recognised in blood smears from acute cases, since apart from size, the piroplasms characteristically form a 'Maltese cross' of four organisms (Fig. 2.94).

Theileria camelensis

Description: Trophozoite forms in the erythrocyte are predominantly round.

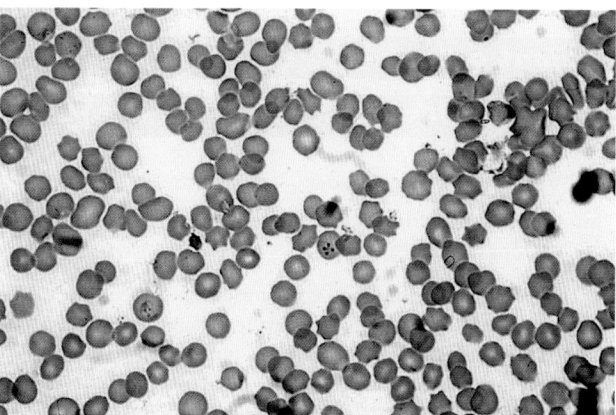

Fig. 2.94 Intraerythrocytic stages of *Theileria equi*. The characteristic 'Maltese cross' of four organisms can be seen within an erythrocyte (bottom centre). (Courtesy of Riccardo Paolo Lia).

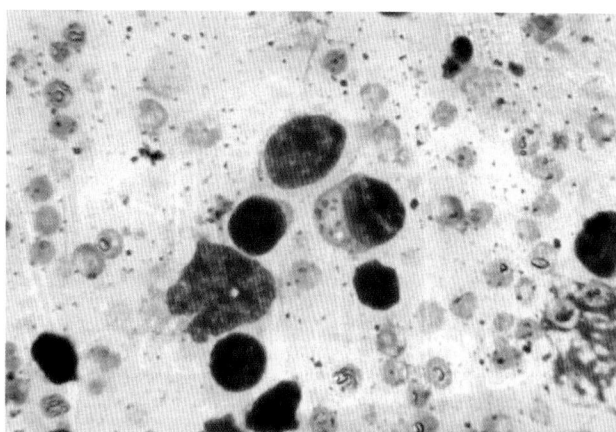

Fig. 2.95 Meront of *Theileria hirci*.

Theileria hirci

Synonym: *Theileria lestoquardi*

Description: Trophozoites are found in lymphocytes and erythrocytes as round (0.6–2 μm in diameter), oval or rod-shaped (1.6 μm long) forms (Fig. 2.95). Binary or quadruple fission takes place in the erythrocytes. Meronts (Koch bodies), averaging 8 μm in diameter but ranging up to 10–20 μm and containing 1–80 granules, are common in the lymphocytes of the spleen and lymph nodes.

Theileria orientalis complex

Synonyms: *Theileria mutans, Theileria buffeli, Theileria sergenti*

Description: Trophozoite forms in erythrocytes are round (1–2 μm diameter), oval (1.5 × 0.6 μm), pyriform or comma-shaped (Fig. 2.96). Binary fission produces two or four daughter cells. There are relatively few Koch bodies (8–20 μm) in the lymphocytes of the spleen and lymph nodes and these contain 1–80 chromatin granules (1–2 μm in diameter).

Life cycle: As for *T. annulata*.

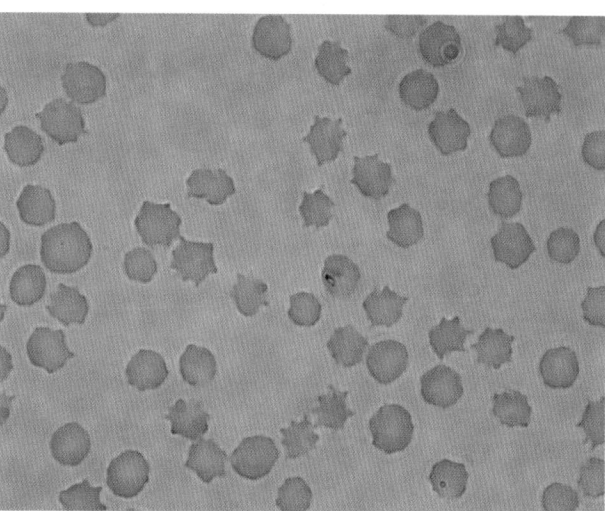

Fig. 2.96 Intraerythrocytic stages of *Theileria orientalis* (*mutans*). (Courtesy of Grazia Carelli).

Theileria ovis

Description: Erythrocytic stages are similar in appearance to *T. hirci* and are found in lymphocytes and erythrocytes as round forms (0.6–2 μm in diameter), oval or rod-shaped (1.6 μm long) but are sparser with less than 2% of erythrocytes infected.

Theileria recondita

Description: Merozoites in the erythrocytes are relatively small, with either rod forms (2 μm) or ring forms (1.22 μm diameter) predominating.

Theileria taurotragi

Synonym: *Cytauxzoon taurotragi*

Description: Erythrocytic forms are similar in appearance to *T. parva*. Trophozoite forms in the erythrocyte are predominantly round to oval, but may also be rod-shaped or comma-shaped (1.2 × 0.5 μm).

Life cycle: As for *T. annulata*.

Theileria velifera

Synonym: *Haematoxenus veliferus*

Description: Trophozoite forms within erythrocytes are pleomorphic but most often small rods 1–2 μm long. The great majority have a rectangular 'veil' 1–3.5 μm extending out from the side.

Life cycle: As for *T. annulata*.

Cytauxzoon

Species of this genus are transmitted by ixodid ticks and infect felids (Table 2.53)

Cytauxzoon felis

Synonym: *Theileria felis*
Description: The single signet-ring shaped forms present within erythrocytes are 1–1.2 μm in diameter. Bipolar oval forms, tetrads and dark-staining 'dots' may also be seen.

Life cycle: The life cycle is poorly understood. Infective sporozoites are injected into the cat from the salivary glands of an infective tick.

Table 2.53 *Cytauxzoon* species.

Species	Hosts	Vector
Cytauxzoon felis (syn. Theileria felis)	Cats, wild felids	Dermacentor variabilis, Amblyomma americanum
Cytauxzoon europaeus	Cats, wildcats	Hard ticks
Cytauxzoon otrantorum	Wildcats	Hard ticks
Cytauxzoon banethi	Wildcats	Hard ticks

Meronts develop primarily within tissue histiocytes in many organs and develop to release merozoites, which invade monocytes and erythrocytes.

Cytauxzoon europaeus, C. otrantorum and *C. banethi* are small intraerythrocytic organisms with a round to oval signet ring shape. The biological life cycle is unknown.

PHYLUM CILIOPHORA

The ciliates of domestic animals all belong to the phylum Ciliophora. Individual organisms have a **micronucleus** containing a normal set of chromosomes which are active in reproduction, and a polyploid **macronucleus**, involved in vegetative functions. Ciliates have either simple cilia or compound **cilia** in at least one stage of their life cycle. Infraciliature are found in the cortex beneath the pellicle composed of ciliary basal granules (**kinetosomes**) and associated fibrils (**kinetodesmata**). Reproduction is by transverse binary fission and sexual reproduction by conjugation, in which there is a transfer of micronuclear material between individuals. Many species of ciliates occur as harmless commensals in the rumen and reticulum of ruminants and the large intestine of equids. The only ciliate of importance in veterinary medicine occurs in the family Balantidiidae.

ORDER VESTIBULIFERIDA

FAMILY BALANTIDIIDAE

The only genus of importance is *Balantioides*, which has an ovoid, ellipsoidal body with elongate macronucleus and a single micronucleus with a cytostome at the base of an anterior vestibulum (see Fig. 2.2). *Balantioides* has worldwide distribution and is found in pigs, monkeys and humans.

Life cycle: Reproduction is by binary fission. Conjugation, a temporary attachment of two individuals during which nuclear material is exchanged, also occurs, after which both cells separate. Eventually, cysts are formed which are passed in the faeces; these have a thick yellowish wall through which the parasite may be seen, and are viable for two weeks at room temperature. Infection of a new host is by ingestion of the cysts.

Balantioides

Balantioides coli

Synonym: *Balantidium coli*

This species infects the large intestine of pigs, humans, camels, monkeys, dogs (rarely) and rats.

Description: An actively motile organism, up to 300 μm, whose pellicle possesses rows of longitudinally arranged cilia (Figs 2.97 and 2.98). At the anterior end there is a funnel-shaped depression, the peristome, which leads to the cytostome or mouth; from this, food particles are passed to vacuoles in the cytoplasm and digested. Internally, there are two nuclei, a macronucleus and adjacent micronucleus, and two contractile vacuoles, which regulate osmotic pressure. Cysts are spherical to ovoid, 40–60 μm in diameter (Fig. 2.99).

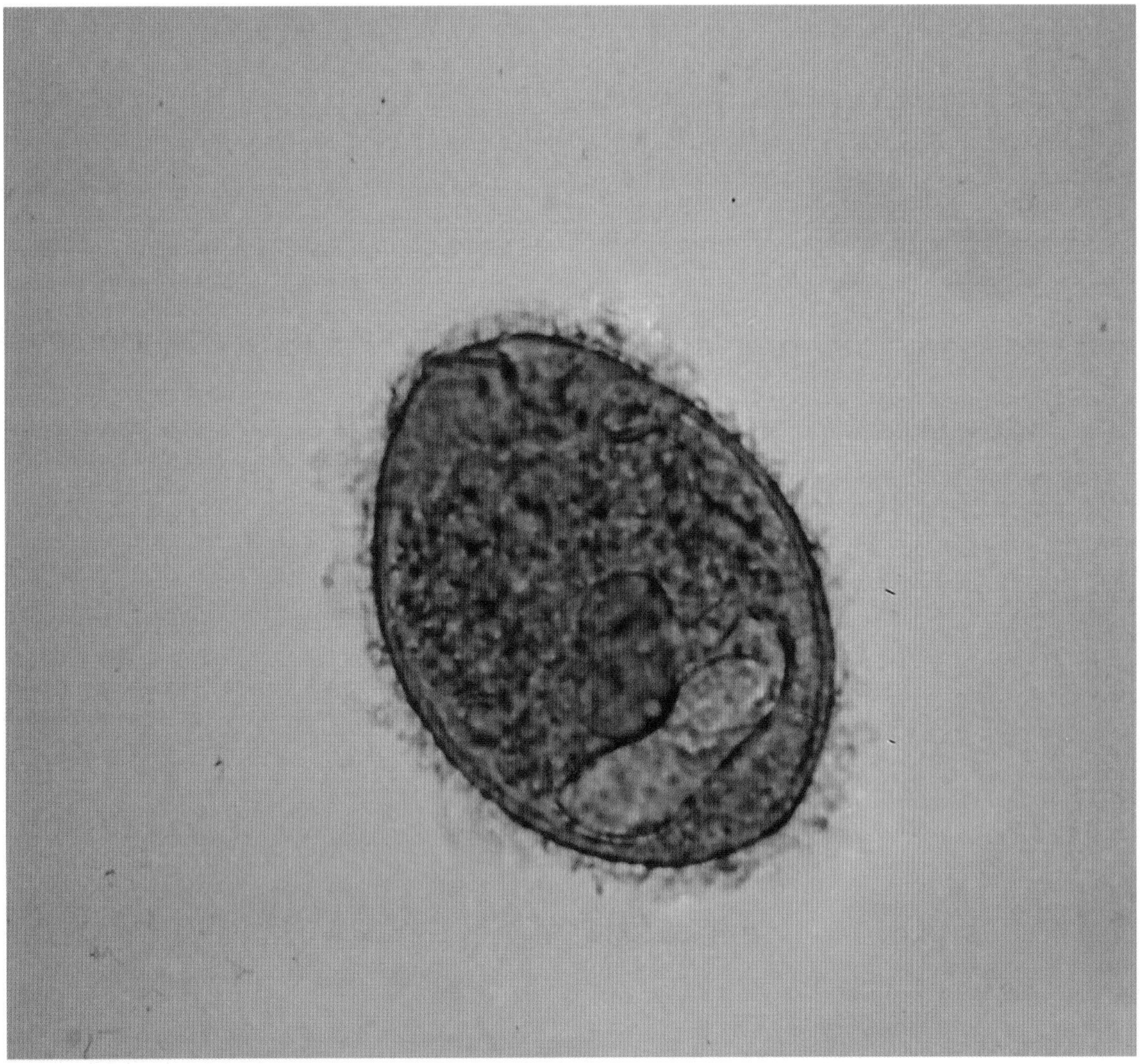

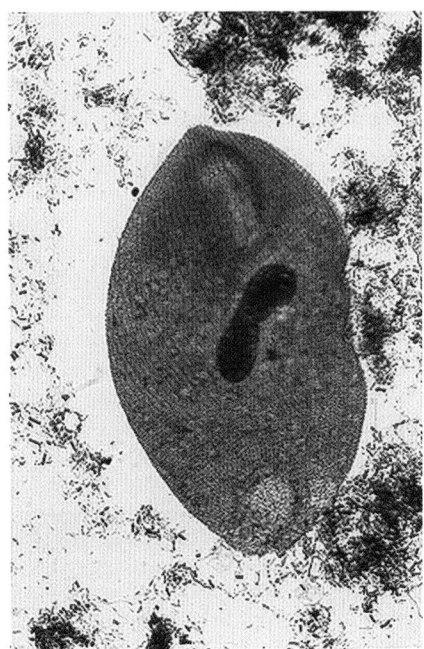

Fig. 2.97 *Balantioides coli* trophozoite.

Fig. 2.98 *Balantioides coli*.

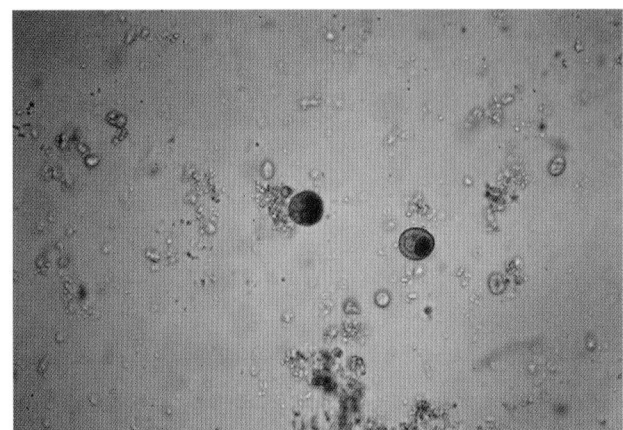

Fig. 2.99 *Balantioides coli* cysts.

FAMILY PYCNOTRICHIDAE

This family contains the genus *Buxtonella*, which has an ovoid, uniformly ciliated body with a prominent curved groove and a cyathostome near the anterior end. *Buxtonella* has worldwide distribution and is found in the caecum of cattle.

Life cycle: The life cycle has not been described.

Buxtonella

Buxtonella sulcata

This species infects the large intestine of cattle, buffalo, goats, sheep, deer, camels and rarely humans.

Description: The body is ovoid, 100 by 72 μm, and uniformly ciliated with a prominent curved groove bordered by two ridges running from end to end with a cyathostome at the anterior end, and an oval or bean-shaped macronucleus 28 by 14 μm in size.

FAMILY NYCTOTHERIDAE

The genus *Nyctotherus* comprises coprophilic ciliated protozoa with a peristome at the anterior end, ending in a cytostome in the middle of the body. *Nyctotherus* is found in the faeces of various species of chelonia and vegetarian lizards such as iguanas.

MISCELLANEOUS 'PROTOZOAL' ORGANISMS

The organisms described in this section have traditionally been included in veterinary parasitology textbooks. For many of these organisms, the taxonomy still remains complicated and confusing. Their inclusion in this text is for completeness and to aid differentiation from morphologically similar protozoal organisms.

KINGDOM FUNGI

PHYLUM MICROSPORIDIA

All Microspora are obligate intracellular parasites with unicellular spores, the spore possessing an extrusion apparatus and a coiled polar tube, typically filamentous, extending backwards to form a polar cap. Most are parasites of insects.

ORDER MICROSPORIDA

FAMILY UNIKARYONIDAE

The Unikaryonidae have ellipsoidal or oval spores consisting of an external wall, sporoplasm, a coiled polar tube and a polar capsule.

Encephalitozoon

The genus *Encephalitozoon* is of minor significance in veterinary medicine, causing disease in dogs, rabbits, other mammals and humans. Three strains of *Encephalitozoon* have been identified:

strain I ('rabbit strain'), strain II ('rodent strain') and strain III ('dog strain'). Each of the three strains has been reported in humans and infections in animals may therefore pose a potential zoonotic risk.

Life cycle: The infective spore stages are highly resistant and can survive for many years. When spores are ingested, the polar tube is everted and when fully extended the sporoplasm passes through the tube and is inoculated into the cytoplasm of the host cell. There then follows a phase of multiplication by binary or multiple fission (merogony). This is followed by sporogony to form sporoblasts, which then mature into spores.

Encephalitozoon cuniculi

Synonym: *Nosema cuniculi*

This microsporidian infects the brain, kidneys, heart and lungs of rabbits, dogs, red foxes, blue foxes, silver foxes, cats, mice, rats, humans and monkeys.

Description: Microsporidia are obligate, intracellular, spore-forming protozoa. Trophozoites are 2–2.5 by 0.8–1.2 μm in tissue sections or 4 by 2.5 μm in smears. Spores are about 2 μm long and contain a spirally coiled polar filament with 4–5 coils.

FAMILY ENTEROCYTOZOONIDAE

The Enterocytozoonidae have oval mature spores measuring 0.7–1.1 um and containing a single nucleus, 5–6 coils of the polar filament, a posterior vacuole, an anchoring disc attached to the polar filament and a thick electron-dense wall.

Enterocytozoon

Enterocytozoon is an intestinal microsporidian frequently found in humans but has also been reported in dogs, cats, cattle, pigs and other domestic animals. Its significance in animal hosts is unknown.

Enterocytozoon bieneusi

This species infects the small intestine of dogs, cats, cattles, pigs, rabbits, chickens and turkeys.

Description: Trophozoites range from 1 to 1.5 μm in size. Spores have a double row of polar tubule coils.

PHYLUM ASCOMYCOTA

ORDER PNEUMOCYSTIDALES

FAMILY PNEUMOCYSTIDACEAE

Pneumocystis

Pneumocystis carinii is widely distributed in a wide range of healthy domestic and wild animals. Currently, it is considered to be an opportunistic mycoses of the family Pneumocystidaceae (phylum Ascomycota, class Pneumocystidomycetes) causing infections in humans, non-human primates and monkeys, particularly in the immunocompromised. Its significance in other hosts is not known.

Description: Two major forms of *P. carinii* have been consistently identified from histological and ultrastructural analysis of organisms found in human and rat lungs. These are a trophic form and a larger cyst stage containing eight intracystic stages.

Life cycle: The life cycle of *Pneumocystis* still remains poorly understood. Information is mostly derived from histochemical and ultrastructural analysis of the lung tissue of rodents and infected humans. Current knowledge suggests that the trophic (trophozoite) forms are produced during asexual development. These forms are usually pleomorphic and found in clusters. They appear capable of replicating asexually by binary fission and also replicate sexually by conjugation, producing a diploid zygote, which undergoes meiosis and subsequent mitosis, resulting in the formation of a precyst initially and then an early cyst and eventually a mature cyst. During differentiation of the organism from precyst to mature cyst, eight intracystic spores, or 'daughter cells', are produced. These intracystic spores are subsequently released as the mature cyst ruptures and develop into trophic forms.

KINGDOM CHROMALVEOLATA

PHYLUM HETEROKONTOPHYTA

FAMILY BLASTOCYTIDAE

Blastocystis

Blastocystis was for many years described as a yeast but then considered to be a protozoan in the subphylum Blastocysta, but more latterly is considered to belong to a group of organisms known as heterokonts (Stramenopiles) in the phylum Heterokontophyta (kingdom Chromalveolata). The organism is found in the intestinal tract of humans and in many animals including monkeys, pigs, birds, rodents, snakes and invertebrates (Table 2.54). There appears to be poor host specificity such that species names are now considered redundant and are instead referred to as subtypes (ST1–ST10).

Blastocystis spp.

Description: Vacuolar forms are brightly refractile, of widely variable diameter (4–15 μm) with a thin band of central cytoplasm surrounding a central vacuole (Fig. 2.100). The cyst form is generally smaller in size and has a thick multilayered cyst wall and lacks a central vacuole.

Table 2.54 *Blastocystis* species.

Species	Hosts	Site
Blastocystis spp. (syn. *Blastocystis hominis*)	Humans	Small and large intestine
Blastocystis spp. (syn. *Blastocystis galli*)	Chickens, gallinaceous birds (pheasants, partridges)	Large intestine, caeca

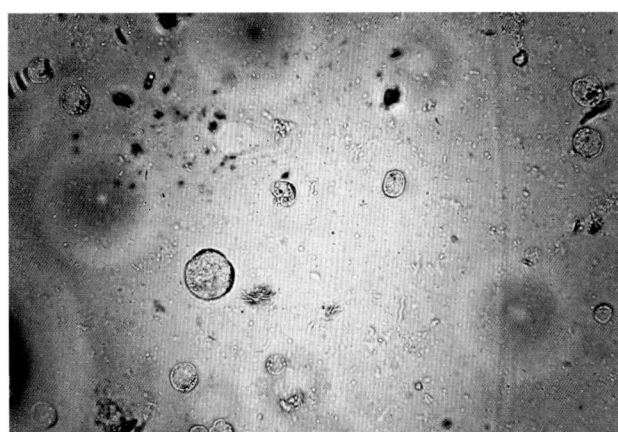

Fig. 2.100 Vacuolar and cyst forms of *Blastocystis* spp. in faeces of red-legged partridge.

KINGDOM BACTERIA

PHYLUM PROTEOBACTERIA

ORDER RICKETTSIALES

Rickettsial organisms are parasitic Gram-negative bacteria, associated with arthropods, which may act as vectors or primary hosts. While the *Rickettsia* are now considered to be in the kingdom Bacteria, for historical reasons they are included in parasitological texts and for this reason mention is made of some genera (Table 2.55).

FAMILY RICKETTSIACEAE

This is the most important family, which in vertebrates are parasites of tissue cells other than erythrocytes and are transmitted by arthropods. The Rickettsieae are capable of infecting suitable vertebrate hosts including humans, who may be the primary host but are more often incidental hosts.

Species of *Rickettsia* are important human pathogens but some species can affect dogs and cats and many have a wildlife reservoir. With the exception of louse-borne typhus and trench fever, all these human infections are zoonoses with no person-to-person or person-to-animal transmission occurring. Three groups can be distinguished within the genus: typhus group, spotted fever group and scrub typhus group.

Rickettsia conorii

Description: Small, pleomorphic, Gram-negative, coccoid, obligatory intracellular organisms infecting endothelial cells of smaller blood vessels.

Life cycle: Ticks become infected with *R. conorii* by feeding on infected small rodents that are the main reservoir of disease. Immature ticks become infected and infection is transmitted transstadially and transovarially to later tick stages, which feed on larger mammals.

Table 2.55 Rickettsial organisms of veterinary importance.

Genus/species	Vector	Hosts	Geographic distribution
Aegyptianella	**Ticks**		
Aegyptianella pullorum	Argas persicus	Chickens, ducks, geese	Southeast Europe, Africa, Asia
Aegyptianella moshkovskii	Argas persicus	Chickens, turkeys, pheasants, wild birds	Africa, India, Southeast Asia, Egypt, Russia
Anaplasma	**Ticks and biting flies**		
Anaplasma centrale	Dermacentor spp., Tabanus, Chrysops spp., Stomoxys, Psorophora spp.	Cattle	Africa, Asia, Australia, southern Europe, North Central and South America
Anaplasma marginale		Cattle	
Anaplasma ovis		Sheep and goats	
Anaplasma phagocytophilum (tick-borne fever)	Ixodes ricinus	Sheep, cattle, dogs, horses, deer, rodents, humans	Probably worldwide. Europe, USA, South America, Australia
Ehrlichia	**Ticks**		
Ehrlichia ruminantium (syn. Cowdria ruminantium) (heartwater)	Amblyomma spp.	Cattle, sheep, goats and other ruminants	Africa, Asia, Africa, Caribbean
Ehrlichia bovis	Hyaloma spp., Amblyomma spp., Rhipicephalus spp.	Cattle, buffalo	Africa, Asia and South America
Ehrlichia canis	Rhipicephalus sanguineus	Dogs	Asia, Europe, Africa, Australia and America
Ehrlichia chaffeensis	Rhipicephalus sanguineus	Dogs, deer, humans	USA
Ehrlichia ewingii	Rhipicephalus sanguineus	Dogs	USA
Ehrlichia equi	Ticks/flies?	Horses	India, Sri Lanka
Ehrlichia ovina	Rhipicephalus spp.	Sheep	North America
Ehrlichia risticii (Potomac horse fever; equine monocytic ehrlichiosis)	Unknown. Trematodes metacercariae/snails/aquatic insects?	Horses	USA
Neorickettsia			
Neorickettsia helminthoeca (salmon poisoning disease)	Trematodes (Nanophyetus salmincola)	Dogs, fish-eating mammals, humans	North America
Rickettsia	**Lice/fleas/ticks/mites**		
Rickettsia akari	Liponyssoides sanguineus	Mice, humans	North America, Russia, Southeast Asia
Rickettsia australis (Queensland tick typhus)	Ixodes holocyclus	Humans	Australia
Rickettsia conorii (boutonneuse fever)	Amblyomma, Hyaloma, Rhipicephalus spp.	Dogs, rats, humans	Africa, Middle East, southern Europe
Rickettsia prowazekii (epidemic typhus)	Pediculus spp.	Humans, flying squirrels	Worldwide
Rickettsia rickettsii (Rocky Mountain spotted fever)	Amblyomma spp., Dermacentor spp., Ixodes spp., Rhipicephalus spp.	Dogs, foxes, raccoons, humans	North and South America
Rickettsia tsutsugamushi	Mites (Leptotrombidium)	Rats, small mammals, birds	Asia, Australia
Rickettsia felis	Fleas	Cats, dogs, humans	North and South America, Europe
Rickettsia typhi (murine typhus)	Fleas (Xenopsylla cheopis)	Rats, humans	Worldwide

Rickettsia felis

Description: Small, pleomorphic, Gram-negative, coccoid, obligatory intracellular organisms infecting endothelial cells of smaller blood vessels.

Life cycle: Fleas become infected with *R. felis* by feeding on infected animals. Infection in the flea is transmitted trans-stadially and transovarially to later stages, and transmission occurs when the adult flea feeds.

Rickettsia rickettsii

Description: Small, pleomorphic, Gram-negative, coccoid, obligatory intracellular organisms infecting endothelial cells of smaller blood vessels.

Life cycle: Ticks become infected with *R. rickettsii* by feeding on infected small rodents that are the main reservoir of disease. Immature ticks become infected and infection is transmitted trans-stadially and transovarially to later tick stages, which feed on larger mammals.

FAMILY ANAPLASMATACEAE

The Anaplasmataceae family includes very small, rickettsia-like bacteria occurring in or on the erythrocytes of vertebrates which are transmitted by arthropods. The genera *Anaplasma*, *Ehrlichia* and *Neoherlichia* include important pathogens of animals.

Anaplasma

The *Anaplasma* genus includes very small (0.3–1 μm diameter) bacteria of the erythrocytes of ruminants which are transmitted biologically by ticks and mechanically by sucking flies, especially tabanids. *Anaplasma phagocytophilum* combo nov. (formerly known as three separate ehrlichiae, *E. phagocytophila*, *E. equi* and

Anaplasma platys [formerly known as *Ehrlichia platys*]) causes canine, equine and human granulocytic ehrlichiosis.

Life cycle: *Anaplasma* are obligate intracellular organisms infecting granulocytes, predominantly neutrophils, appearing within the cytoplasm as membrane-bound vacuoles, and can be transmitted by ticks, and also mechanically by biting flies or contaminated surgical instruments. Once in the blood, the organism enters the red cell by invaginating the cell membrane so that a vacuole is formed; thereafter it divides to form an inclusion body containing up to eight 'initial bodies' packed together (morulae). The inclusion bodies are most numerous during the acute phase of the infection, but some persist for years afterwards. The organisms spend part of their normal life cycle within the tick and are transmitted trans-stadially. As the tick vector feeds on a wide range of vertebrate animals, transmission of the infectious agent may take place to multiple host species.

Anaplasma phagocytophilum

Description: Blood smears stained with Giemsa or Wright stain reveal one or more loose aggregates (morulae or inclusion bodies, 1.5–5 mm in diameter) of blue-grey to dark blue coccoid, coccobacillary or pleomorphic organisms within the cytoplasm of neutrophils (Fig. 2.101).

Anaplasma marginale

Description: In Giemsa-stained blood smears, the organisms of *A. marginale* are seen as small, round, dark red 'inclusion bodies', approximately 0.3–1 μm, within the red cell (Fig. 2.102). Often there is only one organism in a red cell and characteristically this lies at the outer margin; however, these two features are not constant.

Anaplasma centrale

Description: As for *A. marginale*, except that the organisms are commonly found in the centre of the erythrocyte.

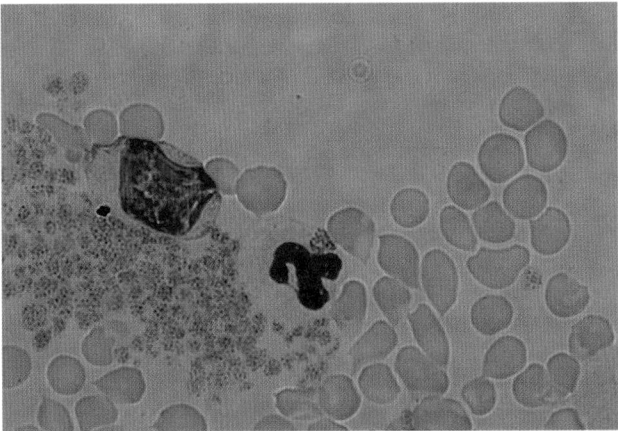

Fig. 2.101 Inclusions of *Anaplasma phagocytophilum*. (Courtesy of Grazia Carelli).

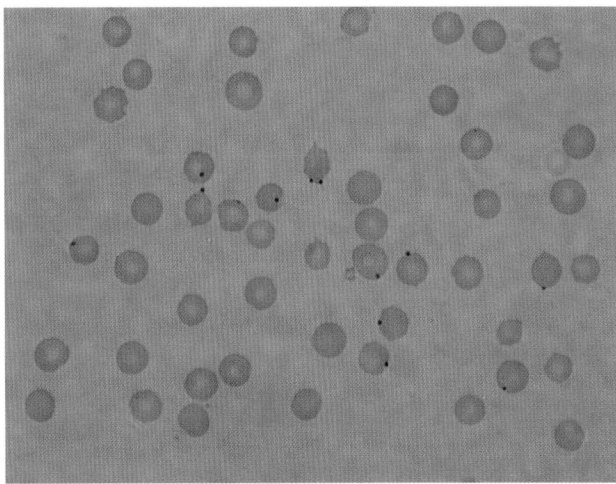

Fig. 2.102 Intraerythrocytic stages of *Anaplasma marginale*. (Courtesy of Grazia Carelli).

Ehrlichia

Ehrlichia spp. are found in leucocytes in the circulating blood and are transmitted by ixodid ticks. Several species of *Ehrlichia* are found in cattle and sheep. *Ehrlichia ruminantium*, which causes heartwater in ruminants, is transmitted by at least five species of *Amblyomma* ticks.

Three species of *Ehrlichia* are important pathogens in dogs. *Ehrlichia canis* and *Ehrlichia chaffeensis* cause canine monocytic ehrlichiosis or tropical canine pancytopaenia; *E. ewingii* causes canine granulocytic ehrlichiosis. *Ehrlichia risticii* is the cause of Potomac horse fever.

Ehrlichia bovis

Description: Round or irregular-shaped intracytoplasmic organisms (2–10 μm in diameter), present in mononuclear cells, particularly monocytes.

Life cycle: Infection is transmitted through the bite of an infected tick. Rickettsiae multiply within monocytes, forming morulae. The incubation period is reported to be 15–18 days.

Ehrlichia canis (canine monocytic ehrlichiosis, tropical canine pancytopenia)

Description: *Ehrlichia canis* is a small, pleomorphic, Gram-negative, coccoid, obligatory intracellular bacterium that parasitises circulating monocytes, intracytoplasmically in clusters (morulae). The earliest stages are small elementary bodies 0.2–0.4 μm in diameter, followed by slightly larger initial bodies 0.5–4 μm in diameter, and finally even larger inclusion bodies 4–6 μm in diameter. The organisms stain blue with Romanowsky stain, light red with Machiavello stain and brown-black by silver stain.

Life cycle: Infection is transmitted to the dog through the bite of an infected *Rhipicephalus sanguineus* tick. Transmission in the tick occurs trans-stadially but not transovarially. Larvae and nymphs become infected while feeding on bacteriaemic dogs and transmit the infection to the host after moulting to nymphs and adults, respectively.

Ehrlichia chaffeensis (canine monocytic ehrlichiosis)

Description: *Ehrlichia chaffeensis* is a small, pleomorphic, Gram-negative, coccoid, obligatory intracellular bacterium that parasitises circulating monocytes and macrophages, intracytoplasmically in clusters (morulae).

Ehrlichia ewingii

Description: *Ehrlichia ewingii* is a small, pleomorphic, Gram-negative, coccoid, obligatory intracellular bacterium that parasitises circulating neutrophils and eosinophils, intracytoplasmically in clusters (morulae).

Life cycle: Infection is transmitted to the dog through the bite of an infected *Amblyomma americanum* tick. Transmission in the tick occurs trans-stadially but not transovarially. Larvae and nymphs become infected while feeding on rickettsaemic dogs and transmit the infection to the host after moulting to nymphs and adults, respectively.

Ehrlichia ruminantium (heartwater)

Synonym: *Cowdria ruminantium*

Description: Organisms are seen as close-packed colonies consisting of less than 10 to many hundred cocci. The organism varies in size from 0.2 to greater than 1.5 μm. The diameter of individual organisms in a given cluster is rather uniform but groups are very pleomorphic. The small granules tend to be coccoid, with larger ones looking like rings, horseshoes, rods and irregular masses.

Life cycle: *Ehrlichia ruminantium* is transmitted by at least five species of *Amblyomma* ticks. In the ruminant host, it is first found in reticuloendothelial cells and then parasitises vascular endothelial cells. Division is by binary fission and it produces morula-like colonies in the cytoplasm of infected cells.

Neorickettsia risticii (Potomac horse fever)

Synonym: *Ehrlichia risticii*

Description: *Neorickettsia risticii* is a Gram-negative obligate intracellular bacterium, 0.6–1.5 μm in size, with a tropism for monocytes. The organism is not visible in monocytes in blood smears from clinical cases.

Life cycle: Details of the life cycle are incomplete but infection to horses appears to involve ingestion of metacercarial stages of trematodes or inadvertent ingestion of aquatic insect stages.

Neorickettsia helminthoeca

This bacterium is the agent of 'salmon poisoning', which frequently produces severe and fatal infections in dogs, foxes and other animals.

Aegyptianella

The genus *Aegyptianella*, previously included in the Anaplasmataceae but currently considered as *incertae sedis*, infects a wide range of wild and domestic birds in the warmer parts of the world and has been recorded from Africa, Asia and southern Europe.

Life cycle: The life cycle is simple, with multiplication of the organisms within erythrocytes. The main vectors are ticks of the genus *Argas*.

Aegyptianella pullorum

Description: *Anaplasma*-like bodies of various sizes are found in the cytoplasm of erythrocytes. The organisms occur as initial bodies followed by development forms and marginal bodies ('signet ring') in the cytoplasm of erythrocytes. The early trophozoites or initial bodies occur in erythrocytes, are small (0.5–1 μm) and round to oval. Spherical bodies up to 4 μm containing up to 25 small granules may occur.

Aegyptianella moshkovskii

Description: The organism usually produces 4–6 trophozoites. The early trophozoites within the erythrocytes are small (0.2–0.6 μm). Larger mature forms are 2.1 by 1.4 μm with large oval or irregular forms (0.9–5.3 μm).

ORDER HYPHOMICROBIALES

FAMILY BARTONELLACEAE

Members of the *Bartonellaceae* are pleomorphic bacteria that are distinguished from the Anaplasmataceae by cultural and structural characteristics. The Bartonellaceae family includes the genus *Bartonella* with several species that have been described in wild and domestic mammalian species, including humans, with different species (i.e. *Bartonella henselae*, *Bartonella clarridgeiae*) being zoonotic. Species of *Bartonella quintana* are the cause of trench fever in humans and the disease is transmitted by lice.

ORDER LEGIONELLALES

FAMILY COXIELLACEAE

The genus *Coxiella* has a single species with worldwide distribution and is the cause of Q fever. Infection is enzootic in cattle, sheep and goats and can cause severe disease in humans. The organism is widely disseminated among wild mammals and birds and has been found in ixodid and argasid ticks, gamasid mites and human body lice (*Pediculus*).

PHYLUM FIRMICUTES

ORDER MYCOPLASMATALES

FAMILY MYCOPLASMATACEAE

The genus *Mycoplasma* that belongs to the family Mycoplasmataceae (class *Mollicutes*) contains the haemotropic bacteria split into the haemofelis and haemominutum groups, formerly known as *Haemobartonella* and *Eperythrozoon*, previously included in the family Bartonellaceae. The current taxonomy is based on 16S rRNA and rpoB gene phylogenetic analysis.

Haemofelis group

Mycoplasma haemofelis (syn. *Haemobartonella felis*) is the agent of feline infectious anaemia and has been found in lice, fleas and ticks. Vertical transmission has also been implicated.

Description: Small, pleomorphic, Gram-negative, coccoid, obligatory intracellular organisms infecting erythrocytes.

Haemominutum group

Species of the haemominutum group, formerly *Eperythrozoon*, are generally opportunistic but occasionally with the action of concurrent risk factors responsible for fever, anaemia and weight loss in feline, ruminants and pigs.

Life cycle: Organisms are transmitted by animal aggressive interactions or insect and tick biting. Replication takes place by binary fission or budding on the red blood cell of the vertebrate host.

Mycoplasma wenyonii

Synonym: *Eperythrozoon wenyonii*

Description: Coccoid, ring- or rod-shaped structures on the surface of red cells, blue to purple when stained with Giemsa.

Mycoplasma ovis

Synonym: *Mycoplasma ovis*

Description: Pleomorphic coccobacilli occurring either as eperythrocytic organisms in depressions on the cell surface or free in the plasma (Fig. 2.103). Single comma-shaped or ring-form cocci predominate in light to moderate infections but form irregular complex bodies in severe parasitaemias. Cocci appear light blue with Giemsa or Romanowsky stains.

Mycoplasma suis

Synonym: *Eperythrozoon suis*

Description: Pleomorphic coccobacilli occurring either in depressions on the cell surface of erythrocytes or free in the plasma. Cocci appear light blue with Giemsa or Romanowsky stains.

Life cycle: Organisms are transmitted by biting insects and possibly lice. Replication takes place by binary fission or budding.

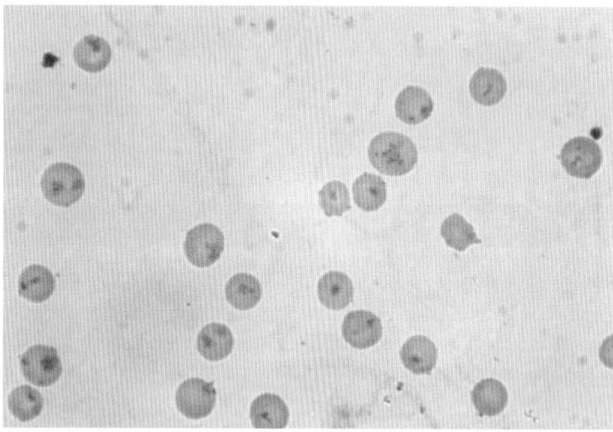

Fig. 2.103 Intraerythrocytic forms of *Mycoplasma ovis*.

CHAPTER 3
Veterinary entomology

Veterinary entomology, in its literal sense, means the study of insects of veterinary importance. This term, however, is commonly used to describe the wider study of all arthropods parasitic on animals (ectoparasites), including arachnids such as ticks and mites.

The association between an arthropod ectoparasite and a vertebrate host may take on a variety of forms. Those parasites that do not need to live or feed on a living host to complete their life cycle, and do so only when suitable hosts are available, are described as **facultative**. Facultative parasites may have only intermittent contact with their hosts, are less host specific and are usually free-living for the major part of their life cycles. In other cases, the parasites may be totally dependent on the host to complete their life cycle, in which case they are described as **obligatory**. Obligatory parasites live in continuous association with their host and in many cases are highly host specific. The biology of both obligate and facultative ectoparasites is considered in this chapter. Guides to identification are provided in Chapter 4 and their clinical impact, epidemiology and treatment are dealt with in their most relevant host-specific chapter.

PHYLUM ARTHROPODA

The phylum Arthropoda contains over 80% of all known animal species, with almost a million species described, and consists of invertebrates whose major characteristics are a hard chitinous exoskeleton, a segmented body and jointed limbs (Fig. 3.1).

CLASSIFICATION

There are two major classes of arthropods of veterinary importance: the Insecta and Arachnida. The **Insecta** have three pairs of legs, the head, thorax and abdomen are distinct, and they have a single pair of antennae. In **Arachnida** (belonging to the subphylum Chelicerata), the adults have four pairs of legs and the body is divided into the gnathosoma (mouthparts) and idiosoma (fused cephalothorax and abdomen); there are no antennae.

A third group of arthropods, the **Pentastomida**, commonly known as Tongue worms, is of lesser veterinary importance. Molecular studies suggest that they may be a degenerate subclass of **Crustacea**. All are obligate parasites and the adults are found in the respiratory passages of vertebrates and superficially resemble annelid worms.

STRUCTURE AND FUNCTION

Segmentation

Arthropods are **metameric**, i.e. the body is divided primitively into segments. However, within a number of arthropod classes, particularly the arachnids, there has been a tendency for segmentation to become greatly reduced and in many of the mites, for example, it has almost disappeared. Segments have become fused into functional groups, known as **tagma**, such as the head, thorax and to a lesser

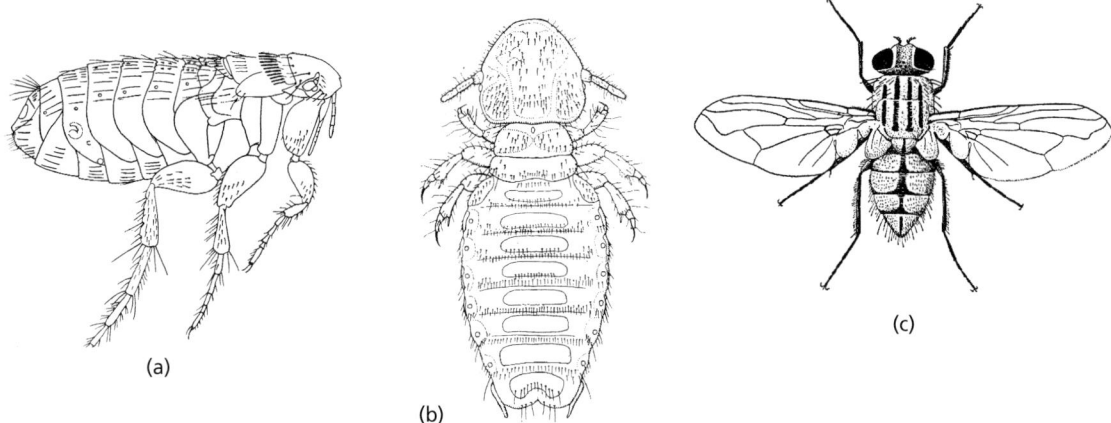

Fig. 3.1 (a) Flea (Siphonaptera), (b) louse (Psocodea [Phthiraptera]) and (c) adult fly (Diptera) showing the general morphological features of insect ectoparasites.

Veterinary Parasitology, Fifth Edition. Domenico Otranto and Richard Wall.
© 2024 John Wiley & Sons Ltd. Published 2024 by John Wiley & Sons Ltd.

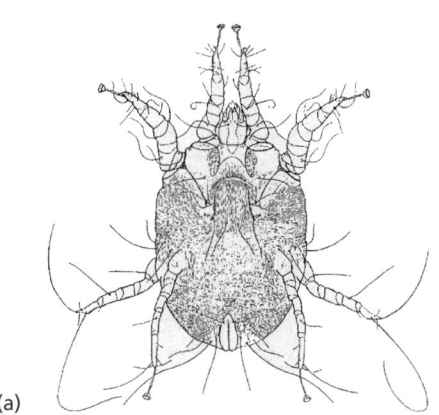

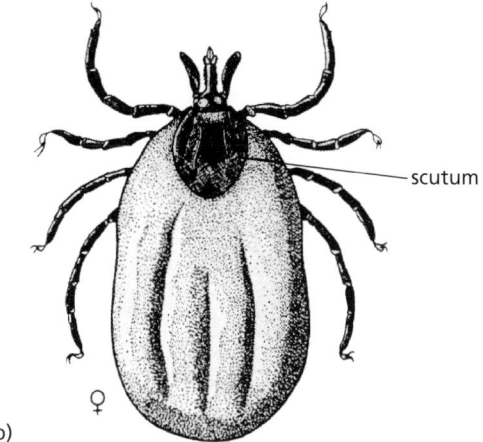

scutum

♀

(a)   (b)

Fig. 3.2 A mite (a) and tick (b) showing the general morphological features of arachnid ectoparasites. (Baker *et al.*, 1956/National Pest Control Association.)

extent the abdomen. Each group of segments is specialised for functions different from those of the other parts of the body (Fig. 3.2).

Exoskeleton

The **exoskeleton** is the outer covering, which provides support and protection to the living tissues of arthropods. The exoskeleton is non-cellular. Instead, it is composed of a number of layers of **cuticle**, which are secreted by a single outer cellular layer of the body known as the **epidermis** (Fig. 3.3). The outer layer of cuticle, the **epicuticle**, is composed largely of proteins and, in many arthropods, is covered by a waxy layer. The next two layers are the outer **exocuticle** and the inner **endocuticle**. Both are composed of a protein and a polysaccharide called **chitin**, which has long fibrous molecules containing nitrogen. For extra strength the exocuticle may be tanned or **sclerotised**. This is where proteins, interwoven between bundles of chitin strands, become tightly cross-linked, giving it extra strength. The sclerotised cuticle is hard and dark in colour.

The cuticle is often penetrated by fine pore canals, which allow the passage of secretions from the epidermis to the surface. The cuticle has many outgrowths in the form of scales, spines, hairs and bristles, many of which are sensory in function.

Movement is made possible by the division of the cuticle into separate plates, called **sclerites**. Plates are connected by **intersegmental** or **articular membranes**, where the cuticle is soft and flexible (Fig. 3.4). The muscles attach on the inside of the exoskeleton to rod-like invaginations of the cuticle called **apodemes**. The cuticle of many larval arthropods is also largely soft, flexible, pale and unsclerotised.

Appendages

Primitively, each arthropod segment bears a pair of leg-like appendages. However, the number of appendages has frequently been modified through loss or structural differentiation. In insects, there are always three pairs of legs in the adult stage. In mites and tick,s there are three pairs of legs in the larval stage and four pairs in the nymphal and adult stages. The cuticular exoskeleton of the legs is divided into tube-like segments connected to one another by soft articular membranes, creating joints at each junction.

Gas exchange

In some small arthropods, the exoskeleton is thin and lacks a waxy epicuticle. For these animals, oxygen and carbon dioxide simply diffuse directly across the cuticle. However, this method of gas

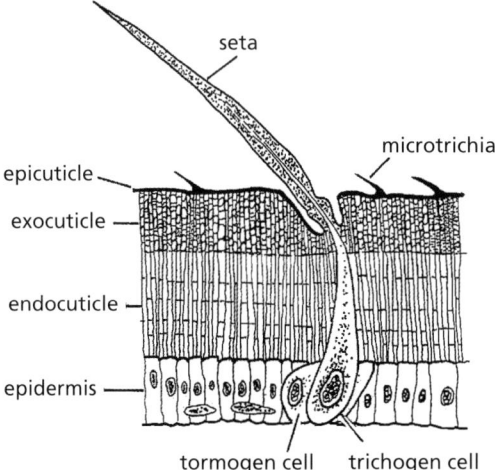

Fig. 3.3 Diagrammatic section through the arthropod integument.

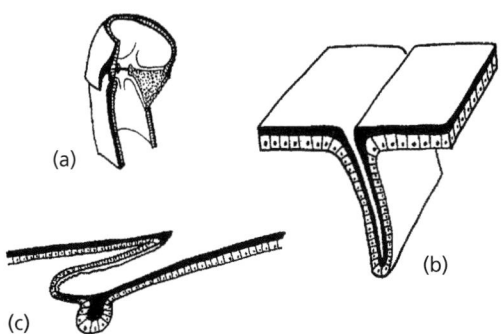

Fig. 3.4 (a) Articulation of a generalised arthropod leg joint. (b) A multicellular apodeme. (c) Intersegmental articulation, showing intersegmental membrane folded beneath the exoskeleton. (Adapted from Snodgrass, 1935.)

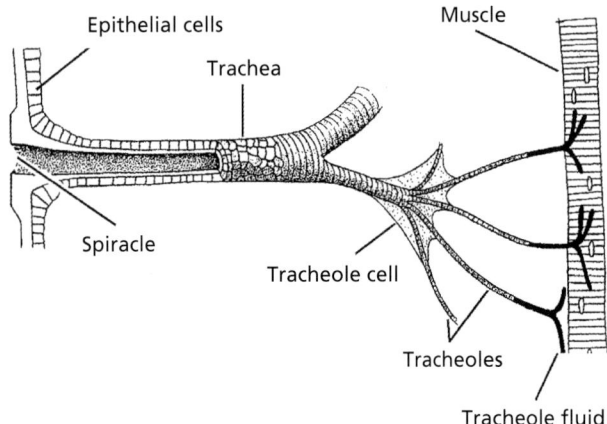

Fig. 3.5 A spiracle, trachea and tracheoles. (Adapted from Snodgrass, 1935.)

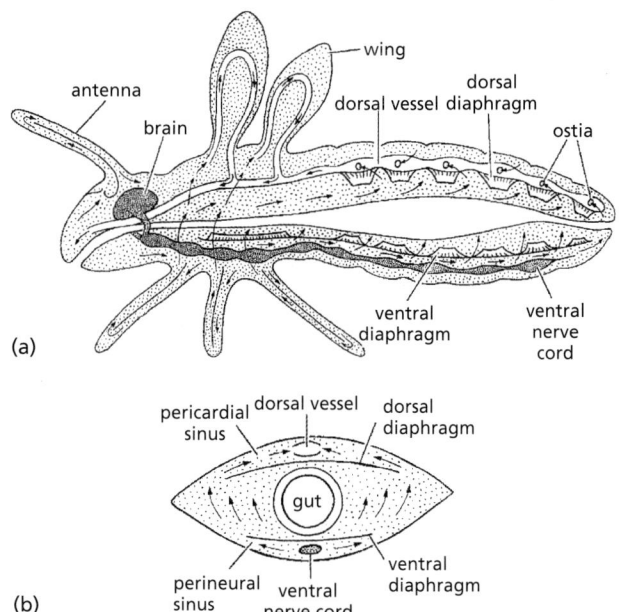

Fig. 3.6 Generalised arthropod circulatory system. (a) Longitudinal section through the body. (b) Transverse section through the abdomen. (From Gullan and Cranston, 1994, after Wigglesworth, 1972.)

exchange is only functional over very short distances and for very small animals restricted to humid environments. In most of the terrestrial groups of arthropod ectoparasites, the protective cuticle is punctured by a number of openings to allow gas exchange. In the insects these openings are called **spiracles**; in the mites and ticks they are usually called **stigmata** (Fig. 3.5).

Typically, spiracles or stigmata open into cuticle-lined, air-conducting tubes called **tracheae**, which form longitudinal and transverse tracheal trunks that interconnect among the segments. The tracheae branch repeatedly as they extend to all parts of the body. The branches of the tracheae end within the cells of muscles and other tissues in extremely fine **tracheoles**, which are the principal sites of gas exchange. The ends of the tracheoles contain fluid and are usually less than 1 µm in diameter. Tracheoles are particularly numerous in tissues with high oxygen requirements.

Oxygen enters through the respiratory openings and passes down the tracheae, usually in smaller arthropods by diffusion along a concentration gradient. Carbon dioxide and (in terrestrial insects) water vapour move in the opposite direction. Reducing water loss is a major problem for most terrestrial arthropods and for them, gas exchange is often a compromise between getting enough oxygen into the body while making sure that they do not desiccate. Hence in periods of inactivity, the respiratory openings are often kept closed by valves which open only periodically. In large and highly mobile insects, active pumping movements of the thorax and/or abdomen may be used to help ventilate the outer parts of the tracheal system.

Circulatory system

The arthropod circulatory system is relatively simple, consisting of a series of central cavities or sinuses, called a **haemocoel** (Fig. 3.6). The haemocoel contains blood, called **haemolymph**, in which hormones are transported, nutrients are distributed from the gut and wastes removed via the excretory organs. The haemolymph is not usually involved in gas exchange and in most parasitic arthropods there is no respiratory pigment (however, some exceptions do exist, for example in *Gasterophilus* larvae which live in the extremely oxygen-deficient environment of the host's gut).

In most mites, the circulatory system consists only of a network of sinuses and circulation results from contraction of body muscles.

Insects, on the other hand, have a functional equivalent of the heart, the **dorsal vessel**. This is essentially a tube running along the length of the body. The dorsal vessel is open at its anterior end, closed at its posterior end and perforated by pairs of lateral openings called **ostia**. The ostia only permit a one-way flow of haemolymph into the dorsal vessel. The dorsal vessel pumps haemolymph forward, eventually into sinuses of the haemocoel in the head. Haemolymph then percolates back through the haemocoel, until it is again moved into the dorsal vessel through the ostia.

Nervous system

Arthropods have a complex nervous system associated with the well-developed sense organs, such as eyes and antennae, and behaviour that is often highly elaborate. The central nervous system consists of a dorsal brain in the head which is connected by a pair of nerves which run around the foregut to a series of ventral nerve cord ganglia.

Digestive system

The gut of an arthropod is essentially a simple tube that runs from mouth to anus. However, the precise shape of the gut may vary considerably between arthropods, depending on the nature of their diet.

The gut is divided into three sections: foregut, midgut and hindgut (**Fig. 3.7**). The foregut and hindgut are lined with cuticle. In fluid-feeding arthropods, there are prominent muscles that attach to the walls of the pharynx to form a pump. The foregut is concerned primarily with the ingestion and storage of food, the latter usually taking place in the **crop**. Between the foregut and the midgut is a valve called the **proventriculus** or **gizzard**. The midgut is the principal site of digestion and absorption. It has a cellular lining,

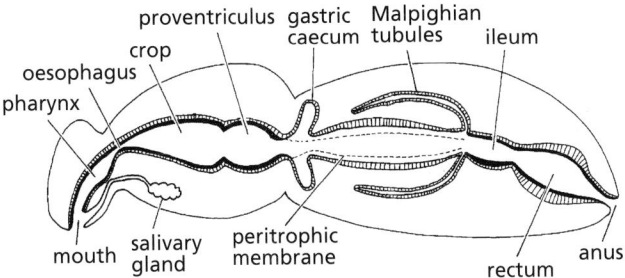

Fig. 3.7 Digestive tract of a generalised arthropod, showing the foregut, midgut and hindgut. The cuticular linings of the foregut and hindgut are indicated by thickened lines.

which secretes digestive enzymes. Absorption of the products of digestion takes place largely in the anterior of the midgut, in large outpockets called **gastric caecae**. The hindgut terminates in an expanded region, the **rectum**, which functions in the absorption of water and the formation of faeces. Nitrogenous wastes are removed from the haemolymph by long thin projections called the **Malpighian tubules**, which extend into the haemocoel and open into the gut at the junction of the midgut and hindgut. In mites and ticks, the gut follows a broadly similar plan but may be simplified, often with only one pair of Malpighian tubules.

Arthropod sense organs

The sensory receptors of arthropods are usually associated with modifications of the chitinous exoskeleton. The most common type of receptor is associated with hairs, bristles and setae. Bristles may act as mechanoreceptors, with movement triggering the receptor at its base. Alternatively, the bristle may carry a range of chemoreceptors, which may be sensitive to specific cues such as carbon dioxide or temperature. The sensory hairs and bristles are distributed most densely at particular locations such as the antennae or legs.

Most arthropods have eyes but these can vary greatly in complexity. Simple eyes, known as **stemmata** and consisting of only a few sensory cells, are found in many larval insects. More complex **ocelli**, which contain between one and 1000 sensory cells and an overlying corneal lens, are found in some larval and many adult insects. These simple eyes do not form images but are very sensitive at low light intensities and to changes in light intensity. The most complex type of arthropod eye, known as a compound eye, is large with thousands of long cylindrical units called **ommatidia**, each covered by a translucent cornea, called a **facet**. There is no mechanism for accommodation, the compound eye does not form an effective image and its principal function is in detecting movement. In the females of some species of insect, the eyes are distinctly separated (**dichoptic**) while in the males they may be very close together (**holoptic**). Ocelli and compound eyes may both occur in the same animal. In some arthropods, such as the mites, ticks and lice, eyes may be greatly reduced or absent. In others, such as some blood-sucking flies, where sight is important in locating their hosts, the eyes are well developed.

Reproductive system

In most arthropods, the sexes are separate and mating is usually required for the production of fertile eggs. The female reproductive system is composed of a pair of **ovaries**. Each ovary is divided into egg tubes, or **ovarioles**. The ovarioles lead, via the **oviduct**, to an **ovipositor**. Most arthropods lay eggs but some retain the eggs which hatch within the oviduct, and live larvae may be deposited at various stages of development.

The male reproductive system is usually composed of a pair of **testes**, each subdivided into a set of sperm tubes, leading to the vas deferens and the external genitalia, with a penis or **aedeagus**. Accessory glands produce secretions that may form a packet called a **spermatophore**, which encloses the sperm and protects it during insemination.

Sperm may be delivered directly to the female during copulation or, in some species of mite, the spermatophore is deposited on the ground and the female is induced to walk over and pick up the spermatophore with her genital opening. In ticks, the spermatophore is inserted into the female genital opening by the male's mouthparts. Sperm are usually stored by the female in organs called **spermathecae**. As an ovulated egg passes down the oviduct, it is fertilised by sperm released from the spermathecae.

Moulting

To grow, arthropods must shed the exoskeleton periodically; this is described as **moulting** or, more properly, **ecdysis**. Before the old exoskeleton is shed, the epidermis secretes a new epicuticle. The new epicuticle is soft and wrinkled at this stage. When the old skeleton is shed, the soft whitish exoskeleton of the newly moulted animal is stretched, often by the ingestion of air or water. Once expanded, sclerotisation occurs, resulting in hardening and darkening of the cuticle. The forms that occur between moults are known as **stages**, or **stadia**, and morphologically distinct life cycle stages are known as **instars**.

CLASS INSECTA

GENERAL MORPHOLOGY AND LIFE CYCLE

Members of the class Insecta can be distinguished from the other arthropods by the presence in the adult of three pairs of legs, a pair of antennae, the broad division of the body into three sections, the head, thorax and abdomen, and the presence of external mouthparts (Entognatha).

The head carries the main sensory organs: the single pair of antennae, a pair of compound eyes and often a number of ocelli. The mouth is surrounded by mouthparts, which are very variable in form. In the ancestral form, represented by living insects such as cockroaches and grasshoppers, the mouthparts are composed of the following elements (Fig. 3.8). The **labrum** is a hinged plate attached to the front of the head by the clypeus. The paired **mandibles** (jaws) and **maxillae** (secondary jaws) have areas of their surfaces adapted for cutting, slashing or grinding. The maxillae may also carry maxillary palps, which are sensory in function and used to handle and taste the food. A **hypopharynx**, arising from the floor of the mouth, may be considered in some ways to act as a tongue and is usually associated with a **salivary duct** leading from the salivary gland. The salivary duct allows saliva, which may contain digestive enzymes, anticoagulants or other chemo-active compounds, to be delivered to the feeding site. Finally, a **labium** usually bears two sensory labial palps, but these may be extensively modified, especially in flies. Insect mouthparts show a remarkable variety of specialisation, related to their diets.

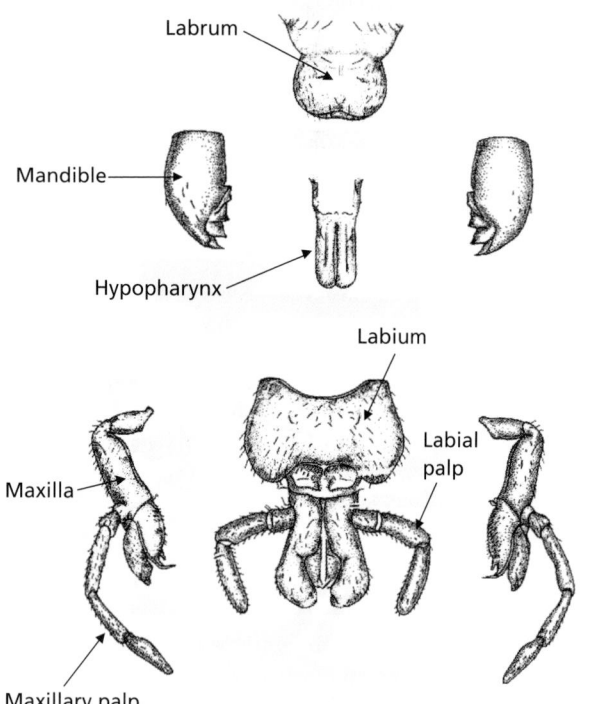

Fig. 3.8 Mouthparts of a generalised omnivorous insect.

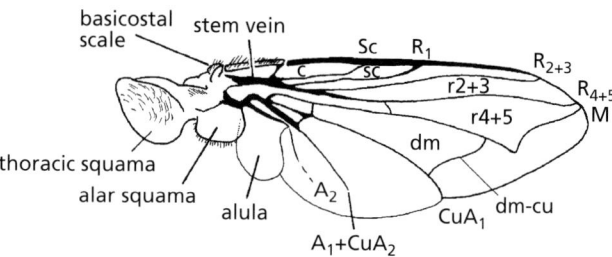

Fig. 3.10 The wing veins and cells of the calliphorid dipteran *Calliphora vicina*.

The thorax is composed of three fused segments: **prothorax**, **mesothorax** and **metathorax**. The prothorax is often greatly reduced in size. On each of these segments there is a single pair of legs. Each leg is composed of six segments. The basal section of the leg articulating with the body is the **coxa**, which is followed by a short triangular **trochanter**. There then follows the **femur**, the **tibia**, one to five segments of the **tarsus**, the tarsomeres and finally the **pretarsus** composed of claws and ridged pads. Between the claws there may be two pad-like **pulvilli** surrounding a central bristle or pad, known as the **empodium** (Fig. 3.9). The legs of insects are generally adapted for walking or running but some are modified for specialised functions, such as jumping (fleas) or clinging to the hairs of their host's body (lice).

In the adult, most orders of insect have two pairs of wings articulating with the mesothorax and metathorax. Winged insects are described as **pterygotes**. Some orders of primitive insects do not possess wings (**apterygotes**), while others such as the fleas and lice, which once had wings, have lost them completely (secondarily

wingless). Others, such as some of the hippoboscids, have wings for only a short time as adults, after which they are shed.

The wing consists of a network of sclerotised veins, which enclose regions of thin transparent cuticle called **cells**. The veins act as a framework to brace and stabilise the wing and may carry trachaea, haemolymph and nerves in the newly emerged adult. Connection to the haemocoel is important in the newly emerged adult insect because changes in blood pressure allow the wing to be expanded. However, the connections to the main body cavity are eventually cut as the adult ages, making the wing increasingly brittle. The arrangement of the veins tends to be characteristic of various groups of insect species and so is important in identification and taxonomy (Fig. 3.10).

In several groups of insects, such as beetles (Coleoptera), the front wings have been modified to various degrees as protective coverings for the hindwings and abdomen and are known as **elytra**. In the true flies (Diptera), the hindwings have been reduced to form a pair of club-like **halteres**, which are used as stabilising organs to assist in flight.

The abdomen is composed primitively of 11 segments, although the 10th and 11th segments are usually small and not externally visible and the 11th segment has been lost in most advanced groups. The genital ducts open ventrally on segment 8 or 9 of the abdomen and these segments often bear external organs that assist in reproduction. The genitalia are composed of structures which probably originated from simple abdominal appendages. In the male, the basic external genitalia consist of one or two pairs of claspers, which grasp the female in copulation, and the penis (aedeagus). However, there is considerable variation in the precise shape of the male genitalia in various groups of insect and these differences may be important in the identification of species. In the female, there may be a specialised **appendicular ovipositor**, composed of appendages on the terminal segments of the abdomen, or the tip of the abdomen may be elongated at the time of oviposition to form a more simple **substitutional ovipositor**.

Within the class Insecta there are generally considered to be 30 orders (although the precise number may vary depending on which classification system is used), of which only three, the flies (Diptera), fleas (Siphonaptera) and lice (Psocodea [Phthiraptera]), are of major veterinary importance.

Insect life cycles

In the most primitive wingless insects, there is no substantive change in body form over the life cycle, there is no **metamorphosis**, and these insects are described as **ametabolous**.

In most winged insect orders, the juvenile stadia broadly resemble the adult except that the genitalia and wings are not developed. The juveniles, usually called **nymphs**, make a new cuticle and shed

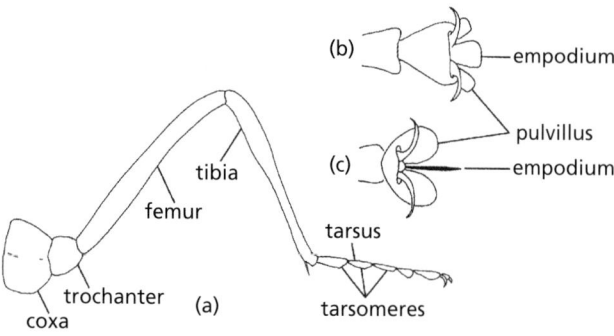

Fig. 3.9 The segments of the leg (a), and the empodium and pulvilli of typical adult tabanid (b) and muscid (c) Diptera.

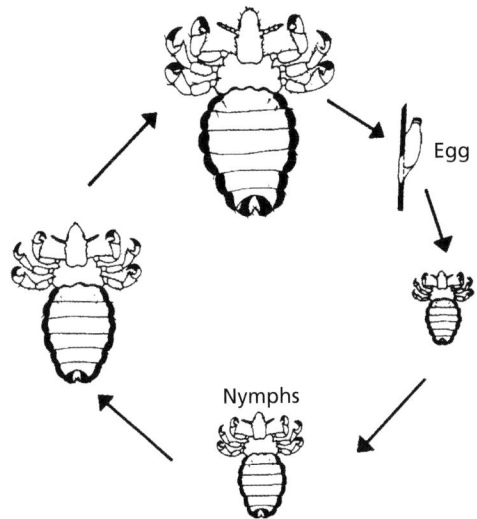

Fig. 3.11 Life cycle of a generalised louse displaying hemimetabolous metamorphosis and passing through three nymphal stages prior to emergence as a reproductive adult.

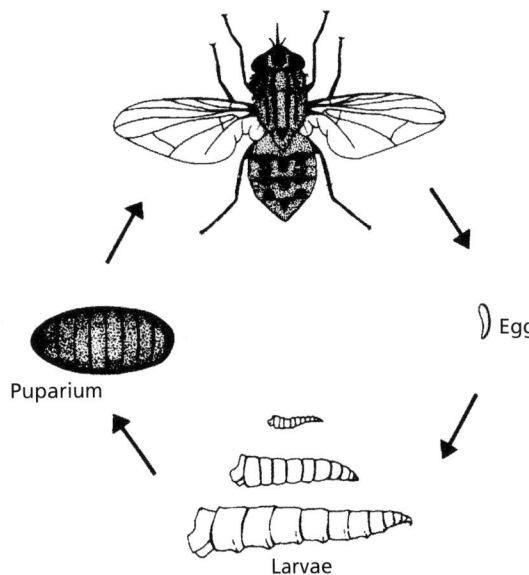

Fig. 3.12 Life cycle of a fly, *Stomoxys calcitrans*, displaying holometabolous metamorphosis, with the egg giving rise to maggot-like larva, pupa and finally reproductive adult.

the old one at intervals throughout development, typically four or five times, increasing in size before the emergence of the adult. This is often described as a simple life cycle with incomplete or partial metamorphosis, known as **hemimetabolous development** (Fig. 3.11).

In other, more advanced insects, the juvenile and adult stages are morphologically dissimilar. The juvenile instar, which may be referred to as a **larva**, **maggot**, **grub** or **caterpillar**, is concerned primarily with feeding and growth. In contrast, the adult, or **imago**, has become the specialised reproductive and dispersal life cycle stage. To reach the adult form, the larva must undergo complete metamorphosis, during which the entire body is reorganised and reconstructed. The transformation between juvenile and adult is made possible by the incorporation of a **pupal** stage, which acts as a bridge between juvenile and adult. The pupa does not feed and is generally (but not always) immobile. However, it is metabolically very active as old larval tissues and organs are lost or remoulded and replaced by adult organs. This pattern of development is described as a **complex life cycle** with **holometabolous development** (Fig. 3.12).

ORDER DIPTERA

The Diptera are the true flies; this order is one of the largest in the class Insecta, with over 120 000 described species. They have only one pair of wings, the hind pair having been reduced to become club-like **halteres**, which vibrate and provide inertia, giving sensory information that helps the insect to maintain stable flight. All species of Diptera have a complex life cycle with complete metamorphosis. As a result, dipterous flies can be parasites as larvae or adults, but they are rarely parasites in both life cycle stages. The adults of many members of this order are also important vectors of disease or nuisance pests.

The Diptera is usually considered to have two suborders: the Nematocera with slender multisegmented antennae and the Brachycera, stouter bodied flies with an antenna consisting of eight or fewer flagellum segments. However, the relationships between the families of Diptera are not completely resolved and the suborder Nematocera is generally thought to be paraphyletic (i.e. not including all the descendants of a common ancestor).

SUBORDER NEMATOCERA

Flies of the suborder Nematocera (thread-horns) are usually small, slender and delicate with long filamentous antennae composed of many articulating segments (Fig. 3.13). The wings are often long and narrow, with conspicuous longitudinal veins (Fig. 3.14). The palps are usually pendulous, though not in mosquitoes, and are

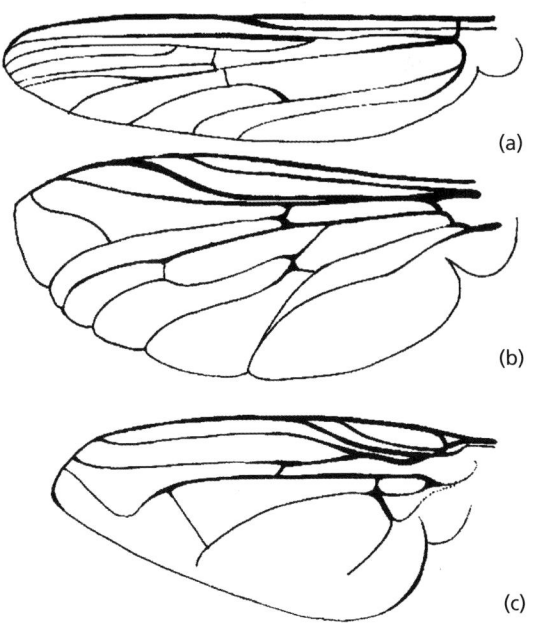

Fig. 3.13 Variations in wing venation found in typical (a) nematocerous, (b) tabanid and (c) muscid Diptera.

232

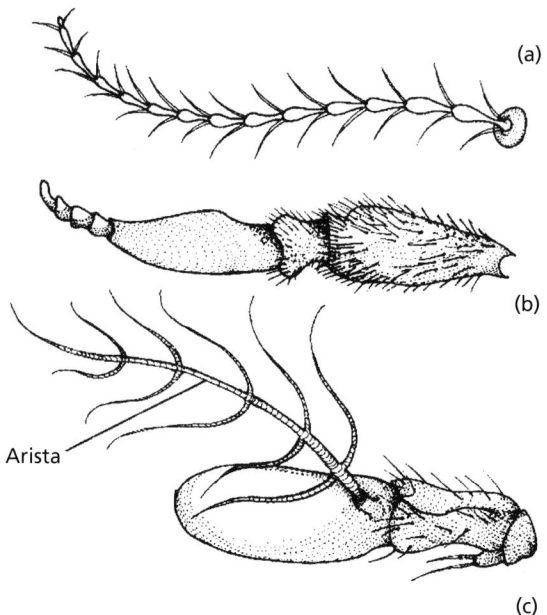

Fig. 3.14 Variations in the structure of the antennae found in typical (a) nematocerous, (b) tabanid and (c) muscid Diptera.

usually composed of four or five segments. Usually, only the females blood feed and have piercing/sucking mouthparts. Eggs are laid in or near water and develop into aquatic larvae and pupae; both of these stages have recognisable heads and are mobile.

The labium forms a protective sheath for the other mouthparts, known collectively as the stylets, and ends in two small sensory labella (Fig. 3.15). Inside the labium lies the labrum which is curled inwards to the edges so that it almost forms a complete tube. The gap in the labrum is closed by the very fine paired mandibles to form a food canal. Behind the mandibles lies the slender hypopharynx, bearing the salivary canal, and behind this are the paired maxillae (laciniae). Both the mandibles and maxillae are finely toothed towards their tips. At the base of the mouthparts is a single pair of sensory maxillary palps. The structure of these mouthparts is essentially similar in all families of blood-feeding Nematocera. However, they are greatly elongated in the mosquitoes.

FAMILY CERATOPOGONIDAE

This family consists of very small flies, commonly known as Biting midges. The females feed on humans and animals and are known to transmit various viruses, protozoa and helminths. The only important genus from a veterinary standpoint is the genus *Culicoides*, of which over 1000 species have been described. Midges feed on birds or mammals, inflicting a painful bite and transmitting many disease pathogens. Most importantly, they act as vectors of more than 50 arboviruses.

Culicoides

Description: *Culicoides* midge adults are 1.5–5 mm in length with the thorax humped over a small head (Fig. 3.16). The wings are generally mottled in pattern, and at rest are held like a closed pair of scissors over the grey or brownish-black abdomen. The legs are relatively short, particularly the forelegs, and the small mouthparts hang vertically. The short piercing proboscis consists of a

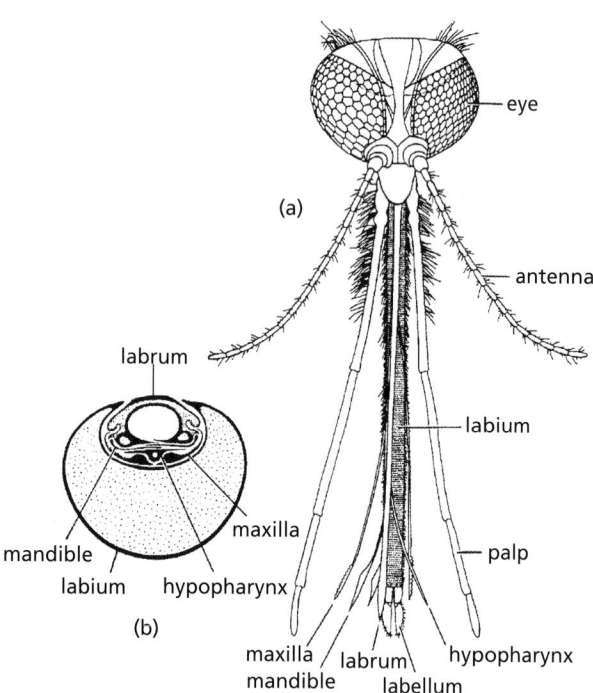

Fig. 3.15 Mouthparts of a mosquito (Diptera: Nematocera): (a) anterior view; (b) transverse section. (From Gullan and Cranston, 1994.)

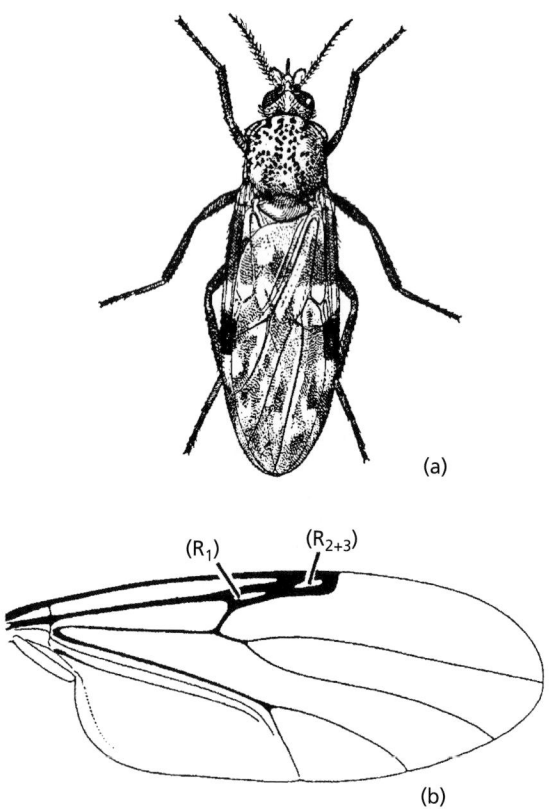

Fig. 3.16 (a) Adult female *Culicoides nubeculosus* at rest. (b) Wing venation typical of species of *Culicoides*, showing the two elongate radial cells. (Edwards *et al.*, 1939/Smithsonian Libraries.)

sharp labrum, two maxillae, two mandibles, a hypopharynx and a fleshy labium, which does not enter the skin during feeding by the adult female. In the male, the long antennae are feathery or plumose, whereas those of the female possess only short hairs and are known as pilose antennae. Microscopic hairs cover the wings. Ceratopogonids have a forked medial vein (M_1, M_2) and species of the genus *Culicoides* usually have a distinct pattern of radial cells on their wings (Fig. 3.16).

Life cycle: The eggs, which are brown or black, are cylindrical or banana-shaped and 0.5 mm in length. Eggs are laid in damp marshy ground or in decaying vegetable matter near water. Hatching occurs in 2–9 days depending on the species and temperature, but temperate species may overwinter as eggs. There are four larval stages characterised by having small dark heads, segmented bodies and terminal anal gills. They have a serpentine swimming action in water and feed on decaying vegetation. Larval development is complete in warm countries in 14–25 days, but in temperate areas this may be delayed for periods of up to seven months. The less active brown pupae, 2–4 mm long, are found at the surface or edges of water and are characterised by a pair of respiratory trumpets on the cephalothorax and a pair of terminal horns that enable the pupa to move. Adult flies emerge from the pupae in 3–10 days. Only females blood feed and inflict a painful bite. Adult *Culicoides* are not strong fliers and are usually found close to larval habitats in small and inconspicuous swarms. Adult *Culicoides* feed especially in dull humid weather and tend to be crepuscular and nocturnal. Females are attracted to the smell and warmth of their hosts and different species may be host specific to varying degrees.

For clinical information see Chapter 10.

For clinical information see Chapter 10.

FAMILY SIMULIIDAE

Of the 12 genera belonging to this family of small flies, *Simulium* is the most important. Commonly referred to as 'Blackflies' or 'buffalo gnats', they have a wide host range, feeding on a great variety of mammals and birds and causing annoyance particularly in livestock due to their painful bites. In humans, however, they are most important as vectors of *Onchocerca volvulus*, the filarioid nematode that causes 'river blindness' in Africa and Central and South America. More than 1700 species of blackflies have been described worldwide, although only 10–20% of these are regarded as pests of humans and their animals.

Simulium

Description: As their common names indicate, these flies are usually black with a humped thorax. The adults are 1.5–5 mm in length and relatively stout-bodied, with broad colourless wings that show indistinct wing veins and are held at rest like the closed blades of a pair of scissors. The wings are short, typically 1.5–6.5 mm long, broad with a large anal lobe, and have veins that are thickened at the anterior margin of the wing (**Fig. 3.17**). The first abdominal tergite is modified to form a prominent basal scale, fringed with fine hairs. Morphologically, adult male and female flies are similar but can be differentiated by the fact that in the female, the eyes are distinctly separated (dichoptic), whereas in males the eyes are very close together (holoptic) with characteristic enlarged ommatidia in the

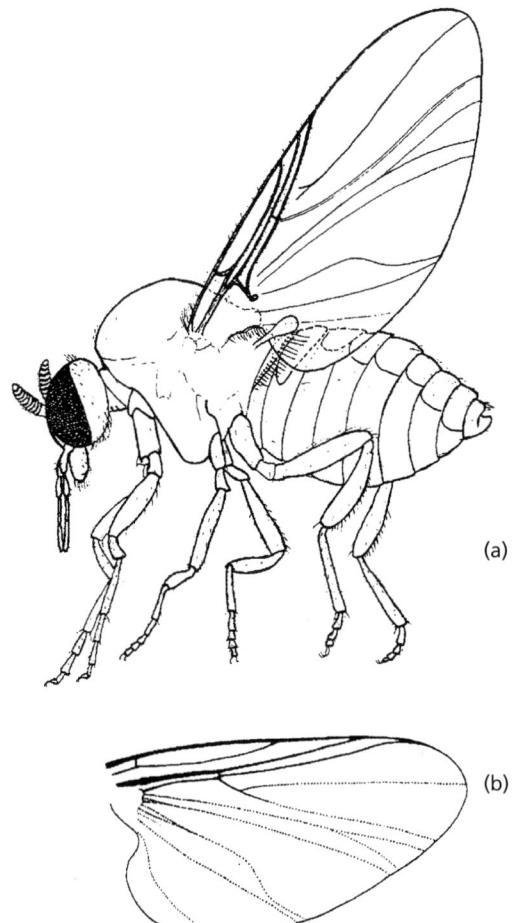

Fig. 3.17 (a) Adult female *Simulium*. (b) Wing venation typical of *Simulium*, showing the large anal lobe and crowding of the veins towards the leading edge. (From Smart, 1943.)

upper part of the eye. This may help males to locate females against the blue backdrop of the sky. Compared with other closely related flies, the antennae, although segmented, are relatively short, stout and devoid of bristles. The mouthparts resemble those of the biting midges except for the presence of conspicuous segmented maxillary palps. The body is covered with short golden or silvery hairs. They are found worldwide except in New Zealand, Hawaii and some minor island groups.

Life cycle: Eggs, 0.1–0.4 mm in length, are laid in sticky masses of 150–600 on partially submerged stones or vegetation in fast-flowing water. Hatching takes only a few days in warm conditions, but may take weeks in temperate areas and in some species the eggs can overwinter. There may be up to eight larval stadia. The mature larvae are 5–13 mm long, light coloured and poorly segmented, and are distinguishable by a blackish head, which bears a prominent pair of feeding brushes (Fig. 3.18). The body is swollen posteriorly and just below the head is an appendage called the proleg, which bears hooks. Larvae normally remain attached to submerged vegetation or rocks by a circlet of posterior hooks, but may change their position in a looping manner by alternate use of the proleg and the posterior hooks. The larvae remain in areas of fast-flowing current, since they require highly oxygenated water to survive. They use the water current to passively filter feed on suspended debris and bacteria. In deoxygenated water, the larvae detach from their silken

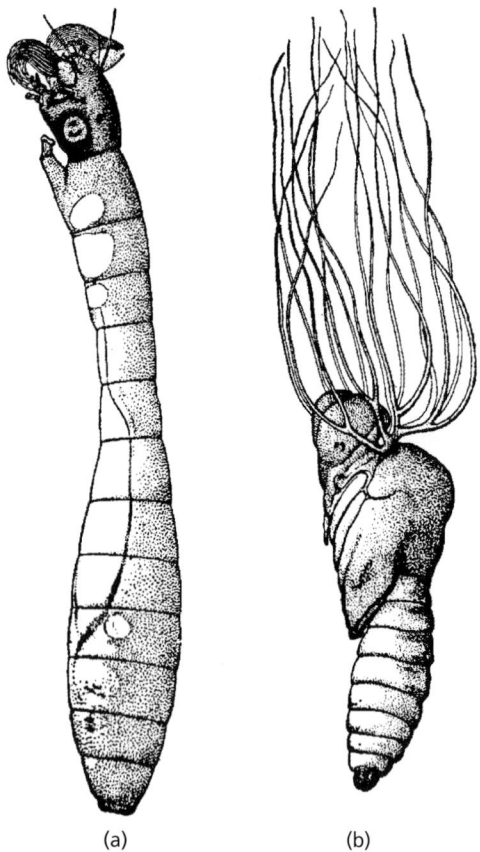

(a)   (b)

Fig. 3.18 Immature stages of Simuliidae: (a) larva; (b) pupa. (Castellani and Chalmers, 1910/Castellani.)

pads and drift downstream. Larval maturation takes from several weeks to several months, and in some species larvae can overwinter. Mature larvae pupate in a slipper-shaped brownish cocoon fixed to submerged objects. The pupa has prominent respiratory gills projecting from the cocoon. In the final stages of pupation, a film of air is secreted between the developing adult and the pupal cuticle. When the pupal case splits, the emerging adult rises to the surface in a bubble of air and is able to fly away immediately. The pupal period is normally 2–6 days and a characteristic feature of many species is that there is simultaneous mass emergence of the adult flies, which take flight from the surface of the water. The duration of the life cycle from egg to adult is variable, depending on the species and water temperature. Typical longevity for adult blackflies ranges from 2–3 weeks to as long as 85 days. Adult flies feed on plant nectar but in most species, females require a blood meal to obtain the protein necessary to mature their eggs.

For clinical information see Chapter 8.

FAMILY PSYCHODIDAE

The flies of this family are called 'sand flies', with *Phlebotomus* the main genus of veterinary importance in the Old World and *Lutzomyia* in the New World. Both genera are important as vectors of *Leishmania*. Since, in some areas of the world, the term 'sand flies' includes some biting midges and blackflies, a better term is 'phlebotomine sand flies'. They are blood-feeding flies that feed on a wide range of mammals, reptiles, birds and humans, and bite

areas of exposed skin such as the ears, eyelids, nose, feet and tail. They are widely distributed in the tropics, subtropics and the Mediterranean area. Most species prefer semi-arid and savannah regions to forests.

Phlebotomus and *Lutzomyia*

Description, adult: These small flies range from about 1.5 to 3 mm long and are characterised by their hairy appearance, large black eyes and long legs (Fig. 3.19). The wings, which unlike those of other biting flies are lanceolate in outline, are also covered in hairs and are held erect over the body at rest. As in many other nematoceran flies, the mouthparts are of short to medium length, hang downwards and are adapted for piercing and sucking. The maxillary palps are relatively conspicuous and consist of five segments. In both sexes the antennae are long, 16-segmented, filamentous and covered in fine setae.

The abdomen has 10 segments, with the terminal ones (last three in females and last four in males) forming the genital apparatus. In the female, the ninth segment is bifurcate and surrounds the genital opening while the tenth segment is small and hosts the anal opening. In the male, the seventh and eighth segments are invaginated in each other, while the ninth and tenth segments form the reproductive apparatus. The latter presents three pairs of appendages: the first pair comprises coxite and stilus (featuring five spines), the second includes the parameres, that envelop the two filamentous sheaths of the penis.

Description, larvae: The mature larva is greyish-white with a dark head. The head carries chewing mouthparts which are used to feed on decaying organic matter. The antennae are small. The abdominal segments bear hairs and ventral unsegmented leg-like structures

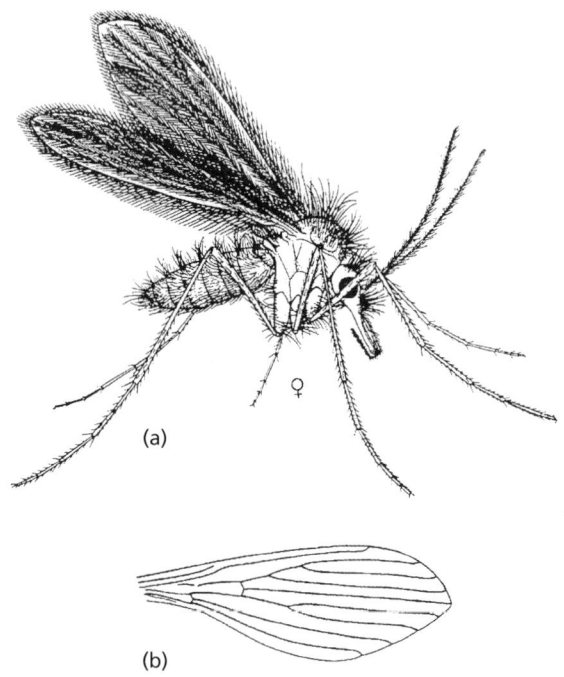

(a)

(b)

Fig. 3.19 (a) Adult female sand fly, *Phlebotomus papatasi*. (b) Wing venation typical of species of *Phlebotomus* (Psychodidae). (From Smart, 1943.)

(pseudopods), which are used in locomotion. A characteristic feature of phlebotomine larvae is the presence of long caudal setae, one pair in first-stage larvae and two pairs in second-, third- and fourth-stage larvae.

Life cycle: Up to 100 ovoid, 0.3–0.4 mm long, brown or black eggs may be laid at each oviposition in small cracks or holes in the ground, the floors of animal houses or in leaf litter. Although they are not laid in water, the eggs need moist conditions for survival, as do the larvae and pupae. A minimum temperature of 15 °C is required for egg development. Under optimal conditions, the eggs can hatch in 1–2 weeks but this may be prolonged in cold weather.

The larvae, which resemble small caterpillars, scavenge on organic matter and can survive flooding. There are four larval stages, maturation taking three weeks to several months, depending on species, temperature and food availability. In more temperate regions, these flies overwinter as mature larvae which are 4–6 mm in length, have a well-developed black head with eyespots, and a segmented greyish body, which is covered in bristles. The pupae attach themselves to the substrate in an erect position with the exuviae of the last larval instar attached at the caudal end. The adults emerge from pupation after 1–2 weeks. The whole life cycle takes 30–100 days, or even longer in cool weather. See **life cycle 41**.

For clinical information see Chapter 12.

LIFE CYCLE 41. LIFE CYCLE OF SAND FLIES (PHLEBOTOMINAE)

Sand flies are relatively small insects, with a sandy-coloured body covered with fine setae, large and black eyes and long legs (1). The female requires a blood meal from a vertebrate host for egg maturation to occur (2). At each oviposition, about 100 elongated, brownish-blackish eggs may be deposited (3). Preferential sites of oviposition are ravines and potholes, cracks and crevices where the terrestrial larvae have a stable temperatures and relative darkness, and feed on decomposing organic material (e.g. fungi, decomposing arthropods, animal faeces and decaying leaves). After hatching, the first-stage larvae (4) dig through the organic material; after four moults (within three weeks to some months according to species, temperature and nutrient availability), the fourth-stage larvae (5) reach 4–6 mm in length and become greyish in colour, segmented and covered in setae, and feature a prominent black head. The adults emerge from the pupae (6) after 1–2 weeks.

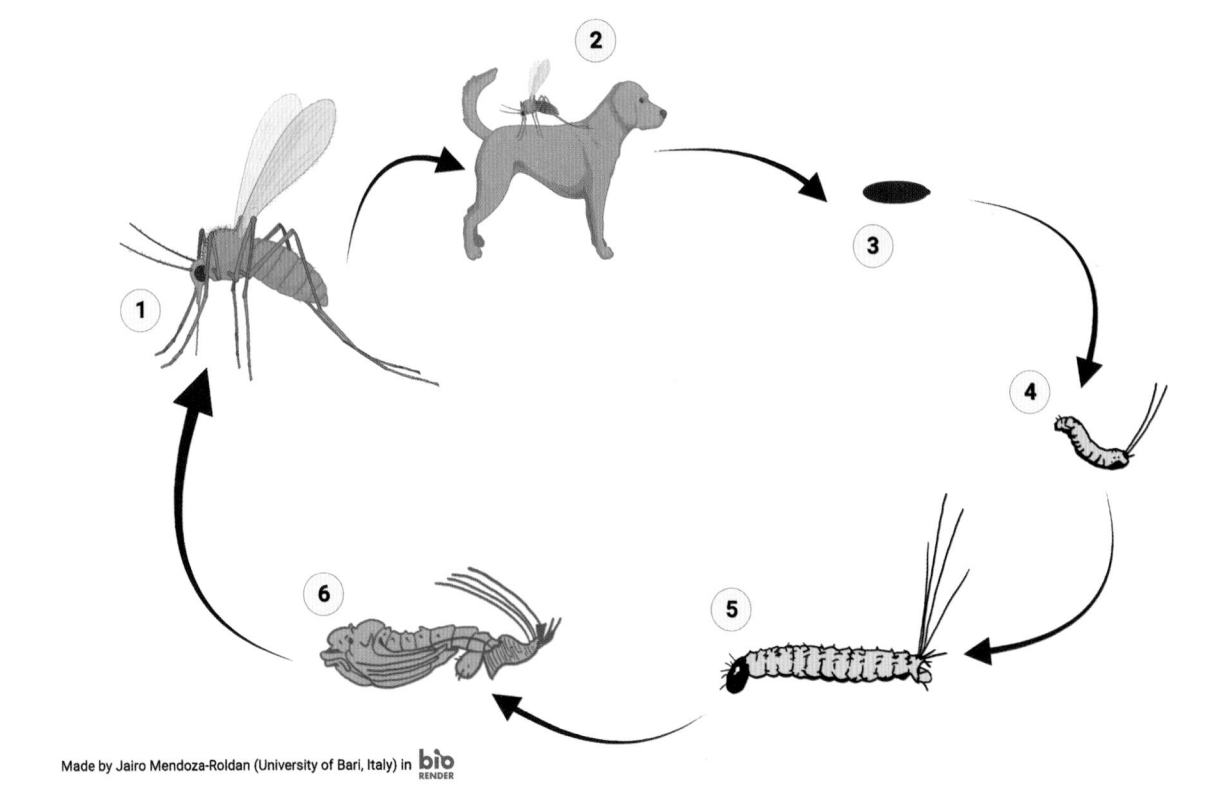

Made by Jairo Mendoza-Roldan (University of Bari, Italy) in bio RENDER

FAMILY CULICIDAE

The Culicidae are the mosquitoes, with over 3000 species described. They are small slender flies with long legs (Fig. 3.20). The main genera of importance are *Anopheles*, *Aedes* and *Culex*.

Their bites are a severe nuisance to humans and animals, commonly causing inflammatory skin reactions and mild allergic responses to their salivary secretions when they bite; while more severe allergic reactions have been reported, anaphylaxis is rare. They can also cause serious adverse impacts on animal herds attacked by extraordinary numbers of blood-seeking mosquitoes. However, the main medical and veterinary importance relies on their role as vectors of disease-causing pathogens; they are principally important as vectors of malaria (*Plasmodium* spp.), filarial nematodes and viruses. Transmission of the canine heartworm, *Dirofilaria immitis*, may be of particular significance, mainly in the tropics and subtropics, where it infests dogs, other canids and rarely cats. Some pathogens can be transmitted mechanically by mosquitoes, the principal disease example being the myxoma virus that is spread among rabbits primarily by mosquitoes in Australia (although in Europe the principal vector of myxomatosis is the flea *Spilopsyllus cuniculi*). Primarily because of their importance as vectors of human malaria, there is a vast literature on their classification, behaviour and control, but the family is of relatively limited veterinary significance. See **Life cycle 42**.

For clinical information see Chapter 12.

Description: Mosquitoes vary from 2 to 10 mm in length and the adults have slender bodies, prominent eyes and long legs (Fig. 3.20c). The long narrow wings are held crossed flat over the abdomen at rest and bear scales, which project as a fringe on the posterior margin. The mouthparts consist of a conspicuous, forward-projecting, elongated proboscis adapted for piercing and sucking. Individual elements comprise a long U-shaped, fleshy labium containing paired maxillae, mandibles and a hypopharynx, which carries a salivary duct that delivers anticoagulant into the host's tissues. The labrum forms the roof of the proboscis. All the elements, with the exception of the labium, enter the skin during feeding by the females, forming a tube through which blood is sucked. In the non-parasitic males, the maxillae and mandibles are reduced or absent. The maxillary palps of different species are variable in length and morphology. Both sexes have long, filamentous, segmented antennae, pilose in females and plumose in males.

Life cycle: The larvae of all species are aquatic and occur in a wide variety of habitats, ranging from extensive areas such as marshes to smaller areas such as the edge of permanent pools, marshes, puddles, flooded tree-holes and even, for some species, temporary water-filled containers. However, they are usually absent from large tracts of uninterrupted water, such as lakes, and from fast-flowing streams or rivers. Mosquito larvae are known as 'wrigglers' and require 3–20 days to develop through four stadia. Hatching is temperature dependent and occurs after several days or weeks, but in some temperate species eggs may overwinter. All four larval stages are aquatic. There is a distinct head with one pair of antennae, compound eyes and prominent mouth brushes, used in feeding on organic material (Fig. 3.20a). Maturation of larvae can extend from one week to several months, and several species overwinter as larvae in temperate areas.

With the final larval moult, the pupal stage occurs. Mosquito pupae (known as 'tumblers') usually remain at the water surface, but when disturbed can be highly mobile. All mosquito pupae are aquatic, motile and comma-shaped, with a distinct cephalothorax that bears a pair of respiratory trumpets (Fig. 3.20b). The tegument of the cephalothorax is transparent and the eyes, legs and other structures of the developing adult are readily visible. The tapering abdominal segments have short hairs, and terminally there is a pair of oval paddle-like extensions, which enable the pupa to move up and down in the water. Generally, the pupal stage is short, only a few days in the tropics and several weeks or longer in temperate regions. The adult emerges through a dorsal split in the pupal tegument. Adults usually only fly up to a few hundred metres from their

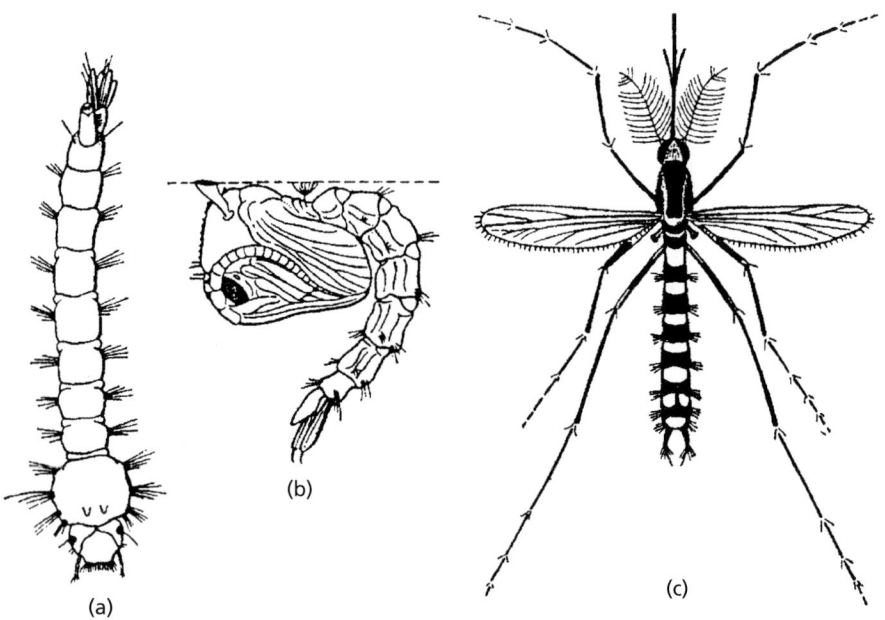

Fig. 3.20 *Aedes atropalpus*: (a) larva; (b) pupa; (c) adult. (From Eidmann and Kuhlhorn, 1970.)

LIFE CYCLE 42. LIFE CYCLE OF CULICIDAE

Mosquitoes have a narrow body, prominent eyes and long legs. The wings are long and covered in scales that, when in resting position, are flattened and crossed over the body. The genera *Anopheles* (1), *Aedes* (2) and *Culex* (3) are of greatest medical and veterinary importance from a global perspective. Females require a blood meal from a vertebrate host to mature eggs. The gravid female oviposits up to 300 eggs on water surfaces, either individually (*Anopheles*) (4) or in floating masses (*Culex*) (5). Conversely, *Aedes* females deposit individual eggs near temporary water pools (6). After hatching, which is determined by conditions of temperature and humidity, aquatic larvae emerge from the eggs. The larvae have a large head with antennae, compound eyes and prominent buccal brushes for prehension, and breathe through a pair of spiracles located on the second to last segment. *Anopheles* larvae (7) position themselves horizontally to the water surface, unlike those of *Aedes* and *Culex* (8) which position themselves obliquely or almost vertically. Pupae of all species are aquatic and characterised by a comma-shaped body, with separate cephalothorax featuring respiratory appendages (9). In tropical areas, the pupal stage is short-lived and adults emerge after only a few days, while in temperate areas, a few weeks are necessary for adults to emerge.

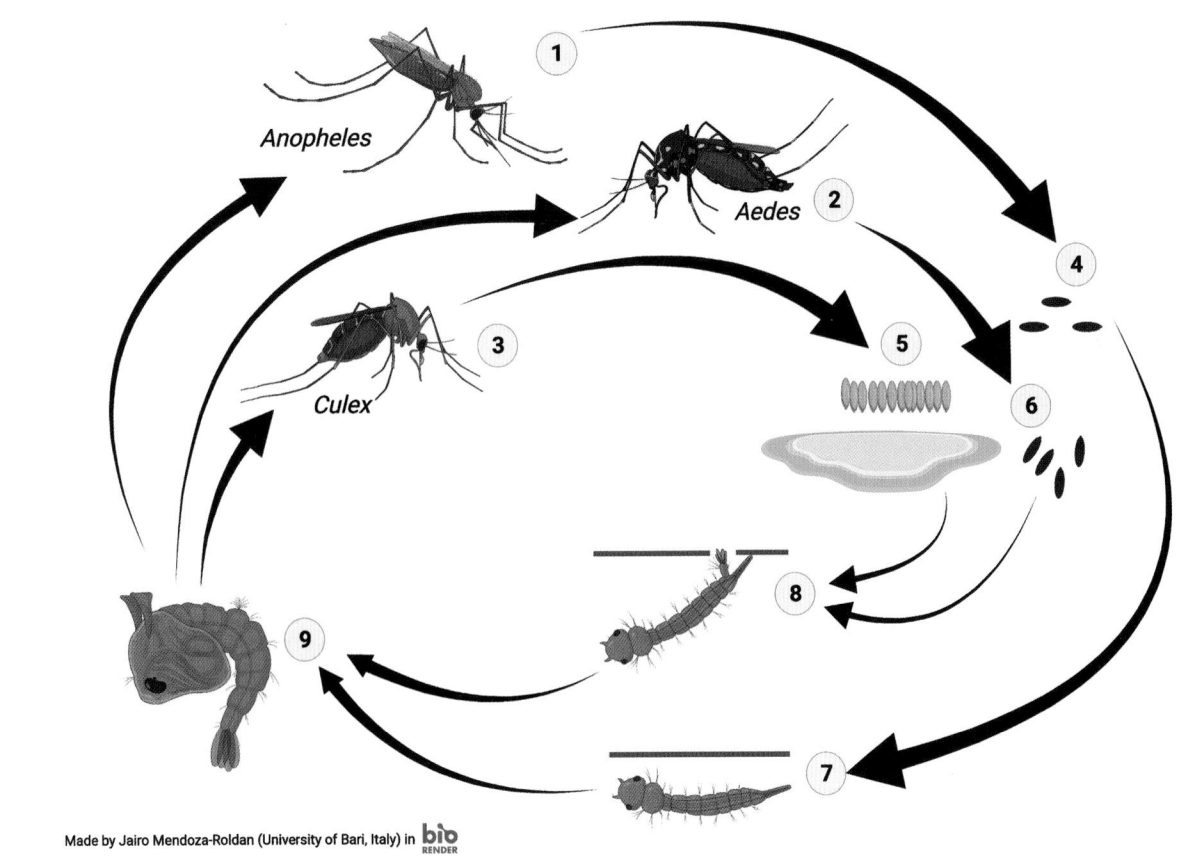

Made by Jairo Mendoza-Roldan (University of Bari, Italy) in **bⁱo** RENDER

breeding sites, but may be dispersed long distances by winds. Although the lifespan of adult flies is generally short, some species can overwinter by hibernating.

When adult mosquitoes emerge from the pupal case, they crawl to a nearby object, where they harden their cuticle and inflate their wings. Mating normally occurs within 24 hours of emergence and is completed in flight. One insemination is usually sufficient for the fertilisation of all eggs. For normal activity and flight, mosquitoes feed on nectar and plant juices, but females are anautogenous – they need an initial blood meal to develop their ovaries and must feed again between each egg batch matured. A female mosquito will live for an average of 2–3 weeks, while the male's lifespan is shorter.

Mosquitoes are nocturnal or crepuscular feeders with a wide host range. Host selection is extremely opportunistic and is largely influenced by the relative abundance of hosts found in the habitat. Host location is achieved using a range of olfactory and visual cues, orientation to wind direction and body warmth. Oviposition begins as soon as a suitable site is located. Adult mosquitoes are strong fliers.

SUBFAMILY CULICINAE

Aedes and *Culex*

Description: The culicine adult rests with its body angled and its abdomen directed towards the surface. The palps of female culicine mosquitoes are usually only about one-quarter the length of the proboscis.

Life cycle: After a blood meal, the gravid female lays up to 300 eggs singly on the surface of water. The eggs are dark coloured, either elongate or ovoid, and cannot survive desiccation. Most species of *Aedes* lay their eggs on moist substrates rather than on the water itself, where they mature and await adequate water to stimulate hatching. In some cases, the eggs may remain viable for up to three years. Despite some degree of temperature tolerance, freezing and high temperatures (in excess of 40 °C) will kill most eggs.

In species of the genus *Culex*, eggs are laid in groups forming 'egg-rafts'. A female *Culex* mosquito may lay a raft of eggs every third night during its lifetime, hence oviposition typically occurs around six or seven times. When the eggs mature, they will hatch into larvae regardless of the availability of water. Hatching is temperature dependent and occurs after several days to weeks, but in some temperate species eggs may overwinter.

All four larval stages are aquatic and the larvae take in air through a pair of spiracles situated at the end the respiratory siphon.

SUBFAMILY ANOPHELINAE

Anopheles spp.

Description: Living anopheline adults can readily be distinguished from culicines, such as *Aedes* and *Culex*, when resting on a flat surface. On landing, anopheline mosquitoes rest with the proboscis, head, thorax and abdomen in one straight line at an angle to the surface. The palps of female anopheline mosquitoes are as long and straight as the proboscis. The abdomen of *Anopheles* bears hairs but not scales.

Life cycle: The eggs are dark-coloured and boat-shaped and possess characteristic lateral floats that prevent them from sinking and maintain their orientation in the water. Such eggs usually hatch within 2–3 days and cannot survive desiccation. Most larvae of *Anopheles* lie parallel to the water surface and take in air through a pair of spiracles on the penultimate abdominal segment.

SUBORDER BRACHYCERA

The Brachycera ("brachy" = "short", "cera" = "antenna") is the second major suborder of the Diptera. Their most distinguishing characteristics in the adult are reduced antennal segmentation with fewer than eight flagellum segments and two or fewer palpal segments. The suborder is extremely diverse. Brachycera contains four infraorders: Stratiomyomorpha, Xylophagomorpha, Tabanomorpha and Muscomorpha. The last two contain species of veterinary importance.

Within the Tabanomorpha, the Tabanidae is one of the largest families of Diptera, containing an estimated 8000 species divided into about 30 genera, only three of which are of major veterinary importance: *Tabanus* (horse flies), *Haematopota* and *Chrysops* (deer flies). Species of the genus *Tabanus* are found worldwide; the *Haematopota* are largely Palaearctic, Afro-tropical and Oriental in distribution; species of the genus *Chrysops* are largely Holarctic and Oriental.

Within the Muscomorpha, the subsection Calyptratae includes the flies of veterinary interest. The Calyptratae includes flies which possess a calypter (squamae) that covers the halteres and includes three superfamilies: **Muscoidea**, **Hippoboscoidea** and **Oestroidea**. The Muscoidea and Hippoboscoidea each contain two families of veterinary interest, the **Muscidae** and **Fanniidae** and the **Hippoboscidae** and **Glossinidae**, respectively. The superfamily Oestroidea contains three families of veterinary interest, **Oestridae**, **Calliphoridae** and **Sarcophagidae**, species of which are primarily associated with **myiasis**, the infestation of the tissues of a living host with fly larvae.

The appearance of the adult flies *Musca domestica*, *Stomoxys calcitrans* and *Haematobia* (*Lyperosia*) spp. is shown in Fig. 3.21.

Adult flies that feed on blood, sweat, skin secretions, tears, saliva, urine or faeces of domestic animals may do this either by puncturing the skin directly, in which case they are known as biting flies, or by scavenging at the surface of the skin, wounds or body orifices, in which case they may be classified as non-biting or nuisance flies. These flies may act as biological and mechanical vectors for a range of disease pathogens. Mechanical transmission may be exacerbated by the fact that some fly species inflict extremely painful bites and are therefore frequently disturbed by the host while blood feeding. As a result, the flies are forced to move from host to host over a short period, thereby increasing their potential for mechanical disease transmission.

There are two basic functional types of mouthparts seen in adult biting or nuisance flies of veterinary interest. Sponging mouthparts are used for feeding on liquid films. Such mouthparts are found in groups such as the house flies, blowflies and face flies. Biting mouthparts are

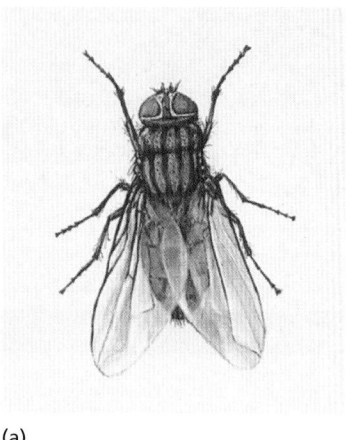
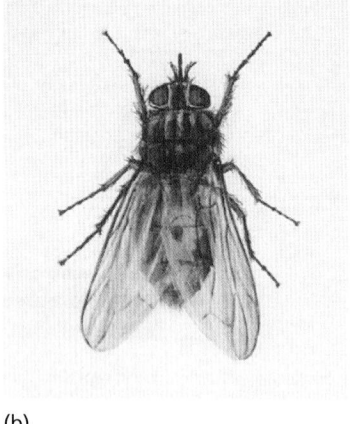
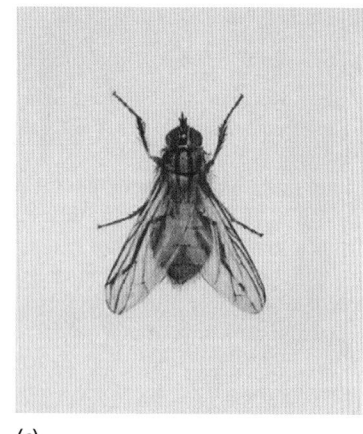

(a)   (b)   (c)

Fig. 3.21 Adult flies: (a) *Musca domestica*; (b) *Stomoxys calcitrans*; (c) *Haematobia* (*Lyperosia*) spp.

used for puncturing the skin and drinking blood. They occur in groups such as the stable flies, horn flies and tsetse flies.

In the sponging-type mouthparts, as seen in the house fly, the proboscis is an elongate feeding tube, composed of a basal **rostrum** bearing the maxillary palps, a median flexible **haustellum**, composed of the labium and flap-like labrum, and apical **labella** (Fig. 3.22). Mandibles and maxillae are absent. The labrum and hypopharynx lie within the flexible anterior gutter in the labium. The labella are sponging organs, the inner surface of which is lined by grooves called **pseudotracheae**. The grooves lead towards the **oral aperture**, known as the **prestomum**. When feeding, the labella are expanded by blood pressure and opened to expose their inner surface. They are then applied to the liquid film. Liquid flows into and along the grooves by capillary action and then is drawn up the food canal by muscular pumping action. At rest, the inner surfaces of the labella are in close contact and kept moist by secretions from the labial salivary glands.

The house fly proboscis is jointed and can be withdrawn into the head capsule when not in use by retraction of the rostrum. There are a number of minute teeth surrounding the prestomum, which can be used directly to rasp at the food. These teeth may be well developed and important in the feeding of various species of Muscidae, for example *Hydrotaea irritans*. The ancestral Diptera probably had sponging mouthparts as described, without mandibles and maxillae. However, a number of species, such as stable flies and tsetse flies, have evolved a blood-sucking capability and show modifications of the basic house fly mouthparts that reflect this behaviour.

In blood-feeding Muscidae, the labella have been reduced in size and the pseudotracheae have been replaced by sharp teeth. The labium has been lengthened and surrounds the labrum and hypopharynx (Fig. 3.23). The rostrum is reduced and the rigid haustellum cannot be retracted. In feeding, the teeth of the labella cut into the skin. The entire labium and the labrum–hypopharynx, forming the food canal, are inserted into the wound. Saliva passes down a duct in the hypopharynx and blood is sucked up the food canal. Variations on this general pattern range from the robust mouthparts of stable flies to the delicate mouthparts of tsetse flies.

The larvae have a poorly defined head, and are mobile and worm-like, often being referred to as 'maggots' (Fig. 3.24).

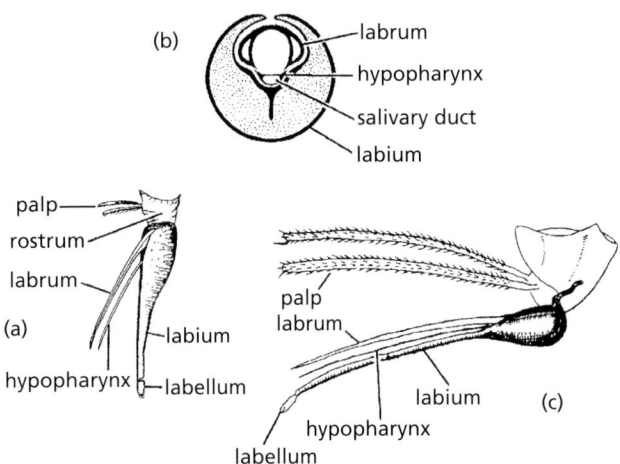

Fig. 3.23 Mouthparts of a stable fly in (a) lateral view and (b) cross-section. (c) Proboscis and palps of a tsetse fly. (From Newstead *et al.*, 1924.)

The mature larva moults to become a pupa, on or in the ground, within a hard pupal case formed from the last larval integument, which is not shed and which is known as a puparium. The pupa is usually immobile.

FAMILY TABANIDAE

Species of Tabanidae are often known as horse flies, deer flies or clegs. These are large flies with stout antennae often consisting of only three segments, the last segment frequently bearing annulations (Fig. 3.25). The maxillary palps are usually held forwards and cross-veins are present on the wings. The females use their slashing/

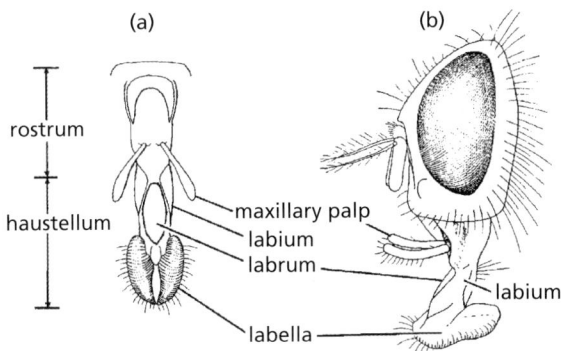

Fig. 3.22 The head and mouthparts of an adult house fly in (a) anterior and (b) lateral views. The mandibles and maxillae have been lost, the labrum reduced and the labial palps expanded to form two large fleshy labella. The labella are covered by a series of fine grooves, called pseudotracheae, along which liquid flows to the oral aperture by capillary action. The labium is flexible and the mouthparts can be retracted into the head. (Adapted from Snodgrass, 1935.)

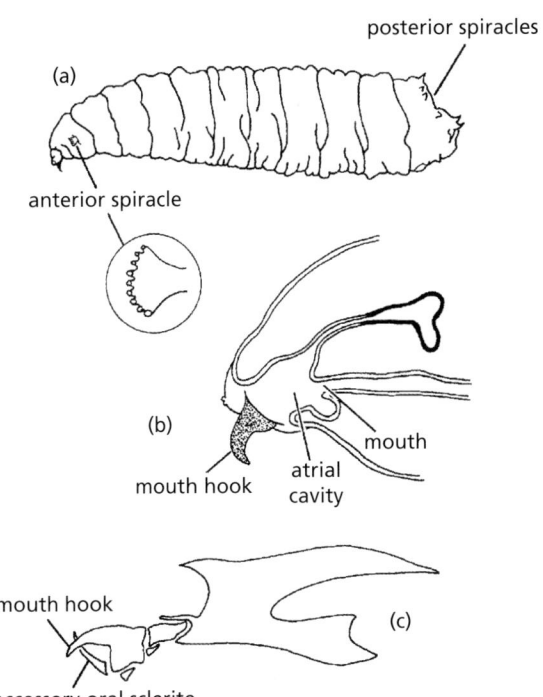

Fig. 3.24 Structure of a fly larva. (a) Lateral view with detail of anterior spiracle. (Adapted from Hall and Smith, 1993). (b) Transverse section through the head and mouthparts. (c) Cephalopharyngeal skeleton.

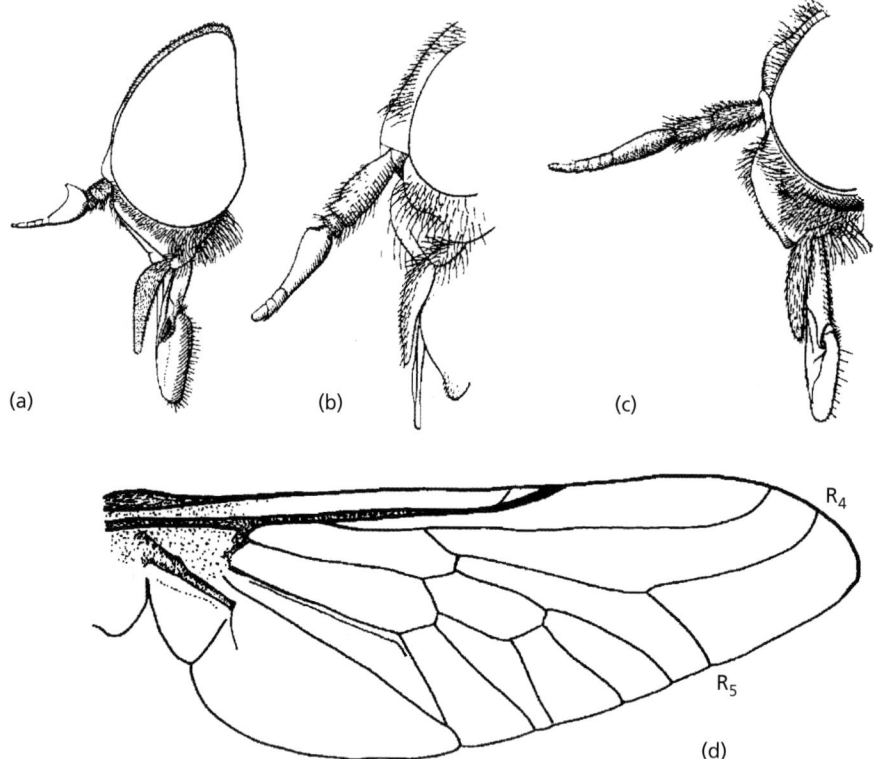

(a)   (b)   (c)

(d)

Fig. 3.25 Antennae of (a) *Tabanus*, (b) *Haematopota* and (c) *Chrysops*. (d) Wing venation of Tabanidae. (From Smart, 1943.)

sponging mouthparts to pierce the skin of their host and then feed on the pool of blood created. The pain caused by their bites leads to interrupted feeding and as a consequence, flies may feed on a succession of hosts and are therefore important in the mechanical transmission of pathogens such as trypanosomes.

The eggs are laid on vegetation overhanging mud or shallow water, and hatch into large carnivorous larvae with ill-defined but usually retractile heads. Like the Nematocera, both larvae and pupae are mobile and aquatic, and are usually found in mud. These powerful flies may disperse many kilometres from their breeding areas and are most active during hot sunny days.

For clinical information see Chapter 10.

Tabanus, Chrysops and Haematopota

Description, adult: These are medium to large biting flies, up to 25 mm in length, with wingspans of up to 65 mm. The head is large and the proboscis prominent. They are generally dark-coloured, but may have various stripes or patches of colour on the abdomen or thorax and even the large eyes, which are dichoptic in the female and holoptic in the male, may be coloured. The coloration of the wings and the short, stout, three-segmented antennae, which have no arista, is useful in differentiating the three major genera of Tabanidae (Fig. 3.25).

The mouthparts, which are adapted for slashing/sponging, are short and strong and always point downwards (Fig. 3.26). Most prominent is the stout labium, which is grooved dorsally to incorporate the other mouthparts, collectively termed the biting fascicle. The labium is also expanded terminally as paired large labella, which carry tubes called pseudotracheae, through which blood or

fluid from wounds is aspirated. The biting fascicle, which creates the wound, consists of six elements: the upper sharp labrum, the hypopharynx with its salivary duct, paired rasp-like maxillae and paired broad-pointed mandibles. Male flies have no mandibles and therefore cannot feed on blood. They instead feed on honeydew and the juice of flowers.

Description, larvae: Larvae are spindle-shaped and off-white in colour and clearly segmented. The cuticle has distinct longitudinal striations. Mature larvae may be 15–30 mm in length. There is a distinct head capsule and strong biting mandibles. Abdominal segments have unsegmented leg-like structures (pseudopods) for locomotion (four pairs in *Tabanus* and three pairs in *Chrysops*). A distinct posterior respiratory siphon is usually present, which may be greatly elongated.

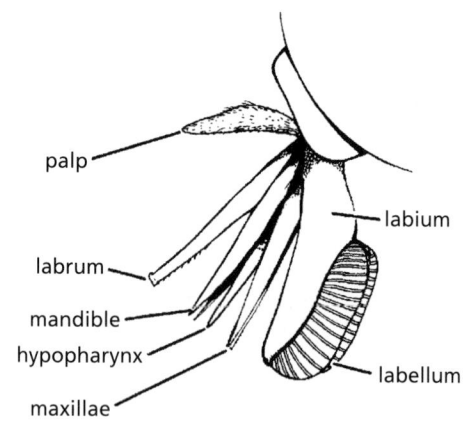

Fig. 3.26 Slashing and sponging mouthparts of a female tabanid fly.

Life cycle: After a blood meal, the female lays batches of 100–1000 creamy white or greyish cigar-shaped eggs, 1–2.5 mm long, on the underside of vegetation or on stones, generally in muddy or marshy areas. The eggs hatch in 1–2 weeks, using a special spine to exit the egg case, and the cylindrical, poorly differentiated larvae drop into the mud or water. The larvae are 1–6 mm in length and have 11 segments. They are recognised as tabanids by their small black retractable heads and the prominent raised rings around the segments, most of which bear pseudopods. They also have a structure in the last segment, unique to tabanid larvae, known as Graber's organ, the function of which may be sensory. They are sluggish and feed either by scavenging on decaying organic matter or by predation on small arthropods, including other tabanid larvae. Optimally, larval development takes three months but, if overwintering occurs, may extend for up to three years.

The subcylindrical pupa is brown, the abdominal segments are movable and the anterior part of the appendages of the adult can be distinguished. Mature larvae pupate while partially buried in mud or soil and the adult fly emerges after 1–3 weeks. In most species, males complete their pupation before females. After emergence, the male pursues the female and mating, initiated in the air, is completed on the ground. Adults are strong fliers and are usually diurnal. The whole life cycle takes a minimum of 4–5 months, or longer if larval development is prolonged.

Populations of adult flies show seasonal fluctuations in both temperate and tropical areas. In temperate climates, adults die in the autumn and are replaced by new populations the following spring and summer, whereas in tropical areas their numbers are merely reduced during the dry season with an increase at the start of the rainy season.

Although the female flies feed mostly on blood from their hosts, if a suitable host is unavailable they will consume honeydew and plant sap (the major food source of males which lack mandibles). They typically bite a number of times in different places before they are replete and the wounds created continue to bleed and may attract other flies. Adults feed approximately every three hours during the day and between feeding rest on the underside of leaves or on stones or trees.

Tabanus (horse flies)

Species of the genus *Tabanus* have transparent wings. Also useful in generic differentiation are the characteristics of the short, stout, three-segmented antennae, which have no arista. The first two antennal segments are small and the terminal segment has a tooth-like projection on its basal part and four annulations (Fig. 3.25a).

Chrysops (horse flies, deer flies)

Chrysops have dark banded wings, which are divergent when at rest. The wing venation is characteristic, especially the branching of the fourth longitudinal vein (Fig. 3.25d).

Haematopota (horse flies, clegs)

Haematopota have characteristically mottled wings that are held divergent when at rest. The first antennal segment is large and the second segment narrower, while the terminal segment has three annulations (Fig. 3.25b).

FAMILY MUSCIDAE

This family comprises many biting and non-biting genera, the latter commonly referred to as Nuisance flies. As a group, they may be responsible for 'fly worry' in livestock and a number of species are vectors of important bacterial, helminth and protozoal diseases of animals. The major genera of veterinary importance include *Musca* (house flies and related flies), *Stomoxys* (stable fly), *Haematobia* (horn flies, buffalo flies) and *Hydrotaea* (sweat and head flies).

Musca

The genus *Musca* contains about 60 species, of which the house fly, *Musca domestica*, and the face fly, *Musca autumnalis*, are of particular importance. *Musca sorbens*, the bazaar fly, is widespread throughout Africa and Asia, and *Musca vetustissima*, the bush fly, is an important pest in Australia. Adults are non-metallic, dull black, grey or brown flies (Fig. 3.27a). The detailed wing venation is of taxonomic importance in the differentiation of *Musca* from similar flies belonging to other genera such as *Fannia*, *Morellia* and *Muscina* and in the identification of different *Musca* species. In flies of this genus, the wing vein M is deflected forward at a strong bend and ends at the wing edge near to the end of wing vein R_{4+5}, with the distance between the two ends not more than the length of cross vein r-m (Fig. 3.27b).

For clinical information see Chapter 8.

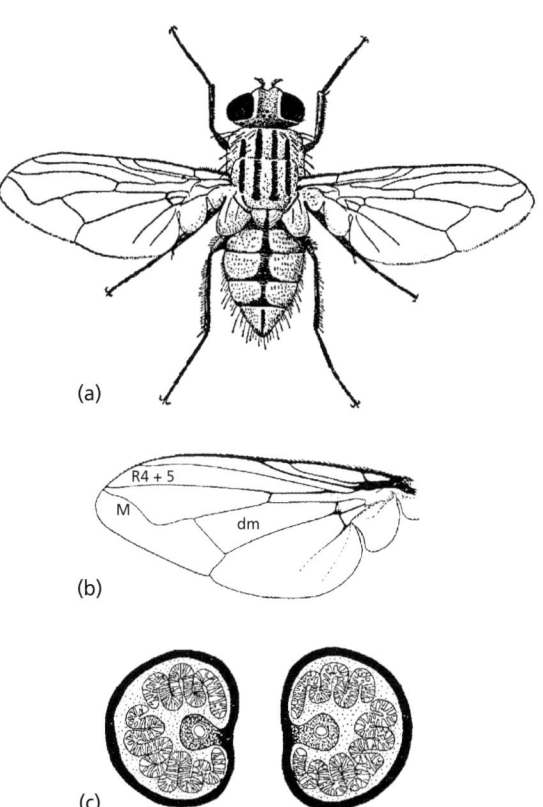

(a)

(b)

(c)

Fig. 3.27 (a) Female house fly, *Musca domestica*. (b) Wing venation typical of species of *Musca*, showing the strongly bent vein M ending close to R_{4+5}. (c) Posterior spiracles of a third-stage larva. (Adapted from Smart, 1943.)

Musca domestica (house fly)

Description: Female adults of *Musca domestica* are 6–8 mm in length, male adults are 5–6 mm, and they vary in colour from light to dark grey. The thorax is usually grey with four dark longitudinal stripes, and there is a sharp upward bend in the fourth longitudinal wing vein (Fig. 3.27a). The abdomen has a yellow-brown background colour with a black median longitudinal stripe. The eyes are reddish and the space between them can be used to determine the sex of a specimen, since in females it is almost twice as broad as in males. The aristae are bilaterally plumose at the tip.

Life cycle: Female flies lay batches of up to 150 creamy white, banana-shaped eggs, approximately 1 mm long, in wet faeces or rotting organic material. The dorsal surface of the eggs has two curved, rib-like thickenings. Batches of eggs are laid at 3–4-day intervals throughout life. The eggs hatch (under optimal temperatures) in 12–24 hours to produce whitish coloured, segmented, cylindrical larvae with a pair of small anterior mouth hooks. High manure moisture favours their survival. At the posterior end of the larvae there are paired respiratory spiracles, the shape and structure of which allow generic and specific differentiation (Fig. 3.27c). The three larval stages feed on decomposing organic material and mature to 10–15 mm in length in 3–7 days under suitable conditions. Optimal temperatures for larval development are 30–37 °C, although as the larvae mature, their temperature tolerance increases. Mature larvae then move to drier areas around the larval habitat and pupate, forming a rigid and dark-brown barrel-shaped puparium or 'pupal case'. The adult fly emerges after 3–26 days, depending on temperature. Mating and oviposition take place a few days after emergence. Total development time from egg to adult fly may be as little as eight days at 35 °C, but is extended at lower temperatures. In temperate areas, a small proportion of pupae or larvae may survive the winter but more frequently, the flies overwinter as hibernating adults.

Musca autumnalis (face fly)

Musca autumnalis feeds on secretions from the eyes, nose and mouth of cattle, as well as on wounds left by biting flies. The species is widely distributed throughout Europe, central Asia and parts of Africa and, since its introduction in the 1950s, can now be found throughout North America.

Description: *Musca autumnalis* is very similar to *M. domestica* in size and appearance, although the abdomen of the female is darker, while in the male tergites 2 and 3 are typically yellowish-orange along the sides. Female adults of *Musca autumnalis* are 6–8 mm in length, male adults 5–6 mm, and they vary in colour from light to dark grey. The thorax is usually grey with four dark longitudinal stripes, and there is a sharp upward bend in the fourth longitudinal wing vein. The abdomen is a yellowish-brown background colour with a black median longitudinal stripe. The eyes are reddish and the space between them can be used to determine the sex of a specimen, since in females it is almost twice as broad as in males. The aristae are bilaterally plumose at the tip. The eggs of *M. autumnalis* bear a terminal respiratory horn.

Life cycle: this fly congregates in large numbers around the faces of cattle. It feeds on secretions from the eyes, nose and mouth as well as blood from wounds left by other flies, such as tabanids. It lays its eggs just beneath the surface of fresh cattle manure within about 15 minutes of the dung pats being deposited. The eggs of *M. autumnalis* are about 3 mm in length and possess a short respiratory stalk. They are arranged so that the respiratory stalk of each egg projects above the surface of the pat. Like *M. domestica*, the larvae pass throughout three stages within approximately one week, before entering the surrounding soil and pupariating to form a whitish-coloured puparium. Summer generations require about two weeks to complete a life cycle. This allows several generations in any one season. Face flies prefer bright sunshine and usually do not follow cattle into barns or heavy shade. Adults are strong fliers and can move between widely separated herds. Face flies overwinter as adults, in response to short photoperiods, aggregating in overwintering sites such as farm buildings.

Musca sorbens and Musca vetustissma

Musca sorbens and *M. vetustissma* are nuisance flies that may be responsible for the mechanical transmission of a variety of important pathogens and parasites.

Description: Adult flies have two broad longitudinal stripes on the thorax and the first abdominal segment is black. Adult flies are grey in colour with two stripes on the dorsal thorax; wing vein M_{1+2} bent forwards at an angle and reaching R_{4+5}.

Musca crassirostris

Musca crassirostris is not an obligatory parasite, but can feed on a wide variety of animal secretions and is especially attracted to wounds. Adult flies may use the prestomal teeth to rasp the skin and draw blood, which is then ingested. This species may act as a mechanical vector for a wide variety of viral and bacterial diseases and protozoan and metazoan parasites.

Description: Adult flies are about 5.5–7.5 mm in length and vary in colour from light to dark grey. There are four distinct dark longitudinal stripes on the thorax and the greyish abdomen has various light and dark markings.

Life cycle: *Musca crassirostris* is not an obligatory parasite, but can feed on a wide variety of animal secretions and is especially attracted to wounds. Female flies lay batches of up to 100 eggs in faeces or rotting organic material. Eggs hatch to produce whitish, segmented, cylindrical larvae (maggots). The three larval stages feed on decomposing organic material and mature within 3–7 days under suitable conditions. These then move to drier areas around the larval habitat and pupate. The adult fly emerges after 3–26 days, depending on temperature.

Stomoxys

This genus contains about 18 species, of which the most common is *Stomoxys calictrans*. *Stomoxys niger* and *S. sitiens* may replace *S. calcitrans* as important pests in Afro-tropical regions and parts of Asia. Although they can be localised pests, they are not of great significance as vectors of disease. Nonetheless, their bites are painful and they pester dogs and can have a huge economic impact on the health and productivity of cattle, being one of the most widespread and economically important pests to attack cattle.

Life cycle: Both male and female flies feed on blood. The female lays batches of 25–50 eggs, resembling those of house flies, in manure and moist decaying vegetable matter, such as hay and straw contaminated with urine. The eggs are yellowish-white with a longitudinal groove on one side, and measure approximately 1 mm in length. Eggs hatch in 1–4 days, or longer in cold weather, and the larvae develop in 6–30 days. Pupation occurs in the drier parts of the breeding material and takes 6–9 days or longer in cold weather. Optimal conditions for pupariation involve complete darkness and a temperature of about 27 °C. The puparia are brown and about 6 mm in length. The complete life cycle from egg to adult fly may take 12–60 days depending mainly on temperature.

After emergence, the adult females require several blood meals before the ovaries mature and egg laying can start (usually after about nine days). If deprived of a blood meal in the first few days after emergence, ovarian development is delayed and females produce fewer, smaller eggs. In temperate areas, flies may overwinter as larvae or pupae, whereas in tropical climates breeding is continuous throughout the year.

Stable flies may double their body weight during feeding. After a blood meal, flies move to a resting site on structures such as barn walls, fences or trees.

Stomoxys calcitrans (stable fly)

Description, adult: Superficially, *Stomoxys calcitrans* resembles the house fly *M. domestica*, being similar in size (about 7–8 mm in length) and grey with four longitudinal dark stripes on the thorax. Its abdomen, however, is shorter and broader than that of *M. domestica*, with three dark spots on the second and third abdominal segments. The wing vein M_{1+2} curves gently forwards and the R_{cell} is open, ending at or behind the apex of the wing. Probably the simplest method of distinguishing stable flies from *M. domestica* and other genera of non-biting muscid flies is by examination of the proboscis, which in *Stomoxys* is conspicuous and forward projecting (Fig. 3.28a). Stable flies can be distinguished from biting muscid flies of the genus *Haematobia* by the larger size and much shorter palps of the former.

Description, larvae: Larvae of *Stomoxys* can be identified by examination of the posterior spiracles, which are relatively well separated; each has three S-shaped slits.

Haematobia

Grey-black blood-sucking flies which resemble the stable fly in appearance. There are two common species in temperate areas: the horn fly, *Haematobia irritans* (syn. *Lyperosia irritans*), found in Europe and the USA, and *H. stimulans* in Europe only. *Haematobia exigua* (buffalo fly) occurs in Asia, China and Australia, and *H. minuta* in Africa. The genus *Lyperosia* is synonymous. They can have a huge economic impact on the health and productivity of cattle, and are one of the most widespread and economically important pests of cattle.

Life cycle: In contrast to other muscids, these flies generally remain on their hosts, leaving only to fly to another host or, in the case of females, to lay eggs in freshly passed faeces. Eggs are laid in groups of 4–6, usually in the fresh faeces or in the soil immediately beneath it. These hatch quickly if the humidity is sufficiently high; larvae may mature in as little as four days given adequate moisture and temperatures of around 27 °C. Low temperatures and dry conditions delay larval development and kill the eggs. The pupal period is around 6–8 days and on emergence, the adult flies seek and remain on their cattle hosts. Horn flies overwinter as pupae in the soil below cowpats, emerging as adults the following spring.

Haematobia irritans (horn fly)

Subspecies: *Haematobia irritans irritans, Haematobia irritans exigua*

Synonym: *Lyperosia irritans*

This small blood-feeding fly often feeds at the base of the horns, back, shoulders and belly, primarily on cattle. It also occasionally attacks horses, sheep and dogs. It is found worldwide, particularly in Europe, the USA and Australia.

Description, adult: The adults are 3–4 mm in length and are usually grey, often with several dark stripes on the thorax. They are the smallest of the blood-sucking muscids. Unlike *Musca*, the proboscis is held forwards and unlike *Stomoxys*, the palps are stout and as long as the proboscis (Fig. 3.28c). In *Haematobia irritans*, the palps are dark greyish. Eggs are 1–1.5 mm long and are laid in fresh faeces.

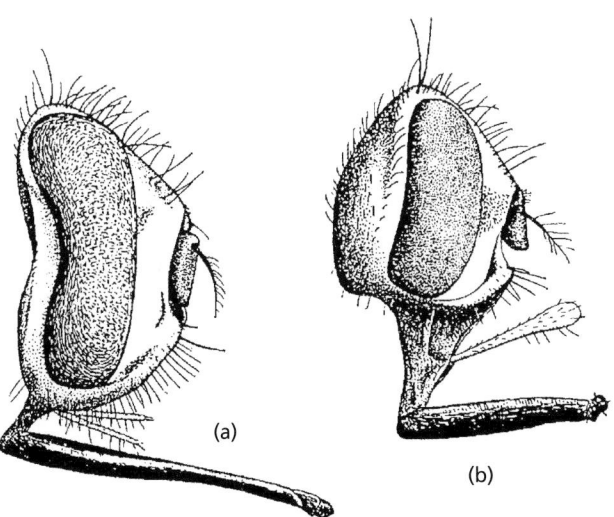

(a)

(b)

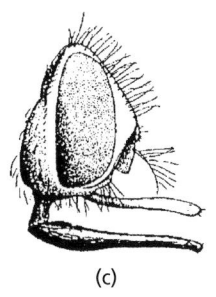

(c)

Fig. 3.28 Lateral views of the heads of blood-sucking Muscidae: (a) *Stomoxys calcitrans*; (b) *Haematobia stimulans*; (c) *Haematobia irritans*. (Edwards *et al.*, 1939/Smithsonian Libraries.)

Description, larvae: The cylindrical larvae are yellow-white and generally about 7 mm long with two D-shaped posterior spiracles. Puparia are dull reddish-brown and 3–4 mm long.

Haematobia minuta

Synonym: *Lyperosia minuta*

This blood feeding fly is found on cattle and buffalo in Africa. It is usually found on the withers, back and sides and occasionally the belly in hot weather.

Description: The adults are up to 4 mm in length. They are usually grey, often with several dark stripes on the thorax.

Haematobia stimulans

Synonym: *Haematobosca irritans*

This blood-feeding fly feeds primarily on cattle and is largely found in Europe.

Description adult: Slightly smaller than *Stomoxys calcitrans* at about 6 mm in length. They are usually grey, often with several dark stripes on the thorax. In *H. stimulans*, the palps are yellow in colour, whereas in *H. irritans* they are dark grey (Fig. 3.28b). The eggs are reddish-brown and lack a terminal horn.

Description, larvae: The larvae are cylindrical and yellow-white in colour. They measure approximately 7 mm in length and have two D-shaped posterior spiracles. Puparia are dull reddish-brown and 3–4 mm long.

Hydrotaea

The sweat or head flies closely resemble *Musca*. The genus contains one important species, *Hydrotaea irritans*, the sheep head fly.

Life cycle: Adult flies prefer still conditions and are found near woodlands and plantations, with peak numbers occurring in midsummer. Eggs are laid in decaying vegetation or faeces; they hatch and develop into mature larvae by the autumn. Each female produces one or two batches of about 30 eggs in its lifetime. Third-stage larvae may be predatory on other larvae. These larvae then go into diapause (a temporary cessation of development) until the following spring when pupation and development are completed, with emergence of a new generation of adults in early summer. Hence, there is only one generation of head flies each year, with peak numbers occurring in midsummer.

Hydrotaea irritans (sheep head fly)

Hydrotaea irritans is widespread throughout northern Europe, but not believed to be present in North America. They feed on the tears, saliva, sweat and wounds of cattle, sheep and horses.

Description: *Hydrotaea irritans* is generally similar in size and appearance to the various species of *Musca*, with adults measuring 4–7 mm in length. It is characterised by an olive-green abdomen and an orange-yellow coloration at the base of the wings. The thorax is black with grey patches.

FAMILY FANNIIDAE

The family contains about 250 species, of which species of the genus *Fannia* are of importance as nuisance pests of livestock.

Fannia

Species of *Fannia* generally resemble house flies in appearance but are more slender and smaller at about 4–6 mm in length. The fourth longitudinal vein is straight (not bent as in the house fly) (Fig. 3.29a).

Life cycle: *Fannia* breed in a wide range of decomposing organic material, particularly the excrement of chickens, humans, horses and cows. The life cycle is typical, with three larval stages followed (Fig. 3.29b) by the pupa and adult. The complete life cycle requires 15–30 days.

Fannia canicularis

Description: *Fannia canicularis* is greyish to almost black in colour, possessing three dark longitudinal stripes on the dorsal thorax. The palps are black. The aristae are bare.

Fannia scalaris

Description: As for *F. canicularis* except the halteres are yellow.

Fannia benjamini

Description: As for *F. canicularis* except the palps are yellow. *Fannia benjamini* may represent a complex of a number of closely related species.

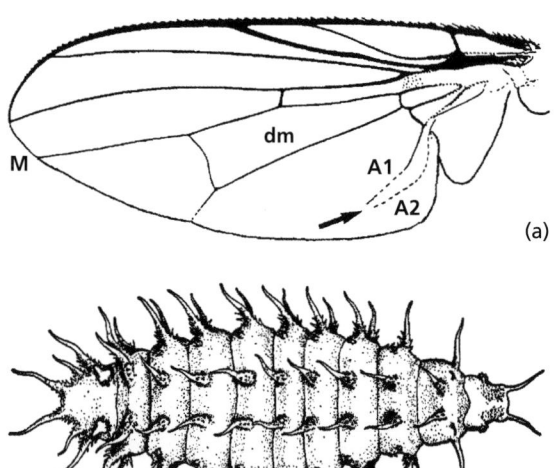

Fig. 3.29 (a) Wing venation typical of species of *Fannia* showing the characteristic convergence of the anal veins. (b) Third-stage larva of the lesser house fly *Fannia canicularis*. (Zumpt, 1965/Butterworths.)

FAMILY HIPPOBOSCIDAE

The Hipposcidae (keds and forest flies) are unusual in being flattened dorsoventrally and having an indistinctly segmented abdomen, which is generally soft and leathery. They have piercing blood-sucking mouthparts, are parasitic on mammals and birds and have strong claws on the feet, which allow them to cling to hair or feathers. There are about 200 species in the family and they tend to be either permanent ectoparasites or remain on their hosts for long periods. The four major genera of veterinary importance are *Hippobosca*, *Melophagus*, *Lipoptena* and *Pseudolynchia*. The hipposcids have relatively robust legs, consisting of an enlarged femur, a flattened tibia and short compact tarsi with one or more basal teeth. Species that parasitise mammals can be distinguished from those that parasitise birds by their shorter and stouter legs and heavier tarsal claws. These species are primarily a nuisance and a cause of disturbance, but they may be mechanical vectors of pathogens.

For clinical information see Chapter 9.

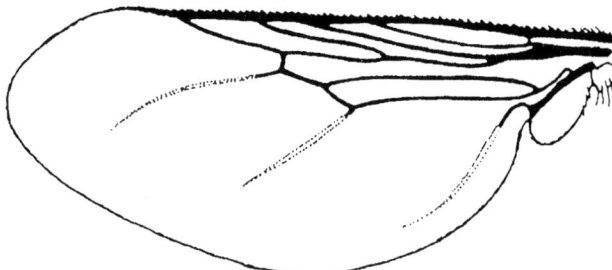

Fig. 3.30 Wing venation typical of species of *Hippobosca* showing the characteristic crowding of the veins into the leading half of the wings. (Zumpt, 1965/Butterworths.)

five or six larvae in its lifetime. These larvae pupate almost immediately. When pupation is completed, the newly emerged winged adults locate a suitable host animal on which they blood feed, remaining on the host for long periods. In temperate areas, flies are most abundant in the summer months.

Hippobosca

Several species of this genus are common parasites of cattle and horses in many parts of the world, where their biting and blood feeding may be extremely damaging (Table 3.1). The flies are about 1 cm long and have a reddish-brown colour. There are two wings, the veins of which are crowded together towards the anterior border.

Hippobosca equina (forest fly, louse fly)

Hippobosca equina feeds primarily on horses but also cattle, although will bite a range of wild and domestic animal hosts; it is found in in Europe and parts of Asia and Africa.

Description: Adult flies are approximately 10 mm in length and are generally pale reddish-brown with yellow spots on the indistinctly segmented abdomen. They have one pair of wings, the veins of which are crowded together towards the anterior margin (Fig. 3.30). The major part of the piercing proboscis is usually retracted under the head, except during feeding. Forest flies remain on their hosts for long periods and their preferred feeding sites are the perineum and between the hindlegs. Both sexes of adult are blood feeders. The larvae are rarely seen and measure about 5 mm in length.

Life cycle: Gravid female flies leave their hosts and deposit mature larvae singly in dry soil or humus. Each female can produce only

Hippobosca camelina

Hippobosca camelina feeds primarily on camels in Europe and parts of Asia and Africa but they can also feed on goats, sheep, cattle, wild animals and humans. It is a vector of a range of pathogens including African trypanosomes and *Anaplasma*.

Description: Adult flies are approximately 10 mm in length and are generally pale reddish-brown with yellow spots on the indistinctly segmented abdomen. They have one pair of wings, the veins of which are crowded together towards the anterior margin. Both sexes of adult are blood feeders.

Life cycle: Gravid female flies mature a single larva within the oviduct. When fully developed, the mature third-stage larva is larviposited on the host. These larvae drop to the ground and pupate almost immediately When pupation is completed, the newly emerged winged adults locate a suitable host animal on which they blood feed, remaining on the host for long periods. Each female produces only five or six larvae in its lifetime.

Other species of *Hippobosca* of importance are listed in Table 3.2.

Melophagus

Members of the genus *Melophagus* are wingless biting flies, of which *Melophagus ovinus* (the sheep ked) is the most important species.

Table 3.1 *Hippobosca* species of veterinary importance.

Species	Common name	Hosts
Hippobosca equina	Forest fly, horse louse fly	Mainly horses and cattle, but other domestic animals and birds may be attacked
Hippobosca camelina	Camel fly	Camels
Hippobosca maculata	Horse and cattle louse fly	Mainly horses and cattle
Hippobosca variegata	Horse louse fly	Horses and cattle
Hippobosca rufipes	Cattle louse fly	Cattle
Hippobosca longipennis	Dog fly	Dogs and wild carnivores

Table 3.2 Other *Hippobosca* species of importance.

Species	Common name	Hosts	Geographical distribution
Hippobosca maculata	Horse and cattle louse fly	Mainly horses and cattle	Tropics and subtropics, particularly India and Africa
Hippobosca variegata	Horse louse fly	Horses and cattle	Tropical Africa
Hippobosca rufipes	Cattle louse fly	Cattle	Africa
Hippobosca longipennis	Dog fly	Dogs and wild carnivores	East and North Africa; parts of the Mediterranean region

Melophagus ovinus (sheep ked)

Life cycle: Keds are permanent ectoparasites and live for several months feeding on the blood of sheep and sometimes goats. A single egg is ovulated at a time. The egg hatches inside the body of the female and the larva is retained and nourished within the female during its three larval stages, until it is fully developed. The mature larvae produced by the females adhere to the wool. These are immobile and pupate immediately, the 3–4 mm long, brown pupae easily visible on the fleece. The pupae are fully formed within 12 hours of larviposition and are resistant to treatment. Adult keds emerge in approximately three weeks in summer, but this period may be extended considerably during winter. Copulation occurs 3–4 days after emergence from the pupa, and females are able to produce offspring 14 days after emergence. Although one mating provides sufficient sperm for a lifetime, repeated matings usually occur when multiple males are present. A female produces between 10 and 20 larvae in its lifetime. Ked populations build up slowly since each female produces only one larva every 10–12 days, up to a total of 15. Adults can only live for short periods off their hosts.

Description: Hairy, brown, wingless 'degenerate' fly, approximately 5–8 mm long with a short head and broad, dorsoventrally flattened, brownish thorax and abdomen (Fig. 3.31). The abdomen is indistinctly segmented and is generally soft and leathery. Both sexes are completely wingless and even the halteres are absent. They have piercing blood-sucking mouthparts and strong legs provided with claws that enable them to cling on to wool and hair.

Lipoptena

The deer keds, *Lipoptena cervi* in Europe and Asia and *Lipoptena depressa* in North America, are common parasites of deer. Adults are winged on emergence but shed their wings on finding a suitable

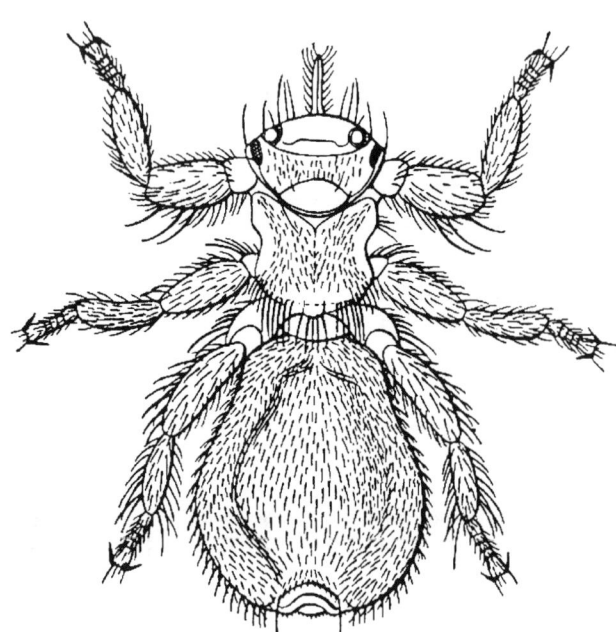

Fig. 3.31 The sheep ked, *Melophagus ovinus*.

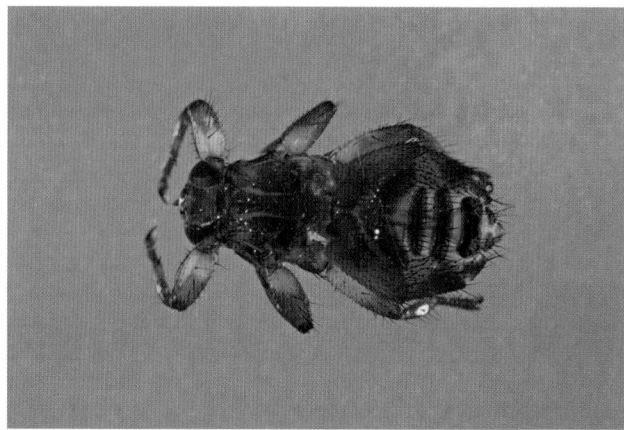

Fig. 3.32 Deer ked, *Lipoptena cervi* (note that the wings have been shed).

host (Fig. 3.32). The wingless adults can be differentiated from *Melophagus* by the presence of halteres.

Life cycle: Like all hippoboscids, adult female flies larviposit single, fully developed third-stage larvae while on the host. Pupae fall to the ground. Following pupation, the newly emerged adult must find a suitable host, feed and mate. Both sexes are blood feeders.

Pseudolynchia

A genus of louse flies, which are parasites of birds.

Life cycle: Gravid female flies mature larvae singly. Each female can produce only five or six larvae in its lifetime. These larvae pupate almost immediately after larviposition. When pupation is completed, the newly emerged winged adults locate a suitable host animal on which they blood feed, remaining on the host for long periods. In temperate areas, flies are most abundant in the summer months.

Pseudolynchia canariensis

Pseudolynchia canariensis is the pigeon louse fly, found on pigeons, doves and other birds.

Description: Adult flies are approximately 10 mm in length and are generally pale reddish-brown with yellow spots on the indistinctly segmented abdomen. They have one pair of wings, the veins of which are crowded together towards the anterior margin. Both sexes of adult are blood feeders.

FAMILY GLOSSINIDAE

The sole genus in the family Glossinidae is *Glossina*, species of which are known as tsetse flies. They are confined to a belt of tropical Africa extending from the southern Sahara in the north (latitude 5° N) to Zimbabwe and Mozambique in the south (latitude 20–30° S). Both sexes feed exclusively on the blood of vertebrates and are of importance as vectors of trypanosomiasis in animals and humans.

The 23 known species and eight subspecies of tsetse can be divided into three groups, each with different habits and requirements. The *Glossina palpalis* group are riverine species that feed primarily on reptiles and ungulates. Flies of the *G. morsitans* group are savannah and dry thorn-bush species and feed mainly on large animals. Members of the *G. fusca* group occur in the rainforest, preferring dense shade and riverine thickets. Key species in the *fusca* and *palpalis* groups include *G. palpalis*, *G. austeni*, *G. fuscipes* and *G. tachinoides*, while key species in the *morsitans* group include *G. morsitans* and *G. palidipes*.

For clinical information see Chapter 8.

Glossina spp. (tsetse flies)

Description: In general, adult tsetse are narrow-bodied, yellow to dark-brown flies, 6–15 mm in length, and have a long, rigid, forward-projecting proboscis (Fig. 3.33a). When at rest, the wings are held over the abdomen like a closed pair of scissors. The thorax is a dull greenish-brown colour and is marked with inconspicuous stripes and spots. The abdomen is brown, with six segments that are visible form the dorsal aspect (Fig. 3.33a). Tsetse flies are easily distinguished from all other flies by the characteristic hatchet-shaped medial cell in the wings (Fig. 3.33b). The antenna has a large third segment, with an arista that bears 17–29 dorsal branching hairs.

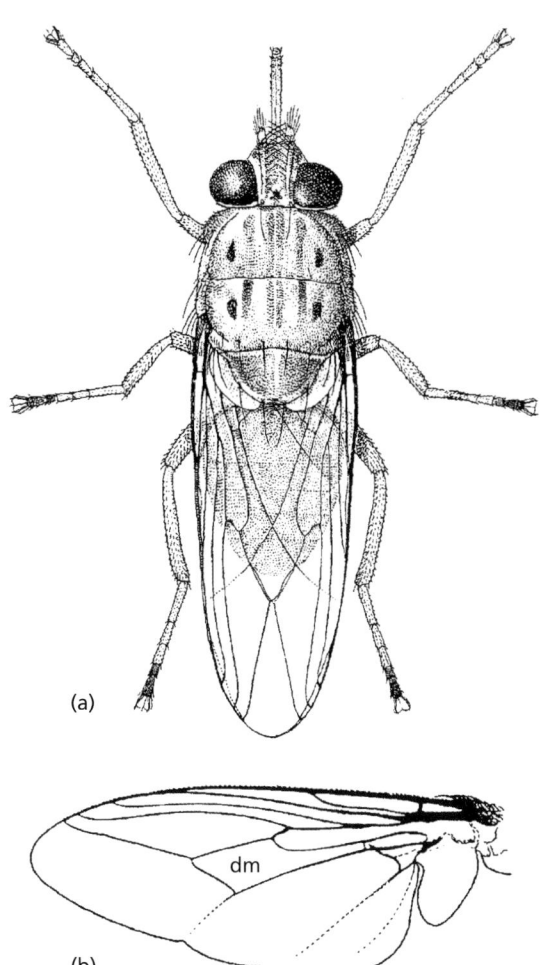

(a)

(b)

Fig. 3.33 (a) Male tsetse fly, *Glossina longipennis*. (b) Wing venation typical of species of *Glossina* showing the characteristic hatchet shape of the cell dm. (Zumpt, 1965/Butterworths.)

There are no maxillae or mandibles in the mouthparts of tsetse flies and the long proboscis is adapted for piercing and sucking. The proboscis is composed of a lower U-shaped labium with rasp-like labella terminally and an upper, narrower labrum, which together create a food channel. Within this food channel sits the slender hypopharynx that carries saliva and anticoagulant down into the wound formed during feeding. The proboscis is held horizontally between long palps, which are of an even thickness throughout.

Life cycle: Both male and female flies suck blood and although the various species of tsetse may have some host preferences, generally they will feed on a wide variety of animals.

The females, in contrast to other muscids, are viviparous. They ovulate a single egg at a time. The fertilised egg is retained in the oviduct, where it hatches after about four days at 25 °C. The larva is retained in the common oviduct (uterus) where it is nourished with secretions from the highly specialised accessory glands. Maturation in the uterus from fertilised egg to the mobile, 8–10 mm long, third-stage larva takes approximately 10 days. At this stage the larva is creamy white, segmented and posteriorly has a pair of prominent dark ear-shaped protuberances known as polypneustic lobes. During the development of the third-stage larva, these lobes protrude from the posterior abdomen of the adult female and have a respiratory function similar to the posterior spiracles of other muscid larvae.

When mature, the larva is deposited on the ground by the adult female, usually into characteristic areas of bare sandy soil under shade. After deposition, the larva wriggles into loose soil to a depth of a few centimetres and forms a rigid, dark-brown, barrel-shaped puparium within 1–2 hours. The pupal period is relatively long, taking 4–5 weeks, or even more in cool weather. On emergence, the adult is unable to fly until its wings have expanded. It takes at least a week for the complete endocuticle to be secreted and for the exocuticle to harden fully. The female fly may require several blood meals over a period of 16–20 days before producing her first larva. Once fully active, the adult flies feed every 2–3 days and the first larviposition occurs 9–12 days after emergence.

Breeding generally continues throughout the year, with peak fly numbers occurring at the end of the rainy season. The longevity of adult flies in nature is variable, ranging from a few days to several months.

Glossina fusca group

Description: Males are characterised by free superior claspers, without a membrane between them. Females have five genital plates, one dorsal pair, one anal pair and a single median sternal plate.

Glossina palpalis group

Description: The superior claspers in the males are connected by a thin membrane deeply divided medially. Females have six genital plates, one dorsal pair, one anal pair, one single median sternal plate and a small mediodorsal plate.

Glossina morsitans group

Description: The superior claspers in the male are completely joined by a membrane and are fused distally. In the female, there is a pair of fused anal plates and a median sternal plate, but the dorsal plates are usually absent.

FAMILY CALLIPHORIDAE

The Calliphoridae, known as blowflies, are a large family, composed of over 1000 species divided between 150 genera. At least 80 species have been recorded as causing traumatic myiasis (infestation of the tissues of a living vertebrate host by fly larvae). The fly larvae feed directly on the host's necrotic or living tissue. The hosts are usually mammals, occasionally birds and, less commonly, amphibians or reptiles.

Myiasis species are found largely in five important genera: *Cochliomyia*, *Chrysomya*, *Cordylobia*, *Lucilia* and *Calliphora* (Fig. 3.34). The genera *Protophormia* and *Phormia* also each contain a single species of importance. Most of these species are either primary or secondary facultative invaders. The screwworms, *Chrysomya bezziana* and *Cochliomyia hominivorax*, and the flies of

the genus *Cordylobia* (*Cordylobia anthropophaga* and *C. rodhaini*) are the only calliphorid species that are obligate agents of myiasis.

Members of this family are medium to large flies, almost all of which have a metallic blue or green sheen. The larvae are usually clearly segmented, pointed anteriorly and truncated posteriorly. However, this shape may be modified, with the larvae of some species being barrel-like or, occasionally, flattened. The cuticle is typically pale and soft, but is often covered by spines or scales arranged in circular bands. Although legless, in some species the body may have a number of fleshy protuberances, which aid in locomotion. The true head is completely invaginated into the thorax. The functional mouth is at the inner end of the preoral cavity, from which a pair of darkened mouth hooks protrudes. The mouth hooks are part of a complex structure known as the cephalopharyngeal skeleton, to which muscles are attached. There is a pair of anterior

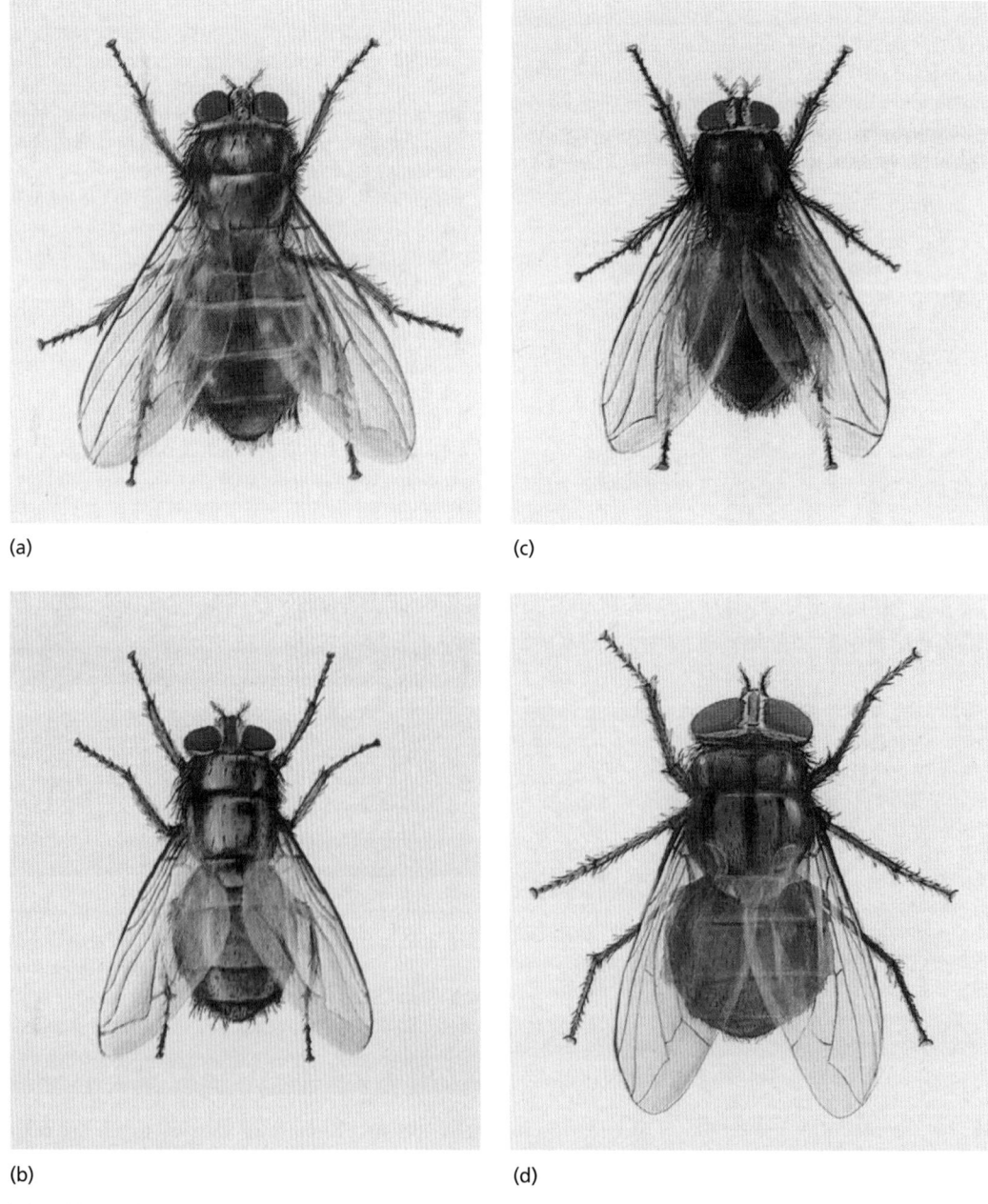

(a)

(b)

(c)

(d)

Fig. 3.34 Adult flies: (a) *Calliphora* spp.; (b) *Lucilia* spp.; (c) *Phormia* spp.; (d) *Cochliomyia* spp.

spiracles on the prothoracic segment, immediately behind the head, and a pair of posterior spiracles on the 12th segment. The structure of the posterior spiracles is of great taxonomic importance. They usually consist of a pair of sclerotised spiracular plates with slits or pores in the surface for gaseous exchange.

Life cycle: A small number of species are obligate agents of myiasis, i.e. they require a living host for larval development. Adult females deposit approximately 200 eggs at a time on the host and the larvae hatch after 12–24 hours, moult once after 12–18 hours and a second time about 30 hours later. They feed for 3–4 days and then move to the soil to pupate for seven days to several weeks depending on temperature. However, the vast majority of species are facultative agents of myiasis. In the latter case, adult flies oviposit primarily in carrion, but may also act as secondary invaders of myiases on live mammals. The life cycle is identical to the obligate species, with three larval stages and the final larval stage migrating from the feeding site prior to pupation.

For clinical information relating to screwworms, see Chapter 8 and for blowflies, Chapter 9.

Cochliomyia hominivorax

Synonym: *Callitroga hominivorax*

Commonly known as the New World screwworm, *Cochliomyia hominivorax* is a primary obligate agent of myiasis most commonly affecting cattle but may also infest pigs and horses and where predisposed, any mammal may be infested, including humans. It occurs primarily in tropical areas of southern and central America and the Caribbean islands. Its range formerly extended north into Mexico and the southern states of North America, from where it has now been eradicated.

Description, adult: The adult fly has a deep greenish-blue metallic colour with a yellow, orange or reddish face and three dark stripes on the dorsal surface of its thorax.

Description, larvae: The mature larvae measure 15 mm in length and have bands of spines around the body segments. The tracheal trunks leading from the posterior spiracles have a dark pigmentation extending forwards as far as the ninth or tenth segment (Fig. 3.35). This pigmentation is most conspicuous in fresh specimens.

Life cycle: *Cochliomyia hominivorax* is an obligate parasite and cannot complete its life cycle on carrion. Female flies oviposit at the edge of wounds or in body orifices, in clusters of 150–300 eggs. Shearing, castration or dehorning wounds are common oviposition sites, as are the navels of newly born calves. Even wounds the size of a tick bite are reported to be sufficient to attract oviposition. The flies lay batches of this size every 2–3 days during adult life, which is on average 7–10 days in length. The larvae hatch in 10–12 hours and penetrate into the tissues, which they liquefy, and extend the lesion considerably. The wound may begin to emit a foul-smelling liquid, attracting other female *C. hominivorax* and secondary agents of myiasis. The larvae become mature in 5–7 days, after which they leave the host to pupate in the ground. The pupal period lasts for between three days and several weeks, depending on temperature. There is no true diapause stage and *C. hominivorax* cannot survive over winter in cool temperate habitats. The entire life cycle may be completed in 24 days in optimum conditions.

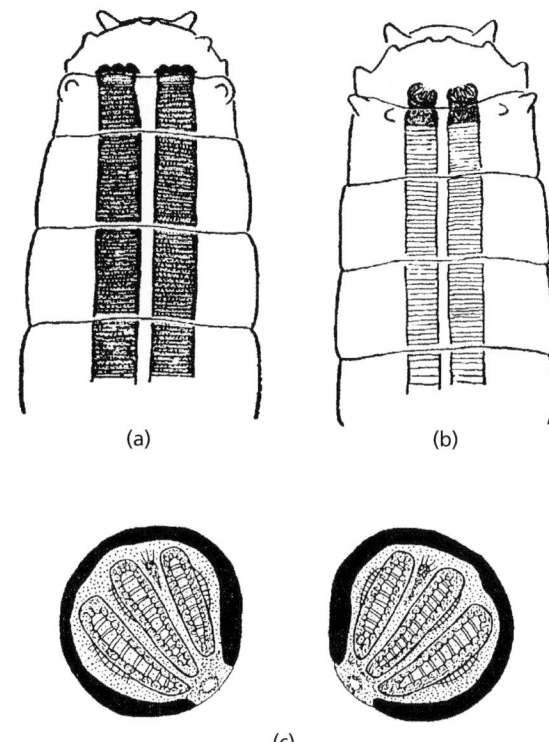

(a)   (b)

(c)

Fig. 3.35 (a) Pigmented dorsal tracheal trunks of larvae of *Cochliomyia hominivorax*. (b) Unpigmented dorsal tracheal trunks and (c) Posterior spiracles of *Cochliomyia macellaria*. (Zumpt, 1965/Butterworths.)

Cochliomyia macellaria

Synonym: *Callitroga macellaria*

Known as the secondary screwworm, this species commonly affects cattle but may also infect a range of other mammals, including humans. It is found throughout the Neotropical and Nearctic regions, from Canada to Argentina, but is more abundant in tropical parts of its range.

Description, adult: These blue-green flies have longitudinal stripes on the thorax and orange-brown eyes. Adults are extremely similar in appearance to *C. hominivorax*, but possess a number of white spots on the last segment of the abdomen.

Description, larvae: The larvae may be distinguished from those of *C. hominivorax* by the absence of pigmented tracheal trunks leading from small posterior spiracles (Fig. 3.35).

Life cycle: *Cochliomyia macellaria* is a ubiquitous carrion breeder. However, it can act as a secondary invader of myiasis.

Chrysomya bezziana

Commonly known as the Old World screwworm, this primary obligate agent of myiasis infests a range of mammals including cattle, sheep, dogs and occasionally humans. It occurs primarily in tropical areas: Africa and southern Asia including India, the Arabian Peninsula, Southeast Asia, the Indonesian and Philippine islands, and New Guinea.

Description, adult: These stout blue-green flies have four longitudinal black stripes on the prescutum, orange-brown eyes and a pale coloured face. They have dark legs and white thoracic squamae. The anterior spiracle is dark orange or black-brown. The adult flies measure 8–10 mm in length.

Description, larvae: The first-stage larvae are creamy white and measure about 1.5 mm in length. The second- and third-stage larvae are 4–9 mm and 18 mm in length, respectively, and are similar in appearance, each segment carrying a broad encircling belt of strongly developed spines (Fig. 3.36).

Life cycle: *Chrysomya bezziana* is an obligate agent of myiasis. Gravid females are attracted to fresh open wounds and body orifices on any warm-blooded animal. Even small wounds resulting from thorn scratches and tick bites may be sufficient to attract oviposition. *Chrysomya bezziana* commonly infests the umbilicus of newborn calves. The female lays batches of 100–300 eggs on the dry perimeter around the wound. Each female produces several batches of eggs in her lifetime of about nine days. The eggs hatch within 10–20 hours at 37 °C and first-stage larvae begin to feed in the open wound or moist tissue, often penetrating deep into the host tissue.

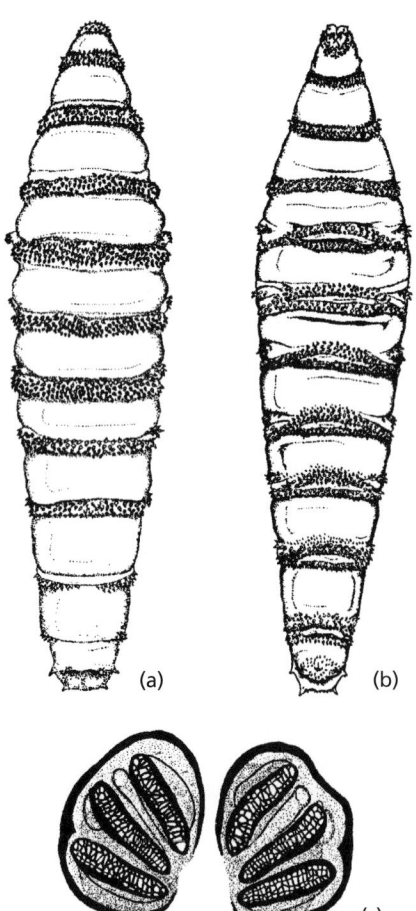

Fig. 3.36 Third-stage larva of *Chrysomya bezziana*: (a) dorsal view; (b) ventral view; (c) posterior peritremes. (Zumpt, 1965/Butterworths.)

Chrysomya megacephala

Chrysomya megacephala, known as the Oriental latrine fly, oviposits primarily in carrion but may also act as a secondary agent of myiases on live mammals. It occurs in the Australasian and Oriental regions. However, this species has been introduced inadvertently into the New World and entered Brazil around 1975. Since then, it has dispersed rapidly to reach Central and North America.

Description, adult: Adults are medium-sized, stout, blue-green flies with longitudinal stripes on the thorax and orange-brown eyes. *Chrysomya megacephala* can be distinguished from *Lucilia* by the broad bands on its rounder abdomen and by its black forelegs (Fig. 3.37). The face is pale coloured. The anterior spiracle of the thorax of adults is dark coloured.

Description, larvae: The larvae are about 18 mm in length. They have hooked mouthparts and bands of small spines on each segment. There are 4–6 projections on the anterior spiracle with fleshy projections on the last segment only.

Life cycle: Females lay batches of up to 250–300 eggs on carcasses, faeces and other decomposing matter. The entire egg-to-adult life cycle takes about eight days at 30 °C. *Chrysomya megacephala* is commonly called the Oriental latrine fly because of its habit of breeding in faeces as well as on carrion and other decomposing organic matter. It may occur in large numbers around latrines and may also become a nuisance in slaughterhouses, confined animal facilities and open-air meat and fish markets.

Chrysomya rufifacies

Chrysomya rufifacies, knows as the hairy maggot blowfly, is a secondary agent of myiasis. It is an Australasian and Oriental species of tropical origin. This species and *C. albiceps* were inadvertently introduced into the Neotropical region in the 1970s and 1980s where, at a dispersal rate estimated at 1.8–3.2 km/day, they have quickly spread and become established throughout much of North and South America.

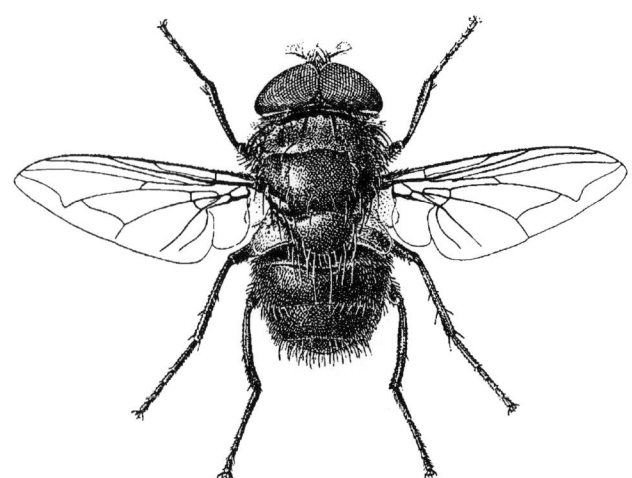

Fig. 3.37 Adult male of *Chrysomya megacephala*. (From Shtakelbergh, 1956.)

Description, adult: These bluish-green flies have longitudinal stripes on the thorax and orange-brown eyes. The hind margins of the abdominal segments have blackish bands and the anterior spiracle is white or pale yellow.

Description, larvae: The larvae bear a number of thorn-like fleshy projections on most of the body segments, which give these species their common name of 'hairy maggot blowflies'. These projections become longer on the dorsal and lateral parts of the body. The larvae of *Chrysomya rufifacies* may be distinguished from those of *C. albiceps* by the presence of small spines on the stalks of the projections (Fig. 3.38).

Life cycle: Flies oviposit primarily in carrion, but may also act as secondary invaders of myiases on live mammals. The larvae of this species will actively feed on other larvae in carcasses.

Chrysomya albiceps

A carrion-breeding blowfly, similar to *Chrysomya rufifacies*, that may occur as a secondary agent of myiasis. Originally found in Africa, southern Europe, the Mediterranean and Asia, it has now spread to Central and South America.

Description, adult: These bluish-green flies have longitudinal stripes on the thorax and orange-brown eyes. The hind margins of the abdominal segments have blackish bands and the anterior spiracle is white or pale yellow.

Description, larvae: The larvae are similar to those of *C. rufifacies* but can be distinguished by the absence of small spines on the stalks of the projections.

Life cycle: Flies oviposit primarily in carrion, but may also act as secondary invaders of myiases on live mammals. This species thrives in warm humid conditions, at temperatures above 17 °C but below 38 °C.

Cordylobia anthropophaga

Cordylobia anthropophaga, known as the tumbu, mango or putzi fly, is an obligate agent of myiasis of mammals (including humans) common in East and Central Africa. It is thought that the primary hosts of *C. anthropophaga* are rodents and that the flies have become secondarily adapted to parasitise many other animal species, including humans. Dogs are particularly important clinical hosts.

Description, adult: The adult fly is stout, yellow-brown and 8–12 mm in length. It has a yellow face and legs and two black marks on the thorax. Adult flies feed on decaying fruits, carrion and faeces and have large, fully developed mouthparts. The arista of the antenna has setae on both sides. The thoracic squamae are without setae and the stem vein of the wing is without bristles.

Description, larvae: Third-stage larvae are 12–28 mm in length and are densely, but incompletely, covered with small, backwardly directed, single-toothed spines. The posterior spiracles have three slightly sinuous slits and a weakly sclerotised peritreme (Fig. 3.39).

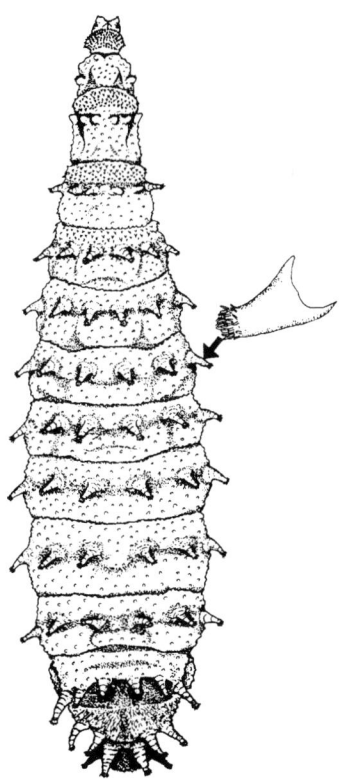

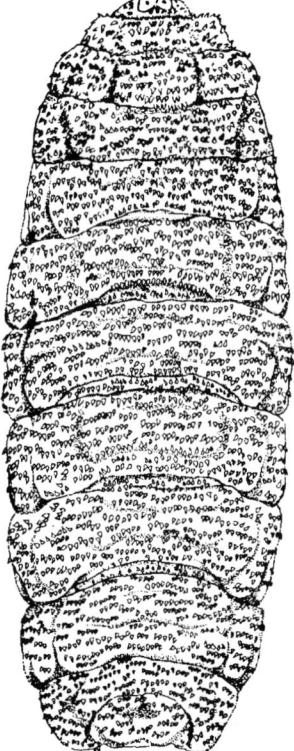

Fig. 3.38 Third-stage larva of *Chrysomya rufifacies*. Inset shows presence of small spines on the stalks of the projections. (Zumpt, 1965/Butterworths.)

Fig. 3.39 Third-stage larva of *Cordylobia anthropophaga*. (Zumpt, 1965/Butterworths.)

Life cycle: The eggs are deposited singly in dry, sandy, shaded areas where animals lie, particularly areas contaminated with host urine or faeces. Females may also be attracted to dry, urine-soiled clothing. Eggs are laid in early morning or late evening. Up to 500 eggs are laid per female over their lifespan of 2–3 weeks. The eggs hatch after 2–4 days and the first-stage larvae wait in the dry substrate for a host. The larvae can remain alive, without feeding, for 9–15 days, hidden just beneath the soil surface. A sudden rise in temperature, vibration or carbon dioxide, which might signify the presence of a host, activates the larvae. They attach to the host and immediately burrow into the skin. Larvae develop beneath the skin and produce a swelling approximately 10 mm in diameter at the point of entry. The swelling has a hole in the centre through which the larva breathes. The swellings may be found anywhere on the host animal's body but are most commonly found on ventral parts. The three larval stages are completed in the host and, when mature (7–15 days after infection), the larvae emerge out of this hole and pupate on the ground in surface debris. Adult flies emerge from the pupae after 3–4 weeks.

Cordylobia rodhaini

Description, adult: The Lund fly closely resembles *C. anthropophaga* but is larger, measuring 12.5 mm in length. The adult is a stout yellow-brown fly with a yellow face and legs and two black marks on the thorax. Adult flies feed on decaying fruits, carrion and faeces and have large, fully developed mouthparts. The arista of the antenna has setae on both sides. The thoracic squamae are without setae and the stem vein of the wing is without bristles.

Description, larvae: Third-stage larvae are 12–28 mm in length and are densely, but incompletely, covered with small, backwardly directed, single-toothed spines. The posterior spiracles are markedly tortuous.

Lucilia

There are at least 27 species of *Lucilia*, known colloquially as 'greenbottles'; however, only two species, *L. sericata* and *L. cuprina*, are of major clinical significance as primary facultative agents of cutaneous myiasis, particularly in sheep.

Lucilia sericata is more common in cool-temperate habitats, such as Europe, and was probably originally endemic to the Palaearctic. *Lucilia cuprina* may originally have been either Afro-tropical or Oriental and replaces *L. sericata* in warm-temperate and subtropical habitats. However, as a result of natural patterns of movement and artificial dispersal by humans and livestock in the past few hundred years, both species may be found worldwide.

Lucilia cuprina is not established in Europe, although it has been recorded occasionally from southern Spain and North Africa. *Lucilia cuprina* was probably introduced into Australia towards the middle or end of the nineteenth century and it is now the dominant sheep myiasis species for mainland Australia and Tasmania, present in 90–99% of fly strike cases. In the early 1980s *L. cuprina* was discovered in New Zealand and was most probably introduced from Australia. Now, in most areas of New Zealand, particularly northern areas, it appears to be displacing *L. sericata* to become the most important primary cause of fly strike in sheep. *Lucilia cuprina* is also the primary myiasis fly of sheep in southern Africa. Although

this species has been known in South Africa since 1830, little sheep strike was recorded until the early decades of the twentieth century, possibly as a result of the introduction of more susceptible Merino breeds or changes in husbandry practices. In North America, *L. cuprina* is known to be present, although it does not appear to be important in sheep myiasis.

There are believed to be two subspecies of *L. cuprina*: *L. c. cuprina* is distributed throughout the Neotropical, Oriental and southern Nearctic regions, while *L. c. dorsalis* is found throughout the sub-Saharan, Afro-tropical and Australasian regions. However, the two subspecies interbreed readily in the laboratory and intermediate forms are believed to be common. The simple division into two subspecies is therefore certainly an oversimplification of the complex pattern of genetic variation that occurs between populations of *L. cuprina*.

Lucilia sericata and Lucilia cuprina

Description, adult: Adult *Lucilia* blowflies measure up to 10 mm in length and are characterised by a metallic greenish to bronze sheen (Fig. 3.40; see also Fig. 3.34b). The adults are characterised by the presence of a bare stem vein, bare squamae and three pairs of post-sutural, dorsocentral bristles on the thorax. The sexes are very similar in appearance but may be distinguished by the distance between the eyes, which are almost touching anteriorly in males and separated in females.

Adult *Lucilia sericata* and *L. cuprina* may be distinguished from most other species of *Lucilia* by the presence of a pale creamy-white

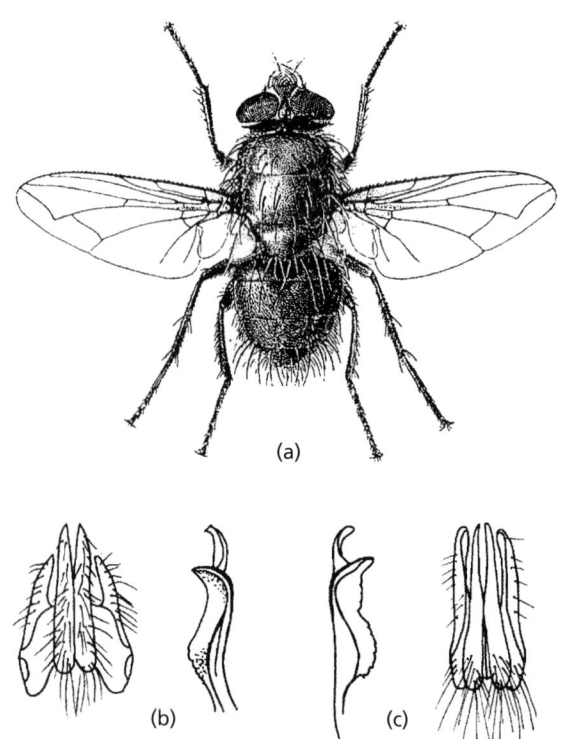

Fig. 3.40 (a) Adult *Lucilia sericata*. (From Shtakelbergh, 1956.) (b,c) Male genitalia (aedeagus in lateral view and forceps in dorsal view) of (b) *Lucilia sericata* and (c) *Lucilia cuprina*. (From Aubertin, 1933. Reproduced with permission from John Wiley & Sons.)

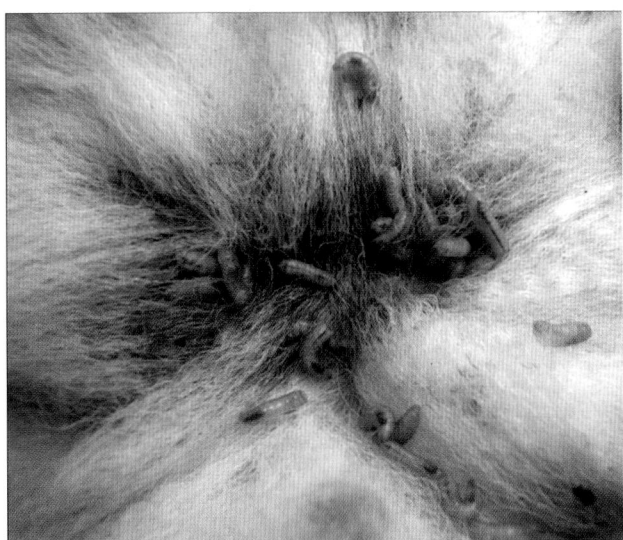

Fig. 3.41 Larvae (maggots) of the blowfly *Lucilia sericata*.

basicostal scale at the base of the wing, three postsutural acrostichal bristles on the thorax and one anterodorsal bristle on the tibia of the middle leg. However, definitive identification to species can only be confirmed using a small number of subtle morphological features, such as the colour of the fore femur, the number of paravertical setae present on the back of the head and, most reliably, the shape of the male genitalia (Fig. 3.40).

Description, larvae: Larvae are smooth, segmented and measure 10–14 mm in length (Fig. 3.41). They possess a pair of oral hooks at the anterior extremity, and at the posterior peritremes bearing spiracles (Fig. 3.42).

Life cycle: *Lucilia* are anautogenous and females must obtain a protein meal before maturing their eggs. When protein is freely available, the gravid female blowfly lays clusters of 225–250 yellowish-cream eggs on wounds, soiled fleece or dead animals, attracted by the odour of the decomposing matter. The eggs hatch into larvae in about 12–24 hours. The larvae then feed, grow rapidly and moult twice to become fully mature maggots in three days. The larvae usually feed superficially on the epidermis and lymphatic exudates, or on necrotic tissue. They will only begin to feed on healthy tissue in crowded conditions. The mouth hooks are used to macerate the tissues, and digestion occurs extraorally by means of amylase in the saliva and proteolytic enzymes in the larval excreta. Mature larvae drop to the ground and pupate in the soil. The pupal stage is completed in 3–7 days in summer. Adult flies can live for about seven days. The time required to complete the life cycle from egg to adult

is highly dependent on the ambient temperature but is usually 4–6 weeks. See **life cycle 43**.

Calliphora

There are numerous species in this genus, known colloquially as 'bluebottles'. The two most important species are *Calliphora vicina* and *C. vomitoria*.

Description: The larvae are smooth, segmented and measure 10–14 mm in length. They possess a pair of oral hooks at the anterior extremity, spiracles on the anterior segment and, posteriorly, spiracular plates. The arrangement of the posterior spiracles on these plates serves to differentiate the species.

Life cycle: Flies oviposit primarily in carrion, but may also act as secondary invaders of myiases on live mammals. The gravid female lays clusters of 100–200 yellowish-cream eggs. The eggs hatch into larvae and the larvae then feed, grow rapidly and moult twice to become fully mature maggots. When they have completed feeding, third-stage larvae migrate to the ground and pupate. Following pupation, the adult female fly must obtain a protein meal and mate.

Calliphora vicina

Synonym: *Calliphora erythrocephala*

In addition to acting as a secondary invader of myiases, *C. vicina* has occasionally been recorded laying eggs on living small mammals. Attempts to induce primary sheep strike by *C. vicina* have proved unsuccessful and it has been suggested that this species may be physiologically unable to infest sound sheep, either because the sheep body temperature is fatally high or because larvae are unable to feed on the animal tissues without the prior activity of *Lucilia* larvae.

Description, adult: Bluebottles are stout and characterised by a metallic blue sheen on the body. The thoracic squamae have long dark hair on the upper surface. *Calliphora vicina* has yellow-orange jowls with black hairs.

Description, larvae: Larvae are smooth, segmented and measure 10–14 mm in length. The posterior spiracles are in a closed peritreme (Fig. 3.43a).

Calliphora vomitoria

Description, adult: As for *Calliphora vicina* but distinguished by having black jowls with predominantly reddish hairs.

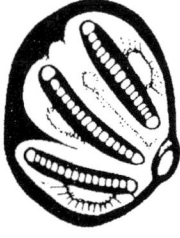
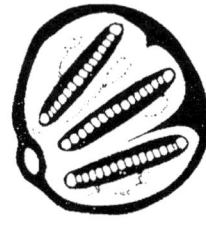
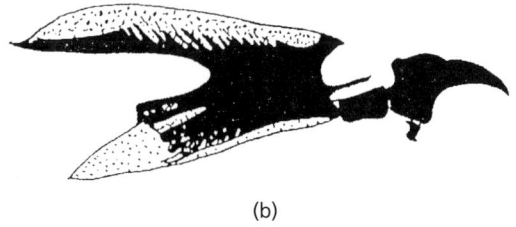

(a)   (b)

Fig. 3.42 *Lucilia sericata*: (a) posterior peritremes; (b) cephalopharyngeal skeleton. (Zumpt, 1965/Butterworths.)

LIFE CYCLE 43. LIFE CYCLE OF *LUCILIA* SPP.

Lucilia cuprina and *L. sericata* are the two most important species of facultative ectoparasite that cause cutaneous myiasis, principally in sheep. Adult females (1) oviposit approximately 225–250 cream-coloured eggs in masses close to the skin of their host, often in areas soiled by faeces or urine (2). The eggs hatch in about 12–24 hours and the larvae move to the skin where they start to feed. There are three larval stages, and larval growth and development require about 72 hours (3). Mature larvae cease feeding, drop off the host's body (4) and pupate (5) in the soil. Adults emerge in 2–3 weeks, depending on ambient temperature.

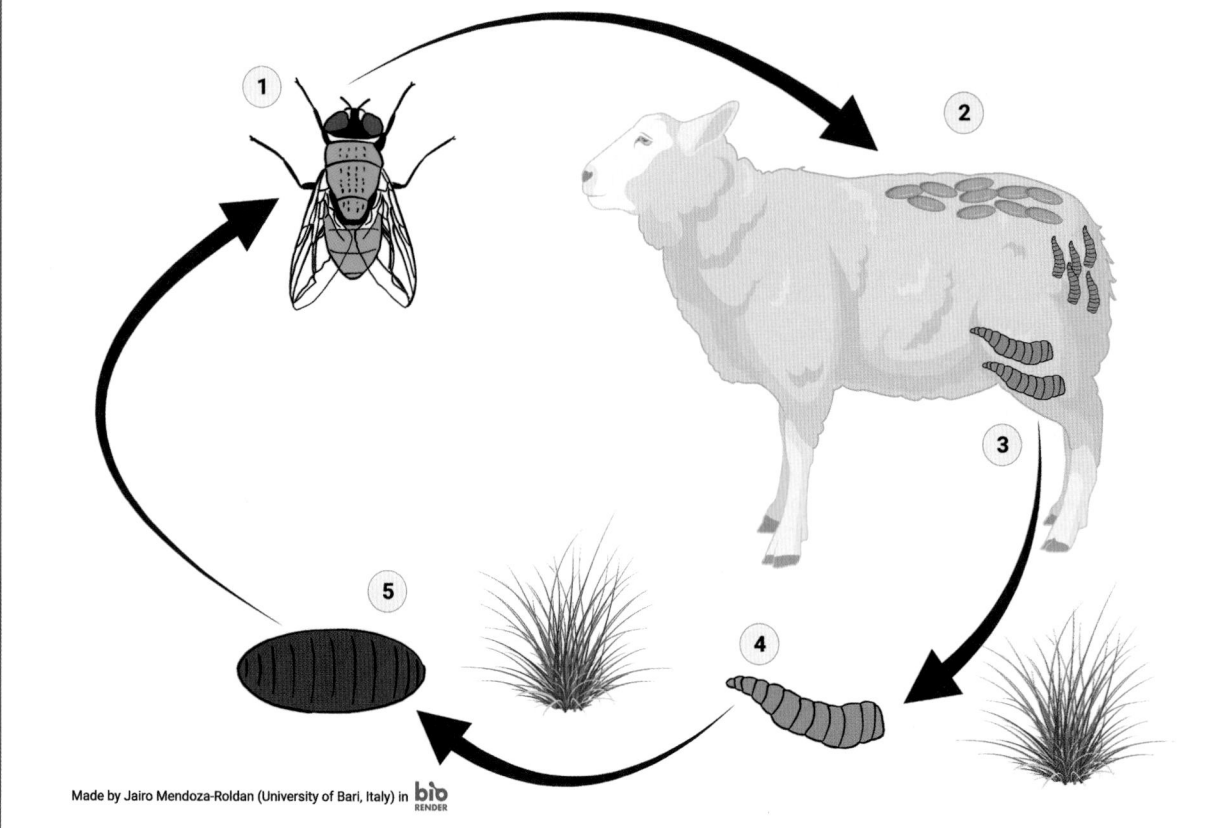

Made by Jairo Mendoza-Roldan (University of Bari, Italy) in **bio**RENDER

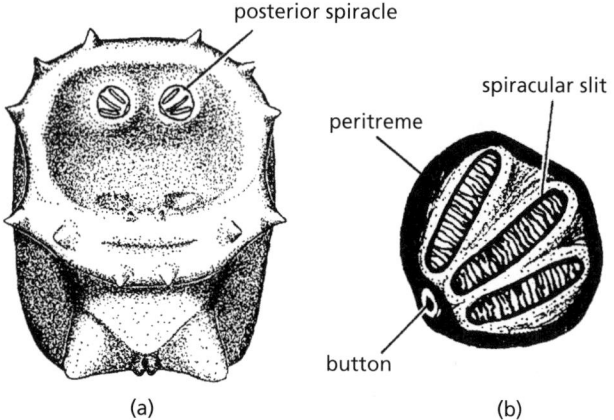

Fig. 3.43 (a) Posterior view of the last abdominal segment of *Calliphora vicina* and (b) detail of the posterior spiracles of a third-stage larva of *C. vomitoria*. (Zumpt, 1965/Butterworths.)

Calliphora augur

Description, adult: The adult *Calliphora augur* is predominantly brown or brown-yellow in colour with a patch of metallic-coloured blue on the medial abdomen. The adult body is approximately 11 mm in length.

Calliphora albifrontalis

Synonym: *Calliphora australis*

Description, adult: In the adult *Calliphora albifrontalis*, the thorax is non-metallic blue-black in colour but the abdomen is predominantly brown or brown-yellow.

Calliphora nociva

Synonym: *Calliphora dubia*

Description, adult: The adult *Calliphora nociva* is predominantly brown or brown-yellow in colour and closely resembles *C. augur* except for the colour patch on the abdomen, which is a much brighter blue on *C. nociva* than on *C. augur. Calliphora nociva* displaces *C. augur* in Western Australia.

Calliphora stygia

Synonyms: *Pollenia stygia, Calliphora laemica*

Calliphora stygia is a large native Australasian blowfly. It is adapted to cooler conditions than other Australasian blowflies and occurs in largest numbers in spring and autumn, but may be found on sunny days in winter as well. This adaptation to the cold gives it an advantage on carrion during the cooler months, and in spring in particular, many thousands of these flies can develop from carcasses. In summer, high temperatures and competition from species such as *Chrysomya rufifacies* reduce its abundance and *C. stygia* becomes scarce. In Western Australia, *C. stygia* is displaced by the very similar *Calliphora albifrontalis*.

Description, adult: The adult has a grey thorax and a yellow-brown mottled abdomen.

Phormia and Protophormia

These two genera are closely related and each contains a single species of interest, *Phormia regina* and *Protophormia terraenovae*. Adult flies are black in colour with an overlying metallic blue-green sheen and may be known colloquially as 'blackbottles'. The third-stage larvae of both species are characterised by strongly developed, fairly pointed tubercles on the posterior face of the last segment. Both species are generally considered to be strongly cold-adapted and are widespread in more northerly regions of both the Nearctic and the Palaearctic.

Phormia regina

Description, adult: *Phormia regina* is a black-coloured blowfly, with an overlying metallic blue-green sheen. This species is very similar to *Protophormia terraenovae* in appearance. In *Phormia regina*, the anterior spiracle is yellow or orange and stands out clearly against the dark background colour of the thorax.

Description, larvae: The third-stage larvae of *P. regina* are characterised by strongly developed, fairly pointed tubercles on the posterior face of the last segment. The tubercles on the upper margin of the last segment are shorter than those of *P. terraenovae*, and are less than half the width of the posterior spiracle in length (Fig. 3.44b). There are no dorsal spines on the posterior margins of segment 10.

Life cycle: Flies oviposit primarily in carrion, but may also act as secondary invaders of myiases on live mammals. The gravid female lays clusters of 100–200 yellowish-cream eggs. The eggs hatch into larvae which then feed, grow rapidly and moult twice to become fully mature maggots. These then migrate to the ground and pupate. Following pupation, the adult female fly must obtain a protein meal and mate. Adult flies can live for approximately 30 days.

Protophormia terraenovae

Description, adult: *Protophormia terraenovae* is a black-coloured blowfly with an overlying metallic blue-green sheen. This species is very similar to *Phormia regina* in appearance. In *P. terraenovae* the anterior thoracic spiracle is black or black-brown and is difficult to distinguish from the general body colour.

Description, larvae: The third-stage larvae of *P. terraenovae* (as with *P. regina*) are characterised by strongly developed, fairly pointed tubercles on the posterior face of the last segment. The tubercles on the upper margin of the last segment are longer than half the width of a posterior spiracle (Fig. 3.44a). The larvae of *P. terraenovae* also possess dorsal spines on the posterior margins of segment 10 (Fig. 3.44c).

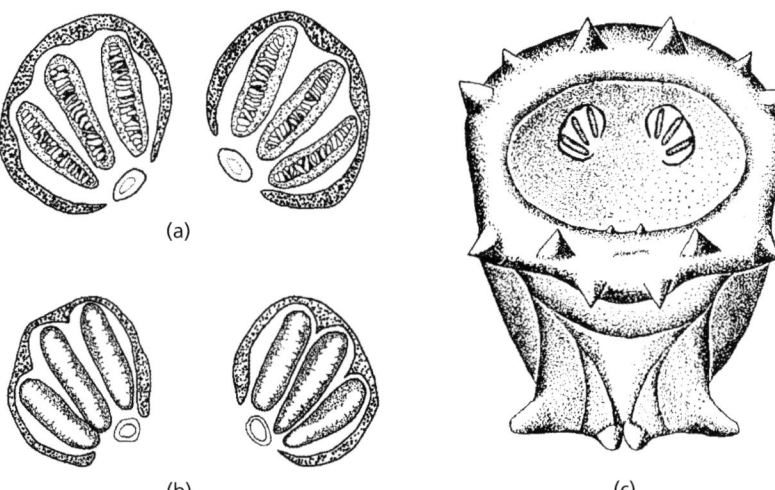

(a)

(b)

(c)

Fig. 3.44 Posterior spiracles of third-stage larvae of (a) *Protophormia terraenovae* and (b) *Phormia regina*. (c) Tubercles on the posterior face of the last segment of third-stage *Protophormia terraenovae*. (Zumpt, 1965/Butterworths.)

FAMILY SARCOPHAGIDAE

The family Sarcophagidae, known as flesh flies, contains over 2000 species in 400 genera. Most species of Sarcophagidae are of no veterinary importance, breeding in excrement, carrion and other decomposing organic matter. The principal genus containing species which act as important agents of veterinary myiasis is *Wohlfahrtia*. Members of the genus *Sarcophaga* may occasionally infest wounds.

Wohlfahrtia

The most economically important species is *Wohlfahrtia magnifica* found throughout the Mediterranean basin, eastern and central Europe and part of Asia. This is an obligate agent of traumatic myiasis. Other species include *Wohlfahrtia vigil* in North America and *W. nubia*, which is a facultative species that breeds in carrion or living hosts in North Africa and the Middle East where it can be locally important, particularly in camels. *Wohlfahrtia opaca* (formerly *W. meigeni*) behaves in North America in a similar manner to *W. vigil*, causing a furuncular, boil-like myiasis in smaller animals.

Wohlfahrtia magnifica

Description, adult: The adult flies are large, measuring 8–14 mm in length, with elongated bodies. They are grey in colour and have three distinct longitudinal thoracic stripes (Fig. 3.45a). The abdomen is clearly marked with black spots (Fig. 3.45c). The flies have numerous bristles covering the body and long black legs. The arista of the antennae does not possess setae.

Description, larvae: Larvae possess strongly developed oral hooks.

Life cycle: *Wohlfahrtia magnifica* is an obligate agent of myiasis. Female flies deposit 120–170 first-stage larvae on the host, in wounds or next to body orifices. The larvae feed and mature in 5–7 days, moulting twice, before leaving the wound and dropping to the ground where they pupate.

Wohlfahrtia nuba

Description, adult: The adult flies are large, 8–14 mm in length, with elongated bodies, longitudinal black thoracic stripes and a grey and black tessellated abdomen.

Life cycle: *Wohlfahrtia nuba* oviposits primarily in carrion but may also act as a secondary invader of myiases on live mammals in North Africa and the Near East. Females deposit live first-stage larvae rather than eggs. When fully mature, the third-stage larvae leave the feeding site to pupate in the ground.

Wohlfahrtia vigil

Description, adult: The adult flies are large, 8–14 mm in length, with elongated bodies, longitudinal black thoracic stripes and a grey and black tessellated abdomen.

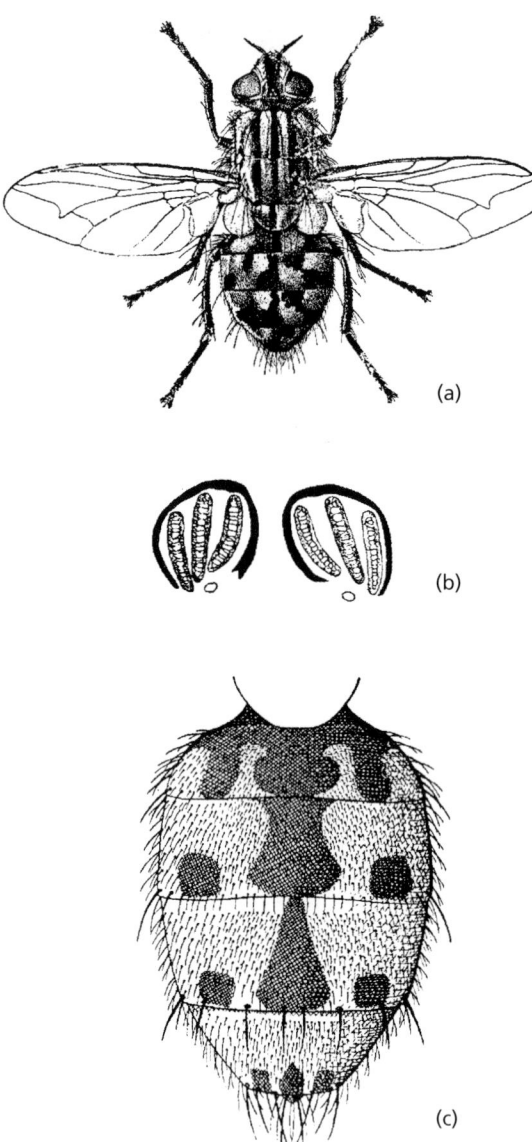

Fig. 3.45 (a) Adult of the flesh fly *Sarcophaga carnaria*. (Castellani and Chalmers, 1910/Castellani.) (b,c) *Wohlfahrtia magnifica*: posterior spiracles deeply sunk in a cavity (b) and abdomen of adult (c). (From Smart, 1943.)

Life cycle: The adult female of *Wohlfahrtia vigil* deposits active maggots on the host, often in wounds, body orifices or existing myiases. However, the larvae can penetrate intact skin if it is thin and tender; hence young animals tend to be most affected. Groups of larvae may be observed in boil-like swellings under the skin. The larvae feed and grow, moulting twice, before leaving the host and dropping to the ground where they pupate.

Wohlfahrtia meigeni

Description, adult: The adult flies are large, 8–14 mm in length, with elongated bodies, longitudinal black thoracic stripes and a grey and black tessellated abdomen.

Sarcophaga

Most species of the genus *Sarcophaga* are of no veterinary importance, breeding in excrement, carrion and other decomposing organic matter, but some species may occasionally infest wounds. One of the more widely distributed species is *Sarcophaga haemorrhoidalis*.

Life cycle: All Sarcophagidae are larviparous: the ovulated eggs are retained within the oviduct of the adult female and batches of 30–200 larvae are deposited shortly after the eggs hatch. The larvae of *Sarcophaga* are normally associated with carrion but may occasionally infest wounds. They may extend the injury, increasing the severity of the infestation.

Sarcophaga haemorrhoidalis

Description, adult: Adults flies are grey-black, non-metallic, medium to large flies with prominent stripes on the thorax and a checkered abdominal pattern.

FAMILY OESTRIDAE

This is an important family consisting of several genera of large, usually hairy flies whose larvae are parasites of animals. All are obligate agents of myiasis, showing a high degree of host specificity. The adults have primitive non-functional mouthparts. However, their larvae spend their entire period of larval growth and development feeding within their vertebrate hosts, causing nasopharyngeal, digestive tract or dermal–furuncular myiases. The larvae are characterised by posterior spiracular plates containing numerous small pores.

The Oestridae contains about 150 species, known as the bots and warbles. There are four subfamilies of importance: **Oestrinae**, **Gasterophilinae**, **Hypodermatinae** and **Cuterebrinae**.

SUBFAMILY OESTRINAE

The subfamily Oestrinae contains one genus of major importance, *Oestrus*, and four genera of lesser importance, *Gedoelstia*, *Rhinoestrus*, *Cephenomyia* and *Cephalopina*. Oestrinae species of veterinary importance are listed in Table 3.3.

Oestrus ovis (nasal bot fly)

Oestrus ovis is an obligate agent of nasal myiasis in sheep found worldwide in the Palearctic region.

Description, adult: Greyish-brown flies about 12 mm long, with small black spots on the abdomen and a covering of short brown hairs (Fig. 3.46). The head is broad, with small eyes, and the frons, scutellum and dorsal thorax bear small wart-like protuberances. The segments of the antennae are small and the arista bare. The mouthparts are reduced to small knobs. The characteristic wing venation has a strongly bent M vein joining the R_{4+5} vein before the wing margin.

For clinical information see Chapter 9.

Table 3.3 Oestrinae species of veterinary importance.

Species	Hosts	Site
Oestrus ovis	Sheep and goat, ibex, camel, rarely humans	Nasal passages
Gedoelstia hassleri	Wild ruminants, occasionally sheep, cattle	Nasopaharynx
Rhinoestrus purpureus	Horse, donkey, rarely human	Nasal passages
Pharyngomyia picta	Red deer (*Cervus elaphus*), sika deer (*Cervus nippon*), fallow deer (*Dama dama*), roe deer (*Capreolus capreolus*)	Nasal passages
Cephenemyia trompe	Reindeer (*Rangifer tarandus*), moose, caribou	Nasopharynx
Cephenemyia auribarbis	Reindeer, caribou, red deer; fallow deer; mule deer (*Odocoileus hemionus*), white-tailed deer (*Odocoileus* spp.)	Nasopharynx
Cephenemyia phobifer	Mule deer	Nasopharynx
Cephenemyia stimulator	Roe deer	Nasopharynx
Cephenemyia jellisoni	Moose (*Alces alces*), elk (*Cervus elaphus*)	Nasopharynx
Cephalopina titillator	Camel	Nasopharynx

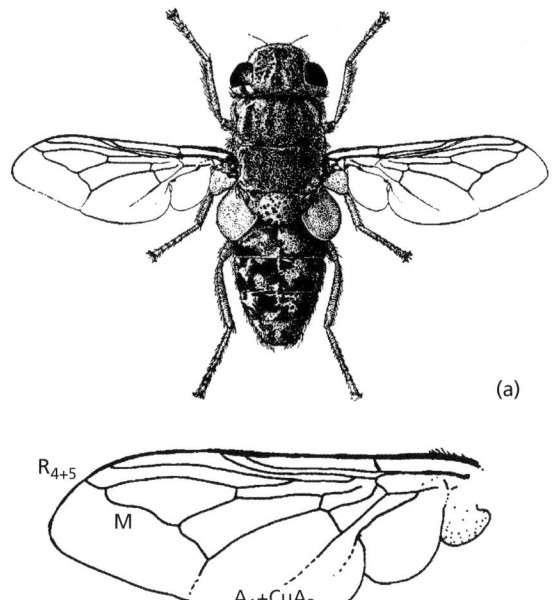

(a)

(b)

Fig. 3.46 (a) Adult female *Oestrus ovis* and (b) wing venation typical of *Oestrus* showing the strongly bent vein M joining R_{4+5} before the wing margin. (Castellani and Chalmers, 1910/Castellani.)

Description, larvae: Mature larvae in the nasal passages are about 30 mm long, yellowish-white and tapering anteriorly. Each segment has a dark transverse band dorsally (Fig. 3.47). They have large black oral hooks, connected to an internal cephalopharyngeal skeleton. The ventral surface bears rows of small spines.

Life cycle: The females are viviparous and infect the sheep by squirting a jet of liquid containing larvae at the nostrils during flight, which delivers up to 25 larvae at a time. The newly deposited L_1 are about 1 mm long and migrate through the nasal passages to the frontal sinuses, feeding on the mucus that is secreted in response to the

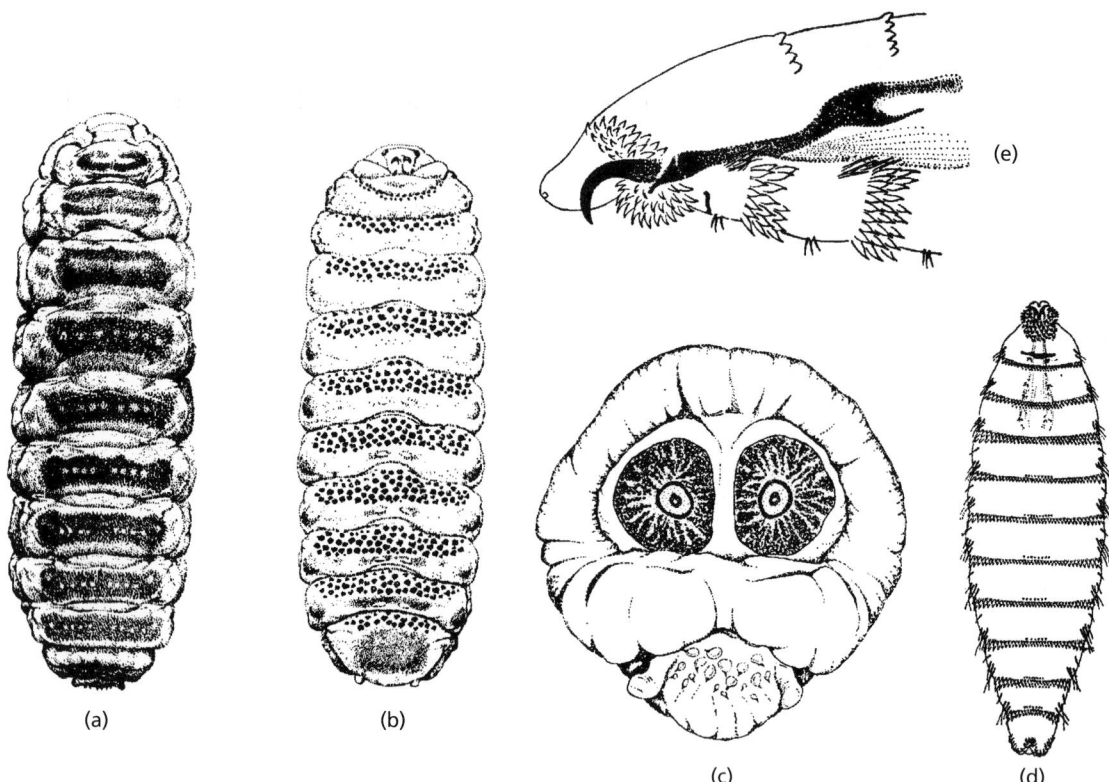

Fig. 3.47 *Oestrus ovis*: (a) dorsal view and (b) ventral view of third-stage larva; (c) posterior view of third-stage larva; (d) first-stage larva; (e) mouthparts of first-stage larva in lateral view. (Zumpt, 1965/Butterworths.)

stimulation of larval movement. Larvae attach themselves to the mucous membrane using oral hooks, which cause irritation. The first moult occurs in the nasal passages, and the L_2 crawl into the frontal sinuses where the final moult to third-stage larvae takes place. In the sinuses, the larvae complete their growth and then migrate back to the nostrils, from where they are sneezed to the ground. Larvae pupate in the ground and pupation lasts for 3–9 weeks.

The larvae remain in the nasal passages for a variable period, ranging from two weeks in summer to nine months during colder seasons. Where flies are active throughout the year, two or three generations are possible, but in cool or cold weather the small L_1 and L_2 become dormant and remain in recesses of the nasal passages over winter. They move to the frontal sinuses only in the warmer spring weather, and then complete their development into the L_3, which emerge from the nostrils and pupate on the ground to give a further generation of adults. The females survive only two weeks but during this time, each can deposit up to 500 larvae in the nasal passages of sheep. See **life cycle 44**.

Gedoelstia hassleri and Gedoelstia cristata

Flies of the genus *Gedoelstia* cause ophthalmomyiasis primarily in wild ruminants in southern Africa but may occasionally cause problems in domestic livestock.

Description, adult: Large robust flies up to 18 mm in length. The head of the adult is reddish-yellow with dark brown spots. The

thorax is rusty-brown in colour with a pattern of glossy black lines. The abdomen is brown with large black lateral patches and a series of large tubercles with sharply pointed tips.

Description, larvae: The third-stage larvae are ovoid, up to 20 mm in length and may be distinguished from all other oestrids by a vertical slit in the posterior peritremes or a vertical suture if the spiracle is closed.

Life cycle: The larvae are deposited by the adult flies in the cornea or conjunctiva of the eyes of the natural hosts, and travel by a vascular route via the optic nerve tract to the nasopharynx where they mature, thus showing some affinity with *Cephenemyia*. Some larvae appear to include the lungs in this migration.

Rhinoestrus purpureus

Larvae of *Rhinoestrus purpureus* cause nasal myiases of equids in the Mediterranean, Middle East and Asia.

Description, adult: A relatively small fly, 8–11 mm in length. The anterior thorax is characterised by a number of glossy black stripes. The head, thorax and abdomen are covered with small wart-like protuberances and a covering of short yellow-brown hairs. The head is broad, with small eyes. The legs are red and yellow-brown. The mouthparts are reduced to small knobs.

Description, larvae: The larvae resemble those of *Oestrus ovis* except that they have strongly recurved mouth hooks and a single row of 8–12 terminal hooklets. There are three larval stages, approximately 1, 3.5 and 20 mm in length respectively.

LIFE CYCLE 44. LIFE CYCLE OF *OESTRUS OVIS* AND *RHINOESTRUS PURPUREUS*

Adult females of *Oestrus ovis* (1) squirt batches of larvae into the nostrils of the host (2, 3). At each attack, up to 25 larvae can be deposited at any one time. The first-stage larvae (L_1) appear whitish-coloured, oval in shape and ~1 mm long (3). Once in the nasal cavities, they rapidly attach to the mucosa using prominent buccal hooks, and penetrate the nasal cavities where they feed on mucus; the larvae continue their migration towards the nasal passages. The first moult from L_1 to L_2 occurs in the nasal cavities, whereas the second (L_2 to L_3) occurs in the frontal sinuses (4). At this stage, the larvae are 20–30 mm long and 7–10 mm in diameter. Once developed, the larvae exit the nasal cavities and the nostrils and leave the host (5). Once on the ground, the L_3 pupates (6) and the adult emerges. The life cycle of *Rhinoestrus purpureus* (7), infecting equines (8), is similar to that of *O. ovis*. The infection causes irritation of the nasal cavities and the pharynx, and lesions of the olfactory nerves.

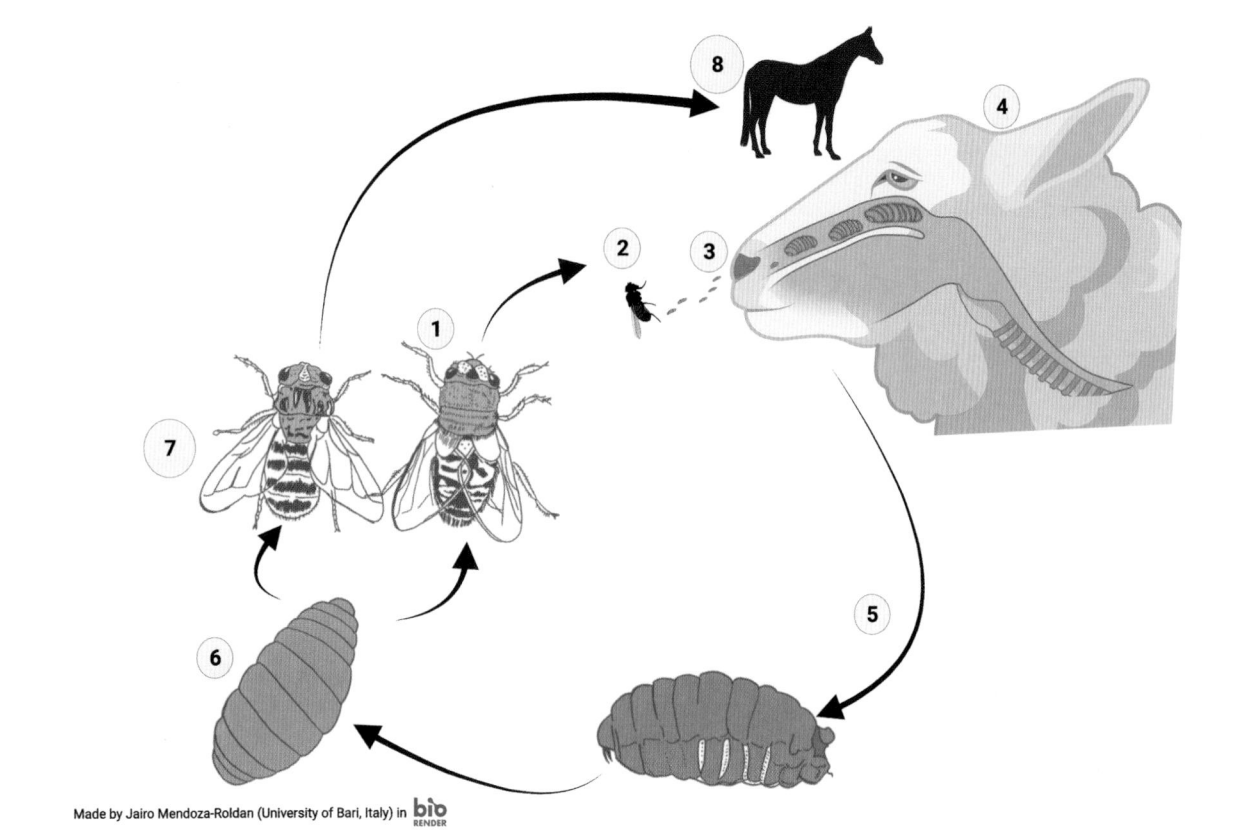

Made by Jairo Mendoza-Roldan (University of Bari, Italy) in **bio**RENDER

Life cycle: The female fly produces 700–800 larvae which are expelled in batches of up to 40 into the nostrils of the hosts. First-stage larvae remain in the nasal cavities before moving to the pharyngeal area where they moult to become second- and then third-stage larvae. The rate of development varies considerably depending on location. Third-stage larvae are expelled and pupate in the ground.

Cephenemyia trompe (reindeer throat bot)

Description, adult: The adult is bee-like in appearance, 14–16 mm in length and covered in long yellowish and black hairs overlying a shining black body.

Description, larvae: Developing larvae are white, while fully developed larvae are about 25–40 mm long and yellowish-brown. The entire larval body is covered by bands of short spines on both sides and narrows posteriorly.

Life cycle: The adult flies are active from June to September and, like *Oestrus*, the females are viviparous. The fly hovers close to the animal, then darts in and ejects larvae in fluid into the nostrils of the host animal. The larvae migrate to the retropharyngeal pouches. There they become attached in clusters and develop. Further development occurs in the nasopharynx, as the larvae migrate to and crowd in the retropharyngeal pouches that lie on either side of the throat at the base of the tongue. Fully developed third-stage larvae, which may be 40 mm in length, crawl to the anterior nasal passages and are sneezed out. Pupation occurs on the ground under surface debris. The pupation period is about four weeks. The adult flies have no mouthparts for feeding so they are short-lived and mate shortly after emerging.

Cephalopina titillator

Description, adult: The adult fly measures 8–10 mm in length. It is relatively robust and has a powdery grey appearance. The head is large, orange above and yellow below. The eyes are broadly separated, especially in the female. The thorax is reddish-brown, with a black pattern. The abdomen has irregular black blotches and white hair and the legs are yellow.

Description, larvae: The first-stage larvae are about 0.7 mm in length and have long spines on the lateral edges of the segments. Third instars are about 25–35 mm in length, and characterised by smooth fleshy lobes on each segment and large mouth hooks.

Life cycle: Eggs are laid around the nasal area. Larvae hatch and migrate into the nasal cavity, frontal sinus and pharynx of their host, where they take several months to feed and moult. When mature, the larvae make their way back to the nose, considerably irritating the host (usually a camel), in the process. As a result, they are sneezed out onto the ground, and from here the larvae burrow into the ground and pupate. Pupation takes about 25 days.

SUBFAMILY GASTEROPHILINAE

The subfamily Gasterophilinae contains a single genus of importance, *Gasterophilus*, which are obligate parasites of horses, donkeys, zebras, elephants and rhinoceroses. Eight species are recognised in total, six of which are of interest as veterinary parasites of equids.

Description, adult: Bot flies are robust dark flies 10–15 mm in length. The body is densely covered with yellowish hairs. In the female, the ovipositor is strong and protruberant. The wings of adult *Gasterophilus* characteristically have no cross-vein dm-cu (Fig. 3.48).

Description, larvae: When mature and present in the stomach or passed in faeces, the larvae are cylindrical, 16–20 mm long and reddish-orange with posterior spiracles (Fig. 3.49). Differentiation of mature larvae of the various species can be made on mouth

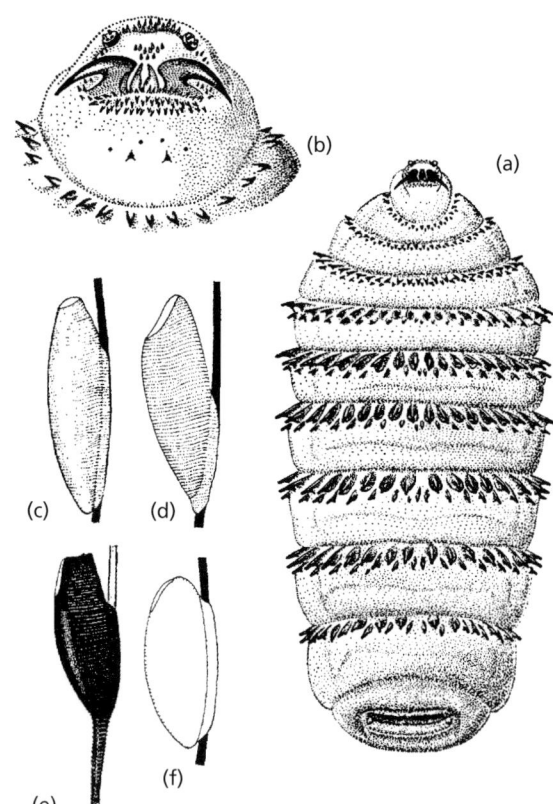

Fig. 3.49 (a) Third-stage larva of *Gasterophilus intestinalis*. (b) Ventral view of pseudocephalon of *G. pecorum*. Eggs of (c) *G. nasalis*; (d) *G. intestinalis*; (e) *G. haemorrhoidalis*; (f) *G. inermis*. (**Zumpt, 1965/Butterworths.**)

hooks (Fig. 3.49b) and the numbers and distribution of the spines present on various segments (Fig. 3.50).

Life cycle: The life cycles of the various species differ only slightly; key differences are highlighted in the following sections. See **life cycle 45**.

For clinical information see Chapter 10.

Gasterophilus haemorrhoidalis

Description, larvae: The spines on the ventral surface of the larval segments are arranged in two rows. The head segment has only lateral groups of denticles and the dorsal row of spines on the eighth segment is not broadly interrupted medially. The mouth hooks are

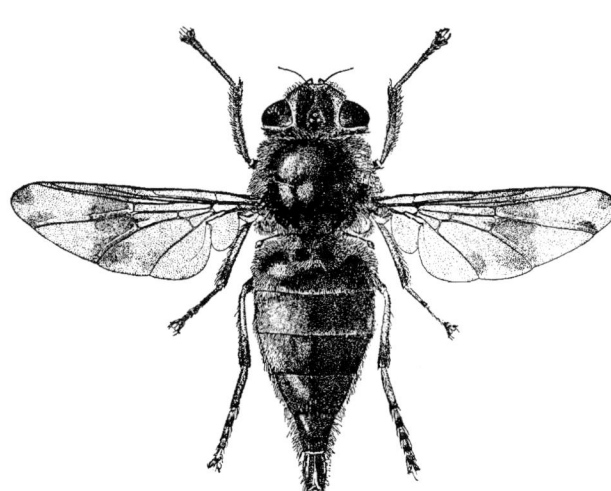

Fig. 3.48 Adult female *Gasterophilus intestinalis*. (Castellani and Chalmers, 1910/Castellani.)

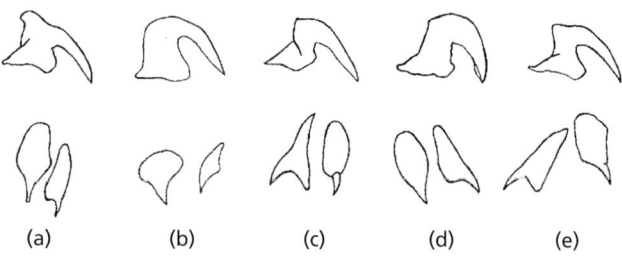

Fig. 3.50 Mouth hooks (top) and ventral spines (bottom) of the fifth segment of (a) *Gasterophilus intestinalis*; (b) *G. inermis*; (c) *G. nasalis*; (d) *G. haemorrhoidalis*; (e) *G. pecorum*. (Zumpt, 1965/Butterworths.)

LIFE CYCLE 45. LIFE CYCLE OF *GASTEROPHILUS* SPP.

Gasterophilus females (1) deposit conical-shaped eggs in different sites depending on species: on the forelimbs and shoulders (*Gasterophilus intestinalis*), on the perilabial area or near the nostrils (*G. haemorrhoidalis* and *G. inermis*) or in some cases (e.g. *G. pecorum*) on grass stems (2). After hatching, first-stage larvae reach the mouth, either actively or via grooming. From the oral mucosa, the first-stage larvae travel through the pharynx and the oesophagus to the cardia of the stomach (3), using a pair of sclerotised mouth hooks to burrow through the tissues. Eventually, in the case of *G. intestinalis*, they attach to areas of the gastric mucosa. The larvae of other *Gasterophilus* species travel to the pylorus, duodenum and rectum, where they remain for the rest of their parasitic life. First-stage larvae (4) develop to second- (5) and third-stage larvae (6). After ~10 months, the third-stage larvae detach from the mucosa and reach the external environment with the faeces. Here, they moult into pupae (7), from which adults subsequently emerge.

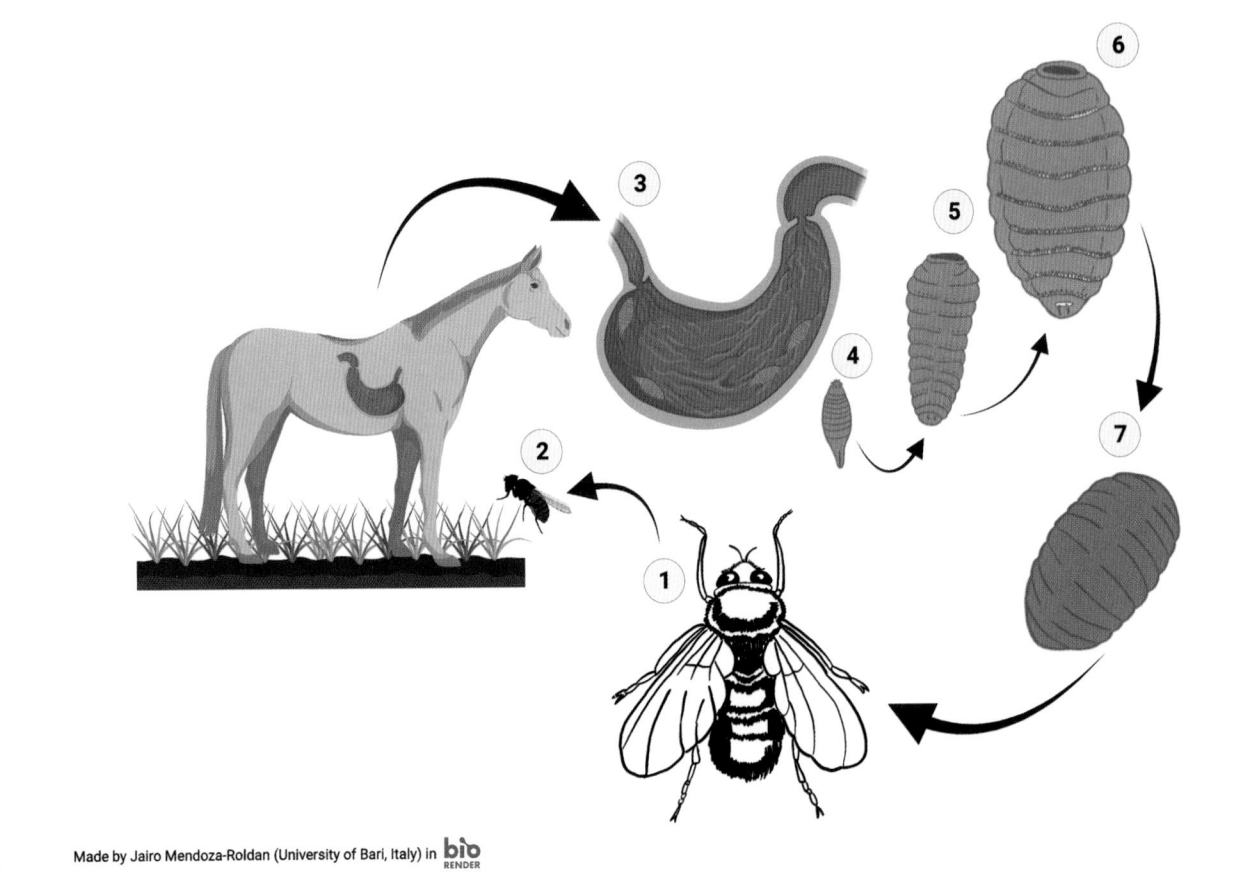

Made by Jairo Mendoza-Roldan (University of Bari, Italy) in **bio**RENDER

uniformly curved dorsally and directed laterally, and the body spines are sharply pointed (Fig. 3.50d).

Life cycle: *Gasterophilus haemorrhoidalis* lays batches of 150–200 eggs around the lips. The adult flies have a short lifespan and females can deposit all their eggs within 2–3 hours if the weather is mild and a suitable host is available. The eggs are easily seen (length 1–2 mm) and are usually black in colour (Fig. 3.49e). They either hatch spontaneously in about five days or are stimulated to do so by warmth, which may be generated during licking and self-grooming. Larvae either crawl into the mouth or are transferred to the tongue during licking. The larvae can burrow into the epidermis of the lips and from there migrate into the mouth. These then penetrate the tongue or buccal mucosa and burrow through these tissues for several weeks while feeding, before moulting and passing via the pharynx and oesophagus to the stomach where they attach to the gastric epithelium.

The larvae remain and develop in the stomach for periods of 10–12 months. When mature in the following spring or early summer, they detach and are passed in the faeces. In this species, the larvae reattach in the rectum for a few days before being passed out. Pupation takes place on the ground and after 1–2 months the adult flies emerge. These do not feed, and live for only a few days or weeks, during which time they mate and lay eggs. If suitable hosts are unavailable, the flies move to high points to aggregate and mate, following which the females initiate a longer-distance search for hosts. There is therefore only one generation of flies per year in temperate areas.

Gasterophilus inermis

Description, larvae: Spines on the ventral surface of the larval segments are arranged in two rows. The head segment has only lateral groups of denticles and the dorsal row of spines on the eighth segment are not broadly interrupted medially. The mouth hooks are strongly curved, with their tips directed backwards and approaching the base; body spines are sharply pointed (Fig. 3.50b). Body segment 3 has three complete rows of spines, and body segment 11 has one row of spines interrupted by a broad median gap.

Life cycle: The adult female lays up to 300 eggs on the cheeks and around the mouth of the host animal. These are each attached individually to the base of a hair in these regions. The eggs are 1–2 mm in length and usually creamy white in colour (Fig. 3.49f). The life cycle is essentially similar to that of *G. haemorrhoidalis*.

Gasterophilus intestinalis

Description, larvae: The mouth hooks are not uniformly curved dorsally and have a shallow depression. The body spines have blunt tips (Fig. 3.50a).

Gasterophilus intestinalis

Description, larvae: The mouth hooks are not uniformly curved dorsally, and have a shallow depression. The body spines have blunt tips (Fig. 3.50a).

Life cycle: *Gasterophilus intestinalis* eggs are laid on the hairs of the forelegs and shoulders. Several eggs may be glued to each hair and up to 1000 eggs may be deposited by a female *G. intestinalis* during its lifetime of only a few days. The eggs are 1–2 mm in length and usually creamy white in colour (Fig. 3.49d). Larvae penetrate the tongue or buccal mucosa at the anterior end of the tongue where they excavate galleries in the subepithelial layer of the mucous membrane. The larvae wander in these tissues for several weeks before exiting the tongue and moulting. Second-stage larvae attach for a few days to the sides of the pharynx, before moving to the oesophageal portion of the stomach where they cluster at the boundary of glandular and non-glandular epithelium. The larvae remain and develop in this site for periods of 10–12 months.

Gasterophilus nasalis

Description, larvae: *Gasterophilus nasalis* larvae have spines on the ventral surface of the larval segments arranged in a single row. The first three body segments are more or less conical and the third segment has a dorsal row of spines and sometimes ventral spines (Fig. 3.50c).

Life cycle: The throat bot fly, *G. nasalis*, lays its eggs in the intermandibular area. Eggs are laid in batches of up to 500, usually with one egg attached per hair (Fig. 3.49c). The larvae burrow into the spaces around the teeth and between the teeth and gums. This may result in the development of pus sockets and necrosis in the gums. The first larval stage lasts 18–24 days, following which larvae moult and second-stage larvae move via the pharynx and oesophagus to the stomach, where they attach to the gastric epithelium. In the

stomach, the yellow *G. nasalis* larvae attach around the pylorus and sometimes the duodenum, where they remain for 10–12 months.

Gasterophilus nigricornis

Description, larvae: Spines on the ventral surface of the larval segments are arranged in a single row. The first three body segments are more or less cylindrical, showing sharp constrictions posteriorly, and the third segment is without spines dorsally or ventrally.

Life cycle: Female flies alight on the host's cheek to oviposit. The larvae hatch in 3–9 days and burrow directly into the skin. They then burrow to the corner of the mouth and penetrate the mucous membranes inside the cheek. Once they have reached the central part of the cheek (about 20–30 days after hatching), they moult and leave the mucous membranes. The second-stage larvae are then swallowed, following which they attach themselves to the wall of the duodenum and remain there for 10–12 months.

Gasterophilus pecorum

Description, larvae: Larvae have spines on the ventral surface of the larval segments, which are arranged in two rows. The head segment has two lateral groups of denticles and one central group, the latter situated between the antennal lobes and mouth hooks. The dorsal rows of spines are broadly interrupted medially on the seventh and eighth segments. Segments 10 and 11 have no spines (Fig. 3.50e).

Life cycle: Adult *G. pecorum* are most active in late summer and, unlike other species, the dark-coloured eggs are laid on pasture and are ingested by horses during grazing. Up to 2000 eggs are laid in batches of 10–115. The eggs are highly resistant and the developed larva may remain viable for months within its egg until ingested by horses. In the mouth, the eggs hatch within 3–5 minutes. First-stage larvae immediately penetrate the mucous membrane of the lips, gums, cheeks, tongue and hard palate and burrow towards the root of the tongue and soft palate where they may remain for 9–10 months until fully developed. They may also be swallowed and settle in the walls of the pharynx, oesophagus or stomach. When mature in the following spring or early summer, the larvae detach and are passed in the faeces.

SUBFAMILY HYPODERMATINAE

The subfamily Hypodermatinae contains one genus of major importance, *Hypoderma* (warble flies or cattle grubs), and a second less widespread genus, *Przhevalskiana* (goat warbles). The genus *Hypoderma* contains six species of veterinary importance. Two species, *H. bovis* and *H. lineatum*, are parasites primarily of cattle, whereas *H. diana*, *H. actaeon*, *H. tarandi* and *H. sinense* affect roe deer, red deer, reindeer and yak, respectively.

Hypoderma

Description, adult: The adults are large and the abdomen is covered with yellow-orange hairs giving them a bee-like appearance (Fig. 3.51). The adults have no functional mouthparts.

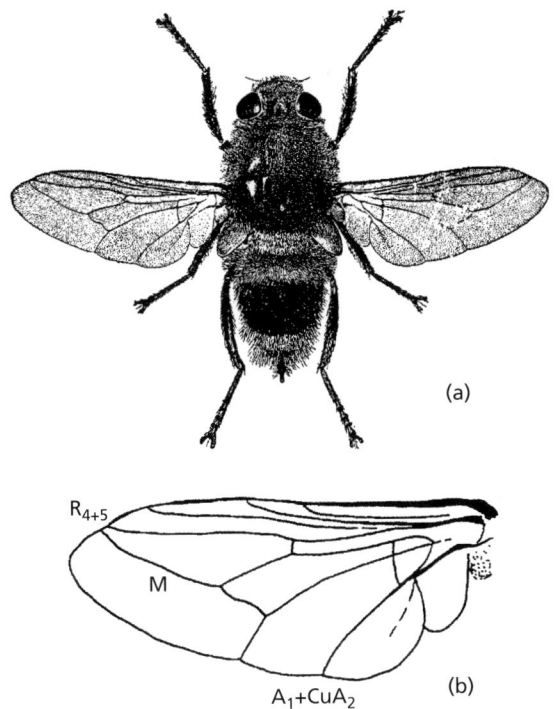

Fig. 3.51 (a) Adult female of *Hypoderma bovis*. (Castellani and Chalmers, 1910/Castellani.) (b) Wing venation typical of *Hypoderma* showing the strongly bent vein M not joining R_{4+5} before the wing margin and vein A_1+CuA_2 reaching the wing margin.

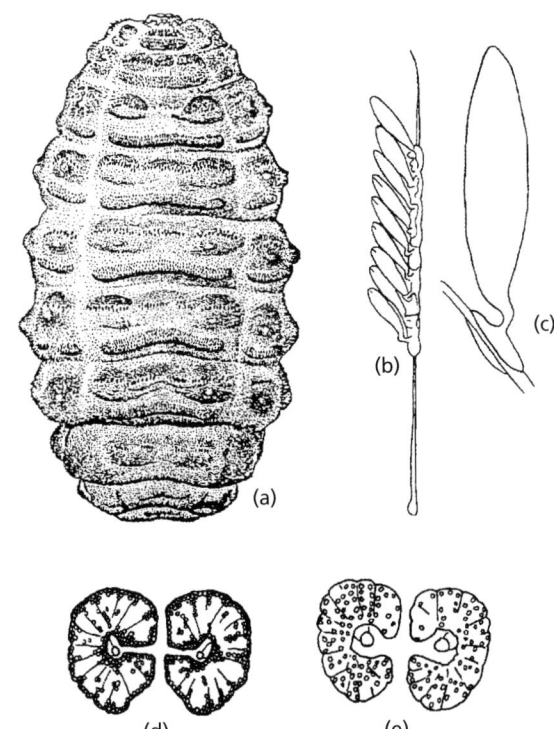

Fig. 3.52 (a) Third-stage larva of *Hypoderma bovis*. Eggs of (b) *H. lineatum* and (c) *H. bovis*. Posterior spiracles of third-stage larvae of (d) *H. bovis* and (e) *H. lineatum*. (Zumpt, 1965/Butterworths.)

For clinical information see Chapter 8.

Description, larvae: Mature larvae are thick and somewhat barrel-shaped, tapering anteriorly (Fig. 3.52a). When mature, they are 25–30 mm long, and most segments bear short spines. The colour is dirty white when newly emerged from the host but rapidly turns to dark brown; the pupa is almost black. The third-stage larvae of the two species of *Hypoderma* that commonly parasitise cattle (*H. bovis* and *H. lineatum*) may be distinguished from other species of *Hypoderma* by examination of the posterior spiracular plate, which is completely surrounded by small spines. The cattle species may be further distinguished as follows: in *H. bovis*, the posterior spiracular plate surrounding the button has a narrow funnel-like channel, whereas in *H. lineatum* it has a broad channel (Fig. 3.52d,e and Table 3.4).

Life cycle: The adult flies are active only in warm weather, and in the northern hemisphere the peak period is usually in June and July. The females attach their eggs to hairs on the lower parts of the body and on the legs above the hocks (Fig. 3.52b,c). The eggs are 1 mm long and are fixed to the hairs using small terminal clasps (Fig. 3.52). One female may lay 100 or more eggs on an individual host. There is no fly activity below approximately 18 °C.

The first-stage larvae, which are less than 1 mm long, hatch in a few days and crawl down the hairs, penetrate the hair follicles and migrate in the body, following species-specific pathways (see following sections). The use of paired mouth hooks and the secretion of proteolytic enzymes aid migration. The larvae feed as they travel to the species-specific resting sites, which are reached in late autumn, where they spend the winter. The moult to the second stage occurs at this resting site. During this stage they grow to

Table 3.4 Summary of differences between the *Hypoderma* which parasitise cattle.

Feature	Hypoderma bovis	Hypoderma lineatum
Adult length	15 mm	13 mm
Eggs laid	Singly	In batches
Larval morphology	Posterior spiracular plate surrounding the button has a narrow funnel-like channel	Posterior spiracular plate surrounding the button has a broad channel
Migration path	Along nerves	Between the fascial planes of muscles and along connective tissue
Overwintering site	Epidural fat of the spinal cord	Submucosa of the oesophagus

12–16 mm. In February and March, migration is resumed and the L_2 arrive under the skin of the back. Here they moult to the L_3 stage, which can be palpated as distinct swellings ('warbles'). The L_3 makes a cutaneous perforation and the larvae breathe by applying their spiracles to the aperture. A fully grown third-stage larva measures 27–28 mm in length. After about 4–6 weeks in this site, they emerge in May–June and fall to the ground, where they pupate under leaves and loose vegetation for about five weeks. The adults then emerge, copulate and the females lay their eggs and die, all within 1–2 weeks. Oviposition can take place as soon as 24 hours after emergence from the puparium. The precise timings and duration of events in the life cycle will vary depending on latitude and ambient temperature. See **life cycle 46**.

Hypoderma spp. of veterinary importance are described in Table 3.5.

LIFE CYCLE 46. LIFE CYCLE OF *HYPODERMA* SPP.

During the summer months, females of *Hypoderma bovis* and *H. lineatum* lay one or 5–7 eggs, respectively, on individual hairs of the legs, abdomen, hips and chest of cattle (2). The eggs hatch into first-stage larvae that produce collagenolytic enzymes that allow them to penetrate the hair follicles and subsequently migrate through the internal organs of the host (3). Larvae of *H. bovis* follow the peripheral nerves, traverse the extradural adipose tissue of the lumbar and sacral segments of the spine and the bone marrow canal to penetrate the subcutaneous tissue of the back of the animal, where they establish (4). Larvae of *H. lineatum* penetrate the skin of the chest and travel through the oesophagus, mediastinum and chest wall to reach the subcutaneous tissue of the back (5). Here, first-stage larvae of both species form nodules, known as warbles (especially in late winter and early spring), and moult to second- and third-stage larvae (6). The latter release lytic enzymes that they have stored throughout their migration to form respiratory holes through which they leave the host to pupate in the external environment (7). The whole life cycle in cattle takes 8–10 months, while emergence of adult flies from the puparia takes 30–45 days, depending on external temperatures.

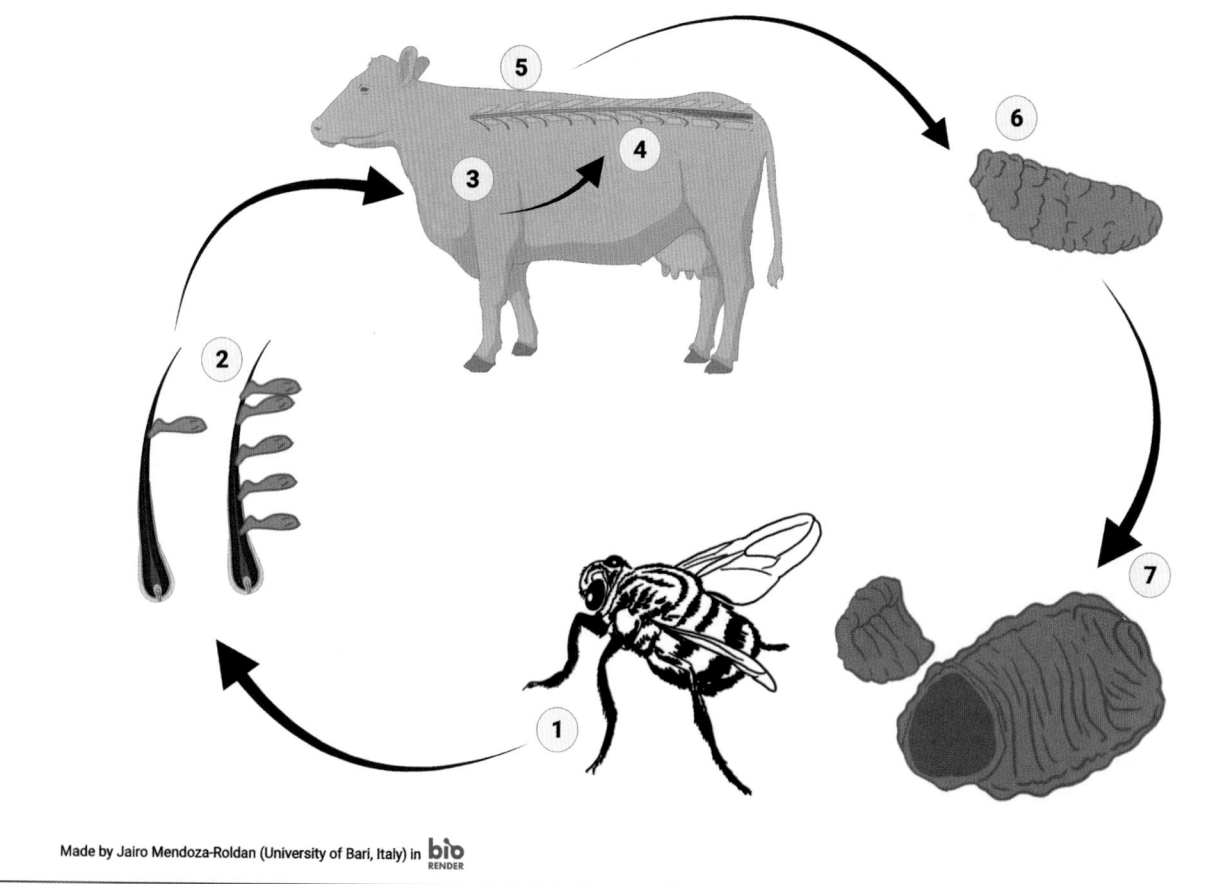

Made by Jairo Mendoza-Roldan (University of Bari, Italy) in **bio**RENDER

Table 3.5 *Hypoderma* of veterinary importance.

Species	Hosts	Site
Hypoderma bovis	Cattle	L_1, epidural fat; L_3, subcutaneous skin
Hypoderma lineatum	Cattle	L_1, oesophagus; L_3, subcutaneous skin
Hypoderma diana	Deer, occasionally horse, sheep	L_1, epidural fat; L_3, subcutaneous skin
Hypoderma tarandi (syn. *Oedemagena tarandi*)	Reindeer, caribou, rarely dog, horse	All larval stages in subcutaneous connective tissue
Hyoderma actaeon	Deer	Not known
Hypoderma sinense	Yak	Not known

Hypoderma bovis (warble fly)

Description, adult: Adult female *Hypoderma bovis* are about 15 mm in length and bee-like in appearance; the abdomen is covered with yellow-orange hairs with a broad band of black hairs around the middle. The hairs on the head and the anterior part of the thorax are greenish-yellow.

Life cycle: Characteristic features of the life cycle of *H. bovis* include that it attaches its eggs singly to hairs on the lower parts of the body (Fig. 3.52c). Following penetration through the skin, the larvae migrate along nerves until they reach the epidural fat of the spine in the region of the thoracic and lumbar vertebrae, where they overwinter.

Hypoderma lineatum (warble fly, heel fly)

Description, adult: Adult female *Hypoderma lineatum* are about 13 mm in length and bee-like in appearance; the abdomen is covered with yellow-orange hairs with a broad band of black hairs around the middle. The hairs on the head and the anterior part of the thorax are yellowish-white.

Life cycle: Characteristic features of the life cycle of *H. lineatum* include that it attaches its eggs in rows of six or more on individual hairs below the hocks (Fig. 3.52b). Following penetration of the skin, the larvae migrate between the fascial planes of muscles and along connective tissue, towards the region of the diaphragm. Eventually they reach the submucosa of the oesophagus where they spend the winter. Adult *H. lineatum* also usually emerge about one month before *H. bovis*.

Hypoderma diana

Description, adult: Adult female *Hypoderma diana* are about 15 mm and similar in appearance to cattle warble flies.

Description, larvae: The larvae are relatively host specific and live as subcutaneous parasites of deer. Mature larvae are thick and somewhat barrel-shaped, tapering anteriorly, and are 25–30 mm in length. Most segments bear short spines and the inner margins of the channels of the posterior peritremes are divergent. Larvae are dirty white in colour when newly emerged from the host, but rapidly turn dark brown. The pupa is almost black.

Life cycle: Females emerge with all their eggs fully developed. They have a relatively short lifespan in which they do not feed, and are able to mate and oviposit soon after emergence. Mating takes place off the host at aggregation points where females are intercepted in flight. The female flies lay between 300 and 600 eggs on the lower regions of the legs and lower body of the host animal, where they are glued to the hairs.

The first-stage larvae are less than 1 mm in length, hatch within a week and crawl down the hairs, burrowing either directly into the skin or into the hair follicles. The larvae then continue to burrow beneath the skin. *Hypoderma diana* migrates below the skin along nerves to the spinal cord. After about four months, usually by autumn, larvae reach the epidural fat of the spine in the region of the thoracic and lumbar vertebrae, where they overwinter.

The following spring, migration is not resumed until about nine months after oviposition when the larvae reach the skin of the back. A characteristic small swelling ('warble') is formed and a small hole is cut to the surface. A cystic nodule then begins to form around each larva. The larva reverses its position and rests with its two posterior spiracles close to the opening in the warble, allowing the larva to breathe. In this location, the larva moults twice, during which time it grows rapidly, more than doubling in length. Larval migration and growth take place in the host until April. The larvae then drop off the host animal and pupate in soil. The fly emerges after approximately 36 days.

The duration of pupation depends on ambient temperature and ground cover; higher pupal survival occurs when there is at least some grass cover and where the ground does not freeze.

Hypoderma tarandi (reindeer warble fly)

Synonym: *Oedemagena tarandi*

Description, adult: Large flies, about 15–18 mm, similar in appearance to *H. bovis*.

Description, larvae: Mature larvae are up to 3 cm in length. The posterior peritremes are heavily sclerotised, and have a broad interior channel leading to the lumen.

Life cycle: The life cycle of *Hypoderma tarandi* resembles that of other species in the genus *Hypoderma*. They are active in July and August, each female laying between 500 and 700 eggs, which are attached to the downy undercoat rather than the outer hair. The flanks, legs and rump are preferential laying sites. After approximately six days, the egg hatches on the skin and the larva then burrows into and under the skin. Unlike other *Hypoderma*, however, the L_1 migrates directly to the back in the subcutaneous connective tissue via the spine. When the larva comes to rest in about September to October, a swelling (warble) is created around it where it feeds on the animal's blood and body fluids. The L_3 makes a cutaneous perforation and the larvae breathe by applying their spiracles to the aperture. When growth is completed in the spring, the larva leaves the reindeer through its air hole and drops to the ground to pupate. It then emerges as an adult fly, completing the cycle.

Przhevalskiana silenus

The goat warble, *Przhevalskiana silenus* is common in the Mediterranean region.

Description, adult: The adult flies are 8–14 mm in length, have large eyes, a grey thorax and grey tessellated abdomen.

Description, larvae: The third-stage larvae are large (up to 25 mm in length), club-shaped, tapering towards the posterior end, with a pair of posterior spiracles. The body is composed of 11 segments with small spines at the conjunction of segments.

Life cycle: The life cycle of this species is similar in many ways to that of *Hypoderma*, the third-stage larva occurring under the skin of the back. After mating, the adult females lay about 100 black oval eggs that are about 0.8 mm in length. One to four eggs are glued on each hair. The first-stage larvae hatch from the eggs in 5–6 days and penetrate the skin into the subcutaneous tissue. They then migrate in the subcutis directly to the back. However, there is no resting site as seen with *Hypoderma*. Larvae reach the subcutaneous tissue of the host's back and flanks between the end of December and the beginning of February. Here they feed, grow and moult into their second and third stages, causing the characteristic warble swelling at the skin surface. The third-stage larva may be 15–18 mm in length and dark-coloured. The L_3 makes a cutaneous perforation, through which the larvae breathe by applying their spiracles to the aperture. When fully mature, in about February to April, the L_3 drops to the ground and pupates. The period required for pupation depends on weather conditions. The adults are active from April to June, lack mouthparts and survive only 5–10 days on resources accumulated during the larval period.

SUBFAMILY CUTEREBRINAE

The subfamily Cuterebrinae contains two genera of interest: *Cuterebra* and *Dermatobia*.

Cuterebra spp.

Species of the genus *Cuterebra* are largely parasites of rodents and rabbits but occasionally infest dogs and cats.

Description, adult: The adults are large flies (up to 30 mm in length) covered by dense short hairs, and have a blue-black abdomen. They have small non-functional mouthparts and do not feed as adults.

Description, larvae: Larvae have strongly curved mouth hooks and numerous strong body spines.

Life cycle: Females lay eggs on the ground near or within the entrance of host nests, or on grass near trails used by hosts. These are picked up by the passing host. The larvae enter the body, directly through the skin or through one of the orifices such as the nose, and then migrate subdermally. At their final, species-specific resting site the larvae eventually form a warble-like swelling. In rodents, the warble is often formed near the anus, scrotum or tail. Larval development may require 3–7 weeks. When mature, the larvae leave the host and drop to the ground where they pupate.

Dermatobia

The genus *Dermatobia* contains a single species of importance, *Dermatobia hominis*, which infests domestic animals and humans. This is a neotropical species, distributed from southern Mexico through Argentina, and inhabits wooded areas along forest margins of river valleys and lowlands. It is variously known as torsalo, the human bot fly or the American warble fly.

Dermatobia hominis (torsalo fly)

Description, adult: The adult *Dermatobia* fly resembles *Calliphora* in appearance, the short broad abdomen having a bluish metallic sheen, but there are only vestigial mouthparts covered by a flap. The female measures approximately 12 mm in length. Adults have a yellow-orange head and legs, and the thorax possesses a sparse covering of short setae. The arista of the antennae has setae on the outer side only.

Description, larvae: Mature larvae measure up to 25 mm long and are somewhat oval. They have 2–3 rows of strong spines on most of the segments. Larvae are narrowed at the posterior end, particularly the second-stage larva. The third-stage larva is more oval in shape with prominent flower-like anterior spiracles and posterior spiracles located in a small deep cleft (Fig. 3.53).

Life cycle: *Dermatobia* is most common in forest and bush regions, the latter known in many parts of South America as the 'monte'. The adult flies do not feed; instead nourishment is derived from food stores accumulated during the larval stages. The female has a sedentary habit, resting on leaves until oviposition is imminent, when she catches an insect (usually a mosquito) and attaches

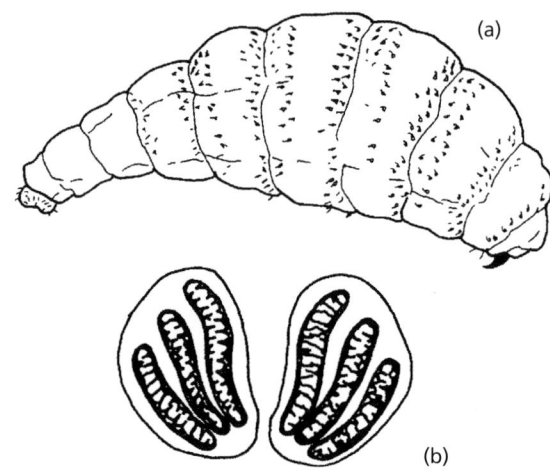

Fig. 3.53 *Dermatobia hominis*: (a) third-stage larva; (b) posterior spiracles.

a batch of up to 25 eggs to the underside of its abdomen or thorax. While attached to this transport host, the L_1 develop within the eggs in about a week, but do not hatch until the carrier insect lands on a warm-blooded animal to feed. The first-stage larvae hatch in response to the sudden temperature rise near the host's body. The larvae then penetrate the skin (often through the opening made by the transport fly) and migrate to the subcutis, where they develop to L_3 and breathe through a skin perforation in the fashion of *Hypoderma*. The larvae do not wander. The mature larvae emerge after about three months and pupate on the ground for a further month before the adult flies emerge. There may be up to three generations each year.

ORDER PSOCODEA (PHTHIRAPTERA)

The classification of lice has undergone considerable recent reorganisation and is likely to change further in the near future as a result of ongoing phylogenetic research. Today, the parasitic lice are grouped with the bark lice and book lice in the Order Psocodea. The parasitic lice form a monophyletic group described as the Phthiraptera, sometimes referred to as an infraorder, but the exact taxonomic status of this grouping is uncertain.

There are about 3500 species of Phthiraptera of which only about 20–30 are of major economic importance. The Phthiraptera was traditionally divided into two clades, the sucking lice (Anoplura) and the chewing lice (Mallophaga) (Fig. 3.54). Mallophaga literally means 'wool eating' but Mallophaga is not a monophyletic group. However, more recently four clades have been recognised: the Anoplura (sucking lice occurring on mammals only), Rhynchophthirina (including just two African species, one of which parasitses elephants and the other warthogs), Ischnocera (mostly chewing lice of birds, but with one family parasitising mammals) and the Amblycera (chewing lice, common on birds but also occurring on South American and Australian mammals). The description 'biting lice' is a misnomer and should be avoided, because all lice bite.

All the parasitic lice are permanent obligate ectoparasites that are highly host specific, many species even being localised on specific anatomical areas of their host. Clinical information relating to each species of veterinary importance can be found within the relevant

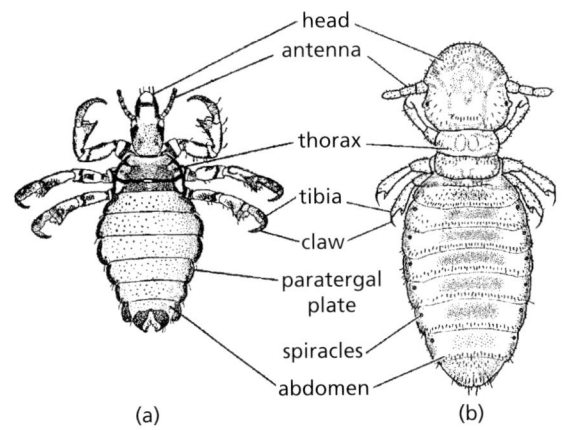

Fig. 3.54 Dorsal view of adult female (a) sucking louse *Haematopinus* (from Smart, 1943) and (b) chewing louse *Bovicola* (from Gullan and Cranston, 1994).

host chapter. They usually only leave their host to transfer to a new one. They are small insects, about 0.5–8 mm in length, dorsoventrally flattened with stout legs and claws for clinging tightly to fur, hair and feathers. All lice are wingless but this is a secondary adaptation to the parasitic lifestyle, and lice are thought to be derived originally from winged ancestors. They feed on epidermal tissue debris, parts of feathers, sebaceous secretions and blood. They usually vary in colour from pale beige to dark grey, but they may darken considerably on feeding. Most are blind, but a few species have simple photosensitive eye spots.

LOUSE LIFE CYCLES

Most lice have very similar life cycles. During a lifespan of about one month the female lays 20–200 operculate eggs ('nits'). These are usually whitish, and are glued to the hair or feathers where they may be seen with the naked eye (Fig. 3.55). From the egg hatches a nymph, which is similar to, though much smaller than, the adult. After three moults the fully grown adult is present. The whole cycle from egg to adult usually takes 2–3 weeks.

Lice that suck blood have piercing mouthparts, whereas lice that chew on skin, hair and feathers are equipped with mouthparts for cutting and grinding. Those on mammals ingest the outer layers of the hair shafts, dermal scales and blood scabs; the bird lice also feed

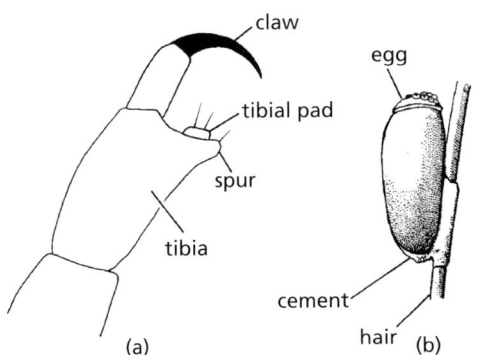

Fig. 3.55 Anopluran louse, *Haematopinus*: detail of (a) the tarsus and claw and (b) an egg attached to a hair. (From Smart, 1943.)

on skin scales and scabs but unlike the mammalian species, they can digest keratin so that they also eat feathers and down.

Heavy louse infestation is generally known as **pediculosis** (although more correctly this term refers specifically to human infestation with lice of the genus *Pediculus*). Some species of lice may act as intermediate hosts to the tapeworm *Dipylidium caninum*. However, despite this, lice are predominantly of veterinary interest because of the direct damage they can cause to their hosts, rather than as vectors. Hence, the effect of lice infestation is usually a function of their density. A small number of lice may present no problem and in fact may be considered as a normal part of the skin fauna. However, louse populations can increase dramatically, reaching high densities. Such heavy louse infestations may cause pruritus, alopecia, excoriation and self-wounding. The disturbance caused may result in lethargy and loss of weight gain or reduced egg production in birds. Severe infestation with sucking lice may cause anaemia. Heavy infestations are usually associated with young animals or older animals in poor health, or those kept in unhygienic conditions.

Transfer of lice from animal to animal or from herd to herd is usually by direct physical contact. Because lice do not survive for long off their host, the potential for animals to pick up infestations from dirty housing is limited, although it cannot be ignored. Occasionally, lice may also be transferred between animals by attachment to flies (phoresy).

In temperate habitats, louse populations are dynamic and exhibit pronounced seasonal fluctuations. The seasonal increase in louse populations may be exacerbated by winter housing, if the animals are in poor condition and particularly if animals are deprived of the opportunity to groom themselves properly. Louse infestation may also be indicative of some other underlying problem, such as malnutrition or chronic disease.

SUBORDER ANOPLURA

Anoplura are small insects, ranging from less than 0.5 to 8 mm in length in the adult; about 2 mm is an average length. The antennae are usually five-segmented; the eyes are reduced and usually absent, and there are no ocelli. The three thoracic segments are fused. The legs have only a single tarsal segment and a single claw; when the claw is retracted it makes contact with a thumb-like process on the tibia (the enclosed space having the diameter of the hairs of the host) and enables the louse to maintain firm attachment to an active host. There is one pair of spiracles (mesothoracic) on the thorax, and six pairs (segments 3–8) on the abdomen, which has nine segments in all.

The mouthparts are highly specialised and are not visible externally. They are highly adapted for piercing the skin of hosts. They are composed of three stylets in a ventral pouch which form a set of fine cutting structures. During feeding, the stylets are used to puncture the skin and blood is sucked into the mouth. The mouthparts have no palps and are usually retracted into the head when not in use so that all that can be seen of them is their outline in the head or their tips protruding.

The suborder Anoplura contains several families, two of which are of major importance in veterinary medicine: Haematopinidae and Linognathidae. The Microthoraciidae contains species that are of importance in camelids. The Polyplacidae and Hoploperidae contain species which are parasites of rodents. The Echinophthiridae contains species which are parasites of marine mammals and the Neolinagnathidae, of which there are only two species, are parasites of elephant shrews. Two other families of medical interest are the Pediculidae and Pthiridae.

FAMILY HAEMATOPINIDAE

The family Haematopinidae contains the genus *Haematopinus*, which is one of the primary genera of veterinary importance, species of which are among the largest lice of domestic mammals, up to 0.5 cm in length, found in cattle, pigs and horses.

Haematopinus

Twenty-six species have been described in the genus *Haematopinus*. All species are large lice, about 4–5 mm and possess prominent angular processes (ocular points or temporal angles) behind the antennae. The legs are of similar size, each terminating in a single large claw that opposes the tibial spur. Distinct sclerotised paratergal plates are visible on abdominal segments 2 or 3 to 8.

Haematopinus species of veterinary importance are listed in Table 3.6.

Haematopinus eurysternus (short-nosed louse)

Description: *Haematopinus eurysternus* is one of the largest lice of domestic mammals, measuring 3.4–4.8 mm in length. The louse is broad in shape with a short pointed head (Fig. 3.56). The head and thorax are yellow or greyish-brown and the abdomen blue-grey with a dark stripe on each side. The hard-shelled eggs are opaque and white and are pointed at their base.

Life cycle: Adult lice live for 10–15 days and when mature, females lay one egg per day for approximately two weeks. The eggs are glued to the hairs or bristles of the host and hatch in 1–2 weeks. The emerging nymphs resemble the adult louse except in size. Nymphs moult to become adults about 14 days after hatching. The female lice begin to lay eggs after feeding and mating.

Haematopinus quadripertusus (tail louse)

Description: *Haematopinus quadripertusus* is a large eyeless louse about 4–5 mm in length. It has a dark, well-developed thoracic

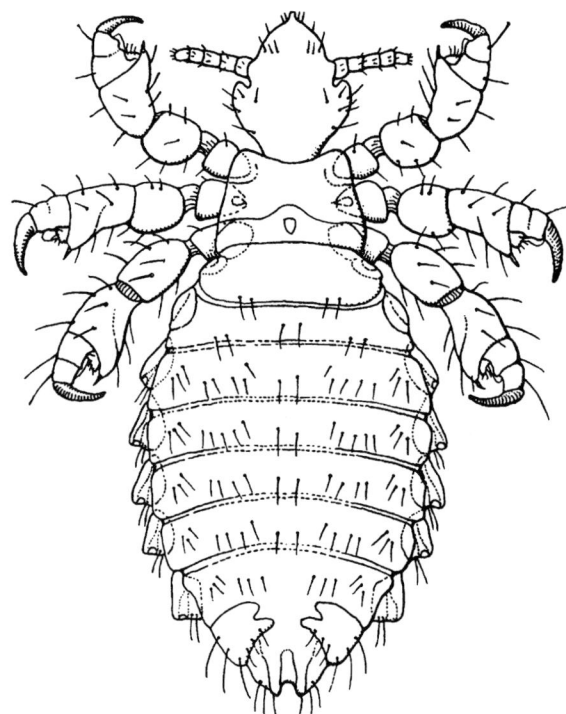

Fig. 3.56 Dorsal view of adult *Haematopinus*. (From Seguy, 1944.)

sternal plate. The legs are of similar sizes, each terminating in a single large claw that opposes the tibial spur.

Life cycle: During a lifespan of about a month, the female lays 50–100 operculate eggs ('nits') at a rate of 1–6 eggs per day. These are usually whitish, and are glued to the hair or feathers where they may be seen with the naked eye. The eggs of this louse are usually deposited on the tail hairs, which become matted with eggs in severe infestations. In very severe cases, the tail head may be shed. The eggs hatch after 9–25 days depending on climatic conditions. Nymphs disperse over the entire body surface of the host, but adults are most commonly found on the tail head. After three nymphal moults, over a period of about 12 days, the fully mature reproductive adult is present. Within four days, after feeding and mating, the adult female begins to lay eggs. The whole cycle from egg to adult takes 2–3 weeks.

Haematopinus tuberculatus (buffalo louse)

Synonym: *Haematopinus bufalieuropaei*

Description: A large louse measuring about 5.5 mm in length, with prominent ocular points but without eyes.

Haematopinus suis (hog louse)

Description: *Haematopinus suis* is a large greyish-brown louse with brown and black markings, measuring 5–6 mm in length. The head is long and with long mouthparts adapted for sucking blood. It has prominent angular processes, known as ocular points or temporal angles, located behind the antennae. Eyes are absent. The thoracic sternal plate is dark and well developed.

Table 3.6 *Haematopinus* species of veterinary importance.

Species	Hosts	Site
Haematopinus eurysternus	Cattle	Skin, poll, base of horns, ears, eyes and nostrils, occasionally tail switch
Haematopinus quadripertusus	Zebu, cattle	Tail and perineum
Haematopinus tuberculatus (syn. *Haematopinus bufalieuropaei*)	Buffalo, cattle	Skin, back, neck and horn base
Haematopinus suis	Pig	Skin, skin folds of the neck and jowl, flanks, insides of the legs
Haematopinus asini	Horse, donkey	Skin of head, neck, back, brisket and between the legs

Life cycle: Female lice lay 1–6 eggs per day. These are deposited singly, and are glued to the hairs on the lower parts of the body and in skinfolds on the neck, and on or in the ears, where they may be seen with the naked eye. The eggs hatch within 13–15 days. The emerging nymphs resemble the adult louse except in size. In about 12 days, the nymphs mature into adults and within four days, after feeding and mating, the female lice begin to lay eggs. The entire life cycle, from egg to adult, takes place on the host and is completed in 2–3 weeks. Adults may live for up to 40 days but cannot survive for more than a few days off the host. Between six and 15 generations may be completed per year, depending on environmental conditions.

Haematopinus asini (horse sucking louse)

Description: *Haematopinus asini* is 3–3.5 mm long and yellow-brown as an adult. The lice have three pairs of legs and a long narrow head with piercing mouthparts adapted for sucking blood and tissue fluids. The lice are found only on equines.

Life cycle: The lifespan of the adult louse is about one month, during which time the female lays operculate eggs at a rate of 1–6 eggs per day. These are usually whitish and are glued to the hair where they may be seen with the naked eye. They hatch in 1–2 weeks. Nymphs grow and moult over a period of about 12 days until the fully grown adult is present. After feeding and mating, the female lice may begin to lay eggs. Adults die after approximately 10–15 days of oviposition, and an average of around 24 eggs are laid per female. The whole cycle from egg to adult takes 3–4 weeks.

FAMILY LINOGNATHIDAE

There are two genera of veterinary importance in the family Linognathidae: *Linognathus* and *Solenopotes*. Members of this family are distinguished by the absence of eyes and ocular points. Most species of *Linognathus* are found on Artiodactyla, and a few on carnivores.

Linognathus

More than 60 species of *Linognathus* have been described, of which six are found on domestic animals (Table 3.7). Lice belonging to this genus do not have eyes or ocular points. The second and third pairs of legs are larger than the first pair and end in stout claws. The thoracic sternal plate is weakly developed or absent. Species differentiation is generally based on host and location on the body.

Linognathus vituli (long-nosed cattle louse)

Description: Bluish-black medium-sized lice with an elongated pointed head and body, approximately 2.5 mm in length (Fig. 3.57). There are no eyes or ocular points. Forelegs are small. Midlegs and hindlegs are larger with a large claw and tibial spur. There are two rows of setae on each segment. The thoracic sternal plate is weakly developed or absent. These lice are gregarious in habit, forming dense isolated clusters. While feeding, they extend their bodies in an upright position.

Life cycle: During a lifespan of about a month, the female lays a number of operculate eggs at a rate of about one egg per day. These are usually whitish, and are glued to the hair where they may be seen with the naked eye. The eggs hatch within 10–15 days. The nymph is similar in appearance to the adult though much smaller. The nymph increases in size as it moults through three instars, to eventually become an adult. The whole cycle from egg to adult takes 2–3 weeks.

Linognathus ovillus (long-nosed sheep louse)

Description: This sucking louse is bluish-black with a long narrow head and slender body. It measures approximately 2.5 mm in length.

Life cycle: Adult females lay a single egg per day. Eggs hatch in 10–15 days, giving rise to nymphs that require about two weeks to pass through three nymphal stages. The egg-to-adult life cycle requires about 20–40 days.

Table 3.7 *Linognathus* species of veterinary importance.

Species	Hosts	Site
Linognathus vituli	Cattle	Skin, head, neck and dewlap
Linognathus africanus	Goat, occasionally sheep	Skin, face
Linognathus ovillus	Sheep	Skin, mainly on face
Linognathus pedalis	Sheep	Skin, abdomen, legs, feet, scrotum
Linognathus stenopsis	Goat	Skin, head, neck, body
Linognathus setosus	Dog	Skin, head, neck, ears

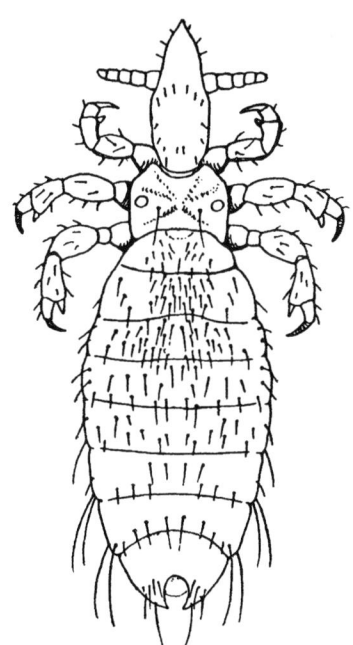

Fig. 3.57 Dorsal view of adult female *Linognathus*. (From Seguy, 1944.)

Linognathus pedalis (sheep foot louse)

Description: The foot louse *Linognathus pedalis* is bluish-grey, with a long pointed head and can reach up to 2 mm in length when fully engorged.

Life cycle: See *L. ovillus.*

Linognathus stenopsis (goat sucking louse)

Description: *Linognathus stenopsis* is up to 2 mm long when fully fed, with a long pointed head.

Life cycle: See *L. ovillus.*

Linognathus africanus (African sheep louse)

Description: Female lice are around 2.2 mm long and males 1.7 mm.

Life cycle: See *L. ovillus.*

Linognathus setosus (dog sucking louse)

Description: This species of louse is up to 2 mm long when fully fed, with a long pointed head. It does not have eyes or ocular points. The second and third pairs of legs are larger than the first pair and end in stout claws. The thoracic sternal plate is absent or if present is weakly developed. Paratergal plates are absent from the abdomen.

Life cycle: Adult females lay a single egg per day. Eggs hatch in 10–15 days, giving rise to nymphs that require about two weeks to pass through three nymphal stages. The egg-to-adult life cycle requires about 20–40 days.

Solenopotes

Description: Eyes and ocular points are absent and the lice have a short rostrum. There are no paratergal plates on the abdomen. The second and third pairs of legs are larger than the first pair and end in stout claws. These lice may be distinguished from the genus *Linognathus* by the presence of abdominal spiracles set on slightly sclerotised tubercles, which project slightly from each abdominal segment (Fig. 3.58). Also, in contrast to species of *Linognathus*, the thoracic sternal plate is distinct. *Solenopotes* species of veterinary importance are listed in Table 3.8.

Solenopotes capillatus

Description: Small bluish lice which tend to occur in clusters on the neck, head, shoulders, dewlap, back and tail. At 1.2–1.5 mm in length, *Solenopotes capillatus* is the smallest of the anopluran lice found on cattle.

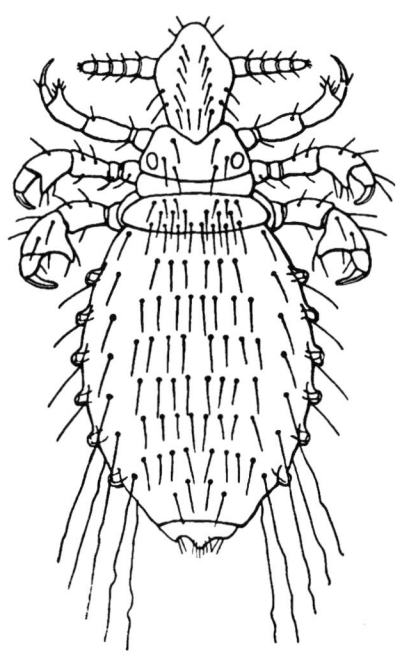

Fig. 3.58 Dorsal view of adult female *Solenopotes*. (From Seguy, 1944.)

Table 3.8 *Solenopotes* species of veterinary importance.

Species	Hosts	Site
Solenopotes capillatus	Cattle	Skin, neck, head, shoulders, dewlap, back, tail
Solenopotes burmeisteri	Red deer, sika deer	Skin, head, neck, shoulders
Solenopotes ferrisi	Elk	Skin, head, neck, shoulders
Solenopotes capreoli	Roe deer	Skin, head, neck, shoulders
Solenopotes muntiacus	Muntjac deer	Skin, head, neck, shoulders
Solenopotes tarandi	Reindeer, caribou	Skin, head, neck, shoulders
Solenopotes binipilosus	White-tailed deer, mule deer	Skin, head, neck, shoulders

Table 3.9 *Microthoracius* species of veterinary importance.

Species	Hosts	Site
Microthoracius mazzai	Llama, alpaca	Skin, neck
Microthoracius animor	Guanaco, llama, vicuna	Skin, neck
Microthoracius praelongiceps	Guanaco, llama, vicuna	Skin, neck
Microthoracius cameli	Camel	Skin, flanks, head, neck, withers

Life cycle: Females lay 1–2 eggs per day, and oviposition usually causes the hairs on which eggs are laid to bend. Eggs hatch after about 10 days and lice moult three times before reaching adulthood 11 days later. The egg-to-adult life cycle requires about five weeks.

FAMILY MICROTHORACIIDAE

This family contains four species of the genus *Microthoracius*. Three species parasitise llamas, and a fourth species is a parasite of camels (Table 3.9).

Microthoracius

Members of this family have a long spindle-shaped head with clypeal segments much shorter than the antenna–ocular segments. Eyes are evident and the antennae generally have five segments. Legs are similar in shape and size with pointed claws and a thick apical bristle.

Life cycle: The life cycle is typical, with eggs giving rise to three nymphal stages followed by the reproductive adult. The life cycle may be completed in as little as two weeks, and adults may live for up to six weeks.

Microthoracius mazzai (llama louse)

Description: *Microthoracius mazzai* has a very characteristic elongated, spindle-shaped head that is almost as long as its swollen rounded abdomen. The entire body is 1–2 mm in length.

Life cycle: The life cycle is typical, with eggs giving rise to three nymphal stages followed by the reproductive adult. The life cycle may be completed in as little as two weeks, and adults may live for up to six weeks.

Microthoracius cameli (camel sucking louse)

Description: *Microthoracius cameli* has a very characteristic elongated, spindle-shaped head that is almost as long as its swollen rounded abdomen. The entire body is 1–2 mm in length.

Life cycle: The life cycle is typical, with eggs giving rise to three nymphal stages followed by the reproductive adult. However, little precise detail is known.

FAMILY POLYPLACIDAE

Lice of the genus *Polyplax* infest rodents and may cause problems in laboratory colonies (Table 3.10). *Haemodipsus* is found on rabbits and hares and may be involved in the transmission of tularaemia in wild lagomorphs.

Polyplax

These lice are slender, 0.6–1.5 mm in length and yellow-brown in colour (Fig. 3.59). The head bears prominent five-segmented antennae, no eyes and no ocular points. There is a distinct sternal plate on the ventral surface of the thorax. The forelegs are small and the hindlegs are large with large claws and tibial spurs. The abdomen has 7–13 dorsal plates and approximately seven lateral plates on each side.

Table 3.10 *Polyplax* species of veterinary importance.

Species	Hosts	Site
Polyplax spinulosa	Rat	Fur
Polyplax serrata	Mouse	Fur

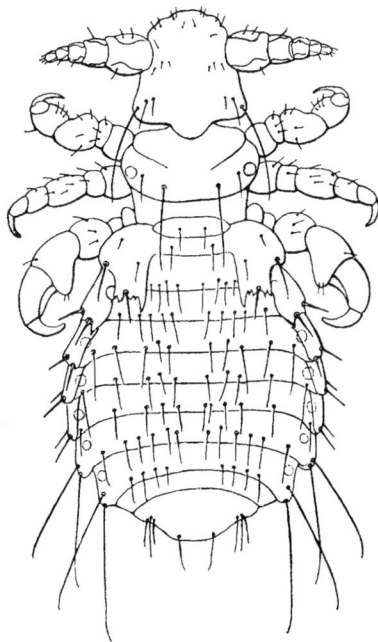

Fig. 3.59 Adult female *Polyplax* in dorsal view.

Life cycle: The lice spend their entire life cycle in the host and transmission occurs by direct contact. The eggs hatch in about 5–6 days to give rise to three nymphal stages, followed by the reproductive adult. The first nymphal stage is found on the entire body, while older stages are found predominantly on the front of the body. The entire life cycle is completed in about two weeks.

Polyplax spinulosa and Polyplax serrata

Description: The species are differentiated by the shape of the ventral thoracic plate. In *P. spinulosa* the ventral plate is triangular while in *P. serrata* it is pentagonal in shape.

FAMILY PEDICINIDAE

Lice of the genus *Pedicinus* are found on species of Old World monkeys.

FAMILY PEDICULIDAE

Lice of the genus *Pediculus*, which includes the human body louse (*P. humanus humanus*) and head louse (*P. humanus capitis*), are found on primates.

FAMILY PTHIRIDAE

Lice of the genus *Pthirus*, which includes the human crab louse (*P. pubis*), are found on primates.

SUBORDER AMBLYCERA

Amblycera are ectoparasites of birds, marsupials and New World mammals. Adults are medium-sized or relatively large lice, usually 2–3 mm in length. They have large rounded heads on which the eyes are reduced or absent. They are chewing lice with mouthparts consisting of distinct mandibles on the ventral surface and a pair of 2–4-segmented maxillary palps. The four-segmented antennae are protected in antennal grooves, so that only the last segment is visible. The Amblycera contains six families, of which the Menoponidae, Boopidae, Gyropidae and Trimenoponidae are of relevance to veterinary medicine.

FAMILY MENOPONIDAE

Several genera are of veterinary importance on birds. *Menacanthus* can cause severe anaemia and is the most pathogenic louse of adult domestic hens and cage birds, in particular canaries. *Menopon* is found mainly on the domestic hen but it will spread to other fowl, such as turkeys and ducks, which are in contact. *Holomenopon*, *Ciconiphilus* and *Trinoton* are found on ducks; *Amyrsidea* and *Mecanthus* are found on gamebirds.

Menacanthus

The taxonomy of this genus is highly uncertain, with over 100 species described, although recent studies have synonymised dozens of species. *Menacanthus* species of veterinary importance are listed in Table 3.11. This genus includes the chicken body louse or yellow body louse, *Menacanthus stramineus*, which is a relatively large pathogenic species.

Menacanthus stramineus (yellow body louse, chicken body louse)

Description: Adult males measure approximately 2.8 mm in length and the female 3.3 mm. The head is almost triangular in shape and the ventral portion of the front of the head is armed with a pair of spine-like processes. The palps and four-segmented antennae are distinct. The antennae are club-shaped and mostly concealed beneath the head. The flattened abdomen is elongated and broadly rounded posteriorly with two dorsal rows of setae on each abdominal segment. There are three pairs of short, two-clawed legs (Fig. 3.60). The eggs have characteristic filaments on the anterior half of the shell and on the operculum.

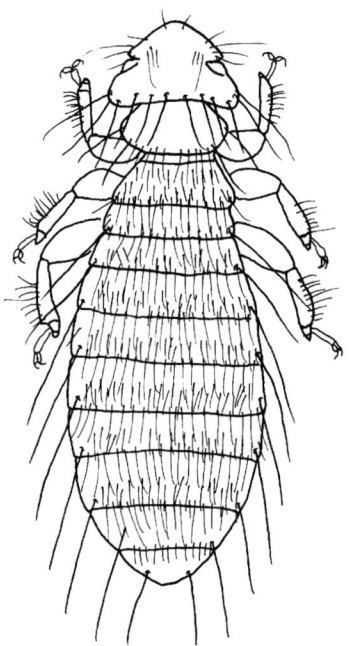

Fig. 3.60 Adult *Menacanthus stramineus* (dorsal view).

Menopon

Species of the genus *Menopon* are feather lice found on chickens and other domestic birds (**Table 3.12**).

Menopon gallinae (shaft louse)

Description: Pale yellow, rapidly moving louse. It is a small louse; adults measure approximately 2 mm in length. *Menopon gallinae* has small palps and a pair of four-segmented antennae, folded into grooves in the head. The abdomen is tapered posteriorly in the female but rounded in the male and has a sparse covering of small to medium-length setae on its dorsal surface (Fig. 3.61).

Menopon leucoxanthum

Description: A small, rapidly moving louse that especially favours the preen gland, inhibiting production of the oily secretion and causing 'wet feather'.

Life cycle: The nymph moults three times over 2–3 weeks before giving rise to the reproductive adult. Individuals are highly mobile and move rapidly.

Table 3.11 *Menacanthus* species of veterinary importance.

Species	Hosts	Site
Menacanthus stramineus	Chicken, turkey, guinea fowl, peafowl, pheasant, quail, cage birds (canary)	Skin, breast, thighs, vent, wings and head
Menacanthus layali	Gamebirds	Skin, body

Table 3.12 *Menopon* species of veterinary importance.

Species	Hosts	Site
Menopon gallinae	Chicken, turkey, duck, pigeon	Thigh and breast feathers
Menopon leucoxanthum (syn. *Holomenopon leucoxanthum*)	Duck	Feathers, especially preen gland
Menopon pallens	Gamebirds	Thigh and breast feathers

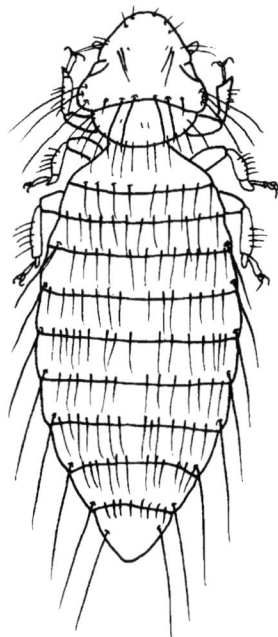

Fig. 3.61 Adult *Menopon gallinae* (dorsal view).

FAMILY BOOPIDAE

Members of this family occur on marsupials. *Heterodoxus* may be of importance on dogs and other Canidae.

Heterodoxus

Species in the genus *Heterodoxus* are primarily parasites of kangaroos and wallabies in Australia and New Guinea. The ancestor of the dog louse, *Heterodoxus spiniger*, presumably colonised dingos after their transport to Australia by early humans. From the dingo, the louse transferred to domestic dogs and from there the louse spread to other parts of the world.

Heterodoxus spiniger

Description: *Heterodoxus spiniger* is a large, slender, yellowish coloured louse. Adults are about 5 mm in length, with a dense covering of thick, medium and long setae (Fig. 3.62). It can easily be distinguished from other lice infesting domestic mammals since the tarsi end in two claws, as opposed to one in the Anoplura and Trichodectidae.

Life cycle: The life cycle is typical, with eggs giving rise to three nymphal stages followed by the reproductive adult. However, little detail is known.

FAMILY GYROPIDAE

Gyropus and *Gliricola* may be important in guinea pigs; *Aotiella* is found on primates. Species of this family may be distinguished from other families of chewing lice because the tarsi of the midlegs and hindlegs have either one or no claws.

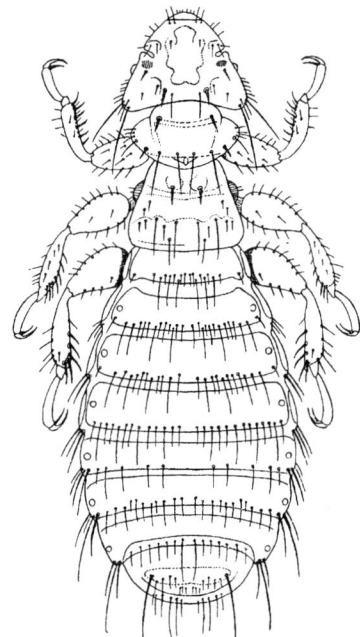

Fig. 3.62 Adult female *Heterodoxus spiniger* in ventral view. (From Seguy, 1944.)

Gyropus ovalis (guinea pig louse)

Description: *Gyropus ovalis* is a chewing louse with club-shaped antennae positioned within grooves in the head. The head is broad and rounded with four-segmented maxillary palps and stout mandibles. The body is pale yellow in colour, oval in shape and 1–1.5 mm in length and has eight abdominal segments (Fig. 3.63).

Life cycle: The life cycle is typical, with eggs giving rise to three nymphal stages followed by the reproductive adult. However, little precise detail is known.

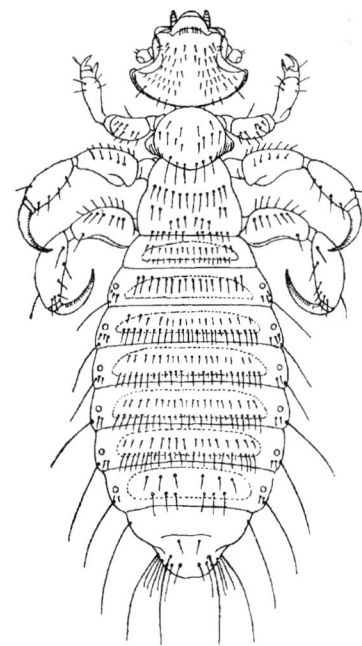

Fig. 3.63 Adult female *Gyropus ovalis*. (From Seguy, 1944.)

Gliricola porcelli (guinea pig louse)

Description: A very similar species to *Gyropus ovalis*. However, *G. porcelli* is a slender yellow louse, typically measuring 1–2 mm in length and 0.3–0.4 mm in width (Fig. 3.64). The head is longer than it is wide and is rounded posteriorly. The maxillary palps have two segments. Antennae are four-segmented with pedicellate terminal segments and are almost concealed by the antennal fossae. The five pairs of abdominal spiracles are located ventrally within distinct sclerotised spiracular plates. The stout legs are modified for grasping hair but have no tarsal claws. A ventral furrow on the abdomen aids attachment to hair.

FAMILY TRIMENOPONIDAE

Trimenopon is found on guinea pigs.

Trimenopon hispidum

Description: Similar in appearance to *Gyropus ovalis* but *Trimenopon hispidum* has five abdominal segments compared to *G. ovalis* with eight.

SUBORDER ISCHNOCERA

The Ischnocera includes five families, three of which, the Philopteridae on domestic birds and mammals and the Trichodectidae and Bovicoliidae on mammals, are of major veterinary importance.

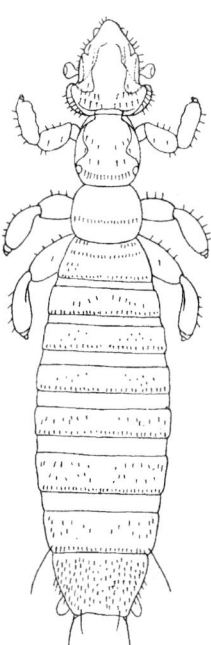

Fig. 3.64 Adult female *Gliricola porcelli*. (From Seguy, 1944.)

FAMILY PHILOPTERIDAE

The family Philopteridae contains the genera *Cuclotogaster*, *Lipeurus*, *Struthiolipeurus*, *Meinertzhageniella* and *Columbicola* and the large genera *Goniodes*, *Goniocotes*, species of which are important parasites of domestic birds (Table 3.13). Other species of lesser importance belong to the genera *Anaticola*, *Acidoproctus*, *Anatoecus* and *Ornithobius*, which are found on ducks, geese and other waterfowl; *Lagopoecus*, which are found on gamebirds; *Struthiolipeurus* found on ostrich; *Tricholipeurus* found on deer; and *Trichophilopterus* found on primates. Only key species are described in more detail below. The Philopteridae have five-segmented antennae and paired claws on the tarsi.

Cuclotogaster heterographus (head louse)

The poultry head louse *Cuclotogaster heterographus* is an important widespread species.

Description: *Cuclotogaster heterographus* has a rounded body with a large slender head that is rounded at the front (Fig. 3.65). Adult males measure approximately 2.5 mm and females 2.6 mm in length. The first segment of the antennae of males is long and thick and bears a posterior process. The abdomen is elongate in the male and barrel-shaped in the female, with dark brown lateral tergal plates. Three long bristles project from each side of the dorsal surface of the head and the five-segmented antennae are fully exposed. Each leg has two tarsal claws.

Lipeurus caponis (wing louse)

A grey, slow-moving louse found close to the skin on the underside of the large wing feathers.

Description: *Lipeurus caponis* is an elongated narrow species, about 2.2 mm in length and 0.3 mm in width (Fig. 3.66). The head is long and rounded at the front, and the antennae are five-segmented and

Table 3.13 Species of *Cuclotogaster*, *Lipeurus*, *Struthiolipeurus*, *Meinertzhageniella* and *Columbicola* of veterinary importance.

Species	Hosts	Site
Cuclotogaster heterographus	Chicken, other poultry	Skin, feathers, head and neck
Cuclotogaster obsuricor	Gamebirds	Skin, feathers, head and neck
Lipeurus caponis	Chicken, pheasant	Skin, wing and tail feathers
Lipeurus maculosus	Gamebirds	Skin, wing and tail feathers
Struthiolipeurus struthionis	Ostrich	Skin, wing and tail feathers
Struthiolipeurus nandu	Ostrich	Skin, wing and tail feathers
Struthiolipeurus stresmanni	Ostrich	Skin, wing and tail feathers
Struthiolipeurus rheae	Ostrich	Skin, wing and tail feathers
Meinertzhageniella lata	Rhea	Skin, wing and tail feathers
Meinertzhageniella schubarti	Rhea	Skin, wing and tail feathers
Dahlemhornia asymmetrica	Emu	Skin, wing and tail feathers
Columbicola columbae	Pigeon, dove	Skin, wings, head, neck

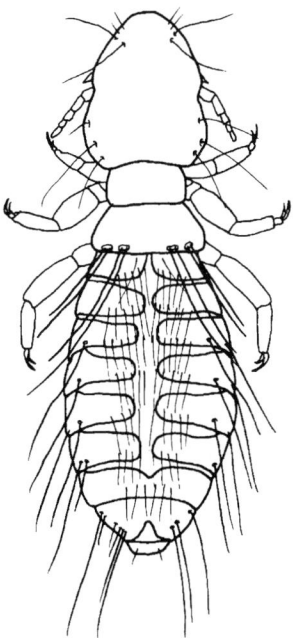

Fig. 3.65 Adult female *Cuclotogaster heterographus* (dorsal view).

fully exposed. The legs are narrow and bear two tarsal claws. Characteristically, the hindlegs are about twice as long as the first two pairs of legs. There are characteristic small angular projections on the head in front of the antennae. There are relatively few dorsal hairs on the abdomen.

Struthiolipeurus

Narrow-bodied lice with large heads found close to the skin on the underside of the large wing feathers of ostrich.

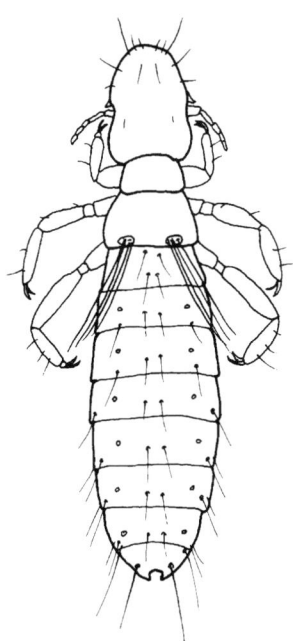

Fig. 3.66 Adult *Lipeurus caponis* (dorsal view).

Life cycle: The biology of these lice has not been fully studied, but is thought to be typical: egg, several nymphal stages and adult requiring about one month for completion. Eggs are deposited on feather barbs.

Goniodes

Goniodes species of veterinary importance are listed in Table 3.14.

Description: These are very large brown lice, with males measuring 3–4 mm and females around 5 mm in length. They have a broad head, which is concave posteriorly, producing marked angular corners at the posterior margins. The head bears two large bristles, which project from each side of its dorsal surface. The antennae have five segments and are fully exposed. Each leg has two tarsal claws.

Life cycle: During a lifespan of about a month, the female lays 200–300 operculate eggs. These are usually whitish and are glued to the hair or feathers, where they may be seen with the naked eye. The eggs hatch within 4–7 days and the lice spend their entire life cycle on the host, feeding on feather debris. The nymph that hatches from the egg is similar to, though much smaller than, the adult. The nymph moults three times over 2–3 weeks before giving rise to the reproductive adult.

Goniodes gigas (large chicken louse)

Description: Very large brown lice occurring on the body and feathers of the fowl. Males measure 3–4 mm and females 5 mm in length.

Goniodes dissimilis (brown chicken louse)

Description: *Goniodes dissimilis* is a large louse about 3 mm in length and brown in colour (Fig. 3.67).

Goniodes meleagridis

Description: These lice are characterised by broad mandibles located ventrally on the head, short antennae (3–5 segments) and a dorsoventrally flattened body. They are large, the adults reaching up to 5 mm in length.

Table 3.14 *Goniodes* species of veterinary importance.

Species	Hosts	Site
Goniodes gigas	Chicken, pheasant, guinea fowl	Skin and body feathers
Goniodes dissimilis	Chicken	Skin and body feathers
Goniodes meleagridis	Turkey	Skin and body feathers
Goniodes colchici	Gamebirds	Skin and body feathers
Goniodes dispar	Gamebirds	Skin and body feathers
Goniodes pavonis	Peafowl	Skin and body feathers

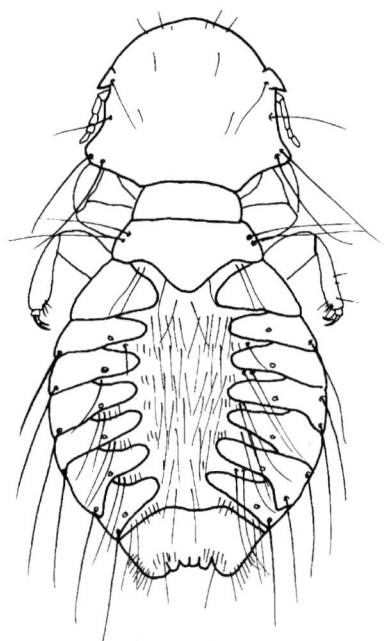

Fig. 3.67 Adult female *Goniodes dissimilis* (dorsal view).

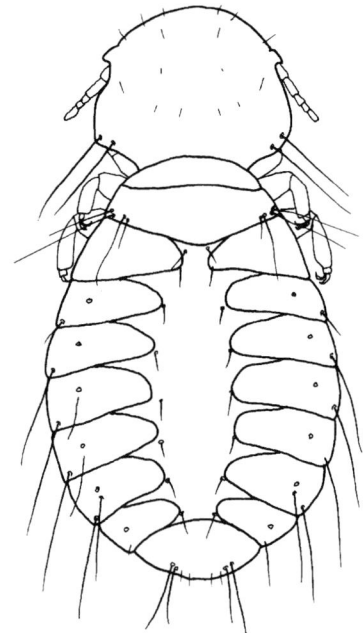

Fig. 3.68 Adult female *Goniocotes gallinae* (dorsal view).

Goniocotes

This genus includes the poultry fluff louse, *Goniocotes gallinae*. *Goniocotes* species of veterinary importance are listed in Table 3.15.

Goniocotes gallinae (fluff louse)

Description: *Goniocotes gallinae* is one of the smallest lice found on poultry, at about 0.7–1.3 mm in length. It has a pale yellow, almost circular body (**Fig. 3.68**). The head is rounded and carries two large bristles projecting from each side of its dorsal surface. The antennae are five-segmented, fully exposed and the same in both sexes. There are two tarsal claws on each leg and few hairs on the dorsal abdomen.

Columbicola

The genus *Columbicola* includes 82 species affecting pigeons and doves. Members of this genus are slender elongate lice, with most species showing sexual dimorphism of the antennae, with males having a much enlarged scape and distally expanded third segment. The head has a distinct bilobed dorso-anterior head plate with a pair of forward-directed broad medio-anterior setae. *Columbicola columbae* is a pale yellow slender louse usually 2–3 mm in length.

Table 3.15 *Goniocotes* species of veterinary importance.

Species	Hosts	Site
Goniocotes gallinae	Chicken	Feathers
Goniocotes chryocephalus	Gamebirds	Feathers
Goniocotes obscurus	Gamebirds	Feathers
Goniocotes microthorax	Gamebirds	Feathers

The head of the male has a long pair of medio-posterior setae extending beyond the posterior margin.

Life cycle: Eggs of this species are usually attached to the feathers close to the skin. There are three nymphal stages similar to, though much smaller than, the adult. Development of the final stage gives rise to the fully mature reproductive adult.

The family Trichodectidae contains the genera *Felicola*, the sole species of louse found on cats; *Trichodectes*, found on dogs and primates; and *Eutrichophilus* and *Cebidicola*, found on primates.

Felicola

Species belonging to this genus are found on members of the cat family and include *Felicola subrostratus*, the only species that commonly occurs on cats.

Life cycle: Eggs are laid on the cat fur and hatch in 10–20 days. The adult stage is reached within 2–3 weeks and the egg-to-adult life cycle requires about 30–40 days.

Felicola subrostratus (cat biting louse)

Description: This louse is beige or yellow in colour, with transverse brown bands. Adults are an average of 1–1.5 mm in length. The shape of the head is very characteristic, being triangular and pointed anteriorly (Fig. 3.69). Ventrally there is a median longitudinal groove on the head, which fits around the individual hairs of the host. The antennae have three segments, are fully exposed and are similar in both sexes. The legs are small, slender and end in single

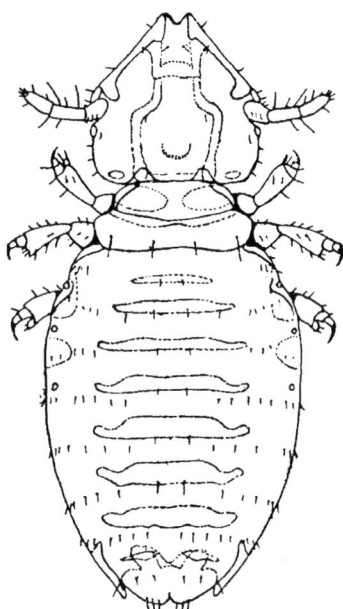

Fig. 3.69 Adult female *Felicola subrostratus* in ventral view. (From Seguy, 1944.)

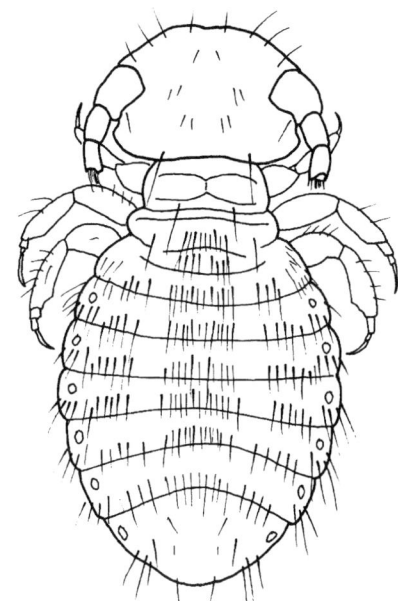

Fig. 3.70 Adult female *Trichodectes canis* in ventral view. (From Seguy, 1944.)

claws. The abdomen has only three pairs of spiracles and is smooth with few setae.

Trichodectes

Species belonging to this genus are found on members of the dog family. The single species of veterinary importance, *Trichodectis canis*, is commonly found on domestic dogs.

Trichodectes canis (dog biting louse)

Description: *Trichodectes canis* is a small, broad, yellowish-coloured louse (Fig. 3.70). It is 1–2 mm in length, with dark markings. The head is broader than long and the antennae are three-segmented, short and exposed. The legs are stout and their tarsi bear single claws, with which they tightly grasp the hair of their host. The abdomen has six pairs of spiracles on segments 2–6, and many rows of large thick setae.

Life cycle: *Trichodectes canis* commonly infests the head, neck and tail regions, where it attaches to the base of a hair using its claws or mandibles. The female lays several eggs per day for approximately 30 days. Eggs hatch in 1–2 weeks and give rise to three nymphal stages. The nymphs mature into reproductive adults within about two weeks. The egg-to-adult life cycle requires about 30–40 days. See **life cycle 47**.

FAMILY BOVICOLIDAE

The family Bovicolidae contains the genus *Bovicola* (formerly *Damalinia*), found on cattle, sheep, horses and deer. *Werneckiella*, sometimes described as a genus, but here described as a subgenus of

Bovicola, contains the species *Bovicola* (*Werneckiella*) *ocellatus* found on donkeys.

Bovicola

This genus includes a number of morphologically similar host-specific species of lice on domestic animals (Table 3.16).

Bovicola ovis

Synonym: *Damalinia ovis*

Description: These chewing lice are up to 3 mm long, reddish-brown in colour, with a relatively large head that is as wide as the body and rounded anteriorly. The mouthparts are ventral. *Bovicola* have three-segmented antennae and a single claw on each tarsus.

Life cycle: Female lice live about one month and lay 1–3 operculate eggs per day. The eggs are usually whitish, and are glued to the hair where they may be seen with the naked eye. *Bovicola ovis* prefers areas close to the skin such as the back, neck and shoulder, but is highly mobile and severe infestations will spread over the whole body. It is estimated to take about 20 weeks for a population of *B. ovis* on a sheep to increase from 5000 to half a million, under favourable conditions. A nymph hatches from the egg; nymphs are similar to, though much smaller than, the adult. The nymph moults twice, at 5–9-day intervals, until eventually moulting to become an adult. The whole cycle from egg to adult takes 2–3 weeks.

The mouthparts of these lice are adapted for biting and chewing the outer layers of the hair shafts, dermal scales and blood scabs. *Bovicola ovis* is capable of rapid population expansion and this is thought to be aided by their ability to change from sexual to asexual reproduction by parthenogenesis (although this has not yet been demonstrated definitively). Hence, highly female-biased sex ratios may be common in a growing population.

LIFE CYCLE 47. LIFE CYCLE OF *TRICHODECTES CANIS*

Trichodectes canis live permanently on the cutaneous surface and the fur of the dog (1). Females lay eggs (nits) on the hair shaft (2), to which they are glued by a sticky substance that forms an anchor.

From the nits, nymphs hatch within one week (3) and then develop through three stages (4, 5) to become adults (1). The life cycle takes 2–3 weeks.

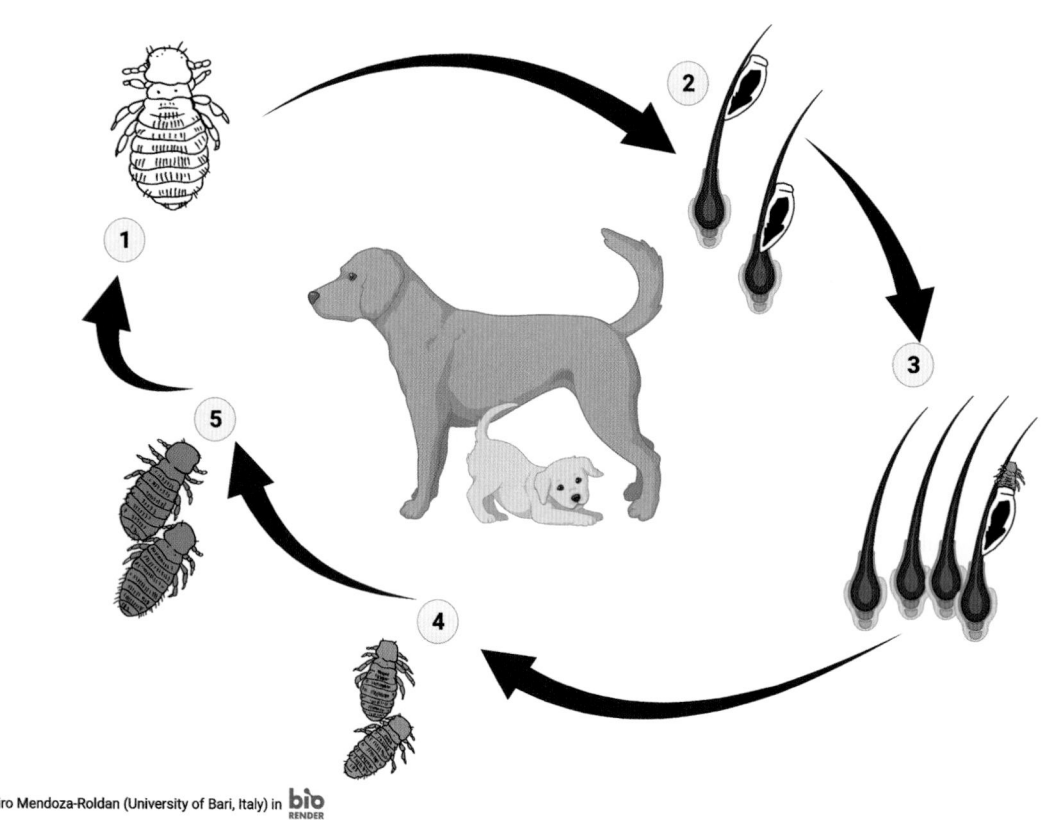

Made by Jairo Mendoza-Roldan (University of Bari, Italy) in **bio**RENDER

Table 3.16 *Bovicola* species of veterinary importance.

Species	Hosts	Site
Bovicola ovis (syn. *Damalinia ovis*)	Sheep	Skin, mainly on the back and upper parts of the body
Bovicola caprae (syn. *Damalinia caprae*)	Goat	Skin, head, back and flanks
Bovicola limbata (syn. *Damalinia limbata*)	Goat (angora)	Skin, back and flanks
Bovicola bovis (syn. *Damalinia bovis*)	Cattle	Skin, head, poll, forehead, neck, shoulders, back, rump, and occasionally the tail switch
Bovicola equi (syn. *Damalinia equi*, *Trichodectes parumpilosus*, *Werneckiella equi equi*)	Horse	Skin, neck, flank, tail base
Bovicola (*Werneckiella*) *ocellatus*	Donkey	Skin, face, neck, back, flanks
Bovicola tibialis	Deer (fallow)	Skin, neck, back, flanks
Bovicola mayeri	Deer (roe)	Skin, neck, back, flanks
Bovicola maai	Deer (sika)	Skin, neck, back, flanks
Bovicola forticula	Deer (muntjac)	Skin, neck, back, flanks

Bovicola bovis (red louse, cattle chewing louse)

Synonym: *Damalinia bovis*

Description: *Bovicola bovis* are a reddish-brown in colour with dark transverse bands on the abdomen. Adult lice are up to 2 mm long and 0.35–0.55 mm in width. The head is relatively large, as wide as the body, and is rounded anteriorly (Fig. 3.71). The mouthparts are ventral and are adapted for chewing. The legs are slender and are adapted for moving among the hair. The claws, on each leg, are small. The nymphs also have lighter sclerotisation and less distinct banding than adult lice. The nymph is similar in appearance though much smaller than the adult.

Life cycle: During a lifespan of about a month, the female lays an egg every two days on average. These eggs are usually whitish, and are glued singly to the hair shaft where they may be seen with the naked eye. The eggs hatch after 7–10 days and each nymphal instar lasts 5–6 days. After three nymphal stages, the nymph moults again

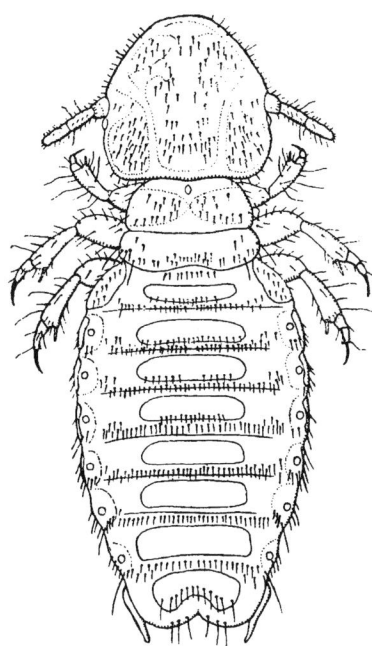

Fig. 3.71 Dorsal view of adult female *Bovicola bovis*. (From Seguy, 1944.)

to become an adult. The whole cycle from egg to adult takes 2–3 weeks. Adults may live for up to 10 weeks. *Bovicola bovis* is also believed to be capable of increasing its rate of population growth by parthenogenesis. As a result, highly female-biased sex ratios may be commonly found in a growing population.

Bovicola equi (horse louse)

Synonyms: *Damalinia equi, Trichodectes parumpilosus, Werneckiella equi equi*

Description: These lice are up to 1–2 mm long and reddish-brown in colour. The relatively large head is as wide as the wingless body, and rounded anteriorly. The mouthparts are ventral. This species has a three-segmented antenna and a single claw on the tarsi.

Life cycle: Female lice lay one egg approximately every day, glued singly on to a hair shaft. The eggs are usually whitish and may be seen with the naked eye. Females avoid ovipositing on the coarse hairs of the mane and tail, instead preferring finer hairs on the side of the neck, the flanks and the tail base. In severe cases the infestation may cover most of the body. The egg hatches into a nymph that is similar in appearance to the adult, though the nymph is much smaller, with lighter sclerotisation and less distinct banding. The cycle from egg to adult takes 3–4 weeks.

SUBORDER RHYNCHOPHTHIRINA

The Rhynchophthirina is a very small suborder including just two species, which are parasites of elephants and warthogs.

ORDER SIPHONAPTERA

Fleas (Siphonaptera) are small, wingless, obligate blood-feeding insects. Both sexes are blood feeders and only the adults are parasitic. The order is relatively small, with about 2500 described

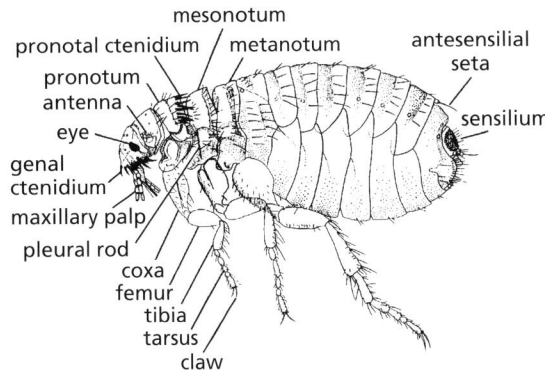

Fig. 3.72 Morphological features of an adult flea. (From Gullan and Cranston, 1994.)

species, almost all of which are morphologically extremely similar. Over 95% of flea species are ectoparasites of mammals, while the others are parasites of birds.

Fleas (Fig. 3.72) are dark-brown wingless insects, usually between 1 and 6 mm in length, with females being larger than males. The body colour may vary from light brown to black. The body is laterally compressed with a glossy surface, allowing easy movement through hairs and feathers. Eyes, when present, are simply dark photosensitive spots and the antennae, which are short and club-like, are recessed into the head. The third pair of legs is much longer than the others, an adaptation for jumping. The head and first segment of the thorax (pronotum) may bear ventral (genal) or posterior (pronotal) rows of dark spines called ctenidia or 'combs', and these are important features used in identification (Table 3.17).

Many species of flea are able to parasitise a range of hosts. This, combined with their mobility, which allows them to move easily between hosts, makes them parasites of considerable medical and veterinary importance and makes them difficult to control.

Once on their host, fleas feed daily or every other day. Females require significantly more blood than males and an initial blood meal is required to start egg production. Blood feeding may have a range of damaging effects on the host animal, causing inflammation, pruritus or anaemia. Fleas may also act as vectors of bacteria, protozoa, viruses and tapeworms. However, in veterinary entomology, fleas are probably of most importance as a cause of cutaneous hypersensitivity reactions. Though most important in dogs, cats and poultry, their readiness to parasitise humans as alternative hosts gives the fleas of these domestic animals a relevance in public health. Ruminants, horses and pigs do not have their own species of fleas.

For clinical information see the relevant host chapter.

Table 3.17 Morphological differentiation of fleas based on presence or absence of pronotal and genal combs.

No combs present	Pronotal combs only	Both pronotal and genal combs	
		Few combs	Several combs
Xenopsylla cheopis	*Nosopsyllus fasciatus*	*Archaeopsylla erinacei*	*Ctenocephalides felis*
Pulex irritans	*Ceratophyllus gallinae*		*Ctenocephalides canis*
Echidnophaga gallinacea			*Spilopsyllus cuniculi* *Leptopsylla segnis*

FLEA LIFE CYCLES

Fleas are holometabolous and go through four life-cycle stages: egg, larva, pupa and adult (Fig. 3.73). The ovoid eggs have smooth surfaces and may be laid on the ground or on the host, from which they soon drop off. Hatching occurs in two days to two weeks, depending on the temperature of the surroundings. The larvae are maggot-like, with a distinct, brownish head, and body segments bear a circlet of backwardly directed bristles that, together with the anal struts on the last segment, enable the larva to move. There are no appendages. They have chewing mouthparts and feed on organic debris (skin, fur or feathers) but also particularly on the faeces of the adult fleas, which contain blood and give the larvae a reddish colour. The larva moults twice, the final stage being about 5–10 mm long, and then spins a cocoon, from which the adult emerges. Moulting and pupation are dependent on the ambient temperature and humidity. Under ideal conditions, the entire cycle may take only 18 days to complete, although it can range from six to 12 months.

Two broad trends in flea life cycles can be seen. A simple association with the nest habitat is preserved in many species of the family Ceratophyllidae, characterised by infrequent and brief associations with the host and often considerable adult movement between hosts and nests. In contrast, many species of the family Pulicidae show prolonged adult associations with the host. However, within these broad categories, a high degree of variation may exist. A few genera remain permanently attached throughout adult life. These are the burrowing, or 'stickfast', fleas, whose females are embedded in the skin, within nodules. Only the posterior part of these fleas communicates with the surface, allowing the eggs or larvae to drop to the ground and develop in the usual manner.

There are generally considered to be 15 or 16 families and 239 genera. Only two families contain species of veterinary importance: the **Ceratophyllidae** and the **Pulicidae**.

FAMILY CERATOPHYLLIDAE

The Ceratophyllidae is a large family containing over 500 species, of which about 80 are parasites of birds and the remainder are parasites of rodents.

Nosopsyllus

Species in this genus are parasites of rodents, including squirrels, with the one cosmopolitan species of veterinary significance, the northern rat flea *Nosopsyllus fasciatus*.

Nosopsyllus fasciatus (northern rat flea)

Description: The flea is elongated, about 3–4 mm in length and has a pronotal comb with 18–20 spines. A genal comb is absent (Fig. 3.74). Eyes are present and the head carries a row of three setae below the eye. The frontal tubercle on the head of both sexes is conspicuous. There are three or four bristles on the inner surface of the hind femur.

Life cycle: The life cycle is typical: egg, three larval stages, pupa and adult. Life-cycle development may be completed at temperatures as low as 5 °C. Larval stages are found only in the nest or burrow. The larvae of this species may pursue and solicit faecal blood meals from adult fleas. The larvae grasp the adult in the region of the sensilium using their large mandibles. Adults respond by defecating stored semi-liquid blood, which is then imbibed by the larvae directly from the anus.

Ceratophyllus

Ceratophyllus parasitises mainly squirrels and other rodents, but contains species of veterinary importance that feed on poultry and other birds. *Ceratophyllus* species of veterinary importance are listed in Table 3.18.

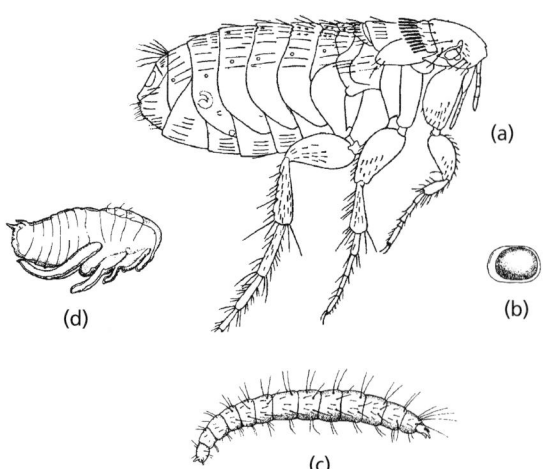

Fig. 3.73 Life cycle of a typical flea: (a) adult; (b) egg; (c) larva; (d) pupa. (Adapted from Seguy, 1944.)

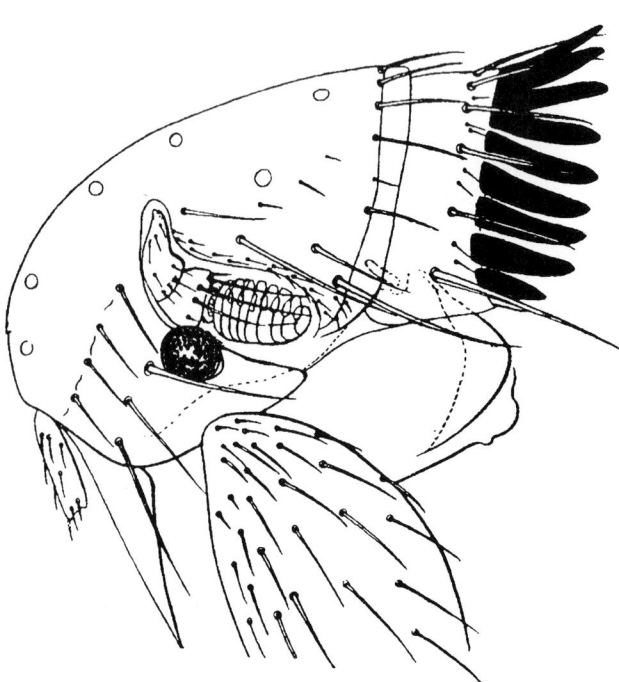

Fig. 3.74 The northern rat flea, *Nosopsyllus fasciatus*, male head. (Adapted from Smart, 1943.)

Table 3.18 *Ceratophyllus* species of veterinary importance.

Species	Hosts	Site
Ceratophyllus gallinae	Poultry, wild birds	Skin
Ceratophyllus niger	Poultry, dog, cat, rat, human	Skin
Ceratophyllus columbae	Pigeon	Skin

Life cycle: The life cycle is typical: egg, three larval stages, pupa and adult. Unlike most other fleas, which often remain on the host and feed for long periods, chicken and pigeon fleas spend most of their time in the nest of the host, and only move onto the birds to feed for short periods. The larvae feed on detritus among the nest material, droppings and undigested blood from the adult faeces. The larval stages are completed in a few weeks, before the pupal cocoon is spun. The flea overwinters in the cocoon and emerges in an old nest in spring as temperatures rise. Large numbers may occur in the nests of passerine birds and they may complete their life cycle during the period of nest occupation by these birds. Work has shown a negative correlation between flea abundance and mean body mass of the brood being parasitised.

If the nest is reused by birds the following year, the newly emerged adults will locate the new hosts, feed and continue the cycle. If the nest is not reused, the newly emerged adults will make their way to the nest entrance, where they may be able to attach to a bird that is examining the old nest as a potential nest site. Alternatively, they may climb up trees and bushes, where they stop periodically and face the brightest source of light, jumping in response to a shadow passing in front of the light.

Ceratophyllus gallinae

Description: Adults of *Ceratophyllus gallinae* are typically 2–2.5 mm long with no antennal fossae. Eyes are present. There is a pronotal comb, carrying more than 24 spines, while the genal comb is absent (Fig. 3.75). There is a lateral row of 4–6 bristles on the inner surface of the hind femur and there are no spines on the basal section of the legs.

Ceratophyllus niger

Description: The genal comb is absent and the pronotal comb has more than 24 spines. Eyes are present and the head bears a row of three strong setae below the eye.

FAMILY PULICIDAE

The Pulicidae are parasites of a range of mammals with worldwide distribution. Genera of veterinary importance include *Ctenocephalides* (dog and cat fleas), *Spilopsyllus, Echidnophaga, Pulex, Xenopsylla, Archaeopsylla* and *Tunga*. See **life cycle 48**.

Ctenocephalides

The genus contains 11 species which are primarily parasites of carnivores, though some species are found on hares and ground squirrels. The two primary *Ctenocephalides* species of veterinary

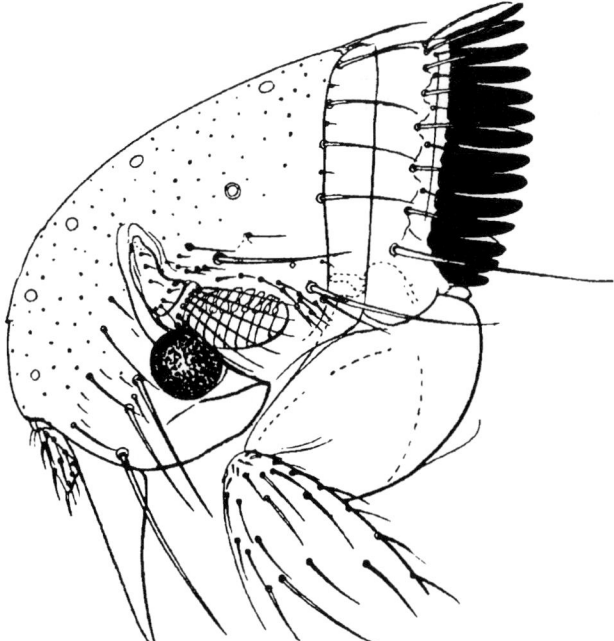

Fig. 3.75 Head and pronotum of a female chicken flea, *Ceratophyllus*. (Adapted from Smart, 1943.)

importance are *C. felis* and *C. canis*. *Ctenocephalides* fleas can be vectors of plague and are intermediate hosts of the tapeworm *Dipylidium caninum*.

Ctenocephalides felis

Subspecies: *Ctenocephalides felis felis, Ctenocephalides felis strongylus, Ctenocephalides felis damarensi, Ctenocephalides felis orientalis*

Description: Cat fleas are dark brown-black, with laterally compressed bodies which have a glossy surface. Females typically measure 2.5 mm in length; males are smaller, sometimes less than 1 mm in length. Eyes are simply dark photosensitive spots and the antennae, which are short and club-like, are recessed into the head. In the female *C. f. felis*, the head is twice as long as high and pointed anteriorly (Fig. 3.76). In the male *C. f. felis*, the head is as long as wide but is also slightly elongate anteriorly. The third pair of legs is much longer than the others and, coupled to elaborate internal musculature, provide an adaptation for jumping to locate the host. The genal comb consists of 7–8 spines and the pronotal comb about 16 spines. The teeth of the genal comb are all about the same length. On the dorsal border of the hind (metathoracic) tibia in both sexes of *C. f. felis*, there are only six notches bearing setae. Between the postmedian and apical long setae, there is a short subapical spine.

Life cycle: Both sexes are blood feeders and only the adults are parasitic. Once on its host, *C. f. felis* tends to become a permanent resident. Within 24–48 hours of the first blood meal, females begin to oviposit. The pearly white ovoid eggs (Fig. 3.77), which measure 0.5 mm in length, have smooth surfaces and may be laid on the ground or on the host, from which they soon drop off. In the laboratory, an adult female *C. f. felis* can produce an average of about 30 eggs per day and a maximum of 50 eggs per day, over a lifespan of about 50–100 days. However, on a cat, the average lifespan is

LIFE CYCLE 48. LIFE CYCLE OF FLEAS (PULICIDAE)

Adults (1) mate on the host and, following a blood meal, females lay eggs on the fur of the host and excrete faeces containing undigested blood from the blood meal. Faeces and eggs fall to the ground, often in the bedding or nest, where the latter hatch (2) into first-stage larvae. Larvae feed on organic matter and mainly on the dry faeces of adult fleas (3). The larvae moult to second and third stages (4). Eventually, when fully grown, the larvae form a cocoon (5) which becomes covered by environmental debris (organic and inorganic material) and moult to become a pupa (5). After a varying length of time, the adult emerges from the cocoon in the presence of mechanical stimuli (e.g. ground vibrations due to the movement of animals).

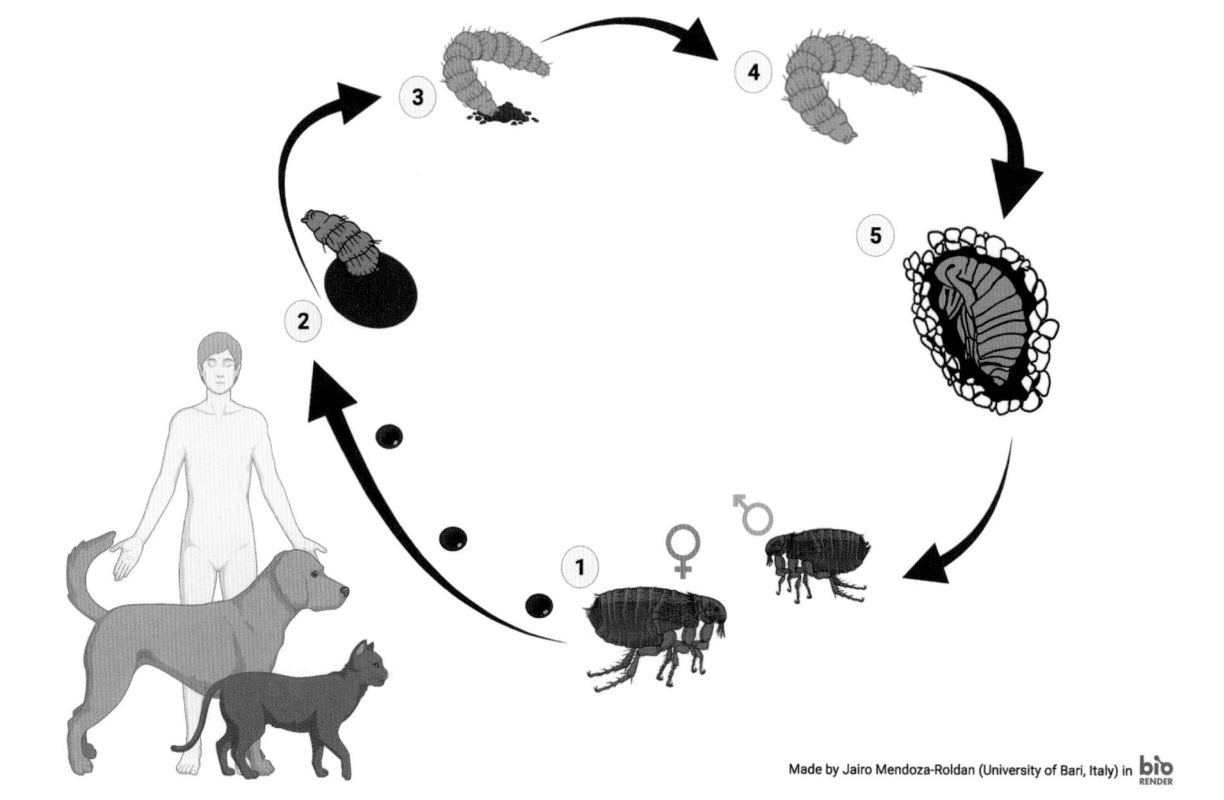

Made by Jairo Mendoza-Roldan (University of Bari, Italy) in bio RENDER

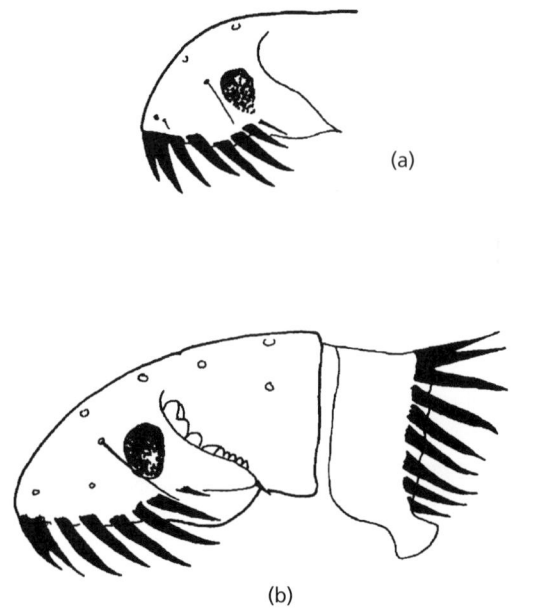

Fig. 3.76 The cat flea, *Ctenocephalides felis felis*: (a) front of male head; (b) female head and pronotum; (c) hind tibia.

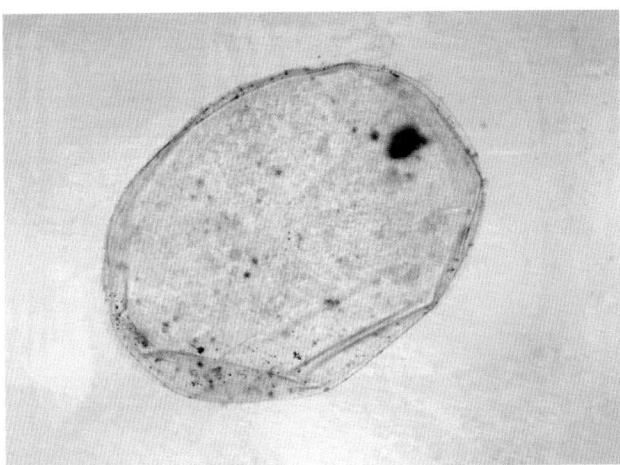

Fig. 3.77 Flea egg.

probably substantially lower than this, possibly less than one week. The rate of oviposition is highest at times of day when cats normally rest, in the early morning and late afternoon. As a result, flea eggs are concentrated at host resting sites rather than over the large areas they roam. The eggs cannot withstand major climatic variations, particularly in temperature and humidity. Only those eggs that fall into an appropriate environment will ultimately develop into adults. At 70% relative humidity and 35 °C, 50% of eggs hatch within 1.5 days. At 70% relative humidity and 15 °C, it takes six days for 50% of eggs to hatch. Eggs cannot survive below 50% relative humidity. Hatching occurs in two days to two weeks, depending on the temperature of the surroundings.

The creamy yellow larvae are elongate, slender and maggot-like (Fig. 3.78); each segment carries a ring of bristles. The last abdominal segment bears two hooked processes called anal struts, which are used for gripping in locomotion. They have chewing mouthparts and feed on debris and on the faeces of the adult fleas, which contain blood and give the larvae a reddish colour.

Within the host's bedding, den or lair, the larvae of *C. f. felis* exist in a protected environment, with relatively high humidity, buffered from the extreme fluctuations of ambient temperatures and provided with detritus and a source of adult flea faecal blood. The larvae have limited powers of movement (probably less than 20 cm before pupation) and crawl about their environment largely at random, but they are negatively phototactic and positively geotactic. In the domestic environment, this behaviour often takes them to the base of carpets where they can encounter food and are sheltered from light and mechanical damage.

The larva moults twice, the final stage being about 5 mm long. At 24 °C and 75% relative humidity, the duration of the three larval stages is about one week, but in unfavourable conditions larvae may develop more slowly. At 13 °C and 75% relative humidity larval development takes about five weeks, though the larval cycle can take up to 200 days. Larvae will only survive at temperatures between 13 and 35 °C. They are extremely susceptible to desiccation and mortality is high below 50% relative humidity.

When fully developed, the mature third-stage larva empties its gut and spins a thin silk cocoon. This process requires a vertical surface against which they can align themselves. Fragments of detritus adhere to the cocoon, giving it some degree of camouflage. The larva pupates within the cocoon. At 24 °C and 78% relative humidity, the duration of the pupal stage is about 8–9 days. If the pupal stage is disturbed, the larvae will either spin another cocoon or develop into naked pupae, showing that the cocoon is not essential for development into an adult. When fully developed, adults emerge from the pupal cuticle but may remain within the cocoon. Adults may remain in this state for up to 140 days at 11 °C and 75% relative humidity. At cooler temperatures, fully formed fleas may remain in their cocoons for up to 12 months.

The areas within a building with the necessary humidity for egg and larval development are limited. Sites outdoors are even less common and flea larvae cannot develop in arid areas exposed to the hot sun. If found outside, they typically inhabit the top few millimetres of soil.

Emergence of the adult from the cocoon is triggered by stimuli such as mechanical pressure, vibrations or heat. Adult emergence may be extremely rapid, when provided with appropriate conditions. The ability to remain within the cocoon for extended periods is essential for a species such as *C. f. felis* since its mobile hosts may only return to the lair or bedding at infrequent intervals. The fully formed adults begin to feed almost as soon as they are on their host, though they can survive for several days without feeding, provided the relative humidity is above about 60%. Within 36 hours of adult emergence, most females will have mated. Females will mate with several males and egg laying begins 24–48 hours after the first blood meal.

Within 10 minutes of feeding, adults begin to produce faeces. Partially digested host blood forms a large component of the flea faeces. The faeces quickly dry into reddish-black faecal pellets known as 'flea dirt'.

It is important to recognise that most of the flea's life cycle is spent away from the host. This includes not only the eggs, larvae and cocoon but also, if necessary, the adult flea.

Ctenocephalides canis

Description: The dog flea, *C. canis*, is closely related and is morphologically very similar to the cat flea *C. f. felis*, although they cannot interbreed and are therefore truly distinct species. The head of the female dog flea is more rounded on its upper and anterior surface than that of the cat flea and less than twice as long as high. Like *C. f. felis*, the dog flea has both genal and pronotal combs. The genal comb consists of 7–8 spines and the pronotal comb about 16 spines. However, in both female and male *C. canis* the first spine of the genal comb is shorter than the rest. On the dorsal border of the hind

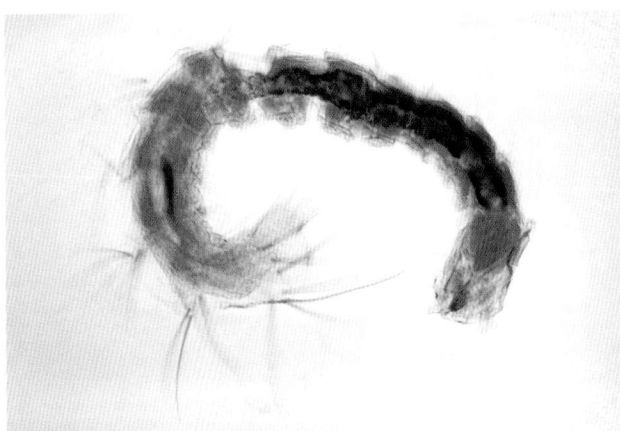

Fig. 3.78 Flea larva.

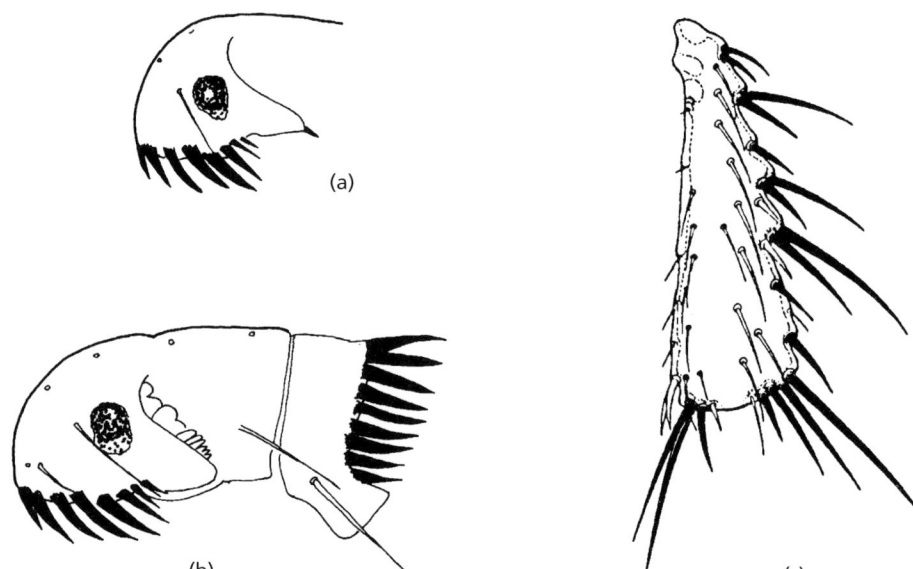

Fig. 3.79 The dog flea, *Ctenocephalides canis*: (a) front of male head; (b) female head and pronotum; (c) hind tibia.

(metathoracic) tibia in both sexes of *C. canis* there are eight notches bearing stout setae (**Fig. 3.79**).

Life cycle: The life cycle of *C. canis* (egg, veriform larva, pupa and adult) is very similar to that of *C. f. felis*. Egg production commences two days after the male and female arrive on the dog. Eggs and larvae do not survive at temperatures of over 35 °C, preferring a temperature range between 13 and 32 °C and relative humidity between 50% and 90%. In these conditions, even unfed adults can survive for many weeks. Pupae may remain dormant for a year or more, yet are able to hatch in 30 seconds when cues, such as vibration, indicate the presence of a suitable host. In an appropriate environment the total life cycle may take as little as three weeks.

Spilopsyllus

This genus includes the rabbit flea, *Spilopsyllus cuniculi*, which is a common vector of myxomatosis.

Spilopsyllus cuniculi (rabbit flea)

Description: The rabbit flea, *S. cuniculi*, has both pronotal and genal combs, the latter being composed of 4–6 oblique spines. Adults are dark brown and females are, on average, 1 mm in length; males are slightly smaller. Eyes are present and the frons at the front of the head is rounded with the frontal tubercle conspicuous. There are two stout spines beneath the eye (Fig. 3.80).

Life cycle: The rabbit flea, *S. cuniculi*, occurs largely on the ears. It is more sedentary than most other species of flea and remains for long periods with its mouthparts embedded in the host. The life cycle of this species is believed to be mediated by host hormones imbibed with the host blood. The presence of progesterones inhibits or delays flea maturation. Following mating, the adult female rabbit ovulates and, about 10 days before parturition, the levels of oestrogens and corticosteroids in the blood increase. These hormones cause the fleas to attach tightly to their host and stimulate development of the eggs of the female flea. Reproductive hormones

of the pregnant female host stimulate maturation of the ovaries and oocytes of feeding female fleas and testicular development in males. These fleas can only reproduce after feeding on a pregnant doe. This serves to synchronise the life cycles of the flea and its host and results in the emergence of adult fleas at the same time as a new litter of host animals is born.

The adult fleas become ready to mate when the litter is born: an air-borne kairomone emanating from the newborn rabbits and their urine boosts copulation. The hormones of the host also cause adult fleas to increase the rate of feeding and defecation by about five times. This provides an abundance of food in the burrow for the newly hatched larvae. Oviposition occurs soon after adults have transferred onto the newborn young. The larvae feed on organic matter in the nest debris and mature 15–45 days later when they infest the host littermates before they disperse from the burrow.

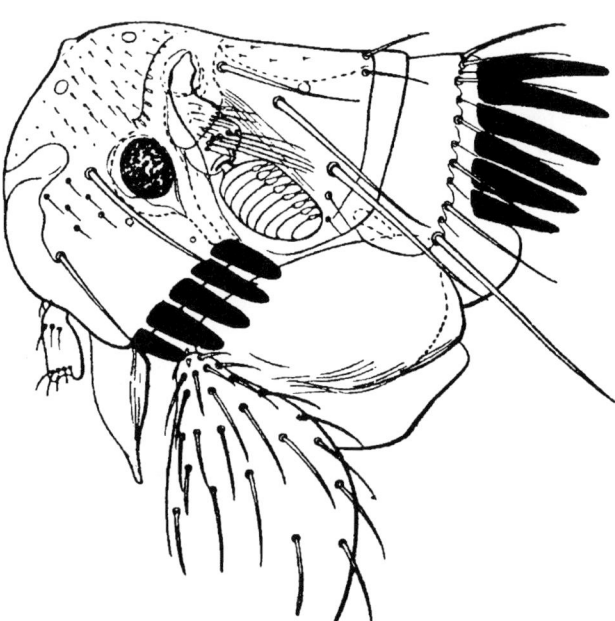

Fig. 3.80 Head and pronotum of the rabbit flea, *Spilopsyllus cuniculi*.

Populations of *S. cuniculi* may increase dramatically during the rabbit breeding season. Adult female fleas on bucks or non-pregnant does are more mobile and will move to pregnant does if able. The rise in ear temperature during rabbit mating will also stimulate movement of fleas from one rabbit to another.

Echidnophaga

The genus *Echidnophaga* includes some 21 species of fleas and includes the cosmopolitan sticktight flea, *Echidnophaga gallinacea*, which occurs on a wide range of birds and mammals.

Echidnophaga gallinacea (sticktight flea)

The sticktight flea *Echidnophaga gallinacea* is a burrowing flea important mainly in domestic poultry, but may also infest cats, dogs, rabbits and humans. These fleas are most common in tropical areas throughout the world, but may also be found in many subtropical and temperate habitats

Description: The adult sticktight flea is small; females are commonly about 2 mm in length and males are less than 1 mm in length. The head is sharply angled at the front (frons). There are no genal or pronotal combs (Fig. 3.81). On the head behind the antenna, there are two setae and, in the female, usually a well-developed occipital lobe. The thoracic segments are narrowed dorsally. Spiracles are present on the second and third abdominal segments. The mouthparts appear large, extending the length of the forecoxae, and project from the head conspicuously. The maxillary laciniae are broad and coarsely serrated. On the anteroventral surface of each hind coxa, there are three rows of minute spiniform bristles.

Life cycle: After host location, females aggregate on bare areas, often the head, comb or wattles. Newly emerged adults are active and move towards sunlight, which helps them accumulate on the wattles of cocks or hens. After feeding, females burrow into the skin where they attach firmly with their mouthparts. Each female may remain attached for 2–6 weeks. Copulation then takes place. The skin around the point of attachment may become ulcerated. The female begins oviposition an average of 6–10 days after attachment, at a rate of about 1–4 eggs per day. Eggs are laid in the ulceration or dropped to the ground. If laid in the ulceration, larvae hatch, emerge from the skin and drop to the ground to complete their development. The incubation period may last 4–14 days, though typically it takes 6–8 days. Eggs fail to survive temperatures of 43 °C and above. The larvae feed on chicken manure and develop through three larval stages over a period of 14–31 days. The pupal period generally requires around 9–19 days and the entire life cycle may be completed in 30–60 days. Adults generally locate a new host and attach within about 5–8 days after emergence.

Pulex irritans

Description: The human flea, *Pulex irritans*, has neither genal nor pronotal combs. The outer margin of the head is smoothly rounded and there is a pair of eyes (Fig. 3.82). This species can be distinguished from *Xenopsylla cheopis* by the presence of the single ocular bristle below the eye and the absence of a row of bristles along the rear margin of the head. The metacoxae have a patch of short spines on the inner side. The maxillary laciniae extend about halfway down the forecoxae.

Life cycle: The life cycle is typical: egg, three larval stages, pupa and adult. It is thought that originally the principal hosts of this species were pigs. Each adult female *P. irritans* lays around 400 eggs. It can

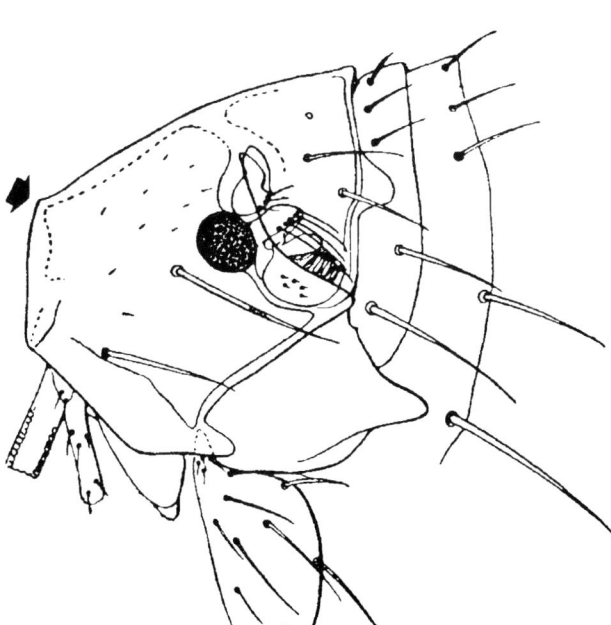

Fig. 3.81 The sticktight flea, *Echidnophaga gallinacea*, female head and thorax (arrow marks angulation of the frons). (Adapted from Smart, 1943.)

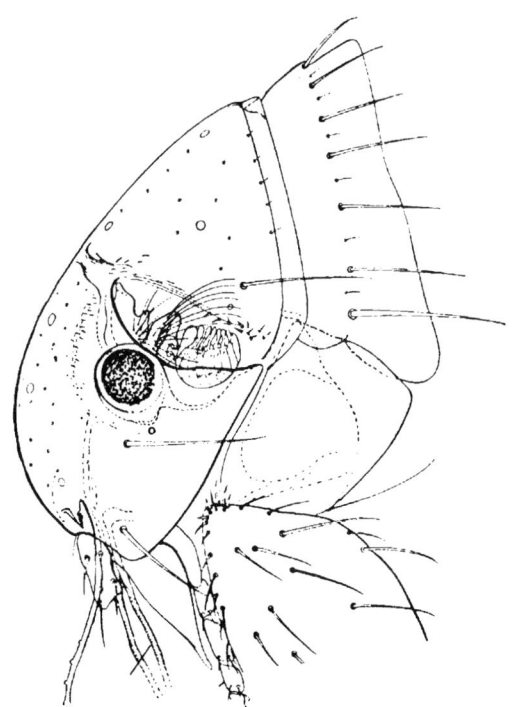

Fig. 3.82 The human flea, *Pulex irritans*, male head and pronotum. (Adapted from Smart, 1943.)

occur worldwide, but it is now uncommon in the USA and most of northern Europe.

Pulex simulans

Description: Similar to *P. irritans* but the laciniae extend for at least three-quarters the length of the forecoxae.

Xenopsylla

The genus *Xenopsylla* contains over 77 species, which are fleas of rats. The Oriental rat flea, *Xenopsylla cheopis*, is the chief vector of *Yersinia pestis*, the causative agent of plague in humans.

Xenopsylla cheopis (Oriental rat flea)

The Oriental or black rat flea *Xenopsylla cheopis* most commonly infests rats but may also infest mice, cottontail rabbits and ground squirrels. It is found worldwide and its distribution largely follows that of its primary host the black rat, *Rattus rattus*. It is one of the most abundant fleas in the southern states of the USA. It is particularly common in urban areas.

Description: *Xenopsylla cheopis* resembles *Pulex irritans* in that both genal and pronotal combs are absent (Fig. 3.83). The head is smoothly rounded anteriorly. The flea has a light amber coloration. The maxillary laciniae reach nearly to the end of the forecoxae. Eyes are present, yet it can only see very bright light. Immediately behind the eyes are two short antennae. The segments of the thorax appear relatively large and the pleural ridge is present in the mesopleuron of the thorax. There is a conspicuous row of bristles along the rear margin of the head and a stout ocular bristle in front of the eye.

Life cycle: The life cycle of *X. cheopis* is typical: egg, three larval stages, pupa and adult. Eggs are usually laid in the environment rather than on the animal host. Eggs are laid in batches of about 3–25 a day, with a female laying 300–1000 eggs over a lifespan that may range from 10 days to more than a year. Eggs hatch after about five days (range 2–14 days depending on local conditions). The larva that emerges avoids light and feeds actively on organic debris. The duration of the larval stage depends on local conditions. The most important environmental variable is humidity and larvae may die if they move outside a narrow range. Humidities above 60–70% and temperatures above 12 °C are required for life-cycle development in this species. The larval period may last 12–84 days, and the pupal and pharate adult period in the cocoon 7–182 days, depending on the availability of a suitable host. Adults may survive for up to 100 days if a host is available, and up to 38 days without food, if humidity is high. Adult males and females can take several blood meals a day. If the host dies, the flea moves almost immediately to find a new one.

Archaeopsylla

The single species *Archaeopsylla erinacei* is a common species on hedgehogs in Europe and North America and can transfer to dogs and cats.

Archaeopsylla erinacei (hedgehog flea)

Description: Adults are easily recognised, being 2–3.5 mm long with a genal comb of 1–3 short spines and a pronotal comb of one short spine (Fig. 3.84).

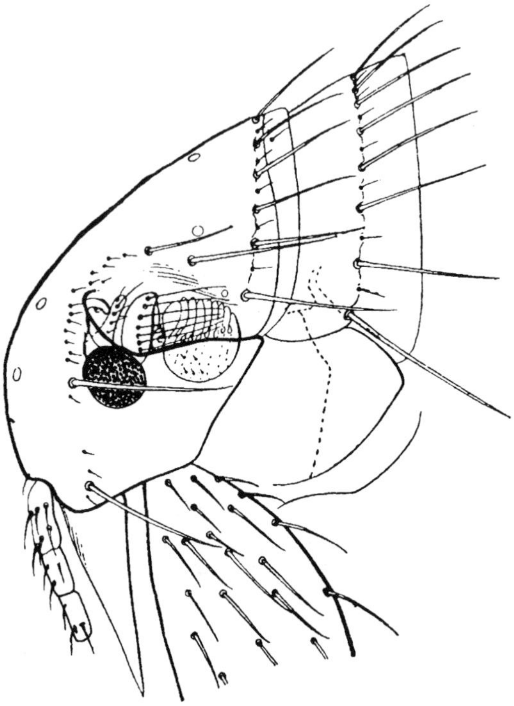

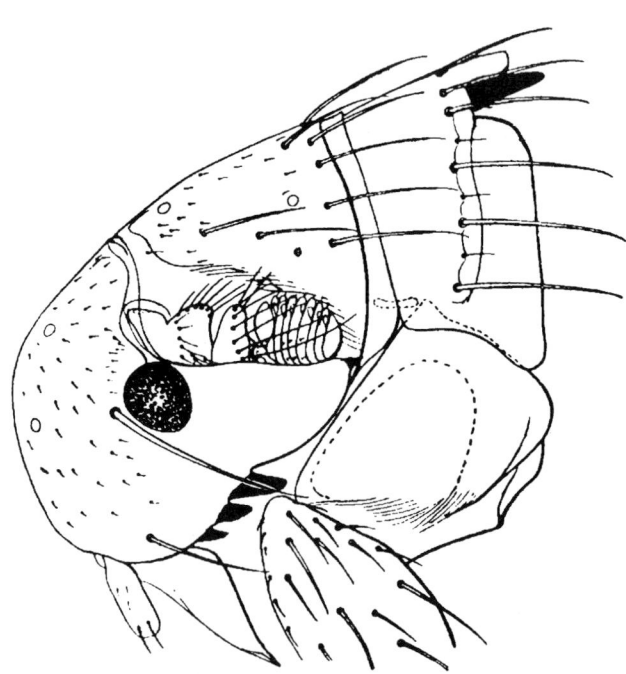

Fig. 3.83 The Oriental rat flea, *Xenopsylla cheopis*, male head. (Adapted from Smart, 1943.)

Fig. 3.84 The hedgehog flea, *Archaeopsylla erinacei*, female head. (Adapted from Smart, 1943.)

Life cycle: The life cycle is typical: egg, three larval stages, pupa and adult. Before the female can begin ovipositing, she needs to feed on the host several times. Once on its host, *A. erinacei* tends to become a permanent resident.

Tunga

Species of this genus, often assigned their own family Tungidae in the superfamily Pulicoidea, are parasites of edentates (armadillos, anteaters), livestock, rodents and humans. *Tunga penetrans*, the jigger or chigger flea, causes tungosis in humans.

Tunga penetrans

Description: *Tunga penetrans* has no combs and no spiniform bristles on the metathoracic coxae. The head is angular and has an acute frontal angle. The thorax is short and reddish-brown. The female is about 1 mm long before a blood meal but may increase to a length of up to 7 mm when gravid. The male flea is smaller, about 0.5 mm long, and never embeds in the host.

Life cycle: The fertilised female slashes the skin of the host with her mouthparts and then burrows into the wound, inserting her head and body until only the last two abdominal segments are exposed. Host skin proliferates and covers the flea, all bar the last abdominal segments. A free-living, mobile, adult male mates with the embedded female. The male possesses one of the longest intromittent organs relative to body size in the animal kingdom and mates from an inverted position. The female remains attached, feeding on host fluids and greatly expanding the size of the abdomen. The female often expands 80-fold to reach the size of a pea after 8–10 days. The embedded female produces a nodular swelling leaving only a small opening to the outside through which up to 200 eggs are passed and drop to the ground. The eggs hatch in 3–4 days, and the fleas moult through two larval stages. The entire life cycle requires about 17 days.

FAMILY LEPTOPSYLLIDAE

Leptopsylla

Leptopsylla segnis (mouse flea)

The European mouse flea, *Leptopsylla segnis*, is found on house mice, rats and other wild rodents and has occasionally been reported on cats and dogs.

Description: In the adult fleas there are both genal and pronotal combs and the genal comb contains only four spines.

Life cycle: The life cycle is typical: egg, three larval stages, pupa and adult. Eggs and larvae are found in the host's nest and the adults are obligate blood feeders on the host animal. The adult fleas live for approximately 20 days on the host. The entire life cycle may be completed in 3–4 weeks under ideal conditions or two years under adverse conditions.

ORDER HEMIPTERA

This order includes a large number of plant lice and bugs of considerable economic importance. Only a small number of species are of veterinary importance.

FAMILY CIMICIDAE

Cimex

Bed bugs of the genus *Cimex* are blood-feeding temporary ectoparasites of birds and mammals, including humans. Two species are of particular importance: *Cimex lectularius* is a cosmopolitan species of temperate and subtropical regions feeding on humans, bats, chickens and other domestic animals; *Cimex hemipterus* is tropicopolitan and subtropical, and feeds on humans and chickens.

Description: Bed bugs have oval flattened bodies. The forewings are reduced to hemelytral pads and the hindwings are absent. The adult bed bug measures 5–7 mm when unfed, with females being slightly larger than males. They are generally red-brown in colour, although they appear darker following a blood meal (Fig. 3.85). The head bears long four-segmented antennae, of which the last three segments are long and slender, and a pair of widely separated compound eyes placed laterally at the sides of the head; there are no ocelli. The labium has three obvious segments and is reflected backwards under the head, reaching as far as the coxae of the first pair of legs. The abdomen is 11-segmented, with segments 2–9 being easily recognisable dorsally. When the bed bug engorges, the abdomen increases greatly in volume. There are seven pairs of spiracles located ventrally on abdominal segments 2–8. Nymphs are smaller than adults, lack mature genitalia, but also blood feed.

The distinguishing morphological differences between the two species of importance are the broader prothorax (located behind the head) of *Cimex lectularius* compared with *Cimex hemipterus* and that *Cimex hemipterus* is about 25% longer than *C. lectularius*.

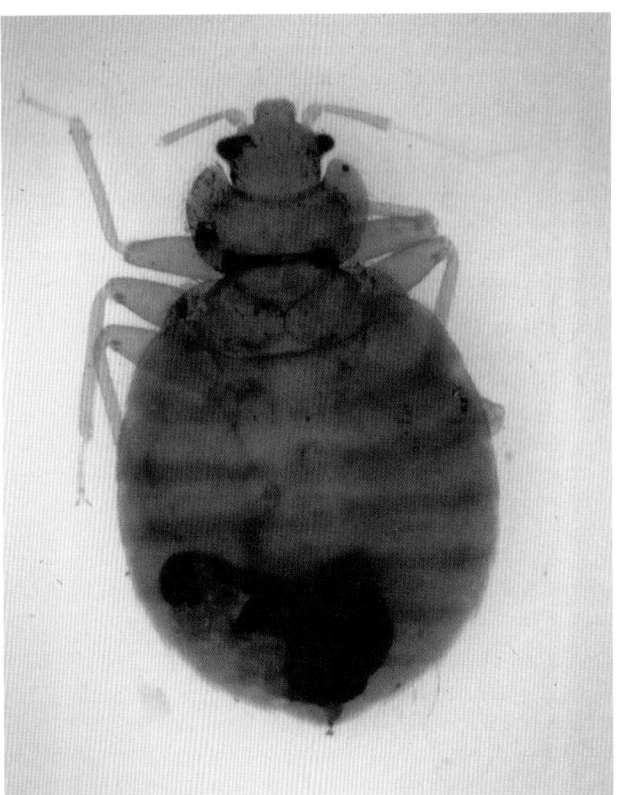

Fig. 3.85 *Cimex* (bed bug).

Life cycle: There are some minor differences between the species but, for *C. lectularius*, eggs are laid on rough rather than smooth surfaces and generally inserted into cracks and crevices. They are laid individually and held in place by transparent cement. The eggs are cream in colour, approximately 1 mm in length and less than 0.5 mm in breadth. The eggs are fertilised while still in the ovary, and embryos undergo some development before being laid. At 22 °C, eggs take 10–12 days to hatch, and the shortest time for development is 4–5 days at 30–35 °C. Hatching does not occur at 37 °C or above or below 13°C, although eggs can remain viable for short periods (less than three months) as the temperature approaches 0 °C. In temperate climates, eggs laid in the autumn are likely to have died before the temperature rises above the threshold in spring, except in houses with heating.

There are five juvenile stages, with each stage requiring at least one blood meal (often two) to moult to the next stage. Nymphs will feed within 24 hours of emergence or of moulting to the next instar. Time for development through the instars is very similar for the first four, but the fifth is usually somewhat longer. The length of the life cycle is very dependent on ambient temperature. The entire nymphal development can take 6–8 weeks at 22 °C, after which the adults can live up to around six months, but at 30 °C development from egg to adult can be completed in three weeks and overall lifespan is shorter.

Cimicidae are widespread in the northern hemisphere. No bird-feeding cimicids occur in tropical Africa or Central America and no native cimicids occur in Australia.

FAMILY REDUVIIDAE

Triatome or cone-nose bugs, sometimes called kissing or assassin bugs, of the genera *Rhodnius*, *Triatoma* and *Panstrongylus* are blood feeders on a wide range of wild and domestic animals, including dogs, cats, cattle, sheep, goats and humans. Over 100 species are found in South and Central America and the southern and midwestern USA, predominantly in the tropical regions. They are vectors of the protozoan parasite *Trypanosoma cruzi* which causes Chagas disease in South America. Important species include *Triatoma infestans* and *Rhodnius prolixus*. However, five species of *Linshcosteus* are found in India and seven species of *Triatoma* are found in Southeast Asia and one in Africa.

Description: The adult reduviid bugs range in length from 10 to 40 mm; the majority of species are around 20–30 mm in length. They are usually dark brown to black in colour, with contrasting patterns of red, orange or yellow marks around the edge of the abdomen. The body is flattened and elongated. The forewings have a hardened basal section and a distal membranous section and overlie the entirely membranous hindwings. The antennae are elbowed with four segments. They also have a piercing proboscis that is three-segmented, tapered and slender and bent back under the body when not in use. Nymphs are smaller than adults, lack mature genitalia or wings, but also blood feed.

Life cycle: All species are nocturnal, obligate, blood-feeding bugs. Gravid females start to lay eggs about two weeks after mating. They then lay one or two eggs daily, each female producing about 200 eggs in total. Each egg is about 2 mm in length. Eggs hatch about two weeks after oviposition, although this is temperature dependent. There are five nymphal stages, all of which blood feed. The entire egg

to adult life cycle may take 2–3 months, but more usually 1–2 years.

Feeding is initiated by chemical and physical cues. Carbon dioxide causes increased activity and heat stimulates probing. When probing is initiated, the rostrum is swung forward and the mandibular stylets are used to cut through the skin and then anchor the mouthparts. The maxillary stylets probe for a blood vessel and saliva, containing an anticoagulant, passes down the salivary canal while blood is pumped up the food canal. Feeding may take between three and 30 minutes. After engorging, the rostrum is removed from the host and the bug defecates, after which it crawls away to find shelter.

CLASS ARACHNIDA

Members of the class Arachnida are a highly diverse group of largely carnivorous terrestrial arthropods. The arachnids do not possess antennae or wings and they have only simple eyes. In this class there is only one group of major veterinary importance, the subclass Acari (sometimes also called Acarina), containing the mites and ticks.

The subclass Acari is an extremely diverse and abundant assembly; over 25 000 species have been described to date. They are usually small, averaging about 1 mm in length. However, some ticks may be over 3 cm in length. Segmentation is inconspicuous or absent and the sections of the body are broadly fused, so that the body appears simple and sack-like.

The first pair of appendages, called **chelicerae**, is positioned in front of the mouth and is used in feeding. The second pair of appendages appears behind the mouth and is composed of **palps**. Their precise structure and function vary from order to order. The palps are usually short sensory structures associated with the chelicerae. Together, the chelicerae and palps form a structure called the **gnathosoma**. The body posterior to the gnathosoma is known as the **idiosoma** (Fig. 3.86). In the adult, the idiosoma is subdivided

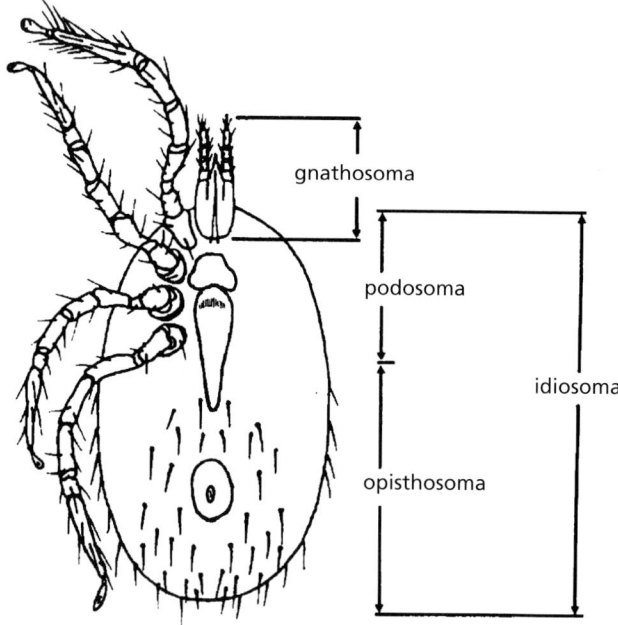

Fig. 3.86 Divisions of the body of a generalised mite.

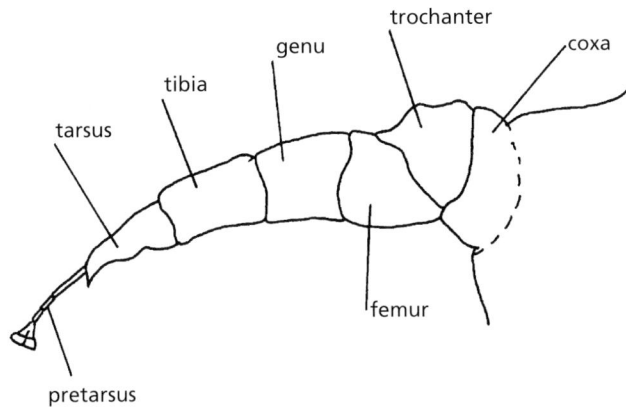

Fig. 3.87 Divisions of the leg of a generalised mite.

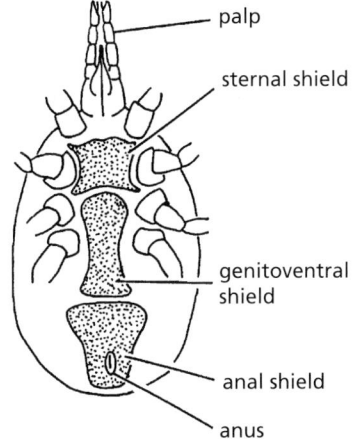

Fig. 3.88 Ventral shields of a generalised mesostigmatid mite.

into the region that carries the legs, the **podosoma**, and the area behind the last pair of legs, the **opisthosoma**. The legs are six-segmented and each is attached to the podosoma at the **coxa**, also known as the epimere. This is then followed by the trochanter, femur, genu, tibia and tarsus, ending in a pair of claws and a pad-like pulvillus (Fig. 3.87).

THE MITES

The classification of mites is complex and subject to ongoing revision as a result of molecular studies. Generally, there are considered to be two main lineages of extant mites: the superorders Parasitiformes and Acariformes.

The Parasitiformes possess 1–4 pairs of lateral stigmata posterior to the coxae of the second pair of legs and the coxae are usually free. The Parasitiformes include the ticks, described as the Ixodida or Metastigmata, and the parasitic mites, described as the Mesostigmata or Gamesid mites.

The Acariformes do not have visible stigmata posterior to the coxae of the second pair of legs and the coxae are often fused to the ventral body wall. The Acariformes include the mite-like mites, the Sarcoptiformes and Trombidiformes, which include the the Astigmata and Prostigmata, respectively. The terms 'metastigmata', 'mesostigmata', 'astigmata' and 'prostigmata' relate to the position of the respiratory openings on the body and provide a convenient, if taxonomically imperfect, way of distinguishing these four groups of mites of parasitic importance.

For clinical information see the relevant host chapter.

The ectoparasitic mites of mammals and birds largely inhabit the skin, where they feed on blood, lymph, skin debris or sebaceous secretions, which they ingest by puncturing the skin, scavenging from the skin surface or imbibing from epidermal lesions. Most ectoparasitic mites spend their entire lives in intimate contact with their host, so that transmission from host to host is primarily by physical contact. Infestation by mites is called **acariasis** and can result in severe dermatitis, known as **mange**, which may cause significant welfare problems and economic losses. Some mites may be intermediate hosts of anoplocephalid cestodes, including *Anoplocephala*, *Moniezia* and *Stilesia*.

Parasitic mites are small, most being less than 0.5 mm long, though a few blood-sucking species may attain several millimetres when fully engorged. The body is unsegmented but can show various sutures and grooves. The body is divided into two sections, the

gnathosoma and idiosoma. The idiosoma may be soft, wrinkled and unsclerotised. However, many mites may have two or more sclerotised dorsal shields and two or three ventral shields: the **sternal**, **genitoventral** and **anal** shields (Fig. 3.88). These may be important features for mite identification. The genitoventral shield, located between the last two (posterior) pairs of legs, bears the genital orifice.

The gnathosoma is a highly specialised feeding apparatus bearing a pair of sensory palps and a pair of chelicerae, the latter sometimes bearing claw-like or stylet-like **chelae** at their tips (Fig. 3.89). Between the chelicerae is the **buccal cone**, both of which fit within a socket-like chamber formed by enlarged coxae of the palps, ventrally and laterally, and by a dorsal projection of the body wall called the **rostrum**.

In the mesostigmatic mites, the fused expanded coxal segments of the palps at the base of the gnathosoma are known as the **basal capituli**, from which protrudes the hypostome (but which is not toothed as in the ticks). The palps are one- or two-segmented in most astigmatic and prostigmatic mites, and five- or six-segmented in the Mesostigmata. The last segment of the palps usually carries a **palpal claw** or **apotele**.

Nymphal and adult mites have four pairs of legs arranged in two sets of anterior and posterior legs. Larval mites have three pairs of legs. The first pairs of legs are often modified to form

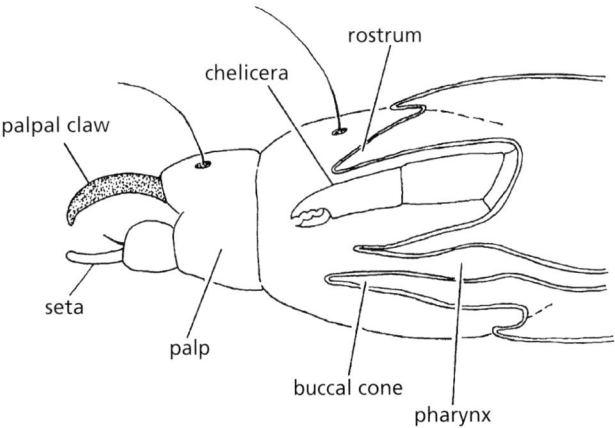

Fig. 3.89 Longitudinal section through the gnathosoma of a generalised mite.

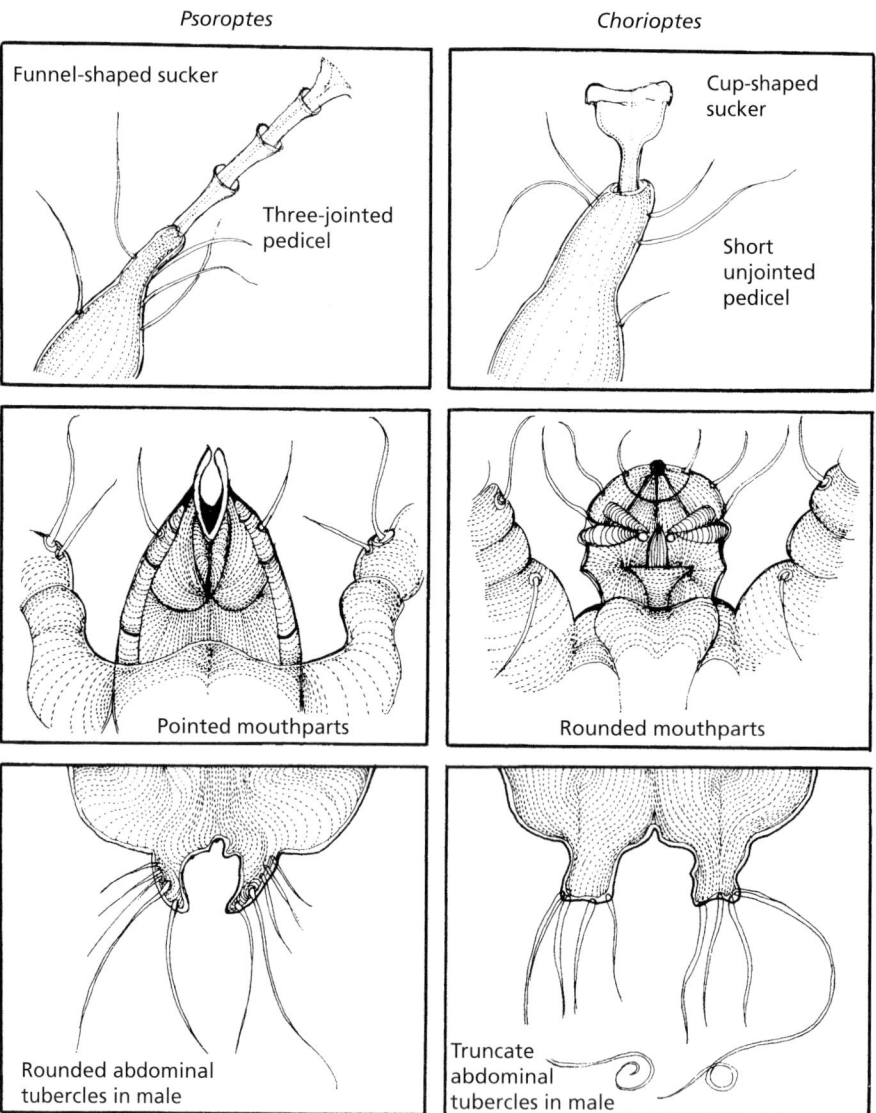

Fig. 3.90 Differential features of *Psoroptes* and *Chorioptes*.

sensory structures and are frequently longer and slender. At the end of the tarsus may be a pretarsus that may bear an **ambulacrum**, usually composed of paired claws, and an **empodium**, which is variable in form and may resemble a pad, sucker, claw or filamentous hair. In some parasitic astigmatic mites, the claws may be absent and replaced by stalked **pretarsi**, which may be expanded terminally into bell or sucker-like **pulvilli** (Figs 3.87 and 3.90).

In many mites, particularly astigmatic mites, gas exchange takes place through the integument. In other mites, gas exchange takes place through 1–4 pairs of stigmata, found on the idiosoma. The presence or absence of stigmata is used for taxonomic purposes. The stigmata in mesostigmatic mites can be associated with elongated processes called **peritremes**.

Eyes are usually absent and hence most mites are blind. Where they are present, however, in groups such as the trombidiformes, the eyes are simple. Hairs, or setae, many of which are sensory in function, cover the idiosoma of many species of mite. The number, position and size of the setae are extremely important in the identification of mite species.

Life cycles

There are four basic life cycle stages: the egg, a six-legged larva, eight-legged nymph and eight-legged adult (Fig. 3.91). These may be further divided into pre-larva, larva, protonymph, deutonymph, tritonymph and adult. There may also be more than one moult in each of these instars. In many Acari, pre-larval and larval instars take place within the egg or have been lost. In others, one or more of the nymphal instars may be omittted.

Although mites, like the ticks, are obligate parasites, they differ in the important respect that most species spend their entire life cycle, from egg to adult, on the host so that transmission is mainly by contact. The life cycle of many parasitic species may be completed in less than four weeks and in some species as little as eight days. Unlike the ticks, once infection is established, pathogenic populations can build up rapidly on an animal without further acquisitions. Female mites produce relatively large eggs from which a small six-legged larva hatches. The larva moults to become an eight-legged nymph. There may be between one and three nymphal stages, known respectively as the protonymph, deutonymph and

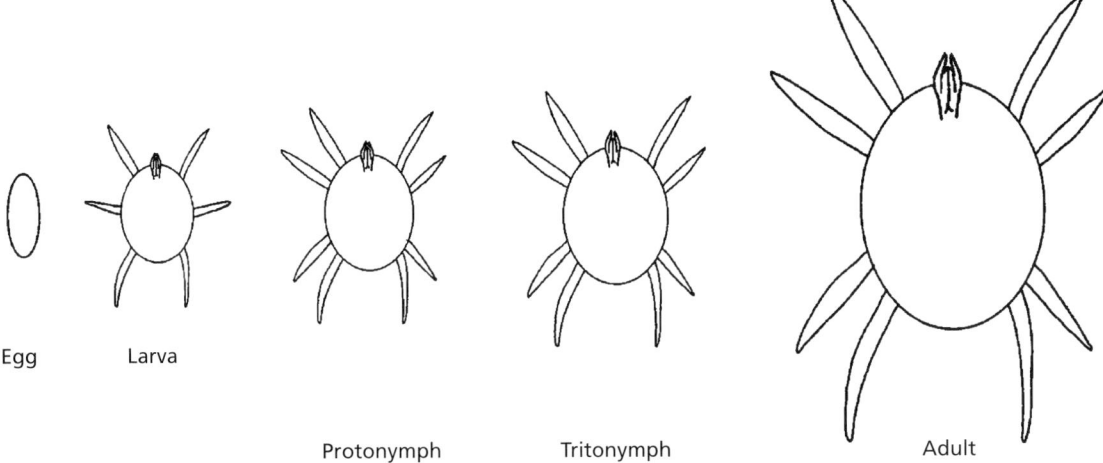

Fig. 3.91 Generalised life cycle of a psoroptid mite.

Egg   Larva   Protonymph   Tritonymph   Adult

tritonymph. In many groups of mites, particularly the Astigmata, one of these nymphal instars, usually the deutonymph, is usually a facultative inactive, dispersal or protective stage, and may be omitted from the life cycle altogether. The tritonymph then moults to become an eight-legged adult.

ORDER SARCOPTIFORMES (ASTIGMATA)

The Astigmata (Order Sarcoptiformes) are a large group of relatively similar mites. They are all weakly sclerotised; stigmata and tracheae are absent and respiration occurs directly through the cuticle. The grouping includes the families **Sarcoptidae**, **Psoroptidae** and **Knemidocoptidae**, which are of major veterinary importance because they contain the most common mite species causing mange and scab. Species of several other families may be important ectoparasites and species of the **Cytoditidae** and **Laminosioptidae** live in the respiratory tracts and muscles of birds and mammals.

FAMILY SARCOPTIDAE

These are burrowing astigmatic mites with circular bodies flattened ventrally and a cuticle covered with fine striations. The coxae are sunk into the body, creating a 'short-leg' appearance with the third and fourth pairs of legs not usually visible when viewed dorsally. The legs have a claw-like empodium with the pulvillus borne on a stalk-like pretarsus. Paired claws on the tarsus are absent. The three genera of veterinary importance are *Sarcoptes*, *Notoedres* and *Trixacarus*.

Sarcoptes

Previously, over 30 species of *Sarcoptes* were described, but today it is generally accepted that there is only one species, *Sarcoptes scabiei*, with a variety of host-adapted strains. Sarcoptid mites are globose mites with a flat ventral surface, the cuticle finely striated and the chelicerae adapted for cutting and paring. Characteristically, the anus is posterior in *Sarcoptes* mites.

Sarcoptes scabiei (sarcoptic mange mite, itch mite)

Description: The adult of this species has a round, ventrally flattened, dorsally convex body (Fig. 3.92). Adult females are 0.3–0.6 mm long and 0.25–0.4 mm wide, while males are smaller, typically up to 0.3 mm long and 0.1–0.2 mm wide. The posterior two pairs of limbs do not extend beyond the body margin. In both sexes, the pretarsi of the first two pairs of legs bear empodial claws and a sucker-like pulvillus, borne on a long stalk-like pretarsus. The sucker-like pulvilli help the mite grip the substrate as it moves. The third and fourth pairs of legs in the female and the third pair of legs

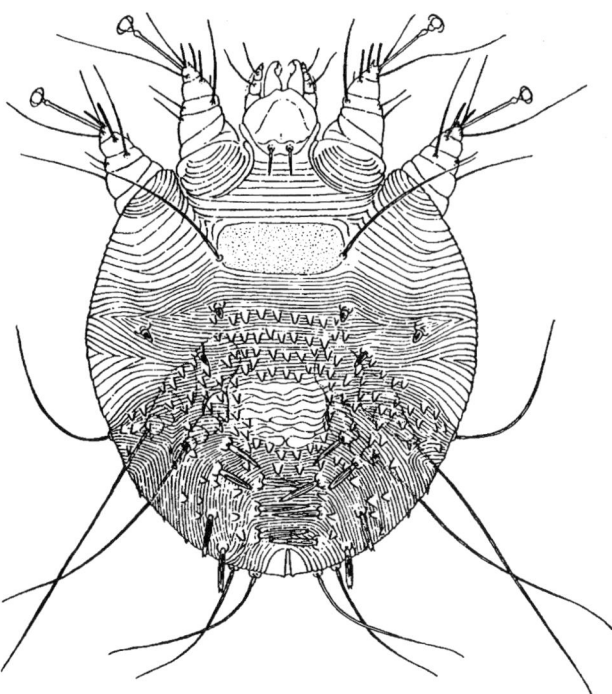

Fig. 3.92 Adult female of *Sarcoptes scabiei*. (Baker *et al.*, 1956/National Pest Control Association.)

in the male end in long setae and lack stalked pulvilli. The mouth-parts have a rounded appearance. These mites have no eyes or stigmata. The dorsal surface of the body of *S. scabiei* is covered with transverse ridges, but also bears a central patch of triangular scales. The dorsal setae are strong and spine-like. The anus is terminal and only slightly dorsal. There are a number of host-adapted varieties of *S. scabiei* that differ subtly in their morphology.

Life cycle: The entire life cycle takes place on the host. Mating probably takes place at the skin surface, following which the female creates a permanent winding burrow, parallel to the skin surface, using her chelicerae and the claw-like empodium on the front two pairs of legs. This burrow may be up to 1 cm in length and burrowing may proceed at up to 5 mm/day. Each tunnel contains only one female, her eggs and faeces. Maturation of the eggs takes 3–4 days, following which the female starts to oviposit 1–3 eggs per day, over a reproductive life of about two months. The eggs, which are oval and about half the length of the adult, are laid singly at the ends of

outpockets, which branch off along the length of these tunnels. Three to four days after oviposition, the six-legged larva hatches from the egg. Most larvae will crawl from the burrow towards the skin surface, while some remain in the tunnels where they continue their development. Two to three days later, the larva moults to become a protonymph. During this time, the larva and nymph find shelter and food in the hair follicles. The protonymph moults to become a tritonymph and again a few days later to become an adult. See **life cycle 49**.

Both adult sexes then start to feed and burrow at the skin surface, creating small pockets of up to 1 mm in length in the skin. Mating occurs on the skin. The male dies shortly after copulation. After fertilisation, female mites wander over the pelage to seek a suitable site for a permanent burrow. Despite their short legs, adults are highly mobile, capable of moving at up to 2.5 cm/min. Within an hour of mating the female begins to excavate her burrow. Females burrow without direction, eating the skin and tissue fluids that result from their excavations. Egg laying begins 4–5 days after completion of the

---

LIFE CYCLE 49. LIFE CYCLE OF *SARCOPTES SCABIEI*

Females of *Sarcoptes scabiei* burrow tunnels through the keratinised layer of the host's epidermis, where they feed on cells and interstitial fluids (1). After mating, females lay eggs in the tunnels dug through the corneal layer of the epidermis (2); these are elliptical in shape and whitish in colour. Larvae hatch within 3–10 days (3) and travel to the surface, where they dig relatively superficial tunnels. Here, they moult to become octopod nymphs (4) and then adults (5) within three weeks of emergence from the egg. After mating, the females burrow new tunnels, thus continuing the life cycle. This mite can infest a range of hosts, including humans.

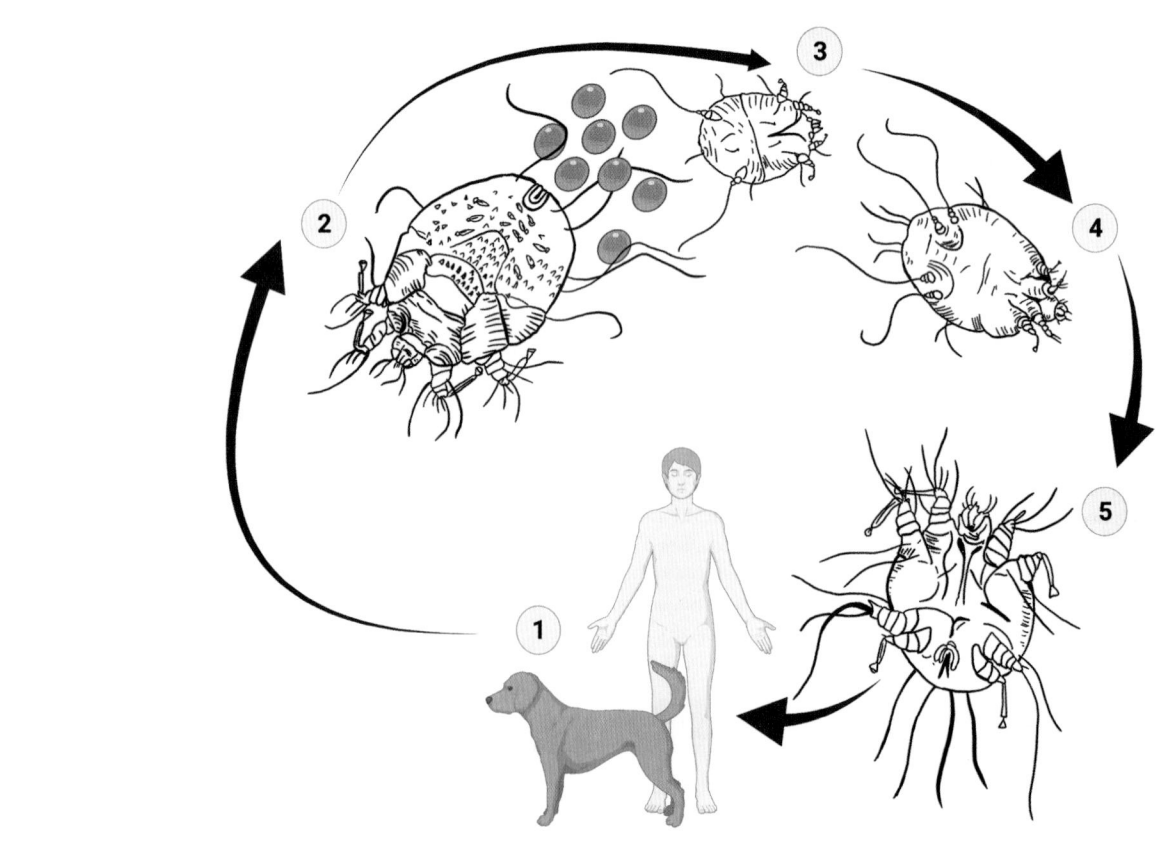

initial permanent winding burrow. Female mites rarely leave their burrows and if removed by scratching, they will attempt to burrow again. The total egg-to-adult life cycle takes between 17 and 21 days, but may be as short as 14 days. During this period, the mortality rate is high, with just 10% of mites that hatch completing their development. During an infection, mite numbers increase rapidly, then decline, leaving a relatively stable mite population.

Notoedres

Mange mites of this genus are found on the ears of mammals. More than 20 species of *Notoedres* have been described, most being parasites of tropical bats. Three species are of interest to the veterinary entomologist, and one, *N. cati*, is important. *Notoedres muris* occurs on rats throughout the world, including laboratory colonies, and *N. musculi* infests the house mouse in Europe (Table 3.19). The anus in this genus is dorsal.

Notoedres cati (notoedric mange mite)

Description: *Notoedres* closely resembles *Sarcoptes*, with a circular outline and short legs with long unjointed pedicels, but it is distinguished by its concentric 'thumbprint' striations and absence of spines (Fig. 3.93). The dorsal scales are rounded and arranged transversely. This species is also smaller than *S. scabiei*; females are about 225 μm in length and males about 150 μm, with a short square rostrum. The anal opening is distinctly dorsal and not posterior. Females have suckers on legs 1 and 2.

Life cycle: Similar to that of *Sarcoptes*, except that the females in the dermis are usually found in aggregations. The fertilised female creates a winding burrow or tunnel in the upper layers of the epidermis, feeding on liquid oozing from the damaged tissues. The eggs are laid in these tunnels, hatch in 3–5 days, and the six-legged larvae crawl on to the skin surface. These larvae, in turn, burrow into the superficial layers of the skin to create small 'moulting pockets', in which the moults to nymph and adult are completed. Development from egg to adult takes 6–10 days. The adult male then emerges and seeks a female either on the skin surface or in a moulting pocket. After fertilisation, the females either produce new tunnels or extend the moulting pocket. New hosts are infected by contact, presumably from transferral of larvae, which are present more superficially than the other stages.

Notoedres muris (rat ear mange mite)

Description: Female mites are larger than *N. cati* (330–440 μm) and lack dorsal idiosomal denticles.

Table 3.19 *Notoedres* species of veterinary importance.

Species	Hosts	Site
Notoedres cati (syn. Notoedres cuniculi)	Cat, rabbit, but may infest dogs, wild cats, foxes, canids and civets, human	Ears
Notoedres muris	Rat, wild rodents	Ears, nose, tail, genitalia, limbs
Notoedres musculi	House mouse	Ears, nose, tail, genitalia, limbs

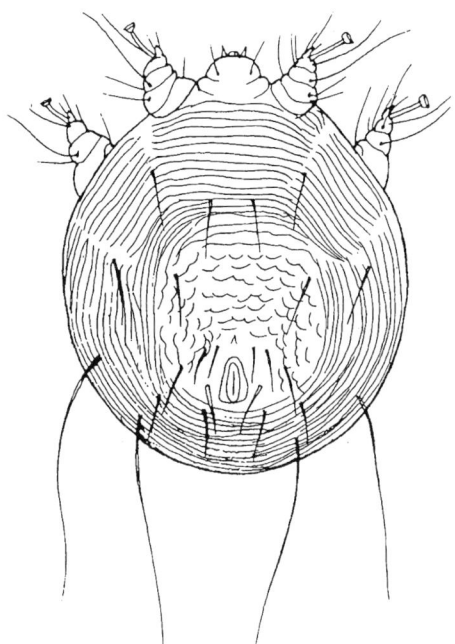

Fig. 3.93 Adult female *Notoedres cati* in dorsal view.

Trixacarus

The single species, *Trixacarus caviae*, is commonly found on guinea pigs.

Trixacarus caviae (guinea pig mite)

Synonym: *Caviacoptes caviae*

Description: *Trixacarus caviae* superficially resembles *S. scabiei*. The dorsal striations of the idiosoma of *T. caviae* are similar to those of *S. scabiei*. However, the dorsal scales, which break the striations, are more sharply pointed and the dorsal setae are simple and not spine-like. Like *N. cati*, the anus is located on the dorsal surface. *Trixacarus caviae* is also smaller than *S. scabiei* and similar in size to *N. cati*; females are about 240 μm in length and 230 μm in breadth (Fig. 3.94).

Life cycle: The life cycle is believed to be similar to that of *S. scabiei*.

FAMILY PSOROPTIDAE

These are oval-bodied, non-burrowing, astigmatic mites. The legs are longer than those of the burrowing mites and the third and fourth pairs of legs are usually visible from above. Males have a pair of copulatory suckers, which engage the copulatory tubicles of the female tritonymph. The three genera of veterinary importance are *Psoroptes*, *Chorioptes* and *Otodectes*.

Psoroptes

Mites of the genus *Psoroptes* are non-burrowing, with adult females up to 0.75 mm in length and adult males 0.55 mm in length. The body is oval in shape and all legs project beyond the

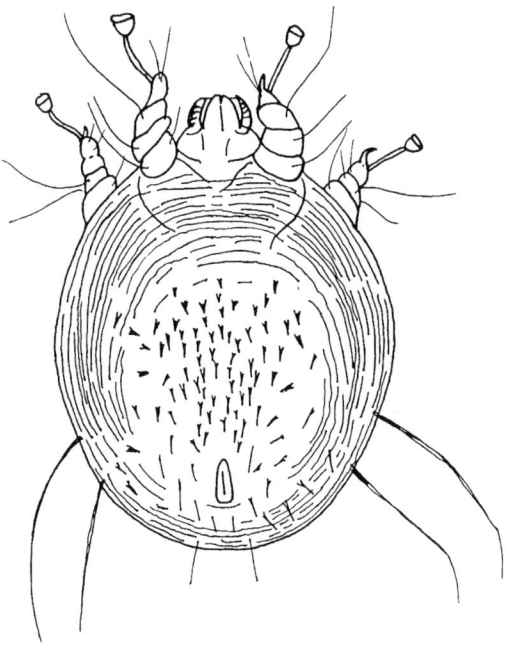

Fig. 3.94 Adult female of *Trixacarus caviae* (dorsal view).

body margin. The most important recognition features are the pointed mouthparts and the three-jointed pretarsi (pedicels) bearing funnel-shaped suckers (pulvilli) (Fig. 3.90). The taxonomy of the mites in this genus is confused, with mites located in different parts of the body or on different hosts traditionally given different species names; however, little good evidence exists to support this nomenclature. In part, the difficulty arises because the mites are usually separated morphologically on the length of the opisthosomal setae in males, but this character is highly variable within and between different host-derived populations and the mean length of the setae is known to decrease with the age

of a body lesion. To date, genetic differences detected to date between host-derived populations of *Psoroptes* are minimal.

Psoroptes ovis (scab mite)

Synonyms: *Psoroptes aucheniae, Psoroptes bovis, Psoroptes cervinus, Psoroptes communis* var. *ovis, Psoroptes equi*

Description: Mites of the genus *Psoroptes* are non-burrowing mites, up to 0.75 mm in length and oval in shape (Fig. 3.95). All the legs project beyond the body margin. Its most important recognition features are the pointed mouthparts and the three-jointed pretarsi (pedicels) bearing funnel-shaped suckers (pulvilli) (Fig. 3.90). Adult females have jointed pretarsi and pulvilli on the first, second and fourth pairs of legs and long whip-like setae on the third pair. In contrast, the smaller adult males, which are recognisable by their copulatory suckers and paired posterior lobes, have pulvilli on the first three pairs of legs and setae on the fourth pair. The legs of adult females are approximately the same length, whereas in males the fourth pair is extremely short.

Life cycle: The eggs of *P. ovis* are relatively large, about 250 μm in length, and oval. The hexapod larva which hatches from the egg is about 330 μm long. The larva moults into a protonymph, the protonymph moults into a tritonymph and the tritonymph moults to become an adult. Egg, larval, protonymph and tritonymph stages and the adult pre-oviposition period each require a minimum of two days to be completed, giving a mean egg-to-adult time of about 10 days.

Adult males attach to female tritonymphs, and occasionally protonymphs, and remain attached until the females moult for the final time, at which point insemination occurs.

Adult females produce eggs at a rate of about 2–3 per day on average. The median life expectancy for an adult female *P. ovis* is about 16 days, during which it will have laid about 40–50 eggs. Populations of *P. ovis* on a host may therefore grow quickly, doubling every six days or so. See **life cycle 50**.

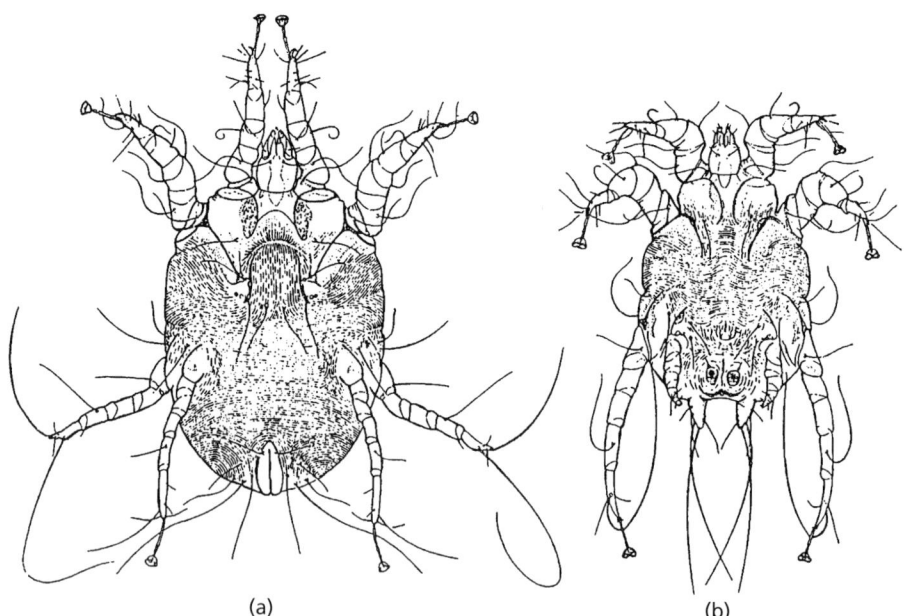

Fig. 3.95 Adult *Psoroptes ovis*, ventral views: (a) female, (b) male. (Baker *et al.*, 1956/National Pest Control Association.)

(a)   (b)

LIFE CYCLE 50. LIFE CYCLE OF *PSOROPTES OVIS*

Psoroptes ovis is a non-burrowing mite. Females lay whitish eggs (2) near the margins of the lesion on the skin of its host. After 2–3 days, hexapod larvae hatch (3, 4); these moult into octopod protonymphs and then tritonymphs (5) in about four days and subsequently into adults (1). The developmental cycle is short, taking only about 12 days. Mites spread on the body of the host by migrating away from the initial papular lesion.

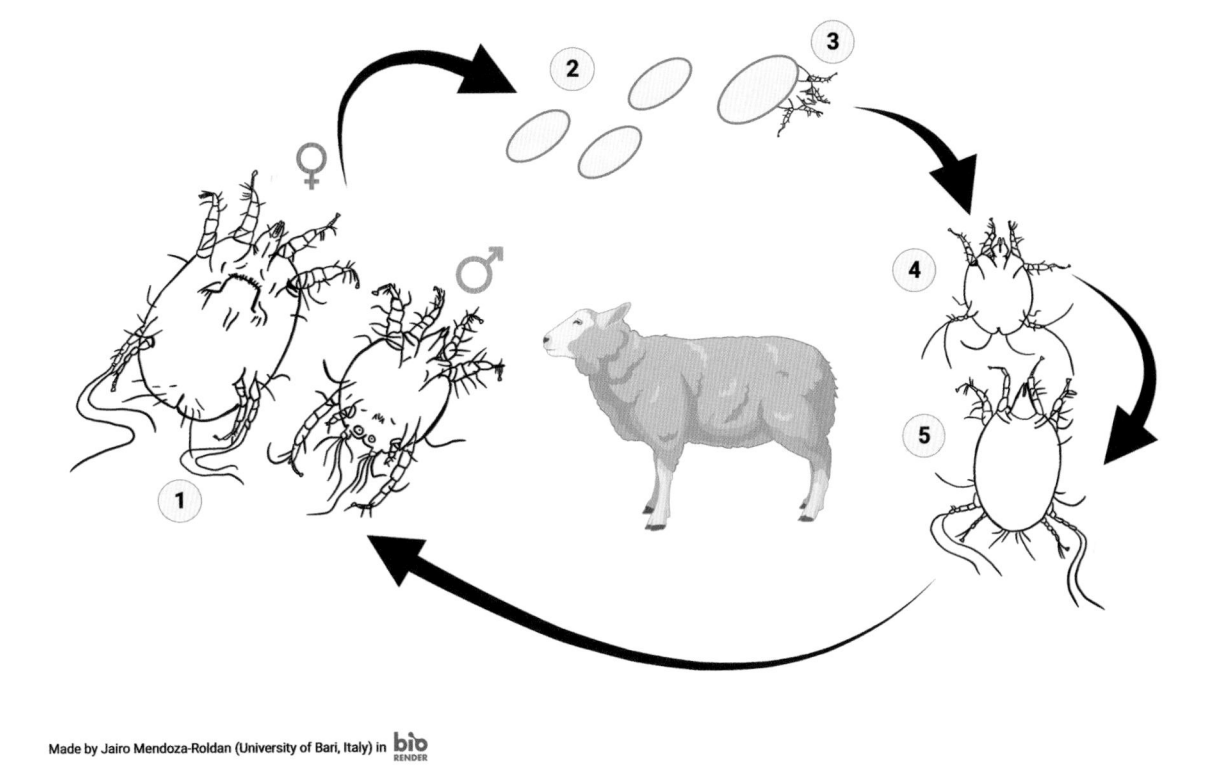

Psoroptes cuniculi (ear mite)

Description: Mites described as *P. cuniculi* are found only in the ear of their host. The species status of *P. cuniculi* remains in question and it has been argued that it should be synomymised with *P. ovis*. In adults of mites described as *P. cuniculi*, the outer opisthosomal setae are, on average, slightly shorter than those seen in *P. ovis*.

Life cycle: The eggs of *P. cuniculi* are relatively large (about 250 μm in length) and oval. The hexapod larva, which hatches from the egg, is about 330 μm long. The larva moults into a protonymph, the protonymph moults into a tritonymph and the tritonymph moults to become an adult. Egg, larval, protonymph and tritonymph stages and the adult pre-oviposition period each require a minimum of two days to be completed, giving a mean egg-to-adult time of about 10 days.

Psoroptes natalensis

Description: Very similar to *P. ovis* but it is believed that *P. natalensis* can be distinguished morphologically by the length and spatulate shape of the fourth outer opisthosomal seta of the male.

However, the precise species status of *P. natalensis* remains to be confirmed.

Chorioptes

Chorioptic mange is the most common form of mange in horses and cattle; it may also be common in goats, llamas and alpacas. Detailed studies of *Chorioptes* have suggested that two distinct species exist, *Chorioptes bovis* and *Chorioptes texanus*, separated by differences in the lengths of the posterior setae of adult males. Both are found infesting the body of their host, but no clear host preference appears to exist between *C. bovis* and *C. texanus*. No behavioural differences in their parasitic behaviour have been recorded. A third species, found within the ear canal of reindeer and moose, may also exist but has not yet been named. The names *Chorioptes ovis*, *Chorioptes equi*, *Chorioptes caprae* and *Chorioptes cuniculi* used to describe the chorioptic mites found on sheep, horses, goats and rabbits, respectively, are now all thought to be synonyms of *C. bovis* or *C. texanus*.

Adult female *Chorioptes* are about 300 μm in length, considerably smaller than *Psoroptes ovis*. *Chorioptes* do not have jointed pretarsi;

their pretarsi are shorter than in *Psoroptes* and the sucker-like pulvillus is more cup-shaped (Fig. 3.90), as opposed to trumpet-shaped in *Psoroptes*.

Chorioptes bovis (chorioptic mange mite, barn itch mite)

Synonyms: *Chorioptes caprae, Chorioptes cuniculi, Chorioptes equi, Chorioptes ovis, Chorioptes japonensis*

Description: In the adult female, tarsi I, II and IV have short-stalked pretarsi and tarsi III have a pair of long, terminal, whip-like setae. The first and second pairs of legs are stronger than the others and the fourth pair has long slender tarsi. In the male, all legs possess short-stalked pretarsi and pulvilli. However, the fourth pair is extremely short, not extending beyond the body margin. Male *C. bovis* are characterised by a very long opisthosomal seta 1 (ae) and short spatulate setae 2 (l4 and d5), on well-developed posterior lobes (Fig. 3.96). The mouthparts are distinctly rounder and the abdominal tubercles of the male are noticeably more truncate than those of *Psoroptes*.

Life cycle: The life cycle is typical: egg, hexapod larva, followed by octopod protonymph, tritonymph and adult. All developmental stages occur on the host. The complete egg-to-adult life cycle takes about three weeks. Eggs are deposited at a rate of one per day and are attached to the host skin. Adult females produce 15–20 eggs and live for 2–3 weeks. *Chorioptes bovis* has mouthparts which are adapted for chewing skin debris. Mites may survive for up to three weeks off the host, allowing transmission from housing and bedding as well as by direct contact.

Chorioptes texanus (chorioptic mange mite)

Description: Identical to *C. bovis*, except for differing lengths of opisthosomal setae; in *C. texanus*, setae 2 (l4 and d5) are longer and

narrower than in *C. bovis*, but most of the other setae are shorter and this is particularly the case for seta 1 (ae).

Life cycle: Believed to be identical to that of *C. bovis*.

Otodectes

Contains the single species, *Otodectes cynotis*, which is an ear mite of dogs, cats and other animals.

Life cycle: The life cycle is typical: egg, hexapod larva, followed by octopod protonymph, tritonymph and adult. All developmental stages occur on the host. The complete egg-to-adult life cycle takes about three weeks. Eggs are deposited at a rate of one per day and are attached to the host skin. Adult females produce 15–20 eggs and live for 2–3 weeks. Like *Chorioptes*, this mite feeds superficially on skin debris.

Otodectes cynotis (ear mite)

Description: *Otodectes* resembles *Psoroptes* and *Chorioptes* in general conformation, having an ovoid body and projecting legs (Fig. 3.97). Like *Chorioptes*, however, it is smaller than *Psoroptes* and does not have jointed pretarsi. The sucker-like pulvillus is cup-shaped, as opposed to trumpet-shaped in *Psoroptes*. In the adult female, the first two pairs of legs carry short, stalked pretarsi, while the third and fourth pairs of legs have a pair of terminal whip-like setae. The fourth pair is much reduced. The genital opening is transverse. In males, all four pairs of legs carry short, stalked pretarsi and pulvilli, but the posterior processes are small.

FAMILY KNEMIDOCOPTIDAE

Twelve species of the genus *Knemidocoptes* (*Neocnemidocoptes*) have been described, of which five are of veterinary importance on poultry and domestic birds.

Knemidocoptes

This is the only burrowing genus parasitising domestic birds, and resembles *Sarcoptes* in many respects. *Knemidocoptes* species of veterinary importance are listed in Table 3.20.

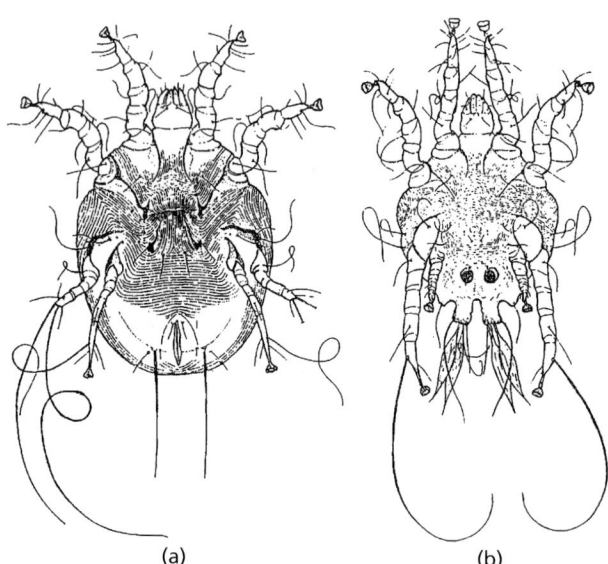

(a)   (b)

Fig. 3.96 Adult *Chorioptes bovis*, ventral views: (a) female, (b) male. (Baker *et al.*, 1956/National Pest Control Association.)

Table 3.20 *Knemidocoptes* species of veterinary importance.

Species	Hosts	Site
Knemidocoptes gallinae (syn. *Cnemidocoptes gallinae*)	Chicken, turkey, pheasant, goose	Feathers
Neocnemidocoptes laevis gallinae (syn. *Knemidocoptes laevis gallinae*)	Chicken, pheasant, partridge	Feathers
Knemidocoptes mutans (syn. *Cnemidocoptes mutans*)	Chicken, turkey	Skin, scales of feet and legs
Knemidocoptes pilae (syn. *Cnemidocoptes pilae*)	Psittacines (budgerigar)	Skin, feather follicles on face, legs, hock
Knemidocoptes jamaicensis	Canary	Legs

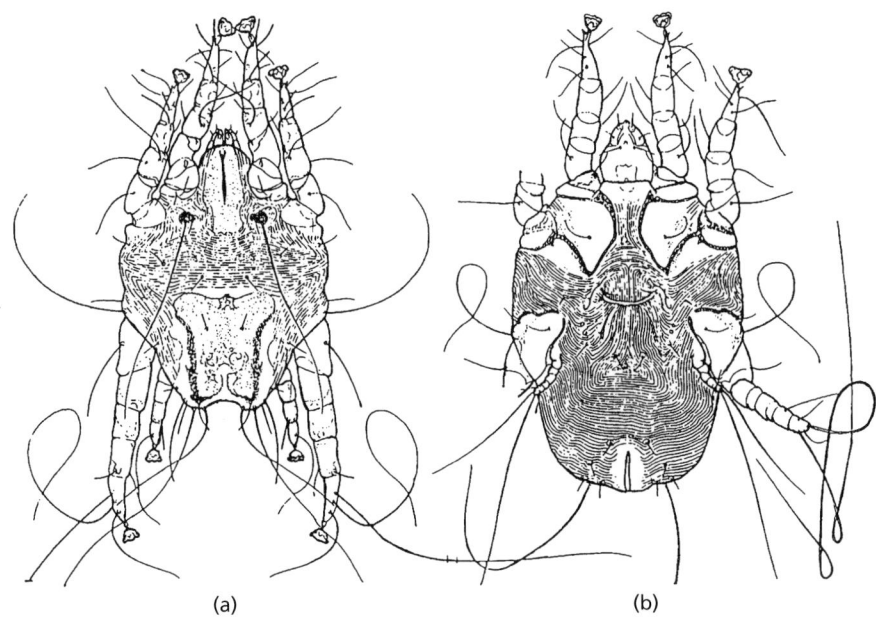

Fig. 3.97 Adult *Otodectes cynotis*: (a) male, dorsal view; (b) female, ventral view. (Baker *et al.*, 1956/National Pest Control Association.)

Life cycle: The fertilised female creates a winding burrow or tunnel in the upper layers of the epidermis, feeding on liquid oozing from the damaged tissues. Females are ovoviviparous, giving birth to live hexapod larvae, which crawl onto the skin surface. These larvae, in turn, burrow into the superficial layers of the skin to create small 'moulting pockets', in which the moults to protonymph, tritonymph and adult are completed. The adult male then emerges and seeks a female either on the skin surface or in a moulting pocket. After fertilisation, the females either produce new tunnels or extend the moulting pocket. The entire life cycle is spent on the host and is completed in 17–21 days.

Knemidocoptes gallinae (depluming itch mite)

Synonym: *Cnemidocoptes gallinae*

Description: The circular body and short stubby legs and the avian host are usually sufficient for generic diagnosis (Fig. 3.98). Although similar in appearance to *Knemidocoptes mutans*, individuals are typically smaller and the pattern of dorsal striations is unbroken.

Neocnemidocoptes laevis gallinae (depluming itch mite)

Synonym: *Knemidocoptes laevis gallinae*

Description: Distinguished from *Knemidocoptes* by having serrated striations on the dorsal surface of the idiostoma, and legs III and IV of the female have a terminal seta which is longer than the leg. The male has a pair of suckers flanking the anus, the posterior limits of apodemes I and II are divergent, and apodemes III and IV are not connected.

Knemidocoptes mutans (scaly leg mite)

Synonym: *Cnemidocoptes mutans*

Description: The general morphology and location on the host are usually sufficient for diagnosis.

Knemidocoptes pilae (scaly face mite)

Synonym: *Cnemidocoptes pilae*

Description: The general morphology and location on the host are usually sufficient for diagnosis. The female mites of *K. pilae* have dorsolateral shields and fused or continuous bases of the setae lateral to the anterior dorsal shield. Male *K. pilae* are characterised by their bilobed pulvillus.

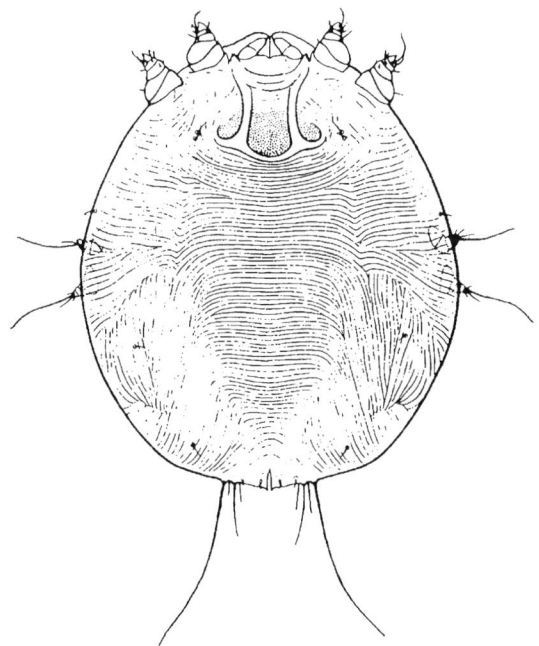

Fig. 3.98 Adult female of *Knemidocoptes gallinae*, dorsal view. (Hirst, 1922/ Springer Nature.)

FAMILY LISTROPHORIDAE

These are parasites of fur-bearing mammals with a distinct dorsal shield, and mouthparts and legs modified for grasping hairs. The genus of veterinary interest is *Leporacarus* (*Listrophorus*).

Leporacarus gibbus (rabbit fur mite)

Synonyms: *Listrophorus gibbus, Listracarus gibbus*

Description: Mites of this species are laterally compressed, brown mites with short legs and a prescapular shield, with a straight anterior margin, that extends over the gnathostoma. The palp coxae are expanded into two overlapping, weakly striated flaps. The legs do not have clasping adaptations, so instead attach to the hair via membranous flaps that arise from the first pair of coxae. Female mites are large and oval with a thumbprint pattern over the body. Males are slightly smaller and have two long adanal processes plus distinct anal suckers.

Life cycle: An obligate parasite, completing all stages of the life cycle (egg, larva, nymph, adult) on the host.

FAMILY MYOCOPTIDAE

Mites of this family were originally a subfamily of the Listrophoridae but are now considered as a separate family. The genus of veterinary interest is *Myocoptes*.

Myocoptes

Myocoptes musculinus (myocoptic mange mite)

Description: These mites are soft-bodied, strongly striated with a distinct dorsal shield, and have mouthparts and legs modified for grasping hairs (Fig. 3.99). Adult female *Myocoptes musculinus* are elongated ventrally, about 300 μm in length, and the propodosomal body striations have spine-like projections. The genital opening is a transverse slit. The anal opening is posterior and ventral. Legs I and II are normal, possessing short-stalked, flap-like pretarsi. Legs III and IV are highly modified for clasping hair. The tibia and tarsus of legs III and IV (female) or III only (male) fold back over enlarged femur and genu. Males are smaller than females, about 190 μm in length, with less pronounced striations and a greatly enlarged fourth pair of legs for grasping the female during copulation. The posterior of the male is bilobed.

Life cycle: *Myocoptes musculinus* spends its entire life on the hair of the host rather than on the skin, feeding at the base of the hair and glueing its eggs to the hairs. The life cycle is typical: egg, hexapod larva, followed by octopod protonymph, tritonymph and adult. All developmental stages occur on the host. The entire life cycle requires around 14 days.

FAMILY CYTODITIDAE

Members of the genus *Cytodites* are found in the respiratory system, lungs and air sacs of chickens, turkeys, canaries and a range of wild birds, and in rodents and bats.

Cytodites

Species belonging to this genus are endoparasites, mainly in the respiratory tract, of birds.

Cytodites nudus (air sac mite)

Description: The mite is oval and about 500 μm long, with a broadly oval idiosoma and smooth cuticle (Fig. 3.100). The chelicerae are absent and the palps are fused to form a soft, sucking organ. Legs are stout and unmodified, ending in a pair of stalked suckers and a pair of small claws.

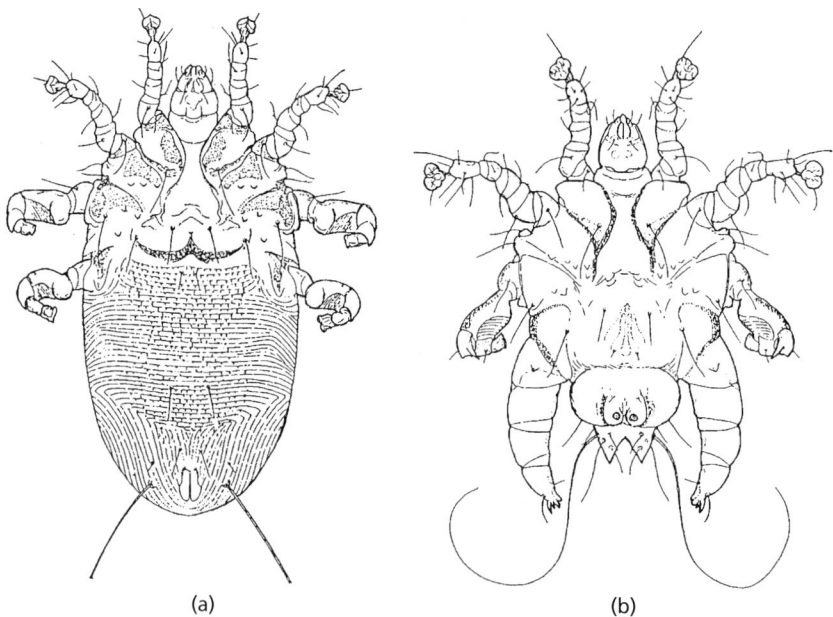

Fig. 3.99 Adults of *Myocoptes musculinus*: (a) female, ventral view; (b) male, ventral view. (Baker *et al.*, 1956/National Pest Control Association.)

(a)   (b)

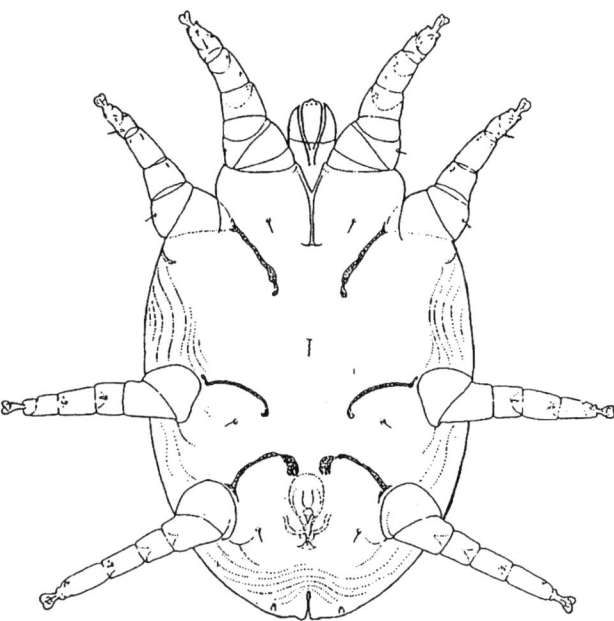

Fig. 3.100 Adult *Cytodites nudus*, ventral view. (Baker *et al.*, 1956/National Pest Control Association.)

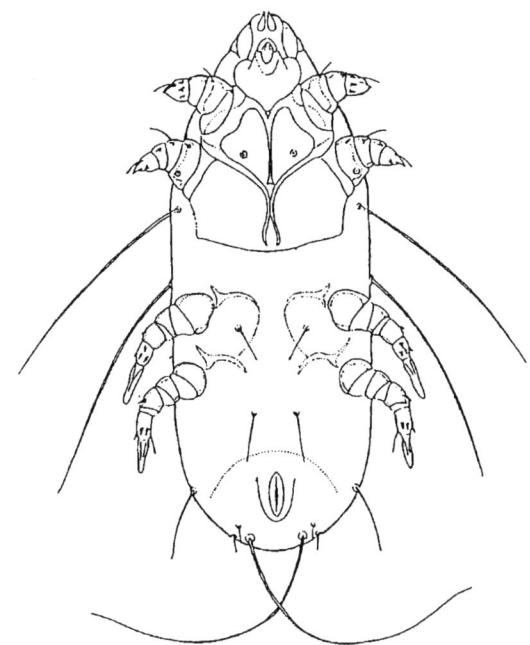

Fig. 3.101 Adult female *Laminosioptes cysticola*, ventral view. (Baker *et al.*, 1956/National Pest Control Association.)

Life cycle: Larval, nymphal and adult stages take place on the surface of the respiratory tract of the host, with the complete life cycle of the mite requiring 14–21 days.

FAMILY LAMINOSIOPTIDAE

Laminosioptes

Laminosioptes are relatively small mites with a smooth elongated body and a few setae, and are subcutaneous parasites of birds.

Laminosioptes cysticola (fowl cyst mite)

Description: This mite is small, approximately 250 μm in length, with a smooth elongated body and few setae. The gnathosoma is small and not visible when viewed from above. The posterior two pairs of legs end in claws and suckerless pedicels, while the anterior two pairs of legs end in claws (Fig. 3.101). The apodemes of coxae II meet in the midline of the idiostoma, then diverge posteriorly.

Life cycle: The life cycle is typical: egg, hexapod larva, followed by octopod protonymph, tritonymph and adult. All developmental stages occur in the host, although complete life-cycle details are lacking.

FAMILY ANALGIDAE

Feather mites of the genus *Megninia* are found on down and contour feathers of the chicken and other captive galliformes. *Megninia* species of veterinary importance are listed in Table 3.21.

Megninia

Table 3.21 *Megninia* species of veterinary importance.

Species	Hosts	Site
Megninia gingylmura	Chicken, galliform birds, pigeon, wild birds	Feathers on body and wings
Megninia cubitalis	Chicken, wild birds	Feathers on body and wings
Megninia ortari	Chicken, wild birds	Feathers on body and wings

Megninia gingylmura (feather mite)

Description: The anterior dorsal shield is narrow with two broad longitudinal bars converging anteriorly. The male has greatly enlarged third legs and large posterior lobes with copulatory suckers. The legs of the female are all of a similar size. Legs I and II have a long anterior spine on the tibia.

Megninia cubitalis (feather mite)

Description: Similar to *M. gingylmura*, except in the female there is a crescent-shaped pregenital sclerite located between apodemes II. Also, the posterior lateral and median pairs of setae near the genital opening are of equal length. In the male, apodemes I are fused into a Y-shape and the anal suckers are flanked by a pair of sclerites.

Megninia ortari (feather mite)

Description: In the female mites, the pregenital sclerite occupies an anterior position between the posterior part of apodeme I. In the male, apodemes I are fused into a Y-shape but there are no sclerites flanking the anal suckers.

FAMILY ATOPOMELIDAE

One species of *Chirodiscoides* has been reported on guinea pigs. Mites of the genus *Listrocarpus* spp. have been reported from primates.

Chirodiscoides

Members of this genus are mainly confined to tropical regions. They were originally a subfamily of the Listrophoridae but are now considered as a separate family. *Chirodiscoides caviae* is found on the fur of guinea pigs.

Chirodiscoides caviae (guinea pig fur mite)

Description: Females of *Chirodiscoides caviae* are about 500 μm and males about 400 μm in length (Fig. 3.102). The gnathosoma is distinctly triangular. The propodosomal sternal shield is strongly striated and used to clasp hairs. The body is flattened dorsoventrally. All legs are slender and well developed, with legs I and II strongly modified for clasping to hair.

Life cycle: *Chirodiscoides caviae* spends its entire life on the hair of the host rather than on the skin, feeding at the base of the hair and glueing its eggs to the hairs. The life cycle is typical: egg, hexapod larva, followed by octopod protonymph, tritonymph and adult. All

developmental stages occur on the host. The entire life cycle requires approximately 14 days.

FAMILY DERMOGLYPHIDAE

Members of the genus *Dermoglyphus* are found on the quills of chickens and cage birds.

Dermoglyphus elongatus (quill mite)

Description: Small elongate mites, the male of which has no posterior lobes or anal suckers on the idiosoma. The apodemes of I and II are fused and the apex of leg IV does not extend beyond the posterior idiosomal margin. *Dermoglyphus elongatus* possesses a dorsal shield that is twice as long in length as in width, has two slender sclerotised bars that curve slightly outwards posteriorly, and has internal setae with separate bases.

Dermoglyphus passerinus (quill mite)

Description: Similar to *D. elongatus* except the dorsal shield is roughly rectangular (length about 1.7 times the width), the sclerotised bars curve slightly inwards and the internal setae have contiguous bases.

FAMILY FREYANIDAE

Members of the genus *Freyana* are found on the quills of chickens and cage birds, particularly the feathers of turkeys (Table 3.22).

Freyana

Table 3.22 *Freyana* species of veterinary importance.

Species	Hosts	Site
Freyana largifolia	Duck	Skin
Freyana anatina	Duck	Skin
Freyana chanayi	Turkey	Skin, feathers

FAMILY EPIDERMOPTIDAE

Bird ked mites cause depluming mange. The genera of interest are *Epidermoptes* and *Rivoltasia*, found on chickens; *Microlichus* found on quail; and *Promyialges* found on passeriform cage and aviary birds. Ked mites also affect hippoboscid flies affecting the bird host.

Epidermoptes bilobatus (ked mite)

Description: These are small mites, approximately 0.4 mm long, with a circular soft body. The idiosoma has a triangular anterior dorsal shield and a posterior dorsal shield, which in the female is roughly square with a concave posterior margin. The idiosoma in the female is rounded posteriorly with one pair of adanal, long

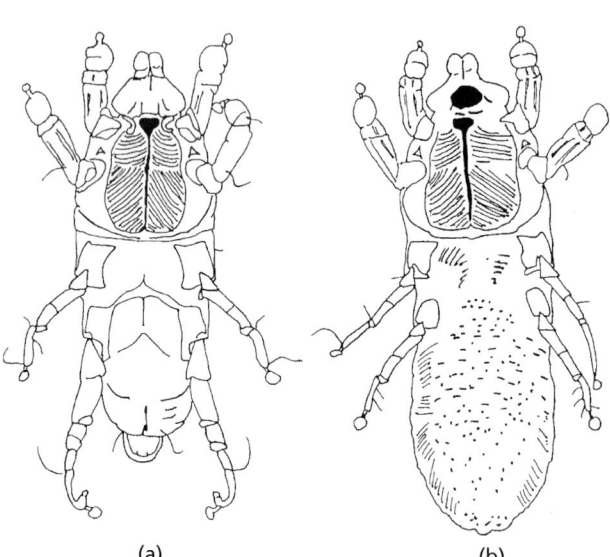

(a)   (b)

Fig. 3.102 Adults of *Chirodiscoides caviae*: (a) male, ventral view; (b) female, ventral view.

setae. Males have a triangular posterior dorsal shield and a pair of adanal suckers.

Rivoltasia bifurcata

Description: Males have long membraneous posterior lobes and female mites have fused pregenital sclerites and apodemes I forming a U-shape. Both sexes have backwardly directed processes on femora III and IV.

Microlichus americanus (ked mite)

Description: Small rounded mites with a triangular anterior dorsal shield and short legs ending in a terminal, recurved, claw-like process on legs I and II. The trochanters of legs III and IV have a ventral flange. In the female mites, the posterior margin of the idiosoma is widely rounded with two pairs of long setae. The posterior shield in the male is triangular and strongly indented, the posterior margin of the idiosoma has two well-formed separated lobes and there are two adanal suckers.

Promyialges macdonaldi (ked mite)

Synonym: *Myialges macdonaldi*

Description: Similar to *Microlichus* but the male is without posterior lobes and anal suckers. In the female, there is a large claw-like process on leg I and the idiosoma narrows to a straight posterior margin with four pairs of thick, spine-like, long setae. The tarsi on legs II–IV in the female and I–IV in the male have a small terminal pointed process.

Lynxacarus radovskyi

Description: a parasite of cats found in the USA and Australasia. The mites are less than 0.5 mm in length, are laterally compressed and found clinging to the hairs. The male mites have greatly enlarged fourth pair of legs. The life cycle is very poorly understood.

FAMILY PTEROLICHIDAE

The two genera of veterinary significance are *Pterolichus*, found on the tail and flight feathers of chickens, and *Sideroferus*, found on the budgerigar.

Pterolichus obtusus (feather mite)

Description: Similar to *Sideroferus* but the apodemes I are free; the female pregenital sclerite is an inverted U-shape and the male has a weakly divided opisthosoma posteriorly, and the legs are all of similar size.

Sideroferus lunula (feather mite)

Synonyms: *Pterolichus lunula, Protolichus lunula, Megninia lunula*

Description: Mites are elongate and both sexes are strongly sclerotised. The males have bifurcated tarsi on the first pair of legs and two long paragenial apodemes extending from the genital region to the posterolateral margins of the body.

FAMILY GABUCINIIDAE

There are several species in this genus, which infest a range of wild birds. Two species of *Gabucinia* are quill mites of ostriches (Table 3.23). These are pale elongated mites, about 0.5 μm in length. The dorsal idiosoma appears patterned or sculpted. The first two pairs of legs protrude anteriorly.

Life cycle: Typical: egg, nymphal stages and reproductive adult. Knowledge of the biology of these quill mites is very limited. Under intensive conditions this parasite is able to multiply rapidly on ostriches, reaching high densities.

FAMILY HYPODERATIDAE

The genus *Hypodectes* is of importance in pigeons, doves and other wild and captive birds. Their life cycle is unusal in that the adults are free-living and non-feeding, and the deutonymph is the main parasitic form present in subcutaneous cysts.

Hypodectes propus

Description: The deutonymph (hypopus) present in subcutaneous cysts is elongate (~1.5 mm long) with parallel sides and very short legs. The adults present in the nest have reduced palps and gnathostoma and in the female reduced chelicerae.

Life cycle: Free-living, nest-inhabiting mite which develops into a 'hypopus' that transiently invades the skin of birds. After leaving the host, the hypopus moults directly into an adult mite.

ORDER TROMBIDIFORMES (PROSTIGMATA)

The Prostigmata (Order Trombidiformes) is a large and diverse group of mites existing in a wide range of forms and occupying various ecological habitats. These prostigmatic mites usually have stigmata, which open on the gnathosoma or the anterior part of the idiosoma, known as the propodosoma. There are over 50 families, of which four contain species of veterinary importance: Demodicidae, Cheyletiellidae, Trombiculidae and Psorergatidae. Other families may be of lesser importance, not as parasites but because of the allergic responses they induce.

Table 3.23 *Gabucinia* species of veterinary importance.

Species	Hosts	Site
Gabucinia sculpturata	Ostrich	Feathers
Gabucinia bicaudatus (syn. *Pterolichus bicaudatus*)	Ostrich	Feathers

The Demodicidae is a family of prostigmatid mites, containing a single genus of veterinary interest, *Demodex*, species of which are found in a wide range of animals including humans.

Species of the genus *Demodex* are highly specialised mites that live in the hair follicles and sebaceous glands of a wide range of wild and domestic animals, including humans. They are believed to form a group of closely related sibling species which are highly specific to particular hosts: *Demodex phylloides* (pig), *Demodex canis* (dog), *Demodex bovis* (cattle), *Demodex equi* (horse), *Demodex musculi* (mouse), *Demodex ratticola* (rat), *Demodex caviae* (guinea pig), *Demodex cati* (cat) and *Demodex folliculorum* and *Demodex brevis* on humans.

Demodex

These are small mites with an elongated cigar-shaped body, up to 0.1–0.4 mm in length, with four pairs of stumpy legs ending in small blunt claws in the adult (Fig. 3.103). Setae are absent from the legs and body. The legs are located at the front of the body, and as such the striated opisthosoma forms at least half the body length. *Demodex* species of veterinary importance are listed in Table 3.24.

Life cycle: *Demodex* spp. usually live as commensals in the skin, and are highly site specific, occupying the hair follicles and sebaceous glands. Females lay 20–24 spindle-shaped eggs in the hair follicle that give rise to hexapod larvae, in which each short leg ends in a single three-pronged claw. Unusually, a second hexapod larval stage follows, in which each leg ends in a pair of three-pronged claws. Octopod protonymph, tritonymph and adult stages then follow. These migrate more deeply into the dermis. One follicle may harbour all life-cycle stages concurrently. The life cycle is completed in 18–24 days. In each follicle or gland, the mites may

Table 3.24 *Demodex* species of veterinary importance.

Species	Hosts	Site
Demodex bovis	Cattle	Skin
Demodex ovis (syn. *Demodex aries*)	Sheep	Skin
Demodex caprae	Goat	Skin
Demodex equi (syn. *Demodex caballi*)	Horse	Skin
Demodex phylloides	Pig	Skin
Demodex canis	Dog	Skin
Demodex cati	Cat	Skin
Demodex gatoi	Cat	Skin
Demodex musculi	Mouse	Skin
Demodex ratticola	Rat	Skin
Demodex caviae	Guinea pig	Skin
Demodex folliculorum	Human	Skin
Demodex brevis	Human	Skin

occur in large numbers in a characteristic head-downward posture. In the newborn and very young, these sites are simple in structure, but later they become compound by outgrowths. The presence of *Demodex* mites much deeper in the dermis than sarcoptids means that they are much less accessible to surface-acting acaricides. Species of *Demodex* are unable to survive off their host. See **life cycle 51**.

The majority of mites in this family are predatory, but several species of mites of the genus *Cheyletiella* are of veterinary and medical importance as ectoparasites of dogs, cats or rabbits that may transfer to humans. The body of the mite, up to 0.4 mm long, has a 'waist' and the palps are greatly enlarged, giving the appearance of an extra pair of legs. The legs terminate in 'combs' instead of claws or suckers.

Cheyletiella

Three very similar species of *Cheyletiella* are of veterinary importance and are common: *Cheyletiella yasguri* on dogs, *C. blakei* on cats and *C. parasitivorax* on rabbits. All three species are morphologically very similar; the solenidion, on the genu of the first pair of legs, is described as globose in *C. parasitivorax*, conical in *C. blakei* and heart-shaped in *C. yasguri* (Fig. 3.104 and Table 3.25). Nevertheless, this feature can vary in individuals and between life-cycle stages, making precise identification difficult. Identification to genus and knowledge of the host is usually sufficient for diagnosis, but it is important to be aware of the potential for cross-transmission of the various species of *Cheyletiella* from other in-contact hosts.

Life cycle: All developmental stages occur on the host animal. Eggs are glued to hairs 2–3 mm above the skin. A pre-larva and then a larva develop within the egg, with fully developed octopod nymphs eventually emerging from the egg. The mites then moult through two nymphal stages before the adult stage is reached. The life cycle is completed in approximately two weeks. The mites live in the hair and fur, only visiting the skin to feed on lymph and other tissue fluids. They feed on these fluids by piercing the epidermis with

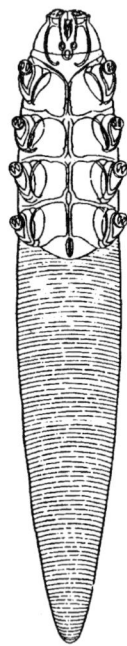

Fig. 3.103 Adult *Demodex* spp., ventral view. (Baker *et al.*, 1956/National Pest Control Association.)

LIFE CYCLE 51. LIFE CYCLE OF *DEMODEX CANIS*

Demodex canis lives permanently in the hair follicles and sebaceous glands of dogs. Adult mites are elongated and cigar-shaped (1), with four pairs of rudimentary legs. Females lay tapered eggs (2) from which hexapod larvae hatch (3) that subsequently moult into octopod nymphs (4) and then into male and female adults. Transmission occurs via direct contact with an infested host, particularly between pups and their dams within the first days of life.

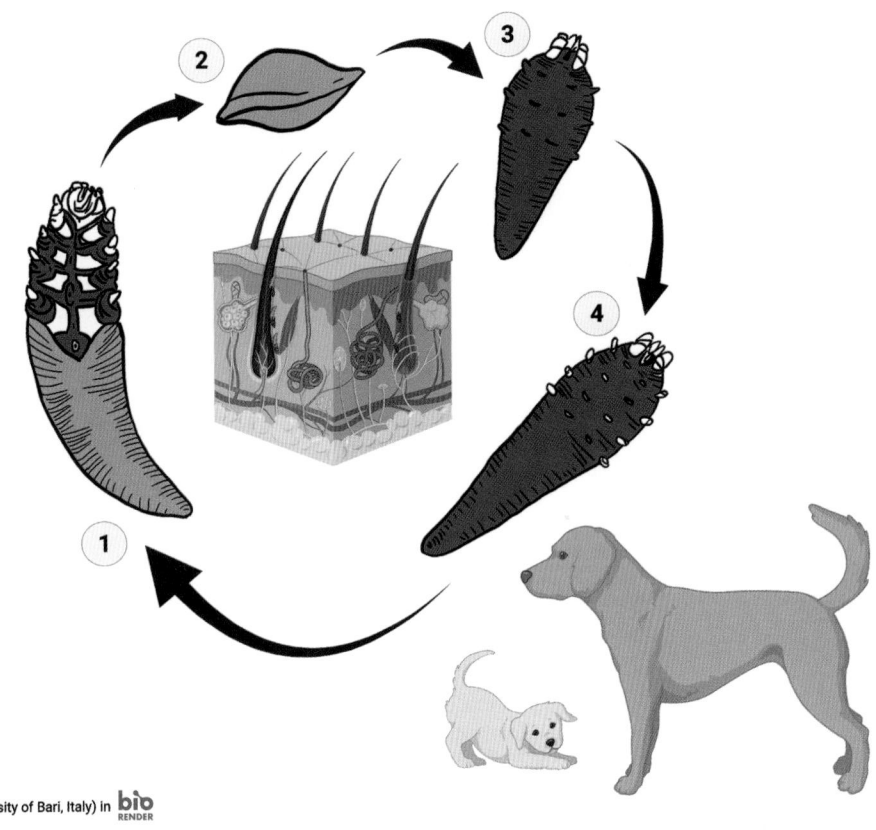

Made by Jairo Mendoza-Roldan (University of Bari, Italy) in **bio** RENDER

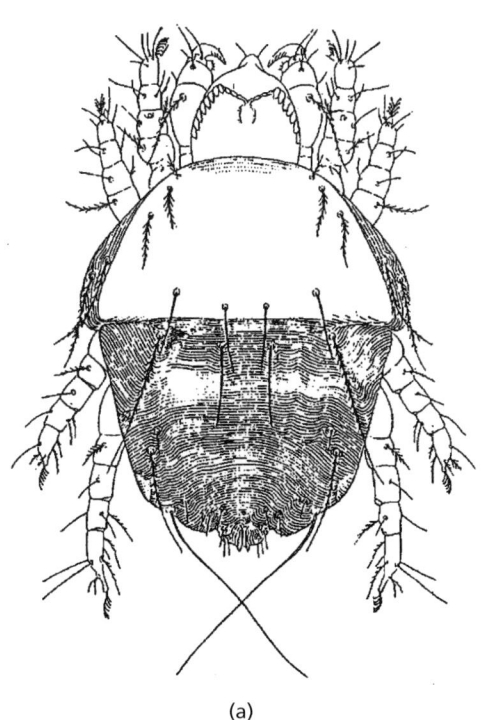

(a)

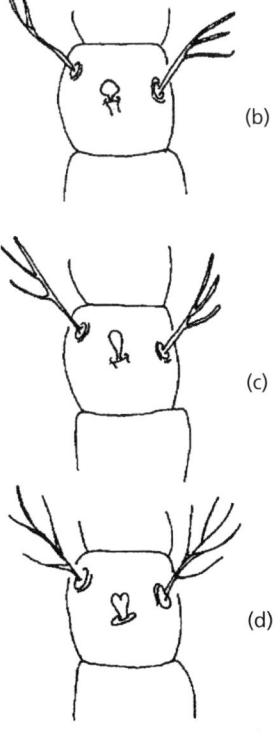

(b)

(c)

(d)

Fig. 3.104 (a) Adult female *Cheyletiella parasitivorax*, dorsal view. (Baker *et al.*, 1956/National Pest Control Association.) (b–d) Genu of the first pair of legs of adult females of (b) *Cheyletiella parasitivorax*, (c) *Cheyletiella blakei* and (d) *Cheyletiella yasguri*.

Table 3.25 *Cheyletiella* species of veterinary importance

Species	Hosts	Site
Cheyletiella parasitivorax	Rabbit, human	Fur
Cheyletiella yasguri	Dog, human	Fur
Cheyletiella blakei	Cat, human	Fur

their stylet-like chelicerae. Adults can survive for at least 10 days off the host without feeding, or longer in cool environments.

Cheyletiella parasitivorax (rabbit fur mite)

Description: Adults are about 400 μm in length and ovoid and have blade-like chelicerae that are used for piercing their host, and short, strong, opposable palps with curved palpal claws. The palpal femur possesses a long serrated dorsal seta. The body tends to be slightly elongated with a 'waist'. The legs are short; tarsal claws are lacking and the empodium is a narrow pad with comb-like pulvilli at the ends of the legs. Adults are highly mobile and are able to move about rapidly. The solenidion, on the genu of the first pair of legs, is described as globose in *C. parasitivorax*.

Cheyletiella yasguri

Description: This species is most easily differentiated from other species by a heart-shaped dorsal solenidion on genu I. Female mites have two small shields behind the anterior dorsal shield. The solenidion, on the genu of the first pair of legs, is heart-shaped.

Cheyletiella blakei

Description: The solenidion, on the genu of the first pair of legs, is conical in *C. blakei*. However, this feature can vary in individuals and between life-cycle stages, making identification difficult.

FAMILY TROMBICULIDAE

Species of the family Trombiculidae are commonly known as Chiggers, red bugs, harvest mites and scrub itch mites. Mites of this family are parasitic only at the larval stage, the nymphs and adults being free-living. More than 1500 species have been described. The mites feed on blood, which they ingest by puncturing the skin. Infestation causes pruritus, erythema and scratching, though there may be considerable individual variation in response. This variation may reflect the development of a hypersensitivity reaction to the mites, which may result in the development of wheals, papules and excoriation leading to hair loss. In some cases, pruritus occasionally may continue long after the larvae have left, and heavy infestations may also induce systemic effects such as fever.

The principal species of veterinary interest are in the genera *Neotrombicula* and *Eutrombicula*. Other lesser genera include *Leptotrombidium*, a vector of scrub typhus (tsutsugamushi fever) in the Far East, and *Neoschongastia*, which can affect chickens, quail and turkeys in North and Central America.

Neotrombicula and Eutrombicula

Species of *Neotrombicula* (harvest mites), which have a wide distribution, mainly in the Old World, and *Eutrombicula*, which occur in North and South America and Australia and whose larvae are known as chiggers, are of veterinary importance (Table 3.26). Larvae of both these genera will parasitise any animal, including humans.

Neotrombicula autumnalis (harvest mites)

Neotrombicula autumnalis are commonly found in clusters on the foot and up the legs of dogs, on the genital area and eyelids of cats, on the face of cattle and horses and on the heads of birds, having been picked up from the grass. They are widespread within Europe.

Description: The hexapod larvae are rounded, red to orange in colour and about 0.2 mm in length (Fig. 3.105). The scutum bears a

Table 3.26 Trombiculidae species of veterinary importance.

Species	Hosts	Site
Neotrombicula autumnalis	Dog, cat, cattle, horse, rabbit and birds, human	Skin, foot, legs, head
Eutrombicula alfreddugesi	Dog, cat, cattle, horse, rabbit, birds	Skin, commonly face, muzzle, thigh and belly
Eutrombicula splendens	Wild mammals, birds, reptiles, poultry, human	Skin, face, feet, legs
Eutrombicula sarcina	Kangaroo, sheep	Skin, face, feet, legs

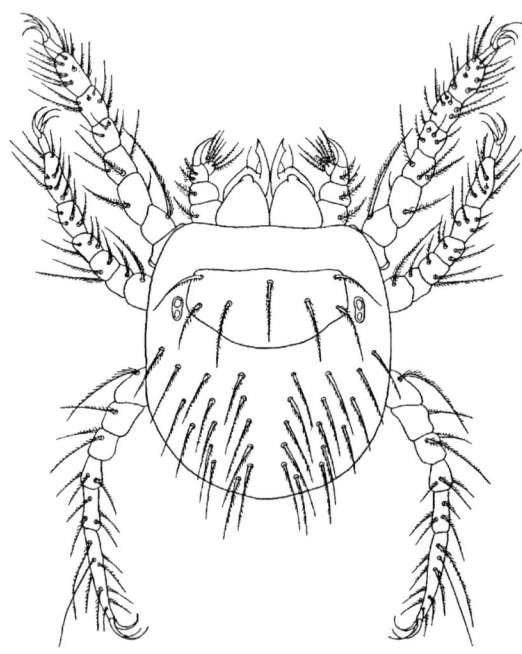

Fig. 3.105 Parasitic larval stage of the harvest mite *Neotrombicula autumnalis*. (From Savory, 1935.)

pair of sensillae and five setae. In *N. autumnalis* the scutum is roughly pentangular and has numerous small punctations. There are two simple eyes on each side of the scutum. The body is covered dorsally with 25–50 relatively long, ciliated, feather-like setae. The chelicerae are flanked by stout five-segmented palps. The palpal femur and genu each bear a single seta. The palpal tibia has three setae and a thumb-like terminal claw, which opposes the palpal tarsus. The palpal claw is three-pronged (trifurcate). Adults and nymphs have a pronounced figure-of-eight shape. They have stigmata, which open at the base of the chelicerae and their bodies are covered with setae. Adults are about 1 mm in length.

Life cycle: They are parasitic only in the larval stage. Female adults lay their spherical eggs in damp but well-drained soil. After about one week, the hexapod larva hatches from the egg and begins to crawl about the soil, eventually climbing an object such as a grass stem. Here it awaits a passing host. Larvae of the species of veterinary interest are not highly host specific and may attach to a variety of domestic animals. The larva attaches itself by its blade-like chelicerae and feeds on the host's serous tissues for several days before falling from the host. After feeding, the larva enters a quiescent stage for a few days as a nymphochrysalis, before moulting to become the active octopod nymph. After a further inactive imagochrysalis nymphal stage, the adult emerges. The nymphal and adult stages are free-living, mobile and predatory. The life cycle typically requires 50–70 days. *Neotrombicula autumnalis* passes through only one generation per year and its abundance is usually strongly seasonal.

Eutrombicula alfreddugesi (chigger mites)

Eutrombicula alfreddugesi will infest a range of hosts including dogs, cats, cattle, horses, rabbits and birds. This species is the most important and widespread of the trombiculid mites of veterinary interest in the New World. It is common from eastern Canada through to South America.

Description: The larvae of *Eutrombicula alfreddugesi*, known as chiggers, are similar in appearance to those of *N. autumnalis*. They are reddish-orange and vary in length between 0.15 mm when not engorged to 0.6 mm when fully fed. However, for the larvae of *E. alfreddugesi* the palpal claws are two-pronged (bifurcate), the scutum is approximately rectangular and 22 dorsal setae are present.

Life cycle: The life cycle is similar to that described for *N. autumnalis*. Adult chiggers are free-living while the immature stages are parasitic. Infestation is most common around the face, muzzle, thigh and belly. The resulting pruritus may persist for several days and is generally a hypersensitivity reaction to the mite saliva, occurring after the individual has detached.

Eutrombicula splendens (chigger mites)

Description: *Eutrombicula splendens* is morphologically similar and frequently sympatric with *E. alfreddugesi*. This species generally occurs in moister habitats than *E. alfreddugesi*, such as swamps and bogs. It is generally confined to the east of North America, from Ontario in Canada to the Gulf States, although it may also be abundant in Florida and parts of Georgia.

Eutrombicula sarcina (scrub itch mites, black soil itch mites)

Eutrombicula sarcina is an important parasite of sheep in Queensland and New South Wales of Australia. Its principal host, however, is the grey kangaroo. These mites prefer areas of savannah and grassland scrub. They may be particularly abundant from November to February, after summer rain. The primary site of infestation is on the leg, resulting in intense irritation.

Description: The parasitic larvae are small (0.2 mm long) round mites with numerous setae.

Leptotrombidium

The larvae (chiggers) feed on rodents, but also occasionally humans and other large mammals. The mites are both vector and reservoir for scrub typhus (*Orientia tsutsugamushi*) infection. *Leptotrombidium* species of veterinary importance are listed in Table 3.27.

Neoschongastia

Larvae of these small mites normally feed on wild animals, birds and reptiles but also attack poultry, causing dermatitis particularly under the wings.

Neoschongastia americana (turkey chigger)

Description: Differentiated from other chigger mites by the presence of a single dorsal tooth on each chelicera, a sunken posterior dorsal shield covered in strations and the shape of the sensilli which are bulbous.

FAMILY PSORERGATIDAE

Two species of the genus *Psorobia* are found on cattle and sheep; the species found on sheep is a major ectoparasite in southern hemisphere countries. The body is almost circular with the legs arranged equidistant around the body circumference, with two pairs of elongate posterior setae in the female adult mite and single pairs in the male. The femur of each leg bears a large, inwardly directed, curved spine.

Life cycle: The life cycle is typical: egg, hexapod larva, followed by octopod protonymph, tritonymph and adult. All developmental stages occur on the host. The egg-to-adult life cycle requires approximately 35 days.

Table 3.27 *Leptotrombidium* species of veterinary importance.

Species	Geographic range
Leptotrombidium akamushi	Japan
Leptotrombidium delicense	China, Thailand, Northern Territory, Australia
Leptotrombidium pallidum	Japan
Leptotrombidium scutellare	Japan

Psorobia ovis (sheep itch mite)

Synonym: *Psorergates ovis*

Description: *Psorobia ovis* is a small mite, roughly circular in form and less than 0.2 mm in diameter (Fig. 3.106). The legs are arranged more or less equidistantly around the body circumference, giving the mite a crude star shape. Larvae of *P. ovis* have short stubby legs. The legs become progressively longer during the nymphal stages until, in the adult, the legs are well developed and the mites become mobile. Adults are about 190 μm long and 160 μm wide. The tarsal claws are simple and the empodium is pad-like. The femur of each leg bears a large, inwardly directed, curved spine. In the adult female, two pairs of long whip-like setae are present posteriorly; in the male there is only a single pair.

Psorobia bovis (cattle itch mite)

Synonym: *Psorergates bos*

Description: Morphologically similae to *Psorobia ovis* but smaller in size (female, 135–145 μm; male, 160 μm).

FAMILY PYEMOTIDAE

These are 'forage' mites found on hay and grain that predate largely on insect larvae, but they can cause dermatitis on animals and humans. Mites of the genus *Pyemotes* are small with elongated bodies, the female mites giving birth to fully formed adults.

Pyemotes tritici (straw itch mite)

Description: Elongate to oval, grey or yellowish mites; females are 220–250 μm but may reach up to 2 mm in diameter when gravid.

Legs are long with II and III widely separated. Tarsus I ends in a hooked claw.

FAMILY MYOBIIDAE

These are small blood-feeding mites found on rodents, bats and insectivores. Species of the genera *Myobia* and *Radfordia* may cause a mild dermatitis of laboratory mice and rats, respectively.

Myobia musculi (mouse fur mite)

Description: The mouse fur mite, *Myobia musculi*, is a small translucent mite, typically around 300 μm in length and 190 μm wide. The body is broadly rounded at the rear with transverse striations on the integument (Fig. 3.107). The gnathosoma is small and simple with stylet-like chelicerae. Between the second, third and fourth pairs of legs there are lateral bulges and each tarsus bears an empodial claw. The anus is dorsal and flanked by a long pair of setae.

Life cycle: The female oviposits in the fur, cementing the eggs to the base of the hairs. Eggs hatch within eight days and the larvae moult four days later. The egg-to-adult life cycle requires a minimum period of 12 days. All stages feed on extracellular fluids.

Radfordia

Mites of this genus are morphologically similar to *M. musculi*, but can be distinguished by the presence of two tarsal claws as opposed to just one (Fig. 3.108). The primary species of *Radfordia* of veterinary importance are *Radfordia affinis* found on mice and *R. ensifera* found on rats.

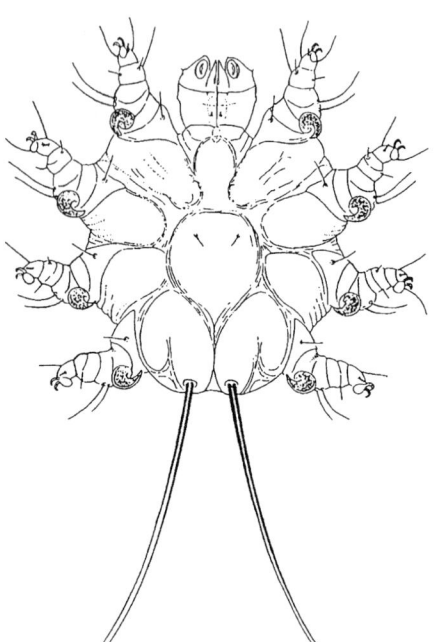

Fig. 3.106 Adult female *Psorobia*. (Baker *et al.*, 1956/National Pest Control Association.)

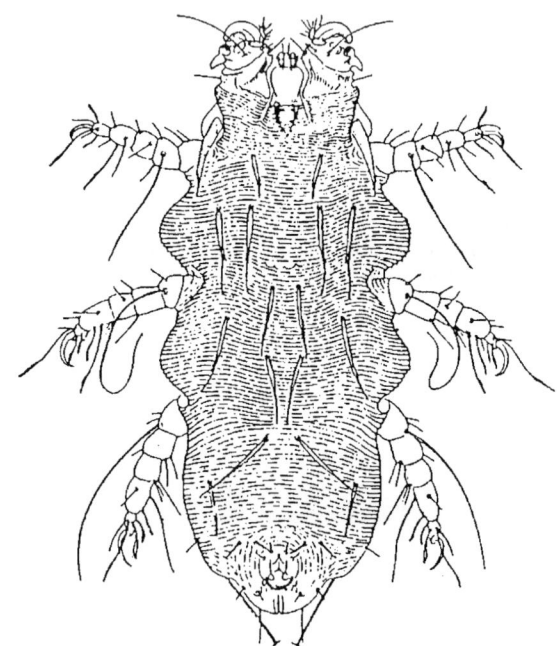

Fig. 3.107 Adult female *Myobia musculi* (dorsal view). (Baker *et al.*, 1956/National Pest Control Association.)

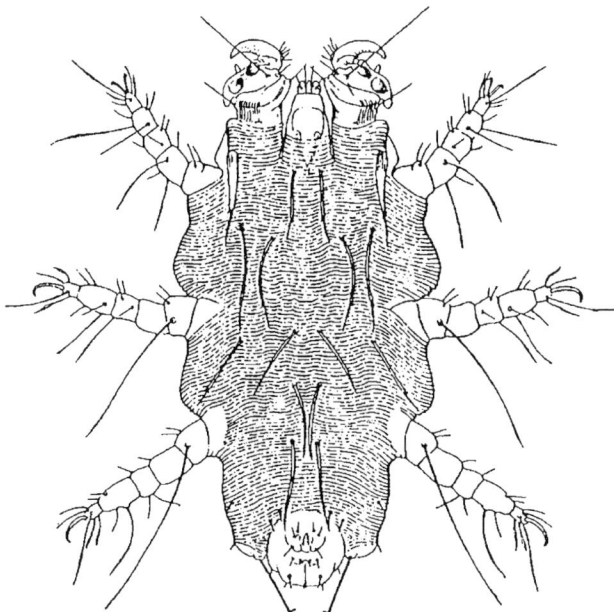

Fig. 3.108 Adult female *Radfordia ensifera* (dorsal view). (Baker *et al.*, 1956/National Pest Control Association.)

Radfordia affinis

Description: Found on rats and identified by the claws on tarsus II, which are equal in size.

Radfordia ensifera

Description: Found on mice and has claws of unequal size on tarsus II.

FAMILY SYRINGOPHILIDAE

Poultry quill mites, *Syringophilus*, feed on tissue fluids of feather follicles causing feather loss.

Syringophilus bipectinatus (quill mite)

Description: Elongate mites, females approximately 600 μm in length and males 500 μm in length; the chelicerae are fused to form a stylophore with pointed posterior margin.

FAMILY OPHIOPTIDAE

These mites are found beneath the scales of snakes.

FAMILY CLOACARIDAE

These mites are found in the cloacal mucosa of reptiles. *Cloacarus* are found in aquatic terrapins.

FAMILY PTERYGOSOMATIDAE

These are parasites of lizards and include the genera *Geckobiella*, *Hirstiella*, *Ixodiderma*, *Pimeliaphilus*, *Scapothrix* and *Zonurobia*.

ORDER MESOSTIGMATA

The Mesostigmata (gamesid mites) are a large group of mites, the majority of which are predatory, but a small number of species are important as ectoparasites of birds and mammals. Mesostigmatid mites have stigmata located above the coxae of the second, third or fourth pairs of legs. They are generally large with usually one large sclerotised shield on the dorsal surface, and a series of smaller shields in the midline of the ventral surface. The legs are long and positioned anteriorly. Some species are host specific but the majority parasitise a range of hosts. There are two main families of veterinary interest, the Dermanyssidae and Macronyssidae, and four families of minor interest: Laelapidae, Halarachinidae, Entonyssidae and Rhinonyssidae.

FAMILY MACRONYSSIDAE

These are relatively large blood-sucking ectoparasites of birds and mammals of which *Ornithonyssus*, in birds, and *Ophionyssus*, in reptiles, are of veterinary importance. Only the protonymph and adult stages blood feed. The mites have relatively long legs and can be seen with the naked eye. The female genital shield and the male holoventral shield taper posteriorly to coxae IV.

Ornithonyssus

Includes the northern fowl mite, *Ornithonyssus sylviarum*, which is capable of transmitting a number of important viral diseases, and *bacoti* (the tropical rat mite). *Ornithonyssus* species of veterinary importance are listed in Table 3.28.

Ornithonyssus sylviarum (northern fowl mite)

Synonyms: *Liponyssus sylviarum, Macronyssus sylviarum*

Description: The adults are relatively large, oval-shaped and 0.75–1 mm in length with long legs that allow it to move rapidly (Fig. 3.109). The body is usually greyish-white, becoming red to

Table 3.28 *Ornithonyssus* species of veterinary importance.

Species	Hosts	Site
Ornithonyssus sylviarum (syn. *Liponyssus sylviarum*, *Macronyssus sylviarum*)	Chicken, poultry, pigeon, wild birds, occasionally mammals, humans	Base of feathers, particularly vent
Ornithonyssus bursa (syn. *Macronyssus bursa*, *Leiognathus bursa*)	Poultry, wild birds	Skin, feathers
Ornithonyssus bacoti (syn. *Liponyssus bacoti*, *Macronyssus bacoti*)	Rodents, cat, human, chicken, wild birds	Skin

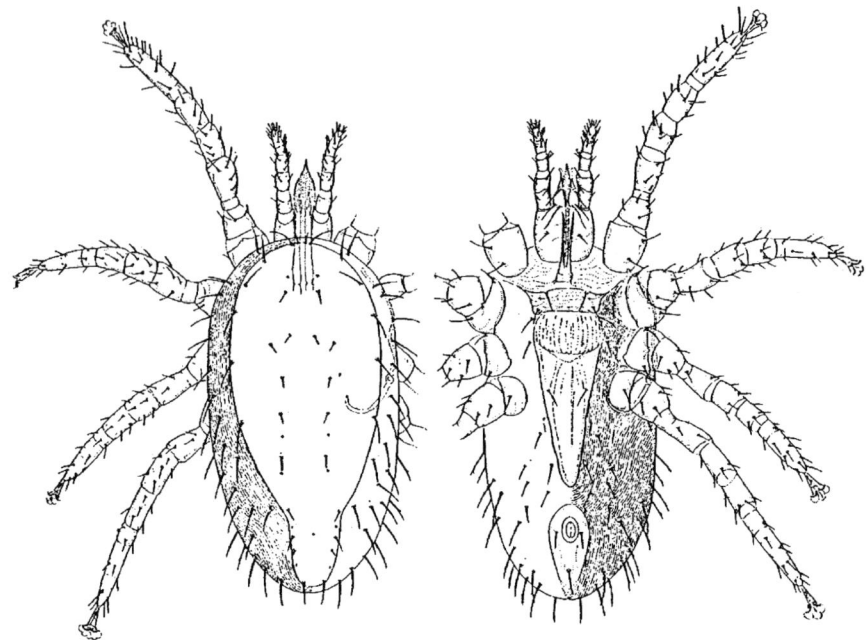

Fig. 3.109 Adult female *Ornithonyssus sylviarum* (northern fowl mite): (left) dorsal view; (right) ventral view. (From Baker *et al.*, 1956.)

black when engorged. A single dorsal shield is wide for two-thirds of its length, then tapers posteriorly to become about half as wide, and is truncated at its posterior margin. The female typically has only two pairs of setae on the sternal shield. The anal shield is relatively large and at least as wide as the genitoventral plate. Three anal setae are present. The chelicerae are elongate and stylet-like. The body carries many long setae and is much more hairy than *Dermanyssus*.

Life cycle: Unlike *Dermanyssus*, *Ornithonyssus* spends its entire life on the bird and can only survive for about 10 days away from a host. The female lays 1–5 sticky whitish-coloured eggs on the host at the base of the feathers, primarily in the vent area, after a blood meal. The eggs hatch within approximately a day to produce hexapod larvae. The larvae do not feed, and moult to become protonymphs. The protonymphs feed on blood from the host, before moulting to become tritonymphs. The tritonymphs do not feed, and moult to the adult stage. The entire life cycle can be completed in 5–12 days under optimal conditions, but usually takes longer. Because of the short generation times, large populations can develop rapidly on the birds.

Ornithonyssus bursa (tropical fowl mite)

Synonyms: *Macronyssus bursa*, *Leiognathus bursa*

Description: Similar to *O. sylviarum*. However, the ventral plate bears three pairs of setae, while in *O. sylviarum* and *Dermanyssus gallinae* only two pairs of setae are present.

Life cycle: Similar to that of *O. sylviarum*.

Ornithonyssus bacoti (tropical rat mite)

Synonyms: *Liponyssus bacoti*, *Macronyssus bacoti*

Description: This rapidly moving, long-legged mite has an oval body, about 1 mm in length. Both sexes feed on blood. The colour varies from white to reddish-black depending on the amount of blood ingested. It is similar in appearance and life cycle to the fowl mite, *Ornithonyssus sylviarum*. However, the female mites bear three pairs of setae on the sternal shield, and the setae on the dorsal shield are as long, or longer, than those on the surrounding cuticle. In the male, the holoventral shield has parallel sides, posterior to coxae IV. The body carries many long setae and is much more hairy than the red mite of poultry, *Dermanyssus gallinae*. The adult female survives for around 70 days, during which it feeds every 2–3 days and lays about 100 eggs.

Life cycle: *Ornithonyssus bacoti* spends its entire life on the host and can only survive for about 10 days away from a host.

Ophionyssus

Parasites of reptiles, the most important species of which, *Ophionyssus natricis* (the reptile mite), is commonly found on snakes and other captive lizards, turtles, crocodiles and other reptiles.

Ophionyssus natricis (reptile mite)

Synonyms: *Ophionyssus serpentium*, *Serpenticola serpentium*

Description: Adults are 0.6–1.3 mm long. Unfed females are yellow-brown; engorged females are dark red, brown or black. The cuticle bears only a few short bristle-like hairs (Fig. 3.110).

Life cycle: The engorged female leaves the host and deposits eggs in cracks and crevices. The eggs hatch in 1–4 days, developing through larva, protonymph and deutonymph stages to the adult. Larvae do not feed but nymphs must feed before moulting to the next stage. The life cycle takes 13–19 days.

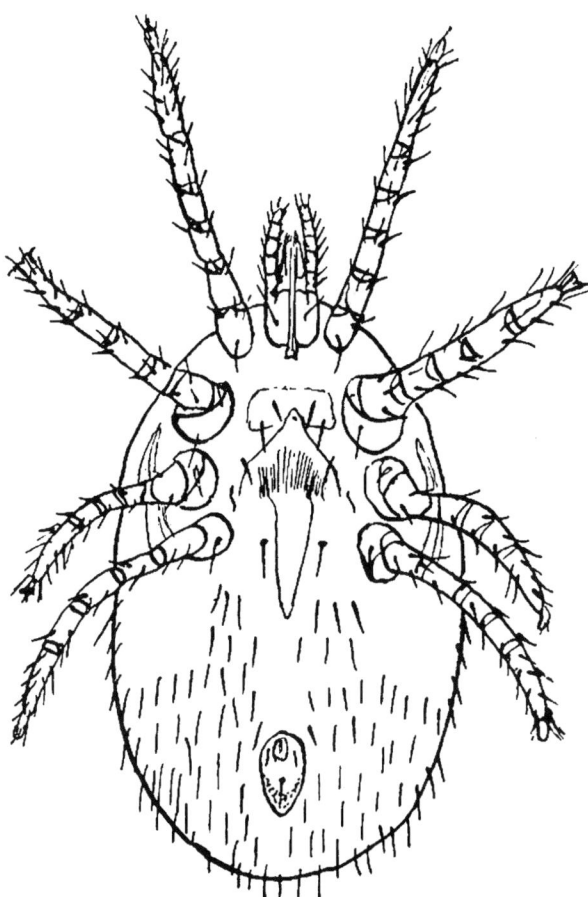

Fig. 3.110 *Ophionyssus natricis*. (Redrawn from Reichenhack-Klinke & Elkan, 1965. Reproduced with permission from Elsevier.)

FAMILY DERMANYSSIDAE

Species of the genus *Dermanyssus* are blood-feeding ectoparasites of birds and mammals. They are large mites with long legs, greyish white, becoming red when engorged. *Liponyssoides*, which affect rodents, are of minor veterinary significance but can act as disease vectors of Q-fever and rickettsial pox to humans.

Dermanyssus

The red mite or chicken mite, *Dermanyssus gallinae*, is one of the most common mites of poultry. It feeds on the blood of fowl, pigeons, cage birds and many other wild birds. It also occasionally bites mammals, including humans, if the usual hosts are unavailable.

Dermanyssus gallinae (poultry red mite)

Description: Adult mites are relatively large at 0.75–1 mm in length, with long legs (Fig. 3.111). The body is usually greyish-white, becoming red to black when engorged. The chelicerae are elongate and stylet-like, and the middle segment in female mites is very slender. A single dorsal shield is present, which tapers posteriorly but is truncated at its posterior margin. The anal shield is relatively large and is at least as wide as the genitoventral plate. Three anal setae are present. In the male, there are small sucker-like projections subterminally on tarsi III and IV.

Life cycle: This mite spends much of its life cycle away from its host, the adult and nymph only visiting birds to feed, mainly at night. The favoured habitats are poultry houses, usually of timber construction, in the crevices of which the eggs are laid. The life

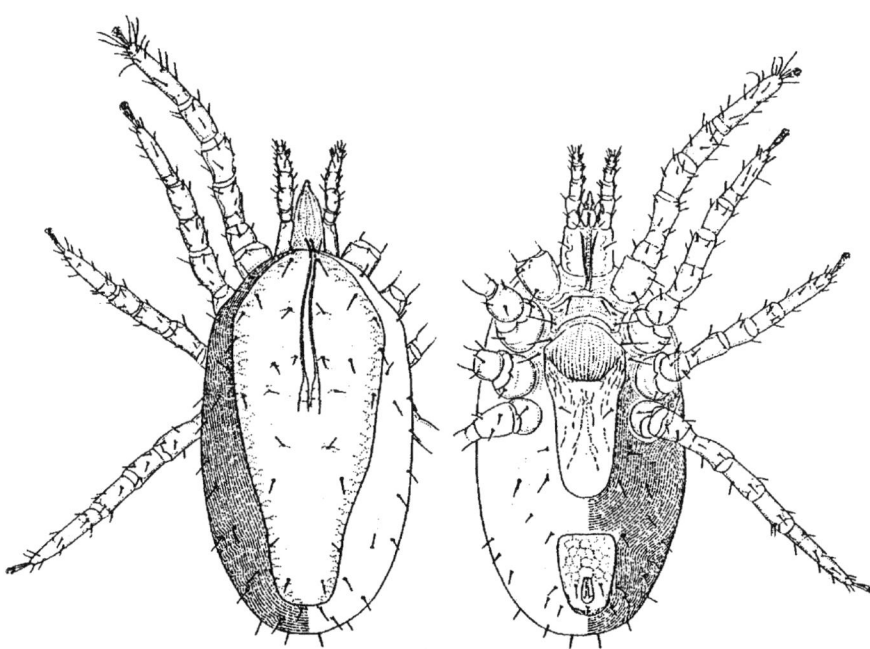

Fig. 3.111 Adult female of the red mite, *Dermanyssus gallinae*: (left) dorsal view; (right) ventral view. (Baker *et al.*, 1956/ National Pest Control Association.)

cycle can be completed in a minimum of a week, allowing large populations to develop rapidly, although during cold weather the cycle is slower. Approximately one day after feeding, batches of eggs are laid in hiding places, detritus or near nests and roosts. Within 2–3 days the eggs hatch into six-legged larvae. The larvae do not feed before moulting, and become octopod protonymphs 1–2 days later. Within another couple of days, they moult again and soon afterward they complete their final moult to become an adult. Both nymphal stages feed, as do the adult mites. The adult can survive for several months without feeding, so a reservoir population can persist in unoccupied poultry houses and aviaries.

FAMILY HALARACHNIDAE

Mites of the subfamily Halarachinae are obligate parasites found in the respiratory tract of mammals. *Pneumonyssoides* is found in the nasal sinuses and nasal passages of dogs. *Pneumonyssus* and *Rhinophaga* are found in the respiratory tract of monkeys. Members of the subfamily Raillietiinae are obligate parasites in the external ears of mammals.

Pneumonyssoides caninum (nasal mite)

Synonym: *Pneumonyssus caninum*

Description: The mites are oval and pale yellow, adults measuring approximately 1–1.5 by 0.6–0.9 mm in length. They have a smooth cuticle with relatively few setae. The mites have a single, irregularly shaped dorsal plate and a small sternal plate. Genital plates are absent in this species and the genital opening is a transverse slit between the coxae of the fourth pair of legs. They have long legs, relative to their body size, which terminate in claws and small chelicerae.

Life cycle: Details of the life history of these mites are not fully known. There appear to be two main life stages, the adult and a six-legged larval stage. There is no nymphal stage in the life cycle of this parasite. The female is ovoviviparous and mature females often contain eggs and it is probable that they give birth to larvae.

Raillietia

Raillietia caprae

Description: Similar to *Pneumonyssoides*, with a heavily patterned holodorsal shield but with a well-developed tritosternum, longer peritremes and the presence of both a genital and sternal shield in the female. This species has a short dorsal shield (500–600 μm) with 17 pairs of setae.

Life cycle: Details of the life history of these mites are not fully known. There appear to be two main life stages, the adult and a six-legged larval stage. There is no nymphal stage in the life cycle of this parasite. The female is ovoviviparous and mature females often contain eggs and it is probable that they give birth to larvae.

Raillietia auris

Description: As for *R. caprae* but with a longer dorsal shield (700–800 μm) with 12 pairs of setae.

FAMILY ENTONYSSIDAE

Mites of the family Entonyssidae are found in the respiratory tract of reptiles. *Entonyssus*, *Entophionyssus* and *Mabuyonyssus* are found in the trachea and lungs of snakes.

FAMILY RHINONYSSIDAE

Most species are parasites of the nasopharynx of birds. *Sternostoma* occurs worldwide and is found in a range of domestic and wild birds, including canaries and budgerigars.

Sternostoma tracheacolum (air sac mite)

The canary lung mite, *Sternosoma tracheacolum*, causes pneumonia and inflammation of the respiratory system in caged and wild birds.

Description: Mites are elongate up to 1 mm in size, with a small gnathosoma and thick legs with claws on II–IV.

FAMILY HAEMOGAMASIDAE

A cosmopolitan family of closely related species – some may be free-living while others are superficial parasites of small mammals, particularly rodents.

Haemogamasus pontiger

Description: Mites are brown in colour, over 1 mm long, covered in many short setae and with long slender legs. Both sexes have a large dorsal shield and in the female there is a sternal shield with a deeply concave posterior margin. The anal shield in female mites is an inverted pear shape with two small median papillae on the anterior margin.

FAMILY LAELAPIDAE

Species of the genera *Haemogamasus*, *Laelaps*, *Androlaelaps*, *Haemolaelaps*, *Echinolaelaps* and *Hirstionyssus* are blood-feeding parasites of rodents and are found worldwide.

Laelaps echidnina (spiny rat mite)

Description: Similar to *Haemogamasus* but with a more circular idiosoma and thicker setae and legs. In the female, there is an opisthogenital shield with a posterior concavity.

Androlaelaps casalis (poultry litter mite)

Androlaelaps casalis, the poultry litter mite or nest mite, can occur in large numbers in chicken house litter.

Description: Similar to *Haemogamasus* but has fewer and mostly paired setae on the dorsal shield and a more tongue-shaped genital shield bearing only one pair of setae. The male holoventral shield has 15 setae, all paired except for the most posterior.

ORDER IXODIDA (METASTIGMATA)

The ticks are obligate blood-feeding ectoparasites of vertebrates, particularly mammals and birds. They are relatively large and long-lived, feeding periodically on large blood meals, often with long intervals between meals. Tick bites may be directly damaging to animals, causing irritation, inflammation or hypersensitivity and, when present in large numbers, anaemia and production losses. The salivary secretions of some ticks may cause toxicosis and paralysis; however, more importantly, when they attach and feed they are capable of transmitting a number of pathogenic viral, bacterial, rickettsial and protozoal diseases.

Ticks belong to two main families, the **Ixodidae** and **Argasidae**. The most important is the Ixodidae, often called the **hard ticks**, because of the presence of a rigid chitinous scutum which covers the entire dorsal surface of the adult male. In the adult female and in the larva and nymph, it extends for only a small area, which permits the abdomen to swell after feeding. The other family is the Argasidae or **soft ticks**, so called because they lack a scutum; included in this family are the bird ticks and the tampans.

For clinical information see the most relevant host chapter.

FAMILY IXODIDAE

Ixodid ticks are important vectors of protozoal, bacterial, viral and rickettsial diseases. The Ixodidae contains about 650 species of ticks. The phylogeny of tick families and genera is undergoing revision and is still not fully resolved, and some genera have been more recently synonymised. *Ixodes* is the largest genus, containing 217 species. Other genera of veterinary importance include *Dermacentor*, *Haemaphysalis*, *Rhipicephalus* (which now subsumes the synonymised genus *Boophilus*), *Hyalomma* and *Amblyomma* (synonymised genus *Aponomma*). However, recently it has also been suggested that ticks in the family Hyalomminae should be subsumed within the Rhipicephalinae, but while acknowledging this likely change here, we will discuss the genus *Hyalomma* separately within this text.

The Ixodidae are relatively large ticks, between 2 and 20 mm in length and flattened dorsoventrally. The enlarged fused coxae of the palps are known as the **basis capituli**, which vary in shape in the different genera. Its ventromedial wall is extended anteriorly to form the **hypostome**, which lies below the chelicerae (Fig. 3.112). The hypostome is armed with rows of backward-facing barbs or teeth, and is used as an anchoring device when the tick feeds. The structure of the hypostome and chelicerae permit the outward flow of saliva and inward flow of host blood. The four-segmented sensory palps and heavily sclerotised chelicerae are anterior and visible from the dorsal surface. On the dorsal surface of the basis capituli, ixodid females have a pair of depressions filled wih tiny pores, known as the **porose area**. Projecting from the posterior corners of the basis capituli may be a pair of projections, called **cornua** on the dorsal surface and **auriculae** on the ventral surface. The presence and shape of these projections may be important in the identification of tick species.

Ixodid ticks have a chitinous dorsal plate or **scutum** (Fig. 3.113), which extends over the whole dorsal surface of the male but covers only a small area behind the gnathosoma in the larva, nymph or female. Other distinguishing features are a series of grooves on the scutum and body and, in some species, a row of notches, called **festoons**, on the posterior border of the body. Chitinous plates are sometimes present on the ventral surface of the males. Some ticks

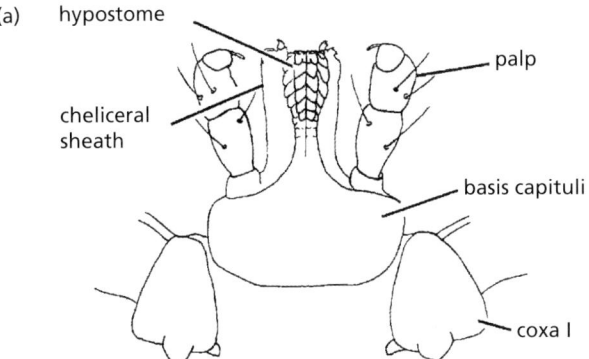

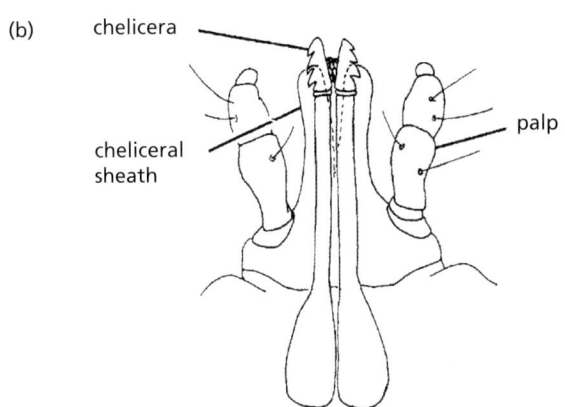

Fig. 3.112 Tick mouthparts: (a) ventral view showing toothed hypostome; (b) dorsal view showing the chelicerae behind the cheliceral sheaths.

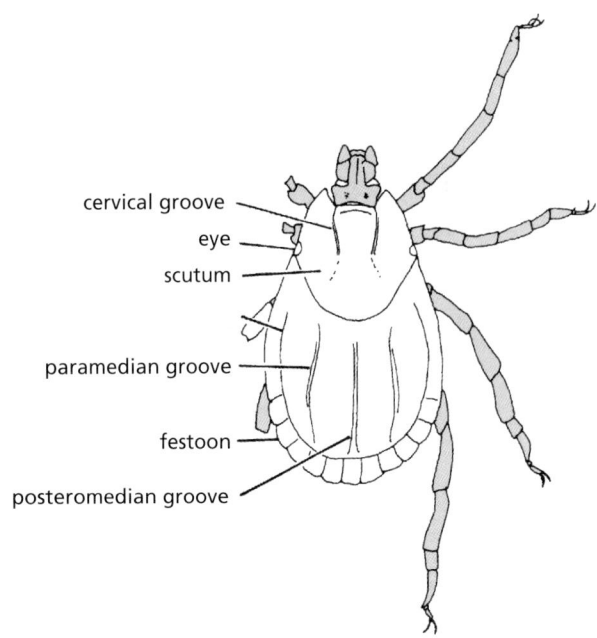

Fig. 3.113 Dorsal view of a generalised female ixodid tick.

have coloured enamel-like areas on the body and these are called 'ornate' ticks.

The coxa of the leg may be armed with internal and external **ventral spurs**; their number and size may be important in species identification (Fig. 3.114). Located on the tarsi of the first pair of

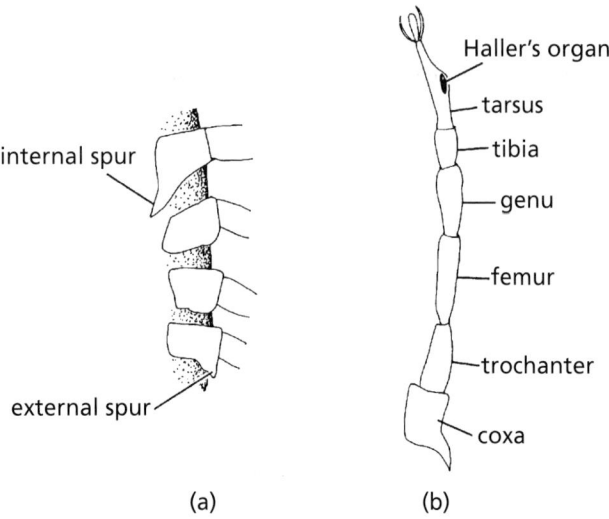

Fig. 3.114 (a) Ventral view of the coxae showing internal and external spurs and (b) segments of the leg of a generalised ixodid tick.

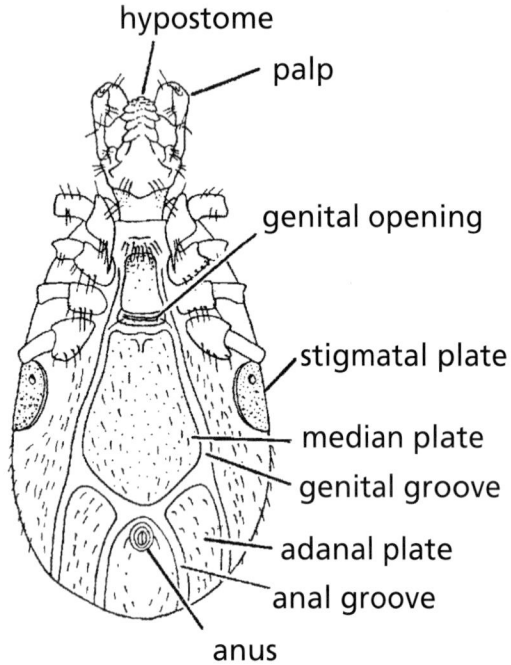

Fig. 3.115 Ventral view of a generalised male ixodid tick.

legs is Haller's organ, which is packed with chemoreceptors used for locating potential hosts. Eyes, when present, are situated on the outside margin of the scutum. Adult and nymphal ticks have a pair of respiratory openings, the **stigmata**, which lead to the tracheae. The stigmata are large and positioned posterior to the coxae of the fourth pair of legs. In adults, the genital opening, the **gonopore**, is situated ventrally behind the gnathosoma, usually at the level of the second pair of legs, and is surrounded by the **genital apron**. A pair of **genital grooves** extend backwards from the gonopore to the **anal groove**, located ventrally and usually posterior to the fourth pair of legs (Fig. 3.115).

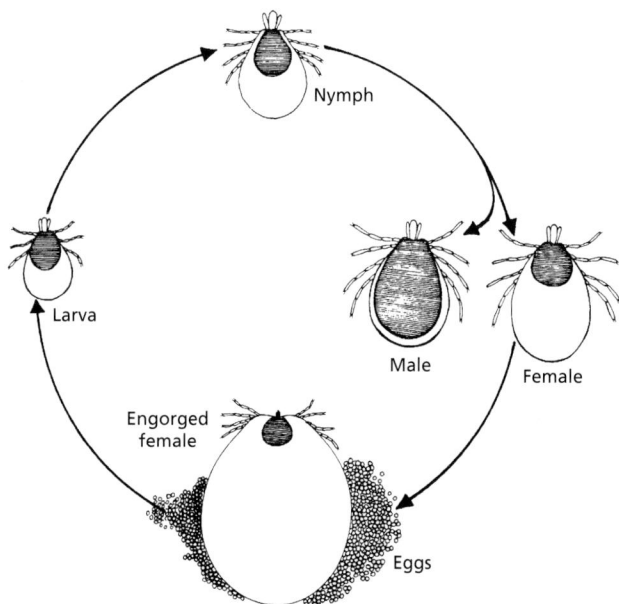

Fig. 3.116 Life cycle of an ixodid tick.

The hard ticks are temporary parasites and most species spend relatively short periods on the host. There is a single hexapod larval stage and a single octopod nymphal stage leading to the reproductive, eight-legged adult stage (Fig. 3.116).

During the passage through these stages, ixodid ticks take a number of large blood meals, interspersed by lengthy free-living periods. They are relatively long-lived and each female may produce several thousand eggs. Most hard ticks are relatively immobile and rather than actively hunting for their hosts, the majority adopt a strategy known as questing, in which they wait at the tips of vegetation for an appropriate host to brush past. Once contact is made, the ticks transfer to the host and then move over the surface to find their preferred attachment sites, such as the ears. Preferred sites for attachment may be highly specific to the particular species of tick.

Ticks have developed a variety of complex life cycles and feeding strategies, which reflect the nature of the habitat that the various species of tick inhabit and the probability of contact with an appropriate host. The number of hosts to which they attach during their parasitic life cycle varies from one to three. Based on this, they are classified as follows.
- **One-host ticks**, where the entire parasitic development from larva to adult takes place on the one host.
- **Two-host ticks**, where larva and nymph occur on one host and the adult on another.
- **Three-host ticks**, where each stage of development takes place on different hosts.

For most, a three-host life cycle has been adopted. Larvae, nymphs and adults all feed on different hosts. Blood feeding typically takes between four and six days, after which they drop to the ground and either moult to the next life-cycle stage or lay eggs. Ticks must then relocate a suitable host to feed and moult again or lay eggs. For a relatively small number of ixodid ticks, about 50 species, which inhabit areas where hosts are scarce and in which lengthy seasonal periods of unfavourable climate occur, two- and one-host feeding strategies have evolved.

In temperate habitats, feeding and generation cycles of hard ticks are closely synchronised with periods of suitable temperature and humidity conditions. Ticks, particularly in the immature stages, are very susceptible to desiccation, particularly when they are active. To minimise drying out, they start questing when saturated with water and return to the humid ground level when dehydrated. Water may also be imbibed by drinking.

In the field, the stability of the microclimate is dependent on factors such as the quantity of herbage or plant debris and the grass species. The various genera of ticks have different thresholds of temperature and humidity within which they are active and feed, and these thresholds govern their distribution. Generally, ticks are most active during the warm season provided there is sufficient rainfall, but in some species the larval and nymphal stages are also active in milder weather. This affects the duration and timing of control programmes.

The long-term control of three-host ticks is geared to the period required for the adult female stage to become fully engorged, which varies from four to 10 days according to the species. If an animal is treated with an acaricide which has a residual effect of, say, three days, it will be at least seven days before any fully engorged female reappears following treatment (i.e. three days residual effect plus a minimum of four days for engorgement). Weekly treatment during the tick season should therefore kill the adult female ticks before they are fully engorged, except in cases of very severe challenge when the treatment interval has to be reduced to 4–5 days.

Theoretically, weekly treatment should also control the larvae and nymphs but in several areas, the peak infestations of larvae and nymphs occur at different seasons to the adult females and the duration of the treatment season has to be extended.

Since many ticks occur on less accessible parts of the body, such as the anus, vulva, groin, scrotum, udder and ear, care must be exercised to ensure that the acaricide is properly applied. Cultivation of land and, in some areas, improved drainage help to reduce the prevalence of tick populations and can be used where more intensive systems of agriculture prevail. Pasture 'spelling', where domestic livestock are removed from pastures for a period of time, has been used in semi-extensive or extensive areas, but often has the disadvantage that ticks can still obtain blood from a wide variety of other hosts.

Ixodes

Ixodes is the largest genus in the family Ixodidae, with about 250 species. They are small inornate ticks that do not have eyes or festoons. The mouthparts are long and are longer in the female than male. The fourth segment of the palps is greatly reduced and bears chemoreceptor sensilla. The second segment of the palps may be restricted at the base, creating a gap between the palp and chelicerae (Fig. 3.117a). Males have several ventral plates, which almost cover the ventral surface. *Ixodes* can be distinguished from other

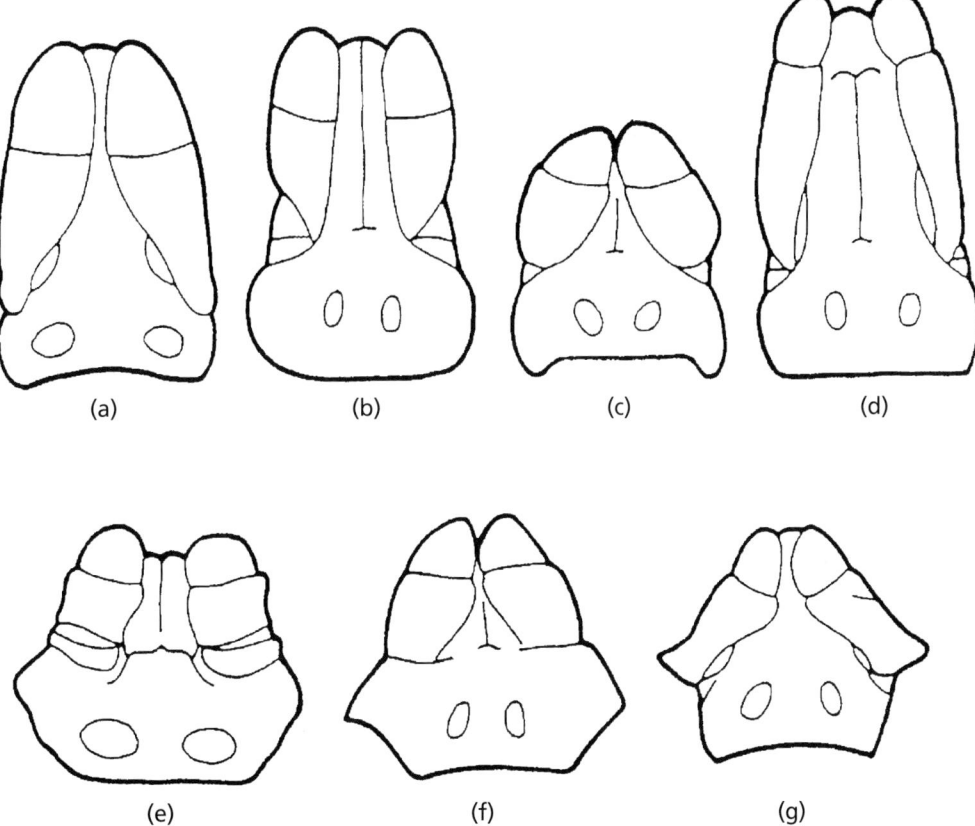

Fig. 3.117 Diagrammatic dorsal view of the gnathosoma of six genera of ixodid ticks: (a) *Ixodes*; (b) *Hyalomma*; (c) *Dermacentor*; (d) *Amblyomma*; (e) *Rhipicephalus* (*Boophilus*); (f) *Rhipicephalus*; (g) *Haemaphysalis*. (From Smart, 1943.)

Table 3.29 *Ixodes* species of veterinary importance.

Species	Hosts	Site
Ixodes ricinus	Sheep, cattle, goat, but can feed on all mammals and birds; juvenile stages may also feed on lizards	Skin
Ixodes canisuga	Dog, fox, sheep, horse and mule	Skin
Ixodes hexagonus	Hedgehog, dog, cat, fox, sheep, horse, mole	Skin
Ixodes holocyclus	Cattle, sheep, goat, dog, cat; all mammals and birds	Skin
Ixodes persulcatus	Sheep, cattle, goat, horse, dog, other mammals, birds and human	Skin
Ixodes rubicundus	Sheep, goat, cattle and wild ungulates	Skin
Ixodes scapularis (syn. *Ixodes dammini*)	Mammals and birds	Skin
Ixodes pacificus	Rodents, lizards and large mammals such as horses, deer and dogs	Skin
Ixodes pilosus	Cattle, sheep, goat, horse, dog, cat and wild ungulates	Skin
Ixodes angustus	Wild mammals, dog	Skin
Ixodes cookie	Wild mammals, dog	Skin
Ixodes kingi	Wild mammals, dog	Skin
Ixodes rugosus	Wild mammals, dog	Skin
Ixodes sculptus	Wild mammals, dog	Skin
Ixodes muris	Wild mammals, dog	Skin
Ixodes texanus	Wild mammals, dog	Skin

ixodid ticks by the anterior position of the anal groove. In other genera of the Ixodidae, the anal groove is either absent or is posterior to the anus. *Ixodes* species of veterinary importance are described in Table 3.29.

Ixodes ricinus (sheep tick, castor bean tick)

Ixodes ricinus is found throughout temperate areas of Europe, Australia, South Africa, Tunisia, Algeria and Asia. It is more common in areas of rough grazing moorland and woodland. This species has never become established in North America. It feeds on a wide range of mammals and birds and is of veterinary importance in sheep and cattle.

Description: The engorged adult female is light grey, up to 1 cm in length and bean shaped (Fig. 3.118). However, when engorged, the legs are not visible when viewed from above. Adult male *Ixodes ricinus* are only 2–3 mm in length, and because they take smaller blood meals than females, the four pairs of legs are readily visible from above. Nymphs resemble the adults but are less than 2 mm in length. The larvae, often described as 'seed ticks' or 'pepper ticks', are less than 1 mm in length and usually yellowish in colour. The tarsi are tapered (Fig. 3.119a) and the posterior internal angle of the first coxa bears a spur, which overlaps the second coxa (Fig. 3.119a).

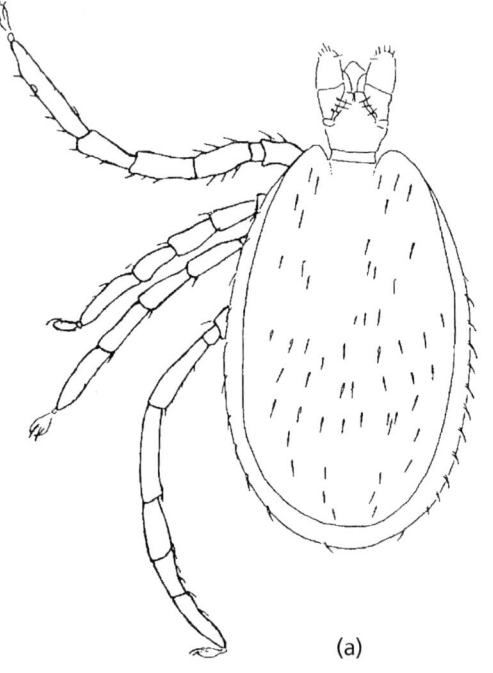
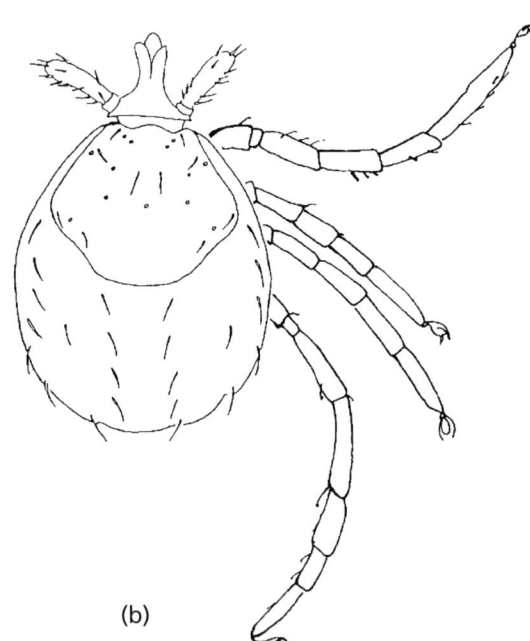

(a)   (b)

Fig. 3.118 Adult *Ixodes ricinus* in dorsal view: (a) male, (b) female. (Arthur, 1962/Springer Nature.)

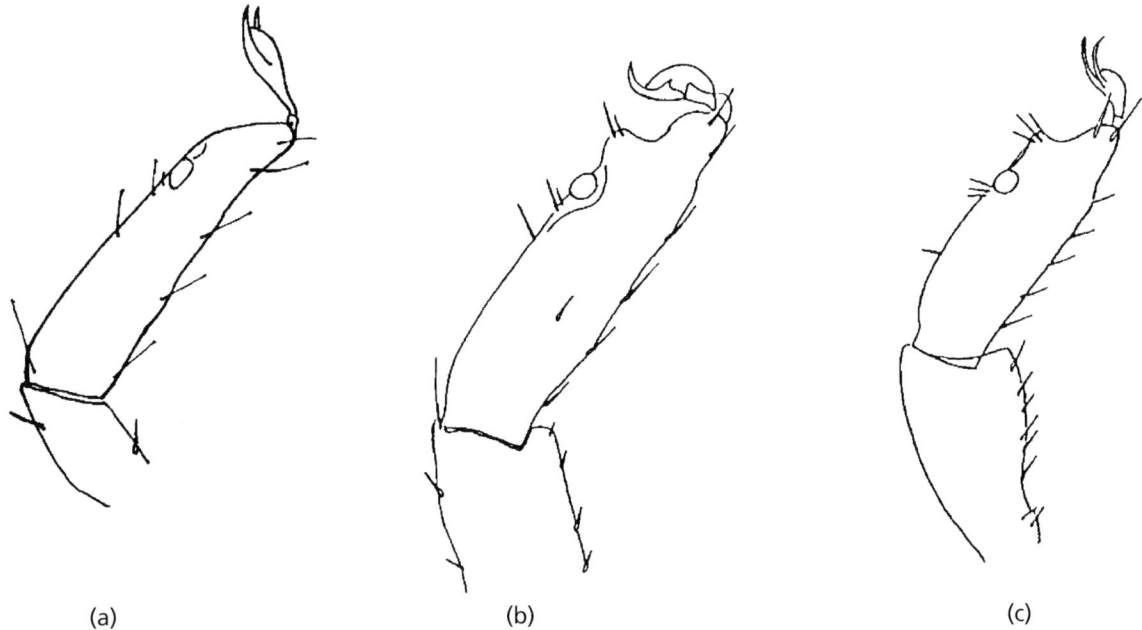

(a)   (b)   (c)

Fig. 3.119 The tarsi of adult male (a) *Ixodes ricinus*, (b) *Ixodes hexagonus* and (c) *Ixodes canisuga*. (Arthur, 1962/Springer Nature.)

Life cycle: *Ixodes ricinus* is a three-host tick and the life cycle requires three years. The tick feeds for only a few days each year, as a larva in the first year, a nymph in the second and an adult in the third. Mating takes place on the host. After attachment, the female is inseminated once and subsequently completes a single large blood meal; in contrast, the males feed intermittently and mate repeatedly. During mating, the male crawls under the female and, after manipulating the female genital opening with its mouthparts, transfers the spermatophore, a sac containing the spermatozoa, into the opening with the aid of his front legs and gnathosoma. Once fertilised, the female subsequently feeds for about 14 days and then drops to the ground to lay several thousand eggs in the soil in sheltered spots, over a period of about 30 days, after which she dies.

The eggs hatch to produce larvae. Larvae begin to quest several days to several weeks after hatching, the precise time depending on temperature and humidity. The larvae climb up the stems of vegetation ready to attach to a passing host. Once a host is located, larvae feed for 3–5 days, increasing their body weight by 10–20 times, then drop back on to the vegetation where they digest their blood meal and moult to become nymphs. The following year, the nymphs begin to seek a new host, again feeding for 3–5 days, before dropping off the host and moulting into the adult stage.

The host on which nymphs feed is usually larger than that of the larvae, typically a bird, rabbit or squirrel. Twelve months later, adults begin to quest for a host, on which they feed and mate. Adults feed for 8–10 days on larger mammals, such as sheep, cattle or deer, and achieve this selection by climbing to different levels in the vegetation while questing.

Although the life cycle takes three years to complete, the larvae, nymphs and adults feed for a total of only 15–20 days and *I. ricinus* is therefore a temporary parasite. Unfed larvae, nymph and adults can survive for many months, entering a state of diapause to assist survival over winter, but the precise period over which they can survive between blood meals depends on temperature and humidity.

Ixodes hexagonus (hedgehog tick)

Ixodes hexagonus is found in Europe and northwest Africa feeding on hedgehogs but also other mammals, particularly cats but also dogs, foxes, sheep and horse.

Description: Adult ticks are red-brown, with legs that may appear somewhat banded in colour. The scutum is broadly hexagonal (hence the name *hexagonus*) and, like *I. ricinus*, the coxae of the first pair of legs bear a spur. However, the spur is smaller than in *I. ricinus* and does not overlap the coxa of the second pair of legs (Fig. 3.120b). When engorged, the female may be up to 8 mm in length. Males are about 3.5–4 mm in length. The tarsi are long (0.8 mm in the female and 0.5 mm in the male) and sharply humped apically (Fig. 3.119b).

Life cycle: *Ixodes hexagonus* is a three-host tick adapted to live with hosts which use burrows or nests. It is primarily a parasite of hedgehogs but may also be found on dogs and other small mammals. The life cycle is similar to that of *I. ricinus*: egg, hexapod larva, octopod nymph and adult, occurring over three years. All life-cycle stages feed on the same host for periods of about eight days. After dropping to the ground, adult females produce 1000–1500 eggs over a period of 19–25 days, before they die. The ticks may be active from early spring to late autumn, but are probably most active during April and May. This species inhabits sheltered habitats such as burrows and kennels and may infest pets in large numbers when they are exposed.

Ixodes canisuga (dog tick)

Ixodes canisuga is found on a range of mammals, particularly dogs, but also foxes, sheep, horses and mules throughout Europe, as far east as Russia.

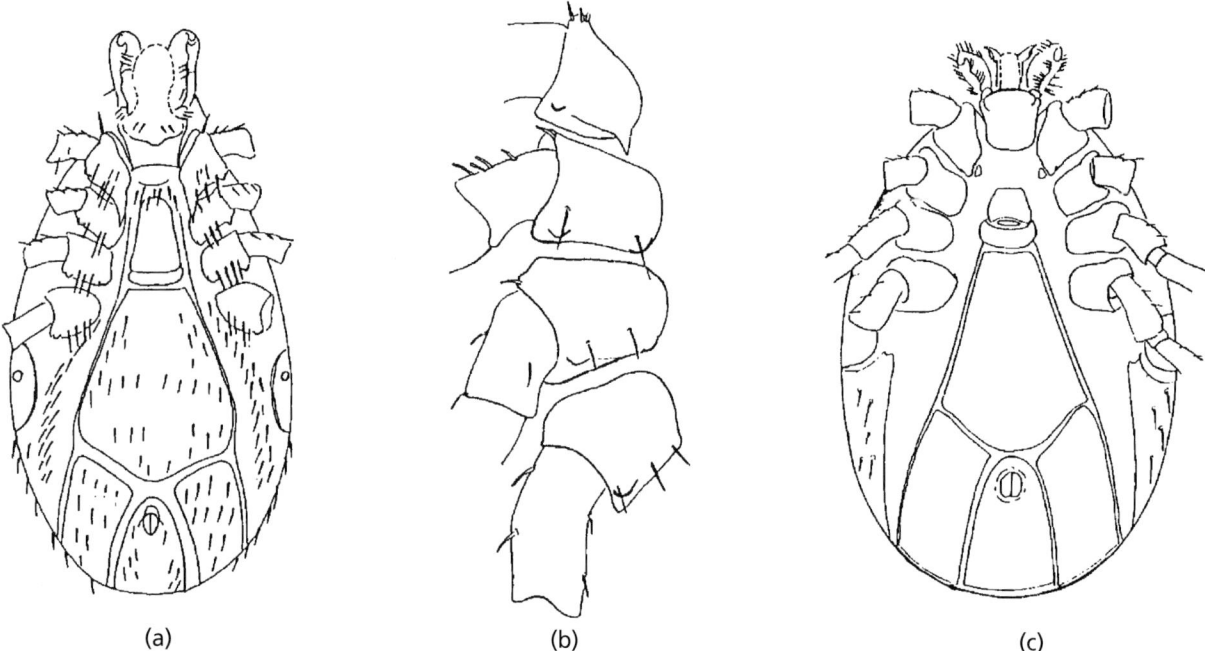

$$(a) \qquad\qquad\qquad\qquad (b) \qquad\qquad\qquad\qquad (c)$$

Fig. 3.120 Ventral view of the coxae of adult male (a) *Ixodes ricinus*, (b) *Ixodes hexagonus* and (c) *Ixodes canisuga*. (Arthur, 1962/Springer Nature.)

Description: *Ixodes canisuga* is an inornate tick, without festoons or eyes. The palps are long and the ventral surface of the male is almost entirely covered with a series of plates (Fig. 3.129c). An anal groove is present anterior to the anus. The engorged adult female is light grey, up to 10 mm in length and bean-shaped, with four pairs of legs. The adult males are only 2–3 mm long and the four pairs of legs are readily visible. *Ixodes canisuga* can be differentiated from *I. ricinus* by the presence of humped tarsi (Fig. 3.120c) and the absence of a spur on the posterior internal angle of the first coxa (Fig. 3.119c). Nymphs resemble the adults and also have four pairs of legs, but are less than 2 mm in size. The larvae ('pepper ticks') are less than 1 mm, usually yellowish in colour and have only three pairs of legs.

Life cycle: *Ixodes canisuga* is a three-host tick and the life cycle requires approximately three years to complete. The tick feeds for only a few days each year, as a larva in the first year, a nymph in the second and an adult in the third. The life cycle is adapted to life in a lair or den. Mating takes place in the den and adult males are only rarely found on the host. Adult females lay relatively small numbers of eggs, probably about 400.

Ixodes holocyclus (paralysis tick)

Ixodes holocyclus is found on cattle, sheep, goat, dog, cat and other mammals and birds throughout Australia.

Description: The Australian paralysis tick is found along the eastern coastline of Australia. Unfed adult females are oval, flat and yellowish in colour and 2–4 mm in length. The palps are long and slender. The anal groove forms a complete oval around the anus; this feature gives the tick its species name *holocyclus* or 'complete

circle'. The marginal groove is well developed and continuous; hairs on the body are small, scattered and most numerous in the region of the marginal fold. Fully engorged adult females may be up to 14 mm in length. The first and last pairs of legs are distinctly darker than the two middle pairs of legs.

Life cycle: This species is a three-host tick. The tick feeds for only a few days each year, as a larva in the first year, a nymph in the second and an adult in the third. Mating takes place on the host. After attachment, the female is inseminated once and subsequently completes her single large blood meal; in contrast, the males feed intermittently and mate repeatedly. Once fertilised, the female subsequently feeds for about 14 days and then drops to the ground to lay several thousand eggs in sheltered spots, after which she dies. The larvae, which hatch from the eggs, will feed for about six days in the following year, then drop to the ground and moult to the nymphal stage. In the third year this stage feeds, drops off and becomes adult. Although the life cycle takes three years to complete, the larvae, nymphs and adults feed for a total of only 26–28 days.

Ixodes persulcatus (taiga tick)

Ixodes persulcatus is commonly found on a range of domestic livestock, dogs and birds throughout eastern Europe, Russia and as far east as Japan.

Description: The taiga tick is morphologically very similar to *I. ricinus*; it is an inornate, red-brown tick, without festoons or eyes. The palps are long and the ventral surface of the male is almost entirely covered with a series of plates. The engorged adult female is light grey and up to 10 mm in length. The major difference is that the female adult *I. persulcatus* has a straight or wavy genital opening rather than arched as in *I. ricinus*.

Life cycle: The taiga tick has a similar life cycle to *I. ricinus*, although adults are rarely active during autumn.

Ixodes rubicundus (Karoo paralysis tick)

Ixodes rubicundus is commonly found on a range of domestic livestock and wild ungulates in southern Africa, particularly the Karrooveld.

Description: Adult ticks have a small internal spine on coxa I and a posterior flap of weakly sclerotised cuticle on coxae I–III. In the male, the ventral ridge on the basis capituli has a central and two smaller lateral lobes and there are two large basal hypostomal teeth. The female scutum has a narrowly rounded posterior margin and flattened oval porose areas.

Life cycle: This is a three-host tick species. The tick feeds for only a few days as a larva, a nymph and an adult. The life cycle of this species takes about two years. Mating takes place on the host. After attachment, the female is inseminated once and subsequently completes her single large blood meal; in contrast, the males feed intermittently and mate repeatedly. Once fertilised, the female subsequently feeds for about 14 days and then drops to the ground to lay several thousand eggs in sheltered spots, after which she dies.

Ixodes scapularis (deer tick, black-legged tick)

Synonym: *Ixodes dammini*

Ixodes scapularis may be found on deer but may also occur on a range of other mammals and birds throughout North America, particularly in and around wooded areas east of the Rocky Mountains.

Description: The identifying characteristics are the black legs, black scutum and long black gnathosoma (capitulum).

Life cycle: This is a three-host tick species. It feeds for only a few days each year, as a larva in the first year, a nymph in the second and an adult in the third. Mating usually takes place on the host. After attachment, the female is inseminated and subsequently completes her single large blood meal. In contrast, the adult males feed intermittently and mate repeatedly. Once fertilised, the female subsequently feeds for about 14 days and then drops to the ground to lay several thousand eggs in sheltered spots, after which she dies. The following year, peak larval activity occurs in August, when larvae attach and feed on a wide variety of mammals and birds, particularly white-footed mice (*Peromyscus leucopus*). After feeding for 3–5 days, engorged larvae drop from the host to the ground where they overwinter before moulting to become a nymph. In May of the following year, larvae moult to become nymphs, which feed on a variety of hosts for 3–4 days. Engorged nymphs then detach and drop to the forest floor where they moult into the adult stage, which becomes active in October. Adult ticks remain active through the winter on days when the ground and ambient temperatures are above freezing. The adult ticks feed on large mammals, primarily white-tailed deer, *Odocoileus virginianus*. Although the life cycle takes three years to complete, the larvae, nymphs and adults feed for a total of only 26–28 days.

Ixodes pacificus (western black-legged tick)

Description: A very similar species to *Ixodes scapularis* found predominantly along the western coast of North America. Adult ticks are red-brown in colour and about 3 mm in size. Larvae and nymphs are smaller and paler in colour.

Dermacentor

Ticks of the genus *Dermacentor* are medium-sized to large ticks, usually with ornate patterning. The palps and mouthparts are short and the basis capituli is rectangular (Fig. 3.112c). Festoons and eyes are present. The coxa of the first pair of legs is divided into two sections in both sexes. Coxae progressively increase in size from I to IV. The males lack ventral plates and, in the adult male, the coxa of the fourth pair of legs is greatly enlarged. Most species of *Dermacentor* are three-host ticks but a few are one-host ticks. The genus is small with about 30 species, most of which are found in the New World. *Dermacentor* species of veterinary importance are listed in Table 3.30. Several of the species are important vectors of pathogens and the salivary secretions of some species may produce tick paralysis.

Dermacentor andersoni (Rocky Mountain wood tick)

Synonym: *Dermacentor venustus*

Dermacentor andersoni are widely distributed throughout the western and central parts of North America from Mexico as far north as British Columbia.

Description: *Dermacentor andersoni* is an ornate tick, with a base colour of brown and a grey pattern (Fig. 3.121). Males are about 2–6 mm in length and females around 3–5 mm in length when unfed and 10–11 mm in length when engorged. The mouthparts are short. The basis capituli is short and broad (Fig. 3.117c). The legs are patterned in the same manner as the body. The coxae of the first pair of legs have well-developed external and internal spurs.

Life cycle: *Dermacentor andersoni* is a three-host tick. Immature stages primarily feed on small rodents, while adults feed largely on wild and domestic herbivores. Mating takes place on the host, following which females lay up to 6500 eggs over about three weeks. The eggs hatch in about one month and the larvae begin to quest. Larvae feed for about five days, before dropping to the ground and moulting to the octopod nymphal stage. One- and two-year population cycles may occur. Eggs hatch in early spring and individuals that are successful in finding hosts pass through their larval stages in spring, their nymphal stages in late summer and then overwinter as adults in a one-year cycle. Nymphs that fail to feed have to overwinter and form a spring-feeding generation of nymphs the following year. Unfed nymphs may survive for up to a year. *Dermacentor andersoni* is most common in areas of scrubby vegetation, since these attract both the small mammals required by the immature stages and the large herbivorous mammals required by the adults.

Table 3.30 *Dermacentor* species of veterinary importance.

Species	Hosts	Site
Dermacentor andersoni (syn. *Dermacentor venustus*)	Rodents, wild and domestic ruminants	Skin
Dermacentor variabilis	Rodents, dog, horse, cattle, human, wild animals	Skin
Dermacentor albipictus	Moose, deer, wild mammals, cattle, horse, human	Skin
Dermacentor reticulatus	Sheep, cattle, dog, horse, pig, human; nymphs and larvae feed on rodents, insectivores and occasionally birds	Skin
Dermacentor marginatus	Sheep, cattle, deer, dog, human, hare and hedgehog; nymphs and larvae feed on rodents, insectivores and birds	Skin
Dermacentor nitens	Horse, cattle, human, many domestic and wild mammals	Skin
Dermacentor silvarum	Cattle, sheep, horse, dog, human	Skin
Dermacentor nuttalli	Rodents, human	Skin
Dermacentor occidentalis	Cattle, horse, wild mammals	Skin

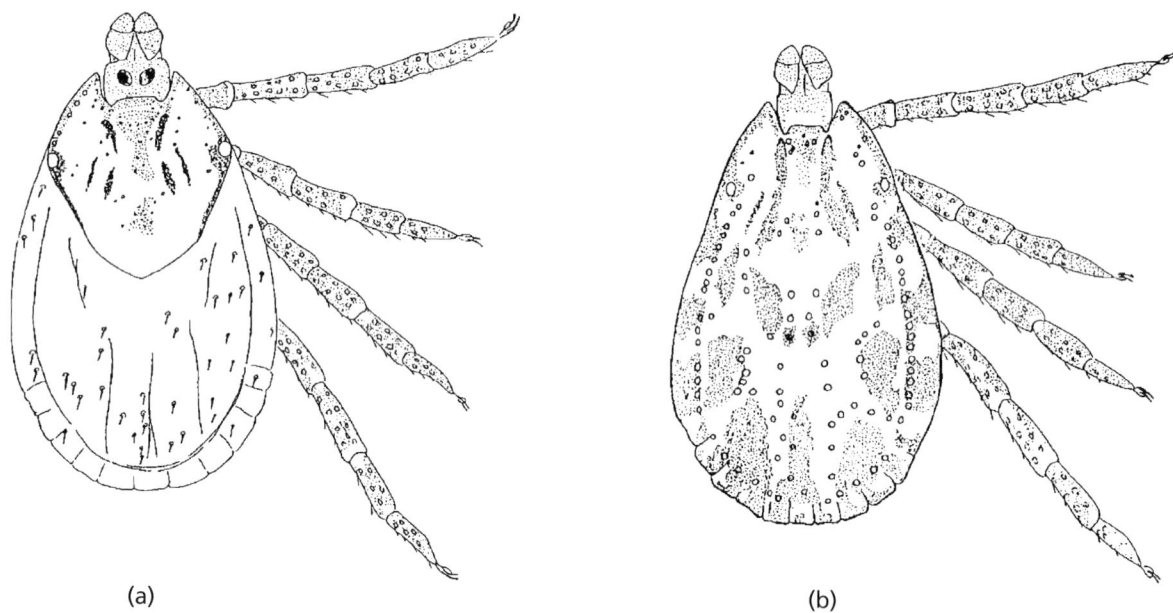

(a)　　　　　　　　　　　　　　　　　(b)

Fig. 3.121 Adult *Dermacentor andersoni*: (a) dorsal view of female; (b) dorsal view of male. (Arthur, 1962/Springer Nature.)

Dermacentor variabilis (American dog tick, wood tick)

Dermacentor variabilis will feed on a wide range of domestic and wild mammals, particularly dogs, horse, cattle and humans, and is found in North America, to the east of the Rocky Mountains.

Description: These are ornate, pale brown and grey ticks with eyes and festoons (Fig. 3.122). The basis capituli is rectangular and the palps short. Adult males are about 3–4 mm in length and adult females about 4 mm in length when unfed and 15 mm in length when engorged. *D. variabilis* can be distinguished by the absence of a posterodorsal spur on palp segment II.

Life cycle: *Dermacentor variabilis* is a three-host tick, feeding once in each of the larval, nymphal and adult life-cycle stages. After each feed, it drops from the host. Mating takes place on the host. Once fertilised, the adult female feeds for 5–27 days before dropping to the ground to lay 4000–6000 eggs in sheltered spots, after which she

dies. Oviposition may last 14–32 days, depending on temperature and humidity. The larvae hatch from the eggs after 20–57 days and feed for between two and 13 days on the host, then drop to the ground and moult to the nymphal stage. This stage feeds over a period of several days, drops off and moults to become an adult. Unfed larvae, nymphs and adults can survive for very long periods of time under appropriate environmental conditions. The larval and nymphal stages feed on wild rodents, particularly the short-tailed meadow mouse (*Microtus* spp.), while the preferred hosts of adults are larger mammals, particularly wild and domestic carnivores.

Dermacentor albipictus (winter tick, moose tick)

Dermacentor albipictus feed particularly on moose, but also on a wide variety of domestic and wild mammals, including horses, cattle and humans. The species is found throughout the northern USA and Canada, particularly in upland and mountainous areas.

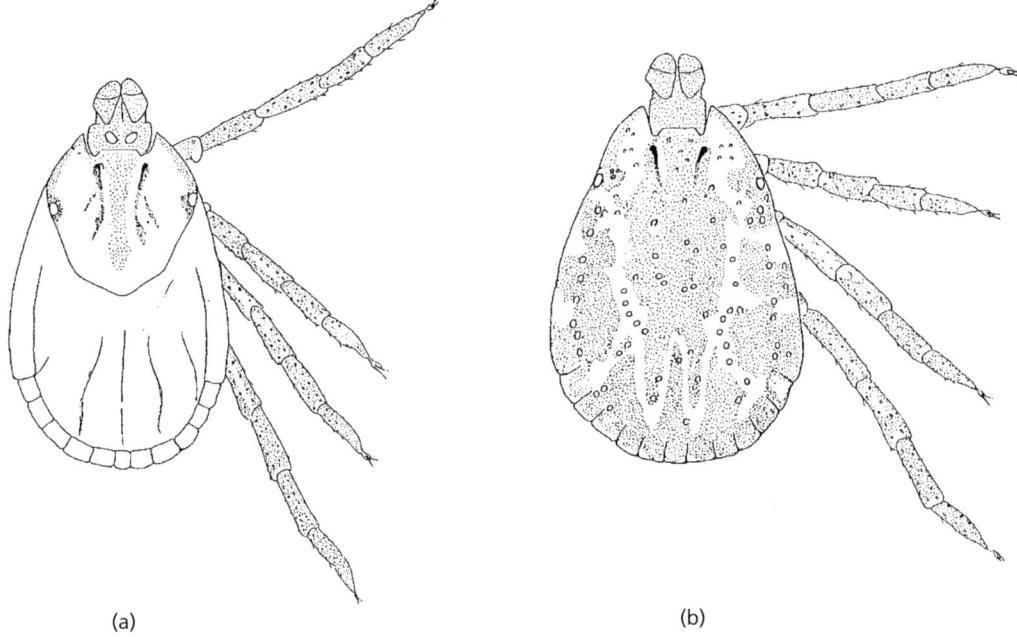

(a)   (b)

Fig. 3.122 Adult *Dermacentor variabilis*: (a) dorsal view of female; (b) dorsal view of male. (Arthur, 1962/Springer Nature.)

Description: The adults are ornately patterned ticks with eyes and festoons present. The basis capituli is rectangular and the palps short. The males lack ventral plates and the coxae of the fourth pair of legs are enlarged. In the adults of both sexes, the coxa of the first pair of legs has an enlarged spur (bidentate), and in the male the coxae increase in size from I to IV.

Life cycle: This is a one-host species of tick. The larva, nymph and adult all attach to, and develop on, a single host. This species feeds only in winter, usually between October and March/April, on horses, deer and related large mammals. The engorged female drops off the host in the spring and lays between 1500 and 4400 eggs over a period of 19–42 days. The eggs hatch within 33–71 days. The larvae remain inactive until autumn when they then attach to a host, feed and moult to the nymph stage in 10–76 days. The nymphs engorge and moult to the adult stage in 10–76 days. Mating takes place on the host. The total period spent on the host is between 28 and 60 days, although unfed larvae can survive for up to 12 months before attachment to the host. Under normal conditions this tick species produces one generation per year.

Dermacentor reticulatus (ornate dog tick, marsh tick, meadow tick, winter tick)

Synonym: *Dermacentor pictus*

Dermacentor reticulatus commonly feeds on sheep, cattle, dogs, horses, pigs and occasionally humans. Nymphs and larvae feed on smaller mammals, such as insectivores and occasionally birds. It is widely distributed in Europe (from the Atlantic coast to Kazakhstan) and Central Africa.

Description: This species is an ornate tick with eyes and festoons present (Fig. 3.123). In both sexes the scutum is usually pale with variegated brown splashes (but coloration may be highly variable). The basis capituli is rectangular and the palps short. The adult

female is 3.8–4.2 mm when unfed and 10 mm in length when engorged. The adult male is approximately 4.2–4.8 mm in length. The males lack ventral plates and the coxae of the fourth pair of legs are enlarged with a narrow tapering external spur. In the adults of both sexes, the coxa of the first pair of legs has an enlarged spur (bidentate). The other coxae have short internal spurs that become progressively smaller in legs II to IV.

Life cycle: *Dermacentor reticulatus* is a three-host tick and the life cycle can be completed in only 1–2 years, depending on environmental conditions. The species feeds once in each of the larval,

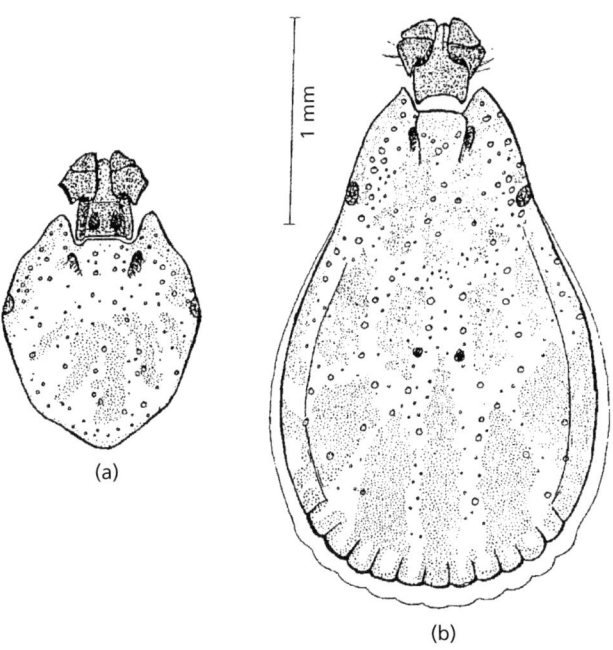

(a)

1 mm

(b)

Fig. 3.123 Dorsal view of the gnathosoma and scutum of adult (a) female and (b) male *Dermacentor reticulatus*. (Arthur, 1962/Springer Nature.)

nymphal and adult life-cycle stages, dropping from a host, moulting and then reacquiring a new host between feeds. Mating takes place on the host and once fertilised, the adult female feeds for 9–15 days, before dropping to the ground to lay approximately 4000 eggs in sheltered spots, after which she dies. Oviposition may last for 6–40 days, depending on temperature and humidity, with oviposition rate peaking on about the fifth day. The larvae hatch from the eggs after 2–3 weeks and feed for approximately two days on the host, then drop to the ground and moult to the nymphal stage. This stage feeds over a period of several days, drops off and moults to become an adult.

Dermacentor marginatus (ornate sheep tick)

Dermacentor marginatus feed largely on sheep but also cattle, deer, horses, dogs, humans, hares and hedgehogs while the nymphs and larvae feed on small mammals and birds. The species is found throughout Europe and North Africa, eastwards to central Asia.

Description: *Dermacentor marginatus* is distinguished from other species of *Dermacentor* by the sclerotised thickening at the base of the dorsal prolongation of the spiracular plate. In the adult, external and internal spurs are present on coxae I, the external spur being slightly shorter than the internal spur. In females the genital aperture forms a narrow V-shape. The engorged adult female may be up to 15 mm in length.

Life cycle: This is a three-host tick.

Dermacentor nitens (tropical horse tick)

Dermacentor nitens feeds on a range of domestic and wild mammals but is of particular veterinary significance as a parasite of horses and sometimes cattle. It is found in the southern regions of North America, Central and South America and the Caribbean.

Description: Male ticks are 2–4 mm long, inornate and appear yellowish-brown in colour. Females are 2–5 mm long. The scutum of female ticks is brownish-yellow in colour, somewhat longer than wide with no discernible pattern, but appears glossy.

Life cycle: This is a one-host tick species; the larva, nymph and adult all attach to, and develop on, a single host. The engorged female drops off the host and lays up to 3500 eggs over a period of 15–37 days. The eggs hatch within 19–39 days. The larvae then attach to the host, feed and moult to the nymph stage in 8–16 days. The nymphs engorge and moult to the adult stage in 7–29 days. Mating takes place on the host. The total period spent on the host is between 26 and 41 days, although unfed larvae can survive for up to 117 days before attachment to the host. Under favourable tropical conditions, this tick species can produce several generations per year.

Dermacentor nuttalli

Dermacentor nuttalli is found throughout Siberia, northern Pakistan, China and Mongolia where it may be an important parasite of cattle, camels and goats.

Description: The basis capituli in the male is broader than long and the ventral spur on palpal segment 3 is lacking. In the female the basis capituli is almost twice as broad as long. The first pair of coxae is small with a relatively broad and bluntly rounded spur. The external spurs on coxae II–IV are approximately equal in length and those of coxae IV do not extend beyond the posterior margin.

Dermacentor occidentalis (Pacific coast tick)

Dermacentor occidentalis is found throughout western USA (Sierra Nevada Mountains and the Pacific coast from Oregon to southern California) where it may be an important parasite of cattle, horses and other domestic animals.

Description: The basis capituli is longer than wide, with the cornua as long as or longer than wide. Sizes of scutal punctations are not greatly disparate and the pearl-grey coloration of the scutum is more extensive than brown.

Life cycle: *Dermacentor occidentalis* is a three-host tick. The tick feeds for only a few days as a larva, a nymph and an adult, each on a different host. Mating takes place on the host. After attachment, the female is inseminated once, subsequently completes her single large blood meal, drops to the ground and lays her eggs.

Haemaphysalis

Ticks of the genus *Haemaphysalis* inhabit humid well-vegetated habitats in Eurasia and tropical Africa. They are three-host ticks, with the larvae and nymphs feeding on small mammals and birds and adults infesting larger mammals and, importantly, livestock. There are about 150 species, found largely in the Old World, with only two species found in the New World. *Haemaphysalis* species of veterinary importance are listed in Table 3.31. Most species of the genus are small, with short mouthparts and a rectangular basis capituli (Fig. 3.117g). The palps are short and broad, usually with lateral projections at the base. Ventral plates are not present in the male. Spiracular plates are rounded or oval in females and rounded or comma-shaped in males. Like *Ixodes* spp., these ticks lack eyes but they differ in having festoons and a posterior anal groove.

Table 3.31 *Haemaphysalis* species of veterinary importance.

Species	Hosts	Site
Haemaphysalis punctata	Cattle, sheep, goat, horse, deer, wolf, bear, bat, birds, rabbit. Larvae: on birds, hedgehogs, rodents and reptiles such as lizards and snakes	Skin
Haemaphysalis leachi	Dog, domestic and wild carnivores, small rodents and occasionally cattle	Skin
Haemaphysalis longicornis	Cattle. All mammals and birds	Skin
Haemaphysalis spinigera	Monkeys, birds and cattle. Larvae and nymphs: small mammals, human	Skin
Haemaphysalis bispinosa	Wide variety of mammals, sheep and cattle	Skin
Haemaphysalis concinna	Variety of mammals, sheep	Skin
Haemaphysalis cinnabarina	Variety of ruminants	Skin
Haemaphysalis leporispalustris	Rabbit, snowshoe hare, birds, rarely feeds on humans	Skin

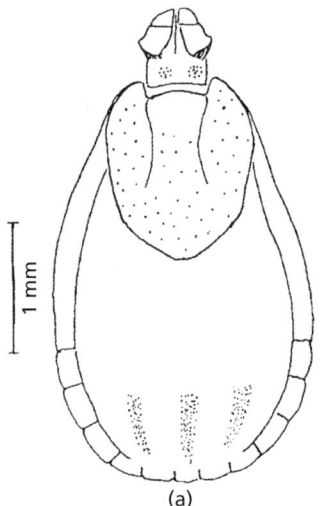 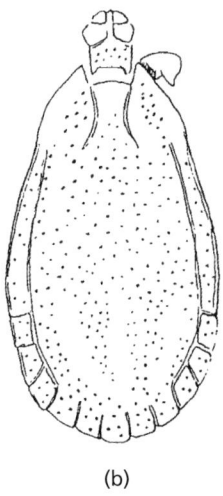 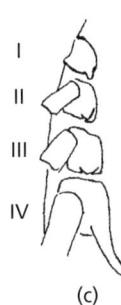

Fig. 3.124 Dorsal view of the gnathosoma and scutum of adult (a) female and (b) male *Haemaphysalis punctata*. (c) Ventral view of the coxae of an adult male. (Arthur, 1962/Springer Nature.)

The identification of more than the major species is beyond the scope of this text and interested readers will need to consult a relevant taxonomic specialist.

Haemaphysalis punctata

Haemaphysalis punctata feeds on a wide range of wild and domestic animals but may be of particular veterinary importance in cattle and sheep. The larvae and nymphs may be found on birds, hedgehogs, rodents and reptiles, such as lizards and snakes. They occur throughout Europe (including southern Scandinavia and Britain), central Asia and North Africa.

Description: Small inornate ticks with festoons; eyes absent (Fig. 3.124). The palps and hypostome are short. The adults of both sexes are about 3 mm in length, the female reaching about 12 mm in length when engorged. However, sexual dimorphism is not pronounced. The basis capituli is rectangular, about twice as broad as long. The sensory palps are short and broad, with the second segment extending beyond the basis capituli. The anal groove is posterior to the anus. The coxae of the first pair of legs have a short blunt internal spur, which is also present on the coxae of the second and third pair of legs and which is enlarged and tapering on the coxae of the fourth pair of legs. In the male the spur may be as long as the coxa.

Life cycle: *Haemaphysalis punctata* is a three-host tick, feeding once in each of the larval, nymphal and adult life-cycle stages. After each blood meal it drops from the host. Engorgement on the host may take 6–30 days to complete. Once fed, each adult female lays 3000–5000 eggs on the ground, over a period of 10 days to seven months. Unfed larvae can survive for up to 10 months, unfed nymphs and adults for 8.5 months.

Haemaphysalis leachi (yellow dog tick)

Haemaphysalis leachi occurs in Africa, Australia and Asia where it is of veterinary importance primarily on dogs and wild carnivores, but also occasionally cattle.

Description: Inornate elongate ticks with 11 festoons; eyes absent. The palps are widely triangular with a basal spur on segment II.

Life cycle: *Haemaphysalis leachi* is a three-host tick, feeding once in each of the larval, nymphal and adult life-cycle stages. After each blood meal it drops from the host.

Haemaphysalis longicornis (Asian long-horned tick, scrub tick, New Zealand cattle tick)

Haemaphysalis longicornis occurs throughout temperate areas of East and Central Asia, including China, Korea and Japan, and has been introduced to Australia, New Zealand and various Pacific islands. This species was reported for the first time in the United States in 2017.

Description: Male ticks have a small internal spur on coxa IV and both sexes have a long internal spur on coxa I.

Life cycle: A three-host tick species. The larvae and nymphs primarily feed on small mammals and birds while adults feed on a wide range of animals, but may be of particular veterinary importance in cattle and sheep although may also be found on goats, cats and dogs. However, if no other hosts are available, each life stage may feed on the same host. Females of this tick can reproduce either sexually or by parthenogenesis. Egg to adult development takes about 90 days, although this depends on temperature and humidity of the environment. Females can produce 900–3000 eggs in a single reproductive event, and as a result, populations of this tick may reach high densities relatively quickly.

Haemaphysalis concinna (bush tick)

Haemaphysalis concinna is found in Eastern, central Europe and Russia east to China where it is of veterinary importance in livestock, particularly sheep.

Description: Similar to *H. punctata* but the female lacks cornua and the male has a long pointed spur on coxa IV.

Haemaphysalis bispinosa (bush tick)

Haemaphysalis bispinosa is found in Asia and Australasia where it is of veterinary importance in livestock, particularly sheep and cattle, but may also be a vector of pathogens for goats, equids and dogs.

Description: Similar to *H. punctata* but has a prominent dorsal spur on the posterior edge of palp segment II.

Life cycle: A three-host tick species. It has been suggested that this tick may reproduce parthenogenetically.

Rhipicephalus

The genus is composed of about 60 species, all of which were originally endemic to the Old World and, for the most part, distributed throughout sub-Saharan Africa. However, many species have now been introduced into a range of new habitats worldwide. They act as important vectors of a number of disease pathogens. They infest a variety of mammals but seldom birds or reptiles. Most species are three-host ticks but some species of the genus are two-host ticks. *Rhipicephalus* species of veterinary importance are listed in Table 3.32.

The basis capituli is hexagonal (Fig. 3.117f) and, in the male, paired plates are found on each side of the anus. They are not ornate. Palps are short and eyes and festoons are usually present. Spiracular plates are comma-shaped. The identification of more than the major species is beyond the scope of this text and interested readers will need to consult a relevant taxonomic specialist.

Rhipicephalus appendiculatus (brown ear tick)

Rhipicephalus appendiculatus feeds on a very wide range of hosts: cattle, horse, sheep, goat, deer, antelope, dogs, rodents and birds. It is found in Africa, south of the Sahara, and occurs particularly in areas with substantial rainfall and shrub cover and it is absent in deserts.

Table 3.32 *Rhipicephalus* species of veterinary importance.

Species	Hosts	Site
Rhipicephalus appendiculatus	Cattle, horse, sheep, goat, deer, antelope, dog, rodents and wide range of mammals and birds	Skin, ears
Rhipicephalus bursa	Cattle, sheep, horse, dog and wide range of mammals and birds	Skin
Rhipicephalus capensis	Cattle, horse, sheep, goat, deer, antelope, dog and wide range of mammals and birds	Skin
Rhipicephalus evertsi	Cattle, sheep, goat, horse, dog and wide range of mammals and birds	Skin
Rhipicephalus sanguineus	Dog, other mammals and birds	Skin, ears, toes
Rhipicephalus pulchellus	Zebra, also infests livestock and game animals	Skin, ears, lower abdomen
Rhipicephalus simus	Dog, wild carnivores, livestock, game animals and humans Larvae and nymphs: burrowing rodents	Skin, ears, lower abdomen

Description: Adult male *R. appendiculatus* are brownish, reddish-brown or very dark, with reddish-brown legs. They vary from 1.8 to 4.4 mm in length. The scutal punctations are scattered and of moderate size; they are evenly dispersed in the centre, but few or none may be found beyond the lateral grooves and in the lateral fields. The cervical grooves are moderately reticulate or non-reticulate. The posteromedian and paramedian grooves are narrow and distinct. The adanal shields are long and have slightly rounded angles, but can be somewhat variable. Adult female ticks are also brown, reddish-brown or very dark. The punctations are small to moderate-sized and are similar to those found in the male. The scutum is approximately equal in length and width; its posterior margin is slightly tapering or abruptly rounded. The lateral grooves are short, poorly defined or absent. The cervical grooves are long and shallow and almost reach the posterolateral margins.

Life cycle: This is a three-host tick.

Rhipicephalus bursa

Rhipicephalus bursa is found in southern Europe and the Mediterranean region, but may reach as far north as central Europe and as far east as Romania. It is the only exophilic species of *Rhipicephalus* and is one of the few species of the genus that occurs in temperate regions. It is found on cattle but also sheep, horse, dogs and occasionally wild mammals, birds and reptiles.

Description: A highly distinctive species. The male has a combination of an anterior spur on coxa I which is visible dorsally, distinct lateral and posterior grooves, and densely punctate scutum and broad adanal plates. The scutum of the female is similar to the conscutum of the male in being densely punctate and without apparent cervical fields. Both sexes have large numbers of setae around the spiracles.

Life cycle: This is a two-host species of tick, with the immature stages commonly infesting the same host and the adults a different host.

Rhipicephalus capensis (Cape brown tick)

Rhipicephalus capensis was originally restricted to the Western Cape Province and southwestern portion of the Northern Cape Province of South Africa where it feeds on wild ungulates, but it has been transported further north to central and East Africa. Adults are of veterinary importance as parasites in cattle but also horse, sheep and goats, and occasionally dogs. There are no records of *R. capensis* causing human parasitism.

Description: This is a morphologically very variable species. Ticks are red-brown in colour, with relatively long, wide and expanding cervical grooves and distinct median and paramedian grooves.

Life cycle: This is thought to be a three-host species of tick. After locating a host, the adult female engorges in 4–21 days. It then drops to the ground where it lays 3000–7000 eggs before dying. The eggs hatch in 28 days to three months, depending on the temperature and climatic conditions. Subsequently, the hexapod larvae locate a suitable host and engorge over a period of 3–6 days. They then drop to the ground before moulting 5–49 days later to become nymphs. The nymphs locate a further host where they engorge over a period of 3–9 days. Nymphs then drop to the ground and moult 10–61 days later to become adults.

Rhipicephalus evertsi (red-legged tick)

Rhipicephalus evertsi is common throughout sub-Saharan Africa, where it feeds on a wide range of domestic and wild hosts, particularly Equidae (horses, donkeys, mules, zebra).

Description: This species can be distinguished from other members of the genus by its red legs. It has a black scutum, which is densely pitted, and in the male leaves a red margin of the opisthosoma uncovered.

Life cycle: This is a two-host species of tick. The larval and nymphal stages engorge on the same host. The female lays approximately 5000–7000 eggs over a period of 6–24 days. These hatch in 4–10 weeks depending on the temperature and climatic conditions. Larvae and nymphs remain on the host for between 10 and 15 days before dropping to the ground. Nymphs then moult after 42–56 days. Subsequently, adults locate a second host, when the adult female engorges in 6–10 days. The larvae and nymphs are commonly found in the ears or the inguinal region, while the adults are mainly found under the tail. Unfed larvae can survive for seven months, while unfed adults can survive for 14 months.

Rhipicephalus sanguineus (brown dog tick, kennel tick)

Rhipicephalus sanguineus occurs worldwide, generally in warmer habitats in both urban and rural areas. It feeds largely on dogs and is often found in the ears and between the toes. This species is believed to have originated in Africa but is now considered to be the most widely distributed tick species in the world.

Description: This species is yellow, reddish or blackish-brown in colour and unfed adults may be 3–4.5 mm in length, although size is highly variable and engorged females may reach a length of 12 mm (Fig. 3.125). The palps and hypostome are short and the basis capituli hexagonal dorsally. The coxa of the first pair of legs has two spurs. The legs may become successively larger from the anterior to the posterior pair. The tarsi of the fourth pair of legs possess a marked ventral tarsal hook. The anal groove encircles only the posterior half of the anus and then extends into a median groove. The males have adanal plates and accessory shields. The six-legged larvae are small and light brown in colour, while the eight-legged nymphs are reddish-brown in colour. Recent taxonomic studies suggest that *Rhipicephalus sanguineus* sensu lato may be a species complex, with morphologically similar but genetically distinct types.

Life cycle: The life cycle is unusual among ticks in that it can be completed entirely indoors, but the species is not exclusively endophilic and it may also survive in outdoor environments. It has a three-host life cycle. Mating takes place on the host. Once fertilised, the female feeds for about 14 days and then drops to the ground to lay approximately 4000 eggs in sheltered spots, after which she dies. Egg masses are likely to be found in above-ground cracks and crevices (e.g. kennel roofs) due to the females' behavioural tendency to crawl upward. The eggs hatch after 17–30 days. The larvae, which hatch from the eggs, will feed for about six days the following year, then drop to the ground and moult to the nymphal stage over a period of 5–23 days. In the third year, this stage feeds for 4–9 days, drops off the host and moults to the adult stage. Under favourable conditions, the life cycle may require as little as 63 days, hence several generations may occur each year. However, under adverse conditions unfed larvae can survive for as long as nine months, unfed nymphs for six months and unfed adults for 19 months. See **life cycle 52**.

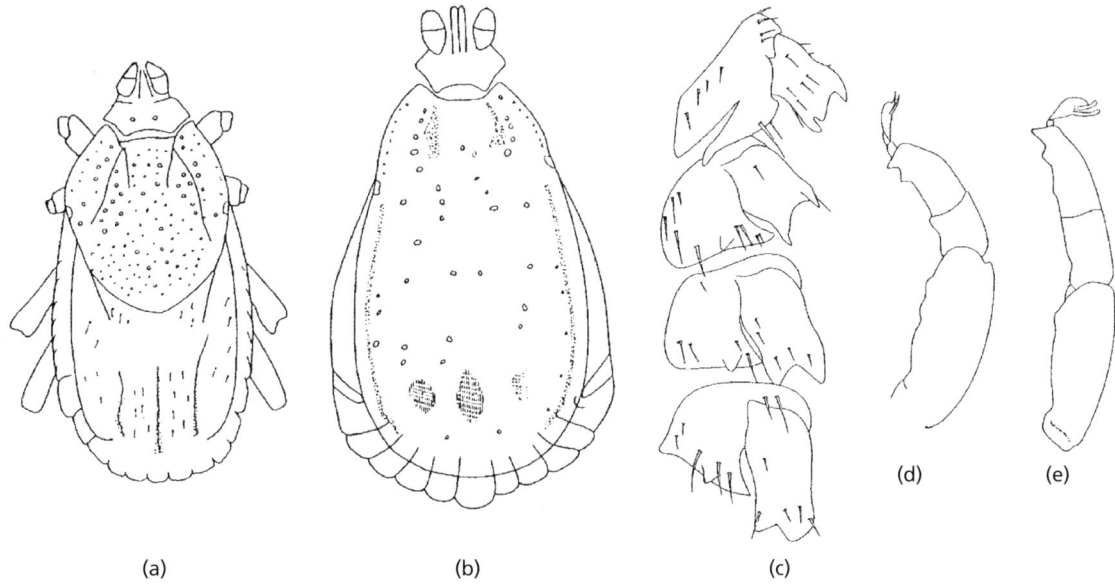

Fig. 3.125 Dorsal view of the gnathosoma and scutum of adult (a) female and (b) male *Rhipicephalus sanguineus*. (c) Ventral view of the coxae and trochanters of an adult male. (d,e) Tarsi and metatarsi of the fourth pair of legs of an adult (d) male and (e) female. (Arthur, 1962/Springer Nature.)

LIFE CYCLE 52. LIFE CYCLE OF *RHIPICEPHALUS SANGUINEUS*

Rhipicephalus sanguineus feeds mostly on dogs. Following a blood meal, the adults mate on the host (1) and the engorged fertilised female drops to the ground where it lays up to 1000–3000 eggs (2) and then dies. Hexapod larvae hatch from the eggs (3). Larvae actively seek out and feed on a new host (4). The engorged larvae drop to the ground and moult to become octopod nymphs (5); these in turn feed on a new host (6) before dropping to the ground and moulting into adults (7). Adults seek out a third and final host, feed (8), and mate on the third host. All three life-cycle stages can feed on the same host and the life cycle can be completed in as little as three months. Humans may be accidental hosts.

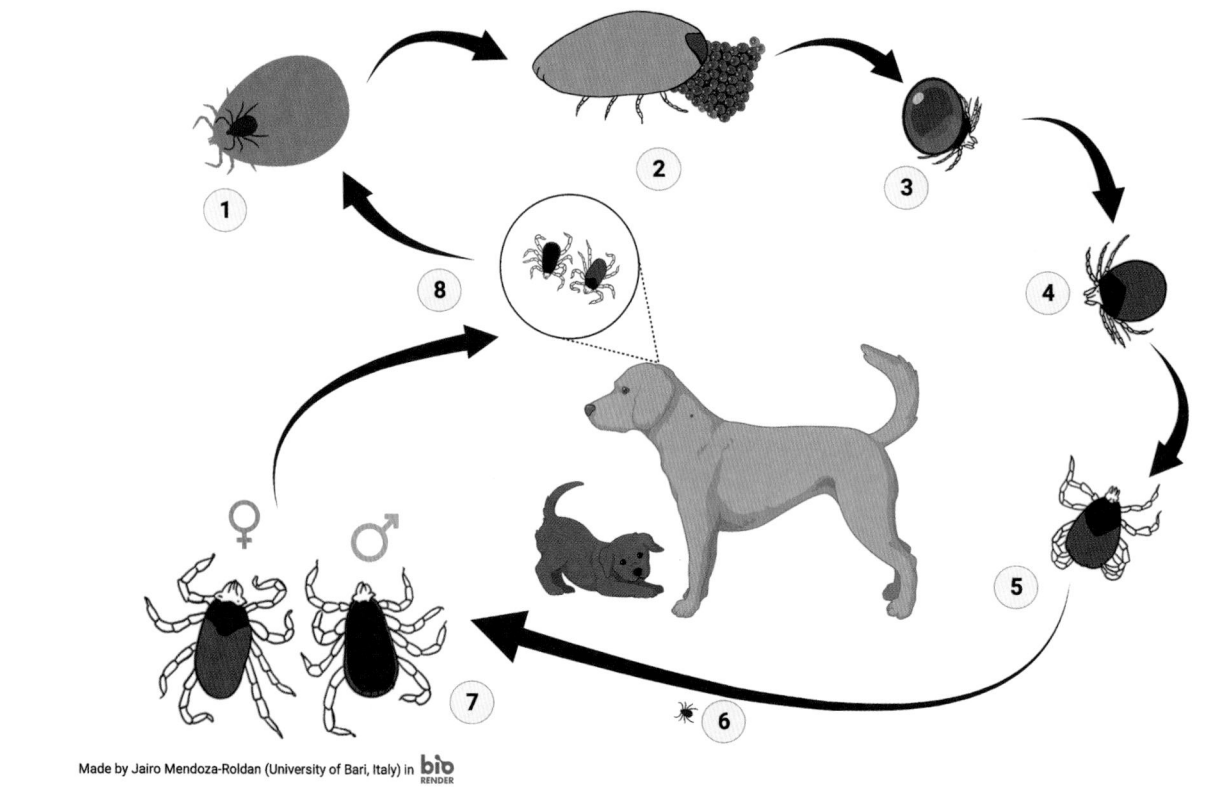

Made by Jairo Mendoza-Roldan (University of Bari, Italy) in **bio**RENDER

Rhipicephalus pulchellus (ivory ornamented tick, zebra tick)

Rhipicephalus pulchellus is found in Africa east of the Rift Valley from southern Ethiopia to Somalia and northeastern Tanzania in savannah habitats with grass, bushes and scattered trees between 300 and 1300 m altitude where the annual rainfall is 250–600 mm. It feeds primarily during wet seasons.

Description: Male ticks have a pattern of stripes of white enamel on a dark brown background over their entire conscutum.

Life cycle: Adults and immatures generally infest the same host; however, immatures also feed on small mammals.

Rhipicephalus simus (glossy tick)

Rhipicephalus simus is found in central and southern Africa. In eastern and northern Africa, *R. simus* is replaced by *R. praetextatus*, which ranges from central Tanzania to Egypt and which is a vector of Thogoto virus. West of the Nile, these species are replaced by *R. senegalensis* and *R. muhsamae*.

Description: Characterised by a shiny black, largely smooth scutum, which in the male has a row of large punctations in the deep marginal groove.

Rhipicephalus (Boophilus)

Ticks of the genus *Boophilus* ('blue ticks') are now considered a subgenus of *Rhipicephalus*, and the name *Rhipicephalus (Boophilus)* is used for the five species in the subgenus for which there is a large amount of literature (Table 3.33). *Rhipicephalus (Boophilus)* species are important as vectors of *Babesia* spp. and *Anaplasma marginale* in cattle in subtropical and tropical countries.

The males have adanal or accessory ventral shields. The basis capituli is hexagonal dorsally. The mouthparts are short and compressed and the palps are ridged dorsally and laterally (Fig. 3.117e). Unfed adults may be only 2 or 3 mm long, reaching lengths of up to 12 mm when engorged. The identification of more than the major species is beyond the scope of this text and interested readers will need to consult a relevant taxonomic specialist.

Table 3.33 Rhipicephalus (Boophilus) species of veterinary importance.

Species	Hosts	Site
Rhipicephalus (Boophilus) annulatus	Cattle, horse, goat, sheep, camel, dog and wide range of mammals and birds	Skin
Rhipicephalus (Boophilus) microplus	Cattle, sheep, goat, wild ungulates	Skin
Rhipicephalus (Boophilus) calcaratus	Cattle, sheep, goat, wild ungulates	Skin
Rhipicephalus (Boophilus) decoloratus	Cattle, horse, donkey, sheep, goat, dog, wild ungulates	Skin

Rhipicephalus (Boophilus) annulatus (blue cattle tick, Texas cattle fever tick)

Rhipicephalus (Boophilus) annulatus is an important vector of pathogens in cattle, but will also infest horses, goats, sheep, camels and dogs. It occurs in central and South America, Africa, Mexico, Eastern Europe and the former USSR, Africa, the Middle East, the Near East, the Mediterranean and Mexico. It has been largely eradicated from North America, but can sometimes be found in Texas or California, in a buffer quarantine zone along the Mexican border.

Description: The internal margin of the first palp article is long and slightly concave, and the spurs and cleft between the spurs on the first coxa of females are less distinct than those of Rhipicephalus (Boophilus) microplus females. The second coxa in females lacks a spur and the males lack a caudal appendage.

Life cycle: This is a one-host tick species. The larva, nymph and adult all attach to, and develop on, a single host. The engorged female drops off the host and lays between 2000 and 3000 eggs over a period of 14–59 days. The larvae hatch after 23–159 days depending on climatic conditions. The larvae then attach to the host, feed and moult to the nymph and then adult stage. Mating takes place on the host. The total period spent on the host is between 15 and 55 days, although unfed larvae can survive for up to eight months before attachment to the host. Two to four generations may occur per year, depending on climatic conditions; the entire life cycle of this species can be completed in six weeks.

Rhipicephalus (Boophilus) microplus (tropical cattle tick, southern cattle tick)

Rhipicephalus (Boophilus) microplus is an important parasite of cattle, sheep, goats and wild ungulates found in Asia, Australia, Mexico, Central and South America, West Indies, South Africa.

Description: Adult ticks have a short straight gnathosoma. The legs are pale cream. The body is oval to rectangular and the scutum is oval and wider at the front. The anal groove is obsolete in the female and is faint in the male and surrounds the anus posteriorly. Coxa I is bifid. The spiracles are circular or oval. The nymphs of this species have an orange-brown scutum. The body is oval and wider at the front. The body colour is brown to blue-grey, with white at the front and sides.

Life cycle: This species is a one-host tick. The larva, nymph and adult all attach to, and develop on, a single host. The engorged female drops off the host and lays between 2000 and 4500 eggs over

a period of 4–44 days. The larvae hatch after 14–146 days depending on climatic conditions. The larvae then attach to the host, feed and moult to the nymph and then adult stages. From the attachment of larvae to engorgement of the adult female requires three weeks. After engorging, females can weigh up to 250 times more than when unfed. Mating takes place on the host. The total period spent on the host is between 17 and 52 days, and the entire life cycle can be completed within two months, although unfed larvae can survive for up to 20 weeks before attachment to the host. Although present all year round, populations reach their peak in summer.

Rhipicephalus (Boophilus) decoloratus (blue tick)

Rhipicephalus (Boophilus) decoloratus is found in cattle-rearing areas worldwide. It has largely been eradicated from North America, but can sometimes be found in Texas or California. It is particularly important in cattle but will also infest horses, goats, sheep, camels and dogs.

Description: The engorged females have slate-blue coloured bodies with pale yellow legs.

Life cycle: This is a one-host tick species. The larva, nymph and adult all attach to, and develop on, a single host. The engorged female drops off the host, then lays and incubates approximately 2500 eggs over a period of 3–6 weeks. The larvae then attach to the host, feed and moult to the nymph and then adult stage. Mating takes place on the host. The total period spent on the host ranges between 21 and 25 days, although unfed larvae can survive for up to seven months before attachment to the host.

Hyalomma

Hyalomma spp. are usually two-host ticks, though some species may use three hosts. They are most commonly found on the legs, udder and tail, or perianal region. There are about 27 valid species; seven species are found in Asia, five in Africa, nine in Asia-Africa and one in Africa-Europe. Hyalomma species of veterinary importance are listed in Table 3.34. They usually inhabit the semi-desert

Table 3.34 Hyalomma species of veterinary importance.

Species	Hosts	Site
Hyalomma anatolicum H. anatolicum anatolicum H. anatolicum excavatum	Cattle, horse, wide range of mammals and birds Rodents; adults on ruminants, horses	Skin, axilla, inguinal region, face, ears
Hyalomma aegyptium	Tortoises (Testudo spp.), lizards, dog, horse	Skin
Hyalomma detritum Hyalomma scupense	Cattle, sheep, goat, horse, wide range of mammals and birds	Skin, axilla, inguinal region, face, ears
Hyalomma dromedarii	Camels, ruminants, horses	Skin, axilla, inguinal region, face, ears
Hyalomma marginatum Hyalomma rufipes Hyalomma turanicum Hyalomma isaaci	Wild herbivores, ruminants, horses Larvae and nymphs: small mammals, birds, lizards	Skin, axilla, inguinal region, face, ears
Hyalomma truncatum	Cattle, sheep, goat, pig, horse, wide range of mammals and birds	Skin, axilla, inguinal region, face, ears
Hyalomma impressum	Cattle, sheep, large African mammals	Skin, axilla, inguinal region, face, ears

lowlands of central Asia, southern Europe and North Africa. They can survive exceptionally cold and dry conditions. Species of *Hyalomma* are medium-sized or large ticks, usually inornate but with banded legs (giving them the common name of the 'bont-legged' ticks). The palps and hypostome are long (Fig. 3.117b), eyes are present and festoons sometimes present. The males have ventral plates on each side of the anus. They are vectors of a wide range of pathogens of veterinary importance.

Hyalomma anatolicum (bont-legged tick)

Hyalomma anatolicum is believed to exist as two subspecies: *Hyalomma anatolicum excavatum* in the central European and Asiatic parts of its range and *Hyalomma anatolicum anatolicum* elsewhere. Some authors have suggested that these should be viewed as separate species. It is of veterinary significance primarily in cattle but will also feed on a range of mammals and birds and it causes tick toxicosis in parts of Africa and the Indian subcontinent.

Description: Usually with banded legs; eyes are present and festoons sometimes present. The palps and hypostome are long. The gnathosoma and coxae are dark, reddish or black-brown. The males have adanal shields. The second segment of the palps is less than twice as long as the third segment, and the scutum has no pattern.

Life cycle: This species is a two- or three-host tick. Larvae acquire a host, feed and moult. Nymphs reattach to the same host soon after moulting. Following engorgement, nymphs drop off the host, moult to the adult stage and then acquire a new second host where they feed. After attachment, mating occurs and the female completes her single large blood meal. Males feed intermittently and mate repeatedly. Once fertilised, the female feeds for about 14 days and then drops to the ground to lay several thousand eggs in sheltered spots, after which she dies. The larvae and nymphs feed on birds and small mammals, and the adults on ruminants and equines. When larvae and nymphs infest smaller mammals, birds or reptiles, the life cycle may become a three-host model.

Hyalomma aegyptium (tortoise tick)

Hyalomma aegyptium feeds on tortoises (*Testudo* spp.) and lizards but may also feed on dogs and horses. It is found throughout southern Europe and southwest Asia.

Description: These are large brown ticks with eyes and long mouthparts. Females 5.5–20 mm; males 3–6 mm. Coxa I has a large divergent spur in females and a prominent, sharply pointed spur in males.

Life cycle: This species is a two-host tick found throughout southern Europe and southwest Asia. The larval and nymphal stages engorge on the same host.

Hyalomma detritum/Hyalomma scupense (bont-legged tick)

In some texts *Hyalomma detritum detritum* and *Hyalomma detritum scupense* are treated as subspecies. However, there are strong arguments that these should be accorded separate species status and this is increasingly accepted. *Hyalomma detritum* is found throughout Africa while *H. scupense* predominates in southwestern Russia and southeastern Europe.

Description: *Hyalomma detritum* is morphologically very similar to *Hyalomma scupense* and the primary difference relates to their life cycle. Both are relatively small and lacking in punctations compared to other *Hyalomma* species. Neither have pale rings on the legs. The legs are yellow to orange coloured in *H. detritum* and relatively long but brown and short in *H. scupense*. The relative thicknesses of the ends of the spiracle plates are distinctive in both sexes: narrow in *H. detritum* and broad in *H. scupense*.

Life cycle: *Hyalomma detritum* is a two-host tick. In contrast, *H. scupense* has a one host life cycle. In *H. detritum* the female lays 5000–7000 eggs over a period of 37–59 days. These hatch in 34–66 days depending on the temperature and climatic conditions. Larvae and nymphs remain on the first host for between 13 and 45 days. Nymphs drop off the host and then moult to become adults. Subsequently, the adult finds a second host where the adult female engorges in 5–6 days. Unfed larvae can survive for 12 months, unfed nymphs for three months and unfed adults for 14 months. *H. scupense* overwinters on the host.

Hyalomma dromedarii (camel tick)

The camel tick *Hyalomma dromedarii* is of veterinary significance primarily in camels, but may also be of importance in ruminants and horses. It is found from India to Africa.

Description: *Hyalomma dromedarii* is usually inornate but with banded legs; eyes are present and festoons are sometimes present. The second segment of the palps is usually less than twice as long as the third segment, and the scutum has no pattern.

Life cycle: This is predominantly a two-host species of tick. Larvae acquire a host, feed and moult. Nymphs reattach to the same host soon after moulting. Following engorgement, nymphs drop off the host, moult to the adult stage and then acquire a new second host where they feed. After attachment, mating occurs and the female completes her single large blood meal. Males feed intermittently and mate repeatedly. Once fertilised, the female feeds for about 14 days and then drops to the ground to lay several thousand eggs in sheltered spots, after which she dies. In some circumstances, a variable life cycle has been reported for *H. dromedarii* with a three-host life cycle observed on sheep or cattle. It appears that the type of host, rearing conditions, density and age of the larvae may influence the life cycle adopted by this species.

Hyalomma marginatum (Mediterranean tick)

Previously there were considered to be four subspecies: *H. marginatum marginatum*, *H. marginatum rufipes*, *H. marginatum turanicum* and *H. marginatum isaaci*. Subsequently, this classification was re-evaluated, leading to the establishment of *H. marginatum*, *H. rufipes*, *H. turanicum* and *H. isaaci* as full species. *Hyalomma marginatum* is found around the Mediterranean basin from Portugal to Iran, the Balkans CIS and northwestern Africa; *H. turanicum* is found in Pakistan, Iran, Arabia and parts of northeastern Africa while *H. isaaci* occurs from Sri Lanka to southern Nepal, Pakistan and northern Afghanistan. Adults feed on wild herbivores and livestock (particularly equines and ruminants). Immature stages primarily parasitise small wild mammals, lizards and birds.

Description: Dark-brown or reddish ticks with pale banded legs. Eyes are present and festoons sometimes present. The palps and hypostome are long. The males have adanal shields. The second segment of the palps is less than twice as long as the third segment, and the scutum has no pattern. Female ticks have a large porose area and punctations on the scutum are small and sparse. In both sexes, coxa I has a long slender external spur.

Life cycle: The members of this species complex have a two-host life cycle, larvae and nymphs remaining and feeding on the same host. The engorged nymphs drop to the ground and moult to become an adult. Subsequently the adult feeds and engorges on a second host. The life cycle takes a minimum of 14 weeks from egg to adult. Adults are active between June and October with peak numbers in July and August.

Hyalomma truncatum (bont-legged tick)

Hyalomma truncatum is of veterinary significance in cattle, sheep, goats, pigs and horses and will also feed on a range of other mammals and birds. It is found throughout Africa south of the Sahara to South Africa, also Nile Valley and southern Arabia.

Description: Reddish-brown to nearly black ticks. The posteromedian and posterolateral spurs on coxa I are long and subequal in length in both sexes. In the female, the genital aperture is wide and deeply rounded.

Life cycle: This species is a two-host tick.

Amblyomma

Members of this genus are large, often highly ornate ticks with long legs, which are often banded. Unfed females are up to 8 mm in length, but when engorged may reach 20 mm in length. Eyes and festoons are present. Males lack ventral plates. They have long mouthparts (Fig. 3.117d) with which they can inflict a deep painful bite that may become secondarily infected. There are about 100 species of *Amblyomma*, largely distributed in tropical and subtropical areas of Africa. However, one important species is found in temperate North America. *Amblyomma* species of veterinary importance are listed in Table 3.35. The identification of more than the major species is beyond the scope of this book and interested readers will need to consult a relevant taxonomic specialist.

Amblyomma americanum (lone star tick)

Amblyomma americanum feeds on a range of wild and domestic animals, and is of particular veterinary significance in cattle. Larvae are most frequently found on wild small mammals. It is widely distributed throughout central and eastern USA.

Description: The lone star tick, *Amblyomma americanum*, is so called because of a single white spot on the scutum of the female

Table 3.35 *Amblyomma* species of veterinary importance.

Species	Hosts	Site
Amblyomma americanum	Wild and domestic animals, particularly cattle; birds. Larvae: small mammals	Skin, ears, flanks, head and ventral abdomen
Amblyomma variegatum	Wide range of mammals, particularly cattle	Skin
Amblyomma cajennense	Wide range of mammals, particularly horses	Skin, lower surface of body, axilla and groin
Amblyomma hebraeum	Wide range of ammals and birds	Skin
Amblyomma gemma	Wide range of mammals, particularly cattle, camels, large herbivores	Skin
Amblyomma maculatum	Wide range of mammals and birds	Skin, ears
Amblyomma pomposum	Mammals, particularly cattle, sheep and goats	Skin
Amblyomma lepidum	Sheep, goats, cattle	Skin
Amblyomma astrion	Buffalo, cattle	Skin
Amblyomma sparsum	Reptiles, tortoise	Skin
Amblyomma marmorium	Tortoise tick	Skin

(Fig. 3.126). These are large, usually ornate ticks the legs of which have bands of colour. Eyes and festoons are present. The palps and hypostome are long, and ventral plates are absent in the males. The engorged female is up to 10 mm in length, bean-shaped and has four pairs of legs. The female is reddish-brown in colour, becoming light grey when engorged. On the scutum are two deep parallel cervical grooves and a large pale spot at its posterior margin. The male is small with two pale symmetrical spots near the hind margin of the body, a pale stripe at each side, and a short oblique pale stripe behind each eye. The males are only 2–3 mm in length, and because of the small idiosoma, the four pairs of legs are readily visible. In both sexes, coxa I has a long external spur and a short internal spur, and the mouthparts are much longer than the basis capituli.

Nymphs resemble the adults and also have four pairs of legs but are less than 2 mm in size, while the larvae ('pepper ticks') are less than 1 mm in length, usually yellowish in colour and have only three pairs of legs.

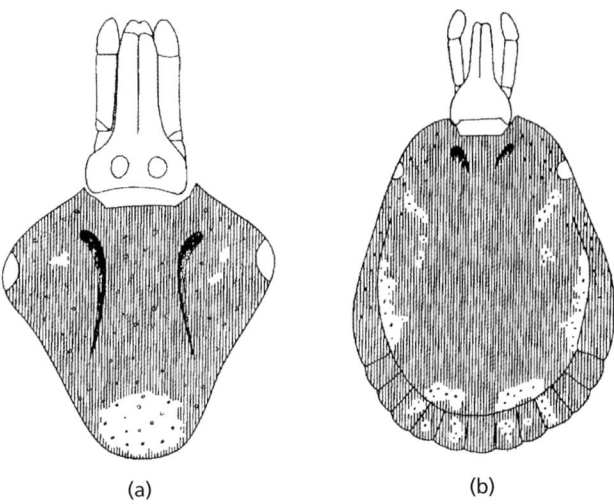

(a) (b)

Fig. 3.126 Dorsal view of the gnathosoma and scutum of adult (a) female and (b) male *Amblyomma americanum*. (Arthur, 1963/Springer Nature.)

Life cycle: The life cycle is typical of a three-host tick. Adult females attach to a host and take a single large blood meal over a period of 3–4 weeks, taking 0.5–2.0 ml of blood, during the course of which they mate once. In contrast, the males feed intermittently and mate repeatedly. Once fertilised, the female drops to the ground to lay several thousand eggs in sheltered spots, after which she dies. The larvae which hatch from the eggs will feed for about six days in the following year, then drop to the ground and moult to the nymphal stage. In the third year this stage feeds, drops off and becomes adult. Although the life cycle takes three years to complete, the larvae, nymphs and adults feed for a total of only 26–28 days. Larvae and nymphs feed on rodents, rabbits and ground-inhabiting birds. Adults feed on larger mammals such as deer, cattle, horses and sheep.

Amblyomma maculatum (Gulf coast tick)

Amblyomma maculatum feeds on a range of mammals and is found in the southern USA, in regions of high temperature and humidity.

Description: Similar to *A. americanum* but it has spurs on the second, third and fourth pairs of legs and more diffuse pale markings on the female ticks.

Amblyomma variegatum (variegated tick, tropical bont tick)

Amblyomma variegatum feeds on a range of mammals but is of particular veterinary significance in cattle and is found throughout Africa.

Description: Female *A. variegatum* are brown with a large pale patch on the posterior scutum, while males are brightly ornamented with orange coloration and a dark-brown border to the idiosoma. Both sexes of *A. variegatum* have hemispherical eyes. *Amblyomma variegatum* (and *A. hebraeum*) can be distinguished from *A. americanum* and *A. cajennense* by the shorter external spur on coxa I, which is closely associated with the internal spur. The scutum sides are straight and the scutum posterior angle is broad. The genital aperture is broadly U-shaped.

Amblyomma cajennense (cayenne tick)

Amblyomma cajennense will feed on a range of mammals but is of particular veterinary importance in horses. It is found throughout South and Central America, southern USA and the Caribbean.

Description: In adults the scutum is usually very ornate, lattice patterned often with bright multicoloured iridescent patterns. There may be pale central patches on the festoons.

Amblyomma hebraeum (bont tick)

Amblyomma hebraeum will feed on a range of hosts but is of particular veterinary significance in livestock and is found throughout Africa.

Description: *Amblyomma hebraeum* is an ornate tick with pink to orange ornamentation and pale rings on the legs. The eyes are slightly convex and close to the margin of the scutum. The scutum sides are convex and the scutum posterior angle is broad. The species has a short external spur on coxa I, which is closely associated with the internal spur.

Amblyomma gemma

Amblyomma gemma feeds on cattle, sheep and goats and is found in Africa, particularly Kenya.

Description: An ornate tick with large amounts of striking pink to orange ornamentation on the dorsal surface. The scutum has straight sides and broad posterior angle. The legs have pale-coloured rings. The eyes are flat and close to the margin of the scutum. In the female tick, the primary punctation on the scutum is localised and small to medium in size. In both male and female ticks, the external spurs on coxae I are medium in length and the internal spurs are short. In the male there is a broad posteromedian stripe.

Aponomma

The genus *Aponomma* has been subsumed with the genus *Amblyomma*. Almost all the *Amblyomma* (*Aponomma*) tick species parasitise reptiles, such as snakes, lizards and tuatara. Four species are adapted to feed on primitive Australian mammals, the monotremes and marsupials.

FAMILY ARGASIDAE

The family Argasidae comprises approximately 218 species, but the classification of many of these species is uncertain. Soft ticks have a leathery and unsclerotised body with a textured surface (Fig. 3.127), which in unfed ticks may be characteristically marked with folds or grooves. The integument is **inornate**. The palps appear somewhat leg-like, with the third and fourth segments equal in size. The gnathosoma is located ventrally and is not visible from the dorsal view in nymphs and adults. When present, the eyes are found in lateral folds above the legs. The stigmata are small and anterior to the coxae of the fourth pair of legs. The legs are similar to those of hard ticks; the pulvilli are usually absent or rudimentary in nymphs and adults, but may be well developed in larvae.

The soft ticks have a multi-host life cycle. The larval stage feeds once before moulting to become a first-stage nymph. There are between two and seven nymphal stages, each of which feeds and then leaves the host before moulting to the next stage. The adult females lay small batches of eggs after each short feed, lasting only a few minutes.

These ticks, unlike the Ixodidae, are drought resistant and capable of living for several years, and are found predominantly in deserts or dry conditions, but living in close proximity to their hosts. There are three genera of veterinary importance: *Argas*, *Otobius* and *Ornithodoros*.

Argasid ticks, which exist in and around animal housing, poultry houses and enclosures, can be controlled by application of an

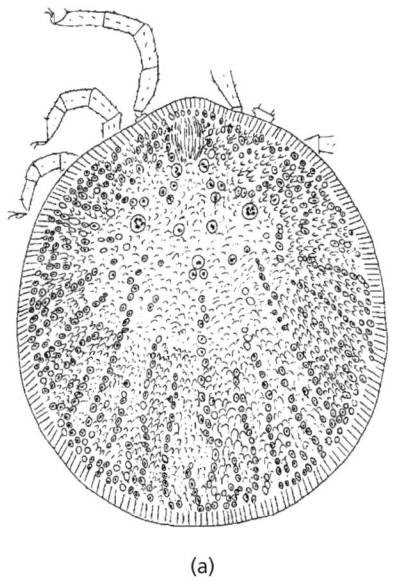
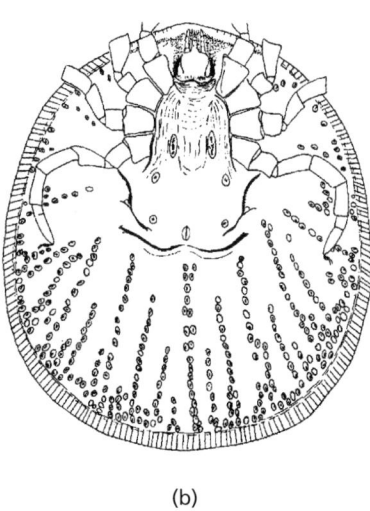

(a)   (b)

Fig. 3.127 An argasid tick, *Argas vespertilonis*: (a) dorsal view of female; (b) ventral view of female. (Arthur, 1963/Springer Nature.)

acaricide to their environment coupled with treatment of the population on the host. Environmental treatment of roosts and poultry houses may be effected using acaricidal sprays or emulsions containing organophosphates and pyrethroids. All niches and crevices in affected buildings should be sprayed, and nesting boxes and perches in poultry houses should also be painted with acaricides. At the same time as premises are treated, birds should be dusted with a suitable acaricide or, in the case of larger animals, sprayed or dipped.

Argas

Species of the genus *Argas* are usually dorsoventrally flattened, with definite margins, which can be seen even when the tick is engorged. The cuticle is wrinkled and leathery. Most species are nocturnal. Sixty-one species have been described in the genus *Argas*, and they are allocated to seven subgenera. Two subgenera, *Argas* and *Persicargas*, parasitise birds; other subgenera are associated with bats and a small number of other mammals, while *Argas* (*Microargas*) *transversus* is a permanent ectoparasite of the Galapagos giant tortoise (*Geochelone elephantopus*). Most species seldom attack humans. Species of this genus are usually found in dry arid habitats. Descriptions of only the major species of veterinary importance are presented (Table 3.36).

Table 3.36 *Argas* species of veterinary importance.

Species	Hosts	Site
Argas persicus	Chicken, turkey and wild birds	Skin
Argas reflexus	Pigeon	Skin
Argas walkerae (syn. *Persicargas walkerae*)	Chicken	Skin, common beneath wings
Argas miniatus	Wild birds	Skin
Argas radiates	Wild birds	Skin
Argas robertsi	Wild birds	Skin
Argas snachezi	Wild birds	Skin

Argas persicus (fowl tick, chicken tick, adobe tick, blue bug)

Argas persicus is of considerable veterinary importance as the most widespread argasid tick feeding on poultry. It is found worldwide, but especially in the tropics.

Description: The unfed adult is pale yellow to reddish-brown, turning slate blue when fed. The female is about 8 mm in length and the male about 5 mm. The margin of the body appears to be composed of irregular quadrangular plates or cells, and no scutum is present. Unlike hard ticks, the four segments of the pedipalps are equal in length. The stigmata are situated on the sides of the body above the third and fourth pairs of legs. The integument is granulated, leathery and wrinkled. The hypostome is notched at the tip (Fig. 3.128f), and the mouthparts are not visible when the tick is viewed from above.

Life cycle: *Argas persicus* is nocturnal and breeds and shelters in cracks and crevices in the structure of poultry houses. Females deposit batches of 25–100 eggs in these cracks and crevices. Up to 700 eggs may be produced by a single female at intervals, each oviposition preceded by a blood meal. After hatching, larvae locate a host and remain attached and feed for several days. After feeding, they detach, leave the host and shelter in the poultry house structure. Several days later they moult to become first-stage nymphs. They then proceed through two or three nymphal stages, interspersed with frequent nightly feeds, before moulting to the adult stage. Adult males and females feed about once a month, but can survive for long periods without a blood meal. Females can become completely engorged within 30–45 minutes. Under favourable conditions the life cycle can be completed in about 30 days. All stages of these ticks remain around the roosting area of poultry, quiescent in the day and actively feeding at night. *Argas persicus* can survive in empty poultry housing for years, and may travel long distances to find their hosts. This tick can undergo rapid increases in abundance, passing through 1–10 generations per year, particularly in areas where birds are present all year round.

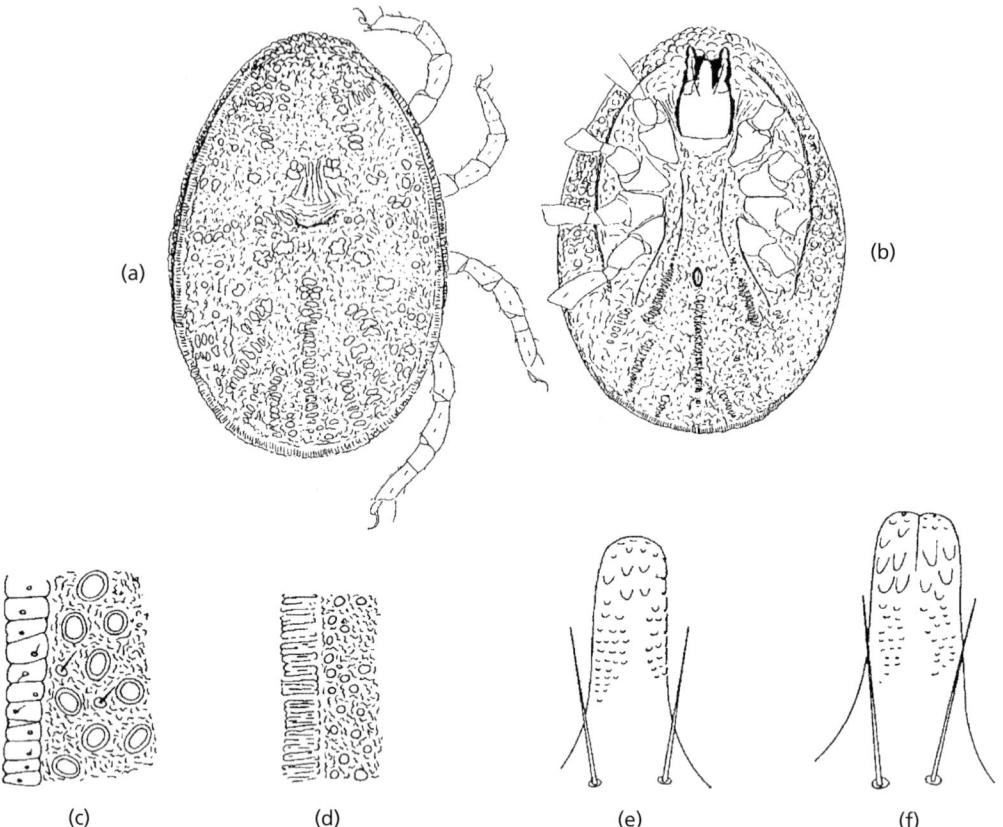

Fig. 3.128 Female *Argas reflexus*: (a) dorsal and (b) ventral view. Margin of (c) *Argas reflexus* and (d) *Argas persicus*. Hypostome of female (e) *Argas reflexus* and (f) *Argas persicus*. (Arthur, 1962/Springer Nature.)

Argas reflexus (pigeon tick)

Argas reflexus is a parasite of pigeons which is abundant in the Middle and Near East, from where it has spread into Europe and most of Asia.

Description: The adult *Argas reflexus* is between 6 and 11 mm in length and may be distinguished from the fowl tick, *Argas persicus*, by its body margin, which is composed of irregular grooves (Fig. 3.128a,b,c,d), and the hypostome, which is not notched apically (Fig. 3.128e). It is reddish-brown in colour with paler legs.

Life cycle: The life cycle is similar to that of *A. persicus*. *Argas reflexus* is nocturnal and breeds and shelters in cracks and crevices in the roost structure. Females deposit batches of 50–100 eggs in these cracks and crevices. After hatching, larvae locate and attach to a host, where they remain and feed for several days. After feeding, they detach, leave the host and shelter in the pigeon lofts or roosts. Several days later they moult to become first-stage nymphs. They then proceed through 2–4 nymphal stadia (with the fewest occurring in cooler temperatures), interspersed with frequent feeds, before moulting to the adult stage. Adult males and females feed about once a month. Females can become completely engorged within 30–45 minutes. All stages of these ticks remain around the roosting area, quiescent in the day and actively feeding at night. *Argas reflexus* can survive in empty roosts for more than a year. The egg-to-adult life cycle can take up to 11 years to complete. Engorged

female ticks diapause during the summer months. If oviposition has already commenced, egg laying stops and resumes the following year without the need for another blood meal.

Argas walkerae (chicken tick, southern fowl tampan)

Argas walkerae is a parasite of chickens found in southern Africa. This species lives in close association with poultry and no wild hosts are known.

Description: In the adults, the dorsal idiosomal discs are arranged more randomly than in *A. persicus*, the cells of the lateral structure vary in shape, and the apex of the hypostome is rounded.

Life cycle: Like most species of this genus: egg, larva, three nymphal stages and adult. It lives in crevices in the poultry house or nest material, moving on to the host to feed.

Ornithodoros

This genus includes approximately 130 known speces, almost all of which are found in tropical and subtropical habitats in both the Old and New Worlds. The genus is probably paraphyletic. Most *Ornithodoros* species are found in Africa, commonly in the burrows

Table 3.37 *Ornithodoros* species of veterinary importance.

Species	Hosts	Site
Ornithodoros savignyi	Most mammals, particularly camels, also cattle, poultry, human	Skin
Ornithodoros moubata (subsp. O. moubata porcinus)	Wide range of mammals: warthog, bushpig, porcupine, pig	Skin
Ornithodoros erraticus (syn. Ornithodoros marocanus)	Small mammals, domestic livestock, pig, human	Skin
Ornithodoros hermsi	Wide range of mammals, particularly rodents	Skin
Ornithodoros parkeri	Wide range of mammals, particularly rodents	Skin
Ornithodoros tholozani	Most mammals, birds and some reptiles	Skin
Ornithodoros turicata	Wide range of mammals, particularly rodents	Skin
Ornithodoros rudis	Wide range of mammals, particularly rodents, human	Skin
Ornithodoros lahorensis	Wild sheep, domestic sheep and goat	Skin
Ornithodoros coriaceus	Cattle, deer, human	Skin

of warthogs and bush pigs, though other species may be found in Central and South America and the Rocky Mountain states of the USA. They are nocturnal and the mouthparts are well developed. The integument has a wrinkled pattern, which runs continuously over the dorsal and ventral surfaces. There is no distinct lateral margin to the body, which appears sac-like. Species of this genus are found largely in habitats such as dens, caves, nests and burrows, and so are not normally problems for most domestic animals. Only the nymphs and adults are parasitic and may be responsible for considerable irritation; heavy infestations can cause mortality of stock from blood loss. Several species of *Ornithodoros* inflict painful bites and may be major vectors of the pathogens responsible for relapsing fever. Descriptions of the major species of veterinary importance are presented (Table 3.37).

Ornithodoros savignyi (sand tampan, eyed tampan)

Ornithodoros savignyi will feed on most mammals but particularly on camels and poultry. It is found throughout Africa, India and the Middle East.

Description: Female ticks are 10–13 mm and males 8–12 mm in length, and rounded when engorged. The cuticle is covered in mammillae of equal size and the dorsal and ventral surfaces are separated by a groove. The sand tampan has two pairs of hemispherical dark eyes located dorsal to coxa I and to coxae III and IV. The leg tarsi and tibiae have distinct dorsal humps and the leg coxae decrease in size posteriorly.

Ornithodoros moubata (eyeless tampan, hut tampan)

The taxonomic position of the two or more known strains of *O. moubata* – *O. moubata porcinus* and *O. moubata moubata* – is not satisfactorily resolved: *O. m. moubata* is hut-dwelling and feeds

on humans and chickens while *O. m. porcinus* lives in burrows and feeds on warthogs, antbears and porcupines. It is likely that they will be reclassified as distinct species following further research.

Description: Members of the *O. moubata* complex are slightly smaller than *O. savignyi*; females are 8–11 mm long but are most easily differentiated by the absence of eyes.

Ornithodoros hermsi

Ornithodoros hermsi is a parasite of small mammals, particularly rodents found in North America (Rocky Mountains and Pacific coast).

Description: *Ornithodoros hermsi* is a pale, sandy coloured soft tick, which appears greyish-blue when engorged. The adult female *O. hermsi* is typically 5–6 mm in length and 3–4 mm wide. The male is morphologically similar, though slightly smaller. It is one of the smallest ticks of the genus *Ornithodoros*.

Life cycle: Females lay batches of approximately 100 eggs in the sand of the host den, cave, nest or burrow and remain with them until they hatch to produce larvae several days later. The larvae remain quiescent until they have moulted to the nymphal stage. There are several nymphal stadia. Both nymphs and adults only feed on their hosts for short periods of time, typically 15–30 minutes. This species is able to survive for long periods without feeding; juvenile stages may live as long as 95 days unfed, and the adults more than seven months.

Otobius

This small genus contains only two species, *Otobius megnini* and *O. lagophilus*, which infest the ear canals of mammals.

Otobius megnini (spinose ear tick)

Otobius megnini commonly infests wild and domestic animals, particularly cattle but also sheep, dogs, horses and occasionally humans. It has spread workldwide and is now found in North and South America, India and southern Africa.

Description: The adult body is rounded posteriorly and slightly attenuated anteriorly (Fig. 3.129). Adult females range in size from 5 to 8 mm in length; males are slightly smaller. They have no lateral sutural line and no distinct margin to the body. Nymphs have spines. In adults, the hypostome is much reduced and the integument is granular. The body has a blue-grey coloration with pale yellow legs and mouthparts. Larvae measure 2–3 mm in length and fully grown engorged nymphs measure 7–10 mm.

Life cycle: This species is a one-host tick. The larval and nymphal stages are parasites of a wide range of mammals, but the adults are not parasitic. Mating takes place off the host, and batches of eggs are laid in sheltered sites such as in cracks and crevices in the walls of animal shelters or under stones or the bark of trees. The larvae hatch within 3–8 weeks and attach to a host animal. They may survive without food for 2–4 months. The preferred predilection site for larvae is deep within the ear. The larvae moult in the ears and

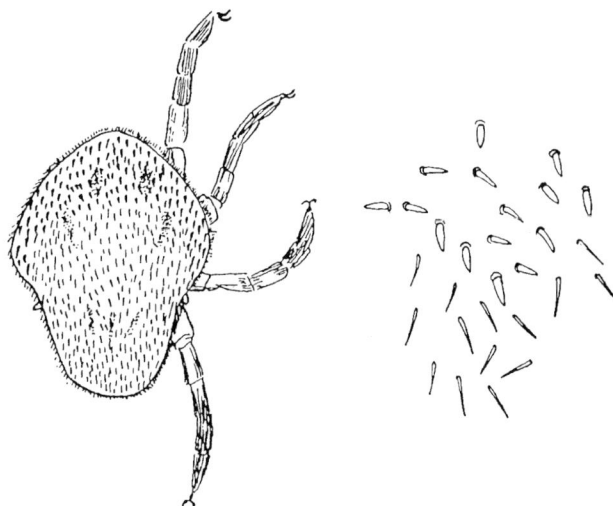

Fig. 3.129 Dorsal view of nymphal *Otobius megnini* and part of the integument showing hairs and spines. (Arthur, 1962/Springer Nature.)

nymphs remain there for 1–7 months. When fully grown and engorged, the nymphs drop off the host and seek dry sheltered sites, where they moult after a few days to become adults. The adults do not feed, and unmated females can survive in empty shelters and stables for over a year. Females lay 500–600 eggs over a period of up to six months.

Otobius lagophilus (rabbit ear tick)

Otobius lagophius commonly infests rabbits and is found in North America and Canada.

Description: The body is rounded at both ends and constricted slightly behind legs IV. The integument is granular with numerous circular pits both dorsally and ventrally, which are more densely arranged than with *O. megnini*. Anterodorsal spines on the nymphs are thick and peg-like in structure.

Life cycle: This species is a one-host tick. Only larvae and nymphs are parasitic.

CLASS CRUSTACEA

The adults of this strange group of about 100 species of aberrant obligate arthropods (subclass Pentastomida; order Porocephalida), often called tongue worms, are found in the respiratory passages and viscera of vertebrates and resemble annelid worms rather than arthropods. The genus *Linguatula* is of some veterinary significance, with adult parasites occurring in the nasal passages and sinuses of dogs, cats, foxes and primates. *Armillifer* is found in the lungs of large snakes but has also been reported in the viscera of primates and humans.

Linguatula

Linguatula serrata (tongue worm)

Description: Males measure up to 20 mm in length while females are 30–130 mm in length. Both sexes are transversely striated, expanded anteriorly and shaped like an elongated tongue. Anteriorly there are five small protuberances, one bearing a small mouth at its extremity, the others bearing tiny claws (Fig. 3.130).

Life cycle: With most pentastomids the life cycle requires an intermediate host. In the case of *Linguatula serrata*, eggs are expelled from the respiratory passage of the host by coughing or sneezing. Eggs are ingested by the herbivorous intermediate host, commonly sheep or cattle or rabbits, and pass into the gut where they hatch. The larva bores through the intestinal wall to the mesenteric glands, liver and lungs. Here, larval development involving a number of moults takes place. The larvae then encyst to develop into the infective nymphal stage. The cysts, about 1 mm in diameter, may be visible in cut surfaces of mesenteric glands. The final host is infected by eating uncooked viscera. Following ingestion, the nymph migrates to the nasal passages where the final moult, mating and egg production occur.

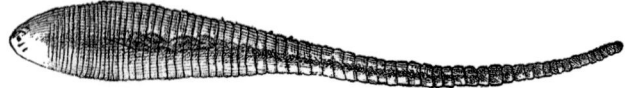

Fig. 3.130 Pentasomid: female *Linguatula serrata*. (Reproduced from Soulsby, 1971/Soulsby.)

CHAPTER 4
Laboratory diagnosis and identification

HELMINTH INFECTIONS

FAECAL EXAMINATION

Although there is much current interest in the use of serology and molecular methods as an aid to the diagnosis of helminthosis, faecal examination for the presence of worm eggs or larvae remains the most common routine aid to diagnosis employed.

COLLECTION OF FAECES

Faecal samples from large animals should preferably be collected from the rectum and examined fresh. If it is difficult to take rectal samples, fresh faeces can be collected from the field or floor, ideally after observing the animal defecating. A plastic glove is suitable for collection, the glove being turned inside out to act as the receptacle. Individual samples are required and for ruminants, a minimum of 10 samples in a herd or flock should be sampled. The wide variation in faecal egg counts (FECs) between animals grazing together in the same field means that random sampling effects have a significant impact on the confidence limits surrounding the estimate of the group mean FEC. Ideally, about 5 g (2–10 g depending on the size of the animal) of faeces should be collected, since this amount is required for some of the concentration methods of examination.

With poultry, representative samples from a number of birds should be collected from different areas of the house or building. For smaller pets a thermometer or glass rod may be used, or faeces collected from the cage or container in which they are housed.

Since eggs embryonate rapidly, the faeces should be stored in the refrigerator unless examination is carried out within a day. The samples can be stored for five days at +4–8 °C; if there is no possibility of analysing the samples within five days of sampling, keep the faecal samples in a vacuum-packed plastic bag (or use anaerobic storage) and store them for up to three weeks in the fridge at +4–8 °C (refrigeration is needed to prevent fungal growth).

METHODS OF EXAMINATION OF FAECES

Several methods are available for preparing faeces for microscopic examination to detect the presence of eggs or larvae. However, whatever method of preparation is used, the slides should first be examined under low power since most eggs can be detected at this magnification. If necessary, higher magnification can then be employed for measurement of the eggs or more detailed morphological differentiation. An eyepiece micrometer is very useful for sizing populations of eggs or larvae.

Direct smear method

A few drops of water plus an equivalent amount of faeces are mixed on a microscope slide. Tilting the slide then allows the lighter eggs to flow away from the heavier debris. A coverslip is placed on the fluid and the preparation is then examined microscopically. It is possible to detect most eggs or larvae by this method, but due to the small amount of faeces used it may only detect relatively heavy infections.

Flotation methods

The basis of any flotation method is that when worm eggs are suspended in a liquid with a specific gravity (s.g.) higher than that of the eggs, the latter will float to the surface. Nematode and cestode eggs float in a liquid with a s.g. of 1.10–1.20; trematode eggs, which are much heavier, require a s.g. of 1.30–1.35.

The flotation solutions (FS) used for nematode and cestode ova are mainly based on sodium chloride (NaCl) or sometimes magnesium sulfate ($MgSO_4$). A saturated solution of these is prepared and stored for a few days and the specific gravity checked prior to usage. In some laboratories a sugar solution of s.g. 1.2 is preferred. For trematode eggs, saturated solutions of zinc chloride ($ZnCl_2$) or zinc sulfate ($ZnSO_4$) with s.g. 1.35 are widely used.

Whatever solutions are employed, the specific gravity should be checked regularly and examination of the solution containing the eggs or larvae made rapidly, otherwise distortion may take place.

Direct flotation

A small amount of fresh faeces (e.g. approximately 2.0 g) is added to 10 ml of the flotation solution and, following thorough mixing, the suspension is poured into a test tube and more flotation solution added to fill the tube to the top. A coverslip is then placed on the surface of the liquid and the tube and coverslip are left standing for 10–15 minutes. The coverslip is then removed vertically and placed on a slide and examined under the microscope. If a centrifuge is available, the flotation of the eggs in the flotation solution may be accelerated by centrifugation. Several commercially available systems, such as Ovassay™ and Ovatec Plus™, use this method for the qualitative examination of faecal samples for the presence of helminth eggs.

Veterinary Parasitology, Fifth Edition. Domenico Otranto and Richard Wall.
© 2024 John Wiley & Sons Ltd. Published 2024 by John Wiley & Sons Ltd.

The use of a filter (gauze or metal sieve) that retains the gross material present in the faeces and subsequent centrifugation of the tube, before forming the meniscus, will help to give a preparation with fewer impurities.

Improved modified McMaster method

This quantitative technique is used where it is desirable to estimate worm burdens by counting the number of eggs or larvae per gram of faeces. A number of McMaster methods have been described, and one of the most commonly used is as follows.

1 Weigh 3.0 g of faeces or, if faeces are diarrhoeic, 3 ml.
2 Break up thoroughly in 42 ml of water in a plastic container. This can be done using a homogeniser if available or in a stoppered bottle containing glass beads.
3 Pour through a fine mesh sieve (aperture 150 μm, or 100 to 1 inch).
4 Collect filtrate, agitate and fill a 15 ml test tube.
5 Centrifuge at 2000 rpm (220 g) for two minutes.
6 Pour off supernatant, agitate sediment and fill tube to previous level with flotation solution.
7 Invert tube six times and remove fluid with pipette to fill both chambers of a McMaster slide (Fig. 4.1). Leave no fluid in the pipette or else pipette rapidly, since the eggs will rise quickly in the flotation fluid.
8 Examine one chamber and multiply the number of eggs or larvae under one grid by 100, or two grids and multiply by 50, to estimate the number of eggs per gram (epg) of faeces.
9 If the total number of eggs in one chamber is counted, then multiply by 30. If both chambers are counted, then multiply by 15.

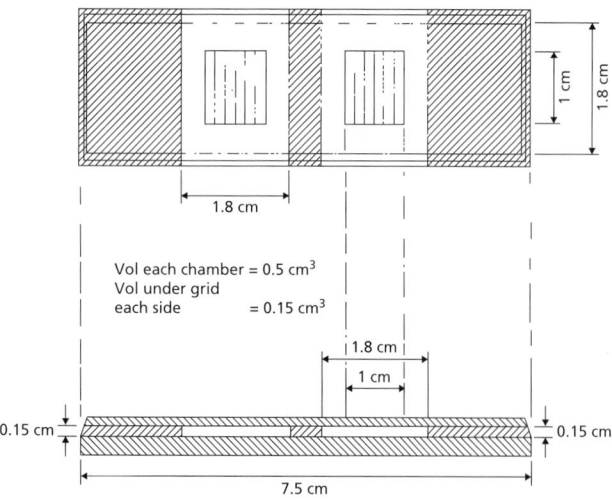

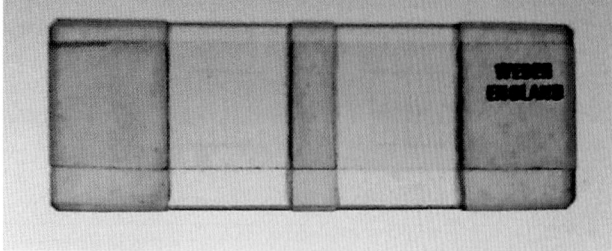

Fig. 4.1 McMaster slide for estimating numbers of nematode eggs in faeces.

The multiplication factor is obtained considering that:
- 3 g of faeces are dissolved in 42 ml
- total volume is 45 ml

    therefore 1 g is in 15 ml and given that the volume under the grid is 0.15 ml, the number of eggs is multiplied by 100 (detection limit = 100 epg). If two grids are examined, multiply by 50 (detection limit = 50 epg).

An abbreviated version of this technique (modified McMaster) is to homogenise the 3 g of faeces in 42 ml of salt solution, sieve and pipette the filtrate directly into the McMaster slide. Although a faster process, the slide contents are more difficult to 'read' because of their dark colour.

Improved sensitivity methods

Centrifugal flotation technique

This method follows the same initial steps described for the improved modified McMaster method.

1 Weight 3 g of faeces and break up thoroughly in 42 ml of water in a plastic container.
2 Pour through a fine mesh sieve (aperture 150 μm).
3 Collect filtrate, agitate and fill a 15 ml test tube.
4 Centrifuge at 2000 rpm (220 g) for two minutes.
5 Pour off supernatant, agitate sediment and fill tube to previous level with saturated NaCl solution.
6 Place the tube in the centrifuge and add further saturated salt until a positive meniscus is formed.
7 A thick 18 × 18 mm coverslip is then placed on the tube, ensuring that no air bubbles are trapped underneath.
8 Centrifuge the tube at 1000 rpm for two minutes.
9 Remove the coverslip by lifting vertically with a deliberate movement.
10 Place the coverslip on a glass slide and count all eggs.
11 By adding 15 ml of filtrate to the centrifuge tube, it will contain the eggs from 1 g of faeces, and if all of these are recovered then the number of eggs counted is equal to the number of eggs per gram. However, about one-sixth of eggs are lost in the process of flotation and a correction factor of ×1.2 should be applied. If x is the capacity of the tube and y the number of eggs seen, then epg = $y × 15/x × 1.2$.

FLOTAC and Mini-FLOTAC techniques

The 'FLOTAC group' includes FLOTAC, Mini-FLOTAC and Fill-FLOTAC devices (Fig. 4.2). The FLOTAC and Mini-FLOTAC techniques permit the simultaneous detection of eggs, larvae, oocysts and cysts of helminths and protozoa in faeces. They can be performed on fresh or preserved (i.e. stored in a fixative) faecal samples. These techniques also ensure safety of technicians as well as environmental protection. The FLOTAC devices are 'closed', thus avoiding contact of faecal samples by lab operators, and they do not use reagents that are harmful for humans or toxic and dangerous to the environment.

FLOTAC

The FLOTAC apparatus has been designed to carry out flotation in a centrifuge, followed by a transverse cut (i.e. translation) of the apical portion of the floating suspension. Several variants of the

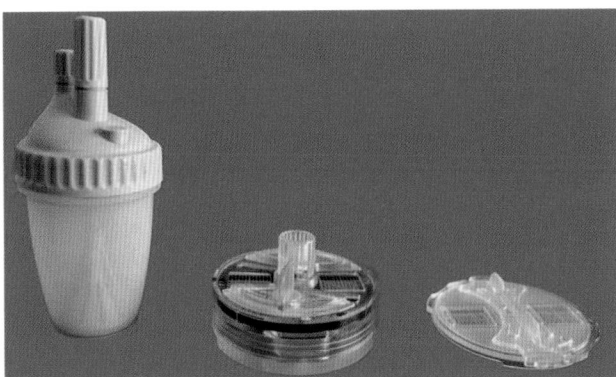

Fig. 4.2 Fill-FLOTAC, FLOTAC and Mini-FLOTAC.

FLOTAC technique are described in the literature: FLOTAC **basic** (1 epg), FLOTAC **dual** (2 epg), FLOTAC **double** (2 epg), FLOTAC **pellet** (different detection limits depending on the weight of the analysed sample). The FLOTAC dual technique is described below. It covers a wide diagnostic range with accuracy and precision because it uses two FS (usually NaCl and ZnSO$_4$) in parallel with the same sample. For the other FLOTAC techniques, please refer to the manuals available at www.parassitologia.unina.it

FLOTAC dual technique (one sample, two different FS).

1 Weigh 10 g of faeces, well-homogenised, into a clean container.
2 Dilute each collected faecal sample in tap water (dilution ratio 1:10); for lower amounts of faeces, the same dilution ratio (1:10) shall be maintained.
3 Homogenise the sample thoroughly (the use of a hand blender is suggested).
4 Filter suspension through a wire mesh (aperture of 250 μm).
5 Transfer two 6 ml aliquots of the filtered suspension into two conic tubes. The two flotation chambers of the FLOTAC apparatus require 5 ml each; an additional 1 ml is necessary to easily fill each flotation chamber.
6 Centrifuge the two tubes for 3 min at 1500 rpm (170 g) at room temperature.
7 After centrifugation, discard the supernatant, leaving only the sediments (pellets) in the tubes.
8 Fill the two tubes with two different FS, up to the previous 6 ml level.
9 Thoroughly homogenise the suspensions (before and between the fillings) and fill the two flotation chambers of the FLOTAC apparatus with the two faecal suspensions: chamber 1 with suspension in NaCl and chamber 2 with suspension in ZnSO$_4$.
10 Close the FLOTAC apparatus and centrifuge for 5 min at 1000 rpm (120 g) at room temperature.

After centrifugation, translate the top parts of the flotation chambers and examine under a microscope.

Mini-FLOTAC

Mini-FLOTAC is a logical evolution of the FLOTAC technique. It is user-friendly, produces highly reproducible results and is particularly useful for monitoring and surveillance, for which large numbers of faecal samples must be rapidly, yet reliably, examined. It is recommended that Mini-FLOTAC be used in combination with Fill-FLOTAC, a kit that protects laboratory personnel against potential biohazards during the preparation (i.e. collection, weighing, homogenisation, filtration and filling of the apparatus) of faecal samples for subsequent microscopic examination. There are two versions of Fill-FLOTAC: Fill-FLOTAC 2, which permits analysis of up to 2 g of faeces (usually used for examination of faeces collected from companion animals and humans), and Fill-FLOTAC 5, which enables analysis of up to 5 g of faeces (usually used for examination of faeces from food-producing animals).

The Mini-FLOTAC apparatus is composed of two physical components (i.e. the base and the reading disc) and two accessories (i.e. the key and the microscope adaptor). The Mini-FLOTAC permits a maximum magnification of 400×.

Several variants of the Mini-FLOTAC technique are described in the literature based on different types of faeces analysed. The Mini-FLOTAC technique used for herbivore samples is reported below. For the other FLOTAC techniques, please refer to the manuals available at www.parassitologia.unina.it

1 Add 45 ml of flotation solution (dilution ratio 1:10) into the Fill-FLOTAC container (the Fill-FLOTAC has a graduate scale).
2 Carefully homogenise the faecal sample by mixing with a wooden spatula, then fill the conical collector (5 g of faeces) of the Fill-FLOTAC.
3 Close the Fill-FLOTAC and homogenise the faecal suspension by pumping the conical collector up and down (10 times) in the container, while turning to the right and left.
4 Put the tip on the lateral hole of the Fill-FLOTAC. Invert the Fill-FLOTAC five times to mix the sample and fill the flotation chambers of the Mini-FLOTAC.
5 After 10 minutes, use the key to turn the reading disc clockwise (about 90°) until the reading disc stops, to separate the floating parasitic elements from the faecal debris. Remove the key and examine the Mini-FLOTAC under a microscope. The multiplication factor used to obtain the number of eggs, larvae, oocysts and cysts per gram of faeces is 5.

Automated systems

Advanced systems based on artificial intelligence and machine learning for helminth egg identification and counting have been developed to reduce human error and time required for reading, thereby increasing diagnostic efficiency. They are mostly based on semi-automated and automated systems combined with image analysis for helminth egg detection. Very few of the automated systems are commercially available (e.g. Parasight System, Telenostic, FECPAKG2, etc.), and most are still in the development phase. In addition, validation studies are needed, as data on the diagnostic performance of these new methods have only been published as proof-of-concept results (e.g. Kubic FLOTAC Microscope).

IDENTIFICATION OF NEMATODE EGGS

The presence of nematode eggs in faeces is a useful aid to diagnosis of worm infections as they can be identified and counted in faecal samples (Figs 4.3–4.11). Strongyle eggs are approximately 60–80 μm long, oval, thin-shelled, contain 4–16 cells and are not easily differentiated; however, eggs of *Trichuris*, *Nematodirus* spp. and *Strongyloides* can be identified and may be counted and reported separately.

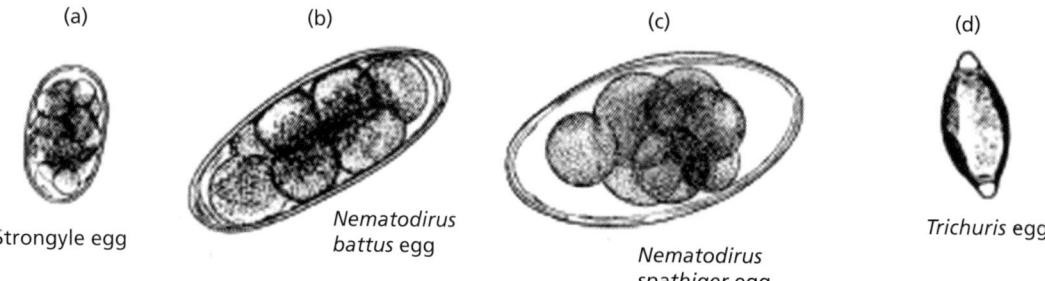

(a)
Strongyle egg
(b)
Nematodirus battus egg
(c)
Nematodirus spathiger egg
(d)
Trichuris egg

Fig. 4.3 Nematode eggs.

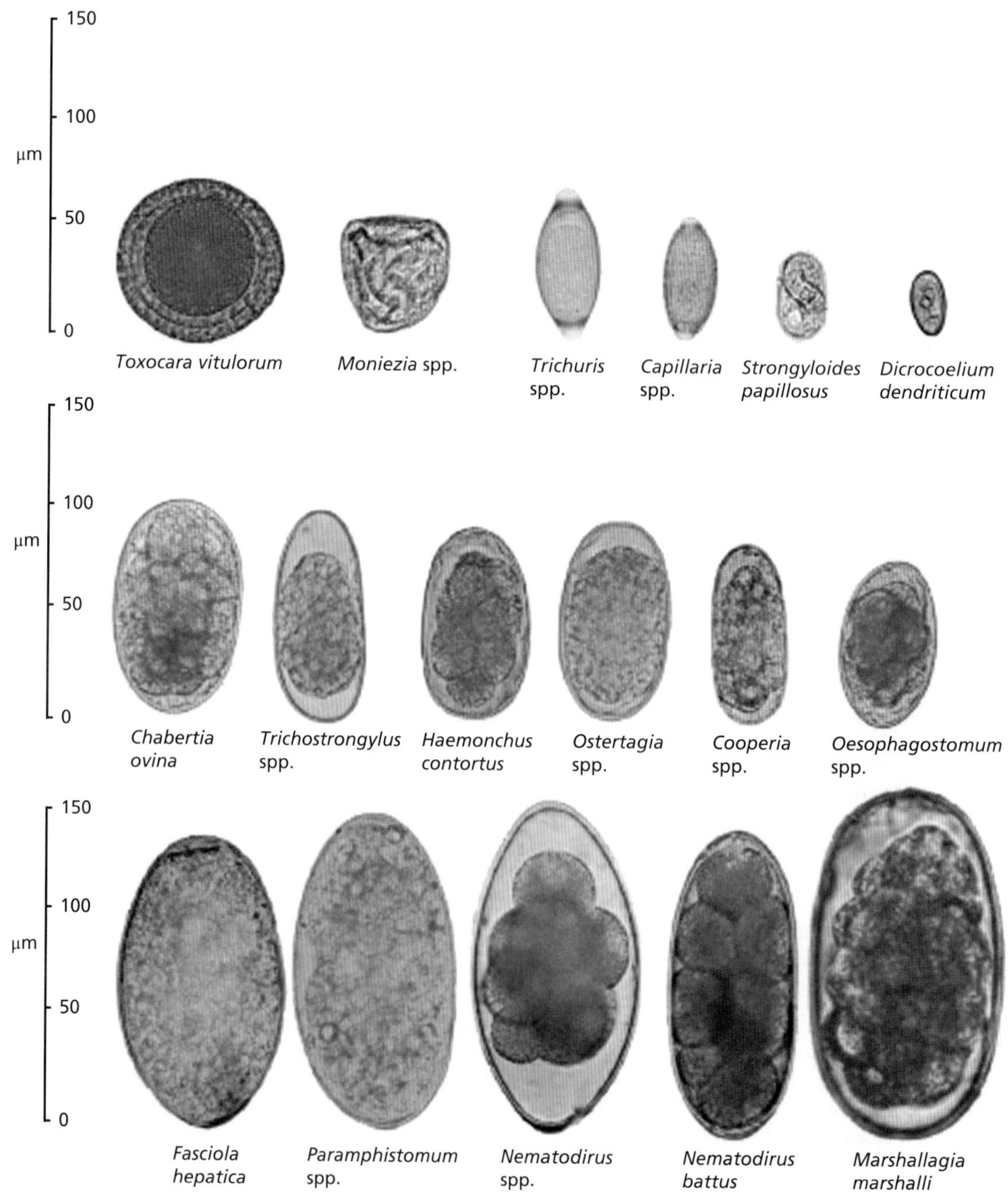

150
100
μm
50
0
Toxocara vitulorum
Moniezia spp.
Trichuris spp.
Capillaria spp.
Strongyloides papillosus
Dicrocoelium dendriticum
150
100
μm
50
0
Chabertia ovina
Trichostrongylus spp.
Haemonchus contortus
Ostertagia spp.
Cooperia spp.
Oesophagostomum spp.
150
100
μm
50
0
Fasciola hepatica
Paramphistomum spp.
Nematodirus spp.
Nematodirus battus
Marshallagia marshalli

Fig. 4.4 Helminth eggs from ruminants.

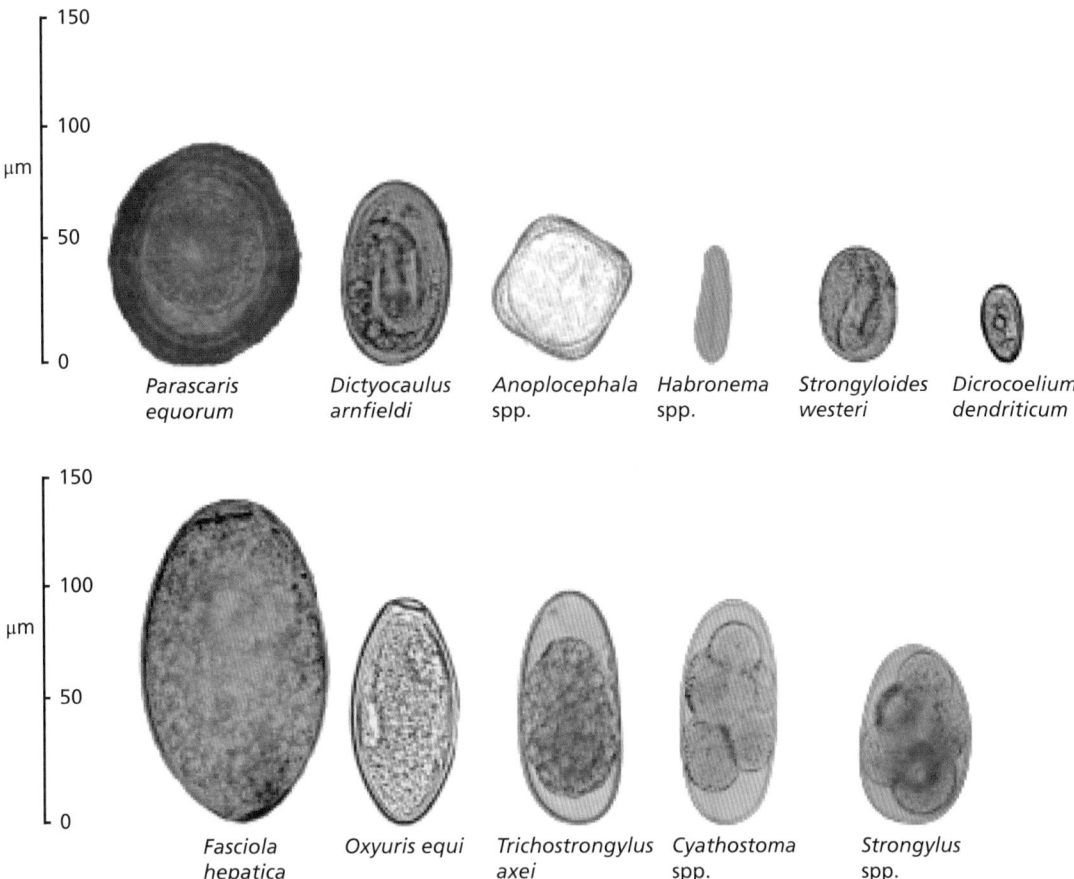

μm

150
100
50
0

| *Parascaris equorum* | *Dictyocaulus arnfieldi* | *Anoplocephala* spp. | *Habronema* spp. | *Strongyloides westeri* | *Dicrocoelium dendriticum* |

μm

150
100
50
0

| *Fasciola hepatica* | *Oxyuris equi* | *Trichostrongylus axei* | *Cyathostoma* spp. | *Strongylus* spp. |

Fig. 4.5 Helminth eggs from horses.

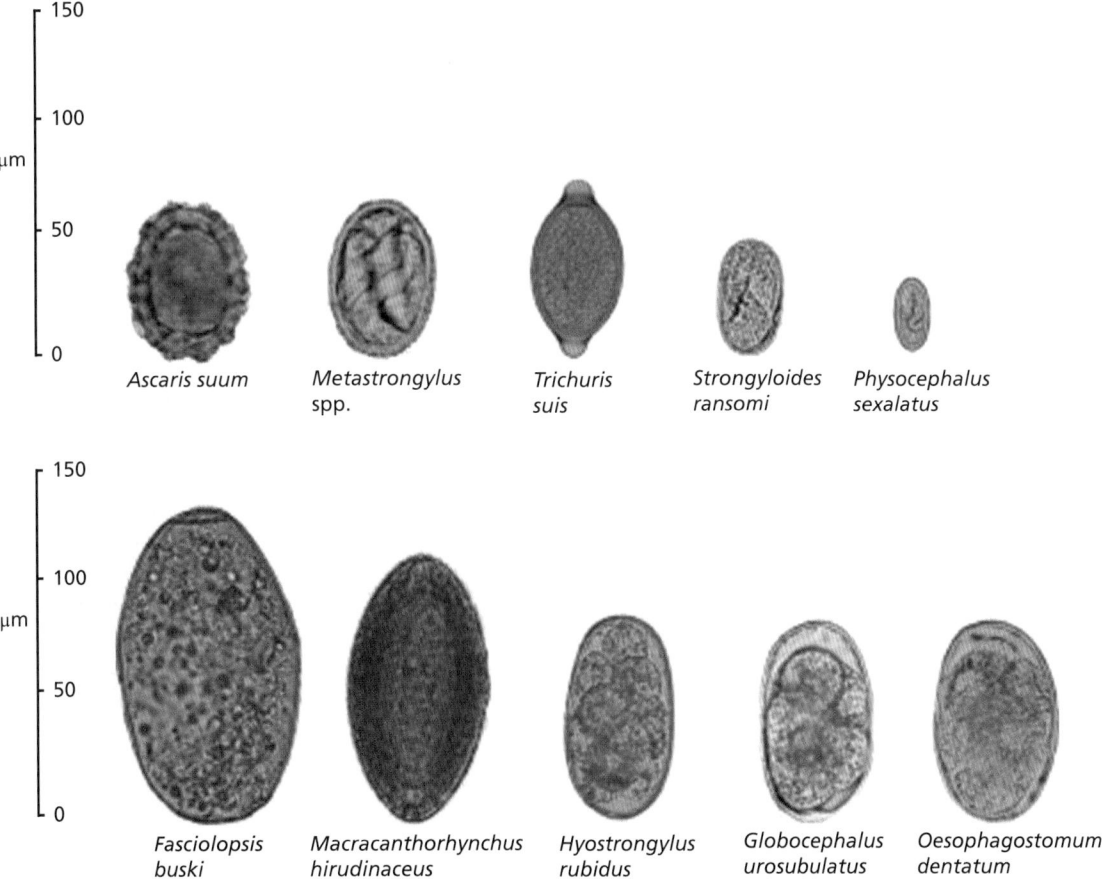

μm

150
100
50
0

| *Ascaris suum* | *Metastrongylus* spp. | *Trichuris suis* | *Strongyloides ransomi* | *Physocephalus sexalatus* |

μm

150
100
50
0

| *Fasciolopsis buski* | *Macracanthorhynchus hirudinaceus* | *Hyostrongylus rubidus* | *Globocephalus urosubulatus* | *Oesophagostomum dentatum* |

Fig. 4.6 Helminth eggs from pigs.

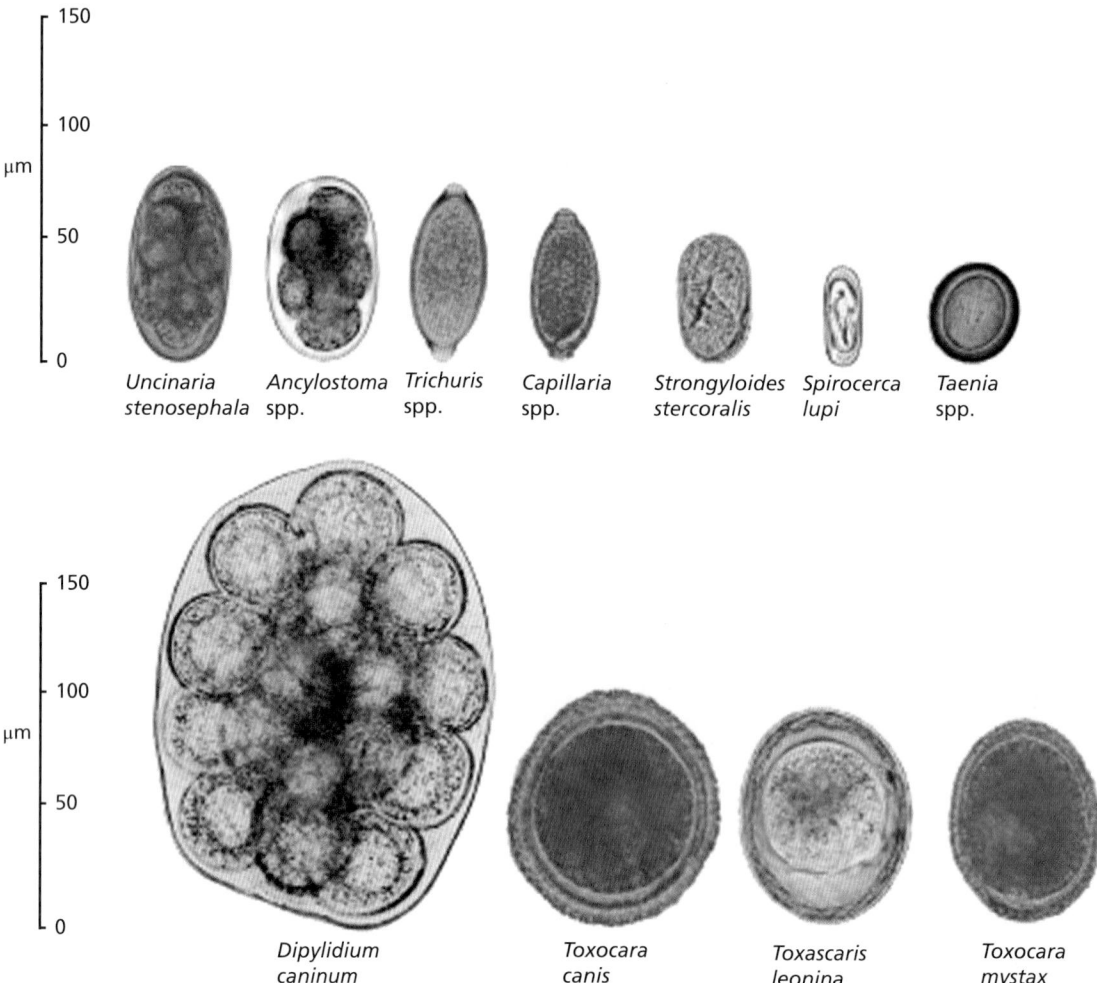

Fig. 4.7 Helminth eggs from dogs and cats.

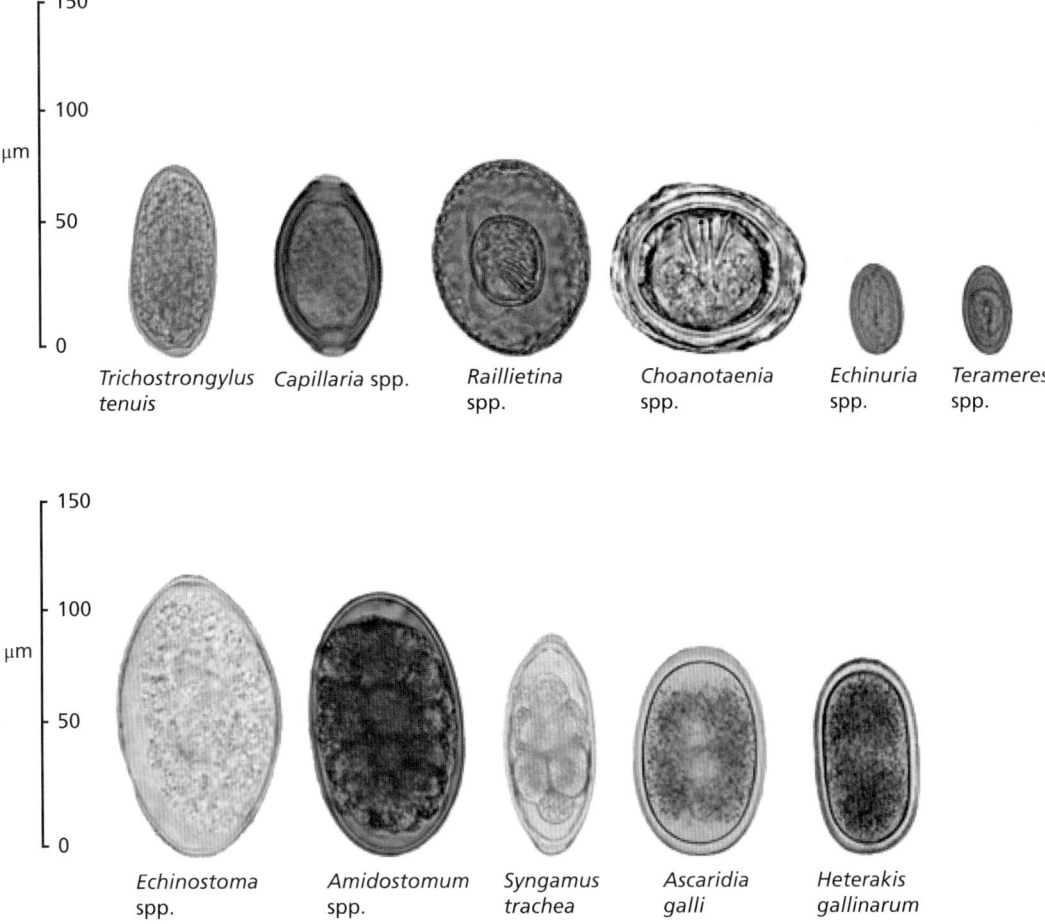

Fig. 4.8 Helminth eggs from poultry.

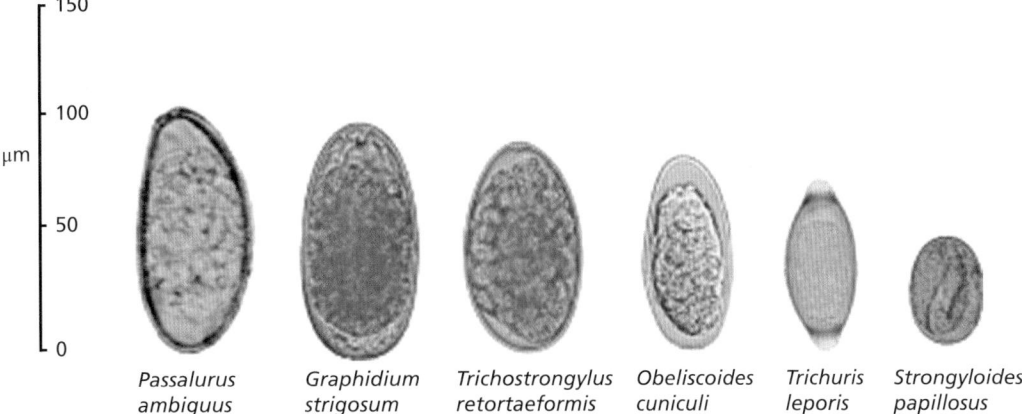

Fig. 4.9 Helminth eggs from rabbits.

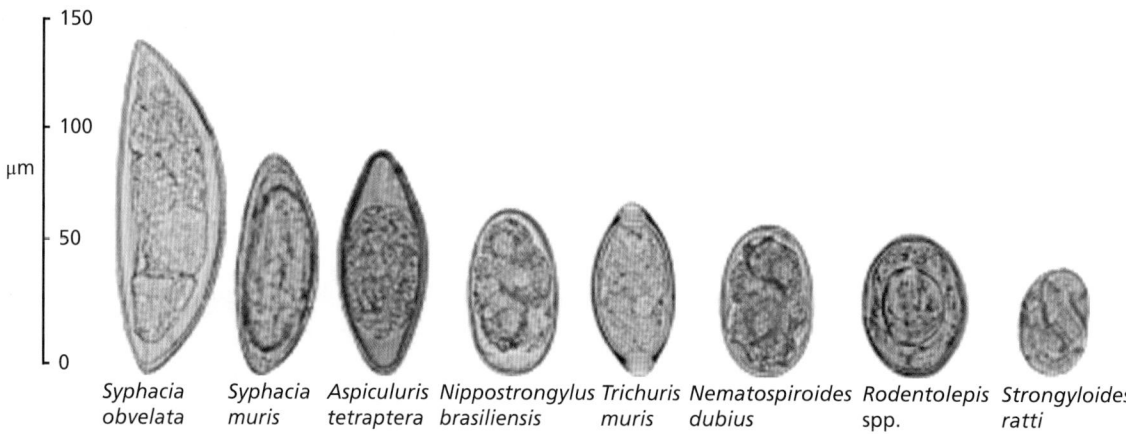

Fig. 4.10 Helminth eggs from rodents.

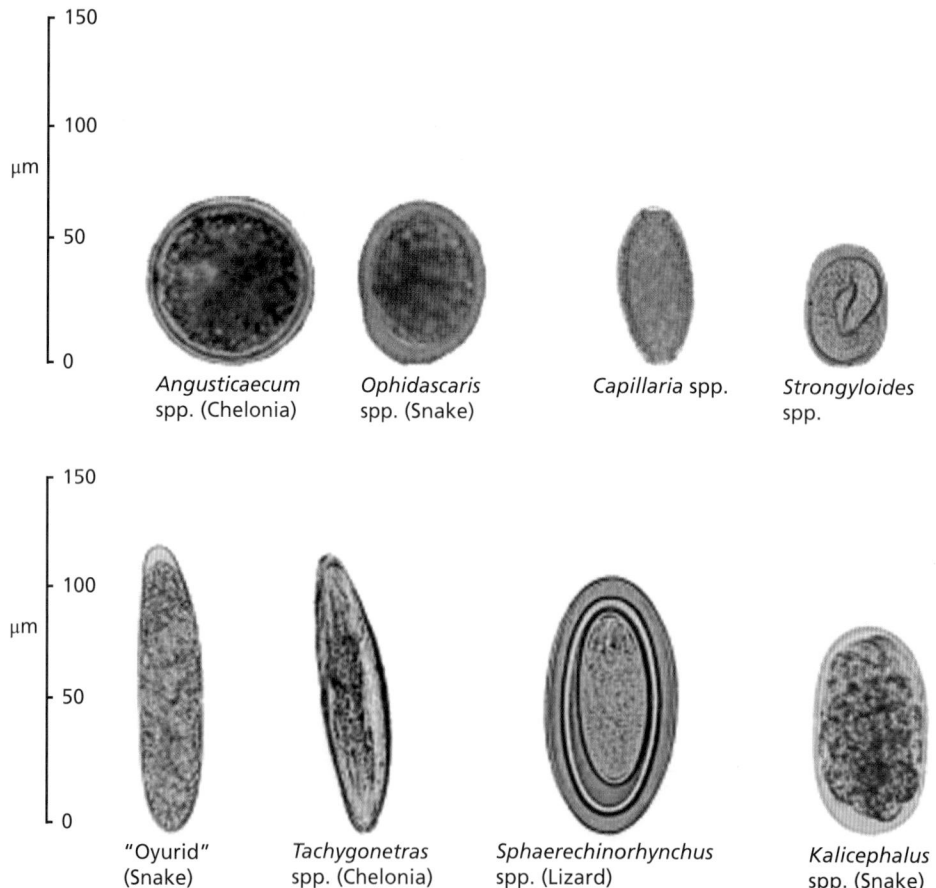

Fig. 4.11 Helminth eggs from reptiles.

Guide to egg count interpretation in ruminants

It is difficult to calculate from the FEC the actual worm population of the host, since many factors influence egg production of worms and the number of eggs also varies with the species. Nevertheless, in ruminants for example, egg counts in excess of 1000 epg are generally considered indicative of heavy infections and those over 500 epg of moderate infection (Tables 4.1 and 4.2). However, a low epg is not necessarily indicative of very low infections, since patency may just be newly established; alternatively, the epg may be affected by developing immunity. The eggs of some species, such as certain ascarids, *Strongyloides*, *Oxyuris*, *Trichuris* and *Capillaria*, can be easily recognised morphologically. However, with the exception of *Nematodirus* spp., the common trichostrongyle eggs require measurement for differentiation.

IDENTIFICATION OF TREMATODE EGGS

While the techniques described will detect the eggs and larvae of most nematodes, cestodes and coccidia, they will not demonstrate trematode eggs, which have a higher specific density. For these, a flotation fluid of higher specific gravity such as a saturated solution of zinc sulfate ($ZnSO_4$) has to be used, or a sedimentation method employed.

Fluke eggs are large, oval and have an operculum at one end. Liver fluke eggs (*Fasciola*) are brown in colour and may need to be differentiated from rumen fluke eggs (*Paramphistomum*, *Calicophoron*, *Cotylophoron*, etc.), whose eggs are much lighter in colour (Fig. 4.4).

Zinc sulfate flotation method for counting fluke eggs

Liver fluke eggs will not float in saturated NaCl solution but will float in saturated $ZnSO_4$ solution, which has a higher specific gravity. The

Table 4.1 Cattle worm egg counts: guide to interpretation.

	Degree of infestation		
Worm species	Light	Moderate	Heavy
Mixed infection	100	200–700	700+
Haemonchus	200	200–500	500+
Ostertagia ostertagi	150		500+
Trichostrongylus spp.	50	50–300	500+
Bunostomum	20	20–100	100+
Cooperia	500	500–3000	3000

Table 4.2 Sheep worm egg counts: guide to interpretation.

	Degree of infestation		
Worm species	Light	Moderate	Heavy
Mixed infection	<250	1000	2000+
Mixed (*H. contortus* absent)	<150	500	1000
Haemonchus contortus	100–2500	2500–8000	8000+
Teladorsagia (*Ostertagia*) *circumcincta*	50–200	200–2000	2000+
Trichostrongylus spp.	100–500	500–2000	2000+
Nematodirus spp.	50–100	100–600	600+
Strongyloides			10 000

procedure is exactly the same as that described for the improved modified McMaster method, with $ZnSO_4$ replacing NaCl.

1. Weigh 3 g of faeces and break up thoroughly in 42 ml of water in a plastic container.
2. Pour through a fine mesh sieve (aperture 250 µm).
3. Collect filtrate, agitate and fill a 15 ml test tube.
4. Centrifuge at 1500 rpm (170 *g*) for two minutes.
5. Pour off supernatant, agitate sediment and fill tube to previous level with saturated $ZnSO_4$ solution.
6. Invert tube six times and remove fluid with pipette to fill both chambers of McMaster slide (one drawback of this method is that the eggs collapse, making identification more difficult, and the collapse may cause the eggs to sink again. This can be prevented with the following steps).
7. Invert tube six times then place the tube in the centrifuge and add further saturated $ZnSO_4$ until a positive meniscus is formed.
8. A thick 18 × 18 mm coverslip is then placed on the tube, ensuring that no air bubble is trapped underneath.
9. Centrifuge the tube at 1000 rpm (120 *g*) for two minutes.
10. Remove the coverslip by lifting vertically with a deliberate movement and wash off into conical tube with about 10 ml of water.
11. Centrifuge the tube at 1500 rpm (170 *g*) for two minutes and siphon off the supernatant and discard.
12. Transfer the sediment in a total volume of about 0.1 ml to a microscope slide. Rinse the tube with a further 0.1 ml water and transfer to slide.
13. Place a 22 × 40 mm coverslip over the fluid and count all eggs. Each egg seen represents 1 epg.

Faecal sedimentation method for fluke eggs

1. Homogenise 3 g (sheep, goats) or 6 g (cattle) of faeces with 50–60 ml of water in a beaker. Agitate or mix the faeces for about 30 seconds until broken down.
2. Sensitivity can be improved by increasing the amount of faeces examined.
3. Add 2 drops of Teepol detergent to the homogenate to improve the release of eggs from faecal material.
4. Pour through a strainer and collect filtrate into beaker or collecting bowl.
5. Strain filtrate through a second screen (~250 µm aperture) into a conical flask.
6. Half fill the beaker with water and wash through the screen into the conical flask.
7. Allow filtrate in the conical flask to sediment for three minutes.
8. Siphon off supernatant with a suction pump, or manually with a large pipette, taking care not to disturb the sediment.
9. Step 7 may be repeated by adding more water to the sediment to further clean the sample.
10. Differentiation of the eggs can be enhanced by adding a couple of drops of methylene blue to the final sediment.
11. The sediment can be examined either in a Petri dish using a dissecting microscope or under a compound microscope by pipetting a small volume onto an ordinary microscope slide with a long coverslip (22 × 40 mm) and repeating until all the sediment has been examined.
12. Scan the Petri dish, or slides, systematically for the presence of fluke eggs.

LARVAL RECOVERY

Lungworm larvae can be recovered from fresh faeces with the Baermann apparatus. This consists of a glass funnel held in a retort stand (Fig. 4.12). A rubber tube, attached to the bottom of the funnel, is constricted by a clip. A sieve (aperture 250 μm) or a double layer of cheesecloth is placed in the wide neck of the funnel, which has been partially filled with water, and a double layer of gauze is placed on top of the sieve. Faeces are placed on the gauze and the funnel is slowly filled with water until the faeces are immersed. Alternatively, faeces are spread on a filter paper, which is then inverted and placed on the sieve. The apparatus is left overnight at room temperature during which the larvae migrate out of the faeces and through the sieve to sediment in the neck of the funnel. The clip on the rubber is then removed and the water in the neck of the funnel collected in a small beaker for microscopic examination in a Petri dish.

Baermann method

1 Weigh 10 g of faeces.
2 The faeces are placed in the centre of a sieve (250 μm). Alternatively, place the faeces in a double layer of cheesecloth that is folded to form a pouch and is closed with either an elastic band or a string. A cocktail stick or rod is then placed under the rubber band or string and the pouch suspended in the funnel.
3 Slowly fill the funnel with lukewarm water until the faeces are immersed.
4 The apparatus is left overnight at room temperature during which the larvae migrate out of the faeces and through the sieve to sediment in the neck of the funnel.
5 The clip on the rubber tubing is then released and the water in the neck of the funnel collected for microscopic examination.
6 The sediment can be examined by drawing off a few millilitres and leaving to sediment for 30 minutes.
7 Alternatively, 5–10 ml can be drawn off into a centrifuge tube and spun at 1500 rpm (170 *g*) for two minutes.
8 The supernatant is then siphoned off and the sediment transferred to a microscope slide.

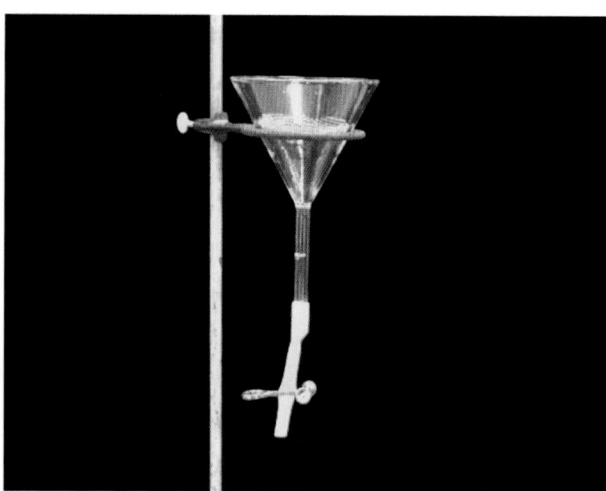

Fig. 4.12 Baermann apparatus. (Taylor et al., 2015/With permission from John Wiley & Sons.)

9 The drops on the slide can be examined without a coverslip for the presence of motile larvae.
A simple adaptation of the above method is to suspend the faeces enclosed in gauze in a wine glass filled with water and leave overnight. The larvae will leave the faeces, migrate through the gauze and settle at the bottom of the glass. After siphoning off the supernatant, the sediment is examined under the low power of the microscope.

Technique for estimating lungworm larvae in faeces (Fig. 4.13)

1 Homogenise 10 g of faeces in approximately 70 ml of water.
2 Pour through a fine mesh sieve (aperture 250 μm) and wash into a collecting bowl until it contains 500–600 ml of filtrate.
3 Transfer the filtrate to a conical beaker and allow to sediment for at least three hours (preferably at 4 °C).
4 Siphon off the supernatant to leave the sediment in a total volume of approximately 60 ml.
5 Divide the sediment evenly between four centrifuge tubes and centrifuge at 1500 rpm (170 *g*) for two minutes.
6 Pour off and discard the supernatant to leave the sediment, which is then thoroughly loosened by gentle agitation.
7 Fill the tubes to within 10 mm of the top with saturated NaCl and invert each tube several times with the thumb over the open end, until the sediment is evenly suspended. Avoid shaking, which leads to the formation of bubbles.
8 Place the tubes in the centrifuge and add saturated NaCl to each tube until a positive meniscus stands above the edge. Place a thick 18 × 18 mm square coverslip on each tube, ensuring that no bubbles are trapped underneath.
9 Centrifuge for two minutes at 1000 rpm (120 *g*).
10 Remove each of the coverslips in turn by lifting vertically with a deliberate movement and wash off any adhering larvae with 2–3 ml of water into a conical centrifuge tube by means of a pipette or plastic wash bottle. This procedure is repeated with the other three coverslips, washing off the larvae into the same conical tube.
11 Centrifuge the conical tube for two minutes at 1500 rpm (170 *g*) and then carefully siphon off the supernatant and discard.
12 Transfer the sediment, which should be in a total volume of approximately 0.1 ml, by pipette to a microscope slide. Rinse the tube with a further 0.1 ml of water and transfer this to the slide.
13 Cover with a 22 × 40 mm coverslip and systematically examine the slide. Because losses amounting to 40% occur during the technique, each larva counted is regarded as representing 0.17 larvae per gram of faeces.

Culture and identification of infective third-stage larvae

The standard method for identifying eggs of trichostrongyle nematodes in faeces is to culture the faeces for 7–10 days and then isolate the third stage (L$_3$) larvae from the faeces. The L$_3$ can then be identified to genus or in some cases species level. Two techniques are widely used for the culture of infective larvae from nematode eggs.

In the first technique, faeces are placed in a jar with a lid and stored in the dark at a temperature of 21–24 °C. The lid should be

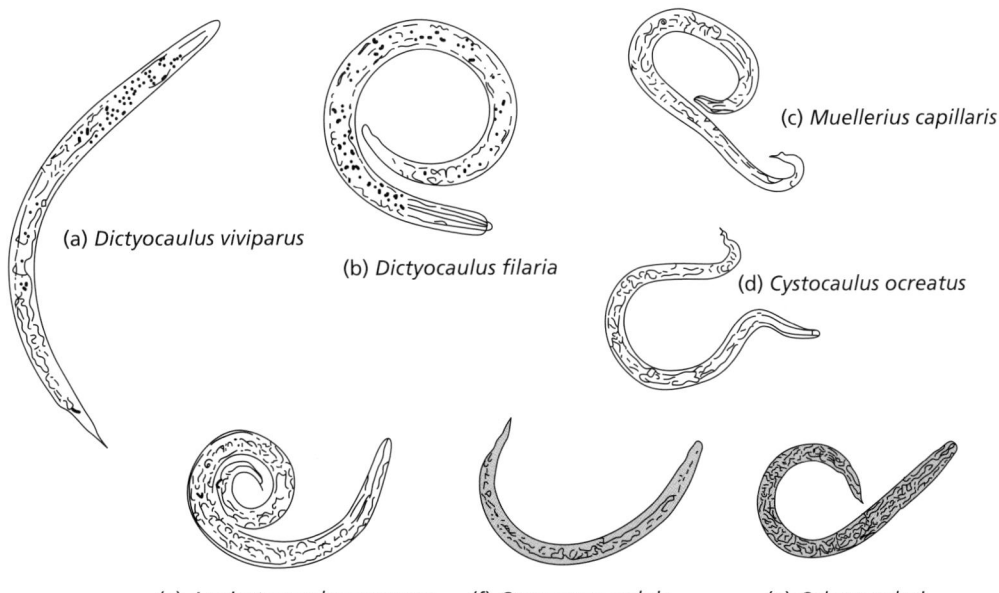

(a) *Dictyocaulus viviparus*

(b) *Dictyocaulus filaria*

(c) *Muellerius capillaris*

(d) *Cystocaulus ocreatus*

(e) *Angiostrongylus vasorum*

(f) *Crenosoma vulpis*

(g) *Oslerus osleri*

Fig. 4.13 First-stage lungworm larvae.

lined with moist filter paper and should not be tightly attached. After 7–10 days of incubation, the jar is filled with water and allowed to stand for 2–3 hours. The larvae will migrate into the water and the latter is poured into a cylinder for sedimentation. The larval suspension can be cleaned and concentrated by using the Baermann apparatus as described and then killed by adding a few drops of Lugol's iodine and examined microscopically.

An alternative method is to spread faeces on the middle third of filter paper placed in a moistened Petri dish. After storage at 21–24 °C for 7–10 days, the dish is flooded with water and the larvae harvested as before.

Ruminant third-stage larval identification

It is often useful to know whether FECs are dominated by worms of one particular genus, particularly on farms where there are worms with high biotic potential, such as *Haemonchus* infections in sheep. If so, larval culture and differentiation can be performed, usually using the faeces from the FEC. This technique takes a further 7–10 days, so results are not available for some time after the FEC is known.

Larval differentiation (Table 4.3; Figs 4.14 and 4.15) requires the hatching of the eggs in the sample, culture (as described above) and subsequent identification of the developed third-stage larvae. Usually, 50 or 100 larvae are counted and the percentage of each genus reported. It should be noted that eggs of each genus do not always hatch at the same rate because of differences in temperature requirements for the different genera. Larval culture results should therefore be used as a general indication of the worm genera present, rather than a precise determination of the proportion of the FEC contributed by each genus. Larvae can be identified in a similar manner for pasture samples (see later).

The technique used is as follows: a small drop of suspension of larvae is placed on a microscope slide and a drop of Gram's iodine added and a coverslip placed over the drops. The iodine kills the larvae and allows for easier identification of the salient features (Fig. 4.15).

RECOVERY OF ADULT NEMATODES

A technique for the collection, counting and identification of adult nematodes from the gastrointestinal tract of ruminants is given in the following list. The procedure is similar for other host species, information on identification being available in the text.

1 As soon as possible after removing the alimentary tract from the body cavity, the abomasal/duodenal junction should be ligatured to prevent transfer of parasites from one site to another.
2 Separate the abomasum, small intestine and large intestine.
3 Open the abomasum along the side of the greater curvature, wash contents into a bucket under running water and make the total volume up to 2–4 l.
4 After thorough mixing, transfer duplicate 200 ml samples to suitably labelled containers and preserve in 10% formalin.
5 Scrape off the abomasal mucosa and digest in a pepsin/HCl mixture at 42 °C for six hours; 200 g of mucosa will require 1 l of mixture. Make the digest up to a volume of 2 or 4 l with cold water and again take duplicate 200 ml samples. Alternatively,

Table 4.3 Key characteristics used in the identification of ruminant nematode third-stage larvae (see Figs 4.14 and 4.15).

Genus	Intestinal cell number	Head characteristics	Sheath tail characteristics
Nematodirus	8	Broad, rounded	Filamentous sheath. Species differentiated by shape of larval tail
Ostertagia/Teladorsagia	16	Squared	Short sheath
Trichostrongylus	16	Tapered	Short sheath
Haemonchus	16	Narrow rounded	Medium offset sheath
Cooperia	16	Squared with refractile bodies	Medium tapering or finely pointed sheath
Bunostomum	16		Short filamentous
Oesophagostomum	32	Broad, rounded	Filamentous sheath
Chabertia	32	Broad, rounded	Filamentous sheath

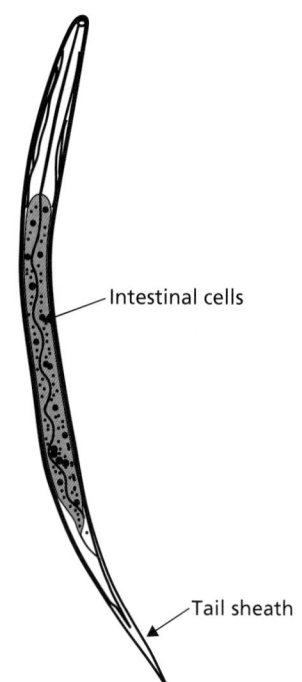

—Intestinal cells

—Tail sheath

Fig. 4.14 Nematode third-stage larva.

the Williams technique may be used. In this, the washed abomasum is placed, mucosal surface down, in a bucket containing several litres of normal saline and maintained at 40 °C for four hours. Subsequently, the abomasum is gently rubbed in a second bucket of warm saline. The saline from both buckets is poured through a sieve (aperture 38 μm, about 600 to 1 inch) and the residue examined.

6 Open the small intestine along its entire length and wash contents into a bucket. Treat as for the abomasal contents, but digestion of mucosal scrapings is usually unnecessary.

7 The contents of the large intestine are washed into a bucket, passed through a coarse mesh sieve (aperture 2–3 mm) and any parasites present collected and formalised.

In this case, visible nematodes, such as *Trichuris*, *Oesophagostomum* and *Chabertia*, may be detected macroscopically. Regarding nematodes of the genus *Skrjabinema*, the material deposited on the filter must be examined at the stereomicroscope.

Worm counting procedure

1 Add 2–3 ml of iodine solution to one of the 200 ml samples.
2 After thorough mixing, transfer 4 ml of suspension to a Petri dish, scored with lines to facilitate counting; add 2–3 ml sodium thiosulfate solution to decolorise the debris. If necessary, worms

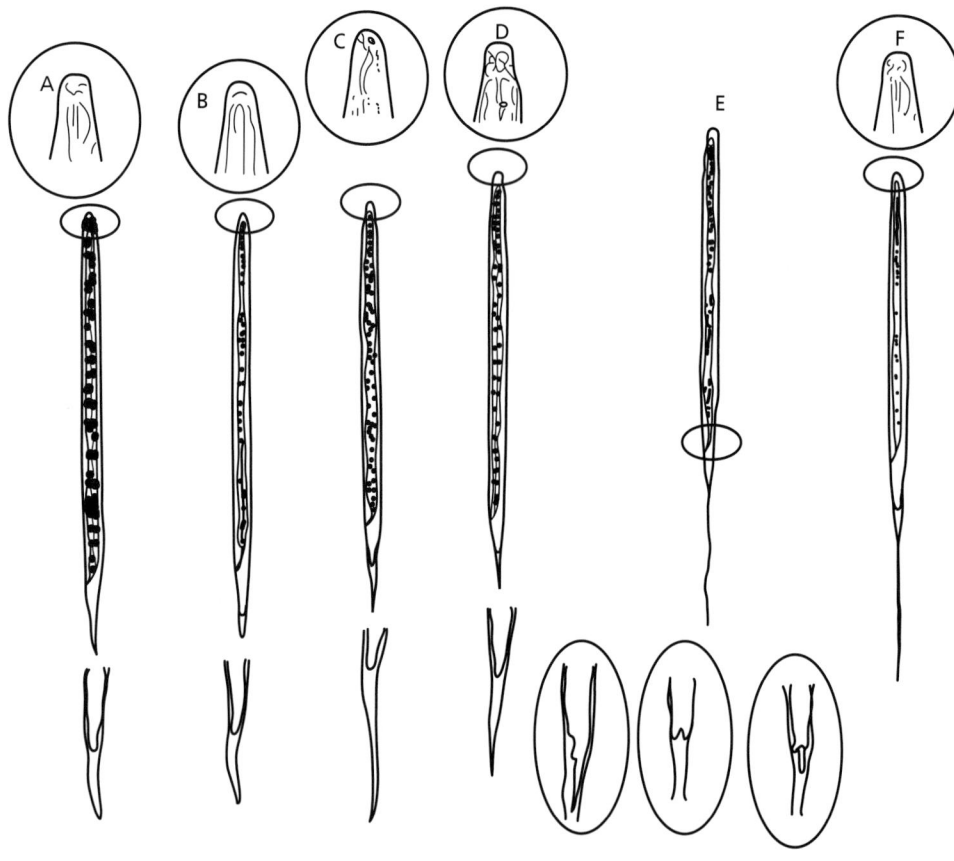

Fig. 4.15 Key to the identification of third-stage larvae of sheep gastrointestinal nematodes:
(A) *Teladorsagia circumcincta*
(B) *Trichostrongylus* spp.
(C) *Haemonchus contortus*
(D) *Cooperia* spp.
(E) *Nematodirus*: (a) *battus*,
(b) *filicollis*, (c) *spathiger*
(F) *Oesophagostomum* spp.

(a) (b) (c)

may be preserved in an aqueous solution of 10% formalin or 70% alcohol. To clear large worms for microscopic examination, immerse in lactophenol for a suitable period prior to examination.

3 Examine for the presence of parasites using a stereoscopic microscope (×12 objective) and identify and count parasites as male, female and larval stages.

KEY TO THE IDENTIFICATION OF GASTROINTESTINAL NEMATODES OF RUMINANTS

Based on the characters described in Table 4.4 (a–c), the following key can be used to differentiate microscopically the genera of some common gastrointestinal nematodes of ruminants.

Body composed of a long filamentous anterior and a short broad posterior region – *Trichuris*

Body not so divided, oesophagus approximately one-third of body length (Fig. 4.16) – *Strongyloides*

Short oesophagus and buccal capsule rudimentary – **Trichostrongyloidea (A)**

Short oesophagus and buccal capsule well developed – **Strongyloidea (B)**

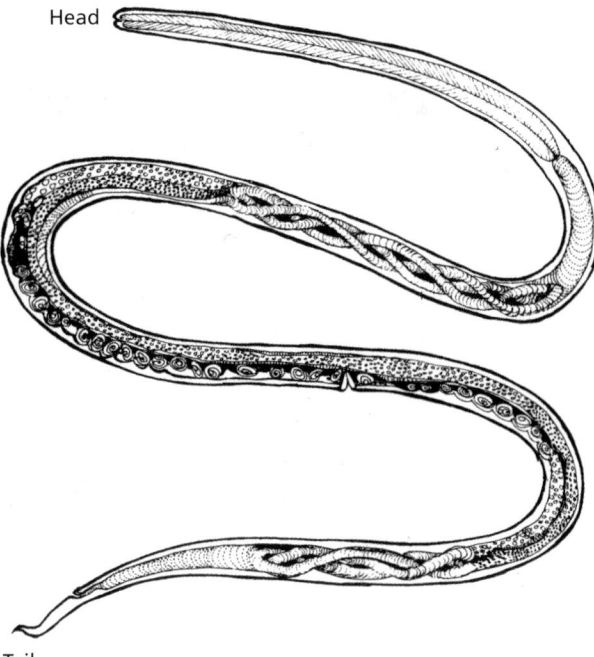

Head

Tail

Fig. 4.16 *Strongyloides* female showing oesophagus approximately one-third length of body.

(A) Trichostrongyloidea

1 Distinct cephalic vesicle (Fig. 4.17). Spicules very long, uniting in a membrane at the tip (Fig. 4.18) – *Nematodirus*

 Cephalic vesicle small (Fig. 4.19). Spicules relatively short and unjoined posteriorly – *Cooperia*

2 No cephalic vesicle. Excretory notch present in both sexes (Fig. 4.20) – *Trichostrongylus*

 Absence of excretory notch – **3**

3 Dorsal lobe of bursa asymmetrical, barbed spicules (Fig. 4.21). Large prominent vulval flap in female (Fig. 4.22) – *Haemonchus*

 Dorsal lobe of bursa is symmetrical (Fig. 4.23). Vulval flap small or absent – *Ostertagia, Teladorsagia*

(B) Strongyloidea

4 Buccal capsule cylindrical (Fig. 4.24) – *Oesophagostomum*

 Buccal capsule well developed – **5**

5 Slight dorsal curvature of head and presence of cutting plates (Fig. 4.25) – *Bunostomum*

 Absence of teeth, rudimentary leaf crowns present (Fig. 4.26) – *Chabertia*

Table 4.4 Guide to adult gastrointestinal nematodes of ruminants.

Table 4.4(a) Abomasal worms.

	Ostertagia spp./*Teladorsagia* spp.	*Trichostrongylus axei*	*Haemonchus contortus*
Mature size	Slender; reddish-brown when fresh	Very small worms, <0.5 cm long, greyish when fresh, tapering to a very fine anterior end	Large worms, reddish when fresh; easily seen, bursa visible with the naked eye
	Male 7–8 mm	Male 3–6 mm	Male 10–20 mm
	Female 9–12 mm	Female 4–8 mm	Female 18–30 mm
Head	Small cervical papillae set more posteriorly; distance from anterior end about five times diameter between papillae Cuticle striations are longitudinal	No cervical papillae Excretory notch visible in oesophageal region Cuticle striations are annular	Prominent large cervical papillae; distance from anterior end about three times the diameter between papillae
Female	Small or no vulval flap. Under high magnification tip of tail shows annular rings. In cattle, female has vulval flap of variable size, but usually skirt-like	Simple genital opening with vulval flap absent; gravid worm contains four or five eggs, pole to pole	In sheep, vulval flap, usually linguiform; gravid worm contains several hundred eggs; ovary coiled around intestine resembling 'barber's pole'. In cattle, vulval flap often bulb-shaped or vestigial
Male tail	Bursal lobes are symmetrical. Spicules vary with species. In sheep species, spicules slender, rod-like (*T. circumcincta*) or stout with branch near middle (*O. trifurcata*). In cattle, male has stout, rod-like spicules with expanded tips (*O. ostertagi*) or very robust spicules, generally rectangular in outline (*O. lyrata*)	Bursal lobes are symmetrical. Spicules unequal in length	Dorsal ray of bursa is asymmetrical. Spicules barbed near tips

Table 4.4(b) Small intestinal worms.

	Trichostrongylus	*Cooperia*	*Nematodirus*	*Strongyloides*	*Bunostomum*
Mature size	Very small worms, ~0.5 cm long, greyish when fresh, tapering to a very fine anterior end	About 0.5 cm long; slender; greyish; comma or watch-spring shape; coiled in one or two tight coils	About 2 cm long; slender; much twisted, often tangled like cottonwool due to twisting of the 'thin neck'	Only females present	About 2 cm long; stout white worms; head bent slightly
	Male 4–5 mm	Male 4–6 mm	Male 10–15 mm		Male 12–17 mm
	Female 5–7 mm	Female 5–7 mm	Female 15–25 mm	Female 3–6 mm	Female 19–26 mm
Other features	Excretory notch present in oesophageal region. Vulval flap absent	Small cephalic vesicle present, giving anterior end a cylindrical appearance; prominent cuticular striations in the oesophageal region	Cephalic vesicle present	Very long oesophagus, one-third to half of total length of the worm	Large buccal cavity has prominent teeth; *B. trigonocephalum* of sheep and goats has one large and two small teeth; *B. phlebotomum* of cattle has two pairs of subventral teeth
Female	Ovejectors present	Body of female swollen at region of vulva	Female tail has prominent spine protruding from a blunt end. Tip of tail is pointed (*N. battus*) or truncate with a small spine (other species). Large eggs present	Ovary and uterus show twisted thread appearance behind oesophagus; ovejectors absent. Eggs expressed from females contain a fully developed larva	
Mail tail	Spicules leaf-shaped (*T. vitrinus*) or with 'step' near tip (*T. colubriformis*)	Male tail has short stout spicules; 'wing' at middle region, bearing striations (*C. curticei*). Spicules of *C. oncophora* have a stout bow-like appearance, with small terminal 'feet'	Male tail has very long slender spicules usually extended beyond the bursa. Bursa shows two sets of parallel rays (*N. battus*) or four sets (other species). Spicules long, slender and fused, with expanded tip which is heart-shaped (*N. battus*); lanceloate (*N. filicollis*); bluntly rounded (*N. spathiger*) (sheep). In cattle, spicules of *N. helvetianus* have a spear-shaped expansion at the tips		*B. trigonocephalum* has short twisted spicules; *B. phlebotomum* has long slender spicules

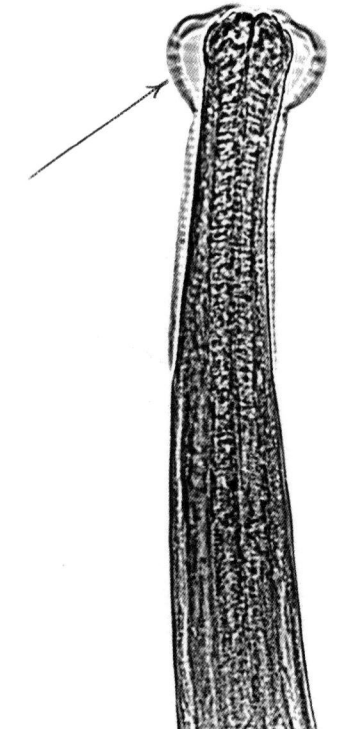

Fig. 4.17 *Nematodirus* cephalic vesicle.

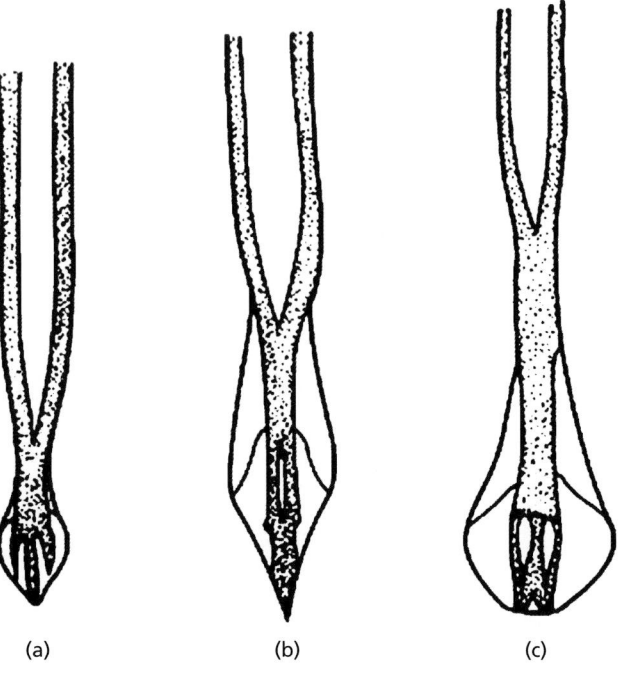

(a)   (b)   (c)

Fig. 4.18 *Nematodirus* fused spicules: (a) *Nematodirus filicollis*, (b) *Nematodirus spathiger* and (c) *Nematodirus battus* from sheep.

Table 4.4(c) Large intestinal worms.

	Trichuris	*Chabertia*	*Oesophagostomum*	*Skrjabinema*
Mature size	Up to 8 cm long; whip-like, with long filamentous anterior part twice as long as posterior part. Called 'whipworm' because of its shape	1.5–2 cm long; large buccal capsule	Up to 2 cm long	Small spindle-shaped worm that is easily overlooked in contents
	Male 50–80 mm	Male 13–14 mm	Male 11–16 mm	Male 3 mm
	Female 35–70 mm	Female 17–20 mm	Female 13–24 mm	Female 6–7 mm
Other features		*Chabertia* has a large bell-shaped buccal cavity that is visible to the naked eye in fresh specimens. There are no teeth in the buccal cavity and rudimentary leaf crowns	Small buccal cavity surrounded by leaf crown. Cephalic vesicle with cervical groove behind it. Leaf crowns and cervical alae often present. Cervical papillae are situated posterior to the oesophagus	Prominent spherical bulb at the posterior of the oesophagus
Female	Female produces barrel-shaped eggs with a transparent plug at each end	Tail of female is bow-shaped		
Male tail	Male has a single spicule in a spinecovered protrusible sheath	Tail of male spirally coiled with one spicule		

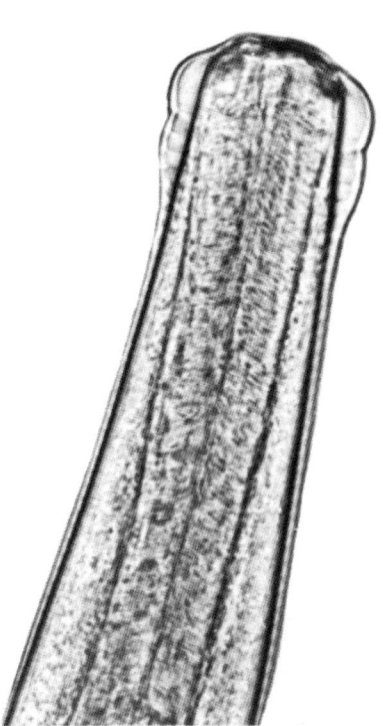

Fig. 4.19 *Cooperia*: head with small cephalic vesicle.

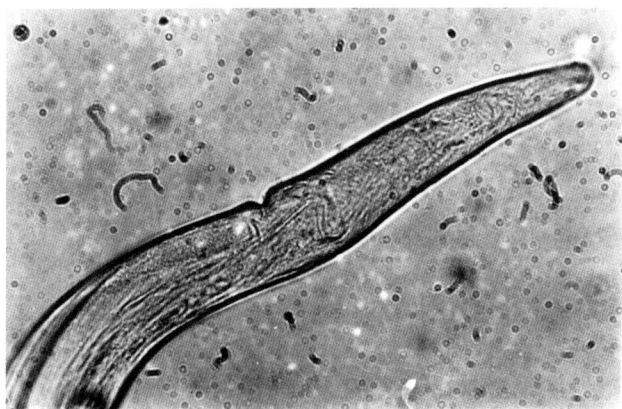

Fig. 4.20 *Trichostrongylus*: head with excretory notch.

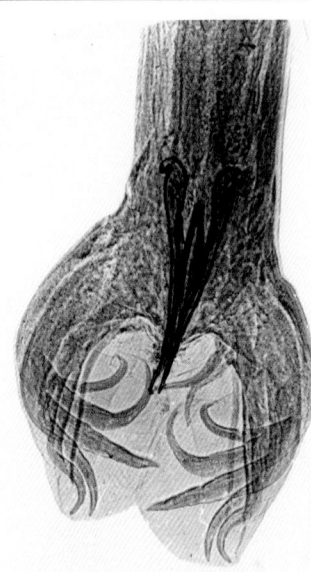

Fig. 4.21 *Haemonchus contortus*: male bursa showing asymmetrical dorsal lobe and barbed spicules.

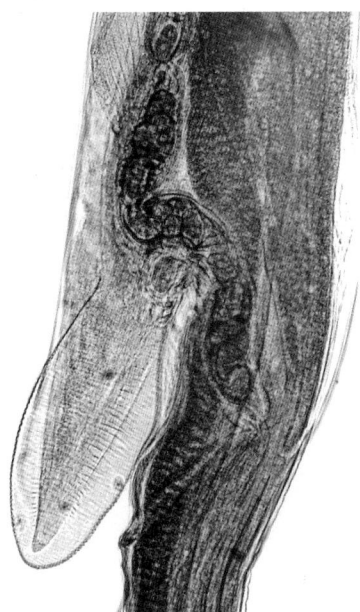

Fig. 4.22 *Haemonchus contortus*: female vulval flap.

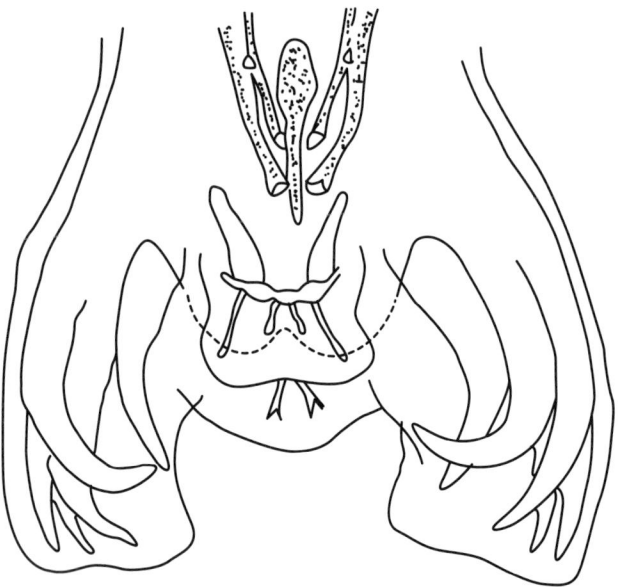

Fig. 4.23 *Ostertagia ostertagi*: male bursa showing symmetrical dorsal lobe.

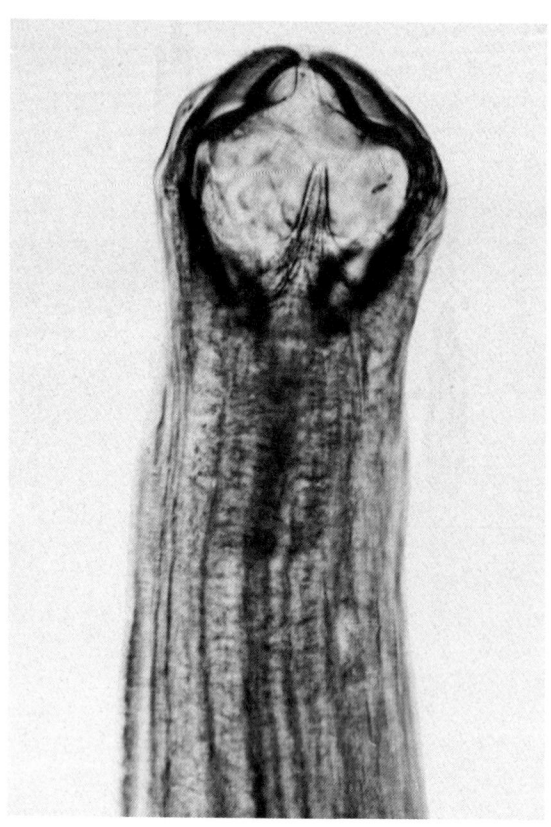

Fig. 4.25 Head of *Bunostomum*.

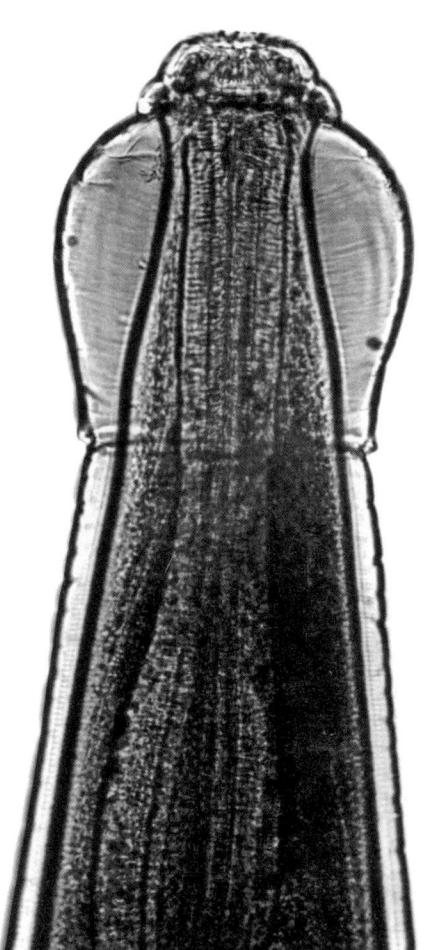

Fig. 4.24 Buccal capsule of *Oesophagostomum*.

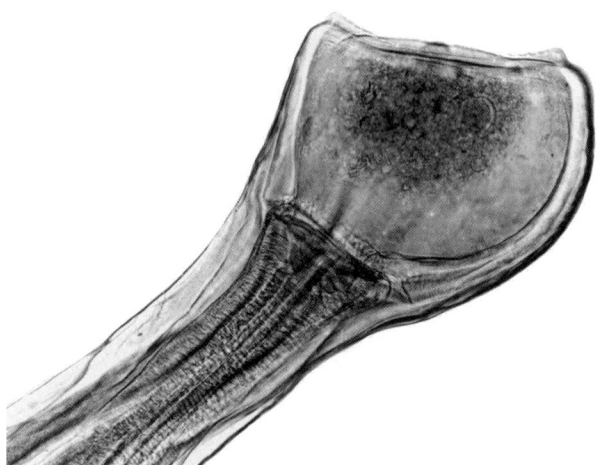

Fig. 4.26 Large buccal capsule of *Chabertia*.

RECOVERY OF ADULT LUNGWORMS

For *Dictyocaulus*, this is best done by opening the air passages starting from the trachea and cutting down to the small bronchi with fine, blunt-pointed scissors. Visible worms are then removed from the opened lungs and transferred to glass beakers containing saline. The worms are best counted immediately, failing which they should be left overnight at 4 °C which will reduce clumping. Additional worms may be recovered if the opened lungs are soaked in warm saline (37 °C) overnight.

Another method is Inderbitzen's modification of the perfusion technique in which the lungs are perfused. The pericardial sac is incised and reflected to expose the pulmonary artery in which a 2 cm incision is made. Rubber tubing is introduced into the artery and fixed *in situ* by double ligatures. The remaining large blood vessels are tied off and water from a mains supply allowed to enter the pulmonary artery. The water ruptures the alveolar and bronchiolar walls, flushes out the bronchial lumina and is expelled from the trachea. The fluid is collected and its contents concentrated by passing through a fine sieve (aperture 38 μm). As before, this is best examined immediately for the presence of adult worms and larvae.

The smaller genera of lungworms of small ruminants are difficult to recover and enumerate, although the Inderbitzen technique may be of value.

RECOVERY OF TREMATODE AND CESTODE PARASITES

For both *Fasciola* and *Dicrocoelium*, the livers are removed and cut into slices approximately 1 cm thick. On squeezing the liver slices, any flukes seen grossly are removed and formalised and the slices immersed in warm water overnight. The gallbladder should also be opened and washed, and any flukes removed.

After soaking, the liver slices are again squeezed, rinsed in clean water and discarded. Both washings are passed through a fine sieve (aperture 100 μm) and the material retained and formalised. In the case of rumen/intestinal paramphistomes, the rumen and first 4 m of the duodenum should be tied off, opened, washed and examined for adherent trematodes.

If the intestinal mucosa is slightly scraped off, the flukes can be collected in a Petri dish and the parasites can thus be counted by the stereomicroscope.

Counts are carried out microscopically, entire flukes plus the numbers of heads and tails being recorded. The highest number of either of the latter is added to the number of entire flukes to give the total count.

Cestodes are usually readily visible in the intestine or liver, but whenever possible these should be removed intact so that, if necessary, the head and the mature and gravid segments are all available for specialist examination. Smaller species (e.g. cestodes of birds or *Echinococcus*) are detected by observation via the stereomicroscope of the mucosal or sediment scraping of the intestinal contents.

In the case of *Echinococcus* in canids, however, the worms are so small that the more detailed examination described in Chapter 12 should be undertaken.

The larval forms of some cestodes (e.g. *Taenia hydatigena*) are found on the liver surface of the intermediate hosts or on the cutting surface of the musculature (e.g. *Taenia saginata* or *Taenia solium*). As for the adult forms, it is necessary, if possible, to remove the intact larva in order to carry out a correct identification.

OTHER AIDS TO DIAGNOSIS OF RUMINANT NEMATODES

Several other techniques are useful aids in the diagnosis of trichostrongyle infections in ruminants. All these techniques should be undertaken in a specialist parasitology laboratory, but a short account is given here of the material required for these tests, the basis of the techniques and how the results may be interpreted.

Lectin-binding assay

The standard method for identifying eggs of trichostrongyle nematodes has been described in the section on culture and identification of infective third-stage larvae, whereby eggs are cultured to third-stage larvae (L_3) and identified to genus after 7–10 days of culture. Although this is the most widely used and best method currently available, it has several shortcomings: it is labour-intensive, time-consuming and requires special training to correctly identify the morphological differences between genera.

A lectin-binding assay has been developed specifically to distinguish *Haemonchus* eggs from other roundworm genera. In this assay, peanut agglutinin (PNA) specifically binds to *Haemonchus* eggs and not those of other trichostrongyle species. By using the lectin conjugated to fluorescein isothiocyanate (FITC), binding to *Haemonchus* eggs can be visualised under ultraviolet (UV) illumination, without having to resort to larval culture and differentiation.

1 Nematode eggs can be extracted from faeces using the sensitive centrifugal flotation technique described in the section above on improved sensitivity methods.
2 Eggs are then cleaned by removing the coverslip and washing the adhering droplet, containing the eggs, into a conical centrifuge tube with phosphate buffered saline (PBS) solution.
3 The volume is made up to 10 ml with PBS and the solution re-centrifuged at 1500 rpm (170 *g*) for two minutes.
4 The supernatant is discarded and the pellet resuspended in 1 m of PNA-FITC.
5 Eggs are then incubated for one hour under constant agitation at room temperature.
6 Samples are washed twice in PBS (as above), and 5 μl of the egg sediment transferred onto a glass slide with 3 μl of fluorescent mounting fluid and then overlaid with a coverslip.
7 Specimens are then examined with a fluorescence microscope using FITC filters. *Haemonchus* eggs have a bright fluorescent green outline.

Plasma pepsinogen test

The estimation of circulating pepsinogen is of value in the diagnosis of abomasal damage, and is especially elevated in cases of ostertagiosis. Elevations also occur with other gastric parasites such as *Trichostrongylus axei*, *Haemonchus contortus* and, in the pig, *Hyostrongylus rubidus*.

The principle of the test, which is best carried out by a diagnostic laboratory, is that the sample of serum or plasma is acidified to pH 2.0, thus activating the inactive zymogen, pepsinogen, to the active proteolytic enzyme, pepsin. This activated pepsin is then allowed to react with a protein substrate (usually bovine serum albumin) and the enzyme concentration calculated in international units (IU) (μmol tyrosine released per 100 ml serum per minute). The tyrosine liberated from the protein substrate by the pepsin is estimated by the blue colour, which is formed when phenolic compounds react with Folin–Ciocalteu reagent. The minimum requirement for the test, as carried out in most laboratories, is 1.5 ml serum or plasma. The anticoagulant used for plasma samples is either EDTA or heparin.

In parasitic gastritis of ruminants due to *Ostertagia* spp. and *T. axei*, the levels of plasma pepsinogen become elevated. In parasite-free animals, the level is less than 1.0 IU of tyrosine; in moderately infected animals, it is between 1.0 and 2.0 IU and in heavily infected animals it usually exceeds 3.0 IU, reaching as high as 10.0 IU or more on occasion. Interpretation is simple in animals during their first 18 months, but thereafter becomes difficult as the level may become elevated when older and immune animals are under challenge. In such cases the absence of the classic clinical signs of diarrhoea and weight loss indicates that there are few adult parasites present. Estimation of circulating pepsinogen is a useful technique not only to evaluate the possible presence of adult parasites, but it has a predictive value even if the parasites have not finished the endogenous cycle and are still at the level of the mucosa at the larval stage. At this stage, the copromicroscopic tests would be negative due to the absence of egg production.

Pasture larval counts

The pasture is the main source of gastrointestinal nematode infestation for ruminants and can be monitored by sampling to detect the presence of third-stage infective larvae. The collection of larvae directly from green forage makes it possible to define the genera and sometimes the species of parasites present, to quantify the number of larval forms per unit area and above all to evaluate the real risk of transmission to animals.

For this technique, samples of grass are plucked from the pasture and placed in a polythene bag, which is then sealed and dispatched to a laboratory for processing. It is important to take a reasonable number of random samples, and one method is to traverse the pasture and remove four grass samples at intervals of about four paces, following a path similar to that of butterfly wings, until approximately 400 have been collected (Fig. 4.27). Another method, primarily for lungworm larvae, is to collect a similar number of samples from the close proximity of faecal pats.

At the laboratory, the grass is thoroughly soaked, washed and dried and the washings containing the larvae passed through a sieve (aperture 38 µm; 600 to 1 inch) to remove fine debris. The material retained on the sieve is then processed by the Baermann method and the infective larvae are identified and counted microscopically under the high power of the microscope. The numbers present are expressed as L_3 per kilogram of dried herbage.

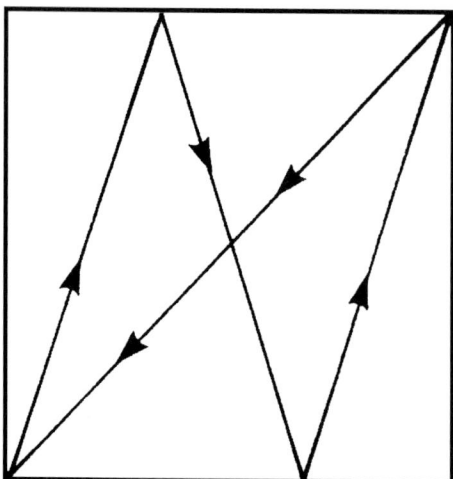

Fig. 4.27 Butterfly route.

Where counts in excess of 1000 L_3/kg of ruminant gastrointestinal trichostrongyles are recorded, the pasture can be regarded as moderately infective, while values of over 5000 L_3/kg can be expected to produce clinical disease in young animals during their first season at grass.

Although this is a useful technique for detecting the level of gastrointestinal nematode L_3 on pastures, it is less valuable for detecting lungworm larvae because of the rapid fluctuations of these larvae on pastures.

A more sophisticated technique, the Jorgensen method, which depends on migration of larvae through an agar medium containing bile, is used in some laboratories for estimating *Dictyocaulus* larval populations on pasture; since most lungworm larvae are concentrated close to faeces, herbage samples should be collected from around faecal deposits. In the present state of knowledge, the detection of any lungworm larvae in herbage samples should be regarded with suspicion and even a negative finding does not necessarily imply that the pasture is free of infection.

Bulk-tank milk tests

Monitoring worm and fluke infections in adult cattle can be used to evaluate the effectiveness of control measures and to target anthelmintic treatments where required. A bulk-tank milk test can be used as a guide to identify those dairy herds with potential to increase milk yield in response to anthelmintic treatment.

Bulk-tank milk test for Ostertagia

This test measures the level of challenge to the herd from stomach worms (*Ostertagia*). Studies have shown the following.
1 Worms reduce milk yield by reducing appetite and the ability of cows to digest forage.
2 The milk yield response following treatment is around 1 kg/cow per day.
3 The financial benefit from worming is maximised when treatment is applied around calving due to:
   a greater daily milk yield response
   b longer duration of milk yield response
   c opportunity to improve reproductive perfomance
   d potential to improve IgG concentrations in colostrum.
Generally, the most appropriate time to collect bulk-tank milk samples for the stomach worm test is in the autumn, prior to housing. A positive treatment response can occur with optical density ratio (ODR) values greater than the cut-off point of 0.5. ODR values >0.8 reflect a high nematode exposure that is likely to be causing significant milk yield losses (Table 4.5).

Bulk-tank milk test for Fasciola

In cattle, fluke infections are generally subclinical, but are considered to produce marked economic effects. Few studies have been conducted to estimate the effect on productivity in adult cattle and control should aim at the reduction of infection to levels that minimise interference on cattle productivity. A positive correlation between *Fasciola*-specific bulk-tank milk antibody levels and herd seroprevalence has been demonstrated and so provides a basis for monitoring herd infection status.

Table 4.5 Guide to the interpretation of *Ostertagia* and fluke bulk-tank milk ELISA.

Ostertagia test result	*Fasciola* test result	Level of infection	What does it mean?	Recommended action
ODR >0.70	ODR >0.70 (3+)	High	Moderate to high exposure of milking cows with probable subclinical effects on health and production	Parasite control in such herds should be reviewed. It is likely that a substantial positive response to anthelmintic treatment of the dairy herd will result
ODR 0.50–0.69	ODR 0.50–0.69 (2+)	Medium	Limited to moderate exposure of milking cows to infection, at levels less likely to have significant impact on the milking herd as a whole	Individual cows may have higher than average levels of infection, with associated effects on health and production, and anthelmintic treatment might be of benefit to them
ODR <0.50	ODR <0.50 (– or +)	Low	Exposure of adult cows to liver fluke or stomach worm is relatively low	No change to parasite control policy indicated. It is unlikely that herd health or production will respond to anthelmintic treatment

Fluke studies have shown that:

1 from a cut-off ODR of 0.5 onwards, there is an average milk yield loss of 0.11 kg/cow per day for each 0.1 unit increase in the bulk-tank milk ELISA result
2 when the bulk-tank milk ODR result exceeds 0.8:
   a it is estimated that for 50% of the cows, the number of inseminations is increased by 75%
   b the average intercalving interval of the herd is prolonged by 4–5 days.

Results should be interpreted in the context of management factors specific to the farm concerned, such as the length of the grazing season, previous anthelmintic treatments and risks from other parasites. Note also that results vary between different laboratories so they should be interpreted in accordance with guidelines provided by the laboratory concerned. Table 4.5 provides some general guidance only.

DNA-BASED METHODS

The main goals of diagnosis in veterinary parasitology are to determine the presence or absence of key pathogenic species and to determine the species composition and resistance status of a given parasite population to antiparasitic drugs. Diagnostic tests to achieve these goals need to be simple, cheap, high-throughput and rapid, in order to encourage uptake in the field.

With veterinary helminths, routine diagnosis still relies heavily on the FEC and microscopic examination of eggs and/or larvae extracted from faecal samples. The morphological identification of nematode eggs and larvae, even to genus level, is a significant diagnostic challenge. In ruminants, for example, with the possible exception of *Nematodirus* whose eggs are morphologically distinct (see Figs 4.3 and 4.4) and *Haemonchus* eggs specifically stained with fluorescent PNA lectin, most trichostrongylid eggs are indistinguishable from one another and require lengthy (7–10 days) coproculture to third-stage larvae to facilitate their identification. Such methods are often labour-intensive and time-consuming and require experienced personnel, making them prohibitively expensive for routine application, whether for use on livestock farms or for large-scale veterinary epidemiological/surveillance purposes.

More recently, a number of immunologically based tests have been developed, such as enzyme-linked immunosorbent assay (ELISA), but many of these are only capable of detecting or measuring a single parasite species per test. Parasitic infections often involve multiple species, genera and even taxa, either simultaneously or as overlapping infections throughout the course of the

parasite season. Species specificity is not usually an issue for immunologically based diagnostic tests; their major limitation is in their ability to detect current infection, because antibody titres can persist long after infection, even after parasites are removed following successful anthelmintic treatment. A further drawback with immunologically based tests is that, with the exception of bulk-tank milk ELISAs, they involve invasive procedures such as blood sampling, which often requires veterinary supervision, to provide the necessary diagnostic sample. As a result, blood sampling for parasite diagnosis is not routine practice in livestock farming and is certainly not economically viable for many farmers.

Any improvement over currently available tests must use the simplest, most convenient source of sample material, be able to cope with multispecies infections, be much more rapid in turn-round time, be sufficiently inexpensive to encourage uptake and, ideally, have potential for pen-side or point-of-care applications.

Potential of DNA-based testing

DNA-based testing has considerable potential for a number of parasite diagnoses, most notably parasite detection and quantification, species identification and resistance detection, which would represent a considerable advancement over existing methodologies. Optimally designed DNA-based methods can be extremely sensitive and specific and can be applied to any parasite life-cycle stage from which DNA can be extracted (eggs, larvae or adults). Moreover, such methods can be readily applied to tiny amounts of starting material, as well as to pooled samples from relatively crude sources (e.g. animal faeces), and they can also operate in a genuine multispecies/multiplex format.

Polymerase chain reaction

Until the advent of polymerase chain reaction (PCR) in the 1980s, most DNA-based diagnostic work was based on radioactive primer/probe hybridisation to DNA targets immobilised on solid supports (e.g. charged nylon membranes) and involved an inherent reliance on gel electrophoresis, radioactive probes and/or X-ray film for detection and quantification. Since then, PCR and PCR-based methods have effectively revolutionised our diagnostic capabilities, especially in the fields of medical virology and bacteriology. Routine application of PCR to medical parasitology has lagged somewhat behind these two disciplines, and its application to veterinary parasitology even more so.

The basic PCR method utilises a thermostable DNA polymerase, usually *Taq* polymerase, to specifically amplify a region of the target DNA, as defined by two opposing nucleotide primers. Under optimal conditions, sequential cycles of DNA template denaturation, primer annealing and extension, achieved through the use of a computer-controlled heating device or 'PCR machine', result in the exponential amplification of the target sequence (Fig. 4.28), such that the PCR product(s) can be visualised through gel electrophoresis or similar methodologies.

A typical PCR reaction comprises a proprietary *Taq* polymerase buffer containing Mg^{2+} ions at the appropriate concentration (this is important for efficient primer/target annealing and can be titrated in the initial optimisation of the PCR assay). The reaction also contains the respective forward and reverse primers, the required nucleotides (A, C, G and T) and the *Taq* polymerase itself. PCR reactions are usually set up as 'mastermixes' and dispensed into the required number of PCR tubes to ensure adequate mixing of reagents and to circumvent problems with pipetting small volumes. Most researchers now utilise commercially available PCR kits to reduce assay-to-assay variability and enhance quality control. The basic PCR method can be made less labour-intensive and achieve higher throughput by the use of multichannel pipettes and microtitre plates, for example.

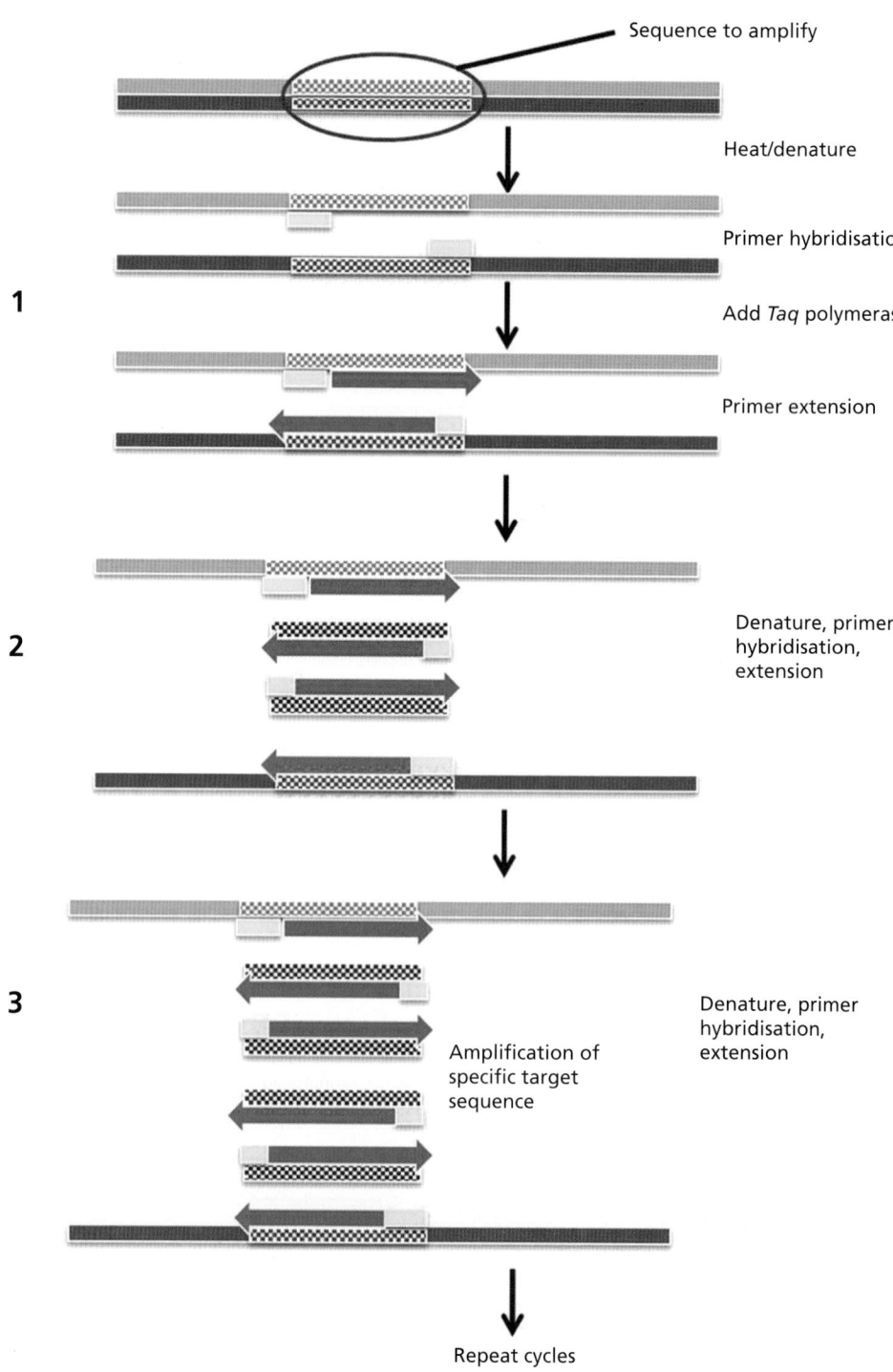

Fig. 4.28 Schematic diagram of PCR. Each cycle of PCR (heating– denaturing, cooling– annealing and extending) doubles the amount of target DNA, increasing the concentration of target DNA exponentially. (Courtesy of Dr P. Skuce, Moredun Research Institute, UK).

PCR reaction mixtures and assays are set up and customised for specific purposes, but a typical conventional PCR reaction protocol is outlined here.

Materials/equipment required

1 PCR machine (thermal cycler).
2 Pipettes and pipette tips (capable of dispensing various volumes, e.g. up to 20 μl, 200 μl, 1 ml, ideally with barrier filters to prevent contamination from aerosol DNA).
3 PCR tubes: thin-walled Eppendorf type.
4 *Taq* polymerase enzyme and proprietary buffer (10×).
5 50 mmol/l stock MgCl₂.
6 10 μmol/l forward and reverse primers.
7 25 μmol/l dNTPs (A, C, G, T).
8 Template DNA.
9 Sterile, nuclease-free H₂O.

PCR primers are typically designed using proprietary primer design software programs or similar algorithms available freely online. Depending on the application, these programs search for unique stretches of DNA sequence on the opposing DNA strands and select forward and reverse primer pairs that are calculated to function optimally under the same PCR conditions. Factors which affect primer, and hence PCR sensitivity and specificity, include the melting temperature (or T_m, the temperature at which double-stranded DNA 'melts' into single strands), primer length (typically 18–22 nucleotides), GC content (ideally ~50%), secondary structure (i.e. predicted loops and/or hairpins that could interfere with primer/target binding), primer dimers (where the primer can bind to itself or its primer partner) and the presence of repetitive sequences (which should be avoided if possible).

Once primers have been designed, the basic PCR must be optimised with respect to the concentration of reagents and the PCR conditions, especially the primer annealing temperature and MgCl₂ concentration, which must be empirically tested. PCR reactions should be set up in separate workstations devoted to DNA template extraction, PCR reaction mastermix, addition of template DNA, thermal cycling and postamplification analysis, respectively. This is to avoid contamination of PCR reagents and mastermixes with previously amplified DNA, which can require lengthy and expensive troubleshooting to resolve. A typical PCR 25 μl reaction mixture is shown in Table 4.6, along with a mastermix to cover 10 × 25 μl reactions.

Table 4.6 A typical PCR 25 μl reaction mixture.

Reagent	Test PCR (μl)	10 × 25 μl mastermix	Final concentrations
10 × buffer (MgCl₂)	2.5	25	1×
50 mmol/l MgCl₂	1	10	2 mmol/l
Forward primer (10 μmol/l)	1	10	0.4 μmol/l
Reverse primer (10 μmol/l)	1	10	0.4 μmol/l
dNTPs (A, C, G, T) @ 2.5 mmol/l	2	20	0.2 mmol/l each
Taq polymerase	0.2	2.0	1.0 unit
Template DNA	1	10 (i.e. 10 × 1 μl)	N/A
ddH₂O	16.3 (i.e. to 25 μl)	163.0	N/A
Total	25	250	N/A

PCR set-up

1 Reagents are assembled in thin-walled PCR tubes, as required. Tubes are capped and contents centrifuged briefly. This is best carried out on ice to prevent primers annealing to template at suboptimal temperatures. This problem has been largely circumvented by the development of 'hot-start' polymerases, which are protected by an antibody until activated at high temperature, typically ~94 °C. This normally results in increased sensitivity, specificity and yield.
2 Tubes are then incubated in a PCR machine programmed with the appropriate thermal cycling conditions. A typical reaction would require 94 °C for two minutes for initial template denaturation, followed by 25–40 cycles of PCR amplification, for example denature at 94 °C for 30 seconds, anneal at 55 °C for 30 seconds, extend at 72 °C for one minute, followed by a 'soak' at 4 °C after thermal cycling.
3 Following PCR, small aliquots (e.g. 5 μl) of the respective PCR products are typically electrophoresed on an agarose gel against a molecular weight marker and photographed under UV illumination. Typical PCR gels are shown in Figs 4.29 and 4.30.

Real-time PCR

A number of modifications to the basic PCR method and developments in PCR-based technologies have taken place over recent years. Most notable of these is a move towards quantitative PCR

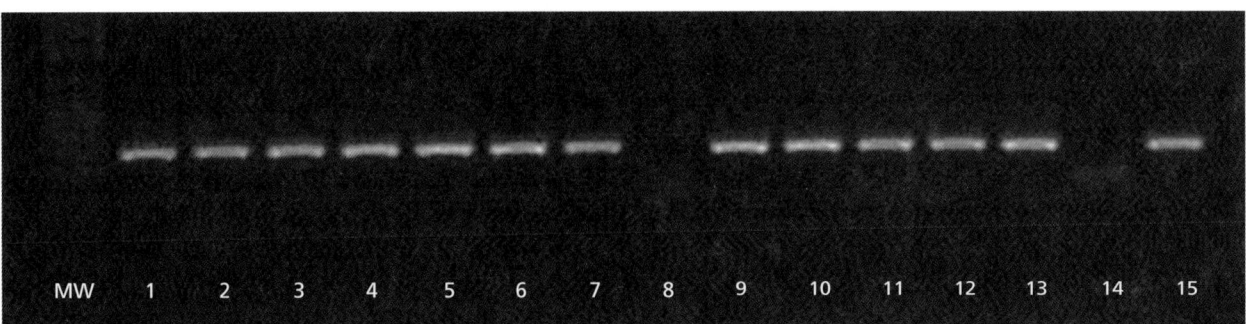

Fig. 4.29 Single-species PCR for sheep gastrointestinal nematodes: screening individual larvae using *Haemonchus contortus*-specific PCR. (Courtesy of Dr L. Melville, Moredun Research Institute, UK).

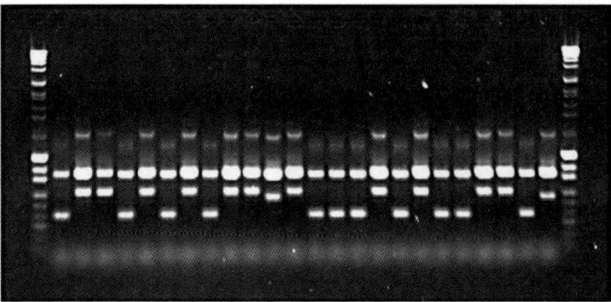

Fig. 4.30 Multiplex PCR for sheep gastrointestinal nematode species identification: the banding patterns indicate species identity of individual larvae. (Courtesy of Dr S.A. Bissett, AgResearch, New Zealand).

applications, where the amplification of PCR product is monitored during the exponential phase in real time (hence the name), rather than the semi-quantitative endpoint of the standard PCR. This has been facilitated by developments in DNA primer and probe chemistry such that the specific PCR product is fluorescently labelled and can be quantified accurately by laser throughout the course of the whole PCR process. Real-time PCR has become the benchmark for accurate and sensitive detection of nucleic acids, and has overcome many of the problems inherent in previous molecular genetic approaches.

Real-time PCR can be achieved through monitoring a build-up of product through intercalation of a fluorochrome dye such as SYBR Green. Alternatively, a primer/probe combination can be used, as in TaqMan™ real-time PCR. Briefly, an oligonucleotide probe, labelled with two fluorescent dyes, is designed to bind within the amplicon specified by the flanking PCR primers. As long as the probe remains intact, the emission of the reporter dye at the 5′ end of the probe is quenched by the fluorescent dye at the 3′ end. However, as the exponential phase of PCR progresses, the polymerase cleaves the probe, resulting in the release of the reporter dye. This is detected within the real-time PCR machine and normalised against a reference standard. The real-time PCR machine then calculates a threshold at which the baseline fluorescence is exceeded. This is defined as the threshold cycle, or C_t, and is directly correlated with the initial quantity of template DNA, i.e. the earlier the fluorescent signal crosses the calculated threshold, the more template DNA was in the sample. The efficiency of primer and probe combinations for real-time PCR must be established and the relative quantification and sensitivity determined through standard curve analysis using serial dilutions of the template DNA (**Fig. 4.31**). The TaqMan and allied real-time PCR method has been extensively used to quantify gene expression and copy number, but also in the detection and quantification of pathogens.

Droplet digital PCR

Droplet digital PCR (ddPCR) combines probe-based PCR (typically TaqMan probes) with a microfluidics analysis platform. In contrast to real-time PCR, ddPCR relies on the analysis of the endpoint of the PCR reaction. Basically, the PCR reaction is subdivided into thousands of small partitions (droplets) by a variety of different available methods. These droplets ideally contain only a single or no template DNA molecule. After PCR, the number of fluorescent droplets is counted using specialised reader instruments. This offers the possibility of determining the number of template molecules by counting the number of droplets with a particular fluorescence and without

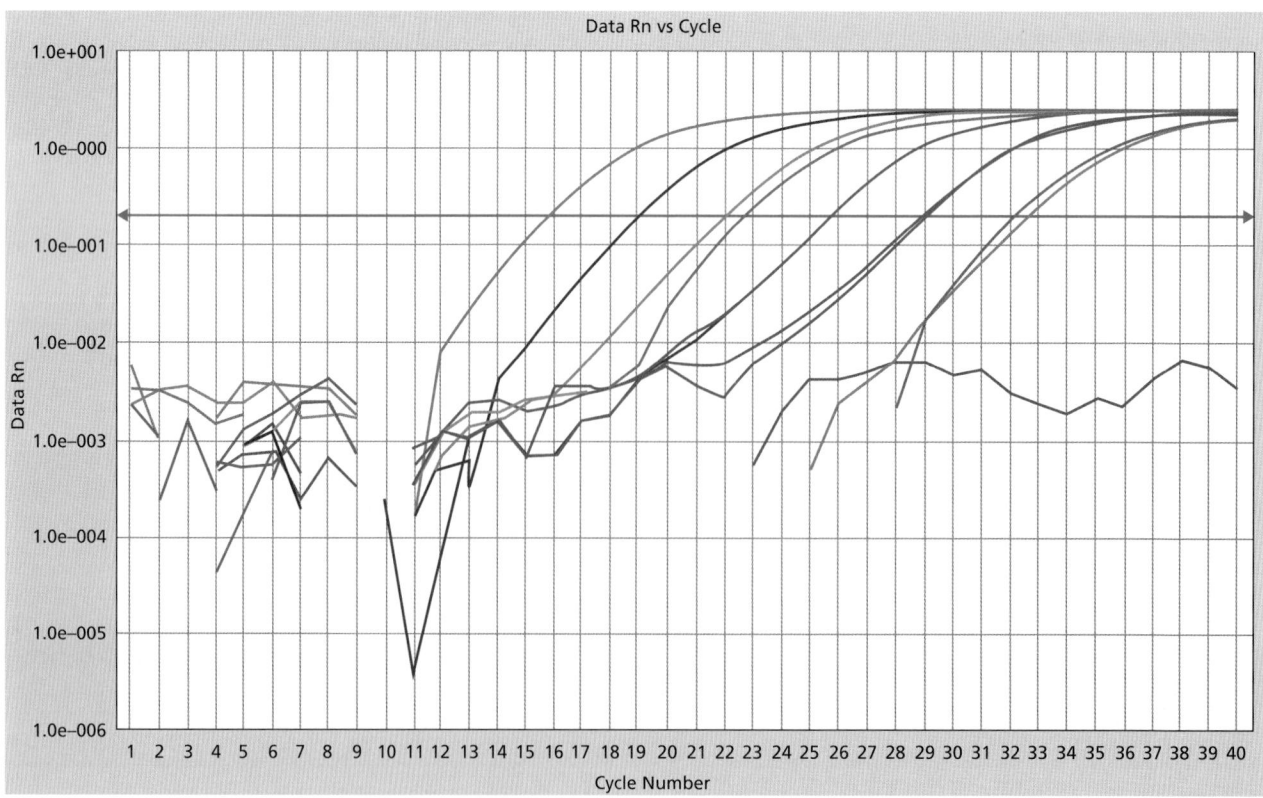

Fig. 4.31 Typical standard curve analysis for real-time PCR. (Courtesy of Dr A. Dicker, Moredun Research Institute, UK).

the need for standard curves. Applying a single primer pair with a single fluorescent probe, ddPCR has been shown to be more sensitive than real-time PCR for the diagnosis of helminth infections. When the template copy number was low, the proportion of positive assays was significantly higher than with qPCR.

The ddPCR approach has advantages when it aims at the simultaneous detection of multiple pathogens. Due to the simple counting method to obtain quantitative data, a direct comparison between multiple species targeted in a single assay is possible and it does not directly rely on factors such as PCR efficacy. Using genus-specific primers and probe sets, it is possible to detect individual and co-infections in faecal samples. Very low copy numbers of one parasite could be reliably detected in the presence of a high abundance of the other.

Challenges for DNA-based diagnosis

PCR-based methods have considerable potential applications within the field of veterinary parasitology but are not without their challenges. One of the main challenges is in DNA template preparation. Tiny amounts of PCR-amplifiable DNA can be extracted from relatively crude samples such as individually lysed parasite eggs or larvae. These can be extracted with relatively simple SDS/NaOH lysis buffers. However, this requires extraction of individual eggs/larvae or cysts/oocysts from faecal samples and/or culturing or excystation, and picking of individual parasites into separate wells/tubes for lysis, which is a time-consuming and labour-intensive process. It would be preferable to extract DNA directly from the faecal sample without any prior extraction of parasite material.

A number of commercial DNA extraction kits have the capability to extract amplifiable DNA from faecal samples but, typically, the amount of DNA in the sample is so small and/or the input of faecal material so large that currently the method is less sensitive than some of the established FEC methods (e.g. McMaster, FLOTAC, Mini-FLOTAC). This is compounded by the fact that *Taq* polymerase is notoriously sensitive to the presence of PCR inhibitors in faecal material.

One possible compromise that has been explored recently is to use PhusionR Hot Start, one of a new generation of polymerase enzymes that are less sensitive to faecal inhibitors, in combination with parasite eggs extracted as a by-product of the routine FEC. These eggs require little or no purification, just a series of freeze–thaw cycles, to release template DNA. This method has been successfully used to detect and quantify gastrointestinal nematode eggs from crude faecal preparations from a number of different host species.

In addition to these technological challenges, the multispecies nature of parasite infections in food-producing and companion animals is a significant challenge to DNA-based diagnosis. This feature, coupled with the extreme genetic variability inherent in parasites, both between and within species, can be both a blessing and a curse in attempting to develop species-specific and/or 'generic' DNA-based tests. This is partly offset by using molecular targets such as subunits within and spacers between the ribosomal RNA (rRNA) genes of key helminth parasites, for example the internal transcribed spacer (ITS)-1 or ITS-2. Such targets comprise a series of highly conserved regions, ideal for placement of universal flanking primer sets, plus regions that are highly variable within and between species for design of species-specific internal primers and/or probes.

Progress to date

PCR-based methods have been shown to provide accurate, sensitive, reproducible and robust diagnostic results from parasitic helminth material and have the potential to support or even replace conventional coprological assays. The early PCR-based assays were designed to provide species-specific detection of individual parasite eggs, larvae and/or adults of gastrointestinal nematode parasites of sheep and were applied to multiple samples in turn. Careful positioning of species-specific primer pairs provided a range of product sizes, which could be pooled and resolved by DNA capillary electrophoresis, thus providing a 'virtual' multiplex readout. However, this was not a genuine multiplex assay in that multiple species could not be detected simultaneously in the same reaction. Genuine multiplex assays have subsequently been developed to identify sheep gastrointestinal nematode stages to species level but these can only realistically be applied to multiple individual parasite samples, which defeats the purpose to some extent. Attempts to analyse pooled samples, either by gel or capillary electrophoresis, invariably result in the loss of certain individual species' PCR products. An equivalent assay designed to discriminate between gastrointestinal nematodes of cattle was much more successful in this regard, possibly due to the lower number of species involved.

Current state of the art

Careful primer and probe design led to the development of a panel of species-specific real-time PCR assays for the key ovine nematodes, including a multiplex real-time PCR assay capable of detecting and quantifying *Haemonchus contortus* and *Teladorsagia circumcincta* in the same reaction. However, attempts to include further key ovine nematode species proved unsuccessful. This obstacle to progress prompted the development of a testing system based on the simultaneous application of multiple species-specific assays in a parallel-plex format. The high speed and throughput of the method are enhanced through the application of robotic systems for the DNA extraction and PCR steps, with the added advantage that the process can be overseen by relatively inexperienced personnel in the testing laboratory. This method offers genuine potential to replace coprological assays for sheep and is now being offered as a commercial service to the livestock sector in Australia.

Available/applicable DNA-based methodologies

Pyrosequencing

Pyrosequencing was developed in the mid-1990s and uses a flexible 'sequencing by synthesis' approach to provide genotyping or short-range DNA sequence data. Pyrosequencing can perform rapid and accurate detection of single-nucleotide polymorphisms (SNPs) from multiple individual samples or determine quantitative allele frequency from pooled material. It can also provide short-range (20–30 bases) *de novo* DNA sequence information.

The method requires initial PCR amplification of the DNA region of interest, using flanking primers, one of which is biotinylated to facilitate subsequent DNA template purification. This is followed by denaturation of purified PCR product into single strands to permit annealing of a specific pyrosequencing primer. This is typically designed to target a particular SNP or polymorphic sequence, which is normally located within about 10 bases of the 3′ end of the pyrosequencing primer. During the pyrosequencing reaction, the respective nucleotides (A, C, G and T) are dispensed in turn (or in order if known). If a nucleotide is successfully incorporated, pyrophosphate is released, which sets off a cascade of enzymatic reactions, leading to the detection of a fluorescent signal by a camera within the pyrosequencer itself. Unincorporated nucleotides are digested by an apyrase enzyme within the pyrosequencing reaction mix. Peak heights on the resultant pyrogram provide a quantitative readout of the nucleotide sequence downstream of the pyrosequencing primer and/or the genotypes of individuals or pools under test (**Fig. 4.32**).

To date, pyrosequencing has been primarily applied to the detection of anthelmintic resistance, specifically benzimidazole resistance in gastrointestinal nematodes of livestock and horses. This is because anthelmintic resistance has a genetic component and the major genetic determinants of benzimidazole resistance are reasonably well understood at the molecular level. With the possible exception of the new amino-acetonitrile derivative monepantel, we do not understand the precise genetic changes associated with resistance to any of the other anthelmintic classes. In most, if not all, nematode parasites, benzimidazole resistance appears to be conferred by the selection of specific mutations (or SNPs) in the coding sequence of the parasite β-tubulin gene. This is most commonly a change at codon 200 from TTC to TAC, which results in a phenylalanine to tyrosine substitution, the so-called F200Y SNP. Other SNPs have been identified at codons 198 (A198E) and 167 (F167Y), but these appear to be less important.

Species-specific benzimidazole resistance pyrosequencing assays have been developed for a number of key sheep nematodes (e.g. *Haemonchus contortus*, *Teladorsagia circumcincta*, *Trichostrongylus* spp., *Nematodirus battus*) and cattle nematodes (e.g. *Ostertagia ostertagi*, *Cooperia oncophora*), as well as a number of equine nematode species. Pyrosequencing assays have been used in the field; for example, an F200Y assay has been used to genotype *Haemonchus contortus* populations in Swedish sheep, and showed good correlation with equivalent FEC reduction test (FECRT) data.

Such assays offer the potential to detect the emergence of anthelmintic resistance, when the frequency of resistance alleles is extremely low, although as yet there are no agreed thresholds to trigger any subsequent management intervention. They also represent excellent research tools to demonstrate the genetic consequences of management strategies (e.g. dose and move, targeted selective treatment) aimed at slowing the spread of anthelmintic resistance. However, if such assays are to find genuine utility in the field, as a proxy or replacement for the FECRT, they must be able to provide allele frequency data from multiple species infections. This remains a significant technological challenge.

This method has its limitations since low amounts of PCR products lead to unreliable signals and thus many of the studies have considered only frequencies of resistant SNPs above 10% as reliable. The ddPCR method has recently been applied for the quantification of SNPs in the isotype 1 β-tubulin gene of a single parasitic nematode, *H. contortus*.

Loop-mediated isothermal amplification

Loop-mediated isothermal amplification (LAMP) is a relatively new DNA-based amplification method that has some potential advantages over PCR-based methods. It relies on the DNA strand displacement activity of *Bst* polymerase and related enzymes, so it does not require thermal cycling, and can be carried out at stable isothermal temperature (Fig. 4.33). This also means fewer requirements for sophisticated equipment, such as gel electrophoresis or thermal cycling machines. These features make LAMP an attractive option for diagnostic/epidemiological studies in the field or for application in less developed countries. The enzyme itself is also significantly less sensitive to faecal inhibitors than *Taq* polymerase and can be several orders of magnitude more sensitive than the equivalent PCR. Furthermore, because a typical LAMP reaction requires a total of six primers, LAMP assays can also be considerably more specific than the equivalent PCR. The exponential build-up of product can be visualised by eye, through turbidity changes in the reaction mixture, or by a colour change following addition of certain dyes or through fluorescence detection under UV light.

Under optimal conditions, LAMP assays can produce visible results within 15–30 minutes, giving the method real potential as a

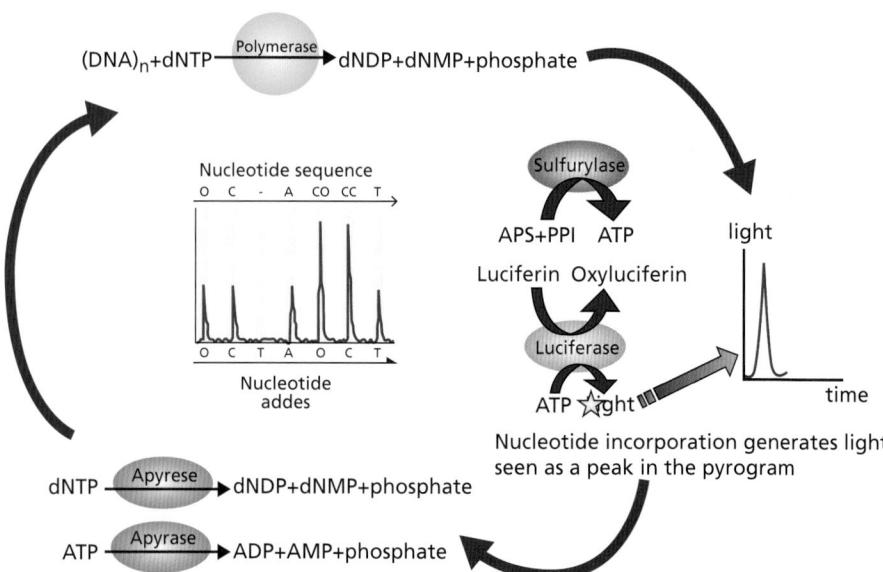

Fig. 4.32 The chemistry behind pyrosequencing and the generation of a pyrogram. (*Source*: www.qiagen.com/resources/technologies/pyrosequencingresource-center/technology-overview. ©QIAGEN, 2014, all rights reserved.)

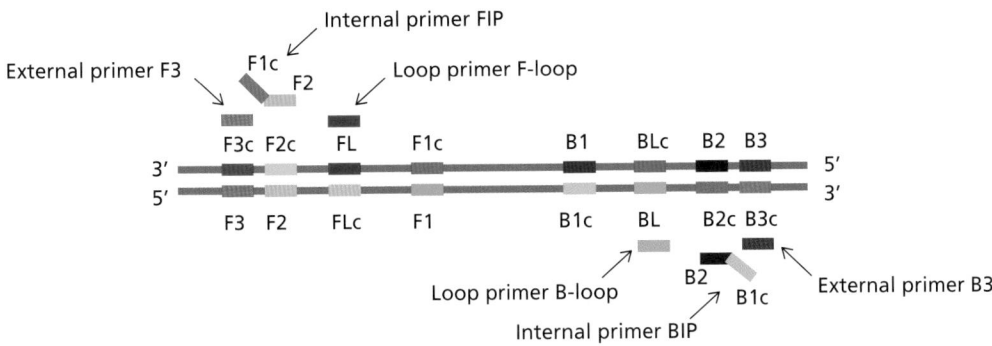

Fig. 4.33 Primer arrangement for loop-mediated isothermal amplification (LAMP). Internal primers (FOP and BIP) each target two primer binding sites (F1 and F2 and B1 and B2, respectively). (Reproduced with permission from Mast Group, Liverpool, UK. Eiken Chemical Co. Ltd.)

pen-side or point-of-care diagnostic test. Moreover, LAMP chemistry can be readily translated onto dipstick or lateral flow-type devices. The product can also be quantified by reading on a turbidity meter, a colorimetric scanner and/or real-time PCR platform. LAMP assays have been reported for the diagnosis of a number of helminth species, for example *Fasciola hepatica*, *Clonorchis sinensis*, *Opisthorchis viverrini* and *Trichinella spiralis*. Careful assay design also allows for presence/absence or quantitative SNP detection for anthelmintic resistance allele frequency studies.

One possible drawback is that the LAMP assay is currently only available in isoplex (i.e. single species format), but research is under way into its multiplexing capability.

Microbead-based detection systems

An example is Luminex®, which is a relatively recent development, combining advances in microfluidics, optics and digital signal processing to provide a flexible multiplex diagnostic platform. The method uses microscopic colour-coded beads (or microspheres), which can be coated with a reagent specific for a given target to allow for capture and laser detection of specific analytes in a sample. Such systems are extremely versatile and can be used to detect and quantify antibody–antigen interactions, enzyme–substrate reactions and nucleic acid primer–probe binding. They can also accommodate multiple analytes (up to 500 at present) in a single sample, and process multiple samples simultaneously in microtitre plate format.

Microbead-based systems are now widely used in medical diagnostic laboratories and a number of proprietary diagnostic assays are available commercially. Their utility has been demonstrated recently in the simultaneous detection and quantification of seven intestinal human parasites from faecal samples. Such systems have not yet been used in veterinary parasitology diagnosis, but their potential to deliver rapid, high-throughput, multiplex assays is currently under evaluation.

DNA sequencing approaches

DNA sequencing has been used in parasite diagnostics for almost 30 years. It has been predominantly used to determine the identity of parasitic nematode specimens using an appropriate taxonomic marker and is often described as DNA barcoding. Species identification of parasitic nematodes using morphological criteria not only requires substantial expertise but can be unreliable when applied to closely related species using eggs and larval stages and often only reliably discriminates to the genus level. Consequently, DNA

sequencing has been used to confirm the species identity of adult nematodes collected from necropsies or from eggs and larvae extracted from faeces of food-producing and companion animals, both in research and in routine diagnostics.

The standard approach has been to amplify an appropriate taxonomic marker locus by PCR and clone and/or directly sequence it by Sanger ('first-generation') sequencing. Different taxonomic markers can be used with their resolution depending on the degree of interspecies and intraspecies sequence variation in the taxonomic group(s) being examined. For example, the nuclear 18S and 28S rDNA coding gene markers are more conserved than the intervening ITS-1 and ITS-2 transcribed spacer regions and mtDNA markers, such as the cytochrome oxidase I (COI) and NADH-ubiquinone oxidoreductase chain 4 (ND4) genes being even less conserved. The choice of taxonomic marker also depends on other factors such as the target sequence length, the ease of sequence alignment and primer design and the availability of references for the species of interest.

Next-generation sequencing

DNA barcoding using Sanger sequencing has been, and still is, valuable for the identification of individual specimens. However, the low scalability has limited its use for many diagnostic or research applications. Nevertheless, the advent of next-generation massively parallel sequencing technologies now allows very large numbers of parasites to be synchronously sequenced at depth in large numbers of samples.

'Next-generation' sequencing (NGS) technologies comprise several high-throughput sequencing approaches based on the concept of massively parallel sequencing ('second generation'). In essence, these new technologies synchronously sequence very large numbers (many millions) of DNA molecules in parallel. Although several different platforms have been developed, Illumina has become the dominant system in recent years. More recently, 'third-generation' massively parallel sequencing has become available which is characterised by the sequencing of individual long strands of nucleic acid in real time. The main third-generation sequencing platforms are Single Molecule Real Time (SMRT) (Pacific Biosciences) and nanopore sequencing (Oxford Nanopore Technologies).

Next-generation sequencing technologies can potentially be used in a variety of ways for gastrointestinal parasite diagnostics. The two main applications of next-generation deep amplicon sequencing in molecular diagnostics of gastrointestinal nematodes of domestic animals to date are ITS-2 rRNA gene metabarcoding for relative quantitation of species present in faecal samples, so-called nemabiome metabarcoding, and the detection and relative quantitation of SNP anthelmintic resistance mutations.

ITS-2 rRNA gene nemabiome metabarcoding methodologies

Nemabiome metabarcoding is essentially large-scale DNA barcoding using massively parallel sequencing technology to allow tens to hundreds of thousands of DNA molecules in a PCR amplicon to be simultaneously sequenced. In doing so, the targeted taxonomic marker is sequenced at depth from a large number of parasites in a sample, not only identifying the parasite species present but also providing information on their relative abundance. Methods for the analysis of the large amount of sequence data generated by short read Illumina ITS-2 rDNA nemabiome metabarcoding are continuously evolving and details are available at www.nemabiome.ca/analysis.html.

DNA-based diagnosis in veterinary parasitology: specific examples

Rumen fluke species identification

For decades, it had been assumed that the predominant rumen fluke species infecting British and Irish livestock was *Paramphistomum cervi*, which is believed to have a natural wildlife host in deer and to favour planorbid aquatic snails as its intermediate molluscan host (see Chapter 1). Genomic DNA extracted from rumen fluke adults, larvae or eggs collected from faecal samples or from *post mortem* material was subjected to PCR, targeting the ITS-2 of the rRNA gene and submitted for DNA sequence analysis. In all cases, the DNA sequences obtained were 100% identical to *Calicophoron daubneyi*, the predominant rumen fluke species found in livestock in mainland Europe. This finding may have implications for rumen fluke epidemiology in Britain and Ireland, as in the rest of Europe, because *C. daubneyi* is known to favour the same mud snail intermediate host, *Galba truncatula*, as liver fluke.

Liver fluke detection in faeces

The detection of acute liver fluke disease, caused by the mass migration of the damaging immature stages, represents a significant diagnostic challenge, especially in sheep. Fluke diagnosis is based mainly around invasive blood tests, looking for biochemical evidence of liver and/or bile duct damage, or the presence of anti-fluke antibodies. These methods are relatively non-specific and can be difficult to interpret. Furthermore, the long prepatent period for fluke, typically 8–12 weeks post infection, means that fluke egg counting is of no practical use in acute fluke cases.

The cELISA has been shown to detect fluke infection several weeks ahead of FEC in experimental challenge models, but this has not yet been observed in the field. However, published evidence suggests that liver fluke DNA, possibly originating from the parasite's gut contents and/or sloughed tegumental material, can be detected in host faeces from as early as two weeks post infection. The method involves targeting a mitochondrial gene using a sensitive nested PCR approach

and with minimal processing of faecal samples. Subsequently, a second liver fluke-specific PCR assay has been developed, based on an ITS-2 sequence, which shows promise in the sensitive detection of flukicide-resistant *Fasciola* populations.

PROTOZOAL INFECTIONS

The laboratory diagnosis of protozoal diseases is often relatively straightforward and well within the scope of the general practitioner, although occasionally it may require specialised techniques and long experience. This section is concerned primarily with the former and supplements the information already given in the general text.

EXAMINATION OF FAECAL SAMPLES FOR COCCIDIA

Faecal oocyst counts can help support the diagnosis of coccidiosis but it is important to identify the species present, as not all species of coccidia are pathogenic. The modified McMaster method, as well as the FLOTAC/Mini-FLOTAC techniques, are the simplest ways of detecting the presence and estimating the number of coccidial oocysts in faeces. The techniques are exactly the same as that described for helminthological diagnosis, although the small size of the oocysts makes microscopic examination more prolonged. If the animal has acute clinical signs of coccidiosis, such as blood-stained faeces, and many thousands of oocysts are present, one may reasonably consider that the diagnosis is confirmed. Unfortunately, with the more pathogenic species of coccidia, clinical signs may appear during the merogonous phase or when oocyst production has just started, so that a negative or low oocyst count does not necessarily indicate that the clinical diagnosis was wrong. The oocyst count is also of little value in the less acute coccidial infections associated with production losses. In general, because of the limitations of the oocyst count, a *post mortem* examination, at least on poultry, is always advisable.

Sometimes, the diagnosis of eimeriosis requires identification of the various species present because of the different pathogenicity attributed to them; in these cases, examination of the characteristics morphometric of the non-sporulated oocysts does not always allow identification of the species. It is therefore necessary to induce sporulation of oocysts themselves to obtain further morphometric details useful for their classification. Oocyst sporulation is obtained by preparation of coprocultures: the faecal sample, supplemented with a solution of 2% potassium dichromate that prevents microbial multiplication, is stored at constant temperature (about 25 °C). Periodically, the material is checked via copromicroscopic examination to check for sporulation.

Descriptive terms used in oocyst identification are shown in Fig. 4.34. Guidelines for the morphological diagnosis of sporulated oocysts from cattle (Fig. 4.35, Table 4.7), sheep (Fig. 4.36, Table 4.8), goats (Fig. 4.37, Table 4.9), pigs (Fig. 4.38, Table 4.10), rabbits (Fig. 4.39, Table 4.11) and chickens and turkeys (Tables 4.12 and 4.13) are given on the following pages. Moreover, for identification of species, evaluation of sporulation time is of great importance.

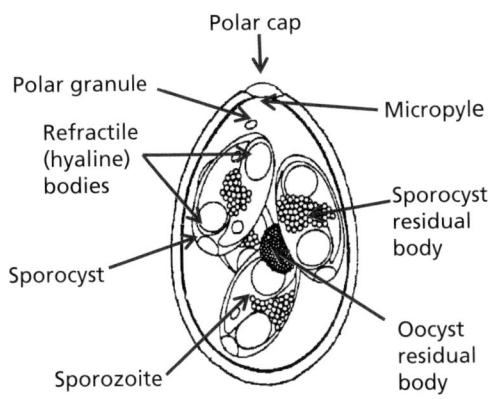

Polar cap

Polar granule

Micropyle

Refractile
(hyaline)
bodies

Sporocyst
residual
body

Sporocyst

Oocyst
residual
body

Sporozoite

Fig. 4.34 Schematic diagram of an *Eimeria* oocyst.

EXAMINATION OF FAECAL SAMPLES FOR OTHER PROTOZOA

For the detection of intestinal protozoa such as *Entamoeba*, *Giardia*, *Balantidium* or *Cryptosporidium*, a small amount of fresh faeces may be mixed with warm saline and examined under a warm-stage microscope for the presence of trophozoites or cysts. However, their identification requires considerable experience and faecal samples preserved in formalin or polyvinyl alcohol should be sent to a specialist laboratory for confirmation. In particular, trophozoites of *Giardia* spp. in samples of diarrhoeal faeces are identified easily and quickly on smears of faecal material, coloured with Giemsa. Instead, concentration techniques are used for detecting *Giardia* and *Entamoeba* cysts. Specifically, the Ridley technique is widely used,

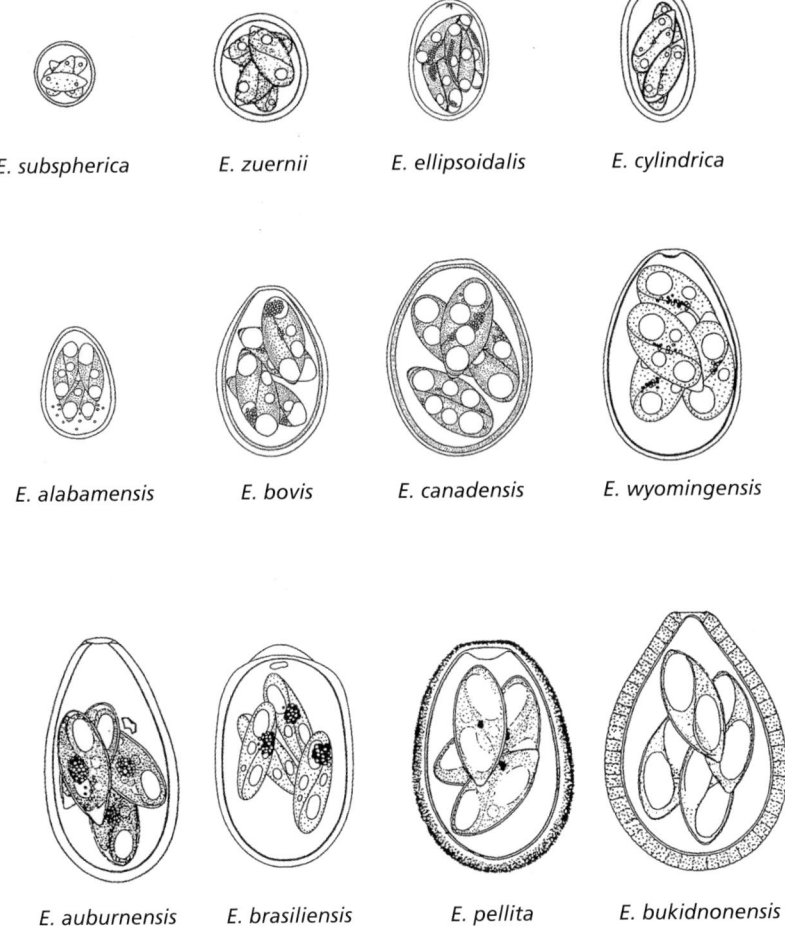

| *E. subspherica* | *E. zuernii* | *E. ellipsoidalis* | *E. cylindrica* |

| *E. alabamensis* | *E. bovis* | *E. canadensis* | *E. wyomingensis* |

| *E. auburnensis* | *E. brasiliensis* | *E. pellita* | *E. bukidnonensis* |

40 µm

Fig. 4.35 Sporulated oocysts of *Eimeria* from cattle.

Table 4.7 Identification key for sporulated oocysts of *Eimeria* from cattle (see Fig. 4.34).

Species	Oocyst description	Mean size (μm)	Sporulation time (days)
Pathogenic species			
Eimeria bovis	Ovoid or subspherical, colourless, and smooth wall with inconspicuous micropyle, no polar granule or oocyst residuum	28 × 20	2–3
E. zuernii	Subspherical, colourless, with no micropyle or oocyst residuum	18 × 16	2–3
E. alabamensis	Usually ovoid with a smooth colourless wall with no micropyle, polar body or residuum	19 × 13	5–8
Non-pathogenic species			
E. auburnensis	Elongated, ovoid, yellowish-brown, with smooth or heavily granulated wall with a micropyle and polar granule, but no oocyst residuum	38 × 23	2–3
E. brasiliensis	Ellipsoidal, yellowish-brown, with a micropyle covered by a distinct polar cap. Polar granules may also be present, but there is no oocyst residuum	37 × 27	12–14
E. bukidnonensis	Pear-shaped or oval, tapering at one pole, yellowish-brown, with a thick, radially striated wall and micropyle. A polar granule may be present but there is no oocyst residuum	49.35	4–7
E. canadensis	Ovoid or ellipsoidal, colourless, or pale yellow, with an inconspicuous micropyle, one or more polar granules and an oocyst residuum	33 × 23	3–4
E. cylindrica	Elongated cylindrical with a colourless smooth wall, no micropyle, and no oocyst residuum	23 × 12	2–3
E. ellipsoidalis	Ellipsoidal to slightly ovoid, colourless, with no discernible micropyle, polar granule or oocyst residuum	23 × 16	2–3
E. pellita	Egg-shaped, very thick, brown wall with evenly distributed protuberances, with a micropyle and polar granule consisting of several rod-like bodies but no oocyst residuum	40 × 28	10–12
E. subspherica	Round or subspherical, colourless, with no micropyle, polar granule or oocyst residuum	11 × 10	4–5
E. wyomingensis	Ovoid, yellowish-brown, with a thick wall, a wide micropyle but no polar granule or oocyst residuum	40 × 28	5–7

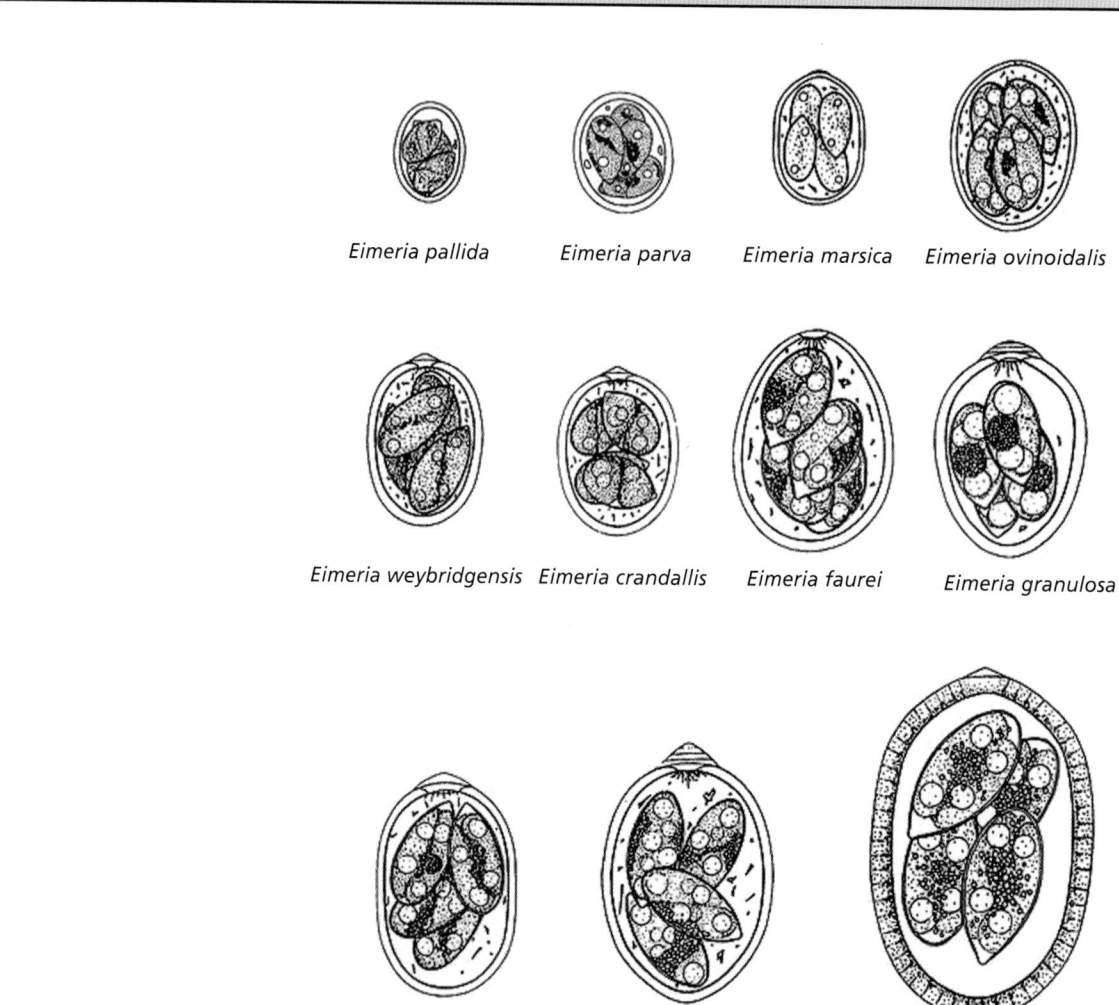

Eimeria pallida   Eimeria parva   Eimeria marsica   Eimeria ovinoidalis

Eimeria weybridgensis Eimeria crandallis   Eimeria faurei   Eimeria granulosa

Eimeria bakuensis   Eimeria ahsata   Eimeria intricata

|— 40 μm —|

Fig. 4.36 Sporulated oocysts of *Eimeria* from sheep.

Table 4.8 Identification key for sporulated oocysts of *Eimeria* from sheep (see Fig. 4.36).

Species	Oocyst description	Mean size (μm)	Sporulation time (days)
Pathogenic species			
Eimeria crandallis	Broadly ellipsoidal or subspherical, with or without polar cap, without oocyst residuum, sporocysts very broad, with sporocyst residuum	22 × 19	1–3
E. ovinoidalis	Ellipsoidal indistinct micropyle, colourless or pale yellow, without oocyst residuum, with sporocyst residuum	23 × 18	1–3
E. ahsata	Ovoid with distinct polar cap, yellowish-brown, no oocyst residuum	33 × 23	2–3
Non-pathogenic species			
E. bakuensis	Ellipsoidal, with polar cap, pale yellowish-brown, without oocyst residuum, with sporocyst residuum	31 × 20	2–4
E. faurei	Ovoid, pale yellowish-brown, without oocyst residuum or sporocyst residuum	32 × 23	1–3
E. granulosa	Urn-shaped with large micropolar cap at broad end, yellowish-brown, without oocyst residuum	29 × 21	3–4
E. intricata	Ellipsoidal, thick and striated wall, brown no oocyst residuum	48 × 34	3–7
E. marsica	Ellipsoidal, with inconspicuous micropyle, colourless or pale yellow, without oocyst or sporocyst residuum	19 × 13	3
E. pallida	Ellipsoidal, thin-walled, colourless to pale yellow, without oocyst residuum, but with sporocyst residuum	14 × 10	1–3
E. parva	Spherical to subspherical, colourless, no oocyst residuum, sporocyst residuum composed of few granules	17 × 14	3–5
E. weybridgensis	Broadly ellipsoidal or subspherical, micropyle with or without polar cap, without oocyst or sporocyst residuum	24 × 17	1–3

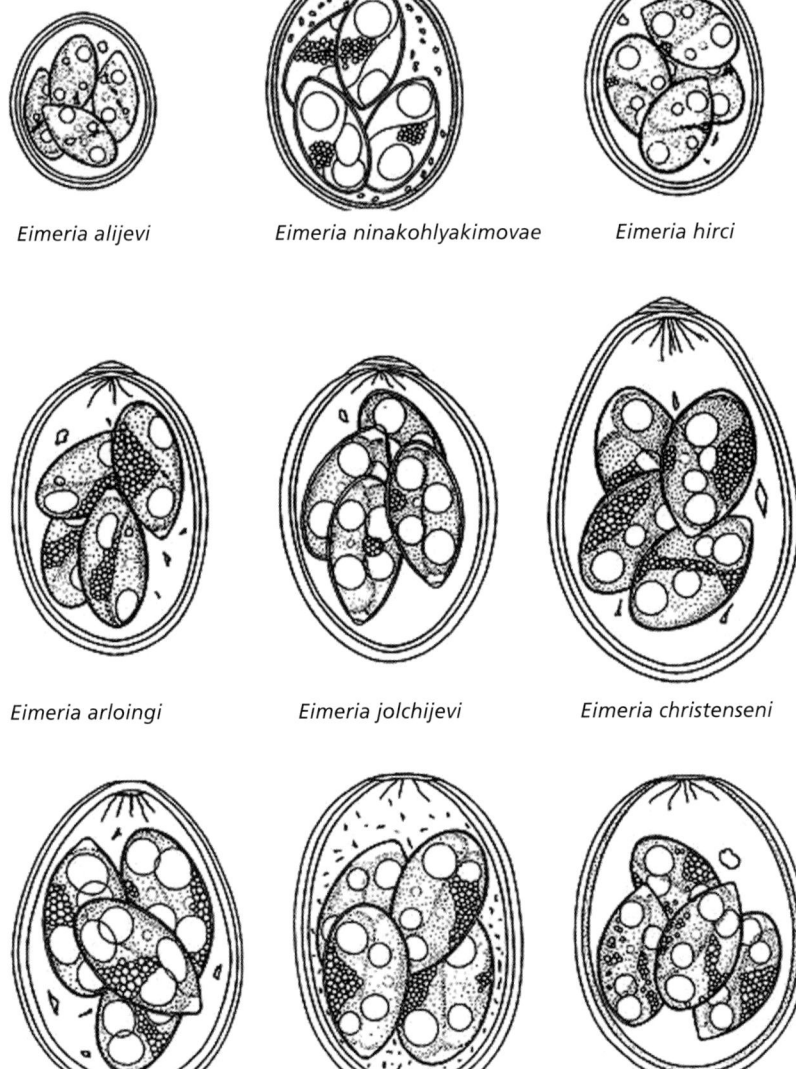

Eimeria alijevi   *Eimeria ninakohlyakimovae*   *Eimeria hirci*

Eimeria arloingi   *Eimeria jolchijevi*   *Eimeria christenseni*

Eimeria aspheronica   *Eimeria caprina*   *Eimeria caprovina*

Fig. 4.37 Sporulated oocysts of *Eimeria* from goats.

Table 4.9 Identification key for sporulated oocysts of *Eimeria* from goats (see Fig. 4.37).

Species	Oocyst description	Mean size (μm)	Sporulation time (days)
Pathogenic species			
Eimeria caprina	Ellipsoidal, dark-brown to brownish-yellow, with micropyle, without oocyst residuum but with sporocyst residuum	32 × 23	2–3
E. ninakohlyakimovae	Ellipsoidal, thin-walled, colourless, micropyle absent or indistinct, without oocyst residuum but with sporocyst residuum	21 × 15	1–4
E. christenseni	Ovoid, thick wall, colourless to pale yellow, with micropyle and polar cap, without oocyst residuum but with sporocyst residuum	38 × 25	6
E. hirci	Roundish oval, light yellow, with micropyle and polar cap, no oocyst residuum, sporocysts broadly oval with small residuum	21 × 16	2–3
Non-pathogenic species			
E. alijevi	Ovoid or ellipsoidal, with inconspicuous micropyle, colourless or pale yellow, without oocyst residuum but with sporocyst residuum	17 × 15	1–5
E. arloingi	Ellipsoidal, thick wall with micropyle and polar cap, without oocyst residuum but with sporocyst residuum	27 × 18	1–2
E. aspheronica	Ovoid, greenish to yellow-brown, with micropyle, without oocyst residuum but with sporocyst residuum	31 × 32	1–2
E. caprovina	Ellipsoidal to subspherical, colourless, with micropyle, without oocyst residuum but with sporocyst residuum	30 × 24	2–3
E. jolchijevi	Ellipsoidal or oval, pale yellow, with micropyle and polar cap, without oocyst residuum but with sporocyst residuum	31 × 22	2–4

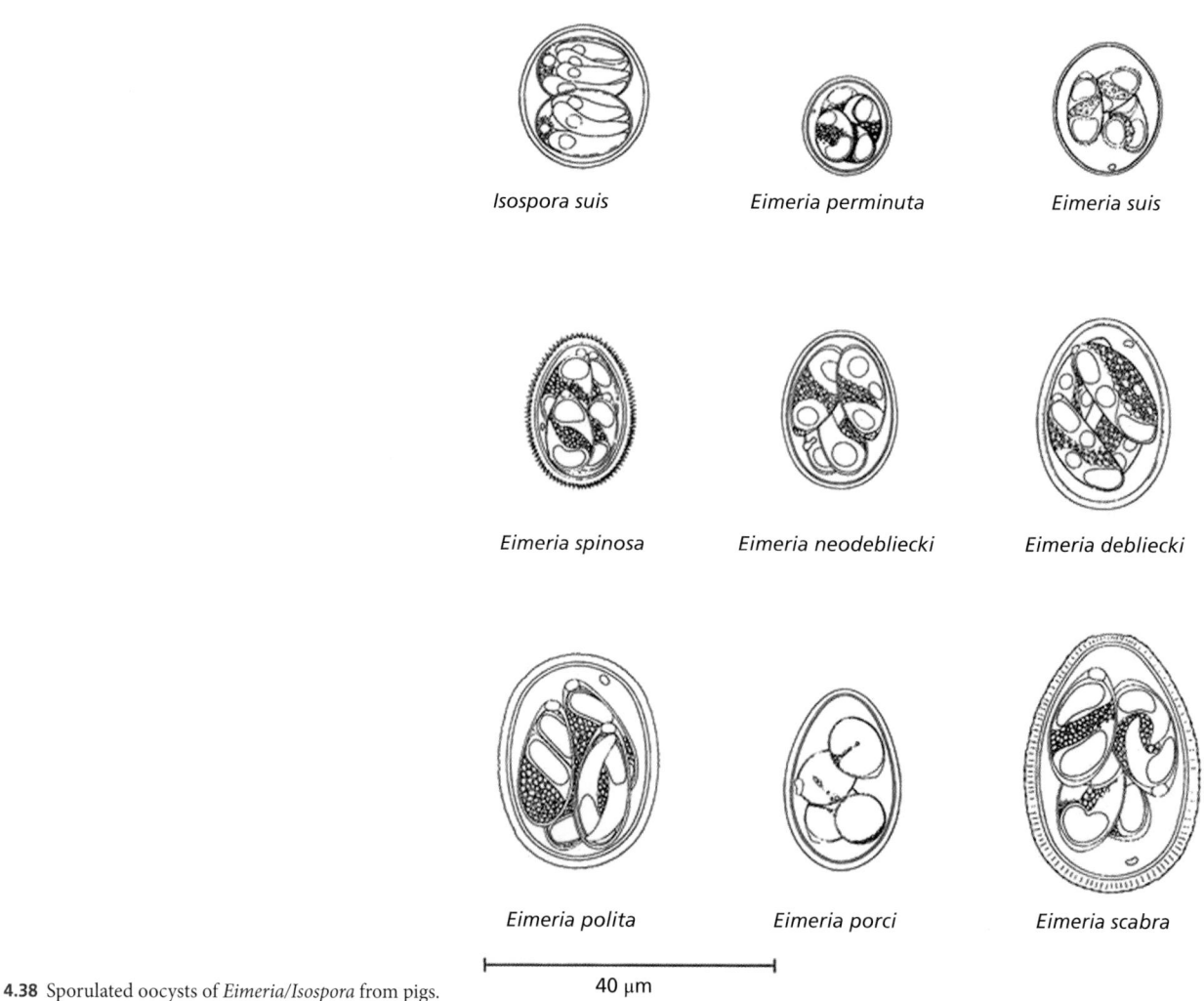

Isospora suis   Eimeria perminuta   Eimeria suis

Eimeria spinosa   Eimeria neodebliecki   Eimeria debliecki

Eimeria polita   Eimeria porci   Eimeria scabra

40 μm

Fig. 4.38 Sporulated oocysts of *Eimeria/Isospora* from pigs.

Table 4.10 Identification key for sporulated oocysts of *Eimeria/Isospora* from pigs (see Fig. 4.38).

Species	Oocyst description	Mean size (μm)	Sporulation time (days)
Isospora suis	Oocysts spherical to subspherical, wall colourless and thin, without a micropyle or residuum and when sporulated contains two sporocysts, each with four sporozoites	21 × 18	1–2
Eimeria perminuta	Ovoid to subspherical, yellow in colour, and wall with a rough surface. A polar granule is present but no micropyle or oocyst residuum	13 × 12	10–12
E. suis	Ellipsoidal, wall smooth and colourless with a polar granule but no micropyle or oocyst residuum	18 × 14	5–6
E. spinosa	Ovoid with a thick, rough, brown wall with long spines. There is a polar granule but no micropyle or oocyst residuum	21 × 16	9–10
E. neodebliecki	Ellipsoid, wall smooth and colourless with no micropyle or oocyst residuum but there is a polar granule	21 × 16	13
E. debliecki	Ellipsoid or ovoid, wall smooth and colourless with no micropyle or oocyst residuum but with a polar granule	19 × 14	5–7
E. polita	Ellipsoidal or broad ovoid with a slightly rough yellowish-brown wall with no micropyle, oocyst residuum, although a polar granule may be present	26 × 18	8–9
E. porci	Ovoid, colourless to yellowish-brown, with an indistinct micropyle, a polar granule but no oocyst residuum	22 × 16	9
E. scabra	Ovoid or ellipsoidal, with a thick rough striated wall, yellow-brown in colour with a micropyle and polar granule, but no oocyst residuum	32 × 23	9–12

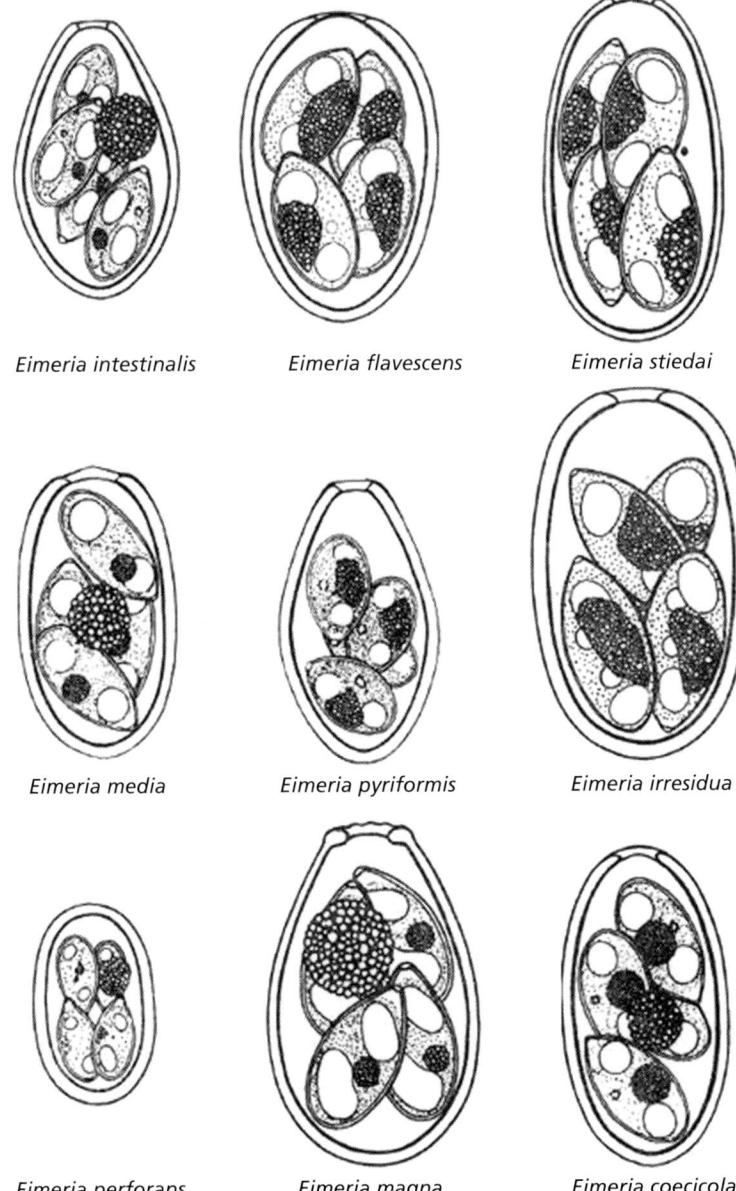

Eimeria intestinalis   Eimeria flavescens   Eimeria stiedai

Eimeria media   Eimeria pyriformis   Eimeria irresidua

Eimeria perforans   Eimeria magna   Eimeria coecicola

Fig. 4.39 Sporulated oocysts of *Eimeria* from rabbits.

Table 4.11 Identification key for sporulated oocysts of *Eimeria* from rabbits (see Fig. 4.39).

Species	Oocyst description	Mean size (μm)	Sporulation time (days)
Highly pathogenic			
Eimeria flavescens	Ovoid, yellowish, with a prominent micropyle at the broad end. There is no polar granule or oocyst residuum	30 × 21	4
E. intestinalis	Pyriform, yellowish-brown, with a micropyle at the narrow end, a large oocyst residuum but no polar granule	27 × 19	3
Pathogenic			
E. stiedae	Slightly ellipsoidal, colourless or pinkish orange, with an inapparent micropyle and no oocyst residuum	37 × 20	2–3
E. media	Ovoid or ellipsoidal, smooth, light pink with a micropyle with a pyramid-shaped protuberance, a medium to large oocyst residuum and no polar granule	31 × 17	2
E. pyriformis	Pyriform, often asymmetrical, yellowish-brown, with a prominent micropyle but no polar granule or oocyst residuum	30 × 18	4
E. irresidua	Ovoid, barrel-shaped, smooth, yellowish, with a wide micropyle; a residuum may be present but there are no polar granules	39 × 23	4
E. magna	Ovoid, dark yellow, truncated at micropylar end with marked collar-like thickening around micropyle, with very large oocyst residuum but no polar granules	36 × 24	2–3
Slight or non-pathogenic			
E. perforans	Ellipsoidal to subrectangular, smooth, colourless with a uniformly thin wall. There is an inconspicuous micropyle and an oocyst residuum but no polar granule	22 × 14	1.5–2
E. exigua	Spherical or subspherical, colourless, with no micropyle, polar granule or oocyst residuum	15 × 14	1
E. vejdovsyi	Elongate or ovoid, micropyle present without collar-like protrusion, and with medium-sized oocyst residuum	32 × 19	2
E. coecicola	Ellipsoidal, light yellow to light brown in colour, with a smooth wall, a distinct micropyle with a slight collar-like protrusion, an oocyst residuum but no polar granule	34 × 20	4

Table 4.12 Identification key for sporulated oocysts of *Eimeria* from chickens.

Species	Oocyst description	Mean size (μm)	Sporulation time (days)
Eimeria acervulina	Ovoid, smooth without a micropyle or residuum but with a polar granule	18 × 14	24
E. brunetti	Ovoid, smooth without a micropyle or residuum but with a polar granule	26 × 22	24–48
E. maxima	Ovoid, yellowish and smooth without a micropyle or residuum but with a polar granule	30 × 20	30–48
E. mitis	Subspherical, smooth without a micropyle or residuum but with a polar granule	16 × 15	18–24
E. necatrix	Ovoid, smooth, colourless without a micropyle or residuum but with a polar granule	20 × 17	18–24
E. praecox	Ovoid, smooth, colourless without a micropyle or residuum but with a polar granule	21 × 17	48
E. tenella	Ovoid, smooth, colourless without a micropyle or residuum but with a polar granule	25 × 19	18–48

Table 4.13 Identification key for sporulated oocysts of *Eimeria* from turkeys.

Species	Oocyst description	Mean size (μm)	Sporulation time (days)
Eimeria adenoides	Ellipsoidal or ovoid, smooth, colourless with a micropyle, one to three polar granules but no oocyst residuum	26 × 17	24
E. dispersa	Ovoid, smooth with no micropyle, polar granule or oocyst residuum	26 × 21	48
E. meleagridis	Ellipsoidal, smooth with no micropyle and no oocyst residuum but with one or two polar granules	23 × 16	15–72
E. meleagrimitis	Subspherical, smooth, colourless with no micropyle or oocyst residuum, but with one to three polar granules	19 × 16	24–72
E. gallapovonis	Ellipsoidal, smooth, colourless without a micropyle or oocyst residuum, but with one polar granule	27 × 17	24
E. innocua	Subspherical, smooth, without a micropyle or polar granules	22 × 21	48
E. subrotunda	Subspherical, smooth, without a micropyle or polar granules	22 × 21	48

characterised by the following stages: 1 gram of stool is emulsified in 10 ml of 4% formaldehyde and filtered, then 3 ml of ethyl ether is added to 9 ml of filtered material. The preparation is stirred by vortex and immediately centrifuged at 2000 rpm (220 *g*) for five minutes. Finally, in the test four layers will be highlighted; the first three must be removed while the sediment is examined under the microscope with the addition of a drop of Lugol's solution.

Cryptosporidium spp. oocysts can be isolated by copromicroscopic flotation examination with saturated NaCl solution (s.g. = 1.20) but the most suitable method, in subjects with clinical symptoms, is the staining of faecal samples. It is possible to use a rapid technique such as that of Heine, which consists in setting up a smear with a very small amount of faecal material amalgamated directly on a slide with an equal quantity of Ziehl–Neelsen carbolfuchsin solution. Then, the preparation is examined under the microscope (1000×) within 10–15 minutes from set-up to avoid overlap oocysts that appear colourless on a reddish background. The carbolfuchsin can be replaced by other dyes of contrast such as malachite green or nigrosin.

Alternatively, a more sensitive technique is used, the modified Ziehl–Neelsen, which uses the acid resistance of *Cryptosporidium* oocysts. The detection limit (analytic sensitivity) of this method is greater than 100 000 oocysts per gram of faeces. A smear of faecal material is fixed in methyl alcohol, coloured with Ziehl–Neelsen carbolfuchsin and subsequently bleached with a 2% sulfuric acid solution. Finally, the smear is subjected to a contrast colour (malachite green or methylene blue). Oocysts appear bright red on a green or blue background. This method, although more complex than rapid staining, allows examination of the preparations even after several days of preparation and easier and more immediate highlighting of oocyst.

In addition, a number of ELISA coproantigen commercial kits have been developed for intestinal protozoa as well as rapid diagnostic tests that employ immunochromatographic methods.

Modified Ziehl–Neelsen method for *Cryptosporidium*

1 Place one drop of saline in the centre of a clean slide (slide washed in methylated spirit and air dried).
2 Add a small sample of faeces and emulsify the sample in the saline by thorough mixing. For liquid faeces, dispense one drop directly onto the slide.
3 Smear faeces on the slide in a wavy pattern to ensure there are thick and thin areas.
4 Either fix the smear by passing through a Bunsen flame twice or air-dry at room temperature and then fix in methanol for three minutes.
5 Immerse the slide in 3% carbolfuchsin and stain for 15 minutes (use a Coplin jar or staining tray).
6 Rinse the slide thoroughly in tap water.
7 Decolorise in 1% acid methanol for 15–20 seconds.
8 Rinse the slide in tap water.
9 Counterstain with 0.4% malachite green for 30 seconds.
10 Rinse the slide in tap water.
11 Air-dry the slide and examine using the ×40 objective lens of a bright-field microscope.
12 To aid identification of oocysts, the smear can be examined under the oil immersion objective lens.

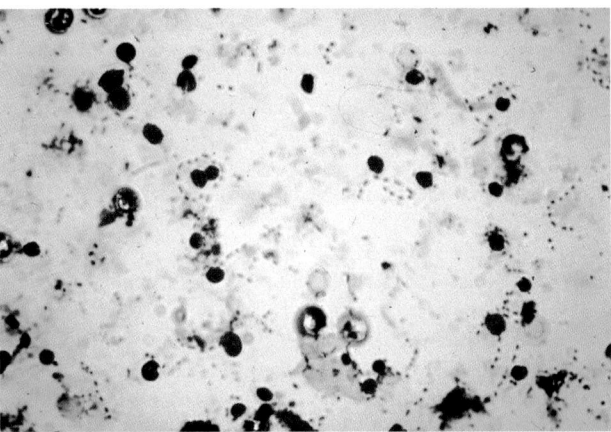

Fig. 4.40 *Cryptosporidium* oocysts (Ziehl–Neelsen stain).

13 Examine the size and shape of the red-stained bodies. *Cryptosporidium* spp. oocysts stain red on a pale green background (Fig. 4.40). The degree and proportion of staining vary with individual oocysts. In addition, the internal structures take up the stain to varying degrees. Some may appear amorphous while others may contain the characteristic crescentic forms of the sporozoites.
14 Oocysts of *Cryptosporidium parvum* are 4–6 μm in diameter.
15 Yeasts and faecal debris stain a dull red. Some bacterial spores may also stain red, but these are too small to cause confusion.
16 A semi-quantitative scoring system can be used based on numbers of oocysts seen. Most clinical infections in calves score 3+ to 4+.

EXAMINATION OF BLOOD AND LYMPH

Thin blood smears stained with Romanowsky dyes, such as Giemsa or Leishmann, and examined under an oil immersion lens are commonly used for the detection of trypanosomes, babesial and theilerial piroplasms, and rickettsial infections such as anaplasmosis, ehrlichiosis and eperythrozoonosis.

On other occasions, needle biopsies of enlarged lymph nodes may be similarly stained for the detection of trypanosomes (especially *Trypanosoma brucei* or *T. vivax*) or theilerial meronts.

Giemsa method

1 Make a thin blood smear and allow to dry.
2 Fix the blood smear with methanol for two minutes.
3 Stain the smear with 15% Giemsa (in buffered distilled water, pH 7.2) for 45 minutes.
4 Rinse the smear under a gentle stream of cold water, drain and allow to air-dry.
5 View under oil using the ×l00 objective lens.

Diff-Quik™ method

1 Make a thin blood smear and allow to dry.
2 Fix the blood smear with methanol for two minutes.

3 Stain as follows: dip the smear into a container of stain A (orange colour) 15 times, each dip lasting one second; immediately switch to stain B (blue colour) and carry out 15 dips, for one second each again. (See Chemicals and Solutions at the end of the chapter for stains details.)

4 Rinse the smear under a gentle stream of cold water to clean the slide, drain, wipe excess moisture from the back of the slide and allow to air-dry.

5 View under oil using the ×100 objective lens.

In trypanosomiasis, the parasitaemia may be light and the chance of a positive diagnosis is increased if a thick blood film, de-haemoglobinised by immersing the slide in water before eosin staining, is used. For this, a drop of fresh blood, with no added anticoagulant, is gently stirred on a slide to cover an area of about 10 mm diameter and allowed to dry. Subsequently, it may be stained by Field's technique as follows.

Field's technique

See section on Chemicals and Solutions at the end of this chapter for details of the solutions.

1 Dip the slide in solution A for 1–3 seconds.
2 Rinse in solution B for 2–3 seconds.
3 Dip the slide in solution C for 1–3 seconds.
4 Rinse in tap water for 2–3 seconds.
5 Stand upright to drain and dry.

This technique is commonly used in large-scale survey work in the field.

A particularly efficient diagnostic technique for trypanosomiasis, described earlier in the text, is the examination, under darkground illumination, of the expressed buffy coat of a microhaematocrit tube for the detection of motile trypanosomes.

The inoculation of mice with fresh blood from suspected cases of *Trypanosoma congolense* or *T. brucei* infection is another common technique practised in the field, despite being more complex. Three days later the tail blood of such mice should be examined and subsequently daily thereafter for about 3–4 weeks to establish if trypanosomes are present.

The detection of specific antibody in a specialist laboratory may also be useful in the diagnosis of several protozoal diseases such as theileriosis, trypanosomiasis (including *T. cruzi* infection), babesiosis, cryptosporidiosis and rickettsial infections such as anaplasmosis and ehrlichiosis. However, a positive result does not necessarily imply the presence of a still active infection, but simply that the animal has at some time been exposed to the pathogen. An exception to this interpretation is the diagnosis of suspected toxoplasmosis in sheep, where rising antibody levels over a period of several weeks are reasonable evidence of recent and active infection.

EXAMINATION OF SKIN

Histological examination is a useful diagnostic tool, also as collateral and/or support, especially in the case of infections and/or infestations caused by reduced, incised into tissues or microscopic parasites (*Sarcocystis, Toxoplasma, Neospora*, etc.).

Histological examination is usually performed on 'suspect' tissue measuring approximately 1 cm in area and 2–3 mm thick and maintained in 10% formalin for a few days. The tissue sample, after dehydration through ascending alcohols, is included in paraffin and then dissected using a microtome for the preparation of histological sections. For the microscopic examination, the histological sections should be stained by different methods (haematoxylin-eosin, trichromic methods, silver impregnations, etc.).

Histological examination of skin biopsies or scrapings from the edges of skin ulcers, suspected to be due to leishmaniosis, may be used to demonstrate the amastigote parasites in the macrophages.

In dourine, caused by *Trypanosoma equiperdum*, fluid extracted from the cutaneous plaques usually offers a better chance of detecting trypanosomes than blood smears.

XENODIAGNOSIS

Although not within the province of the general practitioner, the use of xenodiagnosis as a diagnostic technique should be mentioned. This is used to detect protozoal infections such as babesiosis, thieleriosis or *Trypanosoma cruzi* infection where the parasite cannot be found easily. It involves allowing the correct intermediate host, such as a tick or a haematophagous bug, to feed on the animal. These arthropod vectors have of course to be reared in the laboratory so that they are free from infection. After feeding, the arthropod host is maintained for several weeks to allow any ingested organisms to multiply, after which it is killed and examined for evidence of infection. Although a valuable technique, especially for the detection of carrier states, the method has the disadvantage that the diagnosis may take several weeks.

OTHER DIAGNOSTIC TECHNIQUES

Knott technique

This technique is used mainly for the diagnosis of filarial infections (e.g. *Dirofilaria immitis, D. repens* and *Achantocheilonema reconditum*) in companion animals. For this method, 1 ml of blood can be analysed immediately or after storage with anticoagulant (e.g. EDTA or heparin). The collected blood (1 ml) is mixed with 9 ml of 2% formalin (or tap water) allowing, after agitation for one minute, the lysis of the red blood cells. The conical tube is then centrifuged at 1500–2000 rpm (170–220g) for five minutes, the supernatant is removed and a drop of sediment placed on a slide with a drop of 0.1% methylene blue. The slide is observed under the optical microscope and the microfilariae found subjected to morphometric examination for taxonomic classification (length, width, characteristics of head and tail).

Immunodiagnosis

Antigens and/or antibodies specific to the various classes (especially IgM and IgG, more rarely IgA) may be used, in a specialised laboratory, for the diagnosis of protozoan pathologies such as theileriasis, trypanosomiasis, including infection with *T. cruzi*, babesiosis, cryptosporidiosis, toxoplasmosis,

leishmaniosis and infections from rickettsia such as anaplasmosis and ehrlichiosis. In these cases, a positive result does not necessarily imply the presence of an active infection but simply that the host has at some point come into contact with the pathogen.

However, the use of seroconversion, that is, the assessment of the possible increase of the antibodies in 2–3 weeks after the first blood sampling, represents clear evidence of a recent and active infection.

In any case, the results obtained through immunodiagnostic tests should preferably be compared and interpreted in parallel, where possible, even with a specific parasitological assessment. The immunodiagnosis is not applied solely for diagnostic purposes, but also plays a decisive role in subsequent follow-up after specific therapies, in a prognostic perspective (e.g. canine leishmaniosis).

Depending on the protozoan agent, the methods currently used are different, but the most used are immunofluorescence assay (IFA), ELISA and indirect haemoagglutination (IHA).

Trichinellosis diagnosis

Trichinella infestation in animals usually does not produce an appreciable symptomatology, so *ante mortem* diagnosis takes place mainly through the implementation of immunodiagnosis, such as IFA, for the detection of specific antibodies to antigens of larval cuticular surface, or through ELISA, for the detection of antibodies against soluble antigens. In addition, for the *ante mortem* diagnosis, a muscle biopsy is possible, although not very practical and sensitive. The search for adult nematodes in faeces is difficult because of their small size, and therefore poorly reliable.

The most reliable and therefore widely used diagnostic test is the trichinoscopic examination carried out on the musculature of slaughtered animals. The technique consists in taking muscle samples from different parts of the carcass, which are then compressed between glass plates and examined at the trichinoscope (microscope-like instrument). Other methods include muscle digestion or histological examination. The most sensitive method is the enzymatic digestion of a muscle sample and subsequent identification of the larvae under a microscope. European legislation (No. 2075/2005), which refers to the specific rules applicable to official controls concerning the presence of *Trichinella* in meat of animals regularly slaughtered, reports the methods accredited for the search for larvae, which can also take place through the use of specific equipment (e.g. Stomacher lab-blender 3 500).

Further diagnostic tests can be implemented by bioenzymatic and biomolecular analysis, especially useful for identification of the species.

ECTOPARASITES

Arthropods of veterinary interest are divided into two major groups: the Insecta and the Arachnida. Most are found either in or on the skin, with the exception of the larval stages of some flies, that occur in the somatic tissues of the host. Parasitic insects include flies, lice and fleas, while the two groups of arachnids of veterinary importance are the ticks and mites. In all cases, diagnosis of infection depends primarily on the collection, microscopic examination and identification of the parasite(s) concerned. Photographs are rarely adequate for identification. However, geographic location along with the known range of the parasite, the host species and, in some cases, location on the body are all indicative and should be noted.

DIPTERA

Sampling flies and fly larvae

Adult dipteran flies visiting animals are usually caught by netting, with traps or after being killed by insecticides. Flying insects can be caught with a hand net but the technique depends on the behaviour of the species required. Flies which settle on buildings, animals or plants are best caught with a sweep net. In some situations, continuous sampling may be required and flies can be caught in large numbers by means of traps. There is a wide variety of trap types available. One of the most widely used is the Manitoba-type trap consisting of a tent-like structure of netting held 1 m above the ground below which is suspended a black or red sphere. This may be accompanied by a slow release of carbon dioxide from a box containing dry ice ('cardice') blocks or pellets. Flies which feed or oviposit on carrion or dung can be caught in baited traps. Frequent emptying of traps is important, to avoid deterioration of the samples.

Insect larvae may be collected in areas where animals are housed or directly from animals where the larval stages are parasitic. Special methods are useful in certain cases; warble fly larvae, for example, may be obtained by carefully squeezing from the live animal or from fresh skins at an abattoir. Where insects (or mites) have developmental stages in soil, woodland litter or faeces, various modifications of the Berlese funnel may be used. This consists of a metal funnel with a perforated screen tray inside carrying the litter sample. The funnel is heated and, owing to their increased activity, insect larvae, mites and other arthropods fall through the screen tray into a container. The technique may be more simply adapted to large field samples (e.g. turf or manure) by placing these in wire trays over water. An electric lamp positioned a few centimetres above the tray then provides light and warmth and repels moving arthropods, which again drop through the wire tray into the water.

Identification of the common flies of veterinary interest, at least to genus level, is fairly straightforward, the key characters being described in the guide below. Identification of larvae to genus and species level is rather more specialised and depends on examination of certain features such as the structure of the posterior spiracles. Publications dealing with this may be found in the References and further reading section. The retention of voucher specimens can be important where subsequent verification is required.

Guide to the families of adult Diptera of veterinary importance

1 Insects with one pair of wings on the mesothorax and a pair of club-like halteres on the metathorax **2**

Wingless insects; may be with or without halteres; body divided into head, thorax and abdomen; three pairs of legs; dorsoventrally flattened; brown in colour; 5–8 mm in length; resident on sheep, horses, deer, goats or wild birds (Fig. 4.41) **5**

2 Antennae composed of three segments; third segment usually with an arista (Fig. 4.42c); foot with two pads **3**

Antennae composed of three sections; third antennal section enlarged and composed of 4–8 segments (Fig. 4.42b; Fig. 4.43a,b,c); palps two-jointed with the second segment enlarged; foot with three pads; vein R4+5 forks to form a large 'Y' across the wing tip (Fig. 4.43d); large stout-bodied flies with large eyes... **Tabanidae 12**

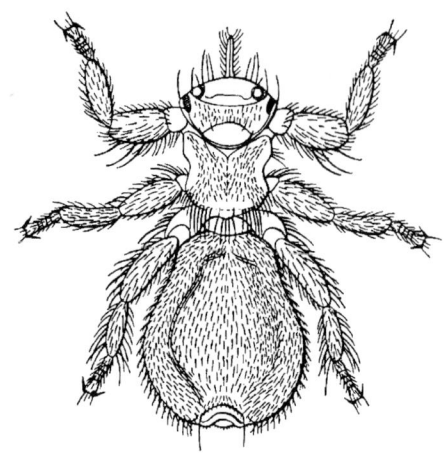

Fig. 4.41 Adult sheep ked, *Melophagus ovinus.*

Antennae long, slender and composed of many articulating segments (Fig. 4.42a); palps composed of 4–5 segments; small slender flies with long narrow wings .... **Nematocera 13**

3 Frons with ptilinal suture, horseshoe-shaped (Fig. 4.44) .... **Schizophora 4**

    Frons without ptilinal suture.................................... **Aschiza**

4 Second antennal segment usually with a groove (Fig. 4.44); thoracic transverse suture strong (Fig. 4.45); thoracic squamae usually well developed (Fig. 4.46) .... **Calypterae 5**

    Second antennal segment usually without a groove; thoracic transverse suture weak; thoracic squamae often vestigial .... **Acalypterae**

5 Thorax broad and dorsoventrally flattened; may appear spider or tick-like; often wingless (Fig. 4.41); wings when present with venation abnormal, with veins crowded into leading half of wing.. **Hippoboscidae**

    Wings with veins not crowded together towards the leading edge; thorax not dorsoventrally flattened **6**

6 Proboscis long, forwardly directed and embraced by long palps; arista with feathery short hairs present only on dorsal side; discal medial cell (dm) of wings characteristically hatchet-shaped (Fig. 4.47); found only in sub-Saharan Africa ....**Glossinidae**

    Discal medial cell of wings widening gradually and more or less regularly from the base.. 7

7 Mouthparts small, usually functionless; head bulbous; antennae small; flies more or less covered with soft hair; larval parasites of vertebrates .... **Oestridae**

    Mouthparts usually well developed; antennae not small; flies with strong bristles.. **8**

8 Hypopleural bristles present (Fig. 4.45b).................................... **9**

    Hypopleural bristles absent.. **11**

9 Postscutellum strongly developed; larval parasitoids of insects .... **Tachinidae**

    Postscutellum weak or absent.. **10**

10 Dull grey appearance; three black stripes on the scutum; abdomen usually with chequered or spotted pattern (Fig. 4.48); larval parasites of vertebrates....................................**Sarcophagidae**

    Metallic, iridescent appearance (blue-black, violet-blue, green); larval parasites of vertebrates .... **Calliphoridae**

11 Wings with vein A$_1$ not reaching the wing edge; strong curved A$_2$ vein the tip of which approaches A$_1$ (Fig. 4.49); aristae bare ....**Fanniidae**

    Wings with vein A$_1$ not reaching the wing edge; A$_2$ vein not strongly curved (Fig.4.49; 4.50); aristae bilaterally plumose to

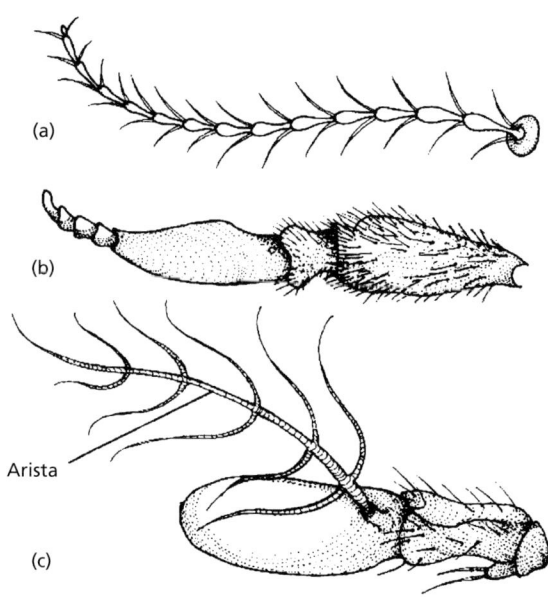

Arista

Fig. 4.42 Variations in the structure of antennae found typically in (a) nematoceran, (b) tabanid and (c) muscid Diptera.

the tip; vein M strongly bent to the margin (Fig. 4.50) ....**Muscidae**

12 Antennal flagellum with four segments (Fig. 4.43b); wings mottled; proboscis shorter than head .... ***Haematopota* spp. (Tabanidae)**

    Antennal flagellum with five segments (Fig. 4.43a); apical spurs on tibiae small and may be hidden by hair; wings usually with costal region dark and a single dark broad transverse band; proboscis shorter than head.............***Chrysops* spp. (Tabanidae)**

    Antennal flagellum with five segments (Fig. 4.43c); no apical spurs on hind tibiae; wings usually clear but may be dark or banded; proboscis shorter than head ....***Tabanus* spp. (Tabanidae)**

13 Small, hairy, moth-like flies; numerous parallel wing veins running to the margin; wings pointed at the tip .... **Psychodidae 14**

    Not like this.. **15**

14 Palps five-segmented; biting mouthparts at least as long as head; antennal segments almost cylindrical; two longitudinal wing veins between radial and medial forks (Fig. 4.51) ....**Phlebotominae**

15 Ten or more veins reaching the wing margin.......................... **16**

    Not more than eight veins reaching the wing margin........ **17**

16 Wing veins and hind margins of wings covered by scales (Fig. 4.52); conspicuous forward-projecting proboscis ....**Culicidae**

17 Wings broad; wing veins thickened at the anterior margin; antennae not hairy; thorax humped; antennae usually with 11 rounded segments; palps long with five segments extending beyond the proboscis; first abdominal tergite with a prominent basal scale fringed with hairs (Fig. 4.53) ....**Simuliidae**

    Wings not particularly broad, antennae hairy..................... **18**

18 Front legs often longer than others; median vein not forked (non-biting midges)...**Chironomidae**

    Front legs not longer than others; wings with median vein forked; antennae with 14–15 visible segments; palps with five segments; female mouthparts short; legs short and stout; two radial cells and cross vein r-m strongly angled in relation to median; at rest wings close flat over abdomen (Fig. 4.54) ....***Culicoides* spp. (Ceratopogonidae)**

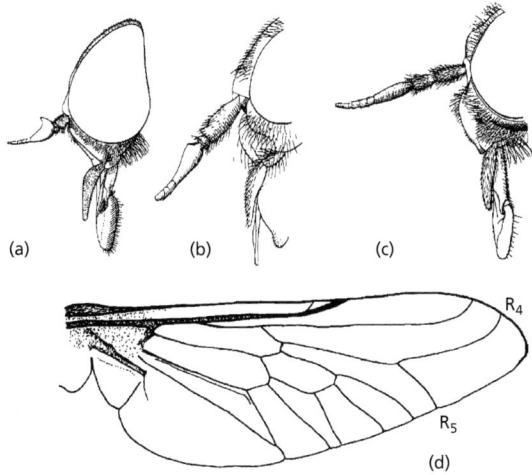

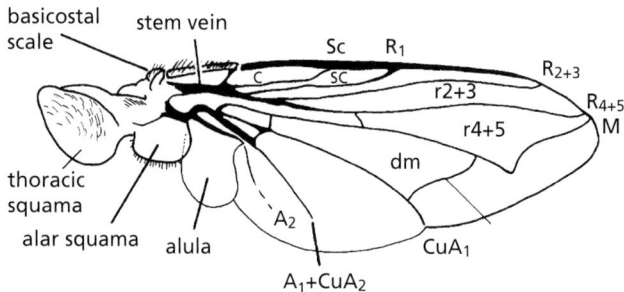

Fig. 4.46 The veins and cells of the wings of a typical calypterate dipteran, *Calliphora vicina*.

Fig. 4.43 Antennae of (a) *Chrysops*, (b) *Haematopota* and (c) *Tabanus*. (d) Wing venation of Tabanidae. (From Smart, 1943.)

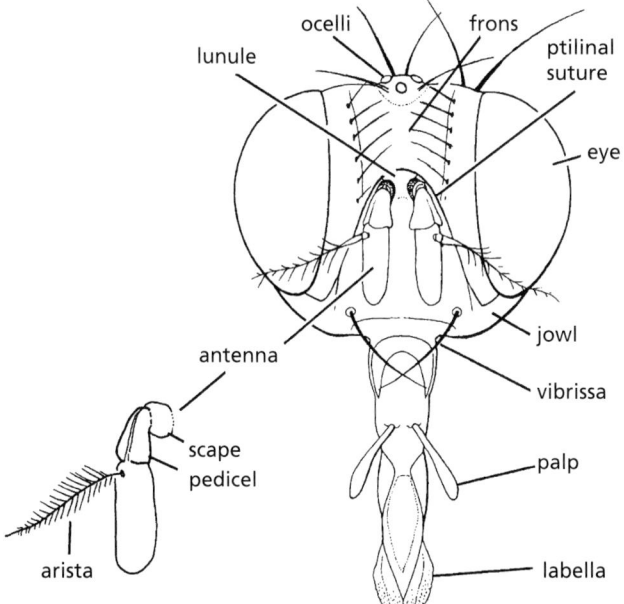

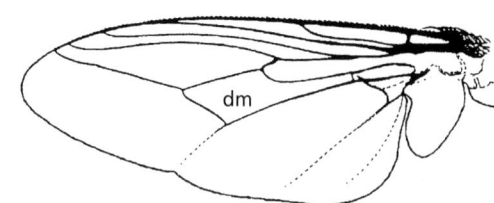

Fig. 4.47 Wing venation typical of species of *Glossina* showing the characteristic hatchet shape of the cell dm.

Fig. 4.44 The principal features of the dichoptic head of a typical adult calypterate dipteran (showing frons with a ptilinal suture). (Redrawn from Smart, 1943.)

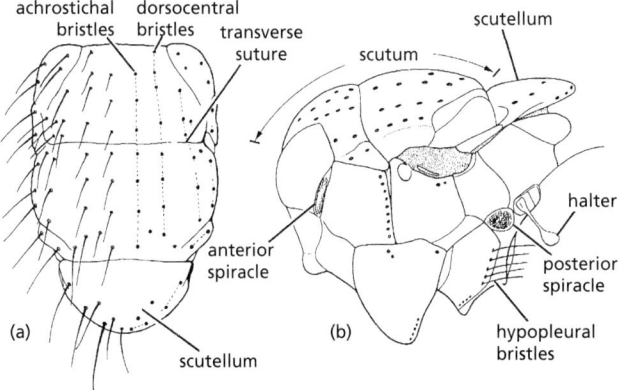

Fig. 4.45 The principal features of the generalised thorax of an adult calypterate dipteran: (a) dorsal view; (b) lateral view. (Redrawn from Smart, 1943.)

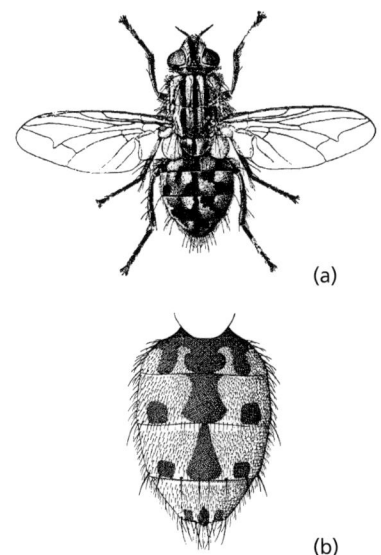

Fig. 4.48 (a) Adult of the flesh fly *Sarcophaga carnaria* (Castellani and Chalmers, 1910/Castellani). (b) *Wohlfahrtia magnifica*, abdomen of adult (from Smart, 1943).

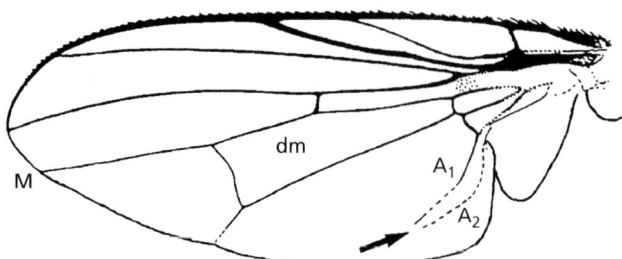

Fig. 4.49 Wing venation typical of species of *Fannia* showing the characteristic convergence of the anal veins.

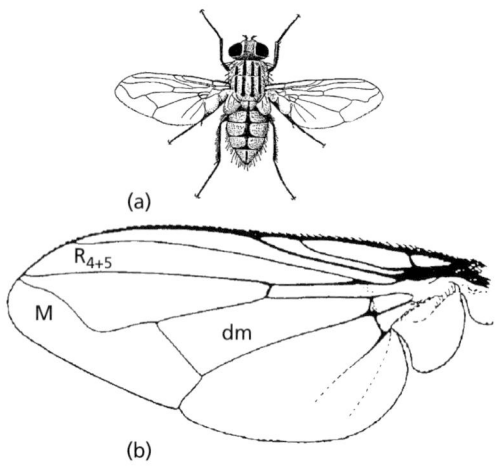

Fig. 4.50 (a) Female house fly, *Musca domestica*. (b) Wing venation typical of species of *Musca* showing the strongly bent vein M ending close to R_{4+5}. (Adapted from Smart, 1943.)

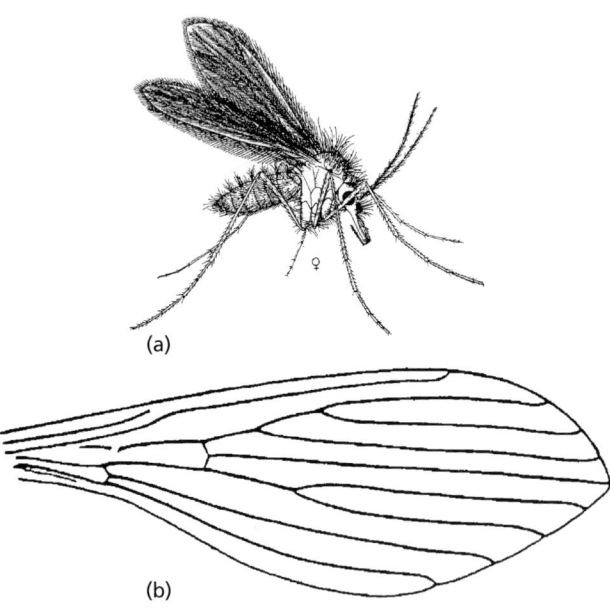

Fig. 4.51 (a) Adult female sand fly, *Phlebotomus papatasi*. (b) Wing venation typical of species of *Phlebotomus* (Psychodidae). (From Smart, 1943.)

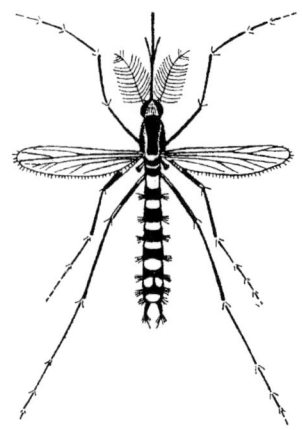

Fig. 4.52 *Aedes atropalpus*: adult. (From Eidmann and Kuhlhorn, 1970).

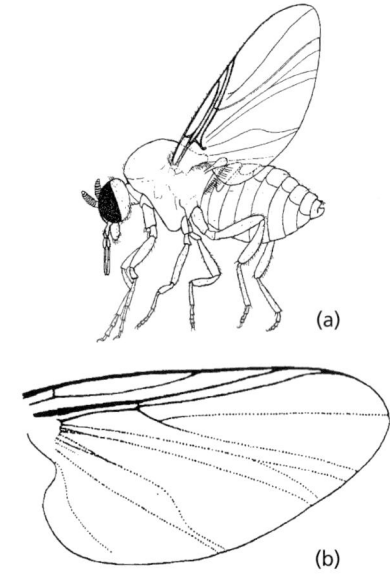

Fig. 4.53 (a) Adult female *Simulium*. (b) Wing venation typical of *Simulium* showing the large anal lobe and crowding of the veins towards the leading edge. (From Smart, 1943.)

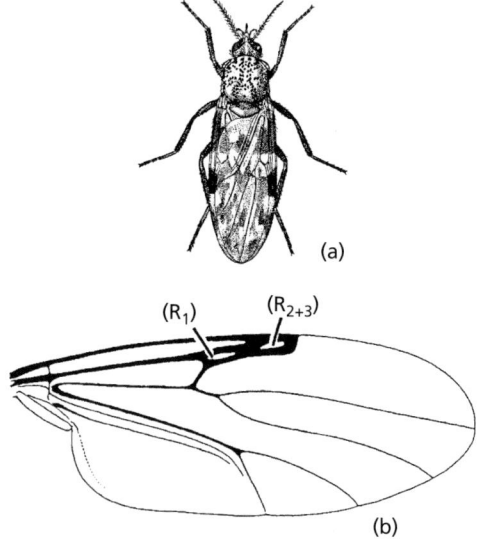

Fig. 4.54 (a) Adult female *Culicoides nebeculosus* at rest. (b) Wing venation typical of species of *Culicoides* showing the two elongate radial cells. (Edwards *et al.*, 1939/Smithsonian Libraries.)

Guide to third-stage larvae causing myiasis in domestic animals

The guide presented below applies specifically to recognition of the third-stage larva. This stage is usually of the longest duration and since the larvae are approaching their maximum size or are beginning to leave the host, is usually the stage when they are most commonly observed. It should be noted that because the external structure of larvae may change over the course of their growth and development, first- and second-stage larvae may not key out appropriately.

1 Body more or less cylindrical; no obvious head capsule ....**Diptera (Muscomorpha) 2**

Fly larvae with an obvious head capsule; rarely found associated with livestock myiasis.....................................**other Diptera**

2 Body with obvious fleshy processes..**3**

Body without fleshy processes..**4**

3 Third-stage larvae large, up to 18 mm long; large, pointed fleshy processes laterally and dorsally (Fig. 4.55); posterior spiracular plate without button (Fig. 4.56); peritremes with a narrow opening; in carrion or secondarily in cutaneous myiasis of sheep; distribution: Afro-tropical, Australasian and Oriental

..............***Chrysomya albiceps*** and ***C. rufifacies*** **(Calliphoridae)**

Third-stage larvae 7–8 mm in length; body flattened, with long processes (Fig. 4.57); posterior spiracles on short stalks on terminal segment; uncommon in livestock myiasis

....**Fanniidae**

4 Posterior spiracles with a large number of small pores or many short intertwining slits arranged radially on each spiracular plate (e.g. Fig. 4.58) **5**

Posterior spiracles with up to three straight or curved slits (e.g. Fig. 4.59)...**7**

5 Mouth hooks well developed, strongly hooked..........................**6**

Mouth hooks poorly developed; third-stage larvae 20–30 mm in length (Fig. 4.60); in subcutaneous swellings or warbles; on cattle or deer.............***Hypoderma*** **spp. (Oestridae)**

6 Body with weak spines in distinct regions; posterior spiracles with many small pores (Fig. 4.58); in nasal myiasis of sheep; distribution worldwide ....***Oestrus ovis*** **(Oestridae)**

Body spines stronger and more evenly distributed; posterior spiracles with many small slits; found in dermal

myiases; in rodents and rabbits; distribution: New World .... ***Cuterebra*** **spp. (Oestridae)**

7 Posterior spiracles with straight or arced slits **8**

Posterior spiracles with serpentine slits; anterior spiracles in the form of membranous stalks bearing finger-like processes; body with obvious spines; furuncular myiases of dogs, rats and humans; distribution: sub-Saharan Africa

....***Cordylobia*** **spp. (Calliphoridae)**

Posterior spiracles with serpentine slits (Fig. 4.61); anterior spiracles not as above; uncommon in livestock myiasis

....**Muscidae**

8 Posterior spiracles sunk in a deep cavity which may conceal them (Fig. 4.62); slits more or less parallel...............................**9**

Posterior spiracles visible, either exposed on surface or set in a ring of tubercles **11**

9 Body with strong spines **10**

Body with short spines; obligate agent of cutaneous myiasis; primarily in sheep and goats; distribution worldwide

....***Wohlfahrtia*** **spp. (Sarcophagidae)**

10 Posterior spiracles with slits bowed outwards at the middle; body oval; found in the pharynx or digestive tract of equids......

....***Gasterophilus*** **spp. (Oestridae)**

Posterior spiracles with slits relatively straight; body enlarged anteriorly and tapering posteriorly (Fig. 4.63); distribution: New World ....***Dermatobia hominis*** **(Oestridae)**

11 Posterior spiracles with straight slits...**12**

Posterior spiracles with arced slits; uncommon in livestock myiasis ....**Muscidae**

12 Posterior spiracles with a fully closed peritremal ring (Fig. 4.64) **13**

Posterior spiracles with an open peritremal ring (Fig. 4.65) **14**

13 Cephalopharyngeal skeleton with pigmented accessory oral sclerite (Fig. 4.66b); distribution worldwide

....***Calliphora*** **spp. (Calliphoridae)**

Cephalopharyngeal skeleton without pigmented accessory oral sclerite (Fig. 4.66a); distribution worldwide

....***Lucilia*** **spp. (Calliphoridae)**

14 Tracheal trunks leading from posterior spiracles without dark pigmentation..**15**

Tracheal trunks leading from posterior spiracles with conspicuous dark pigmentation extending forwards as far as segment 9 or 10 (Fig. 4.65); obligate primary agent of traumatic

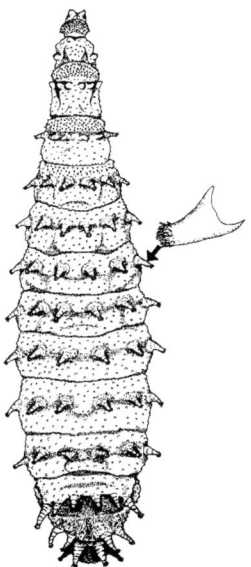

Fig. 4.55 Third-stage larva of *Chrysomya albiceps*. (Zumpt, 1965/Butterworths.)

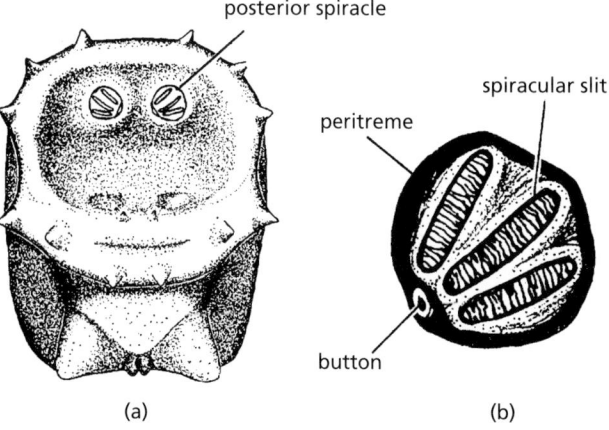

posterior spiracle

spiracular slit

peritreme

button

(a)   (b)

Fig. 4.56 (a) Posterior view of the last abdominal segment of *Calliphora vicina* and (b) detail of the posterior spiracles of a third-stage larva of *Calliphora vomitoria*. (Zumpt, 1965/Butterworths.)

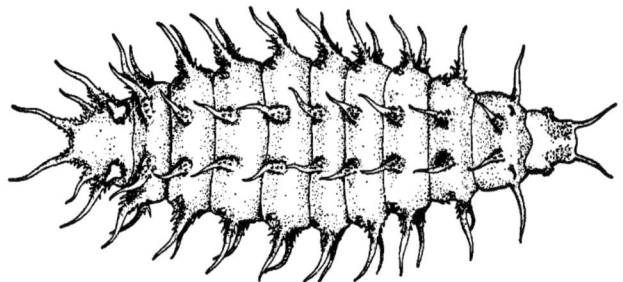

Fig. 4.57 Third-stage larva of the lesser house fly, *Fannia canicularis*. (Zumpt, 1965/Butterworths.)

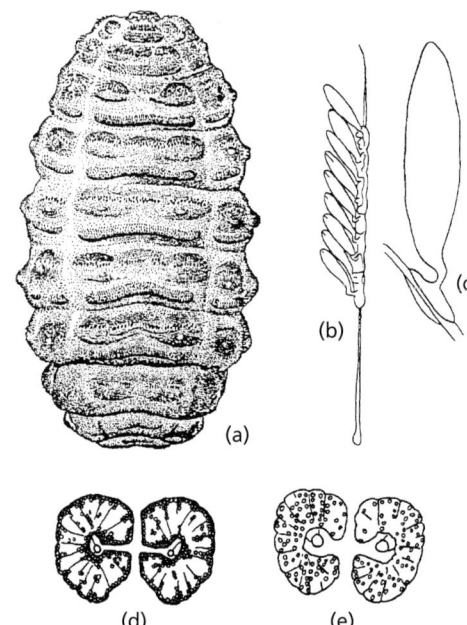

Fig. 4.60 (a) Third-stage larva of *Hypoderma bovis*. Eggs of (b) *H. lineatum* and (c) *H. bovis*. Posterior spiracles of third-stage larvae of (d) *H. bovis* and (e) *H. lineatum*. (From Zumpt, 1965/Butterworths.)

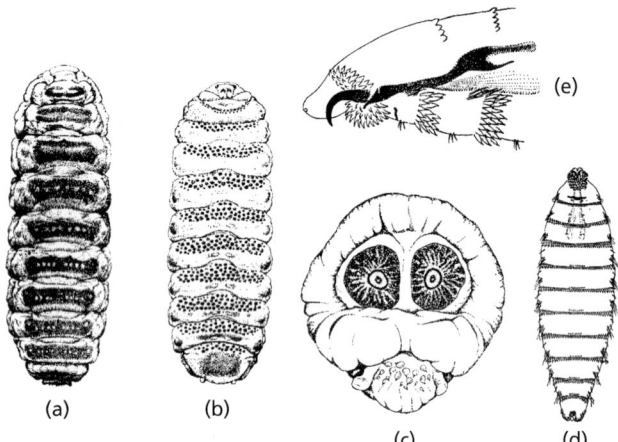

Fig. 4.58 *Oestrus ovis*: (a) ventral and (b) dorsal view of third-stage larva; (c) posterior view of third-stage larva; (d) first-stage larva; (e) mouthparts of first-stage larva in lateral view. (Zumpt, 1965/Butterworths.)

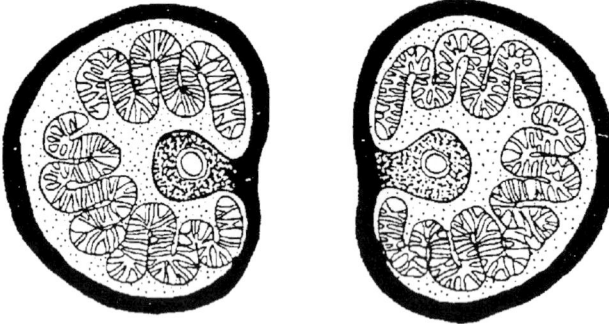

Fig. 4.61 Posterior spiracles of a third-stage larva of the house fly, *Musca domestica*. (Adapted from Smart, 1943.)

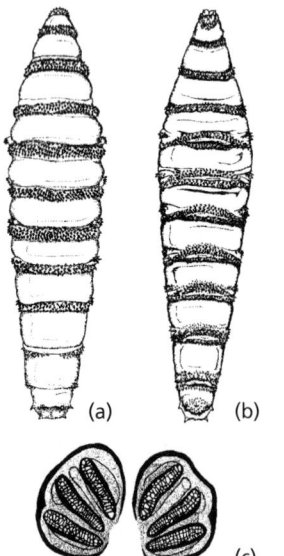

Fig. 4.59 Third-stage larvae of *Chrysomya bezziana*: (a) dorsal view, (b) ventral view and (c) posterior spiracles. (Zumpt, 1965/Butterworths.)

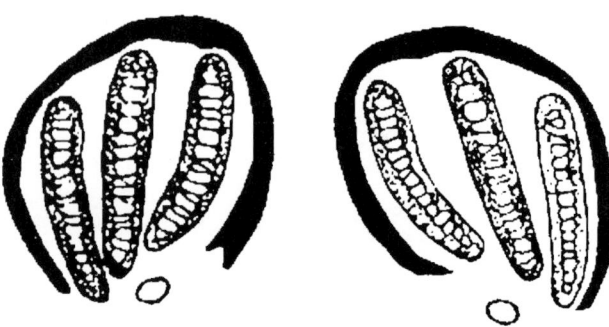

Fig. 4.62 *Wohlfahrtia magnifica*: posterior spiracles deeply sunk in a cavity.

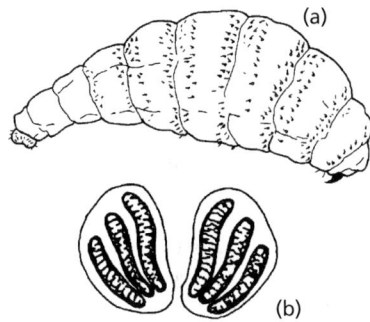

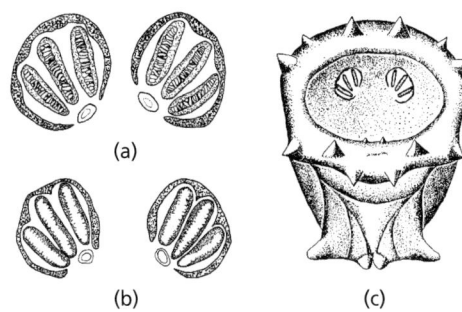

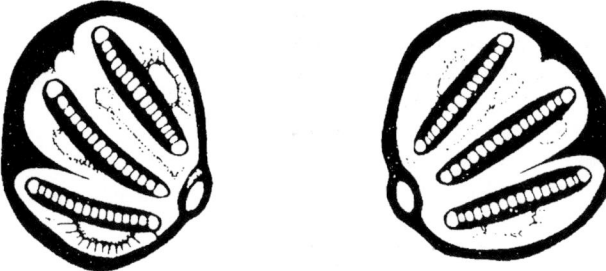

Fig. 4.63 *Dermatobia hominis*: (a) third-stage larva; (b) posterior spiracles.

Fig. 4.67 Posterior spiracles of third-stage larvae of (a) *Protophormia terraenovae* and (b) *Phormia regina*. (c) Tubercles on the posterior face of the last segment of third-stage *Protophormia terraenovae*. (Zumpt, 1965/Butterworths.)

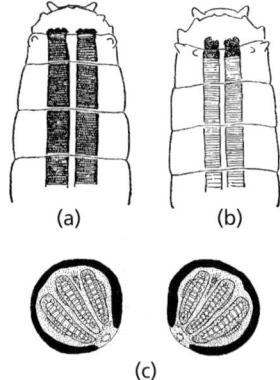

Fig. 4.64 *Lucilia sericata*: posterior peritremes. (Zumpt, 1965/Butterworths.)

livestock myiasis; distribution: Neotropical and Nearctic
.... ***Cochliomyia hominivorax* (Calliphoridae)**

15 Posterior margin of segment 11 with dorsal spines................ **16**

Posterior margin of segment 11 without dorsal spines; a secondary facultative agent of cutaneous livestock myiasis; distribution: Neotropical and Nearctic
.... ***Cochliomyia macellaria* (Calliphoridae)**

16 Posterior spiracles with distinct button **18**

Posterior spiracles without distinct button **17**

17 Body without fleshy processes; segments with belts of strongly developed spines (Fig. 4.59); anterior spiracle with four to six branches; an obligate primary agent of cutaneous livestock myiasis; distribution: Afro-tropical and Oriental
.... ***Chrysomya bezziana* (Calliphoridae)**

Anterior spiracle with 11–13 branches; largely saprophagous; an occasional facultative ectoparasite causing cutaneous myiasis; distribution: Oriental and Australasian
.... ***Chrysomya megacephala* (Calliphoridae)**

18 Posterior margins of segment 10 with dorsal spines; length of the larger tubercles on upper margin of posterior face of terminal segment greater than half the width of a posterior spiracle (Fig. 4.67a,c); causes facultative cutaneous myiasis of cattle, sheep and reindeer; distribution: northern Holarctic
.... ***Protophormia terraenovae* (Calliphoridae)**

Posterior margins of segment 10 without dorsal spines; length of the larger tubercles on upper margin of posterior face of terminal segment less than half the width of a posterior spiracle (Fig. 4.67b); distribution: Holarctic
.... ***Phormia regina* (Calliphoridae)**

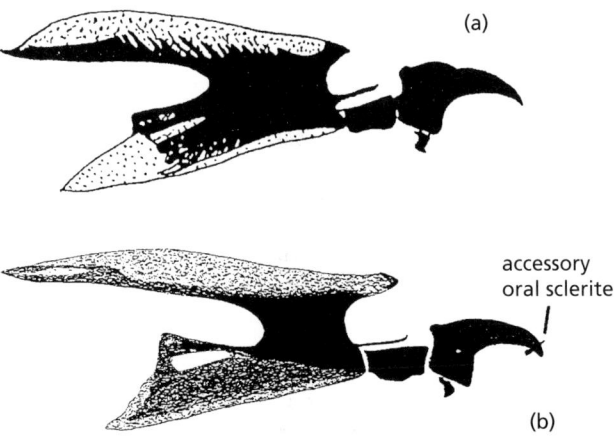

Fig. 4.65 (a) Pigmented dorsal tracheal trunks of *Cochliomyia hominivorax*. (b) Tracheal trunks and (c) posterior spiracles of *Cochliomyia macellaria*. (Zumpt, 1965/Butterworths.)

Guide to the adult Diptera causing myiasis in domestic animals

1 Insects with one pair of wings on the mesothorax and a pair of club-like halteres on the metathorax (Fig. 4.45); antennae composed of three segments, third segment usually with an arista (Fig. 4.44); foot with two pads; frons with ptilinal suture; second antennal segment usually with a groove; thoracic transverse suture strong; thoracic squamae usually well developed (Fig. 4.46)... **Calyptratae (Diptera) 2**

2 Mouthparts small, usually functionless; head bulbous; antennae small; flies more or less covered with soft hair.................... **3**

Mouthparts usually well developed; antennae not small; flies with strong bristles; hypopleural bristles present (Fig. 4.45); postscutellum weak or absent... **7**

accessory oral sclerite

Fig. 4.66 Cephopharyngeal skeleton of (a) *Lucilia sericata* and (b) *Calliphora vicina*.

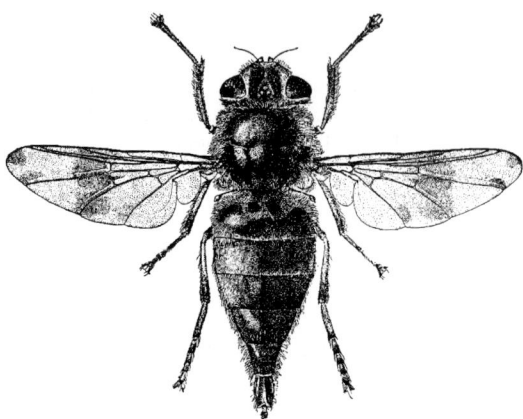

Fig. 4.68 Adult female *Gasterophilus intestinalis*. (Castellani and Chalmers, 1910/Castellani.)

3   Vein M bent towards vein R_{4+5} **4**

   Vein M not bent towards vein R_{4+5}; squamae small; crossvein dm-cu absent; ovipositor strongly developed in female (Fig. 4.68).................................. **Gasterophilus spp. (Oestridae)**

4   Sharp bend of vein M towards vein R_{4+5} but the two do not meet before the margin **5**

   Vein M joins vein R_{4+5} before the margin; vein dm-cu in line with deflection of vein M; vein A_1+CuA_2 does not reach the margin (Fig. 4.69); frons enlarged; frons, scutellum and dorsal thorax bear small wart-like protuberances; eyes small; abdomen brownish black.................................. **Oestrinae (Oestridae)**

5   Blue-black colour .... **Cuterebrinae**

   Not blue-black **6**

6   Vein A_1+CuA_2 reaches the margin; vein dm-cu in line with deflection of vein M (Fig. 4.70); hairy bee-like flies with a light–dark colour pattern; fan of yellow hypopleural hairs; palps absent .... **Hypodermatinae (Oestridae)**

7   Metallic, iridescent appearance (blue-black, violet-blue, green) **8**

   Dull grey appearance; three black stripes on the scutum; abdomen usually with chequered or spotted pattern **13**

   Flies of predominantly reddish-yellow or reddish-brown colour, not metallic; distribution: tropical Africa
   ....*Cordylobia* spp. (Calliphoridae)

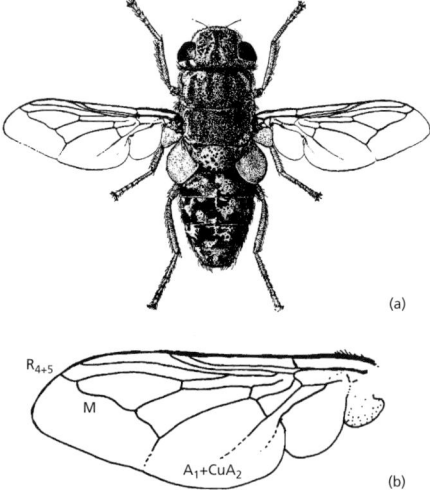

Fig. 4.69 (a) Adult female *Oestrus ovis* and (b) wing venation typical of *Oestrus* showing the strongly bent vein M joining R_{4+5} before the wing margin. (Castellani and Chalmers, 1910/Castellani.)

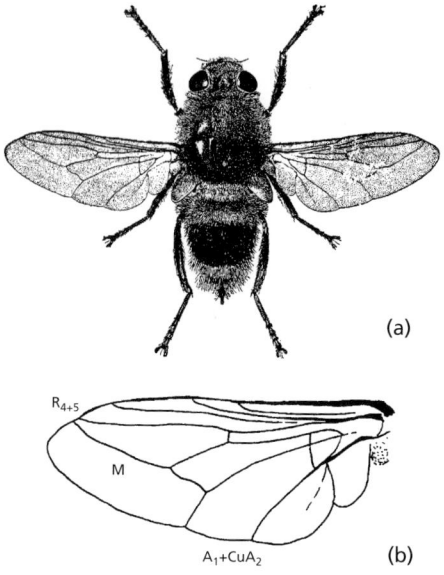

Fig. 4.70 (a) Adult female of *Hypoderma bovis*. (Castellani and Chalmers, 1910/Castellani.) (b) Wing venation typical of *Hypoderma* showing the strongly bent vein M not joining R_{4+5} before the wing margin and vein A_1+CuA_2 reaching the wing margin.

8   Wing with stem vein (base of R) entirely bare (Fig. 4.46)........ **9**

   Wing with stem vein with fine hairs along margin............. **10**

9   Flies with metallic green or coppery green thorax and abdomen (see Fig. 3.34b); thoracic squamae bare; found in cutaneous myiasis, particularly of sheep; distribution worldwide
   ....*Lucilia* spp. (Calliphoridae)

   Flies with black-blue thorax and blue or brown abdomen (see Fig. 3.34a); thoracic squamae with long dark hair on upper surface; may be secondary invaders of cutaneous myiasis; distribution worldwide .... **Calliphora spp. (Calliphoridae)**

10 Head with almost entirely black ground colour and black hair; thoracic squamae bare; alar squamae hairy on outer half or dorsal surface **12**

   Head with ground colour of at least lower half entirely or mainly orange or orange-red and with white, yellow or orange hair; thoracic squamae bare on dorsal surface **11**

11 Thoracic squamae hairy on whole dorsal surface; scutum of thorax without bold black stripes; distribution: Afro-tropical, Oriental, Australasian, southern Palaearctic
   .... **Chrysomya spp. (Calliphoridae)**

   Thoracic squamae hairy only at the base, usually concealed by the alar squamae; scutum of thorax with three bold black stripes (Fig. 3.34d); distribution: Nearctic and Neotropical
   .... **Cochliomyia spp. (Calliphoridae)**

12 Thorax with anterior spiracle black or reddish-brown; alar squamae with obvious dark hair dorsally; distribution: Palaearctic and Nearctic only
   .... **Protophormia spp. (Calliphoridae)**

   Thorax with anterior spiracle yellow or orange; thoracic squamae with white-yellow hair dorsally (Fig. 3.34c); distribution: Palaearctic and Nearctic only
   ....*Phormia* spp. (Calliphoridae)

13 Arista almost bare; abdomen with pattern of black spots (Fig. 4.48b) .... **Wohlfahrtia spp. (Sarcophagidae)**

   Arista with long and conspicuous hairs, at least on the basal half; abdomen with dark and light chequered pattern (Fig. 4.48a) .... **Sarcophaga spp. (Sarcophagidae)**

LICE AND FLEAS

The detection of small ectoparasites such as lice and fleas depends on close examination; in the case of lice, the eggs, commonly known as 'Nits', may also be found attached to the hair or feathers. Fleas may be more difficult to detect, but the finding of flea faeces in the coat, which appear as small dark pieces of grit and which, on contact with moist cottonwool or tissue, produce a red coloration due to ingested blood, allow confirmation of infestation. Collection may be straightforward as in the case of many lice, which may be brushed from the coat or removed by clipping hairs or feathers. Fleas may be removed by combing or brushing the coat. Alternatively, in the case of small animals, the parasites may be readily recovered if the host is placed on a sheet of paper or plastic before being sprayed with an insecticide.

The gross characteristics of biting and sucking lice and a key to the fleas commonly found on domestic animals are described in the following sections.

Guide to the recognition of common lice of veterinary importance

The identification of lice is complex and the features used to describe many genera are obscure. However, because lice in general are highly host specific, in many cases information relating to the species of host and the site of infestation will provide a reliable initial guide to identification. The various species of lice are usually found in all geographical regions of the world in which their host occurs.

1 Head broad, equal or almost equal in width to abdomen........ **2**
   Head elongated, much narrower than abdomen............... **12**
2 Antennae hidden in antennal grooves; antennae four-segmented; maxillary palps present...................... **Amblycera 3**
   Antennae not hidden in grooves; antennae three- to five-segmented; maxillary palps absent .... **Ischnocera 6**
3 On birds.. **4**
   On mammals.. **5**
4 Small lice, adults about 2 mm in length; abdomen with sparse covering of medium-length setae (Fig. 4.71); found on thigh or breast feathers; on birds, especially poultry
   .... *Menopon* **spp. (Menoponidae)**
   Large lice, adults about 3.5 mm in length; abdomen with dense covering of medium-length setae (Fig. 4.72); found on the breast, thighs and around vent; on birds, especially poultry
   .... *Menacanthus* **spp. (Menoponidae)**
5 On guinea pigs; oval abdomen, broad in middle; six pairs of abdominal spiracles are located ventrolaterally within poorly defined spiraclar plates (Fig. 4.73)
   ....*Gyropus* **spp. (Gyropidae)**

On guinea pigs; slender body, with sides of the abdomen parallel; five pairs of abdominal spiracles located ventrally within distinct sclerotised spiraclar plates (Fig. 4.74)
....*Gliricola* **spp. (Gyropidae)**
On dogs; relatively large, adults about 3 mm in length; abdomen with a dense covering of thick, medium and long setae (Fig. 4.75)...................................... *Heterodoxus* **spp. (Boopidae)**
6 On birds; antennae five-segmented; tarsi with paired claws
   .... **Philopteridae 7**
   On mammals; antennae three-segmented; tarsi with single claws .... **Trichodectidae 10**
7 Hindlegs similar in length to first two pairs **8**
   Hindlegs at least twice as long as first two pairs; body long and narrow; head with small narrow projections in front of antennae; first segment of antennae considerably longer than following four segments (Fig. 4.76); on poultry; distribution, worldwide .... *Lipeurus* **spp. (Philopteridae)**
8 Three long bristles projecting from each side of the dorsal surface of the head; rounded body; adult about 2 mm in length (Fig. 4.77); on poultry
   .... *Cuclotogaster* **spp. (Philopteridae)**
   Two long bristles projecting from each side of the dorsal surface of the head **9**
9 Head with prominent angles and a distinct hollow margin posterior to the antennae; adult about 5 mm in length (Fig. 4.78); on poultry.................................... *Goniodes* **spp. (Philopteridae)**
   Head lacking prominent angles; adult about 2 mm in length (Fig. 4.79); on poultry..................... *Goniocotes* **(Philopteridae)**
10 Head rounded anteriorly **11**
   Head sharply angled anteriorly; legs small; abdomen smooth, with only three pairs of spiracles (Fig. 4.80); on cats
   .... *Felicola* **spp. (Trichodectidae)**
11 Setae of abdomen large and thick (Fig. 4.81); on dogs
   .... *Trichodectes* **spp. (Trichodectidae)**
   Setae of abdomen small or of medium length (Fig. 4.82); on mammals .... *Bovicola* **spp. (Trichodectidae)**
12 Distinct ocular points present behind the antennae; all legs of similar size; adult up to 5 mm in length; distinct paratergal plates visible on abdominal segments; ventral surface of the thorax with a dark coloured plate (Fig. 4.83)
   .... *Haematopinus* **spp. (Haematopinidae)**
   No ocular points behind the antennae; forelegs small **13**
13 Two rows of ventral setae on each abdominal segment **14**
   One row of ventral setae on each abdominal segment; paratergal plates absent; spiracles on tubercles which protrude from the abdomen; distinct five-sided sternal plate on the ventral surface of the thorax (Fig. 4.84); on cattle
   .... *Solenopotes* **spp. (Linognathidae)**

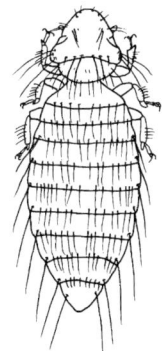

Fig. 4.71 Adult *Menopon gallinae* (dorsal view).

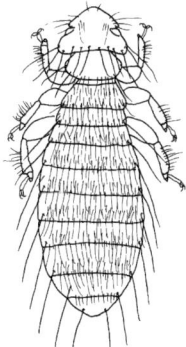

Fig. 4.72 Adult *Menacanthus stramineus* (dorsal view).

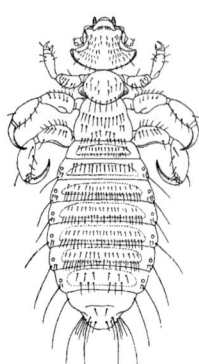

Fig. 4.73 Adult female *Gyropus ovalis*. (From Seguy, 1944.)

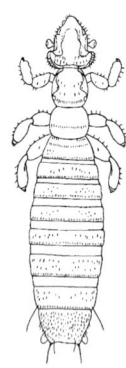

Fig. 4.74 Adult female *Gliricola porcelli*. (From Seguy, 1944.)

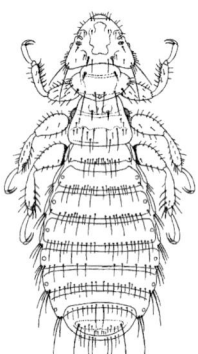

Fig. 4.75 Adult female *Heterodoxus* in ventral view. (From Seguy, 1944.)

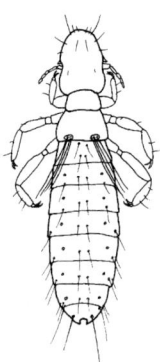

Fig. 4.76 Adult *Lipeurus caponis* (dorsal view).

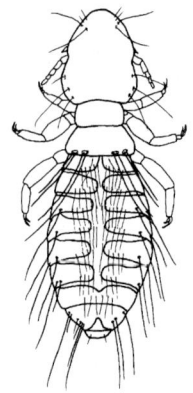

Fig. 4.77 Adult female *Cuclotogaster heterographus* (dorsal view).

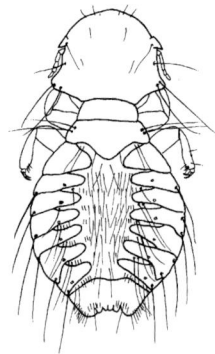

Fig. 4.78 Adult female *Goniodes dissimilis* (dorsal view).

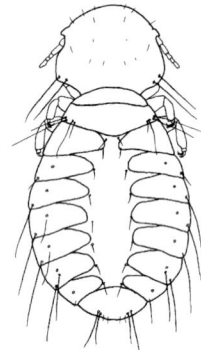

Fig. 4.79 Adult female *Goniocotes gallinae* (dorsal view).

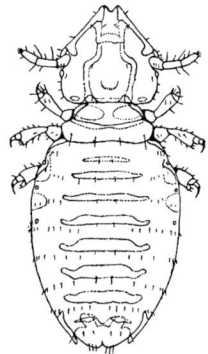

Fig. 4.80 Adult female *Felicola* in ventral view. (From Seguy, 1944.)

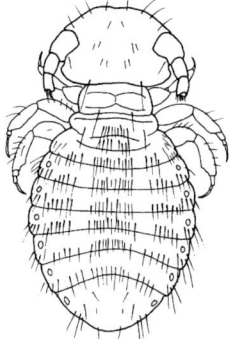

Fig. 4.81 Adult female *Trichodectes* in ventral view. (From Seguy, 1944.)

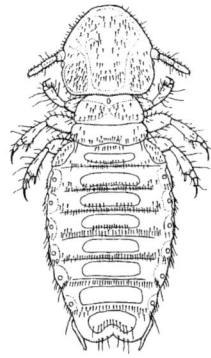

Fig. 4.82 Dorsal view of adult female *Bovicola*. (From Seguy, 1944.)

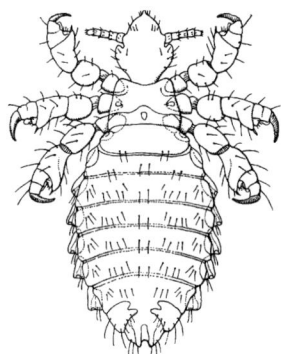

Fig. 4.83 Dorsal view of adult *Haematopinus*. (From Seguy, 1944.)

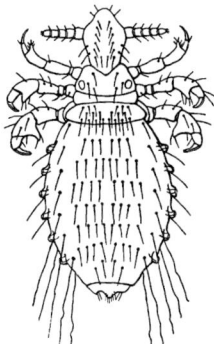

Fig. 4.84 Dorsal view of adult female *Solenopotes*. (From Seguy, 1944.)

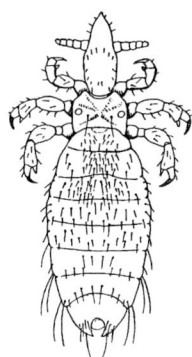

Fig. 4.85 Dorsal view of adult female *Linognathus*. (From Seguy, 1944.)

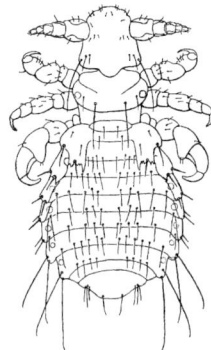

Fig. 4.86 Adult female *Polyplax* in dorsal view.

14 Paratergal plates absent; ventral sternal plate of thorax is narrow or absent (Fig. 4.85); on cattle, sheep, goats and dogs ....*Linognathus* **spp. (Linognathidae)**

Paratergal plates present; ovoid sternal plate on the ventral surface of the thorax (Fig. 4.86); on rodents .... *Polyplax* **spp. (Polyplacidae)**

Guide to the flea species of veterinary importance

The physical differences between flea species and even between families tend to be small and there may be considerable variation between individuals within a species. Identification is therefore often difficult. The following is a general diagnostic guide to the adults of the most common species of veterinary importance found as parasites on domestic and companion animals.

1 Ctenidia absent 2
    Ctenidium present, at least on the pronotum........................ 4
2 Pleural ridge absent.. 3
    Pleural ridge present ....*Xenopsylla cheopis*
3 Frons sharply angled (Fig. 4.87); head behind the antenna with two setae and, in the female, usually with a well-developed occipital lobe; the maxillary laciniae are broad and coarsely serrated; adult females embedded in the skin in aggregations on bare areas; found on birds, especially poultry, also on cats, dogs, rabbits and humans............................ *Echidnophaga gallinacea*
    Frons smoothly rounded; head behind antennae with only one strong seta; conspicuous ocular seta below the eye; a single, much reduced spine on the genal margin (Fig. 4.88); on pigs, badgers, humans... *Pulex irritans*

4 Genal ctenidium present **5**

 Genal ctenidium absent; pronotal ctenidium with 18–20 spines; head with a row of three strong setae below the eye (Fig. 4.89); frontal tubercle on head of both sexes conspicuous; three to four conspicuous bristles on the inner surface of the hind femur; on rodents..............................***Nosopsyllus fasciatus***

 Genal ctenidium absent; pronotal ctenidium with more than 24 spines; head with a row of three strong setae below the eye (Fig. 4.90); on poultry.....................................***Ceratophyllus* spp.**

5 Genal ctenidium formed of eight or nine spines oriented vertically **6**

 Genal ctenidium with four to six oblique spines; frontal tubercle conspicuous on head of both sexes (Fig. 4.91); on rabbits .... ***Spilopsyllus cuniculi***

 Genal ctenidium with three very short oblique spines; single vestigial spine on the genal lobe; single short pronotal spine (Fig. 4.92); on hedgehogs, dogs and cats

 .... ***Archaeopsylla erinacei***

6 Head strongly convex anteriorly in both sexes and not noticeably elongate; hind tibia with eight seta-bearing notches along the dorsal margin (Fig. 4.93); on cats and dogs

 ....***Ctenocephalides canis***

 Head not strongly convex anteriorly and distinctly elongate, especially in the female; hind tibia with six seta-bearing notches along the dorsal margin (Fig. 4.94); on cats and dogs

 ....***Ctenocephalides felis***

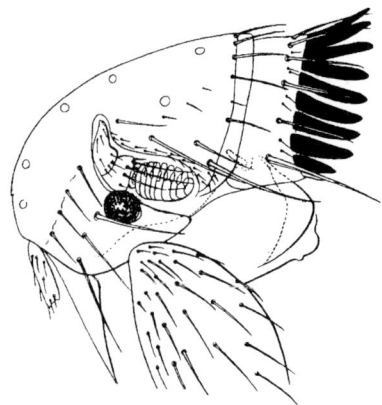

Fig. 4.89 The northern rat flea, *Nosopsyllus fasciatus*: male head. (Adapted from Smart, 1943.)

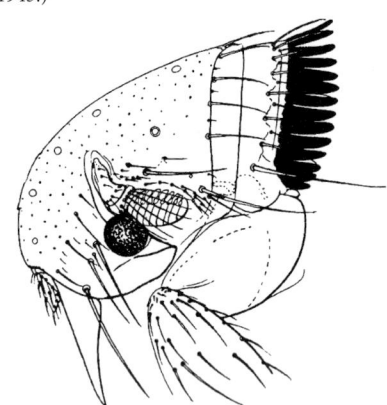

Fig. 4.90 Head and pronotum of a female chicken flea, *Ceratophyllus*. (Adapted from Smart, 1943.)

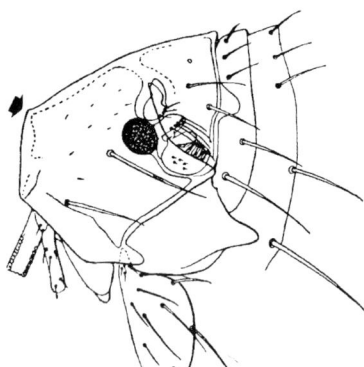

Fig. 4.87 The sticktight flea, *Echidnophaga gallinacea*: female head and thorax (arrow marks angulation of the frons). (Adapted from Smart, 1943.)

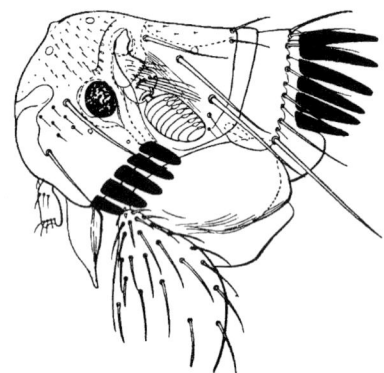

Fig. 4.91 Head and pronotum of the rabbit flea, *Spilopsyllus cuniculi*.

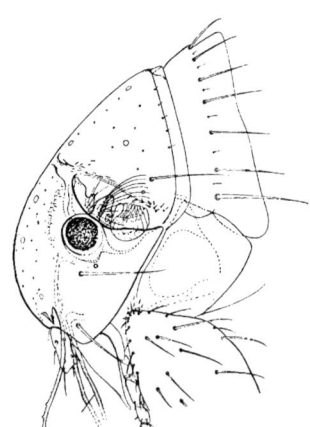

Fig. 4.88 The human flea, *Pulex irritans*: male head and pronotum. (Adapted from Smart, 1943.)

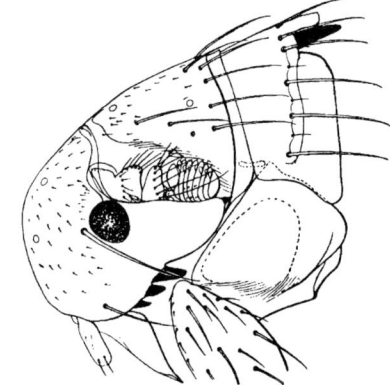

Fig. 4.92 The hedgehog flea, *Archaeopsylla erinacei*: female head. (Adapted from Smart, 1943.)

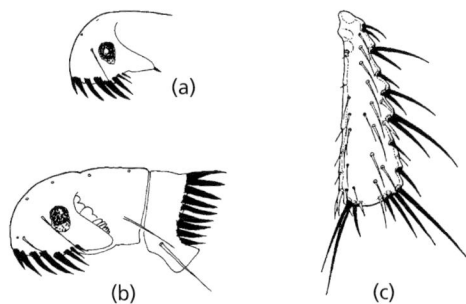

Fig. 4.93 The dog flea, *Ctenocephalides canis*: (a) front of male head; (b) female head and pronotum; (c) hind tibia.

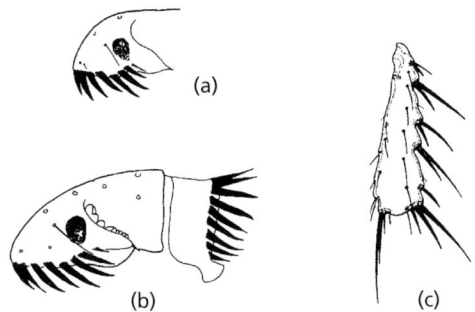

Fig. 4.94 The cat flea, *Ctenocephalides felis felis*: (a) front of male head; (b) female head and pronotum; (c) hind tibia.

TICKS AND MITES

Hypostome of the gnathosoma without backwardly directed barbs. Stigmata present or absent; when present not opening on stigmatal plates; if stigmata lateral to coxae 2 and 3 then with peritremes. Tarsi of first pair of legs without sensory pit............................. **Mites**

　Hypostome of the gnathosoma with backwardly directed barbs. Stigmatal shields present behind coxae of the fourth pair of legs or laterally above the coxae of legs 2 or 3; stigmata without peritremes. Tarsi of the first pair of legs with a sensory pit......................... **Ticks**

Ticks

Feeding or engorged ticks of all three stages (larva, nymph, adult) can be collected by carefully removing them from the host. Care should be taken in their removal since their mouthparts are usually firmly embedded in the skin. Ideally use a tick removal tool. Alternatively, a useful method is to grip the gnathosoma firmly but lightly, by means of forceps, turn the tick over on to its dorsal surface and then pull out sharply, perpendicularly away from the skin. Do not crush the body of the tick. The tick may be persuaded to withdraw its mouthparts if a piece of cotton wool soaked in anaesthetic is placed around it or, alternatively, if something hot is held near its body. On sheep or cattle, the ticks are often found in the axillary and inguinal regions and on the neck or brisket.

　One of the simplest methods used to recover ticks from pasture is to drag a blanket or sheet over the ground to which the unfed ticks attach, as they would to a host. Every 10 m or so, the drag should be turned over and examined for ticks. A white or cream-coloured drag is preferred to a darker colour, as it is easier to find the ticks on the material. Ticks to be kept alive for rearing should be confined in a moisture-saturated atmosphere. A small plug of damp cotton wool, placed in a vial with the ticks, serves this purpose.

Guide to the ticks of veterinary importance

Specific identification of the large variety of tick species that parasitise domestic animals is a specialised task. The guide presented here and the species descriptions given in the following pages are intended as a general guide to the ticks of veterinary interest only. Specialist texts are required for more detailed descriptions of species and their immature stages.

1　Gnathosoma projecting anteriorly and visible when specimen seen from above; scutum present, covering the dorsal surface completely (male) or the anterior portion only (female); stigmatal plates large, situated posteriorly to the coxae of the fourth pair of legs (Figs 4.95 and 4.96) .... **Ixodidae 2**

　Gnathosoma ventral and not visible when adult is viewed from above; scutum absent; dorsal integument leathery; stigmatal plates small, situated anteriorly to the coxae of the fourth pair of legs; eyes, if present, in lateral folds............**Argasidae 11**

2　Anal groove surrounding the anus distinct, both anteriorly and posteriorly (Figs 4.95 and 4.96) .... *Ixodes*

　Anal groove entirely posterior to the anus............................. **3**

3　Eyes absent **4**

　Eyes present.. **5**

4　Palps short and broad, about twice as wide as segment 2 with obvious outer angulation at the base (Figs 4.97g and 4.98) ....*Haemaphysalis*

5　Palps wider than long or, at most, only slightly longer than their width **6**

　Palps much longer than wide.. **10**

6　Basis capituli usually hexagonal dorsally (Fig. 4.97); medium-sized or small ticks, usually without colour patterns................ **7**

　Basis capituli rectangular dorsally (Fig. 4.97c); large ticks with definite colour patterns (Fig. 4.99)................*Dermacentor*

7　Festoons absent; stigmatal plates round or oval; anal groove faint or obsolete **8**

　Festoons present; stigmatal plate with a tail-like protrusion; anal groove distinct.. **9**

8　Palps with dorsal and lateral ridges; male with normal legs ....*Rhipicephalus (Boophilus)*

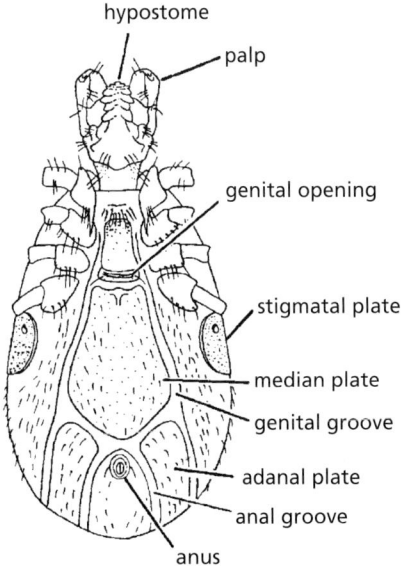

Fig. 4.95 Ventral view of a generalised male ixodid tick.

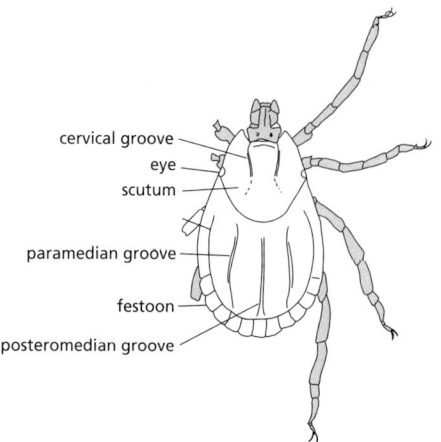

Fig. 4.96 Dorsal view of a generalised female ixodid tick.

9 Basis capituli without pronounced lateral angles (Fig. 4.97f); males with ventral plates; males with coxae of fourth pair of legs normal (Fig. 4.100d) .... ***Rhipicephalus***

10 Palps with second segment less than twice as long as third segment (Fig. 4.97b); scutum without pattern .... ***Hyalomma***

Palps with second segment more than twice as long as third segment (Fig. 4.97d); scutum with pattern; male without ventral plates .... ***Amblyomma***

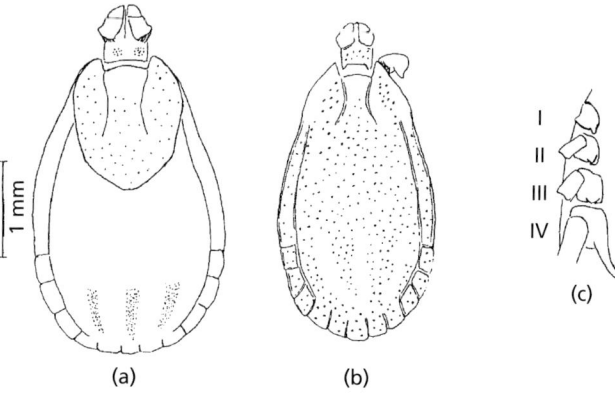

Fig. 4.98 Dorsal view of the gnathosoma and scutum of adult (a) female and (b) male *Haemaphysalis punctata*. (c) Ventral view of the coxae of an adult male. (Arthur, 1962/Springer Nature.)

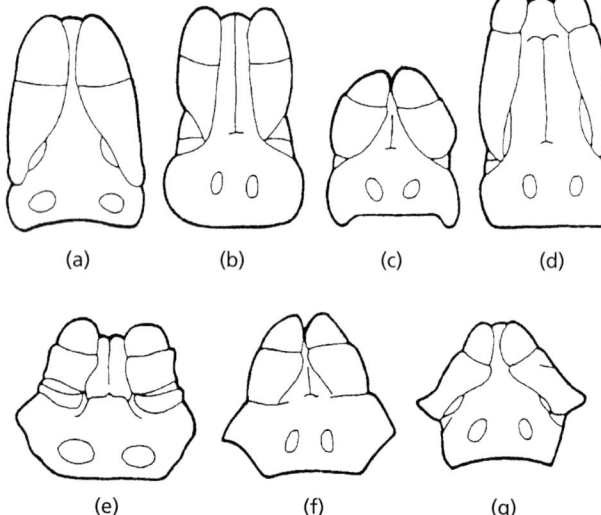

Fig. 4.97 Diagrammatic dorsal view of the gnathosoma of ixodid ticks: (a) *Ixodes*; (b) *Hyalomma*; (c) *Dermacentor*; (d) *Amblyomma*; (e) *Rhipicephalus* (*Boophilus*); (f) *Rhiphicephalus*; (g) *Haemaphysalis*. (From Smart, 1943.)

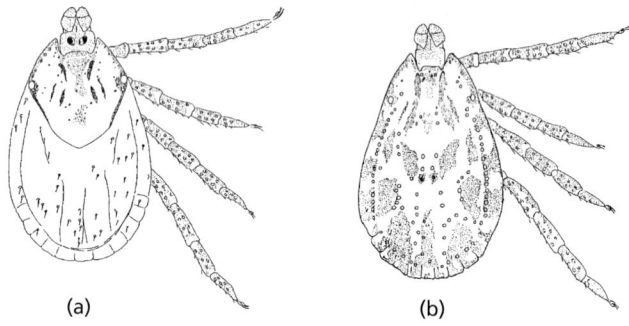

Fig. 4.99 Adult *Dermacentor andersoni*: (a) dorsal view of female; (b) dorsal view of male. (Arthur, 1962/Springer Nature.)

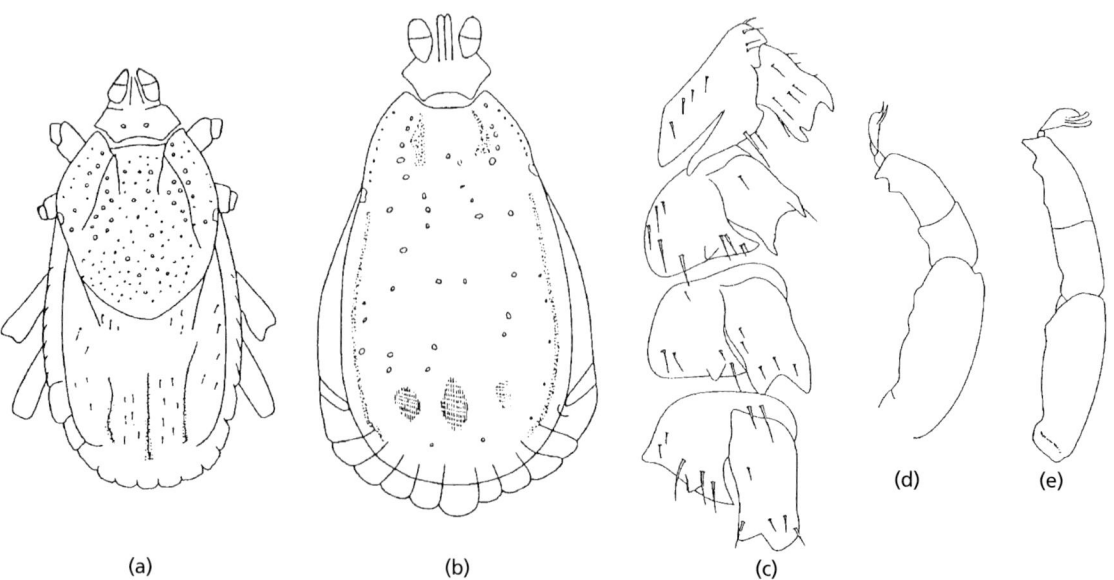

Fig. 4.100 Dorsal view of the gnathosoma and scutum of adult (a) female and (b) male *Rhipicephalus sanguineus*. (c) Ventral view of the coxae and trochanters of an adult male. (d,e) Tarsi and metatarsi of the fourth pair of legs of adult (d) male and (e) female. (Arthur, 1962/Springer Nature.)

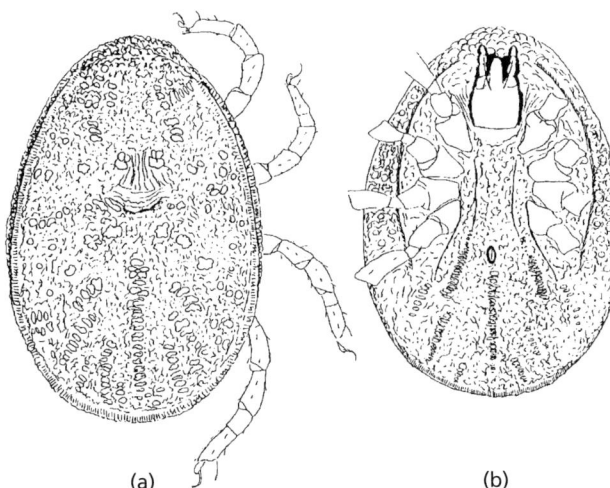

Fig. 4.101 Female *Argas reflexus*: (a) dorsal and (b) ventral view. (Arthur, 1962/Springer Nature.)

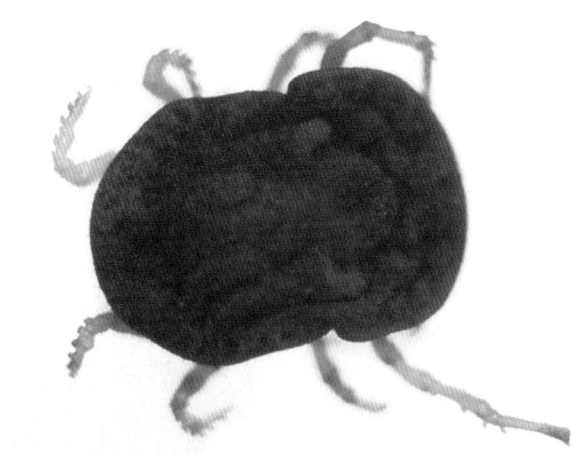

Fig. 4.102 *Ornithodoros* dorsal view.

11 Body periphery undifferentiated, without a definite suture distinguishing the dorsal from ventral surface............................ **12**
    Body surface flattened and usually structurally different from the dorsal surface, with a definite suture distinguishing dorsal and ventral surface (Fig. 4.101) .... ***Argas***
12 Adult integument is granular; hypostome vestigial; nymphal integument spiny; hypostome well developed.............. ***Otobius***
    Adult and nymph integument leathery (Fig. 4.102); hypostome well developed.. ***Ornithodoros***

Mites

Free-living mites often found on animal hair usually originate from food or dust from animal accommodation. The mites can be seen under the microscope and can be recovered by a suitable sieving technique as described for insects.

For parasitic mites present on the animal, visual examination of the hair, fleece or skin may reveal the larger mites such as *Psoroptes*, but in most cases it is necessary to take scrapings for examination in the laboratory. An indication of the presence of mites is the reaction

of the host to scratching or rubbing of the affected skin by the operator: it responds by nibbling the tongue or scratching itself.

Scrapings are taken from the affected areas. The area selected for scraping should be at the edge of a visible lesion and the hair over this area should be clipped away. The presence of unnecessary hair in the sample taken may be an encumbrance, but on occasions it may be useful to examine this for mites or other parasites. The area of skin selected should be the moist part or edge of the lesion. In sarcoptic mange, the scrapings should be taken from the edge of a hairless area or where pruritus or pimples are seen. A drop of lubricating oil such as liquid paraffin is placed on a microscope slide and a clean scalpel blade dipped in the oil before using it to scrape the surface of a fold of affected skin. Scraping should be continued until a slight amount of blood oozes from the skin surface and the material obtained then transferred to the oil on the slide. In animals suspected of chorioptic or psoroptic mange, a sharp scalpel should be used with the blade held at an acute angle, shaving rather than scraping off the outer epidermis together with the hair stumps. The specimen should be transferred or scraped directly into a small tube that can be securely stoppered or into a self-sealing polythene bag.

In the laboratory, scrapings are transferred to a slide, a coverslip then applied and the sample examined under magnification (×100). If during this initial examination no mites are detected, a further sample may be heated on a slide with a drop of 10% caustic potash. After allowing this preparation to clear for 5–10 minutes, it should be re-examined.

Some non-burrowing mites such as *Otodectes* and *Cheyletiella* can be found by close examination. For example, *Otodectes* may be seen either on examination of the external auditory canal using an auroscope or on microscopic examination of ear wax removed by means of a swab; likewise, rigorous brushing of the coat and subsequent microscopic examination of this material will usually confirm infection with *Cheyletiella*. In pustular demodectic mange, the mites are usually abundant and can be demonstrated on examination of the cheesy contents of an expressed or incised pustule. In the case of squamous lesions, a deep scraping is necessary.

Guide to the mite species and families of veterinary importance

The identification of mites can be difficult. However, since mites in general tend to be relatively host specific, a good first practical indication of the likely identity of any species in question can be the species of host and the location of the mite on that host. The following is a general guide to the adults of the most common species and genera of ectoparasitic mites likely to be encountered. It is important to note that this guide is not comprehensive and if in doubt more specialist keys should be used.

1 Stigmata absent posterior to the second pair of legs **2**
    Stigmata present as one lateral pair between the bases of legs II and IV . **3**
2 Legs without claws; palps with two segments; stigmata absent **14**
    Some or all legs with claws; palps with more than two segments; stigmata present or absent, when present they open on the gnathosoma or the anterior part of the idiosoma (Fig. 4.103) **20**
3 Genital plate rudimentary or absent.. **4**
    Genital plate well defined **5**

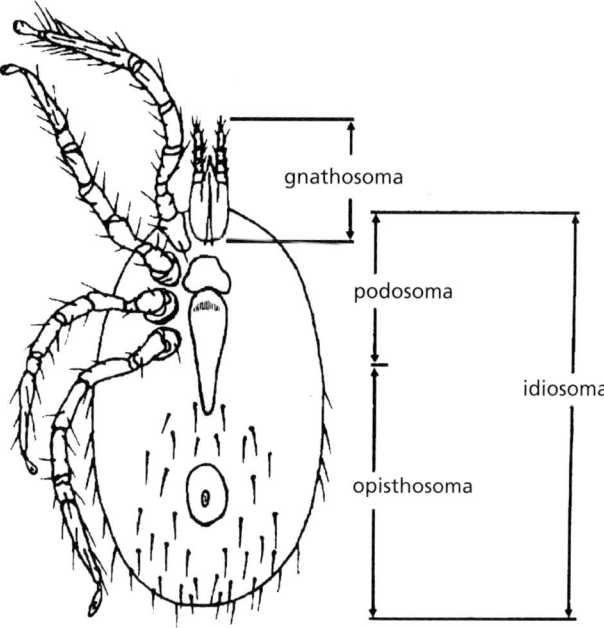

Fig. 4.103 The body of a generalised mite, ventral view.

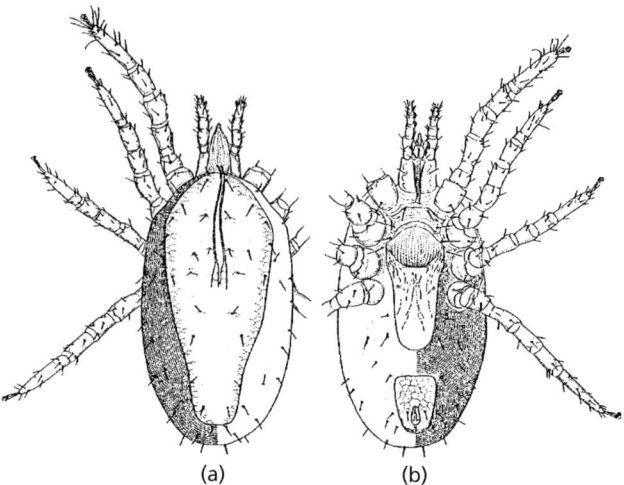

Fig. 4.104 Adult female of the red mite, *Dermanyssus gallinae*: (a) dorsal view; (b) ventral view. (Baker *et al.*, 1956/National Pest Control Association.)

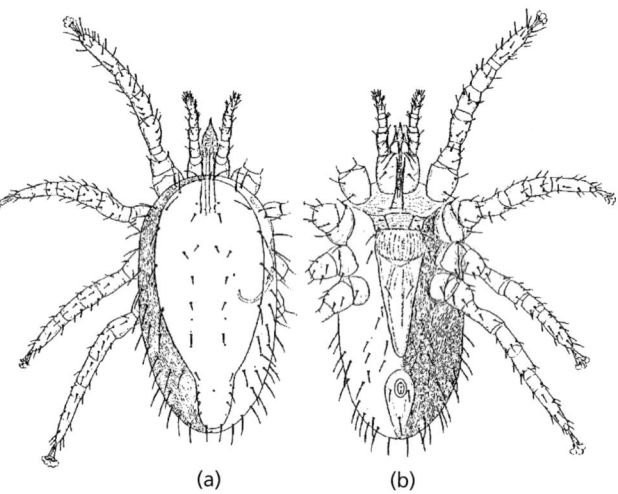

Fig. 4.105 Adult female *Ornithonyssus sylviarum* (northern fowl mite): (a) dorsal view; (b) ventral view. (Baker *et al.*, 1956/National Pest Control Association.)

4 Genital plate present although rudimentary; in lungs of canary .... ***Sternostoma tracheacolum*** (**Rhinonyssidae**)
    Genital plate absent; palps elongated with five segments; in nasal passage of dogs
    .... ***Pneumonyssus caninum*** (**Halarachnidae**)
5 Chelicerae long and whip-like; chelae at tips absent or very small **6**
    Chelicerae not long and whip-like, shorter and stronger; chelae blade-like at tips... **7**
6 Dorsal surface of body with one shield; anal shield not egg-shaped and with anal opening at posterior end (Fig. 4.104); parasite of birds
    ....***Dermanyssus gallinae*** (**Dermanyssidae**)
7 Dorsal shield not nearly covering dorsal body surface; genitoventral shield narrowed posteriorly; chelicerae with toothless chelae... **8**
    Dorsal shield virtually covering dorsal body surface; genitoventral shield not narrowed posteriorly; chelicerae usually with toothed chelae **10**
8 Dorsal shield broad, its setae short **9**
    Dorsal shield narrow and tapering posteriorly, its setae long; parasite of rats, mice, hamsters
    .... ***Ornithonyssus bacoti*** (**Macronyssidae**)
9 Sternal shield with two pairs of setae (Fig. 4.105); parasite of birds...................... ***Ornithonyssus sylviarum*** (**Macronyssidae**)
    Sternal shield with three pairs of setae; parasite of birds
    .... ***Ornithonyssus bursa*** (**Macronyssidae**)
10 Genitoventral shield widened posteriorly, with more than one pair of setae **11**
    Genitoventral shield not widened posteriorly, one pair of setae; on small rodents, weasels and moles
    .... ***Hirstionyssus isabellinus*** (**Laelapidae**)
11 Body densely covered in setae **12**
    Body with few setae (these arranged in transverse rows)
    .... **13**

12 Genitoventral shield with pear-shaped outline; on rodents
    .... ***Haemogamasus pontiger*** (**Laelapidae**)
    Genitoventral shield with large subcircular outline; on rodents .... ***Eulaelaps stabularis*** (**Laelapidae**)
13 Genitoventral shield with concave posterior margin, surrounding anterior part of anal shield; on rodents
    .... ***Laelaps echidninus*** (**Laelapidae**)
14 Legs short and stubby; genital opening of female a transverse slit paralleling body striations; dorsal striations broken by strong pointed scales; dorsal setae strong and spine-like; anus terminal (Fig. 4.106); on mammals
    ....***Sarcoptes scabiei*** (**Sarcoptidae**)
    Dorsal setae not spine-like **15**
    Legs not short and stubby... **17**
15 Anus terminal; tarsi claw-like, with terminal setae **16**
    Anus dorsal; dorsal striations broken by many pointed scales; dorsal setae simple, not spine-like (Fig. 4.107); on rats and guinea pigs .... ***Trixacarus caviae*** (**Sarcoptidae**)
    Anus dorsal; dorsal striations not broken by pointed scales; dorsal setae simple, not spine-like; tarsi with long

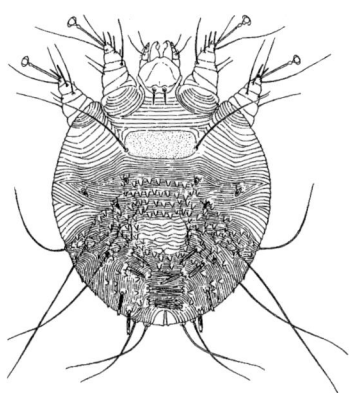

Fig. 4.106 Adult female *Sarcoptes scabiei*, dorsal view. (Baker *et al.*, 1956/ National Pest Control Association.)

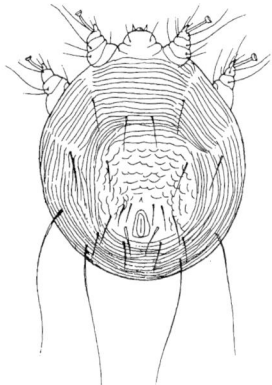

Fig. 4.108 Adult female *Notoedres cati*, dorsal view.

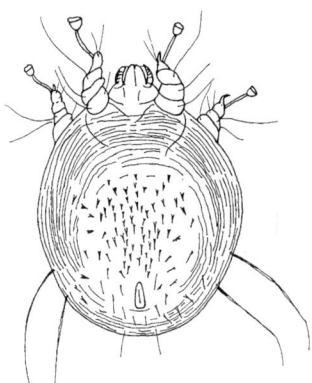

Fig. 4.107 Adult female *Trixacarus caviae*, dorsal view.

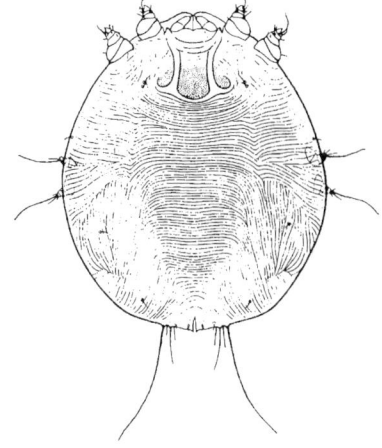

Fig. 4.109 Adult female *Knemidocoptes gallinae*, dorsal view. (Hirst, 1922/ Springer Nature.)

pretarsi on legs I and II (Fig. 4.108); on cats
.... ***Notoedres cati*** **(Sarcoptidae)**

16 Dorsal striations simple, unbroken (Fig. 4.109); on poultry
.... ***Knemidocoptes gallinae*** **(Knemidocoptidae)**

Dorsal striations broken, forming scale-like pattern; on poultry .... ***Knemidocoptes mutans*** **(Knemidocoptidae)**

Dorsal striations broken, forming scale-like pattern; on caged birds...............***Knemidocoptes pilae*** **(Knemidocoptidae)**

17 Pretarsi with short stalks **18**

In the adult female, pretarsi of I, II and IV with three-jointed long stalks; tarsi III with two long terminal whip-like setae; legs of equal sizes; genital opening an inverted 'U'. In the adult male, pretarsi on legs I, II and III with three-jointed long stalks; long setae on legs IV which are smaller than others (Fig. 4.110); on domestic mammals .... ***Psoroptes*** **spp. (Psoroptidae)**

18 In the adult female, tarsi I, II and IV with short-stalked pretarsi; tarsi III with a pair of long terminal whip-like setae; legs I and II stronger than the others; legs III shortest; legs IV with long slender tarsi; genital opening almost a transverse slit. In the adult male all legs with short-stalked pretarsi; fourth pair of legs short (Fig. 4.111); on domestic animals
....***Chorioptes*** **spp. (Psoroptidae)**

Legs I and II with short-stalked pretarsi; legs III and IV with a pair of terminal whip-like setae; legs IV much reduced; genital opening transverse (Fig. 4.112); found in the ears of cats and dogs .... ***Otodectes cynotis*** **(Psoroptidae)**

19 Mouthparts not well developed, reduced; small oval nude mites; all tarsi with pretarsi (Fig. 4.113); in the tissues of birds
.... ***Cytodites nudus*** **(Cytoditidae)**

Mouthparts well developed; elongated mites; body setae long; tarsi I and II claw-like distally; tarsi III and IV with long spatulate pretarsi (Fig. 4.114); in the tissues of birds
.... ***Laminosioptes cysticola*** **(Laminosioptidae)**

20 Body not unusually elongated, with setae.............................**21**

Body unusually elongated and crocodile-like with annulations, without setae (Fig. 4.115); in skin pores of mammals
.... ***Demodex*** **spp. (Demodicidae)**

21 Gnathosoma and palps conspicuous; body with feathery setae; three pairs of legs when attached to host (larval forms) (Fig. 4.116) .... **species of Trombiculidae**

Gnathosoma and palps conspicuous; body not with feathery setae; stigma opening at base of chelicerae...............................**22**

Gnathsoma and palps inconspicuous; body with simple nonfeathery setae; not ectoparasitic
.... ***Pyemotes tritici*** **(Pyemotidae)**

22 Palps with thumb–claw complex... **23**

Palps without thumb–claw complex **24**

23 Chelicerae fused with rostrum to form cone; palps opposable, with large distal claws; peritreme obvious, M-shaped on gnathosoma (Fig. 4.117)

On rabbits..... ***Cheyletiella parasitivorax*** **(Cheyletiellidae)**
On cats .... ***Cheyletiella blakei*** **(Cheyletiellidae)**
On dogs.....................***Cheyletiella yasguri*** **(Cheyletiellidae)**

24 Legs normal, for walking...**25**

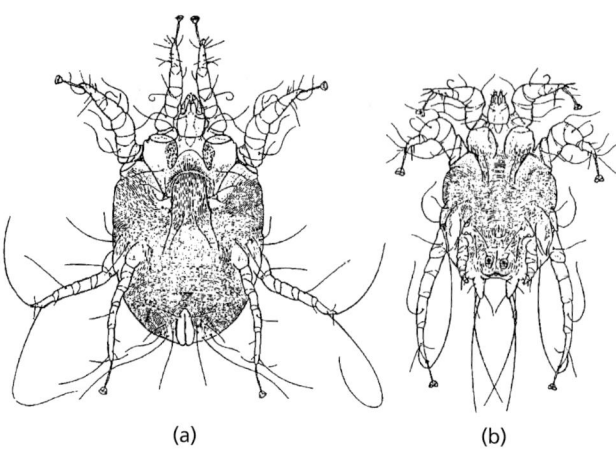

Fig. 4.110 Adult *Psoroptes ovis*, ventral views: (a) female; (b) male. (Baker *et al.*, 1956/National Pest Control Association.)

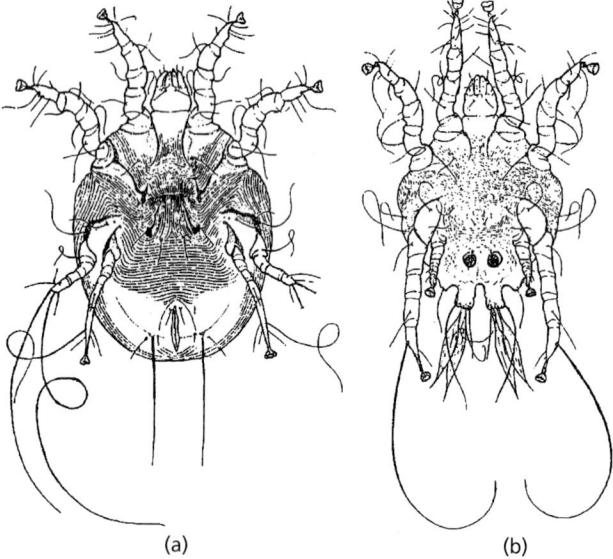

Fig. 4.111 Adult *Chorioptes bovis*, ventral views: (a) female; (b) male. (Baker *et al.*, 1956/National Pest Control Association.)

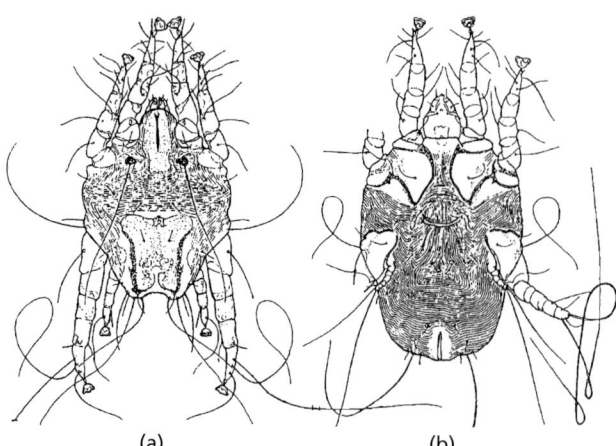

Fig. 4.112 Adult *Otodectes cynotis*: (a) male, dorsal view; (b) female, ventral view. (Baker *et al.*, 1956/National Pest Control Association.)

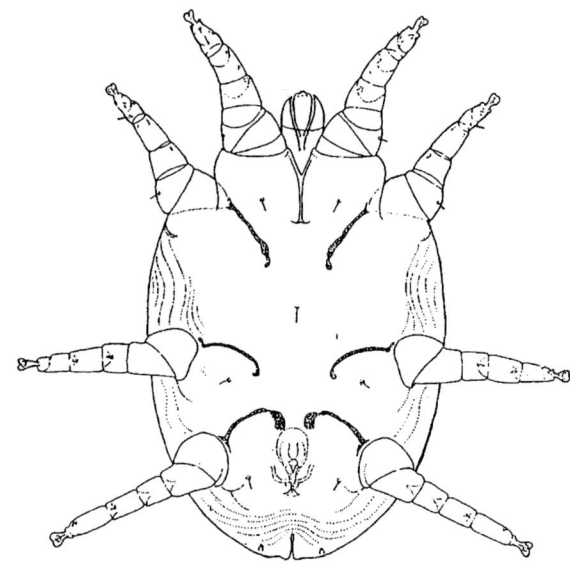

Fig. 4.113 Adult *Cytodites nudus*, ventral view. (Baker *et al.*, 1956/National Pest Control Association.)

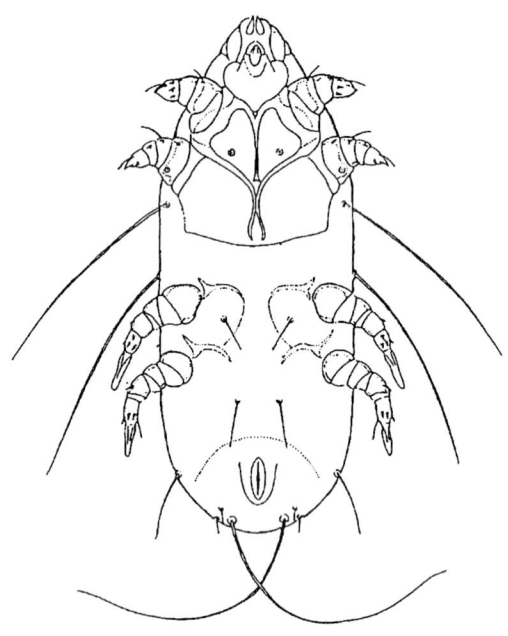

Fig. 4.114 Adult female *Laminosioptes cysticola*, ventral view. (Baker *et al.*, 1956/National Pest Control Association.)

First pair of legs highly modified for clasping hairs of host; body elongate, with transverse striations; on mice and rats .... **Myobidae**

Legs I and II and tarsi IV adapted for clasping hairs (Fig. 4.118); on guinea pigs

.... ***Chirodiscoides caviae* (Listrophoridae)**

Legs III and IV of female modified for clasping hairs (Fig. 4.119); on mice . ***Myocoptes musculinus* (Listrophoridae)**

25 Small round mites with short stubby radiating legs, each with a strong hook; female with two pairs of posterior setae, male with a single pair of posterior setae (Fig. 4.120)

On sheep .... ***Psorobia ovis* (Psorergatidae)**

On cattle .... ***Psorobia bovis* (Psorergatidae)**

On mice .... ***Psorergates simplex* (Psorergatidae)**

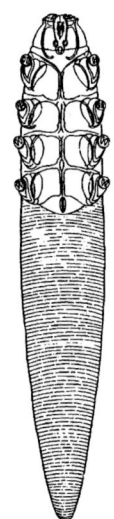

Fig. 4.115 Adult *Demodex* spp., ventral view. (Baker *et al.*, 1956/National Pest Control Association.)

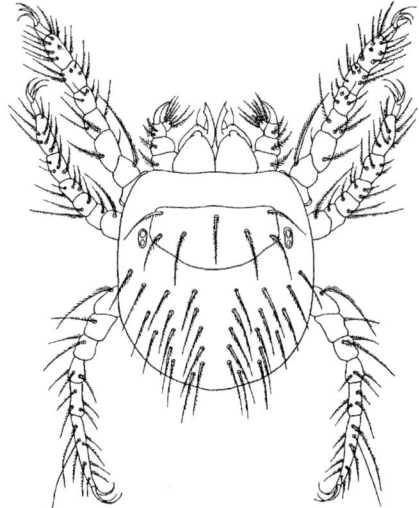

Fig. 4.116 Parasitic larval stage of the harvest mite, *Neotrombicula* (*Trombicula*) *autumnalis*. (Savory, 1935/Edward Arnold.)

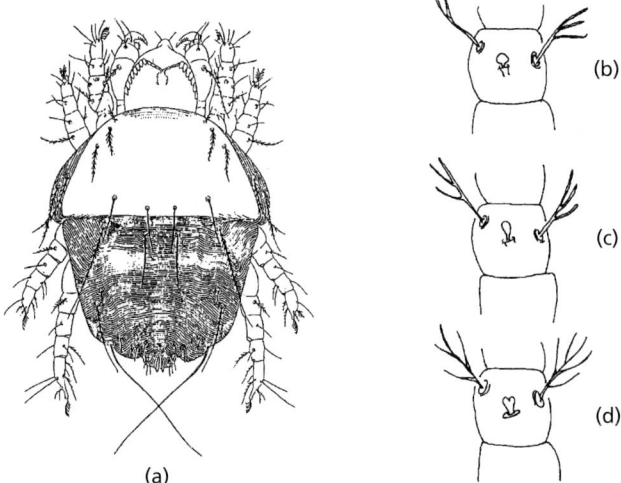

(b)

(c)

(d)

(a)

Fig. 4.117 (a) Adult female *Cheyletiella parasitivorax*, dorsal view. (Baker *et al.*, 1956/National Pest Control Association.) (b–d) Genu of the first pair of legs of adult females of (b) *Cheyletiella parasitivorax*, (c) *Cheyletiella blakei* and (d) *Cheyletiella yasguri*.

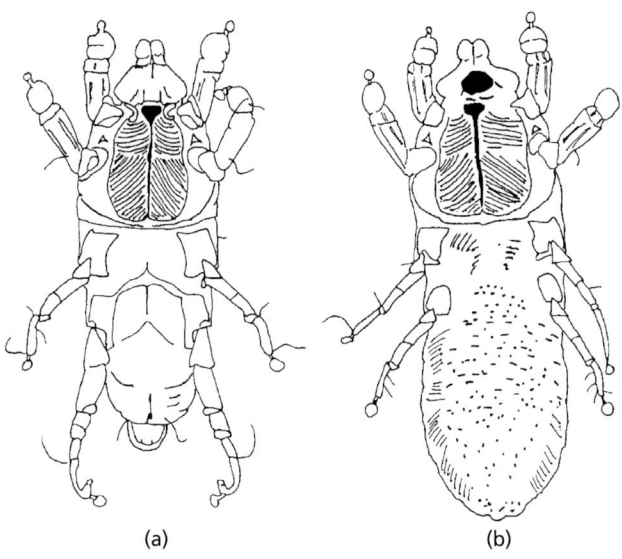

(a)   (b)

Fig. 4.118 Adult *Chirodiscoides caviae*: (a) male, ventral view; (b) female, ventral view.

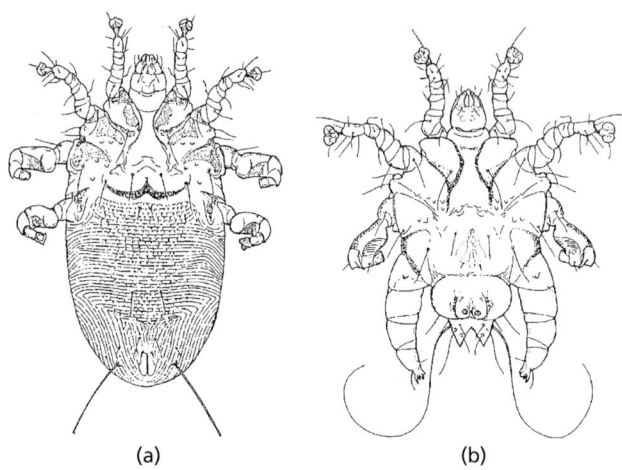

(a)   (b)

Fig. 4.119 Adult *Myocoptes musculinus*: (a) female, ventral view; (b) male, ventral view.

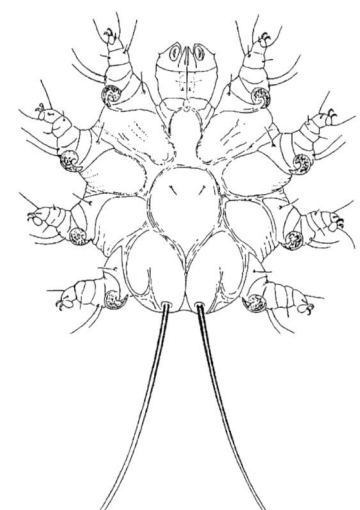

Fig. 4.120 Adult female *Psorobia*. (Baker *et al.*, 1956/National Pest Control Association.)

MOUNTING AND PRESERVATION

It is important that collection details (habitat, locality, date, time and identification) should be noted at the time of collection and entered on a standard label. Large insects should be mounted correctly in an entomological storage box, and should not be left in glass or plastic tubes for more than 24–48 hours, as their condition rapidly deteriorates in humid conditions. If they are allowed to become dry in an open container, subsequent attempts to pin them will result in excessive damage and fragmentation. However, dried specimens can be relaxed to some extent by placing them in a humid atmosphere. A receptacle containing wet cork or cotton wool, with an antifungal agent (e.g. merthiolate), will suffice.

Large insects are normally pinned through the thorax using fine entomological pins. Smaller insects are held by a fine pin inserted in a small block of styrofoam held in turn by a stout main pin. Most small flies including muscids (house fly, stable fly) can be mounted in this way. An alternative method, essential for very small insects such as biting midges (*Simulium*, *Culicoides*), is to attach them to the tip of a card 'point' using a soluble gum.

Small unmounted hard-bodied specimens (e.g. small flies and various insect larvae) are often better preserved for diagnostic and identification purposes if they are kept in 70% alcohol (with 5% glycerine); 10% formalin or 10% formol saline is preferred if they are soft-bodied. Although they will be slow to die, the use of 90% alcohol may be sufficient to kill and preserve soft-bodied insect larvae (e.g. maggots) from general collections of soil- or manure-breeding insects. Various killing fluids have been suggested to overcome these problems. A mixture of four parts 90% ethyl alcohol and one part ethyl acetate is an effective killing and relaxing agent for soft-bodied larvae. The addition of a little glacial acetic acid improves fixation and retains colour. A further fixative which can be used for killing and fixing soft larvae without severe contraction is Peterson's KAA fluid (10 parts 95% ethyl alcohol, 2 parts glacial acetic acid and 1 part kerosene). Preservation should finally be in 70% alcohol.

Small arthropods for microscopic examination on slides may be mounted in the following way.

1   Melted glycerine jelly, and sealed with nail varnish.
2   Berlese's fluid. This clears specimens but delicate insects may deteriorate after a short period.

If little detail can be made out, the specimen can be first cleared by placing it in 10% caustic potash on a slide and warming it for a few minutes or in a tube in a water-bath at 70 °C. A more gentle action can be obtained by leaving the specimen in caustic solution at 37 °C for several hours.

CHEMICALS AND SOLUTIONS

Phosphate buffered saline (10 mmol/l)

1. Dissolve the following in 800 mL distilled H_2O:
   a 8 g of NaCl
   b 0.2 g of KCl
   c 1.44 g of Na_2HPO_4
   d 0.24 g of KH_2PO_4
2. Adjust pH to 7.4 with HCl.
3. Adjust volume to 1 l with additional distilled water.
4. Sterilise by autoclaving.

Potassium bichromate

Dissolve 1 g of potassium bichromate in 100 ml of distilled water.

FLOTATION SOLUTIONS

Saturated salt (NaCl) solution, 1.20 specific gravity

1. Dissolve 400 g NaCl in 1000 ml of water, heat and allow to cool.
2. Decant off solution from any precipitate.

Magnesium sulfate (MgSO₄) solution, 1.28 specific gravity

1. Dissolve 400 g $MgSO_4$ in 1000 ml of boiling water.
2. Add 20 g potassium bichromate to prevent crystallisation.

Sugar (Sheather's) solution, 1.27 specific gravity

1. Dissolve 500 g sugar (sucrose) in 1000 ml boiling water.
2. Add approximately 6 ml of 37% formaldehyde or phenol crystals to prevent mould formation.

Saturated zinc sulfate (ZnSO₄) solution, 1.36 specific gravity

Add 700 g $ZnSO_4$ to 1000 ml of slowly boiling water and allow to cool.

Zinc sulfate (ZnSO₄) solution, 1.20 specific gravity

Add 330 g $ZnSO_4$ to 1000 ml water.

WORM COUNT SOLUTIONS

Pepsin/hydrochloric acid (HCl)

1. Dissolve 80 g of pepsin powder in 3 l of cold water.
2. Add 240 ml concentrated HCl slowly and stir well.
3. Make final volume up to 8 l. Store at 4 °C.

Iodine solution

1. Dissolve 907 g of potassium iodide in 650 ml boiling water.
2. Add 510 g iodine crystals and make up to 1 l.

Sodium thiosulfate solution

Dissolve 100 g of sodium thiosulfate in 5 l of water.

STAINS

Field's technique stains

Solution A

Methylene blue	0.4 g
Azure I	0.25 g
Solution B	250 ml

Solution B

$Na_2HPO_4 \cdot 12H_2O$	25.2 g
KH_2PO_4	12.5 g
Distilled water	1000 ml

Solution C

Eosin	0.5 g
Solution B	250 ml

These solutions do not keep and should be freshly prepared each day.

Ziehl–Neelsen acid-fast stain for *Cryptosporidium*

Strong carbolfuchsin

Dissolve 20 g basic fuchsin in 200 ml absolute methanol. Add 125 ml liquid phenol (GPR [80% w/w in distilled water]) carefully until well mixed. The stock reagent should be stored in a dark cupboard at room temperature. Often the concentration of basic fuchsin can vary within the acceptable range of 1–3%.

1% acid methanol

Add 20 ml hydrochloric acid (GPR/SLR) to 1980 ml of absolute methanol.

0.4% malachite green

Add 2 g malachite green to 480 ml deionised water.

Peanut agglutinin–fluorescein isothiocyanate (PNA-FITC)

Sigma Cat. No. L-7381 lectin from *Arachis hypogaea*, reconstituted at 5 mg per 1 ml PBS.

Diff-Quik stain

Diff-Quik is a commercial Romanowsky-type stain available from a number of suppliers. The kits usually comprise:

Fixative: methanol

Stain A: buffered eosin stain (eosinophilic)

Stain B: buffered Azure B stain (basophilic).

CHAPTER 5

Antiparasitics and resistance

It is not practical to give full efficacy data and methods of application of the large number of drugs currently available against the vast range of parasites of domestic animals. As the number of compounds and their various formulations are continually changing, it is perhaps more appropriate to discuss the use of antiparasitic drugs in general terms, according to the groups of parasites they target. Therefore, in this chapter, antiparasitics are grouped as **anthelmintics**, **antiprotozoals** and **ectoparasiticides**. Details of their use against individual species or groups of parasites have been described under the appropriate sections of the host chapters.

The general guiding principle in the use of all antiparasitic compounds should always be to employ the minimum application frequency necessary to achieve the required clinical outcome. Use should be based on assessed risk to animl health, welfare and husbandry; unnecessary application or overuse should be avoided because it incurs financial costs, promotes resistance and may have adverse impacts on the environment.

ANTHELMINTICS

MODE OF ACTION

The mode of action of many anthelmintics basically depends on interference with essential biochemical processes of the worms or cell integrity, but not, or to a lesser extent, those of the host. Many of the drugs target the nervous system of the parasite, resulting in paralysis and hence expulsion from the host. The nervous system of helminths is well differentiated between species and is very complex in terms of its neurochemicals, possessing many receptor and transmitter interactions that are not found in mammalian hosts. In some cases, the pharmacokinetic properties of the drug within the host result in the parasite being exposed to higher concentrations of the compound than the cells of the host. The major groups of anthelmintics currently in use against nematodes, trematodes and cestodes are shown in Table 5.1.

Benzimidazoles/pro-benzimidazoles (Group 1-BZ)

The benzimidazoles, largely used in veterinary and human medicine against helminthosis, include **thiabendazole**, **parbendazole**, **oxibendazole**, **fenbendazole**, **oxfendazole**, **albendazole**, **triclabendazole** and **ricobendazole** (albendazole oxide). Three other compounds, **febantel**, **netobimin** and **thiophanate** (pro-benzimidazoles), are also included in this group because they are metabolised by the host to active benzimidazoles. Notably, the modification of a particular benzimidazole can affect the pharmacokinetic behaviour of the drug through changes in relative solubility, slowing the elimination of the drug and/or active metabolites. The greater efficacy and wider spectrum of activity of the most recently introduced (second-generation) benzimidazoles

Table 5.1 Anthelmintic groups.

Chemical group	Group code	Nematodes	Trematodes	Cestodes	Ectoparasites
Broad spectrum					
Benzimidazole and pro-benzimidazoles	1-BZ	+	±	±	−
Imidazothiazoles	2-LV	+	−	−	−
Tetrahydropyrimidines		+	−	−	−
Avermectins/milbemycins	3-ML	+	−	−	+
Aminoacetyl derivatives	4-AD	+	−	−	−
Spiroindoles	5-SI	+	−	−	−
Narrow spectrum					
Salicylanilides and substituted phenols		±	+	±	±
Piperazines		±	−	−	−
Arsenicals		+	−	−	−
Others		+	−	+	−

+ effective; ± effective against some species; − ineffective.

Veterinary Parasitology, Fifth Edition. Domenico Otranto and Richard Wall.
© 2024 John Wiley & Sons Ltd. Published 2024 by John Wiley & Sons Ltd.

appear to be due to the relative insolubility of these chemicals, which affects the absorption, transport and excretion of the anthelmintic compound from the host.

Benzimidazoles are poorly soluble and are generally given orally as a suspension. Netobimin can be solubilised and administered via drinking water. Benzimidazoles have also been incorporated into a range of controlled-release devices for use in cattle. All are effective against nematodes affecting domestic animals and have some ovicidal activity. Most are also effective against tapeworms, and some have activity against adult liver fluke (*Fasciola* spp.) in ruminants at increased dose rates and frequency of administrations.

All members of the benzimidazole class have a similar mode of action and interfere with the energetic metabolism of worms by binding to parasite tubulin, a constituent protein present in microtubules and in plasma and mitochondrial membranes. The formation of microtubules is a dynamic process involving the polymerisation of tubulin rings at one end and depolymerisation at the other end. Benzimidazoles bind to β-tubulin, causing capping and inhibition of further microtubule formation, resulting in starvation of the parasite due to inhibition of glucose uptake, protein secretion and microtubule production. There is also a reduction in enzyme activity such as acetylcholinesterase secretion, and carbohydrate catabolism by the fumarate reductase system.

As the mode of action of all the above benzimidazoles is similar (all affecting the β-tubulin receptor protein), extensive cross-resistance occurs between members of this group of drugs. The mode of action of triclabendazole on *Fasciola hepatica* is at present unknown. It appears to have no tubulin-binding properties, unlike other members of this group, and it must therefore act along alternative pathways.

Benzimidazoles have low toxicity, and in some cases can be used at over 10 times the recommended dose rate. Parasite resistance to anthelmintics has most frequently been associated with repeated use of these drugs against nematodes of sheep, goats and horses and in many countries has limited both their effectiveness and use.

Imidazothiazoles/tetrahydropyrimidines (Group 2-LV)

The imidazothiaziole group contains two members, **tetramisole** and **levamisole**. Tetramisole is a racemic mixture of dextro and laevo forms. Levamisole is the levo-isomer, that represents the effective form; therefore the dose rate of levamisole is the half of that of tetramisole, and it has twice the safety index.

Levamisole is used mainly in cattle and sheep and has good activity against a range of gastrointestinal nematodes and is also highly effective against lungworms. Levamisole can be administered orally, by injection or pour-on, combined in a number of products with a specific flukicide (oxyclozanide or triclabendazole) to form a broad-spectrum drench for worms and flukes. Unlike the benzimidazoles, it is not ovicidal. Levamisole is non-teratogenic and is therefore safe to use in pregnant animals. The therapeutic index in relation to other anthelmintics is, however, low. Animals given levamisole may be hyperactive for a few minutes after receiving the therapeutic dose, due to the hyperstimulation of nerve ganglia; toxic signs due to this stimulant effect may manifest as salivation, bradycardia, muscular tremors and, in extreme cases, death

from respiratory failure. Injectable levamisole may cause inflammation at the site of injection.

The drug is rapidly absorbed and excreted, most of the dose being lost from the system within 24 hours of administration. Because of the mode of action of these compounds, nematode paralysis occurs quickly and removal of the worms is rapid. In addition to its anthelmintic properties, levamisole has been shown to stimulate the mammalian immune system by increasing cellular activity. The relationship between the immunostimulatory and nematocidal properties of levamisole is unknown.

Pyrantel and **morantel** are members of the tetrahydropyrimidine group. **Morantel** is used for the treatment of gastrointestinal worms of cattle and sheep but is not effective against mucosal or arrested larval stages (hypobiotic larvae) or against established lungworm infections. Like levamisole, it has no activity against tapeworms and fluke. **Pyrantel** is used for the treatment and control of nematode and tapeworm infections in horses and nematodes in dogs. It is also active against nematodes in ruminants and pigs. Pyrantel salts (tartrate or pamoate) are active against adult and larval stages of large and small strongyles, ascarids and tapeworms (*Anoplocephala* spp.) at double the regular dose, and benzimidazole-resistant strains of cyathostomes in horses. None of these drugs are particularly toxic and they can be used safely in pregnant and young animals.

The imidazothiazoles and tetrahydropyrimidine derivatives act as selective cholinergic agonists, targeting nicotinic acetylcholine receptors of nematodes, initially causing muscle contractions followed by neuromuscular depolarisation, resulting in a rapid reversible spastic paralysis. Paralysed worms are expelled by normal gut peristalsis. These nicotinic acetylcholine receptors are diverse in their location in nematodes (neuromuscular junction, nerve ring and pharynx) and also in their pharmacology and this may explain why resistance to one drug does not necessarily lead to cross-resistance to other related drugs. Studies on neuromuscular nicotinic acetylcholine receptors in *Haemonchus contortus* and *Ascaris suum* have indicated that resistance to levamisole might increase susceptibility to pyrantel and vice versa.

Avermectins/milbemycins (Group 3-ML)

This series of macrocyclic lactone derivatives are fermentation products of the actinomycete *Streptomyces avermitilis* (avermectins) and *Streptomyces cyanogriseus* (milbemycins). Avermectins differ from each other chemically in side-chain substitutions on the lactone ring, while milbemycins differ from the avermectins through the absence of a sugar moiety from the lactone skeleton. The avermectins include **abamectin**, **doramectin**, **eprinomectin**, **selamectin** and **ivermectin**, and are active against a wide range of nematodes and arthropods. **Moxidectin** and **milbemycin oxime** have a similar wide-ranging activity.

The macrocyclic lactones have been shown to have excellent activity, at very low dose rates, not only against a wide range of nematodes but also against certain arthropod parasites and hence are sometimes referred to as endectocides. They are active against adult and larval gastrointestinal roundworms and lungworms of ruminants, horses and pigs, although none of these compounds have activity against tapeworms or liver flukes. Eprinomectin has a zero withdrawal time for meat and milk and is often the drug of choice in lactating dairy cattle. Avermectins are also active against filarial worms (*Parafilaria* spp.) in cattle, microfilariae of *Dirofilaria* spp. in dogs and cats and spiruroid worms, including *Habronema* and *Draschsia*, in horses.

These compounds also have ectoparasiticide activity against warbles (*Hypoderma* spp.) in cattle, sucking lice (*Haematopinus* spp., *Linognathus* spp., *Selenopotes* spp.) and mange mites (*Psoroptes* spp., *Sarcoptes* spp., *Chorioptes* spp.) in cattle, sheep and pigs. More detailed information on the efficacy is provided in the section on ectoparasiticides.

Selamectin is used as a preventive against heartworm disease and is effective against hookworms (*Ancylostoma* spp., *Uncinaria* spp.) and ascarids (*Toxocara* spp., *Toxascaris* spp.) in dogs and cats. Selamectin has been specifically developed for use in dogs and cats and is also active against fleas and mites in these hosts (see section on Ectoparasiticides). It does not appear to exhibit toxicity in ivermectin-sensitive collie dogs, at the recommended dose rates.

Macrocyclic lactones are highly lipophilic and, following administration, are stored in fat tissue from where they are slowly released, metabolised and excreted. Ivermectin is absorbed systemically following oral, subcutaneous or dermal administration, but is absorbed to a greater degree, and has a longer half-life, when given subcutaneously or dermally. A temporary depot appears to occur in the fat and liver, from which there is a slow release. Excretion of the largely unaltered molecule is mainly via the faeces, with less than 2% excreted in the urine (see Chapter 6). The reduced absorption and bioavailability of ivermectin when given orally in ruminants may be due to its metabolism in the rumen. The affinity of these compounds for fat explains their persistence in the body and the extended periods of protection afforded against lungworms and gastric worms in cattle, sheep and goats. Individual variations in these periods of protection reflect differences in drug distribution, metabolism and excretion. In cattle, injectable and pour-on preparations provide protection for up to 42 days for lungworms and 35 days for gastrointestinal worms, depending on the product and formulation. The prolonged half-life of these compounds also determines levels of residues in meat and milk, and subsequent compulsory withdrawal periods following treatment. With the exception of eprinomectin, which has a zero milk withdrawal period, treatment with this class of compounds cannot be given to lactating cattle or during the last two months of pregnancy.

Ivermectin is known to act on γ-aminobutyric acid (GABA) neurotransmission at two or more sites in nematodes, blocking interneuronal stimulation of excitatory motor neurones and thus leading to a flaccid paralysis; the former effect was achieved by stimulating the release of GABA from nerve endings and enhancing the binding of GABA to its receptor on the postsynaptic membrane of an excitatory motor neurone. The enhanced GABA binding results in an increased flow of chloride ions (Cl$^-$) into the cell, leading to hyperpolarisation. In mammals, GABA neurotransmission is confined to the central nervous system; the lack of avermectin effect on the mammalian nervous system, at therapeutic concentrations, is probably because, being a large molecule, it does not readily cross the blood–brain barrier. More recent evidence suggests that the hydrophobic macrocyclic lactones dissolve in the plasma membrane of the cell and bind to glutamate-gated chloride channel receptors at the pore region of the receptor. This binding opens the channel and allows the influx of chloride ions and the resulting hyperpolarisation of the cell causes a flaccid paralysis. This paralysis can occur in body wall muscle, uterine muscle and the pharyngeal muscle.

Amino-acetonitrile derivatives (Group 4-AD)

The anthelmintic molecule **monepantel** has been available since 2010. Its mode of action is similar to the paralysis that occurs with the 2-LV group of anthelmintics but it acts via a previously unknown neuronal nicotinic acetylcholine receptor site (MPTL-1) that is specific to nematodes. When monepantel interferes with this subunit, the receptor allows Na$^+$ and K$^+$ cations freedom to pass through the cell wall, leading to nematode paralysis. There is some evidence that the target receptor ligand may not be acetylcholine but choline. The paralysis could be due to the activation of neurones which control nematode movement or because the choline receptor is expressed also on muscle cells. Monepantel has been shown to be effective against parasites which are resistant to other nicotinic drugs. The safety index of the drug is high.

Spiroindoles (Group 5-SI)

Derquantel is a semi-synthetic derivative of paraherquamide (2-desoxoparaherquamide) that belongs to the family of spiroindoles. Derquantel was launched in 2012 as a 'dual active' product in combination with abamectin (3-ML group). Both active components have similar pharmacokinetic profiles. Derquantel interferes with β-subtype nictotinic acetylcholine receptors, leading to flaccid paralysis in nematodes. This mode of action is different from other chemical groups and as such offers activity against resistant strains of parasites. A study has shown that abamectin and derquantel appear to interact at nicotinic acetylcholine receptors and that the effect of the combination is significantly higher than the predicted additive effect of both drugs at higher acetylcholine concentrations, suggesting a synergism. The combination drench offers a high level of efficacy in killing worms, including those resistant to benzimidazole (1-BZ), levamisole (2-LV) and macrocyclic lactone (3-ML).

Salicylanilides/substituted phenols

The salicylanilides/substituted phenols can be regarded as close analogues and include the **bromsalans, clioxanide, oxyclozanide, brotianide, niclosamide, rafoxanide** and **closantel** (salicylanilides), and **nitroxynil, disophenol, bithionol, hexachlorophene** and **niclofolan** (phenol derivatives). With the exception of niclosamide, the salicylanilides and substituted phenols are usually marketed as flukicides for cattle and sheep, being highly effective against adult and, to a lesser extent, immature flukes (*Fasciola* spp.). Some also possess activity against blood-sucking nematodes such as *Haemonchus* spp. **Disophenol** has been used for treatment of dogs infected with hookworms and is also effective against mature *H. contortus* and may be used in sheep for treatment of benzimidazole-resistant infections. **Niclosamide** is highly effective against tapeworms in cattle, sheep, horses and poultry and possibly against immature paramphistomes in ruminants. In some countries, it is used mainly for the treatment of tapeworms in dogs and cats.

Salicylanilides and substituted phenols appear to be extensively bound to plasma proteins (>99%), which may explain their high efficacy against blood-feeding parasites. Fasciolicidal activity is dependent on the extent to which these drugs persist in the plasma. Rafoxanide and closantel have long plasma half-lives when compared with oxyclozanide. Evidence suggests that the apparent efficacy of these drugs, particularly against immature flukes

(*Fasciola* spp.), may be due more to their persistence in the plasma and the effect they have on maturing adult flukes (once they reach the bile ducts), rather than the effect they have on the immature stages themselves. Young flukes probably ingest mainly liver cells, which contain little amount of anthelmintic. As they grow and migrate through the liver, they cause extensive haemorrhage and come into contact with anthelmintic. Finally, when the flukes reach the bile ducts they are in contact with even greater concentrations of anthelmintic as the bile ducts are important in the excretion of these compounds, as evidenced by the high proportion of these drugs, and their metabolites, excreted in the faeces rather than the urine.

Salicylanilides and substituted phenols uncouple oxidative phosphorylation and therefore decrease the availability of high-energy phosphate compounds such as adenosine triphosphate (ATP) and reduced nicotinamide adenine dinucleotide (NADH⁻) in the mitochondria. They act as protonophores, enabling hydrogen ions to pass through the inner mitochondrial membrane. They have also been shown to inhibit succinate dehydrogenase activity and the fumarate reductase system, which is associated with oxidative phosphorylation. The long half-life of the plasma protein-bound molecules results in a prolonged exposure of the parasites to the drugs.

Plasma binding reduces incorporation of the drugs into host tissues and accounts for the selective parasite toxicity. Looseness of faeces and slight loss of appetite may be seen in some animals after treatment at recommended dose rates. High doses may cause blindness and signs of uncoupled oxidative phosphorylation, such as hyperventilation, hyperthermia, convulsions, tachycardia and ultimately death.

Dichlorophen is a chlorinated phenol and is active against tapeworms (*Dipylidium caninum*, *Taenia* spp.) in dogs and cats. Its mode of action is thought to be similar to that of the salicyclanilides, interfering with oxidative phosphorylation.

Piperazines

Piperazine salts have a narrow spectrum of activity and have been widely used against ascarids, particularly in dogs and cats, acting as an agonist at GABA receptors, thus blocking neuromuscular transmission by hyperpolarisation of the nerve membrane and inducing a flaccid paralysis. Piperazine also inhibits the production of succinate by the parasite, which leads to depletion of energy. Piperazine adipate has been widely used in horses and is effective against adult stages of small strongyles and *Parascaris*. In pigs, the drug is active against *Ascaris suum* and nodular worms *Oesophagostomum* spp. after a single treatment. It has also been widely used in poultry.

Diethylcarbamazine is still marketed in certain parts of the world and is used for the treatment of *Dictyocaulus viviparus* infections in cattle. It is primarily active against immature lungworms. Treatment is relatively impractical since it has to be given for three consecutive days to achieve its effect, and as a result it has been replaced by more modern anthelmintics. The action of diethylcarbamazine on lungworm larvae is thought to induce a flaccid paralysis in the parasite due to hyperpolarisation of neuronal postsynaptic membranes resulting from an increased flow of Cl⁻ into the cell. It can be used as a preventive for heartworm disease when given to dogs in low daily doses throughout the mosquito season and for two months subsequently. The mode of action is incompletely understood, but it is thought to enhance phagocytosis of the microfilariae by the host immune system. However, it is strictly contraindicated in microfilariae-positive dogs because of a possible but rare shock-type reaction that is sometimes fatal, produced by liberation of substances from dying or dead microfilariae following treatment. It has also been reported to be effective against the lungworm *Crenosoma vulpis* of dogs and farmed foxes.

Organophosphates

Several organophosphate compounds (see section on Ectoparasiticides) are active against nematodes, but are becoming less widely available in many countries. Compounds used in the treatment of nematode infections include **coumaphos**, **trichlorphon**, **haloxon** and **dichlorvos**. They act by inhibiting cholinesterase, via phosphorylation of esterification sites, resulting in a build-up of acetylcholine, which leads to neuromuscular spastic paralysis of nematodes and their expulsion. This group of drugs is relatively toxic and has been used most frequently in horses, because of the additional insecticidal action against larvae of horse bots.

Coumaphos has been widely used as an ectoparasitic in livestock. It exhibits a cumulative effect on trichostrongyle nematodes if given in feed daily for one week; there is a good activity against *Haemonchus* spp. and *Cooperia* spp. in cattle and sheep, but it is less effective against *Trichostrongylus* spp., *Ostertagia* spp. and *Oesophagostomum* spp. Anthelmintic activity can be enhanced if the drench passes via the closed oesophageal groove directly to the abomasum, with either sodium bicarbonate in cattle or copper sulfate in sheep. It is also effective against *Capillaria* spp., *Ascaridia* spp. and *Heterakis* spp. in chickens. Coloured breeds of egg-laying hens are more susceptible to the drug than white breeds and birds should not be treated while they are in lay.

Haloxon is still used in many countries for the treatment of nematodes. In cattle, sheep and goats, it is effective against adult *Haemonchus* spp., *Cooperia* spp. in sheep and *Neoascaris* (*Toxocara*) *vitulorum* in cattle. There is a moderate effect against *Ostertagia* spp., *Bunostomum* spp., *Trichostrongylus* spp. and *Oesophagostomum* spp. but little effect against *Nematodirus* spp., *Trichuris* spp. and *Chabertia* spp. It is highly effective against adult stages of *Strongylus vulgaris*, most small strongyles (also benzimidazole-resistant strains), *Parascaris* spp. and *Oxyuris equi* in horses. In pigs, it is active against adult *Ascaris suum* and *Oesophagostomum* spp. but there may be delayed neurotoxicity (posterior paralysis). It is used in some countries in chickens, turkeys, quail and pigeons against *Capillaria* spp. but is ineffective against *Heterakis*. The recommended dose range for birds (50–100 mg/kg) is lethal for geese and possibly waterfowl.

Trichlorphon is effective against adult and immature *Parascaris equorum*, adult pinworms (*Oxyuris equi*), bots (larvae of *Gasterophilus* spp.) and, at higher doses, against large strongyles (*S. vulgaris*) and small strongyles in horses. In some countries, trichlorphon is used in combination with various benzimidazoles, pyrantel pamoate or piperazine/phenothiazine for removal of ascarids, pinworms, small strongyles (cyathostomes) and all three species of large strongyles. It shows good efficacy against adults of *Ascaris* spp., *Trichuris* spp. and *Hyostrongylus* spp. in pigs. At therapeutic doses, there may be mild adverse effects such as transient softening of faeces and mild colic for several hours.

Dichlorvos is an aliphatic organophosphate. It has a similar spectrum of activity to trichlorphon in horses and pigs; formulation in a slow-release resin increases activity against large and small strongyles and safety in pigs. However, the resin pellets, excreted with the faeces of treated animal, are toxic to other animals, especially chickens.

Arsenicals

Thiacetarsamide is an arsenical compound that has been used for many years as an adulticidal drug for treatment of heartworm (*Dirofilaria immitis*) in dogs. Its efficacy varies depending on the sex and age of worm, and there is a risk to treated animals of pulmonary embolism in the first month following treatment. The drug is highly irritant to subcutaneous tissues and is hepatotoxic and nephrotoxic, with mortality during or following therapy related to the degree of clinical manifestation of heartworm disease. It is now no longer available.

Melarsomine dihydrochloride is an arsenical adulticide that can be used for treatment of canine heartworm disease. It is less nephrotoxic and hepatotoxic than thiacetarsamide and has a higher efficacy using a two-dose strategy – a first dose of 2.5 mg/kg and a second administration at the same dose rate after 24 hours. In a patient with a high risk of thromboembolism, a single dose is recommended at 2.5 mg/kg and a second six months later, followed by a third administration after 24 hours. However, before the second treatment, it is recommended to test for circulating antigens released by the nematode female; given that the efficacy of the drug is related to the parasite load and the stage, it may be possible to completely eliminate the parasite after the first treatment. Melarsomine dihydrochloride is generally well tolerated, causing only minor tissue reactions, and is normally administered intramuscularly into the lumbar muscles. The use of this drug is not recommended in cats.

Other drugs

Phenothiazine was the first broad-spectrum anthelmintic and was used for many years but has now virtually disappeared. It is still available in some countries in combination with trichlorphon and piperazine and can be used for treating benzimidazole-resistant strains of small strongyles in horses. The drug is active against adult stages of small strongyles but has little or no effect on large strongyles, immature stages of small strongyles and *Parascaris equorum*. At therapeutic doses there may be side-effects, such as anorexia, muscular weakness, icterus or anaemia, but seldom mortality.

Epsiprantel is an isoquinoline-pyrazine anthelmintic compound active against tapeworm infections in dogs and cats. It is generally formulated and administered with pyrantel pamoate to give a broader range of activity against both roundworms and tapeworms of dogs and cats. It should not be used in kittens and puppies younger than seven weeks old.

Praziquantel is an acylated quinoline-pyrazine and is active against a wide range of adult and larval tapeworms in dogs and cats and at higher dose rates against tapeworms of ruminants. It is the drug of choice against multilocular echinococcosis (*Echinococcus multilocularis*) and is also active against lung flukes (*Paragonimus kellicotti*) and intestinal flukes (*Nanophyetus salmincola*) in dogs. Praziquantel modulates cell membrane permeability, causing spastic paralysis of muscle cells in the parasite and, like a number of other cestodicidal drugs, causes damage to the parasite tegument. It also exhibits activity against trematodes of the genus *Schistosoma*.

Nitroscanate is marketed for treatment of common roundworm and tapeworm infections of dogs. Its use in cats is contraindicated due to adverse side-effects including posterior paralysis, inappetence and vomiting.

Emodepside is a semi-synthetic compound belonging to a group of chemicals called depsipeptides. This anthelmintic requires a voltage-gated ion channel for its activity. The effects are manifested through activation of the SLO-1 gene, which encodes a calcium- and voltage-activated potassium channel. Latrophilin receptors may also be a target for emodepside in some parasites. The effects are often multiple, influencing feeding, locomotion and egg laying by the parasite and leading to paralysis and death. This suggests that more than one target may be activated. Emodepside is active against roundworm, hookworm and certain tapeworm infections in dogs and cats.

Clorsulon is a benzene sulfonamide compound and has been used in the treatment of adult liver fluke (*Fasciola hepatica, F. gigantica*) infections in cattle and sheep. It should be used at the dose rate of 7 mg/kg when orally administered or 2 mg/kg when administered subcutaneously. It does not exhibit activity against young immature stages, but is effective against adult and immature flukes over eight weeks of age. It has been shown to inhibit the glycolytic enzyme phosphoglyceromutase and 2,3-diphosphoglycerate, leading to gradual suppression of motility and paralysis.

ANTHELMINTIC USE

An ideal anthelmintic should possess the following properties.

1 **It should be efficient against all parasitic stages of a particular species**. It is also generally desirable that the spectrum of activity should include members of different genera, for dealing with the equine small and large strongyles, *Oxyuris equi* and *Parascaris equorum*. However, in some circumstances, specific drugs have to be used at different times of year to control infections with parasite with a different epidemiology; for instance, the trichostrongyles responsible for ovine parasitic gastroenteritis and the liver fluke *Fasciola hepatica* require treatment in different periods of the year.

2 **No toxicity or minimal toxicity to the host or at least a wide safety margin**. This is especially important in the treatment of groups of animals such as a flock of sheep, where individual body weights cannot easily be obtained, rather than in the dosing of individual companion animals such as cats or dogs. In addition, the increasing number of antiparasitic drugs that are available without medical prescription or veterinary advice mean that the use of coumpounds with a wide margin of safety is essential to avoid overdosing.

3 In general, an anthelmintic should be **rapidly cleared and excreted by the host**, especially in animals used in meat and milk production. However, in certain circumstances and in certain classes of animals (e.g. dry cattle), drug persistence can be used to prophylactic advantage – for example, the use of closantel to control haemonchosis in sheep. Anthelmintics with long persistence may also have advantages in some specific circumstances, for example in extensively grazed livestock or, in the case of companion aniamals, to increase owner compliance. But these products may substantially increase the rate of selection for resistance and result in peristent excretion of toxic metabolites into the environment (see Chapter 6).

4 Anthelmintics should be **easily administered**, otherwise they will not be readily accepted by owners; different formulations

are available for different domestic animal species. Oral, inject-able and pour-on products are widely used in large and small ruminants. Anthelmintic boluses are also available for cattle and sheep. For horses, oral paste or granular formulations to be mixed with the food are available. For pets, easy administration and acceptance by the animal are important characteristics to be considered, expecially for owner-administered drugs. For dogs and cats, oral (chewable tablets, paste and palatable for-mulations) injectable and spot-on formulations are available.

5 **The cost of an anthelmintic should be reasonable relative to other management costs**. This is of special importance in live-stock where profit margins may be narrow.

Anthelmintics are generally used in two ways: therapeutically, to treat existing infections or clinical outbreaks, or prophylactically, in which the timing of treatment is based on knowledge of the epide-miology. Prophylactic use may be preferable where administration of a drug at selected intervals or continuously over a period can prevent the occurrence of disease.

Therapeutic usage

When used therapeutically, the following factors should be considered.
- If the drug is not active against all parasitic stages, it must at least be effective against the pathogenic stage.
- Use of the anthelmintic should, by successfully removing para-sites, result in cessation of clinical signs of infection, such as diarrhoea and respiratory distress; in other words, there should be a marked clinical improvement and rapid recovery after treatment.

Prophylactic usage

Several points should be considered where anthelmintics are used prophylactically.
- The cost of prophylactic treatment should be justifiable economi-cally, by increased production in food animals or by preventing the occurrence of clinical or subclinical disease in, for example, horses with strongylosis or dogs with heartworm disease.
- The cost–benefit of anthelmintic prophylaxis should stand comparison with the control, which can be achieved by other methods such as pasture management or, for example in the case of dictyocaulosis, by vaccination.
- It is desirable that the use of anthelmintics should not interfere with the development of acquired immunity, since there are reports of outbreaks of disease in older stock that have been over-protected by control measures during their earlier years.
- It is also important that the status of anthelmintic resistance on the farm is known and dosing strategies undertaken to maintain a proportion of the worm population *in refugia*.
- Prolonged prophylactic use of one drug should be avoided as this may encourage the development of anthelmintic resistance.

METHODS OF ADMINISTRATION

Traditionally, anthelmintics have been administered orally or parenterally, usually by subcutaneous injection. Oral administration is common by drenching with liquids or suspensions, or by the incorporation of the drug in the feed or water for farm animals and by the administration of tablets to pets. Paste formulations have been introduced especially for horses. Several compounds have systemic action when applied as pour-on or spot-on formulations to the skin. Methods for injecting compounds directly into the rumen of cattle have also been marketed. Several rumen-dwelling boluses are available, mainly for cattle and to a lesser extent for sheep. Rumen-dwelling boluses are designed to deliver therapeutic doses of anthelmintic at intervals (pulse-release) or low doses over prolonged periods (sustained-release); both prevent the establishment of mature parasite populations and thus limit the contamination of pastures and the occurrence of disease. An apparatus for the delivery of anthelmintics into drinking water at daily or periodic intervals has also been developed.

Combination products

Some products are marketed for cattle and sheep and consist of a mixture of roundworm anthelmintics for the control of multiple-resistant nematode worms. Alternatively, a combination of drugs against roundworms and flukes may be given, but the timing of treatments for roundworms or flukes, whether curative or prophylactic, is often different and the requirement for such combination compounds is therefore limited to situations where both types of parasites are present. Combinations of two or three anthelmintics with different spectra of activity (roundworms, hookworms, heartworm, tapeworms) have proved useful in companion animals where the risk of concurrent infection is high.

Multiple active products

The term 'multiple actives' refers to formulations that are a mixture of two or more distinct anthelmintic classes with a similar spectrum of activity against roundworms only. Multiple active products can be used in sheep or cattle, in an attempt to delay the increase in anthelmintic resistance in those circumstances where the preva-lence of resistant parasites is currently at a low level. The adminis-tration of anthelmintic combinations with a similar spectrum of activity and different mechanisms of action and resistance has been suggested as a potential means of delaying the development of anthelmintic resistance. Multiple actives are commercially available in several countries such as Australia and New Zealand and include dual actives or even triple actives.

There are two main justifications for the use of multiple actives: (i) to enable the effective control of nematodes in the presence of single or multiple drug resistance; and (ii) to slow the development of anthelmintic resistance to the component anthelmintic classes. The rationale for using multiple active formulations to delay the development of resistance was initially inspired by research into insecticide resistance. Results from several modelling studies with insecticides suggested that multiple actives were always more effec-tive at delaying the development of resistance than using the same actives in different patterns of rotation (alternating the use of differ-ent chemical classes) or sequentially (where one chemical class is used exclusively until resistance develops and it is then replaced by a different chemical class), provided certain conditions were met.

Potential pharmacodynamic interactions between co-administered anthelmintics include indifference, antagonism, addi-tive and synergistic effects. An additive effect occurs when the combined effect of two drugs equals the sum of their independent activities measured separately. For example, if co-administered actives have independent modes of action and mechanisms of resistance, nematodes which survive one treatment will be killed by the other, provided they are not multiresistant.

The expected efficacy of a multiple active anthelmintic formulation can be approximated as follows: if two anthelmintics have efficacies a and b, respectively, where efficacy is expressed as the proportion of worms killed, the expected efficacy for the combination, assuming additive effects of the drugs, is given as:

$$\text{Efficacy}(A+B) = \left\{ 1 - \left[(1-a)(1-b) \right] \right\} \times 100$$

The use of multiple active formulations in resistance management is not a panacea and, like all anthelmintic products, maximum benefit will be realised when they are introduced before resistance is detectable and when they are used in accordance with guidelines for sustainable parasite control.

ANTIPROTOZOALS

Unlike other antiparasitic agents, for which a few chemical structural classes exhibit a wide spectrum of biological activity, antiprotozoal activity exists in a wide range of chemical classes, each of which possesses only a narrow spectrum of activity. The classification of antiprotozoal compounds is complex and for the purposes of this chapter, they are divided into eight main groups that are further subdivided on the basis of their structural similarities.

MODE OF ACTION

Antimonials and arsenicals

Antimonials contain the group V metal antimony and have been used extensively for the treatment of leishmaniosis. The antimonials selectively inhibit enzymes that are required for glycolytic and fatty acid oxidation in tissue of amastigotes found within macrophages.

Tartar emetic (**antimony potassium tartrate**) was the first antimonial used for this purpose in cases of human leishmaniosis. It was also used in the treatment of *Trypanosoma congolense congolense* and *T. vivax vivax* infections in cattle and *T. brucei evansi* infections in camels. Extravascular injection causes severe necrosis and the compound has a narrow chemotherapeutic index, resulting in about 6% mortality during routine treatment.

The pentavalent antimony compounds **meglumine antimoniate** (**Glucantime®** or *N*-**methylglucamine antimoniate**), **sodium antimony gluconate** and **sodium stibogluconate** (**Pentostam®**) have been the first-line drugs for the treatment of leishmaniosis in humans and are the principal antimonials used for canine leishmaniosis. The precise chemical structure of these drugs is difficult to identify. *Leishmania infantum* drug tolerance to antimonials, in humans and dogs, is well known, resulting in a high rate of treatment failure and relapse. These drugs may show marked toxic effects such as arthralgia, nephrotoxicity and cardiotoxicity, leading rarely to sudden death.

Antimonials are administered either by intralesional infiltration in simple single cutaneous lesions (in humans) or by subcutaneous injection, in all cases with systemic involvement. Antimony is excreted quickly from the body so that daily treatment is necessary throughout each course of treatment. Meglumine antimoniate and allopurinol given simultaneously have been shown to be effective to maintain dogs in clinical remission. For the treatment of canine leishmaniosis, an alternative approach to meglumine antimoniate is the use of miltefosine (esadecil-phosphocholine) alone or in combination with allopurinol. Miltefosine is a phospholipid analogue; the drug acts against protozoa, interfering with parasite phospholipid metabolism, inhibiting the synthesis of glycol phosphatidylinositol receptors and interrupting the transduction signal acting on phospholipase C and protein kinase C, inducing the apoptosis of the protozoa. In contrast to meglumine antimoniate, which is administered parenterally, miltefosine is given orally. Both drugs should be administered for four weeks, meglumine antimoniate at the dose rate of 50 mg/kg twice a day (or 100 mg/kg once per day), and miltefosine at the dose rate of 2 mg/kg sid.

Arsenicals are substituted benzene arsenic acid salts or esters and have been used in the treatment of trypanosomiasis (**tryparsamide**, **melarsomine**) and coccidiosis (**arsenilic acid**, **roxarsone**). **Melarsomine** is effective against trypanosomes of the *T. brucei* group (*T. b. evansi*). **Roxarsone** was used primarily as a growth promoter but had some activity against *Eimeria tenella* and *E. brunetti* in chickens when used alone or in combination with nitromide or dinitolmide. Arsenicals have a low safety index and have been superseded by comparatively less toxic compounds.

Substituted aromatics

Amidines and diamidines

Pentamidine has the widest spectrum within the group, with activity against *Leishmania*, *Trypanosoma*, *Babesia* and *Pneumocystis*, and is used mainly in human medicine. **Stilbamidine** has been used for the treatment of leishmaniosis. **Amicarbalide** is active against *Babesia* spp. and **diminazene aceturate** is active against both *Babesia* spp. and *Trypanosoma* spp.. Very little is known about the mode of action of this class of compounds. Antiparasitic activity may be related to interference with aerobic glycolysis as well as interference with synthesis of parasite DNA.

Diminazene is highly active against babesiosis in cattle, sheep, pigs, horses and dogs, although the small *Babesia* spp. are generally more refractory to treatment than large ones. There appears to be a wide range of individual animal tolerance to the drug; it is well tolerated in horses at the recommended dose, although higher doses may cause severe side-effects. Various treatment regimens are used for eliminating babesiosis in cattle, horses and dogs. In most cases, the recommended dose is given in divided doses (e.g. 5 mg/kg, twice at 24-hour intervals) to eradicate *Babesia* spp. infections in horses or 1.75 mg/kg twice at 24-hour intervals to reduce or avoid neurotoxic side-effects in horses (lethargy, incoordination and seizures) and dogs (ataxia, opisthotonus, nystagmus, extensor rigidity, coma and even death). Local reactions can occur in cattle and in horses there may be skin sloughing and abscessation following injection. In camels, there may be mortality at the recommended dose rate.

Diminazene is also effective against *T. c. congolense* and *T. v. vivax*, but is less active against *T. b. brucei* and *T. b. evansi* infections and shows no activity against *T. c. simiae*. Widespread use may lead to development of diminazene-resistant *T. v. vivax* and *T. c.*

congolense strains. As a rule, diminazene-resistant strains are susceptible to isometamidium. Trypanosomes resistant to other drugs (except quinapyramine) are commonly susceptible to diminazene.

Phenamidine is used for treating canine and equine babesiosis and has also been used in *Babesia bigemina* infections in cattle. Frequent relapses may occur in *B. gibsoni* infections in dogs. The mechanism of drug action is uncertain but may be similar to that of pentamidine and diminazene.

Arylamides and urea derivatives

These compounds have similar modes of action and act by uncoupling oxidative phosphorylation through inhibition of glycerol phosphate oxidase and glycerol phosphate dehydrogenase, which prevents reoxidation of NADH and decreases ATP synthesis. **Nitolmide** and **dinitolmide** are arylamides (nitrobenzamides) used as coccidiostats in poultry, appearing to affect first-generation meronts; they are active against *Eimeria tenella* and *E. necatrix* infections but have limited activity against *E. acervulina*. Both drugs have been used in combination with roxarsone as in-feed coccidiostats for use in chickens.

Nicarbazin (phenylurea) is also used as a coccidiostat in the control of coccidiosis in chickens and turkeys in shuttle programmes (starter feed only), usually in the winter, and for this reason resistance of coccidia to nicarbazin is not common. It is also used in combination with narasin as it shows synergistic effect with the ionophores. It affects second-generation meronts, impairing oocyst formation and allowing treated birds to develop immunity against coccidia. There may be problems with side-effects, as it can cause increased sensitivity to heat stress during summer, which results in growth depression and mortality in broilers. The drug should not be fed to laying hens because of toxic side-effects (reduced hatchability, interruption of egg laying).

Imidocarb dipropionate is a phenylurea and is the drug of choice for the treatment of babesiosis in cattle, horses and dogs. It appears to act directly on the parasite, leading to an alteration in morphology, and is effective in both treatment and prevention without interfering with the development of immunity.

Ethopabate is an arylamide and has a similar mode of action to the sulfonamides, acting as a *para*-aminobenzoic acid (PABA) agonist, blocking the utilisation of PABA into amino acids and DNA synthesis. It has been administered in combination with amprolium to achieve a broader spectrum of activity for the prophylaxis and treatment of coccidiosis in chickens and turkeys. With chicken coccidia, it has good innate activity against *Eimeria acervulina*, is less active against *E. maxima* and *E. brunetti* and has no activity against *E. tenella*.

Quinuronium sulfate was for many years the drug of choice in treating bovine babesiosis (*B. bigemina*, *B. bovis*, *B. divergens*); it is also active against large *Babesia* of pigs, horses and dogs. The drug has a low therapeutic index and may stimulate the parasympathetic nervous system, resulting in excessive salivation, frequent urination or dyspnoea caused by anticholinesterase activity. The mode of action is unknown.

Sulfonic acids

Suramin and **trypan blue** were amongst the first antiprotozoals. **Suramin** was one of the first antitrypanosomal drugs developed and shows high efficacy against trypanosomes of the subgenus *Trypanozoon* (*T. b. brucei*, *T. b. evansi*, *T. equiperdum*) and is the drug of choice for *T. b. evansi* infections (surra) in camels and horses. The drug inhibits enzymes in the glucose metabolism pathway, preventing reoxidation of NADH and decreased ATP synthesis. It may be toxic in horses, causing oedema of sexual organs, lips and eyelids or painful hoofs. Intramuscular administration can cause severe necrosis at the injection site and suboptimal dosing (<1 g/100 kg) may lead to suramin-resistant strains.

Trypan blue is an azo-naphthalene dye used for the treatment of babesiosis and was the first specific drug with activity against *B. bigemina* in cattle, but its use leads to blue staining of meat and milk, and it has been largely replaced by the diamidines.

Naphthoquinones

Menoctone, **parvaquone** and **buparvaquone** are naphthoquinones with marked antitheilerial activity. They appear to block electron transport at the ubiquinone level. The mechanism of selective toxicity might be due to a difference between parasite and mammalian ubiquinone.

Menoctone was the first drug with high antitheilerial activity, causing marked degeneration in appearance of macroschizonts and suppression of parasitaemia in established *Theileria parva parva* infections in cattle. Its use has now been discontinued.

Parvaquone is highly active against theileriosis (*Theileria p. parva* and *T. annulata*) infections in cattle when treatment is carried out in the early stage of infection, allowing development of protective immunity without apparent clinical signs.

Buparvaquone is an analogue of parvaquone with a substituted alkyl group, and slows down metabolic degradation of the parent compound, increasing efficacy against these species.

Miscellaneous diphenyls

Robenidine is a guanidine derivative and affects the late first-generation and second-stage meronts of *Eimeria* spp. It is both coccidiostatic and coccidiocidal and is used for the treatment of coccidiosis in chickens, turkeys and rabbits. It has a broad spectrum of activity but in rabbits it is active against intestinal *Eimeria* spp. only. It is thought to interfere with energy metabolism by inhibition of respiratory chain phosphorylation and ATPase activity.

Dapsone and **acedapsone** are sulfones active against *Plasmodium* spp. and are generally used in combination products only for treating human malaria. Their mode of action is similar to the sulfonamides, acting as antifolate drugs by blocking the incorporation of PABA to form dihydrofolic acid.

Pyridine derivatives

Decoquinate and **methylbenzoquate** are 4-hydroxyquinolones that act on the sporozoites and first-generation meronts of *Eimeria*, interfering with electron transport at the cytochrome B level and mitochondrial metabolism. Hydroxyquinolines are almost entirely coccidiostatic with activity against sporozoites and trophozoites of all *Eimeria* spp. As single compounds, they have had only limited success because of serious and immediate drug resistance in the field, such that methylbenzoquate-resistant *Eimeria* spp. cannot be controlled by the drug at any level.

Decoquinate has been used for the control of coccidiosis in poultry and is used for the prevention and control of coccidiosis in cattle and sheep. It should not be administered to lactating animals or laying poultry.

Methylbenzoquate is usually administered in combination with clopidol or meticlorpindol, mainly in shuttle or rotation programmes to achieve a broader spectrum of activity for the prophylaxis and treatment of coccidiosis in chickens and turkeys.

Iodoquinol is a 4-hydroxyquinolone that is active against *Entamoeba* spp.

Quinine, **chloroquine**, **hydroxychloroquine**, **primaquine** and **mefloquine** are quinolines used primarily as antimalarial treatments in human medicine, inhibiting electron transport processes by inhibiting pyrimidine synthesis.

Primaquine diphosphate is active against tissue stages of *Plasmodium* spp., but is much less active against erythrocytic stages. It has been shown to be active against *Babesia felis* in cats at 0.5 mg/kg by intramuscular injection, although doses above 1 mg/kg caused mortality. It has also been used in the treatment or prevention of avian malaria (100 mg/kg orally).

Clopidol and **meticlorpindol** are pyridinols and are active against first-generation meronts, arresting sporozoite and trophozoite development; they are effective against all *Eimeria* spp. in chickens, although resistance problems limit their use to shuttle programmes. Both compounds need to be given before or shortly after exposure and are used as a coccidiostats. Clopidol is used in the prevention of coccidiosis in chickens, partridge, guinea fowl, pheasants and rabbits with a high safety index.

Emetine and **dehydroemetine** are isoquinolines with activity against *Entamoeba* spp. The acridine derivative, **quinacrine**, is active against *Plasmodium* spp. and *Giardia* spp. **Acriflavine** hydrochloride is active against *Babesia bigemina* and other large *Babesia*.

Pyrimidine derivatives

Amprolium is structurally similar to thiamine (vitamin B$_1$) and is a competitive thiamine antagonist. Because of the relatively high thiamine requirement of rapidly dividing coccidian cells compared with most host cells, the drug has a high safety margin. Amprolium acts on first-generation meronts, thereby preventing differentiation of merozoites, but has poor activity against some *Eimeria* spp. It is often used in combination with ethopabate but its use has declined in many countries for safety and tolerance reasons in food-producing animals. Amprolium and amprolium plus ethopabate have been used as feed additives for use in chickens, guinea fowl and turkeys for the prevention of coccidiosis, showing activity against *Eimeria tenella* and *E. necatrix*, and to a lesser extent against *E. maxima* of chickens, and also the pathogenic *Eimeria* spp. of turkeys.

Amprolium plus ethopabate have been combined with sulfaquinoxaline and pyrimethamine to extend their activity spectrum and improve efficacy against amprolium-resistant *Eimeria* spp., but such combinations have been discontinued in some countries because of residue problems.

Amprolium and amprolium plus ethopabate have also been used for the treatment and control of coccidiosis in pheasants (but are not active against all *Eimeria* spp.); in lambs and calves; in sows to control disease in suckling pigs before and after farrowing; and in rabbits to control intestinal *Eimeria* spp., but they are ineffective against hepatic coccidiosis in rabbits.

Pyrimethamine and **trimethoprim** are both folate antagonists with activity against *Pneumocystis* and are useful for treating various types of coccidiosis (eimeriosis, toxoplasmosis, sarcocystiosis, neosporosis), malaria and bacterial infections. These compounds target the enzyme dihydrofolate reductase, inhibiting pyrimidine biosynthesis and DNA metabolism, and are usually used in combination with long-acting sulfonamides. As antifolates, they synergise the anticoccidial action of sulfonamides by blocking the same biosynthetic pathway.

Halofuginone is a quinazoline affecting first- and second-generation meronts of *Eimeria* spp. and is used in the control of coccidiosis in chickens and turkeys. The drug has also been shown to possess marked antitheilerial activity in cattle, and is available in some countries for the prevention and treatment of cryptosporidiosis in calves. It has also been shown to be effective against acute sarcosporidiosis in goats and sheep (*Sarcocystis capracanis* and *S. ovicanis*, respectively, at 0.67 mg/kg on two successive days). The therapeutic index of halofuginone is low and overdose may produce severe diarrhoea and cachexia.

Allopurinol is a pyrazolpyrimidine and a xanthine oxidase inhibitor, used alone or in combination with meglumine antimoniate or miltefosine for the treatment of leishmaniosis in dogs.

Aprinocid is no longer available due to the rapid emergence of resistant strains, but it was used as a feed additive for the prevention of coccidiosis in broiler chickens, with a broad spectrum of activity except against *Eimeria tenella*. The compound inhibits sporulation of oocysts and may be coccidiostatic after a short medication period or coccidiocidal after long periods of medication. Arprinocid acts against coccidia by inhibiting hypoxanthine transport.

Phenathridiums

This group of compounds, which includes **isometamidium**, **homidium** and **quinapyramine**, has been used exclusively in the treatment of trypanosomiasis. The mode of action appears to be interference with nucleic acid synthesis by intercalative DNA binding. Other drugs of this series – **pyrithidium**, **phenidium chloride** and **dimidium bromide** – were replaced because of a high incidence of delayed toxicity, including marked liver damage and severe local reaction at the injection site.

Isometamidium is a synthetic hybrid of the diazotised *p*-aminobenzamidine moiety of diminazene molecule linked with homidium chloride. The drug is highly active against *T. v. vivax* infections in ruminants and horses as well as against *T. c. congolense* infections in ruminants, horses and dogs. It is less active against *T. b. brucei* and *T. b. evansi* infections in horses, ruminants, camels and dogs. The recommended dose is usually well tolerated by cattle but intramuscular injection can cause severe local reactions at the injection site. Intravenous injection in horses and camels may avoid local reaction but may cause systemic toxicity (salivation, tachycardia, profuse diarrhoea, hindleg weakness and collapse due to histamine release).

Homidium salts (bromide or chloride) are effective against *T. v. vivax* infections in cattle but less so against *T. c. congolense* and *T. b. brucei*. Their limited protective activity in cattle depends on severity of challenge and may last 3–5 weeks. Homidium can also be used for treating *T. v. vivax* and *T. c. congolense* infections in horses and dogs. Widespread use in cattle resulted in the appearance of resistant *T. c. congolense* strains in East and West Africa. Homidium-resistant trypanosomes can be controlled by diminazene or isometamidium at increased dose rates. The drug is generally well tolerated at the recommended dose and also at higher dose levels but may be irritant at sites of injection. Deep intramuscular injection effectively reduces local irritations. Severe reactions may occur in horses after intramuscular injection, whereas intravenous injection seems to be well tolerated.

Quinapyramine is highly active against *T. c. congolense*, *T. v. vivax*, *T. b. brucei* and *T. b. evansi* and reaches therapeutic levels quickly. The target of action of quinapyramine is protein synthesis, displacing magnesium (Mg^{2+}) ions and polyamines from cytoplasmic ribosomes, leading to extensive loss of ribosomes and condensation of kinetoplast DNA. The drug can cause local and systemic reactions (salivation, shaking, trembling, diarrhoea, collapse) in cattle, horses, dogs and pigs within minutes of treatment. Unexpected acute toxicity and the rapid development of drug-resistant strains of *T. c. congolense* have limited its usefulness in treating trypanosomiasis in cattle. However, the drug seems to be safe and efficient for treating surra (*T. b. evansi*) in camels and horses as well as *T. b. evansi* infections in pigs. Quinapyramine-resistant strains are usually controlled by isometamidium. Quinapyramine is active against suramin-resistant strains of *T. b. evansi* and *T. b. brucei*.

Triazones

Asymmetrical triazones

Diclazuril and **clazuril** are asymmetrical triazones with a broad spectrum of activities against various coccidia in birds and animals at low concentrations (0.5–2 ppm in feed). **Diclazuril** has strong anticoccidial activity and has been developed as a feed additive for the prevention of coccidiosis in chickens and turkeys. It is active against developing first- and second-generation meronts and gamonts of *E. tenella* and other pathogenic *Eimeria* spp. of chickens, but developmental stages most affected by diclazuril vary with the *Eimeria* species. It is highly effective against all stages of *E. tenella* but only against gamont stages of *E. maxima*. Because of the development of resistance, it is used frequently in shuttle programmes. Diclazuril is also used for the treatment of rabbit coccidiosis, showing high activity against hepatic and intestinal coccidiosis, and in the treatment and prevention of coccidiosis in sheep and cattle.

Clazuril has only limited action against some chicken coccidia, but is highly active against coccidiosis in pigeons.

Symmetrical triazones

Toltrazuril is a symmetrical triazone compound and is active against all intracellular stages of coccidia found in chicken, geese, ducks and cattle, sheep, goats and pigs. It is generally used therapeutically for the treatment of outbreaks of coccidiosis. In some species, it can be administered via drinking water and, because of its long residual activity, can be used intermittently to allow the development of protective immunity.

Benzimidazoles

The benzimidazoles have been described in detail in the section on anthelmintics at the beginning of this chapter. Benzimidazoles such as **mebendazole**, **fenbendazole** and **albendazole** are active against

Giardia spp. infections in humans, farm animals and dogs; however, repeat treatments may be necessary to eliminate parasites because of reinfection.

Antibacterials

Sulfonamides

Sulfonamides, such as **sulfadimidine**, **sulfamethoxypyridazine**, **sulfaguanidine**, **sulfaquinoxaline** and **sulfachloropyrazine**, are structural antagonists of *para*-aminobenzoic acid (PABA), which is incorporated into folic acid. They inhibit the conversion of dihydrofolic acid to tetrahydrofolic acid at the dihydropteroate synthase step. Tetrahydrofolate is an important co-factor in many active single-carbon transfer reactions required for the synthesis of certain amino acids, purines and especially the synthesis of deoxythymidylate required for DNA synthesis. Large doses used for therapeutic applications often cause toxicity (haemorrhagic syndrome, kidney damage and growth depression).

Sulfonamides were among the first anticoccidials and are active against first- and second-stage meronts, being coccidiostatic at low doses and coccidiocidal at higher doses. Many of the compounds used in chickens had a broad spectrum of activity against intestinal *Eimeria* spp. but only a moderate effect on *E. tenella* in chickens, but their use has been stopped in many countries. Sulfonamides have also been used in the treatment of coccidiosis in cattle, sheep, pigs, dogs, cats and rabbits. When given in combination with pyrimethamine and other diaminopyrimidines, long-acting sulfonamides (e.g. sulfadoxine or sulfamethoxine) are highly active antibacterials, antimalarials and anticoccidials.

Nitroimidazoles

The nitroimidazoles include **dimetridazole**, **ornidazole**, **ronidazole**, **tinadazole**, **carnidazole** and **metronidazole**, which appear to interfere with RNA synthesis, and **nifursol**, which acts by causing damage to lipids and DNA within the cells.

These compounds exhibit potent activity against trichomonads, *Histomonas* spp., *Spironucleus* spp. and *Giardia* spp., and were the drugs of choice for these infections in turkeys and gamebirds. Ronidazole, dimetridazole and nifursol were used in the treatment of *Histomonas* infections in turkeys and gamebirds (pheasants, partridge); however, because of concerns over mutagenicity, their use has been suspended in many countries. Carnidazole is used for the treatment of trichomoniasis in pigeons. Metronidazole, ornidazole and tinazole are used in humans for the treatment of giardiosis and amoebiosis.

Nitrofurans

The nitrofurans, which include **furazolidone**, **nitrofurazone** and **nitrofurantoin**, are relatively broad-spectrum bactericidal drugs and have coccidiostatic activity; concerns over toxicity and carcinogenicity have restricted their widespread use and they are prohibited in many countries. **Furazolidone** has been used for the prevention and treatment of coccidiosis in chickens, turkeys and pigs and for the treatment of bacterial digestive tract infections and giardiosis. **Nitrofurazone** is active against second-generation meronts of *E. tenella* and *E. necatrix* infections in poultry and has been used for control of coccidiosis in lambs and goat kids.

Ionophores

The polyether ionophores are fermentation products of *Streptomyces* or *Actinomadura*. These are currently the most widely used anticoccidial compounds, mainly for the control of poultry coccidiosis. **Monensin, narasin, salinomycin, maduramicin** and **semduramicin** are 'monovalent' ionophores preferentially binding to the monovalent ions sodium and potassium (Na$^+$, K$^+$), although divalent cations are also bound. **Lasalocid** has the ability to complex divalent cations (Ca^{2+}, Mg^{2+}) and is termed a 'divalent' ionophore. The effect is to destroy cross-membrane ion gradients. They may also block host carbohydrate transport and hence deprive of intracellular parasites of a carbohydrate supply

Ionophores act on the intestinal free forms of coccidian stages (sporozoites, merozoites and gametocytes) when the drug comes into contact with them in the intestinal lumen. These compounds are extremely toxic to horses. Ionophores such as monensin, narasin and salinomycin may cause severe growth retardation when administered with tiamulin, and most of the ionophores may interact with sulfonamides, chloramphenicol and erythromycin.

Monensin has been used extensively in the broiler industry but drug tolerance, as with other ionophores, limits its use to shuttle programmes. It is effective against coccidia in cattle, sheep and rabbits when used prophylactically in feed. Narasin is given in combination with nicarbazine to improve coccidiosis control, and the drug combination may be used in the starter phase of shuttle programmes followed by a different ionophore in the grower–finisher phase.

Salinomycin has broad-spectrum activity and better activity against *E. tenella* and *E. acervulina* than other related ionophores, including drug-tolerant *Eimeria* spp. in the field. In turkeys, it may cause severe toxicity with growth depression, excitement, paralysis of head and legs and death if feed containing recommended or lower doses is given for long periods.

Lasalocid may alter water excretion in treated birds via dietary electrolytes to the extent that wet litter may be a problem at higher drug concentrations. At concentrations of 75 ppm, activity against *E. tenella* is good but it is insufficient against *E. acervulina*. In the field, lasalocid may improve control of coccidiosis where *E. tenella* strains show tolerance to other ionophores.

Macrolide and lincosamide antibiotics

This group of compounds is better known and more widely applied for the treatment of bacterial and fungal infections. The mode of action appears to be inhibition of protein synthesis. **Spiramycin** inhibits protein synthesis by inhibiting the translocation of peptidyl-tRNA. It has been used for the treatment of *Toxoplasma gondii* infections. **Clindamycin** is a lincosamide with a similar mode of action, and has been used to treat *Plasmodium* spp., *Babesia* spp. and *T. gondii* infections. It is considered the antiparasitic of choice for the treatment of clinical toxoplasmosis in cats and dogs.

Amphotericin B is a polyene macrolide antibiotic used mainly as an antifungal agent but is also used as a second-line drug for the treatment of *Leishmania* spp. The drug is extremely nephrotoxic but lipid and unilamellar liposome formulations of amphotericin B have been developed with lower toxicity.

Aminoglycoside antibiotics

Aminoglycoside antibiotics are bactericidal agents widely applied for the treatment of Gram-negative bacterial infections. Aminoglycosides are not absorbed from the gastrointestinal tract and treatment via this route is reserved for the treatment of gastrointestinal infections. **Paromomycin** has activity against *Entamoeba* spp., *Giardia* spp., *Balantidium coli* and *Leishmania* spp.

Tetracycline antibiotics

The tetracyclines are broad-spectrum antibacterials active against a range of Gram-positive and Gram-negative bacteria, but also against the rickettsiales (*Rickettsia* spp., *Ehrlichia* spp., *Anaplasma* spp.), and *Mycoplasma* spp. and *Chlamydia* spp. The mode of action is thought to be via inhibition of protein synthesis.

Oxytetracycline, tetracycline and **chlortetracycline** have similar properties and may be given orally or by intramuscular injection. **Doxycycline** is more lipophilic than the other tetracyclines and is better absorbed orally and penetrates better into the lung and cerebrospinal fluid. Members of this group exhibit the broadest antiprotozoal activity and have been used for the treatment of *Plasmodium* spp., *Balantidium coli*, *Theileria* spp. and *Entamoeba* spp. infections. Oxytetracycline has been shown to control active *Babesia divergens* infections in cattle by continuous administration of 20 mg/kg every four days.

USE OF ANTIPROTOZOALS

The use of antiprotozoals as therapeutic or prophylactic agents is similar to that described for anthelmintics.

METHODS OF ADMINISTRATION

Anticoccidials used for controlling enteric coccidia principally belonging to the genus *Eimeria* are mainly administered in feed. In the poultry industry, it is usual to employ anticoccidials in broiler birds continuously in feed until just before slaughter. In layer replacement stock, pullets are medicated continuously until commencement of egg laying. Continuous use of anticoccidials may lead to ineffective treatment due to drug resistance; as a consequence, various rotational programmes have been developed by the poultry industry to reduce or avoid this problem.

Antiprotozoals are generally used in two ways: therapeutically, to treat existing infections or clinical outbreaks, or prophylactically, in which the timing of treatment is based on knowledge of the epidemiology. Clearly, prophylactic use is preferable where administration of a drug at selected intervals or continuously over a period can prevent the occurrence of disease.

Most other antiprotozoal agents, particularly those targeting haemoprotozoan infections, are given parenterally, by either subcutaneous or intramuscular injection (Table 5.2). Not all trypanocides are available in every country and there is also no guarantee that production of all or any of them will continue for economic reasons.

Table 5.2 Trypanocidal drugs.

Generic name	Dosage rate (mg/kg)	Route	Remarks
Suramin	10	i.v.	Mainly used against *T. evansi* in camels. Some activity against *T. brucei* in camels and *T. equiperdum* in horses
Diminazene aceturate	3.5–7	i.m.	Mainly used in cattle and small ruminants against *T. vivax*, *T. congolense* and *T. brucei*
Homidium bromide	1	i.m.	Mainly used in cattle and small ruminants against *T. vivax*, *T. congolense* and *T. brucei*. Should be dissolved in hot water. Potentially carcinogenic
Homidium chloride	1	i.m.	Mainly used in cattle and small ruminants against *T. vivax*, *T. congolense* and *T. brucei*, but soluble in cold water
Quinapyramine methyl sulfate	5	s.c.	Active against *T. vivax*, *T. congolense* and *T. brucei* in cattle. Now mainly used against *T. evansi* and *T. brucei* in camels and horses; activity against *T. equiperdum* in horses
Isometamidium chloride	0.25–0.5	i.m.	Used mainly in cattle (*T. vivax*, *T. congolense*), as a curative at lower rates, as a prophylactic at higher rates. Also contains homidium and is therefore to be considered as potentially carcinogenic

ECTOPARASITICIDES: INSECTICIDES AND ACARICIDES

MODE OF ACTION

Three main chemical groups have been used historically as the basis of control for the common ectoparasiticides: the organochlorines, the organophosphates and the synthetic pyrethroids. More recently, the isoxazolines have been used increasingly for the control of ticks and fleas in companion animals. Other groups that are also used include the carbamates (primarily in poultry), the formamidines, the triazines, benzylbenzoate and natural plant products such as pyrethrin. The avermectins and milbemycins have also been shown to have activity against a range of ectoparasites and these are increasingly used for ectoparasite control, for example mange in sheep, cattle and pigs. Many compounds affect the growth and development of insects, primarily by replicating or inhibiting the hormones that regulate developmental processes in arthropods. Based on their mode of action, they can be divided into chitin inhibitors, chitin synthesis inhibitors and juvenile hormone analogues. Insect growth regulators (IGRs) are used for flea control in domestic pets and for blowfly control in sheep but have limited use in other host species. For example, lufenuron blocks the formation of larval chitin in fleas and cyromazine disrupts growth regulation in blowfly larvae on sheep.

Organochlorines

Organochlorines are now banned in many countries on the grounds of both human and environmental safety. Organochlorines have persistent impacts in ecosystems, with bioaccumulation and biomagnification in food chains resulting in long-term toxicity. Organochlorines fall into three main groups.

- **Chlorinated ethane derivatives**. This group includes DDT (dichlorodiphenyltrichloroethane), DDE (dichlorodiphenyldichloroethane) and DDD (dicofol, methoxychlor). Chlorinated ethanes cause inhibition of sodium conductance along sensory and motor nerve fibres by holding sodium channels open, resulting in delayed repolarisation of the axonal membrane. This state renders the nerve vulnerable to repetitive discharge from small stimuli that would normally cause an action potential in a fully repolarised neurone.
- **Cyclodienes**. The cyclodienes include chlordane, aldrin, dieldrin, hepatochlor, endrin and tozaphene. They appear to have at least two component modes of action: inhibition of GABA-stimulated Cl$^-$ flux and interference with calcium ion (Ca^{2+}) flux. The resultant inhibitory postsynaptic potential leads to a state of partial depolarisation of the postsynaptic membrane and vulnerability to repeated discharge.
- **Hexachlorocyclohexanes**. This group includes benzene hexachloride (BHC) and its γ-isomer lindane. The mode of action is similar to the cyclodienes, with the drug binding to the picrotoxin side of the GABA receptor, resulting in inhibition of GABA-dependent Cl$^-$ flux into the neurone.

DDT and BHC were used extensively for flystrike control but were subsequently replaced in many countries by the more effective cyclodiene compounds, dieldrin and aldrin. DDT and lindane (BHC) were widely used in dip formulations for the control of sheep scab but the organophosphates and synthetic pyrethroids have largely replaced them. They have the advantage that the effect of the drug persists for a longer time on the coat or fleece of the animal but the disadvantage, at least in food animals, is that they persist in animal tissues. If toxicity occurs, the signs are those of central nervous system (CNS) stimulation with hypersensitivity, followed by increasing muscular spasm progressing to convulsions.

Organophosphates

These include a large number of compounds, of which **chlorfenvinphos, coumaphos, crotoxyphos, crufomate, cythioate, diazinon, dichlofenthion, dichlorvos, fenthion, iodofenphos, malathion, phosmet, propetamphos, ronnel, tetrachlorvinphos** and **trichlorphon** have been among the most used. These can persist in the animal's coat or fleece for periods of several weeks, but residues in animal tissues are relatively short-lived. Some have the ability to act systemically, given parenterally, orally or as a pour-on, but the effective blood levels of these are maintained for only 24 hours. The organophosphates are cholinesterase inhibitors; if acute toxicity occurs, the signs are salivation, dyspnoea, incoordination, muscle tremors and sometimes diarrhoea. There is also concern over the chronic toxicity that may be associated with use of these compounds and which is thought to be the result of inhibition of the enzyme neurotoxic esterase.

Synthetic pyrethroids

The common synthetic pyrethroids in use include **deltamethrin, permethrin, cypermethrin, flumethrin** and **fenvalerate**. The main value of these compounds lies in their repellent effect and since they persist well on the coat or skin, but not in tissue, they are of particular value against parasites which feed on the skin surface, such as lice, some mites and nuisance flies.

Pyrethroids act as neurotoxins on sensory and motor nerves of the neuroendocrine system and CNS of insects. All the pyrethroids are lipophilic and this property helps them to act as contact insecticides. Some have the ability to repel and to 'knock down', i.e. affect flight and balance without causing complete paralysis. Because the synthetic pyrethroids have a strong affinity for sebum, this property has been capitalised upon by incorporating them into ear tags or tail bands. The synthetic pyrethroids are relatively safe but if toxicity does occur, it is expressed in the peripheral nervous system as hypersensitivity and muscle tremors. Pyrethroids should not be used on cats. Synthetic pyrethroids are extremely toxic to fish and aquatic invertebrates and there are environmental concerns over their use.

Carbamates

Carbamate insecticides are closely related to the organophosphates and are anticholinesterases, but unlike organophosphates they appear to induce a spontaneously reversible block of the enzyme acetylcholinesterase without changing it. The two main carbamate compounds in use in veterinary medicine are **carbaryl** and **propoxur**, with **butocarb** and **carbanolate** also used in the control of poultry ectoparasites. Carbaryl has low mammalian toxicity but may be carcinogenic and is often combined with other active ingredients. **Fenoxycarb** is used for flea control and appears to have a mode of action closely related to the juvenile hormone analogues, preventing embryonic development in flea eggs, larval development and adult emergence (see section on Insect growth regulators). It has been formulated with permethrin or chlorpyrifos for use on animals or in liquid concentrate form for environmental flea control.

Avermectins/milbemycins

These compounds are effective at very low-dose levels against certain ectoparasites when given parenterally and in pour-on formulations. They are particularly effective against ectoparasites with tissue stages, such as warbles (*Oestrus* spp., *Hypoderma* spp., *Gasterophilus* spp.), bots and mites, and have good activity against blood-sucking parasites such as lice and one-host ticks. As in nematodes, they are thought to affect cell function by direct action on Cl⁻ channels. They have a very wide safety margin. Some avermectins have a marked residual effect and a single treatment given parenterally is still effective against lice or mites hatching from eggs 3–4 weeks later.

Selamectin is effective against fleas of cats and dogs (*Ctenocephalides* spp.) and prevents flea infestations on dogs and cats for a period of 30 days. It is safe and effective in controlling mite (*Otodectes* spp., *Sarcoptes* spp.) and tick (*Rhipicephalus* spp.) infestations.

Formamidines

The main member of this group is **amitraz**, which acts at octopamine receptor sites in ectoparasites, resulting in neuronal hyperexcitability and death. It is available as a spray or dip for use against mites, lice and ticks in domestic livestock. In cattle, for example, it has been widely used in dips, sprays or pour-on formulations for the control of single-host and multi-host tick species. In dipping baths, it can be stabilised by the addition of calcium hydroxide, and maintained by standard replenishment methods for routine tick control. An alternative method has been the use of total replenishment formulations whereby the dip bath is replenished with the full concentration of amitraz at weekly intervals prior to use. Amitraz has also been shown to have expellent action against attached ticks. It has been shown to be effective in controlling lice and mange in pigs and psoroptic mange in sheep.

In small animals, amitraz is available for topical application for the treatment and control of ticks, and for canine demodicosis (*Demodex canis*) and sarcoptic mange (*Sarcoptes scabiei*). It is contraindicated in horses and in pregnant or nursing bitches and cats, although it has been used at a reduced concentration to treat feline demodicosis. Amitraz is also formulated in collars for tick control in dogs.

Phenylpyrazoles

Fipronil is a phenylpyrazole compound that blocks transmission of signals by the inhibitory neurotransmitter GABA present in insects. The compound binds within the Cl⁻ channel and consequently inhibits the flux of Cl⁻ ions into the nerve cell, resulting in hyperexcitation of the insect nervous system. Fipronil is used worldwide for the treatment and control of flea and tick infestations on dogs and cats and has reported activity against mange mites (*Sarcoptes scabiei*), ear mites (*Otodectes cinotis*), forage mites (*Trombicula* spp., *Cheyletiella* spp.) and dog lice (*Trichodectes* spp.). It is highly lipophilic and diffuses into the sebaceous glands of hair follicles that then act as a reservoir, giving it a long residual activity. Sunlight, immersion in water and bathing do not significantly affect the performance of products containing this compound. There is evidence that fipronil has an extremely rapid knock-down effect which occurs before the fleas have time to feed and hence it may be especially useful in cases of flea allergic dermatitis.

Nitroguanidines and spinosyns

Imidacloprid is a chloronicotinyl insecticide, a synthesised chlorinated derivative of nicotine. It specifically binds to nicotinic acetylcholine receptors in the insect's CNS, leading to inhibition of cholinergic transmission and resulting in paralysis and death. This mode of action is the same as nicotine, which has been used as a natural insecticide for centuries. The favourable selective toxicity of imidacloprid appears to be due to the fact that it only seems to bind to the acetylcholine receptors of insects, having no effect on these receptors in mammals. Its activity appears to be mainly confined to insect parasites and it is available as a spot-on product in many countries for use in dogs and cats for the control of adult fleas, providing protection against reinfestation for up to 4–5 weeks.

Spinosad is a fermentation product of the soil actinomycete *Saccharopolyspora spinosa*, and has been developed in some countries for use on sheep in the control of blowfly strike and lice.

Oxadiazines

Indoxacarb is a pro-insecticide that requires metabolic activation in the target insect to an active metabolite with insecticidal effect. The active metabolite of indoxacarb induces irreversible hyperpolarisation of insect nerve cell membranes, by binding to voltage-gated Na⁺ channels, leading to impaired insect nerve function, feeding cessation, paralysis and death of susceptible insects. Indoxacarb is used for the control of fleas in dogs and cats.

Isoxazolines

The **isoxazolines** (e.g. **afoxolaner, fluralaner, lotilaner, sarolaner**) and the isoxazoline-like tigolaner are a relatively recent class of insecticide that act as non-competitive GABA receptor agonists, binding to Cl⁻ channels in nerve and muscle cells of the target parasites. Isoxazolines are usually given orally or topically and are mainly used for the control of fleas and ticks in companion animals; specific dosages or formulations may provide 3 to 12 months of efficacy against fleas and ticks. Slow release subcutaneous injectable formulations have been developed that give 12 months protection. Their efficacy against mites causing mange in dogs and cats has also been demonstrated and veterinary products containing isoxazolines have been licensed for the treatment of sarcoptic and demodectic mange. In general, isoxazolines have a high margin of safety in cats and dogs, but may occasionally be associated with neurological effects in some dogs, such as muscle tremors, ataxia and seizures.

Insect growth regulators

Several insect growth regulatos (IGRs) are used throughout the world. They constitute a group of chemical compounds that do not kill the target parasite directly but interfere with growth and development. IGRs act mainly on immature stages of the parasite and as such are not usually suitable for the rapid control of established populations of adult parasites. Where parasites show a clear seasonal pattern, IGRs can be applied prior to any anticipated challenge as a preventive measure. Their main advantage is the high specificity against the target pest or parasite while their disadvantage is the relatively slow rate at which they achieve population suppression.

Based on their mode of action, they can be divided into chitin synthesis inhibitors (benzoylphenyl ureas), chitin inhibitors (triazine/pyrimidine derivatives) and juvenile hormone analogues. IGRs are widely used for flea control in domestic pets and for blowfly control in sheep but have limited use in other host species.

Benzoylphenyl ureas

The benzoylphenyl ureas (**diflubenzuron, flufenoxuron, fluazuron, lufenuron** and **triflumuron**) are chitin inhibitors, of which several have been introduced for the control of ectoparasites of veterinary importance. Chitin is a complex aminopolysaccharide and a major component of the insect's cuticle. Around each moult (ecdysis), it has to be newly formed by polymerisation of individual sugar molecules. Chitin molecules, together with proteins, are assembled into chains, which in turn are assembled into microfibrils.

The exact mode of action of the benzoylphenyl ureas is not fully understood. They inhibit chitin synthesis but have no effect on the enzyme chitin synthetase, and it has been suggested that they interfere with the assembly of the chitin chains into microfibrils. When immature insect stages are exposed to these compounds, they are not able to complete ecdysis and as a consequence die during the moulting process. Benzoylphenyl ureas also appear to show a transovarial effect. Exposed adult female insects produce eggs in which the compound is incorporated into the egg nutrient. Egg development proceeds normally but the newly developed larvae are incapable of hatching.

Benzoylphenyl ureas show a broad spectrum of activity against insects but have relatively low efficacy against ticks and mites. The exception to this is fluazuron, which has greater activity against ticks and some mite species. Benzoylphenyl ureas are highly lipophilic molecules and, when administered to the host, build up in the body fat from where they are slowly released into the bloodstream and excreted largely unchanged.

Diflubenzuron and **flufenoxuron** are used for the prevention of blowfly strike (Calliphoridae) in sheep. Diflubenzuron is available in some countries as an emulsifiable concentrate for use as a dip or shower. It is more efficient against first-stage larvae than second and third instars and is therefore recommended as a preventive, providing 12–14 weeks' protection. It may also have potential for controlling a number of major insect pests such as tsetse flies. Fluazuron is available in some countries for use in cattle as a tick development inhibitor. When applied as a pour-on, it provides long-term protection against the one-host tick *Rhipicephalus (Boophilus) microplus*.

Lufenuron is administered orally for the control of fleas of dogs and cats. The drug accumulates in fat tissue, allowing subsequent slow release. Fleas take up the drug through the blood and transfer it to their eggs, which are non-viable within 24 hours of administration. The formation of larval chitin structures is blocked, thereby inhibiting the development of flea larvae and providing environmental control of the flea population. For oral administration, the drug must be administered in the food to allow sufficient time for absorption from the stomach. Injectable treatment is given at six-monthly intervals while oral treatment is given once monthly during summer, commencing two months before fleas become active. As lufenuron has no activity against adult fleas, an insecticide treatment may be required if there is an initial heavy infestation or in cases of severe hypersensitivity. **Triflumuron** is effective against lice and fleas in dogs.

Triazine/pyrimidine derivatives

Triazine and pyrimidine derivatives are closely related compounds that are also chitin inhibitors. They differ from the benzoylphenyl ureas both in chemical structure and in mode of action, in that they appear to alter the deposition of chitin into the cuticle rather than its synthesis.

Cyromazine, a triazine derivative, is effective against blowfly larvae on sheep and lambs and also against other Diptera, such as house flies and mosquitoes. At recommended dose rates, cyromazine shows only limited activity against established strikes and must therefore be used prophylactically before anticipated challenge. Blowflies lay eggs usually on the damp fleece of treated sheep. Although larvae are able to hatch out, the young larvae immediately come into contact with cyromazine, which prevents the moult to second instars. The use of a pour-on preparation of cyromazine has the advantage that efficacy is not dependent on factors such as weather, fleece length and whether the fleece is wet or dry. In addition, the persistence of the drug is such that control can be maintained for up to 13 weeks after a single pour-on application, or longer if applied by dip or shower.

Dicyclanil, a pyrimidine derivative, is highly active against dipteran larvae and is available as a pour-on formulation for blowfly control in sheep in some countries, providing up to 20 weeks' protection.

Juvenile hormone analogues

The juvenile hormone analogues mimic the activity of naturally occurring juvenile hormones and prevent metamorphosis to the adult stage. Once the larva is fully developed, enzymes within the insect's circulatory system destroy endogenous juvenile hormones, and final development occurs to the adult stage. The juvenile hormone analogues bind to juvenile hormone receptor sites but because they are structurally different, are not destroyed by insect esterases. As a consequence, metamorphosis and further development to the adult stage do not proceed.

Methoprene is a terpenoid compound with very low mammalian toxicity that mimics a juvenile insect hormone and is regularly used for flea control. It is sensitive to light and will not persist outdoors. It has been used extensively and successfully in indoor environments and on pets in the form of collars, shampoos, sprays and dips and also as a feed through larvicide for hornfly (*Haematobia irritans*) control on cattle. The other member of this group used for the control of fleas in dogs and cats is **pyriproxyfen**.

Essential oils

There is a growing body of evidence indicating the potential value of essential oils as control agents against a range of arthropod ectoparasites, particularly lice, mites and ticks. Essential oils are blends of approximately 20–80 different plant metabolites that are usually extracted from plants through steam distillation. These metabolites are volatile molecules of low molecular weight. Essential oils usually contain two or three major terpene or terpenoid components, which constitute up to 30% of the oil. Their efficacy is often attributed to the oil's major component(s), although there is also evidence that the various oil components may work in synergy. This may be achieved because some oil components aid cellular accumulation and absorption of other toxic components. Nevertheless, the mode of action of many essential oils or components is largely unknown, although there is evidence of toxic effect on the insect nervous system. Toxicity has been demonstrated following immersion and physical contact with treated surfaces but also after exposure to the vapour of these oils, the latter implying that there is a neurotoxic rather than simply a mechanical pathway in their mode of action. However, because of the volatile nature of essential oils, their residual activity is usually short-lived (around 4–12 hours depending on the substrate treated). Some ovicidal efficacy has been reported, although it is unclear whether this results from neurotoxicity or mechanical suffocation.

Miscellaneous compounds

Piperonyl butoxide (PBO) is a methylenedioxyphenyl compound that has been widely used as a synergistic additive in the control of arthropod pests. It is commonly used as a synergist with natural pyrethrins, the combination having a much greater insecticidal activity than the natural product alone. The degree of potentiation of insecticidal activity is related to the ratio of components in the mixture, such that as the proportion of PBO increases, so the amount of natural pyrethrins required to evoke the same level of kill decreases. The insecticidal activity of other pyrethroids, particularly of knock-down agents, can also be enhanced by the addition of PBO. The enhancement of activity of synthetic pyrethroids is normally less dramatic but PBO may be included in several formulations. PBO inhibits the microsomal enzyme system of some arthropods and has been shown to be effective against some mites. In addition to having low mammalian toxicity and a long record of safety, PBO rapidly degrades in the environment.

Various products from natural sources, as well as synthetic compounds, have been used as insect repellents. These include cinerins, pyrethrins and jasmolins (see Pyrethroids), citronella, indalone, garlic oil, MGK-264, butoxypolypropylene glycol, **DEET** (*N*, *N*-diethyl-meta-toluamide) and **DMP** (dimethylphthalate). The use of repellents is advantageous as legislative and regulatory authorities become more restrictive towards the use of conventional pesticides.

METHODS OF APPLICATION AND USES

Livestock

Traditionally, ectoparasiticides have been applied topically as dusts, sprays, foggers, washes, dips and occasionally used in baits to trap flying insects. However, with the advent of pour-on and spot-on formulations with a systemic effect, the parenteral administration of drugs such as the avermectins and closantel and the use of impregnated ear tags, collars and tail-tags, the methodology of control applications to animals has changed.

Traditional methods

To be successful, the use of insecticides in dusts, sprays or washes usually requires two or more treatments, since even the most diligent application is unlikely to be successful in applying these formulations at the right concentration to all parts of the animal's body. The interval between treatments should be linked to the persistence of the chemical in the skin, hair or wool and to the life cycle of the parasite, further treatment being given prior to completion of another cycle.

Dip baths or spray races containing the necessary concentration of insecticide may be used to control mites, lice and ticks and certain dipterans such as blowflies on sheep on a worldwide basis and on cattle in tropical areas. This technique is more successful in sheep, where the persistence of insecticide is greater in the wool fleece than in the hair coat found in cattle. It is important to remember that the concentration of insecticide in a dip bath is preferentially 'stripped' or removed as sheep or cattle are dipped, and so must be replenished at a higher than initial concentration, sufficient to maintain an adequate concentration of the active ingredient. Most dips are based on the organophosphate group and synthetic pyrethroids. Despite human and environmental safety concerns, some countries have reintroduced organochlorines because of developing resistance to organophosphates.

Insect control in dairies or stables may be aided by the use of various resin strips incorporating the insecticide; dichlorvos and trichlorphon are often used for this purpose. Sometimes baits, containing synthetic pheromones, sugars or hydrolysed yeasts, plus insecticide are spread around animal premises to attract and kill dipterans.

Pour-on, spot-on

Different pour-on and spot-on are available at present and contain organophosphates with a systemic action, such as fenthion or phosmet, the avermectins/milbemycins, the synthetic pyrethroids or isoxazolines. They are recommended for the control of warbles and lice in cattle and lice and keds in sheep. A valuable development is that of pour-on phosmet for the control of sarcoptic mange in pigs and cattle. A single treatment in pigs gives very good results and, if used in sows prior to farrowing, prevents transmission to the litter; two treatments at an interval of 14 days are necessary in cattle. The synthetic pyrethroids are also available as sprays, pour-ons or spot-ons for the treatment of lice and the control of biting and nuisance flies in cattle, sheep and goats.

Ear tags

Ear tags are based primarily on the synthetic pyrethroids and occasionally the organophosphates. They are recommended for the protection of cattle against nuisance flies. The tags are usually made of polyvinylchloride impregnated with the insecticide. When attached to an animal's ear, the insecticide is released from the surface, dissolves in the sebum secreted by the skin and is then spread over the whole body by the normal grooming actions or ear flapping and tail swishing as well as by bodily contact between cattle. Because the insecticide is rapidly bonded to the sebum on the animal's coat, the treatment is rain-fast; also the tag or tail band continues to release a supply of chemical under all climatic conditions. Since the drugs are located in the sebum, they are not absorbed into the tissue so there is no need for a withdrawal period prior to slaughter, nor is it necessary to discard milk. The common synthetic pyrethroids marketed for this purpose are cypermethrin and permethrin. Under conditions of heavy fly challenge, a tag should be inserted in each ear, possibly augmented by a tail band.

Parenteral treatment

The avermectins/milbemycins and closantel may be given parenterally to control some ectoparasites. For example, the endectocides have good activity against warbles, lice, many mites and the one-host tick *Rhipicephalus* (*Boophilus*) *microplus*. Closantel is available in some tropical countries for use against one-host ticks and sucking lice.

Companion or pet animals

Ectoparasiticides of companion animals and pets are mainly used as dusting powders, aerosols, washes/shampoos, spot-on preparations and impregnated collars, while some are available for oral use. They are mainly used for the control of fleas, lice and mange in dogs and cats and for lice, mange and nuisance flies in horses.

Dusting powders

The powders must be distributed well into the animal's fur or hair and, in the case of house pets, into the bedding. The powders commonly used contain pyrethroid-based insecticides with or without the synergist PBO. These are particularly useful for fleas and lice and repeat treatments are generally recommended every 2–3 weeks.

Aerosols and sprays

Although easy to use, some of the noisier sprays can upset pets. Overzealous spraying in confined spaces, such as in a cat basket, may produce toxic effects. Sprays available are generally based on pyrethroids or fipronil, and now rarely, carbamates or a mixture of organophosphates such as dichlorvos plus fenitrothion, or a mixture of the synergist piperonyl butoxide (PBO) with organophosphates or pyrethroids. Depending on the spray, the aerosol container should be held 15–30 cm from the animal and sprayed for up to five seconds for cats and a little longer for dogs. A repeat treatment is often recommended in 7–14 days; however, a single spray application with fipronil can give up to three months' protection against reinfestation with fleas in dogs and cats. The aerosol sprays are very effective for fleas and lice, but several treatments may be necessary for mange mites. The synthetic pyrethroids are also available as a wash or spot-on for horses for the control of flies including midges, which are responsible for 'sweet itch'.

Aerosols containing the insect growth regulator methoprene are available for the control of larval populations of fleas in the environment.

Baths

Different compounds formulated as shampoos, emulsifiable concentrates, wettable agents or creams for the control of fleas, lice and mange mites are available. Most preparations are for dogs and care is needed if they are used for cats. Common ingredients are carbaryl, propoxur and the organophosphate phosmet; amitraz is particularly useful for demodectic mange in dogs. The instructions for bathing should be carefully followed and, where necessary, care taken that the insecticide is properly rinsed from the coat. Organophosphate shampoos should not be used when dogs have insecticidal collars.

Insecticidal collars

Collars are used primarily for flea and biting fly control. Historically, a variety of insecticides such as organophosphates, synthetic pyrethroids and imidacloprid have been used in these collars. Newer insecticide collar formulations contain either deltamethrin or imidacloprid-flumethrin. In the latter, imidacloprid and flumethrin are combined in a slow-release system giving a synergistic effect and the period of protection is claimed to be 7–8 months. They have a pronounced antifeeding effect and these collars are effective at preventing infection with transmissible diseases such as leishmaniosis. With organophosphate collars, occasional problems arise from contact dermatitis and care should be exercised that the animals do not receive other concurrent organophosphate treatments. Apart from collars, impregnated medallions are also available in some countries. Care should be taken with the use of organophosphate collars in pedigree long-haired cats and greyhound dogs due to individual susceptibility.

Oral preparations

Isoxazolines are mainly marketed as oral chewable compounds for dogs and mainly spot ons for cats. This route of adiminstration is one of the most preferred by pet owners and ensures fast and complete adbsorption of the drug.

Spot-ons

Spot-on preparations containing fenthion, deltamethrin, fipronil, imidacloprid, selamectin, and isoxazolines are available for the control of fleas, and ticks and/or mites, on dogs and cats. In horses, lice and areas of mange mite infestation can be treated topically, but the problem of nuisance or pasture flies remains. Spot ons usually provides a sustained efficacy for 1 month. Two categories of spot on formulations are distinguished: i) the spot on with contact activity, the active ingredient diffuses on the skin and is stored in sebum and sebaceous glands, and ii) the spot on with systemic activity after transcutaneous absorption of the actives.

Poultry ectoparasites

The carbamates and the organophosphate malathion are the most widely used. Individual birds are dusted and the insecticide applied in the poultry house, nesting boxes and litter. Cypermethrin is available for the environmental treatment of poultry red mites (*Dermanyssus galline*). Isoxazolines may be used against mites on poultry; the isoxazoline compound is administered through drinking water in two separate doses seven days apart.

PARASITICIDE RESISTANCE

As soon as selective pressure is imposed, such as inducing higher mortality with a parasiticide, those genotypes that are better able to persist and reproduce will inevitably start to increase in frequency in the population. Since resistance is heritable, repeated dosing will therefore select for an increasing proportion of resistant individuals. Resistance mechanisms involve either differences in drug metabolism within the parasite and/or mutations at the binding site of the drug. The prevalence and severity of resistance are increasing and, particularly in livestock, leading to uncontrolled loss of production.

ANTHELMINTIC RESISTANCE

Anthelmintic resistance in small ruminants

Resistance to anthelmintics has been most frequently recorded in sheep and goats (mainly for *Haemonchus* spp. and *Trichostrongylus* spp. in tropical and subtropical regions; *Teladorsagia* spp., occasionally *Cooperia* spp. and *Nematodirus* spp. in temperate areas). This initially involved the benzimidazole group of compounds (1-BZ, benzimidazoles and pro-benzimidazoles) and then the levamisole group (2-LV, levamisole/morantel); more recently, macrocyclic lactone (3-ML, avermectins/milbemycins) resistance has emerged. This sequence of events reflects the period for which these drugs have been available. The severity and prevalence of resistance differ between different geographic locations and between different species of helminths and animal hosts. Resistance can be particularly significant in goats. The highest levels of resistance occur in Australia, South America, South Africa, southern parts of the USA and New Zealand. Resistance to the benzimidazoles, levamisole and some of the macrocyclic lactones is widespread and there are worms which are resistant to all three classes of anthelmintic and in some countries also to some narrow-spectrum drugs.

Resistance has also been reported for some drug combination products. Where recent prevalence studies are available, it has been shown that the level of resistance to some anthelmintics has increased. Of particular concern is that total anthelmintic failure is now prevalent in parts of South America. The situation in Europe differs in that although resistance to the benzimidazoles is high, that for levamisole and the macrocyclic lactones is still comparatively low. However, there are recent reports of isolates with concurrent resistance to 1-BZ, 2-LV and ivermectin (3-ML) but only a few reports of moxidectin resistance.

The differences in the rate of emergence of anthelmintic resistance between these agroclimatic zones are considered to be due to the number of parasite generations and biotic potential of the parasite species involved and also to the proportion of the total population not exposed to the drug (i.e. left *in refugia*). Frequency of treatment and underdosing are considered to be the main causes of benzimidazole and levamisole resistance in *Haemonchus* spp. and *Teladorsagia* spp. The timing of treatments and the presence of larvae *in refugia* may be particularly important in the development of macrocyclic lactone resistance. Trematode resistance to flukicides is currently at lower levels, although there have been increasing reports of triclabendazole resistance in liver fluke (*Fasciola hepatica* and *F. gigantica*) in some countries.

Anthelmintic resistance in cattle nematodes

Although anthelmintic resistance is less frequent in cattle than in sheep and goats, reports of resistance have increased over recent years and the majority involve resistance to the macrocyclic (3-ML) compounds. There is little information to assess the global problem as very few studies have been conducted on the prevalence in cattle. The main species implicated in benzimidazole resistance are *Cooperia* spp., although in some cases *Ostertagia ostertagi*, *Trichostrongylus axei* and *Haemonchus* spp. have also been involved. Reports of macrocyclic lactone resistance mainly involve *Cooperia* spp., which is the dose-limiting species with this class of compounds. Levamisole resistance is not currently common in cattle. Trematode resistance to flukicides is considered to be at a low level and possibly has been selected in sheep and transmitted to cattle where mixed grazing occurs.

Anthelmintic resistance in horse nematodes

Most of the information on anthelmintic resistance in horses originates from the USA and prevalence studies are limited. High levels of resistance to the benzimidazoles (1-BZ) and lower levels to pyrantel (2-LV) exist and the parasites involved are mainly cyathostomins and *Parascaris equorum*. There is evidence that macrocyclic lactone (3-ML) resistance is developing in cyathostomins and is becoming more common and widespread for *P. equorum*.

Resistance management strategies

Studies have shown minimal reversion to susceptibility in highly selected homozygous isolates following withdrawal of the selecting drug and, as a consequence, once resistant worms are present on a livestock enterprise they can be considered as permanent. Therefore, it is important to be able to detect the presence of emerging resistant isolates at an early stage. Unfortunately, the *in vivo* faecal egg count reduction test and the *in vitro* egg hatch assay, larval development assay and larval migration inhibition assay, used to detect the presence of resistant isolates, are time-consuming, insensitive and will only detect resistant parasites when these comprise around 25% of the total population. The use of a discriminating dose of anthelmintic may increase the sensitivity.

There is a need for more convenient tests and robust guidelines for their interpretation to enable uptake by the end-user. New molecular-based probes are more sensitive but to date are only available for the benzimidazoles and are mainly used as research tools. The increasing severity and prevalence of anthelmintic resistance have highlighted the importance of resistance management strategies for the control of nematode infections in livestock. There is an urgent need to change many of the drug treatment strategies, which are known to impose a high level of selection for resistance, and thus preserve the efficacy of current anthelmintics and, most importantly, the two new drugs for use in sheep, monepantel (4-AD) and derquantel (5-SI) often used in combination with the 3-ML drug abamectin. Strategies to delay the development/transmission of anthelmintic resistance are discussed in the section on Treatment, prevention and control of parasitic gastroenteritis in Chapters 8 and 9, but the concept of *refugia* is considered here.

Recently, the concept of leaving enough parasites in the environment that are not exposed to anthelmintic treatment (the principle of *refugia*) has been an area of increased focus. This principle is based on the concept that in order to lower the selection pressure for anthelmintic resistance, any eggs from resistant worms that survive treatment must be diluted by a pool of non-resistant infective larvae. This strategy will reduce the relative contribution of resistant parasites to future worm populations. The application of the concept of maintaining *refugia* from untreated animals requires some alterations to existing management strategies for control of roundworms in livestock farms and, depending on individual circumstances, will usually involve targeted treatment of only a proportion of the stock – often the most highly infected individuals (see below). These treatment approaches aim to create a balance between allowing sufficient larvae to remain unexposed to drug treatment and the inevitable consequence on production performance of a higher worm burden in some animals.

Treatment of the whole flock/herd

In circumstances where treatment of the whole flock/herd is inevitable, then the dosing regimen needs to take into consideration those periods when there is minimal survival of larvae on pasture. Treatment of animals at this time will impose an increased selection for anthelmintic resistance. It may be possible to delay the strategic treatment to those periods in the grazing season when eggs from untreated animals are more likely to develop into infective larvae on

pasture. It may also be possible to provide refugia within a flock/herd by turning animals out after treatment onto 'dirty' pasture for a period to allow any eggs from worms that survived treatment to be diluted. This can be achieved most effectively by moving the more resilient adult treated animals onto 'wormy' pastures rather than the more susceptible younger animals.

Targeted treatments can also be effective. In this approach, an indication of the level of parasitism in the flock, such as regular monitoring for worm eggs in faeces, is used and the whole flock is treated when these reach a predetermined level. A reduction in treatment frequency will lead to a refugia benefit, particularly in situations where animals are exposed to continual larval challenge from pasture. A further potential benefit of this regular monitoring is that additional information on the species of parasites present and their epidemiology will be recorded.

Treatment of a proportion of the flock/herd

One approach is to use indices of animal performance and parasitism to identify those animals in the flock/herd which would most benefit from anthelmintic treatment (i.e. targeted selective treatment) rather than treating the whole group of animals. This approach should maximise the number of parasites which are not exposed to treatment and thus maintain a reservoir of 'susceptible' worms within the overall parasite population on pasture, thus slowing the rate of drug resistance. The indices used vary but include faecal egg counts, the FAMACHA system to assess anaemia in *Haemonchus* spp. infections, serum pepsinogen levels in first-season grazing calves at housing, and production parameters such as liveweight gain, body condition scoring or milk yield.

Recently, a model has been developed which predicts growth rate from the nutritional status of the pasture and size of the animal and highlights any underperforming animals which may benefit from treatment. Recent trials have supported the ability of the targeted selective treatment approach to lower the rate of development of resistance.

The adoption of refugia-based strategies by livestock farmers to reduce the selection pressure for anthelmintic resistance is essential for long-term sustainable parasite control programmes. Unless further new anthelmintic groups are licensed for use in ruminants in the near future, it is essential that the livestock industries adopt control strategies that conserve the efficacy of those compounds which are still effective and of the new 4-AD and 5-SI class of drugs used in sheep. It is encouraging that modelling indicates that in situations where the older anthelmintics still have a reasonably high level of efficacy, the introduction of a new class of anthelmintic may assist in delaying the development of resistance to these older drugs. Other strategies that are directed at increasing the natural effective immune response, such as vaccination, selection of more resistant livestock or the introduction of nutritional supplementation (see Chapter 6), will reduce the overall reliance on anthelmintics.

ANTIPROTOZOAL RESISTANCE

Continuous use of antiprotozoals has also led to ineffective treatment due to drug resistance in the target parasite populations. This is perhaps best exemplified by the situation with anticoccidial compounds. The control of avian coccidiosis (see Chapter 13) has relied almost entirely on chemotherapy, as is evident from the fact that most intensively reared chickens are fed an anticoccidial agent in the diet throughout their period of growth. Feed medication is a convenient and cost-effective method of enabling large numbers of chickens to be reared under intensive conditions. The practice of including drugs in the feed throughout the life of the bird has ensured that few parasites escape the effects of medication. In such an environment, parasites are exposed throughout their life cycle to agents designed for their removal and this has inevitably resulted in the development of resistance.

A succession of chemical compounds has been introduced and has been crucial in the successful control of coccidiosis in the rapidly expanding poultry industries throughout the world. However, the emergence of resistance has been rapid and has limited the useful life of many chemical anticoccidials, although the speed at which resistance develops varies greatly between compounds. With the ionophore antibiotics, which have dominated the scene for the last three decades, resistance has been considerably slower to develop. Nevertheless, resistance to this group has been reported in both Europe and the USA, with cross-resistance occurring notably among the monovalent cation group. Although ionophore-resistant strains may be present, it is possible that the numbers of oocysts are insufficient to cause clinical coccidiosis. Selection pressure is therefore probably lower than with many of the chemical anticoccidials. It has been suggested that this incomplete control of parasite development stimulates production of immunity in the host and this may be a major factor in the effectiveness of ionophores in the field.

Knowledge of the mode of action of anticoccidial compounds is necessary to understand the mechanisms of resistance. Although some information is available on the biochemical pathways inhibited by certain anticoccidial drugs, explanations for their selectivity are either circumstantial or unknown. As in other parasites, the most likely mechanism of resistance involves modification of the target receptor so that its sensitivity to inhibition is decreased. Compounds that share a similar mode of action may also share resistance (cross-resistance). This should be distinguished from multiple resistance in which resistance may be to several drugs with differing modes of action.

It has been shown that parasites resistant to the recommended levels of certain anticoccidial drugs may be suppressed if the concentration of drug is increased. Resistance to these higher concentrations, however, is likely to develop rapidly after further selection. Increasing the concentration of a drug may therefore only be of use in the short term and, furthermore, would not be practical because most anticoccidial drugs are used at levels close to those that are toxic to the chicken.

Resistant strains may emerge if anticoccidial drugs have been employed at concentrations lower than those normally recommended for control. It would therefore appear to be important to maintain adequate drug levels in the field in order to reduce the possibility of selecting resistant strains. A reduction in the use of drugs is desirable since it is generally accepted that the selection of genes for resistance will occur more rapidly as the frequency of treatment is increased. Control of coccidiosis may be achieved by giving drugs intermittently, the objective being to prevent the build-up of infection in a poultry house. However, such a policy would be unacceptable to the poultry industry because of, for example, the impairment of food conversion that would probably result.

The genetics of anticoccidial resistance in *Eimeria* spp. are poorly understood. Most drugs inhibit the asexual stages of the life cycle. Many of the complexities involved in the selection of resistance in diploid organisms, such as the degree of dominance of resistance genes, are absent because these stages are haploid. Any resistant mutants will therefore be immediately selected at the expense of sensitive forms. Asexual division will ensure their rapid multiplication and resistance will swiftly become the dominant phenotype. It has been shown that resistance to certain drugs (e.g. decoquinate, methylbenzoquate) develops rapidly in a single step and may be due to a single mutation, whereas resistance to other drugs, such as amprolium and robenidine, develops more slowly, possibly as a

result of a series of small discrete steps involving successive mutations. Information on the rate at which resistance develops may be helpful in selecting the most appropriate drugs for use in the field.

The control of coccidiosis is likely to continue to depend on chemotherapy, although alternatives, such as immunoprophylaxis, are now established and offer a practical alternative. Until now, as resistance has developed to the older compounds, new ones have been discovered to replace them. It is doubtful whether this situation will continue. It is important therefore that strategies be devised to obtain the best use of existing drugs.

Alternation of drugs (rotation) with different modes of action has been widely advocated in the poultry industry, but this has been based on an empirical, rather than scientific, basis. It is not known for what duration (number of crops) a particular drug should be used before changing to another anticoccidial agent. Alternation of drugs within a single crop (shuttle programmes) has also been widely practised. It has been claimed that this may slow the development of resistance but no evidence to support this contention has been provided. The period of medication for the drugs in a shuttle may be too short to eliminate any resistant forms. Resistant parasites may survive in the litter for the life of the crop and the subsequent use of the same drugs would result in further selection pressure for resistance. A likely result of short periods of alternation between drugs is the development of strains resistant to several drugs (multiple resistance). Vaccines based on live attenuated parasites are now in use as an alternative to medication for the control of coccidiosis. Alternating cycles of planned immunisation and chemotherapy might result in the replacement of drug-resistant parasites by drug-sensitive strains with reduced pathogenicity.

Reversion to sensitivity with older chemical compounds can eventually occur, leading to their reintroduction in control programmes. However, the time interval before a population recovers susceptibility to a drug is likely to be considerably longer than the time taken to acquire resistance. It is also probable that resistance will re-emerge more rapidly if older compounds are reintroduced.

Various combinations of drugs have been employed to extend the spectrum of activity against different species of *Eimeria* spp. rather than prevent the development of resistance (e.g. amprolium and ethopabate). Mixtures have also been used to reduce the risk of toxicity since, in some cases, adequate activity can be obtained with lower doses than if the drugs are used alone (e.g. naracin and nicarbazin). Even where these combination drug mixtures have been used, resistance has developed.

Another area in which resistance has become a problem is in the control of trypanosomiasis. Drug resistance was first noted in trypanosomes to the arsenicals and aromatic compounds. For example, diminazene resistance in *Trypanosoma v. vivax* and *T. c. congolense* strains is now widespread. As a rule, diminazene-resistant strains are susceptible to isometamidium. Widespread use of homidium and quinapyridine in cattle resulted in the appearance of resistant *T. c. congolense* strains in East and West Africa. Homidium-resistant trypanosomes can be controlled by diminazene or isometamidium at increased dose rates. Quinapyramine-resistant strains are usually controlled by isometamidium. Quinapyramine is also active against suramin-resistant strains of *T. b. evansi* and *T. b. brucei*.

INSECTICIDE RESISTANCE

At the recommended doses, modern insecticides are highly effective at removing susceptible individuals, but they can impose strong selection pressure for the development of resistance. The development of resistance may reduce the effectiveness of the treatment applied and

Table 5.3 Insecticide resistance in the major ectoparasites of importance in cattle and sheep. Note in many cases resistance can occur in localised or national populations, and is not necessarily found worldwide.

Family	Species	Primary host	Known resistance
Mites (Acari: Astigmata)	*Sarcoptes scabiei*	Pigs	ML resistance in humans; not yet known in animal parasites
	Psoroptes ovis	Sheep (occasionally cattle)	OP, SP, ML
	Chorioptes bovis	Sheep and cattle	None recorded
Ticks (Acari: Ixodidae)	*Ixodes ricinus*	Sheep and cattle	None recorded
	Ixodes persulcatus	Sheep and cattle	None recorded
	Rhipicephalus sanguineus group, *R. bursa*, *R. turanicus*, *R. appendiculatus*	Sheep and cattle	AM, OP, SP
	Rhipicephalus (Boophilus) annulatus	Sheep and cattle	OC, AM, OP, SP, ML PP
	Hyalomma marginatum	Cattle	None recorded
	Dermacentor reticulatus, D. marginatus	Sheep and cattle	None recorded
	Haemaphysalis punctata	Sheep and cattle	None recorded
Sucking lice (Psocodea: Anoplura)	*Linognathus vituli*	Cattle	None recorded
	Linognathus pedalis, L. ovillus	Sheep	None recorded
	Haematopinus spp.	Cattle	None recorded
	Solenopotes capillatus	Cattle	None recorded
Chewing lice (Psocodea: Ischnocera)	*Bovicola bovis, B. ovis*	Sheep and cattle	OC, OP, SP
Myiasis (Diptera: Calliphoridae)	*Lucilia* spp.	Sheep and cattle	OP, SP, IGR
Myiasis (Diptera: Sarcophagidae)	*Wohlfahrtia magnifica*	Sheep	None recorded
Myiasis (Diptera: Oestridae)	*Oestrus ovis*	Sheep	None recorded
	Hypoderma lineatum, H. bovis	Cattle	None recorded
Fleas: (Siphonaptera: Pulicidae)	*Ctenocephalides felis*	Sheep	Suspected but not yet confirmed

IGR, insect growth regulator; OC, organochlorine; OP, organophosphate; SP, synthetic pyrethroid; AM, Amidenes; ML macrocyclic lactones; PP, Phenylpyrazoles.

thereby increase the frequency of application and the dose required, in turn increasing the costs and adding to the environmental impact.

There are two major variables that determine the rate at which resistance is likely to spread throughout the population: its mechanism of inheritance and the severity of selective pressure (the percentage of susceptible individuals that survive each generation). In general, resistance will spread through a population most rapidly when it is inherited as a single dominant allele and selective pressure is high (meaning very few susceptible individuals escape and reproduce).

When an insect population develops resistance to one pesticide, it may also prove to be resistant to similar compounds that have the same mode of action. This phenomenon, known as class resistance, occurs frequently in insect populations that develop resistance to organophosphate, carbamate or pyrethroid insecticides. In some cases, a population may develop a form of resistance that protects it from compounds in more than one chemical class. This is known as cross-resistance and may result in an insect pest or ectoparasite population that can no longer be controlled with chemical insecticides.

Overall, resistance in the majority of ectoparasite species is not as severe or widespread a problem as that seen in endoparasites (Table 5.3). There are three general approaches that can be used to reduce the rate of resistance development.

1 **Management by saturation** involves heavy or frequent use of a pesticide that is designed to leave absolutely no survivors. It is most effective when the resistant gene is dominant and the target population is small, isolated or living in a limited habitat.

2 **Management by moderation** uses only the minimum control necessary to reduce a population below an acceptable level. This strategy tries to ensure that susceptible genes are never eliminated from the population. It works best when the susceptible trait is dominant over the resistant trait.

3 **Management by multiple attack** involves the use of several control tactics that work in different ways. By rotating insecticides with different modes of action or by alternating chemical with non-chemical control tactics, a pest population is exposed to selective pressures that change from generation to generation.

Clearly, the approach adopted will also depend on the parasite in question, the epidemiology of transmission and the farming environment. Permanent ectoparasites, or highly host-specific species which spend long periods on the host and which have relatively low rates of transmission, such as bot and warble flies, can be susceptible to coordinated programmes of management by saturation because entire populations can be targeted and removed simultaneously. In general, however, for most ectoparasites, management by moderation and management by multiple attack are recommended.

Resistance development may be slowed or even prevented if there is a substantive reservoir of untreated individuals in the population. In addition, it is essential to ensure that the manufacturer's recommendations are scrupulously followed, and that all apparatus is calibrated correctly and working effectively. For farmers wanting to reduce reliance on synthetic insecticides, a range of management practices and non-chemical methods may be utilised in an integrated manner to reduce ectoparasite prevalence (see Chapter 6). One or several techniques may be used but importantly, these should be integrated with each other to form components of a general livestock ectoparasite management programme. Such management is usually based on the use of control technologies which modify some aspect of the parasite's environment, on or off the host, in order to increase pest mortality, reduce fecundity or reduce contact between the pest and host.

CHAPTER 6

Innate and acquired resistance, vaccines and alternative approaches to parasite management

Broadly speaking, resistance to parasitic infections falls into two categories. The first of these, often termed innate resistance, includes species resistance, age resistance and in some cases breed resistance which, by and large, are not immunological in origin. The second category, acquired immunity, is dependent on antigenic stimulation and subsequent humoral and cellular responses.

Although, for reasons explained in this chapter, there are few vaccines available against parasitic diseases, natural expression of acquired immunity plays a highly significant role in protecting animals against infections and in modulating the epidemiology of many parasitic diseases.

INNATE RESISTANCE TO PARASITIC INFECTION

SPECIES RESISTANCE

For a variety of parasitological, physiological and biochemical reasons, many parasites do not develop at all in other than their natural hosts; this is typified by, for example, the remarkable host specificity of the various species of *Eimeria*. In many instances, however, a limited degree of development occurs, although this is not usually associated with clinical signs; for example, some larvae of the cattle parasite *Ostertagia ostertagi* undergo development in sheep, but very few reach the adult stage. However, in these unnatural or aberrant hosts, and especially with parasites which undergo tissue migration, there are occasionally serious consequences, particularly if the migratory route becomes erratic. An example of this is visceral *larva migrans* in children due to *Toxocara canis*, which is associated with hepatomegaly and occasionally ocular and cerebral involvement.

Some parasites, of course, have a very wide host range, *Trichinella spiralis*, *Fasciola hepatica*, *Cryptosporidium parvum* and the asexual stages of *Toxoplasma* being four examples.

AGE RESISTANCE

Many animals become more resistant to primary infections with some parasites as they reach maturity. For example, ascarid infections of animals are most likely to develop to patency if the hosts are a few months old. If hosts are infected at an older age, the parasites either fail to develop or are arrested as larval stages in the tissues; likewise, patent *Strongyloides* infections of ruminants and horses are most commonly seen in very young animals. Sheep of more than three months of age are relatively resistant to *Nematodirus battus* and, in a similar fashion, dogs gradually develop resistance to infection with *Ancylostoma* over their first year of life.

The reasons underlying age resistance are unknown, although it has been suggested that the phenomenon is an indication that the host–parasite relationship has not yet fully evolved. Thus, while the parasite can develop in immature animals, it has not yet completely adapted to the adult.

On the other hand, where age resistance is encountered, most parasitic species seem to have developed an effective countermechanism. Thus, *Ancylostoma caninum*, *Toxocara canis*, *Toxocara mystax*, *Toxocara vitulorum* and *Strongyloides* spp. all survive as larval stages in the tissues of the host, only becoming activated during late pregnancy to infect the young *in utero* or by the transmammary route. In the case of *Nematodirus battus*, the critical hatching requirements for the egg, i.e. prolonged chill followed by a temperature in excess of 10 °C, ensure the parasites' survival as a lamb-to-lamb infection from one season to the next.

Oddly enough, with *Babesia* and *Anaplasma* infection of cattle, there is generally thought to be an inverse age resistance, in that young animals are more resistant than older naive animals.

BREED RESISTANCE

In recent years, there has been considerable practical interest in the fact that some breeds of domestic ruminants are more resistant to certain parasitic infections, such as coccidian protozoa, nematodes, ticks and flies, than other breeds. Probably the best example of this is the phenomenon of trypanotolerance displayed by West African humpless cattle such as the N'dama and West African shorthorn cattle, which survive in areas of heavy trypanosome challenge. The mechanism whereby these cattle control their parasitaemias is still not fully known, although it is thought that immunological responses may play a role.

In helminth infections, it has been shown that Red Masai sheep, indigenous to East Africa, are more resistant to *Haemonchus contortus* infection than some imported breeds studied in that area, while in South Africa it has been reported that the Merino is less susceptible to trichostrongylosis than certain other breeds. In the USA, the Florida Native (Gulf Coast), Barbados Blackbelly and St Croix breeds of sheep are considerably more resistant to *H. contortus* than the Merino or European breeds.

Veterinary Parasitology, Fifth Edition. Domenico Otranto and Richard Wall.
© 2024 John Wiley & Sons Ltd. Published 2024 by John Wiley & Sons Ltd.

Within breeds, haemoglobin genotypes have been shown to reflect differences in susceptibility to *H. contortus* infection in that Merino, Scottish Blackface and Finn Dorset sheep, which are all homozygous for haemoglobin A, develop smaller worm burdens after infection than their haemoglobin B homozygous or heterozygous counterparts. Unfortunately, these genotypic differences in susceptibility often break down under heavy challenge.

Studies within a single breed in Australia have shown that individual Merino lambs may be divided into responders and non-responders on the basis of their immunological response to infection with *Trichostrongylus colubriformis* and that these differences are genetically transferred to the next generation.

The selection of resistant animals could be of great importance, especially in many developing areas of the world, but in practice would be most easily based on some easily recognisable feature such as coat colour rather than be dependent on laboratory tests.

In Australia, resistance to ticks, particularly *Rhipicephalus* (*Boophilus*), has been shown to be influenced by genetics, being high in the humped, *Bos indicus*, Zebu breeds and low in the European, *Bos taurus*, breeds. However, where cattle are 50% Zebu, or greater, in genetic constitution, a high degree of resistance is still possible, allowing a limited use of acaricides.

SELECTION FOR RESISTANCE

An approach to complement other sustainable control measures for parasites in livestock is to breed only from animals which exhibit significantly enhanced levels of innate resistance to parasites in comparison to the mean response of the population and include this trait into selection criteria. There is considerable evidence for extensive genetic variation, both between breeds and within populations of animals, for resistance to internal and external parasites. In sheep, between-flock variation in resistance is often small compared to within-flock variation. Resistance is inherited as a dominant trait, with heritability often exceeding 0.3. An increased resistance to gastrointestinal nematode infections is frequently associated with higher antibody responses, greater levels of T-cell proliferation and increased inflammatory responses.

There has been considerable progress in the last decade in the use of performance-recording schemes and indices of selection that identify those high-producing animals which also exhibit enhanced resistance to internal parasites. Index selection combines production traits (e.g. growth rate, body condition score) under conditions of parasite challenge with markers of parasite burdens such as faecal egg count (FEC) (in some countries a worm FEC service is available) or the FAMACHA index (for those parasites, such as *Haemonchus* spp., that cause anaemia). In general, resistance is assessed in young male animals as they are the major contributors to genetic advancement, and genetic variation within a breed is usually recommended rather than breed substitution. Examples of small ruminants which have been selectively bred for resistance to gastrointestinal nematodes include a *Haemonchus* spp.-resistant Merino sheep flock in New South Wales, Australia; the Rylington Merino, adapted for the winter rainfall regions of western Australia; and a Romney line of sheep in New Zealand. The use of such resistant animals will reduce pasture contamination with worm eggs, and subsequently larval challenge and worm burdens will be lower for all grazing animals, and hence there will be benefits for the whole flock or herd. The outcome will be a reduced effect of parasitism on production and a reduction in the number of drenches required for control.

Concern was initially raised as to whether selection for enhanced resistance to parasites would reduce the genetic gains in other production traits. Evidence suggests that in most cases, livestock which have been bred for resistance to gastrointestinal nematodes are equally as productive over a grazing season as the unselected animals in the flock. Furthermore, there is evidence that animals that are resistant to one species of nematode appear to demonstrate favourable responses to other nematode species and also that this resistance to nematodes has not been gained at the expense of resistance to other diseases.

It is important that breeding for resistance to parasites should be envisaged as a component of an ongoing sustainable parasite control programme and should not be considered in isolation.

ACQUIRED IMMUNITY TO HELMINTH INFECTIONS

Multicellular parasites such as helminths are very complex genetic organisms and because of their physical size, they cannot be consumed by phagocytic cells or destroyed by classic cytotoxic T-cells. The host's immune system has had to devise new approaches to counter invasion by these parasites. These are generally referred to as type 2 immune responses (T-helper 2 or Th2) or the allergy-type immune responses. They are frequently characterised by increases in the concentrations of interleukin (IL)-4 and other Th2-type cytokines, such as IL-5, IL-9, IL-13 and IL-21. These responses are usually characterised by the recruitment and activation of effector cells, such as eosinophils, basophils and mast cells which can produce various type 2 cytokines. There is continual communication between the innate and adaptive components of an active immune response to parasite invasion, with the T-cells evoking signals that increase and modify the function of innate effector cells. The specific effector cells and antibody classes that mediate protection in the host immune responses vary considerably between different parasites. Individual effector cell types may also have multiple functions. Frequently, parasite infestation causes chronic infections and the immune response that develops over a prolonged period can induce pathological changes in tissues. For example, in schistosome infections, antigens shed from eggs can induce a marked Th2-type response that stimulates the development of granulomatous lesions in the liver parenchyma.

Immune responses to helminths are complex, possibly depending on antigenic stimulation by secretory or excretory products released during the development of the L_3 to the adult. For this reason, it has only been possible to develop one or two practical methods of artificial immunisation, of which the radiation-attenuated vaccine against *Dictyocaulus viviparus* is perhaps the best example.

Despite this, there is no doubt that the success of many systems of grazing management depends on the gradual development by cattle and sheep of a naturally acquired degree of immunity to gastrointestinal nematodes. For example, experimental observations have shown that an immune adult sheep may ingest around 50 000 *Teladorsagia* (*Ostertagia*) L_3 daily without showing any clinical signs of parasitic gastritis.

EFFECT OF THE IMMUNE RESPONSE

Dealing first with gastrointestinal and pulmonary nematodes, the effects of the immune response may be grouped under three headings, the sequence reflecting the usual progression of acquired immunity.

1 Initially, the host can attempt to limit reinfection by preventing the migration and establishment of larvae and penetration of the mucosal barrier or, sometimes, by arresting their development at a larval stage. This type of inhibition of development should not be confused with the more common hypobiosis triggered by environmental effects on infective larvae on pasture or, in the present state of knowledge, with the arrested larval development associated with age resistance in, for example, the ascarids.

2 Adults that do develop may be stunted in size or their fecundity may be reduced. The important practical aspect of this mechanism is perhaps not so much the reduced pathogenicity of such worms as the great reduction in pasture contamination with eggs and larvae, which in turn reduces the chance of subsequent reinfection.

3 The development of immunity after a primary infection may be associated with an ability to kill or expel the adult nematodes.

Each of these mechanisms is exemplified in infections of the rat with the trichostrongyloid nematode *Nippostrongylus brasiliensis*, a much-studied laboratory model, which has contributed greatly to the understanding of the mechanisms of host immunity in helminth infection. The infective stage of this parasite is normally a skin penetrator, but in the laboratory is usually injected subcutaneously for convenience. The larvae travel via the bloodstream to the lungs where, having moulted, they pass up the trachea and are swallowed. On reaching the small intestine, they undergo a further moult and become adult, the time elapsing between infection and development to egg-laying adults being 5–6 days. The adult population remains static for about another five days. After this time, the faecal worm egg output drops quickly and the majority of the worms are rapidly expelled from the gut. This expulsion of adult worms, originally known as the 'self-cure' phenomenon, has been shown to be due to an immune response.

If the rats are reinfected, a smaller proportion of the larval dose arrives in the intestine, i.e. their migration is stopped. The few adult worms which do develop in the gut remain stunted and are relatively infertile, and worm expulsion starts earlier and proceeds at a faster rate.

Under natural grazing conditions, larval infections of cattle and sheep are acquired over a period but an approximately similar series of events occurs. For example, calves exposed to *Dictyocaulus viviparus* quite rapidly acquire patent infections, readily recognisable by the clinical signs. After a period of a few weeks, immunity develops and the adult worm burdens are expelled. On subsequent exposure in succeeding years, such animals are highly resistant to challenge, although if this is heavy, clinical signs associated with the reinfection syndrome (i.e. immunological destruction of the invading larvae in the lungs) may be seen. With *Ostertagia* and *Trichostrongylus* infections, the pattern is the same, with the build-up of an infestation of adult worms being followed by their expulsion and subsequent immunity; in later life only small, short-lived, adult infections are established and eventually the infective larvae are expelled without any development at all. However, with gastrointestinal infections in ruminants, the ability to develop good immune responses is often delayed for some months because of immunological unresponsiveness.

The mechanism of immunity to luminal parasites is still not fully understood despite considerable research. This response includes both innate and adaptive components. However, it is generally agreed that such infections stimulate a Th2-type response and produce a state of gut hypersensitivity associated with an increase

in mucosal mast cells in the lamina propria and the production of worm-specific IgE, much of which becomes bound to the surface of the mast cells. The reaction of worm antigen, from an existing infection or from a subsequent challenge, with these sensitised mast cells releases vasoactive amines, which cause an increase in capillary and epithelial permeability and hyperproduction of mucus. Some studies have concluded that these physiological changes simply affect the well-being of the worms by, for example, lowering the oxygen tension of their environment so that they become detached from the mucosa and subsequently expelled. Others have postulated that, in addition, the permeable mucosa allows the 'leakage' of IgG anti-worm antibody from the plasma into the gut lumen, where it has access to the parasites.

Although the majority of helminths induce marked mast cell responses, their role in mediating resistance to infection varies considerably between parasite infections. For example, in rodent models, the presence of mast cells is required for the expulsion of *Trichinella spiralis*, whereas mast cells are not essential for the rejection of *Nippostrongylus brasiliensis*. Additional factors, such as the secretion of specific anti-worm IgA on the mucosal surface and the significance of sensitised T-cells, which are known to promote the differentiation of mast cells, eosinophils and mucus-secreting cells, are also currently under study.

With regard to tissue-invading helminths, the most closely studied have been the schistosomes. Schistosomulae of *Schistosoma mansoni* may be attacked by both eosinophils and macrophages, which attach to the antibody-coated parasite. Eosinophils, especially, attach closely to the parasites where their secretions damage the underlying parasite membrane. Eosinophils release a secondary granule protein and can also produce cytokines (IL-4, IL-13) which can have a regulatory role. Attempts to determine if a similar mechanism exists against *Fasciola hepatica* have indicated that although eosinophils do attach to parts of the tegument of the young fluke, the latter seems able to shed its surface layer to evade damage.

In *Schistosoma* infections, there is an initial Th1-type response to the acute infection that is directed against adult parasites, but following patency and egg deposition in tissues, the response changes to predominantly a Th2-type response. In cases where an effective Th2-type response fails to develop after egg deposition, the outcome is often increased granulomatous inflammation in the tissues and liver parenchyma, induced by the underlying Th1-type response. Thus, the protective Th2-type response minimises the pathological consequences of a Th1-type response and the outcome is often mild granulomas composed of macrophages, lymphocytes and eosinophils.

EVASION OF THE HOST'S IMMUNE RESPONSE

Despite the evidence that animals are able to develop vigorous immune responses to many helminth infections, it is now clear that parasites, in the course of evolution, have capitalised on certain defects in this armoury. This aspect of parasitology is still in its infancy, but four examples of immune evasion are described here.

Neonatal immunological unresponsiveness

This is the inability of young animals to develop a proper immune response to some parasitic infections. For example, calves and lambs fail to develop any useful degree of immunity to reinfection with *Ostertagia* spp. until they have been exposed to constant reinfection for an entire grazing season. Similarly, lambs remain susceptible to *Haemonchus contortus* infection until they are between six and 12 months old. The cause of this unresponsiveness is unknown. However, while calves and lambs ultimately do develop a good immune response to *Ostertagia* or *Teladorsagia* infection, in the sheep/*H. contortus* system the neonatal unresponsiveness is apparently often succeeded by a long period of acquired immunological unresponsiveness; for example, Merino sheep reared from birth in a *Haemonchus*-endemic environment remain susceptible to reinfection throughout their entire lives.

Concomitant immunity

This term is used to describe an immunity which acts against invading larval stages but not against an existing infection. Thus, a host may be infected with adult parasites but has a measure of immunity to further infection. Perhaps the best example is that found with schistosomes, which are covered by a cytoplasmic syncytium that, unlike the chitinous-like cuticle of nematodes, would at first seem to be vulnerable to the action of antibody or cells. However, it has been found that adult schistosomes have the property of being able to incorporate host antigens, such as blood group antigens or host immunoglobulin, on their surface membrane to mask their own foreign antigens.

Concomitant immunity does not appear to operate with *F. hepatica* in sheep, in that they remain susceptible to reinfection. On the other hand, cattle not only expel their primary adult burden of *F. hepatica*, but also develop marked resistance to reinfection. Concomitant immunity also includes the situation where established larval cestodes may survive for years in the tissues of the host, although the latter is completely immune to reinfection. The mechanism is unknown, but it is thought that the established cyst may be masked by host antigen or perhaps secrete an 'anti-complementary' substance which blocks the effect of an immune reaction.

Polyclonal stimulation of immunoglobulin

As well as stimulating the production of specific IgE antibody, helminths 'turn on' the production of large amounts of non-specific IgE. This may help the parasite in two ways. First, if mast cells are coated by non-specific IgE, they are less likely to attract parasite-specific IgE and so will not degranulate when exposed to parasite antigen. Second, the fact that the host is producing immunoglobulin in a non-specific fashion means that specific antibody to the helminth is less likely to be produced in adequate quantity.

Parasite immunomodulation

Despite the diversity of the helminth parasites, they show common ways of evading or manipulating the host immune response to their benefit. They suppress immunopathology by modulating the activity of immune effector cells (different B- and T-cell types) and the expression of a range of cytokines. Thus, distantly related parasites have independently evolved to exploit a range of host immunoregulatory mechanisms to their own advantage and, by invoking generic suppressive pathways, can also suppress bystander responses to allergens and self-antigens. *Fasciola hepatica*, the liver

fluke, is a common parasite of cattle in much of the world and suppresses interferon (IFN)-γ responsiveness in cattle infected with bovine tuberculosis. The determination of blood IFN-γ levels is an important element of tuberculosis testing programmes and it has been suggested that the presence of *F. hepatica* in infected animals could markedly interfere with tuberculosis eradication programmes where tuberculosis incidence and *F. hepatica* infection are both high.

COST OF THE IMMUNE RESPONSE

Sometimes, immune responses are associated with lesions that are damaging to the host. For example, the pathogenic effects of oesophagostomosis are frequently attributable to the intestinal nodules of *Oesophagostomum columbianum*; similarly, the pathogenic effects of schistosomiasis are due to the egg granulomas, the result of cell-mediated reactions, in the liver and bladder.

There is evidence from some studies for a negative genetic interaction between production traits and resistance to parasitism. Sheep which have been selected for their resistance to gastrointestinal nematode infection show a higher incidence of scouring. This may be the result of an increased hypersensitivity to ingested larvae. Indeed, there is now a general consensus that the host's immune responses and immune pathology directly contribute to the impaired productivity observed in parasitised livestock.

Developing and implementing a strong effective immune response against parasite invasion, establishment or subsequent reinfection will utilise essential host resources, in particular protein, since antibodies, cytokines, leukotrienes and effector cellular responses are highly proteinaceous. These effects will be more deleterious in situations where nutrient supply is limited. Thus, in high-production animals on lower planes of nutrition, it may not be desirable to induce a strong immune response. However, these consequences have to be weighed against the need to maintain protection against the potential pathogenic effects of the parasitic infection.

One of the consistent features of many gastrointestinal infections of ruminants is a reduction in voluntary food intake (parasite-induced anorexia), although recent data have shown that the appetite of immunosuppressed parasitised lambs is similar to that of their uninfected controls. This observation might imply that the cascade of events involved in mounting an effective immune response against infection may be partly responsible for the parasite-induced reduction of food intake. Thus, the cost of mounting an effective immune response may outweigh the benefits gained in some situations, although caution is required as these effects may vary between parasite species, host species and genotype.

Longer-term studies would suggest that the lowering of production performance in younger livestock, which often occurs as they are initially acquiring a protective immune response to a gastrointestinal parasite infection, may be offset by the reduction in susceptibility to larval challenge observed in older animals and also the lower infectivity of pastures that results from reduced contamination with nematode eggs.

Now that this complex relationship between the parasite, nutrition and the acquisition of immunity is better understood, it is hoped that in the future the trade-off between the nutrient cost of developing an effective immune response and the economic benefit of maintaining an acceptable level of performance can be addressed in order to maintain the nutrient status of the parasitised animal, particularly in situations where nutrient supply is limited.

ACQUIRED IMMUNITY TO PROTOZOAL INFECTIONS

As might be anticipated from their microscopic size and unicellular state, immunological responses against protozoa are similar to those directed against bacteria. However, the subject is exceedingly complex and the following account is essentially a digest of current information on some of the more important pathogens. As with bacterial infections, immune responses are typically humoral or cell mediated in type and occasionally both are involved. The cell-mediated responses are typically IFN-γ-dominant Th1-type responses which are associated with an increase in the number of cytotoxic CD8$^+$ T-cells, Th1 cells, macrophages and neutrophils.

Trypanosomiasis is a good example of a protozoal disease to which immunity is primarily humoral. Thus, *in vitro*, both IgG and IgM can be shown to lyse or agglutinate trypanosomes and *in vivo* even a small amount of immune serum will clear trypanosomes from the circulation, apparently by facilitating their uptake, through opsonisation, by phagocytic cells. Unfortunately, the phenomenon of antigenic variation, another method of immune evasion, prevents these infections being completely eliminated and typically allows the disease to run a characteristic course of continuous remissions and exacerbations of parasitaemia. It is also likely that the generalised immunosuppression induced by this disease may, sooner or later, limit the responsiveness of the host.

It is also relevant to note that some of the important lesions of trypanosomiasis, such as anaemia, myocarditis and lesions of skeletal muscle, are thought to be attributable to the deposition of trypanosome antigen or immune complexes on these cells, leading to their subsequent destruction by macrophages or lymphocytes, a possible debit effect of the immune response.

Acquired immunity to babesiosis also appears to be mediated by antibody, perhaps acting as an opsonin and facilitating the uptake of infected red cells by splenic macrophages. Antibody is also transferred in the colostrum of the mother to the newborn animal and confers a period of protection against infection.

Finally, in trichomoniasis, antibody, presumably produced by plasma cells in the lamina propria of the uterus and vagina, is present in the mucus secreted by these organs and to a lesser extent in the plasma. This, *in vitro*, kills or agglutinates the trichomonads and is probably the major factor responsible for the self-limiting infections that typically occur in cows.

Of those protozoal infections against which immunity is primarily cell mediated, leishmaniosis is of particular interest in that the amastigotes invade and proliferate in macrophages whose function, paradoxically, is the phagocytosis and destruction of foreign organisms. How they survive in macrophages is unknown, although it has been suggested that they may release substances which inhibit the enzyme activity of lysosomes or that the amastigote surface coat is refractory to lysosomal enzymes. The immunity that develops seems to be cell mediated, perhaps by cytotoxic T-cells destroying infected macrophages or by the soluble products of sensitised T-cells 'activating' macrophages to a point where they are able to destroy their intracellular parasites. Unfortunately, in many cases the efficacy of the immune response and the consequent recovery is delayed or prevented by a variable degree of immunosuppression of uncertain aetiology.

As noted in the preceding paragraphs, sometimes both humoral and cell-mediated reactions are involved in immunity, and this seems to be the situation with coccidiosis, theileriosis and toxoplasmosis.

In coccidiosis, the protective antigens are associated with the developing asexual stages and the expression of immunity is dependent on T-cell activity. It is thought that these function in two ways: first, as helper cells for the production of neutralising antibody against the extracellular sporozoites and merozoites and, second, in a cell-mediated fashion by releasing substances such as lymphokines which inhibit the multiplication of the intracellular stages. The net effect of these two immunological responses is manifested by a reduction in clinical signs and a decrease in oocyst production.

As described earlier, the proliferative stages of theilerial infections are the merogonous stages, which develop in lymphoblasts and divide synchronously with these cells to produce two infected daughter cells. During the course of infection, and provided it is not rapidly fatal, cell-mediated responses are stimulated in the form of cytotoxic T-cells that target the infected lymphoblasts by recognising two antigens on the host surface. One of these is derived from the *Theileria* parasite and the other is a histocompatibility antigen of the host cell. The role of antibodies in protection is less clear, although it has been recently demonstrated, using an *in vitro* test, that an antibody against the sporozoites inoculated by the tick may be highly effective in protection.

In toxoplasmosis also, both humoral and cell-mediated components appear to be involved in the immune response. However, the relative importance of their roles remains to be ascertained, although it is generally believed that antibody formation by the host leads to cessation in the production of tachyzoites and to the development of the latent bradyzoite cyst. It is also believed that recrudescence of tachyzoite activity may occur if the host becomes immunosuppressed as a consequence of therapy or some other disease.

ACQUIRED IMMUNITY TO ARTHROPOD INFESTATIONS

It is known that animals exposed to repeated attacks by some insects gradually develop a degree of acquired immunity. For example, at least in humans, over a period of time the skin reactions to the bites of *Culicoides* and mosquitoes usually decrease in severity. Likewise, after several repeated infestations by blowfly larvae, sheep have been known to develop a degree of resistance to further attack, although this response is short-lived.

A similar sequence of events has been observed with many tick and mite infestations. The immune reaction to ticks, dependent on humoral and cell-mediated components to the oral secretions of the ticks, prevents proper engorgement of the parasites and has serious consequences on their subsequent fertility; dogs that have recovered from sarcoptic mange are usually immune to further infestation. Some sheep infected with psoroptic mange (sheep scab) and which recover may demonstrate a degree of protective immunity to subsequent reinfestation.

Although these immune responses may moderate the clinical significance of some ectoparasitic infestations, the immune response to infestation may result in the unfortunate consequences which often occur when an animal becomes sensitised to arthropod antigens. Examples of this are flea dermatitis in dogs and cats, the pruritus and erythema associated with sarcoptic mange in the dog and pig and with psoroptic mange in sheep and cattle, and 'sweet itch' of horses due to skin hypersensitivity to *Culicoides* bites.

VACCINES

Early approaches that investigated the use of live radiation-attenuated parasite vaccines, which induced a high level of protection against larval challenge, resulted in commercially available vaccines for the bovine lungworm, *Dictyocaulus viviparus*, and also for *Eimeria* infections in poultry. Apart from *D. viviparus*, there are no commercially produced vaccines for the control of helminth infections in ruminants. These encouraging results were experimentally applied to other economically important nematodes of ruminants (notably *T. colubriformis* and *H. contortus*); however, although partially effective in older animals, the vaccines provided an insufficient level of protection or the response was too variable in young animals under field conditions. An irradiated larval vaccine was developed against the dog hookworm *Ancylostoma caninum* that gave a high level of protection in the field but the vaccine was withdrawn from use over concerns with efficacy and storage viability. Early studies to develop a vaccine against liver fluke were hampered by the observation that these parasites do not appear to induce significant immunity in the natural ruminant host, even after repeated exposure to infection.

The increased prevalence of parasites resistant to chemotherapy has led to further investment in vaccine development, particularly those based on recombinant parasite components, and considerable progress has been made over the past two decades in identifying candidate antigens for several important parasite species.

Experimental vaccines have already been developed, for example against *Taenia ovis* infection in sheep, *Babesia canis* in dogs and *Babesia bovis* and *Rhipicephalus (Boophilus) microplus* in cattle. In some cases, these have been commercialised. However, the ongoing commercial success of such vaccines depends not only on their efficacy under field challenge but also on factors such as their ability to deliver effective, low-cost delivery systems that can confer long-acting protection.

Two main approaches have been adopted for vaccine development: those based on 'natural antigens' on the surface of the parasite or excreted/secreted by the parasite which are recognised by the host during the course of infection, and those based on 'hidden' or 'covert' antigens. The latter strategy ignores the mechanisms of natural immunity and directs responses towards molecules located or secreted internally. There have been encouraging advances towards the aim of producing vaccines for the control of several parasitic diseases in the last decade. Recent research has identified protective antigen fractions which have then been enriched and characterised and the genes encoding the active components of many of these have been cloned.

VACCINES FOR HELMINTHS

Natural antigens

Natural antigens are those which are recognised by the host immune system following infection. The following information is not intended to represent a comprehensive list but to highlight some successful natural antigens derived from parasites of veterinary interest.

Surface and somatic antigens

A high level of protective immunity has been demonstrated in sheep vaccinated with fractions derived from the infective larval stage contained within the oncospheres of the cestodes *Taenia* and *Echinococcus* and identification of these protective proteins led initially to effective recombinant antigens for *T. ovis* and *Echinococcus granulosus*. Highly effective recombinant vaccines were subsequently available for vaccination of the intermediate hosts against infections with *Echinococcus multilocularis*, *Taenia solium* and *Taenia saginata*. However, the commercial development of vaccines for *T. ovis* and *T. saginata* was not entirely viable as these tapeworm infections are primarily a zoonotic problem in poor developing countries and are generally of minor economic significance. The economic return and sources of funding need further evaluation.

Excretory/secretory antigens

Parasitic helminths produce and secrete a range of proteins that have a variety of functions. Some enable the parasite to penetrate the host's tissue, while others are involved with the digestion of nutrients or in evasion of the host's immune response. It has been demonstrated that the immune response of the host can impair the function of these proteins and thus lead to worm expulsion and so they have received considerable attention as vaccine antigens.

Highly protective effects have been reported against *H. contortus* using adult worm excretory/secretory (ES) products comprising two proteins of 15 and 24 kDa. However, recombinant versions of these proteins have not been protective. Research conducted over the last two decades has shown that the ES proteases, particularly cysteine proteases, associated with the intestinal surface of ovine nematodes such as *H. contortus* or bovine *Ostertagia ostertagi* are the most effective vaccine components. Other proteases which can mediate vaccine-induced protective immunity in ruminants are the aspartic proteases, metalloproteases, dipeptidyl-peptidases and aminopeptidases and thiol-binding fractions. The mode of action is mainly via induction of antibodies which block enzyme activity, resulting in worm expulsion or impaired fecundity. However, expression of these promising native protease candidates as recombinant vaccines has been unsuccessful, probably as a result of incorrect folding and/or glycosylation of the proteins.

Protective antigens from *Teladorsagia circumcincta*, the major pathogen causing parasitic gastroenteritis in small ruminants in temperate regions, have been identified by studying IgA responses directed at proteins specific to postinfective larvae and also on the basis of their potential immunomodulatory role at the host–parasite interface. Recombinant versions of molecules identified by immunoproteomics, homologous with vaccine candidates in other nematodes, were administered to sheep in a single vaccine formulation with an adjuvant. The animals were subsequently subjected to a repeated challenge infection designed to mimic field conditions. The trial was performed on two occasions. In both trials, vaccinates had much lower mean faecal worm egg outputs and adult worm burdens were reduced by as much as 75% compared to the controls at *post mortem*. These levels of protection indicate that control of parasitic helminths via vaccination with recombinant subunit vaccine cocktails could indeed be an alternative option in the face of multidrug resistance.

Promising vaccines against *F. hepatica* have mostly been based on antigens such as cysteine proteases, leucine aminopeptidase and glutathione *S*-transferase. Cathepsin L cysteine proteases are secretion products from liver flukes that are released throughout the life cycle in the host and facilitate penetration of the parasites through the tissues of the host and are targets for vaccination. High levels of protection (reduced fluke burdens and fewer flukes developing to maturity) have been attained in sheep and cattle against *F. hepatica* using these natural cysteine protease enzymes in vaccine trials. Efficacy was further improved in cattle trials when cathepsin L2 was used in combination with fluke haemoglobin compared with either antigen alone. Recently, field trials of a recombinant cathepsin L1 (rFhCL1) against *F. hepatica* in cattle showed a 48% reduction in fluke burden compared with non-vaccinated controls. Cathepsin B proteases of *Fasciola*, which are predominantly released in the juvenile stage of the life cycle, have also been shown to be promising vaccine targets.

A further potential vaccine candidate for fluke is the fatty acid binding proteins (FABPs), which are thought to play an important role in the uptake of fatty acids from the bloodstream of the mammalian host. FABPs from *F. hepatica* exhibit cross-protection and cross-reaction against *Schistosoma mansoni*. A recombinant version of a FABP (Sm14) from *S. mansoni* reduced the number of liver flukes and limited the histopathological damage to the liver in vaccination trials in sheep against a challenge with *F. hepatica*.

Leucine aminopeptidase, a gut-associated protease isolated from detergent soluble-extract of adult flukes, was successfully used as a vaccine against *F. hepatica* in sheep. Given alone with adjuvant or in combination with the adult stage-specific secreted cathepsin L proteases, it induced high levels of protection in recipient sheep, with vaccinated animals showing an 89% reduction in fluke burden compared with controls. This success has been duplicated with a bacterially produced recombinant protein version of the vaccine.

Considerable progress has been achieved in the area of defining antigenic targets of potential hookworm vaccines. A recombinant haemoglobinase protein, aspartic protease (Ac-APR-1), from the hookworm *Ancylostoma caninum* induces protection in dogs via antibodies that neutralise enzymic activity and thus disrupt blood-feeding activity, resulting in reduced parasite burdens and blood loss. A recombinant glutathione *S*-transferase (Ac-GT-1) also shows efficacy as a vaccine candidate. A further recombinant product, *Ancylostoma* secreted protein (Ac-ASP-2), gave good protection in dogs. The mechanism of protection appears to be directed against the larval stages of the hookworm. The future approach may be to incorporate several potential vaccine antigens, including the promising candidates discussed here, in order to target both the larval and adults stages of hookworms.

Hidden antigens

This approach primarily uses gut membrane proteins from parasites and these are not normally exposed to the host's natural immune system. Injection of these proteins into a host induces high titres of circulating antibody. When a haematophagous parasite ingests blood, these antibodies bind to the surface of the parasite's gut and impair the digestion/absorption of nutrients and the weakened parasite is expelled from the host. This gut membrane approach formed the basis of the recombinant vaccine against *Rhipicephalus* (*Boophilus*) *microplus*, the Australian cattle tick (see details in the section on Ectoparasites).

Early experimental studies with *H. contortus* in sheep, using natural fractions of these gut proteins, have shown that the reduction in the number of eggs passed in faeces can be greater than 80% and worm burdens can be lowered by more than 50% in vaccinated animals when compared to unvaccinated controls. Fractionation of these proteins from adult *H. contortus* showed that two main components are involved: H11 (also known as aminopeptidase N), which contains microsomal aminopeptidases, and H-gal-GP, a gut membrane-associated protein complex containing metalloproteases and aspartyl proteases. Numerous trials conducted over the last two decades with penned sheep have confirmed the efficacy of this approach using native gut membrane proteins.

There has been partial success in applying this 'hidden' antigen approach to non-haematophagous parasites such as *Ostertagia ostertagi* and *Teladorsagia circumcincta*. Despite these encouraging results using natural proteins and the characterisation of the protective antigens, the testing of recombinant versions of these gut membrane proteins has been unsuccessful in vaccine trials, indicating that conformational epitopes are likely to be important in conferring protection. The situation is similar with liver fluke vaccine trials. A natural gut membrane fraction enriched for glutathione *S*-transferases has been shown to lower fluke egg output in faeces and also reduce fluke burdens in both sheep and cattle, although with variable efficiency. However, attempts to vaccinate animals with recombinant versions of these proteins have been unsuccessful.

An important advantage of using 'covert' or hidden antigens in vaccine strategies is that they should be effective in those infections where natural immunity is poorly developed or is ineffective. A possible disadvantage is that immunity is not boosted by infection. However, it has been shown in *H. contortus* infection in lambs that vaccination with hidden gut membrane antigens, which are predominantly proteases and which are not normally recognised by the host during infection, will provide protection and by the time this wanes, sufficient natural immunity will have been acquired. Although considerable progress has been made towards the experimental production of some monovalent vaccines, it is likely to be several years before commercially produced recombinant vaccines are available.

In the light of the problems encountered in expressing the natural proteins in a recombinant form that is immunologically active and protective, attention has focused back on the possibility of using the natural proteins as vaccines. One of the perceived problems with this approach was that large amounts of fresh parasite material were required to produce sufficient quantities of the active fractions. However, once it had been established that the dose of natural antigen required to produce a significant level of protection was actually very small (as low as 5 μg), it became feasible, and a commercial possibility, to extract the relevant integral gut membrane proteins from adult worms collected from animals given booster infections. One example was a field trial where weaner sheep were grazed on pastures contaminated with *H. contortus* and were then vaccinated on three occasions at three-week intervals with the native gut membrane glycoproteins H11 and H-gal-GP in combination. The vaccinated animals showed a significant reduction in their faecal egg counts and also in the severity of anaemia in comparison to that observed in the unvaccinated controls. An experimental vaccine, comprising native integral gut membrane proteins from *H. contortus*, has been shown to confer significant cross-protection in calves against a challenge infection with *Haemonchus placei*.

Recently, the technique for the rapid mass recovery of worms from booster-infected sheep has been markedly improved and this approach has formed the basis for a commercial vaccine, which uses small amounts of native *H. contortus* proteins, purified from the lining of worm intestines. Barbervax® was registered for use in Australia in 2014. This is the first vaccine in the world for a nematode parasite for sheep and it presents a new approach for control of haemonchosis. Currently, trials are being extended into other countries to confirm the commercial potential of this *Haemonchus* vaccine.

It is important to consider that this vaccine strategy will not induce a sterile protection but will lower worm burdens and the faecal egg output sufficiently to be a very useful means of reducing and maintaining a low level of pasture contamination. Mathematical modelling of vaccines that use the hidden antigen approach predicts that a level of protection of around 80% efficacy in 80% of the flock or herd would give a higher level of control than that achieved through an anthelmintic approach.

In conclusion to this whole area of vaccination against helminth parasites, it is considered that the apparent inefficiency of many vaccines, experimentally tested against helminth infections, may be partly due to the focus on only one or two antigens and this invariably produces a fairly narrow antibody response. The most efficient vaccines will undoubtedly need to induce broad Th2-type responses that include strong humoral and cell-mediated constituents.

VACCINES FOR PROTOZOA

A number of vaccines have been on the market for several years or decades to ameliorate the impact of protozoal diseases to the livestock and poultry sectors. The majority of these products are based on live organisms, although more recently there has been increased focus on the development of killed and subunit vaccines. Live organism vaccines are more likely to induce T-cell-mediated immune responses and induce a more potent and longer-lived protective immunity against a challenge infection. Their disadvantage is that many have a fairly short shelf-life and there can be safety issues using live vaccines. They also often require a cold facility for storage and administration.

Live vaccines

Several approaches have been used to produce a protective immune response, including using the native protozoa, attenuated strains, truncated life cycles and chemically abbreviated infections.

Unattenuated vaccines which involve complete life-cycle infections

An example is the control of coccidiosis in poultry using small doses of *Eimeria* species that are sufficiently low as to cause minimal clinical symptoms yet still able to induce a significant level of protection. The first commercial vaccine (CocciVac®) comprised wild-type strains of *Eimeria tenella* oocysts, and over several decades other species of *Eimeria* were introduced to broaden the effectiveness of the vaccine. One disadvantage of this approach was the differences in the levels of pathogenicity induced in inoculated hosts by the live parasites.

Vaccines using virulence-attenuated strains

The safety of the unattenuated approach has been improved through the inclusion of oocysts from natural 'precocious' *Eimeria* strains that exhibit a smaller number of merogenic cycles and hence offer a lower risk of inducing disease. 'Precocious' parasites complete their life cycle more rapidly and exhibit reduced virulence with high immunogenicity and have been developed for the seven species of *Eimeria* in poultry (e.g. Paracox® to protect breeding and laying hens and more recently Eimeriavax® 4m for egg-laying hens and broilers). These vaccines should be administered simultaneously to all individuals and comprise the major type of live attenuated vaccines in use for the control of coccidiosis in poultry.

A further example is the inoculation of cattle with an attenuated strain of *Theileria annulata* for the control of tropical theileriosis. Repeated *in vitro* passaging of the intracellular macroschizont stage of *T. annulata* in tissue culture cell lines resulted in a live attenuated vaccine that has been used in many countries (China, India, North Africa and the Middle East). Continuous passage attenuates the schizont-infected cells so that their pathogenicity is reduced but their infectivity is retained. Cell line immunisation has not been as successful with *Theileria parva* due to histoincompatibility between the cell line and the recipient animal and the fact that *T. parva* and *T. annulata* infect distinct bovine leucocyte populations. Similarly, passage of *Babesia bigemina* and *B. bovis* piroplasms in splenectomised calves resulted in an attenuated strain which is used as a frozen vaccine to reduce the pathogenicity of infection in inoculated cattle.

Vaccines using drug-abbreviated infections

This approach (initiated in the 1970s) has been adopted to limit the losses in cattle arising from East Coast fever in East and Central Africa. Cattle are vaccinated with a defined dose of a cryopreserved wild-type *T. parva* sporozoite stabilate and concurrently given a long-acting tetracycline treatment. The antibiotic slows the rate of schizogony and allows the immune response time to develop. The immunity induced is very strain specific. The main disadvantage is that this approach is expensive for resource-poor farmers. However, a recent collaboration between a small private company and Maasai cattle herders in Tanzania has seen the successful vaccination and treatment of around 500 000 cattle against East Coast fever that lowered the mortality in the herds by up to 95% in some cases. Success was partly due to improved quality control of the vaccine stabilate and the production processes.

Vaccines using parasites which produce a truncated life cycle

This approach is particularly relevant to those parasites that produce cysts within the intermediate hosts. One example is *Toxoplasma gondii* in sheep and goats. The live vaccine comprises tachyzoites attenuated by repeated passage in mice. This attenuated strain (S48) does not form tissue cysts (which contain the bradyzoites) in the intermediate host and is not able to establish a persistent infection. It has also lost the potential to form oocysts in the definitive host, the cat. Thus, the S48 strain is incomplete and undergoes limited multiplication within the intermediate host but is still able to stimulate protective immune responses. This live vaccine confers long-acting immunity (effective protection even at 18 months after inoculation in the absence of further *T. gondii* challenge) against abortion induced by *Toxoplasma* infection in breeding ewes and is available commercially as Toxovax®. This is currently the only commercial vaccine available to help prevent toxoplasmosis.

Killed and subunit vaccines

These vaccines are generally less effective than those using live organisms as they rely mainly on the induction of neutralising antibodies but they can reduce transmission of disease and often can also lower the pathogenic effects of natural infection. The major challenge is to be able to identify and then present relevant parasite antigens to the host's immune system in such a way that they can be processed to induce protective immune responses.

Vaccines using inactivated parasites

Bovilis Neoguard® was a commercial vaccine developed to reduce abortion in pregnant cattle resulting from infection with *Neospora caninum* and was available in the USA, New Zealand and some other countries. This vaccine comprised inactivated whole tachyzoites and inoculation aimed to reduce the transmission of the parasite to the developing fetus. The vaccine has recently been withdrawn from the market by the manufacturer. Although progress has been achieved towards reducing the impact of bovine neosporosis in cattle, a fully effective vaccine needs to prevent disease on primary exposure, reduce vertical transmission and abrogate the clinical signs of infection.

A vaccine is available commercially (GiardiaVax®) to reduce the clinical signs and pathogenesis of *Giardia intestinalis* (syn. *Giardia duodenalis*) infection in dogs and cats. It also lowers the faecal output of oocysts in young vaccinated animals and the period of diarrhoea is of reduced duration. This vaccine is based on disrupting axenically cultured trophozoites from an ovine isolate.

A vaccine has been developed to reduce the pathogenesis of equine protozoal myeloencephalitis in horses caused primarily by infection with *Sarcocystis neurona*. The vaccine is based on chemically inactivated cultured merozoites and has shown to be promising in ameliorating the neurological effects of infection.

Subunit vaccines

A subunit transmission-blocking vaccine which targets the sexual macrogametocyte stages and thus reduces oocyst output has been developed for the control of coccidial infections in poultry. The vaccine (CoxAbic®) comprises affinity-purified antigens from the gametocyte stages of *Eimeria maxima*. It provides a good level of protection across three species of *Eimeria* (*E. maxima*, *E. tenella*, *E. acervulina*) and is administered to laying hens where protection is passed, via the yolk, to their broiler offspring. Unfortunately, it is an expensive vaccine to manufacture and work is ongoing to test whether recombinant forms of the gametocyte proteins are as effective at producing antigenicity as the natural proteins.

A subunit vaccine is available to reduce the severity of clinical disease resulting from canine babesiosis. It contains soluble surface proteins expressed by cultures of *B. canis*. The strain-specific immunity has been broadened in a similar vaccine by the inclusion of *Babesia rossi* antigens.

In South America, two subunit vaccines has been developed for the control of visceral leishmaniosis in dogs caused by *Leishmania infantum*. Leishmune® is based on a surface fucose-mannose-ligand antigen complex and Leish-Tec® is formulated with a recombinant protein A2 and saponin as vaccine adjuvant. These two vaccines have been commercially discontinued. In Europe, there are two commercially available vaccines for the immunisation of dogs. CaniLeish® is a parasite lyophilisate vaccine containing ES proteins of *L. infantum* and adjuvanted with a purified fraction of the *Quilaja saponaria* saponin (QA-21). LetiFend® is a recombinant vaccine based on a chimerical protein (protein Q) formed by five antigenic fragments from four different *L. infantum* proteins (ribosomal proteins LiP2a, LiP2b and LiP0 and the histone H2A), without adjuvant.

VACCINES FOR ECTOPARASITES

An effective vaccine against hypodermosis by the warble, *Hypoderma lineatum*, was developed and patented in the late 1980s but was not commercialised. Using the hidden antigen approach, the first recombinant vaccine was developed in 1994 against the cattle tick *Rhipicephalus* (*Boophilus*) *microplus*, and introduced in Australia under the name TickGARD™. The active antigen was a membrane-bound protein (BM86) from the gut of the tick. A similar vaccine using essentially the same antigen was developed in Cuba, under the trade name Gavac™. In controlled field trials in Cuba, Brazil, Argentina and Mexico, this vaccine showed 55–100% efficacy in the control of *B. microplus* infestations in grazing cattle 12–36 weeks after the first vaccination. However, in order to maintain high levels of circulating antibody, cattle have to be inoculated repeatedly. TickGARD is no longer available commercially and while Gavac is still marketed, efficacy results can be variable. Other tick vaccines include Bovimune Ixovac®, Tick Vac® and Go-Tick®.

The history of vaccine development for ectoparasites demonstrates the importance of economic constraints and that in commercial circumstances, the use of a vaccine for tick control is likely to require more effective vaccines than those developed to date.

Vaccines for the scab mite *Psoroptes ovis* are in experimental development.

NON-CHEMICAL CONTROL

Non-chemical approaches, even though some are still at the research stage of application, include the following.

1 Feeding of nematophagous fungi which can trap larvae in the faeces and thus reduce pasture contamination; the external use of entomophagous fungi.
2 Dietary supplementation with rumen bypass protein or forages rich in condensed tannins, which may increase the supply of protein to the small intestine and thus enhance the rate of acquisition of immunity. Bioactive tanniniferous plants also have direct anthelmintic activity against some gastrointestinal nematodes of small ruminants.
3 Biological actives, such as the external application of plant-derived essential oils against ectoparasites.
4 Use of physical approaches, often involving habitat modification, to reduce populations of insect pests and vectors (particularly the removal of breeding sites such as manure heaps, the use of barriers and the use of traps).

NEMATOPHAGOUS AND ENTOMOPATHOGENIC FUNGI

A potential approach to integrated control strategies is biological control, using the nematode-destroying microfungus *Duddingtonia flagrans*. This is a naturally occurring predacious nematode fungus found in soil and the abundant tough-walled spherical resistant spores (chlamydospores) are capable of surviving passage through the gastrointestinal tract of grazing livestock. Following excretion of fungal spores in faeces and manure, along with nematode eggs, the spores germinate and produce three-dimensional hyphal networks of sticky adhesive filaments during their development which trap the recently hatched free-living larval stages of parasitic nematodes within or around the faeces or faecal pats. The fungus gradually penetrates and digests the trapped nematodes. The advantage of *D. flagrans* is that viable spores are able to germinate rapidly and colonise the faeces and capture free-living larval stages before they have time to migrate out of the faecal mass onto herbage.

Trials have demonstrated that when the spores (chlamydospores) of this fungus are administered daily to grazing livestock over several weeks or months, the pasture infectivity is significantly reduced and hence the intake of larvae is limited and worm burdens of the grazing animals are lowered. These effects have been demonstrated over a wide range of climatic regions and also with many livestock species, including cattle, sheep, goats, horses and pigs. Trials in which fungus was administered continuously showed a significant increase in liveweight gain and production benefits of treated animals compared to those not administered the fungus. The dosages of chlamydospores required to achieve adequate control of parasites vary with the species of livestock.

Field trials have demonstrated the potential for *D. flagrans* to entrap canine *Ancylostoma* spp. infective larvae in soil. There is growing evidence that this approach of feeding nematophagous fungi can provide a useful tool in combination with other non-chemical control systems (previously highlighted) to reduce the loss of productivity attributable to parasitic gastroenteritis, particularly in areas where the prevalence of nematodes resistant to anthelmintics is high. From an environmental viewpoint, the administration of *D. flagrans* does not appear to have a detectable impact on other pasture and soil microorganisms, such as other soil free-living nematodes, microarthropods or earthworms. *D. flagrans* is now available commercially for use in livestock and horses in some parts of the world, to be used in conjunction with a chemical wormer in a formulation to be mixed into feed.

Entomophagous fungi, particularly *Metarhizium anisopliae*, have been shown to be effective against free-living stages of some ectoparasites, such as mites and lice. Fungal spores germinate on the surface of the arthropod after contact and produce hyphae that invade the tissues of the target ectoparasite, resulting in death in 4–5 days. While effective in controlled experimental trials, these entomopathogens have not been commercialised.

DIETARY SUPPLEMENTATION

Protein supplementation

Gastrointestinal nematodes can cause severe pathophysiological effects, such as reduced appetite, lowered efficiency of nutrient utilisation and a change in nutrient metabolism. A framework has been developed which hypothesises that there is a priority for nutrient allocation in parasitised hosts and that supplementation with rumen bypass protein will have beneficial effects, particularly on host resilience to infection. The supplementation of ewes with protein around parturition can reduce or eliminate the phenomenon of the periparturient relaxation in immunity. Protein supplementation is an expensive option and trials in subtropical and tropical regions have shown beneficial effects on the production of livestock using urea–molasses feed-blocks as a source of non-protein nitrogen. This approach is of particular relevance for smallholders farming sheep and browsing goats.

Herbal dewormers

A wide range of plant/herbal dewormers (ethnoveterinary products or phytotherapeutic drugs) are used by smallholder farmers throughout many subtropical/tropical regions of the world. They are usually available locally and can be of low cost. However, in the majority of cases there is a lack of scientific validation of the reported anthelmintic attributes of these plants and extracts.

Sources of material include lichens, ferns, shrubs and trees (*Salix* spp., *Azadirachta indica*, the source of neem, and *Celosia laxa*). Most of these have been used to treat parasitic infections in humans and there are more limited reports on their use in animals. In contrast, a wide variety of herbaceous plants or their extracts have been used for deworming livestock. Some examples (with active ingredient in parentheses) are oil of *Chenopodium anthelminticum* (ascaridole), members of the Asteraceae such as *Artemisia vulgare* (santonin) and Fumariaceae such as *Fumaria parviflora*, common tansy *Tanacetum vulgare* (thujone), tobacco plant *Nicotiana tabacum* and *Nicotiana rustica* (nicotine) and cucumber seeds (cucurbitine). Also, fruits or latex from plants such as papaya, pineapple and fig contain cysteine proteinases which may adversely affect the nematode cuticle.

Some of these potential anthelmintics are toxic in higher concentrations and in order to validate their usefulness, it is essential to isolate, characterise and rigorously test the active molecules in controlled clinical efficacy and safety trials. Indeed, where this approach has been applied, many of these remedies have failed to live up to expectations. Future commercialisation of these non-synthetic anthelmintics may be limited by the problem of obtaining patents for extracts whose nature is widely available in the literature and also by the relatively small global market.

Bioactive forages or nutraceuticals

There has been increased interest in growing specalised crops for the control of nematode infections in grazing ruminants. Although the inclusion of herbs such as caraway, parsley, chicory, chervil, thyme, dill, tansy and wormwood into leys has mainly been of interest to smallholder farmers, there has been wider interest in the use of tanniniferous forages for the control of parasitic nematode infections in small ruminants and more recently this has been extended to include cattle.

These bioactive plants/forages or nutraceuticals contain secondary metabolites, particularly proanthocyanidins (condensed tannins) and flavanols, which have been shown to have a positive effect on host resilience and resistance and are considered likely to bestow their effects on parasite populations at various stages of their life cycle. Examples of those tanniniferous forages adapted to temperate and/or Mediterranean climates are the legumes (Fabaceae), sulla (*Hedysarum coronarium*), lotus major/great trefoil (*Lotus pedunculatus*), birdsfoot trefoil (*Lotus corniculatus*) and sainfoin (*Onobrychis viciifolia*). Chicory (*Cichorium intybus*) is not a tannin-rich plant but possesses sesquiterpene lactones which are considered to exhibit anthelmintic properties. Subtropical and tropical tanniniferous forages include Sericea lespedeza (*Lespedeza cuneata*), which is grown in the southeast of the USA; *Lysiloma latisiliquum* (wild tamarind); *Havardia albicans*; *Acacia gaumeri* in the Caribbean, Central and South America; and *Leucaena leucocephala* and *Zanthoxylum zanthoxyloides*, which have been naturalised in many parts of the tropics. Quebracho, a condensed tannin extracted from the bark of South American trees (*Schinopsis* spp.), has also been shown to exhibit anthelmintic properties and has been used as a model tannin in *in vitro* studies.

These plants and their extracts have shown activity in reducing FECs, worm burdens and/or the fecundity of female parasites in parasitised ruminants. Establishment of infective larvae has also been shown to be reduced in some trials in sheep and goats. Extracts from some of these plants can adversely affect larval feeding behaviour, motility or exsheathment or reduce egg hatching in *in vitro* assays. However, considerable variation in anthelmintic activity against ruminant nematodes has been demonstrated for these plants and extracts, partly as a result of difficulties encountered in standardisation of the tanniniferous polymers or active compounds in the plant material. In addition, the concentration of the active compounds can vary depending on how the plants are cultivated, the growing season and climatic conditions and also the prevailing conditions in the digestive tract.

Tanniniferous plants/extracts may affect parasites through several mechanisms.

1 Condensed tannins bind proteins and therefore may protect them from digestion in the rumen, thus increasing the supply and absorption of digestible protein. Such an additional release of protein can improve the resilience and resistance of the host to nematode infections.

2 It has been demonstrated that some tannins can have a direct anthelmintic effect on established nematode infections *in vivo*. This may be through their ability to form complexes with parasite proteins in the cuticle, digestive or reproductive tract and thus affect essential biological processes.

3 The presence of tannins and/or their breakdown products in faeces has been shown to adversely influence the developmental stages of parasites.

Further studies are required to quantify these effects and also to isolate and characterise the active compounds and their mode of action on the integrity of the parasites.

Although these data on plants or plant extracts present potential alternative approaches to conventional chemotherapy for reducing the impact of parasitism on animal performance, there are many aspects which need to be addressed. Are some of these plants amenable to culture in a variety of differing environments? Can they withstand continuous grazing pressure by livestock and how do they compete in mixed swards and forages? What is their palatability and potential toxicity (particularly those plants which contain alkaloids, glycosides and oxalates)? What is the most appropriate way to use these plants/extracts, curatively or preventively? Pure stands of bioactive forages could be used for short-term grazing as part of a rotational deworming strategy. They could also be harvested, dried and fed strategically to housed animals, either directly or incorporated into feedstuffs, but it would be important to assess the biodegradability of the active components during processing. These options would have a particular use in the niche market of organic farming.

Further development is necessary as although experimental trials have shown some encouraging results with forages, many of the effective plants will not withstand heavy grazing pressure or have a restricted agroclimatic requirement.

TOPICAL APPLCATION OF PLANT-DERIVED BIOACTIVES

There is a growing body of evidence indicating the potential value of essential oils applied to the skin or hair, as control agents against a range of arthropod ectoparasites, particularly lice, mites and ticks. A very wide range of plant oils have been shown to be effective against specific ectoparasites, but tea tree (*Melaleuca alternifolia*), lavender (*Lavandula angustifolia*), thyme (*Thymus vulgaris*) and various members of the mint genus (*Mentha*) appear to be of particular promise.

Essential oils are blends of approximately 20–80 different plant metabolites which are usually extracted through steam distillation. These metabolites are volatile molecules of low molecular weight, usually containing two or three major terpene or terpenoid components, which constitute up to 30% of the oil. Insecticidal and acaracidal efficacy are often attributed to the oil's major component(s), but the various oil components may work in synergy. There is evidence that they have toxic effects on the insect nervous system; for example, terpinen-4-ol inhibits arthropod acetylcholinesterase. In addition, the hydrophobic nature of the oils may simultaneously exert mechanical effects on the parasite through the disruption of the cuticular waxes and spiracle blockage.

The efficacy of essential oils appears to be linked with the vapour pressure to which the ectoparasites are exposed, presumably because this affects the concentration of the volatile components. However, the volatile nature of essential oils also means that their residual activity is usually short-lived. A possible advantage of essential oils over conventional ectoparasite treatments may be their reported ovicidal efficacy.

Usually concentrations of around 5% v/v are required to elicit good clinical effects and care is needed since a range of commercially available shampoo or skin emollient products contain essential oils at subtherapeutic concentrations, largely for cosmetic reasons. The use of essential oils in the control of veterinary ectoparasites is an area which holds considerable potential for the future and research into their application is still at an early stage. One major difficulty is the wide variation in the relative concentrations and standardisation of oil constituents. Experimental trials show good efficacy against lice, mites and ticks but extensive field trials are needed. Nevertheless, commercial products are already available, for example for the control of equine lice.

PHYSICAL APPROACHES

Environmental modification

Simple modification of the environment may reduce pest abundance significantly. For example, many of the fly pests of cattle and horses have larval stages which develop in animal dung or decaying organic refuse. Management of dung is therefore of prime importance in their control and considerable success can be achieved simply by removing dung regularly from pastures or feedlots. Biting and non-biting flies can also be effectively controlled through simple procedures such as the removal of moist bedding and straw, food wastes, heaps of grass cuttings and vegetable refuse in which they breed.

Similarly, changing the suitability of the on-host environment may help reduce the susceptibility of the host to pest attack. With sheep, for example, minimising pasture worm burdens to reduce diarrhoea, tail-docking (amputation of tails) and crutching or dagging (the regular shearing of soiled wool from around the breech) all help to minimise the incidence of myiases by blowflies. These procedures reduce wool soiling and lower the humidity of the on-host environment, thereby reducing the availability of oviposition sites and suitability of the fleece for maggot survival.

High pest abundance, in space or time, can be avoided by appropriate grazing practices which reduce contact with the pest. For example, avoiding low-lying pasture at particular times of the year or simply stabling horses during the morning and evening may prevent or reduce the effects of biting midges during periods of high midge abundance and activity.

Burning has been commonly used in many parts of the world to help manage pasture tick populations. The effects of burning in terms of control are variable, with some studies showing marked reductions in tick abundance and others showing no effect. Burning, however, should generally be avoided because of its contribution to climate warming and the considerable environmental damage done to natural animal and plant communities. Furthermore, the flush of new grass that follows burning may attract greater numbers of grazers, which ultimately may allow the tick population to increase. Ecosystems that are specifically adapted to burning, such as in Australia, may be an exception to this, but care is needed to determine the circumstances in which this management approach might be appropriate.

Barriers

Various types of physical barrier can be employed to protect stock from insect pests. These may be fine mesh screens on windows, plastic strips on milking parlour doors or brow tassels for protection and to help dislodge insects which have alighted on the host. Such techniques may often be used in conjunction with an insecticide.

Trapping

Insects use a complex interaction of olfactory, visual and tactile cues to locate their hosts. If these cues can be identified and isolated, they can be selectively incorporated into trapping device at levels that produce exaggerated responses from the pest species.

Walk-through traps have been developed for the control of *Haematobia irritans*, stable flies and face flies. Commercial traps are widely available for use against tabanids in horse pastures. A screwworm adult suppression system (SWASS) has been used to attract the New World screwworm fly *Cochliomyia hominivorax* in North America. This combined an insecticide (2% dichlorvos) with a synthetic odour cocktail known as 'swormlure' to attract and kill adult flies. Field trials with the SWASS produced a 65–85% reduction in an isolated wild *C. hominivorax* population within three months. However, environmental concerns about the release of large quantities of dichlorvos resulted in the SWASS being largely abandoned as a control technique.

The development of traps for the tsetse fly vectors of trypanosomiasis in Africa has been highly successful, identifying and exploiting appropriate visual shapes and colours in combination with host-mimicking chemical odours to attract and catch flies. Traps baited with synthetic chemicals are also commercially available for the control of sheep blowfly in Australia and New Zealand. Trapping techniques hold considerable promise for future development, but the key determinant of their success is the rate at which adult females are trapped relative to their rate of reproduction, which means that for most insects with a high reproductive rate, high rates of trap catch are required to achieve population suppression.

CHAPTER 7

Epidemiology of parasitic disease and the environmental impacts of its management

THE EPIDEMIOLOGY OF PARASITIC DISEASE

Although the reasons are multiple and often interactive, clinical disease resulting from parasitic infection is a consequence of an interaction between the intensity of infection, the pathogenicity of the parasites and the susceptibility of the host. In the vast majority of cases it occurs for one of five basic reasons.

1 An increase in the numbers of infective stages.
2 Increased development or survival rate of infective stages.
3 An alteration in host susceptibility.
4 The introduction of susceptible stock.
5 The introduction of infection into a clean environment.

INCREASED NUMBERS OF INFECTIVE STAGES

This category usually involves parasitic diseases which occur seasonally. Although more distinct in zones with a wide climatic variation, parasitic diseases may also be observed in zones with minor variations in climate such as the humid tropics. A multiplicity of causes is responsible for the seasonal fluctuations in the numbers and availability of infective stages, and these may be conveniently grouped as factors affecting contamination of the environment and those controlling the development and survival of the free-living stages of the parasites and, where applicable, their intermediate hosts. The level of contamination is influenced by several factors.

Biotic potential

Biotic potential is defined as the capacity of an organism for biological increase, as measured by its fecundity. In population ecology, this is usually described as the basic rate of reproduction, R_o. It is important to note that in infection epidemiology, the term R_o is used to describe the expected number of secondary cases produced by a single infection in a completely susceptible population.

The basic rate of reproduction determines the potential maximum rate of population increase and may vary widely; thus, some nematodes, such as *Haemonchus contortus* and *Ascaris suum*, produce many thousands of eggs daily, while others, like *Trichostrongylus* and *Ostertagia*, produce only a few hundred. Egg production by some external parasites, such as the blowfly *Lucilia sericata* and the tick

Ixodes ricinus, is also very high, whereas tsetse, *Glossina* spp., produce relatively few offspring. The biotic potential of parasites which multiply within either an intermediate or final host is also considerable. For example, the infection of *Galba* (*Lymnaea*) with one miracidium of the trematode *Fasciola hepatica* can give rise to several hundred cercariae. Within the final host, protozoal parasites such as *Eimeria*, because of merogony and gametogony, also give rise to a rapid increase in contamination of the environment.

Stock management

The density of stocking can influence the level of contamination and is particularly important in nematode and cestode infections in which no multiplication of the parasite takes place outside the final host. It has the greatest influence when climatic conditions are optimal for development of the contaminating eggs or larvae, such as in spring and summer in the northern hemisphere. A high stocking density will also favour the spread of ectoparasitic conditions such as pediculosis and sarcoptic mange, where close contact between animals facilitates the spread of infection. This may occur under crowded conditions in cattle yards, or from mother to offspring where, for example, sows and their litters are in close contact. In coccidiosis, where large numbers of oocysts are disseminated, management procedures which encourage the congregation of stock, such as the gathering of lambs around feeding troughs, may lead rapidly to heavy contamination.

In temperate countries, where livestock are stabled during the winter, the date on which they are turned out to graze in spring will influence contamination of pasture with helminth eggs. Since many helminth infective stages which have survived the winter succumb during late spring, the withholding of stock until this time will minimise subsequent infection. Exceptions can occur, as in the case of the intestinal nematode *Nematodirus battus*. With this species, eggs deposited on pasture during the previous grazing season require a period of chill followed by rising temperatures in the spring when a mass hatch of infective larvae occurs. This has evolved to coincide with the availability of young susceptible lambs on pasture.

Immune status of the host

Clearly, the influence of stocking density will be greatest if all the stock are fully susceptible, or if the ratio of susceptible to immune stock is high, as in sheep flocks with a large percentage of twins or in multiple suckled beef herds.

Veterinary Parasitology, Fifth Edition. Domenico Otranto and Richard Wall.
© 2024 John Wiley & Sons Ltd. Published 2024 by John Wiley & Sons Ltd.

However, even where the ratio of adults to juveniles is low, it must be remembered that ewes, sows, female goats and, to a lesser extent, cows become more susceptible to many helminths during late pregnancy and early lactation due to the periparturient relaxation in immunity. In most areas of the world, parturition in grazing animals, synchronised to occur with the climate most favourable to pasture growth, is also the time most suitable for development of the free-living stages of most helminths. Thus, the epidemiological significance of the periparturient relaxation of immunity is that it ensures increased contamination of the environment when the number of susceptible animals is increasing. There is some evidence that resistance to intestinal protozoal infections such as coccidiosis and toxoplasmosis is also lowered during pregnancy and lactation, and so enhances spread of these important infections. On the credit side, host immunity will limit the level of contamination by modifying the development of new infections either by their destruction or arrest at the larval stages, while existing adult worm burdens are either expelled or their egg production is severely curtailed.

While immunity to ectoparasites is less well defined, in cattle it develops against most species of ticks, although in a herd this expression of resistance often inadvertently results in an overdispersed population of ticks with the susceptible young animals carrying most of them. In protozoal diseases, such as babesiosis or theileriosis, the presence of immune adults also limits the likelihood of ticks becoming infected; however, this effect is not absolute since such animals are often silent carriers of these protozoal infections.

Hypobiosis/diapause

These terms are used to describe an interruption in development of a parasite at a specific stage and for periods which may extend to several months. Hypobiosis refers to the arrested development, most usually of nematode larvae, within the host and occurs seasonally, usually at a time when conditions are adverse to the development and survival of the free-living stages. The epidemiological importance of hypobiosis is that the resumption of development of hypobiotic larvae usually occurs when conditions are optimal for free-living development and so results in increased contamination of the environment. There are many examples of seasonal hypobiosis in nematodes, including *Ostertagia/Teladorsagia* infections in ruminants, *Hyostrongylus rubidus* in pigs and cyathostomins in horses. By convention, the term hypobiosis is also often applied to describe overwintering of the larvae of some parasitic flies within their hosts, such as *Oestrus ovis* and *Hypoderma* spp.

The term diapause, most usually applied to the free-living stages of arthropods, is also considered to be an adaptation whereby ectoparasites survive adverse conditions such as cold, by cessation of growth and metabolism. The start of diapause always occurs in advance of the adverse conditions, often triggered by photoperiod, and is associated with physiological change. Diapause usually requires specific conditions, such as a period of cold, for its termination. Diapause must be distinguished from quiescence, which is a cessation of activity or development in immediate response to adverse conditions, such as low temperature, and which resumes immediately the conditions improve. Diapause is most common in temporary arthropod parasites in temperate climates. In these, feeding activity is restricted to the warmer months of the year and

winter survival is often accomplished by a period of diapause. Depending on the extremity of the northern or southern latitudes, this may occur after one or several generations. For example, the head fly *Hydrotoea irritans* in northern latitudes has only one annual cycle and overwinters as a mature larva in diapause. Other insects, such as *Stomoxys calcitrans* or calliphorid blowflies, in these latitudes have three or four generation cycles before entering diapause to overwinter as larvae.

To date, similar phenomena have not been ascribed to protozoa, although there is one report of latent coccidiosis occurring in cattle for which a similar hypothesis has been proposed.

INCREASED DEVELOPMENT OR SURVIVAL RATES OF INFECTIVE STAGES

The factors that affect parasite development and survival are mainly environmental, especially seasonal climatic change and certain management practices. Current changes in the global climate are anticipated to influence the infective stages of many parasites and/or the prevalence of some intermediate hosts. For example, the trend towards warmer wetter seasons has been one factor attributed to the increase in prevalence of *Fasciola hepatica* infection in ruminants in some temperate regions.

The microhabitat

Several environmental factors which affect the microhabitats of free-living parasitic stages are vital for development and survival. Thus, moderate temperatures and high humidity favour the development of most parasites, while cool temperatures slow the rate of development and prolong survival. The microclimate humidity depends, of course, not only on rainfall and temperature but on other elements such as soil structure, vegetation type and drainage.

Soil type influences the growth and species composition of the herbage and this in turn determines the degree to which a layer of 'mat' is formed between the soil and the herbage. The mat is abundant in older pastures and holds a permanent store of moisture in which the relative humidity remains high even after weeks of drought. The presence of this moisture and pockets of air trapped in the mat limits the rate of temperature change and these factors favour the development and survival of helminth larvae, ticks, larval stages of insects and coccidial oocysts. In contrast, the use of rotational cropping of pastures reduces the influence of 'mat' and therefore parasite survival. In the arid tropics, pasture growth is usually negligible, causing a similar effect. In the same way, a high water table is important for the development and survival of intermediate snail vectors of trematodes, such as liver and rumen flukes.

The development and survival of helminth eggs or larvae within faeces are also dependent on temperature and moisture. The host species may also influence this situation since normal cattle faeces remain in their original form for a longer time than, say, sheep or goat pellets. Thus, the moisture content at the centre of a bovine faecal pat remains high for several weeks or even months and so provides shelter for developing larvae until the outside environment is suitable. *Dictyocaulus* larvae may also be distributed with the spores of the fungus *Pilobolus* which grow in bovine faeces, while several species of nematode larvae, including *Oesophagostomum* spp. of pigs, are known to be spread mechanically by some dipteran flies.

Seasonal development

In temperate countries with distinct seasons of summer and winter, there is a limited number of generations and the same is true of countries with distinct dry and wet seasons. In northern Europe, for example, there has generally only been one, or at the most two, parasitic generations of the common trichostrongyle infections of ruminants, since larval development on the pasture occurs only from late spring through to early autumn, the peak levels of infective larvae being present from July until September. This pattern of events has changed in recent years with climate changes to milder and longer seasons. In tropical climates there may be numerous generations per year but even in this case, there are times when conditions for the development and survival of the free-living stages are optimal.

The development of large numbers of infective stages of parasites within distinct seasons is usually followed by a high mortality rate within a few weeks. However, considerable numbers survive for much longer than is commonly realised. For example, in northern Europe, significant numbers of metacercariae of *Fasciola hepatica* and infective larvae of trichostrongyles are capable of surviving for at least nine months. Dipteran fly populations also vary in the number of generations per year. Using the blowflies as an example, there are three or four relatively discrete generations, and therefore higher populations, in southern England, whereas in Scotland there are usually only two, temperature being the limiting factor. In humid tropical or subtropical countries, the development of trichostrongyle larvae or fly populations proceeds throughout most of the year and although this may be slower at certain times, there will be numerous generations per year.

Although the permanent ectoparasites, such as lice or mange mites, live on or in the skin of animals and therefore in a relatively stable environment, this may be affected by the fact that the hair or wool alters in length due to seasonal factors or human intervention. In the northern hemisphere, infestation by these parasites is often highest in the winter when the coat is long, hosts may be in poorest body condition, often as a result of pregnancy, and the microenvironment is humid and temperate.

Apart from the free-living stages of coccidian parasites, which have seasonal requirements similar to those of the trichostrongyles, the prevalence of other protozoan infections is related to the feeding activity of their arthropod vectors. For example, in Britain, babesiosis in cattle occurs at peak times of tick activity in the spring and autumn, although again in recent years climate changes have affected the seasons such that tick activity has become less confined to these times of the year.

Stock management

The availability of helminth infective stages is also affected by certain management practices. Thus, a high density of stocking increases the level of contamination and, by lowering the sward height, enhances the availability of the larval stages largely concentrated in the lower part of the herbage. Also, the scarcity of grass may induce animals to graze closer to faeces than otherwise. However, against this, the microclimate in a short sward is more susceptible to changes in temperature and humidity and so the free-living stages may, on adverse occasions, be particularly vulnerable. This may explain why the helminth burdens of ruminants in close-cropped set-stocked pastures are often less than those in animals on rotated pastures. Similarly, many pasture improvement schemes have direct or indirect effects on arthropod populations. Improved host nutrition results from pasture improvement and helps to maintain host resistance to parasitism. However, pasture improvement, particularly in the tropics, can increase the breeding success of ectoparasites such as ticks. Furthermore, the increased stocking rates on improved pastures may increase the chances of parasites finding a host.

The date of parturition in a flock or herd may also influence the likelihood of parasitic infection. Where livestock are born out of season, the numbers of trichostrongyle infective stages are usually lower and the chance of infection is postponed until the young animals are older and stronger.

ALTERATION IN HOST SUSCEPTIBILITY IN EXISTING INFECTION

For existing infection, this is observed principally in adolescent or adult stock which are harbouring parasite populations below the threshold usually associated with disease and may be explained by various dietary and host factors.

Diet

It has been shown that adequately fed animals are better able to tolerate parasitism than animals on a low plane of nutrition. Thus, ruminants affected with blood-sucking helminths, such as *Haemonchus contortus* or *Fasciola hepatica*, may be able to maintain their haemoglobin levels as long as their iron intake is adequate. However, if their iron reserves become low, their haemopoietic systems become exhausted and they may die. Similarly, cattle may grow at an acceptable rate with moderate trichostrongylid burdens even though some loss of protein is occurring through the alimentary mucosa. However, if there is a change in diet which reduces their protein intake, they are unable to compensate for the loss of protein and lose weight.

These deleterious effects of parasitism, without any change in the level of infection, are not uncommon in outwintered stock or, in the tropics, in animals during a period of drought. Incidentally, the same effect is produced when food intake is not increased during pregnancy and lactation. Good examples of this are the accumulation of lice on poorly fed animals during the winter and the fact that the anaemia caused by ticks is greater in animals on poor nutrition.

Apart from protein and iron, dietary deficiencies in trace elements are also significant. Thus, trichostrongylosis in ruminants is known to impair the absorption of both calcium and phosphorus and, where the dietary intake of these is suboptimal, osteoporosis can occur. Also, the deleterious effects of some abomasal parasites in sheep are greater where there is a cobalt deficiency and, in such animals, levels of parasitism generally considered to be non-pathogenic may be associated with severe diarrhoea and weight loss.

Impact of nutrition on parasite infections

When considering the host's response to parasite challenge, it is convenient to discuss the effects under the headings 'resilience' and 'resistance', although in practice they are inter-related. Resilience refers to the ability of the host to maintain an acceptable level of productivity when subjected to larval challenge or when carrying a significant parasite burden. Resistance describes the ability of the host to limit the establishment, size or fecundity and/or persistence of its parasite population. An animal which is parasitised has the problem of allocating scarce dietary nutrients between essential body functions, such as maintenance, growth and reproduction, and functions induced by parasitic invasion, such as repair of damaged mucosal/tissue barriers, replacement of endogenous protein losses and mounting of an effective immune response in an attempt to limit the parasite population. A **nutrient partitioning framework** has been developed to take account of the differing nutritional requirements of the host during its life and to predict the likely responses to the provision of additional nutrient supplementation during parasite challenge.

Young growing animals

Resilience – animals on a good plane of nutrition are usually better able to maintain their productivity when subjected to parasite challenge. Resilience of growing ruminants has been shown to be markedly improved by the addition of rumen-undegradable protein when they are subjected to challenge with gastrointestinal nematodes. The increased supply of metabolisable protein (MP) partly alleviates the pathophysiological consequences of infection. These effects are usually more dramatic in infections of young naive animals where parasitism often results in severe pathophysiological changes and extensive tissue damage. Other studies have investigated the use of non-protein nitrogen sources. Supplementation with urea–molasses feed-blocks alone will often not completely overcome the adverse effects of parasitism, whereas protein supplementation plus these feed-blocks can increase the resilience of the host. Macrominerals can also influence the resilience of sheep to parasitism. Infection with intestinal nematodes induces phosphorus deficiency and the growth rate of infected lambs can be markedly improved when they are offered diets high in phosphorus.

Resistance

1 **Acquisition phase**. This occurs when the host first encounters parasites and its immune system is recognising the invasion before it can mount an effective immune response. The duration will vary from a few days in the case of some protozoa to several weeks or even months with helminth infections. In the young naive animal, the priority for a scarce nutrient resource will be directed towards the maintenance of body protein (including the maintenance and repair of the gastrointestinal tract and the regulation of blood and plasma proteins and the acquisition of immunity), as these functions have high priority and will ensure that the susceptible animal survives. There is now a body of evidence to indicate that the provision of additional dietary protein to young growing parasitised ruminants has little effect on the early rate of establishment of gastrointestinal nematode infections, although the pathophysiological consequences are usually more severe in animals on lower planes of protein intake.

2 **Expression phase**. This occurs when the host's immune system is responding to limit the existing parasite population and/or the establishment of further infection. During the expression phase of acquired immunity to parasites, it is predicted by the partitioning framework that maintenance of body protein and the requirement for body protein gain (in growing animals) and

maintenance of body protein and reproductive effort (in pregnant/lactating animals) will both have a higher priority for scarce nutrient resources. This being the case, it is anticipated that the benefits of additional MP supplementation on the immune response would be most apparent during the expression phase. Indeed, the main effect of protein supplementation is to increase the rate of acquisition of immunity and increase resistance to reinfection and this has been associated with an enhanced cellular immune response in the gastrointestinal mucosa. It is clear that the provision of additional MP can reduce the establishment of incoming larvae and reduce the fecundity and/or survival of a worm population in young susceptible ruminants. There is evidence that the magnitude of the effect on host resistance is influenced by the level of MP supply and, as predicted from the partitioning framework, is greater in young growing livestock where the demand for protein is higher than that for metabolisable energy. Details of how an increased supply of MP affects the host's immune response to a parasitic infection are poorly understood. However, supplementation with rumen-undegradable protein can enhance the numbers of peripheral/mucosal effector cells involved in the immune response of young sheep infected with gastrointestinal nematodes. Both macronutrients (phosphorus) and micronutrients (molybdenum, copper, cobalt, selenium) can also influence the resistance of livestock to gastrointestinal nematode infection.

Mature reproducing and/or lactating animals

By the time livestock are yearlings, they generally exhibit a protective level of immunity. However, in sheep, and to a lesser extent in cattle, this immunity is reduced in late pregnancy and during lactation (periparturient relaxation of immunity, PPRI) but is restored by the time lambs are weaned.

Resistance – around the periparturient period, the ewe has a high requirement for protein relative to energy and the partitioning framework would suggest that there could be benefits on immune status through the provision of additional rumen-undegradable protein. There is evidence that either direct or indirect manipulation of nutrition can influence the ewe's response to nematode infection at this time. The supply of MP has been shown to be more important than the availability of energy in influencing the response of the periparturient ewe to nematode infection. Removal of lambs at birth or during lactation, which reduces protein demands, has been shown to partially restore the expression of immunity against abomasal parasitism. The addition of rumen-undegradable protein in late pregnancy or early lactation to ewes parasitised with gastrointestinal nematodes can reduce worm fecundity and/or worm populations and enhance local immune responsiveness, the effects being more pronounced in twin-bearing and twin-rearing ewes where the protein demands are higher than for singles. As predicted, the body composition of the ewe has been shown to influence these relationships. There is now considerable evidence to support the view that under conditions where there is a scarcity of MP, the PPRI in the ewe to abomasal nematode infection can be partly alleviated by the provision of an increased supply of MP or by a reduction in the demand for MP. Competition for nutrients, particularly protein, between reproductive processes and the expression of immunity is considered to be a major factor in the phenomenon of PPRI in parasitised ewes.

Influence of nutrition on expression of genotype

Ruminants on similar planes of nutrition show considerable variation in susceptibility to parasitism as a result of genetic variation. Studies with abomasal parasite infections in sheep have shown that the expression of genetic superiority in terms of host resistance (usually measured as reductions in the level of faecal egg count) to infection is not compromised by poor nutrition. It is in situations where the availability of nutrients is low that differences between genotypes are frequently at their greatest and both susceptible and resistant genotypes will usually respond to protein supplementation by showing evidence of increased levels of resistance to infection.

The ability of additional protein supplementation to reduce the pathophysiological consequences of parasite infection in animals on a moderate to high nutritional intake is higher in genetically susceptible than in genetically resistant livestock. Studies in Australia with sheep lines selected for resistance to *H. contortus* have suggested that those lines which exhibit resistance are likely to be directing more of their supply of protein into the immune responses against infection at the expense of channelling protein into production processes such as liveweight gain and wool growth. These genotype-dependent effects will influence the approach to nutrient supplementation.

Pregnancy and lactation

The period of gestation in grazing livestock often coincides with that of inadequate nutrition and is geared to completion at a time when freshly growing pasture becomes available for their newborn progeny. In housed or outwintered livestock, the cost of maintaining an adequate nutritional intake during pregnancy is often high and as a result the nutritional levels are often suboptimal. If this occurs, quite low worm burdens can have a detrimental effect on the food conversion of the dam, which in turn influences fetal growth and subsequently that of the neonate through poor milk production by the dam. This has been clearly illustrated in sows infected with moderate burdens of *Oesophagostomum dentatum* and in ewes infected with helminths such as *Haemonchus* or *Fasciola*.

Steroid therapy

Steroids are widely used in therapy of both humans and animals and it is known that they may alter susceptibility to parasitism. A good example of this is in the cat infected with *Toxoplasma gondii*; excretion of oocysts usually occurs for only about two weeks, but may reappear and be prolonged following the administration of steroids. Egg production by nematodes is also known to increase following steroid treatment and so pasture contamination is increased.

ALTERED SUSCEPTIBILITY TO THE ACQUISITION OF NEW INFECTIONS

Role of intercurrent infections

The interaction of various parasites or a parasite with another pathogen, resulting in exaggerated clinical disease, has been reported on several occasions. For example, in lambs, the nematode *Nematodirus*

battus and the protozoan *Eimeria*; in cattle, the trematode *Fasciola hepatica* and the bacterium *Salmonella dublin*, and also *Fasciola hepatica* and the mange mite *Sarcoptes*; in pigs, the nematode *Trichuris suis* and the spirochaete *Serpula* (*Treponema*) *hyodysenteriae*.

Effect of chemotherapy

In certain instances, immunity to parasites appears to be dependent on the continuing presence of low-threshold infections, commonly called Premunity. If the balance between the host and the immunising infection is disturbed by therapy, then reinfection of the host may occur or, in the case of helminths, an arrested larval population may develop to maturity from the reservoir of infection within the host. Thus, the use of anthelmintics, known to be effective against adult parasites but not arrested nematode larvae, may precipitate development of the latter once the adults are removed; this is known to occur in infections with *Hyostrongylus rubidus* in the pig. Sometimes, also, the overzealous application of anthelmintics in grazing animals will result in the eventual establishment of higher numbers of trichostrongyles than were present prior to treatment. Excessive application of acaricides to control ticks may also lower herd immunity to babesial and theilerial infections, so-called 'enzootic instability'.

Hypersensitivity

In many instances, at least part of the immune response to parasites is associated with a marked IgE response and a hypersensitivity reaction. Where this occurs in the gut, as in intestinal nematode infections, the reaction is associated with increased permeability of the gut to macromolecules such as protein, and this may be a significant factor in immune animals under heavy larval challenge. In sheep, for example, relatively poor growth rates and poor wool production may result. A stunting effect has also been observed in tick-resistant animals which are under constant challenge, while pet animals repeatedly exposed to mite infestations may have severely thickened, hyperaemic and sensitive skin, although only negligible numbers of mites are present.

INTRODUCTION OF SUSCEPTIBLE STOCK

Parasitism may result from the movement of susceptible stock into an infected environment due to the following factors.

Absence of acquired immunity

The common nematode diseases of ruminants provide the best examples of outbreaks of parasitic disease following the movement of calves into infected areas. For example, in western Europe the cattle lungworm, *Dictyocaulus viviparus*, is endemic; the most severe outbreaks are seen in calves born in early spring and turned out in late summer to graze alongside older batches of calves which have grazed from early spring. Overwintered larval populations have cycled in these older calves and when the fresh populations of infective larvae, which develop from these infections, accrue on pasture, the younger calves, with no previous experience of infection, are extremely susceptible. The occurrence of 'cysticercosis storms' in adult cattle, grazed on fields contaminated with eggs of the human tapeworm, *Taenia saginata*, or handled by infected stockmen, are occasionally reported in Europe and the USA. This high degree of susceptibility is due to lack of previous exposure to infection. In contrast, in areas where cysticercosis is endemic, cattle are repeatedly infected and soon acquire solid resistance to reinfection, only the cysts acquired in early life persisting in the muscles.

With protozoal diseases, such as babesiosis, theileriosis, coccidiosis and toxoplasmosis, caution has to be exercised in introducing naive animals into infected areas. In the case of toxoplasmosis, the introduction of female sheep into a flock in which the disease is endemic has to be carefully controlled and these animals should be non-pregnant when purchased and allowed to graze with the flock for some months prior to mating.

Absence of age immunity

A significant age immunity develops against relatively few parasites, and adult stock not previously exposed to many helminth and protozoal infections are at risk if moved into an endemic area. This may be exacerbated if livestock are in poor body condition or on a low plane of nutrition.

Longevity of infective stages

Especially in temperate zones and in parts of the subtropics, the free-living stages of most parasites will survive in the environment or in intermediate hosts for periods sufficiently long to reinfect successive batches of young animals and may cause disease in these animals within a few weeks of exposure.

Influence of genetic factors

Between host species

Most parasites are host specific and this specificity has been utilised in integrated programmes to control gastrointestinal nematodes, such as mixed grazing of sheep and cattle. However, some economically important parasites are capable of infecting a wide range of hosts that vary in their susceptibility to the effects of the parasite. For example, cattle seem able to cope with liver fluke infestations which would cause death in sheep, and goats appear to be very much more susceptible than cattle or sheep to their common gastrointestinal trichostrongyles.

Between breeds

Evidence is accumulating that the susceptibility of various breeds of animals to parasites varies and is genetically determined. For example, some breeds of sheep are more susceptible to the abomasal nematode *Haemonchus contortus* than others; *Bos indicus* breeds of cattle are more resistant to ticks and other haematophagous insects than *Bos taurus* breeds. In Denmark, the black pied cattle are genetically deficient in their cellular immune responses and have proved more susceptible to liver fluke, while the N'dama breed of cattle in West Africa is known to be tolerant to trypanosomiasis. Even within flocks

or herds, individual responders and non-responders, in terms of their ability to develop resistance to internal and external parasites, are usually present and it is recommended by some experts that culling of the poorest responders should take place.

Sex

There is some evidence that entire male animals are more susceptible than females to some helminth infections. This could be of importance in countries where castration is not routinely practised or where androgens are used to fatten castrates or cull cows. Greater infestation of male cattle has also been reported with ticks in some instances.

Populations of parasites

Although this aspect has received scant attention, except in protozoal infections, there is now evidence that there are populations (strains) of helminths and some ectoparasites, such as *Sarcoptes* and *Psoroptes* mites, which vary in infectivity and pathogenicity. In some cases this may be due to the presence of more host-adapted populations. The increasing prevalence of drug-resistant isolates of many parasites is another point which should be considered when disease outbreaks occur in herds, flocks or studs where control measures are routinely applied.

INTRODUCTION OF INFECTION INTO A CLEAN ENVIRONMENT

There are several ways in which a parasite may be introduced into an environment from which it has been eradicated or where it has never been found.

Introduction of new stock

One of the key problems for parasite management is the movement of breeding stock from country to country. Quarantine restrictions and vaccination requirements are stringent in relation to epidemic diseases, but limited or non-existent for parasitic diseases. When infected animals are moved into an area previously free from any given parasite, the infection may cycle, provided suitable conditions exist, and the consequences for the indigenous stock can be extremely serious. Examples of this category include the introduction of *Toxocara vitulorum* into Britain and Ireland, the source of infection being Charolais heifers from mainland Europe with transmission occurring via the dam's milk, and the spread of *Parafilaria bovicola* in Sweden, presumably introduced with cattle or by the inadvertent transportation of muscid intermediate hosts from southern Europe.

In the USA, Australia and Britain, the increased movement of human populations and their pets has seen the spread of a number of diseases of dogs including heartworm, canine babesiosis and ehrlichiosis, infections previously limited to more tropical areas. In some of these situations, competent arthropod vectors suitable for transmission may have already been present in some areas. Psoroptic mange in cattle, originally confined to southern Europe, is now endemic in Belgium and Germany due to trade in breeds of cattle. Protozoal diseases, such as toxoplasmosis, have been introduced into sheep flocks in countries where they were previously absent, by the importation of infected sheep. Babesiosis has also spread where animals carrying infected ticks have moved into non-endemic areas where the ticks were able to become established.

Role of effluent

The transfer of infection from one farm to another via manure has also been reported. Thus, outbreaks of ostertagiosis have occurred on farms following the application of cattle slurry as a fertiliser, while cysticercosis 'storms' due to *Cysticercus bovis* have occurred in cattle following the application of human sewage to pastures. Finally, the application of pig slurry containing ascarid eggs to pastures subsequently grazed by sheep has resulted in pneumonia due to migrating ascarid larvae.

Role of infected vectors

Winged insects transmit a number of helminth and protozoal infections, and these can serve to introduce infection into areas previously free of infection. Migratory birds are known to carry larval or nymphal stages of potentially infected ticks. Occasionally, birds may also mechanically transport infective stages of parasites to a new environment. This has occurred in the Netherlands where the ditches and dykes surrounding reclaimed land have become colonised by *Galba* (*Lymnaea*) snails transported by wild birds. The introduction of livestock lightly infected with *Fasciola hepatica* resulted in the snails becoming infected and, subsequently, outbreaks of clinical fasciolosis.

ENVIRONMENTAL IMPACTS OF PARASITE TREATMENT

LIVESTOCK

Following the treatment of livestock with veterinary parasiticides and insecticides, residues are excreted usually into the dung, but also potentially urine, in concentrations that may be toxic to functionally important, non-target pastureland insects, particularly those that colonise and decompose dung. These residues cause a range of lethal and sublethal effects, the magnitude of which varies with the compound used, mode of administration, concentration and insect species, but also at a landscape level with farm management factors such as the patterns of use and the number of animals treated at any one time. Organic farms have been shown to have significantly greater beetle biomass, diversity and species richness compared to intensively managed farms. A healthy dung decomposer community has been shown to significantly reduce the numbers of nematode larvae on pasture around dung, and thereby contribute to parasitic worm management. Timely burial of dung by beetles may also help to reduce the abundance of dung-breeding nuisance flies.

Particular concern has been associated with the use of macrocyclic lactones (MLs) in this context, although pyrethroid insecticides and some flukicides may also produce similar effects (Table 7.1). The effects are likely to be exacerbated by the use of combination products and long-acting compounds. Loss of pastureland insects may have important damaging ecological effects and the loss of insect dung colonisers in particular may delay dung decomposition, with consequences for nutrient recycling, pasture fertility and the availability of food for other components of the pastureland community. Impacts may be ameliorated in a number of ways.

Table 7.1 Anticipated environmental impact in terrestrial ecosystems of a range of veterinary parasiticide compounds and insecticides used in livestock, based on current data, compiled from a range of sources. The level of concern and rank order will be different in relation to contamination of aquatic ecosystems.

Compound	Anticipated environmental impact
Flukicide (clorsulon – benzenesulphonamide)	LOW
Flukicide (closantel – salicylanilide)	LOW
Antiprotozoal (diclazuril – triazinone)	LOW
Flukicide (nitroxynil)	LOW
Benzamidazole wormers (albendazole, fenbendazole, levamisole, mebendazole, oxfendazole, ricobendazole)	LOW
Flukicide (triclabendazole)	MEDIUM
Pyrethroid insecticide (e.g. deltamethrin)	MEDIUM
Organophosphate insecticide (e.g. diazinon)	MEDIUM
Macrocyclic lactone anthelmintic (moxidectin)	MEDIUM
Macrocyclic lactone anthelmintics (doramectin, eprinomectin, ivermectin, abamectin)	HIGH
Organochlorine[a] insecticides (e.g. DDT, dieldrin, lindane)	HIGH

[a] The use of organochlorines has now been prohibited in most parts of the world.

Risk-based and targeted selective treatment

Treatment of an entire herd or flock may, in many cases, result in unnecessary use of antiparasiticide, because many of the animals treated may have low intensities of parasitic infection. Such treatments leave no refugia for dung-colonising invertebrates and will simultaneously increase the rate of selection for resistance in the parasite population. Best practice approaches involve identifying the animals at highest risk, usually those carrying clinically relevant parasite loads, and targeting treatment at these individuals. This leaves refugia for dung-dwelling insects, reduces treatment costs, allows animals with low intensities of infection to develop acquired immunity and reduces the rate of selection for resistance.

Timing of application

Temperate habitats in particular are characterised by their distinct seasonal changes in climate and photoperiod and strongly seasonal phenology of individual insect species. In tropical habitats, species phenology is often associated with wet and dry seasons, with high rates of emergence at the beginning of the wet season. The impact of parasiticide residues on dung-breeding insects is more severe if it occurs during critical seasonal breeding periods. The synchronised treatment of cattle, for example at spring turn-out in temperate habitats, is particularly likely to adversely affect spring-breeding populations of flies and beetles. Losses early in the insect breeding season will have disproportionately large impacts in terms of population dynamics, compared to losses later in the year. To minimise environmental impacts, where possible, treatments should be focused during times when there is negligible dung-colonising insect activity.

Spatial scale

The impact on parasiticide treatments may extend well outside the treated areas for a distance equal to several daily displacements (the distance moved per day) of the insects in question. It has been recommended that untreated refugia for species should be considered, and that these should be compact blocks at least 25 daily displacements wide.

Mechanical fragmentation

Mechanical fragmentation, through harrowing for example, will serve to break up standing dung in fields and may contribute to the decomposition activity by microorganisms by increasing aeration and surface area. However, this practice is highly damaging to coprophagous insects, especially slow-developing beetle species.

COMPANION ANIMALS

While the effect of the antiparasitic compounds given to livestock are well known, recent concern has been raised about the compounds used to treat cats and dogs for fleas and ticks. The main focus of concern has been on compounds that contain fipronil or the neonicotinoid imidacloprid, since these have been detected in urban freshwater systems where the presumed source is animal treatment. Insufficient data exist to allow assessment of whether the isoxazolines (e.g. afoxolancr, fluralaner, sarolaner, lotilaner) might to present environmental concerns.

The route through which environmental contamination might occur is unclear, although it is presumed to be largely due to direct transfer, when a treated animal enters water or through disposal of partially used product into a drain. At this stage, few data exist to clearly demonstrate such a link or its mechanisms, but good practice would stress the need for a risk-based approach to treatment application to minimise unnecessary use.

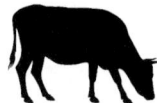

CHAPTER 8

Parasites of cattle

ENDOPARASITES

Parasites of the digestive system

OESOPHAGUS

Gongylonema pulchrum

Gongylonema pulchrum, synonym *Gongylonema scutatum* (Phylum: Nematoda; Class: Chromadorea; Order: Spirurida; Family: Gongylonematidae), commonly known as the Gullet worm, is found worldwide. It is usually localised in the oesophagus and rumen of sheep, goats, cattle, pigs, buffaloes, horses, donkeys, deer, camels and humans. This parasite has coprophagous beetles and cockroaches as intermediate hosts. For more details see **Chapter 9**.

Hypoderma bovis and Hypoderma lineatum

For more details see Parasites of the integument.

RUMEN AND RETICULUM

Gongylonema verrucosum

Gongylonema verrucosum (Phylum: Nematoda; Class: Chromadorea; Order: Spirurida; Family: Gongylonematidae), commonly known as the Rumen gullet worm, is localised in the rumen, reticulum and omasum of cattle, sheep, goats and deer. It occurs in India, South Africa and the USA. This parasite has coprophagous beetles and cockroaches as intermediate hosts. The diagnosis is usually an incidental finding on *post mortem* and the control is neither practical nor necessary.

Epidemiology: Infection is very much dependent on the presence and abundance of the intermediate hosts, principally coprophagous beetles of the genera *Aphodius*, *Onthophagus*, *Blaps* and *Caccobius*.

Clinical signs and pathology: Infection is usually asymptomatic, with adult worms burying in the epithelium of the forestomachs and producing white or red, blood-filled zig-zag tracts in the mucosa.

Paramphistomum and other rumen flukes

Rumen flukes, as their name implies, are mainly parasitic in the forestomachs of ruminants. Their shape is not typical of the trematodes, being conical and thick and fleshy rather than flat. All require a water snail as an intermediate host. There are several genera: *Paramphistomum*, *Cotylophoron*, *Bothriophoron*, *Orthocoelium* and *Gigantocotyle*, of which *Paramphistomum* is the most common and widespread in ruminants. The taxonomy of the paramphistomes is complex and unresolved and many of the species described may be synonymous, being differentiated mainly on size and shape of the suckers.

Epidemiology: Paramphistomosis often depends for its continuous endemicity on permanent water masses, such as lakes and ponds, from which snails are dispersed into previously dry areas by flooding during heavy rains. Paramphistome eggs deposited by animals grazing these areas hatch and infect snails. Subsequent production of cercariae often coincides with receding water levels, making them accessible to grazing ruminants. In other areas, the situation is complicated by the ability of the snails to aestivate on dry pastures and become reactivated on the return of rainfall. A good immunity develops in cattle, and outbreaks are usually confined to young stock. However, adults continue to harbour low burdens of adult parasites and are important reservoirs of infection for snails. In contrast, sheep and goats are relatively susceptible throughout their lives.

Pathogenesis: The adult parasites in the forestomachs are generally well tolerated, even when many thousands are present and feeding on the wall of the rumen or reticulum (Fig. 8.1). Any pathogenic effect is mainly associated with the intestinal phase of the infection, although the presence of adults in the rumen has been reported to cause effects on rumination leading to weight loss and ill-thrift.

Clinical signs: In heavy duodenal infections, the most obvious sign is diarrhoea accompanied by anorexia and intense thirst. Sometimes in cattle there is rectal haemorrhage following a period of prolonged straining. Mortality in acute outbreaks can be as high as 90%.

Pathology: The immature flukes are embedded in the mucosa of the upper ileum and duodenum and are plug feeders, and this can result in severe erosion of the duodenal mucosa. In heavy infections, these cause enteritis characterised by oedema, haemorrhage,

Veterinary Parasitology, Fifth Edition. Domenico Otranto and Richard Wall.
© 2024 John Wiley & Sons Ltd. Published 2024 by John Wiley & Sons Ltd.

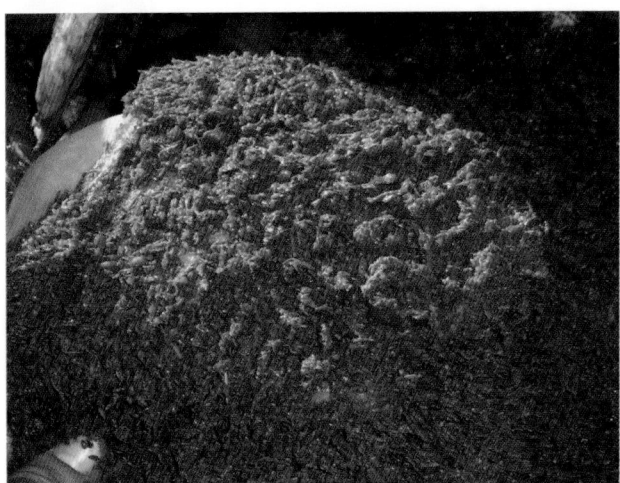

Fig. 8.1 Adult paramphistomes in the rumen.

ulceration and associated anaemia and hypoproteinaemia. At necropsy, the young flukes can be seen as clusters of brownish-pink parasites attached to the duodenal mucosa and occasionally also in the jejunum and abomasum.

Diagnosis: This is based on the clinical signs usually involving young animals in the herd and a history of grazing around snail habitats during a period of dry weather. Faecal examination is of limited value since the acute disease occurs during the prepatent period. However, large numbers of paramphistome eggs can sometimes be present in faeces during acute disease as the intestinal phase may also be accompanied by large numbers of adult flukes in the forestomach. Confirmation can be obtained by *post mortem* examination and recovery of the small pink-coloured immature flukes from the duodenal mucosa and ileal contents.

Control: As in *Fasciola gigantica*, the best control is achieved by providing a piped water supply to troughs and preventing access of animals to natural water. Even then, snails may gain access to watering troughs and regular application of a molluscicide at source or manual removal of snails may be necessary.

Treatment: Resorantel and oxyclozanide, in association with levamisole, are considered the anthelmintics of choice against adult and larval forms of rumen flukes in both cattle and sheep. Studies have also shown that closantel is also effective in cattle at 10 mg/kg, as well as benzimidazoles.

Paramphistomum cervi

Paramphistomum cervi, synonym *Paramphistomum explanatum* (Phylum: Platyhelminthes; Class: Trematoda; Order: Plagiorchiida; Family: Paramphistomatidae), commonly known as the Rumen fluke, is distributed worldwide and found in sheep, goats, deer, buffaloes and antelopes. They complete their biological life cycle in water snails, principally *Planorbis* and *Bulinus*. They are of little veterinary significance in Europe and America, but are occasionally the cause of disease in the tropics and subtropics.

Paramphistomum microbothrium

Paramphistomum microbothrium (Phylum: Platyhelminthes; Class: Trematoda; Order: Plagiorchiida; Family: Paramphistomatidae),

commonly known as the Rumen fluke, is localised in the rumen of cattle, sheep, goats, deer, buffalo and antelopes and occurs in Africa. This parasite has freshwater snails (*Fossaria* spp., *Bulinus* spp.) as intermediate hosts.

Paramphistomum ichikawa

Paramphistomum ichikawa (Phylum: Platyhelminthes; Class: Trematoda; Order: Plagiorchiida; Family: Paramphistomatidae), commonly known as the Rumen fluke, is localised in the rumen of sheep and cattle and occurs in Southeast Asia. This parasite has planorbid snails (*Gyraulus, Helicorbis, Segnetilia*) as intermediate hosts.

Paramphistomum streptocoelium

Paramphistomum streptocoelium, synonyms *Ceylonocotyle streptocoelium*, *Orthocoelium streptocoelium* (Phylum: Platyhelminthes; Class: Trematoda; Order: Plagiorchiida; Family: Paramphistomatidae), commonly known as the Rumen fluke, is localised in the rumen of cattle, sheep, goats and wild ruminants and occurs in Africa. This parasite has freshwater snails (*Glyptanisus* spp.) as intermediate hosts.

Calicophoron daubneyi

Calicophoron daubneyi, synonyms *Paramphistomum daubnei*, *Paramphistomum daubneyi* (Phylum: Platyhelminthes; Class: Trematoda; Order: Plagiorchiida; Family: Paramphistomatidae), commonly known as the Rumen fluke, is localised in the rumen of cattle and goats and occurs largely in Europe (mainly Mediterranean areas but has also been recorded in the UK and Ireland) and parts of Asia. This parasite has freshwater snails (*Omphiscola* spp.) and *Galba truncatula* as intermediate hosts. It is morphologically similar to *P. cervi*, but there is a genital sucker surrounding the genital pore.

Cotylophoron cotylophorum

Cotylophoron cotylophorum, synonym *Paramphistomum cotylophorum* (Phylum: Platyhelminthes; Class: Trematoda; Order: Plagiorchiida; Family: Paramphistomatidae), commonly known as the Rumen fluke, is localised in the rumen and reticulum of cattle, sheep and many other ruminants and occurs in the Indian subcontinent, Australia and several countries except for northern temperate regions. This parasite has freshwater snails (*Bulinus* spp.) as intermediate hosts.

Calicophoron calicophorum

Calicophoron calicophorum, synonym *Paramphistomum calicophorum* (Phylum: Platyhelminthes; Class: Trematoda; Order: Plagiorchiida; Family: Paramphistomatidae), commonly known as the Rumen fluke, is localised in the rumen and reticulum of cattle, sheep and many other ruminants and occurs in the Indian subcontinent, Southeast Asia, Australasia and South Africa. This parasite has freshwater snails as intermediate hosts.

Carmyerius spatiosus

Carmyerius spatiosus, synonym *Gastrothylax spatiosus* (Phylum: Platyhelminthes; Class: Trematoda; Order: Plagiorchiida; Family: Gastrothylacidae), commonly known as the Rumen fluke, is localised in the rumen of cattle and antelopes and occurs in Southeast Asia, India, Africa and America. This parasite has water snails as intermediate hosts.

Carmyerius gregarius

Carmyerius gregarius (Phylum: Platyhelminthes; Class: Trematoda; Order: Plagiorchiida; Family: Gastrothylacidae), commonly known as the Rumen fluke, is localised in the rumen of cattle and buffalo and occurs in India and Africa. This parasite has water snails as intermediate hosts.

Gastrothylax crumenifer

Gastrothylax crumenifer (Phylum: Platyhelminthes; Class: Trematoda; Order: Plagiorchiida; Family: Gastrothylacidae), commonly known as the Rumen fluke, is localised in the rumen and reticulum of cattle, buffalo, sheep and many other ruminants. This fluke is found in the Indian subcontinent, China, Middle East, Africa and parts of Asiatic Russia and Europe.

Fischoederius elongatus

Fischoederius elongatus (Phylum: Platyhelminthes; Class: Trematoda; Order: Plagiorchiida; Family: Gastrothylacidae) is localised in the rumen, duodenum or anterior small intestine of cattle, buffalo, sheep and many other ruminants (accidentally humans) and occurs in Asia. This parasite has water snails as intermediate hosts.

Pathogenesis: Flukes in the rumen usually cause only mild congestion but flukes attached to the duodenum can result in thickening of the mucosa.

Fischoederius cobboldi

Fischoederius cobboldi (Phylum: Platyhelminthes; Class: Trematoda; Order: Plagiorchiida; Family: Gastrothylacidae) is localised in the rumen, duodenum or anterior small intestine of cattle, buffalo, zebu, sheep and many other ruminants. It is found in Asia. This parasite is similar to *F. elongatus* and has water snails as intermediate hosts.

Monocercomonas ruminantium

Monocercomonas ruminantium, synonyms *Trichomonas ruminantium*, *Tritrichomonas ruminantium* (Phylum: Metamonada; Class: Trichomonadea; Order: Trichomonadida; Family: Monocercomonadidae), is a non-pathogenic parasite found worldwide, usually localised in the rumen of cattle and sheep. Transmission presumably occurs by ingestion of trophozoites from faeces or rumen contents and the diagnosis is achieved through the morphological identification of trophozoites. Control and treatment are not required.

Entamoeba bovis

Entamoeba bovis (Phylum: Amoebozoa; Class: Archamoebea; Order: Entamoebida; Family: Entamoebidae) is a non-pathogenic parasite distributed worldwide, usually localised in the rumen of cattle. Diagnosis is achieved through the identification of trophozoites or cysts in large intestinal contents or faeces. Control and treatment are not required.

ABOMASUM

Cattle can be parasitised by over 18 species of gastrointestinal nematodes, with the infection causing parasitic gastroenteritis. The most economically important gastrointestinal nematode in cattle is *Ostertagia ostertagi* and while the diagnosis, epidemiology, treatment and control are described in detail for this parasite, details are similar for other gastrointestinal nematodes. Although treatment for gastrointestinal nematodes is mainly targeted at susceptible first-year grazing animals, more recently there has been a trend to also treat cattle in their second grazing season and in some circumstances even adult animals, particularly where other helminths such as liver fluke and lungworm are present.

Ostertagia ostertagi

Ostertagia ostertagi, synonyms *Ostertagia lyrata*, *Skrjabinagia lyrata* (Phylum: Nematoda; Class: Chromadorea; Order: Rhabditida; Family: Trichostrongylidae), commonly known as the Brown stomach worm, is distributed worldwide and is localised in the abomasum of cattle, deer and very occasionally goats. This parasite is mainly prevalent in temperate climates and in subtropical regions with winter rainfall.

Pathogenesis: Large populations of *O. ostertagi* can induce extensive pathological and biochemical changes and these are maximal when the parasites are emerging from the gastric glands (about 18 days after infection) but may be delayed for several months when arrested larval development occurs.

In heavy infections of 40 000 or more adult worms, the principal effects of these changes are as follows.

1 A reduction in the acidity of the abomasal fluid, the pH increasing from 2.0 to 7.0. This results in a failure to activate pepsinogen to pepsin. There is also a loss of bacteriostatic effect in the abomasum.

2 There is enhanced permeability of the abomasal epithelium to macromolecules.

The results of these changes are leakage of pepsinogen into the circulation, leading to elevated plasma concentrations, and loss of plasma proteins into the gut lumen, eventually leading to hypoalbuminaemia. In addition, in response to the presence of the adult parasites, the zymogen cells secrete increased amounts of pepsin directly into the circulation. Although reduced feed consumption and diarrhoea affect liveweight gain, they do not wholly account for the loss in production. Current evidence suggests that this is primarily because of substantial leakage of endogenous protein into the gastrointestinal tract. Despite some reabsorption, this leads to a

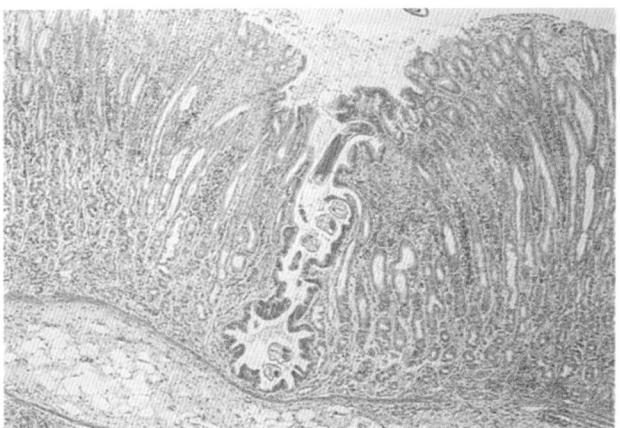

Fig. 8.2 *Ostertagia ostertagi* emerging from a gastric gland.

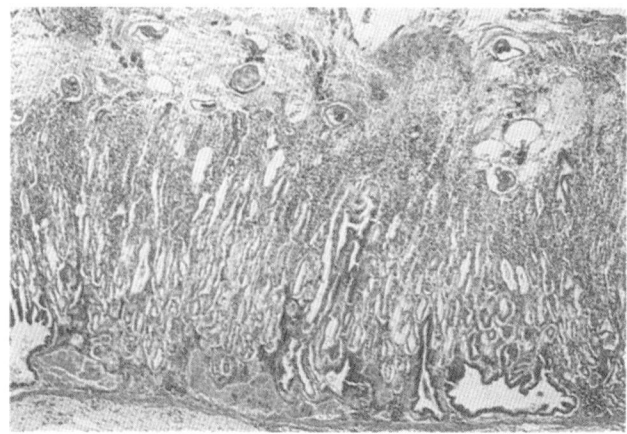

Fig. 8.4 Necrosis of mucosa in severe ostertagiosis.

disturbance in postabsorptive nitrogen and energy metabolism due to the increased demands for the synthesis of vital proteins, such as albumin and the immunoglobulins, which occurs at the expense of muscle protein and fat deposition. The developing parasites cause a reduction in the functional gastric gland mass; in particular the parietal cells, which produce hydrochloric acid, are replaced by rapidly dividing, undifferentiated, non-acid-secreting cells.

Initially, these cellular changes occur in the parasitised gland (Fig. 8.2), but as it becomes distended by the growing worm, these changes spread to the surrounding non-parasitised glands, the end result being a thickened hyperplastic gastric mucosa. Macroscopically, the lesion is a raised nodule with a visible central orifice; in heavy infections these nodules coalesce to produce an effect reminiscent of morocco leather (Fig. 8.3). The abomasal folds are often very oedematous and hyperaemic and sometimes necrosis and sloughing of the mucosal surface occur (Fig. 8.4); the regional lymph nodes are enlarged and reactive.

Clinical signs: Bovine ostertagiosis occurs in two clinical forms. In temperate climates with cold winters, the seasonal occurrence of these is as follows.

- Type I disease is usually seen in calves grazed intensively during their first grazing season, as the result of larvae ingested 3–4 weeks previously; in the northern hemisphere this normally occurs from mid-July onwards. In type I disease, the morbidity is usually

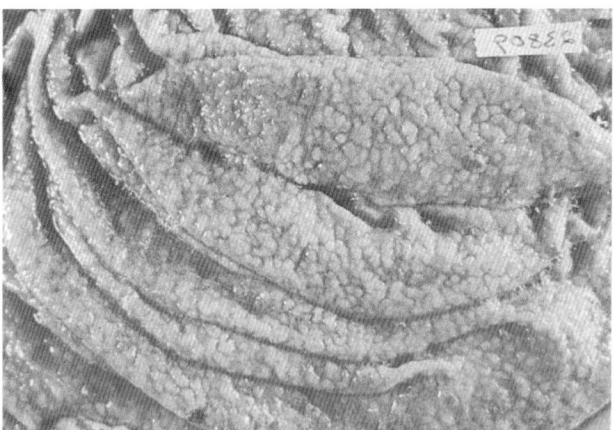

Fig. 8.3 Abomasum showing the characteristic nodules produced by the development of *O. ostertagi* larvae in the gastric glands.

high, often exceeding 75%, but mortality is rare provided treatment is instituted early.
- Type II disease occurs in yearlings, usually in late winter or spring following their first grazing season, and results from the maturation of larvae ingested during the previous autumn and which subsequently become arrested in their development at the EL_4 stage. Hypoalbuminaemia is more marked, often leading to submandibular oedema. In type II the prevalence of clinical disease is comparatively low and often only a proportion of animals in the group are affected; mortality in such animals can be high unless early treatment with an anthelmintic effective against both arrested and developing larval stages is instituted.

The main clinical sign in both type I and type II disease is a profuse watery diarrhoea; in type I disease, where calves are at grass, this is usually persistent and has a characteristic bright green colour. In contrast, in the majority of animals with type II disease, the diarrhoea is often intermittent and anorexia and thirst are usually present. In both forms of the disease, the loss of body weight is considerable during the clinical phase and may reach 20% in 7–10 days.

Diagnosis: In young animals this is based on the following.

1 The clinical signs of inappetence, weight loss and diarrhoea.
2 The season; for example, in Europe type I occurs from July until September and type II from March to May.
3 The grazing history. In type I disease, the calves have usually been set-stocked in one area for several months; in contrast, type II disease often has a typical history of calves being grazed on a field from spring to midsummer, then moved and brought back to the original field in the autumn. Affected farms usually also have a history of ostertagiosis in previous years.
4 Faecal egg counts. In type I disease these are usually more than 1000 eggs per gram (epg) and are a useful aid to diagnosis; in type II the count is highly variable, may even be negative and is of limited value.
5 Plasma pepsinogen levels. In clinically affected animals up to two years old these are usually in excess of 3.0 iu tyrosine (normal levels are 1.0 iu in non-parasitised calves). The test is less reliable in older cattle where high values are not necessarily correlated with large adult worm burdens but, instead, may reflect plasma leakage from a hypersensitive mucosa under heavy larval challenge.
6 *Post mortem* examination. Adult worms can be seen on close inspection of the abomasal surface. Adult worm burdens are

typically in excess of 40 000, although lower numbers are often found in animals which have been diarrhoeic for several days prior to necropsy. Species differentiation is based on the structure of the male spicules (see Table 1.8).

In older animals, laboratory diagnosis is more difficult since faecal egg counts and plasma pepsinogen levels are less reliable. A serum *Ostertagia* enzyme-linked immunosorbent assay (ELISA) has been developed that can detect worm infections in adult milking cattle and this may have a potential effect on milk production. However, the assay can suffer from the disadvantage of cross-reactions with other helminths such as *Dictyocaulus viviparus* and *Fasciola hepatica* where these infections co-exist. A milk ELISA has also been developed to monitor *Ostertagia* antibody levels in adult cattle from individual or from bulk-tank milk samples, with a good level of repeatability. However, milk antibody levels can be influenced by factors such as the age of the cow, stage of lactation and milk yield. Evaluation in the field is currently under way in some countries.

Epidemiology of ostertagiosis in temperate countries of the northern hemisphere

Dairy herds

1 A considerable number of L_3 can survive the winter on pasture and in soil. Sometimes the numbers are sufficient to precipitate type I disease in calves 3–4 weeks after they are turned out to graze in the spring. However, this is unusual and the role of the surviving L_3 is rather to infect calves at a level which produces patent subclinical infection and ensures contamination of the pasture for the rest of the grazing season.

2 A high mortality of overwintered L_3 on the pasture occurs in spring and only negligible numbers can usually be detected by June. This mortality, combined with the dilution effect of the rapidly growing herbage, renders most pastures, not grazed in the spring, safe for grazing after midsummer. However, some L_3 may survive in the soil for at least another year and can subsequently migrate on to the herbage.

3 Eggs deposited in the spring develop slowly to L_3; this rate of development becomes more rapid towards midsummer as temperatures increase and, as a result, the majority of eggs deposited during April to June all reach the infective stage from around mid-July onwards. If sufficient numbers of these L_3 are ingested, the type I disease occurs any time from July until October. Development from egg to L_3 slows during the autumn.

4 As autumn progresses and temperatures decline, an increasing proportion (up to 80%) of the L_3 ingested become inhibited at the early fourth larval stage (EL_4). In late autumn, calves can therefore harbour many thousands of these EL_4 but few developing forms or adults. These infections are generally asymptomatic until maturation of the EL_4 takes place during winter and early spring when type II disease may materialise. Where maturation is not synchronous, clinical signs may not occur but the adult worm burdens which develop can play a significant epidemiological role by contributing to pasture contamination in the spring.

Two factors, one management and one climatic, appear to increase the prevalence of type II ostertagiosis.

1 The practice of grazing calves from May until late July on permanent pasture, then moving these to hay or silage aftermath before returning them to the original grazing in late autumn.

Such pasture will still contain many L_3 and when ingested they will become arrested.

2 In dry summers the L_3 are retained within the crusted faecal pat and cannot migrate on to the pasture until sufficient rainfall occurs. If rainfall is delayed until late autumn, many larvae liberated on to pasture will become arrested following ingestion and so increase the chance of type II disease.

Although primarily a disease of young dairy cattle, ostertagiosis can nevertheless affect groups of older cattle in the herd, particularly if these have had little previous exposure to the parasite.

Acquired immunity is slow to develop and calves do not achieve a significant level of immunity until the end of their first grazing season. Housing over the winter allows the immunity to wane by the following spring and yearlings turned out at that time are partially susceptible to reinfection and so contaminate the pasture with small numbers of eggs. However, immunity is rapidly re-established and any clinical signs which occur are usually of a transient nature. By the second and third years of grazing, adult stock in endemic areas are usually highly immune to reinfection and of little significance in the epidemiology. However, around the periparturient period when immunity wanes, particularly in heifers, there are reports of clinical disease following calving. Burdens of adult *Ostertagia* spp. in dairy cows are usually low and routine treatment of herds at calving should not be required.

Beef herds Although the basic epidemiology in beef herds is similar to that in dairy herds, the influence of immune adult animals grazing alongside susceptible calves has to be considered. Thus, in beef herds where calving takes place in the spring, ostertagiosis is uncommon since egg production by immune adults is low, and the spring mortality of the overwintered L_3 occurs prior to the suckling calves ingesting significant quantities of grass. Consequently, only low numbers of L_3 become available on the pasture later in the year. However, where calving takes place in the autumn or winter, ostertagiosis can be a problem in calves during the following grazing season once they are weaned, the epidemiology then being similar to that for dairy calves.

Epidemiology of ostertagiosis in subtropical and temperate countries in the southern hemisphere

In countries with temperate climates, such as New Zealand, the seasonal pattern is similar to that reported for Europe, with type I disease occurring in the summer and burdens of arrested larvae accumulating in the autumn. In those countries with subtropical climates and winter rainfall, such as parts of southern Australia, southwest Africa and some regions of Argentina, Chile and Brazil, the increase in L_3 population occurs during the winter and outbreaks of type I disease are seen towards the end of the winter period. Arrested larvae accumulate during the spring and where type II disease has been reported, it has occurred in late summer or early autumn. A basically similar pattern of infection is seen in some southern parts of the USA with non-seasonal rainfall, such as Louisiana and Texas. There, larvae accumulate on pasture during winter and arrested development occurs in late winter and early spring with outbreaks of type II disease occurring in late summer or early autumn. The environmental factors which produce arrested larvae in subtropical zones are not yet fully known.

Table 8.1 Risk management of pastures.

	High	Medium	Low
Spring	Grazed by first-year calves in the previous year	Grazed only by adult or yearling cattle the previous year Grazed by beef cows (with or without calves at foot) the previous year	New leys/seeds or forage crops Sheep or conservation only in the previous year
From mid-July	Grazed by first-year calves in the spring	Adult cattle or conservation in the spring Pasture clean at the start of the year and grazed by parasite-naïve calves	Grazed by sheep or conservation only in the first half of the grazing season Forage crops or arable by-products

Control: Traditionally, ostertagiosis has been prevented by routinely treating young cattle with anthelmintics over the period when pasture larval levels are increasing. However, this has the disadvantage that since the calves are under continuous larval challenge, their performance may be impaired. With this system, effective anthelmintic treatment at housing is also necessary using a drug effective against hypobiotic larvae in order to prevent type II disease.

The prevention of ostertagiosis by limiting exposure to infection is a more efficient method of control. This may be achieved by allowing young cattle sufficient exposure to larval infection to stimulate immunity but not sufficient to cause a loss in production. The provision of this 'safe pasture' may be achieved in two ways.

1 Using anthelmintics to limit pasture contamination with eggs during periods when the climate is optimal for development of the free-living larval stages, i.e. spring and summer in temperate climates, autumn and winter in the subtropics.
2 Alternatively, by resting pasture or grazing it with another host, such as sheep, which are not susceptible to *O. ostertagi*, until most of the existing L_3 on the pasture have died out.

Sometimes a combination of these methods is employed. The timing of events in the systems described in Table 8.1 is applicable to the calendar of the northern hemisphere.

Treatment: Type I disease responds well to treatment at the standard dosage rates with any of the modern benzimidazoles, the pro-benzimidazoles (febantel, netobimin and thiophanate), levamisole or the avermectins/milbemycins. All these drugs are effective against developing larvae and adult stages. Following treatment, calves should be moved to pasture which has not been grazed by cattle in the same year. For the successful treatment of type II disease, it is necessary to use drugs which are effective against arrested (hypobiotic) larvae as well as developing larvae and adult stages. Only the modern benzimidazoles (such as albendazole, fenbendazole or oxfendazole) or the avermectins/milbemycins are effective in the treatment of type II disease when used at standard dosage levels, although the pro-benzimidazoles are also effective at higher dose rates. The field where the outbreak originated may be grazed by sheep or rested until the following June. In lactating dairy cattle, topical eprinomectin has the advantage that there is no milk withholding period.

Prophylactic anthelmintic medication Since the crucial period of pasture contamination with *O. ostertagi* eggs is up to mid-July, one of the efficient modern anthelmintics may be given on two or three occasions between turnout in the spring and July to minimise the numbers of eggs deposited on the pasture. For calves going to pasture in early May two treatments, three and six weeks later, are used whereas calves turned out in April require three treatments at intervals of three weeks. Where parenteral or pour-on macrocyclic lactones are used, the interval

after first treatment may be extended to five or eight weeks (the interval depends on the anthelmintic used) due to residual activity against ingested larvae. A long-acting injectable formulation of moxidectin is available in some countries with persistent activity against *O. ostertagi* for around 120 days. Several rumen boluses are available which provide either the sustained release of anthelmintic drugs, at a constant level, over periods of 3–5 months or the pulse release of therapeutic doses of an anthelmintic at intervals of three weeks throughout the grazing season. These are administered to first-season grazing calves at turnout, although some can be administered later in the season, and effectively prevent pasture contamination and the subsequent accumulation of infective larvae. Although offering a high degree of control of gastrointestinal nematodes, there is evidence to suggest that young cattle protected by these boluses, or other highly effective prophylactic drug regimens, are more susceptible to infection in their second year at grass. Boluses can also be used in the second grazing season. One advantage of using boluses is a reduction in handling and hence labour costs. Anthelmintic prophylaxis has the advantage that animals can be grazed throughout the year on the same pasture and is particularly advantageous for the small, heavily stocked farm where grazing is limited.

Anthelmintic treatment and move to safe pasture in mid-July This system, usually referred to as 'dose and move', is based on the knowledge that the annual increase of L_3 occurs after mid-July. Therefore, if calves grazed from early spring are given an anthelmintic treatment in early July and moved immediately to a second pasture such as silage or hay aftermath, the level of infection which develops on the second pasture will be low. The one reservation with this technique is that in certain years the numbers of L_3 that overwinter are sufficient to cause heavy infections in the spring and clinical ostertagiosis can occur in calves in April and May. However, once the dose-and-move system has operated for a few years, this problem is unlikely to arise. In some European countries the same effect has been obtained by delaying the turnout of calves until midsummer. The dose-and-move strategy is considered to select heavily for resistance and the current recommendation for sheep is to delay the move after the dose. Practically, however, this is difficult with calves because of the variations in persistence in activity between macrocyclic lactone products and the timing between treatment intervals. The intention of delaying treatment is to allow any treated calves to become 'lightly' reinfected with susceptible worms before allowing them access to the 'low-risk' pasture. This will ensure that soon after the move, contamination of the 'clean' pasture with eggs from susceptible worms will recommence and reduce the reproductive advantage offered to any resistant parasites surviving treatment. However, it should be possible to plan the availability of aftermaths with turnout and the need for strategic early season worming plans as part of farm health planning initiatives.

Alternate grazing of cattle and sheep   This system ideally utilises a three-year rotation of cattle, sheep and crops. Since the effective lifespan of most *O. ostertagi* L$_3$ is under one year and cross-infection between cattle and sheep in temperate areas is largely limited to *O. leptospicularis*, *Trichostrongylus axei* and occasionally *C. oncophora*, good control of bovine ostertagiosis should, in theory, be achieved. It is particularly applicable to farms with a high proportion of land suitable for cropping or grassland conservation. In marginal or upland areas, reasonable control has been reported using an annual rotation of beef cattle and sheep. The drawback of alternate grazing systems is that they impose a rigorous and inflexible regimen on the use of land. Furthermore, in warmer climates where *Haemonchus* spp. are prevalent, this system can prove dangerous since this very pathogenic genus establishes in both sheep and cattle.

Rotational grazing of adult and young stock   This system involves a continuous rotation of paddocks in which the susceptible younger calves graze ahead of the immune adults and remain long enough in each paddock to remove only the leafy upper herbage. The incoming immune adults then graze the lower, more fibrous echelons of the herbage which contain the majority of the L$_3$. Since the faeces produced by the immune adults contain few if any *O. ostertagi* eggs, the pasture contamination is greatly reduced. The optimal utilisation of permanent grassland and the control of internal parasitism without resort to therapy make it an option for organic systems of production. In single-suckled beef production systems, the grazing of immune cows with their offspring will lower the pasture infectivity levels for the susceptible calves.

Influence of production systems   In northern temperate regions, beef cows normally calve in the spring or autumn. Dairy cows may follow a similar pattern of calving, although in many herds calving occurs all year round. Parasite control in dairy herds reflects the management of the calves, which are usually removed from the dam soon after birth and reared indoors until weaning as heifer replacements. Age and timing of turnout will therefore be influenced by month of birth and availability of pasture. Calving typically occurs in late winter/early spring in spring-calving herds and weaned calves may be turned out onto pasture as early as two months of age in April or May, acquiring infection from overwintering infective larvae and subsequent pasture contamination. With a longer calving period, the calves may be housed until after weaning and then grazed on pasture from midsummer. If the pasture has been grazed by older calves, then they could be exposed to high levels of larval challenge. Calves born in the late summer or autumn may be housed and then enter their second year as mainly parasite-naive livestock and be susceptible to infection after turnout.

Anthelmintic resistance   There are sporadic reports of gastrointestinal nematodes in cattle showing some resistance to benzimidazoles in several countries and a few isolated reports of resistance to the macrocyclic lactones, particularly in *Cooperia* species. However, anthelmintic resistance is considered to be much less of a problem in cattle compared to the situation in sheep and goats. This may be due to less frequent treatment of cattle and also the persistence of faecal pats, which prolong the survival of the free-living larval stages. Despite the current low level of anthelmintic resistance in cattle nematodes, it is advisable to follow guidelines (such as those listed in Table 8.2) devised to limit the development of resistance in cattle.

Table 8.2 Guidelines for the control of gastrointestinal nematodes and use of anthelmintics in cattle (UK COWS recommendations).

Guideline	Comment
1 Work out a control strategy with your veterinarian or adviser	Specialist consultation as part of herd health planning is an increasing requirement on farms. Worm control programmes for cattle will require ongoing consultations
2 Use effective quarantine strategies to prevent the importation of resistant worms in introduced cattle	Bought-in cattle can be a potential route of introducing resistance alleles into a non-closed herd
3 Test for anthelmintic efficacy on your farm	While resistance is still rare in cattle nematodes, treatment failures do occur. It is important to monitor continued efficacy as underdosing can select for anthelmintic resistance
4 Administer anthelmintics effectively	Administer the right dose in the correct way by following the manufacturer's instructions
5 Use anthelmintics only when necessary	Understand the trade-off between tolerating some level of parasitism and minimising selection for anthelmintic resistance. FEC monitoring has an important role
6 Select the appropriate anthelmintic for the task	Target treatment according to parasites (and their stages) present, based on time of year
7 Adopt strategies to preserve susceptible worms on the farm	Aim to reduce selection for anthelmintic resistance when treating adult cattle, immune older animals or when dosing on low contamination pastures
8 Reduce dependence on anthelmintics	Alternative control measures include grazing management using sheep or older immune animals

Notes: *Ostertagia ostertagi* is perhaps the most common cause of parasitic gastritis in cattle. The disease, often simply known as ostertagiosis, typically affects young cattle during their first grazing season, although herd outbreaks and sporadic individual cases have also been reported in adult cattle. *Ostertagia ostertagi* is considered to be a polymorphic species with *Ostertagia lyrata* (syn. *Skrjabinagia*).

Ostertagia leptospicularis

Ostertagia leptospicularis, synonyms *Ostertagia crimensis*, *Skrjabinagia kolchida*, *Grospiculagia podjapolskyi* (Phylum: Nematoda; Class: Chromadorea; Order: Rhabditida; Family: Trichostrongylidae), is localised in the abomasum of roe deer, cattle, sheep and goats and is found in many parts of the world, particularly in Europe and New Zealand. This parasite is considered a polymorphic species with two male morphotypes, *Ostertagia leptospicularis* and *Skrjabinagia kolchida* (*Grospiculagia podjapolskyi*). Details of the pathogenesis, clinical signs, diagnosis, pathology, epidemiology, treatment and control are as for *O. ostertagi*.

Haemonchus contortus

Haemonchus contortus, synonym *Haemonchus placei* (Phylum: Nematoda; Class: Chromadorea; Order: Rhabditida; Family: Trichostrongylidae), is commonly known as the Barber's pole worm. Until recently, the sheep species was called *H. contortus* and the cattle species *H. placei*. However, there is now increasing evidence that these are the single species *H. contortus* with only strain adaptations for cattle and sheep. For more details see Chapter 9.

Trichostrongylus axei

Trichostrongylus axei, synonym *Trichostrongylus extenuatus* (Phylum: Nematoda; Class: Chromadorea; Order: Rhabditida; Family: Trichostrongylidae), is a parasite localised in the abomasum or stomach. For more details, see Chapter 9.

Mecistocirrus digitatus

Mecistocirrus digitatus (Phylum: Nematoda; Class: Chromadorea; Order: Rhabditida; Family: Trichostrongylidae) is localised in the abomasum of cattle, buffalo, sheep and goats (occasionally the stomach of the pig and rarely human) and is found in tropical and subtropical regions, particularly Central America and parts of Asia. In endemic areas, the pathogenesis of this haematophagous parasite is similar to that of *H. contortus* and it is of similar economic importance. For clinical signs, control and treatment, see *H. contortus*.

Cryptosporidium andersoni

Cryptosporidium andersoni, synonym *Cryptosporidium muris* (Phylum: Apicomplexa; Class: Conoidasida; Order: Cryptogregarinorida; Family: Cryptosporidiidae), is generally a non-pathogenic parasite localised in the abomasum of cattle. It is found in the USA, Brazil, UK, Czech Republic, Germany, France, Japan and Iran.

Epidemiology: The epidemiology of infection has not been studied, although it is likely to be similar to that of *Cryptosporidium parvum* in cattle. Many calves are likely to become infected without showing clinical signs but become sources of infection for calves that follow. The primary route of infection is direct animal to animal via the faecal–oral route. Thus, in calves, for example, overcrowding, stress of early weaning, transport and marketing, together with low levels of hygiene, will increase the risk of heavy infections.

Clinical signs and pathology: Usually asymptomatic, although depressed weight gain in calves and milk yields in milking cows have been reported. The presence of the endogenous stages of the parasite leads to destruction of the microvilli of peptic glands, leading to elevated concentrations of plasma pepsinogen.

Diagnosis: Oocysts may be demonstrated using Ziehl–Neelsen stained faecal smears in which the sporozoites appear as bright red granules. Speciation of *Cryptosporidium* is difficult, if not impossible, using conventional techniques. A range of molecular and immunological techniques has been developed that includes the use of immunofluorescence or ELISA. More recently, DNA-based techniques have been used for the molecular characterisation of *Cryptosporidium* species.

Control and treatment: There is no reported treatment. Good hygiene and management are important in preventing disease from cryptosporidiosis. Feed and water containers should be high enough to prevent faecal contamination. Young animals should be given colostrum within the first 24 hours of birth and overstocking and overcrowding should be avoided. Dairy calves should be either isolated in individual pens or kept in similar age groups and cleaned out daily.

Notes: Based on oocyst morphology, *C. muris*-like oocysts have been found in cattle in several countries around the world. Recent molecular characterisations have indicated that all bovine isolates are *C. andersoni*.

SMALL INTESTINE

Cooperia oncophora

Cooperia oncophora (Phylum: Nematoda; Class: Chromadorea; Order: Rhabditida; Family: Cooperidae) is a parasite distributed worldwide and localised in the small intestine of cattle, sheep, goats, deer and camels.

Epidemiology: In temperate areas, this is similar to that of *Ostertagia*. Arrested development (hypobiosis) at the EL_4 stage is a regular feature during late autumn and winter in the northern hemisphere, and in spring and summer in the southern hemisphere. Adult animals usually show few signs of infection but act as carriers, shedding low numbers of eggs in their faeces. In the subtropics, the epidemiology is similar to that of *Haemonchus* though *Cooperia* does not have the same high biotic potential and the L_3 survive rather better under arid conditions. Hypobiosis is also a feature during prolonged dry seasons.

Pathogenesis: *Cooperia oncophora* is generally considered to be a mild pathogen in calves, although in some studies it has been associated with inappetence and poor weight gain. Immunity to reinfection develops after about 8–12 months of exposure to infective larvae.

Clinical signs and pathology: These include loss of appetite and poor weight gain. Occasionally a heavy infection can induce intermittent diarrhoea. Moderate to heavy infections can induce a catarrhal enteritis with localised villous atrophy and oedema of the intestinal mucosa.

Diagnosis: Eggs of *Cooperia* spp. are all very similar morphologically. Faecal culture will allow identification of infective larvae.

Control and treatment: The principles are similar to those applied in bovine ostertagiosis. *Cooperia* is one of the dose-limiting species and one should consult the manufacturer's data sheets for efficacy of anthelmintics against adult and L_4 stages.

Notes: In temperate areas, members of the genus *Cooperia* usually play a secondary role in the pathogenesis of parasitic gastroenteritis of ruminants, although they may be the most numerous trichostrongyle present. However, in some tropical and subtropical areas, some species are responsible for severe enteritis in calves. Three further species of *Cooperia* are found in cattle. Details of the epidemiology, diagnosis, control and treatment are as for *C. oncophora*.

Cooperia punctata

Cooperia punctata (Phylum: Nematoda; Class: Chromadorea; Order: Rhabditida; Family: Cooperidae), commonly known as the Cattle bankrupt worm, is distributed worldwide and localised in the small intestine of cattle and deer.

Pathogenesis: *Cooperia punctata* is a pathogenic parasite since it penetrates the epithelial surface of the small intestine and causes a disruption similar to that of other intestinal trichostrongylid species, which leads to villous atrophy and a reduction in the area available for absorption. In heavy infections, diarrhoea has been reported.

Clinical signs: There is loss of appetite, poor weight gain and diarrhoea, and there may be submandibular oedema.

Cooperia pectinata

Cooperia pectinata (Phylum: Nematoda; Class: Chromadorea; Order: Rhabditida; Family: Cooperidae) is distributed worldwide and localised in the small intestine of cattle and deer. Similar to *C. punctata*, a catarrhal enteritis is often present with loss of appetite, poor weight gain, diarrhoea and, in some cases, submandibular oedema.

Cooperia surnabada

Cooperia surnabada, synonym *Cooperia mcmasteri* (Phylum: Nematoda; Class: Chromadorea; Order: Rhabditida; Family: Cooperidae), is a parasite localised in the small intestine of cattle, sheep and camels and found in parts of Europe, North America and Australia. The infection may cause moderate pathogenicity as the worms penetrate the surface of the small intestine and can induce villous atrophy. For clinical signs and diagnosis, see *C. punctata*; for control and treatment, see *C. oncophora*.

Nematodirus helvetianus

Nematodirus helvetianus (Phylum: Nematoda; Class: Chromadorea; Order: Rhabditida; Family: Molineidae), commonly known as the Thread-necked worm, is distributed worldwide and usually localised in the small intestine of cattle, occasionally sheep, goats and other ruminants.

Epidemiology: The eggs do not usually exhibit delayed hatching. The pattern of infection is similar to that of *Trichostrongylus* species.

Pathogenesis: Although this is similar to that of *Nematodirus battus*, there is some controversy over the extent of the pathogenic effect. *Nematodirus helvetianus* has been incriminated in outbreaks of bovine parasitic gastroenteritis but experimental attempts to reproduce the disease have been unsuccessful.

Clinical signs and pathology: Low to moderate infections may produce no obvious clinical manifestations. In severe infections, diarrhoea can occur during the prepatent period and young animals may become dehydrated. Increased mucus production and focal compression and stunting of villi may occur in the small intestine.

Diagnosis: Examination of faeces will allow the large colourless eggs to be differentiated from those of *N. spathiger*. At necropsy, the tips of the male spicules will allow diagnosis from other *Nematodirus* species.

Control and treatment: Disease due to monospecific *Nematodirus* infections is rarely seen. They are usually part of the worm burden of trichostrongyloid species that are responsible for the syndrome of parasitic gastroenteritis in cattle and as such may be controlled by the measures outlined elsewhere. Several drugs are effective against *Nematodirus* infections: levamisole, an avermectin/milbemycin or one of the modern benzimidazoles. However, *Nematodirus* is one of the dose-limiting species and manufacturer's data sheets should be consulted as there are differences in efficacy against adults and L_4 stages between oral and parenteral administration for some macrocyclic lactones. The response to treatment is usually rapid and if diarrhoea persists, coccidiosis should be considered as a complicating factor.

Bunostomum phlebotomum

Bunostomum phlebotomum, synonym *Monodontus phlebotomum* (Phylum: Nematoda; Class: Chromadorea; Order: Rhabditida; Family: Ancylostomatidae), commonly known as the Cattle hookworm, is distributed worldwide and localised in the anterior jejunum and/or duodenum of cattle.

Epidemiology: Pathogenic infections are more common in the tropics and subtropics and in some areas, such as Nigeria, the highest worm burdens are found at the end of the dry season, apparently due to the maturation of hypobiotic larvae. Young livestock are most susceptible. *Bunostomum phlebotomum* is often a serious pathogen in many regions, such as the southern and mid-western USA, Australia and parts of Africa. In temperate countries, high worm burdens are usually uncommon. The prophylactic dosing regimens adopted for the control of trichostrongyles have contributed to the low prevalence of *Bunostomum*.

Pathogenesis: The adult worms are blood-suckers and infections of 100–500 worms can produce progressive anaemia, hypoalbuminaemia, loss of weight and occasionally diarrhoea. Worm burdens of around 2000 may lead to death in cattle. In stabled cattle, pruritus of the limbs is seen, probably caused by skin penetration by the larvae.

Clinical signs and pathology: There may be inappetence, diarrhoea and emaciation, more frequently seen in young animals. Severe infection can also induce submandibular oedema ('bottle jaw'). *Post mortem* examination often reveals hydrothorax and fluid within the pericardium. Older livestock frequently develop sufficient immunity to limit reinfection and, in many cases, *Bunostomum* is present asymptomatically. In calves, foot stamping and signs of itching may accompany skin penetration by the larvae. The carcass is anaemic and cachexic. Oedema and ascites are seen. The liver is light brown and shows fatty changes. The intestinal contents are haemorrhagic and the mucosa is usually swollen, covered with mucus, and shows numerous lesions resulting from the worms feeding (Fig. 8.5). The parasites may be seen still attached to the mucosa or free in the lumen.

Diagnosis: The clinical signs of anaemia and perhaps diarrhoea in calves are not in themselves pathognomonic of bunostomosis. However, in temperate areas, the epidemiological background may be useful in eliminating the possibility of *Fasciola hepatica* infection. In the tropics, haemonchosis must be considered, possibly originating from hypobiotic larvae. Faecal egg counts are useful in that these are lower than in *Haemonchus* infection while the eggs are more bluntly rounded, with relatively thick sticky shells to which debris is often adhered. For accurate differentiation, larval cultures should be prepared.

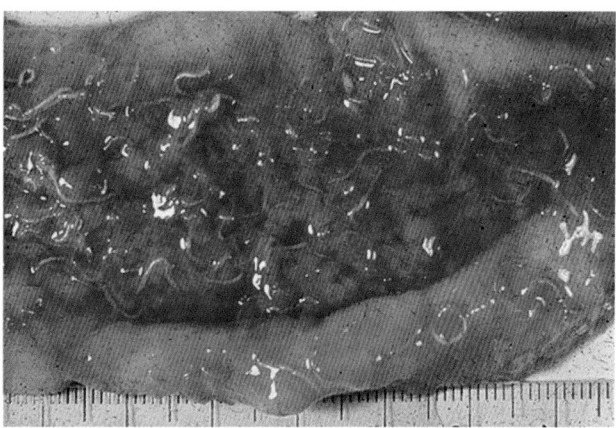

Fig. 8.5 Inflamed and haemorrhagic intestinal mucosa due to the presence of feeding worms (*Bunostomum phlebotomum*).

Control and treatment: A combination of strategic dosing with anthelmintics and pasture management is used in the control of larvae as they are susceptible to desiccation, and the infection is mainly found on permanently or occasionally moist pastures. Avoiding or draining such pastures is an effective control measure. The ground around water troughs should be kept hard and dry, or treated with liberal applications of salt. Stabled cattle should be protected by ensuring the floors and bedding are kept dry and that faeces are removed frequently, and are not allowed to contaminate food and water. Anthelmintics listed for *O. ostertagi* are effective.

Agriostomum vryburgi

Agriostomum vryburgi (Phylum: Nematoda; Class: Chromadorea; Order: Rhabditida; Family: Chabertidae) is localised in the small intestine of cattle and buffalo and found in Asia and South America.

Pathogenesis: The hookworms attach to the mucosa of the anterior small intestine. The pathogenicity, although unknown, presumably depends on its haematophagic habits, inducing anaemia.

Notes: *Agriostomum vryburgi* is a common hookworm of the large intestine throughout its distribution range. Details on the diagnosis, treatment and control are likely to be similar to those for *B. phlebotomum*.

Strongyloides papillosus

Strongyloides papillosus (Phylum: Nematoda; Class: Chromadorea; Order: Rhabditida; Family: Strongyloididae) is distributed worldwide and localised in the small intestine of cattle, sheep, goats and other ruminants such as pigs and rabbits.

Epidemiology: *Strongyloides* infective larvae are not ensheathed and are susceptible to extreme climatic conditions. However, warmth and moisture favour development and allow the accumulation of large numbers of infective stages. For this reason, it can be a major problem in housed calves up to six months of age in some Mediterranean countries. A second major source of infection for the very young animal is the reservoir of larvae in the tissues of their dams and this may lead to clinical strongyloidosis in the first few weeks of life. Successive progeny from the same dam often show heavy infections.

Pathogenesis: Skin penetration by infective larvae may cause an erythematous reaction. Passage of larvae through the lungs has been shown experimentally to result in multiple small haemorrhages visible over most of the lung surfaces. Mature parasites are found in the duodenum and proximal jejunum and if present in large numbers may cause inflammation with oedema and erosion of the epithelium. This results in a catarrhal enteritis with impairment of digestion and absorption.

Clinical signs and pathology: The common clinical signs, usually seen only in very young animals, are diarrhoea, dehydration, anorexia, dullness, loss of weight or reduced growth rate. Adult worms establish in tunnels in the epithelium at the base of the villi in the small intestine. In large numbers, they may cause villous atrophy, with a mixed mononuclear inflammatory cell infiltration of the lamina propria. Crypt epithelium is hyperplastic and there is villous clubbing.

Diagnosis: The clinical signs in very young animals, usually within the first few weeks of life, together with the finding of large numbers of the characteristic eggs or larvae in the faeces, are suggestive of strongyloidosis. However, it should be emphasised that high faecal egg counts may be found in apparently healthy animals.

Control and treatment: Reduction in numbers of free-living larvae by removal of faeces and provision of dry bedding and areas may limit numbers and transmission. Suckling calves should be kept on clean dry areas to prevent infection by skin penetration. Specific control measures for *Strongyloides* infection are rarely required. The benzimidazoles and the avermectins/milbemycins may be used for the treatment of clinical cases.

Toxocara vitulorum

Toxocara vitulorum, synonym *Neoascaris vitulorum* (Phylum: Nematoda; Class: Chromadorea; Order: Ascaridida; Family: Ascarididae), is localised in the small intestine of cattle and buffaloes. It is found in Africa, India and Asia.

Epidemiology: The most important feature is the reservoir of larvae in the tissues of the cow, with subsequent milk-borne transmission ensuring that calves are exposed to infection from the first day of life. The majority of patent infections occur in calves of less than six months of age.

Pathogenesis: The main effects of *T. vitulorum* infection appear to be caused by the adult worms in the intestines of calves up to six months old. Heavy infections are often associated with unthriftiness, catarrhal enteritis and intermittent diarrhoea, and in buffalo calves particularly fatalities may occur. Heavy burdens can be associated with intestinal obstruction and occasionally perforation may occur leading to peritonitis and death.

Clinical signs and pathology: Diarrhoea, poor condition. The pathological effects of adult worms in the intestine are poorly defined. Heavy infections may obstruct the gut and lead to gut perforation. Migration up the bile or pancreatic duct may lead to biliary obstruction and cholangitis.

Diagnosis: In some instances, heavily infected calves may exhale an acetone-like odour. The subglobular eggs, with thick pitted shells, are characteristic in bovine faeces. Egg output in young calves can be very high (>50 000 epg) but patency is short and by around

4–6 months of age calves have expelled most of their adult worm population.

Control and treatment: The prevalence of infection can be dramatically reduced by treatment of calves at three and six weeks of age, preventing developing worms reaching patency. The adult worms are susceptible to a wide range of anthelmintics, including piperazine, levamisole, macrocyclic lactones and the benzimidazoles. Many of these drugs are also effective against developing stages in the intestine.

Capillaria bovis

Capillaria bovis, synonym *Capillaria brevipes* (Phylum: Nematoda; Class: Enoplea; Order: Enoplida; Family: Capillariidae), is distributed worldwide and localised in the small intestine of cattle, sheep and goats. Infection is by ingestion of the larvated eggs and although it occurs commonly in sheep, is usually not of significant clinical concern.

Clinical signs and pathology: No clinical signs have been attributed to infection with this parasite. No associated pathology is known, thus control and treatment are not usually required.

Diagnosis: Because of the non-specific nature of the clinical signs and the fact that, in heavy infections, these may appear before eggs are present in the faeces, diagnosis depends on necropsy and careful examination of the small intestine for the presence of the worms. This may be carried out by microscopic examination of mucosal scrapings squeezed between two glass slides; alternatively, the contents should be gently washed through a fine sieve and the retained material resuspended in water and examined against a black background.

Moniezia benedeni

Moniezia benedeni (Phylum: Platyhelminthes; Class: Cestoda; Order: Cyclophyllidea; Family: Anoplocephalidae) is distributed worldwide and localised in the small intestine of cattle and buffalo. This parasite has forage mites, mainly of the family Oribatidae, as intermediate hosts and is generally regarded as of little pathogenic significance with no clinical signs.

Epidemiology: Infection is common in calves during their first year of life and less common in older animals. A seasonal fluctuation in the incidence of *Moniezia* infection can apparently be related to active periods of the forage mite vectors during the summer in temperate areas. The cysticercoids can overwinter in the mites.

Diagnosis: This is based largely on the presence of mature proglottids in the faeces and the characteristic shape of *Moniezia* eggs (triangular, *M. expansa*; quadrangular, *M. benedeni*) that contain the oncosphere. The eggs of *M. benedeni* are slightly larger than those of *M. expansa* in sheep.

Control and treatment: Ploughing and reseeding, or avoiding the use of the same pastures for young animals in consecutive years, may prove beneficial. In many countries a variety of drugs, including niclosamide, praziquantel, bunamidine and a number of broad-spectrum benzimidazole compounds, which have the advantage of also being active against gastrointestinal nematodes, are available for the treatment of *Moniezia* infection. If this is carried out in calves in late spring, in temperate areas, the numbers of newly infected mites on pasture will be reduced.

Notes: This genus of cestodes is common in ruminants and resembles, in most respects, *Anoplocephala* of the horse. *Moniezia* spp. are the only tapeworms of ruminants in many countries of western Europe.

Thysaniezia ovilla

Thysaniezia ovilla, synonyms *Thysaniezia giardi*, *Helictometra giardi* (Phylum: Platyhelminthes; Class: Cestoda; Order: Cyclophyllidea; Family: Anoplocephalidae), is a non-pathogenic parasite localised in the small intestine of cattle, sheep, goats, camels and wild ruminants and found in southern Africa. Oribatid mites (*Galuma*, *Scheloribates*) and psocids (bark lice, dust lice) are intermediate hosts. Control and treatment of this parasite are as for *Moniezia*, from which it is readily distinguishable based on the shape of mature segments found in the faeces.

The following species have also been reported in cattle. For more details on these species see Chapter 9.

Moniezia expansa

Moniezia expansa (Phylum: Platyhelminthes; Class: Cestoda; Order: Cyclophyllidea; Family: Anoplocephalidae) is localised in the small intestine of sheep, goats and occasionally cattle. This parasite has forage mites, mainly of the family Oribatidae, as intermediate hosts.

Avitellina centripunctata

Avitellina centripunctata (Phylum: Platyhelminthes; Class: Cestoda; Order: Cyclophyllidea; Family: Anoplocephalidae) is localised in the small intestine of sheep, goat, camel and other ruminants and found in Europe, Africa and Asia. This parasite has oribatid mites or psocid lice as intermediate hosts. The infection is usually asymptomatic, being of negligible pathogenicity, similar to *Moniezia* spp.

Thysanosoma actinoides

Thysanosoma actinoides (Phylum: Platyhelminthes; Class: Cestoda; Order: Cyclophyllidea; Family: Anoplocephalidae), commonly known as the Fringed tapeworm, is localised in the small intestine of sheep, cattle and deer and found in North and South America. This parasite has oribatid mites (*Galuma*, *Scheloribates*) and psocids (bark lice, dust lice) as intermediate hosts.

Cymbiforma indica

Cymbiforma indica (Phylum: Platyhelminthes; Class: Trematoda; Order: Plagiorchiida; Family: Notocotylidae) is localised in the gastrointestinal tract of sheep, goats and cattle and is found in India. This parasite has snails as intermediate hosts.

Bovine coccidiosis

At least 20 different species of *Eimeria* are known to infect cattle, of which 13 species are more commonly found. Clinical signs of diarrhoea are associated with the presence of *E. zuernii* or *E. bovis*, which occur in the lower small intestine, caecum and colon. *Eimeria alabamensis* has been reported to cause enteritis in yearling calves in some European countries. Affected animals develop watery diarrhoea, shortly after turnout in the spring on to heavily contaminated pastures previously grazed by calves. The life cycles of the *Eimeria* species are typically coccidian and the general life cycle is described in detail in Chapter 2. Variations in sites of development of meront and gamont stages, and prepatent periods do occur, and where known are described under the respective species.

Epidemiology: Bovine coccidiosis is primarily a disease of young animals, normally occurring in calves between three weeks and six months of age but has been reported in cattle aged one year or more. The disease is usually associated with a previous stressful situation such as shipping, overcrowding, changes in feed, severe weather or concurrent infection with parvovirus. Adult cattle, although possibly the original source of infective oocysts in the environment, are not usually responsible for the heavy levels of contamination encountered. The source is often young calves themselves, which following an initial infection often in the first few days of life may produce millions of oocysts within their own environment. Growing animals may then face potentially lethal doses of infective oocysts three weeks later when their natural resistance is at its lowest. Later-born calves introduced into the same environment are immediately exposed to heavy oocyst challenge. Under unhygienic overcrowded conditions, the young calves will be exposed to and ingest a large proportion of this infection and will develop severe disease and may even die from the infection. If conditions are less crowded and more hygienic, the infective dose ingested will be lower, they may show moderate, slight or no clinical signs and develop immunity to reinfection, but they will in turn have multiplied the infection a million-fold. Stress factors, such a poor milk supply, weaning, cold weather and transport, will reduce any acquired resistance and exacerbate the condition.

A major problem in milking herds (cattle) is that in an attempt to ensure a constant year-round milk supply, births often take place over an extended period of time. If the same pens are used constantly for successive batches, or if young calves are added to a pen already housing older calves, then the later born are immediately exposed to heavy challenge and can show severe coccidiosis in the first few weeks of life. Age is therefore one of the main risk factors. During their first weeks of life, young ruminants are normally protected by passive immunity derived from colostrum. Neonatal animals receiving insufficient intake of colostrum and milk or experiencing periods of stress may start to show clinical signs of disease from about 18 days of age onwards. Adult cattle are usually highly resistant to disease, but not totally resistant to infection. As a result, small numbers of parasites manage to complete their life cycle and usually cause no detectable harm. In the wild or under more natural extensive systems of management, susceptible calves are exposed to only low numbers of oocysts and acquire a protective immunity. Extensive grazing, as occurs under natural conditions in the wild, limits the level of exposure to infective oocysts. Under modern production systems, however, young calves are born into a potentially heavily contaminated environment, and where the numbers of sporulated oocysts are high, disease often occurs.

Traditionally, indoor housing is a high-risk period especially where young calves are heavily stocked and in conditions that favour rapid oocyst sporulation and high numbers of oocysts in the environment. Three management factors are associated with the development of high levels of infection and the development of disease: pens not cleaned on a regular basis, overcrowding in the pens, and pens used to house different age groups.

The season of the year can also play a role in the appearance of coccidiosis. Coccidiosis is common in spring when young calves are born and turned out onto permanent pastures close to the farm buildings. Inclement weather at this time may cause stress at this stage, lowering immunity and precipitating disease. Cold winters favour survival of overwintering oocysts in large enough numbers to represent sufficient disease challenge at turnout in spring; conversely, mild wet springs favour sporulation and rapid accumulation of large numbers of infective oocysts. Autumn-born calves may be born into an already heavily contaminated environment. The effects of coccidial infections may be exacerbated if different species that affect different parts of the gut are present at the same time. Similarly, concurrent infections with other disease-producing agents such as helminths, bacteria and viruses may affect the severity of disease. Interactions between coccidia and parvovirus infection is thought to aggravate coccidiosis in calves.

Most cattle are infected with coccidia during their lives and in the majority of animals, the parasites co-exist and cause minimal damage. Disease usually only occurs if animals are subjected to heavy infection or if their resistance is lowered through stress, poor nutrition or intercurrent disease. The presence of infection does not necessarily lead to the development of clinical signs of disease and in many situations low levels of challenge can actually be beneficial by stimulating protective immune responses in the host.

Pathogenesis: The most pathogenic species of coccidia are those that infect and destroy the crypt cells of the large intestinal mucosa (Table 8.3). This is because the ruminant small intestine is very long, providing a large number of host cells and the potential for enormous parasite replication with minimal damage. If the absorption of nutrients is impaired, the large intestine is, to some extent, capable of compensating. Those species that invade the large intestine are more likely to cause pathological changes, particularly if large numbers of oocysts are ingested over a short period of time. Here, the rate of cellular turnover is much lower and there is no compensation effect from other regions of the gut. In calves that become heavily infected, the mucosa becomes completely denuded,

Table 8.3 Predilection sites and prepatent periods of *Eimeria* species in cattle.

Species	Predilection site	Prepatent period (days)
Eimeria alabamensis	Small and large intestine	6–11
Eimeria auburnensis	Small intestine	16–24
Eimeria bovis	Small and large intestine	16–21
Eimeria brasiliensis	Unknown	?
Eimeria bukidnonensis	Unknown	?
Eimeria canadensis	Unknown	?
Eimeria cylindrica	Unknown	?
Eimeria ellipsoidalis	Small intestine	8–13
Eimeria pellita	Unknown	?
Eimeria subspherica	Unknown	7–18
Eimeria wyomingensis	Unknown	13–15
Eimeria zuernii	Small and large intestine	15–17

resulting in severe haemorrhage and impaired water resorption leading to diarrhoea, dehydration and death. In lighter infections, the effect on the intestinal mucosa is to impair local absorption. Species that develop more superficially in the small intestine cause a change in villous architecture with a reduction in epithelial cell height and a diminution of the brush border, giving the appearance of a 'flat' mucosa. These changes result in a reduction of the surface area available for absorption and consequently reduced feed efficiency.

Clinical signs and pathology: Clinical signs are associated with the presence of the pathogenic species, *E. zuernii* or *E. bovis*, which occur in the lower small intestine, caecum and colon. *Eimeria alabamensis* has been reported to cause enteritis in first-season grazing calves in the first week following turnout in some European countries. Some animals with coccidiosis develop concurrent nervous signs, including tremors, nystagmus, opisthotonus and convulsions. The cause of these symptoms is unknown, although the possibility of the neurological signs being induced by a toxin has been suggested. Clinical signs of coccidiosis include weight loss, anorexia and diarrhoea, often bloody. On *post mortem*, there may be little to see beyond thickening and petechiation of the bowel but mucosal scrapings will reveal masses of gamonts and oocysts. Giant meronts may be seen in the mucosa of the small intestine as pin-point white spots, but unless they are present in vast numbers they cause little harm. The most pathogenic stages are the gamonts.

Host resistance: While animals of all ages are susceptible to infection, younger animals are generally more susceptible to disease. Occasionally, however, acute coccidiosis occurs in much older, even adult cattle with impaired cellular immunity or in those which have been subjected to stress, such as transportation, crowding in feedlot areas, extremes of temperature and weather conditions, changes in environment or severe concurrent infection.

Diagnosis: Diagnosis should be based on history, clinical signs (severe diarrhoea in young calves), *post mortem* findings (inflammation, hyperaemia and thickening of caecum with masses of gamonts and oocysts in scrapings), supported by oocyst counts and speciation to identify pathogenic species. Counts of faecal oocysts identified to species can help to complete the picture, but oocyst numbers may be grossly misleading when considered in isolation. Healthy cattle may pass more than 1 million oocysts per gram of faeces, whereas in animals dying of coccidiosis the count may be less than 10 000 oocysts per gram. For instance, high counts of non-pathogenic species could mask significant numbers of the more pathogenic species and give the impression that the abundant species was the cause. A key to the identification of sporulated oocysts of cattle is provided in Chapter 4 (see Fig. 4.35 and Table 4.7).

Control: Coccidial infections can be reduced through avoidance of overcrowding and stress, and attention to hygiene. Raising of food and water troughs, for example, can help avoid contamination and thus reduce levels of infection. Young animals should be kept off heavily contaminated pastures when they are most susceptible. The control of outbreaks of coccidiosis is a balance between controlling the disease and allowing the development of protective immunity against subsequent oocyst challenge. It should also be remembered that not all species are pathogenic and that immunity is species specific so that exposure to one coccidial species does not confer resistance to another species. Also, exposure to a single infective challenge may confer strong protective immunity with some species

of coccidia, while with others repeated exposure may be required before full protective immunity is acquired. The timing of any treatment intervention is therefore crucial in both preventing severe disease outbreaks and at the same time allowing protective immunity to develop through adequate parasite exposure. To achieve this, it is important to understand the epidemiology of coccidial infections in relation to the different ruminant hosts and the differing systems of production around the world. Using this approach, it is possible to identify within management and husbandry systems periods of stress that may precipitate outbreaks of disease. While appropriate disease prevention methods should always be considered and instigated wherever possible, a more strategic approach to anticoccidial treatment should be applied based on an assessment of disease risks.

Treatment: Outbreaks of clinical coccidiosis can appear suddenly and may prove troublesome to resolve as they often occur on heavily stocked farms, particularly where good husbandry and management are lacking. If deaths are occurring, early confirmation of the diagnosis is vital. Affected cattle should be medicated and moved to uncontaminated pens or pasture as soon as possible. Normally all cattle in a group should be treated, as even those showing no symptoms are likely to be infected. For calves, this would normally be in the form of a single oral drench with either diclazuril or toltrazuril, in countries where these products are both available and licensed for use. Decoquinate can be administered in feed, bearing in mind that not all animals may consume the feed, especially severely affected animals that may be off their feed and dehydrated. Where these products are not available or licensed, then treatment with a sulfonamide such as sulfadimidine or sulfamethoxypyridazine can be considered. Severely infected animals that are diarrhoeic and dehydrated may require oral or intravenous rehydration. Coccidiosis-infected animals may also have concurrent bacterial or parasitic infections that need to be diagnosed and treated with either antibacterial or anthelmintic treatments.

Where non-specific symptoms of weight loss or ill-thrift are present, it is important to investigate all potential causes and seek laboratory confirmation. If coccidiosis is considered significant, much can be done through advice on management and instigation of preventive measures. Batch rearing of animals of similar ages limits the build-up and spread of oocysts and allows targeting of treatment to susceptible age groups during the danger periods.

Eimeria bovis; Eimeria zuernii

For more details see Parasites of the large intestine.

Eimeria alabamensis

Eimeria alabamensis (Phylum: Apicomplexa; Class: Conoidasida; Order: Eucoccidiorida; Family: Eimeriidae) is a parasite localised in the small and large intestine of cattle and is found worldwide, although mainly in Europe. The life cycle is typically coccidian with the developmental stages occurring in the nucleus of epithelial cells. Sporozoites penetrate the intestinal cells as early as day 2 after infection, and meronts are visible in the nucleus 2–8 days post infection. Parasitised cells are usually those at the tips of the villi and multiple invasion of the nucleus may occur. Two generations of meronts have been found: mature first-generation meronts are seen 2–7 days post infection, and mature second-generation meronts 4–7 days post infection. The gametocytes are found in the posterior third of the small intestine and may also occur in the mucous membrane of the caecum and colon in heavy infections. Oocysts may be seen in the cells of the lower ileum as early as six days post infection. The prepatent period is 6–11 days, with a patent period of 1–13 days. Sporulation takes 4–8 days.

Pathogenesis: Particularly pathogenic, attacking the epithelial cells of the jejunum, ileum and, in heavy infections, the caecum and colon.

Clinical signs and pathology: Diarrhoea in calves recently turned out on to permanent paddocks. The calves become depressed and reluctant to rise. From eight days after turnout, 850 000 to several million oocysts per gram faeces are excreted. Growth rate of the calves is adversely affected. Morbidity ranges from 5% to 100% (average 64%) but mortality is generally low. Infection causes catarrhal enteritis in the jejunum, ileum and caecum with petechial haemorrhages. Histologically, there is necrotic inflammation and destruction of epithelial cells. There is an inflammatory response consisting predominantly of mononuclear cells with a few eosinophils and neutrophils. Numerous meronts are seen in the nuclei of villous epithelial cells, with occasional meronts in the upper colon. The mesenteric lymph nodes are enlarged, and parasite stages have been observed in the lymph nodes.

Control: Where infection is suspected to be due to oocysts overwintering on the pasture, the grazing land should be rotated to ensure that calves are not turned out on to potentially heavily infected pasture.

Treatment: Sulfonamides can be used to treat infection. Decoquinate has a prophylactic action against the parasite. Infection with the following species of coccidia present in the small intestine is not usually associated with clinical signs. Specific treatment and control measures are not usually indicated for these species, although they often present as mixed infections. Differentiation is based on oocyst morphology (see Tables 2.18 and 4.7 and Fig. 4.35).

Cryptosporidium parvum

Cryptosporidium parvum (Phylum: Apicomplexa; Class: Conoidasida; Order: Cryptogregarinorida; Family: Cryptosporidiidae) is distributed worldwide and localised in the small intestine of cattle, sheep, goats, horses, deer and humans.

Epidemiology: A variety of mammals act as hosts to *C. parvum* but little is known of the importance of their involvement in transmitting infection to, or maintaining infection in, domestic livestock. In young calves, infection appears to be age related, with seasonal peaks of disease reported to coincide with birth peaks in spring and autumn. The first calves to be born often become infected without showing clinical signs but become sources of infection for calves that follow. Infection spreads rapidly, and later-born calves can become so heavily infected that clinical disease results. In many instances where *Cryptosporidium* is diagnosed in animals, it appears that infections usually originate from the same host species. The primary route of infection is mainly direct animal to animal via the faecal–oral route. Thus, in calves, for example, overcrowding, stress of early weaning, transport and marketing, together with low levels of hygiene, will increase the risk of clinical infections. In lambs,

chilling due to adverse weather conditions in the neonatal period, intercurrent infections or nutritional or mineral deficiencies could exacerbate or increase the likelihood of disease. Infection in these cases is likely to occur via grooming, nuzzling, coprophagy or faecal soiling by direct contact with infected animals. Infection may also occur indirectly through consumption of contaminated foods or environmental sources, including pasture and water.

Clinical signs and pathology: Clinically the disease is characterised by anorexia and diarrhoea, often intermittent, which may result in poor growth rates. Cryptosporidiosis is common in young calves, although the pathogenesis of infection is not clear. It is remarkable in that, unlike other members of the Eimeriidae, *Cryptosporidium* does not enter the cells of the host and lacks host specificity so that cross-infection can occur between domestic animals and humans. The meronts and gamonts develop in a parasitophorous envelope, apparently derived from the microvilli, and so the cell disruption seen with other coccidia does not apparently occur. However, mucosal changes are obvious in the ileum where there is stunting, swelling and eventually fusion of the villi. This has a marked effect on the activity of some of the membrane-bound enzymes.

Diagnosis: Oocysts may be demonstrated using Ziehl–Neelsen stained faecal smears in which the sporozoites appear as bright red granules (Fig. 8.6). Speciation of *Cryptosporidium* is difficult, if not impossible, using conventional techniques. A range of molecular and immunological techniques has been developed that includes the use of immunofluorescence (Fig. 8.7) or ELISA. More recently, DNA-based techniques have been used for the molecular characterisations of *Cryptosporidium* species.

Control: Good hygiene and management are important in preventing disease from cryptosporidiosis. Feed and water containers should be high enough to prevent faecal contamination. Young animals should be given colostrum within the first 24 hours of birth and overstocking and overcrowding should be avoided. Dairy calves should be either isolated in individual pens or kept in similar age groups and cleaned out daily. On calf-rearing farms with recurrent problems, the prophylactic use of halofuginone can be considered by treating for seven days consecutively commencing at 24–48 hours after birth.

Treatment: There is no known treatment, although spiramycin may be of some value. The infection is difficult to control since the

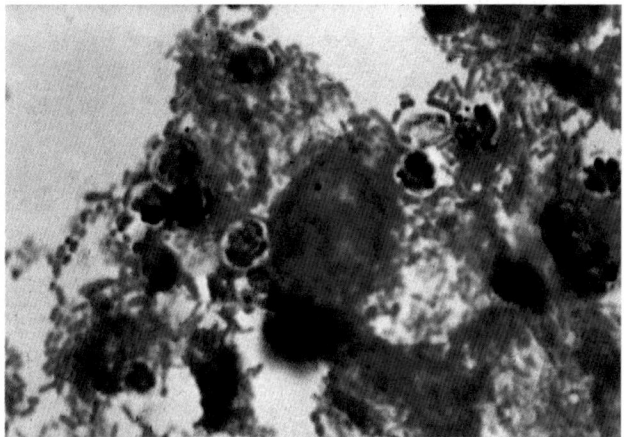

Fig. 8.6 Oocysts of *Cryptosporidium parvum* (Ziehl–Neelsen stain).

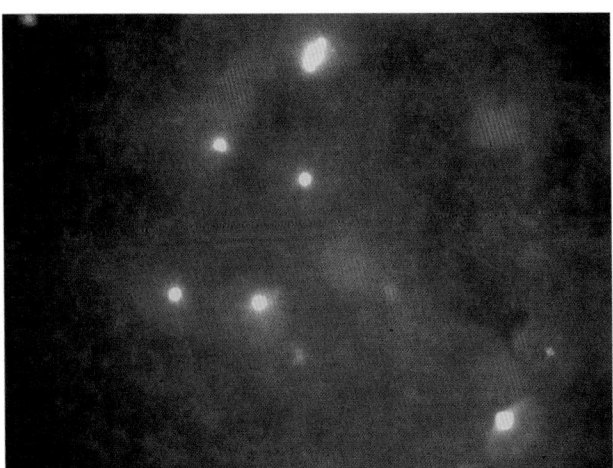

Fig. 8.7 Oocysts of *Cryptosporidium parvum* (immunofluorescent antibody test).

oocysts are highly resistant to most disinfectants except formol-saline and ammonia. Halofuginone is available for the prevention of cryptosporidiosis in calves at a dose rate of 1 mg per 10 kg. Symptomatic treatment may be given in the form of antidiarrhoeals and fluid replacement therapy.

Notes: Recent molecular characterisations have shown that there is extensive host adaptation in *Cryptosporidium* evolution, and many mammals or groups of mammals have host-adapted *Cryptosporidium* genotypes, which differ from each other in both DNA sequences and infectivity. These genotypes are now delineated as distinct species and include, in cattle, *C. parvum*, *C. bovis* (also termed the bovine genotype or genotype 2), *C. ryanae* and *C. ubiquitum*.

Giardia intestinalis

Giardia intestinalis, synonyms *Giardia duodenalis*, *Giardia lamblia*, *Lamblia lamblia* (Phylum: Metamonada; Class: Trepomonadea; Order: Diplomonadida; Family: Giardiidae), is distributed worldwide and localised in the small intestine of humans, cattle, sheep, goats, pigs, horses, alpacas, dogs, cats, guinea pigs and chinchillas.

Epidemiology: Molecular studies have revealed a substantial level of genetic diversity in *G. intestinalis* isolates. Human isolates fall into two major groups (assemblages A and B) with a wide host range in other mammals, and some separate species names may be applicable. Other assemblages may also represent distinct species. Limited epidemiological studies suggest that in animal isolates, direct animal-to-animal contact and faecal soiling are the most likely methods of transmission, although water contamination can also be considered as a possible route. The incidence of these parasites varies but can be assumed to be higher in some species than has been reported. Studies in Canada and the USA indicate levels of infection in cattle of up to 20% in clinically normal animals and 100% infection rates in young diarrhoeic calves.

Pathogenesis: Infections in cattle are often asymptomatic but have been reported to cause diarrhoea in young calves.

Clinical signs and pathology: When disease does occur, the signs often include chronic pasty diarrhoea, weight loss, lethargy and failure to thrive. The diarrhoea may be continuous or intermittent.

There may be villous atrophy, crypt hypertrophy and an increased number of intraepithelial lymphocytes. Trophozoites may be seen between villi, attached by their concave surface to the brush border of epithelial cells.

Diagnosis: *Giardia* cysts can be detected in faeces by a number of methods. Traditional methods of identification involve direct examination of faecal smears, or faecal concentration by formaline-thyl acetate or zinc sulfate methods and subsequent microscopic examination. It is generally recommended that three consecutive samples be examined as cysts are excreted intermittently.

Control and treatment: As infection is transmitted by the faecal–oral route, good hygiene and prevention of faecal contamination of feed and water are essential. There is no recommended treatment for infection in calves. Several benzimidazole anthelmintics (e.g. albendazole, fenbendazole) are effective and may prove to be of benefit.

Notes: The parasite is important because of water-borne outbreaks that have occurred in human populations. Phylogenetic data suggest that *G. intestinalis* is a species complex composed of several species that are host specific. There is still some controversy over the classification of *Giardia* spp. The current molecular classification places isolates into eight distinct assemblages. Some authors give separate specific names to *Giardia* organisms isolated from cattle, for example *Giardia enterica* (Assemblage B), *Giardia bovis* (Assemblage E), although species specificity of many isolates is unknown.

LARGE INTESTINE

Oesophagostomum radiatum

Oesophagostomum radiatum (Phylum: Nematoda; Class: Chromadorea; Order: Rhabditida; Family: Strongylidae), commonly known as the Nodular worm, is distributed worldwide and localised in the large intestine of cattle and buffalo.

Epidemiology: It is not yet known if hypobiosis occurs in *O. radiatum*. It is also capable of overwintering on pasture as L_3. In tropical and subtropical areas *O. radiatum* in cattle is especially important. Cattle develop a good immunity, partly due to age and partly to previous exposure, so that it is primarily a problem in weaned calves.

Pathogenesis: In *O. radiatum* infections in cattle, the pathogenic effect is attributed to the nodules (up to 5.0 mm in diameter) in the intestine and it is one of the most damaging worms to cattle when present in high numbers, with >200 adult worms in calves and >1000 in adult cattle sufficient to produce clinical signs. In the later stages of the disease, anaemia and hypoalbuminaemia develop due to the combined effects of protein loss and leakage of blood through the damaged mucosa.

Clinical signs and pathology: In acute infections, there is anaemia, oedema and diarrhoea. On *post mortem* examination, animals may be pale from anaemia and oedematous from hypoproteinaemia. Colonic lymph nodes are enlarged and the mucosa of the colon is grossly thickened and folded by oedema and increased mixed inflammatory cell infiltrates in the lamina propria. Colonic submucosal lymphoid follicles are large and active. Effusion of tissue fluid and blood cells may be evident through small leaks between cells, or from erosions in glands or on the surface. Although repeated exposure to infective larvae may result in the accumulation of large numbers of fourth-stage worms in nodules, formation of nodules has little pathogenic significance in cattle.

Diagnosis: This is based on clinical signs and *post mortem* examination. The presence of pea-shaped nodules in the intestinal wall on *post mortem* is indicative of nodular worm infection. In the chronic disease, eggs are present and L_3 can be identified following faecal culture.

Control and treatment: While not generally considered highly pathogenic, a combination of strategic dosing with anthelmintics and pasture management, as used in the control of other nematodes, will also help to control *O. radiatum*. Anthelmintic therapy with broad-spectrum anthelmintics (benzimidazoles, levamisole and avermectins/milbemycins) is highly effective.

Trichuris globulosa

Trichuris globulosa, synonym *Trichocephalus globulosa* (Phylum: Nematoda; Class: Enoplea; Order: Enoplida; Family: Trichuridae), commonly known as the Whipworm, is distributed worldwide and localised in the large intestine of cattle, occasionally sheep, goats, camels and other ruminants. Adult nematodes are usually found in the caecum but are only occasionally present in sufficient numbers to be clinically significant.

Epidemiology: The most important feature is the longevity of the eggs, which may survive for 3–4 years. On pasture this is less likely since the eggs tend to be washed into the soil.

Clinical signs and pathology: Most infections are light and asymptomatic. Occasionally, when large numbers of worms are present, they cause a diphtheritic inflammation of the caecal mucosa. Hence, despite the fact that ruminants have a high incidence of light infections, the clinical significance of this genus, especially in ruminants, is generally negligible, although isolated outbreaks have been recorded. In severe cases, the mucosa of the large intestine is inflamed and haemorrhagic with ulceration and formation of diphtheritic membranes.

Diagnosis: Since the clinical signs are not pathognomonic, diagnosis may depend on finding numbers of lemon-shaped *Trichuris* eggs in the faeces. Egg output is often low in *Trichuris* infections.

Control and treatment: Prophylaxis is rarely necessary in ruminants. Benzimidazoles, the avermectins/milbemycins or levamisole by injection are very effective against adult *Trichuris*, but less so against larval stages.

Trichuris discolor

Trichuris discolor (Phylum: Nematoda; Class: Enoplea; Order: Enoplida; Family: Trichuridae), commonly known as the Whipworm, is localised in the large intestine of cattle, buffalo, occasionally sheep and goats. It is found in Europe, Asia and the USA. Details of the life cycle, epidemiology, pathogenesis, clinical signs and pathology, diagnosis, control and treatment are as for *T. globulosa*.

Homalogaster paloniae

Homalogaster paloniae (Phylum: Platyhelminthes; Class: Trematoda; Order: Plagiorchiida; Family: Gastrodiscidae) is generally a non-pathogenic parasite localised in the large intestine of buffalo and cattle and found in Asia and Australasia. This parasite has water snails as intermediate hosts.

Eimeria bovis

Eimeria bovis (Phylum: Apicomplexa; Class: Conoidasida; Order: Eucoccidiorida; Family: Eimeriidae) is distributed worldwide and is localised in the small and large intestine of cattle. There are two asexual generations. The first-generation meronts are in the endothelial cells of the lacteals of the villi in the posterior half of the small intestine, mature at 14–18 days after infection and can be seen grossly as whitish specks in the mucosa. Second-generation meronts occur in the epithelial cells of the caecum and colon, but may extend into the last metre of the small intestine in heavy infections. The sexual stages generally occur in the caecum and colon, but may extend into the ileum in heavy infections; they appear 17 days after infection. The prepatent period is 16–21 days and the patent period usually 5–15 days. The sporulation time is 2–3 days.

Epidemiology: Disease is dependent on conditions that precipitate a massive intake of oocysts, such as overcrowding in unhygienic yards or feedlots. It may also occur at pasture where livestock congregate around water troughs.

Clinical signs and pathology: This is a particularly pathogenic *Eimeria*, attacking the caecum and colon, causing mucosal sloughing and haemorrhage. Clinical signs are characterised by severe enteritis and diarrhoea, or dysentery with tenesmus in heavy infections. The animal may be pyrexic, weak and dehydrated, and if left untreated loses condition and may die. The most severe pathological changes occur in the caecum, colon and terminal 30 cm of the ileum, and are due to the gamonts. The mucosa appears congested, oedematous and thickened with petechiae or diffuse haemorrhages. The gut lumen may contain a large amount of blood. Later in the infection, the mucosa is destroyed and sloughs away. The submucosa may also be lost. If the animal survives, both the mucosa and submucosa regenerate.

Eimeria zuernii

Eimeria zuernii (Phylum: Apicomplexa; Class: Conoidasida; Order: Eucoccidiorida; Family: Eimeriidae) is a parasite distributed worldwide, localised in the small and large intestine of cattle. First-generation meronts are giant meronts and are found in the lamina propria of the lower ileum and mature at 14–16 days after infection, visible as whitish specks in the mucosa; second-generation meronts occur in the epithelial cells of the caecum and proximal colon from about 16 days after infection. The sexual stages generally occur within epithelial cells of the caecum and colon, but may extend into the ileum in heavy infections, appearing 16 days after infection. The prepatent period is 15–17 days and the patent period usually 5–17 days. The sporulation time is 2–10 days.

Pathogenesis: This is the most pathogenic species causing haemorrhagic diarrhoea through erosion and destruction of large areas of the intestinal mucosa. *Eimeria zuernii* is the most common cause of 'winter coccidiosis', which occurs primarily in calves during or following cold or stormy weather in the winter months. The exact aetiology of this syndrome is uncertain.

Clinical signs: In acute infections, *E. zuernii* causes haemorrhagic diarrhoea of calves. At first, the faeces are streaked with blood, but as the diarrhoea becomes more severe, bloody fluid, clots of blood and liquid faeces are passed. Tenesmus and coughing can result in the diarrhoea being spurted out up to 2–3 m. The animal's hindquarters are smeared with red diarrhoea. Secondary infections, especially pneumonia, are common. The acute phase may continue for 3–4 days. If the calf does not die in 7–10 days, it will probably recover. *Eimeria zuernii* may also cause a more chronic form of disease. Diarrhoea is present, but there is little or no blood in the faeces. The animals are emaciated, dehydrated, weak and listless. Their coats are rough, their eyes sunken and their ears droop.

Pathology: Generalised catarrhal enteritis involving both the large and small intestines is present. The lower small intestine, caecum and colon may be filled with semi-fluid haemorrhagic material. Large or small areas of the intestinal mucosa may be eroded and destroyed. The mucous membrane may be thickened with irregular whitish ridges in the large intestine or smooth dull-grey areas in the small intestine or caecum. Diffuse haemorrhages are present in the intestines in acute cases, and petechial haemorrhages are seen in milder cases.

Control and treatment: Prevention is based on good management; in particular, feed troughs and water containers should be moved regularly and bedding kept dry. Treatment of both *E. bovis and E. zuernii* is with a sulfonamide, such as sulfadimidine or sulfamethoxypyridazine, given orally or parenterally and repeated at half the initial dose level on each of the next two days. Alternatively, decoquinate in feed, or diclazuril and toltrazuril given orally may be used.

Flagellate protozoa

The life cycle of the following flagellate protozoa is similar for all species found in cattle. The trophozoites reproduce by longitudinal binary fission, no sexual stages are known and there are no cysts. Transmission is thought to occur by ingestion of trophozoites from faeces. All are considered to be non-pathogenic and are generally only identified from smears taken from the large intestine of fresh carcasses.

Tetratrichomonas buttreyi

Tetratrichomonas buttreyi, synonym *Trichomonas buttreyi* (Phylum: Metamonada; Class: Trichomonadea; Order: Trichomonadida; Family: Trichomonadidae), is distributed worldwide and localised in the caecum and colon of cattle and pigs.

Tritrichomonas enteris

Tritrichomonas enteris (Phylum: Metamonada; Class: Trichomonadea; Order: Trichomonadida; Family: Trichomonadidae) is distributed worldwide and localised in the colon of cattle.

Tetratrichomonas pavlovi

Tetratrichomonas pavlovi, synonyms *Trichomonas bovis*, *Trichomonas pavlovi* (Phylum: Metamonada; Class: Trichomonadea; Order: Trichomonadida; Family: Trichomonadidae), is localised in the caecum of cattle and its geographical distribution is unknown.

Retortamonas ovis

Retortamonas ovis (Phylum: Metamonada; Class: Trepomonadea; Order: Retortamonadida; Family: Retortamonadidae) is a parasite of the large intestine of cattle found worldwide.

Buxtonella sulcata

Buxtonella sulcata (Phylum: Ciliophora; Class: Litostomatea; Order: Vestibuliferida; Family: Pycnotrichidae) is a parasite of the large intestine of cattle found worldwide.

Parasites of the respiratory system

Mammomonogamus laryngeus

Mammomonogamus laryngeus, synonym *Syngamus laryngeus* (Phylum: Nematoda; Class: Chromadorea; Order: Rhabditida; Family: Syngamidae), commonly known as the Gapeworm, is localised in the larynx of cattle, buffalo, goats, sheep, deer and rarely humans and is found in Asia, Central Africa, South America and Caribbean islands. The epidemiology of this parasite is unknown.

Clinical signs and pathology: *Mammomonogamus laryngeus* is not very pathogenic for cattle. Worms attach to the mucosa of the larynx and may cause laryngitis and bronchitis. Therefore, infections are usually asymptomatic but affected animals may cough and lose condition. Calves may develop bronchitis and aspiration pneumonia has been recorded. The pathology is not described.

Diagnosis: This is based on clinical signs and the finding of eggs in the faeces. Disease is probably best confirmed by *post mortem* examination of selected cases, when reddish worms will be found attached to the tracheal mucosa. The infected trachea often contains an increased amount of mucus.

Control and treatment: No preventive or control measures have been described. Successful treatment has not been reported. Benzimidazoles and macrocyclic lactones are likely to be effective.

Notes: This genus, closely related to *Syngamus*, is parasitic in the respiratory passages of mammals. Infection has been reported in humans, causing a laryngo-pharyngeal syndrome.

Mammomonogamus nasicola

Mammomonogamus nasicola, synonyms *Syngamus nasicola*, *Syngamus kingi* (Phylum: Nematoda; Class: Chromadorea; Order: Rhabditida; Family: Syngamidae), is localised in the nasal cavities of sheep, goats, cattle and deer and found in Central and South America, Central Africa and Caribbean islands. For more details on this species see Chapter 9.

Dictyocaulus viviparus

Dictyocaulus viviparus (Phylum: Nematoda; Class: Chromadorea; Order: Rhabditida; Family: Dictyocaulidae), commonly known as the Bovine lungworm, Husk or Hoose, causes a disease known as verminous pneumonia or parasitic bronchitis, and is a parasite of the bronchi and trachea of cattle, buffalo, deer and camels, found worldwide. This parasite is mainly prevalent in temperate climates with a high rainfall.

Epidemiology: Generally, only calves in their first grazing season are clinically affected, since on farms where the disease is endemic older animals have a strong acquired immunity. In endemic areas in the northern hemisphere, infection may persist from year to year in two ways.

1   Overwintered larvae: L_3 may survive on pasture from autumn until late spring in sufficient numbers to initiate infection or occasionally to cause disease.
2   Carrier animals: small numbers of adult worms can persist in the bronchi, particularly in yearlings, until the next grazing season. Chilling of infective larvae before administration to calves will produce arrested L_5; hypobiosis at this stage has also been observed in naturally infected calves in Switzerland, Austria and Canada, although the extent to which this occurs naturally after ingestion of larvae in late autumn and its significance in the transmission of the infection have not yet been fully established.

The dispersal of larvae from the faecal pat appears to be effected by a fungus rather than by simple migration as the infective larvae are relatively inactive. This fungus, *Pilobolus*, is commonly found growing on the surface of bovine faecal pats about one week after deposition. The larvae of *D. viviparus* migrate in large numbers up the stalks of the fungi on to, and even inside, the sporangium or seed capsule (Fig. 8.8). When the sporangium is discharged, it is projected a distance of up to 3 m in still air to land on the surrounding herbage.

Parasitic bronchitis is predominantly a problem in areas such as northern Europe that have a mild climate, high rainfall and abundant permanent grass. Outbreaks of disease occur from June until November, but are most common from July until September. It is not clear why the disease is usually not apparent until calves, turned out to graze in the spring, have been at grass for 2–5 months. One explanation is that the initial infection, acquired from the ingestion of overwintered larvae in May, involves so few worms that neither clinical signs nor immunity is produced; however, sufficient

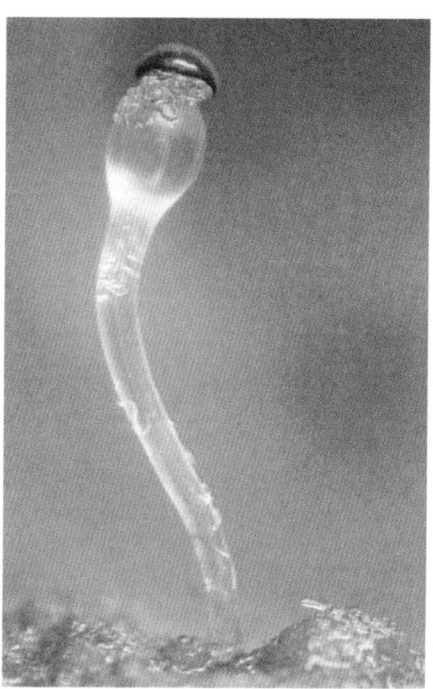

Fig. 8.8 Larvae of *Dictyocaulus viviparus* on the fungus *Pilobolus*.

numbers of larvae are seeded onto the pasture so that by July the numbers of L_3 are sufficient to produce clinical disease. Young calves, added to such a grazing herd in July, may develop clinical disease within 2–3 weeks. An alternative explanation is that L_3 overwinter in the soil and possibly only migrate on to pasture at some point between June and October.

Although dairy or dairy-cross calves are most commonly affected, autumn-born single-suckled beef calves are just as susceptible when turned out to grass in early summer. Spring-born suckled beef calves grazed with their dams until housed or sold do not usually develop clinical signs, although coughing due to a mild infection is common. However, the typical disease may occur in weaned calves grazed until late autumn. Adult cattle can be affected with parasitic bronchitis if they have not had sufficient exposure to lungworm larvae in previous years to develop adequate immunity and are subsequently grazed on heavily contaminated pastures. This is sometimes first seen as a reduction in milk yield with subsequent coughing. In tropical countries, where disease due to *D. viviparus* may occur intermittently, the epidemiology is presumably quite different and probably depends more on pasture contamination by carrier animals, such as may occur during flooding when cattle congregate on damp high areas, rather than on the prolonged survival of infective larvae.

Pathogenesis: Dictyocaulosis is characterised by bronchitis and pneumonia and typically affects young cattle during their first grazing season on permanent or semi-permanent pastures. Pathogenesis may be divided into three phases.

1   Prepatent phase: around days 8–25. This phase starts with the appearance of larvae within the alveoli where they cause alveolitis. This is followed by bronchiolitis and finally bronchitis as the larvae become immature adults and move up the bronchi. Towards the end of this phase, bronchitis develops, characterised by immature lungworms in the airways and by cellular infiltration of the epithelium. Heavily infected animals, whose

lungs contain several thousand developing worms, may die from day 15 onwards due to respiratory failure following the development of severe interstitial emphysema and pulmonary oedema.

2 Patent phase: around days 26–60. This is associated with two main lesions: first, a parasitic bronchitis characterised by the presence of hundreds or even thousands of adult worms in the frothy white mucus in the lumina of the bronchi (Fig. 8.9); and second, the presence of dark-red collapsed areas around infected bronchi (Fig. 8.10). This is a parasitic pneumonia caused by the aspiration of eggs and L₁ into the alveoli.

3 Postpatent phase: around days 61–90. In untreated calves, this is normally the recovery phase after the adult lungworms have been expelled. Although the clinical signs are abating, the bronchi are still inflamed and residual lesions such as bronchial and peribronchial fibrosis may persist for several weeks or months. Eventually the bronchopulmonary system becomes completely normal and coughing ceases. However, in about 25% of animals, which have been heavily infected, there can be a flare-up of clinical signs during this phase that is frequently fatal. This is caused by one of two entities. Most commonly, there is a proliferative lesion so that much of the lung is pink and rubbery and does not collapse when the chest is opened. This, often described as 'epithelialisation', is due to the proliferation of type 2 pneumocytes on the alveoli giving the appearance of a gland-like organ. Gaseous exchange at the alveolar surface is markedly impaired and the lesion is often accompanied by interstitial emphysema and pulmonary oedema. The aetiology is unknown but is thought to be due to the dissolution and aspiration of dead or dying worm material into the alveoli. The clinical syndrome is often termed 'postpatent parasitic bronchitis'. The other cause, usually in animals convalescing indoors, is a superimposed bacterial infection of the imperfectly healed lungs leading to acute interstitial pneumonia.

Clinical signs: Within any affected group, differing degrees of clinical severity are usually apparent. Mildly affected animals cough intermittently, particularly when exercised. Moderately affected animals have frequent bouts of coughing at rest, tachypnoea (60 respirations per minute) and hyperpnoea. Frequently, squeaks and crackles over the posterior lung lobes are heard on auscultation. Severely affected animals show severe tachypnoea (80 respirations per minute) and dyspnoea and frequently adopt the classic 'air hunger' position of mouth breathing with the head and neck outstretched. There is usually a deep harsh cough, squeaks and crackles over the posterior lung lobes, salivation, anorexia and sometimes mild pyrexia. Often the smallest calves are most severely affected. Calves may show clinical signs during the prepatent period and occasionally a massive infection can cause severe dyspnoea of sudden onset often followed by death in 24–48 hours. Most animals gradually recover, although complete return to normality may take weeks or months. However, a proportion of convalescing calves suddenly develop severe respiratory signs, unassociated with pyrexia, which usually terminate fatally 1–4 days later (postpatent parasitic bronchitis).

Pathology: Two phases are recognised.

1 Prepatent phase. Cellular infiltrates of inflammatory cells temporarily plug the lumina of the bronchioles and cause collapse of other groups of alveoli. This lesion is largely responsible for the first clinical signs of tachypnoea and coughing.

2 Patent phase. The bronchial epithelium is hyperplastic and heavily infiltrated by inflammatory cells, particularly eosinophils. Aspirated eggs and larvae quickly provoke dense infiltrates of polymorphs, macrophages and multinucleated giant cells around them (Fig. 8.11). There may be varying degrees of interstitial emphysema and edema.

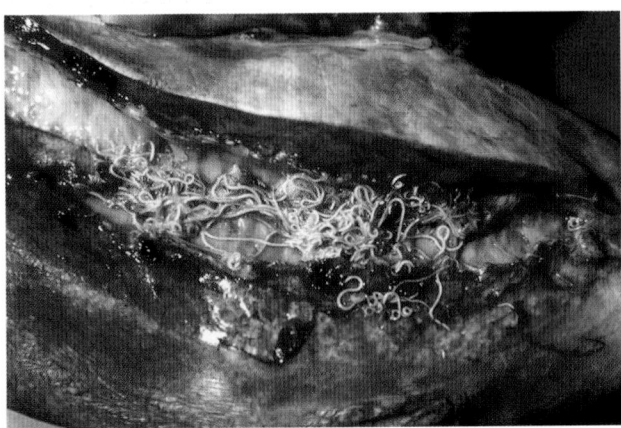

Fig. 8.9 *Dictyocaulus viviparus* worms in the opened bronchi of an infected calf.

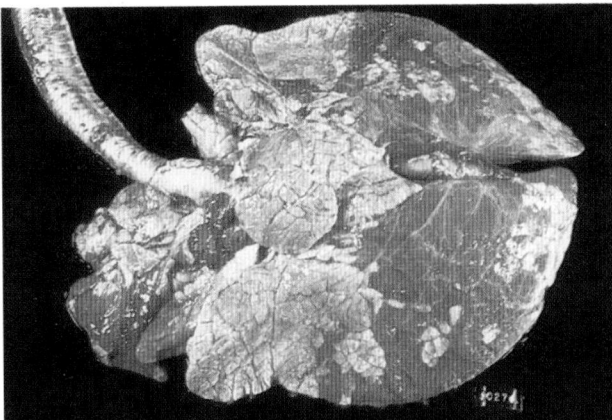

Fig. 8.10 Typical distribution of pneumonic lesions of parasitic bronchitis.

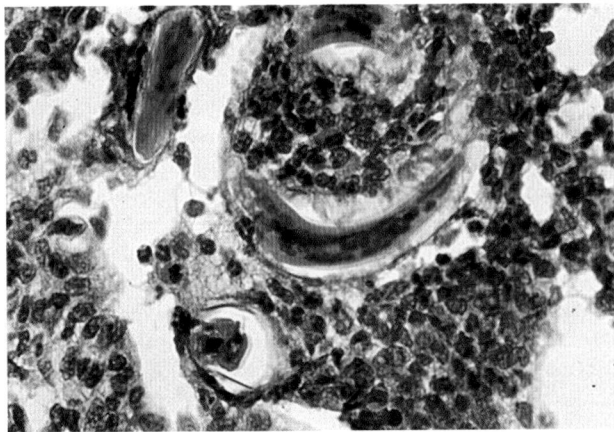

Fig. 8.11 Inflammatory response due to the presence of aspirated eggs and larvae in the bronchioles and alveoli.

Diagnosis: Usually the clinical signs, the time of year and a history of grazing on permanent or semi-permanent pastures are sufficient to enable a diagnosis to be made. Larvae are found (50–1000/g) only in the faeces of patent cases so that faecal samples should be obtained from the rectum of a number of affected individuals. At necropsy, worms will often be apparent in the opened bronchi and their size is diagnostic. A lungworm ELISA can be used to detect antibodies to *D. viviparus*. Seroconversion takes 4–6 weeks and titres persist for 4–7 months. Serology can be helpful in cases of reinfection husk, as it will often detect larval stages. Cross-reactivity can occur with intestinal nematode species so test sensitivity and specificity require validation and setting of appropriate optical density (OD) cut-off values when interpreting results.

Control: The best method of preventing parasitic bronchitis is to immunise all young calves with lungworm vaccine. This live attenuated vaccine is currently only available in parts of Europe and is given orally to calves aged eight weeks or more. Two doses of vaccine are given at an interval of four weeks and, in order to allow a high level of immunity to develop, vaccinated calves should be protected from challenge until two weeks after their second dose. Dairy calves or suckled calves can be vaccinated successfully at grass provided the vaccine is given prior to encountering a significant larval challenge. Although vaccination is effective in preventing clinical disease, it does not completely prevent the establishment of small numbers of lungworms. Consequently, pastures may remain contaminated, albeit at a very low level. For this reason, it is important that all the calves on any farm should be vaccinated whether they go to pasture in the spring or later in the year, and a vaccination programme must be continued annually for each calf crop. Control of parasitic bronchitis in first-year grazing calves has been achieved by the use of prophylactic anthelmintic regimens either by strategic early-season treatments or by the administration of rumen boluses, as recommended in the control of bovine ostertagiosis. The danger of these measures, however, is that through rigorous control in the first grazing season, exposure to lungworm larvae is so curtailed that cattle may remain susceptible to husk during their second season; in such situations it may be advisable to consider vaccination prior to their second year at grass. Because of the unpredictable epidemiology, the technique commonly used in ostertagiosis of 'dose and move' in midsummer does not prevent parasitic bronchitis.

Treatment: The modern benzimidazoles, levamisole or the avermectin/milbemycins have been shown to be highly effective against all stages of lungworms with consequent amelioration of clinical signs. For maximum efficiency, all these drugs should be used as early as possible in the treatment of the disease. Where the disease is severe and well established in a number of calves, one should be aware that anthelmintic treatment, while being the only course available, may exacerbate the clinical signs in one or more animals with a possible fatal termination. Whatever treatment is selected, it is advisable to divide affected calves into two groups, as the prognosis will vary according to the severity of the disease. Those calves which are only coughing and/or tachypnoeic are usually in the prepatent stage of the disease or have a small adult worm burden and treatment of these animals should result in rapid recovery. Calves in this category may not have developed a strong immunity and after treatment should not be returned to grazing which was the source of infection; if this is not possible, parenteral ivermectin, doramectin or moxidectin may be used since their residual effect prevents reinfection for an extended period. Any calves which are dyspnoeic, anorexic and possibly pyrexic should be kept indoors for treatment and further observation. The prognosis must be guarded as a proportion of these animals may not recover while others may remain permanently stunted. In addition to anthelmintics, severely affected animals may require antibiotics if pyrexic and may be in need of hydration if they are not drinking.

Parasitic bronchitis in adult cattle: Parasitic bronchitis is only seen in adult cattle under two circumstances.

1 As a herd phenomenon, or in a particular age group within a herd, if they have failed to acquire immunity through natural challenge in earlier years. Such animals may develop the disease if exposed to heavy larval challenge, as might occur on pasture recently vacated by calves suffering from clinical husk.
2 Disease is occasionally seen where an individual adult is penned in a heavily contaminated calf paddock.

The disease is most commonly encountered in the patent phase, although the other forms have been recognized. In addition to coughing and tachypnoea, a reduction in milk yield in cows is a common presenting sign. In selecting an anthelmintic for treatment, one should consider the withdrawal period of milk for human consumption. Eprinomectin has no withdrawal period for milk.

Reinfection syndrome in parasitic bronchitis: Normally, the natural challenge of adult cattle, yearlings or calves that have acquired immunity to *D. viviparus*, whether by natural exposure or by vaccination, is not associated with clinical signs. Occasionally, however, clinical signs do occur to produce the 'reinfection syndrome', which is usually mild but sometimes severe. It arises when an immune animal is suddenly exposed to a massive larval challenge that reaches the lungs and migrates to the bronchioles, where the larvae are killed by the immune response. The proliferation of lymphoreticular cells around dead larvae causes bronchiolar obstruction and ultimately the formation of a macroscopically visible, greyish-green, lymphoid nodule about 5.0 mm in diameter. Usually, the syndrome is associated with frequent coughing and slight tachypnoea over a period of a few days; less frequently there is marked tachypnoea, hyperpnoea and, in dairy cows, a reduction in milk yield. Deaths rarely occur. It can be difficult to differentiate this syndrome from the early stages of a severe primary infection. The only course of action is treatment with anthelmintics and a change of pasture.

Echinococcus granulosus

For more details see Parasites of the liver.

Pneumocystis carinii

Pneumocystis carinii, synonym *Pneumocystis jiroveci* (Phylum: Ascomycota; Class: Pneumocystidomycetes; Order: Pneumocystidales; Family: Pneumocystidaceae), causes a disease commonly known as Pneumocystosis, and is a fungus of humans, cattle, rats, ferrets, mice, dogs, horses, pigs and rabbits and found worldwide.

Epidemiology: The organism is apparently quite widely distributed in latent form in healthy human individuals, as well as a wide variety of domestic and wild animals. The organism is thought to be transmitted by aerosol, although the natural habitats and modes of transmission of infections in humans are current areas of research.

Pneumocystis DNA has been detected in air and water, suggesting that the free forms of the organism may survive in the environment long enough to infect a susceptible host. However, little information on the means of transmission exists currently. In humans, infections appear to spread between immunosuppressed patients colonised with *Pneumocystis* and immunocompetent individuals transiently parasitised with the organism. Human and non-human *Pneumocystis* species have been shown to be different and host specific, suggesting that zoonotic transmission does not occur. The organism has been reported from a range of animals. In Denmark, examination of lungs from carcasses selected randomly in an abattoir detected *P. carinii* pneumocysts in 3.8% of calves, 3.6% of sheep and 6.7% of pigs. Studies in Japan detected *P. carinii* in cattle and a wide range of other animals. The organism has also been reported to have caused pneumonia in weaning pigs.

Pathogenesis: *Pneumocystis* is one of the major causes of opportunistic mycoses in the immunocompromised, including those with congenital immunodeficiencies, retrovirus infections such as AIDS, and cases receiving immunosuppressive therapy.

Clinical signs and pathology: Infections in animals are generally asymptomatic. In humans, pneumocystosis is observed in four clinical forms: asymptomatic infections, infantile (interstitial plasma cell) pneumonia, pneumonia in immunocompromised host and extrapulmonary infections. Lesions are characterised by a massive plasma cell or histiocyte infiltration of the alveoli in which the organisms may be detected by a silver staining procedure. A foamy eosinophilic material is observed in the lungs during infection. This material is composed of masses of the organism, alveolar macrophages, desquamated epithelial alveolar cells, polymorphonuclear leucocytes and other host cells.

Diagnosis: Gomori's methenamine silver (GMS) and Giemsa stain may be used for microscopic visualisation of *Pneumocystis*. Toluidine blue (TBO) is the most effective for cyst stages while Giemsa stains are used to show trophozoites. Axenic culture methods have been described; however, *in vitro* cultivation, especially from clinical samples, is not always successful. Fluorescence antibody staining techniques can be used to detect both cyst and trophozoite stages of *P. carinii*. A number of polymerase chain reaction (PCR) tests have been reported which amplify specific regions of DNA from *P. carinii* and are approximately 100 times more sensitive than conventional staining techniques.

Control and treatment: Control is difficult given that details of the routes of transmission are unknown. Infection is generally asymptomatic in animals and is only likely to be detected in immunocompromised individuals. Trimethroprim–sulfamethoxazole is the drug of choice for treatment and prophylaxis of *Pneumocystis* infections. Pentamidine and atovaquone are the alternative therapeutic agents in humans.

Notes: Initially reported as a morphological form of *Trypanosoma cruzi*, this microorganism later proved to be a separate genus and was named *Pneumocystis carinii* and classified as a protozoan until the late 1980s. Following further taxonomic revision, *Pneumocystis* is now classified as a fungus, not a protozoan. The taxonomy is still complicated in that *Pneumocystis* from humans and other animals are quite different and there appear to be multiple species in this genus. Genetic variations and DNA sequence polymorphisms are often observed, suggesting the existence of numerous strains even within a single species of *Pneumocystis*.

Parasites of the liver

Fasciola hepatica

Fasciola hepatica (Phylum: Platyhelminthes; Class: Trematoda; Order: Plagiorchiida; Family: Fasciolidae), commonly known as the Liver fluke, is a parasite distributed worldwide and localised in the liver of sheep, cattle, goats, horses, deer, humans and other mammals. This parasite has snails of the genus *Galba* (syn. *Lymnaea*) as intermediate hosts. The most common, *Lymnaea truncatula*, is an amphibious snail with a wide distribution throughout the world. Other important vectors of *F. hepatica* outside Europe are:

L. tomentosa	Australia, New Zealand
L. columella	Central and North America, Australia, New Zealand
L. bulimoides	northern and southern USA and the Caribbean
L. humilis	North America
L. viator	South America
L. diaphena	South America
L. cubensis	South America
L. viridis	China, Papua New Guinea.

For a more detailed description, see entry in Chapter 9.

Pathogenesis: This varies according to the number of metacercariae ingested, the phase of parasitic development in the liver and the species of host involved. Essentially, the pathogenesis is twofold. The first phase occurs during migration in the liver parenchyma and is associated with liver damage and haemorrhage. The second occurs when the parasite is in the bile ducts, and results from the haematophagic activity of the adult flukes and from damage to the biliary mucosa by their cuticular spines. Most studies have been in sheep and the disease in this host is discussed in more detail in Chapter 9. The seasonality of outbreaks described is that which occurs in western Europe. Although acute and subacute disease may occasionally occur under conditions of heavy challenge, especially in young calves, the chronic form of the disease is by far the most important and, as in sheep, is seen in the late winter/early spring. The pathogenesis is similar to that in sheep but has the added features of calcification of the bile ducts and enlargement of the gallbladder. The calcified bile ducts often protrude from the liver surface, giving rise to the term 'pipe-stem liver'. Aberrant migration of the flukes is more common in cattle and encapsulated parasites are often seen in the lungs. On reinfection of adult cows, migration to the fetus has been recorded, resulting in prenatal infection. There is some experimental evidence that fasciolosis increases the susceptibility of cattle to infection with *Salmonella dublin*. *Fasciola* infections may cause a loss of production in milking cows during winter. Clinically, these are difficult to detect since the fluke burdens are usually low and anaemia is not apparent. The main effects are a reduction in milk yield and quality, particularly of the solids-non-fat component.

Clinical signs: In heavy infections in cattle, where anaemia and hypoalbuminaemia are severe, submandibular oedema frequently occurs (Fig. 8.12). With smaller fluke burdens, the clinical effect is minimal and the loss of productivity is difficult to differentiate from inadequate nutrition. It must be emphasised that diarrhoea is not a feature of bovine fasciolosis unless it is complicated by the presence of *Ostertagia* spp. Combined infection with these two parasites has been referred to as the fasciolosis/ostertagiosis complex.

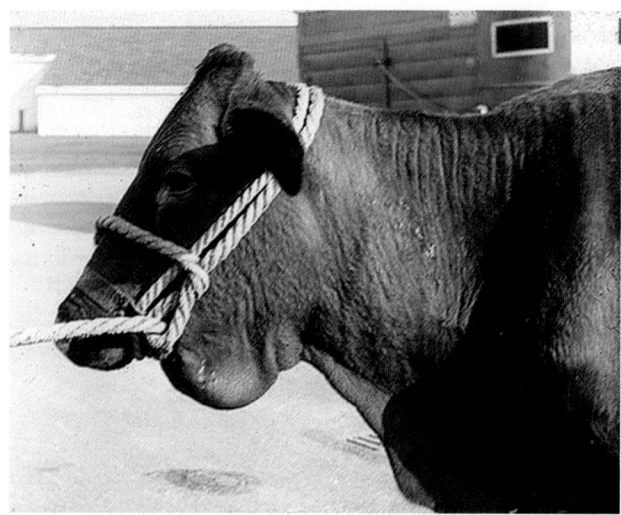

Fig. 8.12 Submandibular oedema in a cow infected with *Fasciola hepatica*.

Pathology: In cattle, the pathogenesis is similar to that seen in sheep with the added features of calcification of the bile ducts and enlargement of the gallbladder. The calcified bile ducts often protrude from the liver surface, giving rise to the term 'pipe-stem liver' (Fig. 8.13). Aberrant migration of flukes is more common in cattle and encapsulated parasites are often seen in the lungs.

Diagnosis: This is based primarily on clinical signs, seasonal occurrence, prevailing weather patterns and a previous history of fasciolosis on the farm or the identification of snail habitats. While diagnosis of ovine fasciolosis should present few problems, especially when a *post mortem* examination is possible, diagnosis of bovine fasciolosis can sometimes prove difficult. In this context, routine haematological tests and examination of faeces for fluke eggs (note that eggs of *Fasciola* are browny-yellow and eggs of Paramphistomidae are colourless) are useful and may be supplemented by other laboratory tests.

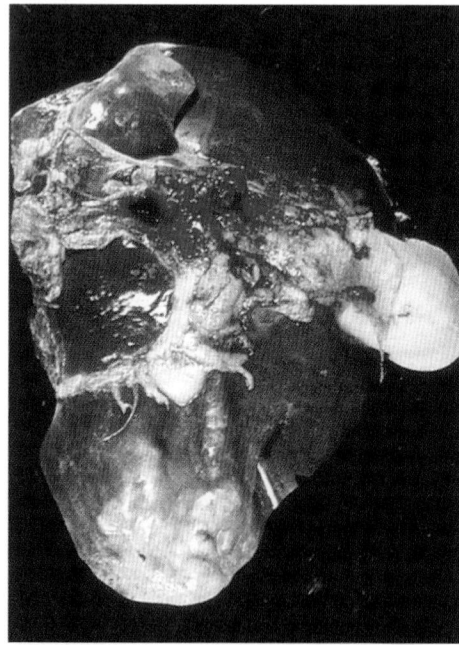

Fig. 8.13 Gross appearance of the liver in bovine fasciolosis.

Table 8.4 Haematological/biochemical parameters in normal and fluke-infected cattle.

Parameter	Normal	Fluke infected
PCV (%)	32 (24–40)	≥20
Eosinophils (%) (× 10³/µl)	2–20 0–2.4	>20%
Glutamate dehydrogenase (GLDH) (iu/l)	2–23	5× normal (50–120) Elevated ≥6 weeks post infection
γ-Glutamyltranspeptidase (GGT) (iu/l)	20–46	Up to 10× normal levels in chronic fluke

Routine haematology will often show the presence of anaemia (normochromic and normocytic) as a result of haemorrhage arising from the direct feeding of the flukes. The packed cell volume (PCV) is also reduced. Fluke infection also leads to an eosinophilia (Table 8.4). Fluke infections lead to a decrease in the albumin/globulin ratio. Hypoalbuminaemia due to protein loss occurs during the parenchymal stage of infection by immature flukes, and also due to the presence of adult fluke in the bile ducts. Globulin levels increase as a result of increased immunoglobulin synthesis.

Serum concentrations of liver-specific enzymes are generally higher in acute liver disease than in chronic liver disease and may be within normal limits in the later stages of subacute or chronic hepatic disease. Glutamate dehydrogenase (GLDH) is released when parenchymal cells are damaged and levels become elevated within the first few weeks of infection. Another enzyme, γ-glutamyltranspeptidase (GGT), indicates damage to the epithelial cells lining the bile ducts; elevation of this enzyme takes place mainly after the flukes reach the bile ducts and raised levels are maintained for a longer period. Interpretation of raised liver enzyme activity can be difficult and careful analysis of laboratory values in conjunction with clinical findings is essential. Detection of antibodies against components of flukes in serum or milk samples can also be undertaken, the ELISA and the passive haemagglutination test being the most reliable.

Antibodies to liver fluke can be detected in serum 2–4 weeks post infection but levels may rise or fall over time. A positive result does not necessarily indicate a current infection but a history of exposure. Serological testing is not widely available and may vary from country to country as to availability for either cattle or sheep. A bulk-tank milk ELISA for cattle gives a positive result when the prevalence in a herd is more than 25%. Interpretation can be difficult as false positives can occur. A coproantigen test is also available which detects fluke proteins in faeces.

Control: Control of fasciolosis may be approached in two ways: by reducing populations of the intermediate snail host or by using anthelmintics (for a more detailed description see entry in Chapter 9). The timing of treatments will depend on the spectrum of activity of the flukicide and it is also important to monitor the need for treatment. The use of meteorological forecasting for fasciolosis is described in detail in Chapter 9. A typical treatment schedule for non-lactating cattle in the northern hemisphere in an average rainfall season would be as follows.

- Dose cattle in autumn with a flukicide that is effective against young immature flukes to reduce liver damage from fluke migration. This is irrespective of whether cattle will be housed or outwintered.
- Dose grazing cattle in winter with a flukicide that is effective against adult flukes and immature stages. Cattle wintered inside

need to be treated after housing (timing of the dose varies with the flukicide used).

- Dose outwintered cattle in spring with a flukicide that is effective against adult stages. This will remove fluke burdens and reduce contamination of pastures with fluke eggs and thus reduce the summer infection of snails.

Dairy cows can be treated at drying-off but particular attention needs to be paid to contraindications relating to both stage of pregnancy and lactation.

Treatment: The older drugs such as carbon tetrachloride, hexachloroethane and hexachlorophene may still be used in some countries, but these have been largely replaced by more efficient and less toxic compounds and only the latter are discussed. At present, there is only one drug, triclabendazole, which will remove the early immature (around two weeks of age in cattle) parenchymal stages. Apart from triclabendazole, the other drugs most commonly used for subacute or chronic fasciolosis are closantel, nitroxynil and oxyclozanide, and several others, such as clorsulon, rafoxanide and niclofolan, are also marketed in some countries. Albendazole, ricobendazole and netobimin are also effective against adult fluke at an increased dosage rate. In lactating cows, where the milk is used for human consumption, the above drugs are either banned or have extended withdrawal periods, and are more usually given during the dry period. An exception is oxyclozanide, which is licensed for use in lactating animals in many countries and has a nil or very short milk-withholding time. At times of the season when the fluke burden predominantly comprises adults, the use of narrow-spectrum flukicides with activity against adult stages only will help to reduce the selection pressure on drugs such as triclabendazole. Combination products with activity against fluke and gastrointestinal nematodes should only be used where both helminths are present. Resistance to flukicides has been reported with triclabendazole use in sheep but is not currently considered to be as significant a problem with fluke in cattle.

Fasciola gigantica

Fasciola gigantica (Phylum: Platyhelminthes; Class: Trematoda; Order: Plagiorchiida; Family: Fasciolidae), commonly known as the Tropical large liver fluke, is localised in the liver of cattle, buffalo, sheep, goats, pigs, camels, deer and humans and found in Africa, Asia, Europe and the USA. This parasite has snails of the genus *Galba* (syn. *Lymnaea*) as intermediate hosts; in southern Europe it is *L. auricularia*, which is also the important species in the southern USA, Middle East and Pacific Islands. Other important vectors of *F. gigantica* are *L. natalensis* in Africa, *L. rufescens*in and *L. acuminata* in the Indian subcontinent, *L. rubiginosa* in Southeast Asia and *L. viridis* in China and Japan. All these snails are primarily aquatic and are found in streams, irrigation channels and marshy swamps. Acute and chronic infection occurs in sheep but only the chronic form predominates in cattle. Like *F. hepatica*, *F. gigantica* is capable of infecting humans.

Epidemiology: The snails that carry the larval stages of *F. gigantica* are primarily aquatic and as a result, the disease is associated with animals grazing on naturally or artificially flooded areas or around permanent water channels or dams. In subtropical or tropical countries with distinct wet and dry seasons, it appears that optimal development of eggs to miracidia occurs at the start of the wet season and development within the snail is complete by the end of the rains. Shedding of cercariae then commences at the start of the dry season when the water level is still high and continues as the water level drops. Under laboratory conditions, a large number of metacercariae simply encyst on the surface of the water rather than on herbage, and under natural conditions this could have a very significant effect on the dissemination of infection. Metacercariae are acquired by animals utilising such areas during the dry season and clinical problems, depending on the rate of infection, occur at the end of that season or at the beginning of the next wet season. Metacercariae encyst on plants under water, such as rice plants, and can survive for up to four months on stored plants, such as rice straw.

Clinical signs and pathology: Clinical signs and pathology are similar to those of *F. hepatica*. In cattle, the pathology is similar to that seen in sheep with the added features of calcification of the bile ducts and enlargement of the gallbladder. The calcified bile ducts often protrude from the liver surface, giving rise to the term 'pipe-stem liver'.

Diagnosis: This is based primarily on clinical signs, seasonal occurrence, prevailing weather patterns and a previous history of fasciolosis on the farm or the identification of snail habitats. Diagnosis can be confirmed by the identification of the typical operculate eggs in faeces samples.

Control: The principles are the same as for the control of *F. hepatica* and are based on the routine use of anthelmintics together with measures to reduce populations of the snail intermediate host. However, there is the important difference that the latter are water snails whose control depends on a different approach from that for the mud snail *G.* (*Lymnaea*) *truncatula*. Routine anthelmintic treatment of animals at seasons when heavy infections of adult flukes accumulate in the host is recommended using a drug effective against adult and immature flukes. This should prevent serious losses in production, but for optimal benefit should be accompanied by snail control. When watering of stock is from a reservoir or stream, complete control can be achieved by fencing the water source and leading a pipe to troughs. To do this effectively from streams, the water may need to be pumped and in remote areas simple water-driven pumps whose power source depends on the water flow have been found useful. It is important that the water troughs be cleaned out regularly since they can become colonised by snails.

Where grazing depends on the dry-season use of marshy areas around receding lakebeds, snail control is difficult. Molluscicides are usually impractical because of the large body of water involved and their possible effect on fish, which may form an important part of the local food supply. Apart from repeated anthelmintic treatment to prevent patency of acquired infections of *F. gigantica*, there is often little one can do. Ideally, such areas are often best suited to irrigation and the growing of cash crops, the profit from which can be used to improve the dry-season food and water supply to cattle.

Treatment: The drugs and dose rates given for the treatment of *F. hepatica* are also generally applicable for the treatment of *F. gigantica*. Triclabendazole is effective against both mature and immature stages of *F. gigantica* in cattle.

Fascioloides magna

Fascioloides magna (Phylum: Platyhelminthes; Class: Trematoda; Order: Plagiorchiida; Family: Fasciolidae), commonly known as the large American liver fluke, is localised in the liver and bile ducts of deer, cattle, sheep, goats, pigs, horses and llamas. It occurs in North

America, central, eastern and southwestern Europe, South Africa and Mexico. This parasite has a variety of freshwater snails, *Fossaria* spp., *Lymnaea* spp. and *Stagnicola* spp., as intermediate hosts.

Epidemiology: The various snail intermediate hosts tend to occur in stagnant semi-permanent water that contains large amounts of dead or dying vegetation, swamp areas, or pools and streams. *Fascioloides magna* is indigenous to North America and is common in Canada and the Great Lakes area where the white-tailed deer and elk are commonly infected. Domestic cattle and sheep become infected when they graze pasture where parasitised deer occur.

Pathogenesis: In deer and cattle, the flukes are frequently encapsulated in thin-walled fibrous cysts in the liver parenchyma and this restricted migration results in low pathogenicity. In cattle and pigs, the flukes may become entrapped in a thick-walled fibrous capsule and there is no connection to the bile ducts and consequently it is rare to find fluke eggs in faeces in these livestock. Sometimes flukes can also be found in calcified cysts. Although haemorrhage and fibrosis may be present in the liver, there is often no obvious clinical sign of infection.

Clinical signs and pathology: In deer and cattle, the parasites can cause hepatic damage on reaching the liver but the flukes rapidly become encapsulated by the host reaction and clinical signs are minimal. In cattle and pigs, thick-walled cysts with fibrous capsules or calcified cysts may be present in the liver.

Diagnosis: This is based primarily on clinical signs and history of contact with grazing deer in known endemic areas. Cysts and the large flukes are usually seen on *post mortem* examination. Faecal examination for the presence of fluke eggs is a useful aid to diagnosis.

Control: Avoid grazing sheep or cattle on areas which are frequented by deer. Elimination of the snail intermediate hosts is difficult due to their varied habitats. Similarly, removal of Cervidae may not be practical. Because of these factors, sheep rearing, particularly, is difficult in areas where the parasite is prevalent.

Treatment: For cattle and sheep, the commonly used flukicides, such as triclabendazole, closantel, clorsulon and albendazole, are effective. Mature *F. magna* are susceptible to oxyclosanide.

Notes: *Fascioloides magna* is primarily a parasite of deer (Cervidae) and is commonly found in white-tailed deer, elk and moose. For more details see Chapter 14.

Dicrocoelium dendriticum

Dicrocoelium dendriticum, synonym *Dicrocoelium lanceolatum* (Phylum: Platyhelminthes; Class: Trematoda; Order: Plagiorchiida; Family: Dicrocoeliidae), is commonly known as the Small lanceolate fluke. It is distributed worldwide (except for South Africa and Australia), localised in the liver of sheep, goats, cattle, deer, rabbits and occasionally horses, dogs and pigs. This parasite requires two intermediate hosts.
  1 Land snails of many genera, principally *Cionella lubrica* in North America and *Zebrina detrita* in Europe. Some 29 other species have been reported to serve as first intermediate hosts, including the genera *Abida*, *Theba*, *Helicella* and *Xerophila*.
  2 Brown ants of the genus *Formica*, frequently *F. fusca*.
For more information on epidemiology, pathogenesis, control and treatment see Chapter 9.

Dicrocoelium hospes

Dicrocoelium hospes (Phylum: Platyhelminthes; Class: Trematoda; Order: Plagiorchiida; Family: Dicrocoeliidae) is a parasite localised in the liver of cattle, oxen and goats (occasionally sheep) and found in parts of Africa.

Gigantocotyle explanatum

Gigantocotyle explanatum, synonyms *Explanatum explanatum*, *Paramphistomum explanatum* (Phylum: Platyhelminthes; Class: Trematoda; Order: Plagiorchiida; Family: Paramphistomatidae), is localised in the liver, intrahepatic ductules, bile ducts, gallbladder and duodenum of cattle, buffalo and other ruminants and occurs in the Indian subcontinent, Southeast Asia, tropical and subtropical regions of the Middle East and Africa. This parasite has snails as intermediate hosts.

Clinical signs and pathology: Large numbers of immature flukes can cause amphistomosis with enteritis that in some cases, particularly young buffalo, can be fatal to the host. The flukes can cause connective tissue proliferation and haemorrhage at the site of attachment, with general wasting of body condition, diarrhoea and loss of weight. There is extensive fibrosis and hyperplasia of the bile ducts and multifocal granulomatous nodules occur over their luminal surface.

Echinococcus granulosus, Echinococcus orteleppi (G5)

Echinococcus granulosus (Phylum: Platyhelminthes; Class: Cestoda; Order: Cyclophyllidea; Family: Taeniidae), commonly known as the Dwarf dog tapeworm, is distributed worldwide and is usually localised in the small intestine of dogs and many wild canids. This parasite has cattle (G5), sheep, camels, pigs, buffalo, deer and humans as intermediate hosts.

Notes: *Echinococcus granulosus* possesses a high degree of genetic divergence and various strains (G1–G10) have been described that show differences in morphology, host range, pathogenicity and geographical distribution. *Echinococcus orteleppi* (the former cattle strain G5) is now recognised as an individual species. For more details on pathology, control and treatment see Chapter 9.

Stilesia hepatica

Stilesia hepatica (Phylum: Platyhelminthes; Class: Cestoda; Order: Cyclophyllidea; Family: Anoplocephalidae) is localised in the bile ducts of sheep, cattle and other ruminants and found in Africa and Asia. This parasite probably has an oribatid mite as intermediate host. For more details see Chapter 9.

Taenia hydatigena

Taenia hydatigena, synonym *Taenia marginata* (Phylum: Platyhelminthes; Class: Cestoda; Order: Cyclophyllidea; Family: Taeniidae), is a parasite distributed worldwide, localised in the small intestine of dogs, foxes, weasels, stoats, polecats, wolves and hyenas. This parasite has sheep, cattle, deer, pigs and horses as intermediate hosts.

Notes: The correct nomenclature for the intermediate host stage is the 'metacestode stage of *Taenia hydatigena*' rather than '*Cysticercus tenuicollis*'. For more details see Chapter 9.

Thysanosoma actinioides

For more details see Parasites of the small intestine.

Parasites of the pancreas

Eurytrema pancreaticum

Eurytrema pancreaticum, synonyms *Distoma pancreaticum*, *Eurytrema ovis* (Phylum: Platyhelminthes; Class: Trematoda; Order: Plagiorchiida; Family: Dicrocoeliidae), commonly known as the Pancreatic fluke, is localised in the pancreatic ducts, rarely bile ducts, of cattle, buffalo, sheep, goats, pigs, camels and humans and occurs in South America, Asia and Europe. This parasite requires two intermediate hosts: (1) land snails, particularly of the genus *Bradybaena*, and (2) grasshoppers of the genus *Conocephalus* or tree crickets (*Oecanthus*).

Clinical signs and pathology: Low to moderate infections produce little effect on the host. Heavy infections may cause a sporadic wasting syndrome and emaciation with no specific signs. Large numbers of flukes can cause dilation and thickening of the pancreatic ducts and extensive fibrosis. Flukes may also be embedded in the pancreatic parenchyma, causing chronic interstitial pancreatitis and there is sometimes a granulomatous reaction around fluke eggs that have penetrated the walls of the ducts.

Diagnosis: Usually reported as an incidental finding at necropsy.

Control and treatment: This is not feasible where the intermediate hosts are endemic. There is no specific treatment for eurytrematosis, although praziquantel 20 mg/kg for two days or albendazole 7–10 mg/kg have been reported to be effective.

Eurytrema coelomaticum

Eurytrema coelomaticum, synonym *Distoma coelomaticum* (Phylum: Platyhelminthes; Class: Trematoda; Order: Plagiorchiida; Family: Dicrocoeliidae), commonly known as the Pancreatic fluke, is localised in the pancreatic ducts and occasionally bile ducts and duodenum of cattle. This parasite is found in eastern Asia and South America. Details of the life cycle, host range, epidemiology, pathogenesis, clinical signs and pathology, diagnosis, control and treatment are as for *E. pancreaticum*.

Thysanosoma actinioides

For more details see Parasites of the small intestine.

Parasites of the circulatory system

Elaeophora poeli

Elaeophora poeli (Phylum: Nematoda; Class: Chromadorea; Order: Spirurida; Family: Onchocercidae) causes a disease commonly known as Large aortic filariosis, and is localised in the blood vessels of cattle, buffalo and zebu. This parasite is found in parts of Africa, Asia and the Far East and it is likely that tabanid flies act as intermediate hosts. Because of the innocuous nature of the infection in cattle, the distribution of the species in these hosts is not completely known.

Pathogenesis: In cattle, nodules, from which the female worms protrude, form on the intima of the vessels but in other animals the adults appear to provoke little reaction.

Clinical signs and pathology: Infection is usually asymptomatic. The main affected area is the thoracic region of the aorta. In light infections, the lesions are found chiefly on the dorsal wall of the aorta, near the openings of the intercostal arteries. In heavy infections, the artery becomes swollen, the wall is thickened and the intima contains fibrous tracts. The raised nodules can measure up to 1 cm in diameter.

Diagnosis: This is not normally required. Infection is usually diagnosed as an incidental finding on *post mortem* examination of thickened blood vessels, or those containing nodules.

Control and treatment: Any reduction in vector numbers will reduce transmission. Treatment is not indicated.

Onchocerca armillata

Onchocerca armillata (Phylum: Nematoda; Class: Chromadorea; Order: Spirurida; Family: Onchocercidae) causes a disease commonly known as Aortic filariosis, and is localised in the aorta of cattle, buffalo, sheep, goats, rarely camels; it is found in parts of Africa, the Middle East and India. This parasite has midges (*Culicoides*) and blackflies (*Simulium*) as intermediate hosts.

Epidemiology: Prevalence is very high; in some regions 80–90% of animals are infected.

Pathogenesis: It is interesting that *O. armillata*, though occurring in a strategically important site in the bovine aorta, is not usually associated with clinical signs. It is usually only discovered at the abattoir, surveys in the Middle East having shown a prevalence as high as 90%.

Clinical signs and pathology: Infection is usually inapparent. *Onchocerca armillata* is found in grossly visible nodules in the intima, media and adventitia of the aorta (Fig. 8.14), and atheromatous plaques are commonly seen on the intima. In chronic infections, the aortic wall is thickened and the intima shows tortuous tunnels with numerous nodules containing yellow caseous fluid and coiled worms. Aortic aneurysms have been noted in about one quarter of infections.

Diagnosis: Typical nodular lesions may be found in the wall of the aorta on *post mortem* examination. Microfilariae may also be found in skin biopsy samples taken from affected areas. The piece of skin

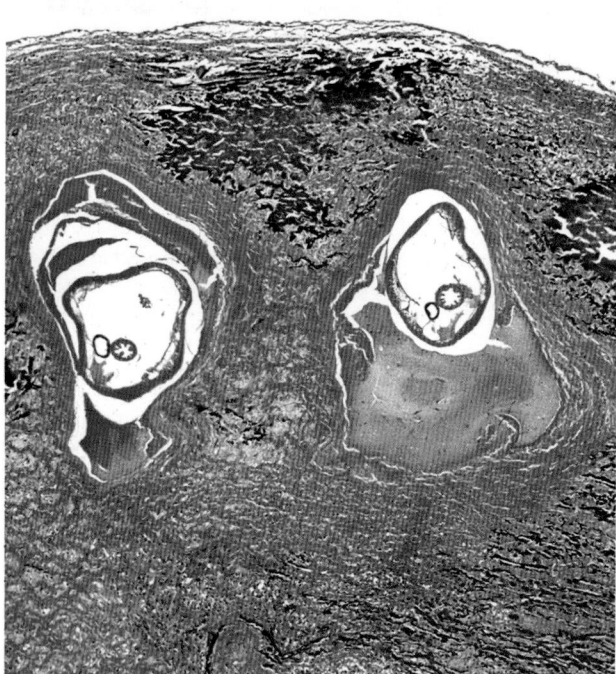

Fig. 8.14 *Onchocerca armillata* within the aorta.

is placed in warm saline and teased to allow emergence of the microfilariae, and is then incubated for about 8–12 hours. The microfilariae are readily recognised by their sinuous movements in a centrifuged sample of the saline. Another option is to scarify the skin of a predilection site and examine the fluid exudate for microfilariae.

Control and treatment: With the ubiquity of the insect vectors there is little possibility of efficient control, though the use of microfilaricides will reduce the numbers of infected flies. In any case, with the relatively innocuous nature of the infection there is unlikely to be any demand for control. Though treatment is rarely indicated, daily administration of diethylcarbamazine over a period of 21 days acts as a microfilaricide, and a single dose of ivermectin is highly efficient in this respect, although the dying microfilariae may provoke local tissue reactions.

Schistosomes

Schistosomes are flukes found in the circulatory system in which the sexes are separate, the small adult female lying permanently in a longitudinal groove, the gynaecophoric canal, in the body of the male. The genus has been divided into four groups – *haematobium*, *indicum*, *mansoni* and *japonicum* – but the genus as currently defined is paraphyletic so revisions are likely.

Haematobium group

Schistosoma bovis

Schistosoma bovis (Phylum: Platyhelminthes; Class: Trematoda; Order: Strigeidida; Family: Schistosomatidae), commonly known as the Blood fluke, causes a disease named bilharziosis and is

localised in the portal, mesenteric and urogenital veins of cattle, sheep, goats and camels. This parasite has snails (*Bulinus contortus*, *B. truncates*, *Physopsis africana*, *P. nasuta*) as intermediate hosts and is found in Africa, the Middle East, southern Asia and southern Europe.

Epidemiology: The epidemiology is totally dependent on water as a medium for infection of both the intermediate and final host. Small streams, irrigation canals, wet savannah and marshy or damp areas are the main snail habitats. Eggs, miracidia and cercariae are short-lived with seasonal transmission directly related to rainfall and temperature. The fact that percutaneous infection may occur encourages infection where livestock are obliged to wade in water. In cattle, high prevalence is usually associated with low numbers of worms, although worm burdens increase with age while egg excretion declines markedly in animals above two years of age due to the development of partial immunity.

Pathogenesis: The young flukes cause some damage during migration but most serious damage is caused by the irritation produced by the parasite eggs in the intestine and the blood-sucking habit of the worms. Acute disease is characterised by diarrhoea and anorexia due to the response to deposition of eggs in the mesenteric veins and their subsequent infiltration in the intestinal mucosa. The presence of the worms in veins of the bladder in cattle may cause damage to the bladder wall and haematuria.

Clinical signs: These are diarrhoea, sometimes blood-stained and containing mucus, anorexia, thirst, anaemia and emaciation. In cattle, the presence of the worms in the vesical veins may cause haematuria.

Pathology: At necropsy during the acute phase of the disease, there are marked haemorrhagic lesions in the mucosa of the intestine but as the disease progresses, the wall of the intestine appears greyish, thickened and oedematous due to confluence of the egg granulomas and the associated inflammatory changes. The liver may be larger than normal, depending on the stage of the disease, and may be markedly cirrhotic in long-standing infections. On microscopic examination, there is pigmentation of the liver and numerous eggs may be found, surrounded by cellular infiltration and fibrous tissue. The spleen may be slightly swollen and lymph glands are usually pigmented.

Diagnosis: This is based mainly on the clinicopathological picture of diarrhoea, wasting and anaemia, coupled with a history of access to natural water sources. The relatively persistent diarrhoea, often blood-stained and containing mucus, may help to differentiate this syndrome from fasciolosis. The demonstration of the characteristic eggs in the faeces or in squash preparations of blood and mucus from the faeces is useful in the period following patency but less useful as egg production drops in the later stages of infection. In general, when schistosomiasis is suspected, diagnosis is best confirmed by a detailed *post mortem* examination which will reveal the lesions and, if the mesentery is stretched, the presence of numerous schistosomes in the veins. In epidemological surveys, serological tests may be of value.

Control: This is similar to that outlined for *F. gigantica* and *Paramphistomum* infections. Since the prevalence of snail populations varies according to temperature, local efforts should be made to identify the months of maximum snail population, and cattle movements planned to avoid their exposure to dangerous stretches of water at these times. When watering of stock is from a reservoir or stream, fencing the water source and leading a pipe to troughs can achieve control. To do this effectively from streams, the water may need to be pumped and in remote areas simple water-driven pumps whose power source depends on the water flow have been found useful. It is important that the water troughs be cleaned out regularly since they can become colonised by snails.

When grazing depends on the dry-season use of marshy areas around receding lakebeds, snail control is difficult. Molluscicides are usually impractical because of the large body of water involved and their possible effect on fish, which may form an important part of the local food supply. Apart from repeated anthelmintic treatment to prevent patency of acquired infections of *Schistosoma*, there is often little one can do. Ideally, such areas are often best suited to irrigation and the growing of cash crops, the profit from which can be used to improve the dry-season food and water supply to cattle.

Treatment: For economic reasons, chemotherapy is not suitable for the control of schistosomiasis in domestic stock except during severe clinical outbreaks. Care has to be exercised in treating clinical cases of schistosomiasis since the dislodgement of the damaged flukes may result in emboli being formed and subsequent occlusion of major mesenteric and portal blood vessels with fatal consequences. Older drugs still used in some areas are the antimonial preparations tartar emetic, antimosan and stibophen, and niridazole and trichlorphon, all of which have to be given over a period of days at high dosage rates. Fatalities associated with the use of these drugs are not uncommon. Praziquantel, which is the drug of choice for treatment of human schistosomiasis, is also effective in ruminants at 15–20 mg/kg *per os* but may be cost-prohibitive.

Schistosoma mattheei

Schistosoma mattheei (Phylum: Platyhelminthes; Class: Trematoda; Order: Strigeidida; Family: Schistosomatidae) is localised in the portal, mesenteric and bladder veins of cattle, sheep, goats, camels, rodents and humans. This parasite has snails (*Bulinus* and *Physopsis* spp.) as intermediate hosts and is found in South and Central Africa and the Middle East.

Notes: Thought to be synonymous with *S. bovis* but differs on morphological and pathological grounds and is restricted to the alimentary canal.

Schistosoma leiperi

Schistosoma leiperi (Phylum: Platyhelminthes; Class: Trematoda; Order: Strigeidida; Family: Schistosomatidae) is localised in the mesenteric veins of antelopes and cattle. This parasite has snails (*Bulinus*) as intermediate hosts and is found in Africa.

Indicum group

Schistosoma indicum

Schistosoma indicum (Phylum: Platyhelminthes; Class: Trematoda; Order: Strigeidida; Family: Schistosomatidae) is localised in the portal, pancreatic, hepatic and mesenteric veins of cattle, sheep, goats, horses, donkeys, camels and buffalo and occurs in India. This parasite has snails (*Indoplanorbis*) as intermediate hosts.

Schistosoma nasale

Schistosoma nasale, synonym *Schistosoma nasalis* (Phylum: Platyhelminthes; Class: Trematoda; Order: Strigeidida; Family: Schistosomatidae), causes what is commonly known as the Snoring disease and is localised in the veins of the nasal mucosa of cattle, goats, sheep, buffalo and horses. This parasite has snails (*Lymnaea luteola*, *L. acuminata*, *Indoplanorbis exustus*) as intermediate hosts and occurs in India, Pakistan and Southeast Asia. Control and treatment are as for *S. bovis*.

Epidemiology: The epidemiology is totally dependent on water as a medium for infection of both the intermediate and final host.

Pathogenesis: In heavy infections there is a copious mucopurulent discharge, snoring and dyspnoea. The main pathogenic effects are associated with the eggs, which cause abscess formation in the mucosa. Fibrous granulomatous growths occur which may occlude the nasal passages.

Clinical signs and pathology: Coryza, sneezing, dyspnoea and snoring. The mucosa of the nasal sinuses is studded with small abscesses that contain the eggs of the worms, and later show much fibrous tissue and proliferating epithelium (Fig. 8.15).

Diagnosis: Infection is confirmed by the presence of the spindle-shaped eggs in the nasal discharge.

Notes: Several other *Schistosoma* species have been reported in cattle. Details on the life cycle, epidemiology, pathogenesis, control and treatment are essentially similar to those for *S. bovis*.

Schistosoma spindale

Schistosoma spindale (Phylum: Platyhelminthes; Class: Trematoda; Order: Strigeidida; Family: Schistosomatidae) is localised in the mesenteric veins of cattle, buffalo, horses, pigs and occasionally dogs and occurs in parts of Asia and the Far East.

Japonicum group

Schistosoma japonicum

Schistosoma japonicum (Phylum: Platyhelminthes; Class: Trematoda; Order: Strigeidida; Family: Schistosomatidae), commonly known as the Blood fluke, causes a disease named bilharziosis, and is localised

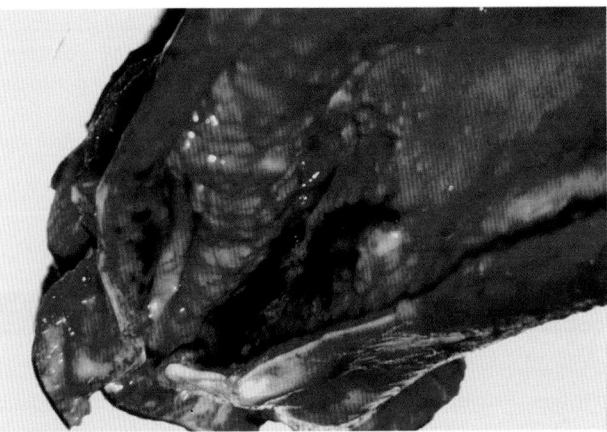

Fig. 8.15 *Schistosoma nasale* lesions in nasal mucosa.

in the portal and mesenteric veins of cattle, horses, sheep, goats, dogs, cats, rabbits, pigs, rodents and humans. This parasite has snails of the genus *Oncomelania* as intermediate hosts and is found in South and East Asia.

Pathogenesis: The penetration of the cercariae through the skin causes dermatitis, which is evident about 24 hours after infection. Passage through the lungs may cause pneumonia in gross infections and abdominal organs such as the liver may become congested during the early stages of the disease due to the arrival of immature worms in the intrahepatic portal blood vessels. The most serious damage is caused by the adult parasites in the egg-laying stage due to the irritation caused by eggs lodged in the tissues, which are forced to find their way through small venules to the epithelium and lumen of the gut. The masses of eggs become surrounded by inflamed areas and an infiltration of leucocytes, particularly eosinophils, gives rise to a rather characteristic type of abscess. The abscesses in the intestinal wall usually burst, discharging their contents into the lumen of the gut and eventually heal, forming scar tissue. In the liver, the abscesses become encapsulated and eventually calcified, a large number of such foci leading to liver enlargement, cirrhosis and ascites. Acute disease, characterised by diarrhoea and anorexia, occurs 7–8 weeks after heavy infection and is entirely due to the inflammatory and granulomatous response to the deposition of eggs in the mesenteric veins and their subsequent infiltration in the intestinal mucosa. Following massive infection, death can occur rapidly, but more usually the clinical signs abate slowly as the infection progresses. As this occurs, there appears to be a partial shift of worms away from the intestinal mucosa and reactions to these migrating parasites and their eggs can occur in the liver. Schistosomiasis is generally considered to be a much more serious and important infection in sheep than in larger ruminants, and even where a high prevalence of the parasite is detected in slaughtered cattle, clinical signs of the disease are seen only rarely. In sheep, anaemia and hypoalbuminaemia have been shown to be prominent during the clinical phase apparently as a result of mucosal haemorrhage, dyshaemopoiesis and an expansion in plasma volume. The significance of low-level infection is not known, but it has been suggested that this may have a considerable effect on productivity. There is experimental evidence of acquired resistance to reinfection by homologous species and, from natural infections, that resistance may develop as a result of prior exposure to a heterologous species.

Clinical signs and pathology: This is similar to that seen in *S. bovis*. Scar tissue and frequent papillomatous growths may be seen on the intestinal mucosa. On sections of the liver, there is also evidence of egg granulomas and of portal fibrosis provoked by eggs which have inadvertently been swept into small portal vessels. The mesentery, mesenteric lymph nodes and spleen are frequently altered due to the presence of abnormal amounts of connective tissue.

Details of the epidemiology, clinical signs, diagnosis, control and treatment are as for *S. bovis*.

Other schistosomes

Schistosoma turkestanica

Schistosoma turkestanica, synonym *Orientobilharzia turkestanicum* (Phylum: Platyhelminthes; Class: Trematoda; Order: Strigeidida; Family: Schistosomatidae), is localised in the mesenteric and small veins of the pancreas and liver of cattle, buffalo, sheep, goats, camels,

horses, donkeys, mules and cats. This parasite has snails (*Lymnaea euphratica*) as intermediate hosts and is found in Asia, the Middle East and parts of Europe.

Pathogenesis: Of little significance in cattle but can produce marked debility in sheep and goats, causing hepatic cirrhosis and nodules in the wall of the intestines. This is often accompanied by loss of body weight in small ruminants.

Trypanosomes

Members of the genus *Trypanosoma* are haemoflagellates of overwhelming importance in cattle in sub-Saharan Africa as a cause of trypanosomosis. See Chapter 2 for general descriptions.

Salivarian trypanosomes

A number of species of *Trypanosoma*, found in domestic and wild animals, are all transmitted cyclically by *Glossina* in much of sub-Saharan Africa. The presence of trypanosomosis precludes the rearing of livestock in many areas, while in others where the vectors are not so numerous, trypanosomosis is often a serious problem, particularly in cattle. The disease, sometimes known as Nagana, is characterised by lymphadenopathy and anaemia accompanied by progressive emaciation and, often, death.

Epidemiology: The vectors are various species of *Glossina* including *G. morsitans*, *G. palpalis*, *G. longipalpis*, *G. pallidipes* and *G. austeni*. *Trypanosoma congolense* can also be transmitted mechanically by other biting flies in tsetse-free areas, although this is uncommon. Since the life cycle of *T. vivax* is short, it is more readily transmitted than other species and mechanical transmission of *T. vivax* by tabanids allows it to spread outside the tsetse belt. The disease can also be transmitted mechanically through contaminated needles and instruments.

The epidemiology depends on three factors: the distribution of the vectors, virulence of the parasite and the response of the host.
- **The vectors**. Of the three groups of tsetse flies (see *Glossina*), the savannah and riverine are the most important since they inhabit areas suitable for grazing and watering. Although the infection rate of *Glossina* with trypanosomes is usually low, ranging from 1% to 20% of the flies, each is infected for life, and their presence in any number makes the rearing of cattle, pigs and horses extremely difficult. Biting flies may act as mechanical vectors, but their significance in Africa is still undefined.
- **The parasites**. Since parasitaemic animals commonly survive for prolonged periods, there are ample opportunities for fly transmission. Perhaps the most important aspect of trypanosomosis which accounts for the persistent parasitaemia is the way in which the parasite evades the immune response of the host. As noted previously, metacyclic and bloodstream trypanosomes possess a glycoprotein coat which is antigenic and provokes the formation of antibodies that cause opsonisation and lysis of the trypanosomes. Unfortunately, by the time the antibody is produced, a proportion of the trypanosomes have altered the chemical composition of their glycoprotein coat and now, displaying a different antigenic surface, are unaffected by the antibody. Those trypanosomes possessing this new **variant antigen** multiply to produce a second wave of parasitaemia; the host produces a second antibody, but again the glycoprotein coat has altered in a number of

trypanosomes so that a third wave of parasitaemia occurs. This process of **antigenic variation** associated with waves and remissions of parasitaemias, often at weekly intervals, may continue for months, usually with a fatal outcome. The repeated switching of the glycoprotein coat is now known to depend on a loosely ordered sequential expression of an undefined number of genes, each coding for a different glycoprotein coat. This, together with the finding that metacyclic trypanosomes may be a mixture of antigenic types, each expressing a different genetic repertoire, explains why domestic animals, even if treated successfully, are often immediately susceptible to reinfection. The complexity of antigens potentially involved has also defeated attempts at vaccination.

• **The hosts**. trypanosomosis is basically an infection of wildlife in which, by and large, it has achieved a *modus vivendi* in that the animal hosts are parasitaemic for prolonged periods but generally remain in good health. This situation is known as **trypanotolerance**. In contrast, rearing of domestic livestock in endemic areas has always been associated with excessive morbidity and mortality, although there is evidence that a degree of adaptation or selection has occurred in several breeds. Thus, in West Africa, small humpless cattle of the *Bos taurus* type, notably the N'Dama, survive and breed in areas of heavy trypanosome challenge despite the absence of control measures (Fig. 8.16). However, their resistance is not absolute and trypanosomosis exacts a heavy toll, particularly in productivity. In other areas of Africa, indigenous breeds of sheep and goats are known to be trypanotolerant, although this may be partly due to their being relatively unattractive hosts for *Glossina*. Precisely how trypanotolerant animals cope with antigenic variation is unknown. It is thought that the control and gradual elimination of their parasitaemias may depend on the possession of a particularly rapid and effective antibody response, although other factors may also be involved.

Pathogenesis: The signs and effects of the various trypanosomes found in domestic animals are more or less similar. The pathogenesis of trypanosomosis may be considered under three headings.

1 **Lymphoid enlargement** and **splenomegaly** develop. This is associated with plasma cell hyperplasia and hypergammaglobulinaemia, which is primarily due to an increase in IgM. Concurrently there is a variable degree of suppression of immune responses to other antigens such as microbial pathogens or vaccines. Ultimately, in infections of long duration, the lymphoid organs and spleen become shrunken due to exhaustion of their cellular elements.

2 **Anaemia** is a cardinal feature of the disease, particularly in cattle, and initially is proportional to the degree of parasitaemia. Anaemia is caused mainly by extravascular haemolysis through erythrophagocytosis in the mononuclear phagocytic systems of the spleen, liver and lungs, but as the disease becomes chronic there may be decreased haemoglobin synthesis. Leucopenia and thrombocytopenia are caused by mechanisms that predispose leucocytes and platelets to phagocytosis. Immunological mechanisms in the pathogenesis lead to extensive proliferation of activated macrophages, which engulf or destroy erythrocytes, leucocytes, platelets and haematopoietic cells. Later, in infections of several months' duration, when the parasitaemia often becomes low and intermittent, the anaemia may resolve to a variable degree. However, in some chronic cases it may persist despite chemotherapy.

3 **Cell degeneration** and **inflammatory infiltrates** occur in many organs, such as the skeletal muscle and the central nervous system (CNS), but perhaps most significantly in the myocardium where there is separation and degeneration of the muscle fibres. The mechanisms underlying these changes are still under study.

Clinical signs: In cattle, the major signs are anaemia, generalised enlargement of the superficial lymph glands (Fig. 8.17), lethargy and progressive loss of bodily condition. Fever and loss of appetite occur intermittently during parasitaemic peaks, the latter becoming marked in the terminal stages of the disease. Typically, the disease is chronic, extending over several months, and usually terminates fatally if untreated. As a herd phenomenon, the growth of young animals is stunted while adults show decreased fertility, and if pregnant may abort or give birth to weak offspring. In the terminal stages, animals become extremely weak, the lymph nodes are reduced in size and there is often a jugular pulse. Death is associated with congestive heart failure due to anaemia and myocarditis. Occasionally, the disease is acute, death occurring within 2–3 weeks of infection preceded by fever, anaemia and widespread haemorrhages.

Pathology: The carcass is often pale and emaciated and there may be oedematous swellings in the lower part of the abdomen and genital organs with serous atrophy of fat. The liver, lymph nodes and

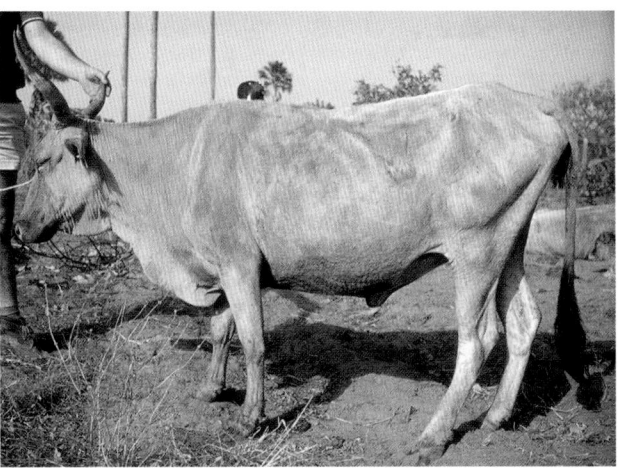

Fig. 8.16 Trypanotolerant N'Dama breed of West Africa.

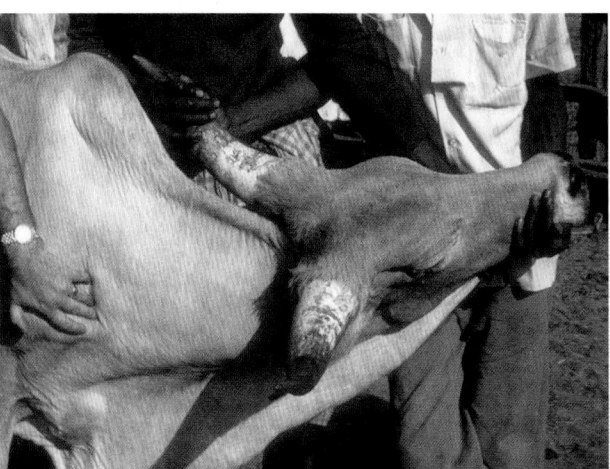

Fig. 8.17 Enlarged prescapular lymph node of zebu with trypanosomosis.

spleen are enlarged and the viscera are congested. Petechiae may appear on lymph nodes, pericardium and intestinal mucosa. The liver is hypertrophic and congested with degeneration and necrosis of the hepatocytes, dilation of blood vessels and parenchymal infiltration of mononuclear cells. A non-suppurative myocarditis, sometimes associated with hydropericarditis, has been reported accompanied by degeneration and necrosis of the myocardial tissue. Other lesions can include glomerulonephritis, renal tubular necrosis, non-suppurative meningo-encephalomyelitis, focal poliomalacia, keratitis, ophthalmitis, orchitis, interstitial pneumonia and bone marrow atrophy. Splenic and lymph node hypertrophy occurs during the acute phase but the lymphoid tissues are usually exhausted and fibrotic in the chronic stage.

Diagnosis: The clinical signs of the disease, although indicative, are not pathognomonic. Confirmation of clinical diagnosis depends on the demonstration of trypanosomes in the blood. If a herd or flock is involved, a representative number of blood samples should be examined, since in individual animals the parasitaemia may be in remission or in long-standing cases may be extremely scanty. Occasionally, when the parasitaemia is massive it is possible to detect motile trypanosomes in fresh smears of blood. More usually, both thick and thin smears of blood are air-dried and examined later. Thick smears, de-haemoglobinised before staining with Giemsa or Leishman's stain, offer a better chance of finding trypanosomes, while the stained thin smears are used for differentiation of the trypanosome species. More sensitive techniques utilise centrifugation in a microhaematocrit tube followed by microscopic examination of the interface between the buffy coat and the plasma; alternatively, the tube may be snapped, the buffy coat expressed onto a slide and the contents examined under dark-ground or phase-contrast microscopy for motile trypanosomes. With these techniques, the PCV is also obtained which is of indirect value in diagnosis if one can eliminate other causes of anaemia, especially helminthosis.

A number of serological tests have been described, including the indirect fluorescent antibody test and ELISA, and have been partially validated but require further evaluation and standardisation.

Trypanosoma brucei brucei

Trypanosoma brucei brucei (Phylum: Euglenozoa; Class: Kinetoplastea; Order: Trypanosomatida; Family: Trypanosomatidae) causes a disease commonly known as Nagana. It is localised in the blood, myocardium, CNS and reproductive tract of cattle, horses, donkeys, zebu, sheep, goats, camels, pigs, dogs, cats and wild game species, particularly antelopes. This protozoon occurs over approximately 10 million km² of sub-Saharan Africa between latitudes 14° N and 29° S.

Pathogenesis: In *T. brucei brucei* infections, the disease is usually more chronic in cattle and animals may survive for several months and may recover.

Treatment: The two drugs in common use are isometamidium and diminazene aceturate. These are usually successful except where trypanosomes have developed resistance to the drug or in some very chronic cases. Treatment should be followed by surveillance since reinfection, followed by clinical signs and parasitaemia, may occur within a week or two. Alternatively, the animal may relapse after chemotherapy, due to a persisting focus of infection in its tissues or because the trypanosomes are drug resistant.

Notes: Antelope are the natural host species and are reservoirs of infection for domestic animals. Horses, mules and donkeys are very susceptible, and the disease is very severe in sheep, goats, camels and dogs (see respective hosts). Other subspecies of *T. brucei* – *T. brucei evansi* and *T. brucei equiperdum* – are described separately under their respective subspecies and definitive hosts. Two other subspecies, *T. brucei gambiense* and *T. brucei rhodesiense*, are important causes of 'sleeping sickness' in humans.

Trypanosoma brucei evansi

Trypanosoma brucei evansi, synonyms *Trypanosoma evansi*, *Trypanosoma equinum* (Phylum: Euglenozoa; Class: Kinetoplastea; Order: Trypanosomatida; Family: Trypanosomatidae), causes a disease commonly known as Surra, El debab, Mbori, Murrina, Mal de Caderas, Doukane or Dioufar or Thaga, and is localised in the blood of horses, donkeys, camels, cattle, zebu, goats, pigs, dogs, water buffalo, elephants, capybaras, tapirs, mongooses, ocelots, deer and other wild animals and laboratory animals. It occurs in North Africa, Central and South America, central and southern Russia and parts of Asia (India, Burma, Malaysia, southern China, Indonesia, Philippines).

Pathogenesis: Domestic species such as cattle, buffalo and pigs are commonly infected, but overt disease is uncommon and their main significance is as reservoirs of infection.

Control and treatment: Suramin or quinapyramine (Trypacide®) are the drugs of choice for treatment and also confer a short period of prophylaxis. For more prolonged protection, a modified quinapyramine known as Trypacide Pro-Salt is also available. Unfortunately, drug resistance, at least to suramin, is not uncommon.

Notes: The original distribution of this parasite coincided with that of the camel, and is often associated with arid desert and semi-arid steppes. For more details see Chapter 10.

Trypanosoma congolense

Trypanosoma congolense (Phylum: Euglenozoa; Class: Kinetoplastea; Order: Trypanosomatida; Family: Trypanosomatidae) causes a disease commonly known as Nagana, Paranagana, Gambia fever, Ghindi or Gobial, and is localised in the blood of cattle, sheep, goats, horses, camels, dogs, pigs, antelopes, giraffes, zebras, elephants and warthogs. It is found in tropical Africa between latitudes 15° N and 25° S.

Pathogenesis: With *T. congolense*, there are many strains which differ markedly in virulence. In cattle, the parasite can cause an acute fatal disease resulting in death in about 10 weeks, a chronic condition with recovery in about one year, or a mild, almost asymptomatic condition. The signs caused by this species are similar to those caused by other trypanosomes, but the CNS is not affected.

Control and treatment: In infected cattle, the two drugs in common use are diminazene aceturate (Berenil®) and homidium salts (Ethidium® and Novidium®). As with *T. brucei*, these drugs are usually successful except where trypanosomes have developed resistance to the drug or in some very chronic cases. Additional comments made for treatment and control of *T. brucei* infections equally apply to *T. congolense*.

Notes: *Trypanosoma congolense congolense* is the most important trypanosome of cattle in tropical Africa. The African disease Nagana is caused by *T. congolense*, often in mixed infection with *T. brucei* and *T. vivax*.

Trypanosoma vivax

Trypanosoma vivax (Phylum: Euglenozoa; Class: Kinetoplastea; Order: Trypanosomatida; Family: Trypanosomatidae) causes a disease commonly known as Nagana or Souma, and is localised in the blood of cattle, sheep, goats, camels, horses, antelopes and giraffes. It is found in Central Africa, West Indies, Central and South America (Brazil, Venezuela, Bolivia, Colombia, Guyana, French Guiana) and Mauritius.

Epidemiology: There are three subspecies.

- *Trypanosoma vivax vivax* causes the disease souma in Africa and is found in mixed infections with *T. congolense* and *T. brucei*.
- *Trypanosoma vivax viennei* occurs in the New World and is transmitted by horse flies. This subspecies occurs in cattle, horses, sheep and goats in northern South America, Central America, West Indies and Mauritius.
- *Trypanosoma vivax uniforme* is similar to *T. vivax vivax* but is smaller, 12–20 μm long (mean 16 μm). It occurs in cattle, sheep, goats and antelopes in Uganda and Zaire, causing a disease similar to that of *T. vivax vivax*.

Pathogenesis: *Trypanosoma vivax* is most important in cattle. Generally, strains of *T. vivax* in West Africa are more pathogenic than ones in East Africa, except for one strain in East Africa that causes acute haemorrhagic disease which is very pathogenic.

Salivarian trypanosomosis control and treatment This currently depends on the control of tsetse flies, discussed under the Tsetse flies (*Glossina* spp.) section, and on the use of drugs (Table 8.5). In cattle, and if necessary in sheep and goats, isometamidium is the drug of choice since it remains in the tissues and has a prophylactic effect for 2–6 months. Otherwise, diminazene may be used as cases arise, these being selected either by clinical examination or on the haematological detection of anaemic animals. To reduce the possible development of drug resistance, it may be advisable periodically to change from one trypanocidal drug to another. To further enhance the effective use of trypanocidal drugs, they may be used as 'sanative' pairs and treatment restricted to individual clinically affected animals. Two important aspects of control are:

- the necessity to protect cattle from a tsetse-free zone while being trekked to market through an area of endemic trypanosomosis

Table 8.5 Drugs used in the treatment and control of Nagana in cattle.

Drug	Recommended dose	Comments
Diminazene aceturate	3–10 mg/kg i.m.	*Trypanosoma brucei, Trypanosoma congolense, Trypanosoma vivax*
Isometamidium	0.25–1 mg/kg i.m.	*Trypanosoma brucei, Trypanosoma congolense, Trypanosoma vivax* Local reaction
Homidium bromide Homidium chloride	1 mg/kg s.c.	*Trypanosoma congolense, Trypanosoma vivax* Prophylaxis for six weeks
Pyrithidium bromide	2–2.5 mg/kg	*Trypanosoma congolense, Trypanosoma vivax* Prophylaxis for four months

- an awareness of the dangers of stocking a tsetse-free ranch with cattle from areas where trypanosomosis is present, as mechanical transmission may cause an outbreak of disease.

In both cases treatment with a trypanocidal drug at an appropriate time is advisable. An alternative approach, using trypanotolerant breeds of ruminants, perhaps combined with judicious drug therapy, may in the future offer a realistic solution in many areas where the disease is endemic and this aspect is currently under intensive study. The treatment is as for *T. congolense*.

Stercorarian trypanosomes

These are relatively large trypanosomes found in the blood of cattle, with faecal transmission by tabanid flies (*Tabanus, Haematopota*).

Trypanosoma theileri

Trypanosoma theileri (Phylum: Euglenozoa; Class: Kinetoplastea; Order: Trypanosomatida; Family: Trypanosomatidae) is a parasite distributed worldwide and localised in the blood of cattle. This parasite is generally considered as non-pathogenic, provoking transient parasitaemias and asymptomatic infections, although under conditions of stress it may cause abortion and even death.

Epidemiology: *Trypanosoma theileri* is transmitted by tabanid flies (*Tabanus, Haematopota*); the worldwide distribution of the trypanosome corresponds to the range and prevalence of its intermediate hosts. The metacyclic trypomastigotes, present in the faeces of the vector, gain access to the blood of their mammalian host by penetrating abraded skin, by contamination of mucous membranes, or following ingestion of the vector when the liberated trypanosomes penetrate the mucosa. Intrauterine infection has been reported.

Diagnosis: Can only be usually diagnosed by incubating blood in culture medium suitable for the multiplication of trypanosomes.

Control and treatment: Not usually required, although general fly control measures may help to limit potential transmission from tabanid flies.

Babesiosis

Babesia are intraerythrocytic parasites of domestic animals and are transmitted by ticks. Babesiosis is particularly severe in naive cattle introduced into endemic areas and is a considerable constraint on livestock development in many parts of the world.

Epidemiology: The epidemiology of the bovine *Babesia* species depends on the interplay of a number of factors.

1 The virulence of the particular species of *Babesia*. *Babesia bigemina* and *B. bovis* in tropical and subtropical regions are highly pathogenic, *B. divergens* in northern Europe is relatively pathogenic, while *B. major* produces only mild and transient anaemia.
2 The age of the host. It is frequently stated that there is an inverse age resistance to *Babesia* infection in that young animals are less susceptible to babesiosis than older animals. The reason for this is not known.
3 The immune status of the host. In endemic areas, the young animal first acquires immunity passively, in the colostrum of

the dam, and as a result often suffers only transient infections with mild clinical signs. However, these infections are apparently sufficient to stimulate active immunity, although recovery is followed by a long period during which they are carriers when, although showing no clinical signs, their blood remains infective to ticks for many months. It used to be thought that this active immunity was dependent on the persistence of the carrier state and the phenomenon was termed 'premunity'. However, it seems unlikely that this is the case since it is now known that such animals may lose their infection, either naturally or by chemotherapy, but still retain a solid immunity.

4 The level of tick challenge. In endemic areas, where there are many infected ticks, the immunity of the host is maintained at a high level through repeated challenge and overt disease is rare. In contrast, where there are few ticks or when they are confined to limited areas, the immune status of the population is low and the young animals receive little if any colostral protection. If, in these circumstances, the number of ticks suddenly increases due to favourable climatic conditions or a reduction in dipping frequency, the incidence of clinical cases may rise sharply. This situation is known as enzootic instability.

5 Stress. In endemic areas, the occasional outbreak of clinical disease, particularly in adult animals, is often associated with some form of stress, such as parturition or the presence of another disease, such as tick-borne fever.

Babesia bigemina

Babesia bigemina (Phylum: Apicomplexa; Class: Aconoidasida; Order: Piroplasmida; Family: Babesiidae) causes a disease commonly known as Texas fever and is localised in the blood of cattle and buffalo. It is found in Australia, Africa, North, Central and South America, Asia and southern Europe.

Epidemiology: *Rhipicephalus* (*Boophilus*) *annulatus*, *Rhipicephalus* (*Boophilus*) *microplus* and *Rhipicephalus* (*Boophilus*) *decoloratus* are the principal vectors of *B. bigemina*. Mechanical transmission is possible, but it is not efficient enough to maintain infection in the absence of specific tick vectors.

Pathogenesis: The rapidly dividing parasites in the red cells produce rapid destruction of the erythrocytes with accompanying haemoglobinaemia, haemoglobinuria and fever. Generally, *B. bigemina* infections are not as virulent as those of *B. bovis*, despite the fact that the parasites may infect 40% of the red cells. Otherwise, the disease is typically biphasic, the acute haemolytic crisis, if not fatal, being followed by a prolonged period of recovery.

Clinical signs: Calves are relatively resistant to infection and do not usually show clinical disease. In older animals, clinical signs can be very severe; however, differences in pathogenicity may occur with various *B. bigemina* isolates associated with different geographical areas. The first sign is usually a high fever with rectal temperatures reaching 41.5 °C (106.7 °F). There is anorexia and ruminal atony. Often the first visible appearance of infection is that the animal isolates itself from the herd, becomes uneasy, seeks shade and may lie down. Cattle may stand with an arched back, have a roughened hair coat and show evidence of dyspnoea and tachycardia. The mucous membranes are first inflamed and reddened but as erythrocytic lysis occurs, they become pallid and show signs of anaemia. Anaemia is a contributory factor to the weakness and loss of

condition seen in cattle that survive the acute phase of the disease. The anaemia may occur very rapidly, with 75% or more of the erythrocytes being destroyed in just a few days. This is usually associated with severe haemoglobinaemia and haemoglobinuria. After onset of fever, the crisis will usually pass within a week, and if the animal survives there is usually severe weight loss, drop in milk production, possible abortion and a protracted recovery. Mortality is extremely variable and may reach 50% or higher, but in the absence of undue stress most animals will survive. The diagnosis is as for *B. bovis*.

Pathology: Acute infections as for *B. bovis*. In cattle that have suffered a more prolonged illness, acute lesions are much less conspicuous. Subepicardial petechial haemorrhages may be present, the carcass is usually emaciated and icteric, the blood is thin and watery, the intermuscular fascia is oedematous, the liver yellowish-brown, and the bile may contain flakes of semi-solid material. The kidneys are pale and often oedematous, and the bladder may contain normal urine, depending on how long after the haemolytic crisis the necropsy is performed. Although the spleen is enlarged, the pulp is firmer than in acute babesiosis.

Control: Specific control measures are not usually necessary for animals born of mothers in endemic areas, since their colostrum-acquired immunity is gradually reinforced by repeated exposure to infection. Indeed, the veterinary importance of babesiosis is chiefly that it acts as a constraint to the introduction of improved livestock from other areas. Areas of enzootic instability also create problems when tick numbers suddenly increase or animals, for some reason, are forced to use an adjacent tick-infested area.

Immunisation, using blood from carrier animals, has been practised for many years in tropical areas, and more recently in Australia; rapidly passaged strains of *Babesia*, which are relatively non-pathogenic, have been widely utilised in live vaccines. In the near future, these may be superseded by adjuvanted vaccines prepared from several recombinant *Babesia* antigens. Otherwise, the control of babesiosis in susceptible animals introduced into endemic areas depends on surveillance for the first few months after their arrival and, if necessary, treatment.

Vaccination of cattle against *B. bigemina* infection is commonly practised in many countries by inoculating blood from donor animals. This is usually obtained from a recently recovered case, any untoward reactions in the 'vaccinates' being controlled by babesicidal drugs. In Australia, the procedure is more sophisticated in that the vaccine is produced from acute infections produced in splenectomised donors. For economy, the blood is collected by exchange transfusion rather than by exsanguination. It is interesting that the rapid passage of the parasite by blood inoculation in splenectomised calves has fortuitously had the very desirable effect of decreasing the virulence of the infection in non-splenectomised calves to the extent that postvaccination surveillance of cattle is frequently not performed. The parasite count of the blood determines the dilution of the latter, which is dispensed in plastic bags, packed in ice and despatched in insulated containers. Each dose of vaccine contains about 10 million parasites. Most of the vaccine is used in cattle under 12 months of age living in conditions of enzootic instability. The degree of protection induced is such that only 1% of vaccinated cattle subsequently develop clinical babesiosis from field challenge, compared with 18% of unvaccinated cattle.

The primary disadvantage of red cell vaccines is their lability and the fact that unless their preparation is carefully supervised, they may spread diseases such as enzootic bovine leucosis. Obviously, there will be no such problem with a vaccine based on recombinant antigens. A regimen of four injections of long-acting oxytetracycline at weekly intervals, administered to naive cattle during their first month of grazing on tick-infested pastures, has been shown to confer prophylaxis against *B. bigemina* during this period, after which the cattle were immune to subsequent challenge.

Treatment: As with *B. bovis*, successful treatment of *B. bigemina* depends on early diagnosis and prompt administration of effective drugs. If medication is administered early, success is the rule, for there are several effective compounds. One of the first successful treatments was trypan blue. This may be used to determine the type of infection present: *B. bigemina* is susceptible to trypan blue treatment whereas *B. bovis* is not. Generally, the small babesias are more resistant to chemotherapy. The most commonly used compounds for treatment are diminazene diaceturate (3–5 mg/kg), imidocarb (1–3 mg/kg) and amicarbalide (5–10 mg/kg); however, the quinuronium and acridine derivatives are also effective where these are available. Treatment of *B. bigemina* is so effective in some instances that radical cures occur that will eventually leave the animal susceptible to reinfection. For this reason, reduced drug levels are sometimes indicated. Imidocarb has been successfully used as a chemoprophylactic that will prevent clinical infection for as long as two months, but will allow mild subclinical infection to occur as the drug level wanes resulting in premunition and immunity.

Notes: *Babesia bigemina*, a large babesia, is of particular interest historically since it was the first protozoan infection of humans or animals demonstrated to have an arthropod intermediate host. This was shown in 1893 by Smith and Kilborne while investigating the cause of the locally known 'Texas fever' in cattle in the USA. The disease has since been eradicated in that country.

Babesia bovis

Babesia bovis, synonym *Babesia argentina* (Phylum: Apicomplexa; Class: Aconoidasida; Order: Piroplasmida; Family: Babesiidae), is localised in the blood of cattle, buffalo and deer. It is found in Australia, Africa, Central and South America, Asia and southern Europe.

Epidemiology: *Babesia bovis* is transmitted by the same ticks that transmit *B. bigemina*, i.e. *Rhipicephalus (Boophilus) annulatus* and *Rhipicephalus (Boophilus) microplus*. The tick *Rhipicephalus (Boophilus) decoloratus*, which is widely distributed in Africa, does not appear to transmit *B. bovis* even though it readily transmits *B. bigemina*. There are reports from Europe of *B. bovis*, for which the vector is thought to be *Ixodes ricinus*.

Pathogenesis: *Babesia bovis* is generally regarded as the most pathogenic of the bovine babesia. Although the classic signs of fever, anaemia and haemoglobinuria occur, the degree of anaemia is disproportional to the parasitaemia since haematocrit levels below 20% may be associated with infections of less than 1% of the red cells. The reason for this is unknown. In addition, *B. bovis* infection is associated with sludging of red cells in the small capillaries. In the cerebrum, this causes blockage of the vessels by clumps of infected red cells, leading to anoxia and tissue damage. The resulting clinical signs of aggression, incoordination or convulsions and depression are invariably fatal. Finally, recent work has indicated that some of the severity of *B. bovis* infection may be associated with the activation of certain plasma components, leading to circulatory stasis, shock and intravascular coagulation.

Clinical signs and pathology: incoordination, convulsions, depression, death. At necropsy, the carcass is pale and jaundiced and the lungs may be oedematous and congested in cattle that have died early in the course of infection. The pericardial sac may contain serosanguineous fluid and subepicardial and subendocardial petechial haemorrhages. The liver is enlarged and icteric and the gallbladder, which may have haemorrhage on the mucous surface, is distended with thick dark-green bile. The spleen is markedly enlarged and has a dark pulpy consistency. The abomasal and intestinal mucosa may be icteric with patches of subserosal haemorrhages (Fig. 8.18). The blood is thin and watery. The urinary bladder is frequently distended, with dark reddish-brown urine. Jaundice is commonly distributed in the connective tissue. The lymph nodes are oedematous and often have petechiation.

Diagnosis: The history and clinical signs of fever, anaemia, jaundice and haemoglobinuria in cattle located in enzootic areas where *Rhipicephalus* spp. ticks occur are usually sufficient to justify a diagnosis of babesiosis. For confirmation, the examination of blood smears stained with Giemsa will reveal the parasites in the red cells. However, once the acute febrile phase has subsided, they are often impossible to find since they are rapidly removed from the circulation. In addition, a technique of brain biopsies has been described that has proven very useful in detecting and diagnosing *B. bovis* infections. The characteristic low parasitaemias in the circulating blood make this technique very useful in improving the chances of seeing the organism. There is a marked concentration of infected erythrocytes in the capillaries of the brain. From each animal, six blood smears should be made, air-dried and fixed in methanol and/or a sample of whole blood in an anticoagulant and serum should be collected. In cases of chronic infection, diagnosis is usually made using a variety of serological tests for the detection of specific antibodies, since the organism disappears or is present in extremely low numbers soon after the acute infection. Presently, immunofluorescence assay is the test of choice in the serological diagnosis of *B. bovis*. Other conditions that should be considered and which may resemble babesiosis are anaplasmosis, trypanosomosis, theileriosis, leptospirosis, bacillary haemoglobinuria, hemotropic mycoplasmosis.

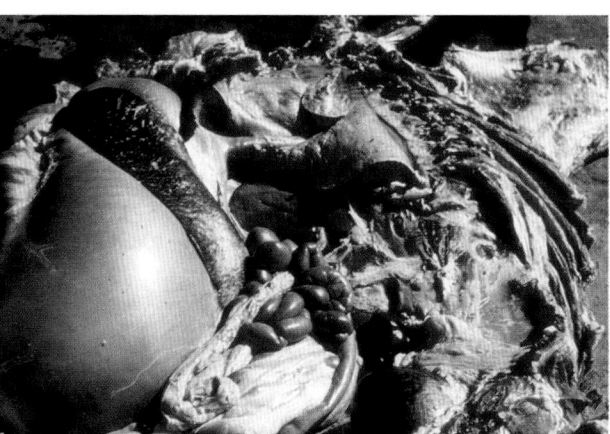

Fig. 8.18 *Post mortem* findings with *Babesia bovis* infections.

Control: The numbers of ticks and therefore the quantum of *Babesia* infection may be reduced by regular spraying or dipping with acaricides. In addition, the selection and breeding of cattle which acquire a high degree of resistance to ticks is practised, particularly in Australia. Widespread use of tick vaccines may also have a significant influence on the incidence of infection in cattle (see control of *B. bigemina*). Repeated passage of *B. bovis* in splenectomised calves results in the attenuation of the organism and for many years this attenuated vaccine has been produced and successfully used in Australia for the prevention of *B. bovis*. In some cattle (older, and producing dairy cows), chemotherapy may be indicated but usually the vaccine may be used without treatment. The development of *in vitro* techniques for the cultivation of *B. bovis* on bovine erythrocytes has led to the isolation of soluble antigens which, when combined with adjuvants, have proven immunogenic. Although they do not prevent infection, these non-infectious vaccines appear to be responsible for moderating the effects of infection. They do not produce as high a level of protection as seen with premunising vaccines but are safe and do not yield carriers. In some instances, these vaccines, although protective against homologous challenge, may not protect against immunological variants. The continuous *in vitro* passage of *B. bovis* has been shown to induce a level of attenuation similar to that seen with passage of the organism in splenectomised calves and infection with this attenuated organism has been reported to prevent clinical infection following a challenge with virulent *B. bovis*. The primary disadvantage of red cell vaccines is their lability and the fact that, unless their preparation is carefully supervised, they may spread diseases such as enzootic bovine leucosis. Obviously, there will be no such problem with a vaccine based on recombinant antigens.

Treatment: Successful treatment depends on early diagnosis and the prompt administration of effective drugs. There is less likelihood of success if treatment is delayed until the animal has been weakened by fever and anaemia. Chemotherapy is generally effective, although *B. bovis* is usually somewhat more difficult to treat than other *Babesia* species, and a second treatment, or slightly increased dose rates, may be desirable. The most commonly used compounds for the treatment of babesiosis are diminazene diacetrate (3–5 mg/kg), imidocarb (1–3 mg/kg) and amicarbalide (5–10 mg/kg); however, the quinuronium and acridine derivatives are also effective where these are available. Trypan blue is not effective against *B. bovis*.

Babesia divergens

Babesia divergens (Phylum: Apicomplexa; Class: Aconoidasida; Order: Piroplasmida; Family: Babesiidae) causes a disease commonly known as Redwater fever, is localised in the blood of cattle and occurs in northern Europe.

Epidemiology: *Babesia divergens* is transmitted by *Ixodes ricinus*, and is widespread and pathogenic, with clinical cases occurring during periods of tick activity, primarily in the spring and autumn. Infection in the tick is transovarially transmitted and the larvae, nymphs and adults of the next generation are all able to transmit infection to cattle.

Pathogenesis: The rapidly dividing parasites in the red cells produce rapid destruction of erythrocytes with accompanying haemoglobinaemia, haemoglobinuria and fever. This may be so acute as to cause death within a few days, during which the PCV falls below 20%. The parasitaemia, which is usually detectable once the clinical signs appear, may involve between 0.2% and 45% of the red cells. Milder forms of the disease, associated with relatively resistant hosts, are characterised by fever, anorexia and perhaps slight jaundice for a period of several days.

Clinical signs and pathology: Typically, the acute disease occurs 1–2 weeks after the tick starts to feed and is characterised by fever and haemoglobinuria ('redwater'). The mucous membranes, at first congested, become jaundiced, the respiratory and pulse rates are increased, the heartbeat is usually very audible, and in cattle ruminal movements cease and abortion may occur. If untreated, death commonly occurs in this phase. Otherwise, convalescence is prolonged, there is loss of weight and milk production and diarrhoea followed by constipation is common. In animals previously exposed to infection, clinical signs may be mild or even inapparent. At necropsy, the carcass is pale and jaundiced, the bile is thick and granular and there may be subepicardial and subendocardial haemorrhages.

Diagnosis: The history and clinical signs are usually sufficient to justify a diagnosis of babesiosis. For confirmation, examination of blood smears stained with Giemsa will reveal parasites in the red cells (Fig. 8.19). However, once the acute febrile phase has subsided, they are often impossible to find since they are rapidly removed from the circulation.

Control: Normally no effort is made to control this infection in endemic areas, although cattle recently introduced require surveillance for some months since, on average, one in four will develop clinical disease and of these, one in six will die if untreated. However, in some parts of mainland Europe, such as the Netherlands, where ticks are confined to rough vegetation on the edge of pastures and on roadsides, it is often possible to take evasive measures. It is thought that red and roe deer are not important reservoir hosts since only mild infections have been experimentally produced in splenectomised deer.

Treatment: Amicarbalide, diminazene aceturate and imidocarb are the most commonly used drugs. Recently, long-acting preparations of oxytetracycline have been shown to have a prophylactic effect against *B. divergens* infection. Imidocarb, due to its persistence in the tissues, has a prophylactic effect for several weeks. During the convalescent phase of the disease, blood transfusions may be valuable, as are drugs designed to stimulate food and water intake.

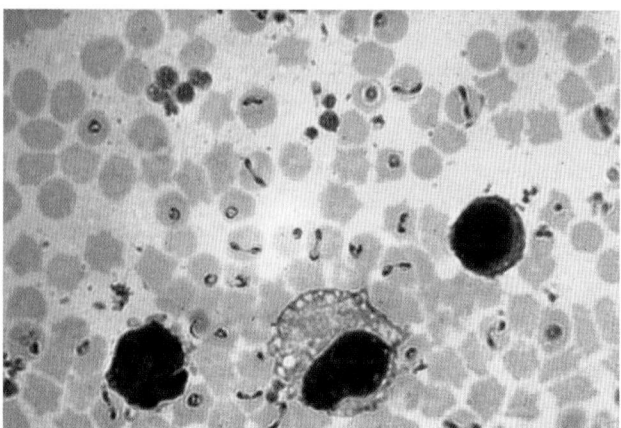

Fig. 8.19 Intraerythrocytic stages of *Babesia divergens*.

Notes: Since 1957, several cases of fatal babesiosis due to *B. divergens* infection have occurred in humans in the former Yugoslavia, Russia, Ireland and Scotland. In each case, the individual had been splenectomised some time previously or was currently undergoing immunosuppressive treatment.

Babesia major

Babesia major (Phylum: Apicomplexa; Class: Aconoidasida; Order: Piroplasmida; Family: Babesiidae) is a mildly pathogenic parasite localised in the blood of cattle. This parasite is transmitted by the three-host tick *Haemaphysalis punctata* and is found in Europe, North Africa and South America.

Clinical signs: Clinical signs with *B. major* are usually inapparent but where symptoms do occur, they are characterised by a haemolytic syndrome with elevated temperature, mild anaemia and haemoglobinuria.

Diagnosis: Examination of blood smears stained with Giemsa will reveal the parasites in the red cells.

Control and treatment: Specific control measures are not usually necessary for animals born of mothers in endemic areas since, as noted previously, their colostrally acquired immunity is gradually reinforced by repeated exposure to infection. Tick numbers may be reduced by regular spraying or dipping with acaricides. The control of infection in susceptible animals introduced into endemic areas depends on surveillance for the first few months after their arrival and, if necessary, treatment. This is not usually required but amicarbalide, diminazene aceturate and imidocarb are effective.

Other species of Babesia in cattle

See Table 8.6.

Theileriosis

Diseases caused by several species of *Theileria* (theileriosis) are a serious constraint to livestock production in Africa, Asia and the Middle East. The parasites, which are tick transmitted, undergo repeated merogony in the lymphocytes, ultimately releasing small merozoites that invade the red cells to become piroplasms.

Theileria are widely distributed in cattle in Africa, Asia, Europe and Australia, have a variety of tick vectors and are associated with infections which range from clinically inapparent to rapidly fatal. Although the speciation of many *Theileria* is still controversial, largely because of their morphological similarity, there are two species of major veterinary importance in cattle. Minor and

Table 8.6 Other species of *Babesia* in cattle.

Species	Hosts	Vectors	Distribution
Babesia jakimovi	Cattle, deer (roe deer, elk, reindeer)	*Ixodes ricinus*	Northern Europe (Siberia)
Babesia ovata	Cattle	*Hyalomma longicornis*	Japan, China
Babesia occultans	Cattle	*Hyalomma marginatum rufipes*	Southern Africa

mildly pathogenic species infecting cattle include *T. velifera* and *T. taurotragi* in Africa, *T. mutans* and the *T. sergenti/orientalis/buffeli* complex.

Theileria parva

Theileria parva (Phylum: Apicomplexa; Class: Aconoidasida; Order: Piroplasmida; Family: Theileriidae) causes disease commonly known as the East Coast fever or corridor fever, and is localised in the blood and lymphatics of cattle and buffalo. It is found in East and Central Africa.

Epidemiology: Since the tick vector, *Rhipicephalus appendiculatus*, is most active following the onset of rain, outbreaks of East Coast fever may be seasonal or, where rainfall is relatively constant, may occur at any time. Fortunately, indigenous cattle reared in endemic areas show a high degree of resistance and although transient mild infection occurs in early life, mortality is negligible. The mechanism of this resistance is unknown. However, such cattle may remain carriers and act as a reservoir of infection for ticks. Susceptible cattle introduced into such areas suffer high mortality, irrespective of age or breed, unless rigid precautions are observed. In areas where survival of the tick vector is marginal, challenge is low and indigenous cattle may have little immunity. Such areas, during a prolonged period of rain, may become ecologically suitable for the survival and proliferation of the ticks, ultimately resulting in disastrous outbreaks of East Coast fever. In some parts of East and Central Africa where populations of cattle and wild African buffalo overlap, there is an additional epidemiological complication due to the presence of a strain of *T. parva* known as *T. parva lawrencei*. This occurs naturally in African buffalo, many of which remain as carriers. The tick vector is also *R. appendiculatus* and in cattle, the disease causes high mortality. Since infected ticks may survive for nearly two years, physical contact between buffalo and cattle need not be close.

Pathogenesis: The sequence of events in a typical acute and fatal infection progresses through three phases, each spanning about one week. The first is the incubation period of about one week when neither parasite nor lesions can be detected. This is followed during the second week by marked hyperplasia and expansion of the infected lymphoblast population, initially in the regional lymph node draining the site of the tick bite and ultimately throughout the body. During the third week, there is a phase of lymphoid depletion and disorganisation associated with massive lymphocytolysis and depressed leucopoiesis. The cause of the lymphocytolysis is unknown, but is due perhaps to the activation of natural killer cells like macrophages.

Theileria parva lawrencei is transmitted from the African buffalo and becomes indistinguishable in its behaviour from *T. parva parva* following several passages in cattle.

Clinical signs: About one week after infection, in a fully susceptible animal, the lymph node draining the area of tick bite, usually the parotid, becomes enlarged and the animal becomes pyrexic (40–41.7 °C, 104–107 °F). Within a few days, there is generalised swelling of the superficial lymph nodes, ears, eyes and submandibular regions. The animal becomes anorexic, shows decreased milk production and rapidly loses condition, ceases rumination, becomes weak with a rapid heartbeat, and petechial haemorrhages may occur under the tongue and on the vulva. Affected animals become emaciated and dyspnoeic and there is terminal diarrhoea, often blood-stained. Recumbency and death almost invariably occur, usually within three weeks of infection. Occasionally, nervous signs, the so-called 'turning sickness', have been reported and attributed to the presence of meronts in cerebral capillaries. Milder infections show a mild fever lasting 3–7 days, listlessness and swelling of superficial lymph nodes.

Pathology: Necropsy during the terminal phase shows lymph nodes to be swollen, with atrophy of the cellular content of the lymph nodes and variable hyperaemia. The spleen is usually enlarged with soft pulp and prominent Malpighian corpuscles. The liver is enlarged, friable and brownish-yellow, with parenchymatous degeneration. The kidneys are either congested or pale brown, with variable numbers of infarcts. The meninges may be slightly congested. The heart is flabby, with petechiae on the epicardium and endocardium. The lungs are often congested and oedematous. There may be hydrothorax and hydropericardium, and the kidney capsule may contain a large amount of serous fluid. There may be petechiae in the visceral and parietal pleura, adrenal cortex, urinary bladder and mediastinum. There are characteristic ulcers 2–5 mm or more in diameter in the abomasum and small and large intestines. Peyer's patches are swollen and the intestinal contents yellowish.

Diagnosis: East Coast fever only occurs where *R. appendiculatus* is present, although occasionally outbreaks outwith such areas have been recorded due to the introduction of tick-infected cattle from an enzootic area. In sick animals, macroschizonts are readily detected in biopsy smears of lymph nodes and in dead animals in impression smears of lymph nodes and spleen. In advanced cases, Giemsa-stained blood smears show piroplasms in the red cells, up to 80% of which may be parasitised. The indirect fluorescent antibody test is of value in detecting cattle which have recovered from East Coast fever.

Control: Traditionally, the control of East Coast fever in areas where improved cattle are raised has relied on legislation to control the movement of cattle, on fencing to prevent access by nomadic cattle and buffalo and on repeated treatment of cattle with acaricides. In areas of high challenge, such treatments may need to be carried out twice weekly in order to kill the tick before the infective sporozoites develop in the salivary glands. This is not only expensive but creates a population of fully susceptible cattle; if the acaricide fails, through human error or the acquisition of acaricide resistance by the ticks, the consequences can be disastrous. Great efforts have been made to develop a suitable vaccine, but these have been thwarted by the complex immunological mechanisms involved in immunity to East Coast fever and by the discovery of immunologically different strains of *T. parva* in the field. However, an 'infection and treatment' regimen that involves the concurrent injection of a virulent stabilate of *T. parva* and long-acting tetracycline has been shown to be successful, although it has not been used on a large scale as yet. Apparently, the tetracycline slows the rate of schizogony, giving the immune response time to develop.

Treatment: Although the tetracyclines have a therapeutic effect if given at the time of infection, they are of no value in the treatment of clinical cases. The drugs of choice in clinical cases of East Coast fever are the naphthaquinone compounds parvaquone and buparvaquone and the anticoccidial drug halofuginone.

Notes: Because of the wide distribution of its tick vector, *Rhipicephalus*, and the fact that infection in cattle introduced into enzootic areas can be associated with a mortality of 100%, *T. parva* infection is an immense obstacle to livestock improvement.

Theileria annulata

Theileria annulata (Phylum: Apicomplexa; Class: Aconoidasida; Order: Piroplasmida; Family: Theileriidae) causes a disease commonly known as Mediterranean theileriosis or Mediterranean coast fever, and is localised in the blood and lymphatics of cattle and domestic buffalo. It is found in Mediterranean countries (Portugal and Spain, the Balkans), the Middle East, the Indian subcontinent and China.

Epidemiology: *Theileria annulata* is transmitted trans-stadially by ticks of the genus *Hyalomma*: *H. detritum* in North Africa; *H. detritum* and *H. excavatum* in the former Soviet states; *H. truncatum* in parts of Africa; *H. dromedarii* in central Asia; *H. excavatum*, *H. turanicum* and *H. marginatum* in Asia Minor; *H. marginatum* in India; and *H. longicornis* in Siberia and the Far East. Like East Coast fever, indigenous cattle in endemic areas are relatively resistant while improved cattle, particularly European breeds, are highly susceptible. However, unlike East Coast fever, the disease in such cattle is not uniformly fatal, although the mortality rate may reach 70%. Congenital infection can occur occasionally in calves.

Pathogenesis: The pathogenesis and clinical signs are initially similar to those of East Coast fever with pyrexia and lymph node enlargement, but in the late stages there is a haemolytic anaemia and often icterus. Convalescence is protracted in those cases that recover.

Clinical signs: In the acute form there is fever (40–41.7 °C, 104–107 °F), inappetence, cessation of rumination, rapid heartbeat, weakness, decreased milk production, swelling of superficial lymph nodes and eyelids, diarrhoea (containing blood and mucus), jaundice and petechial haemorrhages. Affected animals become emaciated and death can occur. In the more chronic form, there is intermittent fever, inappetence, emaciation, anaemia and jaundice.

Pathology: The lymph nodes are often but not always swollen; the spleen is often much enlarged and infarcts are usually present in the kidneys. The lungs are usually oedematous; characteristic ulcers are present in the abomasum and small and large intestines.

Diagnosis: Diagnosis depends on the detection of meronts in both lymph node biopsy specimens and, unlike *T. parva*, in blood smears. A low-grade piroplasm parasitaemia, in the absence of schizonts, is usually indicative of a recovered carrier animal.

Control and treatment: In many areas, the prevention of *T. annulata* infection in imported dairy stock is based on permanent housing. However, this is expensive and there is always the possibility that infected ticks may be brought in with the fodder to cause disease and colonise crevices in the cattle accommodation. In some countries, immunisation with meronts attenuated by prolonged *in vitro* culture has given excellent results. For the treatment see under *T. parva*.

Theileria orientalis **complex**

Theileria orientalis complex, synonyms *Theileria mutans*, *Theileria buffeli*, *Theileria sergenti* (Phylum: Apicomplexa; Class: Aconoidasida; Order: Piroplasmida; Family: Theileriidae), causes a disease commonly known as Benign theileriosis, and is a mildly pathogenic parasite localised in the blood of cattle. It is found in southern Europe, the Middle East, Asia and Australia. Vectors are *Amblyomma variegatum*, *A. cohaerens* and *A. hebraeum*. *Haemaphysalis bispinosa* and *H. bancrofti* are the probable vectors in Australia.

Clinical signs and pathology: Similar in appearance to the mild form of *T. annulata* causing anaemia, with jaundice and lymphadenopathy occasionally present. In acute cases, the spleen and liver are swollen, the lungs may be oedematous and there are characteristic ulcers in the abomasum; infarcts may be present in the kidneys. Macroschizonts may also be found in impression smears of lymph nodes and spleen taken from dead animals.

Diagnosis: Giemsa-stained blood smears may show piroplasms in the red cells, or macroschizonts may be detected in biopsy smears of lymph nodes.

Control and treatment: Tick control methods may be considered, including fencing and dipping or cleaning cattle of ticks, but these are not usually required. Little information is available on treatment, although the drugs of choice in clinical cases are likely to be parvaquone and buparvaquone.

Notes: The taxonomy of benign theileriosis species is complicated and it is now considered that *T. orientalis* is part of a complex with *T. sergenti*, *T. buffeli* and *T. mutans*.

Theileria taurotragi

Theileria taurotragi, synonym *Cytauxzoon taurotragi* (Phylum: Apicomplexa; Class: Aconoidasida; Order: Piroplasmida; Family: Theileriidae), is a mildly pathogenic parasite localised in the blood of cattle and antelopes, particularly elands (*Taurotragi oryx*). This parasite is transmitted by the vectors *R. appendiculatus* and *R. pulchellus* and it is found throughout Africa.

Clinical signs and pathology: Mild transient fever and anaemia. Meront stages have been reported in liver, lung and lymph nodes.

Diagnosis: Presence of erythrocytic forms in blood smears or meronts in lymph node biopsy specimens. *Theileria taurotragi* is morphologically indistinguishable from more pathogenic forms, but generally differentiated on clinical signs and history.

Theileria velifera

Theileria velifera, synonym *Haematoxenus veliferus* (Phylum: Apicomplexa; Class: Aconoidasida; Order: Piroplasmida; Family: Theileriidae), is a non-pathogenic parasite localised in the blood of cattle and zebu, in Africa. This parasite is transmitted by the vectors *Amblyomma variegatum*, *A. lepidu* and *A. hebraeum*.

Diagnosis: Giemsa-stained blood smears may show the characteristic 'veiled' piroplasms in the red cells.

Rickettsia

While the *Rickettsia* are now considered to be in the Kingdom Bacteria, for historical reasons they are included within parasitological texts and for this reason, mention is made below of some genera and species of importance in cattle.

Anaplasma marginale

Anaplasma marginale (Phylum: Proteobacteria; Class: Alphaproteobacteria; Order: Rickettsiales; Family: Anaplasmataceae) is localised in the blood of cattle and wild ruminants. This parasite is transmitted by tick vectors and is found in Africa, southern Europe, Australia, South America, Asia, former Soviet states and the USA.

Epidemiology: The organism is distributed throughout the tropics corresponding to the distribution of the main tick vectors, *Rhipicephalus* (*Boophilus*) *annulatus*, *Rhipicephalus* (*Boophilus*) *decoloratus* and *Rhipicephalus* (*Boophilus*) *microplus*. In the USA, the main tick vectors are *Dermacentor andersoni*, *D. occidentalis* and *D. variabilis*. Horse flies (Tabanidae), stable flies (*Stomoxys*), deer flies (*Chrysops*), horn flies and mosquitoes have also been incriminated as potential vectors. Reservoirs of infection are maintained in carrier cattle and wild ruminants such as deer. Cattle, especially adults, introduced into endemic areas are particularly susceptible, the mortality rate being up to 80%. In contrast, cattle reared in endemic areas are much less susceptible, presumably due to previous exposure when young, although their acquired immunity usually co-exists with a carrier state. This balance may, on occasion, be disturbed and clinical anaplasmosis supervenes when cattle are stressed by other diseases such as babesiosis.

Pathogenesis: Typically, the changes are those of an acute febrile reaction accompanied by a severe haemolytic anaemia. After an incubation period of around four weeks, fever and parasitaemia appear, and as the latter develops, the anaemia becomes more severe so that within a week or so, up to 70% of the erythrocytes are destroyed. The clinical signs are usually very mild in naive cattle under one year old. Thereafter, susceptibility increases so that cattle aged 2–3 years develop typical and often fatal anaplasmosis, while in cattle over three years the disease is often peracute and frequently fatal.

Clinical signs: Clinical signs are attributed to severe anaemia and include depression, weakness, fever, laboured breathing, inappetance, dehydration, constipation and jaundice. The acute stage of the disease is characterised by fever (39.4–41.7 °C, 103–107 °F) that persists for 3–7 days. During the febrile phase there is decreased rumination, dryness of the muzzle, loss of appetite, dullness and depression. Lactating cows show a depression in milk yield and abortion is a common feature in advanced pregnancy. The severity of the disease increases with age, with animals over three years of age showing the peracute and possibly fatal disease.

Pathology: Gross pathological lesions are those usually associated with anaemia. Mucous membranes are jaundiced and there is pallor of the tissues. The spleen is often greatly enlarged with enlarged splenic follicles. The liver may be enlarged with rounded borders. The gallbladder is enlarged and obstructed with dark thick bile. Petechiae may be observed on the epicardium, pericardium, pleura and diaphragm. The lymph glands are enlarged. Microscopically, there is hyperplasia of the bone marrow. The spleen shows a decrease in lymphoblasts and increased vacuolation and degeneration of reticular cells and there is reduction of the white pulp and accumulation of pigment resembling haemosiderin.

Diagnosis: The clinical signs, supplemented if possible by haematocrit estimation and the demonstration of *Anaplasma* inclusions in the red cells, are usually sufficient for diagnosis. For the detection of immune carriers, complement fixation and agglutination tests are available; an indirect fluorescent antibody test and DNA probe have also been developed.

Control: Vaccination of susceptible stock with small quantities of blood containing the mildly pathogenic *A. centrale* or a relatively avirulent strain of *A. marginale* is practised in several countries, any clinical signs in adults being controlled by drugs. In the USA, a killed *A. marginale* vaccine containing erythrocyte stroma is also available. Although all are generally successful in the clinical sense, challenged cattle become carriers and so perpetuate transmission. The killed vaccine has the disadvantage that antibodies produced to the red cell stroma, if transferred in the colostrum, may produce isoerythrolysis in nursing calves. Improved inactivated vaccines are currently under development. Otherwise, control at present depends largely on the reduction of ticks and biting flies.

Treatment: Tetracycline compounds are effective in treatment if given early in the course of the disease and especially before the parasitaemia has reached its peak. More recently, imidocarb has been shown to be effective and may also be used to sterilise carrier animals.

Anaplasma centrale

Anaplasma centrale (Phylum: Proteobacteria; Class: Alphaproteobacteria; Order: Rickettsiales; Family: Anaplasmataceae) is a bacterium found worldwide and is localised in the blood of cattle, wild ruminants and sheep, which probably act as reservoirs of infection. Although similar to *A. marginale*, this bacterium is generally considered less pathogenic. Details on the life cycle, diagnosis, control and treatment are as for *A. marginale*.

Epidemiology: Apart from the various modes of transmission previously described, little information is available. Reservoirs of infection are maintained in carrier cattle and perhaps in wild ruminants or sheep. Cattle, especially adults, introduced into endemic areas are particularly susceptible, the mortality rate being up to 80%. In contrast, cattle reared in endemic areas are much less susceptible, presumably due to previous exposure when young, although their acquired immunity usually co-exists with a carrier state. This balance may, on occasion, be disturbed and clinical anaplasmosis supervenes when cattle are stressed by other diseases such as babesiosis.

Clinical signs: The clinical features include pyrexia, anaemia and often jaundice, anorexia, laboured breathing and, in cows, a severe drop in milk yield or abortion. Occasionally, peracute cases occur, which usually die within a day of the onset of clinical signs.

Pathology: Necropsy at this time often reveals a jaundiced carcass, a grossly enlarged gallbladder and, on section, a liver suffused with bile. The spleen and lymph nodes are enlarged and congested and there are petechial haemorrhages in the heart muscle. The urine, unlike that in babesiosis, is normal in colour. In survivors, recovery is prolonged.

Anaplasma phagocytophilum

Anaplasma phagocytophilum, synonyms *Anaplasma phagocytophila*, *Ehrlichia phagocytophila*, *Cytoecetes phagocytophila* (Phylum: Proteobacteria; Class: Alphaproteobacteria; Order: Rickettsiales;

Family: Anaplasmataceae), causes a disease commonly known as Tick-borne fever, Pasture fever, Canine granulocytic ehrlichiosis, Human granulocytic ehrlichiosis or Equine granulocytic ehrlichiosis, and is localised in the blood of cattle. For more detailed descriptions on epidemiology, pathogenesis, control and treatment, see Chapter 9.

Ehrlichia bovis

Ehrlichia bovis (Phylum: Proteobacteria; Class: Alphaproteobacteria; Order: Rickettsiales; Family: Anaplasmataceae) is localised in the blood of cattle. It is found in Africa, the Middle East (Turkey, Iran), India and Sri Lanka.

Epidemiology: Transmitted by ticks of the genera *Hyalomma*, *Rhipicephalus* and *Amblyomma*. Known vectors are *Hyalomma anatolicum*, *Rhipicephalus appendiculatus*, *Amblyomma cajennense* and possibly *A. variegatum*.

Pathogenesis: Has been associated with acute and fatal disease in some regions of Africa.

Clinical signs and pathology: Affected animals show anorexia, weakness, muscular trembling, drunken gait and bulging eyes. In fatal cases there is hydropericardium, hydrothorax, splenomegaly and swollen lymph nodes. Monocytosis may occur in terminal infections.

Diagnosis: The rickettsiae can be demonstrated by staining blood or organ smears with Giemsa.

Control: Specific control measures have not been reported but tick control may assist in preventing infection with *E. bovis*.

Treatment: Little information is available although, as with other members of this group, tetracyclines may be effective.

Ehrlichia ruminantium

Ehrlichia ruminantium, synonym *Cowdria ruminantium* (Phylum: Proteobacteria; Class: Alphaproteobacteria; Order: Rickettsiales; Family: Anaplasmataceae), causes a disease commonly known as Heartwater, Cowdriosis or Malkopsiekte (Afrikaans), and is localised in the blood of cattle, sheep, goats, buffalo and wild ruminants. This parasite is transmitted by tick vectors and is found in Africa, south of the Sahara, and the Caribbean (Guadeloupe, Marie-Galante and Antigua).

Epidemiology: Distribution of heartwater coincides with that of the *Amblyomma* ticks, which require a warm humid climate and bushy grass. A number of African species of the genus *Amblyomma* (*A. hebraeum*, *A. variegatum*, *A. pomposum*, *A. gemma*, *A. lepidum*, *A. tholloni*, *A. sparsum*, *A. astrion*, *A. cohaerens*, *A. marmoreum*) and American species of *Amblyomma* (*A. maculatum*, *A. cajennense*, *A. dissimile*) are able to transmit infection. Transmission usually appears to be trans-stadial, although transovarian transmission can occur more rarely. The level of infection is often unknown as indigenous domestic and wild animals often show no signs. It is only when susceptible exotic species are introduced that infection becomes apparent. Besides cattle, sheep, goats, Asian buffalo, antelopes and deer are susceptible to infection and disease. Indigenous cattle undergo inapparent infection. Calves under three weeks old, even from susceptible stock, are difficult to infect. Heartwater can occur throughout the year, but incidence declines in the dry season due to reduced tick activity. The incubation period is variable, from seven to 28 days, with fever starting on average after 18 days. Mortality can be up to 60% in exotic breeds but less than 5% in local cattle.

Pathogenesis: In the ruminant host, the organism is first found in reticuloendothelial cells and then parasitises vascular endothelial cells. Division is by binary fission and produces morula-like colonies in the cytoplasm of infected cells. The pathogenesis of the disease is far from clear. Hydropericardium may lead to cardiac insufficiency and hydrothorax and pulmonary oedema to respiratory difficulties. Oedema is often so pronounced in peracute heartwater that it is responsible for sudden death by asphyxia. The occasional sudden fall in plasma volume preceding death has been associated with development of the transudates. Brain lesions are not sufficiently consistent to explain the nervous symptoms.

Clinical signs: The average natural incubation period is two weeks, but can vary from 10 days to one month. In most cases, heartwater is an acute febrile disease, with a sudden rise in body temperature; temperature may exceed 41 °C within 1–2 days. It remains high with small fluctuations and drops shortly before death. A peracute form occurs in exotic breeds introduced into an endemic region. The animal appears clinically normal but on examination has a marked pyrexia. It may then suddenly collapse, go into convulsions and die. Thoracic auscultation will often reveal oedema in the lungs and bronchi. In the acute form, fever is followed by inappetence, sometimes listlessness, diarrhoea (particularly in cattle) and dyspnoea indicative of lung oedema. The course of infection is 3–6 days and consists of pyrexia (often over 41 °C, 106 °F). A mild cough may be heard and, on auscultation, hydrothorax, hydropericardium and lung oedema are noted. A profuse diarrhoea is often present or there may be blood in the faeces. Nervous signs develop gradually. The animal is restless, walks in circles, makes sucking movements and stands rigidly with tremors of the superficial muscles. Cattle may push their head against a wall or present aggressive or anxious behaviour. Finally, the animal falls to the ground, pedalling and exhibiting opisthotonus, nystagmus and chewing movements. The animal usually dies during or following such a nervous attack. In the subacute form, the signs are like those of the acute form but they are much less severe with a transient fever and sometimes diarrhoea. Disease may last for over a week and the animal usually improves gradually but a few cases progress to collapse and death. This is often the most severe form seen in indigenous cattle and those previously infected. In these stocks, symptoms are usually absent.

Pathology: The lesions present are very variable and not pathognomonic. In the peracute form there are few gross lesions, but in some there is marked lung oedema with tracheal and bronchial fluids. In the acute form the most common macroscopic lesions are hydropericardium, hydrothorax, pulmonary oedema, intestinal congestion, oedema of the mediastinal and bronchial lymph nodes, petechiae on the epicardium and endocardium, congestion of the brain and moderate splenomegaly. The liver is often engorged, with the gallbladder distended. The spleen is occasionally enlarged. There may be congestion of the meningeal blood vessels.

Diagnosis: There is no specific method for diagnosis in the living animal. A tentative diagnosis of heartwater is based on the presence of *Amblyomma* vectors, clinical nervous signs and transudates in the pericardium and thorax at *post mortem* examination. Provisional indication can be gained from the history and clinical signs. Lymph node material can be aspirated to examine for vacuoles containing organisms in the cytoplasm of the reticular cells. Serum can be examined using a capillary flocculation test. A number of serological tests have been described but all suffer from false-positive reactions due to cross-reactions with other *Ehrlichia* species. Diagnosis is easier at *post mortem* as the organism can be discerned in brain tissue capillaries that have been fixed in methyl alcohol and stained with Giemsa. Typical colonies of *E. ruminantium* can be observed in brain smears made after death. Slides are examined for the presence of the characteristic colonies. Experience is required to differentiate from other haemoparasites (*Babesia bovis*), certain blood cells (thrombocytes, granulocytes), normal subcellular structures (mitochondria, mast cell granules) or stain artefacts (stain precipitates). The specificity of the reading can be improved by staining formalin-fixed brain sections using immunoperoxidase techniques. Transmission electron microscopy can be used to demonstrate organisms inside a vacuole-like structure, which is surrounded by a membrane in the endothelial cell's cytoplasm. Differential clinical diagnosis should be made with anthrax, theileriosis, anaplasmosis, botulism and, in nervous cases, rabies, tetanus, strychnine poisoning, cerebral theileriosis, cerebral babesiosis and hypomagnesaemia.

Control: Prevention is aimed at controlling the tick vector by dipping cattle at weekly intervals with reliable acaricides. However, ticks of the genus *Amblyomma* are less susceptible than those from other genera. As the tick may transmit infection after 24 hours on the host, better control is obtained by applying acaricide by dipping or spraying every three days. Resistance to organophosphates and arsenic has been reported. Care should also be taken not to introduce *Amblyomma* on infected animals or in forage to uninfected cows. In areas where disease is endemic, most cattle are immune. A carrier state develops after infection and remains for several weeks. Non-infected resistance persists a variable time, lasting from a few months to several years. After this time reinfection can occur. The only method of immunisation is an infection and treatment method using infected blood or homogenised pre-fed infected ticks followed by tetracycline treatment as soon as pyrexia develops.

Treatment: Therapy is most effective when carried out early in disease. Tetracyclines can be used and do not interfere with development of immunity.

Notes: Heartwater is one of the main obstacles to the improvement of livestock productivity in sub-Saharan Africa. It was first recognised as a major disease in southern Africa after the introduction of exotic breeds. Its importance depends to a very large extent on the type of livestock present. There are very few reliable data about its importance in local breeds in endemic areas. However, there is no doubt that in endemic areas, indigenous cattle are far more resistant than exotic or cross-bred cattle, presumably because of natural selection. In contrast, small ruminants in general, and goats in particular, are not always very resistant. The name 'heartwater' was used because hydropericardium was regarded as a pathognomonic lesion of the disease. The disease is still also generally known as 'cowdriosis'.

Mycoplasma wenyonii

Mycoplasma wenyonii, synonym *Eperythrozoon wenyonii* (Phylum: Firmicutes; Class: Mollicutes; Order: Mycoplasmatales; Family: Mycoplasmataceae), is a bacterium distributed worldwide and

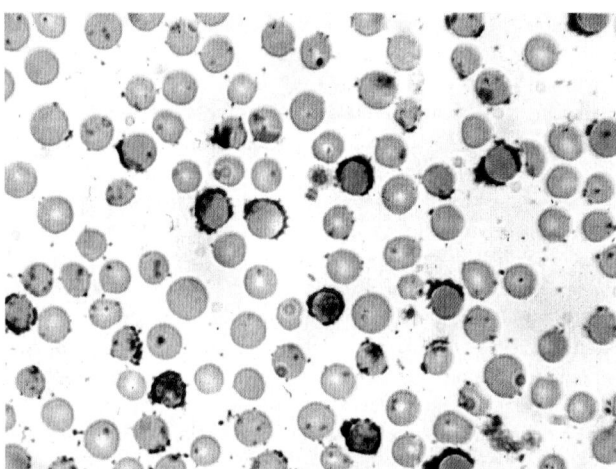

Fig. 8.20 *Mycoplasma wenyonii* on the surface of erythrocytes.

localised in the blood of cattle. Vectors are thought to be involved in transmission but precise details are not known.

Pathogenesis and clinical signs: Typically present on red cells, it produces mild and clinically inapparent infections in a variety of domestic animals throughout the world. *Mycoplasma wenyonii* is occasionally responsible for fever, anaemia and loss of weight.

Diagnosis: Identification of parasites from staining artefacts requires good blood smears and filtered Giemsa stain. They appear as cocci or short rods on the surface of the erythrocytes, often completely surrounding the margin of the red cell (Fig. 8.20). However, the organisms of *Mycoplasma* are relatively loosely attached to the red cell surface and are often found free in the plasma.

Control and treatment: Lack of detailed knowledge on the vectors limits any vector control measures. Susceptible to tetracyclines.

Notes: The taxonomy of this species is subject to much debate and there is a proposal to reclassify it into the bacterial genus *Mycoplasma* (class Mollicutes) based on 16S rRNA gene sequences and phylogenetic analysis.

Rickettsia conorii

Rickettsia conorii (Phylum: Proteobacteria; Class: Alphaproteobacteria; Order: Rickettsiales; Family: Rickettsiaceae) causes the commonly known Boutonneuse fever, Mediterranean spotted fever, Indian tick typhus or East African tick typhus, and is a bacterium distributed worldwide and localised in the blood of cattle. For more detailed descriptions on epidemiology, pathogenesis, control and treatment, see Chapter 12.

Parasites of the nervous system

Taenia multiceps

For more details see Chapter 12.

Thelazia rhodesi

Thelazia rhodesi (Phylum: Nematoda; Class: Chromadorea; Order: Spirurida; Family: Thelaziidae), commonly known as the Cattle eyeworm, is distributed worldwide and localised in the eye, conjunctival sac and lacrimal duct of cattle, buffalo, occasionally sheep, goat and camel. This parasite has muscid flies, particularly *Musca* spp. and *Fannia* spp., as intermediate hosts. Two other species of eyeworm (*T. gulosa* and *T. skrjabini*) are found in cattle. Details are essentially similar to *T. rhodesi*.

Epidemiology: *Thelazia* infections occur seasonally and are linked to periods of maximum fly activity. The parasite can survive in the eye for several years, but since it is only the young adult which is pathogenic, a reservoir of infection may persist in symptomless carrier cattle. Survival of larvae also occurs in the adult stages of flies, which are in diapause, during the winter.

Pathogenesis: Lesions are caused by the serrated cuticle of the worm and most damage results from movement by the active young adults causing lacrimation, followed by conjunctivitis. In heavy infections, the cornea may become cloudy and ulcerated. There is usually complete recovery in about two months, although in some cases areas of corneal opacity can persist. Infection may predispose to infectious keratoconjunctivitis ('pink eye') caused by *Moraxella*.

Clinical signs: Lacrimation, conjunctivitis and photophobia. Flies are usually clustered around the eye because of the excessive secretion. In severe cases, the whole cornea can be opaque and, without treatment, progressive keratitis and ulceration of the cornea may occur.

Pathology: Invasion of the lacrimal gland and ducts may cause inflammation and necrotic exudation leading to occlusion and reduced tear production. Mechanical irritation of the conjunctiva produces inflammation, while damage to the cornea leads to opacity, keratitis and corneal ulceration.

Diagnosis: The presence of a conjunctivitis that is coincident with the season of fly activity is an indication of possible infection. In some cases, the *Thelazia* worms may be seen on the surface of the conjunctiva or in the conjunctival sac. Sometimes eggs or larvae can be recovered from lacrimal secretions. It may be necessary to instil a few drops of local anaesthetic to facilitate manipulation of the third eyelid.

Control and treatment: Prevention is difficult because of the ubiquitous nature of the fly vectors. Fly control measures aimed at protecting the face, such as insecticide-impregnated ear tags, aid in the control of eyeworm infection. Treatment was at one time based on manual removal of the worms under a local anaesthetic, but this is now replaced by administering an effective anthelmintic such as levamisole or an avermectin; the former drug may be applied topically as a 1% aqueous solution.

Thelazia gulosa

Thelazia gulosa, synonym *Thelazia alfortensis* (Phylum: Nematoda; Class: Chromadorea; Order: Spirurida; Family: Thelaziidae), commonly known as the Cattle eyeworm, is probably distributed worldwide and localised in the eye, conjunctival sac and lacrimal duct of cattle.

Thelazia skrjabini

Thelazia skrjabini (Phylum: Nematoda; Class: Chromadorea; Order: Spirurida; Family: Thelaziidae), commonly known as the Cattle eyeworm, is localised in the eye, conjunctival sac and lacrimal duct of cattle and found in North America, parts of Asia and Europe.

Hypoderma bovis

For more details see Parasites of the integument.

Toxoplasma gondii

For more details see Parasites of the locomotory system.

Trypanosoma brucei brucei

For more details see Parasites of the circulatory system.

Parasites of the reproductive/ urogenital system

Stephanurus dentatus

Stephanurus dentatus (Phylum: Nematoda; Class: Chromadorea; Order: Rhabditida; Family: Syngamidae), commonly known as the Pig kidney worm, is localised in the kidney and perirenal fat of pigs, wild boar and rarely cattle, which may occasionally cause severe liver damage in calves grazing on contaminated ground. For a more detailed description see Chapter 11.

Tritrichomonas foetus

Tritrichomonas foetus, synonym *Trichomonas foetus* (Phylum: Metamonada; Class: Trichomonadea; Order: Trichomonadida; Family: Trichomonadidae), is distributed worldwide and localised in the prepuce and uterus of cattle.

Epidemiology: Bulls, once infected, remain so permanently. The organisms inhabit the preputial cavity and transmission to the cow occurs during coitus. From the vagina, the trichomonads reach the uterus via the cervix to produce a low-grade endometritis. Intermittently, organisms are flushed into the vagina, often 2–3 days before oestrus. Infection is usually followed by early abortion, the organisms being found in the amniotic and allantoic fluid. Subsequently, cows appear to 'self-cure' and, in most cases, appear to develop a sterile immunity.

Pathogenesis: In the bull, a preputial discharge associated with small nodules on the preputial and penile membranes may develop shortly after infection. Organisms are present in small numbers in the preputial cavity of bulls, with some concentration in the fornix and around the glans penis. The chronically infected bull shows no gross lesions.

In the cow, the initial lesion is a vaginitis, which can be followed in animals that become pregnant by invasion of the cervix and uterus. Various sequelae can result, including a placentitis leading to early abortion (1–16 weeks), uterine discharge and pyometra. Abortion before the fourth month of pregnancy is the most common sequela and this is normally followed by recovery. Occasionally, the developing fetal membranes are retained, leading to a purulent endometritis, persistent uterine discharge and anoestrus; infrequently the corpus luteum is retained and the cervical seal remains closed, when a massive pyometra develops which visually simulates the appearance of pregnancy. In some cases, despite infection, pregnancy is not terminated by abortion and a normal full-term calf is born.

Clinical signs: In the bull, there are no clinical signs once the infection is established. In the cow, early abortion is a characteristic feature although this is often undetected because of the small size of the fetus and the case may present as one of an irregular oestrous cycle. Other clinical signs are those of purulent endometritis or a closed pyometra and in these cases, the cow may become permanently sterile. On a herd basis, cows exhibit irregular oestrous cycles, uterine discharge, pyometra and early abortion. The cow usually recovers and generally becomes immune, at least for that breeding season, after infection or abortion.

Pathology: Infection in females causes cervicitis and endometritis leading to infertility, abortion or pyometra. The inflammatory changes in the endometrium and cervix are relatively mild and non-specific, although there may be a copious mucopurulent discharge. The exudates may be continuous or intermittent in their discharge, and the number and activity of the trichomonads can vary considerably. Abortions may occur at any time but mainly in the first half of pregnancy. There are no specific fetal lesions, but large numbers of protozoa may be found in the fetal fluids and stomach. The placenta may be covered by white or yellowish flocculent exudates in small amounts, and thickening and haemorrhage without necrosis may be evident on the cotyledons. Pyometra, when it develops, may be copious with watery exudates containing floccules which may be brownish and sticky and contain swarms of trichomonads.

Diagnosis: A tentative diagnosis of trichomoniasis is based on the clinical history, signs of early abortion, repeated returns to service or irregular oestrous cycles. Confirmation depends on the demonstration of organisms in placental fluid, stomach contents of the aborted fetus, uterine washings, pyometra discharge or vaginal mucus. Apart from a problem of infertility, which usually follows the purchase of a mature bull, confirmation of diagnosis depends on demonstration of the organism. Vaginal mucus collected from the anterior end of the vagina by suction into a sterile tube, or preputial washings from the bull, may be examined using a warm-stage microscope for the presence of organisms. The number of organisms varies in different situations. They are numerous in the aborted fetus, in the uterus several days after abortion and, in recently infected cows, they are plentiful in the vaginal mucus 12–20 days after infection. Thereafter, the number of organisms varies according to the phase of the oestrous cycle, being highest 3–7 days after ovulation. In the infected bull *T. foetus* organisms are present in highest numbers on the mucosa of the prepuce and penis, apparently not invading the submucosal tissues. It is generally recommended to allow one week after the last service before taking a preputial sample. Since the organism is often only present intermittently, the examination may need to be repeated several times. Under phase illumination, the number of flagella observed is an important characteristic as this can help to differentiate *T. foetus* from some bovine flagellates that appear similar. Organisms may be cultured *in vitro*, in Diamond's medium, Clausen's medium or *Trichomonas* medium, which is available commercially. A field culture test that allows for growth of the trichomonads and direct microscopic examination without aspiration of the inoculum has been developed in the USA (InPouch® TF). Alternatively, on a herd basis, samples of vaginal mucus may be examined in the laboratory for the presence of specific agglutinins against laboratory cultures of *T. foetus*.

Control and treatment: Artificial insemination from non-infected donors is the only entirely satisfactory method of control. If a return to natural service is contemplated, recovered cows should be disposed of since some may be carriers. Since the disease is self-limiting in the female, only symptomatic treatment and sexual rest for three months is normally necessary. In the bull, slaughter is the best policy, although dimetridazole orally or intravenously has been reported to be effective.

Notes: Normally one might expect the overall prevalence of trichomoniasis to be high, since it is venereally transmitted by bulls, which show no clinical signs. In fact, the advent of supervised schemes of artificial insemination has largely eradicated the disease, and today it is limited to areas where there are many small farms each with their own bulls or to countries where veterinary supervision is limited. In a few early studies, three serotypes were recognised based on agglutination: the '*Belfast*' strain reportedly predominated in Europe, Africa and the USA; the '*Brisbane*' strain in Australia; and the '*Manley*' strain, which has been reported in only a few outbreaks. A morphologically identical organism (*T. suis*) has been identified in pigs, in which it commonly causes asymptomatic infection of the nasal cavity, stomach and intestine (see Chapter 11). This organism is now considered synonymous with *T. foetus*. The organism has also been reported in cats to be associated with large bowel diarrhoea (see Chapter 12).

Neospora caninum

Neospora caninum (Phylum: Apicomplexa; Class: Conoidasida; Order: Eucoccidiorida; Family: Sarcocystidae) is distributed worldwide and localised in the blood of dogs, coyotes, wolves and dingoes. This parasite has cattle, sheep, goats, deer, horses, dogs, foxes, chickens and wild birds as intermediate hosts.

Epidemiology: The dog and other canids are the final host, and can also act as intermediate hosts in prenatal infections. In cattle, infection can be both vertically transmitted from dam to calf *in utero* and lactogenically and naturally transmitted by ingestion of food and water contaminated with dog faeces containing *Neospora caninum* oocysts. *Neospora caninum* is one of the most efficiently transplacentally transmitted parasites and in certain herds it has been found that virtually all calves born alive are infected but without symptoms of infection. Transmission from infected bulls is thought not to occur. The presence of birds on pasture has been correlated with higher infection rates in cattle and birds may be an important link in the transmission of *N. caninum* to other animals. In some countries, there appears to be an increase in abortion rates associated with mild wet seasons. Infections with other disease agents, such as bovine viral diarrhoea, leptospirosis and *Salmonella*, appear to increase the risk or recrudescence of latent infection and are likely to be associated with a higher risk of abortion in infected cows. It is possible for cattle that have previously aborted due to *Neospora* infection to have a repeat abortion, such that infected cows are more likely to abort than non-infected cows. Offspring born alive are likely to be infected themselves and go on to have a higher risk of abortion.

Pathogenesis: *Neospora caninum* is a major cause of abortion in both dairy and beef cattle. Cows of any age can abort from three months of gestation to full term, although most abortions occur at 5–6 months. Fetuses can be born alive or may die *in utero* and be mummified or reabsorbed. Calves that are infected may be born underweight, weak or with neurological symptoms such as ataxia, decreased reflexes and exophthalmia. Infection is thought to reduce milk production in adult dairy cows through its effects on fertility.

Clinical signs and pathology: The infection causes abortion, mummification, weak calves with ataxia, and exophthalmia. Tachyzoites and tissue cysts are found intracellularly in the CNS and retina of affected cattle. Although infection can be found in many organs, the most common site is the brain. Microscopic lesions of non-suppurative encephalitis and myocarditis may be seen in the brain, spinal cord and heart of aborted fetuses. Hepatitis can also be found in epidemic abortions.

Diagnosis: Diagnosis is based on histological examination of freshly aborted fetuses. The lesions in the heart and CNS are significantly characteristic for diagnosis but can be confirmed by immunocytochemistry. An ELISA is commercially available and can be used to test serum samples for *Neospora*-specific antibodies and several PCR-based tests have been reported. Bulk milk sampling can also be used but is generally only useful in herds where more than 10–20% of cows are infected.

Control: Control of *Neospora*-induced abortion in cattle depends on protecting food and water sources from possible contamination with the faeces of any animal and the disposal of aborted fetuses and placentas by incineration. The lack of complete knowledge of both the life cycle and the range of definitive hosts has limited effective control measures but there is a strong argument for the culling of seropositive animals from a herd. Seropositive animals have been shown to suffer a higher risk of abortion than seronegative animals in the herd. Dogs should not be allowed to eat aborted fetuses or fetal membranes, and their faeces should be prevented from contaminating bovine feedstuffs. Where *Neospora* has not previously been isolated in a herd, there are several measures which can be taken to reduce the risk of the disease entering the herd.

- Quarantine and testing of all replacements before entry to the herd to ensure freedom from infection.
- Preventing transmission by keeping dogs away from foodstuffs, and ensuring that dogs have no access to either placentas or aborted fetuses.
- Reducing the risk of water-borne transmission by using a mains water supply and avoiding cattle drinking from stagnant water such as ponds.
- Maintaining good rodent control as some studies have implicated rodents in the spread of disease.

In herds where *Neospora* is present, further methods can be used to reduce the risk of animals aborting.

- Testing and culling: *N. caninum*-infected cows should be considered a reservoir of infection with the potential to transmit the infection to other cows. This can occur either by giving birth to live infected offspring or by environmental contamination.

Although this method of control is effective, it is not always economically realistic. It can be applied as follows:

- test and cull either seropositive or seropositive aborting cows
- test and inseminate seropositive cows with beef semen only; or
- test and exclude the progeny of seropositive cows from breeding.

If testing of cows is carried out and cattle are culled on the basis of these results, it is important to ensure that steps are also taken to prevent infection from the environment. A commercial vaccine (Bovilis® Neoguard) was developed to reduce abortion in pregnant cattle resulting from infection with *N. caninum* and was available in the USA, New Zealand and some other countries. This vaccine comprised inactivated whole tachyzoites and inoculation aimed to reduce the transmission of the parasite to the developing fetus. However, the vaccine has been withdrawn from the market by the manufacturer. There is no effective treatment in cattle.

Trypanosoma brucei brucei

For more details see Parasites of the circulatory system.

Parasites of the locomotory system

Taenia saginata

Taenia saginata, synonym *Taeniarhynchus saginata* (Phylum: Platyhelminthes; Class: Cestoda; Order: Cyclophyllidea; Family: Taeniidae), commonly known as the Beef tapeworm, causes a disease named beef measles and is distributed worldwide and localised in the small intestine of humans. The intermediate stage of the parasite (named *Cysticercus bovis*) has cattle, sheep, goats, deer, horses, dogs, foxes, chickens and wild birds as intermediate hosts, where it is localised in muscle, liver and kidney, posing economic problems to the meat industry and a public health hazard.

Epidemiology: There are two quite distinct epidemiological patterns found in developing countries and developed countries respectively.

- Developing countries. In many parts of Africa, Asia and Latin America, cattle are reared on an extensive scale, human sanitation is poorly developed and cooking fuel is expensive. In these circumstances the incidence of human infection with *T. saginata* is high, in certain areas being well over 20%. Because of this, calves are usually infected in early life, often within the first few days after birth, from infected stockmen whose hands are contaminated with *Taenia* eggs. Prenatal infection of calves may also occur but is rare. Of the cysts which develop, a proportion persist for years even though the host has developed an acquired immunity and is completely resistant to further infection. Based on routine carcass inspection, the infection rate is often around 30–60%, although the real prevalence is considerably higher.
- Developed countries. In areas such as Europe, North America, Australia and New Zealand, the standards of sanitation are high and meat is carefully inspected and generally thoroughly cooked before consumption. In such countries, the prevalence of cysticercosis is low, being less than 1% of carcasses inspected. Occasionally, however, a cysticercosis 'storm', where a high proportion of cattle are infected, has been reported on particular

farms. In Britain and Australia, this has been associated with the use of human sewage on pasture as a fertiliser in the form of sludge, i.e. sedimented or bacterial-digested faeces. Since *T. saginata* eggs may survive for more than 200 days in sludge, the occurrence of these 'storms' is perhaps not surprising. Other causes of a sudden high incidence of infection on particular farms are due to a tapeworm infection in a stockman occurring either as a random event or, as has been reported from feedlots in some of the southern states of the USA, as a result of the use of migrant labour from a country with a high prevalence of infection. As distinct from these 'storms', the cause of the low but persistent prevalence of infection in cattle is obscure, but is thought to be due to the access of cattle to water contaminated with sewage effluents, to the carriage and dispersal of *T. saginata* eggs by birds which frequent sewage works or feed on effluent discharged into rivers or the sea, and to occasional fouling of pasture by itinerant infected individuals. In contrast to the epidemiology in developing countries, cattle of any age are susceptible to infection since they generally possess no acquired immunity. There is also evidence that when cattle are first infected as adults, the longevity of the cysticerci is limited, most being dead within nine months.

Pathogenesis: Although *C. bovis* may occur anywhere in the striated muscles, the predilection sites, at least from the viewpoint of routine meat inspection, are the heart, tongue and masseter and intercostal muscles (Fig. 8.21). Under natural conditions the presence of cysticerci in the muscles of cattle is not associated with clinical signs although, experimentally, calves given massive infections of *T. saginata* eggs have developed severe myocarditis and heart failure associated with developing cysticerci in the heart.

Clinical signs and pathology: In humans, the adult tapeworm may produce diarrhoea and hunger pains, but the infection is usually asymptomatic and is mainly objectionable on aesthetic grounds. Cysticerci start to degenerate 4–6 months after infection and by nine months a substantial number may be dead. With light infections, cysticerci may remain viable for two years or more.

Diagnosis: Individual countries have different regulations regarding the inspection of carcasses, but invariably the masseter muscle, tongue and heart are incised and examined and the intercostal muscles and diaphragm inspected; the triceps muscle is also incised in many countries. The inspection is inevitably a compromise between detection of cysticerci and preservation of the economic value of

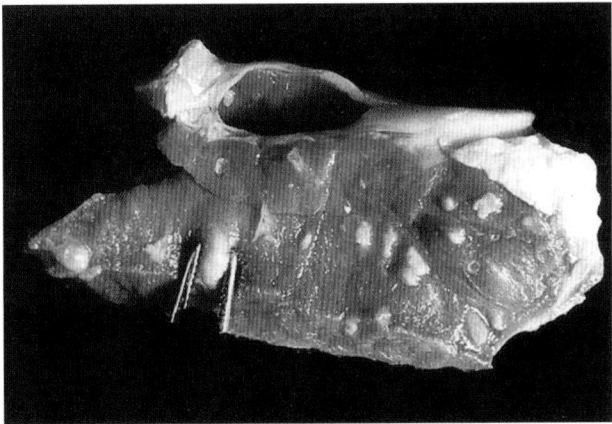

Fig. 8.21 *Cysticercus bovis* in skeletal muscle.

Table 8.7 *Sarcocystis* species found in the muscles of cattle.

Species	Synonym	Definitive host	Pathogenicity (cattle)	Pathogenicity (final host)
Sarcocystis bovicanis	*Sarcocystis cruzi, Sarcocystis fusiformis*	Dogs, coyotes, wolves	+++	0
Sarcocystis bovifelis	*Sarcocystis hirsuto*	Cats	0	0
Sarcocystis bovihominis	*Sarcocystis hominis*	Humans, primates	0	+

0, non-pathogenic; +, mildly pathogenic; +++, severe pathogenicity.

the carcass. Immunoserology has some usefulness for screening infected herds. In humans, the presence of tapeworms is recognised by the passage of proglottids and/or eggs in faeces.

Control and treatment: In developed countries, the control of bovine cysticercosis depends on a high standard of human sanitation, on the general practice of cooking meat thoroughly (the thermal death point of cysticerci is 57 °C) and on compulsory meat inspection. Regulations usually require that infected carcasses are frozen at –10 °C for at least 10 days, which is sufficient to kill the cysticerci although the process reduces the economic value of the meat. Where relatively heavy infections of more than 25 cysticerci are detected, it is usual to destroy the carcass. In agricultural practice, the use of human sludge as a fertiliser should be confined to cultivated fields or those on which cattle will not be grazed for at least two years. In developing countries, the same measures are necessary but are not always economically feasible, and at present the most useful step would appear to be the education of communities in both sanitary hygiene and the thorough cooking of meat. As yet, there is no licensed drug available that will effectively destroy all the cysticerci in the muscle, although praziquantel has shown efficacy in experimental situations.

Onchocerca dukei

Onchocerca dukei (Phylum: Nematoda; Class: Chromadorea; Order: Spirurida; Family: Onchocercidae) is localised in the muscle connective tissue of cattle and is found in Africa. This parasite probably has blackflies (*Simulium*) as intermediate hosts. The infection is asymptomatic and control and treatment are not required.

Epidemiology and pathogenesis: The incidence of infection can be very high in endemic areas, though the parasite is rarely detected. *Onchocerca dukei* is of little clinical or economic importance. Losses may occur by condemnation of localised areas at meat inspection caused by nodular damage.

Diagnosis: Diagnosis is often made at meat inspection. Nodules are found particularly in the thorax and abdomen and may need to be differentiated from *Cysticercus bovis*. Microfilariae may be identified after soaking skin biopsy specimens in physiological saline for 12 hours and staining with Giemsa.

Sarcocystiosis

The previously complex nomenclature for the large number of *Sarcocystis* spp. has largely been discarded by many workers in favour of a new system based on their biology. The new names generally incorporate those of the **intermediate** and **final hosts** in that order. Although unacceptable to systematists, this practice has

the virtue of simplicity. The three species of *Sarcocystis* reported in cattle are summarised in Table 8.7 and described below. Further details are given in Chapter 2.

Epidemiology: Little is known of the epidemiology, but from the high prevalence of symptomless infections observed in abattoirs, it is clear that where dogs or cats are kept in close association with farm animals or their feed, then transmission is likely. Sheepdogs are known to play an important part in the transmission of *S. bovicanis* and farm cats in the transmission of *S. bovifelis* so care should be exercised that only cooked meat is fed to dogs or cats. Acute outbreaks are probably most likely when livestock, which have been reared without dog or cat contact, are subsequently exposed to large numbers of the sporocysts from dog or cat faeces. The longevity of the sporocysts shed in the faeces is not known.

Diagnosis: Most cases of *Sarcocystis* infection are only diagnosed at meat inspection when the grossly visible sarcocysts in the muscle are discovered. However, in heavy infections of cattle, diagnosis is based on the clinical signs and histological demonstration of meronts in the blood vessels of organs such as kidney or heart and the presence of cysts in the muscles at necropsy or biopsy. An indirect haemagglutination test, using bradyzoites as antigen, is also a useful aid to diagnosis; however, the presence of a titre need not imply active lesions of *Sarcocystis*. Also, animals may die prior to a detectable humoral response. In cattle, the degenerative muscle changes closely resemble those of vitamin E/selenium deficiency, although the latter lacks an inflammatory cellular response. Examination of faeces from dogs or cats on the farm for the presence of sporocysts may be helpful in the diagnosis.

Control and treatment: The only control measures possible are those of simple hygiene. Farm dogs and cats should not be housed in, or allowed access to, fodder stores nor should they be allowed to defecate in pens where livestock are housed. It is also important that they are not fed uncooked meat. There is no effective treatment for infection, in either the final or the intermediate host. Where an outbreak occurs in cattle, it has been suggested that the introduction of amprolium (100 mg/kg *per os*, daily over 30 days) into the diet of the animals has a prophylactic effect.

Sarcocystis bovicanis

Sarcocystis bovicanis, synonyms *Sarcocystis cruzi, Sarcocystis fusiformis* (Phylum: Apicomplexa; Class: Conoidasida; Order: Eucoccidiorida; Family: Sarcocystidae), is distributed worldwide and localised in the muscle of dogs, foxes, wolves and coyotes. This parasite has cattle as intermediate hosts.

Pathogenesis: Infection in the final host is normally non-pathogenic, although mild diarrhoea has occasionally been reported. The principal pathogenic effect is attributable to the second stage of merogony in the vascular endothelium. Heavy experimental infections of calves with *S. bovicanis* have resulted in mortality one month later, with necropsy showing petechial haemorrhages in almost every organ, including the heart, together with generalised lymphadenopathy. Experimental infection of adult cows has resulted in abortion. A naturally occurring chronic disease of cattle, Dalmeny disease, has been recognised in Canada, the USA and Britain. This is characterised by emaciation, submandibular oedema, recumbency and exophthalmia; at *post mortem* examination, numerous meronts are found in endothelial cells, and developing sarcocysts in areas of degenerative myositis.

Clinical signs: In heavy infections there is anorexia, fever, anaemia, loss of weight, a disinclination to move and sometimes recumbency. In cattle, there is often a marked loss of hair at the end of the tail. These signs may be accompanied by submandibular oedema, exophthalmia and enlargement of lymph nodes. Abortions may occur in breeding stock.

Pathology: Meronts present in endothelial cells of capillaries in various organs lead to endothelial cell destruction. As the organisms enter muscle, a wide range of change may be encountered. Microscopic inspection of *Sarcocystis*-infected muscle often reveals occasional degenerate parasitic cysts surrounded by variable numbers of inflammatory cells (very few of which are eosinophils) or, at a later stage, macrophages and granulation tissue. Usually there is no muscle fibre degeneration, but there may be thin linear collections of lymphocytes between fibres in the region. The extent of muscle change bears little relationship to the numbers of developing cysts, but generally very low numbers of *Sarcocystis* produce no reaction. As cysts mature, the cyst capsule within the enlarged muscle fibre becomes thicker and more clearly differentiated from the muscle sarcoplasm.

Sarcocystis bovifelis

Sarcocystis bovifelis, synonym *Sarcocystis hirsuta* (Phylum: Apicomplexa; Class: Conoidasida; Order: Eucoccidiorida; Family: Sarcocystidae), is distributed worldwide and localised in the muscle of cats. This parasite has cattle as intermediate hosts.

Pathogenesis: Infections are generally non-pathogenic; any pathogenic effect is attributable to the second stage of merogony in the vascular endothelium.

Clinical signs and pathology: Infections are usually asymptomatic. Heavy infections may occasionally produce anorexia, fever, diarrhoea, anaemia and weight loss. In cattle, the tissue cysts may be visible to the naked eye especially in the oesophagus but are more likely to be detected on histopathology (Fig. 8.22).

Sarcocystis bovihominis

Sarcocystis bovihominis, synonym *Sarcocystis hominis* (Phylum: Apicomplexa; Class: Conoidasida; Order: Eucoccidiorida; Family: Sarcocystidae), is distributed worldwide and localised in the muscle of humans and non-human primates. This parasite has cattle as intermediate hosts and is only slightly pathogenic for calves, if at all.

Clinical signs and pathology: Infection is usually asymptomatic in calves. Sarcocysts are present in striated muscle. Usually there is no

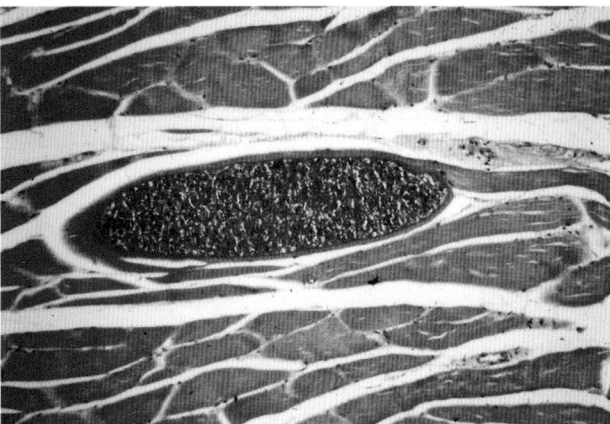
Fig. 8.22 *Sarcocystis bovifelis* in oesophageal muscle.

muscle fibre degeneration, but there may be thin linear collections of lymphocytes between fibres in the region.

Toxoplasma gondii

Toxoplasma gondii (Phylum: Apicomplexa; Class: Conoidasida; Order: Eucoccidiorida; Family: Sarcocystidae) is distributed worldwide and is localised in the muscle, lungs, liver, reproductive system and CNS of cats and other felids. This parasite has any mammal, including humans, and birds as intermediate hosts. In addition, the final host may also be an intermediate host and harbour extraintestinal stages. For more detailed description see Chapter 9.

Epidemiology: The cat plays a central role in the epidemiology of toxoplasmosis and the disease is virtually absent from areas where cats do not occur. Compared with sheep, toxoplasmosis in cattle is relatively uncommon and rarely causes clinical signs.

Pathogenesis: Most *Toxoplasma* infections in cattle are light and consequently asymptomatic. Infections are usually acquired via the digestive tract, and so organisms are disseminated by the lymphatics and portal system with subsequent invasion of various organs and tissues. Pathogenic effects are always related to the extraintestinal phase of development. In heavy infections, the multiplying tachyzoites may produce areas of necrosis in vital organs such as the myocardium, lungs, liver and brain, and during this phase the host can become pyrexic and lymphadenopathy occurs. As the disease progresses bradyzoites are formed, with this chronic phase being usually asymptomatic.

Clinical signs and pathology: There are only a few reports of clinical toxoplasmosis associated with fever, dyspnoea, nervous signs and abortion in cattle. In heavy infections, the multiplying tachyzoites may produce areas of necrosis in vital organs such as the myocardium, lungs, liver and brain.

Control and treatment: Control on farms is more difficult, but where possible animal feedstuffs should be covered to exclude access by cats. No treatment is indicated.

Trypanosoma brucei brucei

For more details see Parasites of the circulatory system.

Parasites of the connective tissue

Several species of *Onchocerca* are found in the connective tissue of cattle and are summarised in Table 8.8.

Onchocerca gutturosa

Onchocerca gutturosa, synonym *Onchocerca lienalis* (Phylum: Nematoda; Class: Chromadorea; Order: Spirurida; Family: Onchocercidae), causes a disease commonly known as Ligamentary onchocercosis, and is distributed worldwide and localised in the connective tissue, ligamentum nuchae and gastrosplenic ligament of cattle. In Australia and North America, the parasite *Onchocerca lienalis* (considered to be synonymous) is found in the gastrosplenic ligament. This parasite has blackflies (*Simulium*) as intermediate hosts and is of little clinical or economic importance. The incidence of infection can be very high in endemic areas, although the parasite is rarely detected.

Species of *Onchocerca* spp. causing bovine onchocercosis are listed in Table 8.8.

Clinical signs and pathology: Infection in cattle is asymptomatic. Adult worms, which are found in pairs, are most frequently located in the ligamentum nuchae adjacent to the thoracic spines and less frequently in the connective tissue on the scapula, humerus and femur. The worms do not stimulate nodule formation but lie loose in the connective tissue and cause no disease or reaction.

Diagnosis: Diagnosis is rarely called for and depends on the finding of microfilariae in skin biopsy samples taken from affected areas (Fig. 8.23). The microfilariae are concentrated in the preferred feeding sites of the vectors, which are the back, ears and neck. The piece of skin is placed in warm saline and teased to allow emergence of the microfilariae, and is then incubated for about 8–12 hours. The microfilariae are readily recognised by their sinuous movements in a centrifuged sample of the saline. Another option is to scarify the skin of a predilection site and examine the fluid exudate for microfilariae.

Control and treatment: With the ubiquity of the insect vectors, there is little possibility of efficient control, though the use of microfilaricides will reduce the numbers of infected flies. In any case, with the relatively innocuous nature of the infection there is unlikely to be any demand for control. No treatment is required.

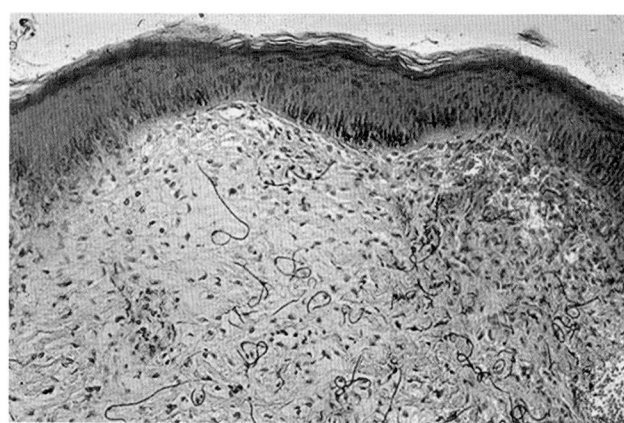

Fig. 8.23 Microfilariae of *Onchocerca gutturosa* in subdermal connective tissue of the back.

Onchocerca gibsoni

Onchocerca gibsoni (Phylum: Nematoda; Class: Chromadorea; Order: Spirurida; Family: Onchocercidae) is localised in the connective tissue of cattle and is found in Africa, Asia and Australasia. This parasite has midges (*Culicoides*) as intermediate hosts. The incidence of infection can be very high in endemic areas.

Pathogenesis: Worms occur in groups ('worm nests') and provoke a fibrous reaction around the coiled worms in muscle tissue (nodules can measure up to 5 cm in diameter). The nodules are often in the brisket and can be responsible for economic loss due to carcass trimming.

Clinical signs and pathology: Affected animals are not clinically ill and show no presenting signs other than subcutaneous nodules at the predilections sites. A nodule forms around the worms with the head becoming fixed and surrounded by fibroblasts. Successive portions of the worm are drawn into the nodule, where they eventually lie coiled up and surrounded by a fibrous tissue capsule, which increases in thickness as the lesion grows older. In older nodules, degeneration of the tissues and calcification of the worms frequently take place. The capsule consists of dense fibrous tissue containing blood vessels, leucocytes and lymph spaces. Microfilariae are common and wander in the lymph spaces. Their presence may lead to thickening of the dermis.

Diagnosis: In active lesions, the presence of worms is readily established on section of the subcutaneous nodules. Microfilariae may also be found in skin biopsy samples taken from affected areas with

Table 8.8 Bovine onchocercosis.

Species	Site	Distribution	Vector	Significance
Onchocerca gutturosa (synonym *Onchocerca lienalis*)	Ligamentum nuchae and other parts of the body	Most parts of the world	*Simulium* spp.	No economic significance
	Gastrosplenic ligaments	Many parts of the world	*Simulium* spp.	No economic significance
Onchocerca gibsoni	Subcutaneous and intermuscular nodules	Africa, Asia, Australasia	*Culicoides* spp.	Carcass trimming
Onchocerca ochengi (synonym *Onchocerca dermata*)	Scrotum, udder, connective tissue	East and West Africa	Unknown	Blemished hides
Onchocerca armillata	Wall of thoracic aorta	Middle East, Africa, India	*Culicoides, Simulium*	No economic significance
Onchocerca dukei	Abdomen, thorax, thighs	West Africa	Unknown *Simulium*?	Confused with *Cysticercus bovis* at meat inspection
Onchocerca cebei (synonym *Onchocerca sweetae*)	Abdomen, thorax, thighs	Far East, Australia	*Culicoides* spp.	Blemished hides

subcutaneous lymph spaces. The microfilariae are concentrated in the preferred feeding sites of the vectors, which for *Culicoides* spp. are usually the shaded lower parts of the trunk, and it is usually recommended that samples be taken from the region of the linea alba. The piece of skin is placed in warm saline and teased to allow emergence of the microfilariae, and is then incubated for about 8–12 hours. The microfilariae are readily recognised by their sinuous movements in a centrifuged sample of the saline. Another option is to scarify the skin of a predilection site and examine the fluid exudate for microfilariae.

Control and treatment: With the ubiquity of the insect vectors, there is little possibility of efficient control, though insect repellents will help reduce insect attack. In any case, with the relatively innocuous nature of the infection there is unlikely to be any demand for control. In the past, treatment has consisted of daily administration of diethylcarbamazine over a period as a microfilaricide, but it now appears that a single dose of ivermectin is highly efficient in this respect, although the dying microfilariae may provoke local tissue reactions. Affected carcasses must be trimmed to remove the nodules.

Onchocerca ochengi

Onchocerca ochengi, synonym *Onchocerca dermatan* (Phylum: Nematoda; Class: Chromadorea; Order: Spirurida; Family: Onchocercidae), is localised in the connective tissue, scrotum and udder of cattle and found in parts of East and West Africa. The intermediate hosts of this parasite are unknown. The incidence of infection can be very high in endemic areas and diagnosis, control and treatment are as for *O. gibsoni*.

Clinical signs and pathology: *Onchocerca ochengi* in the skin causes some economic loss from blemished hides. Affected animals are not clinically ill and show no presenting signs other than subcutaneous nodules at the predilection sites. No pathology is reported.

Parafilaria bovicola

Parafilaria bovicola (Phylum: Nematoda; Class: Chromadorea; Order: Spirurida; Family: Filariidae) causes a disease commonly known as Summer bleeding disease or Verminous nodules, and is localised in the subcutaneous and intermuscular connective tissue of cattle and buffalo. The infection is found in Africa, Asia, southern Europe and Sweden. Muscid flies (*Musca autumnalis* in Europe) act as intermediate hosts of this parasite.

Epidemiology: In Europe, bovine parafilariosis occurs in spring and summer, disappearing in winter, whereas in tropical areas it is seen mainly after the rainy season. A high prevalence of 36% in cattle has been reported from some endemic areas in South Africa and the disease is now present in Sweden, an area previously free from infection. *Parafilaria* infection may be introduced by the importation of cattle from endemic areas, but its spread will depend on the presence of specific fly vectors. It has been estimated in Sweden that one 'bleeding' cow will act as a source of infection for three other animals.

Pathogenesis: Adult worms in the subcutaneous connective tissue induce small inflammatory lesions and haemorrhagic nodules, usually in the upper body regions. When the gravid female punctures the skin to lay her eggs, there is a haemorrhagic exudate or 'bleeding point' which streaks and mats the surrounding hairs and attracts flies. Individual lesions only bleed for a short time and healing is rapid. There is some evidence that exposure to sunlight is required to initiate bleeding of the nodules. At the sites of infection, which are predominantly on the shoulders, withers and thoracic areas, there is inflammation and oedema which, at meat inspection, resemble subcutaneous bruising in early lesions and have a gelatinous greenish-yellow appearance with a metallic odour in longer-standing cases. Sometimes the lesions extend into the intermuscular fascia. The affected areas have to be trimmed at marketing and further economic loss is incurred by rejection or downgrading of the hides.

Clinical signs and pathology: The signs of parafilariosis, such as 'bleeding points' during the warmer seasons, are pathognomonic. Active bleeding lesions are seen most commonly in warm weather, an apparent adaptation to coincide with the presence of the fly intermediate host. The haemorrhagic exudate often streaks the hair and may lead to focal matting. Nodules formed in the cutaneous and intermuscular connective tissue are 1–2 cm in diameter, enlarge in the summer months, burst open and haemorrhage and heal with scarring.

Diagnosis: This is normally based on clinical signs but if laboratory confirmation is required, the small embryonated eggs or microfilariae may be found on examination of fresh exudate from bleeding points. The demonstration of eosinophils in smears taken from lesions is also considered a constant diagnostic feature. Serodiagnosis using an ELISA technique has been developed.

Control: This is difficult because of the long prepatent period during which drugs are thought not to be effective. In Sweden, dairy cattle and particularly heifers at pasture are the main source of infection for *M. autumnalis*, which is an outdoor fly, active in spring and summer. However, infections in young beef cattle are the chief cause of economic loss through carcass damage. Since neither ivermectin nor nitroxynil is effective against immature worms, treatment is only useful for patent infections recognisable by the clinical signs. However, because of restrictions on the use of ivermectin and nitroxynil in lactating cows, these are rarely treated and instead are kept indoors during the period of fly activity. In endemic areas, young beef cattle may be treated with an anthelmintic some time before slaughter as described above. In Sweden, the use of insecticide-impregnated ear tags has been recommended for vector control.

Treatment: Patent infections in beef and non-lactating dairy cattle may be treated with ivermectin, moxidectin or nitroxynil. The former two drugs are given parenterally as a single dose, whereas two doses of nitroxynil are required at an interval of three days. None of these drugs is licensed for use in lactating cattle, when the less effective levamisole may be tried. These drugs produce a marked reduction in bleeding points and, due to resolution of the muscle lesions, a significant reduction in meat condemnation if slaughter is delayed for 70 days after treatment.

Notes: The adults of this genus of primitive filarioids live under the skin where they produce inflammatory lesions or nodules and, during egg laying, haemorrhagic exudates or 'bleeding points' on the skin surface.

Setaria labiato-papillosa

Setaria labiato-papillosa, synonyms *Setaria cervi*, *Setaria altaica*, *Setaria digitata* (Phylum: Nematoda; Class: Chromadorea; Order: Spirurida; Family: Onchocercidae), causes a disease commonly known as Bovine abdominal filariosis, is distributed worldwide and is localised in the peritoneum and pleural cavity of cattle, buffalo, bison, yaks, various deer and antelopes and rarely sheep. This parasite has mosquitoes (*Aedes* and *Culex*) as intermediate hosts.

Epidemiology: Since the worms are usually innocuous, their epidemiology has received little study. The prevalence is higher in warmer countries, where there is longer seasonal activity of the mosquito vectors.

Pathogenesis: The worms in their normal site are usually harmless, occasionally inducing a mild fibrinous peritonitis, and are only discovered at necropsy. *Setaria labiato-papillosa* may have an erratic migration in sheep and goats and enter the spinal canal, causing cerebrospinal setariosis ('lumbar paralysis'), which is irreversible and often fatal; the condition has only been reported in the Middle and Far East.

Clinical signs: There are no clinical signs when the worms are in their normal site, but when nervous tissue is involved there is locomotor disturbance, usually of the hindlimbs, and if the parasites are high in the spinal canal, there may be paraplegia.

Pathology: A mild fibrinous peritonitis may be found on *post mortem*. Migrating larvae affecting the CNS may cause areas of damage seen as brown foci or streaks grossly. The lesions show microcavitation and variable haemorrhage. There is loss of myelin and fragmentation of axons locally with eosinophils, neutrophils and macrophages present along with mild meningitis and vascular cuffing.

Diagnosis: Infection with the adult worms is only accidentally discovered in the living animal by the finding of microfilariae in routine blood smears. In cases of cerebrospinal nematodosis, confirmatory diagnosis is only possible by microscopic examination of the spinal cord, since the parasites exist only as larval forms in their aberrant site.

Control and treatment: This would depend on control of the mosquito vectors, which is unlikely to be applied specifically for this parasite. There is no treatment for setarial paralysis.

Notes: *Setaria labiato-papillosa* has often been referred to as *S. cervi*, although the latter species is considered a parasite of axis deer (*Cervus axis*). The parasite is also considered to be identical to *S. digitatus*, although some consider the latter to be a valid and distinct species.

Setaria digitatus

Setaria digitatus (Phylum: Nematoda; Class: Chromadorea; Order: Spirurida; Family: Onchocercidae) causes a disease commonly known as Kumri and is localised in the peritoneum and pleural cavity of cattle and buffaloes and diffused in Asia. This parasite has mosquitoes (*Armigeres*, *Aedes*, *Anopheles*, *Culex*) as intermediate hosts. Details on the life cycle, epidemiology, control and treatment are as for *S. labiato-papillosa*.

Pathogenesis: The parasites inhabit the thoracic and peritoneal cavities, causing little harm. Immature forms have been reported in the CNS of sheep, goats and horses causing epizootic cerebrospinal nematodosis. Affected animals suffer acute focal encephalomyelomalacia, which causes acute or subacute tetraplegia or paraplegia of the hindlimbs.

Clinical signs and pathology: In aberrant hosts, migrating larvae affecting the CNS may cause areas of damage seen as brown foci or streaks grossly. Acute malacia occurs along the track of the worm such that the lesions show microcavitation and variable haemorrhage. There is loss of myelin and fragmentation of axons locally with eosinophils, neutrophils and macrophages present along with a mild meningitis and vascular cuffing.

Parasites of the integument

Stephanofilaria stilesi

Stephanofilaria stilesi (Phylum: Nematoda; Class: Chromadorea; Order: Spirurida; Family: Filariidae) is localised in the skin of cattle. This parasite has horn flies (*Haematobia irritans* and *H. titillans*) as intermediate hosts and is found in the USA, Japan and Commonwealth of Independent States (CIS).

Epidemiology: In endemic areas the incidence of infection may be as high as 90% and occurrence is to a great extent influenced by the type of herbage. Succulent grazing produces soft moist faeces, which are more suitable breeding sites for the flies than the hard crumbly faeces deposited on sparse dry grazing. Hence, irrigation of pasture may result in an increase in stephanofilariosis. Although the lesions subside in cooler weather, the damage to the hide is permanent and may result in considerable economic loss. Milk yield may be severely diminished from the pain of the lesions and the irritation of cattle by the flies.

Pathogenesis: Lesions begin to appear within two weeks of infection. In this species, the lesions are usually localised to the preferred biting areas of the vectors on the lower abdomen, commonly along the midventral line between the brisket and navel, but also on the udder, scrotum, flanks and ears. The flies feed predominantly along the midventral line of the host and their bites create lesions that permit microfilariae to invade the skin. These lesions are attractive to both species of horn flies as well as non-biting muscids. Adult nematodes occur in the dermis and microfilariae in the dermal papillae of lesions but not in adjacent healthy tissue.

Clinical signs: In endemic regions, granulomatous and ulcerative lesions may be seen on the skin, particularly in the midventral line between the brisket and navel (Fig. 8.24). The dermatitis can be exudative and haemorrhagic.

Pathology: The skin is at first nodular, but later there is papular eruption with an exudate of blood and pus. In the centre of the lesion, there may be sloughing of the skin, but at the margin there is often hyperkeratosis and alopecia. The condition is essentially an exudative, often haemorrhagic, dermatitis that attracts the fly vectors. Sometimes the lesions are exacerbated by secondary bacterial infection.

Diagnosis: Though adult worms and microfilariae are present in the lesions, they are often scarce and many scrapings prove negative.

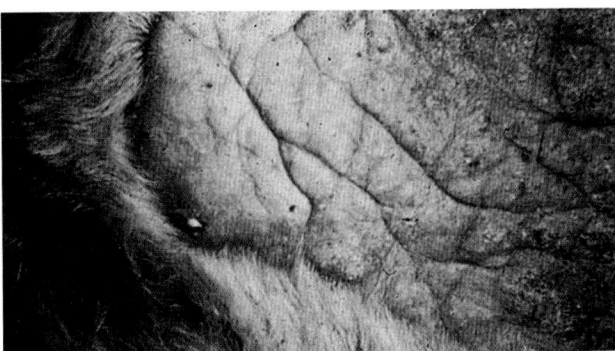

Fig. 8.24 Granulomatous skin on the lower abdomen associated with *Stephanofilaria stilesi*.

Diagnosis is therefore usually presumptive in endemic areas, and is based on the appearance and site of the lesions. Deep skin scrapings macerated in saline will release microfilariae and adult worms. Biopsy sections readily reveal microfilariae and adults.

Control and treatment: Control of horn flies is feasible by the proper handling of manure and the use of insecticides. Macrocyclic lactones applied topically give reported protection against horn flies for periods of up to five weeks. Organophosphate compounds, such as trichlorphon, applied topically as an ointment have proved effective. Levamisole at 9–12 mg/kg by injection followed by daily application of zinc oxide ointment has also been reported as effective. Avermectins have reported activity against larval stages but have no appreciable effect against adult stages.

Stephanofilaria dedoesi

Stephanofilaria dedoesi (Phylum: Nematoda; Class: Chromadorea; Order: Spirurida; Family: Filariidae) is localised in the skin of cattle, in Indonesia.

Clinical signs: Lesions occur mainly on the head, legs and teats of cattle. The dermatitis can be exudative and haemorrhagic. Other filarial species have been reported in cattle and buffalo in India and parts of Asia. The identification of individual species is beyond the scope of this book and interested readers will need to consult a relevant taxonomic specialist.

Parafilaria bovicola

For more details see Parasites of connective tissue.

Dracunculus medinensis

Dracunculus medinensis (Phylum: Nematoda; Class: Chromadorea; Order: Spirurida; Family: Dracunculidae), commonly known as the Guinea worm or Medina worm, is localised in the subcutaneous connective tissue of human and occasionally cattle, horses, dogs, cats and other mammals and is found in Africa, the Middle East and parts of Asia. This parasite has copepod crustaceans (*Cyclops* spp.) as intermediate hosts. A major global eradication programme has reduced the incidence and importance of *D. medinensis*.

Pathogenesis: Following initial infection there are virtually no signs of disease until the gravid adult female emerges in the subcutaneous tissues of the extremities. Pathogenesis is associated with the cutaneous ulcer formation.

Clinical signs and pathology: The migration of the worm to the surface of the skin may induce pruritus and urticaria and a blister on an extremity. Secondary bacterial infection of the ulcer lesion or degeneration of worms can cause marked abscessation. Symptoms of dracunculosis are pathognomonic.

Control and treatment: This is best achieved through the provision of clean drinking water or water that has been adequately sieved to remove any copepods. The worm may be gradually removed through the lesion by winding it round a small stick at a rate of about 2 cm each day or it may be surgically excised. Treatment with thiabendazole or niridazole, administered over several days, might be effective. Ivermectin or albendazole may be useful but efficacy data are lacking.

Besnoitia besnoiti

Besnoitia besnoiti, synonym *Sarcocystis besnoiti* (Phylum: Apicomplexa; Class: Conoidasida; Order: Eucoccidiorida; Family: Sarcocystidae), is a parasite that is distributed worldwide and localised in the skin and conjunctiva of cats and wild cats (lions, cheetahs, leopards). This parasite has cattle, goats and wild ruminants (wildebeest, impala, kudu) as intermediate hosts and is particularly important in tropical and subtropical countries, especially Africa.

Epidemiology: Although infection of cattle is thought to be mainly by ingestion of sporulated oocysts from cat faeces, there is a suggestion that mechanical spread by biting flies feeding on skin lesions of cattle may be another route of transmission.

Pathogenesis: Following infection in cattle, there is a systemic phase accompanied by lymphadenopathy and oedematous swellings in dependent parts of the body. Subsequently, bradyzoites develop in fibroblasts in the dermis, subcutaneous tissues and fascia and in the nasal and laryngeal mucosa. The developing cysts in the skin result in a severe condition characterised by painful subcutaneous swellings and thickenings of the skin, loss of hair and necrosis. Apart from the clinical manifestations, which in severe cases can result in death, there can be considerable economic losses due to condemnation of hides at slaughter.

Clinical signs: Affected animals show skin thickening, swelling, hair loss and skin necrosis. Photophobia, excessive lacrimation and hyperaemia of the sclera are present, and the cornea is studded with whitish elevated specks (pseudocysts).

Pathology: This genus differs from other members of the Sarcocystidae in that the cysts containing bradyzoites are found mainly in fibroblasts in or under the skin. The host cell enlarges and becomes multinucleate as the *Besnoitia* cyst grows within a parasitophorous vacuole, eventually reaching up to 0.6 mm in diameter (see Fig. 2.72).

Diagnosis: Besnoitiosis can be diagnosed by biopsy examination of skin. The spherical encapsulated cysts are pathognomonic. The best method is examination of the scleral conjunctiva where the pseudocysts can be seen macroscopically.

Control and treatment: Limiting contact of domestic cattle with cats can help reduce the incidence of infection. In countries where the disease is endemic in wildlife populations, control is difficult or impossible to achieve and may be limited to the elimination of infected animals. There is no known treatment.

Hypoderma spp.

Hypoderma (Phylum: Arthropoda; Class: Insecta; Order: Diptera; Family: Oestridae), commonly known as Warble flies, are parasitic as larvae in cattle. They may occur erratically in other animals including equines, sheep and, very rarely, humans. They are found throughout the northern hemisphere. However, *Hypoderma* is absent from extreme northern latitudes, including Scandinavia, and it has occasionally been found sparsely south of the equator in Argentina, Chile, Peru and southern Africa following accidental introduction in imported cattle. There are two species of importance in cattle: *Hypoderma bovis* and *Hypoderma lineatum* (Table 8.9).

Epidemiology: The flies occur in the summer, particularly from mid-June to early September. They are most active on warm days, when they lay their eggs on cattle. The flies are limited in dispersal ability and can travel for more than 5 km.

Pathogenesis: By far the most important feature of this genus is the economic loss caused by downgrading and condemnation of hides perforated by larvae. The L_3 under the skin damage the adjacent flesh and this necessitates trimming from the carcass the greenish gelatinous tissue called 'butcher's jelly', also seen in the infested oesophageal submucosal tissues. In addition, the adult flies themselves are responsible for some loss. When they approach animals to lay their eggs, their characteristic buzzing noise, which appears to be instantly recognisable, causes the animals to panic or 'gad', sometimes injuring themselves on posts, barbed wire and other obstacles. Dairy cows show reduced milk yield and beef animals have reduced weight gain as a result of interrupted feeding. This species will pursue animals for some distance, making repeated attacks.

Clinical signs and pathology: Except for poor growth and decreased milk yield in bad cases, the host animals show no appreciable signs until the larvae appear along the back. The presence of L_3 causes characteristic fluid-filled swellings ('warbles') in the dermis of the back, which can be seen and felt (Fig. 8.25). Warble larvae induce a pronounced tissue inflammation. The cellular reaction is predominantly eosinophilic and lymphocytic. The presence of the larvae also induces the production of a thickened connective tissue-lined cavity surrounding the larva, filled with inflammatory cells, particularly

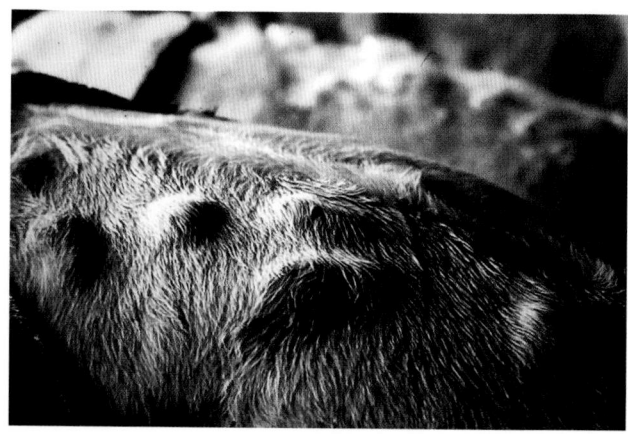

Fig. 8.25 'Warble' larvae of *Hypoderma* spp. on the back of a bovine animal.

eosinophils. If larvae die in the spinal canal, the release of a highly toxic proteolysin may cause paraplegia. Larval death in other regions may, in very rare cases, lead to anaphylaxis in sensitised animals.

Diagnosis: The presence of the larvae under the skin of the back allows diagnosis of warble flies. The eggs may also be found on the hairs of the animals in the summer. Immunodiagnostic tests may be used to detect animals infected with migrating larvae and hence those needing treatment.

Control and treatment: In control schemes in Europe, a single annual treatment is usually recommended, preferably in September, October or November. This is before the larvae of *H. bovis* have reached the spinal canal, so that there is no risk of spinal damage from disintegration of dead larvae. Treatment in the spring when the larvae have left their resting sites and arrived under the skin of the back, although effective in control, is less desirable since the breathing L_3 has then perforated the hide. However, in some countries such as the UK, such treatment is mandatory if warbles are present on the backs of cattle. Successful eradication schemes supported by legislation, such as restriction of cattle movement on infected farms and compulsory treatment in the autumn, have been undertaken on islands such as the UK and Eire. For example, in the UK the prevalence of infected cattle was reduced from around 40% in the 1970s to virtually zero in the 1990s. However, evidence of infection is still encountered occasionally in animals imported into the UK. Other areas that have practised successful eradication, such as Denmark and the Netherlands, are clearly at greater risk of reintroduction. *Hypoderma* are highly susceptible to systemically active organophosphate insecticides and to the macrocyclic lactones abamectin, ivermectin, doramectin, eprinomectin and moxidectin. The organophosphate preparations are applied as pour-ons to the backs of cattle and are absorbed systemically; macrocyclic lactones can be given by subcutaneous injection or pour-on.

ECTOPARASITES

BITING AND NUISANCE FLIES

Biting and nuisance flies (Phylum: Arthropoda; Order: Diptera) are important pests of cattle, through direct blood feeding and through the irritating effects they have on cattle as they attempt to feed on various body fluids and secretions.

Table 8.9 Summary of differences between the *Hypoderma* species which parasitise cattle.

Feature	*Hypoderma bovis*	*Hypoderma lineatum*
Adult length	15 mm	13 mm
Eggs laid	Singly	In batches
Larval morphology	Posterior spiracular plate surrounding the button has a narrow funnel-like channel	Posterior spiracular plate surrounding the button has a broad channel
Migration path	Along nerves	Between the fascial planes of muscles and along connective tissue
Overwintering site	Epidural fat of the spinal cord	Sub mucosa of the oesophagus

Clinical signs: The activity of both biting and non-biting species of fly results in marked defensive behaviour, described as 'fly-worry' in livestock. This is the disturbance caused by the presence and attempted feeding behaviour of flies. Responses by the host may range from dramatic escape behaviour, in which self-injury can occur, to less or increased levels of tail twitching, licking, foot stamping and skin rippling; animals may bunch or seek the shelter of overhanging vegetation. All these changes in behaviour result in reduced time spent feeding and decreased performance. Flies may be observed, often in large numbers, feeding along the back, sides and ventral abdomen, particularly of cattle and horses. Irritation and blood loss can lead to a marked reduction in weight gain.

Diagnosis: Increased levels of disturbance in the host animals; observation of flies on the animals. Precise identification will require microscopic examination of specimens. Identification of the larvae of most species is extremely difficult and, where possible, adults should be collected or samples of live larvae should be retained until adult emergence to confirm the identification, which is more easily accomplished with the adult fly. The detailed description and identification of the larvae of most species are beyond the scope of this text and if identification to species level is required, specimens should be referred to a relevant taxonomic specialist.

Control and treatment: Various types of screens and electrocution grids for buildings are available to reduce fly nuisance, but the best methods of control are those aimed at improving sanitation and reducing breeding places (source reduction). For example, in stables and farms, manure should be removed or stacked in large heaps where the heat of fermentation will kill the developing stages of flies, as well as eggs and larvae of helminths. In addition, insecticides applied to the surface of manure heaps may prove beneficial. A range of insecticides and procedures is available for the control of adult flies. Aerosol space sprays, residual insecticides applied to walls and ceilings and insecticide-impregnated cards and strips may reduce fly numbers indoors. Insecticides may also be incorporated in solid or liquid fly baits, using attractants such as various sugary syrups or hydrolysed yeast and animal proteins. Insecticide dust bags ('back-rubbers') have been used to reduce the numbers of muscid flies associated with fly-worry. These consist of sacking impregnated with or containing insecticide, which is suspended between two posts at a height that allows cattle to rub and thus apply the insecticide to the skin. However, given the high rates of reproduction, high rates of dispersal and multiple generations per year, area-wide control of most dipterous agents of myiasis is impractical. Insecticide-impregnated ear tags, tail bands and halters, mainly containing synthetic pyrethroids, together with pour-on, spot-on and spray preparations, are widely used to reduce fly annoyance in cattle and horses.

FAMILY MUSCIDAE

Musca autumnalis

Musca autumnalis (Phylum: Arthropoda; Class: Insecta; Order: Diptera; Suborder: Brachycera; Family: Muscidae), commonly known as the Face fly, feeds on secretions from the eyes, nose and mouth of cattle, as well as on wounds left by biting flies.

Epidemiology: In northern Europe, *M. autumnalis* may often be the most numerous fly worrying cattle in pasture. The eggs of *M. autumnalis* are usually laid in bovine faeces and if conditions are

suitable, the resultant large fly populations can cause serious annoyance. This can lead to bunching and so interfere with grazing, contributing to reduced production rates.

Pathogenesis: This is often the most numerous of the flies which worry cattle at pasture. These flies are considered to be important in the transmission of infectious bovine keratoconjunctivitis ('pink eye' or New Forest disease) due to *Moraxella bovis*, and they are also intermediate hosts of *Parafilaria bovicola*. Adults are developmental hosts for *Thelazia* (nematodes which live in the conjunctival sac of cattle and horses, causing conjunctivitis, keratitis, photophobia and epiphora).

Notes: *Musca autumnalis* is one of the most important livestock pests to invade North America. Its introduction from Europe was first detected in 1951 in Nova Scotia. From there it spread southward and, by 1959, many cases were being reported on cattle. It now occurs throughout cattle-rearing areas of the USA and Canada.

Musca domestica

Musca domestica (Phylum: Arthropoda; Class: Insecta; Order: Diptera; Suborder: Brachycera; Family: Muscidae), commonly known as the House fly, although not itself a parasite of living animals, is responsible for the transmission of a variety of important diseases and parasites, particularly to humans and a wide variety of domestic animals.

Pathogenesis: House flies, as their name suggests, are closely associated with buildings inhabited by animals and humans. They are not only a source of annoyance, but may also mechanically transmit viruses, bacteria, helminths and protozoa due to their habit of visiting faecal and decaying organic material. Pathogens are either carried on the hairs of the feet and body or regurgitated as salivary vomit during subsequent feeding. A number of *Musca* spp. have been incriminated in the spread of diseases including mastitis, conjunctivitis and anthrax. In humans, they are probably most important in the dissemination of *Shigella* and other enteric bacteria. Eggs of various helminths may be carried by the flies, and they may also act as intermediate hosts of a number of helminths such as *Habronema* spp. and *Raillietina* spp. Deposition of *Habronema* larvae in wounds may give rise to skin lesions commonly termed 'Summer sores' in horses. The house fly, *Musca domestica*, is closely associated with humans, livestock, their buildings and organic wastes. Although it may be of only minor direct annoyance to animals, its potential for transmission of viral and bacterial diseases and protozoan and metazoan parasites is significant.

Musca sorbens

Musca sorbens (Phylum: Arthropoda; Class: Insecta; Order: Diptera; Suborder: Brachycera; Family: Muscidae), commonly known as the Bazaar fly, is a widespread species in Africa, the Pacific islands and Oriental regions, largely replacing *M. domestica* where it occurs, and is an important vector of disease in these regions (see *M. domestica*).

Musca vetustissima

Musca vetustissima (Phylum: Arthropoda; Class: Insecta; Order: Diptera; Suborder: Brachycera; Family: Muscidae), commonly known as the Bush fly, is very closely related to *M. sorbens* and is a common non-biting nuisance fly of humans and livestock in Australia.

Pathogenesis: *Musca vetustissima* has been shown to transmit eye infections and other enteric diseases between animals and humans.

Hydrotaea irritans

Hydrotaea irritans (Phylum: Arthropoda; Class: Insecta; Order: Diptera; Suborder: Brachycera; Family: Muscidae), commonly known as the Sheep head fly, is widespread throughout northern Europe, but not believed to be present in North America. It feeds on the tears, saliva, sweat and wounds of cattle, sheep and horses.

Epidemiology: Although commonly known as the Sheep head fly, this species may be the most numerous muscid species found on cattle and horses. The populations of *Hydrotaea irritans* peak during midsummer. Adult flies prefer still conditions and are associated with permanent, fairly sheltered pastures that border woodlands or plantations.

Pathogenesis: Head flies are attracted to animals and feed on tears, saliva, sweat and wounds, such as those incurred by fighting rams. The mouthparts are adapted for feeding on liquids, but in addition they possess small teeth and the rasping effect of these during feeding leads to skin damage. They are facultative blood feeders and will ingest blood at the edges of wounds if available. Horned breeds of sheep, such as the Swaledale and Scottish blackface, are most susceptible to attack. Swarms of these flies around the head lead to intense irritation and annoyance and result in self-inflicted wounds, which then attract more flies. Clusters of flies feeding at the base of the horns lead to extension of these wounds, and the condition may be confused with blowfly myiasis. Secondary bacterial infection of wounds is common, which may encourage blowfly strike. The economic losses due to head fly infection are difficult to assess, but are thought to be substantial. In cattle, large numbers of *Hydrotaea irritans* have been found on the ventral abdomen and udder and, since the bacteria involved in 'summer mastitis' (*Corynebacterium pyogenes*, *Streptococcus dysgalactiae* and *Peptococcus indolicus*) have been isolated from these flies, there is strong presumptive evidence that they may transmit the disease. In addition, this species has been incriminated in the transmission of infectious bovine keratoconjunctivitis.

Stomoxys calcitrans

Stomoxys calcitrans (Phylum: Arthropoda; Class: Insecta; Order: Diptera; Suborder: Brachycera; Family: Muscidae), commonly known as the Stable fly, is a blood-feeding fly found worldwide that can be a significant pest for cattle but also companion animals, such as dogs.

Epidemiology: Approximately three minutes is required for a blood meal during which time flies may almost double in weight. The bite of stable flies is painful and as such, they are a serious pest of animals. In large numbers, these flies are a great source of annoyance to grazing cattle and in some areas there are estimates of milk and meat production losses of up to 20%. Adult flies live for about one month and are abundant around farm buildings and stables in late summer and autumn in temperate areas. They largely

remain in areas of strong sunlight and they bite mainly out of doors, although they will follow animals inside to feed. They will also enter buildings during rainy weather in the autumn. *Stomoxys calcitrans* are swift fliers but in general do not travel long distances.

Pathogenesis: The salivary secretions of this species may cause toxic reactions with an immunosuppressive effect, rendering the host more susceptible to disease. Stable flies may probe and attempt to feed on a number of hosts in rapid succession. They may therefore act as important mechanical vectors in the transmission of pathogens such as trypanosomes. *Trypanosoma evansi* (causing surra of equines and dogs), *T. equinum* (mal de caderas of equines, cattle, sheep and goats), *T. gambiense* and *T. rhodesiense* (human African trypanosomiasis) and *T. brucei* and *T. vivax* (nagana of equines, cattle, sheep and goats) are all mechanically transmitted by *S. calcitrans*. These flies also act as vectors for anthrax and *Dermatophilus congolensis*. *Stomoxys calcitrans* also serves as an intermediate host of the nematode *Habronema*.

Haematobia irritans

Haematobia irritans (Phylum: Arthropoda; Class: Insecta; Order: Diptera; Family: Muscidae), commonly known as the Horn fly, is a small blood-feeding fly that feeds at the base of the horns, back, shoulders and belly primarily on cattle. They also occasionally attack horses, sheep and dogs.

Epidemiology: Hot humid weather, with a temperature of 23–27 °C and relative humidity of 65–90%, is ideal for horn fly activity. The flies may be more abundant on cattle with dark coats and dark-coloured areas of bicoloured cattle. When temperatures are above 29 °C, flies migrate to the shaded skin of the belly and udder.

Pathogenesis: The adult flies feed on the host animal's blood, causing injury and irritation due to the constant piercing of the skin. Loss of blood due to horn flies can be considerable. In addition, during feeding the horn fly withdraws and reinserts its mouthparts many times, resulting in considerable irritation to the host. Although less important than many other muscid flies in disease transmission, *Haematobia* may transmit *Stephanofilaria*, the skin filarioid of cattle.

Haematobia irritans exigua

Haematobia irritans exigua (Phylum: Arthropoda; Class: Insecta; Order: Diptera; Family: Muscidae), commonly known as the Buffalo fly, feeds particularly on buffalo and cattle, often on the withers, back and sides, and occasionally the belly in hot weather. It is found worldwide, particularly in Asia and Australia. The buffalo fly (*Haematobia irritans exigua*) and the horn fly (*H. irritans irritans*) were once recognised as two separate species. However, they are often regarded as subspecies of *H. irritans*.

Pathogenesis: The buffalo fly has a pronounced effect on the health and productivity of buffalo and cattle. Significant blood loss can occur due to the high densities on the host (often several thousand) and because both sexes feed several times per day. The bites are painful and irritating and may cause feeding lesions. Species of *Haematobia* may transmit *Stephanofilaria*, the skin filarioid of cattle.

Haematobia minuta

Haematobia minuta, synonym *Lyperosia minuta* (Phylum: Arthropoda; Class: Insecta; Order: Diptera; Family: Muscidae), is a small blood-feeding fly that feeds particularly on cattle and buffalo in Africa. It is usually found on the withers, back and sides and occasionally the belly in hot weather.

Pathogenesis: Large numbers of flies cause intense irritation, and the skin wounds made during feeding may attract other muscids and myiasis-producing flies. These flies may have a pronounced effect on the health and productivity of the cattle. Significant blood loss can occur due to the high densities on the host (often several thousand) and also because both sexes feed several times per day. The bites are painful and irritating and may cause feeding lesions. It is difficult to assess the precise economic effect of these flies, but their effective control on grazing cattle can result in significant increases in production. Although less important than many other muscid flies in disease transmission, species of *Haematobia* transmit *Stephanofilaria*, the skin filarioid of cattle and, in some areas, camel trypanosomosis.

Haematobia stimulans

Haematobia stimulans, synonym *Haematobosca stimulans* (Phylum: Arthropoda; Class: Insecta; Order: Diptera; Family: Muscidae), is a blood-feeding fly that feeds primarily on cattle and is largely found in Europe.

Pathogenesis: The bites are painful and irritating and may cause feeding lesions. Although less important than many other muscid flies in disease transmission, species of *Haematobia* transmit *Stephanofilaria*, the skin filarioid of cattle.

Fannia canicularis

Fannia cannicularis (Phylum: Arthropoda; Class: Insecta; Order: Diptera; Family: Fanniidae), commonly known as the Lesser house fly, is a nuisance fly found worldwide, often bothering livestock around the mouth, nose and eyes.

Epidemiology: Flies may be observed feeding on animal faeces, manure piles, garbage and other types of decomposing organic material, and seen attempting to land and feed on the liquid exudates of the eyes, nose and mouth. *Fannia canicularis* is the most cosmopolitan species and is commonly found breeding in animal manure and confined livestock facilities. In contrast to *Musca domestica*, the eggs and larvae of most species of *Fannia* are more susceptible to desiccation. Hence, they are more abundant in semi-liquid sites, especially pools of semi-liquid faeces. Adults are more abundant in the cooler months of spring and autumn, declining in midsummer. Adults of *Fannia* are readily attracted into buildings and adult males are familiar as the flies responsible for the regular triangular flight paths beneath light bulbs or shafts of sunlight from windows in buildings.

Pathogenesis: Species of *Fannia* are of interest as nuisance pests of livestock and humans, especially in caged-layer poultry facilities, cattle confinement areas and dairies. They rarely feed directly from animals; however, the few that do are attracted to smeared faeces, sweat and mucus. Although it may be of only minor direct annoyance to animals, its potential for transmission of viral and bacterial diseases and protozoan and metazoan parasites is of significance, as for *Musca domestica*.

FAMILY SIMULIIDAE

Simulium (Phylum: Arthropoda; Class: Insecta; Order: Diptera; Family: Simuliidae) are commonly known as Blackflies or Buffalo gnats. The adult females feed on the blood of warm-blooded vertebrates, biting all over the body but particularly the head, abdomen and legs. They are found worldwide except New Zealand, Hawaii and some minor island groups.

Epidemiology: Only the adult females blood feed, and different species have different preferred feeding sites and times. Generally, they feed on the legs, abdomen, head and ears, and most species are particularly active during the morning and evening in cloudy, warm weather. Although flies may be active throughout the year, there may be a large increase in their numbers in the tropics during the rainy season. In temperate and arctic regions, the biting nuisance may be seasonal, since adults die in the autumn, with new generations emerging in spring and summer. The adult flies are found in swarms near free-running, well-aerated streams, which are their breeding sites. Some rivers can produce nearly a billion flies per kilometre of riverbed per day. Adults are strong fliers and are highly responsive to carbon dioxide and other host animal odours. They may fly as much as 6.6–13.3 km in search of a host, before returning to the breeding site to commence oviposition.

Pathogenesis: *Simulium* spp. may transmit the viruses causing eastern equine encephalitis and vesicular stomatitis and the avian protozoan *Leucocytozoon*. They also act as vectors for filarioid helminths, such as the nematodes *Onchocerca gutturosa* and *O. dukei* of cattle and *Onchocerca cervicalis* of horses. Bovine and equine onchocercosis produce nodules containing adult worms in various regions of the skin, particularly the withers of cattle, resulting in hide damage. From a medical perspective, Simuliidae are particularly important as vectors of the filarioid nematode *Onchocerca volvulus*, which causes river blindness in humans in Africa and Central and South America.

Clinical signs and pathology: Simulids cause severe irritation to livestock when they occur in large numbers and herds will often stampede. Bites are inflicted on all parts of the body and give rise to vesicles, which burst, exposing the underlying flesh. These skin wounds heal very slowly. In domestic animals, especially cattle, mass attack by these flies may be associated with an acute syndrome characterised by generalised petechial haemorrhages, particularly in areas of fine skin, together with oedema of the larynx and abdominal wall. The painful bites of swarms of *Simulium* may interfere with grazing and cause production loss. In certain areas of central Europe, it is often impossible to graze cattle during the spring due to the activity of these flies. Horses are often affected by the flies feeding inside the ears, and poultry may become anaemic from blood loss when attacked. Even at relatively low population densities, the painful bites may cause considerable disturbance and reduced productivity. Some host animals may suffer from allergic reactions to saliva secreted by the flies as they feed. Certain areas of the tropics are rendered uninhabitable by *Simulium*.

Diagnosis: The attacking swarms of adult flies are characteristic of most *Simulium* species. If the flies are seen on the host animal, they may be collected and identified.

Control and treatment: Blackfly control is extremely difficult since immature larval stages are found in running well-aerated water, often some distance from the farm or housing, and adult flies are capable of flying over 5 km. The most practical control method is the application of insecticides to breeding sites to kill larvae. This technique has been developed for the control of *Simulium* species that are vectors of river blindness in humans in Africa, and entails the repeated application of insecticides to selected watercourses at intervals throughout the year. The insecticide is then carried downstream and kills larvae over long stretches of water. Flies spend limited time on their hosts and are difficult to control using insecticides unless these have rapid killing or repellent activity. Applications of pyrethroid insecticides may give effective, though short-term, local control.

Species of importance: Possibly the most damaging simuliid of temperate latitudes in the New World is *Simulium arcticum* which can be a major livestock pest in western Canada. Populations can reach densities which are high enough to kill cattle. In the USA, *Simulium venustum* and *S. vittatum* may be common and widespread pests of livestock, particularly numerous in June and July. *Simulium pecuarum*, the southern buffalo gnat, may cause losses in cattle in the Mississippi valley. The turkey gnat, *S. meridionale*, is common in southern USA and the Mississippi valley, where it may be a significant pest of poultry. *Simulium equinum*, *S. erythrocephalum* and *S. ornatum* may cause problems in western Europe and *S. kurenze* in Russia. Particularly damaging in central and southern Europe is *S. colombaschense*, which may cause heavy mortality of livestock.

FAMILY GLOSSINIDAE

Glossina spp.

Glossina (Phylum: Arthropoda; Class: Insecta; Order: Diptera; Family: Glossinidae), commonly known as Tsetse flies, feed on the blood of various mammals, reptiles and birds. Tsetse flies are entirely restricted to sub-Saharan Africa.

Epidemiology: The normal hosts of tsetse flies are African wild large mammals and reptiles, which experience few or no ill effects from the presence of the trypanosomes in their blood unless subject to stresses such as starvation. These wild animals act as reservoirs of the disease. When humans or domestic animals become infected, however, the pathogenic effects of the trypanosomes can be debilitating or fatal unless treated.

Pathogenesis: Although the bites of tsetse flies are very painful and cause marked irritation, their main significance is in the transmission of animal and human trypanosomiasis, described as nagana or sleeping sickness, respectively. Flies become infected with protozoan trypanosome parasites during feeding and these then undergo multiplication and maturation within the fly. The fly is then infective to other hosts during subsequent feeding.

Clinical signs: Host animals may scratch and rub bite wound sites, which may result in significant skin trauma. The symptoms of tsetse-transmitted trypanosomosis include hyperthermia, anaemia,

rapid emaciation, oedema of the lower parts of the abdomen and thorax, joints and genitalia, keratitis and nasal discharge. Paralysis may also occur.

Diagnosis: Observation and identification of the adult flies feeding on the host animal. The flies are most active at dawn and dusk.

Control and treatment: In the past, campaigns against tsetse flies to control trypanosomiasis in both humans and animals depended mainly on large-scale killing of the game animals that act as reservoirs of trypanosome infection and as a source of blood for the flies. It was also common to clear large areas of bush in order to destroy the habitats of the adult flies. These methods were fairly successful, but are now largely unacceptable on ecological and economic grounds.

Currently, most anti-tsetse measures rely on the use of insecticides applied from the ground or by aircraft. When the objective is complete eradication of *Glossina*, residual formulations of insecticides are used. It is also essential that the area to be sprayed has economic potential and that agricultural development of the cleared area should proceed contemporaneously. Local eradication of tsetse populations is possible because of the relatively low rate of tsetse reproduction but, because of the inevitable reinvasion of tsetse from surrounding untreated areas, is uneconomic unless the selected area is on the edge of a tsetse belt where the fly population is already under stress because of relatively unfavourable climatic conditions. Advocates of insecticidal spraying argue that, since *Glossina* is highly susceptible to the insecticides used, the sophisticated and selective use of modern chemicals, usually on one occasion only, has no major and permanent effects on the environment. In fact, they point out that the changes in land use which should ensue from successful control are much more significant in this respect.

Populations of tsetse flies have been reduced or eradicated in localised areas by the use of traps. These have the advantages of being cheap, can be used by local communities and are harmless to the environment. They depend on the presentation of a material, such as dark cloth, which attracts the flies and leads into a trap that often incorporates an insecticide. Volatile chemical odours, such as acetone, octenol or phenoloc compounds from cattle urine, placed in or near traps attract flies and increase the number caught. However, traps are relatively difficult to deploy and maintain in densely vegetated areas of bush.

Some breeds of domestic livestock such as N'dama cattle are relatively trypanotolerant. Dipping cattle in pyrethroid insecticides such as deltamethrin can also effectively protect against tsetse feeding. Trypanocidal drugs can be used to treat trypanosome infection.

Notes: Key species in the *fusca* and *palpalis* groups include *G. palpalis*, *G. austeni*, *G. fuscipes* and *G. tachinoides*, while key species in the *morsitans* group include *G. morsitans* and *G. palidipes*.

FAMILY CALLIPHORIDAE

Cochliomyia hominivorax

Cochliomyia hominivorax, synonym *Callitroga hominivoraxix* (Phylum: Arthropoda; Class: Insecta; Order: Diptera; Family: Calliphoridae), commonly known as the New World screwworm, is a primary obligate agent of myiasis, most commonly affecting cattle, but it may also infest pigs and horses and, where predisposed, any mammal may be infested, including humans.

Epidemiology: Adult females have been reported to fly up to 320 km. The infestation can also be spread by the transport of animals and people from infested areas.

Clinical signs and pathology: It may be difficult to see screwworm maggots at the wound surface because only the posterior spiracles are exposed. Larvae of other blowflies such as *Lucilia* do not feed in a vertical position or burrow deep into the wound, but instead feed more superficially. In cattle, infestation initially causes intermittent irritation and pyrexia, followed by the production of a cavernous lesion. The tissue shows progressive liquefaction, necrosis and haemorrhage, before the larvae leave the wound. If untreated, repeated infestation by *C. hominivorax* and secondary fly species may quickly lead to the death of the host within 1–2 weeks.

Diagnosis: Screwworm larvae have distinct dorsal tracheal pigmentation that extends from somatic segment 12 to segment 10 or 9.

Control and treatment: As a result of the economic cost of this pest, large-scale screwworm fly control was initiated in the southeastern states of the USA in 1957–1959. This was achieved by the release of large numbers of male *C. hominivorax* that had been sterilised by radiation. Sterilised males mate with wild females, which are in turn rendered infertile. Subsequent control operations spread the area of sterile male release and by 1980 effective control of *C. hominivorax* in the USA was achieved. Despite a number of sporadic but significant outbreaks, effective control has been maintained. The eradication programme has subsequently been successfully directed against the fly in Mexico, Puerto Rico and as far as Panama.

Notes: In 1988, *C. hominivorax* were discovered in an area 10 km south of Tripoli in Libya. This was the first known established population of this species outside the Americas. The fly quickly spread to infest about 25 000 km². In 1989 there were about 150 cases of myiasis by *C. hominivorax* but by 1990 a total of 12 068 confirmed cases of screwworm fly myiasis were recorded and, at its peak, almost 3000 cases were seen in the single month of September 1990. It was estimated that if unchecked, the infestation could cost the Libyan livestock industry about US$30 million per year and the North African region approximately US$280 million per year. This led to the implementation of a major international control programme, which successfully eradicated the fly from this area, again using the release of sterile males.

Cochliomyia macellaria

Cochliomyia macellaria, synonym *Callitroga macellaria* (Phylum: Arthropoda; Class: Insecta; Order: Diptera; Family: Calliphoridae), is an agent of myiasis in cattle, but may also infest a range of other mammals, including humans.

Epidemiology: *Cochliomyia macellaria* is often attracted to the wounds initiated by *C. hominivorax*. The two species are commonly found together.

Pathogenesis: Mechanical transmission of disease attributed to this species includes botulism in birds, 12 different *Salmonella* types, including *Salmonella typhimurium*, poliomyelitis and swine influenza.

Chrysomya bezziana

Chrysomya bezziana (Phylum: Arthropoda; Class: Insecta; Order: Diptera; Family: Calliphoridae), commonly known as the Old World screwworm, is a primary obligate agent of myiasis that infests a range of mammals, including cattle, sheep, dogs and occasionally humans.

Epidemiology: In temperate regions, screwworm attacks are restricted to the warm seasons, although may occur during mild winters. In the tropics they are continuous. Female screwworms are attracted to all warm-blooded animals. The distance a fly will travel ranges from 10 to 20 km in tropical environments.

Pathogenesis: Infestation by *Chrysomya bezziana* causes intermittent irritation and pyrexia, followed by the production of a cavernous lesion. Infested wounds often have a serosanguineous discharge and sometimes a distinctive foul-smelling odour. Sometimes, there may be large pockets of larvae with only small openings in the skin. The tissue shows progressive liquefaction, necrosis and haemorrhage, before the larvae leave the wound. Animals may die from secondary infection or toxicity in 1–2 weeks if the infestation is not treated.

Clinical signs and pathology: In the first day or two, screwworm infestations are difficult to detect. Often, all that can be seen is slight motion inside the wound. As the larvae feed, the wound gradually enlarges and deepens. Animals infested with screwworms may appear dull, lethargic and separate from the herd. They may cease feeding and show weight loss. Wounds with foul-smelling odour will be observed on inspection; however, it may be difficult to see the maggots at the wound surface because only the posterior spiracles are exposed. Larvae of other blowflies such as *Lucilia* do not feed in a vertical position or burrow deep into the wound, but instead feed more superficially. Screwworms may be particularly difficult to find inside the nasal, anal and vaginal openings.

Diagnosis: The larvae can be found packed deep inside the wound. Screwworms are diagnosed by the removal of the larvae and identification with a dissecting microscope.

Notes: The precise status of *Chrysomya bezziana* as a clinical and economic pest is uncertain, particularly in sub-Saharan Africa, and few studies have been able to obtain quantitative estimates of myiasis incidence and its clinical or economic importance. The absence of livestock throughout much of its range in sub-Saharan Africa, due to the presence of trypanosomosis and its vector the tsetse fly, may substantially limit its economic impact. However, *C. bezziana* has been inadvertently introduced into several countries in the Middle East, and such an introduction is believed to pose a major economic threat to the pastoral industry of Australia.

FAMILY OESTRIDAE

Dermatobia hominis

Dermatobia hominis (Phylum: Arthropoda; Class: Insecta; Order: Diptera; Family: Oestridae), commonly known as the Torsalo, Berne or Human bot fly, is an agent of subdermal myiasis that affects humans, most domestic and wild mammals and many species of birds. It is found throughout Latin America from Mexico to northern Argentina and the island of Trinidad.

Epidemiology: The most common vectors of *D. hominis* larvae are members of the genera *Psorophora*, *Culex* and *Stomoxys*. These flies breed in forests where both domestic and wild animals are commonly parasitised. Humans are usually infected through association with domestic animals; however, non-insect transmission may occur when *D. hominis* eggs are deposited on damp clothes or laundry.

Pathogenesis: The larvae occur in swellings in various parts of the body and these may suppurate and cause severe pain. In Latin America, this condition is often known as 'ura'. *Dermatobia* is a major problem in cattle in South America. Lesions are most numerous on the upper body, neck, back, flanks and tail, and are often grouped together to form large and often purulent swellings. As well as hide damage, the pain and distress of the lesions result in reduced time spent grazing, retarded growth and lowered meat and milk production. The exit holes made by the larvae may also attract myiasis-producing flies, including screwworms. In humans, the most common larval sites are the extremities of the limbs and the scalp. Fatal cerebral damage has occurred in children when larvae have migrated through the fontanelle into the cranial cavity.

Clinical signs: Signs include the swellings and lesions made by larvae. Infected animals show reduced weight gain and milk production.

LICE

Heavy louse infestation is known as pediculosis. Blood-sucking lice have been implicated in the transmission of disease, such as those that transmit rickettsial anaplasmosis; however, lice are predominantly of importance because of the direct damage they cause. This effect is usually a function of their density. A small number of lice may be very common and present no problem. However, louse populations can increase dramatically, reaching high densities. Transfer of lice from animal to animal or from herd to herd is usually by direct physical contact. Because lice do not survive for long off their host, the potential for animals to pick up infestations from dirty housing is limited, although it cannot be ignored. Occasionally, lice may also be transferred between animals by attachment to flies (phoresy).

Epidemiology: In warm countries there is no marked seasonality of bovine pediculosis, but in cold and temperate regions the heaviest infestations are in late winter and early spring, when the coat is at its thickest, giving a sheltered, bulky and humid habitat for optimal multiplication. The most rapid annual increase in louse populations is seen when cattle are winter-housed, and lice can build up in numbers very quickly. In late spring, there is usually an abrupt fall in the numbers of lice, most of the parasites and eggs being shed with the winter coat. Numbers generally remain low throughout the summer, partly because the thinness of the coat provides a restricted habitat, but partly also because high skin surface temperatures and direct sunlight limit multiplication and may even be lethal.

Pathogenesis: Light infestations are usually only discovered accidentally and should not be considered of any pathogenic importance, lice being almost normal inhabitants of the dermis and coat of many cattle, especially in winter. Moderate infestations are associated only with a mild chronic dermatitis, and are well tolerated. In heavier infestations, there is pruritus, with rubbing and licking, but if sucking lice are present in large numbers there may be anaemia and weakness.

Clinical signs and pathology Light infestations are usually only discovered accidentally. In these infections, the lice and eggs are easily found by parting the hair, especially along the back, the lice being next to the skin and the eggs scattered like coarse powder throughout the hair. It is important to remember that a heavy louse infestation may itself be merely a symptom of some other underlying condition such as malnutrition or chronic disease, since debilitated animals do not groom themselves and leave the lice undisturbed. In such animals, the shedding of the winter coat may be delayed for many weeks, retaining large numbers of lice.

Diagnosis: The lice may be seen on the skin. Removal and examination under a light microscope will allow species identification. The eggs are also visible and appear as white specks attached to the hairs.

Control and treatment: The timing and frequency of treatments depend very much on individual circumstances. In many cases, treatment in late autumn or early winter will give adequate control of cattle lice. In Europe, louse control is usually undertaken when cattle are housed for the winter. Because a wide variety of chemical classes are effective, louse control is not difficult to achieve. Insecticide resistance is widespread in lice, and its rapid spread may be linked to the facultative parthenogenesis seen in many louse species. Hence, in an attempt to reduce the risk of selection for resistance, rotation of chemical classes is strongly advised. Treatment of all stock on farm and subsequent initial quarantine and treatment of all newly introduced animals will allow a good degree of louse control to be maintained. The organophosphate insecticides (e.g. chlorfenvinphos, coumaphos, chlorpyrifos, crotoxyphos, trichlorphon, phosmet and propetamphos), usually applied as pour-on or spot-on applications, are effective in killing all lice. However, most insecticides registered for use on cattle are not very active against louse eggs. This means that after treatment eggs can still hatch and continue the infestation. A second treatment is therefore recommended two weeks later to kill newly emerged lice. Pour-on or spot-on synthetic pyrethroids, such as cypermethrin or permethrin, or pour-on avermectins may also be used, although the latter have only limited activity against chewing lice. Essential oils have been shown to be very effective against chewing lice when groomed into the hair.

Bovicola bovis

Bovicola bovis, synonym *Damalinia bovis* (Phylum: Arthropoda; Class: Insecta; Order: Psocodea; Suborder: Ischnocera; Family: Bovicolidae), commonly known as the Red louse or Cattle chewing louse, is a parasite of importance in cattle worldwide. It is most commonly found on the top of the head, especially the curly hair of the poll and forehead, the neck, shoulders, back and rump, and occasionally the tail switch.

Epidemiology: *Bovicola bovis* is one of the most common cattle parasites in Europe and is the only chewing louse found on cattle in the USA. Though it causes less individual damage than sucking lice, it is present in larger numbers and so can be extremely damaging. Infested cattle may show disrupted feeding patterns.

Pathogenesis: The mouthparts of *B. bovis* are equipped for biting and chewing, and these lice feed on the outer layers of the hair shafts, dermal scales and blood scabs. If infestations increase, the lice may spread down the sides and may cover the rest of the body. This louse feeds by scraping away scurf and skin debris from the base of the hairs, causing considerable irritation to the host animal. The skin reaction can cause the hair to loosen and the cattle react to the irritation by rubbing or scratching, which will result in patches of hair being pulled or rubbed off. Scratching may produce wounds or bruises and a roughness to the skin. This may lead to secondary skin infections and skin trauma such as spot and fleck grain loss in the hide, reducing its value.

Haematopinus eurysternus

Haematopinus eurysternus (Phylum: Arthropoda; Class: Insecta; Order: Psocodea; Suborder: Anoplura; Family: Haematopinidae), commonly known as the Short-nosed louse, is found worldwide most commonly on the skin, poll and base of the horns, in the ears and around the eyes and nostrils; even in mild infestations it is found in the tail switch.

Pathogenesis: In severe infestations, the entire region from the base of the horns, over the face (Fig. 8.26) to the base of the tail can be infested.

Notes: This species is more commonly found infesting mature cattle than young animals. In North America, *Haematopinus eurysternus* is more prevalent in the Great Plains and Rocky Mountain regions.

Haematopinus quadripertusus

Haematopinus quadripertusus (Phylum: Arthropoda; Class: Insecta; Order: Psocodea; Suborder: Anoplura; Family: Haematopinidae), commonly known as the Tail louse, occurs worldwide and is most often seen on the tail and perineum of cattle, particularly zebu (*Bos indicus*).

Epidemiology: This species is most commonly found among the long tail hairs at the base of the tail. Unlike other cattle lice,

H. quadripertusus is most abundant during the summer and in warmer climates. The lice are transmitted through direct contact between hosts.

Pathogenesis: *Haematopinus quadripertusus* feeds on host blood using its piercing mouthparts. In severe infestations, the entire region from the base of the horns to the base of the tail can be infested.

Haematopinus tuberculatus

Haematopinus tuberculosus (Phylum: Arthropoda; Class: Insecta; Order: Psocodea; Suborder: Anoplura; Family: Haematopinidae), commonly known as the Buffalo louse, was originally a parasite of buffalo in Africa, but is now also found infesting cattle.

Pathogenesis: Populations build up during the winter when the animal's coat is longer and thicker but it is not generally considered of any great clinical importance.

Linognathus vituli

Linognathus vituli (Phylum: Arthropoda; Class: Insecta; Order: Psocodea; Suborder: Anoplura; Family: Linognathidae), commonly known as the Long-nosed cattle louse, is an important parasite of cattle found worldwide.

Epidemiology: Heaviest infestation occurs in late winter and early spring, commonly on the head and around the eyes (Fig. 8.27).

Pathogenesis: This species is capable of transmitting bovine anaplasmosis, dermatomycosis (ringworm) and theileriosis.

Solenopotes capillatus

Solenopotes capillatus (Phylum: Arthropoda; Class: Insecta; Order: Psocodea; Suborder: Anoplura; Family: Linognathidae), commonly known as the Little blue cattle louse, is found on the skin of neck, head, shoulders, dewlap, back and tail of cattle.

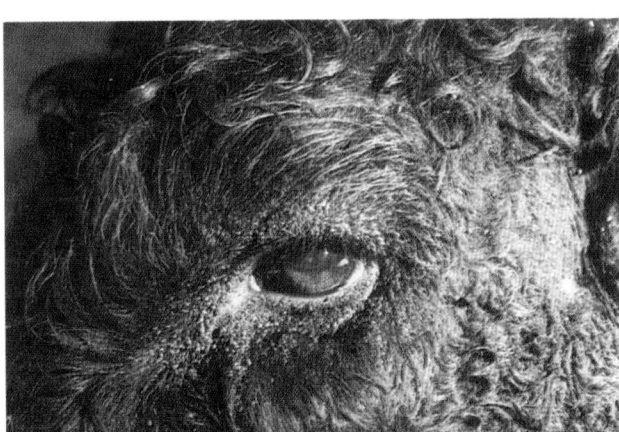

Fig. 8.26 Severe bovine pediculosis due to *Haematopinus eurysternus*.

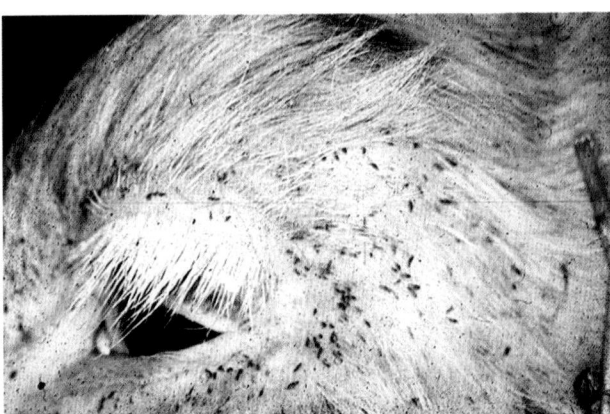

Fig. 8.27 Heavy louse infestation of *Linognathus vituli*.

MITES

The ectoparasitic mites of cattle feed on blood, lymph, skin debris or sebaceous secretions, which they ingest by puncturing the skin, scavenging from the skin surface or imbibing from epidermal lesions. Most ectoparasitic mites spend their entire lives in intimate contact with their host, so that transmission from host to host is primarily by physical contact. Infestation by mites is called acariosis and can result in severe dermatitis, known as mange, which may cause significant welfare problems and economic losses.

Demodex bovis

Demodex bovis (Phylum: Arthropoda; Class: Arachnida; Subclass: Acari; Order: Trombidiformes (Prostigmata); Family: Demodicidae) is localised in the hair follicles and sebaceous glands. It occurs worldwide.

Epidemiology: Probably because of its location deep in the dermis, it is almost impossible to transmit *Demodex* between animals unless there is prolonged contact. Such contact usually only occurs during suckling and as such, it is thought that most infections are acquired in the early weeks of life. The muzzle, neck, withers and back are all common sites of infestation.

Pathogenesis: The most important effect of bovine demodicosis is the formation of many pea-sized nodules, each containing caseous material and several thousand mites, which cause hide damage and economic loss. Although these nodules can be easily seen in smooth-coated animals, they are often undetected in rough-coated cattle until the hide has been dressed. Problems caused by demodicosis in cattle are primarily a result of the damage caused to the hides. In some rare cases demodicosis may become generalised and fatal.

Clinical signs and pathology: Pea-sized nodules containing caseous material and mites, particularly on the withers, lateral neck, back and flanks. Concurrent pyoderma may occur, leading to furunculosis with ulceration and crust formation. In cattle, cutaneous nodules consist of follicular cysts lined with squamous epithelium and filled with waxy keratin squames and mites. Eruption of the cysts on to the skin may form a thick crust; rupture within the dermis may form an abcess or granulomatous reaction.

Diagnosis: For confirmatory diagnosis, deep scrapings are necessary to reach the mites deep in the follicles and glands. This is best achieved by taking a fold of skin, applying a drop of liquid paraffin and scraping until capillary blood appears.

Control and treatment: Control is rarely applied in cattle since there is little incentive for farmers to treat their animals. In many cases, demodicosis spontaneously resolves and treatment is unnecessary. The organophosphate trichlorphon, used on three occasions two days apart, and systemic macrocyclic lactones may be effective.

Notes: Species of the genus *Demodex* are highly specialised mites that live in the hair follicles and sebaceous glands of a wide range of wild and domestic animals, including humans. They are believed to form a group of closely related sibling species that are highly specific to particular hosts: *Demodex phylloides* (pig), *Demodex canis* (dog), *Demodex bovis* (cattle), *Demodex equi* (horse), *Demodex musculi* (mouse), *Demodex ratti* (rat), *Demodex caviae* (guinea pig), *Demodex cati* (cat) and *Demodex folliculorum* and *Demodex brevis* on humans.

In some parts of Australia 95% of hides are damaged, and surveys in the USA have shown one-quarter of the hides to be affected. In Britain 17% of hides have been found to have *Demodex* nodules.

Psorobia bovis

Psorobia bovis, synonym *Psorergates bos* (Phylum: Arthropoda; Class: Arachnida; Subclass: Acari; Order: Trombidiformes (Prostigmata); Family: Psorergatidae), commonly known as the Cattle itch mite, occurs on the skin of cattle. It is found Australia, New Zealand, southern Africa, North and South America. It has not been reported in Europe. This mite has little or no pathogenic effect.

Epidemiology: This mite is not normally considered to be of clinical significance.

Clinical signs and pathology: There are few clinical signs associated with infestations of this mite. Mites may occur on apparently normal skin without causing itching of the host animal. Rarely, the mite may cause alopecia and desquamation, but in the majority of cases there appears to be no recognisable lesion associated with the infection.

Diagnosis: To obtain mites it is necessary, having clipped away a patch of hair, to apply a drop of mineral oil and scrape the skin down to the blood capillary level. The mites themselves are easily identified.

Control and treatment: Regular checks of livestock and treatments will keep infection rate under control. *Psorobia* is relatively unsusceptible to most acaricides, although the formamidine amitraz has recently been shown to be of considerable value. Otherwise, the older arsenic–sulfur preparations may be used. Macrocyclic lactones may be effective.

Psoroptes ovis

Psoroptes ovis, synonyms *Psoroptes communis* var. *ovis, Psoroptes cuniculi, Psoroptes cervinus, Psoroptes bovis, Psoroptes equi* (Phylum: Arthropoda; Class: Arachnida; Subclass: Acari; Order: Sarcoptiformes (Astigmata); Family: Psoroptidae), commonly known as the Sheep scab mite, is found on the skin, particularly the legs, feet, base of tail and udder, but in heavy infestations may spread all over the body.

Pathogenesis: In cattle these mites cause intense pruritus, papules, crusts, excoriation and lichenification (Fig. 8.28). Lesions may cover almost the entire body; secondary bacterial infections are common in severe cases. Death in untreated calves, weight loss, decreased milk production and increased susceptibility to other diseases can occur.

Control and treatment: In cattle, dipping and topical application of non-systemic acaricides, such as the organophosphates (diazinon, coumaphos or phosmet), amitraz or a lime–sulfur dip, may be effective. Dippings should be repeated at two-week intervals. The topical application of flumethrin is also used in some parts of the world. Most treatments are not licensed for use in dairy cattle. Injectable formulations of avermectins (ivermectin and doramectin) and

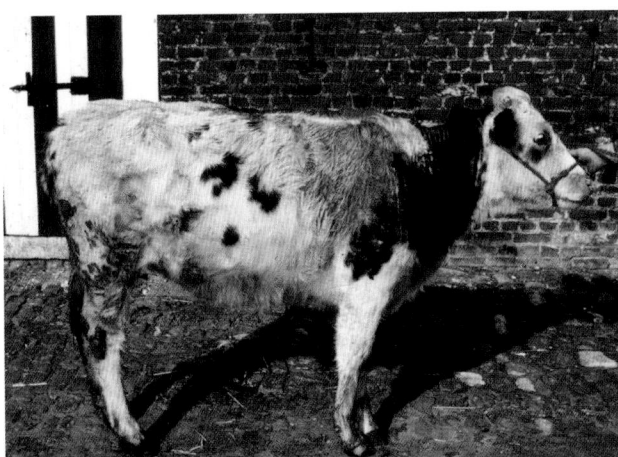

Fig. 8.28 Bovine psoroptic mange.

milbemycins (moxidectin) may be effective, although following treatment with ivermectin the isolation of treated animals for 2–3 weeks after treatment is required to pevent reinfestation. Eprinomectin is available as a pour-on formulation, and is the only macrocyclic lactone that may be used in dairy cattle. Following diagnosis, the treatment of all animals on infected premises and subsequent treatment of all incoming stock are recommended. For a more detailed description see Chapter 9.

Chorioptes bovis

Chorioptes bovis, synonyms *Psoroptes communis* var. *ovis*, *Psoroptes cuniculi*, *Psoroptes cervinus*, *Psoroptes bovis*, *Psoroptes equi* (Phylum: Arthropoda; Class: Arachnida; Subclass: Acari; Order: Sarcoptiformes (Astigmata); Family: Psoroptidae), is found worldwide. This mite will infest a variety of livestock, particularly cattle but also sheep, horses, camelids and goats. They are most commonly found on the legs, feet, base of tail and udder.

Epidemiology: Mite populations are highest in the winter and may regress over summer. It is the most common type of mange in cattle in the USA.

Pathogenesis: In cattle, chorioptic mange occurs most often in housed animals, particularly dairy animals, affecting mainly the neck, tail head, udder and legs. Usually only a few animals in a group are clinically affected. The mites are found more commonly on the hindleg than on the foreleg. It is a mild condition and lesions tend to remain localised, with slow spread. Its importance is economic, the pruritus caused by the mites resulting in rubbing and scratching, with damage to the hide. High infestations have been associated with decreased milk production. The treatment is the same as for sarcoptic mange in cattle.

Clinical signs and pathology: Hosts can be asymptomatic with low densities of mites present and thus act as carriers that transfer the mite to other animals. Host reactions are normally only induced when the numbers increase to thousands of mites per host. Scabs or scales develop on the skin of the lower parts of the body. There is some exudation and crust formation on the legs and lower body, but in most cases this does not spread over a wide area. Infected animals may stamp and scratch infected areas. The majority of the

mites are likely to be found on the lower leg, particularly the pastern and foot. However, in some animals the infestation may become acute and generalised, and closely resemble infestation with *Psoroptes*. The pathology is highly variable, depending on the intensity and duration of infection; subclinical infections are common. Clinically affected animals may have pustular, crusted, scaly and lichenified lesions and alopecia.

Diagnosis: Skin scrapings from the suspect lesions should be taken for microscopic examination.

Control and treatment: Regular checks of livestock and quarantining of infected animals will help to control the frequency and extent of infestations. The dips used for psoroptic mange in cattle are also effective against *Chorioptes*. They should be repeated at two-week intervals. Ivermectin, doramectin, eprinomectin and moxidectin applied topically as a pour-on are also effective against chorioptic mange.

Notes: The names *Chorioptes ovis*, *Chorioptes equi*, *Chorioptes caprae* and *Chorioptes cuniculi* used to describe the chorioptic mites found on sheep, horses, goats and rabbits, respectively, are now all thought to be synonyms of *Chorioptes bovis*.

Sarcoptes scabiei

Sarcoptes scabiei (Phylum: Arthropoda; Class: Arachnida; Subclass: Acari; Order: Sarcoptiformes (Astigmata); Family: Sarcoptidae), commonly kown as the Scabies mite, is found worldwide.

Pathogenesis: Sarcoptic mange is potentially the most severe of the cattle manges, although many cases are mild. Nevertheless, it is being increasingly diagnosed in Britain and in some areas, including Canada and parts of the USA, the disease is notifiable and the entry of cattle carrying *Sarcoptes*, whether clinically affected or not, is not permitted. The mite has partial site preferences, which in the USA have given it the common name of 'neck and tail mange', but it may occur on any part of the body. Mild infections merely show scaly skin with little hair loss, but in severe cases the skin becomes thickened, there is marked loss of hair and crusts form on the less well-haired parts of the body (Fig. 8.29), such as the escutcheon of cows. There is intense pruritus leading to loss of meat and milk production and to hides being downgraded because of damage by scratching and rubbing.

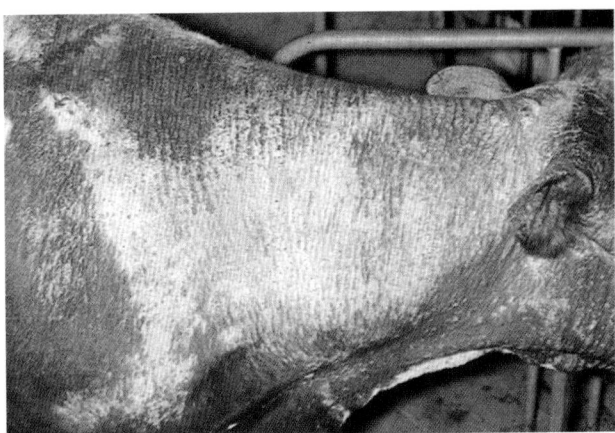

Fig. 8.29 Characteristic lesions of bovine sarcoptic mange.

Control and treatment: Treatment has largely depended on the use of repeated washes or sprays, usually organochlorine insecticides such as γ-hexachlorocyclohexane. However, organochlorine insecticides are not now available in most countries. Systemic macrocyclic lactones may give good results. Alternatively, the application of a pour-on organophosphate such as phosmet, on two occasions at an interval of 14 days, is also effective. Neither macrocyclic lactones nor phosmet are licensed for use in lactating animals whose milk is used for human consumption. The formamidine amitraz is effective against sarcoptic mange in cattle and has withdrawal periods of 24 and 48 hours, respectively, for meat and milk. For further details see Chapter 12.

TICKS

IXODIDAE

Ixodes

Ixodes ricinus

See Chapter 9.

Ixodes holocyclus

Ixodes holocyclus (Phylum: Arthropoda; Class: Arachnida; Order: Ixodida; Family: Ixodidae), commonly known as the Paralysis tick, is found on cattle, sheep, goats, dogs, cats, other mammals and birds throughout Australia.

Epidemiology: This species is most commonly found among low leafy vegetation since this protects it against sun and wind exposure and maintains the high humidity required for development.

Pathogenesis: *Ixodes holocyclus* is the main cause of tick paralysis in Australia. Its paralysing toxin has been reported to affect at least 20 000 domestic animals annually. Although infestations usually consist of relatively few individual ticks, *I. holocyclus* infestations can kill cattle, particularly calves, and small domestic animals. Fifty larvae or five nymphs will kill a 40 g rat, and larger numbers of either can cause paralysis in dogs and cats. Generally, only the adult stage infests cattle, with the worst outbreaks in late winter, spring and summer. *Ixodes holocyclus* is also a vector for *Coxiella burnetii* (Q-fever) and *Rickettsia australis* (Queensland tick typhus).

Ixodes rubicundus

Ixodes rubicundus (Phylum: Arthropoda; Class: Arachnida; Order: Ixodida; Family: Ixodidae), commonly known as the Karoo paralysis tick, is found on a range of domestic livestock and wild ungulates in southern Africa, particularly the Karrooveld.

Pathogenesis: *Ixodes rubicundus*, the Karoo paralysis tick, parasitises domestic stock and wild ungulates in South Africa and may lead to serious losses. Ticks may cause damage at the site of attachment, leading to local injury, which may predispose to secondary bacterial infection. The adult tick produces a toxin that causes paralysis in sheep and goats. Affected animals become paralysed and some may show signs of incoordination and stumbling. Unless ticks are removed, the animal will remain paralysed and die within days. Most affected animals recover within 24–48 hours once the ticks have been removed or animals have been dipped.

Dermacentor

Dermacentor andersoni

Dermacentor andersoni, synonym *Dermacentor venustus* (Phylum: Arthropoda; Class: Arachnida; Order: Ixodida; Family: Ixodidae), commonly known as the Rocky Mountain wood tick, is a three-host tick speces the immature stages of which infest small rodents while the adults infest wild and domestic herbivores. They are widely distributed throughout the western and central parts of North America from Mexico as far north as British Columbia.

Epidemiology: Adult numbers peak in May, then decline by July. Larvae and nymphs appear later and have usually disappeared by late summer. This species is particularly common among damp, grassy, brush-covered areas, since these attract both the small mammals required by the immature stages and the large herbivorous mammals required by the adults. Infection occurs when host animals brush against vegetation harbouring tick larvae.

Pathogenesis: High infestation levels may cause anaemia. *Dermacentor andersoni* may cause tick paralysis, particularly in calves, and may be responsible for the transmission of bovine anaplasmosis, caused by *Anaplasma marginale*. It also transmits the Colorado tick fever virus and the bacteria that cause tularaemia. *Dermacentor andersoni* is the chief vector of *Rickettsia rickettsii* (Rocky Mountain spotted fever) in western USA.

Dermacentor reticulatus

Dermacentor reticulatus, synonym *Dermacentor pictus* (Phylum: Arthropoda; Class: Arachnida; Order: Ixodida; Family: Ixodidae), commonly known as the Marsh tick, Meadow tick, Winter or Ornate dog tick, usually feeds on sheep, cattle, dogs, horses, pigs and occasionally humans. Nymphs and larvae feed on smaller mammals, such as insectivores and occasionally birds. It is widely distributed in Europe (from the Atlantic coast to Kazakhstan) and Central Africa. *Dermacentor reticulatus* is a three-host tick, and the life cycle can be completed in only 1–2 years, depending on environmental conditions.

Pathogenesis: *Dermacentor reticulatus* is a vector for the transmission of a wide range of pathogens. It is particularly important as an ectoparasite of cattle and may be found along their backs in early spring. In cattle, it is a vector for *Babesia divergens* (redwater), *B. ovis*, *Theileria ovis*, *Coxiella burnetii* (Q-fever), *Francisella tularensis* (tularaemia), *Brucella*, *Rickettsia conorii* (boutonneuse fever) and *Anaplasma ovis*. In horses it is a vector of *Babesia caballi*, *Theileria equi* and infectious encephalomyelitis of horses. In dogs it is a vector for *Babesia canis*.

Other species of *Dermacentor* of veterinary importance in cattle are listed in Table 8.10.

Table 8.10 Other species of *Dermacentor* of veterinary importance in cattle.

Species	Distribution	Hosts	Pathogenesis
Dermacentor nutalli	Siberia, northern Pakistan, China, Mongolia	Cattle, camels, goats	*Rickettsia sibirica*
Dermacentor occidentalis	Western USA (Sierra Nevada Mountains and the Pacific coast from Oregon to southern California)	Cattle, horses, other domestic and wild mammals	Anaplasmosis, Colorado tick fever, Q-fever, tularaemia, may cause tick paralysis
Dermacentor silvarum	Asia (central Siberia and northeastern China to Japan)	Cattle, sheep, horses, dogs and humans	*Rickettsia sibirica*, *Babesia bovis*, *B. caballi*, *B. canis*, *Theileria equi*, *T. ovis* and *Anaplasma ovis*

Rhipicephalus

Rhipicephalus appendiculatus

Rhipicephalus appendiculatus (Phylum: Arthropoda; Class: Arachnida; Order: Ixodida; Family: Ixodidae), commonly known as the Brown ear tick, feeds on a very wide range of hosts: cattle, horses, sheep, goats, deer, antelopes, dogs, rodents and birds. It is found in Africa, south of the Sahara.

Epidemiology: This species is a three-host tick and mating take place on the host. Adults and immatures feed in the ears of cattle and other livestock and seasonal activity is closely associated with temperature and rain periods. *Rhipicephalus appendiculatus* is more abundant in cool, shaded, shrubby or woody savannah with at least 60 cm of annual rainfall.

Pathogenesis: This tick is considered a major pest in areas where it is endemic. Heavy infestations on cattle can result in severe damage to the ears and toxaemia. The excess blood excreted by the ticks may attract flies, leading to secondary myiasis. Tick bites may become infected with bacteria. Tick salivary fluids and salivary toxins can produce host reactions such as toxicosis (sweating sickness and tick paralysis). Heavy infestations can result in fatal toxaemia and loss of resistance to other infections as well as severe damage to the host's ears, udder and tail. *Rhipicephalus appendiculatus* is a vector of East Coast fever (*Theileria parva*), *T. lawrencei*, Nairobi sheep disease virus, *Ehrlichia bovis*, *Hepatozoon canis*, *Rickettsia conorii* and Thogoto virus.

Other species of *Rhipicephalus* of veterinary importance in cattle are listed in Table 8.11.

Control and treatment: Weekly dipping during the tick season should kill the adult female ticks before they are engorged, except in cases of very severe challenge when the dipping interval has to be reduced to 4–5 days. Dipping intervals of the latter frequency are also necessary for cattle infested with *R. appendiculatus* in areas where East Coast fever is endemic so that the ticks are killed before the sporozoites of *T. parva* have time to develop to the infective stage in the salivary glands of the tick. Theoretically, weekly dipping should also control the larvae and nymphs but in several areas, the peak infestations of larvae and nymphs occur at different seasons to the adult females and the duration of the dipping season has to be extended.

Rhipicephalus (Boophilus)

Rhipicephalus (Boophilus) annulatus

Rhipicephalus (Boophilus) annulatus (Phylum: Arthropoda; Class: Arachnida; Order: Ixodida; Family: Ixodidae), commonly known as the Blue cattle tick or Texas cattle fever tick, is found in cattle-rearing areas worldwide. It has been largely eradicated from North America, but can sometimes be found in Texas or California. It is particularly important as a vector of pathogens in cattle but will also infest horses, goats, sheep, camels and dogs.

Epidemiology: This is a one-host tick species. Two to four generations may occur per year, depending on climatic conditions; the entire life cycle of this species can be completed in six weeks.

Table 8.11 Other species of *Rhipicephalus* of veterinary importance in cattle.

Species	Distribution	Hosts	Pathogenesis
Rhipicephalus bursa	Southern Europe, reaching central Europe and as far east as Romania	Cattle but also sheep, horses, dogs, occasionally wild ungulates	*Babesia bovis*, *B. ovis*, *B. motasi*, *B. caballi*, *Theileria equi*, *T. ovis*, *Anaplasma marginale*, *A. phagocytophilum*, *Ehrlichia canis*, *Coxiella burnetii*
Rhipicephalus capensis	Sothern Africa (with some report from Central and East Africa)	Cattle but also horses, sheep, goats, deer, antelopes, dogs	East Coast fever (*Theileria parva*) and *Anaplasma marginale*
Rhipicephalus evertsi	Africa, south of the Sahara	Cattle but also horses, sheep, goats, deer, antelopes, dogs	East Coast fever (*Theileria parva*), redwater (*Babesia bigemina*) and *Theileria mutans* in cattle. It also transmits *Borrelia* in various animals, and biliary fever (*Theileria equi*) in horses
Rhipicephalus pulchellus	Africa, east of the Rift Valley from southern Ethiopia to Somalia and northeastern Tanzania	Zebras; also infests livestock and game animals	*Babesia equi*, *Theileria* spp., *Trypanosoma theileri*, *Rickettsia conorii*, several Bunyaviridae (Crimean–Congo haemorrhagic fever virus, Nairobi sheep disease, kajiado, kismayo and dugbe viruses) and Barur virus
Rhipicephalus simus	Central and southern Africa	Dogs, wild carnivores, livestock, game animals and humans. Immature stages feed on the common burrowing savannah rodents	*Anaplasma marginale*, *A. centrale*, *Rickettsia conorii* and *Coxiella burnetii*. It can also cause tick paralysis in humans

Pathogenesis: These ticks are the most important vectors of *Babesia* spp. and *Anaplasma marginale* in cattle in subtropical and tropical countries. *Boophilus annulatus* is an important vector of Texas cattle fever caused by *Babesia bigemina* and *B. bovis*. Skin irritation induces scratching and licking, sometimes leading to secondary infections. Severe infestations may cause anaemia.

Control and treatment: The basis of successful control is to prevent the development of the engorged female ticks and so limit the deposition of large numbers of eggs. Since species of *Boophilus* have a parasitic life cycle that requires 20 days before adult females become fully engorged, an animal dipped with an acaricide that has a residual effect of 3–4 days should not harbour engorged females for at least 24 days (i.e. 20 + 4). In theory, therefore, treatment every 21 days during the tick season should give good control, but since the nymphal stages appear to be less susceptible to most acaricides, a 12-day interval is often necessary between treatments at the beginning of the tick season. The avermectins/milbemycins may play an increasing role in the control of one-host ticks. A single acaricide treatment can destroy all the ticks on an animal but will not prevent reinfestation. Hence, to effect long-term control, cattle that have had direct or presumed contact with *Boophilus* must be dipped at regular intervals for at least a year and the movement of animals into affected farms or ranches should be strictly controlled.

Rhipicephalus (Boophilus) microplus

Rhipicephalus (Boophilus) microplus (Phylum: Arthropoda; Class: Arachnida; Order: Ixodida; Family: Ixodidae), commonly known as the Tropical cattle tick or Southern cattle tick, is an important parasite of cattle, sheep, goats and wild ungulates found in Asia, Australia, Mexico, Central and South America, West Indies and South Africa.

Pathogenesis: *Rhipicephalus (Boophilus) microplus* is widely distributed in the southern hemisphere and the southern states of the USA and is considered one of the most serious external parasites of Australian cattle. This tick species is an important vector for the transmission of *Babesia bigemina* and *Borrelia theileri* in South America, *Anaplasma marginale* in Australia and South America and *Coxiella burnetii* in Australia. Disease transmission can occur throughout all the parasite stages. Disease organisms may be passed transovarially to be transmitted by the next tick generation. Some disease organisms such as *Babesia* spp. may remain in the body of the ticks for as many as five generations even when fed on non-infected, non-susceptible hosts.

Other species of *Rhipicephalus (Boophilus)* of veterinary importance are listed in Table 8.12.

Table 8.12 Other species of *Rhipicephalus (Boophilus)* of veterinary importance.

Species	Distribution	Hosts	Pathogenesis
Rhipicephalus (Boophilus) calcaratus	Asia, North Africa	Cattle but also sheep, goats and wild ungulates	*Babesia bigemina* and *B. bovis* in North Africa and *Anaplasma marginale* in the northern Caucasus
Rhipicephalus (Boophilus) decoloratus	Africa	Cattle but also sheep, goats and wild ungulates	*Babesia bigemina*, *B. ovis* and *Anaplasma marginale* in cattle. It also transmits spirochaetosis (*Borrelia theileri*) in cattle, horses, goats and sheep and *Babesia trautmanni* in pigs in East Africa

Hyalomma

Hyalomma anatolicum

Hyalomma anatolicum (Phylum: Arthropoda; Class: Arachnida; Order: Ixodida; Family: Ixodidae), commonly known as the Bont-legged tick, is a parasite of cattle but will also feed on a range of mammals and birds. It is found in steppe and semi-desert environments from central Asia to Bangladesh, the Middle and Near East, Arabia, southeastern Europe and Africa.

Epidemiology: This species is a two- or three-host tick. Larvae acquire a host, feed and moult. Nymphs reattach to the same host soon after moulting. The larvae and nymphs feed on birds and small mammals, and the adults on ruminants and equines. When larvae and nymphs infest smaller mammals, birds or reptiles, the life cycle may become a three-host model.

Pathogenesis: This genus is mainly responsible for tick toxicosis in parts of Africa and the Indian subcontinent. The 'toxin' produced by the adult tick causes a sweating sickness in ruminants and pigs characterised by widespread hyperaemia of the mucous membranes and a profuse moist eczema. This is a highly damaging tick species. *Hyalomma anatolicum* transmits *Theileria annulata*, *T. equi*, *Babesia caballi*, *Anaplasma marginale*, *Trypanosoma theileri* and at least five arboviruses.

Notes: A closely related species, *H. lusitanicum*, replaces *H. anatolicum* from central Italy to Portugal, Morocco and the Canary Islands. It is believed to be a vector of equine and bovine babesiosis.

Hyalomma excavatum

Hyalomma excavatum, synonym *Hyalomma anatolicum excavatum* (Phylum: Arthropoda; Class: Arachnida; Order: Ixodida; Family: Ixodidae), is commonly known as the Brown ear tick. This species feeds primarily on burrowing rodents, particularly as larvae and nymphs. However, adults will also feed on ruminants and equines, where this species may be of veterinary significance. It is found throughout Africa, Asia Minor and southern Europe.

Pathogenesis: *Hyalomma excavatum* is a vector for the transmission of *Theileria annulata*, causing tropical theileriosis or Mediterranean coast fever in Bovidae species, and of equine and bovine babesiosis.

Hyalomma detritum/Hyalomma scupense

Hyalomma detritum and *Hyalomma scupense* (Phylum: Arthropoda; Class: Arachnida; Order: Ixodida; Family: Ixodidae), commonly known as the Bont-legged tick, are of veterinary importance primarily in cattle, but will also feed on sheep, goats, pigs and horses. In some texts they are treated as subspecies – *H d. detritum* and *H.d. scupense* – but their status as separate species is increasingly accepted. *Hyalomma detritum* is found throughout Africa while *H. scupense* predominates in southwestern Russia and and southeastern Europe.

Pathogenesis: This genus is responsible for tick toxicosis in parts of southern Africa. The 'toxin' produced by the adult tick causes a sweating sickness in ruminants and pigs characterised by widespread hyperaemia of the mucous membranes and a profuse moist eczema.

Hyalomma truncatum

Hyalomma truncatum (Phylum: Arthropoda; Class: Arachnida; Order: Ixodida; Family: Ixodidae), commonly known as the Bont-legged tick, is a two-host tick of veterinary significance on cattle, sheep, goats, pigs and horses and will also feed on a range of other mammals and birds. It is found throughout Africa.

Pathogenesis: This species is responsible for tick toxicosis in parts of southern Africa. The 'toxin' produced by the adult tick causes a sweating sickness in ruminants and pigs characterised by widespread hyperaemia of the mucous membranes and a profuse moist eczema. This species can act as a vector of *Babesia caballi, Theileria equi, T. parva, T. annulata, T. dispar, Coxiella burnetii, Rickettsia bovis* and *R. conorii.*

Amblyomma

Amblyomma americanum

Amblyomma americanum (Phylum: Arthropoda; Class: Arachnida; Order: Ixodida; Family: Ixodidae), commonly known as the Lone Star tick, feeds on a range of wild and domestic animals and is of particular veterinary significance in cattle. Larvae are most frequently found on wild small mammals. It is widely distributed throughout central and eastern USA.

Epidemiology: Larvae and nymphs feed on rodents, rabbits and ground-inhabiting birds. Adults feed on livestock such as cattle, horses and sheep and wild hosts such as deer. Feeding larvae, nymphs and adults are active between early spring and late summer in distinct periods corresponding with the feeding activity of each stage. There is usually a single generation per year. This species is particularly common in wooded areas, where hosts become infected as they brush against vegetation harbouring ticks.

Pathogenesis: This tick is most commonly found on the ears, flanks, head and belly. Tick infestation is irritating and painful, and infestation has been shown to reduce weight gain in cattle. Each female ingests 0.5–2.0 ml of host blood, so large numbers can cause anaemia. Bites may cause tick paralysis. *Amblyomma americanum* is an important vector of *Rickettsia rickettsii* (Rocky Mountain spotted fever) and *Francisella tularensis* (tularaemia). It has also been implicated as a vector of *Borrelia burgdorferi* (Lyme disease), Q-fever, canine ehrlichiosis and human monocytic ehrlichiosis.

Amblyomma maculatum

Amblyomma maculatum (Phylum: Arthropoda; Class: Arachnida; Order: Ixodida; Family: Ixodidae), commonly known as the Gulf Coast tick, feeds on a range of mammals but is of particular veterinary significance in cattle. It is found in the southern USA, in regions of high temperature and humidity.

Pathogenesis: The Gulf Coast tick, *A. maculatum*, is not known to transmit pathogens of disease but does cause severe bites and painful swellings and has been associated with tick paralysis. The wounds created by this species may create a suitable site for screwworm myiasis associated with *Cochliomyia* spp.

Amblyomma variegatum

Amblyomma variegatum (Phylum: Arthropoda; Class: Arachnida; Order: Ixodida; Family: Ixodidae), commonly known as the Variegated or Tropical bont tick, feeds on a range of mammals but is of particular veterinary significance in cattle. It is found throughout Africa.

Pathogenesis: *Amblyomma variegatum* transmits the important disease heartwater in cattle, caused by the rickettsia *Ehrlichia ruminantium*. It also transmits the Nairobi sheep disease virus and Q-fever, caused by *Coxiella burnetii*.

Other *Amblyomma* tick species in cattle are listed in Table 8.13.

Haemaphysalis

Haemaphysalis punctata

Haemaphysalis punctata (Phylum: Arthropoda; Class: Arachnida; Order: Ixodida; Family: Ixodidae) feeds on a wide range of wild and domestic animals, but may be of particular veterinary importance in cattle and sheep. The larvae and nymphs may be found on birds, hedgehogs, rodents and reptiles such as lizards and snakes. They occur throughout Europe (including southern Scandinavia and Britain), central Asia and North Africa.

Epidemiology: *Haemaphysalis punctata* is a three-host tick, feeding once in each of the larval, nymphal and adult life-cycle stages.

Pathogenesis: *Haemaphysalis punctata* is responsible for the transmission of *Babesia major* and *B. bigemina, Theileria mutans* (*T. buffeli/orientalis*), *Anaplasma marginale* and *A. centrale* in

Table 8.13 Other *Amblyomma* tick species in cattle.

Species	Hosts	Geographical distribution	Pathogenesis
Amblyomma hebraeum	Cattle, sheep and goats	Mainly Africa	Heartwater (*Ehrlichia ruminantium*)
Amblyomma gemma	Cattle, sheep and goats	Africa, particularly Kenya	Heartwater (*Ehrlichia ruminantium*)
Amblyomma pomposum	Mammals, particularly cattle, sheep and goats	Africa, mainly western Zambia, southern DRC and Angola	Heartwater (*Ehrlichia ruminantium*)
Amblyomma lepidum	Sheep, goats, cattle	Sudan	Heartwater (*Ehrlichia ruminantium*) and boutonneuse fever (*Rickettsia conorii*)
Amblyomma astrion	Buffalo, cattle	West and Central Africa	Heartwater (*Ehrlichia ruminantium*)
Amblyomma sparsum	Reptiles, tortoises	Sub-Saharan Africa	
Amblyomma marmorium	Tortoises	Sub-Saharan Africa	These species are of particular importance because they are vectors of the rickettsia *Ehrlichia ruminantium*, the causal agent of heartwater in cattle, sheep, goats, deer and buffalo. Infected ticks may be present on imported reptiles, facilitating the transmission of disease into new areas such as the USA

Table 8.14 Other species of *Haemaphysalis* of veterinary importance in cattle.

Species	Distribution	Hosts	Pathogenesis
Haemaphysalis longicornis	Far East and Australasia	Primarily cattle but also occasionally other mammals and birds	
Haemaphysalis bispinosa	Asia and Australasia	Feeds on a range of mammals, including sheep and cattle	*Babesia motasi* and *B. ovis* in sheep and goats, *B. equi* in horses and donkeys and *B. canis* and *B. gibsoni* in dogs

cattle. In sheep, it transmits *Babesia motasi* and the benign *Theileria ovis*. It has also been reported to cause tick paralysis. In addition to transmitting *Anaplasma* and *Babesia* spp., different *H. punctata* populations are infected by tick-borne encephalitis virus, Tribec virus, Bhanja virus and Crimean–Congo haemorrhagic fever virus.

Other species of *Haemaphysalis* of veterinary importance in cattle are listed in Table 8.14.

ARGASIDAE
Otobius megnini

Otobius megnini (Phylum: Arthropoda; Class: Arachnida; Order: Ixodida; Family: Argasidae), commonly known as the Spinose ear tick, usually infests wild and domestic animals, particularly cattle but also sheep, dogs, horses and occasionally humans. It is found in North and South America, India and southern Africa.

Pathogenesis: The larvae and nymphs feed in the external ear canal of the host, producing severe inflammation and a waxy exudate in the ear canals. Secondary bacterial infections can occur, which may extend up the ear canal. Infested hosts may scratch and shake their heads. Scratching can cause local skin trauma and occasionally perforate the eardrum. This can lead to infection, ulceration and in some cases meningitis. In horses, clinical signs may be mistaken for signs of colic.

Ornithodoros erraticus

Ornithodoros erraticus (Phylum: Arthropoda; Class: Arachnida; Order: Ixodida; Family: Argasidae), commonly known as a Sand tampan, is a parasite of small mammals, but is of particular veterinary importance because it will also bite domestic livestock. It is found throughout Europe, Africa and the Middle East.

Pathogenesis: *Ornithodoros erraticus* is a vector of the rickettsial parasite *Coxiella burnetii,* the causative agent of Q-fever in cattle, sheep and goats. It also transmits *Borrelia hispanica* in the Spanish peninsula and adjacent North Africa, and *B. crocidurae* in Africa, the Near East and Central Asia. These are both spirochaetes which cause tick-borne relapsing fever. This species also acts as a reservoir and vector for African swine fever virus and *Babesia*.

HOST–PARASITE CHECKLIST

In the following checklists, the codes listed below apply.

Helminths

N, nematode; T, trematode; C, cestode; A, acanthocephalan.

Arthropods

F, fly; L, louse; S, flea; M, mite; Mx, maxillopod; Ti, tick.

Protozoa

Co, coccidia; Bs, blood sporozoa; Am, amoeba; Fl, flagellate; Ci, ciliate.

Miscellaneous 'protozoal organisms'

B, blastocyst; Mi, microsporidian; My, *Mycoplasma*; P, Pneumocystidomycete; R, *Rickettsia*.

Cattle parasite checklist.

Section/host system	Helminths Parasite	(Super) family	Arthropods Parasite	Family	Protozoa Parasite	Family
Digestive						
Oesophagus	Gongylonema pulchrum	Spiruroidea (N)	Hypoderma bovis	Oestridae (F)	Monocercomonas ruminantium	Monocercomonadidae (Fl)
			Hypoderma lineatum	Oestridae (F)	Entamoeba bovis	Entamoebidae (AM)
Rumen/reticulum	Gongylonema verrucosum	Spiruroidea (N)				
	Gongylonema pulchrum	Spiruroidea (N)				
	Paramphistomum cervi	Paramphistomatidae (T)				
	Calicophoron daubneyi	Paramphistomatidae (T)				
	Paramphistomum microbothrium	Paramphistomatidae (T)				
	Paramphistomum ichikawa	Paramphistomatidae (T)				
	Paramphistomum streptocoelium	Paramphistomatidae (T)				
	Cotylophoron cotylophorum	Paramphistomatidae (T)				
	Calicophoron calicophorum	Paramphistomatidae (T)				
	Gastrothylax crumenifer	Gastrothylacidae (T)				
	Fischoederius elongatus	Gastrothylacidae (T)				
	Fischoederius cobboldi	Gastrothylacidae (T)				
	Carmyerius spatiosus	Gastrothylacidae (T)				
	Carmyerius gregarius	Gastrothylacidae (T)				
Abomasum	Ostertagia ostertagi (lyrata)	Trichostrongyloidea (N)			Cryptosporidium andersoni	Cryptosporidiidae (Co)
	Ostertagia leptospicularis	Trichostrongyloidea (N)				
	Spiculopteragia spiculoptera	Trichostrongyloidea (N)				
	Haemonchus contortus	Trichostrongyloidea (N)				
	Haemonchus similis	Trichostrongyloidea (N)				
	Trichostrongylus axei	Trichostrongyloidea (N)				
	Mecistocirrus digitatus	Trichostrongyloidea (N)				
	Parabronema skrjabini	Spiruroidea (N)				
	Capillaria bilobata	Trichuroidea (N)				
Small intestine	Trichostrongylus colubriformis	Trichostrongyloidea (N)			Eimeria bovis	Eimeriidae (Co)
	Trichostrongylus longispicularis	Trichostrongyloidea (N)			Eimeria zuernii	Eimeriidae (Co)
	Cooperia oncophora	Trichostrongyloidea (N)			Eimeria alabamensis	Eimeriidae (Co)
	Cooperia punctata	Trichostrongyloidea (N)			Eimeria aubernensis	Eimeriidae (Co)
	Cooperia pectinata	Trichostrongyloidea (N)			Eimeria brasiliensis	Eimeriidae (Co)
	Cooperia surnabada	Trichostrongyloidea (N)			Eimeria bukidnonensis	Eimeriidae (Co)
	Nematodirus helvetianus	Trichostrongyloidea (N)			Eimeria canadensis	Eimeriidae (Co)
	Nematodirus battus	Trichostrongyloidea (N)			Eimeria cylindrica	Eimeriidae (Co)
	Nematodirus spathiger	Trichostrongyloidea (N)			Eimeria ellipsoidalis	Eimeriidae (Co)
	Bunostomum phlebotomum	Ancylostomatoidea (N)			Eimeria pellita	Eimeriidae (Co)
	Agriostomum vryburgi	Ancylostomatoidea (N)			Eimeria subspherica	Eimeriidae (Co)
	Strongyloides papillosus	Rhabditoidea (N)			Eimeria wyomingensis	Eimeriidae (Co)
	Toxocara vitulorum	Ascaridoidea (N)			Cryptosporidium parvum	Cryptosporidiidae (Co)
	Capillaria bovis	Trichuroidea (N)			Cryptosporidium ryanae	Cryptosporidiidae (Co)
	Moniezia benedeni	Anoplocephalidae (C)			Cryptosporidium ubiquitum	Cryptosporidiidae (Co)
	Moniezia expansa	Anoplocephalidae (C)			Giardia intestinalis	Giardiidae (Fl)
	Thysaniezia ovilla	Anoplocephalidae (C)				
	Avitellina centripunctata	Anoplocephalidae (C)				
	Stilesia globipunctata	Anoplocephalidae (C)				
	Thysaniezia ovilla	Anoplocephalidae (C)				
	Thysanosoma actinoides	Anoplocephalidae (C)				
	Cymbiforma indica	Notocotylidae (T)				
Caecum	Oesophagostomum radiatum	Trichostrongyloidea (N)			Eimeria zuernii	Eimeriidae (Co)
	Trichuris globulosa	Trichuroidea (N)				
Colon	Trichuris discolor	Trichuroidea (N)			Eimeria bovis	Eimeriidae (Co)
	Homalogaster paloniae	Gastrodiscidae (T)			Tetratrichomonas buttreyi	Trichomonadidae (Fl)
					Tetratrichomonas pavlovi	Trichomonadidae (Fl)
					Tritrichomonas enteris	Trichomonadidae (Fl)
					Retortamonas ovis	Retortamonadidae (Fl)
					Buxtonella sulcata	Pycnotrichidae (Ci)

(Continued)

Cattle parasite checklist. *Continued*

Section/host system	Helminths		Arthropods		Protozoa	
	Parasite	(Super) family	Parasite	Family	Parasite	Family
Respiratory						
Nasal cavities	*Mammomonogamus laryngeus*	Trichostrongyloidea (N)				
Trachea/bronchi	*Mammomonogamus nasicola*	Trichostrongyloidea (N)				
	Schistosoma nasale	Schistosomatidae (T)				
	Dictyocaulus viviparus	Trichostrongyloidea (N)				
Lung	*Echinococcus granulosus*	Taeniidae (C)			*Pneumocystis carinii*	Pneumocystidaceae (P)
Liver	*Fasciola hepatica*	Fasciolidae (T)				
	Fasciola gigantica	Fasciolidae (T)				
	Fascioloides magna	Fasciolidae (T)				
	Dicrocoelium dendriticum	Dicrocoeliidae (T)				
	Dicrocoelium hospes	Dicrocoeliidae (T)				
	Gigantocotyle explanatum	Paramphistomatidae (T)				
	Echinococcus granulosus	Taeniidae (C)				
	Echinococcus ortleppi	Taeniidae (C)				
	Stilesia hepatica	Anoplocephalidae (C)				
	Cysticercus tenuicollis (Taenia hydatigena)	Taeniidae (C)				
	Thysanosoma actinioides	Anoplocephalidae (C)				
Pancreas	*Eurytrema pancreaticum*	Dicrocoeliidae (T)				
	Eurytrema coelomaticum	Dicrocoeliidae (T)				
	Thysanosoma actinioides	Anoplocephalidae (C)				
Circulatory						
Blood	*Schistosoma bovis*	Schistosomatidae (T)			*Trypanosoma brucei brucei*	Trypanosomatidae (Fl)
	Schistosoma mattheei	Schistosomatidae (T)			*Trypanosoma brucei evansi*	Trypanosomatidae (Fl)
	Schistosoma leiperi	Schistosomatidae (T)			*Trypanosoma congolense*	Trypanosomatidae (Fl)
	Schistosoma indicum	Schistosomatidae (T)			*Trypanosoma vivax*	Trypanosomatidae (Fl)
	Schistosoma nasale	Schistosomatidae (T)			*Trypansoma theileri*	Trypanosomatidae (Fl)
	Schistosoma spindale	Schistosomatidae (T)			*Babesia bigemina*	Babesiidae (Bs)
	Schistosoma japonicum	Schistosomatidae (T)			*Babesia bovis*	Babesiidae (Bs)
	Schistosoma turkestanica	Schistosomatidae (T)			*Babesia divergens*	Babesiidae (Bs)
					Babesia major	Babesiidae (Bs)
					Babesia occultans	Babesiidae (Bs)
					Babesia ovata	Babesiidae (Bs)
					Babesia jakimovae	Babesiidae (Bs)
					Theileria parva	Theileriidae (Bs)
					Theileria annulata	Theileriidae (Bs)
					Theileria orientalis complex	Theileriidae (Bs)
					Theileria taurotragi	Theileriidae (Bs)
					Theileria velifera	Theileriidae (Bs)
					Anaplasma marginale	Anaplasmataceae (R)
					Anaplasma centrale	Anaplasmataceae (R)
					Anaplasma phagocytophilum	Anaplasmataceae (R)
					Ehrlichia bovis	Anaplasmataceae (R)
					Ehrlichia ruminantium	Anaplasmataceae (R)
					Rickettsia conorii	Rickettsiaceae (R)
					Mycoplasma wenyonii	Mycoplasmataceae (My)

System	Helminth species	Helminth taxon	Arthropod/mite species	Arthropod/mite taxon	Protozoan species	Protozoan taxon
Blood vessels	*Elaeophora poeli*	Filarioidea (N)			*Toxoplasma gondii*	Sarcocystidae (Co)
	Onchocerca armillata	Filarioidea (N)			*Trypanosoma brucei brucei*	Trypanosomatidae (Fl)
Nervous						
CNS	*Coenurus cerebralis* (metacestode: *Taenia multiceps*)	Taeniidae (C)	*Hypoderma bovis*	Oestridae (F)		
Eye	*Thelazia rhodesi*	Spiruroidea (N)				
	Thelazia gulosa	Spiruroidea (N)				
	Thelazia skrjabini	Spiruroidea (N)				
Ear			*Railietia auris*	Halarachnidae (M)		
Reproductive/urogenital						
	Stepahanurus dentatus	Trichostrongyloidea (N)			*Tritrichomonas foetus*	Trichomonadidae (Fl)
					Neospora caninum	Sarcocystidae (Co)
					Trypanosoma brucei	Trypanosomatidae (Fl)
Locomotory						
Muscle	*Cysticercus bovis* (metacestode: *Taenia saginata*)	Taeniidae (C)			*Sarcocystis bovicanis*	Sarcocystidae (Co)
					Sarcocystis bovifelis	Sarcocystidae (Co)
					Sarcocystis bovihominis	Sarcocystidae (Co)
					Toxoplasma gondii	Sarcocystidae (Co)
Connective tissue						
	Onchocerca gutturosa	Filarioidea (N)				
	Onchocerca gibsoni	Filarioidea (N)				
	Onchocerca ochengi	Filarioidea (N)				
	Onchocerca dukei	Filarioidea (N)				
	Parafilaria bovicola	Filarioidea (N)				
	Setaria labiato-papillosa	Filarioidea (N)				
	Setaria digitatus	Filarioidea (N)				
Subcutaneous	*Parafilaria bovicola*	Filarioidea (N)	*Hypoderma bovis*	Oestridae (F)		
	Dracunculus medinensis	Dracunculidae (N)	*Hypoderma lineatum*	Oestridae (F)		
			Dermatobia hominis	Oestridae (F)		
			Calliphora albifrontis	Calliphoridae (F)		
			Calliphora nociva	Calliphoridae (F)		
			Calliphora stygia	Calliphoridae (F)		
			Calliphora vicina	Calliphoridae (F)		
			Calliphora vomitoria	Calliphoridae (F)		
			Lucilia sericata	Calliphoridae (F)		
			Lucilia cuprina	Calliphoridae (F)		
			Lucilia illustris	Calliphoridae (F)		
			Protophormia terraenovae	Calliphoridae (F)		
			Phormia regina	Calliphoridae (F)		
			Cordylobia anthropophaga	Calliphoridae (F)		
			Cochliomyia hominivorax	Calliphoridae (F)		
			Cochliomyia macellaria	Calliphoridae (F)		
			Chrysomya bezziana	Calliphoridae (F)		
			Chrysomya megacephala	Calliphoridae (F)		
			Wohlfahrtia magnifica	Sarcophagidae (F)		
			Sarcophaga haemorrhoidalis	Sarcophagidae (F)		

(Continued)

Cattle parasite checklist. *Continued*

Section/host system	Helminths		Arthropods		Protozoa	
	Parasite	(Super) family	Parasite	Family	Parasite	Family
Integument						
Skin	*Stephanofilaria stilesi*	Filarioidea (N)	*Bovicola bovis*	Trichodectidae (L)	*Besnoitia besnoiti*	Sarcocystidae (Co)
	Stephanofilaria assamensis	Filarioidea (N)	*Haematopinus eurysternus*	Haematopinidae (L)		
	Stephanofilaria zaheeri	Filarioidea (N)	*Haematopinus quadripertusus*	Haematopinidae (L)		
	Stephanofilaria kaeli	Filarioidea (N)	*Haematopinus tuberculatus*	Haematopinidae (L)		
	Stephanofilaria dedoesi	Filarioidea (N)	*Linognathus vituli*	Linognathidae (L)		
	Stephanofilaria okinawaensis	Filarioidea (N)	*Solenopotes capillatus*	Linognathidae (L)		
			Demodex bovis	Demodicidae (M)		
			Psorobia bovis	Psorergatidae (M)		
			Psoroptes ovis	Psoroptidae (M)		
			Psoroptes natalensis	Psoroptidae (M)		
			Chorioptes bovis	Psoroptidae (M)		
			Sarcoptes scabiei	Sarcoptidae (M)		

Flies of veterinary importance on cattle.

Group	Genus	Species	Family
Blackflies Buffalo gnats	Simulium	spp.	Simuliidae (F)
Blowflies and screwworms	Calliphora	albifrontis nociva stygia vicina vomitoria	Calliphoridae (F)
	Chrysomya	albiceps bezziana megacephala	
	Cochliomyia	hominivorax macellaria	
	Cordylobia	anthropophaga	
	Lucilia	cuprina illustris sericata	
	Phormia	regina	
	Protophormia	terraenovae	
Bot flies	Gedoelstia	haessleri	Oestridae (F)
	Hypoderma	bovis lineatum	
	Dermatobia	hominis	
Flesh flies	Sarcophaga	fusicausa haemorrhoidalis	Sarcophagidae (F)
	Wohlfahrtia	magnifica meigeni vigil	
Hippoboscids	Hippobosca	equina rufipes maculata camelina	Hippoboscidae (F)
Midges	Culicoides	spp.	Ceratopogonidae (F)
Mosquitoes	Aedes Anopheles Culex	spp. spp. spp.	Culicidae (F)
Muscids	Haematobia	irritans exigua	Muscidae (F)
	Musca	autumnalis domestica	
	Stomoxys	calcitrans	
Sand flies	Phlebotomus	spp.	Psychodidae (F)
Tabanids	Chrysops Haematopota Tabanus	spp. spp. spp.	Tabanidae (F)
Tsetse flies	Glossina	fusca morsitans palpalis	Glossinidae (F)

Tick species found on cattle.

Genus	Species	Common name	Family
Ornithodoros	moubata	Eyeless or hut tampan	Argasidae (Ti)
	savignyi	Eyed or sand tampan	
Otobius	megnini	Spinose ear tick	Argasidae (Ti)
Amblyomma	americanum	Lone star tick	Ixodidae (Ti)
	cajennense	Cayenne tick	
	gemma		
	hebraeum	South African bont tick	
	maculatum	Gulf Coast tick	
	pomposum		
	variegatum	Variegated or tropical bont tick	
Dermacentor	andersoni	Rocky Mountain wood tick	Ixodidae (Ti)
	marginatus	Ornate sheep tick	
	nutalli		
	reticulatus	Marsh tick, meadow tick	
	occidentalis	Pacific coast tick	
	silvarium		
	variabilis	American dog tick	
Haemaphysalis	punctata		Ixodidae (Ti)
	concinna	Bush tick	
	bispinosa	Bush tick	
	longicornis	Scrub tick, New Zealand cattle tick	
Hyalomma	anatolicum	Bont-legged tick	Ixodidae (Ti)
	detritum	Bont-legged tick	
	dromedarii	Camel tick	
	excavatum		
	marginatum	Mediterranean tick	
	truncatum	Bont-legged tick	
Ixodes	ricinus	Castor bean or European sheep tick	Ixodidae (Ti)
	holocyclus	Paralysis tick	
	rubicundus	Karoo paralysis tick	
	scapularis	Deer tick, black-legged tick	
Rhipicephalus	appendiculatus	Brown ear tick	Ixodidae (Ti)
	bursa		
	capensis	Cape brown tick	
	evertsi	Red or red-legged tick	
	sanguineus	Brown dog or kennel tick	
	simus	Glossy tick	
Rhipicephalus (Boophilus)	annulatus	Texas cattle fever tick	Ixodidae (Ti)
	decoloratus	Blue tick	
	microplus	Pantropical or southern cattle tick	

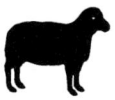

ENDOPARASITES

Parasites of the digestive system

OESOPHAGUS

Gongylonema pulchrum

Gongylonema pulchrum, synonym *Gongylonema scutatum* (Phylum: Nematoda; Class: Chromadorea; Order: Spirurida; Family: Gongylonematidae), commonly known as the Gullet worm, is distributed worldwide and localised in the oesophagus and rumen of sheep, goats, cattle, pigs, buffalo, horses, donkeys, deer, camels and humans. This parasite has coprophagous beetles and cockroaches as intermediate hosts.

Epidemiology: Infection is very much dependent on the presence and abundance of the intermediate hosts, principally coprophagous beetles of the genera *Aphodius*, *Onthophagus*, *Blaps*, *Caccobius* and *Onthophagus*. Humans can acquire infection through direct ingestion of the intermediate host. Also, water can contain infective larvae that have emerged from infected cockroaches in the water source.

Pathogenesis: Infection is usually regarded as non-pathogenic, though it has been associated with a mild chronic oesophagitis in ruminants. *Gongylonema pulchrum* in humans presents as a painful tumour-like area in the oral epithelium or subcutaneous tissues that contains coiled worms.

Clinical signs and pathology: Usually asymptomatic in ruminants. Adult worms bury in the epithelium of the forestomachs, producing white or red, blood-filled zig-zag tracts in the mucosa. Incidental finding on *post mortem* is considered the only diagnostic method available. Control is not practical or necessary.

RUMEN AND RETICULUM

Gongylonema verrucosum

Gongylonema verrucosum (Phylum: Nematoda; Class: Chromadorea; Order: Spirurida; Family: Gongylonematidae), commonly known as the Rumen gullet worm, is localised in the rumen, reticulum and omasum of cattle, sheep, goats and deer, and is distributed in India, South Africa and the USA. This parasite has coprophagous beetles and cockroaches as intermediate hosts. For additional details see Chapter 8.

Paramphistomum and other rumen flukes

Rumen flukes are mainly parasitic in the forestomachs of ruminants. Their shape is not typical of the trematodes, being conical, thick and fleshy rather than flat. All require a water snail as an intermediate host. There are several genera: *Paramphistomum*, *Cotylophoron*, *Bothriophoron*, *Orthocoelium* and *Giganocotyle*, of which *Paramphistomum* is the most common and widespread in ruminants. The taxonomy of the paramphistomes is complex and unresolved and many of the species described may be synonymous, being differentiated mainly on size and shape of the suckers. Details on the pathogenesis, treatment and control of rumen flukes are provided in Chapter 8.

Paramphistomum cervi

Paramphistomum cervi, synonym *Paramphistomum explanatum* (Phylum: Platyhelminthes; Class: Trematoda; Order: Plagiorchiida; Family: Paramphistomatidae), commonly known as the Rumen fluke, is distributed worldwide and localised in the rumen of cattle, sheep, goats, deer, buffaloes and antelopes. They complete their biological life cycle in water snails, principally *Planorbis* and *Bulinus*. They are of little veterinary significance in Europe and America, but are occasionally the cause of disease in the tropics and subtropics.

Gastrothylax crumenifer

Gastrothylax crumenifer (Phylum: Platyhelminthes; Class: Trematoda; Order: Plagiorchiida; Family: Gastrothylacidae), commonly known as the Rumen fluke, is localised in the rumen and reticulum of cattle, buffalo, zebus, sheep and many other ruminants. This fluke is distributed in the Indian subcontinent, China, Middle East, Africa and parts of Asiatic Russia and Europe and the infection mainly causes anaemia.

Veterinary Parasitology, Fifth Edition. Domenico Otranto and Richard Wall.
© 2024 John Wiley & Sons Ltd. Published 2024 by John Wiley & Sons Ltd.

Fischoederius elongatus

Fischoederius elongatus (Phylum: Platyhelminthes; Class: Trematoda; Order: Plagiorchiida; Family: Gastrothylacidae) is localised in the rumen, duodenum or anterior small intestine of cattle, buffalo, zebus, sheep and many other ruminants. It can accidentally infect humans and is distributed in Asia. This parasite is similar to *Fischoederius cobboldi*.

Pathogenesis: Flukes in the rumen usually cause only mild congestion but flukes attached to the duodenum can result in thickening of the mucosa.

Monocercomonas ruminantium

Monocercomonas ruminantium, synonyms *Trichomonas ruminantium*, *Tritrichomonas ruminantium* (Phylum: Metamonada; Class Trichomonadea; Order: Tricomonadida; Family: Monocercomonadidae), is a protozoan distributed worldwide and localised in the rumen of cattle and sheep. It is not considered to be pathogenic and transmission presumably occurs by ingestion of trophozoites from faeces or rumen contents. Diagnosis is performed through the identification of trophozoites based on morphological examination.

ABOMASUM

Teladorsagia circumcincta

Teladorsagia circumcincta, synonym *Ostertagia circumcincta* (Phylum: Nematoda; Class: Chromadorea; Order: Rhabditida; Family: Trichostrongylidae), commonly known as the Brown stomach worm, is distributed worldwide and localised in the abomasum of sheep, goats and deer. *Teladorsagia circumcincta* is considered a polymorphic species with at least two male morphs, *Teladorsagia circumcincta* and *Ostertagia trifurcata*, and possibly a third, *Teladorsagia davtiani*. The females cannot be differentiated but are distinguishable from other ostertagian females. Based on ITS-2 sequence analysis, *Ostertagia trifurcata* and *Teladorsagia davtiani* belong to a single species, *T. circumcincta*.

Epidemiology: In sheep, *T. circumcincta* is responsible for outbreaks of clinical disease, particularly in lambs. In Europe, a clinical syndrome analogous to type I bovine ostertagiosis occurs from August to October; thereafter arrested development of many ingested larvae occurs and a type II syndrome has been occasionally reported in late winter and early spring, especially in young adults. In subtropical areas with winter rainfall, outbreaks of disease occur primarily in late winter.

Temperate regions   In Europe, the herbage numbers of *T. circumcincta* L_3 increase markedly from midsummer onwards and this is when most disease appears. These larvae are derived mainly from eggs passed in the faeces of ewes during the periparturient period, from about two weeks prior to lambing until about six weeks after lambing. Eggs passed by lambs, from worm burdens which have accrued from the ingestion of overwintered larvae, also contribute to pasture contamination. It is these eggs deposited in the first half of the grazing season from April to June which give rise to

the potentially dangerous populations of L_3 from July to October. If ingested prior to October, the majority of these larvae mature in three weeks; thereafter, many become arrested in development for several months and may precipitate type II disease when they mature. Immunity is acquired slowly and usually requires exposure over two grazing seasons before significant resistance to infection develops. Subsequently, adult ewes harbour only very low populations of *Teladorsagia* except during the annual periparturient rise (PPR).

Subtropical regions   The epidemiology in subtropical areas is basically similar to that in temperate zones, except that the seasonal timing of events is different. In many of these areas, lambing is geared to an increase in the growth of pasture, which occurs with the onset of rain in late autumn or winter. This coincides with conditions which are favourable to the development of the free-living stages of *Teladorsagia* and so infective larvae accumulate during the winter to cause clinical problems or production loss in the second half of the winter; arrested larval development occurs at the end of the winter or early spring. The sources of pasture contamination are again the ewes, during the PPR, and the lambs, following ingestion of larvae that have survived the summer. The relative importance of these sources in any country varies according to the conditions during the adverse period for larval survival. Where the summer is very dry and hot, the longevity of L_3 is reduced, except in areas with shade, and these can act as reservoirs of infection until the following winter. Although L_3 can persist in sheep faeces during adverse weather conditions, the protection is probably less than that afforded by the more abundant bovine faecal pat.

Ostertagia trifurcata   In temperate regions, this is similar to *T. circumcincta*. In tropical and subtropical zones where the summer is very dry and hot, the longevity of L_3 is reduced, except in areas with shade, and these can act as reservoirs of infection until the following winter. Although L_3 can persist in sheep faeces during adverse weather conditions, the protection is probably less than that afforded by the more abundant bovine faecal pat. In winter rainfall areas, the numbers of *Ostertagia* and *Teladorsagia* larvae on pasture reach a maximum in late winter and decline markedly through spring into summer as the pastures dry out.

Pathogenesis: In clinical infections, this resembles the situation in cattle and similar lesions are present at necropsy, although the Morocco leather appearance of the abomasal surface seen in cattle is not common in sheep and goats. In subclinical infections, it has been shown under both experimental and natural conditions that *T. circumcincta* causes a marked depression in appetite and this, together with loss of plasma protein into the gastrointestinal tract and sloughed intestinal epithelium, results in interference with the postabsorptive metabolism of protein. In lambs with moderate infections of *T. circumcincta*, carcass evaluation can show poor protein and fat deposition. Skeletal growth can also be impaired.

Clinical signs and pathology: The most frequent clinical sign is a marked loss of weight. Diarrhoea is intermittent and although stained hindquarters are common, the fluid faeces that characterise bovine ostertagiosis are less frequently seen. The pathology is similar to that described for *O. ostertagi* in cattle. The developing parasites cause distension of parasitised gastric glands, leading to a thickened hyperplastic gastric mucosa similar to that seen in cattle (see Fig. 8.3). In heavy infections, these nodules coalesce and the abomasal folds are often very oedematous and hyperaemic.

Diagnosis: This is based on clinical signs, seasonality of infection and faecal egg counts and, if possible, *post mortem* examination, when the characteristic lesions can be seen in the abomasum. Plasma pepsinogen levels are above the normal of about 0.8 iu tyrosine and usually exceed 2.0 iu in sheep with heavy infections.

Control and treatment: For control, see section on control and treatment of parasitic gastroenteritis in sheep. Many of the anthelmintics recommended for sheep are not registered for use in goats. Where goat milk or milk products are used for human consumption, milk-withholding periods for different drugs should be observed. Thiabendazole has antifungal properties and should not be used when milk is processed for cheese. Ovine teladorsagiosis often responds well to treatment with any of the modern benzimidazoles or pro-benzimidazoles, levamisole (which in sheep is effective against arrested larvae), the avermectins/milbemycins or the recently introduced monepantel and derquantel (in combination with abamectin). However, the widespread prevalence of isolates of *T. circumcincta* that are resistant to the benzimidazoles, and increasingly resistant to levamisole and macrocyclic lactones, dictates that farmers must monitor the resistance status of their flocks to ensure that an effective anthelmintic is used. Treated lambs should preferably be moved to safer pasture, but one which contains infective larvae *in refugia*; if this is not possible, treatment may have to be repeated at six-weekly intervals until the pasture larval levels decrease in late autumn.

Control and treatment of parasitic gastroenteritis in sheep

The recommendations outlined here are applicable to temperate areas of the northern hemisphere, but the principles can be adapted to local conditions in other regions. Although the control of parasitic gastroenteritis (PGE) in sheep is based on the same principles as those described for *O. ostertagi* in cattle, its practice is somewhat different for the following reasons.

1 The PPR (periparturient rise in faecal egg counts) is very marked in ewes and is the most important cause of pasture contamination with nematode eggs in the spring.
2 PGE in sheep is generally associated with a variety of nematode genera with differing epidemiological characteristics.
3 Most sheep graze throughout their lives so that pasture contamination with nematode eggs and the intake of infective larvae are almost continuous and modified only by climatic restrictions.
4 Anthelmintic resistance is now widespread throughout many sheep-rearing areas of the world and therefore strategies are required to manage existing resistance and/or to limit the further development of resistant isolates. In Britain, for example, guidelines for the use of anthelmintics in sustainable control strategies for sheep in northern temperate areas have been produced (Sustainable Control of Parasites in Sheep or SCOPS; available at www.scops.org.uk) and are outlined in Table 9.1. The key factors which define the rate of development of anthelmintic resistance, on which the SCOPS principles are based, are summarised directly from the guidelines:
   • the proportion of worms on a farm that carry resistant alleles
   • the frequency of anthelmintic use
   • the efficacy of each treatment

Table 9.1 SCOPS guidelines.

1. Work out a control strategy with your veterinarian or adviser. The need for specialist consultation is greater now than ever before. Decisions about the judicious use of anthelmintics in worm control programmes are complex, and will require ongoing consultations
2. Use effective quarantine strategies to prevent the importation of resistant worms in introduced sheep and goats. Introduction of resistance alleles is considered a major cause of anthelmintic resistance in UK flocks. The recommended treatments also prevent the importation of *Haemonchus contortus*
3. Test for anthelmintic resistance on your farm. Knowing which products (chemical groups) are effective in a flock is fundamental to an effective control strategy
4. Administer anthelmintics effectively. Administer the right dose in the correct way, and exploit opportunities to enhance drug efficacy to ensure maximum kill rates
5. Use anthelmintics only when necessary. Understand the trade-off between tolerating some level of parasitism and minimising selection for anthelmintic resistance. Faecal egg count monitoring has an important role
6. Select the appropriate anthelmintic for the task. Consider narrow-spectrum treatments whenever possible. Alternate chemical groups in appropriate ways
7. Adopt strategies to preserve susceptible worms on the farm. Aim to reduce the heavy selection for anthelmintic resistance imposed when treating sheep with strong acquired immunity or when dosing on to low contamination pastures
8. Reduce dependence on anthelmintics. Use alternative control measures when possible. These include grazing management, risk assessment and using rams that have been selected for resistance to nematodes

Source: Adapted from Abbott *et al.* (2012).

• the proportion of the total worm population in the animal at the time of treatment
• the speed with which any surviving parasites are subsequently diluted with unselected parasites *in refugia*.

In fat lamb production systems, because of the short period between birth and marketing, treatments for PGE are generally given preventively rather than as specific therapeutic interventions to treat disease outbreaks. However, when necessary, treatment with any of the benzimidazoles, levamisole, an avermectin/ milbemycin or the new drugs monepantel and the dual-active derquantel–abamectin will remove adult worms and developing stages, unless resistance to some of the older drugs is present in the flock. Treatment with these two new compounds should be used strategically and integrated into parasite control options for the farm, along with existing anthelmintics where these still possess a reasonably high level of efficacy. Following treatment, lambs can be moved to pasture not grazed by sheep that year, but it is important that these pastures have sufficient levels of larvae *in refugia* to dilute any larvae arising from eggs of worms that have survived treatment. The occasional outbreaks of type II teladorsagiosis (ostertagiosis) in young adult sheep in the spring may be treated with the same anthelmintics. Unlike *O. ostertagi* in calves, the arrested stages of the common sheep nematodes are susceptible to the benzimidazoles and levamisole.

Summary of guidelines for the control of gastrointestinal nematodes and use of anthelmintics in sheep and goats

Anthelmintic usage

1 **Use anthelmintics sparingly**. This will reduce the selection pressure for further development of drug resistance. Effective

monitoring of faecal egg counts is integral to this approach. This strategy is discussed more fully under treatment of ewes and lambs.

2 **Use anthelmintics effectively**. It is important to check the dosing equipment regularly and to apply correct techniques to maximise the efficacy of the drug and also to ensure that the drug is stored according to the manufacturer's recommendations. It is important to read the instructions for injectable products as the injection site can vary depending on whether the drug is long-acting or whether it is administered subcutaneously or intramuscularly. Sheep should be dosed at the rate recommended for the heaviest animal in a subgroup to reduce the likelihood of underdosing.

3 **Monitor for anthelmintic resistance**. It is essential to ensure that the drug to be administered will be effective. The resistance status of each family of anthelmintic should be assessed on the farm.

4 **Use the appropriate anthelmintic**. In some situations, it may be possible to target treatment by using a narrow-spectrum drug, for example closantel against a specific infection dominated by *Haemonchus* or a benzimidazole against *Nematodirus*. Avoidance of a broad-spectrum drug in these circumstances will reduce the selection pressure on this family of anthelmintics. Annual rotation of anthelmintic families can be useful, especially where resistance to the macrocyclic lactones is absent or at a very low level. This strategy will have minimal impact where multiple resistance is firmly established.

Control strategies (see also Chapter 6)

1 **Use effective quarantine procedures**. It is essential to treat all sheep and goats imported onto the home farm effectively in order to prevent the introduction of anthelmintic-resistant worms. This may involve the introduction of new livestock or the return of stock that has been temporarily grazed away from the main farm on other pastures. If any resistant worms survive the quarantine treatment, then their numbers should be so low that the emergence of anthelmintic resistance will be greatly delayed. This may be difficult on farms with resistance to all three families of drugs. The recent availability in some countries of the new 4-AD class of anthelmintic (i.e. monepantel) and the new dual-active containing both derquantel (5-SI) and abamectin (3-ML) provides new drug choices for this treatment dose. A narrow-spectrum product may also be useful in some circumstances. In many northern temperate areas, resistance is mainly to the benzimidazoles, with some resistance to levamisole and emerging resistance to the macrocyclic lactones. In these circumstances, the SCOPS guidelines recommend the treatment of all imported sheep either **sequentially** with a moxidectin anthelmintic (3-ML) and monepantel (4-AD) or with a **single treatment** using the new dual-active product derquantel–abamectin. Treated animals should be held off pasture for 24–48 hours to allow any worm eggs in the alimentary tract to pass out in the faeces.

2 **Use strategies to conserve susceptible worms**. The aim is to lower the selection pressure for development of resistance which occurs when sheep are treated and moved on to pasture with low contamination or when immune animals are treated. Two approaches are appropriate. First, do not move treated sheep immediately on to low-contamination pasture as any worms which survive treatment will not be diluted by large numbers of more susceptible parasites. Instead, delay moving the sheep from contaminated pasture after dosing to allow them to become lightly reinfected and then move them onto the 'cleaner' grazing. Second, leave a proportion (about 10%) of the flock untreated so that some animals will shed eggs on to the low-contamination pasture. There is inevitably a trade-off between the potential to reduce selection for resistance versus some loss of productivity.

3 **Use strategies that reduce the reliance on anthelmintics**. Approaches which integrate grazing management will reduce the exposure to infective larvae, and thus reduce the adverse effects of infection on productivity, while allowing sufficient exposure to induce a measure of acquired immunity. This strategy is considered in more detail in the following sections.

In selecting the best method of prophylaxis, much depends on whether the farm consists primarily of permanent pasture or has pastures which are rotated with crops so that new leys or hay and silage aftermaths are available each year.

Prophylaxis on farms consisting of mainly permanent pasture

On such farms, control may be obtained either by anthelmintic prophylaxis or by alternate grazing on an annual basis with cattle and sheep. The former is the only feasible method where the farm stock is primarily sheep, while the latter can be used where cattle and sheep are both present in reasonable proportions.

Prophylaxis by anthelmintics Intensive chemoprophylaxis is not a long-term option for the sustainable control of ovine and caprine PGE.

1 **Adult sheep at tupping**. At this time, most ewes in good body condition will be carrying low worm burdens as they will have a strong acquired immunity. Treatment at this period can significantly select for anthelmintic resistance. It is therefore recommended that only mature ewes with a low body condition score or immature ewes are dosed around tupping. Use an anthelmintic which is effective against arrested larval stages.

2 **Adult sheep at lambing**. The most important source of infection for the lamb crop is undoubtedly the increase in nematode eggs in ewe faeces during the PPR and prophylaxis will only be efficient if this is kept to a minimum. Effective anthelmintic therapy of ewes during the fourth month of pregnancy should eliminate most of the worm burdens present at this time, including arrested larval stages and in the case of ewes on extensive grazing, where nutritional status is frequently low, this treatment often results in improved general body condition. Treatment around lambing or turnout, and again 4–5 weeks later, will significantly reduce the ewe contribution to pasture contamination, but it may also increase the selection for drug resistance. To reduce the selection pressure, it has been suggested that ewes are dosed early in the lactation period to allow them to become reinfected before a high level of immunity is re-established. In addition, leaving a proportion of the ewes untreated will allow the pasture to be contaminated with unselected parasites. However, both of these approaches could increase the risk of disease in the lamb crop later in the season. Where ewes are inwintered or housed for a period before lambing, dose them on entry to the shed. Following turnout on to contaminated pasture, they may require further treatment in

about 4–5 weeks. An alternative to the gathering of ewes for these treatments is to provide anthelmintic incorporated in a feed or energy block during the periparturient period. The results obtained with the latter system appear to be best when the ewes are contained in small paddocks or fields, as the uptake of drug is less consistent under extensive grazing systems. Rumen boluses designed for the slow release of anthelmintics over a prolonged period are available in some countries for sheep and are recommended for use in ewes during the periparturient period to eliminate worm egg output. Young adults and rams should also be treated at these times.

3 **Lambs**. Treatment for *Nematodirus battus* infection is considered separately under the relevant section. In general, lambs should be treated at weaning, and where possible moved to 'safe' pastures, i.e. those not grazed by sheep since the previous year. Where such grazing is not available, prophylactic treatments (using a levamisole, benzimidazole, pro-benzimidazole or avermectin/milbemycin product) should be repeated until autumn or marketing. Where anthelmintic resistance has been confirmed to one or more of these drugs, their use should either be discontinued or targeted at known specific and susceptible worm populations, and the introduction of the new 4-AD or 5-SI family of anthelmintics should be considered where these drugs are available. The number of treatments will vary depending on the stocking rate, and levels of challenge that the lambs experience between weaning and marketing, for those under more intensive conditions. In order to reduce unnecessary dosing of lambs, it is recommended that faecal egg counts are monitored to predict the need for treatment.

The prophylactic programmes outlined are relatively costly in terms of drugs and labour but are currently the only practicable options available where the enterprise is heavily dependent on one animal species.

Prophylaxis by alternate grazing of sheep and cattle

On farms where sheep and cattle are both present in significant numbers, effective control is theoretically possible by alternating the grazing of pasture on an annual basis with each host, due to the relative insusceptibility of cattle to sheep nematodes and vice versa. However, *Nematodirus battus* can infect young susceptible calves and this may inadvertently contaminate pasture which is being prepared for next season's lambs. In practice, control is best achieved by exchanging, in the spring, pastures grazed by sheep and beef cattle over the previous year, preferably combined with anthelmintic treatment at the time of exchange.

Prophylaxis on farms with alternative grazing

In these mostly intensive farms, rotation of crops and grass is often a feature, and therefore new leys and hay and silage aftermaths are available as safe pastures each year and can be reserved for susceptible stock. In such a situation, control should be based on a combination of grazing management and anthelmintic prophylaxis.

1 **Prophylaxis by grazing management and anthelmintics**. Good control is possible with only one annual anthelmintic treatment of ewes when they leave the lambing field. This will terminate the PPR in faecal egg counts prior to moving the ewes and lambs to a safe pasture. At weaning, the lambs should be moved to another safe pasture and an anthelmintic treatment of the lambs at this time is good policy. A second system

has been devised for farms where arable crops, sheep and cattle are major components and involves a three-year rotation of cattle, sheep and crops. With this system, the aftermath grazing available after cropping may be used for weaned calves and weaned lambs. It has been suggested that anthelmintic prophylaxis can be disposed of completely under this system, but clinical PGE has sometimes occurred when treatment has been omitted. As anthelmintics may not remove all the worms present and some cattle nematodes can infect sheep and vice versa, and because a few infective larvae on the pasture can survive for beyond two years, it is advisable to give at least one annual spring treatment to all stock prior to moving to new pastures, following current advice not to move treated lambs immediately after treatment and to also leave a proportion undosed in order to reduce the pressures on selection for anthelmintic resistance.

2 **Prophylaxis by grazing management alone**. Systems using strip or creep grazing, which limit the return of sheep to pastures until the contamination has declined to a low level, have been used with some success but are costly in terms of labour and fencing. A system where sheep are rapidly rotated through a series of paddocks has been used for the control of *Haemonchus* in set tropical areas. Sheep only graze a paddock for 3.5–4 days and are then moved to the next paddock. A short grazing time is required to prevent autoinfection. Return to the original paddock must not occur at an interval of less than five weeks. Under the hot humid environment, the infective larvae are very active and die out rapidly on the herbage.

Ostertagia leptospicularis

Ostertagia leptospicularis, synonyms *Ostertagia crimensis*, *Skrjabinagia kolchida*, *Grosspiculagia podjapolskyi* (Phylum: Nematoda; Class: Chromadorea; Order: Rhabditida; Family: Trichostrongylidae), is localised in the abomasum of deer (roe deer), cattle, sheep, goats and camels. This parasite is distributed in many parts of the world, particularly Europe and New Zealand (for more details see Chapter 8).

Marshallagia marshalli

Marshallagia marshalli, synonyms *Ostertagia marshalli*, *Ostertagia tricuspis* (Phylum: Nematoda; Class: Chromadorea; Order: Rhabditida; Family: Trichostrongylidae), is localised in the abomasum of sheep, goats, deer, camels and wild small ruminants. This parasite is distributed in the tropics and subtropics including southern Europe, USA, South America, India and Russia. Wild ruminants serve as an important reservoir of infection. Generally, *M. marshalli* is not considered to be an important pathogen.

Diagnosis: Adults are readily identified based on the structure of the male spicules. Eggs are recognised in faecal samples by their large size.

Control and treatment: Anthelmintics used to treat other gastrointestinal nematodes are likely to be effective.

Notes: Other species include *M. mongolica*, which is found in the abomasum of sheep, goats and camels in parts of Mongolia, and *M. schikhobalovi* and *M. dentispicularis*, which occur in sheep in Russia.

Haemonchus contortus

Haemonchus contortus, synonym *Haemonchus placei* (see Notes) (Phylum: Nematoda; Class: Chromadorea; Order: Rhabditida; Family: Trichostrongylidae), commonly known as the Barber's pole worm, is distributed worldwide, though it is most important in tropical and subtropical areas. This parasite is localised in the abomasum of sheep, goats, cattle, deer, camels and llamas.

Epidemiology: The epidemiology of *H. contortus* is best considered separately, depending on whether it occurs in tropical and subtropical or in temperate areas.

Tropical and subtropical areas Because larval development of *H. contortus* occurs optimally at relatively high temperatures, haemonchosis is primarily a disease of sheep in warm climates. However, since high humidity, at least in the microclimate of the faeces and herbage, is also essential for larval development and survival, the frequency and severity of outbreaks of disease are largely dependent on the rainfall in any particular area. Given these climatic conditions, the sudden occurrence of acute clinical haemonchosis appears to depend on two further factors. First, the high faecal worm egg output of between 2000 and 20 000 epg, even in moderate infections, means that massive pasture populations of L_3 may appear very quickly. Second, in contrast to many other helminth infections, there is little evidence that sheep in endemic areas develop an effective acquired immunity to *Haemonchus*, so that there is continuous contamination of the pasture. In certain areas of the tropics and subtropics, such as Australia, Brazil, the Middle East and Nigeria, survival of the parasite is also associated with the ability of *H. contortus* larvae to undergo hypobiosis. Although the trigger for this phenomenon is unknown, hypobiosis occurs at the start of a prolonged dry season and permits the parasite to survive in the host as arrested L_4 instead of maturing and producing eggs, which would inevitably fail to develop on the arid pasture. Resumption of development occurs just before the onset of seasonal rains. In other tropical areas such as East Africa, no significant degree of hypobiosis has been observed and this may be due to more frequent rainfall in these areas making such an evolutionary development unnecessary. The survival of *H. contortus* infection on tropical pastures is variable depending on the climate and degree of shade, but the infective larvae are relatively resistant to desiccation and some may survive for 1–3 months on pasture or in faeces. In areas of endemic haemonchosis, it has often been observed that after the advent of a period of heavy rain, the faecal worm egg counts of sheep infected with *H. contortus* drop sharply to near zero levels due to the expulsion of the major part of the adult worm burden. This event is commonly termed the self-cure phenomenon, and has been reproduced experimentally by superimposing an infection of *H. contortus* larvae on an existing adult infection in the abomasum. The expulsion of the adult worm population is considered to be the consequence of an immediate-type hypersensitivity reaction to antigens derived from the developing larvae. It is thought that a similar mechanism operates in the naturally occurring self-cure when large numbers of larvae mature to the infective stage on pasture after rain. Although this phenomenon has an immunological mechanism, it is not necessarily associated with protection against reinfection since the larval challenge often develops to maturity. Another explanation of the self-cure phenomenon as it occurs in the field is based on the observation that it may happen in lambs and adults contemporaneously

and on pasture with insignificant numbers of infective larvae. This suggests that the phenomenon may also be caused, in some nonspecific way, by the ingestion of fresh growing grass. Whatever the cause, self-cure is probably of mutual benefit to both host and parasite. The former gains a temporary respite from persistent blood loss while the ageing parasite population is eventually replaced by a vigorous young generation.

Temperate areas In the British Isles, the Netherlands and presumably in other parts of northern Europe and in Canada, which are among the least favourable areas for the survival of *H. contortus*, the epidemiology is different from that of tropical zones. From the information available, infections seem to develop in two ways. Perhaps most common is the single annual cycle. Infective larvae, which have developed from eggs deposited by ewes in the spring, are ingested by ewes and lambs in early summer. The majority of this worm population become arrested in the abomasum as EL_4, and does not complete development until the following spring. During the period of maturation of these hypobiotic larvae, clinical signs of acute haemonchosis may occur and in the ewe this often coincides with lambing. The epidemiology is unknown, but is perhaps associated with pasture contamination by that proportion of ingested larvae which did not undergo hypobiosis in early summer.

Pathogenesis: Essentially, the pathogenesis of haemonchosis is that of an acute haemorrhagic anaemia due to the blood-sucking habits of the worms. Each worm removes about 0.05 ml of blood per day by ingestion and seepage from the lesions, so that a sheep with 5000 *H. contortus* may lose about 250 ml daily. In acute haemonchosis, anaemia becomes apparent about two weeks after infection and is characterised by a progressive and dramatic fall in the packed red cell volume. During the subsequent weeks, the haematocrit usually stabilises at a low level, but only at the expense of a twofold to threefold compensatory expansion of erythropoiesis. However, due to the continual loss of iron and protein into the gastrointestinal tract and increasing inappetence, the marrow eventually becomes exhausted and the haematocrit falls still further before death occurs. When ewes are affected, the consequent agalactia may result in the death of the suckling lambs. Less commonly, in heavier infections of up to 30 000 worms, apparently healthy sheep may die suddenly from severe haemorrhagic gastritis (Fig. 9.1). This is termed hyperacute haemonchosis.

Perhaps as important as acute haemonchosis in tropical areas is the lesser known syndrome of chronic haemonchosis. This develops during a prolonged dry season when reinfection is negligible but the pasture becomes deficient in nutrients. Over such a period, the continual loss of blood from small persisting burdens of several hundred worms is sufficient to produce clinical signs associated primarily with loss of weight, weakness and inappetence rather than marked anaemia.

Clinical signs and pathology: In hyperacute cases, sheep die suddenly from haemorrhagic gastritis. Acute haemonchosis is characterised by anaemia (Fig. 9.2), variable degrees of oedema, of which the submandibular form and ascites are most easily recognised, lethargy, dark-coloured faeces and falling wool. Diarrhoea is not generally a feature. Chronic haemonchosis is associated with progressive weight loss and weakness, neither severe anaemia nor gross oedema being present. At necropsy in cases of acute haemonchosis, there may be between 2000 and 20 000 worms present on the abomasal mucosa, which shows numerous small haemorrhagic lesions.

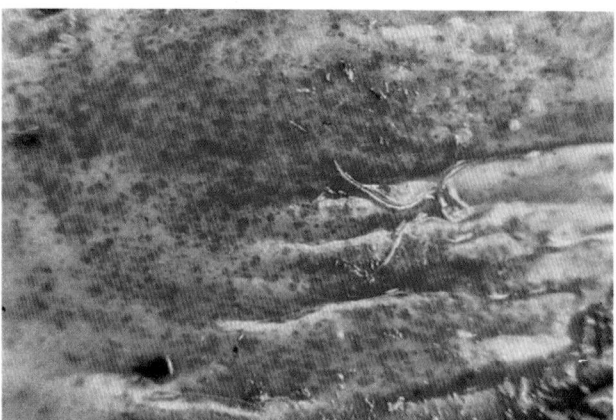

Fig. 9.1 Abomasal haemorrhages in acute haemonchosis.

The abomasal contents are fluid and dark brown due to the presence of altered blood. The carcass is pale and oedematous and the red marrow has expanded from the epiphyses into the medullary cavity.

Diagnosis: The history and clinical signs are often sufficient for the diagnosis of the acute syndrome especially if supported by faecal worm egg counts. Necropsy, paying attention to both the abomasum and the marrow changes in the long bones, is also useful. Changes are usually evident in both, although in sheep which have just undergone 'self-cure' (see section on Epidemiology) or are in a terminal stage of the disease, the bulk of the worm burden may have been lost from the abomasum. In hyperacute haemonchosis, only the abomasum may show changes since death may have occurred so rapidly that marrow changes are minimal. The diagnosis of chronic haemonchosis is more difficult because of the concurrent presence of poor nutrition and confirmation may have to depend on the gradual disappearance of the syndrome after anthelmintic treatment.

Control and treatment: In the tropics and subtropics, control varies depending on the duration and number of periods in the year when rainfall and temperature permit high pasture levels of *H. contortus* larvae to develop. At such times it may be necessary to use an anthelmintic at intervals of 2–4 weeks, depending on the degree of challenge. Sheep should also be treated at least once at the start of the

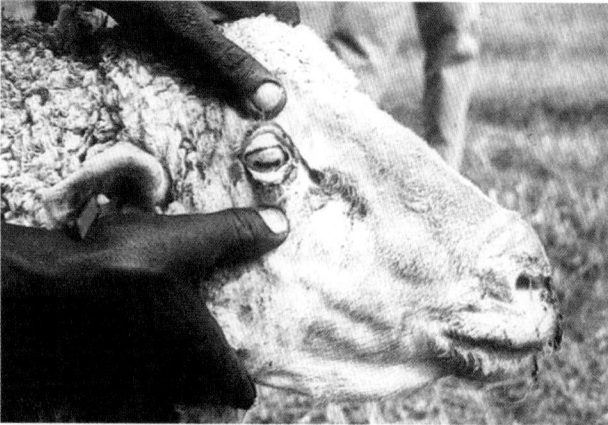

Fig. 9.2 Anaemia and submandibular oedema characteristic of haemonchosis.

dry season and preferably also before the start of prolonged rain to remove persisting hypobiotic larvae whose development could pose a future threat. For this purpose, one of the modern benzimidazoles or an avermectin/milbemycin is recommended. In some wool-producing areas where *Haemonchus* is endemic, closantel, which has a residual prophylactic effect, may be used. Because of long withdrawal periods, this is of more limited use in meat-producing animals. Apart from anthelmintic prophylaxis, some studies, especially in Kenya, have indicated the potential value of some indigenous breeds of sheep which seem to be naturally highly resistant to *H. contortus* infection. Presumably such breeds could be of value in developing areas of the world where veterinary surveillance is poor. Rapid rotation through a series of paddocks can be effective in certain wet tropical areas (for details see discussion of prophylaxis by grazing management alone in the section on Treatment and control of parasitic gastroenteritis in sheep). In temperate areas, the measures outlined for the control of PGE in sheep are usually sufficient to pre-empt outbreaks of haemonchosis. Currently, trials are in progress to determine the efficacy of both a recombinant vaccine based on a membrane glycoprotein of intestinal microvilli, and on native antigens, for the control of parasitic stages of *H. contortus*. When an acute outbreak has occurred, the sheep should be treated with one of the benzimidazoles, levamisole, an avermectin/milbemycin or a salicylanilide (closantel) and moved to pasture not recently grazed by sheep. When the original pasture is grazed again, prophylactic measures should be undertaken, as enough larvae may have survived to institute a fresh cycle of infection. Chronic haemonchosis is dealt with in a similar fashion. If possible, the new pasture should have a good nutritional value; alternatively, some supplementary feeding may be given.

Notes: Until recently, the sheep species was called *H. contortus* and the cattle species *H. placei*. However, there is now increasing evidence that these are the single species *H. contortus* with only strain adaptations for cattle and sheep.

Trichostrongylus axei

Trichostrongylus axei, synonym *Trichostrongylus extenuates* (Phylum: Nematoda; Class: Chromadorea; Order: Rhabditida; Family: Trichostrongylidae), commonly known as the Stomach hairworm, is distributed worldwide and localised in the abomasum or stomach of cattle, sheep, goats, deer, horses, donkeys, pigs and occasionally humans.

Epidemiology: The embryonated eggs and infective L_3 of *T. axei* can survive under adverse conditions. Larval numbers increase on pasture in late summer/autumn, often giving rise to clinical problems during the winter and early spring. Immunity is slowly acquired and age immunity is not well developed.

Pathogenesis: The extent of the lesions in the abomasum or stomach is dependent on the size of the worm population. Small irregular areas showing diffuse congestion and whitish-grey, raised, circular lesions may be present in the pyloric and fundic regions. These lesions are about 1–2 cm in diameter and have been termed plaques or ringworm lesions (Fig. 9.3). In heavy infections, shallow ulcers may be seen. The changes induced in the gastric mucosa are similar to those of *Ostertagia*, with an increase in pH and increased permeability of the mucosa leading to an increase in plasma pepsinogen concentration and hypoalbuminaemia.

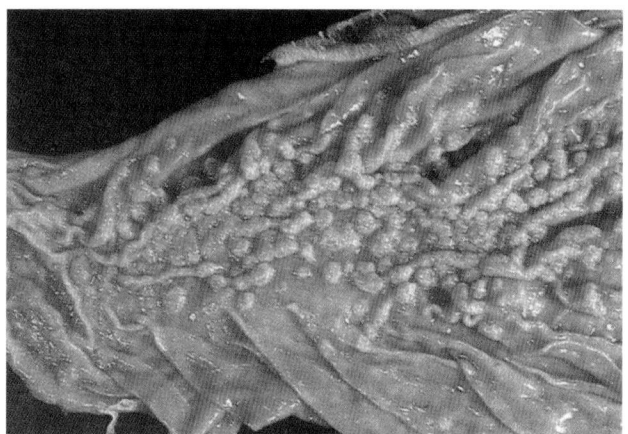

Fig. 9.3 Raised plaques in abomasum due to *Trichostrongylus axei*.

Clinical signs and pathology: The principal clinical signs in heavy infections are rapid weight loss and diarrhoea. At lower levels of infection, inappetence and poor growth rates, sometimes accompanied by soft faeces, are the common signs. In sheep, there is often extensive desquamation of the superficial epithelium of the mucosa. A mucoid hyperplasia is seen in the plaques and in longer established infections there may be shallow ulcers in the neck regions of the glands. Cellular infiltration of the lamina propria occurs, particularly an influx of eosinophils and lymphocytes. In most cases there is not a marked reduction in the number of parietal or zymogen cells. Over time, infection can lead to a chronic proliferative inflammation and shallow depressed ulcers may be present.

Diagnosis: This is based on clinical signs, seasonal occurrence of disease and, if possible, lesions at *post mortem* examination. Faecal egg counts are a useful aid to diagnosis, although faecal cultures are necessary for generic identification of larvae. At necropsy, *T. axei* is easily identified from washings and digests of the abomasum or stomach.

Control and treatment: See section on treatment and control of parasitic gastroenteritis in sheep.

Parabronema skrjabini

Parabronema skrjabini (Phylum: Nematoda; Class: Chromadorea; Order: Spirurida; Family: Habronematidae) is localised in the abomasum of sheep, goats, cattle and camels, and is distributed in Central and East Africa, Asia and some Mediterranean countries, notably Cyprus. This parasite has muscid flies of the genera *Stomoxys* and *Lyperosia* as intermediate hosts. The infection is seasonal, related to the activity of the fly vectors.

Clinical signs and pathology: *Parabronema* is usually regarded as non-pathogenic, although it can cause nodular lesions in the abomasal wall. An abomasitis may be found and lesions may become nodular. Abomasal worms may be found in abomasal scrapings on *post mortem*.

Control and treatment: Any measures to reduce fly populations will be beneficial, whereas treatment is normally not required.

Notes: This genus in ruminants is equivalent to *Habronema* in equines.

Eimeria gilruthi

Eimeria gilruthi, synonym *Globidium gilruthi* (Phylum: Apicomplexa; Class: Conoidasida; Order: Eucoccidiorida; Family: Eimeriidae), is a parasite localised in the abomasum of sheep and goats. Abomasal coccidiosis attributed to *Eimeria* (*Globidium*) *gilruthi* infection is sporadically reported in sheep and goats from different parts of the world. Infections are generally believed to be incidental and are characterised by the presence of giant meronts within the mucosa of the abomasum and, less commonly, the duodenum. The absence of oocysts and sexual tissue stages suggests that sheep may be abnormal hosts for *E. gilruthi*, with infections resulting in one or more generations of merogony in the abomasum, but without progression to gametogony.

SMALL INTESTINE

Trichostrongylus spp.

Species of *Trichostrongylus* (Phylum: Nematoda; Class: Chromadorea; Order: Rhabditida; Family: Trichostrongylidae) are small, light brownish-red, hair-like worms, and are difficult to see with the naked eye. *Trichostrongylus* spp. is rarely a primary pathogen in temperate areas, but is usually a component of parasitic gastroenteritis in ruminants. By contrast, in the subtropics it is one of the most important causes of PGE.

Epidemiology: The embryonated eggs and infective L_3 of *Trichostrongylus* can survive under adverse conditions. In temperate areas the L_3 survive the winter, occasionally in sufficient numbers to precipitate clinical disease in the spring, but more commonly larval numbers increase on pasture in summer and autumn, giving rise to clinical problems during these seasons. Hypobiosis plays an important part in the epidemiology, the seasonal occurrence being similar to that of *Ostertagia* spp. In contrast to other trichostrongyles, hypobiosis occurs at the L_3 stage although their role in outbreaks of disease has not been fully established. In the southern hemisphere, larvae accumulate in late winter and outbreaks are usually seen in spring. In Australia and Africa, following a period of drought, the advent of rain has been shown to rehydrate large numbers of apparently desiccated L_3 (anhydrobiosis) which then become active and rapidly available to grazing animals. *Trichostrongylus colubriformis* also survives adverse environmental conditions as adult parasites within the host and these can persist for many months. Immunity to *Trichostrongylus*, as in *Ostertagia*, is slowly acquired and in sheep, and probably goats, it wanes during the periparturient period.

Diagnosis: This is based on clinical signs, seasonal occurrence of disease and, if possible, lesions at *post mortem* examination. Faecal egg counts are a useful aid to diagnosis, although faecal cultures are necessary for generic identification of larvae. At necropsy, the small intestine is often inflamed and the mucosa thickened with an increase in mucus. There may be flattened red areas that are demarcated from the surrounding mucosa. Digestion of the gut in warm physiological saline for 2–3 hours will release the small hair-like worms for examination.

Pathology: Microscopically, there is villous atrophy and fusion of villi with elongation and dilation of the intestinal crypts and an increase in the number of mucus-secreting goblet cells. This is accompanied by marked cellular infiltration of the lamina propria, in particular an increase in eosinophils. Intraepithelial globule leucocytes are numerous, often in the more normal surrounding areas of the mucosa.

Control and treatment: See section on treatment and control of parasitic gastroenteritis in sheep. This is as described for ostertagiosis and PGE in sheep.

Trichostrongylus colubriformis

Trichostrongylus colubriformis, synonym *Trichostrongylus instabilis* (Phylum: Nematoda; Class: Chromadorea; Order: Rhabditida; Family: Trichostrongylidae), commonly known as the Black scour or Bankrupt worm, is distributed worldwide and localised in the duodenum and anterior small intestine of sheep, goats, cattle, camels and occasionally pigs and humans. Although *T. colubriformis* occurs in temperate regions, it is mainly a parasite of subtropical and tropical zones.

Pathogenesis: Following ingestion, the larvae penetrate the mucosa and developing worms are located in superficial channels sited just beneath the surface epithelium and parallel with the luminal surface, but above the lamina propria. When the subepithelial tunnels containing the developing worms rupture to liberate the young worms about 10–12 days after infection, there is considerable haemorrhage and oedema and plasma proteins are lost into the lumen of the gut, leading to hypoalbuminaemia and hypoproteinaemia. Grossly there is an enteritis, particularly in the duodenum; the villi become distorted and flattened and the mucosa is inflamed, oedematous and covered in mucus. However, many areas may superficially appear normal. Where parasites are congregated within a small area, erosion of the mucosal surface is apparent with severe villous atrophy (Fig. 9.4). In heavy infections, diarrhoea occurs and this, together with the loss of plasma protein into the lumen of the intestine and an increase in turnover of the intestinal epithelium, leads to an impairment in protein metabolism for growth and is reflected as weight loss. Reduced deposition of body protein, calcium and phosphorus and efficiency of food utilisation may occur. Heavy infections can induce osteoporosis and osteomalacia of the skeleton.

Clinical signs: The principal clinical signs in heavy infections are rapid weight loss and diarrhoea, often dark-coloured. Deaths can be high, particularly if animals are also malnourished and they receive a high larval challenge over a short period. At lower levels of infection, inappetence and poor growth rates, sometimes accompanied by soft faeces, are the common signs. It is often difficult to distinguish the effects of low infections from malnutrition.

Trichostrongylus vitrinus

Trichostrongylus vitrinus (Phylum: Nematoda; Class: Chromadorea; Order: Rhabditida; Family: Trichostrongylidae), commonly known as the Black scour worm, is a parasite localised in the duodenum and small intestine of sheep, goats, deer, camels, occasionally pigs and humans, in mainly temperate regions of the world.

Pathogenesis: The macroscopic lesions in the intestine are similar to those described for *T. colubriformis*, although they tend not to be as extensive and appear to resolve earlier, possibly being indicative of an earlier expulsion of worms than with *T. colubriformis*. Frequently, shallow red depressed areas, demarcated from the more normal-coloured surrounding mucosa, are present on the surface of the intestine. These have been termed 'finger-print' lesions. These affected areas are devoid of villi, or the villi appear as rounded protuberances, and numerous worms are embedded in the surface mucosa (Fig. 9.5). Infection can induce similar adverse effects on protein and mineral metabolism to those described for *T. colubriformis*.

Clinical signs: The principal clinical signs in heavy infections are weight loss and diarrhoea. At lower levels of infection, inappetence and poor growth rates, sometimes accompanied by soft faeces, are the common signs.

Trichostrongylus longispicularis

Trichostrongylus longispicularis (Phylum: Nematoda; Class: Chromadorea; Order: Rhabditida; Family: Trichostrongylidae) is a parasite of the small intestine of cattle, sheep, goats, deer, camels and llamas. It infects ruminants in Australia and cattle in America and parts of Europe. The adults are similar in size to *T. colubriformis*. There are a number of other species of *Trichostrongylus* found in the small intestine of sheep and goats (*T. rugatus*, *T. falculatus*, *T. probolurus*, *T. drepanoformis* and *T. capricola*). These have a more local distribution. The species in rabbits, *T. retortaeformis* and *T. affinus*, have occasionally been recovered from small ruminants.

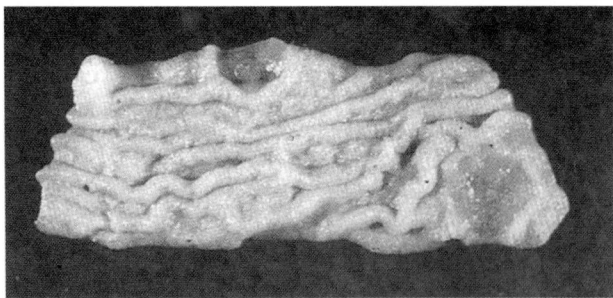

Fig. 9.4 Erosions characteristic of intestinal trichostrongylosis.

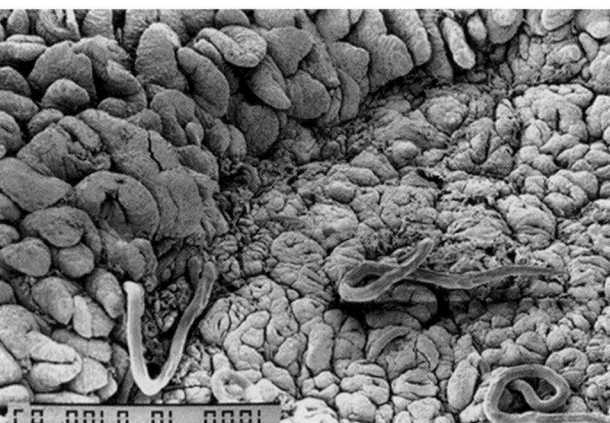

Fig. 9.5 Scanning electron micrograph of small intestine showing villous atrophy in areas where *Trichostrongylus* worms are present.

Cooperia curticei

Cooperia curticei (Phylum: Nematoda; Class: Chromadorea; Order: Rhabditida; Family: Cooperidae) is localised in the small intestine of sheep, goats and deer and distributed worldwide. In temperate areas, members of the genus *Cooperia* usually play a secondary role in the pathogenesis of PGE of small ruminants, although they may be the most numerous trichostrongyle present.

Epidemiology: In temperate areas, this is similar to that of *Teladorsagia*. Hypobiosis at the L_4 is a regular feature during late autumn and winter in the northern hemisphere, and spring and summer in the southern hemisphere. Generally, first-year grazing animals are most likely to accumulate moderate worm populations. Exposure to infective pasture enables animals to acquire a good level of immunity and as adults they usually show few clinical signs of infection but act as carriers, shedding low numbers of eggs in their faeces. Infective larvae survive well on pasture, being tolerant of cold conditions.

Pathogenesis: *Cooperia curticei* is generally considered to be a mild pathogen in lambs and kids, although in some studies it has been associated with inappetence and poor weight gains. A partial immunity to reinfection develops after about 8–12 months of exposure to infective larvae.

Clinical signs and pathology: Low to moderate infections are often asymptomatic but heavy worm burdens can lead to loss of appetite and poor growth rates. *Cooperia* do not tunnel into the epithelium but coil among the intestinal villi, causing adjacent villous atrophy. In heavy infections there is more widespread villous atrophy in the small intestine leading to loss of brush border enzymes and digestive disturbance.

Diagnosis: Eggs of *Cooperia* spp. are all very similar morphologically. Faecal culture will allow identification of infective larvae.

Control and treatment: Control is similar to that recommended for *Teladorsagia*. The principles used for the treatment of the infection are similar to those applied in PGE in sheep. *Cooperia* is one of the dose-limiting species and one should consult the manufacturer's data sheets for efficacy of anthelmintics against adult and L_4.

Nematodirus battus

Nematodirus battus (Phylum: Nematoda; Class: Chromadorea; Order: Rhabditida; Family: Molineidae), commonly known as the Thread-necked worm, is localised in the small intestine of sheep, goats, camelids and occasionally cattle (calves). *Nematodirus battus* is most important in the British Isles, but also occurs in a number of European countries (Norway, Sweden, Netherlands) and parts of USA and Canada.

Epidemiology: The three most important features of the epidemiology of *N. battus* infections are as follows.

1 The capacity of the free-living stages, particularly the egg containing the L_3, to survive on pasture, some for up to two years.
2 The critical hatching requirements of most eggs, which ensure the appearance of large numbers of L_3 on the pasture simultaneously, usually in May and June. Although the flush of larvae on the pasture may be an annual event, the appearance of clinical nematodirosis is not: if the flush of L_3 is early, the suckling lambs may not be consuming sufficient grass to acquire large numbers of L_3; if it is late, the lambs may be old enough to resist the larval challenge. There is some evidence that there is an age resistance to *N. battus*, which commences when lambs are about three months old. However, susceptible lambs of 6–7 months can have considerable *N. battus* burdens and it is therefore doubtful if this age immunity is absolute.
3 The negligible role played by the ewe in the annual cycling of *N. battus*, which can thus be considered a lamb-to-lamb disease with usually only one generation of parasites each year in the spring, although in some years an autumn generation of parasites may be seen. Adult sheep often have a few *N. battus* eggs in their faeces, but these are insufficient to precipitate a larval flush, although they are enough to ensure the persistence of infection on the pastures. In management systems that involve both sheep and cattle, young calves can become infected when they graze pasture that carried lambs the previous spring.

Pathogenesis: Nematodirosis, due to *N. battus* infection, is an example of a parasitic disease where the principal pathogenic effect is attributable to the larval stages. Following ingestion of large numbers of L_3, there is disruption of the intestinal mucosa, particularly in the ileum, although the majority of developing stages are found on the mucosal surface. Development through L_4 to L_5 is complete by 10–12 days from infection and this coincides with severe damage to the villi and erosion of the mucosa leading to villous atrophy. The ability of the intestine to exchange fluids and nutrients is grossly impaired, and with the onset of diarrhoea the lamb rapidly becomes dehydrated.

Clinical signs: In severe infections, yellow-green diarrhoea is the most prominent clinical sign and can occur during the prepatent period. As dehydration proceeds, the affected animals become thirsty and in infected flocks the ewes continue to graze, apparently unaffected by the larval challenge, while their inappetent and diarrhoeic lambs congregate round drinking places. At necropsy, the carcass has a dehydrated appearance and there is often an acute enteritis. The intertwining of the thin twisted worms in the intestine can produce an appearance similar to that of cotton wool. Mortalities can be high in untreated animals. Concurrent infection with pathogenic species of coccidia can exacerbate the severity of disease.

Pathology: Gross pathological changes may be limited to fluid mucoid contents in the upper small intestine with occasional hyperaemia of the mucosa of the duodenum with excess mucus on the surface. Worm counts may reveal tangled cottony masses of elongate, coiled nematodes. The presence of large numbers of larvae is associated with villous atrophy and fusion, while crypts may appear elongate and dilated. Local erosions may occur if villous atrophy is severe and on histopathology there is a mixed inflammatory response with large numbers of lymphocytes, plasma cells and eosinophils in the lamina propria.

Diagnosis: Because the clinical signs appear during the prepatent period, faecal egg counts are of little value in early diagnosis, which is best made on grazing history, clinical signs and, if possible, a *post mortem* examination. Nematodirosis should be differentiated from coccidiosis.

Control: Because of the annual hatching of *N. battus* eggs in spring, the disease can be controlled by avoiding the grazing of successive lamb crops on the same pasture. Where such alternative grazing is not available each year, control can be achieved by anthelmintic prophylaxis, the timing of treatments being based on the knowledge that the peak time for the appearance of *N. battus* L_3 is May to early June. Ideally, dosing should be at three-week intervals over May and June and it is unwise to await the appearance of clinical signs of diarrhoea before administering the drugs. Forecasting systems are based primarily on soil temperature in the early spring which can predict the likely severity of nematodirosis. In years when the forecast predicts severe disease, three treatments are recommended during May and June; in other years two treatments in May should suffice.

Treatment: Several drugs are effective against *Nematodirus* infections: levamisole, an avermectin/milbemycin or one of the modern benzimidazoles. However, *Nematodirus* is one of the dose-limiting species and the manufacturer's data sheet should be consulted as there are differences in efficacy against adults and L_4 stages between oral and parenteral administration for some macrocyclic lactones. The response to treatment is usually rapid and, if diarrhoea persists, coccidiosis should be considered as a complicating factor. As anthelmintic resistance is rare in *Nematodirus* species, it may be advisable to use a benzimidazole against specific *Nematodirus* infection and in this way reduce the selection pressure on the other families of drugs.

Nematodirus filicollis

Nematodirus filicollis (Phylum: Nematoda; Class: Chromadorea; Order: Rhabditida; Family: Molineidae), commonly known as the Thread-necked worm, is localised in the small intestine of sheep, goats and occasionally cattle and deer. Though it is distributed worldwide, it is more prevalent in temperate zones.

Epidemiology: The hatch of L_3 from the eggs occurs over a more prolonged period than with *N. battus*, and numbers of infective larvae accumulate on pasture and often peak in late autumn to early winter. More than one annual generation is possible. Although *N. filicollis* has been associated with outbreaks of nematodirosis in small ruminants, it is more common to find it in conjunction with the other trichostrongyles that contribute to ovine PGE.

Clinical signs and pathology: Low to moderate infections may produce no obvious clinical manifestations. In severe infections, diarrhoea can occur during the prepatent period and young animals may become dehydrated. Third-stage larvae enter the deep layers of the mucosa, penetrating into the crypts. Larvae emerge as fourth- or fifth-stage larvae and coil among the villi with their posterior ends protruding into the lumen. The presence of large numbers of worms leads to the development of villous atrophy, crypt dilation and elongation. If villous atrophy is severe, the worms may not be able to maintain their position in the intestine.

Diagnosis: Examination of faeces will enable the colourless eggs to be differentiated from the brown eggs of *N. battus*. At necropsy, the tips of the male spicules will allow diagnosis from other *Nematodirus* species.

Control and treatment: For control see *Nematodirus battus*. Disease due to monospecific *N. filicollis* infections is rarely seen. They are usually part of the worm burden of trichostrongyloid species that are responsible for the syndrome of PGE in sheep and as such may be controlled by the measures outlined elsewhere.

Nematodirus spathiger

Nematodirus spathiger (Phylum: Nematoda; Class: Chromadorea; Order: Rhabditida; Family: Molineidae), commonly known as the Thread-necked worm, is a cosmopolitan parasite of the small intestine of sheep, goats and occasionally cattle and other ruminants. For control and treatment, see *Nematodirus battus*.

Epidemiology: The eggs do not usually exhibit delayed hatching, and the pattern of infection is similar to that of *Trichostrongylus* species.

Clinical signs and pathology: Low to moderate infections may produce no obvious clinical manifestations. In severe infections, diarrhoea can occur during the prepatent period and young animals may become dehydrated. Pathology is the same as for *N. filicollis*.

Diagnosis: Examination of faeces will enable the colourless eggs to be differentiated from the brown eggs of *N. battus*. At necropsy, the tips of the male spicules will allow diagnosis from other *Nematodirus* species.

Bunostomum trigonocephalum

Bunostomum trigonocephalum, synonym *Monodontus trigonocephalum* (Phylum: Nematoda; Class: Chromadorea; Order: Rhabditida; Family: Ancylostomatidae), commonly known as the Hookworm, is localised in the small intestine of cattle, sheep, goats and deer. This parasite is distributed worldwide, but it is of more economic importance in warm climates.

Epidemiology: Pathogenic infections are more common in the tropics and subtropics and, in some areas, the highest worm burdens are found at the end of the dry season, apparently due to the maturation of hypobiotic larvae. Young animals are most susceptible. In temperate countries, high worm burdens are usually uncommon. The prophylactic dosing regimens adopted for the control of trichostrongyles have contributed to the low prevalence of *Bunostomum*.

Pathogenesis: The adult worms are bloodsuckers and infections of 100–500 worms can produce progressive anaemia, hypoalbuminaemia, loss of weight and occasionally diarrhoea. Worm burdens of around 600 may lead to death in sheep.

Clinical signs and pathology: The main clinical signs are progressive anaemia, with associated changes in the blood picture, hydraemia and oedema, which show particularly as submandibular oedema ('bottle jaw'). The animals become weak and emaciated and the appetite usually decreases. The skin is dry and the wool of sheep falls out in irregular patches. Diarrhoea may occur, and the faeces may be dark because of altered blood pigments. Collapse and death may occur. The carcass is anaemic and cachexic. Oedema and ascites are seen. The liver is light brown and shows fatty changes. The intestinal contents are haemorrhagic and the mucosa is usually swollen, covered with mucus and shows numerous lesions resulting from the worms feeding. The parasites may be seen still attached to the mucosa or free in the lumen.

Diagnosis: The clinical signs of anaemia and perhaps diarrhoea in young sheep are not in themselves pathognomonic of bunostomosis. However, in temperate areas, the epidemiological background may be useful in eliminating the possibility of *Fasciola hepatica* infection. In the tropics, haemonchosis must be considered, possibly originating from hypobiotic larvae. Faecal worm egg counts are useful in that these are lower than in *Haemonchus* infection, while the eggs are more bluntly rounded, with relatively thick sticky shells to which debris is often adherent. For accurate differentiation, larval cultures should be prepared.

Control and treatment: A combination of strategic dosing with anthelmintics and pasture management as used in the control of ovine PGE is effective. Larvae are susceptible to desiccation, and the infection is mainly found on permanently or occasionally moist pastures. Avoiding or draining such pastures is an effective control measure. The ground around water troughs should be kept hard and dry, or treated with liberal applications of salt. Housed sheep and goats should be protected by ensuring the floors and bedding are kept dry and that faeces are removed frequently and are not allowed to contaminate food and water. The prophylactic anthelmintic regimens advocated for other gastrointestinal nematodes are usually sufficient.

Gaigeria pachyscalis

Gaigeria pachyscalis (Phylum: Nematoda; Class: Chromadorea; Order: Rhabditida; Family: Ancylostomatidae), commonly known as the Hookworm, is localised in the duodenum and small intestine of sheep, goats and wild ruminants, and distributed in South America, South Africa, Indonesia and parts of Asia. Control and treatment are as for *B. trigonocephalum*.

Pathogenesis: The parasite is a voracious bloodsucker; as few as 100–200 worms are sufficient to produce death in sheep within a few weeks.

Clinical signs and pathology: The infection may cause severe anaemia and death. The pathology is similar to that described for *B. trigonocephalum*.

Diagnosis: Demonstration of the characteristic large eggs in the faeces.

Strongyloides papillosus

Strongyloides papillosus (Phylum: Nematoda; Class: Chromadorea; Order: Rhabditida; Family: Strongyloididae), commonly known as the Threadworm, is distributed worldwide and localised in the small intestine of sheep, goats, cattle, other ruminants, pigs and rabbits. For more details on pathogenesis, epidemiology, treatment and control, see Chapter 8.

Capillaria longipes

Capillaria longipes (Phylum: Nematoda; Class: Enoplea; Order: Enoplida; Family: Capillariidae) is distributed worldwide and localised in the small intestine of sheep, goats and occasionally cattle. Infection occurs by ingestion of the larvated eggs and is common in sheep though not significant. It is considered of low pathogenicity and of little veterinary significance, thus does not requiring any specific treatment.

Diagnosis: Because of the non-specific nature of the clinical signs and the fact that, in heavy infections, these may appear before

Capillaria eggs are present in the faeces, diagnosis depends on necropsy and careful examination of the small intestine for the presence of the worms. This may be carried out by microscopic examination of mucosal scrapings squeezed between two glass slides; alternatively, the contents should be gently washed through a fine sieve and the retained material resuspended in water and examined against a black background.

Moniezia expansa

Moniezia expansa (Phylum: Platyhelminthes; Class: Cestoda; Order: Cyclophyllidea; Family: Anoplocephalidae) is distributed worldwide and localised in the small intestine of sheep, goats and occasionally cattle. They complete their biological life cycle in free-living forage mites, mainly of the family Oribatidae.

Epidemiology: Infection is common in lambs, kids and calves during their first year of life and less common in older animals. A seasonal fluctuation in the incidence of *Moniezia* infection can apparently be related to active periods of the forage mite vectors during the summer in temperate areas. The cysticercoids can overwinter in the mites.

Pathogenesis: Although generally regarded as of little pathogenic significance, there are several reports, especially from Eastern Europe and New Zealand, of heavy infections causing unthriftiness, diarrhoea and even intestinal obstruction. However, *Moniezia* infections are so obvious, both in life, because of the presence of proglottids in the faeces, and at necropsy, that other causes of ill health may be overlooked. It is interesting that experimental studies have failed to demonstrate substantial clinical effects even with fairly heavy worm burdens.

Clinical signs and pathology: While a great variety of clinical signs, including unthriftiness, diarrhoea, respiratory signs and even convulsions, have been attributed to *Moniezia*, infections are generally symptomless. Subclinical effects remain to be established. Little pathology is associated with the presence of light infections. Heavy infections may produce a solid mass of tapeworms that may occlude the intestinal lumen.

Diagnosis: This is based largely on the presence of mature proglottids in the faeces and the characteristic shape of *Moniezia* eggs (triangular, *M. expansa*; quadrangular, *M. benedeni*) that contain the oncosphere. The eggs of *M. benedeni* are slightly larger than those of *M. expansa*.

Control and treatment: Ploughing and reseeding, or avoiding the use of the same pastures for young animals in consecutive years, may prove beneficial. In many countries, several drugs, including niclosamide, praziquantel, bunamidine and a number of broad-spectrum benzimidazole compounds, which have the advantage of also being active against gastrointestinal nematodes, are available for the treatment of *Moniezia* infection. If this is carried out in lambs and calves in late spring, in temperate areas, the numbers of newly infected mites on pasture will be reduced.

Notes: This genus of cestodes is common in ruminants and resembles, in most respects, *Anoplocephala* of the horse. *Moniezia* spp. are the only tapeworms of ruminants in many countries of Western Europe. Other species of tapeworms are found in the small intestine of sheep and goats. Many of the details are essentially similar to *Moniezia*.

Avitellina centripunctata

Avitellina centripunctata, synonym *Avitellina woodlandi* (Phylum: Platyhelminthes; Class: Cestoda; Order: Cyclophyllidea; Family: Anoplocephalidae), is localised in the small intestine of sheep, goats, camels and other ruminants and distributed in Europe, Africa and Asia. The parasite intermediate hosts are thought to be oribatid mites or psocid lice. It is of negligible pathogenicity, similar to that of *Moniezia* spp.

Notes: Several minor species of *Avitellina* occur. *A. goughi* and *A. chalmersi* are found mainly in sheep in Asia and Africa and *A. tatia* occurs in goats in the Indian subcontinent. These species have more than one parauterine organ in each proglottid.

Stilesia globipunctata

Stilesia globipunctata (Phylum: Platyhelminthes; Class: Cestoda; Order: Cyclophyllidea; Family: Anoplocephalidae) is a parasite of the small intestine of sheep, goats, cattle and other ruminants. They are distributed in southern Europe, Africa and Asia and complete their biological life cycle in oribatid mites and psocid lice. These parasites are generally considered of low pathogenicity, although severe infection has been reported to cause death.

Clinical signs and pathology: Though the infection is normally asymptomatic, nodules and desquamation may occur in the jejunum where the scoleces of the immature tapeworms penetrate the epithelium. The scolex and anterior proglottids are embedded within the nodule, the posterior proglottids being free in the lumen of the intestine.

Treatment: Treatment is rarely called for, but praziquantel administered at 8–15 mg/kg has proved effective.

Thysaniezia ovilla

Thysaniezia ovilla, synonyms *Thysaniezia giardi*, *Helictometra giardi* (Phylum: Platyhelminthes; Class: Cestoda; Order: Cyclophyllidea; Family: Anoplocephalidae), is localised in the small intestine of cattle, sheep, goats, camels and wild ruminants and distributed in southern Africa. This parasite has oribatid mites (*Galuma*, *Scheloribates*) and psocids (bark lice, dust lice) as intermediate hosts. It is considered non-pathogenic.

Diagnosis: The mature segments are found in the faeces and readily distinguishable from those of *Moniezia*.

Thysanosoma actinoides

Thysanosoma actinoides (Phylum: Platyhelminthes; Class: Cestoda; Order: Cyclophyllidea; Family: Anoplocephalidae), commonly known as the Fringed tapeworm, is localised in the small intestine, bile and pancreatic duct of cattle, sheep and deer. This parasite has oribatid mites (*Galuma*, *Scheloribates*) and psocids (bark lice, book lice and dust lice) as intermediate hosts. Infection is commonly found in sheep, cattle and deer in the western USA and parts of South America.

Pathogenesis and clinical signs: Generally, not considered pathogenic. Blockage of the bile or pancreatic ducts may occur, resulting in digestive disorders and unthriftiness.

Diagnosis: Identification of the mature segments and eggs in the faeces.

Cymbiforma indica

Cymbiforma indica, synonym *Ogmocotyle indica* (Phylum: Platyhelminthes; Class: Trematoda; Order: Plagiorchiida; Family: Notocotylidae), is localised in the gastrointestinal tract, particularly the duodenum of sheep, goats and cattle, and is distributed in India. This parasite has snails as intermediate hosts. Generally not considered pathogenic, despite heavy infections are frequently reported.

Skrjabinotrema ovis

Skrjabinotrema ovis (Phylum: Platyhelminthes; Class: Trematoda; Order: Strigeidida; Family: Brachylaemidae) is localised in the small intestine of sheep and distributed in China, Russia and the eastern CIS. This parasite has snails as intermediate hosts. Heavy infections may cause catarrhal enteritis.

Sheep coccidia

Fifteen species of *Eimeria* have been identified in sheep, of which 11 species are commonly identified based on oocyst morphology (Table 9.2; see also Table 4.8 and Fig. 4.36). Each stage of individual coccidial species has its preferences as to which cells and which parts of the gut it infects. Those infecting the posterior part of the intestine tend to be more harmful. Although the majority of sheep, particularly those under one year old, carry coccidia, only two species (*E. crandallis* and *E. ovinoidalis*) are known to be highly pathogenic. It was thought for many years that the species of *Eimeria* affecting sheep and goats were the same. However, cross-transmission studies have shown that although morphologically similar, coccidia in small ruminants are host specific and cross-infection between sheep and goats does not occur. The following general descriptions apply to sheep and goat *Eimeria*.

Epidemiology: Coccidia are normally present in animals of all ages and usually cause no clinical signs, as immunity is quickly acquired

Table 9.2 Predilection sites and prepatent periods of *Eimeria* species in sheep.

Species	Predilection site	Prepatent period (days)
Eimeria ahsata	Small intestine	18–30
Eimeria bakuensis	Small intestine	18–29
Eimeria crandallis	Small and large intestine	15–20
Eimeria faurei	Small and large intestine	13–15
Eimeria granulosa	Unknown	?
Eimeria intricata	Small and large intestine	23–27
Eimeria marsica	Unknown	14–16
Eimeria ovinoidalis	Small and large intestine	12–15
Eimeria pallida	Unknown	?
Eimeria parva	Small and large intestine	12–14
Eimeria weybridgensis	Small intestine	23–33

and maintained by continuous exposure to reinfection. However, intensification may alter the delicate balance between immunity and disease with serious consequences for young animals. Coccidiosis is one of the most important diseases of lambs, particularly in their first few months of life. While coccidial infection is common, the presence of infection does not necessarily lead to the development of clinical signs of disease and, in many situations, low levels of challenge can actually be beneficial by stimulating protective immune responses in the host. Development of disease is dependent on a number of factors, in particular husbandry and management. Adult animals are highly resistant to the disease, but not totally resistant to infection. As a result, small numbers of parasites manage to complete their life cycle and usually cause no detectable harm. In the wild or under more natural, extensive systems of management, susceptible animals are exposed to only low numbers of oocysts and acquire a protective immunity. Extensive grazing, as occurs under natural conditions in the wild, limits the level of exposure to infective oocysts. Under modern production systems, however, lambs or kids are born into a potentially heavily contaminated environment, and where the numbers of sporulated oocysts are high, disease often occurs. Three management factors are associated with the development of high levels of infection and the development of disease: pens not cleaned on a regular basis; overcrowding in the pens; pens used to house different age groups. Adults, although possibly the original source of infective oocysts in the environment, are not usually responsible for the heavy levels of contamination encountered. The source is often the lambs themselves, which following an initial infection in the first few days of life may produce millions of oocysts within their own environment. Growing animals may then face potentially lethal doses of infective oocysts three weeks later when their natural resistance is at its lowest. Later-born animals introduced into the same environment are immediately exposed to heavy oocyst challenge. Under unhygienic, overcrowded conditions, the lambs will be exposed to, and ingest a large proportion of, this infection and will develop severe disease and may even die. If conditions are less crowded and more hygienic, the infective dose ingested will be lower, they may show moderate, slight or no clinical signs and develop an immunity to reinfection, but they in turn will have multiplied the infection a million-fold. Stress factors, such as poor milk supply, weaning, cold weather and transport, will reduce any acquired resistance and exacerbate the condition. Colostrum provides passive immunity to coccidiosis during the first few weeks of life. Thereafter, susceptibility to coccidial infections has been found to increase progressively. Subsequently, animals acquire resistance to coccidia as a result of active immunity. While animals of all ages are susceptible to infection, younger animals are generally more susceptible to disease. The majority of lambs will probably become infected during the first few months of life and may or may not show signs of disease. Those that reach adulthood are highly resistant to the pathogenic effects of the parasites but may continue to harbour small numbers throughout their lives. Occasionally, acute coccidiosis occurs in adult animals with impaired cellular immunity or in those which have been subjected to stress, such as dietary changes, prolonged travel, extremes of temperature and weather conditions, changes in environment or severe concurrent infection. An animal's nutritional status and mineral and vitamin deficiencies can also influence resistance to infection. Suckling animals, in addition to benefiting from colostral intake, may forage less and hence pick up fewer oocysts from pasture. Well-nourished animals may simply be able to fight off infection more readily.

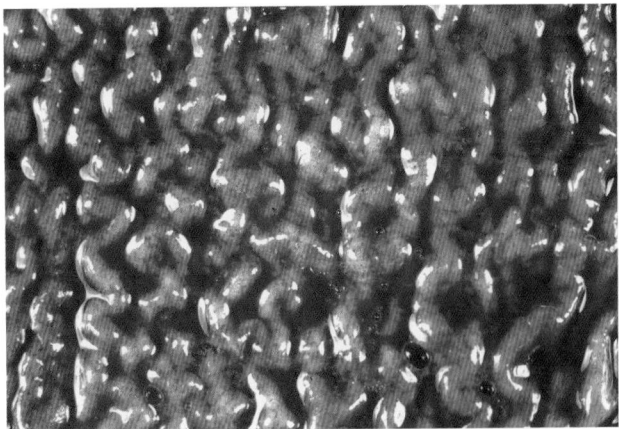

Fig. 9.6 Haemorrhagic mucosa due to infection with *Eimeria ovinoidalis*.

Pathogenesis: The most pathogenic species of coccidia are those that infect and destroy the crypt cells of the large intestinal mucosa. This is because the ruminant small intestine is very long, providing a large number of host cells and the potential for enormous parasite replication with minimal damage. If the absorption of nutrients is impaired, the large intestine is, to some extent, capable of compensating. Those species that invade the large intestine are more likely to cause pathological changes, particularly if large numbers of oocysts are ingested over a short period of time. Here, the rate of cellular turnover is much lower and there is no compensation effect from other regions of the gut. In lambs or kids that become heavily infected, the mucosa becomes completely denuded, resulting in severe haemorrhage (Fig. 9.6) and impaired water resorption, leading to diarrhoea, dehydration and death. In lighter infections, the effect on the intestinal mucosa is to impair local absorption. Species that develop more superficially in the small intestine cause a change in villous architecture with a reduction in epithelial cell height and a diminution of the brush border, giving the appearance of a 'flat' mucosa. These changes result in a reduction of the surface area available for absorption and consequently a reduced feed efficiency.

Clinical signs and pathology: Clinical signs vary, from loss of pellet formation to weight loss, anorexia and diarrhoea (with or without blood) (Fig. 9.7). On *post mortem*, there may be little to see beyond thickening and petechiation of the bowel but mucosal scrapings will reveal masses of gamonts and oocysts. Giant meronts may be seen in the mucosa of the small intestine as pin-point white spots (Fig. 9.8), but unless they are in vast numbers, they cause little harm. The most pathogenic stages are the gamonts (Fig. 9.9).

Diagnosis: Diagnosis should be based on history, clinical signs (severe diarrhoea in young animals), *post mortem* findings (inflammation, hyperaemia and thickening of the caecum with masses of gamonts and oocysts in scrapings) supported by oocyst counts and speciation to identify pathogenic species. Counts of faecal oocysts identified to species can help to complete the picture, but oocyst numbers may be grossly misleading when considered in isolation. Healthy animals may pass more than a million oocysts per gram of faeces, whereas in animals dying of coccidiosis, the count may be less than 10 000 oocysts per gram of faeces. High counts of non-pathogenic species could mask significant numbers of the more pathogenic species, for instance, and give the impression that the abundant species were the cause.

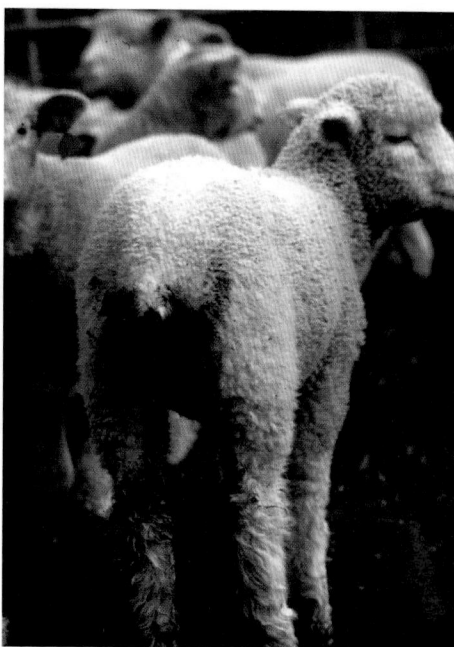

Fig. 9.7 Clinically affected lamb with coccidiosis.

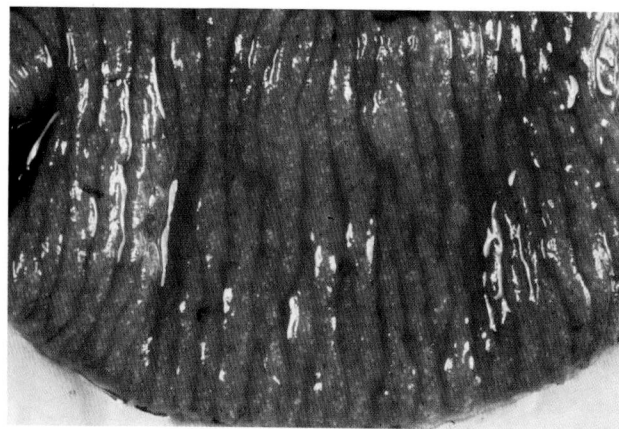

Fig. 9.8 *Eimeria ovinoidalis.* Large intestinal mucosa with 'giant' meronts visible as pin-point white spots.

Control and treatment: Animals particularly at risk from coccidiosis are those kept indoors on damp bedding or those on contaminated heavily stocked pastures, particularly in cold wet weather. The incidence of disease can be reduced through avoidance of overcrowding and stress, and attention to hygiene. Regularly moving food and water troughs, and raising or covering them to prevent faecal contamination, can help reduce the levels of infection. It is good practice to clean and disinfect all buildings between groups of sheep or provide clean pasture for animals turned out to grass. Steam cleaning or pressure washing helps remove faecal debris and it is important to use a disinfectant that claims activity against coccidial oocysts, as not all disinfectants will kill oocysts. Ammonia-based disinfectants are normally used, although other disinfectants containing chlorophenol (chlorom-cresol) are also effective. Young animals should be kept off heavily contaminated pastures when they are most susceptible. Good feeding of dams prior to parturition and creep feeding of their progeny will also help to boost resistance to coccidiosis. Coccidiosis in young lambs at pasture has become a significant problem, particularly with increased stocking densities and reduced availability of pasture for sheep. In early weaning lamb flocks kept indoors, then disease can be anticipated in housed lambs aged 2–3 weeks post weaning. Strategic treatments in these situations usually comprise in-feed decoquinate, or diclazuril or toltrazuril, administered prior to identified periods of risk. The timing of such treatments should be based on the farm history, prevailing management and husbandry systems, and knowledge of the epidemiology of the disease. Intervention treatments should aim to limit disease signs but not prevent sufficient exposure to coccidial oocysts that lead to the development of protective immunity. Outbreaks of clinical coccidiosis can appear suddenly and may prove troublesome to resolve as they often occur on heavily stocked farms, particularly where good husbandry and management are lacking. If deaths are occurring, early confirmation of the diagnosis is vital and should be based on history, *post mortem* examination and intestinal smears. Affected animals should be medicated and moved to uncontaminated pens or pasture as soon as possible. Normally, all lambs in a group should be treated, as even those showing no symptoms are likely

to be infected. Appearance of clinical symptoms will require treatment with an appropriate anticoccidial product. This would normally be in the form of a single oral drench with either diclazuril or toltrazuril, in countries where these products are both available and licensed for use. Decoquinate can be administered in feed, bearing in mind that not all lambs may consume the feed, especially severely affected animals that may be off their feed and dehydrated. Where these products are not available or licensed, then treatment with a sulfonamide such as sulfadimidine or sulfamethoxypyridazine can be considered. Severely infected animals that are diarrhoeic and dehydrated may require oral or intravenous rehydration. Where non-specific symptoms of weight loss or ill-thrift are present, it is important to investigate all potential causes and seek laboratory confirmation. If coccidiosis is considered significant, much can be done through advice on management and instigation of preventive measures outlined earlier. Batch rearing of animals of similar ages limits the build-up and spread of oocysts and allows targeting of treatment to susceptible age groups during the danger periods.

Eimeria ahsata

Eimeria ahsata (Phylum: Apicomplexa; Class: Conoidasida; Order: Eucoccidiorida; Family: Eimeriidae) is a protozoan distributed worldwide and localised in the small intestine of sheep.

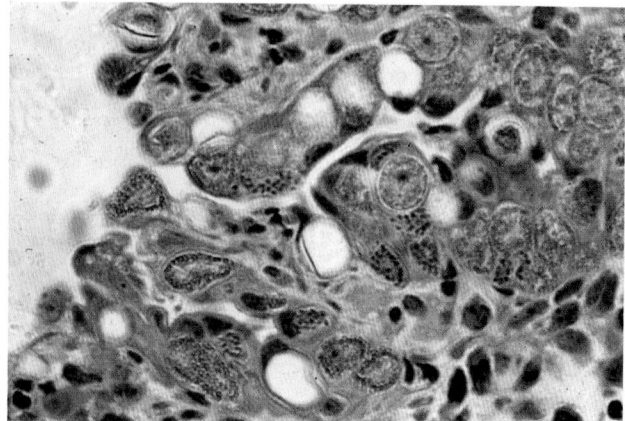

Fig. 9.9 Macrogamonts of *Eimeria ovinoidalis.*

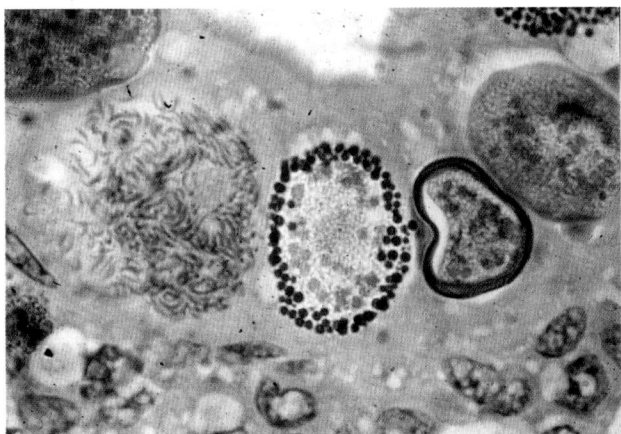

Fig. 9.10 Gamonts of *Eimeria ahsata* within epithelial crypt cells.

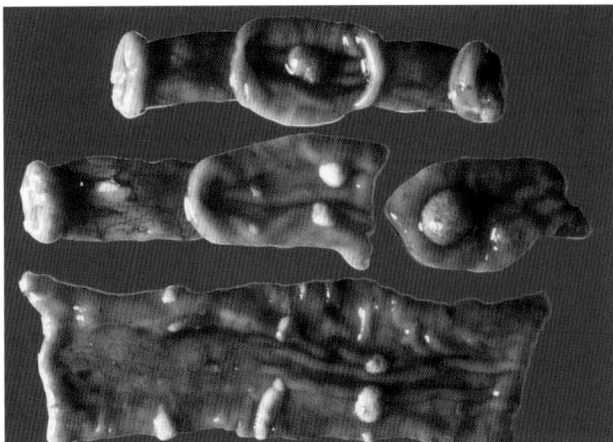

Fig. 9.11 *Eimeria bakuensis* polyps in the small intestine.

First-generation meronts are localised along the length of the small intestine, but mainly in the jejunum. Second-generation meronts appear in the cytoplasm of epithelial cells 15–20 days after infection. The gamonts appear at 11 days post infection, suggesting that merogony and gametogony run parallel for a time. Most sexual stages develop in epithelial cells of the crypts (Fig. 9.10). The prepatent period is 18–21 days and the patent period is 10–12 days. Sporulation time is 2–3 days.

Pathogenesis and pathology: Not considered to be pathogenic, although there have been some reports of *E. ahsata* causing diarrhoea, inappetence, weight loss and even death. Thickening of the wall of the ileum, especially anteriorly, with inflammation of Peyer's patches has been reported.

Eimeria bakuensis

Eimeria bakuensis, synonym *Eimeria ovina* (Phylum: Apicomplexa; Class: Conoidasida; Order: Eucoccidiorida; Family: Eimeriidae), is a protozoan distributed worldwide and localised in the small intestine of sheep. There appears to be only one asexual generation. The meronts are found in the endothelial cells lining the central lacteals of the small intestinal villi and mature 13–21 days after infection. The sexual stages are found in the epithelial cells of the small intestinal villi. Synchronous division of the parasites occurs. The microgamonts contain a large residual mass. The sporulation time is 2–4 days. The prepatent period is 19–29 days and the patent period around 10 days.

Pathology: Papilloma-like lesions may occur in the small intestine, usually as a sequela to gametocyte formation, but these are not of great pathogenic significance. A few small, slightly haemorrhagic areas are seen scattered throughout the lining of the small intestine and thick white opaque patches, composed of groups of heavily parasitised villi, are present leading to the formation of polyps (Fig. 9.11).

Diagnosis: The presence of polyps containing large numbers of gamonts and oocysts is indicative of *E. bakuensis* infection. Oocysts are prevalent in the faeces of sheep of all ages, and coccidiosis cannot be diagnosed solely by finding oocysts. Peak oocyst counts above 1 million per gram of faeces have been reported in clinically healthy lambs.

Goat coccidia

Fourteen species of coccidia have been identified in goats, of which nine species are commonly identified based on oocyst morphology and predilection site (Table 9.3; see also Table 4.9 and Fig. 4.37). *Eimeria ninakohlyakimovae* and *E. caprina* cause widespread denudation of the mucosa in the upper and lower large intestine in young kids. *Eimeria arloingi* is probably the most commonly encountered coccidia causing polyp formation and focal hyperplasia of the mucosa. Other species that are considered pathogenic in goats are *E. christenseni* and *E. hirci*.

Epidemiology: Management factors associated with the development of high levels of infection and the development of disease are overcrowding, dirty conditions and repeat use of rearing pens for different age groups of young goats. If the same pens are used constantly for successive batches, or if young goats are added to a pen already housing older animals, then the later-born animals are immediately exposed to heavy challenge and can show severe coccidiosis in the first few weeks of life. On heavily stocked and overgrazed pastures, levels of contamination may be high, leading to disease. A major problem in milking goat herds is that, in an attempt to ensure a constant year-round milk supply, births often take place over an extended period of time. If the same pens are used constantly for successive batches, or if young kids are added to a pen already housing older animals, then the later-born kids are immediately exposed to heavy challenge and can show severe coccidiosis in the first few weeks of life.

Table 9.3 Predilection sites and prepatent periods of *Eimeria* species in goats.

Species	Predilection site	Prepatent period (days)
Eimeria alijevi	Small and large intestine	7–12
Eimeria aspheronica	Unknown	14–17
Eimeria arloingi	Small intestine	14–17
Eimeria caprina	Small and large intestine	17–20
Eimeria caprovina	Unknown	14–20
Eimeria christenseni	Small intestine	14–23
Eimeria hirci	Unknown	13–16
Eimeria jolchijevi	Unknown	14–17
Eimeria ninakohlyakimovae	Small and large intestine	10–13

Clinical signs: Clinical signs for *E. christenseni*, *E. hirci*, *E. ninakohlya-kimovae* and *E. caprina* (see details in section on Large intestine) are similar. Infection leads to loss of appetite, unthriftiness and profuse diarrhoea, often containing streaks of blood. If left untreated, these animals may continue to scour and eventually die of dehydration.

Diagnosis: Diagnosis is based on history, age, *post mortem* lesions and faecal examination for oocysts. The latter may be present in very large numbers in both healthy and diseased animals so that *post mortem* or oocyst differentiation is advisable.

Control and treatment: Good management and hygiene practices (regular moving of feed and water troughs), avoidance of overcrowding and stress, batch rearing and feeding of dams prior to parturition can all help to reduce the incidence of infection. While the same compounds used for the treatment and control of coccidiosis in sheep should be effective in goats, little information is available on the efficacy of these compounds in goats. Sulfonamides, decoquinate or diclazuril may be effective if disease is suspected.

Eimeria christenseni

Eimeria christenseni (Phylum: Apicomplexa; Class: Conoidasida; Order: Eucoccidiorida; Family: Eimeriidae) is a protozoan distributed worldwide and localised in the small intestine of goats. This species is one of the more pathogenic in young goats, infection causing desquamation of the mucosa and superficial necrosis. First-generation meronts are situated in the endothelial cells of the lacteals of the jejunum and ileum, and in the lamina propria and lymph vessels of the submucosa and mesenteric lymph nodes. Second-generation meronts occur 16 days after infection, mostly in epithelial cells of the crypts, and less often in those of the villi in the small intestine and also in the sinuses of the mesenteric lymph nodes. Gamonts are present in the epithelial cells of the villi and the crypts of the small intestine from 16 days after infection. The prepatent period is 14–23 days and the patent period is 3–30+ days. The sporulation time is 3–6 days.

Pathology: Focal aggregates of coccidia, particularly gamonts and oocysts, occur in the jejunum and ileum and are associated with local infiltration by lymphocytes and plasma cells, epithelial necrosis and submucosal oedema. Superficial desquamation of the mucosa and superficial necrosis are also present. The capillaries are congested and there are petechial haemorrhages. The cellular reaction in the submucosa consists of lymphocytes, macrophages, plasma cells, neutrophils and eosinophils. In the lymph nodes, there is oedema and perivascular infiltration by lymphocytes. There are white foci in the intestine consisting essentially of masses of macrogametes, microgamonts and oocysts in the epithelial cells of the tips and sides of the villi and in the crypts.

Eimeria hirci

Eimeria hirci (Phylum: Apicomplexa; Class: Conoidasida; Order: Eucoccidiorida; Family: Eimeriidae) is a protozoan of goats and distributed presumably worldwide. Details of the life cycle are not known. The prepatent period is 13–16 days and the patent period is 5–14 days. The sporulation time is 1–3 days.

Pathogenesis: This species is considered pathogenic but lesions and pathology have not been described in detail.

Eimeria alijevi

Eimeria alijevi (Phylum: Apicomplexa; Class: Conoidasida; Order: Eucoccidiorida; Family: Eimeriidae) is localised in the small and large intestine of goats and distributed worldwide. The life cycle is typically coccidian with first-generation meronts sited in the epithelial cells of the villi in the middle part of the small intestine. Smaller second-generation meronts occur within crypts of the small intestine. Gamonts and oocysts are in the epithelial cells of the colon, caecum and posterior small intestine. The prepatent period is 7–12 days and the patent period is 6–18 days. Sporulation time is 1–5 days.

Eimeria arloingi

Eimeria arloingi (Phylum: Apicomplexa; Class: Conoidasida; Order: Eucoccidiorida; Family: Eimeriidae) is a protozoan distributed worldwide and localised in the small intestine of goats. There are two generations of meronts, with the mature first-generation meronts occurring in the endothelial cells of the lacteals of the villi, in Peyer's patches in the duodenum, jejunum and ileum, and also in the sinuses of the mesenteric lymph nodes draining these regions. These mature 9–12 days after infection. Second-generation meronts lie in the epithelial cells of the villi and the crypts of the small intestine and are mature at about 12 days post infection. Gamonts are found 11–26 days after infection in the epithelial cells lining the crypts and the villi of the jejunum and ileum. The prepatent period is 14–17 days and the patent period 14–15 days. Sporulation time is 1–4 days.

Pathogenesis: Papilloma-like lesions or polyps may occur in the small intestine, usually as a sequela to gametocyte formation, but these are not of great pathogenic significance.

Pathology: A few, small, slightly haemorrhagic areas are seen scattered throughout the lining of the small intestine and thick white opaque patches composed of groups of heavily parasitised villi are present leading to the formation of polyps.

Eimeria caprovina

Eimeria caprovina (Phylum: Apicomplexa; Class: Conoidasida; Order: Eucoccidiorida; Family: Eimeriidae) is a protozoan of goats and distributed in North America and Europe. Details of the life cycle are not known. The prepatent period is 14–20 days and patent period is 4–9 days. Sporulation time is 2–3 days.

Eimeria jolchijevi

Eimeria jolchijevi (Phylum: Apicomplexa; Class: Conoidasida; Order: Eucoccidiorida; Family: Eimeriidae) is a protozoan of goats distributed worldwide. Details of the life cycle are not known. The prepatent period is 14–17 days and patent period 3–10 days. Sporulation time is 2–4 days.

Other protozoa

Cryptosporidium parvum

Cryptosporidium parvum (Phylum: Apicomplexa; Class: Conoidasida; Order: Cryptogregarinorida; Family: Cryptosporidiidae) is a protozoan distributed worldwide and localised in the small intestine of cattle, sheep, goats, horses, deer and humans.

Epidemiology: A variety of mammals act as hosts to *C. parvum* but little is known of the importance of their involvement in transmitting infection to, or maintaining infection in, domestic livestock. In young lambs infection appears to be age related, with seasonal peaks of disease reported to coincide with birth peaks in spring and autumn. The primary route of infection is mainly direct animal to animal via the faecal–oral route. In lambs, chilling due to adverse weather conditions in the neonatal period, intercurrent infections or nutritional or mineral deficiencies could exacerbate or increase the likelihood of disease. Infection in these cases is likely to occur through grooming, nuzzling, coprophagy or faecal soiling by direct contact with infected animals. Infection may also occur indirectly through consumption of contaminated foods or environmental sources including pasture and water. For more details see Chapter 8.

Giardia intestinalis

Giardia intestinalis, synonyms *Giardia duodenalis*, *Giardia lamblia*, *Lamblia lamblia* (Phylum: Metamonada; Class: Trepomonadea; Order: Diplomonadida; Family: Giardiidae), is a protozoan distributed worldwide and localised in the small intestine of humans, cattle, sheep, goats, pigs, horses, alpacas, dogs, cats, guinea pigs and chinchillas. Infections in sheep are considered non-pathogenic. For more details see Chapter 8.

LARGE INTESTINE

Oesophagostomum columbianum

Oesophagostomum columbianum (Phylum: Nematoda; Class: Chromadorea; Order: Rhabditida; Family: Strongylidae), commonly known as the Nodular worm, is localised in the large intestine of sheep, goats, camels and wild ruminants. This parasite is distributed worldwide but more important in tropical and subtropical areas.

Epidemiology: In tropical and subtropical areas, *O. columbianum* is especially important in sheep. The prolonged survival of the L_4 within the nodules in the gut wall and the lack of an effective immunity made control difficult until the advent of effective anthelmintics.

Pathogenesis: In the intestine, *O. columbianum* L_3 migrate deep into the mucosa, provoking an inflammatory response with the formation of nodules, which are visible to the naked eye. On reinfection, this response is more marked, the nodules reaching 2 cm in diameter and containing greenish eosinophilic pus and an L_4. When the L_4 emerge, there may be ulceration of the mucosa. Diarrhoea occurs coincident with emergence about a week after primary infection and from several months to a year after reinfection. In heavy infections, there may be ulcerative colitis and the disease runs a chronic debilitating course with effects on the production of wool and mutton. The nodules in the gut wall also render the intestines useless for processing as sausage skins and surgical suture material.

Clinical signs: In acute infections, severe dark-green fetid diarrhoea is the main clinical sign and there is usually a rapid loss of weight, emaciation, prostration and death in young animals. In chronic infections, there is inappetence and emaciation with intermittent diarrhoea and anaemia.

Pathology: On *post mortem*, the carcass is emaciated, the mesenteric lymph nodes are enlarged and the colonic mucosa is thickened, congested and covered by a layer of mucus in which the worms are scattered. There is hyperplasia of goblet cells and the lamina propria contains a heavy mixed inflammatory infiltrate with eosinophils, lymphocytes and plasma cells. Nodules caused by histotropic L_4, mainly in the large intestine, are 0.5–3 cm in diameter and comprise a central caseous or mineralised core surrounded by a thin, fibrous, encapsulating stroma. Microscopically, the nematode or its remnants are present among a mass of necrotic debris in which eosinophils are prominent. Giant cells and macophages may surround the necrotic material. Similar nodules may be found in liver, lungs, mesentery and mesenteric lymph nodes. Those in the deeper layers of the gut project from the serosal surface ('pimply gut') and may cause adhesion to adjacent loops of gut or to other organs, and rarely may incite intussusception or peritonitis. In most cases, however, nodules are incidental findings at necropsy. They are probably the response to histotropic L_4 in hosts sensitised by L_3, or the result of prior infection. The nodules caused by the histotropic L_3 consist of small concentrations of suppurative exudate, which resolve as minor foci of granulomatous inflammation after evacuation of the larvae.

Diagnosis: This is based on clinical signs and *post mortem* examination. Since the acute disease occurs within the prepatent period, eggs of *Oesophagostomum* spp. are not usually present in the faeces. In the chronic disease, eggs are present and L_3 can be identified following faecal culture.

Control and treatment: A combination of strategic dosing with anthelmintics and pasture management, as used in the control of other nematodes, will also help to control *O. columbianum*. Anthelmintic therapy with broad-spectrum anthelmintics (benzimidazoles, levamisole and avermectins/milbemycins) is highly effective.

Notes: The more pathogenic species in sheep occur in the subtropics and tropics and are associated with nodule formation in the intestine.

Oesophagostomum venulosum

Oesophagostomum venulosum, synonym *Oesophagostomum virginimembrum* (Phylum: Nematoda; Class: Chromadorea; Order: Rhabditida; Family: Strongylidae), commonly known as the Large bowel worm, is distributed worldwide and localised in the large intestine of sheep, goats, camels and wild ruminants.

Epidemiology: The basic epidemiology of *O. venulosum* is similar to that of other trichostrongylid infections of sheep and further details on the life cycle are given in Chapter 1. In temperate areas, there is evidence that *O. venulosum* undergoes hypobiosis at the L_4

stage in sheep during autumn and winter, and that this is the principal manner in which this species survives until the next spring. The species is also capable of overwintering on pasture as L_3.

Clinical signs and pathology: Generally considered nonpathogenic, it is not associated with clinical signs. *Oesophagostomum venulosum* seldom causes significant nodule formation (cf. *O. columbianum*) and when it does, the nodules are small and mainly confined to the caecum and colon.

Diagnosis: Diagnosis of gastrointestinal nematodes is generally based on clinical signs, grazing history, *post mortem* findings and faecal egg counts. Faecal worm egg counts are not that useful, as the eggs of *O. venulosum* are difficult to differentiate from other trichostrongyle eggs. For accurate differentiation, larval cultures should be prepared.

Control and treatment: As for *O. columbianum*

Notes: *Oesophagostomum virginimembrum* is specific to the dromedary camel but is considered synonymous with *O. venulosum*. Other species of *Oesophagostomum* have been reported in sheep and goats. Little is known of their pathogenesis and treatment is not usually indicated.

Chabertia ovina

Chabertia ovina (Phylum: Nematoda; Class: Chromadorea; Order: Rhabditida; Family: Chabertidae), commonly known as the Large-mouthed bowel worm, is localised in the large intestine of sheep, goats, occasionally deer, cattle and other ruminants. This parasite is distributed worldwide but more prevalent in temperate regions.

Epidemiology: In temperate areas, L_3 are capable of surviving the winter. The parasite may also overwinter in the host as hypobiotic L_4 in the wall of the intestine, emerging in the late winter and early spring. Although outbreaks of chabertiosis have been recorded in goats and sheep in Europe, the disease is more important in the winter rainfall areas of Australasia and South Africa.

Pathogenesis: *Chabertia ovina* is present, usually in low numbers, in the majority of sheep and goats. It contributes to the syndrome of PGE and only occasionally occurs in sufficient numbers to cause clinical disease on its own. The major pathogenic effect is caused by the L_5 and by mature adults; these attach to the mucosa of the colon via their buccal capsules and then feed by ingesting large plugs of tissue, resulting in local haemorrhage and loss of protein through the damaged mucosa. A burden of around 300 worms is considered pathogenic and in severe outbreaks the effects become evident during the late prepatent period. The wall of the colon becomes oedematous, congested and thickened with small haemorrhages at the sites of worm attachment.

Clinical signs and pathology: Moderate infections are usually asymptomatic. In severe infections, diarrhoea, which may contain blood and mucus and in which worms may be found, is the most common clinical sign. The sheep become anaemic and hypoalbuminaemic and can suffer severe weight loss. There are petechial haemorrhages in the mucosa of the colon due to immatures, and immature and adult worms are found in the gut lumen.

Diagnosis: Since much of the pathogenic effect occurs within the prepatent period, the faecal egg count may be very low. However, during the diarrhoeic phase, the worms may be expelled and are easily recognised. At necropsy, diagnosis is generally based on the lesions since the worm burden may be negligible following the expulsion of worms in the faeces, although in some cases worms may be observed attached to the mucosa of the colon.

Control and treatment: The control is similar to that for other strongylid intestinal nematodes. Treatment involves anthelmintic therapy with broad-spectrum anthelmintics (benzimidazoles, levamisole and avermectins/milbemycins) and is highly effective.

Skrjabinema ovis

Skrjabinema ovis, synonym *Oxyuris ovis* (Phylum: Nematoda; Class: Chromadorea; Order: Oxyurida; Family: Oxyuridae), commonly known as the Pinworm, is distributed worldwide and localised in the caecum and colon of sheep and goats. Infection occurs by ingestion, either through nuzzling or suckling, or through intake of the larvated eggs in grass, hay or bedding.

Clinical signs and pathology: These pinworms have rarely been incriminated as a cause of disease and are usually recognised only at necropsy with no associated pathology.

Diagnosis: Identification of the worms on *post mortem*, or the larvated eggs in faeces.

Control and treatment: Not usually required.

Trichuris ovis

Trichuris ovis, synonym *Trichocephalus ovis* (Phylum: Nematoda; Class: Enoplea; Order: Enoplida; Family: Trichuridae), commonly known as the Whipworm, is distributed worldwide and localised in the large intestines of sheep, goats, occasionally cattle and other ruminants.

Epidemiology: The most important feature is the longevity of the eggs, which may survive for 3–4 years. On pasture, this is less likely since the eggs tend to be washed into the soil.

Pathogenesis: Most infections are light and asymptomatic. Occasionally, when large numbers of worms are present, they cause a haemorrhagic colitis and/or a diphtheritic inflammation of the caecal mucosa. This results from the subepithelial location and continuous movement of the anterior end to the whipworm as it searches for blood and fluid.

Clinical signs and pathology: Despite the fact that ruminants have a high incidence of light infections, the clinical significance of this genus, especially in ruminants, is generally negligible although isolated outbreaks have been recorded. In heavy infections there may be a mucohaemorrhagic typhlitis.

Diagnosis: Since the clinical signs are not pathognomonic, diagnosis may depend on finding numbers of lemon-shaped *Trichuris* eggs in the faeces. Egg output is often low in *Trichuris* infections. However, since clinical signs may occur during the prepatent period, diagnosis in food animals may depend on necropsy.

Control and treatment: Prophylaxis is rarely necessary in ruminants. In ruminants, the benzimidazoles, avermectins/milbemycins or levamisole by injection are very effective against adult *Trichuris*, but less so against larval stages.

Notes: The adults are usually found in the caecum but are only occasionally present in sufficient numbers to be clinically significant. Other species of *Trichuris* are found less commonly in sheep and goats.

Eimeria crandallis

Eimeria crandallis (Phylum: Apicomplexa; Class: Conoidasida; Order: Eucoccidiorida; Family: Eimeriidae) is a protozoan distributed worldwide and localised in the small and large intestine of sheep. First-generation meronts appear on day 3 after infection and are mature by day 10. Second-generation meronts appear at day 10–12 after infection in the cytoplasm of epithelial cells of the small intestine and caecum. Most lie at the base of the crypts and contain 5–9 merozoites. Progamonts appear in the nuclei of the epithelial cells in the crypts and villi of the jejunum, ileum and caecum at 11–16 days after infection. The progamonts divide synchronously. By day 16, the progamonts on the villi mature into gamonts, and enlarge and move into the cytoplasm above the nucleus where they differentiate into macrogamonts and microgamonts. The progamonts in the crypts mature from day 18. The prepatent period is 13–20 days and sporulation time is 1–3 days.

Pathogenesis: The pathogenic lesions are mainly in the ileum, caecum and colon where gametogony of *E. crandallis* occurs. Large numbers of gamonts cause local haemorrhage and oedema, and villous atrophy may be a sequela resulting in malabsorption. Infection is a particular problem in very young lambs, especially if their immune status is poor or they have been colostrum deprived. Light infections produce a very strong immunity.

Pathology: In heavily infected lambs at around 10 days after infection, there is whitish discoloration of the mucosa due to masses of first-generation meronts, and this is apparent through the serosa (Fig. 9.12). From the onset of diarrhoea there is hyperaemia and thickening of the wall of the small intestine, increasing in severity towards the caecum. Gamonts are found in scrapings from these areas. In heavy infections, the caecum and colon may be similarly affected. Histologically, there is leucocyte infiltration with loss of villous epithelium associated with first- and second-generation meronts in the small intestine. There is resulting villous atrophy and the crypt epithelium is also affected, resulting in loss of crypts

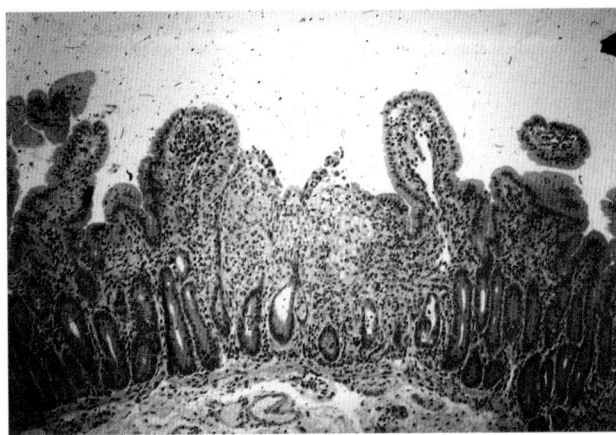

Fig. 9.13 *Eimeria crandallis* infection of the intestinal mucosa showing inflammatory response and villous atrophy.

(Fig. 9.13). From day 11 after infection, progamonts can be detected in the small and large intestines. Infected crypts are hyperplastic with large basophilic enterocytes and reduced goblet cell numbers. Damage to the mucosa and epithelial sloughing may lead to the presence of intestinal 'casts' in the faeces (Fig. 9.14).

Eimeria ovinoidalis

Eimeria ovinoidalis (Phylum: Apicomplexa; Class: Conoidasida; Order: Eucoccidiorida; Family: Eimeriidae) is a protozoan distributed worldwide and localised in the small and large intestines of sheep. Following ingestion of sporulated oocysts, eight sporozoites emerge from each oocyst into the small intestine and penetrate cells in the intestinal mucosa. The parasites undergo at least one asexual multiplication within the mucosa, giving rise to merozoites within meronts. The first-generation meronts are very large (100–300 µm) and may be visible to the naked eye as pinpoint white spots on the mucosa. These mature in the small intestine lamina propria nine days after infection, and give rise to a second generation of meronts that are much smaller than the first. Second-generation meronts lie in epithelial cells lining the crypts of the large intestine, maturing 10–11 days after infection. From this last meront generation,

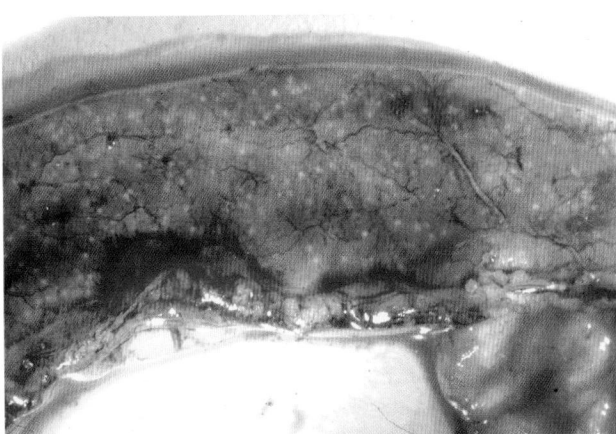

Fig. 9.12 Section of small intestine with numerous first-generation meronts of *Eimeria crandallis* visible through the serosal surface.

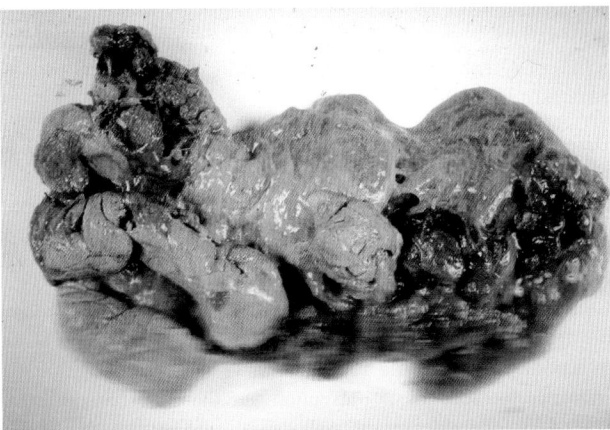

Fig. 9.14 Lamb faeces containing mucus and fragments of sloughed mucosa.

merozoites emerge which give rise to the sexual forms (gamonts), which in turn form oocysts that pass out in the faeces. Once outside, the oocysts sporulate, i.e. they undergo two divisions to produce four sporocysts, each containing two sporozoites. Only the sporulated oocysts are infective. If ingested by a susceptible host, the sporozoites emerge and start the cycle again. The prepatent period is 12–15 days and the patent period is 7–28 days. Sporulation time is 1–3 days.

Epidemiology: In spring-lambing flocks in Western Europe, infection of lambs results both from oocysts which have survived the winter and from those produced by earlier born lambs. Lambs are usually affected between four and eight weeks of age, with peak infection around six weeks. The outbreaks reported have occurred where ewes and lambs were housed in unhygienic conditions or grazed intensively. The feeding of concentrates in stationary troughs, around which heavy contamination with oocysts has occurred, can also be a precipitating factor. In the USA, coccidiosis occurs when older lambs are confined in feedlots after weaning.

Pathogenesis: The pathogenic lesions are mainly in the caecum and colon where second-stage merogony and gametogony of *E. ovinoidalis* occur. Petechial haemorrhages appear in the small intestine 3–7 days after infection. The small intestine may become thickened and inflamed. The giant first-generation meronts which form in the mucosa of the small intestine 10 days after infection cause leucocyte and macrophage infiltration, crypt hyperplasia and epithelial loss. There is extensive haemorrhage in the posterior small intestine of severely affected lambs by day 15 after infection. The caecum and upper part of the small intestine become thickened and oedematous, and are haemorrhagic by day 19. The gamonts result in loss of crypt and surface epithelium, leading to a denuded mucosa. The lesions cause local haemorrhage and oedema, and villous atrophy may be a sequela resulting in malabsorption.

Clinical signs and pathology: Clinical signs for both *E. crandallis* and *E. ovinoidalis* are similar. The first sign that coccidiosis may be affecting a flock is that lambs may not be thriving as expected. Several lambs may have a tucked-up and open-fleeced appearance with a few showing faecal staining around the hindquarters due to diarrhoea (see Fig. 9.9). Lambs eventually lose their appetite and become weak and unthrifty. As the disease progresses, some lambs show profuse watery diarrhoea, often containing streaks of blood. If left untreated, these animals may continue to scour and eventually die of dehydration. On *post mortem* examination, the caecum is usually inflamed, empty and contracted, with a hyperaemic, oedematous and thickened wall. In some cases, the mucosa may be haemorrhagic. Other lesions are more specific but are not usually associated with clinical signs.

Diagnosis: Diagnosis is based on the management history, the age of the lambs, *post mortem* lesions, faecal examination for oocysts and oocyst speciation. Oocysts may be present in very large numbers in both healthy and diseased lambs so that a necropsy is always advisable.

Control and treatment: Decoquinate, diclazuril or toltrazuril are the drugs generally used for the prevention and treatment of these infections. Monensin and amprolium have also been used in some countries for coccidiosis prevention but their use has declined. Several sulfonamides, such as sulfadimidine, sulfamethoxypyridazine, sulfadiazine, sulfadoxine and sulfatroxazole, were used for the treatment of infected animals but in many countries are no

longer licensed for treatment of coccidial infections in ruminants. All animals in a group should be treated and dehydrated animals may require oral or intravenous rehydration. Where non-specific symptoms of weight loss or ill-thrift are present, it is important to investigate all potential causes and seek laboratory confirmation. Good management and hygiene practices, by regular moving of feed and water troughs, avoidance of overcrowding and stress, batch rearing, feeding of dams prior to parturition and creep feeding, will reduce the incidence of infection. Further details on control are provided in the section on Sheep coccidia.

Eimeria caprina

Eimeria caprina (Phylum: Apicomplexa; Class: Conoidasida; Order: Eucoccidiorida; Family: Eimeriidae) is a protozoan distributed worldwide and localised in the small and large intestines of goats. Details of the life cycle are not known. The prepatent period is 17–20 days and the patent period 3–6 days. Sporulation time is 2–3 days.

Pathogenesis and clinical signs: This species is considered pathogenic but lesions and pathology have not been described in detail. The clinical signs for *E. ninakohlyakimovae* and *E. caprina* are generally similar. Infection leads to loss of appetite, unthriftiness and profuse diarrhoea, often containing streaks of blood. If left untreated, these animals may continue to scour and eventually die of dehydration.

Flagellate protozoa

The life cycle of flagellate protozoa is similar for all species found in sheep and goats. The trophozoites reproduce by longitudinal binary fission. No sexual stages are known and there are no cysts. Transmission is thought to occur by ingestion of trophozoites from faeces. All are considered to be non-pathogenic and are generally only identified from smears taken from the large intestine of fresh carcasses.

Retortamonas ovis

Retortamonas ovis (Phylum: Metamonada; Class: Trepomonadea; Order: Retortamonadida; Family: Retortamonadidae) is a protozoan distributed worldwide and localised in the large intestine of sheep and cattle.

Parasites of the respiratory system

Mammomonogamus nasicola

Mammomonogamus nasicola, synonym *Syngamus nasicola* (Phylum: Nematoda; Class: Chromadorea; Order: Rhabditida; Family: Syngamidae), is localised in the nasal cavities of sheep, goats, cattle and deer. It is distributed in Central and South America, Central Africa and Caribbean islands. Infections are usually asymptomatic but heavy infections cause irritation of the nasal mucosa, sneezing and nasal discharges. The diagnosis is based on clinical signs and the finding of eggs in the faeces or adult worms on *post mortem*.

Control and treatment: No preventive or control measures have been described. Successful treatment has not been reported. Benzimidazoles and macrocyclic lactones are likely to be effective.

Notes: This genus, closely related to *Syngamus*, is parasitic in the respiratory passages of mammals. Infection has been reported in human and causes a laryngopharyngeal syndrome.

Mammomonogamus laryngeus

Mammomonogamus laryngeus, synonym *Syngamus laryngeus* (Phylum: Nematoda; Class: Chromadorea; Order: Rhabditida; Family: Syngamidae), commonly known as the Gapeworm, is localised in the larynx of cattle, buffalo, goats, sheep, deer and rarely humans. This parasite is distributed in Asia, Central Africa, South America and Caribbean islands. For more details of this species see Chapter 8.

Oestrus ovis

Oestrus ovis (Phylum: Arthropoda; Class: Insecta; Order: Diptera; Family: Oestridae), commonly known as the Sheep nasal bot, is a parasite localised in the nasal passages of primarily sheep and goats, but also ibexes, camels and, occasionally, humans. Although originally Palaearctic, it is now found in all sheep-farming areas of the world, having been spread with sheep as they were transported worldwide.

Epidemiology: The adult flies occur from spring to autumn and are particularly active during the summer months. However, in warm climates they may even be active in winter. In southern Europe, three generation peaks in *O. ovis* populations have been recorded in March–April, June–July and September–October. More commonly, however, there are only two generations per year, with adults present in late spring and late summer. Geographically, infestation prevalence tends to be highly localised. The flies hide in warm corners and crevices and in the early morning can be seen sitting on walls and objects in the sun.

Pathogenesis: Most infections are light, with only an average of 2–20 larvae being present in the frontal sinus of infested animals at any one time. Sheep show nasal discharge and sneezing, and rub their noses on fixed objects. In the rare heavier infections, there is unthriftiness and sheep may circle and show lack of coordination, these signs being termed 'false gid'. If a larva dies in the sinuses, there may be secondary bacterial invasion and cerebral involvement. This may occur if larvae crawl into small cavities and are unable to leave when fully grown. Occasionally the larvae may penetrate the bones of the skull and enter the cerebral cavity. The larvae and the thickening of the nasal mucosa may impair respiration. Changes in the nasal tissues of infected sheep include catarrh, infiltration of inflammatory cells and squamous metaplasia, characterised by conversion of secretory epithelium to stratified squamous type. Immune responses by the host to infestation by *O. ovis* have been recorded. However, the most important effects are due to the activity of the adult flies. When they approach sheep to deposit larvae, the animals panic, stamp their feet, bunch together and press their nostrils into each other's fleeces and against the ground. There may be several attacks each day, so that feeding is interrupted and animals may fail to gain weight. *Oestrus* can occasionally also infect

humans. Larvae are usually deposited near the eyes, where a catarrhal conjunctivitis may result, or around the lips, leading to a stomatitis. Such larvae never fully develop.

Clinical signs and pathology: Infested animals present nasal discharge, rubbing, sneezing, unthriftiness, circling and lack of coordination. Secondary bacterial infections are common. In addition to mechanical damage to the tissues, infestation induces a marked hypersensitivity reaction in which there is an increase in the numbers of serous mast cells and eosinophils and increased production of IgE. Interstitial pneumonia may develop during the course of ovine oestrosis, marked by increases in the numbers of oesinophils and mast cells in the lung parenchyma, mainly in the peribronchial region. This pathology is probably caused by permanent antigenic stimulation during infection, aspirated larval antigen inducing pulmonary sensitisation.

Diagnosis: Although the clinical signs may assist in diagnosis, infestations of *O. ovis* must be differentiated from other conditions with similar symptoms. Occasionally a larva may be found on the ground after a severe sneezing attack, but often a positive diagnosis can only be made at necropsy.

Control and treatment: Should a control scheme be necessary, flock treatment should be given twice a year, the first at the beginning of summer to kill newly acquired larvae and the second in midwinter to kill any overwintering larvae. Fly repellents may be used but so far these have shown limited success. Where the numbers of larvae are small, it may not be economically viable to treat. However, in heavy infections, closantel, nitroxynil and the endectocides ivermectin, doramectin and moxidectin are highly effective, as are the organophosphates trichlorphon and dichlorvos.

Gedoelstia spp.

Gedoelstia spp. (Phylum: Arthropoda; Class: Insecta; Order: Diptera; Family: Oestridae), commonly known as the Sheep nasal bot, is a parasite localised in the nasopharynx of sheep, occasionally cattle, horses and antelopes and distributed in southern Africa.

Epidemiology: Flocks may have a 30% morbidity, of which one-third will die, and in some areas sheep farming has had to be abandoned and replaced by cattle farming because of this parasite.

Pathogenesis: In the normal wildlife hosts, larvae appear to cause little pathological damage, although there are reports of loss of coordination. The infection becomes of veterinary importance when domestic ruminants are grazed close to, or among, the wild hosts. In sheep, the larvae usually penetrate through the eye or enter via the nose. The larvae then migrate, arresting eventually in the brain, ocular tissues, nasal cavities or heart. It is in the eye that the signs are most prominent, with glaucoma, extrusion and even rupture of the eyeball.

Clinical signs and pathology: In southern Africa this oestrid fly is responsible for an oculovascular myiasis, causing extrusion of the eyeball in sheep and, rarely, cattle. In domestic hosts, three main forms of infestation are distinguished: ophthalmic, encephalitic and cardiac, characterised by thrombophlebitis and thromboencarditis with encephalomalacia, from vascular thrombosis. Myocardial, pulmonary and renal infarction may also occur.

Diagnosis: First-stage larvae may occasionally be observed on the cornea, but often a positive diagnosis can only be made at necropsy.

Control and treatment: Domestic stock can safely graze with antelope during winter, when the flies are inactive (June–August). They should be removed from such areas in early spring when flies begin to emerge from puparia with the rising temperature. Organophosphates such as trichlorphon are effective against the larvae, and flock treatment will reduce the blindness and mortality. Topical application of 0.25% cypermethrin spray to the eye has been used effectively to kill first-stage larvae.

Dictyocaulus filaria

Dictyocaulus filaria (Phylum: Nematoda; Class: Chromadorea; Order: Rhabditida; Family: Dictyocaulidae), commonly known as the Sheep lungworm, is localised in the lungs of sheep, goats and a few wild ruminants and distributed worldwide.

Epidemiology: Although this parasite is prevalent worldwide, it is only responsible for sporadic outbreaks of disease in temperate countries such as the UK and North America. It occurs more frequently as a clinical problem in Eastern Europe and some Mediterranean countries, the Middle East and India. In temperate areas, the epidemiology is similar to that of *D. viviparus* in that both the survival of overwintered larvae on pasture and the role of the ewe and doe as carriers are significant factors in the persistence of infection on pasture from year to year in endemic areas. In ewes, it is likely that the parasites are present largely as hypobiotic larvae in the lungs during each winter and mature in the spring. Development to the L_3 only occurs during the period from spring to autumn. In lambs and kids, patent infections first occur in early summer, but the heaviest infections are usually seen in autumn. The prevalence of infection is lower in adult animals and their larval output smaller. Infective L_3 can migrate from the faeces without the need for fungal dispersion. It is likely that only two cycles of the parasite occur during each grazing season. In warmer climates, where conditions are often unsuitable for larval survival, the carrier animal is probably a more important source of pasture contamination and outbreaks of disease in young susceptible animals are most likely to occur after a period of prolonged rain around weaning. Goats are often more susceptible to infection than sheep and can disseminate infection when both are grazed together.

Pathogenesis: Similar to that of *D. viviparus*, infection leading to a catarrhal bronchitis (Fig. 9.15). However, since the number of lungworms in individual animals is generally low, the widespread lesions associated with the bovine infection are not common.

Clinical signs and pathology: The most common signs are coughing and unthriftiness which, in endemic areas, are usually confined to young animals. In more severe cases, dyspnoea, tachypnoea and a tenacious nasal discharge are also present. These signs may be accompanied by diarrhoea or anaemia due to concurrent gastrointestinal trichostrongylosis or fasciolosis. In severe cases, pulmonary oedema and emphysema may occur and the lung surface may be studded with purulent areas of secondary bacterial infection.

Diagnosis: This is based on history and clinical signs, but should be confirmed by examination of fresh faeces taken from a large proportion of the flock. The L_1 resembles that of *D. viviparus* but has a

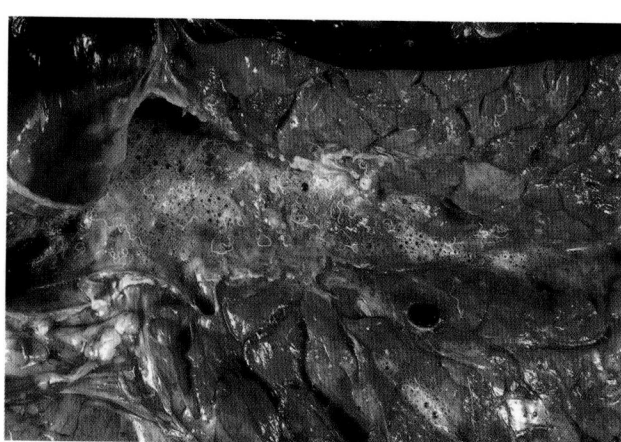

Fig. 9.15 *Dictyocaulus filaria* in the bronchus of an infected sheep.

characteristic cuticular knob at the anterior extremity and dark granulation of the intestinal cells. It is differentiated from other ovine lungworms by its larger size and blunt-ended tail (see Fig. 1.59a).

Control and treatment: When necessary to apply specific control measures, it is suggested that the flock should be treated annually with a suitable anthelmintic in late pregnancy. The ewes and lambs should then be grazed on pasture which, in temperate areas at least, should not have been used by sheep during the previous year. Where sporadic outbreaks occur, the affected animals, or preferably the whole flock, should be gathered, treated with a suitable anthelmintic (see *Dictyocaulus viviparus*) and then, if possible, moved to fresh pasture. The prophylactic regimens of control currently recommended for the control of gastrointestinal nematodes in sheep will, in normal years, be effective to a large extent in suppressing *D. filaria* infection.

Notes: This species, the most important lungworm of sheep and goats, is commonly associated with a chronic syndrome of coughing and unthriftiness, which usually affects lambs and kids.

Protostrongylus rufescens

Protostrongylus rufescens (Phylum: Nematoda; Class: Chromadorea; Order: Rhabditida; Family: Protostrongylidae), commonly known as the Red lungworm, is localised in the small bronchioles of sheep, goats, deer and wild small ruminants and distributed in Europe, Africa, Australia and North America. This parasite has snails (*Helicella, Theba, Abida, Zebrina, Arianta*) as intermediate hosts.

Epidemiology: *Protostrongylus*, whose intermediate host range is restricted to certain species of snail, has a lower prevalence than *Muellerius* although its geographic range is just as wide. Additional factors which play a part in ensuring the endemicity of these worms are, first, the ability of the L_1 to survive for months in faecal pellets and, second, the persistence of the L_3 in the intermediate host for the lifetime of the mollusc. Also important in this respect are the long periods of patency and the apparent inability of the final host to develop acquired immunity, so that adult sheep have the heaviest infections and the highest prevalence.

Pathogenesis: The worms live in the small bronchioles where they produce irritation and local areas of inflammation develop, leading

Table 9.4 Other protostrongylid species in sheep.

Species	Distribution
Protostrongylus skrjabini	Eastern Europe and Russia
Protostrongylus stilesi	USA
Protostrongylus rushi	USA
Protostrongylus brevispiculum	USA
Protostrongylus davtiani	USA

to small foci of lobular pneumonia. The number of nodules on the lung surface may relate to the intensity of infection.

Clinical signs and pathology: Pneumonic signs have rarely been observed and infections are almost always inapparent, being identified only at necropsy. In *Protostrongylus* infection, there is a somewhat larger area of lung involvement than with *Muellerius* infection; occlusion of the small bronchioles by worms causes the lesser branches that occur toward the lung surface to be filled with eggs, larvae and cellular debris. The affected alveolar and bronchial epithelium is desquamated, blood vessels are occluded and cellular infiltration and proliferation of connective tissue occurs. This results in a small area of lobular pneumonia and the grey-yellowish lesion has a roughly conical form, with the base on the surface of the lung.

Diagnosis: The presence of infection is usually noted only during routine faecal examination. The L_1 are first differentiated from those of *Dictyocaulus filaria* by the absence of an anterior protoplasmic knob and then on the individual characters of the larval tail.

Control and treatment: Because of the ubiquity of the molluscan intermediate hosts, and the fact that the L_3 can survive as long as the molluscs, specific control is difficult but fortunately rarely necessary. In some enterprises, it may be practical to reduce snail numbers through the liming of pastures. The modern benzimidazoles, levamisole, ivermectin and moxidectin have been shown to be effective. However, higher dose rates or repeated treatments may be necessary for high efficacy. Other *Protostrongylus* species reported in sheep are shown in Table 9.4.

Muellerius capillaris

Muellerius capillaris (Phylum: Nematoda; Class: Chromadorea; Order: Rhabditida; Family: Protostrongylidae), commonly known as the Nodular lungworm, is localised in the lungs of sheep, goats, deer and wild small ruminants. This parasite has snails (*Helix*, *Succinea*) and slugs (*Limax*, *Agriolimax*, *Arion*) as intermediate hosts and is distributed worldwide except for arctic and subarctic regions.

Epidemiology: *Muellerius* is by far the most common genus of sheep lungworm, and in many temperate areas such as Britain, the eastern states of the USA and the winter rainfall regions of Australia, almost all sheep carry the infection; the extensive distribution and high prevalence are partly attributable to its wide range of intermediate hosts and the ability of larvae to overwinter in the molluscs. Prevalence of infection tends to increase with age. Additional factors which play a part in ensuring the endemicity of these worms are, first, the ability of the L_1 to survive for months in faecal pellets and, second, the persistence of the L_3 in the intermediate host for

the lifetime of the mollusc. Also important in this respect are the long periods of patency and the apparent inability of the final host to develop acquired immunity, so that adult sheep have the heaviest infections and the highest prevalence. Wild small ruminants are frequently heavily infected and could transmit protostrongylids to grazing sheep and goats under some management systems.

Pathogenesis: Although there can be extensive emphysemic nodules, pneumonic signs have rarely been observed and infections are usually inapparent, being identified only at necropsy. Sometimes mild infections are accompanied by sporadic coughing. Heavy infections may predispose the lungs to secondary bacterial infection. In goats, heavy infection with *M. capillaris* can induce coughing and dyspnoea and occasionally pneumonia.

Clinical signs and pathology: The infection is generally asymptomatic but occasional coughing and dyspnoea are reported in heavy infections. *Muellerius* is frequently associated with small, spherical, nodular, focal lesions that occur most commonly near, or on, the lung surface, and on palpation have the feel and size of lead shot. Nodules containing single worms are almost imperceptible, and the visible ones enclose several of the tiny worms as well as eggs and larvae. Occasionally, larger greyish nodules, up to 2 cm in diameter, are apparent and sometimes the nodules are calcified. The nodules consist of necrotic masses, resulting from the degeneration of accumulated leucocytes and pulmonary tissue, and they are surrounded by connective tissue and occasional giant cells. Adjoining pulmonary tissue may be hyperaemic and the alveoli become filled with cells and debris.

Diagnosis: The presence of infection is usually noted only during routine faecal examination. The L_1 are first differentiated from those of *Dictyocaulus filaria* by the absence of an anterior protoplasmic knob and then on the individual characters of the larval tail. Frequently, several species of small nodular lungworms may be present.

Control and treatment: As for *Protostrongylus rufescens*.

The following metastrongylid worms all inhabit the lungs, but none is a major pathogen and, though common, they are of little economic importance compared with the other helminth parasites of sheep and goats. Although there are several different genera and species, they are sufficiently similar in behaviour to be considered together.

Cystocaulus ocreatus

Cystocaulus ocreatus (Phylum: Nematoda; Class: Chromadorea; Order: Rhabditida; Family: Protostrongylidae), commonly known as the Small lungworm, is localised in the lungs of sheep, goats, deer and wild small ruminants and distributed worldwide. This parasite has snails (*Helicella*, *Helix*, *Theba*, *Cepaea*, *Monacha*) as intermediate hosts.

Epidemiology: *Cystocaulus*, whose intermediate host range is restricted to certain species of snail, has a lower prevalence than *Muellerius* although its geographic range is just as wide. Additional factors which play a part in ensuring the endemicity of these worms are, first, the ability of the L_1 to survive for months in faecal pellets and, second, the persistence of the L_3 in the intermediate host for the lifetime of the mollusc. Also important in this respect are the long periods of patency and the apparent inability of the final host to develop acquired immunity, so that adult sheep have the heaviest infections and the highest prevalence.

Pathogenesis: The worms live in the small bronchioles where they produce irritation, and local areas of inflammation develop, leading to small foci of lobular pneumonia; the number of nodules on the lung surface may relate to the intensity of infection.

Clinical signs and pathology: Pneumonic signs have rarely been observed, and infections are almost always inapparent, being identified only at necropsy. In *Cystocaulus* infections, occlusion of the small bronchioles by worms causes the lesser branches that occur toward the lung surface to be filled with eggs, larvae and cellular debris. The affected alveolar and bronchial epithelium is desquamated, blood vessels are occluded and cellular infiltration and proliferation of connective tissue occur. This results in a small area of lobular pneumonia and the dark-brown to black lesion has a roughly conical form, with the base on the surface of the lung.

Diagnosis: The presence of infection is usually noted only during routine faecal examination. The L$_1$ are first differentiated from those of *Dictyocaulus filaria* by the absence of an anterior protoplasmic knob and then on the individual characters of the larval tail.

Control and treatment: As for *Protostrongylus rufescens*.

Notes: A second species, *C. nigrescens*, is found in eastern Russia and Europe.

Neostrongylus linearis

Neostrongylus linearis (Phylum: Nematoda; Class: Chromadorea; Order: Rhabditida; Family: Protostrongylidae), commonly known as the Small lungworm, is localised in the lungs and distributed in Central Europe and the Middle East. Control and treatment are as for *Protostrongylus rufescens*.

Echinococcus granulosus

Echinococcus granulosus (Phylum: Platyhelminthes; Class: Cestoda; Order: Cyclophyllidea; Family: Taeniidae), commonly known as the Dwarf dog tapeworm or Hydatidosis, is localised mainly in the liver and lungs (intermediate hosts) and small intestine (definitive host) of dogs and many wild canids and distributed worldwide. This parasite has domestic and wild ruminants, human and non-human primates, pigs and lagomorphs as intermediate hosts; however, horses and donkeys are resistant.

Epidemiology: Only a few countries, notably Iceland and Eire, are free from *E. granulosus*. It is customary to consider the epidemiology as being based on two cycles, pastoral and sylvatic. In the pastoral cycle, the dog is always involved, being infected by feeding on ruminant offal containing hydatid cysts. The domestic intermediate host will vary according to the local husbandry but the most important is the sheep, which appears to be the natural intermediate host, scolices from these animals being the most highly infective for dogs. In parts of the Middle East, the camel is the main reservoir of hydatids, while in northern Europe and northern Russia it is the reindeer. The pastoral cycle is the primary source of hydatidosis in humans, infection being by accidental ingestion of oncospheres from the coats of dogs, or from vegetables and other foodstuffs

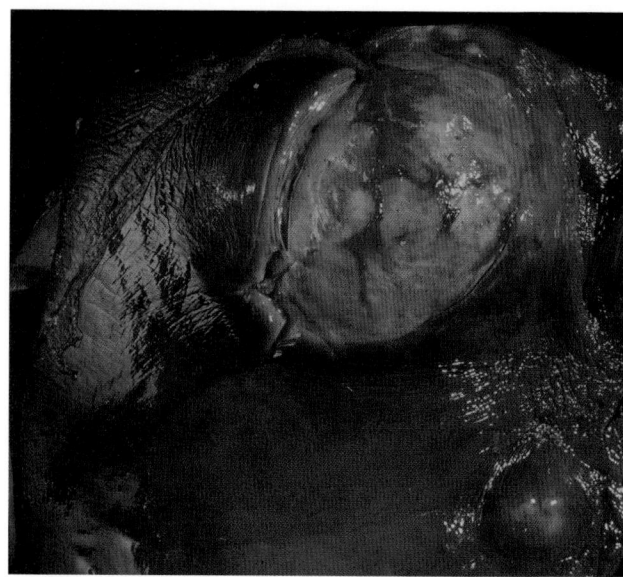

Fig. 9.16 Hydatid cysts of *Echinococcus granulosus* in the lung.

contaminated by dog faeces. The sylvatic cycle occurs in wild canids and ruminants and is based on predation or carrion feeding. It is less important as a source of human infection, except in hunting communities where the infection may be introduced to domestic dogs by the feeding of viscera of wild ruminants.

Pathogenesis: In domestic animals the hydatid in the lungs or liver (Figs 9.16 and 9.17) is usually tolerated without any clinical signs, and the majority of infections are only revealed at the abattoir. Where oncospheres have been carried in the circulation to other sites, such as the kidney, pancreas, central nervous system (CNS) or marrow cavity of long bones, pressure by the growing cyst may cause a variety of clinical signs. In contrast, when humans are involved as intermediate hosts, the hydatid in its pulmonary or hepatic site is often of pathogenic significance. One or both lungs may be affected, causing respiratory symptoms, and if several hydatids are present in the liver, there may be gross abdominal distension. If a cyst should rupture, there is a risk of death from anaphylaxis; if the person survives, released daughter cysts may resume development in other regions of the body.

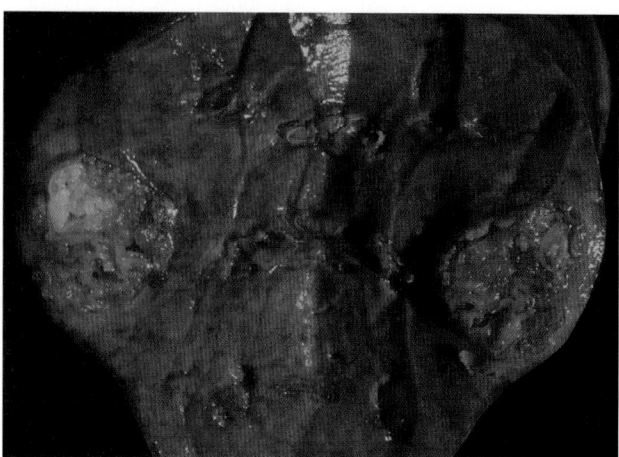

Fig. 9.17 Hydatid cyst of *Echinococcus granulosus* in the liver.

Clinical signs and pathology: Infection in cattle or sheep is generally not associated with clinical signs. Human infection can result in respiratory distress or abdominal enlargement, depending on whether the lungs or liver are infected. In sheep, about 70% of hydatids occur in the lungs, about 25% in the liver and the remainder in other organs.

Diagnosis: The presence of hydatids as a clinical entity is rarely suspected in domestic animals, and specific diagnosis is never necessary.

Control and treatment: Control is based on the regular treatment of dogs to eliminate the adult tapeworms and on the prevention of infection in dogs by exclusion from their diet of animal material containing hydatids. This is achieved by denying dogs access to abattoirs and, where possible, by proper disposal of sheep carcasses on farms. In some countries these measures have been supported by legislation, with penalties when they are disregarded. In countries where no specific measures for hydatid control exist, it has been found that an incidental benefit from the destruction of stray dogs for rabies control has been a great reduction in the incidence of hydatid infection in humans. A recombinant DNA vaccine has been developed for *E. granulosus* but it requires further refinement for practical application and is currently not available commercially. There is no treatment in sheep.

Notes: Considerable phenotypic and genetic variability has been observed within the species *E. granulosus* and several strains have been identified based on molecular genotyping. New data demonstrate that '*E. granulosus*' is an assembly of several, rather diverse strains and genotypes (designated G1–G10) that show fundamental differences not only in their epidemiology but also in their pathogenicity to humans.

Parasites of the liver

Fasciola hepatica

Fasciola hepatica (Phylum: Platyhelminthes; Class: Trematoda; Order: Plagiorchiida; Family: Fasciolidae), commonly known as the Liver fluke, is localised in the liver of sheep, cattle, goats, horses, deer, humans and other mammals. *Fasciola hepatica* is distributed worldwide, although discontinuous, according to the presence of snails of the genus *Galba* (formerly *Lymnaea*), which act as intermediate hosts.

Epidemiology: There are three main factors influencing the production of the large numbers of metacercariae necessary for outbreaks of fasciolosis.

1 **Availability of suitable snail habitats**: *Galba truncatula* prefers wet mud to free water, and permanent habitats include the banks of ditches or streams, marshy areas and the edges of small ponds. Following heavy rainfall or flooding, temporary habitats may be provided by hoof marks, wheel ruts or rain ponds. Fields with clumps of rushes are often suspect sites. Although a slightly acid pH environment is optimal for *G. truncatula*, excessively acid pH levels are detrimental, such as occur in peat bogs and areas of sphagnum moss.

2 **Temperature**: A mean day/night temperature of 10 °C or above is necessary both for snails to breed and for the development of *F. hepatica* within the snail, and all activity ceases at 5 °C. This

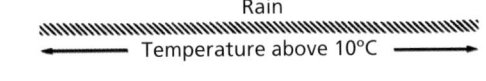
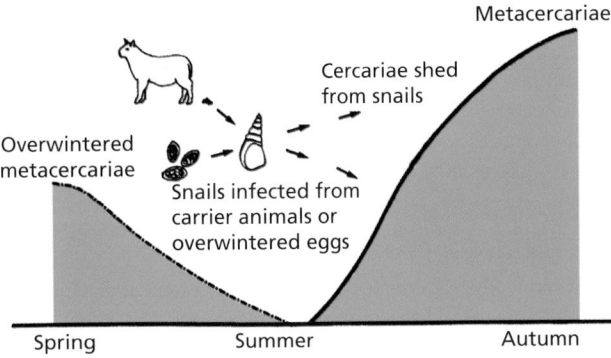

Fig. 9.18 Summer infection of snails.

is also the minimum range for the development and hatching of *F. hepatica* eggs. However, it is only when temperatures rise to 15 °C and are maintained above that level that a significant multiplication of snails and fluke larval stages ensues.

3 **Moisture**: The ideal moisture conditions for snail breeding and the development of *F. hepatica* within snails are provided when rainfall exceeds transpiration and field saturation is attained. Such conditions are also essential for the development of fluke eggs, for miracidia searching for snails and for the dispersal of cercariae being shed from the snails.

In temperate countries such as Britain, these factors usually only exist from May to October. A marked increase in numbers of metacercariae on pasture is therefore possible during two periods. First, from what is known as the summer infection of snails, in which metacercariae appear on pasture from August to October (Fig. 9.18). These snail infections arise from miracidia that have hatched from eggs either excreted in the spring/early summer by infected animals or which have survived the winter in an undeveloped state. Development in the snail occurs during the summer and the cercariae are shed from August until October. Alternatively, infections arise from the winter infection of snails, in which metacercariae appear on the pasture in May to June (Fig. 9.19). These are derived

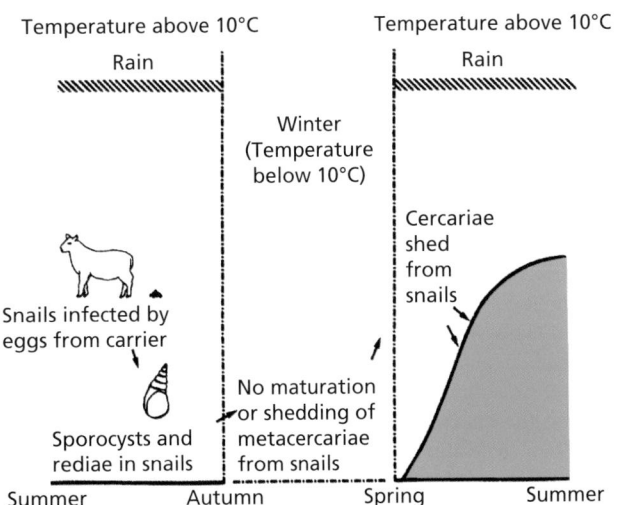

Fig. 9.19 Winter infection of snails.

from snails which were infected the previous autumn, and in which larval development had temporarily ceased during the period of winter hibernation of the snail host and recommenced in the spring. Both *F. hepatica* eggs and metacercariae can survive over winter and play important roles in the epidemiology. The presence of metacercariae on pasture in early spring results in eggs being available by midsummer, when snail breeding is optimal. However, survival of metacercariae is poor under conditions of high temperatures and drought and they rapidly lose their infectivity during processes such as silage making, although they may survive for several months on hay.

In most European countries, the summer infection of snails is the more important and an increase in the numbers of metacercariae occurs annually from August to October. The extent of this increase is highest in years when summer rainfall is heavy. The winter infection of snails is much less important, but occasionally gives rise to large numbers of metacercariae in late spring and early summer, particularly when the preceding months have been unduly wet.

Circulating antibodies to *F. hepatica* are readily detectable in sheep, but there is no evidence that, under field conditions, sheep ever become immune to reinfection with *F. hepatica*, and in the absence of treatment, the flukes will live as long as the sheep. Severe outbreaks of ovine fasciolosis frequently involve adult sheep which have been previously exposed to infection. In contrast, although outbreaks do occur in young cattle, more usually an acquired immunity gradually develops; this limits the lifespan of the primary infection, slows the migration of secondary infection and eventually reduces the numbers of flukes established. Thus, in endemic areas, adult cattle often appear unaffected clinically whereas severe losses from fasciolosis may be occurring in adult sheep.

Finally, it should be remembered that *F. hepatica* can infect a wide range of mammals, including horses, donkeys, deer, pigs and rabbits, and it is possible that on occasions these hosts may act as reservoirs of infection. Humans may also become infected, especially from the consumption of watercress from unfenced beds.

Most of the above comments on the ecology of *G. truncatula* also apply to the other amphibian species of *Galba* which transmit the parasite. Differentiation of *Galba/Lymnaea* species is a specialist task and is usually based on morphological characteristics, although biochemical and immunological methods are now also employed. Note also that taxonomic revisions have resulted in reclassification of many of these species. In warmer areas, such as the southern USA or Australia, the sequence of events has a different seasonality, but the epidemiological principles are the same. For example, in both Texas and Louisiana, snail activity is maximal during the cooler months of autumn, with peak numbers of metacercariae appearing in the winter. The situation differs with *G. tomentosa* which, although classed as an amphibian snail, is well adapted to aquatic life in swampy areas or irrigation channels and therefore temperature is the most important controlling biological factor. Thus, in most of eastern Australia, *G. tomentosa* continues to produce egg masses throughout the year, although the rate of reproduction is controlled by temperature and is at its lowest during the winter. The lower winter temperatures also delay hatching of fluke eggs and larval development in the snail so that large numbers of metacercariae first appear in late spring. During the summer and autumn, there is a second wave of metacercarial production derived from new generations of snails. *Galba tomentosa* can extend its range by floating/drifting on water currents. There is some evidence that the prevalence of fasciolosis in hot countries is higher after several months of drought, possibly because the animals congregate around areas of water conservation and so the chances of snails becoming infected are increased.

Ecology of Galba ***species in temperate climates***   Since *G. truncatula* is the most widespread and important species involved in the transmission of *F. hepatica*, it is discussed here in detail. *Galba truncatula* is a small snail, the adults being about 1 cm in length. The shell is usually dark brown and has a turreted appearance, being coiled in a series of spiral whorls. When held with the turret upright and the aperture facing the observer, the latter is approximately half the length of the snail and is on the right-hand side, and there are 4.5 whorls. The snails are amphibious and although they spend hours in shallow water, they periodically emerge onto surrounding mud. They commonly inhabit drainage ditches and poorly drained land. They are capable of withstanding summer drought or winter freezing for several months by, respectively, aestivating or hibernating deep in the mud. Optimal conditions include a slightly acid pH environment and a slowly moving water medium to carry away waste products. They feed mostly on algae and the optimum temperature range for development is 15–22 °C; below 5 °C development ceases. In Britain, for example, snails breed continuously from May to October, each snail being capable of producing up to 100 000 descendants over three months.

Treatment: The older drugs, such as carbon tetrachloride, hexachlorethane and hexachlorophene, may still be used in some countries but these have been largely replaced by more efficient and less toxic compounds and only the latter will be discussed.

- **Acute ovine fasciolosis**. Until fairly recently, treatment was not highly successful due to the inefficiency of the older drugs against the early parenchymal stages. However, efficient drugs are now available and the one of choice is triclabendazole, which removes all developing stages over two days old in sheep. Other drugs are closantel and nitroxynil, which will remove flukes over 4–6 weeks old. A single dose of triclabendazole accompanied with a move to fluke-free pasture or a well-drained recently cultivated field should usually be adequate treatment. With closantel or nitroxynil, a second treatment may be necessary 4–6 weeks after moving to fluke-free ground. Where sheep cannot be moved to clean ground, treatment should be repeated at three-weekly intervals until six weeks after deaths have ceased.
- **Subacute ovine fasciolosis**. The drugs recommended for acute fasciolosis can be used against older flukes responsible for subacute fasciolosis. Movement to fluke-free pasture is again advisable following treatment, and where this is not possible treatment should be repeated at four and eight weeks to eliminate maturing flukes. In addition to the above drugs, brotianide (available in some countries) is also effective.
- **Chronic ovine fasciolosis**. Outbreaks of chronic fasciolosis can be successfully treated with a single dose of any of a range of drugs (nitroxynil, closantel, oxyclozanide and triclabendazole) and following treatment the anaemia usually regresses within 2–3 weeks. The roundworm anthelmintics albendazole, ricobendazole and netobimin are also effective against adult flukes, albeit at increased dosage rates.

Frequent treatment with flukicides which belong to the same chemical group or with the same anthelmintic season after season may enhance the development of drug-resistant flukes. Flukes resistant to triclabendazole have been reported in a number of countries. It is advisable to plan a control strategy which incorporates a change of flukicides from year to year, although the spectrum of activity of the drugs also needs to be considered.

Pathogenesis: This varies according to the number of metacercariae ingested, the phase of parasitic development in the liver and the species of host involved. Essentially, the pathogenesis is twofold. The first phase occurs during migration in the liver parenchyma and is associated with liver damage and haemorrhage. The second occurs when the parasite is in the bile ducts and results from the haematophagic activity of the adult flukes and from damage to the biliary mucosa by their cuticular spines. Most studies have been in sheep and the disease in this host is discussed in detail.

The seasonality of outbreaks is that which occurs in Western Europe. Fasciolosis in sheep may be acute, subacute or chronic. The acute disease is the less common type and occurs 2–6 weeks after the ingestion of large numbers of metacercariae, usually over 2000, and is due to extensive destruction of the liver parenchyma and the severe haemorrhage which results when the young flukes, simultaneously migrating in the liver parenchyma, rupture blood vessels. Outbreaks of acute fasciolosis may be complicated by concurrent infections with *Clostridium novyi*, resulting in clostridial necrotic hepatitis ('black disease'), although this is less common nowadays because of widespread vaccination against clostridial diseases. In the subacute disease, metacercariae are ingested over a longer period and while some have reached the bile ducts, where they cause a cholangitis, others are still migrating through the liver parenchyma, causing lesions less severe than, but similar to, those of the acute disease; thus the liver is enlarged with numerous necrotic or haemorrhagic tracts visible on the surface and in the substance. Subcapsular haemorrhages are usually evident but rupture of these is rare. This form of the disease, occurring 6–10 weeks after ingestion of approximately 500–1500 metacercariae, also appears in the late autumn and winter. It presents as a rapid and severe haemorrhagic anaemia with hypoalbuminaemia and, if untreated, can result in a high mortality rate. However, it is not so rapidly fatal as the acute condition and affected sheep may show clinical signs for 1–2 weeks prior to death; these include a rapid loss of condition, reduced appetite, a marked pallor of the mucous membranes and an enlarged and palpable liver. Submandibular oedema and ascites may be present. Chronic fasciolosis, which is seen mainly in late winter/early spring, is the most common form of the disease. It occurs 4–5 months after the ingestion of moderate numbers (200–500) of metacercariae. The principal pathogenic effects are anaemia and hypoalbuminaemia and more than 0.5 ml blood per fluke can be lost into the bile ducts each day. Additional loss of plasma proteins occurs by leakage through the hyperplastic biliary mucosa and the pathogenic effect is exacerbated if the sheep is on a low plane of nutrition.

Clinical signs: Outbreaks of acute fasciolosis in sheep are generally presented as sudden deaths during autumn and early winter. On examination of the remainder of the flock, affected animals are weak, with pale mucous membranes and dyspnoea; in some instances, they will have palpably enlarged livers associated with abdominal pain and ascites and often are reluctant to move. Clinically, chronic fasciolosis is characterised by a progressive loss of condition, progressive weakness, lowered appetite and the development of anaemia and hypoalbuminaemia, which can result in emaciation, an open brittle fleece, pallor of the mucous membranes, submandibular oedema ('bottle jaw') (Fig. 9.20) and ascites. The anaemia is hypochromic and macrocytic with an accompanying

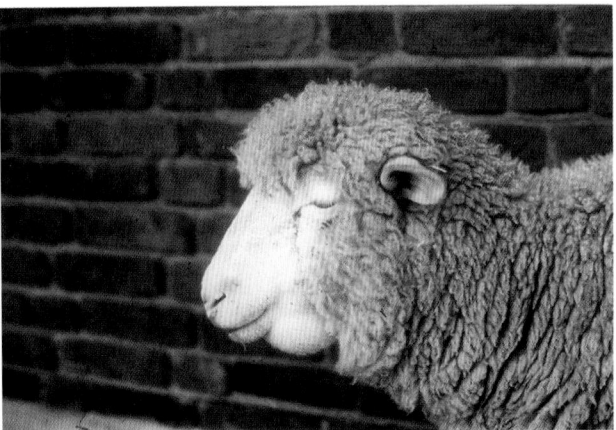

Fig. 9.20 Submandibular oedema ('bottle jaw') associated with chronic fluke infection.

eosinophilia. *Fasciola* eggs can be demonstrated in the faeces. In light infections, the clinical effect may not be readily discernible but the parasites can have a significant effect on production due to impairment of appetite and to their effect on the postabsorptive metabolism of protein, carbohydrates and minerals.

Pathology: In acute fluke disease in sheep, at necropsy the liver is enlarged, friable, haemorrhagic and honeycombed with the tracts of migrating flukes (Fig. 9.21). The surface, particularly over the ventral lobe, is frequently covered with a fibrinous exudate. Subcapsular haemorrhages are common and these may rupture so that a quantity of blood-stained fluid is often present in the abdominal cavity (Fig. 9.22). In the subacute form, the liver is enlarged with numerous necrotic or haemorrhagic tracts visible on the surface and in the substance. Subcapsular haemorrhages are usually evident, but rupture of these is rare. In the chronic form, the liver has an irregular outline and is pale and firm, the ventral lobe being most affected and reduced in size. The bile ducts are distended and frequently contain numerous adult flukes. The liver pathology is characterised by hepatic fibrosis and hyperplastic cholangitis (Fig. 9.23). Several different types of fibrosis are present. The first to occur is postnecrotic scarring found mainly in the ventral lobe and associated with the healing of fluke tracts. The second, often termed ischaemic fibrosis, is a sequela of infarction caused by damage and

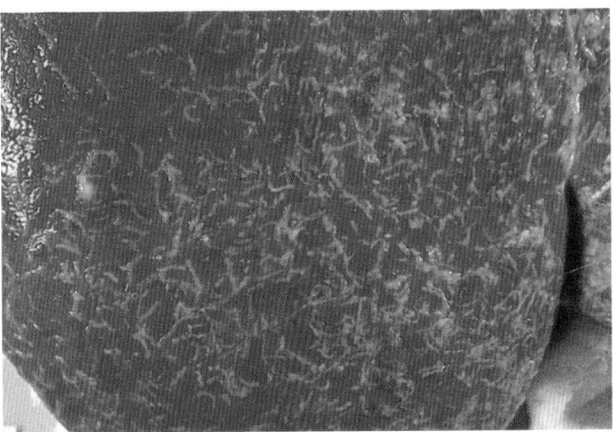

Fig. 9.21 Liver lesions associated with acute ovine fasciolosis.

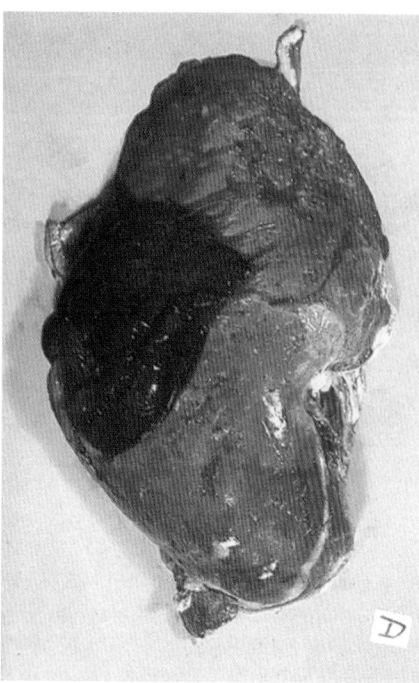

Fig. 9.22 Massive subcapsular haemorrhage frequently seen in acute ovine fasciolosis.

Table 9.5 Haematological/biochemical parameters in normal and fluke-infected sheep.

Parameter	Normal	Fluke infected
PCV (%)	35 (27–45)	≥6
Eosinophils		
(%)	0–10	>10
(×10₃/µl)	0–1	
Protein (g/l)	60–79	<55
Albumin (g/l)	28–34	10–20
Globulin (g/l)	32–43	65–80
Glutamate dehydrogenase (GLDH) (iu/l)	2–10	30× normal (150–300) Elevated ≥4 weeks post infection
γ-Glutamyltranspeptidase (GGT) (iu/l)	0–32	25× normal levels in chronic fluke

thrombosis of large vessels. Third, a peribiliary fibrosis develops when the flukes reach the small bile ducts. Sometimes fluke eggs provoke a granuloma-like reaction, which can result in obliteration of the affected bile ducts. The hyperplastic cholangitis in the larger bile ducts arises from the severe erosion and necrosis of the mucosa caused by the feeding mature flukes.

Diagnosis: This is based primarily on clinical signs, seasonal occurrence, prevailing weather patterns and a previous history of fasciolosis on the farm or the identification of snail habitats. Diagnosis of ovine fasciolosis should present few problems, especially when a *post mortem* examination is possible. Routine haematological tests

and examination of faeces for fluke eggs (note that eggs of *Fasciola* are brown-yellow and eggs of Paramphistomidae are colourless) are useful and may be supplemented by two other laboratory tests. Routine haematology will often show the presence of anaemia (normochromic and normocytic) as a result of haemorrhage resultant from the direct feeding of the flukes. The packed cell volume (PCV) is also reduced. Fluke infection also leads to an eosinophilia (Table 9.5). Fluke infections lead to a decrease in the albumin/globulin ratio. Hypoalbuminaemia due to protein loss occurs both during the parenchymal stage of infection by immature flukes and because of the presence of adult fluke in the bile ducts. Globulin levels increase as a result of increased immunoglobulin synthesis. Serum concentrations of liver-specific enzymes are generally higher in acute liver disease than in chronic liver disease and may be within normal limits in the later stages of subacute or chronic hepatic disease. Glutamate dehydrogenase (GLDH) is released when parenchymal cells are damaged and levels become elevated within the first few weeks of infection. Another enzyme, γ-glutamyltranspeptidase (GGT), indicates damage to the epithelial cells lining the bile ducts; elevation of this enzyme takes place mainly after the flukes reach the bile ducts and raised levels are maintained for a longer period. Interpretation of raised liver enzyme activity can be difficult and careful interpretation of laboratory values in conjunction with clinical findings is essential. Detection of antibodies against components of flukes in serum samples can also be undertaken, the enzyme-linked immunosorbent assay (ELISA) and the passive haemagglutination test being the most reliable. Antibodies to liver fluke can be detected in serum 2–4 weeks post infection but levels may rise or fall over time. A positive result does not necessarily indicate a current infection but a history of exposure. Serological testing is not widely available and may vary from country to country as to availability for either cattle or sheep.

Control: Control of fasciolosis may be approached in two ways: by reducing populations of the intermediate snail host or by using anthelmintics.

Reduction of snail populations   Before any scheme of snail control is undertaken, a survey of the area for snail habitats should be made to determine whether these are localised or widespread. The best long-term method of reducing mud snail populations such as *G. truncatula* is drainage, since it ensures permanent destruction of snail habitats. However, farmers are often hesitant to undertake

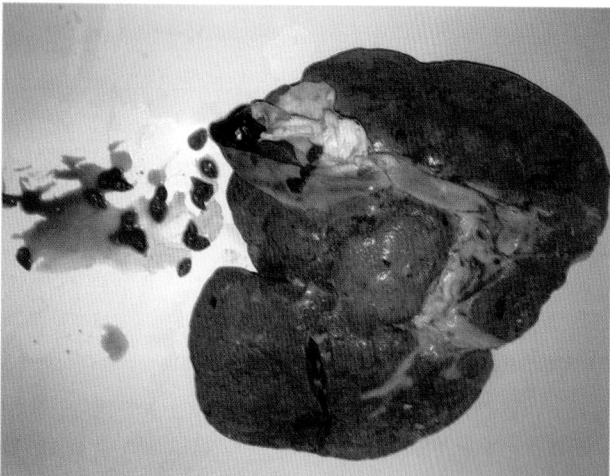

Fig. 9.23 Liver showing lesions of chronic fasciolosis characterised by hepatic fibrosis and cholangitis.

expensive drainage schemes, although in some countries special drainage grants are available. When the snail habitat is limited, a simple method of control is to fence off this area or treat annually with a molluscicide, copper sulfate being the most widely used. Although more efficient molluscicides such as *N*-tritylmorpholine have been developed, none are now generally available, or used, because of environmental concerns. In Europe, experimental evidence indicated that a molluscicide could be applied either in the spring (May), to kill snail populations prior to the commencement of breeding, or in summer (July/August) to kill infected snails. The spring application should ensure better contact with the snails because pasture growth is limited, but in practice this is often impractical because the saturated nature of the habitat makes vehicular access difficult. In the summer, this is less of a problem, although molluscicide–snail contact may be reduced because of the increase in herbage growth. The application of a molluscicide should be combined with anthelmintic treatment to remove existing fluke populations and thus the contamination of habitats with eggs. When the intermediate snail host is aquatic, such as *G. tomentosa*, good control is possible by adding a molluscicide such as *N*-tritylmorpholine or niclosamide to the water habitat of the snail, but there are many environmental objections to the use of molluscicides in water or irrigation channels, and rapid recolonisation of snail habitats can occur.

Use of anthelmintics The prophylactic use of fluke anthelmintics is aimed at the following.
1 Reducing pasture contamination by fluke eggs at a time most suitable for their development, i.e. April to August.
2 Removing fluke populations at a time of heavy burdens or at a period of nutritional and pregnancy stress to the animal. To achieve these objectives, the following control programme for sheep in the British Isles is recommended for years with normal or below average rainfall. Since the timing of treatments is based on the fact that most metacercariae appear in autumn and early winter, it may require modification for use in other areas.
   a In late April/early May, treat all adult sheep with a drug effective against adult stages. At this time, products containing both a fasciolicide and a drug effective against nematodes that contribute to the PPR in faecal egg counts in ewes may be used.
   b In October, treat the entire flock using a drug effective against parenchymal stages, such as triclabendazole or closantel.
   c In January, treat the flock with any drug effective against immature and adult stages.
   d In wet years, further doses may be necessary. In June, 4–6 weeks after the April/May dose, all adult sheep should be treated with a drug effective against adult and late immature flukes. In October/November, four weeks after the early October dose, treat all sheep with a drug effective against parenchymal stages.
   e The precise timing of the spring and autumn treatments will depend on lambing and service dates.

Meteorological forecasting of fasciolosis The life cycle of the liver fluke and the prevalence of fasciolosis are dependent on climate. This has led to the development of forecasting systems in Britain and Northern Ireland, for example, based on meteorological data, which estimate the likely timing and severity of the disease. In several Western European countries, these forecasts are used as the basis for annual control programmes. Two different formulae have been developed.
1 Estimation of 'ground surface wetness', which is the critical factor affecting the summer infection of snails, using the formula $M = n (R - P + 5)$, where M is the month, R is the monthly rainfall in inches (1 inch = 2.54 cm), P is evapotranspiration in inches and n is the number of wet days per month. A value of 100 or more per month is optimal for parasite development and therefore values of more than 100 are registered as 100. The formula is applied over the months when temperatures are suitable for snail breeding and parasite development, i.e. May–October in Europe, and the monthly values summated to give a seasonal index or Mt value. Since temperatures are generally lower in May and October in northern hemisphere countries, the values for these months are halved prior to summation. Where Mt exceeds 450, the prevalence of fasciolosis is likely to be high. The forecast is used to issue an early warning of disease by calculating data from May to August so that control measures can be introduced prior to shedding of cercariae. The disadvantage of the forecast is that it may overestimate the prevalence where there is an autumn drought or underestimate the likely prevalence where the presence of drainage ditches allows the parasite life cycle to be maintained in dry summers. Although this technique is mainly applied to the summer infection of snails, it is also used for forecasting the winter infection of snails by summating the values for August, September and October; if these exceed 250 and the following May or June has a high rainfall, then fasciolosis is forecast for the area.
2 'Wet day' forecast. This compares the prevalence of fasciolosis over a number of years with the number of rain-days during the summers of these years. In essence, widespread fasciolosis is associated with 12 wet days (over 1.0 mm of rainfall) per month from June to September where temperatures do not fall below the seasonal normal. Computer-based forecast systems have also been developed.

Fasciola gigantica

Fasciola gigantica (Phylum: Platyhelminthes; Class: Trematoda; Order: Plagiorchiida; Family: Fasciolidae), commonly known as the Tropical large liver fluke, is localised in the liver of cattle, buffalo, sheep, goats, pigs, camels, deer and humans, and distributed in Africa, Asia and tropical regions. This parasite has snails of the genus *Galba* as intermediate hosts.

Epidemiology: The various snail intermediate hosts tend to occur in stagnant semi-permanent water that contains large amounts of dead or dying vegetation, swamp areas, or pools and streams. *Fascioloides magna* is indigenous to North America and is common in Canada and the Great Lakes areas where the white-tailed deer and elk are commonly infected. Domestic cattle and sheep become infected when they graze pasture where parasitised deer occur.

Pathology: In acute infections in sheep, the liver is enlarged, friable, haemorrhagic and honeycombed with the tracts of migrating flukes. In the chronic form, the liver has an irregular outline and is pale and firm, the ventral lobe being most affected and reduced in size. The liver pathology is characterised by hepatic fibrosis and hyperplastic cholangitis. The hyperplastic cholangitis in the larger bile ducts arises from the severe erosion and necrosis of the mucosa caused by the feeding mature flukes.

Treatment: For acute fluke infections in sheep, the drug of choice is triclabendazole. Other drugs include closantel and nitroxynil, which will remove flukes over four weeks old. Outbreaks of chronic fasciolosis can be successfully treated with a single dose of any of a range of drugs (nitroxynil, brotianide, closantel, oxyclozanide and triclabendazole). For more details see Chapter 8.

Fascioloides magna

Fascioloides magna (Phylum: Platyhelminthes; Class: Trematoda; Order: Plagiorchiida; Family: Fasciolidae), commonly known as the Large American liver fluke, is localised in the liver and occasionally bile ducts of deer, cattle, sheep, goats, pigs and horses. This fluke has snails of the genus *Galba* as intermediate hosts and it mainly occurs in North America, central, eastern and southwestern Europe, South Africa and Mexico.

Pathogenesis: In contrast to the situation in deer and cattle, in sheep and goats the host response is negligible and the continual migration of the flukes through the liver parenchyma leads to haemorrhage, hepatitis and fibrosis. Occasionally flukes may be found in the lungs and peritoneal cavity. Infection can be fatal in sheep and goats.

Clinical signs and pathology: Infection in sheep and goats may cause sudden death. In sheep and goats, the young immature flukes generally fail to mature and the presence of migratory flukes in the liver parenchyma leads to haemorrhage, hepatitis and fibrosis. Occasionally flukes may be found in the lungs and peritoneal cavity.

Diagnosis: This is based primarily on clinical signs, and history of contact with grazing deer in known endemic areas. Large flukes, and the presence of cysts, are usually seen on *post mortem*. Faecal examination for the presence of fluke eggs is not a useful aid to diagnosis as *F. magna* infection is frequently non-patent in sheep and goats.

Control and treatment: Control is performed by not grazing sheep or cattle in areas which are frequented by deer. Elimination of the snail intermediate hosts is difficult due to their varied habitats. Similarly, removal of Cervidae may not be practical. Because of these factors, sheep rearing in particular is difficult in areas where the parasite is prevalent. For cattle and sheep, the commonly used flukicides, such as triclabendazole, closantel, clorsulon and albendazole, are effective. Mature *F. magna* are susceptible to oxyclosanide.

Notes: *Fascioloides magna* is primarily a parasite of deer (Cervidae) and is commonly found in white-tailed deer (*Odocoileus virginianus*), elk and moose. For more details see Chapter 14.

Dicrocoelium dendriticum

Dicrocoelium dendriticum, synonym *Dicrocoelium lanceolatum* (Phylum: Platyhelminthes; Class: Trematoda; Order: Plagiorchiida; Family: Dicrocoeliidae), commonly known as the Small lanceolate fluke, is localised in the liver of sheep, goats, cattle, deer, rabbits and occasionally horses and pigs. This small fluke is distributed worldwide except for South Africa and Australia. In Europe, the prevalence is high but in the British Isles prevalence is low, being confined to small foci throughout the country. This parasite has land snails of many genera, principally *Cionella lubrica* in North America and *Zebrina detrita* in Europe, as intermediate hosts. Some 29 other species have been reported to serve as first intermediate hosts, including the genera *Abida*, *Theba*, *Helicella* and *Xerophila*. Brown ants of the genus *Formica*, frequently *F. fusca*, are the second intermediate hosts.

Epidemiology: There are two important features that differentiate the epidemiology of *Dicrocoelium* from that of *Fasciola*.

1 The intermediate hosts are independent of water and are evenly distributed on the terrain.
2 The egg can survive for months on dry pasture, presenting a reservoir additional to that in the intermediate and final hosts.

Pathogenesis: Although several thousand *D. dendriticum* are commonly found in the bile ducts, the livers are relatively normal; this is presumably due to the absence of a migratory phase. However, in heavier infections there is fibrosis of the smaller bile ducts and extensive cirrhosis can occur and sometimes the bile ducts become markedly distended. Condemnation of livers at slaughter may cause severe economic losses among cattle herds and sheep flocks.

Clinical signs and pathology: In many instances clinical signs are absent. Anaemia, oedema, emaciation and reduced wool growth have been reported in severe cases. Infected livers are relatively normal; this is presumably due to the absence of a migratory phase. However, in heavier infections there is fibrosis of the smaller bile ducts and extensive cirrhosis can occur and sometimes the bile ducts become markedly distended (Fig. 9.24).

Diagnosis: This is entirely based on faecal examination for eggs and necropsy examination of the bile ducts for the presence of flukes.

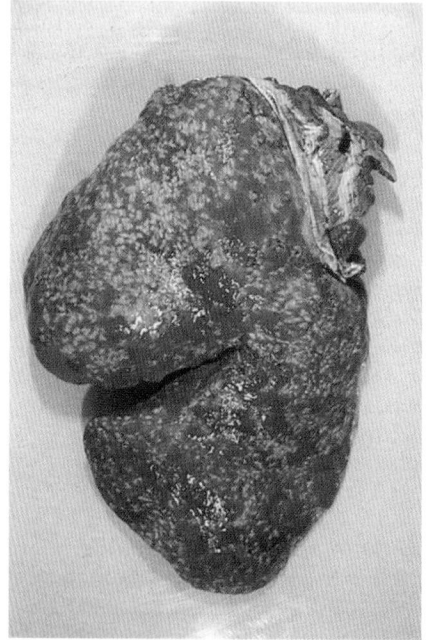

Fig. 9.24 Liver lesions caused by severe *Dicrocoelium dendriticum*.

Control and treatment: Control of this infection is difficult because of the longevity of *D. dendriticum* eggs, the wide distribution of the intermediate hosts and the number of reservoir hosts. Control depends almost entirely on regular anthelmintic treatment. Many flukicides show no activity against *D. dendriticum* when administered at the recommended fluke dose rates. Netobimin has been shown to be highly effective at a dose rate of 20 mg/kg. Albendazole, given orally at 20 mg/kg, is very effective, as is praziquantel at 50 mg/kg. Other drugs such as fenbendazole are also effective, but at very high dose rates (50 mg/kg).

Dicrocoelium hospes

Dicrocoelium hospes (Phylum: Platyhelminthes; Class: Trematoda; Order: Plagiorchiida; Family: Dicrocoeliidae) is localised in the liver of cattle, and occasionally sheep and goats, and distributed in parts of Africa. It is essentially similar to *D. dendriticum*.

Stilesia hepatica

Stilesia hepatica (Phylum: Platyhelminthes; Class: Cestoda; Order: Cyclophyllidea; Family: Anoplocephalidae) is a parasite of the bile ducts of sheep and other ruminants. It is distributed in Africa and Asia and probably has an oribatid mite as intermediate host.

Epidemiology: *Stilesia hepatica* is very common in sheep and other ruminants.

Clinical signs and pathology: Generally considered to be of low pathogenicity, infection is usually asymptomatic. No significant lesions are induced despite large numbers of parasites almost occluding the bile ducts.

Diagnosis: Identification of eggs or proglottids in the faeces.

Control and treatment: Treatment is rarely necessary, but praziquantel administered at 8–15 mg/kg has proved effective.

Notes: Large numbers of these tapeworms are often found in the bile ducts of sheep at slaughter and although they cause neither clinical signs nor significant hepatic pathology, the liver condemnations are a source of considerable economic loss, on aesthetic grounds.

Taenia hydatigena (metacestode)

Taenia hydatigena, synonyms *Taenia marginata*, *Cysticercus tenuicollis* (Phylum: Platyhelminthes; Class: Cestoda; Order: Cyclophyllidea; Family: Taeniidae), is distributed worldwide and localised in the abdominal cavity and liver of sheep, goats, cattle, deer, pigs and horses (intermediate hosts), and small intestine of dogs, foxes, weasels, stoats, polecats, wolves and hyenas (definitive hosts).

Epidemiology: Ruminants are infected by grazing pasture and forages contaminated with dog faeces harbouring eggs of *T. hydatigena*. A wolf and reindeer cycle exists in northern latitudes in which the metacestodes are found in the liver of the intermediate host and dogs can be infected as definitive hosts.

Pathogenesis: Heavy infections in young lambs can lead to hepatitis and death. Occasionally, also, the developing cysticerci are killed

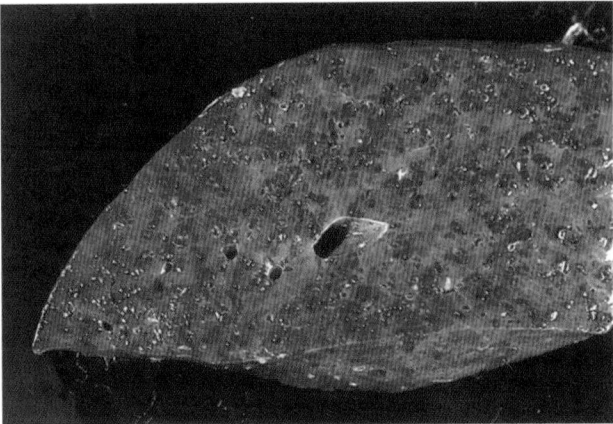

Fig. 9.25 Hepatitis cysticercosa caused by massive infection with *Taenia hydatigena*.

in the liver, presumably in sheep previously exposed to infection; in these cases the subcapsular surface of the liver is studded with greenish nodules of around 1 cm in diameter. Severe infection of the liver or tissues may result in liver/carcass condemnation at slaughter. The mature cysticerci in the peritoneal cavity are usually benign. Concomitant immunity can occur in the intermediate host, allowing metacestodes, acquired from a primary infection, to survive in the host, although the host is resistant to reinfection. Infrequently, large numbers of developing cysticerci migrate contemporaneously in the liver of the sheep or pig producing hepatitis cysticercosa, a condition whose gross pathology resembles acute fasciolosis and which is often fatal (Fig. 9.25).

Clinical signs and pathology: Loss of condition, emaciation and ascites may be present. The main lesions are seen in the liver, which exhibits a number of dark red foci and streaking, and young cysticerci may be found in migratory tracts. Metacestode stages are frequently found attached to the omentum, intestinal mesentery and the serosal surface of abdominal organs, especially the liver, in the intermediate ruminant hosts (Fig. 9.26).

Diagnosis: Chronic infection in sheep is usually confirmed at meat inspection where the large larval cysts are observed on the mesentery, omentum and abdominal organs. The liver of animals that have died as a result of acute infestation may contain haemorrhagic tracts and developing metacestodes.

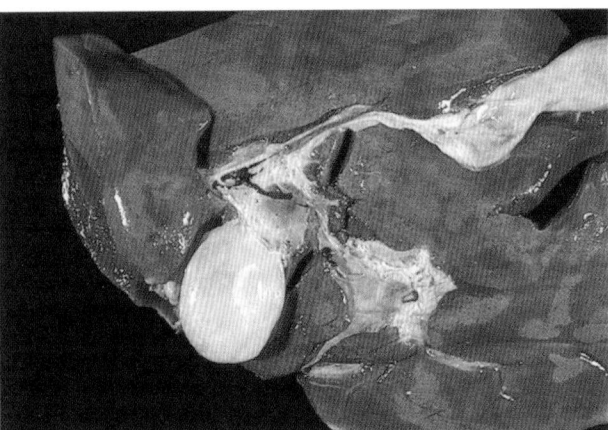

Fig. 9.26 Large fluid-filled *Taenia hydatigena* attached to liver.

Control and treatment: This is similar to that of other taeniids and involves control of infection in the definitive host and the burial or disposal of ruminant carcasses and offal. No practical treatment is available for the intermediate host.

Notes: The correct nomenclature for the intermediate host stage is 'metacestode stage of *Taenia hydatigena*' rather than '*Cysticercus tenuicollis*'.

Echinococcus granulosus

For more details see Parasites of the respiratory system.

Ascaris suum

Ascaris suum (Phylum: Nematoda; Class: Chromadorea; Order: Ascaridida; Family: Ascarididae), commonly known as the Large roundworm or White spot, is localised in the small intestine of pigs, wild boar, rarely sheep, cattle and humans.

Pathogenesis: In sheep and occasionally cattle, migrating ascarids can cause eosinophilic granulomas and interstitial hepatitis and fibrosis with heavy eosinophilic infiltrates in the livers of sheep grazing contaminated areas. In heavy infections where death ensues, the lungs are moderately consolidated, with alveolar and interstitial emphysema and interlobular oedema.

Pathology: Microscopically, there is thickening of the alveolar septae, and effusion of fluid and macrophages into the alveoli. Larvae present within alveoli and bronchioles provoke an acute bronchiolitis.

Parasites of the pancreas

Eurytrema pancreaticum

Eurytrema pancreaticum, synonyms *Distoma pancreaticum*, *Eurytrema ovis*, (Phylum: Platyhelminthes; Class: Trematoda; Order: Plagiorchiida; Family: Dicrocoeliidae), commonly known as the Pancreatic fluke, is localised in the pancreatic ducts, rarely the bile ducts of cattle, buffalo, sheep, goats, pigs, camels, humans and non-human primates. It is distributed in South America, Asia and Europe. This parasite has land snails, particularly of the genus *Bradybaena*, and grasshoppers of the genus *Conocephalus* or tree crickets (*Oecanthus*) as intermediate hosts.

Control and treatment: This is not feasible where the intermediate hosts are endemic. There is no specific treatment for eurytrematosis, although praziquantel at 20 mg/kg for two days or albendazole at 7.5 mg/kg have been reported to be effective.

Eurytrema coelomaticum

Eurytrema coelomaticum, synonym *Distoma coelomaticum* (Phylum: Platyhelminthes; Class: Trematoda; Order: Plagiorchiida; Family: Dicrocoeliidae), commonly known as the Pancreatic fluke, is localised in the pancreatic ducts and occasionally the bile ducts and duodenum. This parasite is distributed in eastern Asia and South America. For more details of these species see Chapter 8.

Parasites of the circulatory system

Elaeophora schneideri

Elaeophora schneideri (Phylum: Nematoda; Class: Chromadorea; Order: Spirurida; Family: Onchocercidae) causes a disease commonly known as Filarial dermatosis, and is localised in the blood vessels of sheep, goat and deer (elk, moose, mule deer). It is distributed around western and southern USA. This parasite has tabanid flies as the intermediate host.

Epidemiology: The natural hosts appear to be deer of the *Odocoileus* spp. (white-tail and mule deer) and in these, the infection is clinically inapparent. However, in American elk (*Cervus canadensis*), thrombosis due to the worms often results in necrosis of the muzzle, ears and optic nerves, resulting in severe facial damage, blindness and frequently death.

Pathogenesis: In *E. schneideri* infection in sheep, the circulating microfilariae are associated with a facial dermatitis, 'sorehead', in which a granulomatous inflammation of the skin occurs accompanied by intense pruritus. Occasionally the feet are also affected. This appears in the summer months. In severe cases there may be self-injury from rubbing, with abrasion, bleeding and scab formation. Lesions may alternate between periods of activity and inactivity. Lesions ultimately resolve with healing of the skin and regrowth of wool. It is thought that the natural hosts of *E. schneideri* are deer, in which the infection is asymptomatic, and that sheep may be abnormal hosts.

Clinical signs and pathology: Only the seasonal facial dermatitis in sheep is recognised as a clinical indication of elaeophorosis. The usual skin lesion seen in sheep is 5–10 cm in diameter, usually on the poll, although lesions may appear on the coronary band. Ischaemic chorioretinitis due to occlusive vasculitis has been reported in elk due to the circulating microfilariae.

Diagnosis: Only in sheep is diagnosis required, and though the obvious method is by examination of a skin biopsy, microfilariae are often scarce in samples and diagnosis is usually presumptive based on the locality, facial lesions and seasonal appearance of the dermatitis.

Control and treatment: Any reduction in vector numbers will reduce transmission.

Notes: These worms inhabit large blood vessels but are only of local importance.

Onchocerca armillata

Onchocerca armillata (Phylum: Nematoda; Class: Chromadorea; Order: Spirurida; Family: Onchocercidae) causes a disease commonly known as Aortic filariosis, and is localised in the aorta of cattle, sheep, goats and rarely camels.

Schistosomes

Schistosomes are flukes found in the circulatory system. The sexes are separate, the small adult female lying permanently in a longitudinal groove, the gynaecophoric canal, in the body of the male.

The genus has been divided into four groups – *haematobium*, *indicum*, *mansoni* and *japonicum* – but the genus as currently defined is paraphyletic so revisions are likely.

Haematobium group

Schistosoma bovis

Schistosoma bovis (Phylum: Platyhelminthes; Class: Trematoda; Order: Strigeidida; Family: Schistosomatidae), commonly known as the Blood fluke, causes a disease commonly known as Bilharziosis and is localised in the portal, mesenteric and urogenital veins of cattle, sheep and goats. The infection is distributed in Africa, Middle East, southern Asia and southern Europe. This parasite has snails (*Bulinus contortus, B. truncates, Physopsis africana, P. nasuta*) as intermediate hosts.

Notes: *Schistosoma mattheei* is thought to be synonymous with *S. bovis* but differs on morphological and pathological grounds and is restricted to the alimentary canal. It is distributed in South and Central Africa and the Middle East where it may infect cattle, sheep, goats and humans.

Indicum group

Schistosoma indicum

Schistosoma indicum (Phylum: Platyhelminthes; Class: Trematoda; Order: Strigeidida; Family: Schistosomatidae), commonly known as the Blood fluke, causes a disease commonly known as Bilharziosis and is localised in the portal, pancreatic, hepatic and mesenteric veins of cattle, sheep, goats, horses, donkeys and camels. The infection is distributed in India. This parasite has snails (*Indoplanorbis* spp.) as intermediate hosts.

Schistosoma nasale

Schistosoma nasale, synonym *Schistosoma nasalis* (Phylum: Platyhelminthes; Class: Trematoda; Order: Strigeidida; Family: Schistosomatidae), causes a condition commonly known as the Snoring disease, and is localised in the veins of the nasal mucosa of cattle, goats, sheep, buffalo and horses. This parasite has snails (*Galba luteola, L. acuminata, Indoplanorbis exustus*) as intermediate hosts and is distributed in India, Pakistan and Southeast Asia.

Japonicum group

Schistosoma japonicum

Schistosoma japonicum (Phylum: Platyhelminthes; Class: Trematoda; Order: Strigeidida; Family: Schistosomatidae), commonly known as the Blood fluke, causes a disease commonly known as Bilharziosis and is localised in the portal and mesenteric veins of cattle, horses, sheep, goats, dogs, cats, rabbits, pigs and humans. This infection is distributed in South and East Asia. This parasite has snails belonging to the genus *Oncomelania* as intermediate hosts.

Trypanosomes

Members of the genus *Trypanosoma* are haemoflagellates of overwhelming importance in cattle in sub-Saharan Africa but also occur in sheep and goats. See Chapter 2 for general and detailed descriptions of individual species of trypanosomes, and Chapter 8 for detailed descriptions on pathogenesis, epidemiology, treatment and trypanosome control.

Trypanosoma brucei brucei

Trypanosoma brucei brucei (Phylum: Euglenozoa; Class: Kinetoplastea; Order: Trypanosomatida; Family: Trypanosomatidae) causes a disease commonly known as Nagana, and is localised in the blood of cattle, horses, donkeys, sheep, goats, camels, pigs, dogs, cats and wild game species. This *Trypanosoma* is distributed in sub-Saharan Africa.

Treatment: The two drugs in common use in cattle are isometamidium and diminazene aceturate and both should be suitable for use in sheep and goats. These are usually successful except where trypanosomes have developed resistance to the drug or in some very chronic cases. Treatment should be followed by surveillance, since reinfection followed by clinical signs and parasitaemia may occur within a week or two. Alternatively, the animal may relapse after chemotherapy, due to a persisting focus of infection in its tissues or because the trypanosomes are drug resistant.

Trypanosoma brucei evansi

Trypanosoma brucei evansi, synonyms *Trypanosoma evansi*, *Trypanosoma equinum* (Phylum: Euglenozoa; Class: Kinetoplastea; Order: Trypanosomatida; Family: Trypanosomatidae), causes a disease commonly known as Surra, El debab, Mbori, Murrina, Mal de caderas, Doukane, Dioufar or Thaga, and is localised in the blood of horses, donkeys, camels, cattle, goats, pigs, dogs, water buffalo, elephants, capybaras, tapirs, mongooses, ocelots, deer and other wild animals. Many laboratory and wild animals can be infected experimentally. This protozoan is distributed in North Africa, Central and South America, central and southern Russia and parts of Asia (India, Myanmar, Malaysia, southern China, Indonesia, Philippines).

Trypanosoma congolense

Trypanosoma congolense (Phylum: Euglenozoa; Class: Kinetoplastea; Order: Trypanosomatida; Family: Trypanosomatidae) causes a disease commonly known as Nagana, Paranagana, Gambia fever, Ghindi or Gobial, and is localised in the blood of cattle, sheep, goats, horses, camels, dogs and pigs. Reservoir hosts include antelopes, giraffes, zebras, elephants and warthogs and the disease is distributed in sub-Saharan Africa.

Treatment: In infected cattle, the two drugs in common use are diminazene aceturate (Berenil®) and homidium salts (Ethidium® and Novidium®) and are appropriate for use in sheep and goats infected with *T. congolense*. As with *T. brucei*, these drugs are usually successful except where trypanosomes have developed resistance to the drug or in some very chronic cases.

Trypanosoma vivax

Trypanosoma vivax (Phylum: Euglenozoa; Class: Kinetoplastea; Order: Trypanosomatida; Family: Trypanosomatidae) causes a disease commonly known as Nagana and Souma, and is localised in the blood of cattle, sheep, goats, camels and horses. Antelopes and giraffes are reservoirs. This parasite is distributed in Central Africa, West Indies, Central and South America (Brazil, Venezuela, Bolivia, Colombia, Guyana, French Guiana) and Mauritius. For more details of these species see Chapter 8.

Treatment: As for *T. congolense*.

Trypanosoma simiae

Trypanosoma simiae, synonyms *Trypanosoma congolense simiae*, *Trypanosoma rodhaini*, *Trypanosoma porci* (Phylum: Euglenozoa; Class: Kinetoplastea; Order: Trypanosomatida; Family: Trypanosomatidae), is localised in the blood of pigs, camels, sheep and goats, and is distributed in Central Africa. For more details see Chapter 11.

Stercorarian trypanosomes

These are relatively large trypanosomes found in the blood with faecal transmission by keds.

Trypanosoma melophagium

Trypanosoma melophagium (Phylum: Euglenozoa; Class: Kinetoplastea; Order: Trypanosomatida; Family: Trypanosomatidae) is distributed worldwide and localised in the blood of sheep, goat and cattle.

Epidemiology: Trypomastigotes are transmitted by the sheep ked, *Melophagus ovinus*, and epimastigote and amastigote forms in the midgut multiply by binary fission. Epimastigote forms change into small metacyclic trypomastigotes forms in the hindgut. Sheep are infected when they bite into the keds and the trypomastigotes are released and pass through the intact mucosa. It has been suggested that replication does not occur in the sheep. Infection is linked to the presence and abundance of ked infections.

Diagnosis: Infections in the blood are so sparse they can only be detected by culture in a selective medium.

Control: Not required, although general ectoparasite control strategies effective against keds will also control infection levels of the trypanosome.

Babesiosis

For details on the epidemiology of babesiosis, see Chapter 8. Control measures are essentially similar and require control of tick vectors. Topical application of acaricides may provide some level of protection but may be difficult in sheep, expensive, and may have a negative cost–benefit. Under certain conditions, it may be more beneficial to attain endemic stability, allowing early infection and development of immunity.

Babesia motasi

Babesia motasi (Phylum: Apicomplexa; Class: Aconoidasida; Order: Piroplasmida; Family: Babesiidae) is localised in the blood of sheep and goats, and distributed in southern Europe, Middle East, the former Soviet Union, Southeast Asia and Africa.

Epidemiology: This protozoan is transmitted by ticks of the genus *Haemaphysalis* (*H. punctata*, *H. otophila*), *Dermacentor* (*D. silvarum*) and *Rhipicephalus* (*R. bursa*).

Pathogenesis: Strains of *B. motasi* from Europe produce a mild clinical response characterised by fever and anaemia but alone are rarely responsible for significant death losses. Strains from the Mediterranean basin may be more pathogenic and some strains are transmissible to goats, but this is not a consistent observation.

Clinical signs and pathology: Disease may be acute or chronic. Animals show pyrexia, prostration, marked anaemia and haemoglobinuria in the acute form, and may die. There are no characteristic signs in the chronic disease. In pathogenic infections, the principal lesions include splenomegaly with soft dark red splenic pulp and prominent splenic corpuscles. The liver is enlarged and yellowish-brown and the gallbladder is distended with thick dark bile. The mucosa of the abomasum and intestine, and the subcutaneous, subserous and intramuscular connective tissues are oedematous and icteric with patches of haemorrhage. The blood is thin and watery, and the plasma tinged with red.

Diagnosis and treatment: Examination of blood smears, stained with Giemsa, will reveal the parasites in the red cells. Diminazene aceturate is effective against *B. motasi*.

Babesia ovis

Babesia ovis (Phylum: Apicomplexa; Class: Aconoidasida; Order: Piroplasmida; Family: Babesiidae) is localised in the blood of sheep and goats. It is distributed in southern Europe, former Soviet States, Middle East and Asia.

Epidemiology: *Rhipicephalus bursa* has been shown to be a vector for this parasite, and *Ixodes ricinus*, *Ixodes persulcatus* and *Dermacentor reticulatus* are suspected vectors.

Pathogenesis: Infections occur as a pathogenic entity in southern Europe and the Middle East but are generally mild in indigenous sheep, with severe clinical signs occurring in animals introduced from a non-endemic area. Death, if it occurs, is due to organ failure which, in turn, is due not only to destruction of the erythrocytes with resultant anaemia, oedema and icterus, but also to the clogging of capillaries of various organs by parasitised cells and free parasites. The stasis from this sludging causes degeneration of the endothelial cells of the small blood vessels, anoxia, accumulation of toxic metabolic products, capillary fragility and eventual perivascular escape of erythrocytes and macroscopic haemorrhage.

Clinical signs and pathology: The clinical signs of infection include anaemia, jaundice, oedema and haemoglobinuria. Infections are often mild and often are inapparent. In pathogenic infections, the principal lesions include splenomegaly with soft dark red splenic pulp and prominent splenic corpuscles. The liver is enlarged and yellowish-brown and the gallbladder is distended with thick dark bile. The mucosa of the abomasum and intestine, and the

Table 9.6 *Theileria* species reported in sheep and goats.

Species	Disease	Tick vectors	Hosts	Distribution
Theileria hirci (synonym *Theileria lestoquardi*)	Malignant theileriosis	*Rhipicephalus bursa, Hyalomma anatolicum*	Sheep, goats	Southern Europe, Middle East, Asia, North and East Africa
Theileria ovis	Benign theileriosis	*Rhipicephalus bursa* in Mediterranean basin; *Rhipicephalus evertsi* in Africa	Sheep, goats	Europe, Africa, Asia, India
Theileria recondite	Non-pathogenic	*Haemaphysalis punctata*	Sheep, goats, deer	Western Europe (Germany, UK)
Theileria separate	Non-pathogenic	*Rhipicephalus evertsi*	Sheep, goats	Sub-Saharan Africa
Theileira spp.	Pathogenic	*Haemaphysalis* spp.	Sheep	China

subcutaneous, subserous and intramuscular connective tissues are oedematous and icteric with patches of haemorrhage. The blood is thin and watery, and the plasma tinged with red.

Diagnosis and treatment: Examination of blood smears, stained with Giemsa, will reveal the parasites in the red cells. Usually less than 0.6% of the erythrocytes are infected. Diminazene aceturate is effective against *B. ovis*. Quinuronium sulfate is still used in some countries.

Theileriosis

Theileria spp. are widely distributed in cattle and sheep in Africa, Asia, Europe and Australia, have a variety of tick vectors, and are associated with infections that range from clinically inapparent to rapidly fatal. Although the speciation of many *Theileria* is still controversial, largely because of their morphological similarity, there are two species of major veterinary importance in sheep (Table 9.6).

Theileria hirci

Theileria hirci, synonym *Theileria lestoquardi* (Phylum: Apicomplexa; Class: Aconoidasida; Order: Piroplasmida; Family: Theileriidae), causes a disease commonly known as Malignant theileriosis of small ruminants, and is localised in the blood, lymph nodes and spleen of sheep and goats. It is transmitted by tick vectors, such as *Rhipicephalus bursa* and *Hyalomma anatolicum*, being distributed in southern Europe, Middle East, Asia, North and East Africa.

Pathogenesis: This *Theileria* is highly pathogenic, causing an acute and highly fatal disease in adult sheep and goats with mortalities of 46–100%. The infection is mild in young lambs and kids due to maternal immunity. An acute form is more common, but subacute and chronic forms have been observed.

Clinical signs and pathology: In the acute form there is fever (40–41.7 °C, 104–107 °F), inappetence, cessation of rumination, rapid heartbeat, weakness, swelling of superficial lymph nodes and eyelids, diarrhoea (containing blood and mucus) and jaundice, and haemorrhage in submucous, subserous and subcutaneous tissues may occur. Affected animals become emaciated and death occurs. In chronic infections there is intermittent fever, inappetence, emaciation, anaemia and jaundice. The lymph nodes are always swollen, the liver usually swollen, the spleen markedly enlarged and the lungs oedematous. Infarcts are often present in the kidneys, and there are petechiae on the mucosa of the abomasum and irregularly disseminated red patches on the intestinal mucosa.

Diagnosis: Diagnosis depends on the detection of meronts in blood smears, lymph node biopsies or lymph node or spleen smears on *post mortem*.

Control and treatment: Tick control measures can be considered for controlling disease. Topical application of acaricides may provide some level of protection but may be difficult in sheep, expensive, and may have a negative cost–benefit. A single injection of parvaquone at a dose rate of 20 mg/kg i.m., or buparvaquone at 2.5 mg/kg given on two occasions, are effective. A single dose of halofuginone at 1.2 mg/kg orally is also reported to be effective.

Notes: Causes significant losses in small ruminant populations in the Mediterranean and North African regions.

Theileria ovis

Theileria ovis (Phylum: Apicomplexa; Class: Aconoidasida; Order: Piroplasmida; Family: Theileriidae) causes a disease commonly known as Benign theileriosis of small ruminants, is localised in the blood and lymph nodes of sheep and goats, and distributed in Europe, Africa, Asia and India. It is transmitted by *Rhipicephalus bursa* ticks in the Mediterranean basin and by *Rhipicephalus evertsi* in Africa.

Pathogenesis: The pathogenicity and mortality are low although prevalence may be very high in endemic areas.

Clinical signs: The infection is usually mild and clinically inapparent and therefore control and treatment are not usually required.

Diagnosis: Demonstration of the parasites in stained blood or lymph node smears. The organism is indistinguishable from *T. hirci* but the small number of parasites present and the lack of pathogenicity help to differentiate them.

Rickettsia

Although *Rickettsia* are now considered to be in the kingdom Bacteria, for historical reasons they are included within parasitological texts and for this reason mention is made of some genera and species of importance in sheep and goats.

Anaplasma phagocytophilum

Anaplasma phagocytophilum, synonyms *Anaplasma phagocytophila*, *Ehrlichia phagocytophila*, *Ehrlichia equi* (Phylum: Proteobacteria; Class: Alphaproteobacteria; Order: Rickettsiales; Family: Anaplasmataceae), causes a disease commonly known as Tick-borne fever, Pasture fever,

Canine granulocytic ehrlichiosis, Human granulocytic ehrlichiosis or Equine granulocytic ehrlichiosis, and is localised in the blood of sheep, cattle, dogs, horses, deer and rodents, and distributed worldwide.

Epidemiology: Rodents, as well as domestic and wild ruminants (sheep and deer), have been reported as reservoir hosts of *A. phagocytophilum* in Europe. The predominant reservoir host varies depending on the local natural and agricultural landscape. The vector of *A. phagocytophilum* in Europe is the common sheep tick, *Ixodes ricinus*. In endemic areas, the prevalence of infection in young hill lambs is virtually 100%.

Pathogenesis: Organisms enter the dermis via a tick bite and are then spread via the blood and/or lymph and localise in mature granulocytes, mainly in neutrophils but also in eosinophils, of the peripheral blood. However, it is not clear whether they invade mature cells or precursor cells within the myelopoietic system. After endocytosis, multiplication occurs within cytoplasmic phagosomes and the organisms can be found in many organs (e.g. spleen, lungs and liver). The veterinary significance of tick-borne fever in sheep is threefold. First, although the disease in itself is transient, its occurrence in very young lambs on rough upland pastures may lead to death through inability to maintain contact with the dam. Second, the disease, possibly because of the associated leucopenia, predisposes lambs to louping ill, tick pyaemia (enzootic staphylococcosis) and pasteurellosis. Finally, the occurrence of the disease in adult sheep or cattle newly introduced into an endemic area may cause abortion or temporary sterility in males, possibly as consequences of the pyrexia. Both animals and humans can be co-infected with various *Anaplasma*, *Ehrlichia*, *Borrelia*, *Bartonella*, *Rickettsia*, *Babesia* and arboviral species. Infection with any of these organisms causes a wide range of clinical and pathological abnormalities, ranging in severity from asymptomatic infection to death. The risk of acquiring one or more tick-borne infections may be dependent on the prevalence of multi-infected vectors. For example, *A. phagocytophilum* and *Borrelia burgdorferi* share both reservoir hosts and vectors, and in geographical areas where tick-borne fever is endemic, borreliosis is also prevalent.

Clinical signs and pathology: In sheep, following an incubation period of seven days there is fever, dullness and inappetence, which persist for around 10 days. During this time, although leucopenia is marked, the characteristic 'morula' inclusions may be seen in a variable proportion of the polymorphonuclear leucocytes present. Recovery is usually uneventful, although such animals remain carriers for many months. The disease is characterised by haematological changes typified by thrombocytopenia and leucopenia. The leucopenia is a result of early lymphopenia later accompanied by neutropenia. Thrombocytopenia is one of the most consistent haematological abnormalities in infected dogs. It may be moderate to severe and persists for a few days before returning to normal. Biochemical abnormalities may include mildly elevated serum alkaline phosphatase and alanine aminotransferase activities.

Diagnosis: Tick-borne fever should be considered when an animal presents with an acute febrile illness in an endemic geographic area. Stained blood smears should be examined and, with Wright's stain, morulae typically appear as dark blue, irregularly stained densities in the cytoplasm of neutrophils. The colour of the morulae is usually darker than that of the cell nucleus. Morulae are often sparse and difficult to detect and a negative blood smear cannot rule out *A. phagocytophilum* infection. Specific diagnostic tests include the indirect fluorescent antibody test (IFAT), immunoblot analyses, ELISA and polymerase chain reaction (PCR) analyses. The most widely accepted diagnostic criterion is a fourfold change in titre by IFAT. However, cross-reactivity may occur with other members of the genera *Anaplasma* and *Ehrlichia*.

Control and treatment: In sheep, prophylaxis depends on tick control. Treatment of tick-borne fever in sheep is rarely indicated. When tick pyaemia in lambs is a problem, one or two prophylactic injections of long-acting oxytetracycline protect against infection for 2–3 weeks. Doxycycline 5–10 mg/kg for three weeks appears to be the most effective regimen for treating infections in dogs and cats. Severe disease may require treatment for longer periods. The most common side-effects of doxycycline treatment are nausea and vomiting, which are avoided by administering the drug with food.

Notes: The newly reclassified *Anaplasma phagocytophilum* combo nov. (formerly known as three separate ehrlichiae, *E. phagocytophila*, *E. equi* and *Anaplasma platys* [formerly known as *E. platys*]) causes canine, equine and human granulocytic ehrlichiosis.

Mycoplasma ovis

Mycoplasma ovis, synonym of *Mycoplasma ovis* (Phylum: Firmicutes; Class: Mollicutes; Order: Mycoplasmatales; Family: Mycoplasmataceae), is a pathogen distributed worldwide and localised in the blood of sheep and goats.

Epidemiology: *Mycoplasma ovis* is transmitted by stable flies (*Stomoxys calcitrans*) and keds (*Melophagus ovinus*) and in the tropics and subtropics by mosquitoes (*Aedes camptorhynchus*, *Anopheles annulipes*, *Culex annulirostris*) and ticks (*Haemaphysalis plumbeum* and *Rhipicephalus bursa*). Transplacental infection is also thought to occur.

Pathogenesis: Most infections are normally benign, but *E. ovis* is occasionally responsible for fever, anaemia and loss of weight. The onset of clinical signs is insidious. Lambs infected at about 2–3 months of age show growth retardation and are slow to reach sexual maturity.

Clinical signs and pathology: Disease in lambs is mild and limited to vague ill-thrift. Initial haematological changes are a fall in PCV, total erythrocytes and haemoglobin and as the parasitaemia drops there is gradual development of an autoimmune haemolytic anaemia. Platelet counts are reduced and prothrombin times are prolonged.

Diagnosis: Identification from staining artefacts requires good blood smears and filtered Giemsa stain. The organisms appear as cocci or short rods on the surface of the erythrocytes, often completely surrounding the margin of the red cell. However, the organisms of *Mycoplasma* are relatively loosely attached to the red cell surface and are often found free in the plasma.

Control and treatment: Tetracyclines should be effective but control is not usually practical or necessary.

Notes: The taxonomy of this species is subject to much debate and this genus has now been reclassified into the bacterial genus *Mycoplasma* (class Mollicutes) based on 16S rRNA gene sequences and phylogenetic analysis.

Parasites of the nervous system

Taenia multiceps

Taenia multiceps, synonym *Multiceps multiceps* (Phylum: Platyhelminthes; Class: Cestoda; Order: Cyclophyllidea; Family: Taeniidae), is a cestode distributed worldwide, whose larval form is known as *Coenurus cerebralis*. The larval stage causes a disease commonly known as Gid, Sturdy, Staggers or Coenurosis, and it is localised in the brain and spinal cord of sheep, cattle, deer, pigs, horses, camels, humans and non-human primates (intermediate hosts). The adult tapeworm is present in the small intestine of dogs, foxes, coyotes and jackals (final hosts).

Epidemiology: Where livestock, particularly sheep, have access to grazing land that is contaminated with infective dog faeces, then there is a risk of larval migration of the metacestode stage into the CNS.

Pathogenesis: The coenurus takes about eight months to mature in the CNS and as it develops, it causes damage to the brain tissue, resulting in neurological disturbances. These cysts can cause pressure atrophy, which may lead to perforation of the skull. When cysts locate in the spinal cord, the resulting pressure can lead to paresis of the hindlimbs. Although an acute form of coenurosis can occur, chronic disease is more frequently identified. Acute disease is likely to occur when sheep are grazed on pasture heavily contaminated with faeces from untreated dogs. The migration of large numbers of larval stages through the brain can rapidly lead to neurological dysfunction and death. Chronic disease presents as a progressive focal lesion of the brain, with signs of neurological dysfunction appearing about 3–6 months from initial infection, and is usually seen in sheep of 6–24 months of age. Coenurosis is much less common in cattle.

Clinical signs and pathology: Clinical signs can be acute or chronic and depend on the location and size of the cyst or cysts and include circling behaviour, visual defects and peculiarities in gait, stumbling, uncoordinated movements, hyperaesthesia or paraplegia. As the infection progresses animals may become anorexic and lose weight and death may result. The clinical syndrome is often known as 'gid' or 'staggers', in which the animal holds its head to one side and turns in a circle to the affected side. The cyst or cysts are mainly located in one cerebral hemisphere and occur less frequently in the cerebellum and spinal cord (Fig. 9.27). The growth of the cysts within the brain or skull causes pressure atrophy of adjacent cerebral tissue. The migration of large numbers of immature stages in the brain of lambs can lead to acute meningoencephalitis. In acute cases of coenurosis, pale yellow tracts are frequently present on the surface of the brain. They are composed of necrotic tissue with marked cellular infiltration. In chronic coenurosis there may be compression of brain tissue by the developing cyst and the increased intracranial pressure can result in local softening of the bones of the skull, either above the cyst or in other areas.

Diagnosis: It is difficult to diagnose infection in sheep or goats unless obvious neurological signs are apparent. Even then, other organisms, such as *Listeria monocytogenes*, *Oestrus ovis* and louping ill, should be considered in any evaluation of acute coenurosis. Most diagnoses are made at *post mortem*. Where cysts are located on the surface of the brain, it is sometimes possible to palpate the local softening of the frontal bones of the skull (Fig. 9.27).

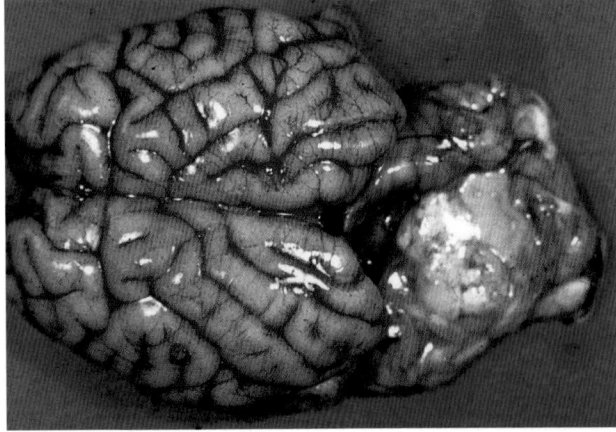

Fig. 9.27 *Coenurus cerebralis* cyst on the surface of the cerebellum from an infected sheep.

Control: This can be achieved by ensuring that dogs, in particular sheepdogs, do not have access to the heads of slaughtered or dead sheep or goats. It is essential that all sheep carcasses are buried as soon as possible. In areas where coenurosis is endemic, the regular deworming of dogs with an effective anthelmintic every 6–8 weeks will reduce the contamination into the environment and, by breaking the sheep–dog cycle, may lead to eradication of the disease. Foxes are not thought to be an important final host for *T. multiceps*.

Treatment: Surgical removal is possible if the cyst is situated on the brain surface. This may be detected by local softening of the skull or by detailed neurological examination. However, for many cases there is no treatment.

Parasites of the reproductive/urogenital system

Toxoplasma gondii

Toxoplasma gondii (Phylum: Apicomplexa; Class: Conoidasida; Order: Eucoccidiorida; Family: Sarcocystidae) is localised in the muscle, lung, liver, reproductive system, CNS and placenta of the intermediate hosts represented by any mammal species, including humans, or birds. Note that the definitive host, the cat and other felids, may also be intermediate hosts and harbour extraintestinal stages.

Epidemiology: The cat plays a central role in the epidemiology of toxoplasmosis and the disease is virtually absent from areas where cats do not occur. It is difficult to explain the widespread prevalence of toxoplasmosis in ruminants, particularly sheep, in view of the relatively low number of oocysts shed into the environment. It has been suggested that pregnant ewes are most commonly infected during periods of concentrate feeding prior to 'tupping' or lambing, the stored food having been contaminated with cat faeces in which millions of oocysts may be present. Further spread of oocysts may occur via coprophagous insects, which can contaminate vegetables, meat and animal fodder. It has been suggested that venereal transmission can occur in sheep.

Pathogenesis: Infections are usually acquired via the digestive tract, and so organisms are disseminated by the lymphatics and

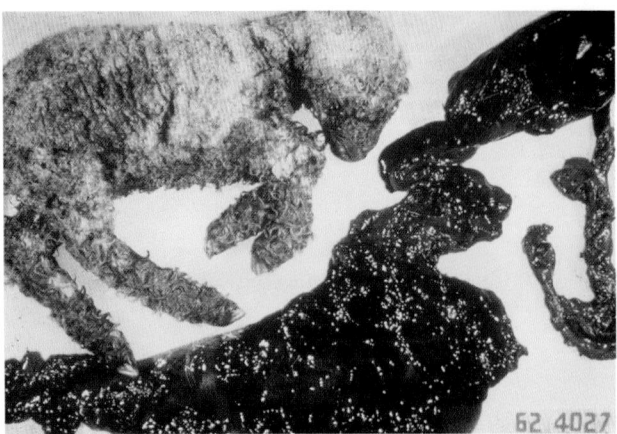

Fig. 9.28 *Toxoplasma gondii*: aborted foetus and necrotic placenta.

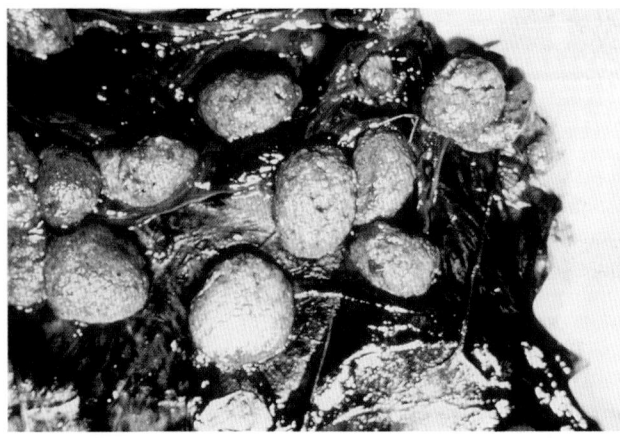

Fig. 9.29 Cotyledons of aborted placenta showing white focal lesions.

portal system with subsequent invasion of various organs and tissues. Pathogenic effects are always related to the extraintestinal phase of development. In heavy infections, the multiplying tachyzoites may produce areas of necrosis in vital organs such as the myocardium, lungs, liver and brain; during this phase the host can become pyrexic and lymphadenopathy occurs. As the disease progresses, bradyzoites are formed, this chronic phase being usually asymptomatic. In pregnant animals, exposed for the first time to *T. gondii* infection, congenital disease may occur. The predominant lesions are found in the CNS, although other tissues may be affected. Thus, retinochoroiditis is a frequent lesion in congenital toxoplasmosis.

Clinical signs and pathology: Undoubtedly, the most important role of toxoplasmosis, particularly in sheep, is its association with abortion in ewes and perinatal mortality in lambs (Fig. 9.28). If infection of the ewe occurs early in gestation (<55 days), there is death and expulsion of the small fetus, which is seldom observed. If infection occurs in mid-gestation, abortion is more readily detected, the organisms being found in the typical white lesions, 2.0 mm in diameter, in the cotyledons of the placenta and in fetal tissues; alternatively, the dead fetus may be retained, mummified and expelled later. If the fetus survives *in utero*, the lamb may be stillborn or, if alive, weak. Ewes that abort due to *T. gondii* in one year usually lamb normally in subsequent years. In heavy infections, the multiplying tachyzoites may produce areas of necrosis in vital organs such as the myocardium, lungs, liver and brain. In sheep abortions, characteristically the placental intercotyledonary membranes are normal but white foci of necrosis, approximately 2–3 mm in diameter, may be visible in the cotyledons (Fig. 9.29). Microscopically, these foci appear as areas of coagulative necrosis that are relatively free of inflammation. Inflammation, when present, is non-suppurative. *Toxoplasma* tachyzoites are seen only rarely in association with these foci, usually at the periphery of the lesion. Examination of the brain may reveal focal microgliosis. The lesions often have a small central focus of necrosis that might be mineralised. Focal leucomalacia in cerebral white matter, due to anoxia arising from placental pathology, is often present. Focal microgliosis is more specific, as leucomalacia reflects placental damage, but may occur in other conditions such as border disease or rarely ovine chlamydiosis.

Diagnosis: Tachyzoites of *T. gondii* are often difficult to find in tissue sections, but are more likely to be present in sections of brain

and placenta. Identification can be confirmed by immunohistochemistry, while PCR may be used to identify parasite DNA in tissues. Several serological tests have been developed, of which the dye test is the longest established serological method and in many ways represents the gold standard, at least in humans. The dye test uses live virulent *Toxoplasma* tachyzoites, a complement-like 'accessory factor' and test serum. When specific antibody acts on the tachyzoites, the latter do not stain uniformly with alkaline methylene blue. The test has proven unreliable in some species. The IFAT gives titres comparable with the dye test but is safer as it uses killed tachyzoites and can be used to differentiate IgM and IgG antibodies. Other tests for the detection of *Toxoplasma* antibodies include a direct agglutination test, a latex agglutination test and an ELISA.

Abortion in sheep and goats due to *T. gondii* must be differentiated from other infectious causes of abortion, including infections with *Chlamydophila abortus* (enzootic abortion), *Coxiella burnetii* (Q-fever), *Brucella melitensis*, *Campylobacter fetus fetus*, *Salmonella* spp., border disease and the viruses that cause bluetongue, Wesselsbron disease and Akabane disease.

Control and treatment: On farms, control is difficult but where possible, animal feedstuffs should be covered to exclude access by cats and insects. Monensin and decoquinate have also been administered to ewes in mid-pregnancy in attempts to control abortion due to toxoplasmosis. Sheep that abort following toxoplasmosis usually lamb normally in subsequent years. It has often been advised that such sheep should be mixed with replacement stock some weeks before mating in the hope that these will become naturally infected and develop immunity before becoming pregnant. Presumably, the value of this technique depends on the replacements being exposed to circumstances similar to those of the initial outbreak. It is sometimes also advised to mix replacement stock with ewes at the time of the outbreak of abortion in order to facilitate transmission of infection. This is extremely unwise, since other causes of abortion, notably the agent of enzootic abortion of ewes, if also present, may affect the replacement stock and be responsible for abortion in subsequent years. Fortunately, a vaccine is now available for sheep, which is less of a 'hit or miss' than the above techniques. This is a live vaccine consisting of tachyzoites attenuated by repeated passage in mice. The strain used has lost the capacity to form tissue cysts and therefore the potential to form oocysts in cats. It is usually recommended to vaccinate the whole flock initially and thereafter only annual vaccination of replacements. The vaccine consists of 104–106 tachyzoites and is given as a single dose intramuscularly at least three weeks prior to tupping.

Parasites of the locomotory system

Taenia ovis

Taenia ovis (Phylum: Platyhelminthes; Class: Cestoda; Order: Cyclophyllidea; Family: Taeniidae) is a cestode distributed worldwide, whose larval form is known as *Cysticercus ovis*. The infection is also known as ovine cysticercosis, sheep measles or sheep bladder worm. It is localised in the muscles of sheep and goats (intermediate hosts) and small intestine of dogs, foxes and wild carnivores (final/ definitive hosts). This parasite has sheep and goats as intermediate hosts.

Epidemiology: Ruminants are infected by grazing pasture and forages contaminated with dog or fox faeces harbouring eggs of *T. ovis*. The thick-walled eggs can survive on pasture for up to six months under ideal weather conditions.

Pathogenesis: Ovine cysticercosis is primarily important because of aesthetic objections to the appearance of the cysts in sheep meat and, in consequence, it can be a significant cause of economic loss through condemnation at meat inspection.

Clinical signs and pathology: Adult tapeworms normally induce only mild symptoms in the host and are considered of little pathogenic importance. Infected intermediate hosts do not usually show clinical signs of disease. Sheep can develop a strong acquired immunity to reinfection but this immunity does not have a major impact on existing cysts. The mature, ovoid, white cysticerci are grossly visible in the cardiac and skeletal musculature of sheep and goats. Commonly, the cysticerci are degenerate with a green or cream caseous or calcified centre.

Diagnosis: Diagnosis in sheep and goats is by identification of cysts at meat inspection. Cysts may be present in the heart, tongue, cheek muscles, diaphragm and skeletal muscles (Fig. 9.30).

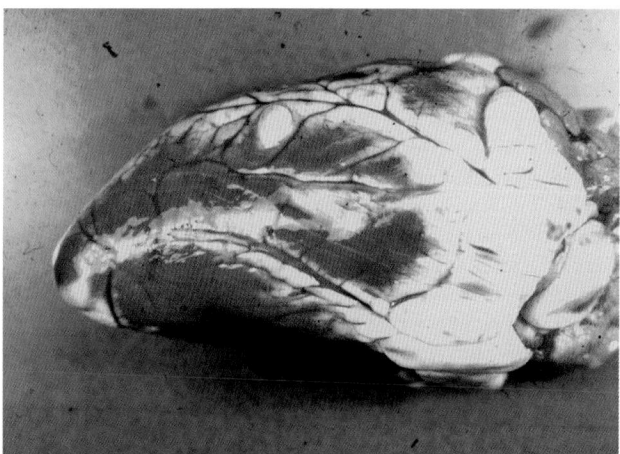

Fig. 9.30 *Cysticercus ovis* in sheep heart.

Control and treatment: Regular treatment of dogs with an effective anthelmintic will reduce contamination of the environment. Dogs should be denied access to raw sheep and goat meat and carcasses. A highly protective recombinant vaccine is available in some countries. No practical treatment is available for the intermediate host.

Notes: The correct nomenclature for the intermediate host stage is 'metacestode stage of *Taenia ovis*' rather than '*Cysticercus ovis*'.

Toxoplasma gondii

For more details see Parasites of the reproductive/urogenital system.

Sarcocystosis

Sarcocystis is one of the most prevalent parasites of livestock. The parasites derive their name from the intramuscular cyst stage (sarcocyst) present in the intermediate (prey) host. The nomenclature used in this book incorporates the names of the intermediate and final hosts in that order. *Sarcocystis* species affecting sheep and goats are host specific for their intermediate hosts and family specific for their final hosts. Further general details on nomenclature, diagnosis and epidemiology are given in Chapters 2 and 8.

There is no effective treatment for infection, either in the final or in the intermediate host. Where an outbreak occurs in sheep or goats, it has been suggested that the introduction of amprolium into the diet of the animals has a prophylactic effect. Amprolium and halofuginone (0.66 mg/kg orally on two consecutive days) may be used in sheep to avoid clinical disease after infection. The only control measures possible are those of simple hygiene. Farm dogs should not be housed in, or allowed access to, fodder stores nor should they be allowed to defecate in pens where livestock are housed. It is also important that they are not fed uncooked meat.

Sarcocystis ovicanis

Sarcocystis ovicanis, synonyms *Sarcocystis tenella*, *Isospora bigemina* (Phylum: Apicomplexa; Class: Conoidasida; Order: Eucoccidiorida; Family: Sarcocystidae), is a protozoan distributed worldwide and localised in the muscle of dogs. This parasite has sheep as intermediate hosts.

Pathogenesis: In the sheep intermediate host, the principal pathogenic effect is attributable to the second stage of merogony in the vascular endothelium. *Sarcocystis ovicanis* is highly pathogenic for lambs, reportedly causing severe myositis and encephalomyelitis in lambs in several countries, and has been incriminated as the cause of abortion in ewes. Generally, however, clinical signs are rarely observed in *Sarcocystis* infection and the most significant effect is the presence of cysts in the muscles resulting in downgrading or condemnation of carcasses. While the dog-borne species were thought to be of primary importance in this context, there is increasing evidence that cat-borne species are also responsible for lesions in meat.

Clinical signs: In heavy infections in sheep, there is anorexia, fever, anaemia, loss of weight, a disinclination to move and sometimes recumbency; in lambs a dog-sitting posture has been recorded. Abortions may occur in breeding stock.

Pathology: In sheep, meronts present in endothelial cells of capillaries in various organs lead to endothelial cell destruction. As the organisms enter muscle, a wide range of change may be encountered. Microscopic inspection of *Sarcocystis*-infected muscle often reveals occasional degenerate parasitic cysts surrounded by variable numbers of inflammatory cells (very few of which are eosinophils) or, at a later stage, macrophages and granulation tissue. Usually there is no muscle fibre degeneration, but there may be thin linear collections of lymphocytes between fibres in the region. The extent of muscle change bears little relationship to the numbers of developing cysts, but generally very low numbers of *Sarcocystis* produce no reaction. As cysts mature, the cyst capsule within the enlarged muscle fibre becomes thicker and more clearly differentiated from the muscle sarcoplasm.

Sarcocystis ovifelis

Sarcocystis ovifelis, synonyms *Sarcocystis gigantea*, *Sarcocystis medusiformis*, *Isospora bigemina* (Phylum: Apicomplexa; Class: Conoidasida; Order: Eucoccidiorida; Family: Sarcocystidae), is a protozoan distributed worldwide and localised in the muscle of cats. This parasite has sheep as intermediate hosts.

Pathogenesis: Infection in the final host is normally non-pathogenic, although mild diarrhoea has occasionally been reported. Generally, however, clinical signs are rarely observed in *Sarcocystis* infection and the most significant effect is the presence of cysts in the muscles resulting in downgrading or condemnation of carcasses.

Clinical signs and pathology: Infection is usually asymptomatic but may occasionally cause a febrile illness. In sheep, the tissue cysts may just be visible to the naked eye, especially in the oesophagus and tongue, but are more likely to be detected on histopathology.

Sarcocystis capracanis

Sarcocystis capracanis (Phylum: Apicomplexa; Class: Conoidasida; Order: Eucoccidiorida; Family: Sarcocystidae) is a protozoan distributed worldwide and localised in the muscle of dogs, foxes and wolves. This parasite has goats as intermediate hosts.

Pathogenesis: In goats, the merogony stages in the vascular endothelium are pathogenic for the goat and can cause abortion and death. Generally, however, clinical signs are rarely observed in *Sarcocystis* infection and the most significant effect is the presence of cysts in the muscles resulting in downgrading or condemnation of carcasses.

Clinical signs: In heavy infections in goats, there is anorexia, fever, anaemia, loss of weight, a disinclination to move and sometimes recumbency. Abortions may occur in breeding stock.

Pathology: Similar to that described for *S. ovicanis* in sheep.

Sarcocystis hircicanis

Sarcocystis hircicanis (Phylum: Apicomplexa; Class: Conoidasida; Order: Eucoccidiorida; Family: Sarcocystidae) is a protozoan localised in the muscle of dogs, foxes and wolves, and distributed in Europe and Asia. This protozoan has goats as intermediate hosts. The pathogenesis, clinical signs and pathology are similar to *S. capracanis*.

Sarcocystis hircifelis

Sarcocystis hircifelis, synonym *Sarcocystis moulei* (Phylum: Apicomplexa; Class: Conoidasida; Order: Eucoccidiorida; Family: Sarcocystidae), is a protozoan localised in the muscle of cats (definitive host) and is distributed worldwide. This protozoan has goats as intermediate hosts. The infection is usually asymptomatic.

Parasites of the integument

Besnoitia besnoiti

Besnoitia besnoiti (Phylum: Apicomplexa; Class: Conoidasida; Order: Eucoccidiorida; Family: Sarcocystidae) is distributed worldwide, although important in tropical and subtropical countries, especially in Africa. This protozoan is localised in the skin and conjunctiva of cats and wild cats (lions, cheetahs, leopards). Cattle, goats and wild ruminants (wildebeest, impala, kudu) represent intermediate hosts. For further details on pathogenesis, diagnosis, treatment and control see Chapter 8.

Przhevalskiana silenus

Przhevalskiana silenus, synonyms *Hypoderma ageratum*, *Hypoderma crossi*, *Przhevalskiana ageratum* (Phylum: Arthropoda; Class: Insecta; Order: Diptera; Family: Oestridae), commonly known as the Goat warble, is distributed throughout Asia, Middle East, North Africa and southern Europe. It is found in the subcutaneous connective tissue of domestic goats and, less commonly, sheep, with gazelles as wild reservoirs over much of its range.

Epidemiology: Younger animals appear to be more prone to infestation than older animals. Flock prevalences of between 30% and 90% have been reported in goat herds in southern Italy and Greece, with mean intensities of about five larvae per animal.

Pathogenesis: Heavy infestations can result in loss of weight and reduction in milk production; however, the chief importance of *Przhevalskiana* is in hide damage.

Clinical signs and pathology: Symptoms depend on the intensity of infestation and the number of larvae in the subcutaneous tissue. Generally, hosts are restless and reduce feeding, and significantly infested animals lose condition. Except for poor growth and decreased milk yield in cases of heavy infestation, the host animals show no appreciable signs until the larvae and characteristic 'warbles' appear at the skin surface. The pathology is variable and depends on the intensity of infestation. Histologically, a fibrous thick-walled cavity is formed around the third-stage larva by granulation tissue, surrounded by a hyalinised and eosinophilic cuff. After granulocyte infiltration there may be a second infiltration by lymphocytes, plasma cells, macrophages and giant cells.

Diagnosis: The presence of the larvae in swellings under the skin, detected by palpation, allows diagnosis. Respiratory holes at the centre of each swelling, with associated reddish dried exudate, may be observed. The eggs may also be found on the hairs of the animals in the summer. Serological diagnosis has been demonstrated to be effective.

Control and treatment: A programme incorporating a single annual treatment of macrocyclic lactone should form the basis of effective goat warble fly infestation control in areas where the disease is prevalent. Organophosphate insecticides such as trichlorphon appear to be less effective when used to treat goat warble fly infestation than for bovine hypodermosis. However, the macrocyclic lactones abamectin, ivermectin, doramectin, eprinomectin and moxidectin have been shown to be highly effective against *P. silenus* infestation.

Notes: Limited geographical distribution, but locally of veterinary importance.

Hypoderma diana

Hypoderma diana (Phylum: Arthropoda; Class: Insecta; Order: Diptera; Family: Oestridae), commonly known as the Deer warble, largely infests deer but is occasionally found in horses and sheep. It does not infect cattle. Larvae are usually localised in the subcutaneous connective tissue.

ECTOPARASITES

FLIES

Melophagus ovinus

Melophagus ovinus (Phylum: Arthropoda; Class: Insecta; Order: Diptera; Family: Hippoboscidae), commonly known as the Sheep ked, is found on the skin, often on the neck, shoulders and belly. It occurs worldwide, but is most common in temperate areas.

Epidemiology: Keds are permanent ectoparasites. The spread of sheep keds is largely through contact, and the movement of keds from ewes to lambs is an important route of infestation. Within a flock, transfer occurs when sheep keds move to the tips of the fleece in response to increasing air temperature. Air temperature must usually be 21 °C or above before many keds are observed on the surface of the fleece. Consequently, transfer between animals is more likely, and occurs more rapidly, in summer than in winter. Sheep with dense, long or clotted fleeces are more likely to spread the infection because the keds come to the surface of such fleeces. Heavy infestations of keds are most commonly seen in autumn and winter. Poorly fed animals or those that are not sufficiently protected against cold weather are most liable to suffer from keds, and the parasites are particularly common towards the end of winter.

Pathogenesis: Since keds suck blood, heavy infections may lead to loss of condition and anaemia. Inflammation leads to pruritus, biting, rubbing, wool loss and a vertical ridging of the skin known as 'cockle'. *Melophagus ovinus* is also responsible for an allergic dermatitis in sheep characterised by small nodules on the grain layer of the skin, reduced weight gain and darkened patches at the affected site. They are spread by contact and long-wooled breeds appear to be particularly susceptible. *Melophagus ovinus* is the vector of the non-pathogenic *Trypanosoma melophagium*. If the sheep eats a ked, the metacyclic stages may penetrate the buccal mucosa.

Clinical signs: Intense irritation from infestation causes sheep to rub, bite and scratch themselves, tearing the fleece. Heavy infestation may cause anaemia. The piercing mouthparts of keds create open wounds susceptible to further bacterial and parasitic infections. The faeces of the keds produce stains in the coat that do not wash out readily.

Diagnosis: Adults and pupae may be seen on the host animal, most frequently around the ribs.

Control and treatment: Specific measures are rarely undertaken, since the routine use of insecticides for the control of blowflies and ticks usually also results in the efficient control of keds. Organophosphates and pyrethroids applied as dips, sprays or pour-on formulations are highly effective at treating *M. ovinus* infestations. Pupae are resistant to treatment but shearing removes pupae and adults.

Notes: The sheep ked is of considerable economic importance and is generally regarded as one of the most damaging ectoparasites of sheep in North and South America. The overall losses in the USA due to keds have been estimated to be about US$40 million per year.

FLY STRIKE (MYIASIS)

Myiasis is the infestation of the organs or tissues of host animals by the larval stages of dipterous flies, usually known as maggots or grubs. The fly larvae feed directly on the host's necrotic or living tissue. A small number of species are obligate ectoparasites and must have a living host to complete their development (see this chapter for *Oestrus* and Chapter 8 for obligate calliphorid agents of myiasis). However, the majority that are of importance in sheep are facultative parasites and these can develop in both living and dead organic matter. The facultative species can be subdivided into primary and secondary facultative species. The primary species usually adopt an ectoparasitic habit and are capable of initiating myiasis, but may occasionally live as saprophages in decaying organic matter and animal carcasses. The secondary facultative ectoparasites normally live as saprophages and usually cannot initiate a myiasis; they may secondarily invade pre-existing infestations.

Epidemiology: The epidemiology of cutaneous myiasis in sheep depends on factors that affect the prevalence of blowflies and those which affect host susceptibility. The three principal factors are as follows.

1 **Temperature.** High ambient temperatures allow elevated levels of fly activity and, provided the relative humidity is also high, favour the creation of suitable areas of microclimate in the fleece that attract the adult flies to lay their eggs. In temperate areas, the rising temperatures of late spring allow overwintering larvae to complete their development and the first wave of adult blowflies to emerge. Ambient temperature then determines the number of generations and hence the maximum abundance of flies over the summer.

2 **Rainfall.** Persistent rain can make the fleece more attractive to the adult female flies, stimulate oviposition and increase the survival of eggs and first-stage larvae, which require areas of high humidity in the wool to persist.

3 **Host susceptibility**. This is increased where putrefactive odours, often resulting from the bacterial decomposition of organic matter, develop in the fleece. The most common causes of this are soiling of the hindquarters due to diarrhoea, bacterial fleece rot and injuries due to fighting, especially on the head in rams. Long fleece, long tails and wrinkled skinfolds in some breeds may also increase host susceptibility. Footrot, caused by two anaerobic Gram-negative bacteria, *Bacteroides nodosus* and *Fusobacterium necrophorum*, is also an important predisposing factor leading to foot strike.

Clinical signs: Infestations resulting from small numbers of larvae may be tolerated well by sheep; nothing can be seen until the fleece is parted, revealing the damaged skin and the larvae. Heavily affected sheep are anorexic, appear dull and usually stand away from the main flock. The fleece in the affected area is darker, has a damp appearance and a foul odour.

Diagnosis: This is based on clinical signs and recognition of the larvae in lesions.

Pathogenesis: Infestations resulting from a single batch of eggs may be tolerated well by sheep, produce few clinical signs and be difficult to detect without detailed examination. When the larvae cease feeding and leave the host, the lesions created by such small infestations heal well and usually without complications. However, the odour of an existing infestation may attract more blowflies and induce further oviposition; the high humidity at an active strike lesion may also enhance egg and larval survival. Hence, once infested, sheep become far more likely to receive multiple strikes (Fig. 9.31). At the initial lesion site there may be alopecia and underlying scar tissue formation, while the lesion spreads from its margins as further ovipositions occur and waves of larvae feed under the surrounding wool (Fig. 9.32). The irritation and distress caused by the expanding lesion are extremely debilitating and sheep can rapidly lose condition.

Control and treatment: This should be based largely on the prophylactic treatment of sheep with insecticides. The problems

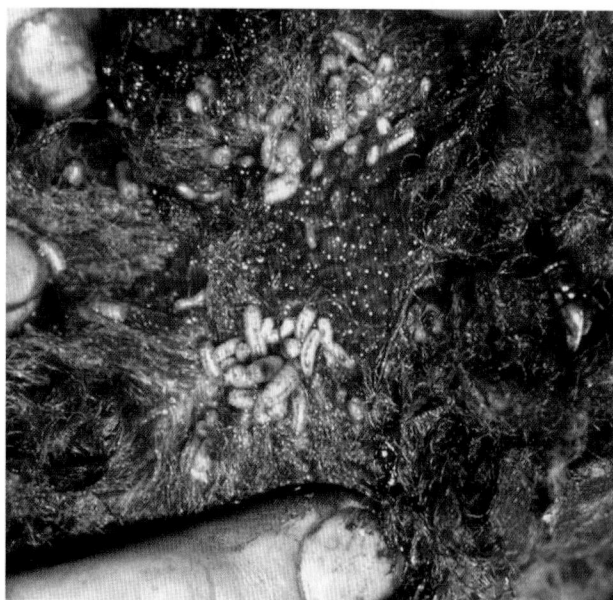

Fig. 9.31 Blowfly strike of sheep by larvae of *Lucilia sericata*.

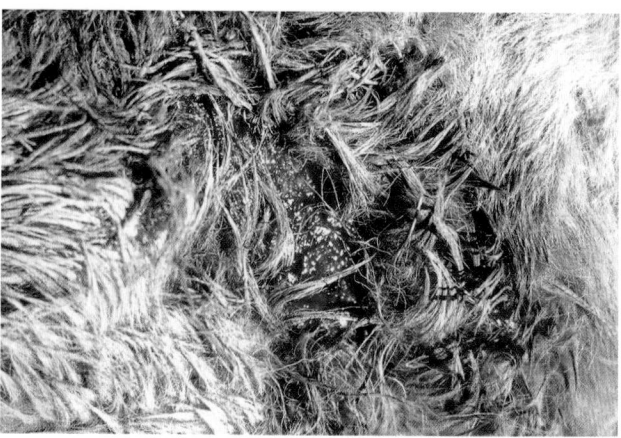

Fig. 9.32 Inflamed and damaged skin caused by feeding blowfly larvae.

associated with this are the relatively short period spent by the larvae that cause facultative myiasis on the sheep, the repeated infestations (which occur throughout the season) and the rapidity with which severe damage occurs. Any insecticide used must therefore not only kill the larvae but also persist in the fleece. Organophosphate and pyrethroid insecticides may give effective protection for up to 10 weeks. Application of these insecticides is made by hand spraying, plunge dipping, in a spray race or by jetting. In the northern hemisphere, two annual treatments, usually in May and August, should give protection for the whole of the fly season, but the timing and number of treatments needed are entirely dependent on the residual activity of the product used. The insect growth inhibitor dicyclanil gives excellent protection for up 12–20 weeks after a single application. These chemicals are applied as a spray or pour-on, ideally before the anticipated seasonal challenge.

Other measures that should be taken to aid control are the prevention of diarrhoea by effective worm control and the removal of excess wool from the groin and perineal area to prevent soiling, a technique known as crutching. Shearing reduces strike risk in ewes and the docking of lamb tails will also significantly reduce the risk of breech strike. Appropriate disposal of carcasses, which otherwise offer an excellent alternative breeding place for blowflies, is also recommended. Once the problem is diagnosed, all affected sheep should be separated and the area surrounding the lesion clipped. Where possible, larvae should be removed and killed; larvae that are more than 24 hours old that are allowed to drop from the lesion will survive and subsequently emerge as adults. The lesion should be dressed with a suitable preparation of dilute insecticide, such as diazinon, cypermethrin or deltamethrin.

Lucilia

Two species, *L. sericata* and *L. cuprina*, are important primary facultative agents of myiasis.

Lucilia sericata

Lucilia sericata, synonym *Phaenicia sericata* (Phylum: Arthropoda; Class: Insecta; Order: Diptera; Family: Calliphoridae), commonly known as a Greenbottle or Sheep blowfly, is found superficially in lesions on the skin. Originally *Lucilia sericata* was probably endemic to the Palaearctic but as a result of natural patterns of movement and artificial dispersal by humans and livestock in the past few hundred years, the species is now found worldwide. *Lucilia sericata* is more common in cool–temperate habitats, such as Europe, and is often replaced by the closely related *Lucilia cuprina* in warm–temperate and subtropical habitats.

Epidemiology: The risk of myiasis by *L. sericata* has been shown to increase with increasing flock size and stocking density, and to decrease with increasing farm altitude. Initially in spring, unshorn adults may be most at risk. Immediately following shearing, the risk of strike in adult sheep is considerably reduced. However, the susceptibility of strike in lambs increases, peaking in late summer as their fleeces grow and as populations of pasture nematodes increase, against which they have no acquired immunity, leading to diarrhoea and faecal soiling. In temperate areas under summer conditions, up to four generations may develop per year. In these areas, the final generation overwinters in the soil as larvae, to emerge as adults in the following spring. The precise timing of spring emergence and the growth of the population are highly temperature dependent. In warmer climates, the number of generations per annum is greater and up to nine or 10 have been recorded in southern Africa and Australia. The period of risk is more prolonged in warm, moist weather.

Pathogenesis: Blowfly strike by *L. sericata* occurs most commonly in the perineal and tail-head region and is strongly associated with the accumulation of faeces in wool around the anus and tail. There is little recorded involvement of dermatitis in predisposing sheep to strike by *L. sericata* in northern Europe. Following initial strike by *L. sericata*, secondary blowfly species may also invade the site of infestation. These secondary invaders include other species of *Lucilia*, *Calliphora* spp. and, in some regions, *Chrysomya* spp. *Lucilia sericata* adults may act as passive vectors of *Mycobacterium avium avium*, *M. a. paratuberculosis* and *M. a. hominissuis*.

Notes: *Lucilia sericata* is the most important agent of sheep myiasis throughout northern Europe and was first recorded as an ectoparasite in England in the fifteenth century. *Lucilia sericata* arrived in New Zealand over 100 years ago and soon established itself as the primary myiasis fly in the country, occurring in 75% of all cases of sheep strike. However, now *L. cuprina* appears to be displacing *L. sericata* to become the most important primary cause of fly strike in sheep in New Zealand.

Lucilia cuprina

Lucilia cuprina, synonyms *Phaenicia cuprina*, *Phaenicia pallescens* (Phylum: Arthropoda; Class: Insecta; Order: Diptera; Family: Calliphoridae), is commonly known as the Australian sheep blowfly. It is thought that the original distribution of *Lucilia cuprina* may have been either Afro-tropical or Oriental. However, as a result of natural patterns of movement and artificial dispersal by humans and livestock in the past few hundred years, the species is now found worldwide, although in general *L. cuprina* occurs in warm–temperate and subtropical habitats. There are believed to be two subspecies: *L. c. cuprina* is distributed throughout the Neotropical, Oriental and southern Nearctic regions, while *L. c. dorsalis* is found throughout the sub-Saharan, Afro-tropical and Australasian regions. However, the two subspecies interbreed readily in the laboratory and intermediate forms are believed to be common. The simple division into two subspecies is therefore certainly an oversimplification of the complex pattern of genetic variation that occurs between populations of *L. cuprina*.

Epidemiology: In warmer parts of its range, nine or 10 generations per year have been recorded and *L. cuprina* may be active all year round in some parts of its range.

Pathogenesis: In Australia and New Zealand, body strike caused by *L. cuprina* is frequently the main form of myiasis. Body strike occurs most commonly around the shoulders and back region and is frequently associated with the incidence of bacterial dermatophilosis caused by the bacterium *Dermatophilus congolensis*. Body strike in Australasia is also often associated with bacterial fleece rot, a superficial dermatitis induced by moisture and proliferation of the bacterium *Pseudomonas aeruginosa* on the skin, resulting in a matted band of discoloured fleece. It is possible that dermatophilosis and fleece rot act synergistically in attracting blowflies and their subsequent oviposition. However, where the Merino breed is prevalent, breech and tail strike may also be common due to the conformation of this breed and the wrinkled skin in the breech area that favours the accumulation of urine and faeces. Following initial strike by *Lucilia cuprina*, a variety of secondary species may also invade the site of infestation. They frequently extend the injury, rendering the strike one of great severity. These secondary invaders include *Calliphora* spp. and *Chrysomya* spp. *Lucilia cuprina* is suspected of spreading diseases such as gastroenteritis and anthrax among host animals.

Notes: *Lucilia cuprina* is absent from most of Europe, although it has been recorded from southern Spain and North Africa. *Lucilia cuprina* was probably introduced into Australia towards the middle or end of the nineteenth century and it is now the dominant sheep myiasis species for mainland Australia and Tasmania, being present in 90–99% of fly strike cases. In the early 1980s *L. cuprina* was discovered in New Zealand and was most probably introduced from Australia. Now, despite its low abundance, in northern areas of New Zealand it appears to be displacing *L. sericata* to become the most important primary cause of fly strike in sheep. *Lucilia cuprina* is also the primary myiasis fly of sheep in southern Africa. Although this species had been known in South Africa since 1830, little sheep strike was recorded until the early decades of the twentieth century, possibly as a result of the introduction of more susceptible Merino breeds or changes in husbandry practices. In North America, *L. cuprina* is known to be present, although it does not appear to be economically important in sheep myiasis.

Secondary myiasis blowflies

Species of the genera *Calliphora*, *Phormia* and *Protophormia* (Phylum: Arthropoda; Class: Insecta, Order: Diptera, Family: Calliphoridae) are usually secondary invaders of carrion and most commonly breed in carrion (Table 9.7).

Epidemiology: Secondary flies usually follow an initial strike by a primary fly such as *Lucilia cuprina* and invade the site of infestation. They frequently extend the injury, increasing the severity of the strike.

Clinical signs: Diagnosis, pathology, epidemiology, treatment and control are as for *Lucilia*.

Table 9.7 Secondary agents of blowfly myiasis.

Species	Common name	Hosts	Geographical distribution
Chrysomya megacephala	Oriental latrine fly	Warm-blooded animals	Worldwide
Chrysomya rufifacies	Hairy maggot blowfly	Warm-blooded animals	Worldwide
Chrysomya albiceps	Hairy maggot blowfly	Warm-blooded animals	Worldwide
Calliphora augur	Lesser brown blowfly, blue-bodied blowfly	Mainly sheep	Mainly eastern Australia
Calliphora albifrontalis	Western Australian brown blowfly	Mainly sheep	Australia
Calliphora nociva	Lesser brown blowfly	Mainly sheep	Mainly Western Australia
Calliphora stygia	Eastern golden-haired blowfly	Mainly sheep	Australia
Calliphora vicina	Blubottle	Mainly sheep	Worldwide
Calliphora vomitoria	Bluebottle	Mainly sheep	Worldwide
Phormia regina	Blackbottle, black blowfly	Mainly sheep	Northern Canada, USA, Europe, Scandinavia, Russia
Protophormia terraenovae	Blackbottle	Mainly sheep but may also be a serious pest of cattle and reindeer	Northern Canada, USA, Europe, Scandinavia, Russia

Pathogenesis: When involved in myiasis, secondary blowflies are attracted by the odour of the infestation and their larvae extend and deepen the lesion. The irritation and distress caused by the lesion are extremely debilitating and the host animal can rapidly lose condition. The latter is often the first obvious sign of strike as the lesion occurs at the skin surface and is sometimes observed only on close examination.

LICE

Heavy louse infestation is known as pediculosis. Blood-sucking lice have been implicated in the transmission of disease; however, lice are predominantly of importance because of the direct damage they cause. This effect is usually a function of their density. A small number of lice is very common and presents no problem. However, louse populations can increase dramatically, reaching high densities. Transfer of lice from animal to animal, from flock to flock or herd to herd is usually by direct physical contact. Because lice do not survive for long off their host, the potential for animals to pick up infestations from dirty housing is limited, although it cannot be ignored. Occasionally, lice may also be transferred between animals by attachment to flies (phoresy).

Epidemiology: Generally, for the transfer of louse infestation, close bodily contact is necessary. Transmission occurs when sheep or goats are brought together as in sale yards, and especially when animals are housed for the winter, since the heavy fleece or coat provides habitats that are readily colonised by lice. Adult lice positioned near the tip of the wool fibre or hair are passed on to the new host as it brushes past an infested animal. In sheep, it can take a single infested animal just four months to infest the entire flock. Lice populations peak in spring and lambs may be particularly susceptible to infestation.

Diagnosis: The lice and their eggs may be seen within the hair and on the skin when the coat is parted. The lice may be removed and identified under a light microscope.

Pathology: The pathology of louse infestation is extremely variable. Infestations may induce alopecia, irritation, papulocrustous dermatitis and self-excoriation. Sucking lice may cause anaemia.

Control and treatment: Insecticide resistance is widespread in lice, and its rapid spread may be linked to the facultative parthenogenesis seen in many louse species. Hence, in an attempt to reduce the risk of selection for resistance, rotation of chemical classes is strongly advised. A good degree of louse control can be achieved by shearing because solar radiation and dehydration reduce the hatch rate of louse eggs. Subsequently, another good management procedure is to treat sheep immediately after shearing, which ensures a greater proportion of lice come into contact with insecticide and reduces the volume of chemical necessary to achieve this. If ewes are dipped during early pregnancy, the risk that they will still be louse infested at lambing is reduced, as is the chance of the lambs becoming infested. Dipping the lambs then results in the flock becoming as nearly louse free as possible. The ewe lambs, when old enough to be mated, should not then be in a position to so readily infest their progeny. This could lead to a situation where treatment is necessary less frequently, assuming that there is a residual louse population as is commonly the case. In sheep, several topical insecticides, such as amidine, amitraz or organophosphates (e.g. chlorfenvinphos, coumaphos, chlorpyrifos, crotoxyphos, trichlorphon, phosmet and propetamphos), applied in dips or sprays are effective but are becoming more limited in their availability in some countries due to safety and environmental concerns. Two treatments, 14 days apart, may be required. Topical applications of the pour-on pyrethroid cypermethrin, the spot-on deltamethrin and the insect growth regulator triflumuron have also been shown to be effective. The pyrethroids, which act by diffusion over the body surface in the sebum and give protection for 8–14 weeks, are probably the treatment of choice. Macrocyclic lactones (ivermectin, doramectin and moxidectin) may also be used, although they have only limited activity against chewing lice. Essential oils have been shown to be very effective against chewing lice when groomed into the fleece. The situation for goats is different in that few treatments have been specifically evaluated for use in goats and pour-on treatments may be less effective because of the variability in hair fibres found on different goat breeds.

Bovicola ovis

Bovicola ovis, synonym *Damalinia ovis* (Phylum: Arthropoda; Class: Insecta; Order: Psocodea; Family: Bovicolidae), is distributed worldwide. This insect is found on the skin, mainly on the back and upper parts of the body of sheep, although in heavy infestations lice may be found over the entire body.

Table 9.8 Other lice of goats.

Species name	Family	Distribution	Hosts
Bovicola ovis (synonym *Damalinia caprae*)	Bovicolidae	Worldwide	Goats
Bovicola limbata (synonym *Damalinia limbata*)	Bovicolidae	Worldwide	Goats (Angora)

Epidemiology: *Bovicola ovis* is very active, roaming in the wool. It is susceptible to high temperatures but is also intolerant of moisture. In a damp fleece, with a relative humidity of more than 90%, it will die in six hours, and when covered by water it will drown in an hour.

For other lice of goats, see Table 9.8.

Pathogenesis: *Bovicola* may cause intense irritation, resulting in rubbing and scratching, with matting and loss of hair, involving almost the whole body in extreme cases. The scratching animal may tear or pull out the fleece and exuded serum from bite wounds may cause wool matting and discoloration. Wounds may attract blowflies. Lice reduce the quality of wool and can reduce wool production if left uncontrolled.

Clinical signs: Restlessness, rubbing and damage to the coat would suggest that lice are present, and when the hair is parted the parasites will be found. Lice appear as small yellowish specks in the hair and the small pale eggs are readily found scattered throughout the coat.

Linognathus ovillus

Linognathus ovillus (Phylum: Arthropoda; Class: Insecta; Order: Psocodea; Family: Linognathidae) is commonly known as the Long-nosed louse or Sheep face louse. It is distributed worldwide but is particularly common in Australia and New Zealand. This insect is found mainly on the face of sheep.

Pathogenesis: Lice cause sheep to rub and scratch, sometimes to the point of denuding areas of skin. Infestation by *Linognathus* spp. results in a chronic dermatitis characterised by constant irritation and rubbing and biting of the fleece. Because they are blood feeders, anaemia is common where high populations of lice exist. Anaemia may predispose animals to respiratory or other diseases. *Linognathus ovillus* is a known vector of *Mycoplasma ovis* in sheep.

Clinical signs: *Linognathus ovillus* is mainly found on the face of sheep but at high densities may spread over the entire body (Fig. 9.33). Infested animals will stamp their feet or bite the infested areas. Sheep infested with lice have a ragged appearance, often with tags of wool hanging from the fleece. Newly infested sheep are very sensitive to lice. Others which have had lice for long periods can develop quite severe infestations but show few signs. Often lousy wool has a yellow colour due to a heavy suint and skin secretions.

Linognathus pedalis

Linognathus pedalis (Phylum: Arthropoda; Class: Insecta; Order: Psocodea; Family: Linognathidae), commonly known as the Sheep foot louse, is found on the legs, belly and feet of sheep. It occurs

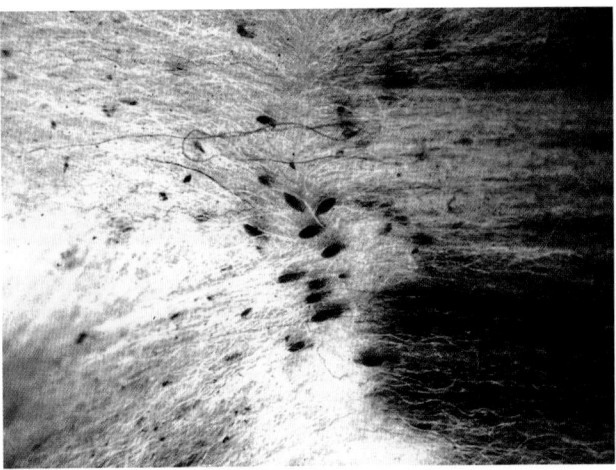

Fig. 9.33 Infestation of sucking lice, *Linognathus ovillus*.

Table 9.9 Lice of importance in goats.

Species name	Family	Distribution	Hosts
Bovicola ovis (synonym *Damalinia caprae*)	Trichodectidae	Worldwide	Goats
Bovicola limbata (synonym *Damalinia limbata*)	Trichodectidae	Worldwide	Goats (Angora)
Linognathus stenopsis	Linognathidae	Worldwide	Goats
Linognathus africanus	Linognathidae	Africa, although probably now worldwide	Goats, occasionally sheep

most commonly in the USA, South America, South Africa and Australasia.

Epidemiology: In its normal habitat on the legs, it is exposed to great fluctuations in temperature and, having adapted to survive in these conditions, it is one of the few lice which can live away from the host's body and is viable on pasture for about a week. As a consequence of this, infestations may be picked up off contaminated pasture.

For other lice of importance in goats, see Table 9.9.

Pathogenesis: On the host, *L. pedalis* is more sedentary than *L. ovillus* and tends to occur in aggregations in its preferred sites, which are the more lightly wooled areas of the body such as the legs, belly and feet. However, at high densities both species may spread over the entire body. Infestation by *Linognathus* results in a chronic dermatitis characterised by constant irritation and rubbing and biting of the fleece. Because they are blood feeders, anaemia may occur where very high populations of lice exist. Anaemia may predispose animals to respiratory or other diseases.

Clinical signs: See *L. ovillus*. In Merinos and other heavily wooled breeds, it is usually first detected at crutching.

MITES

The ectoparasitic mites of sheep and goats feed on blood, lymph, skin debris or sebaceous secretions, which they ingest by puncturing the skin, scavenging from the skin surface or imbibing from epidermal lesions. Most ectoparasitic mites spend their entire lives associated with their host, so that transmission from host to host is primarily by physical contact. Infestation by mites is called acariosis and can result in severe dermatitis, known as mange, which may cause significant welfare problems and economic losses.

Demodex ovis

Demodex ovis, synonym *Demodex ariae* (Phylum: Arthropoda; Class: Arachnida; Order: Trombidiformes (Prostigmata); Family: Demodicidae), is distributed worldwide. This mite is localised in the hair follicles and sebaceous glands, most commonly on the face of sheep.

Epidemiology: Probably because of its location deep in the dermis, it is very difficult to transmit *Demodex* between animals unless there is prolonged contact. In nature such contact only occurs during suckling and it is thought that most infections are acquired in the early weeks of life. Transmission appears to occur during the earlier days of suckling.

Pathogenesis: This form of mange is rare in sheep and is of little economic importance, as it is confined to the face region and mild in character. Large numbers of mites may cause hide damage.

Clinical signs and pathology: Ovine demodectic mange is uncommon. Clinical signs include alopecia and scaling, especially on the face, neck and shoulders. Lesions may be papular, nodular and, rarely, pustular. The mites in sebaceous glands occasionally induce folliculitis or furunculosis.

Diagnosis: For confirmatory diagnosis, deep scrapings are necessary to reach the mites deep in the follicles and glands. This is best achieved by taking a fold of skin, applying a drop of liquid paraffin, and scraping until capillary blood appears.

Control and treatment: Control is rarely applied. In many cases, demodicosis spontaneously resolves and treatment is unnecessary. Systemic macrocyclic lactones may be effective.

Notes: Species of the genus *Demodex* are highly specialised mites that live in the hair follicles and sebaceous glands of a wide range of wild and domestic animals, including humans. They are believed to form a group of closely related sibling species that are highly specific to particular hosts: *Demodex phylloides* (pig), *Demodex canis* (dog), *Demodex bovis* (cattle), *Demodex equi* (horse), *Demodex musculi* (mouse), *Demodex ratti* (rat), *Demodex caviae* (guinea pig), *Demodex cati* (cat) and *Demodex folliculorum* and *Demodex brevis* (human). Various morphological variations may be seen on a host; these are sometimes, probably incorrectly, ascribed separate species status.

Demodex caprae

Demodex caprae, synonym *Demodex ariae* (Phylum: Arthropoda; Class: Arachnida; Order: Trombidiformes (Prostigmata); Family: Demodicidae), is distributed worldwide. This mite is localised in the hair follicles and sebaceous glands of goats.

Epidemiology: Probably because of its location deep in the dermis, it is very difficult to transmit *Demodex* between animals unless there is prolonged contact. Such contact usually only occurs during

suckling and as such, it is thought that most infections are acquired in the early weeks of life. The muzzle, neck, withers and back are common sites of infestation.

Pathogenesis: The disease is similar to that in cattle. The initial lesions on the face and neck extend to the chest and flanks and may eventually involve the whole body, with the formation of cutaneous nodules of up to 20 mm in diameter containing yellowish caseous material with large numbers of mites. This form of mange is rarely debilitating, and is of greatest importance as a cause of downgrading or condemnation of goat skins.

Clinical signs and pathology: Pea-sized nodules containing caseous material and mites, particularly on the withers, lateral neck, back and flanks. Concurrent pyoderma may occur, leading to furunculosis with ulceration and crust formation. Cutaneous nodules consist of follicular cysts lined with squamous epithelium and filled with waxy keratin squames and mites. Eruption of the cysts onto the skin may form a thick crust; rupture within the dermis may form an abscess or granulomatous reaction.

Diagnosis: For confirmatory diagnosis, deep scrapings are necessary to reach the mites deep in the follicles and glands. This is best achieved by taking a fold of skin, applying a drop of liquid paraffin, and scraping until capillary blood appears.

Control and treatment: Control is rarely applied. In many cases, demodicosis spontaneously resolves and treatment is unnecessary. The organophosphate trichlorphon, used on three occasions two days apart, and systemic macrocyclic lactones may be effective.

Psoroptes ovis

Psoroptes ovis, synonyms *Psoroptes communis* var. *ovis*, *Psoroptes cuniculi*, *Psoroptes cervinus*, *Psoroptes bovis*, *Psoroptes equi*, *Psoroptes aucheniae* (Phylum: Arthropoda; Class: Arachnida; Order: Sarcoptiformes (Astigmata); Family: Psoroptidae), is commonly known as the Sheep scab mite. It is distributed worldwide, particularly in Europe and South America, but not Australia or New Zealand. This insect is found on the skin of sheep, cattle, goats, horses, rabbits and camelids.

Epidemiology: Transmission is primarily through physical contact and the majority of sheep become infected while the mites are active and multiplying. However, transmission may also occur via the environment. The length of time a mite can survive off its host is strongly affected by ambient temperature and humidity, but at low temperatures (<15 °C) and high humidity (>75%), survival may be in excess of 18 days, allowing transmission from housing, bedding or contaminated machinery such as shearing equipment. Time of year may have an important impact on off-host survival. This has important implications for the potential for transmission from the environment to new hosts, transmission risk usually being considerably greater in the winter. The period when the mite infestation has declined, either as a response to environmental conditions or the host's immune response, is also very significant in the epidemiology of the disease. Sheep that appear to be uninfested but which carry small populations of mites may be introduced to healthy flocks and subsequently initiate outbreaks.

Pathogenesis: The mites are non-burrowing and feed superficially on a lipid emulsion of skin cells, bacteria and lymph on the host skin, produced as a result of a hypersensitivity reaction to the

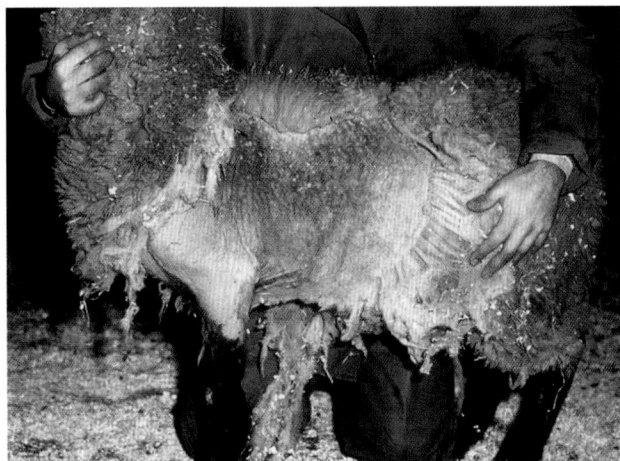

Fig. 9.34 Sheep with psoroptic mange. (Courtesy of Eduardo Berriatua).

presence of antigenic mite faecal material. This hypersensitivity causes inflammation, surface exudation, scale and crust formation, with excoriation (scratching) due to self-trauma. Infestation is described as psoroptic mange or sheep scab (Fig. 9.34). The serous exudate produced in response to the mites dries on the skin to form a dry yellow crust, surrounded by a border of inflamed skin covered in a moist crust. Mites are found on the moist skin at the edge of the lesion, which extends rapidly and may take as little as 6–8 weeks to cover three-quarters of the host's skin. Eventually the crust lifts off as the new fleece grows. Infestation in sheep leads to severe pruritus, wool loss, restlessness, biting and scratching of infested areas, weight loss, reduced weight gain and, in some cases, death. When handled, infested sheep may demonstrate a 'nibble reflex', characterised by lip smacking and protrusion of the tongue; others may show epileptiform fits lasting 5–10 minutes. In sheep, lesions may occur on any part of the body, but are particularly obvious on the neck, shoulders, back and flanks. In severe cases, the skin may be excoriated, lichenified and secondarily infected, with numerous thick-walled abscesses of between 5 and 20 mm in diameter. Sheep scab can affect sheep of all ages but may be particularly severe in young lambs and sheep in poor condition. The incidence of the disease varies according to season. In warm weather, mite populations may decline, leaving residual populations in sites such as the axilla, groin, infraorbital fossa and inner surface of the pinna and auditory canal during spring, summer and early autumn. Populations of *Psoroptes* may also be found localised in the ears of sheep, causing chronic irritation, often associated with haematomas, head shaking and scratching.

Clinical signs and pathology: The earliest phase following infection is seen as a zone of inflammation with the appearance of small vesicles and serous exudate. As the lesion spreads, the centre becomes dry and covered by a yellow crust while the borders, in which the mites are multiplying, are moist. Scab lesions occur most frequently around the shoulders and back. The first visible sign is usually a patch of lighter wool but as the area of damage enlarges, the sheep responds to the intense itching associated with mite activity by rubbing and scratching against fence posts and other objects, so that the wool becomes ragged and stained, and is shed from large areas. In addition to wool loss, the sheep may become restless and preoccupied in scratching. As a result, weight gains may

be impaired in growing animals, while in adults there may be weight loss. The mite faeces and its flora, shed cuticle and enzymes in the peritrophic membrane that surrounds the faecal pellets induce a rapid profound inflammatory response by the host. Histopathology includes subcorneal eosinophilic pustules and a dermal infiltrate composed of eosinophils, neutrophils, macrophages and lymphocytes, accompanied by mast cell hyperplasia. There is pronounced dermal oedema.

Diagnosis: Another non-burrowing mite, *Chorioptes*, can be common in sheep, and it is essential that this less pathogenic mite should be differentiated from the more pathogenic *Psoroptes*. The important differential features are shown in Fig. 3.92. Although relatively easy to identify the active disease within a flock, the latent lesions make it more difficult to declare a flock free of infection. Particular attention should be paid to the areas in which these lesions are found. A sample may be obtained from skin scrapings taken around the lesion; this can then be examined microscopically.

Control and treatment: Because of its short life cycle of about 10 days, there is very rapid increase in abundance on a host which facilitates quick transmission between hosts. This has led to legislative control in many countries since the economic consequences of uncontrolled sheep scab are serious. For example, the disease was presumed to have been eradicated from the UK in 1952, there having been no notifications of outbreaks for a number of years; it reappeared in 1972, most probably having been introduced on subclinically infected imported sheep and very rapidly spread to flocks throughout the UK. It was eradicated from Australia and New Zealand many years ago, but remains notifiable in these countries. Legislation in support of control is based on inspection of flocks, limitation of movement of sheep in, and from, areas in which the infection has been diagnosed, and compulsory treatment of all sheep at prescribed times.

A common source of infection of a flock is through the introduction of new animals. These must be checked over thoroughly and subjected to a quarantine period if possible. Common grazing, where flocks mix together, is another important transmission route and where this is practised, control is particularly difficult unless all owners coordinate their treatment activities.

Plunge dipping with organophosphate insecticide is generally recommended for sheep scab control. Sheep should remain in the bath for at least one minute, and the head should be immersed at least twice. They should be held in clean pens before dipping and it is customary to hold them in draining pens for a time afterwards to conserve dip and assist in its proper disposal. Modern acaricides have been developed which have an affinity for wool grease, so that as a succession of sheep go through the bath, the acaricide is gradually 'stripped out' and manufacturers give directions for replenishment after a specified number of sheep have been dipped. Other methods of applying acaricide, such as showering, have not been shown to be effective against scab mites. In most countries in which control is practised, only specified acaricides are permitted for use in dips. For many years only γ-hexachlorocyclohexane (HCH) was used, but this has been largely replaced by the organophosphates diazinon and propetamphos, which in addition to giving the required persistence in the fleece are rapidly detoxified and excreted from tissues. The synthetic pyrethroids flumethrin and α-cypermethrin were licensed for the control of sheep scab but due to concerns over health and safety their use has declined in many countries. Two treatments with injectable ivermectin 200 μg/kg at an interval of seven days have given complete clearance of *P. ovis*. Additionally, doramectin 300 μg/kg or moxidectin 200 μg/kg give control following a single injection; all are now licensed in several countries for this purpose. However, resistance in *P. ovis* to macrocyclic lactones has been detected both in Europe and South America and, given the importance of these compounds for the control of endoparasites, the use of MLs against scab mites is to be avoided where possible.

Notes: The taxonomy of the mites in this genus is confused, with mites located in different parts of the body or on different hosts traditionally given different species names; however, little good evidence exists to support this nomenclature.

Psorobia ovis

Psorobia ovis, synonym *Psorergates ovis* (Phylum: Arthropoda; Class: Arachnida; Order: Trombidiformes (Prostigmata); Family: Psorergatidae), is commonly known as the Sheep itch mite. It occurs in Australia, New Zealand, southern Africa, North and South America. It has not been reported in Europe. This mite is found on skin, all over the body of sheep, particularly fine-wooled breeds such as the Merino.

Epidemiology: The adult mites are spread by direct contact between hosts and are most often transferred between shorn sheep. Mites are generally found at higher densities in winter and spring. *Psorobia ovis* is very sensitive to desiccation, can only survive for 24–48 hours off the host and only the adults are mobile. As a consequence of these factors, the spread of infestation through a flock is generally slow and is most evident during the winter months.

Pathogenesis: Infection is most common in fine-wool breeds such as the Merino and Corriedale and is acquired by contact when the wool is short; as the fleece lengthens, it presents a barrier to the transfer of mites. The spread of the mite population is very slow, and infestation is rarely found in animals less than six months old. The animal may be three years or more before the whole fleece area is affected. Although a non-burrowing mite, *Psorobia* attacks the skin itself, living in the superficial layers and causing chronic irritation and skin thickening. The earliest signs are small pale areas of wool on the shoulders, body and flanks, which gradually extend over the rest of the fleece, with irritation increasing as the mite population grows. Sheep rub, bite and chew their wool, which becomes ragged, with loose strands trailing from the sides of the body. In long-standing cases, large patches of wool may be lost. The fleece itself contains much scurf and has a slightly yellowish hue, while the staple is very dry and easily broken. Microscopically, there is a hyperkeratosis and marked desquamation, with the deeper superficial layers showing round cell infiltration and eosinophilia in the immediate vicinity of the parasite. In severe cases the whole fleece, which is difficult to shear because of its matted consistency, must be discarded. In less severely affected sheep and especially in older animals (which have become tolerant of the itch because of their thickened damaged skin), fleeces are downgraded.

Clinical signs and pathology: These parasites are severely irritating, causing host animals to rub and bite at their fleece. The fleece may be weakened and the wool may break easily. Infection induces pruritus; light dry scabs may be present.

Diagnosis: To obtain mites, it is necessary, having clipped away a patch of wool, to apply a drop of mineral oil and scrape the skin down to the blood capillary level. The mites themselves are easily identified using a microscope. The absence of mites in a single scraping is not sufficient evidence for a negative diagnosis.

Control and treatment: Sheep should be dipped soon after shearing. Annual dipping after shearing will suppress the mite population, keeping the infestation rate low but rarely eradicating it completely.

Psorobia is relatively unsusceptible to most acaricides, although the formamidine amitraz and lime–sulfur dips have been shown to be of considerable value. Otherwise, the older arsenic–sulfur preparations may be used. Macrocyclic lactones are highly effective against this species, with a single treatment usually killing all the mites.

Sarcoptes scabiei

Sarcoptes scabiei (Phylum: Arthropoda; Class: Arachnida; Order: Sarcoptiformes (Astigmata); Family: Sarcoptidae) is commonly known as the Scabies mite. It is usually found in the skin and will infest sheep and goats.

Pathogenesis, sheep: The mites, unlike the non-burrowing mites of the genus *Psoroptes*, are generally found in regions without wool, such as the face, ears, axillae and groin, and spread slowly. Affected areas are at first erythematous and scurfy. The intense pruritus characteristic of sarcoptic mange is present, and sheep scratch and rub the head, body and legs against trees, posts and walls. Because of the itch, sheep are almost continuously restless and are unable to graze, so that there is progressive emaciation. In haired sheep, the whole body may be affected. Sarcoptic mange has a wide geographic distribution in many sheep-raising areas of the world, such as the Middle East. In Africa it occurs in the local breeds of haired sheep and, because of hide damage, is of considerable economic importance, more than a million sheepskins being exported from the region annually. Sarcoptic mange of sheep in Britain has not been encountered for more than 30 years.

Pathogenesis, goats: This form of mange in goats is worldwide in distribution but is of greatest economic importance in areas where the goat is the basic domestic ruminant, such as India and West Africa. In goats, the condition is often chronic, and may have been present simply as 'skin disease' for many months before definitive diagnosis has been made. As in other sarcoptic infections, the main signs are irritation with encrustations, loss of hair and excoriation from rubbing and scratching. In long-standing cases the skin becomes thickened and nodules may develop on the less well-haired parts of the skin, including the muzzle, around the eyes and inside the ears.

Treatment: In sheep, treatment and control are similar to those described for the more common psoroptic mange. In goats, repeated treatment is often necessary, sometimes over several months in long-standing cases. Although not licensed for the treatment of milking goats, a single injection of systemic macrocyclic lactone may be effective. Corticosteroid therapy has been reported to aid recovery as it suppresses the pruritus. For further details see Chapter 11.

Chorioptes bovis

Chorioptes bovis, synonyms *Chorioptes ovis*, *Chorioptes equi*, *Chorioptes caprae*, *Chorioptes cuniculi*, *Chorioptes japonensis* (Phylum: Arthropoda; Class: Arachnida; Order: Sarcoptiformes (Astigmata); Family: Psoroptidae), is found superficially on the skin, particularly the legs, feet, base of tail and udder. It will infest a wide range of livestock.

Pathogenesis: In sheep, the mites are found mainly on the legs and feet and though very common, little harm is caused. When clinical cases do occur, they are typically in the form of foot mange, affecting the forefeet. The mites cluster about the accessory digits and along the coronary border of the outer claws, causing crusting below the accessory digits and in the interdigital spaces. Lambs are thought to become infected by contact with the legs of the ewe. In some cases, there may be spread from the limbs to the face and other regions and, in occasional severe cases, pustular dermatitis (with wrinkling and thickening of the skin) may occur. It has been noted in New Zealand that when the mange spreads to the scrotum, the thickened and inflamed skin allows the scrotal temperature to remain high, resulting in testicular atrophy and cessation of spermatogenesis. Infected rams have impaired reproductive ability or sterility, though their general health is not affected. The condition is not irreversible; semen production and fertility return to normal after successful mange treatment. Prevalence of leg and scrotal mange is usually highest in the autumn and winter months, and declines in spring. In goats, the mites occur mostly on the forefeet around the accessory digits and claws. However, they may also occur higher on the foot and on the pastern. The lesions produced are relatively mild. Infestation rates of *C. bovis* tend to be higher in goats than sheep, with up to 80–90% of goats in individual herds being parasitised.

Control and treatment: Chorioptic mange in sheep is easily treated by dipping or by local treatment with a suitable acaricide. Macrocyclic lactones are an effective treatment against chorioptic mange. Crotoxyphos (0.25%) applied as a spray can also be used to treat infestations. In goats, a suitable acaricidal wash, scrubbed on to the lesions on two occasions 14 days apart, is effective.

Notes: The names *Chorioptes ovis*, *Chorioptes equi*, *Chorioptes caprae* and *Chorioptes cuniculi* used to describe the chorioptic mites found on sheep, horses, goats and rabbits, respectively, are now all thought to be synonyms of *Chorioptes bovis*. For further details see Chapter 8.

Eutrombicula sarcina

Eutrombicula sarcina (Phylum: Arthropoda; Class: Arachnida; Order: Trombidiformes (Prostigmata); Family: Trombiculidae), commonly known as the Scrub itch mite or Black soil itch mite, is an important parasite of sheep in Queensland and New South Wales of Australia. Its principal host, however, is the grey kangaroo.

These mites prefer areas of savannah and grassland scrub. They may be particularly abundant from November to February, after summer rain. The primary site of infestation is on the leg, resulting in intense irritation.

TICKS

Ixodes ricinus (Phylum: Arthropoda; Class: Arachnida; Order: Ixodida; Family: Ixodidae), commonly known as the Sheep tick, Castor bean tick or Forest tick, is found throughout temperate areas of Europe, Australia, South Africa, North Africa and Asia. This species has never become established in North America. It feeds on a wide range of mammals and birds and is also of veterinary importance in sheep, cattle, dogs and cats.

Pathogenesis: *Ixodes* ticks ingest blood and, occasionally, heavy infestations can cause anaemia. Tick bites may damage the host at the site of attachment, causing local injury which may predispose to secondary bacterial infection. The lesions caused during feeding may predispose to myiasis. Also, at slaughter the value of the hide or fleece may be reduced. Most significant of all, this tick transmits a range of pathogens. In Western Europe, in cattle it transmits *Babesia divergens* and *B. bovis*, the causes of redwater fever, and *Anaplasma marginale*, the cause of anaplasmosis. In sheep and cattle, it transmits the virus that causes louping ill and the rickettsia responsible for tick-borne fever. It is also associated with tick pyaemia, caused by *Staphylococcus aureus*, in lambs in Britain and Norway. Ixodid ticks also transmit *Borrelia burgdorferi*, the spirochaete responsible for Lyme disease in humans. *Ixodes ricinus* has been reported to cause tick paralysis and act as a vector for Czechoslovakian encephalitis, Russian spring–summer encephalitis and *Coxiella burnetii*. This tick may also transmit Bukhovinian haemorrhagic fever.

Diagnosis: The adult ticks, particularly the engorged females, are easily seen on the skin, the predilection sites being the face, ears, axilla and inguinal region. Usually, small inflamed nodules are also seen in these areas. Ticks may be collected from the host or directly from the environment and microscopic examination used to identify individual species.

Clinical signs and pathology: There are no obvious signs of tick infestation other than the presence of the parasites and the local skin reactions to their bites. Ticks are also important vectors of protozoal, bacterial, viral and rickettsial diseases. The local reaction to tick bites varies considerably; commonly small granulomatous reactions may form at the site of tick bites, consisting of a mixed inflammatory cell response with fibrosis.

Control and treatment: The control of ixodid ticks is largely based on the use of chemical acaricides applied either by total immersion in a dipping bath or in the form of a spray, shower, spot-on or slow-release ear tags. A wide variety of formulations of organophosphate (e.g. malathion, chlorpyrifos, fenthion, dichlorvos, cythoate, diazinon, propetamphos, phosmet) and pyrethroid insecticides (e.g. permethrin, deltamethrin) are available for application as sprays, dips, spot-on or showers. Macrocyclic lactones or closantel given by the parenteral route have also been shown to be a useful aid in control of ticks. Where severely parasitised animals require individual treatment, special formulations of acaricides suspended in a greasy base may be applied to affected areas.

Dermacentor marginatus

Dermacentor marginatus (Phylum: Arthropoda; Class: Arachnida; Order: Ixodida; Family: Ixodidae), commonly known as the Ornate sheep tick, feeds as an adult largely on sheep, cattle, deer, dogs, humans, hares and hedgehogs, while the nymphs and larvae feed on small mammals and birds. The species is found throughout Europe and North Africa, eastwards to central Asia.

Pathogenesis: This species is a vector for a wide range of diseases: in dogs, *Babesia canis*; in cattle, *B. divergens*; in sheep, *B. ovis*, *Theileria ovis* and *Anaplasma ovis*; in horses, *B. caballi*, *Theileria equi* and infectious encephalomyelitis; also *Coxiella burnetii* (Q-fever), *Francisella tularensis* (tularaemia), *Brucella* spp. and *Rickettsia conorii* (boutonneuse fever).

HOST–PARASITE CHECKLISTS

In the following checklists, the codes listed below apply.

Helminths

N, nematode; T, trematode; C, cestode; A, acanthocephalan.

Arthropods

F, fly; L, louse; S, flea; M, mite; Mx, maxillopod; Ti, tick.

Protozoa

Co, coccidia; Bs, blood sporozoa; Am, amoeba; Fl, flagellate; Ci, ciliate.

Miscellaneous 'protozoal organisms'

B, blastocyst; Mi, microsporidian; My, *Mycoplasma*; P, Pneumocystidomycete; R, *Rickettsia*.

Sheep parasite checklist.

Section/host system	Helminths Parasite	Helminths (Super) family	Arthropods Parasite	Arthropods Family	Protozoa Parasite	Protozoa Family
Digestive						
Oesophagus	Gongylonema pulchrum	Spiruroidea (N)				
Rumen/reticulum	Gongylonema verrucosum	Spiruroidea (N)			Monocercomonas ruminantium	Monocercomonadidae (Fl)
	Gongylonema monnigi	Spiruroidea (N)				
	Paramphistomum cervi	Paramphistomatidae (T)				
	Paramphistomum microbothrium	Paramphistomatidae (T)				
	Paramphistomum ichikawa	Paramphistomatidae (T)				
	Paramphistomum streptocoelium	Paramphistomatidae (T)				
	Cotylophoron cotylophorum	Paramphistomatidae (T)				
	Calicophoron calicophorum	Paramphistomatidae (T)				
	Gastrothylax crumenifer	Gastrothylacidae (T)				
	Fischoederius elongatus	Gastrothylacidae (T)				
	Fischoederius cobboldi	Gastrothylacidae (T)				
Abomasum	Teladorsagia circumcincta	Trichostrongyloidea (N)			Eimeria gilruthi	Eimeriidae (Co)
	Ostertagia leptospicularis	Trichostrongyloidea (N)				
	Marshallagia marshalli	Trichostrongyloidea (N)				
	Haemonchus contortus	Trichostrongyloidea (N)				
	Trichostrongylus axei	Trichostrongyloidea (N)				
	Parabronema skrjabini	Spiruroidea (N)				
Small intestine	Trichostrongylus colubriformis	Trichostrongyloidea (N)			Eimeria crandallis	Eimeriidae (Co)
	Trichostrongylus vitrinus	Trichostrongyloidea (N)			Eimeria ovinoidalis	Eimeriidae (Co)
	Trichostrongylus longispicularis	Trichostrongyloidea (N)			Eimeria ahsata	Eimeriidae (Co)
	Cooperia curticei	Trichostrongyloidea (N)			Eimeria bakuensis	Eimeriidae (Co)
	Cooperia surnabada	Trichostrongyloidea (N)			Eimeria faurei	Eimeriidae (Co)
	Nematodirus filicollis	Trichostrongyloidea (N)			Eimeria granulosa	Eimeriidae (Co)
	Nematodirus battus	Trichostrongyloidea (N)			Eimeria intricata	Eimeriidae (Co)
	Nematodirus spathiger	Trichostrongyloidea (N)			Eimeria marsica	Eimeriidae (Co)
	Bunostomum trigonocephalum	Ancylostomatoidea (N)			Eimeria parva	Eimeriidae (Co)
	Gaigeria pachyscalis	Ancylostomatoidea (N)			Eimeria pallida	Eimeriidae (Co)
	Strongyloides papillosus	Strongyloidoidea (N)			Eimeria weybridgensis	Eimeriidae (Co)
	Capillaria longipes	Trichuroidea (N)			Eimeria punctata	Eimeriidae (Co)
	Moniezia expansa	Anoplocephalidae (C)			Cryptosporidium parvum	Cryptosporidiidae (Co)
	Avitellina centripunctata	Anoplocephalidae (C)			Cryptosporidium xiaoi	Cryptosporidiidae (Co)
	Avitellina goughi	Anoplocephalidae (C)			Giardia intestinalis	Giardiidae (Fl)
	Avitellina chalmersi	Anoplocephalidae (C)				
	Avitellina tatia	Anoplocephalidae (C)				
	Stilesia globipunctata	Anoplocephalidae (C)				
	Thysaniezia ovilla	Anoplocephalidae (C)				
	Thysanosoma actinoides	Anoplocephalidae (C)				
	Cymbiforma indica	Notocotylidae (T)				
	Skrjabinotrema ovis	Brachylaemidae (T)				
Caecum, colon	Oesophagostomum columbianum	Strongyloidea (N)			Eimeria crandallis	Eimeriidae (Co)
	Oesophagostomum venulosum	Strongyloidea (N)			Eimeria ovinoidalis	Eimeriidae (Co)
	Oesophagostomum multifoliatum	Strongyloidea (N)			Retortamonas ovis	Retortamonadorididae (Fl)
	Oesophagostomum asperum	Strongyloidea (N)			Tetratrichomonas ovis	Trichomonadidae (Fl)
	Chabertia ovina	Strongyloidea (N)			Entamoeba ovis	Entamoebidae (Am)
	Skrjabinema ovis	Oxyuroidea (N)				
	Skrjabinema alata	Oxyuroidea (N)				
	Trichuris ovis	Trichuroidea (N)				
	Trichuris skrjabini	Trichuroidea (N)				
	Trichuris discolor	Trichuroidea (N)				

(Continued)

Sheep parasite checklist. *Continued*

Section/host system	Helminths		Arthropods		Protozoa	
	Parasite	(Super) family	Parasite	Family	Parasite	Family
Respiratory						
Nasal cavities	*Mammomonogamus nasicola*	Strongyloidea (N)	*Oestrus ovis*	Oestridae (F)		
			Gedoelstia cristata	Oestridae (F)		
			Gedoelstia haessleri	Oestridae (F)		
Larynx	*Mammomonogamus laryngeus*	Strongyloidea (N)				
Trachea, bronchi	*Dictyocaulus filaria*	Trichostrongyloidea (N)				
Lung	*Muellerius capillaris*	Metastrongyloidea (N)				
	Protostrongylus rufescens	Metastrongyloidea (N)				
	Protostrongylus brevispeculum	Metastrongyloidea (N)				
	Protostrongylus skrjabini	Metastrongyloidea (N)				
	Protostrongylus rushi	Metastrongyloidea (N)				
	Protostrongylus davtiani	Metastrongyloidea (N)				
	Protostrongylus stilesi	Metastrongyloidea (N)				
	Cystocaulus ocreatus	Metastrongyloidea (N)				
	Cystocaulus nigrescens	Metastrongyloidea (N)				
	Neostrongylus linearis	Metastrongyloidea (N)				
	Spiculocaulus austriacus	Metastrongyloidea (N)				
	Varestrongylus schulzi	Metastrongyloidea (N)				
	Echinococcus granulosus	Taeniidae (C)				
Liver						
	Fasciola hepatica	Fasciolidae (T)				
	Fasciola gigantica	Fasciolidae (T)				
	Fascioloides magna	Fasciolidae (T)				
	Dicrocoelium dendriticum	Dicrocoeliidae (T)				
	Dicrocoelium hospes	Dicrocoeliidae (T)				
	Stilesia hepatica	Anoplocephalidae (C)				
	Thysanosoma actinioides	Anoplocephalidae (C)				
	Cysticercus tenuicollis (metacestode: *Taenia hydatigena*)	Taeniidae (C)				
	Echinococcus granulosus	Taeniidae (C)				
	Ascaris suum	Ascaridoidea (N)				
Pancreas						
	Eurytrema pancreaticum	Dicrocoeliidae (T)				
	Eurytrema coelomaticum	Dicrocoeliidae (T)				
	Eurytrema ovis	Dicrocoeliidae (T)				
Circulatory						
Blood	*Schistosoma bovis*	Schistosomatidae (T)			*Trypanosoma brucei brucei*	Trypanosomatidae (Fl)
	Schistosoma mattheei	Schistosomatidae (T)			*Trypanosoma congolense*	Trypanosomatidae (Fl)
	Schistosoma indicum	Schistosomatidae (T)			*Trypanosoma simiae*	Trypanosomatidae (Fl)
	Schistosoma nasale	Schistosomatidae (T)			*Trypanosoma vivax*	Trypanosomatidae (Fl)
	Schistosoma japonicum	Schistosomatidae (T)			*Trypansoma melophagium*	Trypanosomatidae (Fl)
	Schistosoma turkestanicum	Schistosomatidae (T)			*Babesia motasi*	Babesiidae (Bs)
	(*Orientobilharzia turkestanicum*)				*Babesia ovis*	Babesiidae (Bs)
					Theileria hirci	Theileriidae (Bs)
					Theileria ovis	Theileriidae (Bs)
					Theileria recondita	Theileriidae (Bs)
					Theileria separata	Theileriidae (Bs)
					Anaplasma phagocytophilum	Anaplasmataceae (R)
					Anaplasma ovis	Anaplasmataceae (R)
					Ehrlichia ruminantium	Anaplasmataceae (R)
					Rickettsia conorii	Rickettsiaceae (R)
					Mycoplasma ovis	Mycoplasmataceae (My)

Location	Species	Family (code)
Blood vessels	Elaeophora schneideri	Filarioidea (N)
	Onchocerca armillata	Filarioidea (N)
Nervous		
CNS	Coenurus cerebralis (metacestode: Taenia multiceps)	Taeniidae (C)
	Gedoelstia cristata	Oestridae (F)
	Gedoelstia haessleri	Oestridae (F)
	Toxoplasma gondii	Sarcocystidae (Co)
Ear	Gedoelstia cristata	Oestridae (F)
	Gedoelstia haessleri	Oestridae (F)
Ear	Raillietia caprae	Halarachnidae (M)
Reproductive/urogenital	Toxoplasma gondii	Sarcocystidae (Co)
Locomotory		
Muscle	Cysticercus ovis (metacestode: Taenia ovis)	Taeniidae (C)
	Toxoplasma gondii	Sarcocystidae (Co)
	Sarcocystis ovicanis	Sarcocystidae (Co)
	Sarcocystis ovifelis	Sarcocystidae (Co)
Connective tissue		
Subcutaneous	Przhevalskiana silensis	Oestridae (F)
	Dermatobia hominis	Oestridae (F)
	Hypoderma diana	Oestridae (F)
	Calliphora augur	Calliphoridae (F)
	Calliphora albifrontalis	Calliphoridae (F)
	Calliphora nociva	Calliphoridae (F)
	Calliphora stygia	Calliphoridae (F)
	Calliphora vicina	Calliphoridae (F)
	Calliphora vomitoria	Calliphoridae (F)
	Lucilia sericata	Calliphoridae (F)
	Lucilia cuprina	Calliphoridae (F)
	Protophormia terraenovae	Calliphoridae (F)
	Phormia regina	Calliphoridae (F)
	Cordylobia anthrophaga	Calliphoridae (F)
	Cochliomyia hominivorax	Calliphoridae (F)
	Cochliomyia macellaria	Calliphoridae (F)
	Chrysomya bezziana	Calliphoridae (F)
	Chrysomya megacephala	Calliphoridae (F)
	Wohlfahrtia magnifica	Sarcophagidae (F)
	Wohlfahrtia meigeni	Sarcophagidae (F)
	Wohlfahrtia vigil	Sarcophagidae (F)
Integument		
Skin	Linognathus ovillus	Linognathidae (L)
	Linognathus pedalis	Linognathidae (L)
	Linognathus africanus	Linognathidae (L)
	Bovicola ovis	Bovicolidae (L)
	Melophagus ovinus	Hippoboscidae (L)
	Demodex ovis	Demodicidae (M)
	Psoroptes ovis	Psoroptidae (M)
	Chorioptes bovis	Psoroptidae (M)
	Psorobia ovis	Psorergatidae (M)
	Sarcoptes scabiei	Sarcoptidae (M)

The following species of flies and ticks are found on sheep. More detailed descriptions are found in Chapter 3.

Flies of veterinary importance on sheep.

Group	Genus	Species	Family
Blackflies Buffalo gnats	*Simulium*	spp.	Simuliidae (F)
Blowflies and screwworms	*Calliphora*	*albifrontis* *nociva* *stygia* *vicina* *vomitoria*	Calliphoridae (F)
	Chrysomya	*albiceps* *bezziana* *megacephala*	
	Cochliomyia	*hominivorax* *macellaria*	
	Cordylobia	*anthropophaga*	
	Lucilia	*cuprina* *illustris* *sericata*	
	Phormia	*regina*	
	Protophormia	*terraenovae*	
Bot flies	*Dermatobia*	*hominis*	Oestridae (F)
	Gedoelstia	*haessleri*	
	Oestrus	*ovis*	
	Przhevalskiana	*aegagri silenus*	
Flesh flies	*Sarcophaga*	*fusicausa* *haemorrhoidalis*	Sarcophagidae (F)
	Wohlfahrtia	*magnifica* *meigeni* *vigil*	
Hippoboscids	*Hippobosca*	*equina* *rufipes* *maculata*	Hippoboscidae (F)
Midges	*Culicoides*	spp.	Ceratopogonidae (F)
Mosquitoes	*Aedes*	spp.	Culicidae (F)
	Anopheles	spp.	
	Culex	spp.	
Muscids	*Hydrotaea*	*irritans*	Muscidae (F)
	Musca	*autumnalis* *domestica*	
	Stomoxys	*calcitrans*	
Sand flies	*Phlebotomus*	spp.	Psychodidae (F)
Tabanids	*Chrysops*	spp.	Tabanidae (F)
	Haematopota	spp.	
	Tabanus	spp.	
Tsetse flies	*Glossina*	*fusca* *morsitans* *palplalis*	Glossinidae (F)

Tick species found on sheep.

Genus	Species	Common name	Family
Ornithodoros	*moubata*	Eyeless or hut tampan	Argasidae (Ti)
	savignyi	Eyed or sand tampan	
Otobius	*megnini*	Spinose ear tick	Argasidae (Ti)
Amblyomma	*americanum*	Lone Star tick	Ixodidae (Ti)
	cajennense	Cayenne tick	
	gemma		
	hebraeum	South African bont tick	
	maculatum	Gulf Coast tick	
	pomposum		
	variegatum	Variegated or tropical bont tick	
Dermacentor	*andersoni*	Rocky Mountain wood tick	Ixodidae (Ti)
	marginatus	Ornate sheep tick	
	reticulatus	Marsh tick, meadow tick	
	occidentalis	Pacific Coast tick	
	variabilis	American dog tick, wood tick	
Haemaphysalis	*punctata*		Ixodidae (Ti)
	concinna	Bush tick	
	bispinosa	Bush tick	
	longicornis	Scrub tick, New Zealand cattle tick	
Hyalomma	*detritum*	Bont-legged tick	Ixodidae (Ti)
	dromedarii	Camel tick	
	marginatum	Mediterranean tick	
	truncatum	Bont-legged tick	
Ixodes	*ricinus*	Castor bean or European sheep tick	Ixodidae (Ti)
	holocyclus	Paralysis tick	
	rubicundus	Karoo paralysis tick	
	scapularis	Deer tick, black-legged tick	
Rhipicephalus	*appendiculatus*	Brown ear tick	Ixodidae (Ti)
	bursa		
	capensis	Cape brown tick	
	evertsi	Red or red-legged tick	
	sanguineus	Brown dog or kennel tick	
	simus	Glossy tick	
Rhipicephalus (*Boophilus*)	*annulatus*	Blue cattle tick, Texas cattle fever tick	Ixodidae (Ti)
	decoloratus	Blue tick	
	microplus	Pantropical or southern cattle tick	

Goat parasite checklist.

	Helminths		Arthropods		Protozoa	
Section/host system	Parasite	(Super) family	Parasite	Family	Parasite	Family
Digestive						
Oesophagus	Gongylonema pulchrum	Spiruroidea (N)				
Rumen/reticulum	Gongylonema verrucosum	Spiruroidea (N)			Monocercomonoides caprae	Polymastigidae (Fl)
	Gongylonema monnigi	Spiruroidea (N)				
	Paramphistomum cervi	Paramphistomatidae (T)				
	Calicophoron daubneyi	Paramphistomatidae (T)				
	Paramphistomum microbothrium	Paramphistomatidae (T)				
	Paramphistomum streptocoelium	Paramphistomatidae (T)				
	Cotylophoron cotylophorum	Paramphistomatidae (T)				
Abomasum	Teladorsagia circumcincta	Trichostrongyloidea (N)			Eimeria gilruthi	Eimeriidae (Co)
	Ostertagia leptospicularis	Trichostrongyloidea (N)				
	Marshallagia marshalli	Trichostrongyloidea (N)				
	Haemonchus contortus	Trichostrongyloidea (N)				
	Trichostrongylus axei	Trichostrongyloidea (N)				
	Parabronema skrjabini	Spiruriodea (N)				
Small intestine	Trichostrongylus colubriformis	Trichostrongyloidea (N)			Eimeria ninakohlyakimovae	Eimeriidae (Co)
	Trichostrongylus vitrinus	Trichostrongyloidea (N)			Eimeria alijevi	Eimeriidae (Co)
	Trichostrongylus longispicularis	Trichostrongyloidea (N)			Eimeria arloingi	Eimeriidae (Co)
	Cooperia curticei	Trichostrongyloidea (N)			Eimeria aspheronica	Eimeriidae (Co)
	Cooperia surnabada	Trichostrongyloidea (N)			Eimeria caprina	Eimeriidae (Co)
	Nematodirus filicollis	Trichostrongyloidea (N)			Eimeria caprovina	Eimeriidae (Co)
	Nematodirus battus	Trichostrongyloidea (N)			Eimeria christenseni	Eimeriidae (Co)
	Nematodirus spathiger	Trichostrongyloidea (N)			Eimeria hirci	Eimeriidae (Co)
	Bunostomum trigonocephalum	Ancylostomatoidea (N)			Eimeria jolchijevi	Eimeriidae (Co)
	Gaigeria pachyscalis	Ancylostomatoidea (N)			Eimeria capralis	Eimeriidae (Co)
	Strongyloides papillosus	Strongyloidoidea (N)			Eimeria masseyensis	Eimeriidae (Co)
	Capillaria longipes	Trichuroidea (N)			Eimeria charlestoni	Eimeriidae (Co)
	Moniezia expansa	Anoplocephalidae (C)			Eimeria punctata	Eimeriidae (Co)
	Avitellina centripunctata	Anoplocephalidae (C)			Eimeria pallida	Eimeriidae (Co)
	Avitellina goughi	Anoplocephalidae (C)			Cryptosporidium parvum	Cryptosporidiidae (Co)
	Avitellina chalmersi	Anoplocephalidae (C)			Cryptosporidium xiaoi	Cryptosporidiidae (Co)
	Avitellina tatia	Anoplocephalidae (C)			Giardia intestinalis	Giardiidae (Fl)
	Stilesia globipunctata	Anoplocephalidae (C)				
	Thysaniezia ovilla	Anoplocephalidae (C)				
	Cymbiforma indica	Notocotylidae (T)				
Caecum, colon	Oesophagostomum columbianum	Strongyloidea (N)			Eimeria ninakohlyakimovae	Eimeriidae (Co)
	Oesophagostomum venulosum	Strongyloidea (N)			Eimeria caprina	Eimeriidae (Co)
	Oesophagostomum multifoliatum	Strongyloidea (N)			Retortamonas ovis	Retortamonadoridae (Fl)
	Oesophagostomum asperum	Strongyloidea (N)			Tetratrichomonas ovis	Trichomonadidae (Fl)
	Chabertia ovina	Trichostrongyloidea (N)			Entamoeba ovis	Entamoebidae (Am)
	Skrjabinema ovis	Oxyuroidea (N)			Entamoeba wenyonii	Entamoebidae (Am)
	Skrjabinema caprae	Oxyuroidea (N)				
	Trichuris ovis	Trichuroidea (N)				
	Trichuris skrjabini	Trichuroidea (N)				
	Trichuris discolor	Trichuroidea (N)				

(Continued)

Goat parasite checklist. *Continued*

Section/host system	Helminths		Arthropods		Protozoa	
	Parasite	(Super)family	Parasite	Family	Parasite	Family
Respiratory						
Nasal cavities	*Mammomonogamus nasicola*	Strongyloidea (N)	*Oestrus ovis*	Oestridae (F)		
			Gedoelstia cristata	Oestridae (F)		
			Gedoelstia haessleri	Oestridae (F)		
Larynx	*Mammomonogamus laryngeus*	Strongyloidea (N)				
Trachea, bronchi	*Dictyocaulus filaria*	Trichostrongyloidea (N)				
Lung	*Muellerius capillaris*	Metastrongyloidea (N)				
	Protostrongylus rufescens	Metastrongyloidea (N)				
	Protostrongylus brevispeculum	Metastrongyloidea (N)				
	Protostrongylus skrjabini	Metastrongyloidea (N)				
	Protostrongylus rushi	Metastrongyloidea (N)				
	Protostrongylus davtiani	Metastrongyloidea (N)				
	Cystocaulus ocreatus	Metastrongyloidea (N)				
	Cystocaulus nigrescens	Metastrongyloidea (N)				
	Neostrongylus linearis	Metastrongyloidea (N)				
	Spiculocaulus austriacus	Metastrongyloidea (N)				
	Varestrongylus schulzi	Metastrongyloidea (N)				
	Echinococcus granulosus	Taeniidae (C)				
Liver						
	Fasciola hepatica	Fasciolidae (T)				
	Fasciola gigantica	Fasciolidae (T)				
	Fascioloides magna	Fasciolidae (T)				
	Dicrocoelium dendriticum	Dicrocoeliidae (T)				
	Dicrocoelium hospes	Dicrocoeliidae (T)				
	Stilesia hepatica	Anoplocephalidae (C)				
	Cysticercus tenuicollis (metacestode: *Taenia hydatigena*)	Taeniidae (C)				
	Echinococcus granulosus	Taeniidae (C)				
Pancreas						
	Eurytrema pancreaticum	Dicrocoeliidae (T)				
Circulatory						
Blood	*Schistosoma bovis*	Schistosomatidae (T)			*Trypanosoma brucei brucei*	Trypanosomatidae (Fl)
	Schistosoma mattheei	Schistosomatidae (T)			*Trypanosoma brucei evansi*	Trypanosomatidae (Fl)
	Schistosoma indicum	Schistosomatidae (T)			*Trypanosoma congolense*	Trypanosomatidae (Fl)
	Schistosoma nasale	Schistosomatidae (T)			*Trypanosoma simiae*	Trypanosomatidae (Fl)
	Schistosoma japonicum	Schistosomatidae (T)			*Trypanosoma vivax*	Trypanosomatidae (Fl)
	Schistosoma turkestanicum	Schistosomatidae (T)			*Trypansoma melophagium*	Trypanosomatidae (Fl)
					Babesia motasi	Babesiidae (Bs)
					Babesia ovis	Babesiidae (Bs)
					Theileria hirci	Theileriidae (Bs)
					Theileria ovis	Theileriidae (Bs)
					Theileria recondita	Theileriidae (Bs)
					Theileria separata	Theileriidae (Bs)
					Anaplasma ovis	Anaplasmataceae (R)
					Ehrlichia ruminantium	Anaplasmataceae (R)
					Rickettsia conorii	Rickettsiaceae (R)
					Mycoplasma ovis	Mycoplasmataceae (My)
Blood vessels	*Elaeophora schneideri*	Filarioidea (N)				
	Onchocerca armillata	Filarioidea (N)				

System	Organ/Site	Parasite	Family (code)
Nervous			
	CNS	*Coenurus cerebralis* (metacestode: *Taenia multiceps*)	Taeniidae (C)
		Gedoelstia cristata	Oestridae (F)
		Gedoelstia haessleri	Oestridae (F)
		Toxoplasma gondii	Sarcocystidae (Col)
	Eye	*Gedoelstia cristata*	Oestridae (F)
		Gedoelstia haessleri	Oestridae (F)
	Ear	*Raillietia caprae*	Halarachnidae (M)
Reproductive/urogenital		*Toxoplasma gondii*	Sarcocystidae (Co)
Locomotory			
	Muscle	*Cysticercus ovis* (metacestode: *Taenia ovis*)	Taeniidae (C)
		Toxoplasma gondii	Sarcocystidae (Co)
		Sarcocystis capracanis	Sarcocystidae (Co)
		Sarcocystis hircicanis	Sarcocystidae (Co)
		Sarcocystis hircifelis	Sarcocystidae (Co
Connective tissue			
	Subcutaneous	*Besnoitia besnoiti*	Sarcocystidae (Co)
		Przhevalskiana silensis	Oestridae (F)
		Calliphora augur	Calliphoridae (I)
		Calliphora albifrontis	Calliphoridae (F)
		Calliphora nociva	Calliphoridae (F)
		Calliphora stygia	Calliphoridae (F)
		Calliphora vicina	Calliphoridae (F)
		Calliphora vomitoria	Calliphoridae (F)
		Lucilia cuprina	Calliphoridae (F)
		Lucilia sericata	Calliphoridae (F)
		Protophormia terraenovae	Calliphoridae (F)
		Phormia regina	Calliphoridae (F)
		Cordylobia anthropophaga	Calliphoridae (F)
		Cochliomyia hominivorax	Calliphoridae (F)
		Cochliomyia macellaria	Calliphoridae (F)
		Chrysomya bezziana	Calliphoridae (F)
		Chrysomya megacephala	Calliphoridae (F)
		Wohlfahrtia magnifica	Sarcophagidae (F)
		Wohlfahrtia meigeni	Sarcophagidae (F)
		Wohlfahrtia vigil	Sarcophagidae (F)
		Dermatobia hominis	Oestridae (F)
Integument			
	Skin	*Bovicola caprae*	Bovicolidae (L)
		Bovicola limbata	Bovicolidae (L)
		Linognathus stenopsis	Linognathidae (L)
		Linognathus africanus	Linognathidae (L)
		Demodex caprae	Demodicidae (M)
		Sarcoptes scabiei	Sarcoptidae (M)
		Psoroptes ovis	Psoroptidae (M)
		Chorioptes bovis	Psoroptidae (M)

The following species of flies and ticks are found on goats. More detailed descriptions are found in Chapter 3.

Flies of veterinary importance on goats.

Group	Genus	Species	Family
Blackflies Buffalo gnats	Simulium	spp.	Simuliidae (F)
Blowflies and screwworms	Calliphora	albifrontis nociva stygia vicina vomitoria	Calliphoridae (F)
	Chrysomya	albiceps bezziana megacephala	
	Cochliomyia	hominivorax macellaria	
	Cordylobia	anthropophaga	
	Lucilia	cuprina illustris sericata	
	Phormia	regina	
	Protophormia	terraenovae	
Bot flies	Dermatobia	hominis	Oestridae (F)
	Gedoelstia	haessleri	
	Oestrus	ovis	
	Przhevalskiana	aegagri silenus	
Flesh flies	Sarcophaga	fusicausa haemorrhoidalis	Sarcophagidae (F)
	Wohlfahrtia	magnifica meigeni vigil	
Hippoboscids	Hippobosca	equina rufipes maculata	Hippoboscidae (F)
Midges	Culicoides	spp.	Ceratopogonidae (F)
Mosquitoes	Aedes	spp.	Culicidae (F)
	Anopheles	spp.	
	Culex	spp.	
Muscids	Hydrotaea	irritans	Muscidae (F)
	Musca	autumnalis domestica	
	Stomoxys	calcitrans	
Sand flies	Phlebotomus	spp.	Psychodidae (F)
Tabanids	Chrysops	spp.	Tabanidae (F)
	Haematopota	spp.	
	Tabanus	spp.	
Tsetse flies	Glossina	fusca morsitans palpalis	Glossinidae (F)

Tick species found on goats.

Genus	Species	Common name	Family
Ornithodoros	moubata	Eyeless or hut tampan	Argasidae (Ti)
	savignyi	Eyed or sand tampan	
Otobius	megnini	Spinose ear tick	Argasidae (Ti)
Amblyomma	americanum	Lone Star tick	Ixodidae (Ti)
	cajennense	Cayenne tick	
	gemma		
	hebraeum	South African bont tick	
	maculatum	Gulf Coast tick	
	pomposum		
	variegatum	Variegated or tropical bont tick	
Dermacentor	andersoni	Rocky Mountain wood tick	Ixodidae (Ti)
	marginatus	Ornate sheep tick	
	reticulatus	Marsh tick	
	occidentalis	Pacific Coast tick	
	variabilis	American dog tick	
Haemaphysalis	punctata		Ixodidae (Ti)
	concinna	Bush tick	
	bispinosa	Bush tick	
	longicornis	Scrub tick, New Zealand cattle tick	
Hyalomma	detritum	Bont-legged tick	Ixodidae (Ti)
	dromedarii	Camel tick	
	marginatum	Mediterranean tick	
	truncatum	Bont-legged tick	
Ixodes	ricinus	Castor bean or European sheep tick	Ixodidae (Ti)
	holocyclus	Paralysis tick	
	rubicundus	Karoo paralysis tick	
	scapularis	Deer tick, black-legged tick	
Rhipicephalus	appendiculatus	Brown ear tick	Ixodidae (Ti)
	bursa		
	capensis	Cape brown tick	
	evertsi	Red or red-legged tick	
	sanguineus	Brown dog or kennel tick	
	simus	Glossy tick	
Rhipicephalus (Boophilus)	annulatus	Texas cattle fever tick	Ixodidae (Ti)
	decoloratus	Blue tick	
	microplus	Pantropical or southern cattle tick	

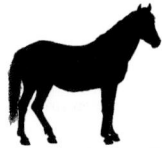
ENDOPARASITES

Parasites of the digestive system

STOMACH

Members of the genus *Habronema*, and the closely related genus *Draschia*, are parasites localised in the stomach of horses. *Habronema* inhabits the mucous layer of the gastric mucosa and may cause a catarrhal gastritis but is not considered an important pathogen, while *Draschia* parasitises the fundic region of the stomach wall and provokes the formation of large fibrous nodules that are occasionally significant. The chief importance of these parasites is as a cause of cutaneous habronematidosis or 'summer sores' in warm countries. The seasonality of cutaneous lesions is related to the activity of the fly vectors.

Control: Obviously, any measures taken to prevent injuries and control fly populations will be beneficial. Stacking manure and using insecticides during the day, for example, limit fly populations and attack. Skin wounds should be treated with either fly repellents or a combination of antiseptic and insecticide.

Treatment: A number of modern broad-spectrum anthelmintics including oxfendazole, oxibendazole, albendazole and the macrocyclic lactones have been shown to have activity against the adult parasites in the stomach. Cutaneous lesions are best treated with ivermectin. The use of insect repellents has some benefit and radiation therapy and cryosurgery have been used in more chronic cases.

Draschia megastoma

Draschia megastoma, synonym *Habronema megastoma* (Phylum: Nematoda; Class: Chromadorea; Order: Spirurida; Family: Habronematidae), is distributed worldwide and localised in the fundic region of the stomach wall of horses and other equines. This worm has dipteran flies of the genera *Musca*, *Stomoxys* and *Haematobia* as intermediate hosts.

Pathogenesis: In the stomach, the worms live in colonies in the mucosa around which develop large nodular fibrous tumour-like lesions (Fig. 10.1). These occur in the fundus region and seem to be well tolerated unless they protrude into the lumen sufficiently to interfere mechanically with stomach function or, more rarely, cause abscessation or perforation when the lesions become secondarily

infected with pyogenic bacteria. *Draschia megastoma* can cause a skin reaction, cutaneous habronematidosis or 'summer sores', when larvae are deposited on broken skin or open wounds by infected flies.

Clinical signs and pathology: The presence of adult worms in the stomach causes very little clinical disturbance. Cutaneous habronematidosis presents as intense itching of the affected skin. Non-healing granulomatous lesions, raised above the surface of the skin, may be a feature (see *Habronema*). Adult worms burrow into the submucosa of the stomach producing large tumour-like nodules filled with a creamy pus-like substance, causing the mucosa to protrude into the gastric lumen. The worms provoke a surrounding granulomatous reaction, which contains a central core of necrotic and cellular debris and large numbers of eosinophils. Burrowing larvae in the conjunctivae cause an ulcerative weeping lesion at the medial canthus, which becomes progressively more nodular as the lesion becomes more granulomatous. Mineralised granules, caseous debris and larvae may be found in the lesion. Larvae in the skin cause lesions that are rapidly progressive and proliferative in nature, comprising ulcerated masses of granulation tissue that haemorrhages readily. Lesions may be single or multiple and range in size from 5 to 15 cm. On section, the lesions are caseous and histologically there are aggregates of eosinophils scattered throughout the connective tissue, which contains a few macrophages and multinucleate giant cells surrounding degenerating larvae. The surface of the lesion is usually covered with a fibronecrotic exudate overlying a highly vascular granulation tissue infiltrated with neutrophils.

Diagnosis: Usually only low numbers of eggs or larvae are present in the faeces. Eggs may be demonstrated in gastric lavage taken via a stomach tube. Sometimes larvae can be identified in the small granulomatous skin lesions.

Habronema microstoma

Habronema microstoma, synonym *Habronema majus* (Phylum: Nematoda; Class: Chromadorea; Order: Spirurida; Family: Habronematidae), is distributed worldwide and localised in the mucous layer of the gastric mucosa of horses and other equines. This worm has dipteran flies of the genera *Musca*, *Stomoxys* and *Haematobia* as intermediate hosts.

Pathogenesis: The adult *Habronema* in the stomach may cause a mild catarrhal gastritis with excess mucus production. Nodules are not usually present. More important are the granulomatous lesions

Veterinary Parasitology, Fifth Edition. Domenico Otranto and Richard Wall.
© 2024 John Wiley & Sons Ltd. Published 2024 by John Wiley & Sons Ltd.

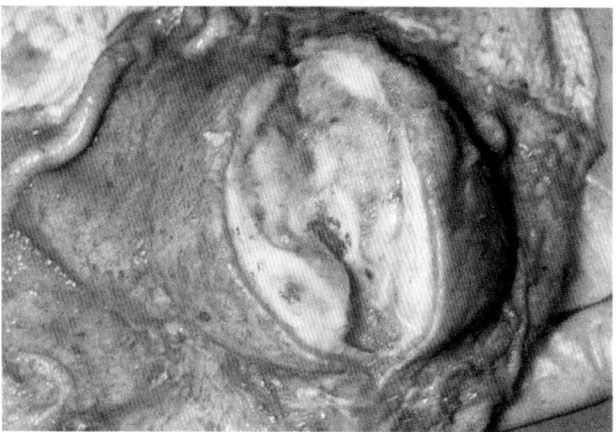

Fig. 10.1 Large nodular tumour-like lesion in the stomach induced by *Draschia megastoma* infection.

of cutaneous habronematidosis, commonly known as 'Summer sores', and the persistent conjunctivitis with nodular thickening and ulceration of the eyelids associated with invasion of the eyes. Larvae have also been found associated with small lung abscesses.

Clinical signs: Clinical signs are usually absent in gastric habronematidosis. Lesions of cutaneous habronematidosis are most common in areas of the body susceptible to injury and occur during the fly season in warm humid countries, although they also occur in temperate regions.

Pathology: During the early stages, there is intense itching of the infected wound or abrasion, which may cause further self-inflicted damage. Subsequently, a reddish-brown, non-healing, cauliflower-like granuloma develops that protrudes above the level of the surrounding skin and may be up to 8 cm in diameter (Fig. 10.2). These lesions are known as 'summer sores' in acute cases. Later, the lesion may become more chronic, fibrous and inactive but will not heal until the advent of cooler weather when fly activity ceases. Invasion of the eye produces a persistent conjunctivitis with nodular ulcers, especially at the medial canthus. Sometimes larvae invade the skin of the prepuce and glans penis of stallions. Adult worms in the mucosa of the stomach have been associated with a mild ulceration. Burrowing larvae in the conjunctivae cause an ulcerative

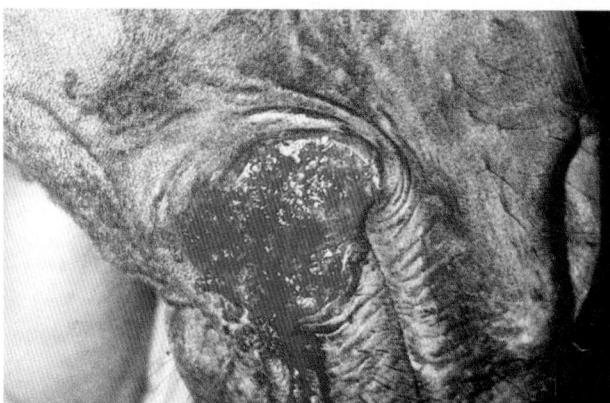

Fig. 10.2 Ulcerated granuloma ('summer sore') on commissure of lips of a horse due to cutaneous habronematidosis.

weeping lesion at the medial canthus, which becomes progressively more nodular as the lesion becomes more granulomatous.

Diagnosis: This is based on the finding of non-healing, reddish cutaneous granulomas. The larvae, recognised by spiny knobs on their tails, may be found in material from these lesions. Gastric infection is not easily diagnosed since *Habronema* eggs and larvae are not readily demonstrable in the faeces by routine techniques.

Habronema muscae

Habronema muscae (Phylum: Nematoda; Class: Chromadorea; Order: Spirurida; Family: Habronematidae) is distributed worldwide and localised in the mucous layer of the gastric mucosa of horses and other equines. This worm has dipteran flies of the genera *Musca*, *Stomoxys* and *Haematobia* (*Lyperosia*) as intermediate hosts.

Trichostrongylus axei

Trichostrongylus axei, synonym *Trichostrongylus extenuatus*, (Phylum: Nematoda; Class: Chromadorea; Order: Rhabditida; Family: Trichostrongylidae), commonly known as the Stomach hairworm, is distributed worldwide and localised in the stomach of cattle, sheep, goats, deer, horses, donkeys, pigs and occasionally humans.

Clinical signs and pathology: *Trichostrongylus axei* is responsible for gastritis in horses. In the host, initial lesions are circumscribed areas of hyperaemia in the gastric mucosa, which progress to catarrhal or lymphocytic inflammation and erosion of the epithelium. This may be associated with necrosis. Over time, infection can lead to a chronic proliferative inflammation and shallow depressed ulcers may be present.

Control and treatment: These are described under control and treatment of strongylosis in horses.

Gasterophilus

Gasterophilus (Phylum: Arthropoda; Class: Insecta; Order: Diptera; Family: Oestridae) are commonly known as Bots. They are obligate parasites of horses, donkeys, mules, zebras, elephants and rhinoceroses. Nine species are recognised in total, six of which are of interest as veterinary parasites of equids. All species of *Gasterophilus* were originally restricted to the Palaearctic and Afro-tropical regions but three species, *Gasterophilus nasalis*, *G. haemorrhoidalis* and *G. intestinalis*, have been inadvertently introduced into the New World. Adult flies are most active during late summer.

Pathogenesis: The presence of larvae in the buccal cavity may lead to stomatitis with ulceration of the tongue. On attachment by their oral hooks to the stomach lining, larvae provoke an inflammatory reaction with the formation of funnel-shaped ulcers surrounded by a rim of hyperplastic epithelium (Fig. 10.3). These are commonly seen at *post mortem* examination of horses in areas of high fly prevalence and although dramatic in appearance, their true pathogenic significance remains obscure.

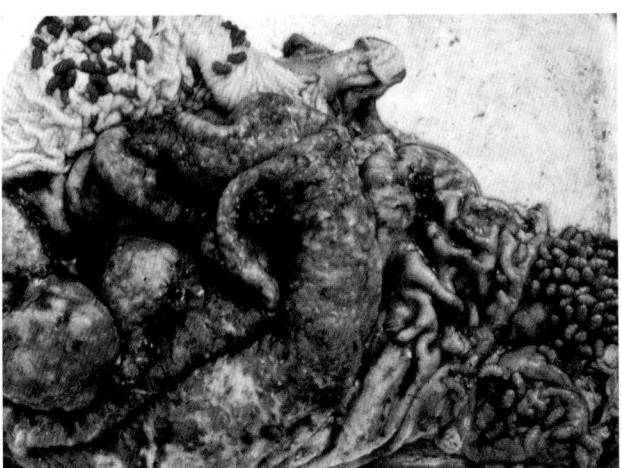

Fig. 10.3 *Gasterophilus* larvae in the stomach of a horse.

Clinical signs and pathology: Burrowing of the first-stage larvae in the mouth lining, tongue and gums can produce pus pockets, loosen teeth and cause loss of appetite in the host. Larvae attached to the gastrointestinal mucosa cause inflammation and ulceration. The adult fly can cause irritation and intense avoidance reactions when hovering around the host and laying eggs on the skin. Ovipositing females may be tenacious, laying eggs on mobile as well as stationary animals. Females will pursue galloping horses and immediately resume oviposition when the horse stops. The burrowing of first- and second-stage *Gasterophilus* larvae in the tissues of the tongue and mouth may result in lesions, the appearance of which is dependent on the degree of burrowing activity. Active tunnelling removes virtually all tissue in the path of the larvae, including nerves and capillaries, leading to haemorrhage and exocytosis into the tunnels, which fill with erythrocytes mixed with macrophages, lymphocytes and some eosinophils. The tunnels may become infected with bacteria, which result in microabscesses composed of clotted erythrocytes, bacteria, disintegrating epithelial cells and large numbers of neutrophils. Cells surrounding the tunnel exhibit pyknosis and epithelial hydropic degeneration and became separated from each other. Interdental gingiva invaded by larvae appear hyperaemic and denuded of epithelia. Recession and ulceration of the gingiva produce periodontal pockets. Extensive invasion by larvae leads to compound periodontal pockets. The attachment of third-stage larvae results in ulceration at the site of attachment with intense fibrosis below the ulcer. The cephalic portions of embedded larvae become surrounded by a cellular exudate containing erythrocytes and mononuclear cells.

Diagnosis: The adult flies may be visible and recognisable on and around the host. The eggs are also easily recognisable on the host and may be identified by colour and location. Damage to the mouth and tongue may be detected. The presence of larval parasites in the stomach is difficult to identify except by observation of the larvae in faeces.

Control and treatment: The most effective means of control of this parasite is to remove the eggs from the host's coat. This requires, where possible, daily examination of the animal, paying particular attention to the area around the lips. If eggs are found during the summer and autumn, subsequent infection can be prevented by vigorously sponging with warm water containing an insecticide. The warmth stimulates hatching and the insecticide kills the newly hatched larvae. From the life cycle, it is clear that in temperate areas during the winter, almost the entire *Gasterophilus* population will be present as larvae in the stomach, since adult fly activity ceases with the advent of the first frosts in autumn. A single treatment during the winter should therefore effectively break the cycle. In certain areas where adult fly activity is prolonged by mild conditions, additional treatments may be required.

Despite the lack of understanding of the pathogenic effect of bots, treatment is usually recommended as owners are concerned when larvae appear in the faeces. Treatment, however, does reduce fly populations and thus the fly worry associated with egg laying. The most widely used specific drugs included trichlorphon and dichlorvos, but these have generally been replaced by broad-spectrum macrocyclic lactone compounds such as ivermectin and moxidectin.

Gasterophilus haemorrhoidalis

Gasterophilus haemorrhoidalis (Phylum: Arthropoda; Class: Insecta; Order: Diptera; Family: Oestridae), commonly known as the Horse bot fly, is usually localised in the stomach of horses and donkeys worldwide.

Gasterophilus inermis

Gasterophilus inermis (Phylum: Arthropoda; Class: Insecta; Order: Diptera; Family: Oestridae), commonly known as the Horse bot fly, is usually localised in the stomach of horses, donkeys and zebras. It is found in northern Europe, northern Asia and Africa.

Gasterophilus intestinalis

Gasterophilus intestinalis (Phylum: Arthropoda; Class: Insecta; Order: Diptera; Family: Oestridae), commonly known as the Horse bot fly, is usually localised in the stomach of horses and donkeys worldwide.

Gasterophilus nasalis

Gasterophilus nasalis (Phylum: Arthropoda; Class: Insecta; Order: Diptera; Family: Oestridae), commonly known as the Horse nasal bot fly, is usually localised in the stomach of horses, donkeys and zebras. It is found worldwide but particularly in the Holarctic.

Gasterophilus nigricornis

Gasterophilus nigricornis (Phylum: Arthropoda; Class: Insecta; Order: Diptera; Family: Oestridae), commonly known as the Broad-bellied horse bot, is usually localised in the duodenum of horses and donkeys. It is found throughout the Middle East, southern Russia and China.

Gasterophilus pecorum

Gasterophilus pecorum (Phylum: Arthropoda; Class: Insecta; Order: Diptera; Family: Oestridae), commonly known as the Dark-winged horse bot, is usually localised in the mouth, tongue, oesophagus or stomach of horses and donkeys. It is found throughout Europe, Africa and Asia.

Pathogenesis: *Gasterophilus pecorum* is the most pathogenic species in the genus. Large numbers of attached larvae can cause inflammation, hinder swallowing and may eventually lead to death resulting from constriction of the oesophagus.

Clinical signs: Burrowing of the first-stage larvae in the mouth lining, tongue and gums can produce pus pockets, loosen teeth and cause loss of appetite in the host. Large numbers of attached larvae can cause inflammation and choking and hinder swallowing.

Diagnosis: Larvae present in the pharynx can usually be seen on direct inspection. Larvae further down the digestive tract can only be detected by observation of the mature detached larvae in faeces.

SMALL INTESTINE

Strongyloides westeri

Strongyloides westeri (Phylum: Nematoda; Class: Chromadorea; Order: Rhabditida; Family: Strongyloididae), commonly known as the Threadworm, is distributed worldwide and localised in the small intestine of horses, donkeys, zebras and rarely pigs.

Epidemiology: Infections are very common, especially in warm and humid environments. *Strongyloides* infective larvae are not ensheathed and are susceptible to extreme climatic conditions. However, warmth and moisture favour development and allow the accumulation of large numbers of infective stages. A second major source of infection for the very young animal is the reservoir of larvae in the tissues of their dams and this may lead to clinical strongyloidosis in foals in the first few weeks of life. Successive progeny from the same dam often show heavy infections.

Pathogenesis: Mature parasites are found in the duodenum and proximal jejunum and if present in large numbers, may cause inflammation with oedema and erosion of the epithelium. This results in catarrhal enteritis with impairment of digestion and absorption. Migration of larvae through the lungs can cause severe haemorrhage and respiratory distress. Skin penetration may result in irritation and dermatitis.

Clinical signs and pathology: Foals with heavy burdens show acute diarrhoea, weakness and emaciation. Older animals may harbour large burdens without showing clinical signs. Adult worms establish in tunnels in the epithelium at the base of the villi in the small intestine. In large numbers, they may cause villous atrophy, with a mixed mononuclear inflammatory cell infiltration of the lamina propria. Crypt epithelium is hyperplastic and there is villous clubbing.

Diagnosis: The clinical signs in very young animals, usually within the first few weeks of life, together with the finding of large numbers of the characteristic eggs or larvae in the faeces are suggestive of strongyloidosis. It should be emphasised, however, that high faecal egg counts may be found in apparently healthy animals. The dam of an infected foal will often not pass any eggs in faeces even though she is the source of infection through her milk.

Control and treatment: Specific control measures for infection are rarely necessary. Not all anthelmintics show high efficacy, but most of the modern benzimidazoles are effective. Macrocyclic lactones are effective against adult worms. Reduction in numbers of free-living larvae by removal of faeces and provision of dry bedding and areas may limit numbers and transmission. On stud farms, foals are often given an anthelmintic treatment against *S. westeri* at 1–2 weeks of age.

Parascaris equorum

Parascaris equorum, synonyms *Ascaris equorum* and *Ascaris megacephala* (Phylum: Nematoda; Class: Chromadorea; Order: Ascaridida; Family: Ascarididae), is distributed worldwide and localised in the small intestine of horses, donkeys and zebras.

Epidemiology: Infection with *P. equorum* is common throughout the world and is a major cause of unthriftiness in young foals. There are two important factors in the epidemiology of infection. First is the high fecundity of the adult female parasite, some infected foals passing millions of eggs in the faeces each day. Second, the extreme resistance of the egg in the environment ensures its persistence for several years. The sticky nature of the outer shell may also facilitate passive spread of eggs, adhering to the udder and teats of the pregnant mare. In the northern hemisphere, summer temperatures are such that many eggs become infective at a time when a population of susceptible foals is present. The infection acquired by these foals results in further contamination of pasture with eggs, which may survive during several subsequent grazing seasons. Although mature horses may harbour a few adult worms and act as carriers, heavy burdens are usually confined to yearlings and to foals, which become infected from the first month or so of life; infection is maintained largely by seasonal transmission between these groups of young animals. Exposed foals often develop immunity, resulting in partial or total loss of the worm population.

Pathogenesis: During the migratory phase of experimental infections, up to four weeks following infection, the major signs are frequent coughing accompanied in some cases by a greyish nasal discharge, although the foals remain bright and alert. Light intestinal infections are well tolerated, but moderate to heavy infections will cause unthriftiness in young animals with poor growth rates, dull coats and lassitude. A wide variety of other clinical signs, including fever, nervous disturbances and colic, has been attributed to field cases of parascariosis, but these have not been observed in experimental studies.

Clinical signs: Adult worms in heavy infections can cause severe enteritis resulting in alternating constipation and foul-smelling diarrhoea. Large numbers of larvae may cause coughing, with fever and anorexia. The hair coat may be dull and the animal appears malnourished.

Pathology: Gross changes are provoked in the liver and lungs by migrating *P. equorum* larvae. In the liver, larvae cause focal haemorrhages and eosinophilic tracts that resolve, leaving whitish areas of fibrosis. Larval migration in the lungs also leads to haemorrhage and infiltration by eosinophils, which are later replaced by accumulations of lymphocytes, while subpleural greyish-green lymphocytic nodules develop around dead or dying larvae; these nodules are more numerous following reinfections. These liver and lung lesions are usually of little pathological significance. Although the presence of worms in the small intestine (Fig. 10.4) is not associated with any specific lesions, heavy infections have occasionally been reported as a cause of impaction and perforation leading to peritonitis. Adult worms may cause catarrhal enteritis and intermittent diarrhoea.

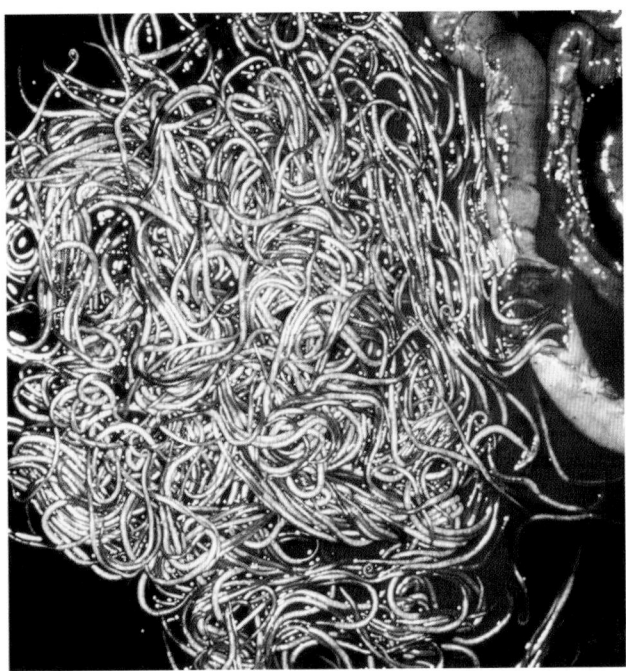

Fig. 10.4 *Parascaris equorum* from the intestine of an infected horse.

However, under experimental conditions, unthriftiness is a major sign and despite maintaining a good appetite, infected foals lose weight and may become emaciated. Competition between a large mass of parasites and the host for nutrients may be the underlying cause of this weight loss.

Diagnosis: This depends on clinical signs and the presence of spherical, thick, brownish, rough-shelled eggs on faecal examination. Occasionally, atypical thick-walled eggs are seen that lack the dark outer shell. If disease due to prepatent infection is suspected, faecal examination having proved negative, diagnosis may be confirmed by administration of an anthelmintic when large numbers of immature worms may be observed in the faeces.

Control and treatment: Since transmission is largely on a foal-to-foal basis, it is good policy to avoid using the same paddocks for nursing mares and their foals in successive years. Treatment should start when foals are about eight weeks old and be repeated at appropriate intervals, depending on the anthelmintic used. As the eggs are highly resistant to desiccation and most chemical disinfectants, regular removal of manure and bedding from stables and steam cleaning are recommended. Benzimidazoles (e.g. fenbendazole, oxfendazole, oxibendazole), pyrantel, ivermectin and moxidectin have all been shown to be effective against adult and larval stages when given orally. However, there are recent reports of suspected resistance of *P. equorum* to moxidectin and ivermectin, some worms remaining after treatment.

Notes: Infection with *P. equorum* is common throughout the world and is a major cause of unthriftiness in young foals.

Tapeworms

Several tapeworm species are found in horses, donkeys and other equines. Intermediate hosts for all species are forage mites of the family Oribatidae, in which the intermediate cysticercoid stages are found. Horses of all ages may be affected, but clinical cases have been reported mainly in animals up to 3–4 years of age.

Diagnosis: Where clinical signs occur, they may be difficult to differentiate from more common causes of unthriftiness and digestive upsets. However, it may be possible to confirm the presence of *Anoplocephala* by demonstration of the typical eggs on faecal examination or on *post mortem*. An enzyme-linked immunosorbent assay (ELISA) can be used to detect IgG to these parasites. A saliva antibody test has recently also become available.

Control: Control is difficult, since forage mites are widespread on pasture. Treatment with an effective anthelmintic before the animals enter new grazing may help to control *Anoplocephala* infections in areas where problems have arisen.

Treatment: Specific treatment for *Anoplocephala* infection is rarely called for but a number of compounds have been reported as effective, including pyrantel at increased dosage rates (38 mg/kg). Praziquantel at 1 mg/kg is also effective.

Anoplocephala perfoliata

Anoplocephala perfoliata (Phylum: Platyhelminthes; Class: Cestoda; Order: Cyclophyllidea; Family: Anoplocephalidae) is distributed worldwide and localised in the terminal ileum and caecum of equines.

Pathogenesis: *Anoplocephala perfoliata* has been considered to be relatively non-pathogenic but there is increasing evidence that heavy infections may cause severe clinical signs and may even prove fatal. *Anoplocephala perfoliata* is usually found around the ileocaecal junction (Fig. 10.5) and causes ulceration of the mucosa at its site of attachment and inflammation and thickening of the intestinal wall; these lesions have been incriminated as a cause of intussusception of the ileum into the caecum. Cases of intestinal obstruction and perforation of the intestinal wall have been recorded associated with massive infections.

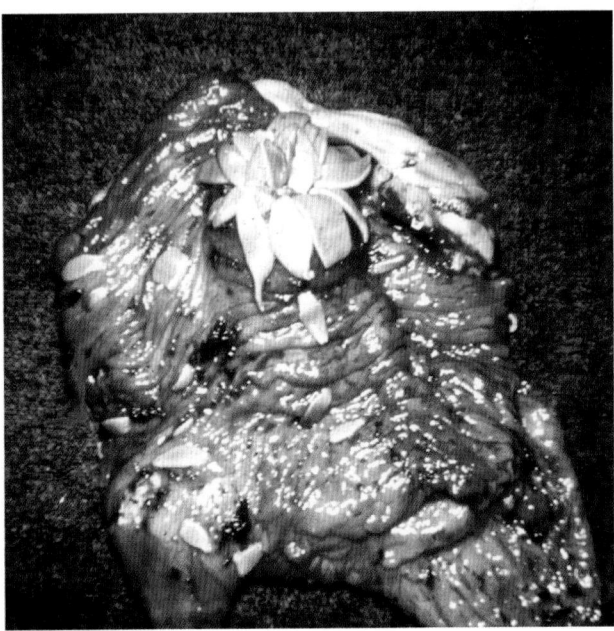

Fig. 10.5 *Anoplocephala perfoliata* tapeworms around the ileocaecal junction.

Clinical signs and pathology: In most infections there are no clinical signs. However, when there are significant pathological changes in the intestine, there may be unthriftiness, enteritis and colic. Perforation of the intestine will prove rapidly fatal. The mucosa at the site of attachment may be inflamed, thickened and ulcerated, particularly in the area of the ileocaecal junction where it may lead to partial or fatal occlusion of the ileocaecal orifice.

Anoplocephala magna

Anoplocephala magna (Phylum: Platyhelminthes; Class: Cestoda; Order: Cyclophyllidea; Family: Anoplocephalidae), commonly known as the Dwarf equine tapeworm, is distributed worldwide and localised in the small intestine and rarely stomach of equines.

Pathogenesis: Heavy infections of *A. magna* may cause catarrhal, haemorrhagic or ulcerative enteritis. Cases of intestinal obstruction, colic and perforation of the intestinal wall have been recorded associated with massive infections.

Clinical signs and pathology: Clinical signs are rare, but the infection can cause diarrhoea and colic. The mucosa at the site of attachment may be inflamed, thickened and ulcerated.

Paranoplocephala mamillana

Paranoplocephala mamillana, synonym *Anoplocephaloides mamillana* (Phylum: Platyhelminthes; Class: Cestoda; Order: Cyclophyllidea; Family: Anoplocephalidae), is distributed worldwide and localised in the small intestine and rarely stomach of equines, of all ages.

Clinical signs and pathology: *Paranoplocephala* is usually considered to be relatively non-pathogenic and in most infections there are no clinical signs. Infection is rarely associated with lesions but occasionally the site of attachment is inflamed and slightly ulcerated.

Diagnosis: It may be possible to confirm the presence of *Paranoplocephala* by the demonstration of the typical eggs on faecal examination or on *post mortem*.

Coccidiosis

Several species of coccidia have been reported from horses. Few details are available on the life cycles, pathogenesis and epidemiology. Similarly, little is known about treatment and control of equine coccidiosis but, by analogy with other hosts, sulfonamides can be tried. Prevention is based on good management and hygiene. Young animals should be kept off heavily contaminated pastures when they are most susceptible. Good feeding of dams prior to parturition and rearing animals of similar ages together limits the build-up and spread of oocysts.

Eimeria leuckarti

Eimeria leuckarti, synonym *Globidium leuckarti* (Phylum: Apicomplexa; Class: Conoidasida; Order: Eucoccidiorida; Family: Eimeriidae), is distributed worldwide and localised in the small

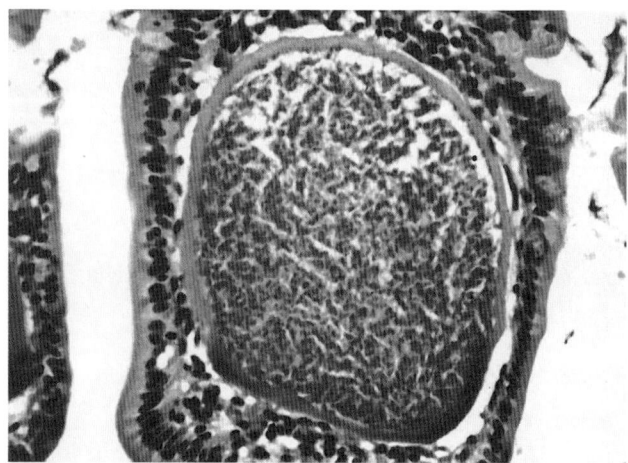

Fig. 10.6 'Giant' meront of *Eimeria leuckarti*.

intestine of horses and donkeys. Complete details of the life cycle are not known and merogony stages have not been described. Early gamonts are found in the cells of the lamina propria of the small intestine. The prepatent period is 15–33 days and sporulation time is 15–41 days.

Pathology: This parasite has been incriminated as the cause of intermittent diarrhoea and provokes marked inflammatory changes in the mucosa and disruption of villous architecture due to the presence of large meront stages (Fig. 10.6).

Diagnosis: Diagnosis is difficult. Because of the heavy nature of the oocysts, sedimentation techniques should be employed or, if flotation is used, a concentrated sugar solution is necessary.

Eimeria solipedum

Eimeria solipedum (Phylum: Apicomplexa; Class: Conoidasida; Order: Eucoccidiorida; Family: Eimeriidae) is localised in the small intestine of horses and donkeys and occurs in Russia and the Commonwealth of Independent States (CIS). Almost 10% of horses in the former Soviet Union (now Russia and CIS) have been found to be infected. This *Eimeria* has been reported to cause intermittent diarrhoea and is diagnosed through the identification of oocysts from faecal samples.

Other protozoa

Cryptosporidium parvum

Cryptosporidium parvum (Phylum: Apicomplexa; Class: Conoidasida; Order: Cryptogregarinorida; Family: Cryptosporidiidae) is distributed worldwide and localised in the small intestine of cattle, sheep, goats, horses, deer and humans (for more details see Chapter 8).

Epidemiology: Several mammals act as hosts to *C. parvum*, but little is known of the importance of their involvement in transmitting infection to, or maintaining infection in, domestic livestock. In the UK, surveys in horses have shown the presence of *C. parvum* in 28% of thoroughbred foals, although there was no association between infection and diarrhoea. Subsequent studies have demonstrated the genotype in horses to be genotype 2.

Clinical signs: Cryptosporidiosis has been reported in immuno-deficient foals as a cause of anorexia and diarrhoea.

Treatment: There is no known effective drug therapy. Where cryptosporidiosis is diagnosed, supportive treatment, in the form of antidiarrhoeals and fluids, is usually sufficient. For more details see Chapter 8.

Giardia intestinalis

Giardia intestinalis, synonyms *Giardia duodenalis*, *Giardia lamblia* or *Lamblia lamblia* (Phylum: Metamonada; Class: Trepomonadea; Order: Diplomonadida; Family: Giardiidae), is distributed worldwide and localised in the small intestine of humans, cattle, sheep, goats, pigs, horses, alpacas, dogs, cats, guinea pigs and chinchillas (for more details see Chapter 8).

Pathogenesis: Infection in horses is considered non-pathogenic with no clinical signs.

Notes: There is still controversy over the classification of *Giardia* spp. The current molecular classification places isolates into eight distinct assemblages. Some authors give separate specific names to organisms isolated from different hosts, although species specificity of many isolates is unknown. Phylogenetic data suggest that *G. intestinalis* is a species complex composed of several species that are host specific. For more details see Chapter 8.

LARGE INTESTINE

Large strongyles

Members of the genus *Strongylus* live in the large intestine of horses and donkeys and, with *Triodontophorus*, are commonly known as the Large strongyles. Since members of these genera form only one component of the total parasitic burden of the large intestine of the horse, general aspects on their epidemiology, treatment and control are described under the general introduction to small strongyles. Diagnosis of these migratory species is difficult during the migratory prepatent phase and is based on grazing history and clinical signs. Because of the long prepatent period, clinically apparent strongylosis may be associated with no, or low, faecal egg counts. Species or generic diagnosis is not usually required but may be undertaken by specialist laboratories based on morphology of larvae or adult worms.

Strongylus edentatus

Strongylus edentatus, synonym *Alfortia edentates* (Phylum: Nematoda; Class: Chromadorea; Order: Rhabditida; Family: Strongylidae), commonly known as the Large strongyle, is distributed worldwide and localised in the large intestine of horses and donkeys.

Pathogenesis: In *S. edentatus* infection, there are gross changes in the liver associated with early larval migration, but these rarely result in clinical signs. Similarly, the haemorrhages and fluid-filled nodules which accompany later larval development in subperitoneal tissues rarely result in clinical signs. For details of the pathogenesis of infection with adult worms, see *S. vulgaris*.

Clinical signs and pathology: This infection may cause diarrhoea, fever, oedema, anorexia, depression and weight loss. Haemorrhagic tracts may be produced in the hepatic parenchyma from migrating larvae and parenchymal scars of fibrous tissue on the hepatic capsule are often found on *post mortem*. Migrating larvae may also elicit subperitoneal haematomas, haemorrhage, peritonitis and omental adhesions. In the gut wall, they may form nodules and haemorrhagic foci.

Strongylus equinus

Strongylus equinus (Phylum: Nematoda; Class: Chromadorea; Order: Rhabditida; Family: Strongylidae), commonly known as the Large strongyle, is distributed worldwide and localised in the large intestine of horses and donkeys. This parasite is relatively less prevalent and abundant than other members of the genus.

Pathogenesis: Despite the invasive behaviour of the parasitic larval stages, little specific pathogenic effect can be attributed to them. There has been little work on the pathogenesis of migrating larvae of *S. equinus*. For details of the pathogenesis of infection with adult worms, see *S. vulgaris*.

Clinical signs and pathology: This infection may cause diarrhoea, fever, oedema, anorexia, depression and weight loss. Haemorrhagic tracts may be produced in the hepatic parenchyma from migrating larvae and parenchymal scars of fibrous tissue on the hepatic capsule are often found on *post mortem*. Omental adhesions may also be a sequela to larval migration. In the gut wall, they may form nodules and haemorrhagic foci.

Strongylus vulgaris

Strongylus vulgaris, synonym *Delafondia vulgaris* (Phylum: Nematoda; Class: Chromadorea; Order: Rhabditida; Family: Strongylidae), commonly known as the Large strongyle, is distributed worldwide and localised in the large intestine of horses and donkeys.

Pathogenesis: *Strongylus vulgaris* is now much less common than it was 20–30 years ago in many countries but is still the most significant and pathogenic nematode parasitic in horses. Larval forms cause endoarteritis in the mesenteric circulation, resulting in colic and thromboembolic infarction of the large bowel, while the adults cause anaemia and ill-thrift. Much of the information concerning *S. vulgaris* has been derived from experimental infection of foals. A few weeks after infection with several hundred L_3, a clinical syndrome of fever, inappetence and dullness occurs, sometimes accompanied by colic. At necropsy, these signs are associated with arteritis and thrombosis of intestinal blood vessels, with subsequent infarction and necrosis of areas of bowel. However, a syndrome of such severity is not commonly reported in foals under natural conditions, probably because larval intake is continuous during grazing; it has been shown experimentally that foals may tolerate large numbers of larvae administered in small doses over a long period. Maximum adult burdens are usually 100–200 worms.

The pathogenesis of infection with adult worms is associated with damage to the large intestinal mucosa due to the feeding habits of the worms and, to some extent, the disruption caused by emergence of young adults into the intestine following completion of

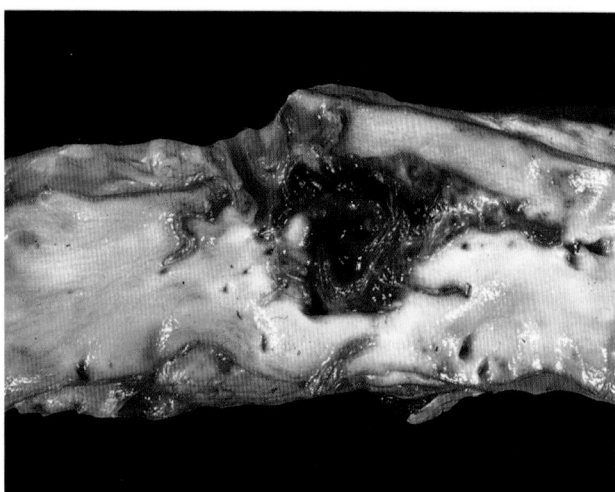

Fig. 10.7 *Strongylus vulgaris* larvae in the cranial mesenteric artery.

their parasitic larval development. These worms have large buccal capsules and feed by ingestion of plugs of mucosa as they move over the surface of the intestine. Although the worms appear to feed entirely on mucosal material, the incidental damage to blood vessels can cause considerable haemorrhage. Ulcers, which result from these bites, eventually heal, leaving small circular scars. The effects of infection with the adult worms have not been quantified, but the gross damage and subsequent loss of blood and tissue fluids are certainly partly responsible for the unthriftiness and anaemia associated with intestinal helminthosis in the horse. As *S. vulgaris* is approximately half the size of *S. edentatus* and *S. equinus*, the blood-feeding losses may not be as severe.

Clinical signs and pathology: Clinical signs are characterised by anaemia, poor condition and performance, varying degrees of colic, temporary lameness, intestinal stasis, rarely intestinal rupture and death. Lesions due to migrating larvae are most common in the cranial mesenteric artery and its main branches (Fig. 10.7) and consist of thrombus formation provoked by larval damage to the endothelium, together with marked inflammation and thickening of the arterial wall (Fig. 10.8). True aneurysms with dilation and thinning of the arterial wall, although uncommon, may be found, especially in animals which have experienced repeated infection. The arterial lesions heal quite markedly following treatment with anthelmintics, such as the macrocyclic lactones.

Diagnosis: Colic due to verminous arteritis may be associated with a palpable, painful enlargement at the root of the mesentery.

Triodontophorus

Members of the genus *Triodontophorus* (i.e. *Triodontophorus brevicauda, Triodontophorus minor, Triodontophorus nipponicus, Triodontophorus serratus, Triodontophorus tenuicollis*) are non-migratory large strongyles frequently found in large numbers in the colon and contribute to the deleterious effects of mixed strongyle infection.

Pathogenesis: Like the other horse strongyles, the pathogenic effect of these worms is damage to the large intestinal mucosa from the feeding habits of the adult parasites. The base of the buccal cavity contains small teeth (see Fig. 1.42).

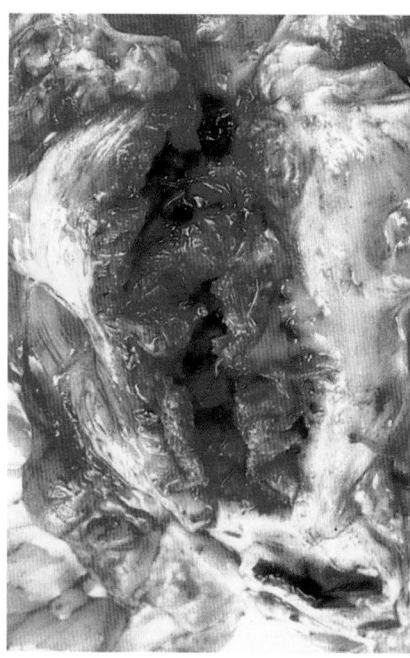

Fig. 10.8 Arteritis and thrombosis of cranial mesenteric artery caused by *Strongylus vulgaris* infection.

Clinical signs and pathology: The infection may cause loss of condition, anaemia, weakness and diarrhoea. Feeding worms lead to the formation of ulcers in the right dorsal colon. The ulcers may be deep and haemorrhagic and bunches of worms may be attached to them (Fig. 10.9).

Cyathostomins (small strongyles)

The group 'small strongyles' embraces over 40 species, popularly known as trichonemes, cyathostomes or cyathostomins. Small strongyles are extremely prevalent, and grazing horses usually carry a mixed burden of large and small strongyles. Fifteen species of small strongyles are commonly present in large numbers in horses. For many years, there has been a great deal of confusion in the classification of this group of parasites and in a new revision it has been

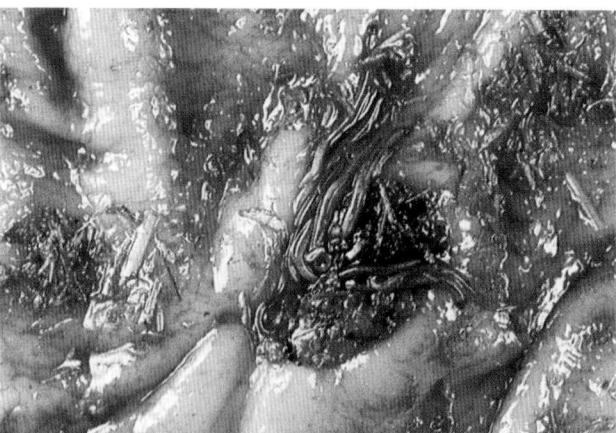

Fig. 10.9 *Triodontophorus tenuicollis* adults feeding around the periphery of an ulcer in the ventral colon.

Table 10.1 Cyathostomin species of the genera *Cyathostomum*, *Cylicocyclus*, *Cylicodontophorus* and *Cylicostephanus*.

Cyathostomum	Cylicocyclus	Cylicodontophorus	Cylicostaphanus
alveatum	adersi	bicoronatus	asymetricus
catinatum	auriculatus	euproctus	bidentatus
coronatum	brevicapsulatus	mettami	calicatus
labiatum	elongatus		goldi
labratum	insigne		hybridus
montgomeryi	largocapsulatus		longibursatus
pateratum	leptostomus		minutus
saginatum	maturmurai		ornatus
tetracanthrum	nassatus		poculatus
	radiatus		skrjabini
	triramosus		
	ultrajectinus		

Table 10.2 Geographical distribution of *Cyathostomum* spp.

Species	Distribution	Comments
Cyathostomum alveatum	Africa, Asia, Europe	Rare
Cyathostomum catinatum	Cosmopolitan	Very common
Cyathostomum coronatum	Cosmopolitan	Common
Cyathostomum labiatum	Cosmopolitan	Common
Cyathostomum labratum	Cosmopolitan	Common
Cyathostomum montgomeryi	Africa	Rare. In zebras, horses and mules
Cyathostomum pateratum	Cosmopolitan	Common
Cyathostomum saginatum	Europe, Asia	Rare
Cyathostomum tetracanthrum	Cosmopolitan	Rare

Table 10.3 Geographical distribution of *Cylicocyclus* spp.

Species	Distribution	Comments
Cylicocyclus adersi	Africa, Asia	Rare
Cylicocyclus auriculatus	Africa, Asia, America	Rare
Cylicocyclus brevicapsulatus	Africa, Asia, Europe, North America	Very rare
Cylicocyclus elongatus	Cosmopolitan	Common
Cylicocyclus insigne	Cosmopolitan	Very common
Cylicocyclus largocapsulatus	Asia	Very rare
Cylicocyclus leptostomus	Africa, Asia, Europe, North America	Common
Cylicocyclus maturmurai	Asia	Very rare
Cylicocyclus nassatus	Cosmopolitan	Very common
Cylicocyclus radiatus	Cosmopolitan	Rare
Cyliococyclus triramosus	Africa, Asia, Europe, North America	Rare
Cylicocyclus ultrajectinus	Cosmopolitan	Common

Table 10.4 Geographical distribution of *Cylicodontophorus* spp.

Species	Distribution	Comments
Cylicodontophorus bicoronatus	Cosmopolitan	Common
Cylicodontophorus euproctus	Cosmopolitan	Rare
Cylicodontophorus mettami	Africa, Europe, Asia	Very rare

Table 10.5 Geographical distribution of *Cylicostephanus* spp.

Species	Distribution	Comments
Cylicostephanus asymetricus	Africa, Asia, Europe, North America	Very rare
Cylicostephanus bidentatus	Europe, North America	Very rare
Cylicostephanus calicatus	Cosmopolitan	Very common
Cylicostephanus goldi	Cosmopolitan	Common
Cylicostephanus hybridus	Asia, Europe	Rare
Cylicostephanus longibursatus	Cosmopolitan	Very common
Cylicostephanus minutus	Cosmopolitan	Very common
Cylicostephanus ornatus	Asia, Europe	Rare
Cylicostephanus poculatus	Cosmopolitan	Rare
Cylicostephanus skrjabini	Asia	Rare

proposed that the genus *Trichonema* be discarded and replaced by four main genera, namely *Cyathostomum*, *Cylicocyclus*, *Cylicodontophorus* and *Cylicostephanus*, these being collectively referred to as cyathostomes or, more recently, cyathostomins. More detailed descriptions of the individual species within these genera, as listed in Table 10.1, are provided in Chapter 1. Other genera of unknown significance included in this group are *Poteriostomum*, *Craterostomum* and *Oesophagodontus*. Since the majority of species involved are similar, both morphologically and behaviourally, they will be referred to in this text as cyathostomins or 'small strongyles'. Details on the geographical distribution of these species are reported in Tables 10.2–10.5.

Epidemiology: Strongylosis is most frequently a problem in young horses reared on permanent horse pastures, although cases of severe disease may occur in adult animals kept in suburban paddocks and subjected to overcrowding and poor management. Although the preparasitic larval requirements of horse strongyles are similar to those of the trichostrongyles of ruminants, adult horses, unlike cattle, may carry substantial worm burdens and therefore have a considerable influence on the epidemiology of infection. Thus, there are two sources of infection during the grazing season in temperate areas. First, there are infective larvae that developed during the previous grazing season and which have survived on pasture over winter. The second and probably more important source of infective larvae is the eggs passed in the current grazing season by horses, including nursing mares, sharing the same grazing area. Pasture larval levels increase markedly during the summer months when environmental conditions are optimal

for rapid development of eggs to L_3 and may lead to the accumulation of large infections in the autumn. At present, there is little evidence for a consistent periparturient rise in faecal egg output in breeding mares due to a relaxation of immunity, since the egg rise in the spring occurs in both breeding and non-breeding animals and is often unrelated to parturition. There is increasing evidence that many cyathostome L_3 ingested during the autumn show a degree of hypobiosis and remain in the large intestinal mucosa until the following spring. Mass emergence of these larvae results in the severe clinical signs described previously.

Clinical signs and pathology: The major clinical signs associated with heavy infections in animals up to 2–3 years of age are unthriftiness, anaemia and sometimes diarrhoea. Marked clinical signs are less common in older animals, although general performance may be impaired. In temperate countries, an acute syndrome of catarrhal and/or haemorrhagic enteritis with severe diarrhoea, leading to emaciation and in some cases death, in horses and ponies in the

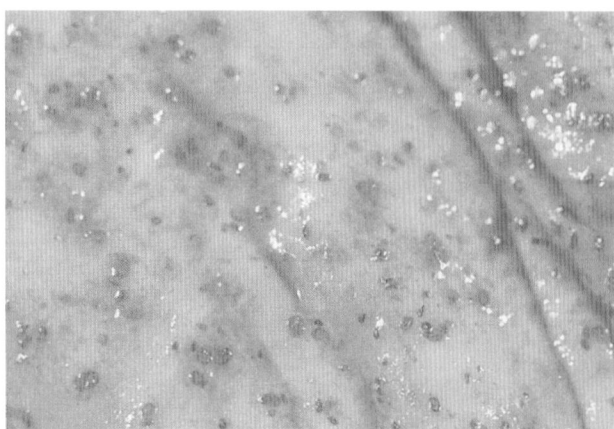

Fig. 10.10 Developing small strongyle larvae in the mucosa of the caecum.

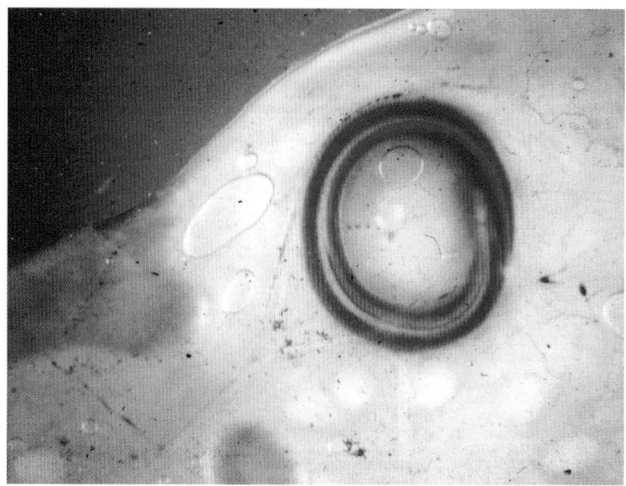

Fig. 10.11 Cyathostomin larva in the mucosa of the caecum visualised by transmural illumination.

spring has been reported; this is associated with the simultaneous mass emergence of cyathostome L_4 from the intestinal mucosa and submucosa. This may have aetiological and epidemiological similarities to type II ostertagiosis in young cattle and is often referred to as acute larval cyathostomosis.

Parasitic larval development of most species takes place entirely in the mucosa of the caecum and colon, but a few penetrate the muscularis and develop in the submucosa. The entry of larval cyathostomes (Fig. 10.10) into the lumina of the tubular glands generally provokes an inflammatory response together with marked goblet cell hypertrophy. Emergence of the bright red L_4 into the gut lumen appears to be associated with massive infiltration of the gut mucosa with eosinophils. Many thousand L_4 may be present, but their pathogenic significance has been little studied. There are, however, reports of heavy natural infections of adult worms and larvae associated with catarrhal and haemorrhagic enteritis, with thickening and oedema of the mucosa, especially in animals of six months to three years of age. Mature parasites are frequently present in large numbers in the lumen of the large intestine; during feeding, those species with small buccal capsules take in only glandular epithelium, while large species may damage deeper layers of the mucosa. Although the erosions caused by individual parasites may be slight, when large numbers are present a desquamative enteritis may result.

Diagnosis: Diagnosis is based on the grazing history and clinical signs of loss of condition and anaemia. Although the finding of typical oval thin-shelled strongyle eggs on faecal examination may be a useful aid to diagnosis, it is important to remember that substantial worm burdens may be associated with faecal egg counts of only a few hundred eggs per gram (epg) due to low fecundity of adult worms, the long prepatent period or the presence of many immature parasites. Frequently, the majority of eggs passed in the faeces of grazing horses will be Cyathostominae (small strongyles) as they are usually present in larger numbers than the Strongylinae (large strongyles). On *post mortem*, it may be possible to visualise the L_4 larvae in the intestinal mucosa using the transmural illumination technique (Fig. 10.11). On some occasions when heavy cyathostome infections in the spring cause severe diarrhoea, thousands of bright red cyathostome L_4, apparently unable to establish, may be present in the faeces (Fig. 10.12).

Control and treatment: Since horses of any age can become infected and excrete eggs, all grazing animals over two months of

age should be treated every 4–8 weeks with an effective broad-spectrum anthelmintic. This regimen will also control infections with other intestinal parasites such as *Parascaris equorum* and *Oxyuris equi*. Any new animals joining a treated group should receive an anthelmintic and be isolated for 48–72 hours before being introduced. If possible, a paddock rotation system should be adopted so that nursing mares and their foals do not graze the same area in successive years. Avoid overstocking.

If horses are housed in the winter, treatment at that time with an anthelmintic effective against larval cyathostomes will reduce the risk of disease due to their mass emergence in the spring. There is evidence that some species of cyathostomes are becoming resistant to benzimidazole compounds, pyrantel and piperazine, and to avoid this it is suggested that these should be used strategically, alternated with chemically unrelated anthelmintics on an annual or six-monthly basis. Faecal samples from groups of horses should be examined at regular intervals to monitor drug efficiency. Selective chemotherapy, targeted at those horses with high faecal egg counts, would reduce the overall usage of anthelmintic and may reduce the selection pressure for development of resistant worms.

The introduction of pasture management techniques may be feasible for some enterprises, such as pasture cleaning twice a week

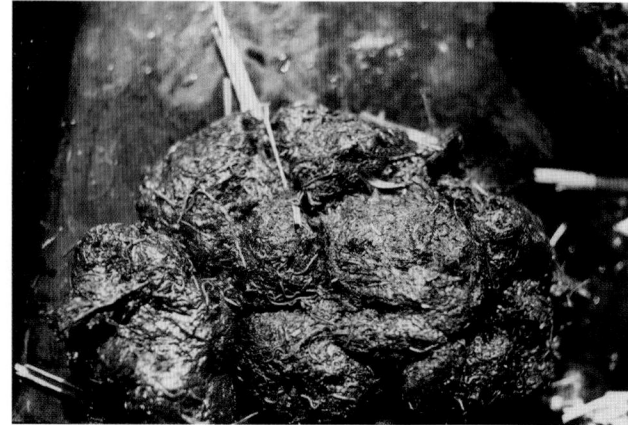

Fig. 10.12 Small strongyles in fresh faeces.

(vacuuming or sweeping) or the alternate grazing of pasture by ruminant livestock.

Treatment for clinical strongylosis should not be necessary if prophylactic measures are adequate. Several broad-spectrum anthelmintics, including the benzimidazoles, pyrantel and the aver-mectins/milbemycins (macrocyclic lactones), are effective in removing lumen-dwelling adult and larval strongyles and these are usually marketed as in-feed or oral preparations. The macrocyclic lactones have the additional advantage of activity against larvae of horse bot flies (*Gasterophilus* spp.), which develop in the stomach. Some modern benzimidazoles and macrocyclic lactones are also efficient against both developing cyathostome larvae in the gut wall and some migrating stages of the large strongyles.

Oxyuris equi

Oxyuris equi (Phylum: Nematoda; Class: Chromadorea; Order: Oxyurida; Family: Oxyuridae), commonly known as the Equine pinworm or Rat-tail, is distributed worldwide and localised in the caecum, colon and rectum of horses and donkeys.

Epidemiology: Although the infective stage may be reached on the skin, more often flakes of material containing eggs are dispersed in the environment by the animal rubbing on stable fittings, fencing posts or other solid objects. Heavy burdens may build up in horses in infected stables and there appears to be little immunity to reinfection.

Pathogenesis: Most of the pathogenic effects of *O. equi* in the intestine are due to the feeding habits of the L_4, which result in small erosions of the mucosa; in heavy infections, these may be widespread and accompanied by an inflammatory response. Normally, a more important effect is the perineal irritation and anal pruritus caused by the adult females during egg laying and the adhesive egg masses. The resultant dull hair coat and loss of hair, as the horse rubs its tail against solid objects to relieve itching, is known as 'rat-tail'.

Clinical signs and pathology: The presence of parasites in the intestine rarely causes any clinical signs. However, intense pruritus around the anus causes the animal to rub on available solid objects, resulting in broken hairs, bare patches and inflammation, scarification and scaling of the skin over the rump and tail head. The intense itching often leads to restlessness and impaired feeding, causing some loss of condition. Small erosions may occur in the mucosa in heavy infections accompanied by a mixed inflammatory cell response.

Diagnosis: This is based on signs of anal pruritus and tail rubbing and the finding of greyish-yellow egg masses on the perineal skin (Fig. 10.13). The large white long-tailed female worms are often seen in the faeces (Fig. 10.14), having been dislodged while laying their eggs. *Oxyuris equi* eggs are rarely found on faecal examination of samples taken from the rectum but may be observed in material from the perineum or taken from the ground. The condition needs to be differentiated from mange.

Control and treatment: A high standard of stable hygiene should be observed, such as the frequent removal of bedding and the provision of feeding racks and water troughs that cannot easily be contaminated by bedding. Immature and adult *O. equi* are susceptible to many broad-spectrum anthelmintics and should be controlled by

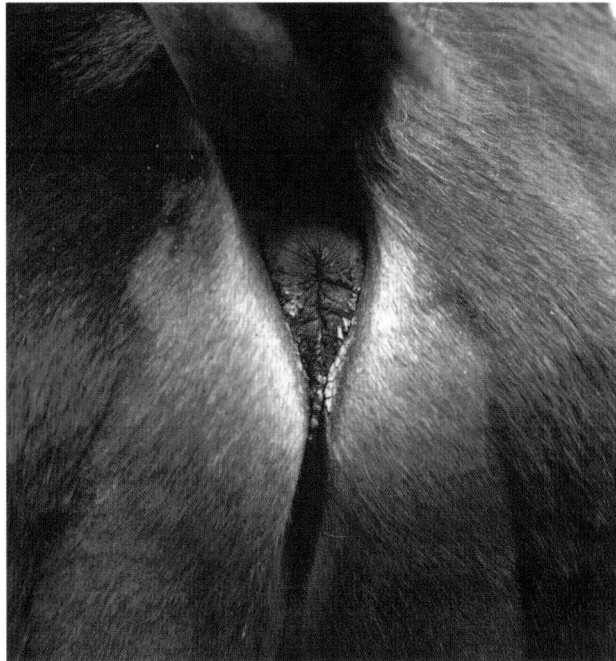

Fig. 10.13 Clumps of *Oxyuris equi* eggs around the rectum of a horse.

routine chemotherapy for the more important horse parasites. Effective anthelmintics include ivermectin, moxidectin, the benzimidazoles (fenbendazole, oxfendazole, oxibendazole) and pyrantel. Newly acquired horses should be treated routinely. Where animals are showing clinical signs, the perineal skin and underside of the tail should be frequently cleaned (about every four days) using a disposable cloth to remove the egg masses prior to their development to L_3 larvae, in addition to anthelmintic treatment.

Notes: Infection with the horse pinworm, *Oxyuris equi*, is extremely common. Although of limited pathogenic significance in the intestine, the female parasites may cause an intense anal pruritus during the process of egg laying.

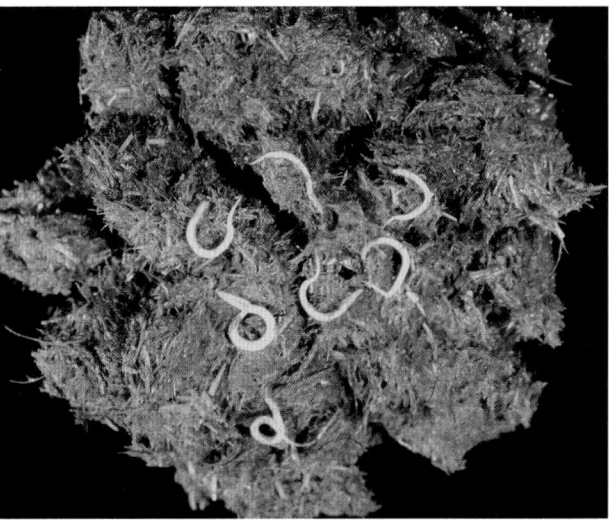

Fig. 10.14 Adult *Oxyuris equi* worms in faeces.

Probstmayria vivipara

Probstmayria vivipara (Phylum: Nematoda; Class: Chromadorea; Order: Oxyurida; Family: Kathlaniidae), commonly known as the Small equine pinworm, is localised in the colon of horses and various equids and probably distributed worldwide, except for some regions of western Europe. The transmission is probably via coprophagia.

Pathogenesis: It is generally considered to be non-pathogenic; although millions of these pinworms may be present, they have never given rise to any clinical signs.

Diagnosis: First-stage larvae may be found in the faeces or larvae and adult worms may be found on necropsy.

Control and treatment: Control is usually not required. The parasite is susceptible to most modern anthelmintics.

Intestinal flukes

Several species of intestinal flukes belonging to the genera *Gastrodiscus* and *Pseudodiscus* are found in the large intestine of horses. Intermediate hosts are snails. Infection is acquired by ingesting the intermediate hosts with vegetation.

Clinical signs and pathology: Adult flukes cause little damage to the intestine. Disease is usually caused by large numbers of immature flukes. Mild infections are subclinical, whereas heavy infections are accompanied by diarrhoea, anaemia, oedema, emaciation and marked weakness. Immature flukes are embedded in the mucosa, causing haemorrhage and necrosis. In heavy infections, there may be catarrhal and haemorrhagic enteritis.

Diagnosis: Diagnosis is based on the presence of eggs in faeces or immature flukes in fluid faeces.

Control and treatment: Wet pastures or swamps where the intermediate hosts are found should be avoided. Flukicidal drugs, such as nitroxynil, oxyclozanide, closantel, triclabendazole or albendazole and netobimin, are active against the adult flukes; triclabendazole 10 mg/kg or closantel 7 mg/kg are active against immature flukes.

Parasites of the respiratory system

Rhinoestrus purpureus

Rhinoestrus purpureus (Phylum: Arthropoda; Class: Insecta: Order: Diptera; Family: Oestridae), commonly known as the Horse nasal bot fly, is localised in the nasal passages of horses, donkeys and occasionally humans. It is found in Russia, Ukraine and Central Asia.

Epidemiology: Adults are on the wing in midsummer. Usually only one generation per year occurs, although a second may be observed in some areas.

Pathogenesis: This species is a serious veterinary problem in areas such as Russia, and infestation by large numbers of larvae in the throat may result in a high level of mortality. Catarrh, infiltration of inflammatory cells and squamous metaplasia, characterised by conversion of secretory epithelium to stratified squamous type, may be observed. Immune responses by the host to infestation may be recorded.

Clinical signs and pathology: Nasal discharge, rubbing, sneezing, unthriftiness, circling and lack of coordination. Secondary bacterial infections are common.

Diagnosis: Larvae may be observed in the nasal cavities, throat and base of the tongue.

Control and treatment: Area-wide control may be impractical; herd treatment may be given twice a year, the first at the beginning of summer to kill newly acquired larvae, and the second in midwinter to kill any overwintering larvae. Where the numbers of larvae are small, it may not be economically viable to treat. However, in heavy infections, closantel, nitroxynil and the endectocides ivermectin, doramectin and moxidectin are highly effective, as are the organophosphates trichlorphon and dichlorvos.

Dictyocaulus arnfieldi

Dictyocaulus arnfieldi (Phylum: Nematoda; Class: Chromadorea; Order: Rhabditida; Family: Dictyocaulidae), commonly known as the Equine lungworm, is distributed worldwide and localised in the lungs of donkeys, other equids and occasionally horses.

Epidemiology: Donkeys acquire infection as foals and yearlings and tend to remain infected, presumably through re-exposure, all their lives. Horses are thought to acquire infection mainly from pastures contaminated by donkeys during the summer months. Most commonly, this occurs when donkeys are grazed as companion animals with horses. However, natural infection in horses can occur in the absence of donkeys. In horses, the prevalence of *D. arnfieldi* is difficult to establish since infections only occasionally achieve patency. *Pilobolus* fungi may play a role in the dissemination of *D. arnfieldi* larvae from faeces, as in *D. viviparus*.

Clinical signs and pathology: The characteristic lesion is similar in both horses and donkeys and is somewhat different from bovine parasitic bronchitis. Despite the prevalence of patent *D. arnfieldi* infection in donkeys, overt clinical signs are rarely seen; however, on close examination slight hyperpnoea and harsh lung sounds may be detected. This absence of significant clinical abnormality may be partly a reflection of the fact that donkeys are rarely required to perform sustained exercise. Infection is much less prevalent in horses. However, patent infections may develop in foals and these are not usually associated with clinical signs. In older horses, infections rarely become patent but are often associated with persistent coughing, nasal discharge and an increased respiratory rate. In the caudal lung lobes particularly, there are raised circumscribed areas of over-inflated pulmonary tissue 3–5 cm in diameter. On section, at the centre of each lesion is a small bronchus containing lungworms and mucopurulent exudate. Microscopically, the epithelium is hyperplastic with an increase in the size and number of mucus-secreting cells while the lamina propria is heavily infiltrated and often surrounded by inflammatory cells, predominantly lymphocytes.

Diagnosis: In donkeys, patent infections are common and L_1 are readily recovered from fresh faeces. In horses, although a history of donkey contact and clinical signs may be suggestive of *D. arnfieldi* infection, it is often not possible to confirm a diagnosis by demonstrating larvae in the faeces, as many infections do not reach patency. In practice, a presumptive diagnosis of lungworm infection in horses is often only possible in retrospect, when resolution of the clinical signs occurs after treatment.

Control and treatment: Ideally, horses and donkeys should not be grazed together but if they are, it is advisable to treat the donkeys, preferably in the spring, with a suitable anthelmintic. A similar regimen should be practised in donkey studs and visiting animals should be isolated in separate paddocks. Successful treatment of both horses and donkeys has been reported using ivermectin or some benzimidazoles, such as fenbendazole and mebendazole.

Echinococcus equinus

For more details see Parasites of the liver.

Parasites of the liver

Fasciola hepatica

Fasciola hepatica (Phylum: Platyhelminthes; Class: Trematoda; Order: Plagiorchiida; Family: Fasciolidae), commonly known as the Liver fluke, is distributed worldwide and localised in the liver of sheep, cattle, goats, horses, deer, humans and other mammals. This parasite has snails of the genus *Galba* as intermediate hosts (for more details see Chapter 9).

Echinococcus equinus

Echinococcus equinus, synonym *Echinococcus granulosus* (Phylum: Platyhelminthes; Class: Cestoda; Order: Cyclophyllidea; Family: Taeniidae), commonly known as the Dwarf dog tapeworm, causes a disease called hydatidosis and is localised mainly in liver and lungs of intermediate hosts (i.e. horses, donkeys) and small intestine of definitive hosts (dogs, foxes). This parasite occurs mainly in Europe.

Epidemiology: Equine hydatidosis is mostly common in Europe, and in other parts of the world most cases have been recorded in imported European horses. The strain is highly specific for the horse and the eggs do not develop in sheep. The domestic dog and red fox are the final hosts, and the cycle in countries of high prevalence depends on access by dogs to infected equine viscera. On mainland Europe, the most likely source is offal from horse abattoirs; in Britain the viscera of hunting horses, which are fed to foxhounds. The horse strain does not appear to be infective to humans.

Pathogenesis and clinical signs: Infection in horses is generally not associated with clinical signs.

Control and treatment: Control is based on the regular treatment of dogs to eliminate the adult tapeworms and on the prevention of infection in dogs by exclusion from their diet of animal material containing hydatids. This is achieved by denying dogs access to abattoirs and, where possible, by proper disposal of equine viscera. In some countries these measures have been supported by legislation, with penalties when they are disregarded. No treatment is necessary in horses.

Notes: Considerable phenotypic and genetic variability has been observed within the species *E. granulosus* and several strains have been identified based on molecular genotyping. New data demonstrate that '*E. granulosus*' is an assembly of several, rather diverse strains and genotypes (designated G1–G10) that show fundamental differences, not only in their epidemiology but also in their pathogenicity to humans. *Echinococcus equinus* was formerly known as the horse strain (G4) of *E. granulosus*.

Parasites of the circulatory system

Elaeophora bohmi

Elaeophora bohmi (Phylum: Nematoda; Class: Chromadorea; Order: Spirurida; Family: Onchocercidae) is localised in the blood vessels of horses and other equids and is distributed in Europe (in particular Austria) and Middle East (Iran). This parasite has tabanids and other flies as intermediate hosts. Because of the innocuous nature of the infection in equines, the distribution of the species in these hosts is not completely known.

Pathogenesis: Found in the large veins and arteries, often of lower limbs where they usually induce very little pathological reaction.

Clinical signs and pathology: Infection is usually asymptomatic. Severe infection can cause thickening of the wall of arteries and veins, commonly those in the extremities, and nodules containing calcified worms may be present. The parasites selectively involve the media of the vessels, with the fibrous reaction that develops sometimes causing stenosis of the lumen. The worms are coiled and entwined among the tissue layers, provoking parasitic granulomas with intense eosinophilic and macrophage infiltration. In longstanding infections, the nodular and fibrous thickenings are visible in the vessel walls.

Diagnosis: This is not normally required. Infection is usually diagnosed as an incidental finding on *post mortem* examination of thickened blood vessels, or those containing nodules.

Control and treatment: Any reduction in vector numbers will reduce transmission. Treatment is unknown, although repeated administration of diethylcarbamazine is effective, but the risk of fatalities from the presence of dead worms in the arteries should be recognised.

Schistosomes

Schistosomes are flukes found in the circulatory system. The sexes are separate, the small adult female lying permanently in a longitudinal groove, the gynaecophoric canal, in the body of the male. The genus has been divided into four groups – *haematobium*, *indicum*, *mansoni* and *japonicum* – but the genus as currently defined is paraphyletic so revisions are likely.

Indicum group

Schistosoma nasale

Schistosoma nasale, synonym *Schistosoma nasalis* (Phylum: Platyhelminthes; Class: Trematoda; Order: Strigeidida; Family: Schistosomatidae), causes a condition commonly known as the Snoring disease, is localised in the nasal mucosa veins of cattle, goats, sheep, buffalo and horses and occurs in India, Pakistan and Southeast Asia. This parasite has snails (*Galba luteola*, *G. acuminata*, *Indoplanorbis exustus*) as intermediate hosts.

Epidemiology: The epidemiology is totally dependent on water as a medium for infection of both the intermediate and final hosts.

Pathogenesis: In heavy infections there is a copious mucopurulent discharge, snoring and dyspnoea. The main pathogenic effects are associated with the eggs, which cause abscess formation in the mucosa. Fibrous granulomatous growths occur which may occlude the nasal passages.

Clinical signs and pathology: Coryza, sneezing, dyspnoea and snoring. The mucosa of the nasal sinuses is studded with small abscesses that contain the eggs of the worms, and later show much fibrous tissue and proliferating epithelium.

Diagnosis: Infection is confirmed by the presence of the spindle-shaped eggs in the nasal discharge.

Japonicum group

Schistosoma japonicum

Schistosoma japonicum (Phylum: Platyhelminthes; Class: Trematoda; Order: Strigeidida; Family: Schistosomatidae), commonly known as the Blood fluke, causes a disease commonly known as Bilharziosis, and is localised in the portal and mesenteric veins of cattle, horses, sheep, goats, dogs, cats, rabbits, pigs, rodents and humans. This parasite occurs in South and East Asia and has snails belonging to the genus *Oncomelania* as intermediate hosts.

Trypanosomes

See Chapter 2 (Family Trypanosomatidae) for a general description and Chapter 8 for detailed descriptions of individual species of trypanosomes and their control.

Trypanosoma brucei brucei

Trypanosoma brucei brucei (Phylum: Euglenozoa; Class: Kinetoplastea; Order: Trypanosomatida; Family: Trypanosomatidae) causes a disease commonly known as Nagana, is localised in the blood but also myocardium, central nervous system (CNS) and reproductive tract of cattle, horses, donkeys, zebu, sheep, goats, camels, pigs, dogs, cats and wild game species and occurs in sub-Saharan Africa.

Pathogenesis: In horses, *T. brucei brucei* infections may be acute or chronic, often accompanied by oedema of the limbs and genitalia.

Table 10.6 Drugs used in the treatment of *Trypanosoma brucei brucei* infection.

Drug	Recommended dose	Comments
Diminazene aceturate	3–10 mg/kg i.m.	Ruminants, pigs, horses. Contraindicated in dogs and camels
Isometamidium	0.25–1 mg/kg i.m.	Ruminants, horses, dogs. Local reaction
Quinapyramine sulfate	3–5 mg/kg i.m.	Horses only. Banned in ruminants
Quinapyramine methylsulfate	5 mg/kg s.c.	Dogs
Suramin	7–10 mg/kg i.m. or i.v.	Horses, camels. Local and systemic reactions

Treatment: Horses are particularly susceptible to *T. brucei brucei* and suramin and quinapyramine methylsulfate are the drugs of choice (Table 10.6). Diminazene is relatively toxic to horses. Despite treatment, relapse from CNS infection is likely.

Trypanosoma brucei evansi

Trypanosoma brucei evansi, synonyms *Trypanosoma evansi* or *Trypanosoma equinum* (Phylum: Euglenozoa; Class: Kinetoplastea; Order: Trypanosomatida; Family: Trypanosomatidae), causes a disease commonly known as Surra, El debab, Mbori, Murrina, Mal de caderas, Doukane or Dioufar thaga, and is localised in blood of horses, donkeys, camels, cattle, zebu, goats, pigs, dogs, water buffalo, elephants, capybaras, tapirs, mongooses, ocelots, deer and other wild animals. Many laboratory and wild animals can be infected experimentally. This parasite occurs in North Africa, Central and South America, central and southern Russia and parts of Asia (India, Myanmar, Malaysia, southern China, Indonesia, Philippines); it is mechanically transmitted by biting insects.

Epidemiology: This species, although closely related to the salivarian trypanosome *T. brucei brucei*, is mechanically transmitted by biting insects; the common vectors are horse flies (*Tabanus*) but *Stomoxys*, *Haematopota* and *Lyperosia* can also transmit the infection. No cyclical development occurs in the vector, with the trypanosomes remaining in the proboscis. In Central and South America, the vampire bat is a vector and can transmit the disease (murrina).

Pathogenesis: Depending on the virulence of the strain and the susceptibility of the individual host, the disease may be acute in horses, camels and dogs. Other domestic species, such as cattle, buffalo and pig, are commonly infected but overt disease is uncommon, and their main significance is as reservoirs of infection. The syndrome is similar to that caused by the tsetse-transmitted trypanosomes. Anaemia is caused mainly by extravascular haemolysis through erythrophagocytosis in the mononuclear phagocytic systems of the spleen, liver and lungs; as the disease becomes chronic, there may be decreased haemoglobin synthesis. Leucopenia and thrombocytopenia are caused by mechanisms that predispose leucocytes and platelets to phagocytosis. Immunological mechanisms in the pathogenesis lead to extensive proliferation of activated macrophages, which engulf or destroy erythrocytes, leucocytes, platelets and haematopoietic cells.

Clinical signs: All domestic animals are susceptible, but the disease is only fatal in horses, camels and dogs. The disease is manifested by pyrexia, progressive anaemia, loss of condition and depression. Recurrent episodes of fever occur during the course of disease. Oedematous swellings, ranging from cutaneous plaques to frank oedema of the ventral abdomen and genitalia, and petechial haemorrhages of the serous membranes are often observed. Abortions have been reported in buffalo in Asia. Nervous signs may occur and include circling, incoordination, staggering, head pressing, paraplegia, paralysis and prostration.

Pathology: The carcass is often pale and emaciated and there may be oedematous swellings in the lower part of the abdomen and genital organs with serous atrophy of fat. The liver, lymph nodes and spleen are enlarged, and the viscera are congested. Petechiae may appear on lymph nodes, pericardium and intestinal mucosa. The liver is hypertrophic and congested, with degeneration and necrosis of the hepatocytes, dilation of blood vessels and parenchymal infiltration of mononuclear cells. A non-suppurative myocarditis, sometimes associated with hydropericarditis, has been reported, accompanied by degeneration and necrosis of the myocardial tissue. Other lesions can include glomerulonephritis, renal tubular necrosis, non-suppurative meningoencephalomyelitis, focal poliomalacia, keratitis, ophthalmitis, orchitis, interstitial pneumonia and bone marrow atrophy. Splenic and lymph node hypertrophy occur during the acute phase, but the lymphoid tissues are usually exhausted and fibrotic in the chronic stage.

Diagnosis: The clinical signs of the disease, although indicative, are not pathognomonic. Confirmation of clinical diagnosis depends on the demonstration of trypanosomes in the blood; if a herd or flock is involved, a representative number of blood samples should be examined since, in individual animals, the parasitaemia may be in remission or in long-standing cases may be extremely scanty. Occasionally, when the parasitaemia is massive, it is possible to detect motile trypanosomes in fresh smears of blood. More usually, both thick and thin smears of blood are air-dried and examined later. Thick smears, de-haemoglobinised before staining with Giemsa or Leishman's stain, offer a better chance of finding trypanosomes, while the stained thin smears are used for differentiation of the trypanosome species. More sensitive techniques utilise centrifugation in a microhaematocrit tube followed by microscopic examination of the interface between the buffy coat and the plasma; alternatively, the tube may be snapped, the buffy coat expressed on to a slide, and the contents examined under dark-ground or phase-contrast microscopy for motile trypanosomes. With these techniques, the packed red cell volume is also obtained which is of indirect value in diagnosis if one can eliminate other causes of anaemia, especially helminthosis. A number of serological tests have been described, including the indirect fluorescent antibody test (IFAT) and ELISA, and have been partially validated but require further evaluation and standardisation.

Control and treatment: Suramin or quinapyramine (Trypacide®) are the drugs of choice for treatment and also confer a short period of prophylaxis. For more prolonged protection, a modified quinapyramine known as Trypacide Pro-Salt is also available. Unfortunately, drug resistance, at least to suramin, is not uncommon.

Notes: The original distribution of this parasite coincided with that of the camel and is often associated with arid deserts and semi-arid steppes.

Table 10.7 Drugs used in the treatment of *Trypanosoma congolense congolense* infection.

Drug	Recommended dose	Comments
Diminazene aceturate	3–5 mg/kg i.m.	Ruminants, pigs, horses. Contraindicated in dogs and camels
Homidium bromide Homidium chloride	1 mg/kg s.c.	Cattle, sheep, goats and horses. Prophylaxis for six weeks
Isometamidium	0.25–1 mg/kg i.m.	Ruminants, horses, dogs. Local reaction
Pyrithidium bromide	2–2.5 mg/kg i.m.	Cattle, sheep, horses, donkeys. Prophylaxis for four months

Trypanosoma congolense

Trypanosoma congolense (Phylum: Euglenozoa; Class: Kinetoplastea; Order: Trypanosomatida; Family: Trypanosomatidae) causes a disease commonly known as Nagana, Paranagana, Gambia fever, Ghindi or Gobial, and is localised in the blood of cattle, sheep, goats, horses, camels, dogs and pigs. This parasite occurs in sub-Saharan Africa and has antelopes, giraffes, zebras, elephants and warthogs as reservoir hosts.

Pathogenesis: The signs caused by this species are similar to those caused by other trypanosomes, but the CNS is not affected. Anaemia is caused mainly by extravascular haemolysis through erythrophagocytosis in the mononuclear phagocytic systems of the spleen, liver and lungs but as the disease becomes chronic, there may be decreased haemoglobin synthesis. Leucopenia and thrombocytopenia are caused by mechanisms that predispose leucocytes and platelets to phagocytosis. Immunological mechanisms in the pathogenesis lead to extensive proliferation of activated macrophages, which engulf or destroy erythrocytes, leucocytes, platelets and haematopoietic cells.

Clinical signs: Symptoms include intermittent fever, anaemia, oedema of the limbs and dependent parts, progressive weakness and loss of condition.

Treatment: Homidium salts, isometamidium and pyrithidium can be used for treatment. Diminazene is relatively toxic to horses (Table 10.7).

Babesiosis/theileriosis

Two species, the small *Theileria equi* (formerly *Babesia equi*) and the large *B. caballi*, are of importance in horses.

Babesia caballi

Babesia caballi (Phylum: Apicomplexa; Class: Aconoidasida; Order: Piroplasmida; Family: Babesiidae) is localised in the blood of horses and donkeys and its distribution is related to the presence of ticks: Europe, Asia, Africa, South and Central America, southern USA and Australia.

Epidemiology: *Babesia caballi* is transmitted by a variety of tick species, including *Dermacentor*, *Hyalomma* and *Rhipicephalus*. Tick vectors include *Dermacentor reticulatus*, *D. variabilis*, *D. albipictus*,

D. silvarum, D. nitens, Hyalomma excavatum, H. scupense, Rhipicephalus bursa, R. sanguineus and others according to geographical location. Young animals are less susceptible than old ones. Recovered horses may remain carriers for 10 months to four years.

Pathogenesis: Death, if it occurs, is a result of organ failure, which in turn is due not only to destruction of the erythrocytes, with resultant anaemia, oedema and icterus, but also to the clogging of the capillaries of various organs by parasitised cells and free parasites. The stasis from this sludging causes degeneration of the endothelial cells of the small blood vessels, anoxia, accumulation of toxic metabolic products, capillary fragility and eventual perivascular escape of erythrocytes and macroscopic haemorrhage. The incubation period is 6–10 days.

Clinical signs and pathology: The disease may be chronic or acute, and in either case can be mild or fatal. Haemoglobinuria is rare but fever, anaemia and icterus are present. Gastroenteritis is common. Locomotor signs are usually present and posterior paralysis may occur. Principal lesions include splenomegaly with soft dark red splenic pulp and prominent splenic corpuscles. The liver is enlarged and yellowish-brown and the gallbladder is distended with thick dark bile. The mucosa of the intestine is oedematous and icteric with patches of haemorrhage. Subcutaneous, subserous and intramuscular connective tissues are oedematous and icteric. The blood is thin and watery, and the plasma tinged with red.

Diagnosis: Examination of blood smears, stained with Romanowsky stains such as Giemsa, will reveal the parasites in the red cells. Species identification is essential with regard to choice of therapeutic drugs. The paired merozoites joined at their posterior ends are considered to be a diagnostic feature of *B. caballi*. Examinations should be made as early as possible, since the parasites begin to disappear from the peripheral blood after the fifth day. The complement fixation test (CFT) is the primary screening test used for horses travelling between countries. Because the CFT may not identify all infected animals, especially those that have been treated, and because of anti-complementary reactions produced by some sera, the IFAT is used as a supplementary test. Test sera are inactivated for 30 minutes at 60 °C and tested in dilutions of 1:5 to 1:5120. A lysis of 50% is recorded as positive, with the titre being the greatest serum dilution giving 50% lysis. A titre of 1:5 is regarded as positive. Anti-complementary samples are examined by the IFAT, with which the recognition of a strong positive reaction is relatively simple, but any differentiation between weak positive and negative reactions requires considerable experience in interpretation. Each sample of serum is tested against an antigen of *B. caballi*. Test, positive and negative control sera are diluted from 1:80 to 1:1280. Sera diluted 1:80 or more that show strong fluorescence are usually considered to be positive, although due consideration is also given to the patterns of fluorescence of the positive and negative controls.

Control and treatment: Immunity in horses after infection lasts for more than one year and horses are therefore protected in enzootic areas even with the seasonal fluctuation of the tick population. Tick control is essential. Special attention should be paid to the ears, region under the tail and between the hindlegs. Horses introduced into endemic areas are very susceptible and should therefore receive special attention. Treatment of equine piroplasmosis is based on a combination of supportive and symptomatic treatment as well as chemotherapy. Supportive treatment is essential in the treatment of acute disease and may include blood transfusion, fluid therapy, vitamins and good nutrition. The chemotherapy of babesiosis in

Table 10.8 Drugs used in the treatment of *Babesia caballi* infection.

Drug	Recommended dose	Frequency	Comments
Imidocarb dipropionate	2–3 mg/kg i.m.	Two doses at 24-hour interval	Pain at injection site
Diminazene aceturate	5 mg/kg i.m.	Two doses at 24-hour interval	Low therapeutic index
Amicarbalide di-isethionate	9–10 mg/kg i.m.	Single or repeat at 24 hours	Low therapeutic index

horses is difficult and, due to the toxicity of most effective drugs, care must be taken in the administration of the correct dosage. The most commonly used drugs for chemotherapy of equine piroplasmosis are as follows (Table 10.8).
- Imidocarb dipropionate, given intramuscularly at 2–3 mg/kg body weight in doses 24 hours apart, will usually be sufficient for sterilisation of *B. caballi* infections.
- Amicarbalide di-isethionate produces clinical recovery at a dose rate of 9–10 mg/kg as a single dose, or as a divided dose over 24 hours. High doses may reportedly cause pronounced side-effects.
- Diminazene aceturate 5 mg/kg given twice at 24-hour intervals produces clinical recovery.

Theileria equi

Theileria equi, synonyms *Babesia equi*, *Nuttalia equi* (Phylum: Apicomplexa; Class: Aconoidasida; Order: Piroplasmida; Family: Theileriidae), is localised in the blood of horses and donkeys.

Epidemiology: *Theileria equi* is transmitted by a variety of tick species, including *Dermacentor*, *Hyalomma* and *Rhipicephalus*. Vectors are *Dermacentor reticulatus*, *D. albipictus*, *Hyalomma marginatum* (*H. detritum*), *H. scupense*, *Rhipicephalus bursa* in Russia and former Soviet states; *R. evertsi* in equatorial Africa; *H. anatolicum* and *H. marginatum* in Greece; *H. dromedarii* and *R. sanguineus* in central Asia. The vectors in the USA include *D. variabilis*, *D. albipictus*, *D. (Anocentor) nitens* and *R. sanguineus*; and in South America *D. (A.) nitens*.

Pathogenesis: Death, if it occurs, is a result of organ failure, which in turn is due not only to destruction of the erythrocytes, with resultant anaemia, oedema and icterus, but also to the clogging of the capillaries of various organs by parasitised cells and free parasites. The stasis from this sludging causes degeneration of the endothelial cells of the small blood vessels, anoxia, accumulation of toxic metabolic products, capillary fragility and eventual perivascular escape of erythrocytes and macroscopic haemorrhage.

Clinical signs and pathology: The incubation period following an infective tick bite is 10–21 days. The first sign of disease is a rise in temperature followed by listlessness, depression, marked thirst, inappetence, lacrimation and blepharitis. The most characteristic sign is icterus. There is marked anaemia and more than half the erythrocytes are often destroyed, leading to haemoglobinuria. Oedema of the head, legs and ventral part of the body is sometimes present, although posterior paralysis, sometimes seen in *B. caballi* infection, is absent. Affected animals are constipated and pass small hard balls of faeces covered with yellow mucus. The animals lose condition fairly rapidly and may become extremely emaciated.

Haemorrhages are present on the mucosa of the nasal passages, vagina and third eyelid. The disease lasts 7–12 days but may be peracute, with death occurring in 1–2 days, or may be chronic and last for weeks. Mortality is usually about 10% but may reach 50%. Recovery is slow.

Emaciation, icterus, anaemia and oedema are seen at *post mortem* examination. There are accumulations of fluid in the pericardial sac and body cavities, and the fat is gelatinous and yellow. The spleen is enlarged, with soft dark brown pulp. The lymph nodes are swollen and sometimes inflamed. The liver is swollen, engorged and brownish-yellow, and the hepatic lobules are yellow in the centre and greenish-yellow round the edges. The kidneys are pale yellow and may contain petechial haemorrhages. There are petechial or ecchymotic haemorrhages on the mucosa of the intestine and stomach.

Diagnosis: Examination of blood smears, stained with Romanowsky stains such as Giemsa, will reveal the parasites in the red cells. Species identification is essential with regard to choice of therapeutic drugs. The tetrad or Maltese cross arrangement is a diagnostic feature of *T. equi* (see Fig. 2.94). Examinations should be made as early as possible since the parasites begin to disappear from the peripheral blood after the fifth day.

The CFT is the primary screening test used for horses travelling between countries. Because the CFT may not identify all infected animals, especially those that have been treated, and because of anti-complementary reactions produced by some sera, the IFAT is used as a supplementary test. Test sera are inactivated for 30 minutes at 60 °C and tested in dilutions of 1:5 to 1:5120. A lysis of 50% is recorded as positive, with the titre being the greatest serum dilution giving 50% lysis. A titre of 1:5 is regarded as positive.

Anti-complementary samples are examined by the IFAT, with which the recognition of a strong positive reaction is relatively simple, but any differentiation between weak positive and negative reactions requires considerable experience in interpretation. Each sample of serum is tested against an antigen of *T. equi*. Test, positive and negative control sera are diluted from 1:80 to 1:1280. Sera diluted 1:80 or more that show strong fluorescence are usually considered to be positive, although due consideration is also given to the patterns of fluorescence of the positive and negative controls.

Treatment: Imidocarb dipropionate given intramuscularly at 2–3 mg/kg body weight in doses 24 hours apart will bring about recovery from *T. equi* infections, but not sterilisation of infection. The use of four doses of 4 mg/kg body weight at 72-hour intervals is reported to sterilise *T. equi* infections, but this high-dose therapy may cause severe side-effects, such as extreme restlessness, sweating and signs of abdominal pain. Treated horses may become seronegative to CFT but remain positive to IFAT and infective to tick vectors. Treatment with amicarbalide di-isethionate produces clinical recovery at a dose of 9–10 mg/kg as a single dose, or as a divided dose over 24 hours. High doses may reportedly cause pronounced side-effects. Diminazene aceturate 6–12 mg/kg body weight given twice in a 48-hour period may be required for clinical recovery (Table 10.9).

Notes: There is no cross-immunity between *T. equi* and *B. caballi*. Young animals are less seriously affected than adults and mixed infections of these parasites can occur.

Table 10.9 Drugs used in the treatment of *Theileria equi* infection.

Drug	Recommended dose	Frequency	Comments
Imidocarb dipropionate	2–3 mg/kg i.m. or 4 mg/kg	Two doses at 24-hour interval or four doses at 72-hour interval for sterility	Pain at injection site
Diminazene aceturate	6–12 mg/kg i.m.	Two doses at 48-hour interval	Low therapeutic index
Amicarbalide di-isethionate	9–10 mg/kg i.m.	Single or repeat at 24 hours	Low therapeutic index

Neorickettsia risticii

Neorickettsia risticii, synonym *Ehrlichia risticii* (Phylum: Proteobacteria; Class: Alphaproteobacteria; Order: Rickettsiales; Family: Anaplasmataceae), causes a disease commonly known as Equine monocytic ehrlichiosis, Potomac horse fever, Ditch fever, Shasta River crud or Equine ehrlichial colitis. It is an obligate intracellular bacterium localised in the reproductive tract of horses, rarely dogs and cats and occurs in the USA.

Epidemiology: The disease is seen in spring, summer and early autumn and is associated with pastures bordering creeks or rivers. *Neorickettsia risticii* has been identified in freshwater snails and isolated from trematodes released from the snails. DNA has been detected in 13 species of immature and adult caddisflies (Trichoptera), mayflies (Ephemeroptera), damselflies (Odonata, Zygoptera), dragonflies (Odonata, Anisoptera) and stoneflies (Plecoptera). Transmission studies using *N. risticii*-infected caddisflies have reproduced the clinical disease. One route of exposure is believed to be inadvertent ingestion of aquatic insects that carry *N. risticii* in the metacercarial stage of a trematode. The incubation period is 10–18 days. Clinically ill horses are not contagious and can be housed with susceptible horses.

Pathogenesis: Potomac horse fever is an acute enterocolitis syndrome producing mild colic, fever and diarrhoea in horses of all ages, as well as abortion in pregnant mares. Following ingestion within the insect or trematode, the organism is taken up by cells of the monocyte/macrophage series and the organisms accumulate in the reticuloendothelial cells in the wall of the large colon. The infection of enterocytes of the small and large intestine results in acute colitis, which is one of the principal clinical signs. Other signs vary from transient mild fever to severe diarrhoea, which become apparent after 12–18 days. Colic of variable severity and abdominal distension may precede the onset of diarrhoea in about 25% of cases. As well as blood and lymphoid tissue, the organisms have been detected in macrophages, crypt endothelial cells and mast cells in the wall of the colon, caecum and small intestine, where it is thought that a localised endotoxaemia may lead to electrolyte imbalance. A bluish 'toxic ring' surrounding the teeth may be present and affected horses may also exhibit mild to moderate tachypnoea and tachycardia. Mild to severe laminitis has been reported following the onset of diarrhoea. Infection has also been associated with abortion in mares.

Clinical signs and pathology: Fever, depression, leucopenia, dehydration, laminitis and diarrhoea. On *post mortem*, there are few or no gross pathological changes although histological changes include focal degeneration of endothelial cells in the colon, leading to small ulcerative lesions and patchy hyperaemia in the large intestine. There is marked depletion of goblet cells and dilation of intestinal crypts.

Diagnosis: A provisional diagnosis is often based on the presence of typical clinical signs and the seasonal and geographic occurrence of the disease. Examination of peripheral blood smears is of no value as infected monocytes are present in small numbers in the blood. A definitive diagnosis should be based on isolation or detection of *N. risticii* from the blood or faeces of infected horses. Although serological tests such as IFAT or ELISA exist, serological testing is of limited value as a diagnostic tool, although many infected horses have high antibody titres at the time of infection. Because of the high prevalence of false-positive titres, interpretation of the IFAT in individual horses is difficult. Isolation of the agent in cell culture, although possible, is time-consuming and not routinely available in many diagnostic laboratories. A recently developed real-time polymerase chain reaction (PCR) assay allows the detection of *N. risticii* DNA within two hours, making this a much more feasible test for routine diagnostic examination. To enhance the chances of detection of *N. risticii*, the assay should be performed on a blood as well as a faecal sample, as the presence of the organism in blood and faeces may not necessarily coincide.

Control and treatment: Several inactivated whole-cell vaccines based on the same strain of *N. risticii* are commercially available, although they are only marginally protective in the field. Reduction of snail numbers in rivers and ditches may be attempted to lessen sources of infection. Oxytetracycline administered at a dose of 6.6 mg/kg i.v. for five days is highly effective if given early in the clinical course of the disease. Supportive therapy with fluids, electrolytes, non-steroidal anti-inflammatory drugs (NSAIDs) and antidiarrhoeals may also be indicated in animals exhibiting signs of enterocolitis. Laminitis, if it develops, is usually severe and often refractory to treatment.

Notes: The causative agent, formerly known as *Ehrlichia risticii*, has recently been renamed *Neorickettsia risticii* because of its lesser genetic relationships to other *Ehrlichia* groups.

Anaplasma phagocytophilum

Anaplasma phagocytophilum, synonym *Ehrlichia equi* (Phylum: Proteobacteria; Class: Alphaproteobacteria; Order: Rickettsiales; Family: Anaplasmataceae), causes a disease commonly known as Equine granulocytic ehrlichiosis. It is an obligate intracellular bacterium localised in the blood of sheep, cattle, dogs, horses, deer, rodents and humans and occurs in the USA, South America and Europe.

Epidemiology: In endemic areas the disease is seasonal, occurring during periods of peak tick activity. In the USA, transmission to horses is by the tick *Ixodes pacificus* (western black-legged tick).

Pathogenesis: Equine granulocytic ehrlichiosis is an infectious, non-contagious, seasonal disease. Severity of signs varies with age of the animal and duration of the illness. Signs may be mild. Horses less than one year old may have a fever only. Horses 1–3 years old develop fever, depression, mild limb oedema and ataxia. Adults exhibit the characteristic signs of fever, partial anorexia, depression, reluctance to move, limb oedema, petechiation and jaundice. The fever, which is highest during the first 1–3 days (39.5–40 °C),

persists for 6–12 days. Rarely, myocardial vasculitis may cause transient ventricular arrhythmias. Any concurrent infection can be exacerbated. Cytoplasmic inclusion bodies are few during the first 48 hours and increase to 30–40% of circulating neutrophils at days 3–5 of infection.

Clinical signs and pathology: Fever, depression, limb oedema, jaundice and ataxia. Gross petechiation, ecchymoses and oedema develop in the subcutis and fascia. Vasculitis is regional, with the subcutis and fascia of the legs predominantly affected.

Diagnosis: Demonstration of the characteristic cytoplasmic inclusion bodies in blood smears is diagnostic. PCR can detect *A. phagocytophilum* DNA in unclotted blood or buffy coat smears. An IFAT can detect rising antibody titres to *A. phagocytophilum*.

Control and treatment: Recovered horses are solidly immune for more than two years. There is no vaccine. Oxytetracycline and tetracycline 7 mg/kg i.v. for eight days has eliminated the infection. Horses with severe ataxia and oedema may benefit from short-term corticosteroid treatment (dexamethasone 20 mg for 2–3 days).

Notes: The causal riskettsial agent was initially termed *Ehrlichia equi* but, based on DNA sequence relationships, the organism is now referred to as *Anaplasma phagocytophilum*.

Parasites of the nervous system

Thelazia lacrymalis

Thelazia lacrymalis (Phylum: Nematoda; Class: Chromadorea; Order: Spirurida; Family: Thelaziidae), commonly known as the Equine eyeworm, is localised in the eye, conjunctival sac and lacrimal duct of horses and other equids. This parasite is found in Europe, North and South America and parts of Asia and has muscid flies, particularly *Musca*, *Fannia* and *Morellia*, as intermediate hosts.

Epidemiology: *Thelazia lacrymalis* is very common in some areas and infestation occurs seasonally, linked to periods of maximum fly activity. The parasite can survive in the eye for several years, but since it is only the young adult that is pathogenic, a reservoir of infection may persist in symptomless carrier animals. Only heavy infections cause symptoms. Survival of larvae also occurs in the pupal stages of flies during the winter.

Pathogenesis: In many hosts, moderate eyeworm infection causes little pathogenic disease. Lesions are caused by the serrated cuticle of the worm and most damage results from movement by the active young adults, causing lacrimation, followed by conjunctivitis. In heavy infections, the cornea may become cloudy and ulcerated. There is usually complete recovery in about two months, although in some cases areas of corneal opacity can persist. Infection may predispose the host to secondary bacterial infection.

Clinical signs and pathology: Often infection can be inapparent, but heavy infestations can cause lacrimation, conjunctivitis and photophobia. Flies are usually clustered around the eye because of the excessive secretion. In severe cases the eyes may be swollen, with keratitis and corneal ulceration with a purulent exudate. Invasion of the lacrimal gland and ducts may cause inflammation and necrotic exudation leading to occlusion and reduced tear production. Mechanical irritation of the conjunctiva produces inflammation, while damage to the cornea leads to opacity, keratitis and corneal ulceration.

Diagnosis: This is based on observation of the parasites in the conjunctival sac. Examination of the lacrimal secretion may reveal first-stage larvae.

Control and treatment: Prevention is difficult because of the ubiquitous nature of the fly vectors. Fly control measures aimed at protecting the face, such as headbands, aid in the control of eyeworm infection. Fenbendazole 10 mg/kg orally for five days is effective. Ivermectin given directly into the conjunctival sac may also have some effect but is not effective when given orally. Mechanical removal with forceps following the application of an ocular local anaesthetic is also useful. In cases of secondary bacterial infection, the use of antibiotic eye preparations may be indicated.

Halicephalobus delitrix

Halicephalobus delitrix, synonyms *Micronema delatrix* and *Halicephalobus gingivalis* (Phylum: Nematoda; Class: Chromadorea; Order: Rhabditida; Family: Panagrolaimidae), is a parasite that has been found in the brain, spinal cord, meninges and granulomatous tissues of the nares and maxilla of horses. It can also infect humans.

Pathogenesis: This saprophagous free-living nematode inhabits decaying organic matter, such as manure, and can be highly pathogenic.

Toxoplasma gondii

For more details see Parasites of the locomotory system.

Sarcocystis neurona

Sarcocystis neurona (Phylum: Apicomplexa; Class: Conoidasida; Order: Eucoccidiorida; Family: Sarcocystidae) causes a disease commonly known as Equine protozoal myeloencephalitis, and is localised in the brain and spinal cord of horses (intermediate hosts). This parasite has opossums (*Didelphis virginiana*) as final hosts and occurs in North, Central and South America. Armadillos, skunks, raccoons, sea otters, seals and domestic cats have all been implicated in the life cycle, but their significance is not known.

Epidemiology: The North American opossum is thought to be one definitive host with transmission to horses via sporocysts in faeces. The life cycle may also involve opossums scavenging on bird carcasses containing an identical organism, *Sarcocystis falcatula*, a parasite of several North American bird species. In this respect, horses may be acting as an abnormal aberrant host. The disease is sporadic, although multiple cases have been reported on farms or racing establishments but there is no evidence of horse-to-horse transmission. The disease occurs most frequently in young adult breeding stock.

Clinical signs and pathology: The organism causes wide-ranging neurological signs associated with infection of any part of the CNS. Clinical signs include circling, cranial nerve signs of muscle atrophy, facial paralysis, unilateral vestibular disease, cervical spinal cord disease (wobbler syndrome), monoplegia with muscle atrophy, gait abnormalities, pruritus and cauda equina syndrome. There is focal discoloration, haemorrhage and malacia of CNS tissue. On histopathology, the parasites are found in association with mixed inflammatory cellular responses and neuronal degeneration. Meronts in various stages of maturation, or free merozoites, are commonly seen within the cytoplasm of neurones or macrophages, neutrophils, eosinophils, more rarely capillary endothelial cells and myelinated axons.

Diagnosis: Diagnosis is based on clinical signs, analysis of cerebrospinal fluid, response to antiprotozoal therapy and negative response to corticosteroid therapy. *Post mortem* diagnosis is confirmed by demonstration of the organisms in CNS lesions. A Western blot test for *S. neurona* antibody in cerebrospinal fluid has been developed.

Control and treatment: The source of the infection is probably opossum faeces so measures to prevent feed contamination should be considered. A vaccine based on chemically inactivated cultured merozoites has shown promise in ameliorating the neurological effects of infection. The treatment of choice appears to be trimethoprim-sulfadiazine 15 mg/kg twice daily combined with pyrimethamine 0.25 mg/kg daily in feed. This may be followed by intermittent therapy with the same drugs at 20 mg/kg and 1 mg/kg, respectively, once every 1–2 weeks.

Parasites of the reproductive/urogenital system

Trypanosoma equiperdum

Trypanosoma equiperdum (Phylum: Euglenozoa; Class: Kinetoplastea; Order: Trypanosomatida; Family: Trypanosomatidae) causes a disease commonly known as Dourine. It is localised in the reproductive tract of horses and donkeys and occurs in the Mediterranean basin, South Africa, Middle East and South America.

Epidemiology: *Trypanosoma equiperdum* is the only trypanosome that is not transmitted by an invertebrate vector. Organisms present in the equine reproductive tract are transmitted during coitus and very rarely by biting flies. As trypanosomes are not continually present in the genital tract throughout the course of the disease, transmission of the infection does not necessarily take place at every copulation involving an infected animal. Transmission of infection from mare to foal can occur via the mucosa, such as the conjunctiva. Mares' milk has been shown to be infectious. *Trypanosoma equiperdum* occurs in donkeys but the disease is asymptomatic. Oedema on the genitals is not obvious and skin plaques only occur in less than 10% of infected donkeys. Sperm and vaginal discharges contain large numbers of parasites and are therefore a significant reservoir of the pathogen.

Pathogenesis: The disease is marked by stages of exacerbation, tolerance or relapse that vary in duration and which may occur once or several times before death or recovery. The signs most frequently noted are pyrexia, tumefaction and local oedema of the genitalia and mammary glands, oedematous cutaneous eruptions, knuckling of the joints, incoordination, facial paralysis, ocular lesions, anaemia and emaciation. A pathognomonic sign is the oedematous plaque consisting of an elevated lesion in the skin, up to 5–8 cm in diameter and

1 cm thick. The plaques usually appear over the ribs, although they may occur anywhere on the body, and usually persist for 3–7 days. They are not a constant feature. In long-standing cases, the external genitalia may be fibrosed. The incubation period is 2–12 weeks and the disease runs a chronic course over six months to two years.

Clinical signs and pathology: The first sign is oedema of the genitalia and there is slight fever, inappetence and a mucous discharge from the urethra and vagina. Circumscribed areas of the mucosa of the vulva or penis may become depigmented. The second stage of the disease is characterised by urticaria and appears after 4–6 weeks. Circular, sharply circumscribed urticarial plaques about 3 cm in diameter arise on the sides of the body, remain for 3–4 days and then disappear. The plaques may develop again later. Muscular paralysis develops, beginning with the muscles of the nostrils and neck, extending to the hindlimbs and finally to the rest of the body. The animal shows incoordination and then complete paralysis. Dourine is usually fatal unless treated, but mild strains of the parasite may occur in some regions. At *post mortem* examination, gelatinous exudates are present under the skin. In the stallion, the scrotum, sheath and testicular tunica are thickened and infiltrated. In some cases, the testes are fibrosed and may be unrecognisable. In the mare, the vulva, vaginal mucosa, uterus, bladder and mammary glands may be thickened with gelatinous infiltration. The lymph nodes, particularly in the abdominal cavity, are hypertrophied, softened and, in some cases, haemorrhagic. There is pronounced anaemia and oedematous infiltration of the perineal tissues and ventral abdominal wall, and hydrothorax, hydropericardium and ascites are often pronounced. The spinal cord of animals with paraplegia is often soft, pulpy and discoloured, particularly in the lumbar and sacral regions.

Diagnosis: Demonstration of the trypanosomes from the urethral or vaginal discharges, the skin plaques or the peripheral blood is generally not possible, although centrifugation of these fluids may help to find the pathogens. The clinical disease is typical in endemic areas to allow diagnosis. Infected animals can be detected with the CFT but cross-reactions with *T. evansi* and *T. brucei* are common. An IFAT is used as a confirmatory test for dourine or to resolve inconclusive results obtained by CFT.

Control and treatment: Strict control of breeding and movements of horses together with quarantine and slaughter in clinical outbreaks has a marked effect on the incidence of disease. Detection and slaughter of carrier equines lead to eventual eradication. In-contact animals are declared free after three consecutive monthly negative CFTs. Quinapyramine sulfate (3–5 mg/kg s.c.) is one of the few compounds effective against *T. equiperdum*. In many countries, chemotherapy is prohibited, and strict border controls are required before importation of horses and donkeys.

Notes: *Trypanosoma equiperdum* causes the most important venereal disease in horses and is responsible for great losses wherever it occurs. Animals other than equids can be infected experimentally. Rat-adapted strains can be maintained indefinitely; infected rat blood can be satisfactorily cryopreserved. Antigens for serological tests are commonly produced from infected laboratory rats.

Klossiella equi

Klossiella equi (Phylum: Apicomplexa; Class: Conoidasida; Order: Eucoccidiorida; Family: Klossiellidae) is distributed worldwide and localised in the kidney of horses, donkeys and zebras. Sporocysts are passed in the urine and infection takes place by ingestion of the sporulated sporocysts. This species is apparently quite common throughout the world but seldom reported.

Pathogenesis, clinical signs and pathology: Non-pathogenic and not usually associated with clinical signs. Only heavily parasitised kidneys have gross lesions, which appear as tiny grey foci on the cortical surface. Microscopically, these foci are areas of necrosis, with perivascular infiltration of inflammatory cells, especially lymphocytes, with an increase in interstitial fibroblasts.

Diagnosis: Sporocysts may be detected in urine sediments or trophozoite stages may be found on *post mortem* in the kidney. The site and location are pathognomonic.

Control and treatment: Not required.

Parasites of the locomotory system

Trichinella spiralis

Trichinella spiralis, synonym *Trichina spiralis* (Phylum: Nematoda; Class: Enoplea; Order: Enoplida; Family: Trichinellidae), commonly known as the Muscle worm, is localised in the small intestine and muscle of pigs, rats, horses, humans and most mammals. This parasite occurs worldwide, with the apparent exceptions of Australia, Denmark and Great Britain (for more details see Chapter 11).

Toxoplasma gondii

Toxoplasma gondii (Phylum: Apicomplexa; Class: Conoidasida; Order: Eucoccidiorida; Family: Sarcocystidae) is localised in the muscle, lung, liver, reproductive system and CNS of horses but there are few, if any, clinical reports of the disease (for more details see Chapter 9).

Sarcocystiosis

Sarcocystis is one of the most prevalent parasites of grazing animals.

Epidemiology: Little is known of the epidemiology, but from the high prevalence of symptomless infections observed in abattoirs, it is clear that where dogs are kept in close association with horses or their feed, then transmission is likely. Acute outbreaks are probably most likely when horses which have been reared without dog contact are subsequently exposed to large numbers of the sporocysts from dog faeces. The longevity of the sporocysts shed in the faeces is not known.

Pathology: For the two species reported in horses, microscopic inspection has revealed minimal host reaction in infected tissues.

Diagnosis: Most cases of *Sarcocystis* infection in horses are only revealed at *post mortem*, when the grossly visible sarcocysts in the muscle are discovered. Examination of faeces from dogs on the farm for the presence of sporocysts may be helpful in the diagnosis.

Control and treatment: The only control measures possible are those of simple hygiene. Farm dogs should not be housed in, or allowed access to, fodder stores, nor should they be allowed to defecate in pens where horses are housed. It is also important that they are not fed uncooked meat. There is no effective treatment for *Sarcocystis* infection in horses.

Sarcocystis fayeri

Sarcocystis fayeri (Phylum: Apicomplexa; Class: Conoidasida; Order: Eucoccidiorida; Family: Sarcocystidae) is distributed worldwide and localised in the muscle of horses (intermediate hosts). This parasite has dogs as final hosts.

Pathogenesis: Few pathogenic effects are associated with *S. fayeri* in the horse, although a few cases of severe myositis and myalgia have been reported.

Parasites of the integument

Onchocerca reticulata

Onchocerca reticulata (Phylum: Nematoda; Class: Chromadorea; Order: Spirurida; Family: Onchocercidae) causes a disease commonly known as Kasen summer mange or Equine dhobie itch. It is distributed worldwide and localised in the connective tissue, flexor tendons and suspensory fetlock ligament of horses and donkeys. This parasite has *Culicoides* spp. (biting midges) as intermediate hosts. Although onchocercosis is an important filarial infection in human medicine, most species in domestic animals are relatively harmless.

Epidemiology: The general prevalence of equine onchocercosis is high, most surveys in the USA having shown rates of more than 50%, though the highest so far recorded in Britain is 23%. The accumulation of microfilariae in the definitive host is highest during the seasons of greatest midge activity.

Pathogenesis: The connective tissue of the flexor tendons and suspensory ligament of the fetlocks is the preferential site. Following inoculation of L_3 by the midge vector *Culicoides*, the arrival of the parasites in their final site results in host reaction in the form of a painless diffuse swelling. This gradually increases in size to become a palpable soft lump, and then regresses to leave a calcified focus, the skin over the area remaining intact. In the lower limbs, the reaction to the presence of the parasite leads to the formation of soft painless swellings succeeded by small fibrous nodules.

Clinical signs and pathology: Apart from the initial mild reaction, no clinical signs attributable to the adult worms have been demonstrated. The microfilariae are reported to cause a chronic dermatitis of horses, being severe in summer and disappearing during the winter. The ventral skin lesions are indistinguishable from those of *Culicoides* sensitivity. Gross lesions include alopecia, scaling, crusting and leucoderma. Secondary excoriations and ulcerative dermatitis are induced by self-trauma.

Diagnosis: Infection may be confirmed by examination of thick skin sections taken from the predilection sites. The piece of skin is placed in warm saline for about 8–12 hours and teased to allow emergence of the microfilariae. These are readily recognised by their sinuous movements in a centrifuged sample of the saline. Fluid from scarified skin can also be examined for the presence of microfilariae.

Control and treatment: Control is usually not required. Ivermectin has good activity against the microfilariae stages and will provide relief in cases of onchocercal dermatitis. Insecticidal sprays or repellents may reduce attacks by biting midges.

Notes: Although onchocercosis is an important filarial infection in human medicine, most species in domestic animals are relatively harmless.

Parafilaria multipapillosa

Parafilaria multipapillosa, synonym *Filaria haemorrhagica* (Phylum: Nematoda; Class: Chromadorea; Order: Spirurida; Family: Filariidae), causes a disease commonly known as the summer bleeding disease or summer sores. It is localised in the subcutaneous and intermuscular connective tissue of horses and donkeys and occurs in North Africa, eastern and southern Europe, Asia and South America. This parasite has horn flies, *Haematobia atripalpis* and other *Haematobia* spp. in Europe as intermediate hosts.

Epidemiology: The disease is usually only apparent in the warmer seasons in temperate regions, whereas in hot tropical areas lesions are often seen after the rainy season. Although the condition tends to disappear in cold weather, it will periodically reappear during warmer months for up to four years in individual animals.

Pathogenesis: Infection results in the formation of subcutaneous nodules, which break open and ooze blood (Fig. 10.15). Their distribution in the harness areas may make the animals unsuitable for work.

Clinical signs and pathology: Clinically, the condition is characterised by matting of the hair due to blood and tissue fluid exudates from ruptured nodules. The lesions are more prominent in the summer and particularly when the animals are hot, so that they appear to be 'sweating blood'. Occasionally, lesions are mistaken for

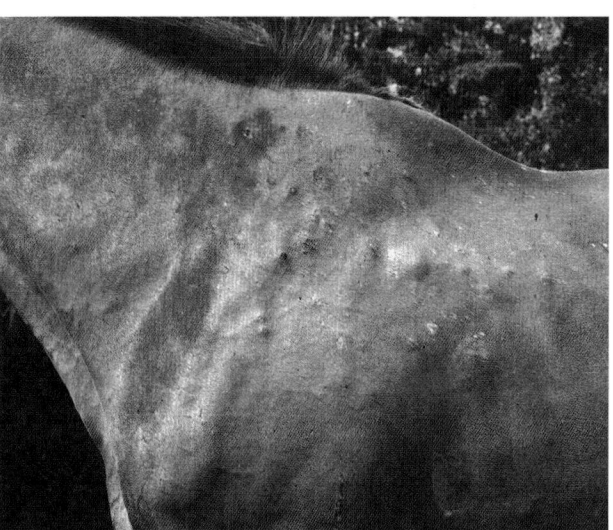

Fig. 10.15 Flank of a horse showing subcutaneous nodules induced by *Parafilaria multipapillosa*.

injuries caused by thorns and barbed wire. Nodules formed in the cutaneous and intermuscular connective tissue are 1–2 cm in diameter, enlarge in the summer months, burst open and haemorrhage and heal by scarring.

Diagnosis: The presence of nodules in the skin ('bleeding points') is pathognomonic. Larvated eggs or microfilariae can be demonstrated by microscopic examination of smears taken from the haemorrhagic exudate of fresh lesions. An ELISA is also available in some countries for serodiagnosis.

Control and treatment: Fly control measures will be beneficial. The treatment is difficult, but oral ivermectin or moxidectin may be tried.

Setaria equina

Setaria equina (Phylum: Nematoda; Class: Chromadorea; Order: Spirurida; Family: Onchocercidae), commonly known as the Abdominal worm, is distributed worldwide and localised in the peritoneum and pleural cavity of horses and donkeys. This worm has mosquitoes as intermediate hosts.

Epidemiology: Since the worms are usually innocuous, their epidemiology has received little study. The prevalence is higher in warmer countries, where there is longer seasonal activity of the mosquito vectors.

Pathogenesis: The adult worms live in the abdominal body cavity. Occasionally, the adults invade the lungs and eyes. The worms in their normal site are usually harmless and are only discovered at necropsy. Migrating larvae can cause an encephalomyelitis in horses and can also invade the eye and induce blindness.

Clinical signs and pathology: There are no clinical signs when the worms are in their normal site but when nervous tissue is involved, there is locomotor disturbance and in severe cases lumbar paralysis. Migrating larvae affecting the CNS may cause areas of damage seen grossly as brown foci or streaks. The lesions show microcavitation and variable haemorrhage. There is loss of myelin and fragmentation of axons locally, with eosinophils, neutrophils and macrophages present along with a mild meningitis and vascular cuffing.

Diagnosis: Infection with the adult worms is only accidentally discovered in the living animal by the finding of microfilariae in routine blood smears. In cases of cerebrospinal setariosis, confirmatory diagnosis is only possible by microscopic examination of the spinal cord, since the parasites exist only as larval forms in their aberrant site.

Control and treatment: Control would depend on control of the mosquito vectors, which is unlikely to be applied specifically for this parasite. There is no treatment for setarial paralysis. Ivermectin has been reported to be effective against adult *S. equina*.

Notes: The members of this genus are usually harmless inhabitants of the peritoneal and pleural cavities.

Hypoderma diana

Hypoderma diana (Phylum: Arthropoda; Class: Insecta; Order: Diptera; Family: Oestridae), commonly known as the Deer warble,

is found as larvae within the subcutaneous connective tissue. Its primary hosts are deer, but it may occasionally infest horses and sheep; it does not infest cattle.

ECTOPARASITES

FLIES

Culicoides

Culicoides (Phylum: Arthropoda; Class: Insecta; Order: Diptera; Suborder: Nematocera; Family: Ceratopogonidae), commonly known as Biting midges, are blood-feeding flies. They feed on a wide range of domestic animals and humans and are found worldwide.

Epidemiology: *Culicoides* adults are crepuscular or nocturnal feeders, that may be particularly active in dull humid weather. Flight activity can be influenced by temperature, light intensity, lunar cycles, relative humidity, wind velocity and other weather conditions. The mean flight distance by *Culicoides* females is about 2 km, although males travel shorter distances. However, wind dispersal may be important in long-distance movement. Adult *Culicoides* are usually found close to larval habitats in small and inconspicuous swarms. Females are attracted to the smell and warmth of their hosts, and different species may be host specific to varying degrees; for example, *C. brevitarsis* feeds mainly on cattle and *C. imicola* on horses. There are a large number of species of *Culicoides* of varying importance as nuisance pests and vectors. Of particular note in Europe and Asia are *Culicoides pulicaris*, *C. obsoletus* (a complex of four separate species), *C. impunctatus* and *C. sibirica*. *Culicoides imicola* is found throughout Africa and southern Europe and is the key vector of African horse sickness and bluetongue virus. In North America, *C. furens* and *C. denningi* inflict painful bites and *C. variipennis* is the primary vector of bluetongue virus.

Pathogenesis: In large numbers, biting midges can be a serious source of irritation and annoyance to livestock. The main areas affected are usually the head and neck. The biting of midges has been linked to an immediate-type hypersensitivity reaction which causes an intensely pruritic skin disease of horses, described as seasonal equine pruritic dermatitis. Symptoms include pruritus, crusting and alopecia of the face, ears, withers, mane, rump and tail. The lesions are exacerbated by self-trauma and scratching, resulting in hyperpigmentation and skin thickening. This is one of the most common allergic skin diseases in horses worldwide; it is known as 'sweet itch' in the UK and 'Queensland itch' in Australia. In the UK, the disease is particularly a problem of native ponies and the tendency to develop a hypersensitivity reaction is likely to be inherited.

Several species are involved in this condition: *C. pulicaris* in Europe, *C. robertsi* in Australia and *C. insignis*, *C. stelifer* and *C. venustus* in the USA. *Culicoides* biting midges act as vectors of more than 50 arboviruses, which are transmitted across their broad host range, including those responsible for the important livestock diseases causing bluetongue in sheep, African horse sickness, bovine ephemeral fever and, in the USA, eastern equine encephalitis. Species of *Culicoides* may act as mechanical vectors for the filarioid nematodes *Onchocerca cervicalis* to horses and several species of protozoa (*Haemoproteus*, *Leucocytozoon*) to poultry and other birds.

Clinical signs and pathology: The host animal's reaction to a bite of a *Culicoides* midge typically consists of a localised stinging or burning sensation and a well-defined reddened area around the bite site. These may remain itchy from a few minutes to 2–3 days and will cause the host animal to rub and scratch at the area.

Diagnosis: The bite of the adult flies leaves a characteristic reddened area and may remain itchy for several days. Flies may be seen on the host animal.

Control and treatment: Flies spend limited time on their hosts and are difficult to control using insecticides unless these have rapid killing or repellent ability. Applications of pyrethroid insecticides may give effective, though short-term, local control. However, control is difficult because of the usually extensive breeding habitat and depends on the destruction of breeding sites by drainage or spraying with insecticides. Repellents or screens may be used but the latter have to be sufficiently fine to reduce airflow, so screens impregnated with insecticides (originally designed to exclude larger flies) have been recommended instead. For 'sweet itch', antihistamine treatment may give immediate relief and the regular application of synthetic pyrethroid dressings may help prevent recurrence of the condition. It is also recommended that susceptible animals be housed when fly activity is maximal, usually in late afternoon and early morning.

Notes: African horse sickness is caused by a retrovirus (AHSV) and is among the most lethal of equine diseases. It frequently causes mortality rates in excess of 90%. It is enzootic in Africa. A series of epizootics in Spain and Portugal from 1987 to the present have resulted in the deaths of over 3000 equines. *Culicoides imicola* is one of the members of the genus able to transmit the virus and occurs widely in Spain, Portugal and southern Greece. Eastern equine encephalitis is a viral disease of horses and humans found only in the New World. It is caused by a species of the *Alphavirus* genus which is part of the Togaviridae. The disease is present throughout North and South America as far south as Argentina. The wild reservoir hosts are birds, and the primary midge vector is *Culicoides melanura*.

Tabanidae

Tabanus, *Chrysops* and *Haematopota* (Phylum: Arthropoda; Class: Insecta; Order: Diptera; Suborder: Brachycera; Family: Tabanidae) are commonly known as the Horse fly or Deer fly. The adult females of *Tabanus* locate their prey mainly by sight and their bites are deep and painful. They feed every 3–4 days, causing a great deal of annoyance. The pain caused by their bites leads to interrupted feeding and as a consequence, flies may feed on a succession of hosts. They are therefore important in the mechanical transmission of a range of pathogens that cause diseases, such as anthrax, pasteurellosis, trypanosomiasis, anaplasmosis and the human filarial disease loaosis. In North America in particular, several species of the genus *Tabanus* are especially important pests. These include *T. atratus* (the black horse fly), *T. lineola* and *T. similis* in the eastern states. In the western USA, *T. punctifer* and *T. sulcifrons* are of particular importance. Other common species are *T. quinquevittatus* and *T. nigrovittatus*, which are well known in North America as 'creenheads'.

Chrysops species are responsible for the mechanical transmission of several diseases and pathogens. *Chrysops discalis* is a vector of

Pasteurella tularensis in North America. *Chrysops dimidiata* (the mango fly) and *C. siacea* are intermediate hosts of the filarioid nematode loa loa. A number of *Chrysops* species also transmit carious species of *Trypanosoma*, such as *T. evansi*, the causative agent of surra in equines and dogs, *T. equinum*, the cause of mal de caderas of equines, *T. simiae* of pigs, *T. vivax* and *T. brucei* which cause nagana of equines, cattle, sheep and other ungulates, and *T. gambiense* and *T. rhodesiense* which cause human African trypanosomiasis. *Haematopota* species may feed on a number of hosts in rapid succession. They may therefore act as important mechanical vectors in the transmission of pathogens that cause disease, such as anthrax, pasteurellosis, trypanosomosis, anaplasmosis and the human filarial disease loaosis.

Hippoboscidae

Hippobosca equina

Hippobosca equina (Phylum: Arthropoda; Class: Insecta; Order: Diptera; Family: Hippoboscidae), commonly known as the Forest fly or Horse louse fly, is a blood-feeding fly, commonly found on the perineum and between the hind legs of horses.

Epidemiology: The adult flies are most abundant on the host during the summer months and attack more frequently in sunny weather.

Pathogenesis: This species is primarily a nuisance and a cause of disturbance. Since they pierce the skin to suck blood, they may be mechanical vectors of blood parasites such as the non-pathogenic *Trypanosoma theileri* in cattle, piroplasmosis of horses, Q-fever and other types of rickettsioses. They may also transmit *Haemoproteus* species to birds.

LICE

Bovicola equi

Bovicola equi, synonyms *Damalinia equi*, *Trichodectes parumpilosus*, *Werneckiella equi equi* (Phylum: Arthropoda; Class: Insecta; Order: Psocodea; Suborder: Ischnocera; Family: Bovicolidae), is commonly known as the Horse louse. This species occurs worldwide.

Epidemiology: The mouthparts of *B. equi* are adapted for biting and chewing, and allow them to feed on the outer layers of the hair shafts, dermal scales and blood scabs. They also feed on the exudates resulting from their irritant effect. *Bovicola equi* is capable of rapid population expansion.

Equine pediculosis spreads by contact and via contaminated grooming equipment, blankets, rugs and saddlery. Severe infestations spread over the entire body, and the numbers are greatest in winter and early spring when the winter coat is at its most dense. Longer-haired animals and breeds are more prone to infestation by this species. As in cattle, the shedding of the winter coat is important in ridding animals of the greater part of their louse burden in spring. In hot countries, the skin temperature of the animal's back may be high enough to kill lice in the exposed, fine-coated areas.

Pathogenesis: *Bovicola equi* may cause intense irritation, resulting in rubbing and scratching, with matting and loss of hair and sometimes self-excoriation, involving almost the entire body in extreme cases. It is possible that heavy louse infestations in equines are themselves symptomatic of some other disorder, such as disease or, more likely, simple neglect. If neglected and left ungroomed, the undisturbed louse population will multiply more rapidly. In addition, animals in a debilitated condition will fail to shed their winter coats and hence retain very large numbers of lice. This species may act as a vector of the pathogen that causes equine infectious anaemia.

Clinical signs and pathology: Restlessness, rubbing and damage to the coat will suggest that lice are present, and when the hair is parted the parasites will be found. *Bovicola equi* appears as small yellowish specks in the hair, and the small pale eggs are readily found scattered throughout the coat. Other symptoms include a rough coat, skin infections, loss of hair and weight loss. The pathology of louse infestation is extremely variable. Infestations may induce alopecia, dermal irritation, papulocrustous dermatitis and self-excoriation.

Diagnosis: The lice and their eggs may be seen within the hair and on the skin when the coat is parted. The lice may be removed and identified under a light microscope.

Control and treatment: Currently pyrethroid-based insecticides, applied as non-systemic pour-on formulations, are usually used to control lice as many older drugs are no longer available. All the horses in the establishment should be treated. Because eggs are relatively resistant to insecticides, treatment should be repeated every 7–14 days to kill newly hatched lice. Systemic treatments, such as the avermectins, are not approved for treatment of lice on horses. Essential oils (such as tea tree or lavender oil), at a 5% (v/v) concentration, groomed into the coat may be highly effective in reducing equine louse infestations. Grooming equipment should be scalded, blankets and rugs thoroughly washed and saddlery thoroughly cleaned. Ideally, animals should have individual grooming equipment and saddlery should not be interchanged, but this may not be economically feasible within some establishments. Regular and thorough grooming is important for good control.

Haematopinus asini

Haematopinus asini (Phylum: Arthropoda; Class: Insecta; Order: Psocodea; Suborder: Anoplura; Family: Haematopinidae), commonly known as the Horse sucking louse, is distributed worldwide and infests horses and donkeys.

Epidemiology: In normal light infestations, lice occupy sites in the dense hair of the mane, the base of the tail, the submaxillary space and also on the fetlocks of rough-legged breeds. From these sites, spread occurs over the whole body, and the numbers are greatest in winter and early spring when the winter coat is at its most dense. As in cattle, the shedding of the winter coat is important to rid animals of the greater part of their louse burden in spring. In hot conditions, the skin temperature of the animal's back may be high enough to kill lice in the exposed, fine-coated areas. Equine pediculosis spreads by contact and via contaminated grooming equipment, blankets, rugs and saddlery.

Pathogenesis: On horses, *H. asini* is most commonly found on the head, neck, back and inner surface of the upper legs. Symptoms include heavy dandruff and greasy skin and eventually bald spots with raw red centres. Light infestations may be asymptomatic but if present in sufficient numbers, they have been known to cause anaemia, weight loss and loss of vitality and appetite. Outbreaks of equine lice tend to be more frequent in the early spring, since the accumulated dirt in the barn and tack room, plus dander from the shedding of winter coats, provides an ideal environment for them. In horses, lice are often associated with poor grooming and management. Thin, aged, stressed or physically compromised horses seem to be more susceptible. Heavy lice infestations may in themselves be symptomatic of some other disorder such as disease or, more likely, simple neglect. Animals in a debilitated condition may harbour very large numbers of lice and the louse population will rapidly multiply on neglected ungroomed animals.

Clinical signs and pathology: *Haematopinus* spp. irritate their hosts by taking small but frequent blood meals. Each time they feed, they puncture the skin in a different place. As in other animals, equine lice may cause intense irritation, resulting in rubbing and scratching, with matting and loss of hair and sometimes excoriation, involving almost the whole body in extreme cases. Animals are restless and lose condition, and in heavy *Haematopinus* infestations there may also be anaemia. Loss of condition and weight may increase the susceptibility of the host animal to other diseases. The pathology of louse infestation is extremely variable. Low infestations may induce alopecia, irritation, papulocrustous dermatitis and self-excoriation. The blood feeding of *Haematopinus* may cause anaemia.

Diagnosis: Restlessness, rubbing and damage to the coat would suggest that lice are present, and when the hair is parted the parasites will be found. These lice are large and yellow-brown, and very easily seen, and in temperate countries on warm sunny days will often move on to the surface of the coat.

Control and treatment: As for *B. equi*.

MITES

Demodex equi

Demodex equi (Phylum: Arthropoda; Class: Arachnida; Subclass: Acari; Order: Trombidiformes (Prostigmata); Family: Demodicidae) is distributed worldwide, but not reported in Australia. It is localised in the hair follicles and sebaceous glands of horses and donkeys.

Epidemiology: Probably because of its location deep in the dermis, it is difficult to transmit *Demodex* between animals unless there is prolonged contact. Such contact occurs most commonly at suckling.

Pathogenesis: In the horse, demodectic mange is rare but may occur as either the squamous or pustular type, affecting initially the muzzle, forehead and periocular area.

Clinical signs and pathology: Lesions in horses, evident as patchy alopecia and scaling with or without papules and pustules, or as nodules, usually begin on the head and neck but may rapidly spread to involve most of the body. Lesions are seen largely on the face, shoulders, neck and limbs. Pruritus is absent. Demodicosis in horses has been reported in association with chronic corticosteroid treatment.

Diagnosis: For confirmatory diagnosis, deep scrapings are necessary to reach the mites deep in the follicles and glands. This is best achieved by taking a fold of skin, applying a drop of liquid paraffin, and scraping until capillary blood appears.

Control and treatment: There is little information regarding the treatment of equine demodicosis. Investigation and treatment of underlying systemic disease should be performed. Amitraz is contraindicated in horses because it can cause severe colic and death. Control is not usually required

Notes: A second species, *Demodex caballi*, which infests the eyelids and muzzle, has been described in horses; whether this is a true species or a morphological variant has not been established.

Sarcoptes scabiei

Sarcoptes scabiei (Phylum: Arthropoda; Class: Arachnida; Subclass: Acari; Order: Sarcoptiformes (Astigmata); Family: Sarcoptidae), commonly known as the Scabies mite, is distributed worldwide and found on the skin of equids.

Clinical signs and pathology: When present, sacrcoptic mange can be severe. There may be intense pruritus due to hypersensitivity. Early lesions appear on the head, neck and shoulders as small papules and vesicles that later develop into crusts. As alopecia and crusting spread, the skin becomes lichenified, forming folds. If untreated, lesions may extend over the whole body, leading to emaciation, general weakness and anorexia.

Control and treatment: If suspected, organophosphate insecticides or lime-sulfur solution can be applied by spray or dipping. Treatment should be repeated at 12–14-day intervals at least 3–4 times. Alternatively, the oral administration of ivermectin or moxidectin 200 µg/kg can be attempted. Several treatments are required, 2–3 weeks apart, and it is important to treat all contact animals.

Notes: This mange is now uncommon in horses. In Britain, for example, only two cases have been recorded since 1948. In both cases there was strong evidence that the infection had been acquired from other domestic species.

More detailed description can be found in the section on Ectoparasites in Chapters 3 and 11.

Psoroptes ovis

Psoroptes ovis, synonyms *Psoroptes equi*, *Psoroptes cuniculi*, *Psoroptes cervinus*, *Psoroptes bovis* (Phylum: Arthropoda; Class: Arachnida; Subclass: Acari; Order: Sarcoptiformes (Astigmata); Family: Psoroptidae), commonly known as the Mange mite, is distributed worldwide and found on the skin of equids.

Pathogenesis: Infestation is rare in horses. When present, pruritic lesions may be seen on thickly haired regions of the body, such as under the forelock and mane, at the base of the tail, between the hind legs and in the axillae. Lesions start as papules and alopecia and develop into thick haemorrhagic crusts.

Control and treatment: As for sarcoptic mange.

More detailed description can be found in Chapter 3 and the section on Ectoparasites in Chapter 9.

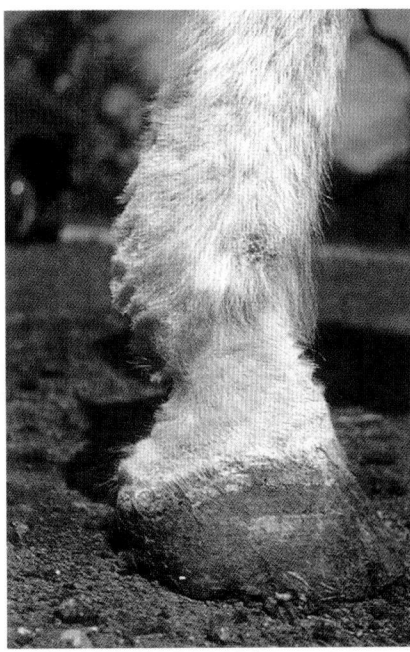

Fig. 10.16 Characteristic leg lesions of chorioptic mange in a horse.

Chorioptes bovis

Chorioptes bovis, synonyms *Chorioptes ovis*, *Chorioptes equi*, *Chorioptes caprae*, *Chorioptes cuniculi* (Phylum: Arthropoda; Class: Arachnida; Subclass: Acari; Order: Sarcoptiformes (Astigmata); Family: Psoroptidae), commonly known as the Mange mite, is distributed worldwide.

Pathogenesis: In horses, chorioptic mange due to *C. bovis* is occasionally observed. The mites are usually restricted to the pasterns, occur as crusty lesions with thickened skin on the legs below the knees and hocks, and are most prevalent in rough-legged animals and in those with heavy feather (Fig. 10.16). Although the mites are active only superficially, their movement causes irritation and restlessness, especially at night when animals are housed, and minor injuries may occur in the fetlock region from kicking against walls.

Notes: The names *Chorioptes ovis*, *Chorioptes equi*, *Chorioptes caprae* and *Chorioptes cuniculi* used to describe the chorioptic mites found on sheep, horses, goats and rabbits, respectively, are now all thought to be synonyms of *Chorioptes bovis*.

More detailed description can be found in Chapter 3 and the section on Ectoparasites in Chapter 8.

TICKS

Dermacentor nitens

Dermacentor nitens (Phylum: Arthropoda; Class: Arachnida; Order: Ixodida; Family: Ixodidae), commonly known as the Tropical horse tick, feeds on a range of domestic and wild mammals but is of particular veterinary significance as a parasite of horses and sometimes cattle. It is found in the southern regions of North America, Central and South America and the Caribbean.

Epidemiology: This is a one-host tick species; the larva, nymph and adult all attach to, and develop on, a single host. Under favourable tropical conditions this tick species can produce several generations per year.

Pathogenesis: Heavy burdens may lead to suppuration of the ears, and bite wounds may predispose the host to oviposition by screwworm flies. *Dermacentor nitens* is an important vector of *Babesia caballi*, resulting in equine babesiosis. It is able to transmit this pathogen transovarially to successive generations, and is important in the horse racing industry.

Amblyomma cajennense

Amblyomma cajennense (Phylum: Arthropoda; Class: Arachnida; Order: Ixodida; Family: Ixodidae), commonly known as the Cayenne tick, will feed on a range of mammals but is of particular veterinary importance in horses. It is found throughout South and Central America, southern USA and the Caribbean.

Pathogenesis: *Amblyomma cajennense* is an important tick in South America, the bites caused by this genus being particularly painful, probably due to the long mouthparts. In severe cases in South America this species has been reported to cause fever and weakness in cattle. The wounds caused by this tick may create a suitable site for screwworm myiasis associated with *Cochliomyia* spp. This species transmits spotted fever in South America as well as *Leptospira pomona*.

HOST–PARASITE CHECKLISTS

In the following checklists, the codes listed below apply.

Helminths

N, nematode; T, trematode; C, cestode; A, acanthocephalan.

Arthropods

F, fly; L, louse; S, flea; M, mite; Mx, maxillopod; Ti, tick.

Protozoa

Co, coccidia; Bs, blood sporozoa; Am, amoeba; Fl, flagellate; Ci, ciliate.

Miscellaneous 'protozoal organisms'

B, blastocyst; Mi, microsporidian; My, *Mycoplasma*; P, Pneumocystidomycete; R, *Rickettsia*.

Horse parasite checklist.

Section/host system	Helminths		Arthropods		Protozoa	
	Parasite	(Super) family	Parasite	Family	Parasite	Family
Digestive						
Mouth, oesophagus			*Gasterophilus pecorum*	Oestridae (F)	*Entamoeba equibuccalis*	Entamoebidae (Am)
Stomach	*Draschia megastoma*	Spiruroidea (N)	*Gasterophilus haemorrhoidalis*	Oestridae (F)		
	Habronema microstoma	Spiruroidea (N)	*Gasterophilus inermis*	Oestridae (F)		
	Habronema muscae	Spiruroidea (N)	*Gasterophilus intestinalis*	Oestridae (F)		
	Trichostrongylus axei	Trichostrongyloidea (N)	*Gasterophilus nasalis*	Oestridae (F)		
			Gasterophilus pecorum	Oestridae (F)		
Small intestine	*Strongyloides westeri*	Strongyloidoidea (N)	*Gasterophilus nigricornis*	Oestridae (F)	*Eimeria leuckarti*	Eimeriidae (Co)
	Parascaris equorum	Ascaridoidea (N)			*Eimeria solipedum*	Eimeriidae (Co)
	Anoplocephala perfoliata	Anoplocephalidae (C)			*Eimeria uniungulati*	Eimeriidae (Co)
	Anoplocephala magna	Anoplocephalidae (C)			*Cryptosporidium parvum*	Cryptosporidiidae (Co)
	Paranoplocephala mamillana	Anoplocephalidae (C)			*Giardia intestinalis*	Giardiidae (Fl)
Caecum, colon	*Cyathostomum alveatum*	Strongyloidea (N)			*Entamoeba gedoelsti*	Entamoebidae (Am)
	Cyathostomum catinatum	Strongyloidea (N)			*Entamoeba equi*	Entamoebidae (Am)
	Cyathostomum coronatum	Strongyloidea (N)				
	Cyathostomum labiatum	Strongyloidea (N)				
	Cyathostomum labratum	Strongyloidea (N)				
	Cyathostomum montgomeryi	Strongyloidea (N)				
	Cyathostomum pateratum	Strongyloidea (N)				
	Cyathostomum saginatum	Strongyloidea (N)				
	Cyathostomum tetracanthrum	Strongyloidea (N)				
	Cylicocyclus adersi	Strongyloidea (N)				
	Cylicocyclus auriculatus	Strongyloidea (N)				
	Cylicocyclus brevicapsulatus	Strongyloidea (N)				
	Cylicocyclus elongatus	Strongyloidea (N)				
	Cylicocyclus insigne	Strongyloidea (N)				
	Cylicocyclus largocapsulatus	Strongyloidea (N)				
	Cylicocyclus leptostomus	Strongyloidea (N)				
	Cylicocyclus maturmurai	Strongyloidea (N)				
	Cylicocyclus nassatus	Strongyloidea (N)				
	Cylicocyclus radiatus	Strongyloidea (N)				
	Cylicocyclus triramosus	Strongyloidea (N)				
	Cylicocyclus ultrajectinus	Strongyloidea (N)				
	Cylicodontophorus bicoronatus	Strongyloidea (N)				
	Cylicodontophorus euproctus	Strongyloidea (N)				
	Cylicodontophorus mettami	Strongyloidea (N)				
	Cylicostephanus asymetricus	Strongyloidea (N)				
	Cylicostephanus bidentatus	Strongyloidea (N)				
	Cylicostephanus calicatus	Strongyloidea (N)				
	Cylicostephanus goldi	Strongyloidea (N)				
	Cylicostephanus hybridus	Strongyloidea (N)				
	Cylicostephanus longibursatus	Strongyloidea (N)				
	Cylicostephanus minutus	Strongyloidea (N)				
	Cylicostephanus ornatus	Strongyloidea (N)				
	Cylicostephanus poculatus	Strongyloidea (N)				
	Cylicostephanus skrjabini	Strongyloidea (N)				
	Poteriostomum imparidentatum	Strongyloidea (N)				
	Poteriostomum ratzii	Strongyloidea (N)				
	Craterostomum acuticaudatum	Strongyloidea (N)				
	Craterostomum tenuicauda	Strongyloidea (N)				

(Continued)

Horse parasite checklist. *Continued*

Section/host system	Helminths		Arthropods		Protozoa	
	Parasite	(Super) family	Parasite	Family	Parasite	Family
	Oesophagodontus robustus	Strongyloidea (N)				
	Strongylus edentatus	Strongyloidea (N)				
	Strongylus equinus	Strongyloidea (N)				
	Strongylus vulgaris	Strongyloidea (N)				
	Triodontophorus brevicauda	Strongyloidea (N)				
	Triodontophorus minor	Strongyloidea (N)				
	Triodontophorus nipponicus	Strongyloidea (N)				
	Triodontophorus serratus	Strongyloidea (N)				
	Triodontophorus tenuicollis	Strongyloidea (N)				
	Oxyuris equi	Oxyuroidea (N)				
	Probstmayria vivipara	Oxyuroidea (N)				
	Gastrodiscus aegyptiacus	Gastrodiscidae (T)				
	Gastrodiscus secundus	Gastrodiscidae (T)				
	Pseudodiscus collinsi	Paramphistomatidae (T)				
	Anoplocephala perfoliata	Anoplocephalidae (C)				
Respiratory						
Nose			*Rhinoestrus purpureus*	Oestridae (F)		
Trachea, bronchi	*Dictyocaulus arnfieldi*	Trichostrongyloidea (N)				
Lung	*Echinococcus equinus*	Taeniidae (C)				
Liver	*Fasciola hepatica*	Fasciolidae (T)				
	Echinococcus equinus	Taeniidae (C)				
Pancreas						
Circulatory						
Blood	*Schistosoma japonicum*	Schistosomatidae (T)			*Trypanosoma brucei brucei*	Trypanosomatidae (Fl)
	Schistosoma nasale	Schistosomatidae (T)			*Trypanosoma brucei evansi*	Trypanosomatidae (Fl)
	Schistosoma indicum	Schistosomatidae (T)			*Trypanosoma congolense congolense*	Trypanosomatidae (Fl)
	Schistosoma spindale	Schistosomatidae (T)			*Babesia caballi*	Babesiidae (Bs)
	Schistosoma turkestanicum	Schistosomatidae (T)			*Theileria equi*	Theileriidae (Bs)
					Neorickettsia risticii	Anaplasmataceae (R)
					Anaplasma phagocytophilum	Anaplasmataceae (R)
Blood vessels	*Elaeophora bohmi*	Filarioidea (N)				
Nervous						
CNS	*Halicephalobus (Micronema) delitrix*	Rhabditoidea (N)			*Toxoplasma gondii*	Sarcocystidae (Co)
					Sarcocystis neurona	Sarcocystidae (Co)
Eye	*Thelazia lacrymalis*	Spiruroidea (N)				

Location	Species	Taxon (Type)
Reproductive/urogenital		
Kidneys	Trypanosoma equiperdum	Trypanosomatidae (Fl)
	Klossiella equi	Klossiellidae (Co)
Locomotory		
Muscle	Trichinella spiralis	Trichinelloidea (N)
	Toxoplasma gondii	Sarcocystidae (Co)
	Sarcocystis equicanis	Sarcocystidae (Co)
	Sarcocystis fayeri	Sarcocystidae (Co)
Connective tissue		
Subcutaneous	Onchocerca reticulata	Filarioidea (N)
	Parafilaria multipapillosa	Filarioidea (N)
	Setaria equina	Filarioidea (N)
	Dracunculus medinensis	Dracuncululoidea (N)
	Cordylobia anthropophaga	Calliphoridae (F)
	Cochliomyia hominivorax	Calliphoridae (F)
	Cochliomyia macellaria	Calliphoridae (F)
	Chrysomya bezziana	Calliphoridae (F)
	Chrysomya megacephala	Calliphoridae (F)
	Wohlfahrtia magnifica	Sarcophagidae (F)
	Wohlfahrtia meigeni	Sarcophagidae (F)
	Wohlfahrtia vigil	Sarcophagidae (F)
	Dermatobia hominis	Oestridae (F)
	Hypoderma diana	Oestridae (F)
Integument		
Skin	Rhabditis (Pelodera) spp.	Rhabditoidea (N)
	Hippobosca equina	Hippoboscidae (F)
	Bovicola equi	Trichodectidae (L)
	Haematopinus asini	Linognathidae (L)
	Demodex equi	Demodicidae (M)
	Sarcoptes scabiei	Sarcoptidae (M)
	Psoroptes ovis	Psoroptidae (M)
	Chorioptes bovis	Psoroptidae (M)

The following species of flies and ticks are found on horses. More detailed descriptions are found in Chapter 3.

Flies of veterinary importance on horses.

Group	Genus	Species	Family
Blackflies Buffalo gnats	*Simulium*	spp.	Simuliidae (F)
Bot flies	*Dermatobia*	*hominis*	Oestridae (F)
Flesh flies	*Sarcophaga*	*fusicausa haemorrhoidalis*	Sarcophagidae (F)
	Wohlfahrtia	*magnifica meigeni vigil*	
Midges	*Culicoides*	spp.	Ceratopogonidae (F)
Mosquitoes	*Aedes*	spp.	Culicidae (F)
	Anopheles	spp.	
	Culex	spp.	
Muscids	*Hydrotaea*	*irritans*	Muscidae (F)
	Musca	*autumnalis domestica*	
	Stomoxys	*calcitrans*	
Sand flies	*Phlebotomus*	spp.	Psychodidae (F)
Screwworms and blowflies	*Chrysomya*	*albiceps bezziana megacephala*	Calliphoridae (F)
	Cochliomyia	*hominivorax macellaria*	
	Cordylobia	*anthropophaga*	
Tabanids	*Chrysops*	spp.	Tabanidae (F)
	Haematopota	spp.	
	Tabanus	spp.	

Tick species found on horses.

Genus	Species	Common name	Family
Ornithodoros	*moubata*	Eyeless or hut tampan	Argasidae (Ti)
	savignyi	Eyed or sand tampan	
Amblyomma	*cajennense*	Cayenne tick	Ixodidae (Ti)
	hebraeum	Bont tick	
	maculatum	Gulf Coast tick	
	variegatum	Tropical bont tick	
Dermacentor	*albipictus*	Winter or moose tick	Ixodidae (Ti)
	andersoni	Rocky Mountain wood tick	
	nitens	Tropical horse tick	
	occidentalis	Pacific Coast tick	
	reticulatus	Marsh tick	
	silvarum		
Haemaphysalis	*punctata*		Ixodidae (Ti)
Hyalomma	*anatolicum*	Bont-legged tick	Ixodidae (Ti)
	detritum	Bont-legged tick	
	excavatum	Brown ear tick	
	marginatum	Mediterranean *Hyalomma*	
	truncatum	Bont-legged tick	
Ixodes	*ricinus*	Castor bean or European sheep tick	Ixodidae (Ti)
	holocyclus	Paralysis tick	
	rubicundus	Karoo paralysis tick	
	scapularis	Shoulder tick	
Rhipicephalus (*Boophilus*)	*appendiculatus*	Brown ear tick	Ixodidae (Ti)
	bursa		
	capensis	Cape brown tick	
	evertsi	Red or red-legged tick	
	sanguineus	Brown dog or kennel tick	

CHAPTER 11
Parasites of pigs

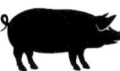

ENDOPARASITES

Parasites of the digestive system

OESOPHAGUS

Gongylonema pulchrum

For more details see Chapter 9.

STOMACH

Hyostrongylus rubidus

Hyostrongylus rubidus (Phylum: Nematoda; Class: Chromadorea; Order: Rhabditida; Family: Trichostrongylidae), commonly known as the Red stomach worm, is a parasite distributed worldwide and localised in the stomach of pigs, wild boars and occasionally rabbits.

Epidemiology: Because of the preparasitic larval requirements, infection is confined to pigs with access to pasture or those kept in straw yards. It is therefore more common in breeding stock, particularly gilts. The free-living larvae are particularly sensitive to desiccation and low temperatures. The epidemiology, at least in temperate zones, is similar to that of *Ostertagia* in ruminants, with seasonal hypobiosis a feature. Adult pigs often act as a reservoir of infection.

Pathogenesis: Similar to ostertagiosis, with penetration of the gastric glands by the L_3 and replacement of the parietal cells by rapidly dividing undifferentiated cells which proliferate to give rise to nodules on the mucosal surface. The pH becomes elevated in heavy infections and there is an increase in mucus production and a catarrhal gastritis. Sometimes there is ulceration and haemorrhage of the nodular lesions (Fig. 11.1), but more commonly light infections occur, and these are associated with decreased appetite and poor feed conversion rates.

Clinical signs and pathology: Light infections are often asymptomatic. Heavy infections can lead to inappetence, vomiting, anaemia and loss of condition and body weight. Diarrhoea may or may not occur. During the course of larval development, there is dilation of infected gastric glands and hyperplasia of the glandular epithelium of both infected and neighbouring glands. The lamina propria is oedematous with infiltration by lymphocytes, plasma cells and eosinophils. Larvae are found in the gastric glands, with adults mainly on the surface. During the course of development, the hyperplasia causes the formation of pale nodules, which may become confluent in heavy infections, leading to the formation of a thickened convoluted mucosa. There may be focal or diffusely eroded areas and occasionally ulceration of the glandular mucosa.

Diagnosis: This is based on a history of access to permanent pig pastures and the clinical signs. Confirmatory diagnosis is by examination of faeces for eggs; larval identification following faecal culture may be necessary, particularly to differentiate *Hyostrongylus* from *Oesophagostomum*. At necropsy, the small reddish worms can be seen in the mucous exudates on the gastric mucosa. Other stomach worms, the spiruroid nematodes, are larger (>13 mm).

Control and treatment: When *Hyostrongylus* infection is diagnosed, particularly in breeding stock, it is important to use a drug such as a modern benzimidazole or a macrocyclic lactone, which will remove hypobiotic larvae. The same principles apply as for the control of parasitic gastroenteritis in ruminants. For example, in temperate areas there should be an annual rotation of pasture with other livestock or crops. The timing of the move to other pastures may be dependent on other farming activities; if it can be delayed until October or later and accompanied by an anthelmintic treatment, then eggs from any worms which survive the treatment are unlikely to develop due to the unfavourable winter temperatures. A second treatment, again using a modern benzimidazole or a macrocyclic lactone, is recommended 3–4 weeks later to remove any residual infection. It may be advantageous to treat pregnant pigs before farrowing.

Notes: This parasite is responsible for a chronic gastritis in pigs, particularly gilts and sows.

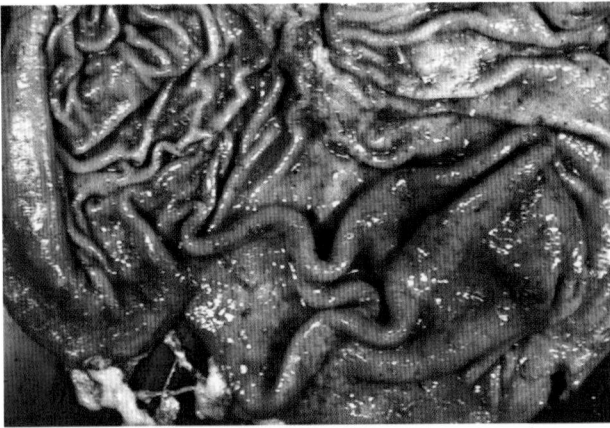

Fig. 11.1 Inflamed pig stomach infected with *Hyostrongylus rubidus*.

Veterinary Parasitology, Fifth Edition. Domenico Otranto and Richard Wall.
© 2024 John Wiley & Sons Ltd. Published 2024 by John Wiley & Sons Ltd.

Ollulanus tricuspis

Ollulanus tricuspis (Phylum: Nematoda; Class: Chromadorea; Order: Rhabditida; Family: Molineidae) is localised in the stomach of cats, wild felids and occasionally in pigs, foxes and domestic dogs. This parasite occurs mainly in Europe, North and South America, Australasia and the Middle East.

Epidemiology: The parasite is common in some parts of the world, particularly in cat colonies and cats that roam. The parasite can replicate in the stomach without any need for external egg or larval phases and can spread via vomit. The disease spreads mainly among starving stray cats and from them to other hosts.

Clinical signs and pathology: The infection causes occasional vomiting and emaciation. The worms lie beneath the mucus on the surface of the stomach, or partly in the gastric glands, and their presence may lead to mucosal lymphoid hyperplasia and elevated numbers of globule leucocytes in the gastric epithelium. Heavy infections result in hyperplasia of the gastric glands, causing the stomach mucosa to become convoluted and thrown into folds.

Diagnosis: Diagnosis of ollulanosis is seldom made because of their small size and lack of eggs and larvae in the faeces. Examination of vomit, following an emetic, for the presence of worms is a useful approach. At necropsy, recovery and identification of the very small worms from the gastric mucosa should lead to a diagnosis.

Control and treatment: Control is mainly achieved through the implementation of good hygiene procedures and prevention of contact with cats. Treatment is not reported in the pig, although benzimidazoles or ivermectin should be effective.

Ascarops strongylina

Ascarops strongylina, synonym *Arduenna strongylina* (Phylum: Nematoda; Class: Chromadorea; Order: Spirurida; Family: Spirocercidae), is a parasite distributed worldwide and localised in the stomach of pigs and wild boar. This parasite has coprophagous beetles (*Aphodius*, *Onthophagus*, *Gymnopleurus*) as intermediate hosts, thus the infection is more prevalent in outdoor pigs at pasture.

Clinical signs and pathology: Clinical signs are usually absent, although in heavy infections softening of faeces and inappetence may occur. The main effect is a catarrhal gastritis, particularly in young animals. On *post mortem*, the gastric mucosa is sometimes reddened and oedematous.

Diagnosis: Diagnosis of a particular genus is difficult by faecal examination, but the presence of the small elongate eggs in the faeces of animals showing signs of gastritis will give a tentative indication of spiruroidosis.

Control and treatment: Not usually required.

Gnathostoma hispidum

Gnathostoma hispidum (Phylum: Nematoda; Class: Chromadorea; Order: Spirurida; Family: Ganthostomatidae) is localised in the stomach of pigs and rarely humans and is distributed in Europe,

Asia and Africa. This parasite has *Cyclops* spp. and related freshwater crustaceans as intermediate hosts.

Epidemiology: It should be noted that the final hosts are also eligible second intermediate hosts, so that, for example, the pig may harbour L_3 in its liver and muscles as well as adult worms in its stomach.

Pathogenesis: The most obvious effect of gnathostomiasis is the presence of fibrous growths on the stomach wall. Ulceration and necrosis of the stomach wall are often present. In some cases, a number of larvae will migrate from the stomach to other organs, most commonly the liver, in which they burrow, leaving necrotic tracks in the parenchyma. It occurs erratically in humans as a cause of visceral *larva migrans*.

Clinical signs and pathology: *Gnathostoma* infection is usually inapparent. Severe infections may produce a marked gastritis leading to inappetence and weight loss. Fibrous growths are of variable size, the largest being 3–4 cm in diameter, and are cavitated, amounting to thick-walled cysts containing several worms and fluid.

Diagnosis: The infection in the living animal can only be diagnosed by the finding of the greenish oval eggs, which have a thin cap at one pole, in the faeces. Often, however, eggs are not present in faeces.

Control and treatment: With the ubiquity of the first and second intermediate hosts, complete control cannot be achieved, but partial limitation is possible by thorough cooking of all food. Treatment has not been fully investigated.

Physocephalus sexalatus

Physocephalus sexalatus (Phylum: Nematoda; Class: Chromadorea; Order: Spirurida; Family: Spirocercidae) is localised in the stomach of pigs, camels and occasionally rabbits and hares. This parasite is widely distributed in many parts of the world and has coprophagous beetles as intermediate hosts. Infection occurs where the intermediate hosts are plentiful. Transmission may also occur through paratenic hosts, such as amphibians or birds.

Pathogenesis: The parasites lie on the surface of the stomach wall under a layer of mucus. *Physocephalus sexalatus* is not severely pathogenic, the main effect being a catarrhal gastritis, particularly in young piglets.

Clinical signs and pathology: In many infections, obvious clinical signs are absent; in heavy infections, softening of faeces and inappetence may occur. At necropsy, the gastric mucosa is sometimes reddened and oedematous. The tiny worms can be seen in the mucus covering the gastric mucosa.

Diagnosis: As for other spiruroid parasites.

Control and treatment: Measures that restrict dung beetle populations feeding on pig faeces will be beneficial. Treatment is not reported.

Notes: *Physocephalus sexalatus* is not considered to be of great economic or pathogenic importance.

Simondsia paradoxa

Simondsia paradoxa, synonym *Spiroptera cesticillus* (Phylum: Nematoda; Class: Chromadorea; Order: Spirurida; Family: Spirocercidae), is localised in the stomach of pigs and occasionally rabbits and hares. This parasite is predominantly distributed in tropical and subtropical regions but occurs also in parts of Europe and has beetles as intermediate hosts. Infection is likely to be more common in outdoor pigs where the intermediate hosts are more abundant.

Pathogenesis: *Simondsia paradoxa* is not severely pathogenic, the main effect being a catarrhal gastritis. In addition, there can be some fibrous reaction around the nodules in the stomach wall.

Clinical signs and pathology: Infections are usually asymptomatic. Females are present in nodules 6–8 mm in diameter.

Diagnosis: Diagnosis of a particular genus is difficult by faecal examination, but the presence of the small elongate eggs in the faeces of animals showing signs of gastritis will give a tentative indication of spiruroidosis.

Control and treatment: Attempts to control these spiruroids are unlikely to be successful because of the ready availability of the intermediate hosts. Treatment is generally not considered.

Trichostrongylus axei

Trichostrongylus axei, synonym *Trichostrongylus extenuatus* (Phylum: Nematoda; Class: Chromadorea; Order: Rhabditida; Family: Trichostrongylidae), commonly known as the Stomach hairworm, is a parasite distributed worldwide and localised in the stomach of cattle, sheep, goats, deer, horses, donkeys, pigs and occasionally humans. *Trichostrongylus axei* may occasionally be found in the stomach of pigs but is considered to be of minor importance.

SMALL INTESTINE

Globocephalus urosubulatus

Globocephalus urosubulatus, synonyms *Globocephalus longemucronatus* and *Globocephalus samoensis* (Phylum: Nematoda; Class: Chromadorea; Order: Rhabditida; Family: Ancylostomatidae), commonly known as the Pig hookworm, is localised in the small intestine of pigs and wild boar, and occurs in North and South America, Europe, Africa and Asia.

Pathogenesis: Not known but thought to be generally of little pathological significance, although heavy infections may affect piglets severely.

Clinical signs and pathology: Generally asymptomatic, although heavily infected piglets may be anaemic and show weight loss and emaciation. The pathology is not described.

Diagnosis: Identification of eggs in the faeces, or adult worms found in the small intestine on *post mortem*.

Control and treatment: Frequent removal of faeces and bedding on dry straw or concrete will help reduce the risk of infection. Most modern benzimidazoles and macrocyclic lactones are likely to be effective.

Ascaris suum

Ascaris suum (Phylum: Nematoda; Class: Chromadorea; Order: Ascaridida; Family: Ascarididae), commonly known as the Large roundworm or white spot, is a parasite distributed worldwide and localised in the small intestine of pigs, wild boar, rarely sheep, cattle and humans.

Epidemiology: Young suckling piglets can become infected early after birth through the ingestion of embryonated eggs that are attached to the underbelly of the sow. Prevalence of infection is usually highest in pigs of around 3–6 months of age. A partial age immunity operates in pigs from about four months of age onwards and this, coupled with the fact that the worms themselves have a limited lifespan of several months, would suggest that the main source of infection is the highly resistant egg on the ground, a common characteristic of the ascaridoids. Hence 'milk spot', which is economically very important since it is a cause of much liver condemnation, presents a continuous problem in some pig establishments.

This condition has been widely noted to have a distinct seasonality of occurrence, appearing in greatest incidence in temperate areas during the warm summer months and almost disappearing when the temperatures of autumn, winter and spring are too low to allow development of eggs to the infective stage. Also, earthworms are generally more active and available during the summer months.

Sows and boars act as reservoirs of light infection. *Ascaris suum* may occasionally infect cattle, causing an acute, atypical, interstitial pneumonia that may prove fatal. In most reported cases, the cattle have had access to housing previously occupied by pigs, sometimes several years before, or to land fertilised with pig manure. In lambs, *A. suum* may also be a cause of clinical pneumonia as well as 'milk spot' lesions, resulting in condemnation of livers. In most cases lambs have been grazed on land fertilised with pig manure or slurry, such pasture remaining infective for lambs even after ploughing and cropping. Young adults of *A. suum* are occasionally found in the small intestine of sheep. There are a few recorded cases of patent *A. suum* infection in humans but cross-infection is not of epidemiological significance.

Pathogenesis: The migrating larval stages in large numbers may cause numerous small haemorrhages, emphysema and a transient pneumonia, but it is now recognised that many cases of so-called '*Ascaris* pneumonia' may be attributable to other infections, or to piglet anaemia. In the liver, the migrating larvae can cause 'milk spot' or 'white spot', which appears as cloudy whitish spots of up to 1 cm in diameter on the surface of the liver and represents the fibrous repair of inflammatory reactions to the passage of larvae in the livers of previously sensitised pigs (Fig. 11.2). Livers showing 'milk spot' lesions may be condemned at meat inspection. The adult worms in the intestine cause little apparent damage to the mucosa but occasionally, if large numbers are present, there may be obstruction, and rarely a worm may migrate into the bile duct, causing obstructive jaundice and carcass condemnation. Experimental infections have shown that in young pigs, the important effect of alimentary ascariosis is economic, with poor feed conversion and slower weight gains, leading to an extension of the fattening period by 6–8 weeks.

Clinical signs: The main effect of the adult worms in pigs is to cause production loss in terms of diminished weight gain. Otherwise, clinical signs are absent except in the occasional case of intestinal or biliary obstruction. Heavy infections may increase the susceptibility of young pigs to other bacterial and viral pathogens. In piglets under four months old, larval activity during the pulmonary phase of migration may cause a clinically evident pneumonia, which is usually transient and rapidly resolving. In sheep and cattle exposed to contaminated grazing, there may be acute dyspnoea,

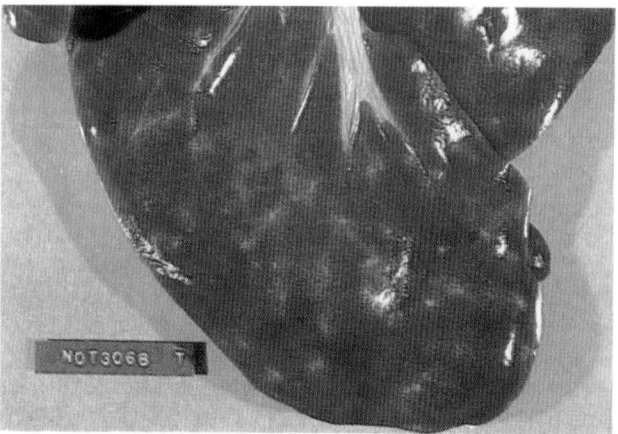

Fig. 11.2 Milk spot lesions in the liver associated with *Ascaris suum*.

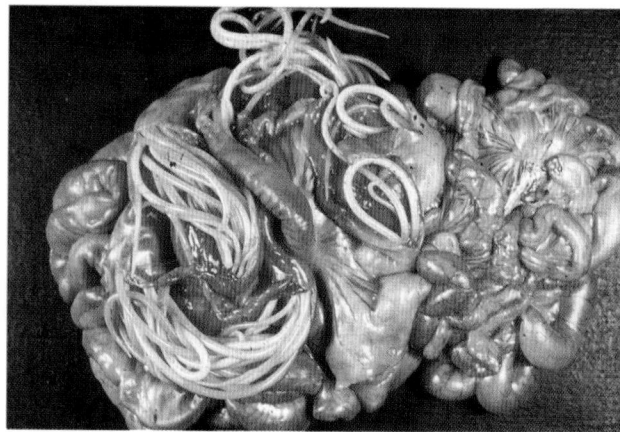

Fig. 11.3 A knot of *Ascaris suum* in the small intestine of an infected pig.

tachypnoea and coughing following acute challenge with migrating larvae in the lungs.

Pathology: Larval migration induces lesions in the liver and lungs. In the lungs, gross lesions are limited largely to numerous focal haemorrhages scattered over and through the pulmonary parenchyma. There may be some oedema, congestion and alveolar emphysema. Microscopically, there is an eosinophilic bronchiolitis. Bronchioles are surrounded by macrophages and eosinophils, and the bronchiolar wall is infiltrated by eosinophils, which are also present, with necrotic debris, in the lumen. Larvae are usually readily found in tissue sections and may be present in alveoli, alveolar ducts, bronchioles or bronchi, and in more chronic cases are found within eosinophilic granulomas. Lesions in the liver result in considerable economic loss from condemnation at meat inspection. Haemorrhagic tracks are present near portal areas and throughout lobules, visible through the capsule as pinpoint red areas, sometimes slightly depressed and surrounded by a narrow pale zone. These lesions collapse, healing by fibrosis, which extends around portal tracts and extends out more diffusely, emphasising lobular outlines. Granulomatous foci containing giant cells, macrophages and eosinophils may centre on the remnants of larvae trapped and destroyed in the liver. The inflammatory infiltrates in livers of animals exposed to larval ascarids may become severe and diffuse, and this is reflected in the gross appearance of the liver, which has extensive 'milk spots' and prominent definition of lobules. The liver is firm, and heavy scars may become confluent, obliterating some lobules and extending out to exaggerate interlobular septa throughout the liver.

Diagnosis: Diagnosis is based on clinical signs, history of disease and, in infections with the adult worm, on the presence in faeces of the yellow-brown ovoid eggs with thick mamillated shells. Being dense, the eggs float more readily in saturated solutions of zinc sulfate or magnesium sulfate than in the saturated sodium chloride solution that is used in most faecal examination techniques. Low counts of *A. suum* eggs in faeces (<200 eggs per gram) may represent false positives due to the coprophagic activity of pigs. At necropsy, the large worms in the small intestine are easy to recognise.

The pathogenicity of adult ascarids in the intestine is poorly defined. Heavy infections may obstruct the gut, being visible as rope-like masses through the intestinal wall (Fig. 11.3). Ascarids may occasionally pass to the stomach and be vomited or migrate up the pancreatic or bile ducts. Sometimes biliary obstruction and icterus, or

purulent cholangitis, may ensue. Rarely, intestinal perforation occurs. On histology, there may be substantial hypertrophy of the muscularis externa and elongation of the crypts of Lieberkuhn, though height of villi is not significantly reduced. Hypertrophy and exhaustion of the goblet cell population and increased infiltrates of eosinophils and mast cells are also observed in infected intestines.

Control and treatment: In the past, elaborate control systems have been designed for ascariosis in pigs but with the appearance of highly effective anthelmintics, these labour-intensive systems are rarely used. The chief problem in control is the great survival capacity of the eggs. In housed pigs, strict hygiene in feeding and bedding, with frequent hosing/steam cleaning of walls, floors and feeding troughs, will limit the risk of infection. Some disinfectants and chemical solutions will limit infectivity. In pigs on free range, the problem is greater and where there is serious ascariosis it may be necessary to discontinue the use of paddocks for several years, since the eggs can survive cultivation. It is good practice to treat in-pig sows at entry to the farrowing pen, and young pigs should receive anthelmintic treatment when purchased or on entry to the finishing house and eight weeks later; boars should be treated every 3–6 months. Washing of the skin of sows prior to their removal to the farrowing pen should reduce contamination with embryonated eggs. The intestinal stages are susceptible to most of the anthelmintics in current use in pigs, and the majority of these, such as the benzimidazoles, are given in the feed over several days. In cases of suspected *Ascaris* pneumonia, injectable levamisole and ivermectin may be more convenient. For 3–4 days after treatment, the faeces should be removed from the pens and destroyed, as they will often contain large numbers of eggs and expelled/disintegrating worms.

Notes: The type species, *Ascaris lumbricoides*, occurs in humans and at one time it was not differentiated from *A. suum*, so that the pig was thought to present a zoonotic risk for humans. With species distinction now possible, *A. lumbricoides* is accepted as specific for humans and some species of primates.

Strongyloides ransomi

Strongyloides ransomi (Phylum: Nematoda; Class: Chromadorea; Order: Rhabditida; Family: Strongyloididae), commonly known as the Threadworm, is a parasite distributed worldwide and localised in the small intestine of pigs.

Epidemiology: *Strongyloides* infective larvae are not ensheathed and are susceptible to extreme climatic conditions. However, warmth and moisture favour development and allow the accumulation of large numbers of infective stages. Adult breeding stock may be infected with dormant larvae in their subcutaneous fat. Pregnancy and farrowing appear to stimulate the re-emergence of these larvae, which then may infect piglets via the colostrum. This appears to be the major route of infection in young piglets and, in only seven days after birth, piglets may be passing eggs in their faeces.

Pathogenesis: Skin penetration by infective larvae may cause an erythematous reaction. Mature parasites are found in the duodenum and proximal jejunum and, if present in large numbers, may cause inflammation with oedema and erosion of the epithelium. This results in catarrhal enteritis with impairment of digestion and absorption. Infection in young piglets can result in retarded growth.

Clinical signs and pathology: In light infections, animals show no clinical signs. In heavy infections, there is bloody diarrhoea, anaemia, anorexia and emaciation, and sudden death may occur. During the migratory phase, there may be coughing, abdominal pain and vomiting. The adult female worms burrow into the intestinal wall and establish in tunnels in the epithelium at the base of the villi in the small intestine, causing an inflammatory response. In large numbers they may cause villous atrophy, with a mixed mononuclear inflammatory cell infiltration of the lamina propria. Crypt epithelium is hyperplastic and there is villous clubbing.

Diagnosis: Demonstration of larvated eggs in faeces or the adults in scrapings from the intestine on *post mortem* is diagnostic.

Control and treatment: Specific control measures for *Strongyloides* infection are rarely called for. The benzimidazoles, levamisole and the macrocyclic lactones may be used for the treatment of clinical cases and a single dose of ivermectin 4–16 days prior to farrowing has been shown to suppress larval excretion in the milk of sows. Strict hygiene and cleaning of pens before farrowing help limit levels of infection. Treating the sows before farrowing can also help reduce infections in piglets.

Trichinella spiralis

Trichinella spiralis (Phylum: Nematoda; Class: Enoplea; Order: Enoplida; Family: Trichinellidae), commonly known as the Muscle worm, is localised in the small intestine and muscle of pigs, rats, horses, humans and most mammals. This parasite is found worldwide, with the apparent exceptions of Australia, Denmark and the UK.

Epidemiology: It is important to realise that trichinellosis is basically an infection of animals in the wild and that the involvement of humans in these circumstances is accidental.

The epidemiology of trichinellosis depends on two factors. First, animals may become infected from a wide variety of sources, predation and cannibalism being perhaps the most common. Others include feeding on carrion, since the encapsulated larvae are capable of surviving for several months in decomposing flesh, and the ingestion of fresh faeces from animals with a patent infection. It is also thought that transport hosts, such as crustaceans and fish, feeding on drowned terrestrial animals, may account for infection in some aquatic mammals such as seals.

The second factor is the wide host range of the parasite, infecting various carnivores and omnivorous mammals. In temperate areas, rodents, brown bears, badgers and wild pigs are most commonly involved; in the Arctic, polar bears, wolfes and foxes; in the tropics, lions, leopards, bushpigs, hyenas, jackals and warthogs. In these sylvatic or feral cycles, humans and their animals are only occasionally involved. For example, the consumption of polar bear meat may cause infection in Inuit and sled-dogs, while in Europe the hunting and subsequent ingestion of wild pigs may also produce disease in humans and their companion animals.

The domestic or synanthropic cycle in the human and the pig is an 'artificial' zoonosis largely created by feeding pigs on food waste containing the flesh of infected pigs; more recently, tail biting in pigs has been shown to be a mode of transmission. Rats in piggeries also maintain a secondary cycle, which may on occasion pass to pigs or vice versa from the ingestion of infected flesh or faeces. Infection in humans is acquired from the ingestion of raw or inadequately cooked pork or its by-products, such as sausages, ham and salami. It is also important to realise that smoking, drying or curing pork does not necessarily kill larvae in pork products. Horse meat has increasingly been implicated in the transmission of *Trichinella* to humans.

In areas such as Poland, Germany and the USA, human trichinosis acquired from pork has, until recently, been an important zoonosis. Over the past few decades, prohibition of feeding uncooked food waste to pigs, improved meat inspection and public awareness have greatly diminished the significance of the problem. In Britain and other countries in Europe and in the USA, the numbers of outbreaks are few and sporadic. The decreasing prevalence is also reflected in the fact that inapparent infection in humans, as shown by the presence of *T. spiralis* larvae in muscle samples at necropsy, has decreased from 10% to not recorded in Britain, and from 20% to under 5% in the USA over the past 60 years.

Pathogenesis: The adults occur in the glandular crypts of the proximal small intestine and their larvae in the striated muscles; the diaphragmatic, intercostal and masseter muscles and the tongue are considered to be the main predilection sites. Infection in domestic animals is invariably light, and clinical signs do not occur. However, when hundreds of larvae are ingested, as occasionally happens in humans and presumably also in predatory animals in the wild, including cats and dogs, the intestinal infection is often associated with catarrhal enteritis and diarrhoea, and 1–2 weeks later the massive larval invasion of the muscles causes acute myositis, fever, eosinophilia and myocarditis. Periorbital oedema and ascites are also common in humans, sometimes accompanied by vomiting, diarrhoea, fever and myocarditis. Unless treated with an anthelmintic and anti-inflammatory drug, such infections may frequently be fatal as a consequence of paralysis of respiratory muscles, but in persons who survive this phase the clinical signs start to abate after 2–3 weeks.

Clinical signs and pathology: These are variable and depend on the host and the level of infection. Signs are usually non-specific and resemble those of other diseases, such as diarrhoea, fever, muscular pain, dyspnoea and peripheral eosinophilia. *Trichinella spiralis* infection in young pigs can induce inappetence, weakness and diarrhoea. Older pigs are generally more tolerant of infection.

The adults occur in the glandular crypts of the proximal small intestine where there is little associated pathology. Larvae are found in the striated muscles, with the diaphragmatic, intercostal and masseter muscles and the tongue considered to be the main predilection sites. On microscopic examination, the larvae lie in a bulging clear segment of muscle fibre, which may be loosely encircled by eosinophils, lymphocytes, plasma cells and macrophages. In a heavy infection, a large proportion of the muscle fibres in the predilection muscles may be infected with larvae and surrounded by reactive zones. As the cellular reaction subsides, muscle fibres surrounded by the larvae have the appearance of a fibrous capsule. Once larvae become encysted, there is muscle fibre degeneration and mineralisation, which does not appear to affect larval viability, as larvae can survive for up to 20 years.

Diagnosis: This is not relevant in live domestic animals. At meat inspection, heavy larval infections may occasionally be just seen with the naked eye as tiny greyish-white spots. For routine purposes, small samples of pig muscle (taken from the preferential predilection sites) of about 1 g are squeezed between glass plates, the apparatus being called a compressorium, and examined for the presence of larvae by direct low-power microscopic examination or projection onto a screen using a trichinoscope. Alternatively, small portions of diaphragm tissue may be digested in pepsin/HCl and the sediment examined microscopically for the presence of larvae (Fig. 11.4). The digestion method is now the preferred approach in most countries as it is less expensive and labour-intensive to perform. For mass screening purposes, designed to determine the incidence of trichinellosis in pigs within regions or for some high-volume slaughterhouses, immunodiagnostic tests have been used. Of these, the antibody detection enzyme-linked immunosorbent assay (ELISA) or enzyme immunoassay appears to be the test of choice.

Control: Probably the most important factor in the control of trichinellosis is a legal requirement that swill or waste human food intended for consumption by pigs must be boiled (100 °C for 30 minutes). In fact, this practice is mandatory in many countries to limit the potential spread of other diseases, such as foot and mouth disease and swine fever.

Other essential steps include the following.
1 Meat inspection plays an essential role in monitoring the detection of infected carcasses. Such carcasses must be condemned.
2 Measures to eliminate rodents and other wild animals from piggeries and slaughterhouses.

3 Preventing exposure of pigs to dead animal carcasses, particularly those of rats and other pigs.
4 Regulations to ensure that larvae in pork are destroyed by cooking or freezing. In the USA, for example, any pork or pork products, other than fresh pork, must be treated by heating or freezing before marketing and it is likely also that irradiation might soon be introduced as a further method of control.
5 Consumer education, and particularly the recognition that pork or pork products or the flesh of carnivorous game should be thoroughly cooked before consumption. It is worth noting that the larvae of *Trichinella nativa* that occur in wild carnivores and seals in some arctic and subarctic regions are very resistant to freezing.

Treatment: Although rarely called for in animals, the adult worms and the larvae in muscles are susceptible to several of the benzimidazole anthelmintics, such as in-feed treatment with flubendazole in pigs.

Notes: The taxonomy of the genus has been controversial until very recently. It is composed of several sibling species that cannot be differentiated morphologically but molecular typing, and other criteria, have now identified eight species of *Trichinella* (for more details see Table 1.47).

Macracanthorhynchus hirudinaceus

Macracanthorhynchus hirudinaceus (Phylum: Acanthocephala; Class: Archiacanthocephala; Order: Oligacanthorhynchida; Family: Oligacanthorhynchidae), commonly known as the Thorny-headed worm, is localised in the duodenum and proximal small intestine of pigs, wild boar, occasionally dogs, wild carnivores and humans. This parasite is found worldwide but is absent from certain areas, for example parts of Western Europe, and has various dung beetles and water beetles as intermediate hosts.

Epidemiology: Infection is seasonal, being partly dependent on the availability of the intermediate hosts. The eggs are able to remain viable in the environment for several years. Infection tends to be more prevalent in pigs of around 1–2 years of age.

Clinical signs and pathology: Low or mild infections are not very pathogenic, but heavy infections may cause inappetence, retarded growth rates and emaciation.

Diagnosis: This is based on finding the typical eggs in the faeces. At necropsy, the worms superficially appear similar to *Ascaris suum* but when placed in water, the spiny proboscis is protruded, thus aiding differentiation. *Macracanthorhynchus hirudinaceus* penetrates deep into the intestinal wall with its proboscis and produces inflammation and may provoke granuloma formation at the site of attachment in the wall of the duodenum and small intestine. Heavy infections may induce a catarrhal enteritis and, rarely, penetration of the intestinal wall, which can result in a fatal peritonitis.

Control and treatment: Pigs should be prevented from access to the intermediate hosts. In modern management systems, this may be easily achieved but where pigs are kept in small sties, the faeces should be regularly removed to reduce the prevalence of the dung beetle intermediate hosts. Although there is little information on treatment, levamisole, ivermectin and doramectin are reported to be effective.

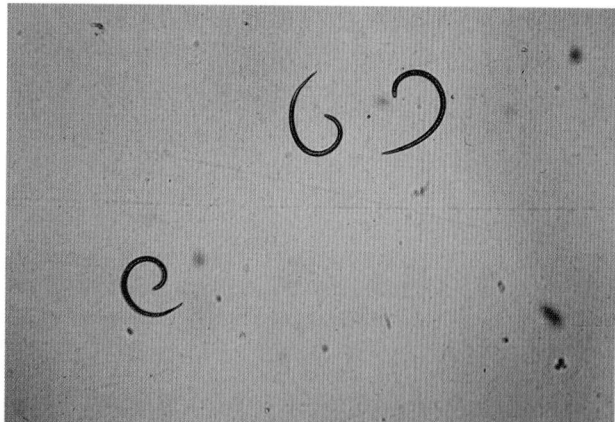

Fig. 11.4 Larvae of *Trichinella spiralis* following digestion in pepsin/HCl.

Fasciolopsis buski

Fasciolopsis buski (Phylum: Platyhelminthes; Class: Trematoda; Order: Plagiorchiida; Family: Fasciolidae) is localised in the small intestine of pigs, dogs and humans. This parasite is distributed in India, Pakistan, Southeast Asia and China and has flat spiral-shelled freshwater snails of *Planorbis*, *Hippeutis* and *Segmentina* species as intermediate host.

Epidemiology: The intermediate snail hosts feed on certain plants, namely water caltrop (*Trapa natans*) and water chestnut (*Eleocharis tuberosa*), which are cultivated for food and often fertilised with human faeces. The cercariae encyst on the tubers or nuts of these plants, and cause infection if eaten raw. Pigs also become infected through eating these plants.

Pathogenesis: The parasite is mainly of importance as a cause of disease in humans. It is located in the small intestine where it can cause severe ulceration of the intestinal mucosa in heavy infections in humans. Lesions are less severe in the pig and dog.

Clinical signs and pathology: Infection causes abdominal pain, diarrhoea, oedema, ascites and occasionally intestinal obstruction leading to malnutrition and death in humans. Symptoms are less severe in pigs and dogs. Heavier infections produce ulceration of the intestinal mucosa.

Diagnosis: Diagnosis is confirmed by faecal identification of the eggs, which have to be differentiated from those of *Fasciola* spp.

Control and treatment: The disease is easily preventable by avoiding raw or uncooked aquatic plants in endemic areas. The introduction of good sanitation facilities limits contamination of local watercourses and ponds. Albendazole (10 mg/kg) and praziquantel (15 mg/kg) are both effective.

Notes: *Fasciolopsis buski* is primarily a parasite of humans, but can occur in the pig and dog, which may act as reservoir hosts.

Postharmostomum suis

Postharmostomum suis (Phylum: Platyhelminthes; Class: Trematoda; Order: Strigeidida; Family: Brachylaemidae) is localised in the small intestine of pigs and is found in North Africa. This parasite has land snails, particularly species of *Xerophilia*, as intermediate hosts. The parasite ingests blood but is not considered to be very pathogenic.

Coccidiosis

Although some 10 species of coccidia have been described from pigs, their importance is not clear. *Cystoisospora suis* is a cause of a naturally occurring severe enteritis in young piglets aged 1–2 weeks. *Eimeria deblieki* has been described as causing clinical disease and severe pathology; *Eimeria polita*, *E. scabra* and *E. spinosa* cause moderate to mild diarrhoea in piglets (Table 11.1).

The source of infection appears to be oocysts produced by the sow during the periparturient period, the piglets becoming initially infected by coprophagia; the second phase of diarrhoea is initiated by reinvasion from tissue stages. Diagnosis of the condition is difficult unless *post mortem* material is available since clinical signs

Table 11.1 Predilection sites and prepatent periods of coccidia species in pigs.

Species	Predilection site	Prepatent period (days)
Cystoisospora suis (syn. *Isospora suis*)	Small intestine	5
Eimeria deblieki	Small intestine	6–7
Eimeria polita	Small intestine	7–8
Eimeria scabra	Small and large intestine	7–11
Eimeria spinosa	Small intestine	7
Eimeria porci	Small intestine	5–7
Eimeria neodebliecki	Unknown	10
Eimeria perminuta	Unknown	?
Eimeria suis	Unknown	10

occur prior to the shedding of oocysts and are very similar to those caused by other pathogens, such as rotavirus.

Diagnosis of coccidial infections is based on history and clinical signs and, in patent infections, on the presence of oocysts of the pathogenic species in the faeces. Oocysts may not be shed during the diarrhoeal phase so faecal counts are not always of value.

Control of coccidiosis is based on reducing environmental contamination by improved hygiene. Pens should be kept clean and dry. Ammonia-based disinfectants can be used after thoroughly cleaning farrowing pens by high-pressure hosing or steam disinfection. Overcrowding of piglets and faecal contamination of food and water should be avoided. Prevention has been achieved by the in-feed administration of amprolium to sows during the periparturient period, from one week prior to farrowing until three weeks post farrowing, where such treatments are still licensed or approved.

Treatment for all species of *Eimeria* (and *Cystoisospora*) has generally relied on the use of a sulfonamide-trimethoprim product combined with electrolyte and fluid therapy. Treatment with several anticoccidial drugs, such as halofuginone, salinomycin, toltrazuril and diclazuril given orally to affected animals, has been reported to be effective, although such treatments may not be licensed or approved in many countries.

Cystoisospora suis

Cystoisospora suis, synonym *Isospora suis* (Phylum: Apicomplexa; Class: Conoidasida; Order: Eucoccidiorida; Family: Sarcocystidae), is a parasite distributed worldwide and localised in the small intestine of pigs.

Pathogenesis: Infection can occur in all types of farrowing facilities and under all types of management systems. Piglets with clinical infection develop a characteristic non-haemorrhagic disease that is unresponsive to routine antibiotic therapy. Scours tend to occur in individuals from about six days of age, but most of the litter scours at 8–10 days of age. The diarrhoea ranges from white to pasty cream faeces through to a watery diarrhoea. Affected piglets tend to be stunted and hairy. Severely affected piglets become dehydrated, continue to suckle but weight gains are reduced. Mortality is generally low to moderate. *Cystoisospora suis* can cause infection on its own or in combination with other enteropathogens, such as enterotoxigenic *Escherichia coli*, rotavirus and transmissible gastroenteritis virus.

Clinical signs and pathology: The main clinical sign is diarrhoea, often biphasic, which varies in its severity from white to pasty

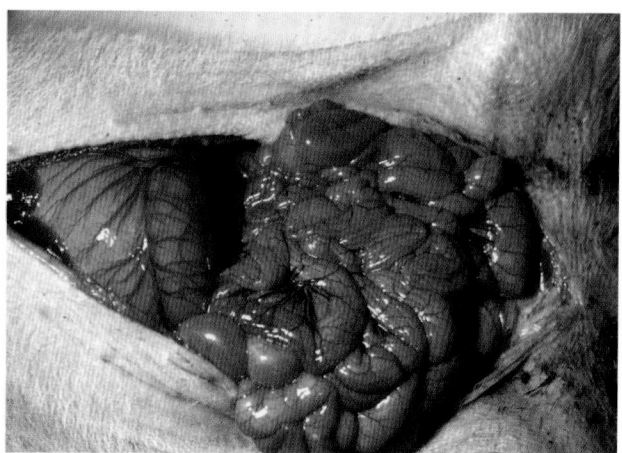

Fig. 11.5 *Cystoisospora suis* infection in a piglet.

cream faeces through to a watery diarrhoea. Lesions caused by *C. suis* in young piglets are present in the jejunum and ileum and are associated with the development stages of the parasite. The affected intestine is inflamed and reddened (Fig. 11.5). Microscopic changes include villous atrophy, villous fusion, crypt hyperplasia and necrotic enteritis.

Diagnosis: Diagnosis of the condition is difficult unless *post mortem* material is available, since clinical signs occur prior to the shedding of oocysts and are very similar to those caused by other pathogens such as rotavirus.

Treatment: Treatment with toltrazuril (1 ml of 5% suspension) given orally to affected piglets at four days of age has proved effective.

Eimeria debliecki

Eimeria debliecki (Phylum: Apicomplexa; Class: Conoidasida; Order: Eucoccidiorida; Family: Eimeriidae) is a parasite distributed worldwide and localised in the small intestine of pigs. The endogenous stages are located in the distal part of the columnar epithelial cells of the tips of the villi in the small intestine posterior to the bile duct. First-generation meronts mature at two days and second-generation meronts at four days; gamonts mature about five days after infection. The prepatent period is 6–7 days and the patent period approximately five days. Oocyst sporulation time is 5–7 days.

Clinical signs and pathology: *Eimeria debliecki* has been described as causing clinical disease and severe pathology, with diarrhoea, inappetence, emaciation, depressed growth and occasional mortality in young piglets. Older animals are seldom, if ever, affected. Catarrhal inflammation of the jejunum is seen. On *post mortem*, there may be enteritis and large numbers of meronts and gamonts may be found in mucosal scrapings. On histopathology, there may be villous atrophy, villous fusion and crypt hyperplasia.

Eimeria polita

Eimeria polita (Phylum: Apicomplexa; Class: Conoidasida; Order: Eucoccidiorida; Family: Eimeriidae) is a parasite distributed worldwide and localised in the small intestine of pigs. The endogenous

stages occur in the epithelium at the tips of the villi in the jejunum and ileum. There are thought to be two generations of meronts. Gamonts and gametes are found in the same area of the intestine and mature 8–9 days after infection. The prepatent period is 7–8 days and the patent period 6–8 days.

Clinical signs and pathology: *Eimeria polita* is thought to be moderately pathogenic. Mixed infections are common and several coccidial species may be involved in causing diarrhoea in young piglets. Heavy infections may cause diarrhoea, inappetence, weight loss, unthriftiness, dehydration and death. On *post mortem*, there may be enteritis and large numbers of meronts and gamonts may be found in mucosal scrapings. On histopathology, there may be villous atrophy, villous fusion and crypt hyperplasia.

Eimeria scabra

Eimeria scabra (Phylum: Apicomplexa; Class: Conoidasida; Order: Eucoccidiorida; Family: Eimeriidae) is a parasite distributed worldwide and localised in the small intestine of pigs. It is not generally considered pathogenic, but it may cause mild diarrhoea in piglets. The endogenous stages are found in the epithelial cells of the villi and the necks of the crypts in the posterior small intestine, and also in the caecum and colon. There are three generations of meronts. The first-generation meronts mature at three days, second-generation meronts mature at five days and a third generation of meronts matures seven days after infection. The prepatent period is 7–11 days and the patent period 4–8 days. Sporulation time is 9–12 days.

Clinical signs and pathology: Occasional diarrhoea. On *post mortem*, there may be enteritis and large numbers of meronts and gamonts may be found in mucosal scrapings. On histopathology, there may be villous atrophy, villous fusion and crypt hyperplasia.

Eimeria spinosa

Eimeria spinosa (Phylum: Apicomplexa; Class: Conoidasida; Order: Eucoccidiorida; Family: Eimeriidae) is a parasite distributed worldwide and localised in the small intestine of pigs. All the endogenous stages are found in the villous epithelial cells of the jejunum and ileum. The number of meront generations is not known. The prepatent period is seven days. The sporulation time is 9–10 days.

Clinical signs and pathology: *Eimeria spinosa* has been described as causing clinical disease in young piglets, with diarrhoea, inappetence, emaciation, depressed growth and occasional mortality. Older animals are generally not affected.

Eimeria porci, *E. neodebliecki*, *E. perminuta* and *E. suis* found in pigs are considered non-pathogenic. Oocyst descriptions of these *Eimeria* species, including diagrammatic drawings, are provided in Chapter 4.

Cryptosporidium parvum

Cryptosporidium parvum (Phylum: Apicomplexa; Class: Conoidasida; Order: Cryptogregarinorida; Family: Cryptosporidiidae) is a parasite distributed worldwide and localised in the small intestine of cattle, sheep, goats, horses, pigs, deer and humans (further details of *C. parvum* are given in Chapter 8).

Epidemiology: The epidemiology of infection has not been studied although it is likely to be similar to *C. parvum* infection in other hosts. Piglets are likely to become infected without showing clinical signs but become sources of infection for other piglets that follow. The primary route of infection is direct animal to animal via the faecal–oral route.

Clinical signs and pathology: Most pig cryptosporidial infections are asymptomatic, with the majority of infections occurring in pigs aged 6–12 weeks. Clinically, the disease is characterised by anorexia and diarrhoea, often intermittent, which may result in poor growth rates. Vomiting and diarrhoea have been reported in young piglets with combined rotavirus and *Cryptosporidium* infections. The meronts and gamonts develop in a parasitophorous envelope apparently derived from the microvilli and so the cell disruption seen in other coccidia does not apparently occur. However, mucosal changes are obvious in the ileum where there is stunting, swelling and eventually fusion of the villi. This has a marked effect on the activity of some of the membrane-bound enzymes.

Notes: Recent molecular characterisations have shown that there is extensive host adaptation in *Cryptosporidium* evolution, and many mammals or groups of mammals have host-adapted *Cryptosporidium* genotypes that differ from each other in both DNA sequence and infectivity. Genetic and biological studies have identified two distinct host-adapted strains of *Cryptosporidium* in pigs. Pig genotype I is now considered to be *Cryptosporidium suis*.

Giardia intestinalis

Giardia intestinalis, synonyms *Giardia duodenalis, Giardia lamblia* and *Lamblia lamblia* (Phylum: Metamonada; Class: Trepomonadea; Order: Diplomonadida; Family: Giardiidae), is a parasite distributed worldwide and localised in the small intestine of humans, cattle, sheep, goats, pigs, horses, alpacas, dogs, cats, guinea pigs and chinchillas (further details of this species are given in Chapters 2 and 8). Infection in pigs is considered non-pathogenic.

Notes: The current molecular classification places isolates into eight distinct assemblages. Some authors give separate specific names to organisms isolated from different hosts, although species specificity of many isolates is unknown. Phylogenetic data suggest that *G. intestinalis* is a species complex composed of several species that are host specific.

LARGE INTESTINE

Oesophagostomum

Six species of *Oesophagostomum* have been described from pigs, of which the most commonly encountered species is *O. dentatum* (Table 11.2).

Oesophagostomum dentatum

Oesophagostomum dentatum (Phylum: Nematoda; Class: Chromadorea; Order: Rhabditida; Family: Strongylidae), commonly known as the Nodular worm, is a parasite distributed worldwide and localised in the large intestine of pigs.

Table 11.2 Species of *Oesophagostomum*.

Species	Host	Geographical distribution
Oesophagostomum dentatum	Pigs	Worldwide
Oesophagostomum quadrispinulatum	Pigs, wild boar	Worldwide
Oesophagostomum brevicaudum	Pigs	North America
Oesophagostomum longicaudatum	Pigs	Europe
Oesophagostomum georgianum	Pigs	North America
Oesophagostomum granatensis	Pigs	Europe

Epidemiology: Infection is more prevalent in older pigs, which are generally less susceptible to the pathogenic effects than younger pigs. Survival of free-living L_3 on the pasture and hypobiotic L_4 in the host occur during autumn and winter; the hypobiotic larvae complete their development in the spring, often coincident with farrowing. Transmission may also occur by flies, which can carry L_3 on their legs.

Pathogenesis: *Oesophagostomum* infections in the pig are not often associated with clinical disease. Occasional diarrhoea, depression in weight gain and poor food conversion may occur, especially during the period of emergence of larvae and maturation of worms in the lumen of the large intestine. Burdens of about 3000–20 000 adult worms are associated with subclinical disease experimentally. Occasionally, infection with *Oesophagostomum*, particularly mucosal damage precipitated by larval encystment, may predispose to necrotic enteritis in association with anaerobic flora and perhaps *Balantioides*.

Clinical signs and pathology: Pregnant sows show inappetence, become very thin, and following farrowing milk production is reduced, with effects on litter performance. In heavy infections, there is thickening of the large intestinal wall with catarrhal enteritis. Nodule formation with *O. dentatum* is small compared with other species.

Diagnosis: It is based on *post mortem* findings and faecal egg counts. Mixed infections with nodular worms and *Hyostrongylus* occur frequently in pigs at pasture and their eggs are difficult to distinguish, requiring faecal culture to distinguish L_3.

Control and treatment: Infections with *Oesophagostomum* are more likely to occur in outdoor pigs kept on pasture. Good management practices, such as provision of clean pastures, rotation, mixed or alternate grazing and strategic dosing regimens, should be considered. Adult worms are susceptible to benzimidazoles, levamisole and macrocyclic lactones. Anthelmintic treatment does not always affect the larvae within the nodules and repeat treatments several weeks apart are required to reduce the worm population.

Trichuris suis

Trichuris suis (Phylum: Nematoda; Class: Enoplea; Order: Enoplida; Family: Trichuridae), commonly known as the Whipworm, is a parasite distributed worldwide and localised in the large intestine of pigs and wild boar.

Epidemiology: The most important feature is the longevity of the eggs, which may survive for three or even four years as a reservoir of infection in piggeries. Generally, pigs of around 2–4 months of age are the most heavily infected.

Pathogenesis: Most infections are light and asymptomatic. Occasionally, when large numbers of worms are present, they cause a haemorrhagic colitis and/or a diphtheritic inflammation of the caecal mucosa. This results from the subepithelial location and continuous movement of the anterior end of the whipworm as it searches for blood and fluid. In pigs, heavy infections are thought to facilitate the invasion of potentially pathogenic spirochaetes.

Clinical signs and pathology: Despite the fact that pigs have a high incidence of light infections, the clinical significance of this genus is generally negligible, although isolated outbreaks have been recorded. Sporadic disease due to heavy infection is occasionally seen and is associated with an acute or chronic inflammation of the caecal mucosa with watery diarrhoea that often contains blood. Anaemia may be present. In severe cases, the mucosa of the large intestine is inflamed and haemorrhagic with ulceration and formation of diphtheritic membranes.

Diagnosis: Since the clinical signs are not pathognomonic, diagnosis may depend on finding numbers of lemon-shaped *Trichuris* eggs in the faeces. However, since clinical signs may occur during the prepatent period, diagnosis in food animals may depend on necropsy.

Control and treatment: Prophylaxis is rarely necessary. Attention should be given to areas where eggs might continue to survive for long periods. Such areas should be thoroughly cleaned and disinfected or sterilised by wet or dry heat. The benzimidazoles or levamisole by injection are effective against adult *Trichuris*, but less so against the larval stage. Some benzimidazoles need to be administered over several days. Doramectin is also effective, as is in-feed medication with dichlorvos (where available).

Notes: The adults are usually found in the caecum but are only occasionally present in sufficient numbers to be clinically significant.

Intestinal flukes

Several species of intestinal fluke belonging to the genera *Gastrodiscus* and *Gastrodiscoides* have been reported in pigs. Further details on the life cycle, epidemiology, treatment and control of intestinal flukes are provided in Chapter 10.

Gastrodiscus aegyptiacus

Gastrodiscus aegyptiacus (Phylum: Platyhelminthes; Class: Trematoda; Order: Plagiorchiida; Family: Gastrodiscidae), commonly known as the Intestinal fluke, is localised in the small and large intestines of horses, pigs, warthogs and humans. The intermediate hosts are snails of the genera *Bulinus* and *Cleopatra* and it is distributed in Africa and India.

Gastrodiscus hominis

Gastrodiscus hominis (Phylum: Platyhelminthes; Class: Trematoda; Order: Plagiorchiida; Family: Gastrodiscidae), commonly known as the Intestinal fluke, is localised in the large intestine of pigs and humans and is distributed in Asia.

Flagellate protozoa

Flagellate protozoa are commonly found in pig faeces but are generally considered non-pathogenic. The life cycle is similar for all species found in pigs. Transmission is thought to occur by ingestion of trophozoites from faeces. All are generally only identified from smears taken from the large intestine of fresh carcasses.

Tritrichomonas suis

Tritrichomonas suis, synonyms *Trichomonas suis* and *Tritrichomonas foetus* (Phylum: Metamonada; Class: Trichomonadea; Order: Trichomonadida; Family: Trichomonadidae), is a parasite distributed worldwide and localised in the nasal passages, stomach, caecum and colon of pigs. It occurs commonly and is considered non-pathogenic. The organism can cause abortion in sows when experimentally introduced into the reproductive tract.

Notes: *Tritrichomonas suis* is now thought to be synonymous with *Tritrichomonas foetus*, which has been found worldwide and is an important cause of infertility, abortion and endometritis in cattle (see Chapter 8). *Tritrichomonas foetus* is also associated with large bowel diarrhoea in cats (see Chapter 12).

Chilomastix mesnili

Chilomastix mesnili, synonyms *Chilomastix suis*, *Chilomastix hominis* and *Macrostoma mesnili* (Phylum: Metamonada; Class: Trepomonadea; Order: Retortamonadida; Family: Retortamonadorididae), is a parasite distributed worldwide and localised in the caecum and colon of humans, apes (chimpanzee, orangutan), monkeys (macaques) and pigs, being non-pathogenic.

Other intestinal protozoa

Entamoeba suis

Entamoeba suis (Phylum: Amoebozoa; Class: Archamoeba; Order: Entamoebida; Family: Entamoebidae) is a non-pathogenic parasite distributed worldwide and localised in the large intestine of pigs.

Diagnosis: Identification of trophozoites or cysts in large intestinal contents or faeces.

Control and treatment: Not required.

Iodamoeba buetschlii

Iodamoeba buetschlii, synonyms *Iodamoeba wenyonii*, *Iodamoeba suis*, *Entamoeba williamsi* and *Endolimax williamsi* (Phylum: Amoebozoa; Class: Archamoebea; Order: Entamoebida; Family: Entamoebidae), is a parasite distributed worldwide and localised in the large intestine of pigs, humans, apes (chimpanzee, gorilla) and monkeys. It is non-pathogenic.

Notes: *Iodamoeba buetschlii* is the most common amoeba found in pigs and is also commonly found in monkeys and humans.

Endolimax nana

Endolimax nana, synonyms *Amoeba limax*, *Entamoeba nana*, *Endolimax intestinalis*, *Endolimax suis* and *Endolimax ratti* (Phylum: Amoebozoa; Class: Archamoebea; Order: Entamoebida; Family: Entamoebidae), is a parasite distributed worldwide and localised in the large intestine of pigs, humans, apes (chimpanzee, gorilla) and monkeys. It is non-pathogenic.

Notes: *Endolimax nana* is common in humans, primates and pigs.

Balantioides coli

Balantioides coli (Phylum: Ciliophora; Class: Litostomatea; Order: Vestibuliferida; Family: Balantidiidae) is a parasite distributed worldwide and it is localised in the large intestine of pigs, humans, camels, monkeys, dogs (rarely) and rats.

Epidemiology: *Balantioides coli* probably exists as a commensal in the large intestine of most pigs. Humans may occasionally become clinically affected through contamination of foodstuffs or hands with pig faeces. Transmission occurs by ingestion of cysts or trophozoites. The cysts are resistant to environmental conditions and can survive for weeks in pig faeces. The pig is the usual source of infection for humans and dogs.

Pathogenesis: Normally non-pathogenic, these protozoa may, for reasons unknown, occasionally cause ulceration of the mucosa and accompanying dysentery in the pig. *Balantioides* may be a secondary invader within lesions of the large intestine.

Clinical signs and pathology: Occasionally it causes diarrhoea or dysentery. The organisms are found in enormous numbers in the lumen of the large intestine with normal caecal mucosa (Fig. 11.6). However, the organism may be found within mucosal ulcers initiated

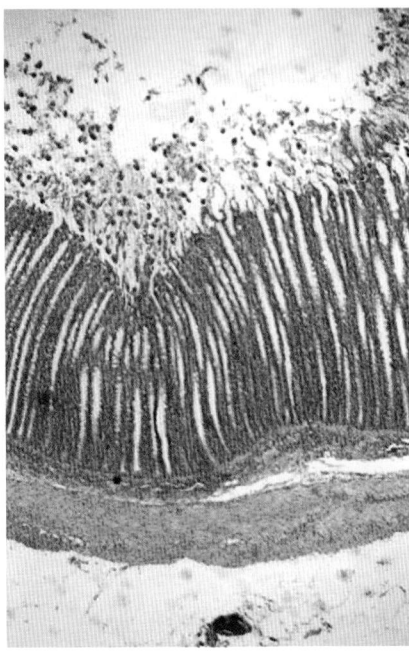

Fig. 11.6 Large numbers of *Balantioides coli* in the lumen of the large intestine.

by other infections. It produces hyaluronidase, which might help to enlarge the lesions by attacking the intercellular ground substance.

Diagnosis: *Balantioides* is easily recognised by microscopic examination of intestinal contents or by histological examination of intestinal lesions.

Control and treatment: Routine hygiene measures to prevent ingestion of cysts or faeces should prevent infection. Tetracyclines are effective.

Parasites of the respiratory system

NASAL PASSAGES

Tritrichomonas suis

For more details see section on Large intestine.

LUNGS

Metastrongylus spp.

Epidemiology: Metastrongylosis shows a characteristic age distribution, being most prevalent in pigs of 4–7 months old. It can be of high prevalence in wild boar. The parasite is common in most countries, although outbreaks of disease do not often occur, probably due to the fact that most systems of pig husbandry do not allow ready access to earthworms by pigs. Although it is often suggested that *Metastrongylus* may transmit some of the porcine viruses and may enhance the effect of pathogens already present in the lungs, the role of the worm is not conclusively proven.

Pathogenesis: The adult worms are found in the lumen of small bronchi and bronchioles, especially those of the posterior lobes of the lungs, and provoke a chronic catarrhal and eosinophilic bronchiolitis and bronchitis. Purulent staphylococcal infection in the lungs has been noted in many cases of metastrongylosis. The worms are also believed to be responsible for the occasional transmission of swine influenza virus, but conclusive proof is not available.

Clinical signs and pathology: Most infections are light and asymptomatic, particularly in older pigs. However, in heavy infections in young animals, coughing can be marked and is accompanied by dyspnoea and nasal discharge. Secondary bacterial infection may complicate the signs, inducing inappetence and loss of weight. During the prepatent period, areas of pulmonary consolidation, bronchial muscular hypertrophy and peribronchial lymphoid hyperplasia develop, often accompanied by areas of overinflation. When the worms are mature, and eggs are aspirated into the smaller air passages and parenchyma, consolidation increases and emphysema is more marked. Hypersecretion of bronchiolar mucus also occurs during this stage. About six weeks after infection, chronic bronchitis and emphysema are established and small greyish nodules may be found in the posterior part of the diaphragmatic lobes; these may aggregate to form larger areas and are slow to resolve.

Diagnosis: For faecal examination, saturated magnesium sulfate should be used as the flotation solution because of the heavy density of the eggs. The small, rough-shelled, larvated eggs are characteristic, but it should be noted that *Metastrongylus* is often present in normal pigs, and pulmonary signs may be due to microbial infection rather than lungworms. Egg output may be sporadic in older pigs. The disease is most often encountered in pigs on pasture, though an occasional outbreak has occurred in yarded pigs. Disease history and clinical signs are also an aid to diagnosis.

Control and treatment: When pig husbandry is based on pasture, control is extremely difficult because of the ubiquity and longevity of the earthworm intermediate host. On farms where severe outbreaks have occurred, pigs should be housed, dosed and the infected pasture cultivated or grazed with other livestock. Many anthelmintics, including the modern benzimidazoles, levamisole and the macrocyclic lactones, are highly effective.

Metastrongylus apri

Metastrongylus apri, synonym *Metastrongylus elongatus* (Phylum: Nematoda; Class: Chromadorea; Order: Rhabditida; Family: Metastrongylidae), commonly known as the Pig lungworm, is a parasite distributed worldwide and localised in the lung of pigs and wild boars, but it has been recorded also in sheep, deer and in other ruminants. This parasite has earthworms (i.e. *Lumbricus terrestris*, *Lumbricus rubellus*, *Diplocardia* spp., *Eisenia austriaca*, *Dendrobaena rubida*, *Helodrilus foetidus* and *Helodrilus caliginosus*) as intermediate hosts.

Metastrongylus pudendotectus

Metastrongylus pudendotectus, synonym *Metastrongylus brevivaginatus* (Phylum: Nematoda; Class: Chromadorea; Order: Rhabditida; Family: Metastrongylidae), commonly known as the Pig lungworm, is a parasite distributed worldwide and localised in the lung of pigs and wild boars. This parasite has earthworms (i.e. *Lumbricus terrestris*, *L. rubellus*) as intermediate hosts.

Echinococcus granulosus

For more details see Parasites of the liver.

Parasites of the liver

Ascaris suum

For more details on 'milk spot' liver caused by migrating larvae, see section on Small intestine.

Toxocara canis

Migrating larvae of this species can also cause 'milk spot' liver in pigs. For more details see Chapter 12.

Fasciola hepatica

Fasciola hepatica (Phylum: Platyhelminthes; Class: Trematoda; Order: Plagiorchiida; Family: Fasciolidae), commonly known as the Liver fluke, is a parasite distributed worldwide and localised in the liver of sheep, cattle, goats, horses, deer, humans and other mammals. This parasite has snails of the genus *Galba* as intermediate hosts (for more details see Chapter 9).

Fasciola gigantica

Fasciola gigantica (Phylum: Platyhelminthes; Class: Trematoda; Order: Plagiorchiida; Family: Fasciolidae), commonly known as the Tropical large liver fluke, is localised in the liver of cattle, buffalo, sheep, goats, pigs, camels, deer and humans. This parasite is found in Africa and Asia and has snails of the genus *Galba* as intermediate hosts (for more details see Chapter 9).

Echinococcus granulosus

Echinococcus granulosus (Phylum: Platyhelminthes; Class: Cestoda; Order: Cyclophyllidea; Family: Taeniidae), commonly known as the Dwarf dog tapeworm, causes a disease named as hydatidosis, is a parasite distributed worldwide, and is localised mainly in the liver and lungs of intermediate hosts (i.e. domestic and wild ruminants, humans, primates, pigs and lagomorphs) and small intestine of definitive hosts (dogs and many wild canids) (for more details see Chapter 9).

Pathogenesis: Hydatid cysts generally cause no clinical signs in pigs. Pressure atrophy of the liver and ascites may be found in heavy infections. Dyspnoea and coughing may be observed in heavily infected lungs.

Taenia hydatigena (metacestode)

Taenia hydatigena, synonyms *Taenia marginata* and *Cysticercus tenuicollis* (Phylum: Platyhelminthes; Class: Cestoda; Order: Cyclophyllidea; Family: Taeniidae), is a parasite distributed worldwide and localised mainly in the abdominal cavity and liver of intermediate hosts (i.e. sheep, cattle, deer, pigs and horses) and small intestine of definitive hosts (dogs, foxes, weasels, stoats, polecats, wolves and hyenas) (for more details see Chapter 9).

Notes: The correct nomenclature for the intermediate host stage is 'metacestode stage of *Taenia hydatigena*' rather than '*Cysticercus tenuicollis*'.

Parasites of the pancreas

Eurytrema pancreaticum

Eurytrema pancreaticum, synonyms *Distoma pancreaticum* and *Eurytrema ovis* (Phylum: Platyhelminthes; Class: Trematoda; Order: Plagiorchiida; Family: Dicrocoeliidae), commonly known as the Pancreatic fluke, is localised in the pancreatic ducts and occasionally the bile ducts or duodenum of cattle, buffalo, sheep, goats, pigs, camels and humans. This parasite is found in eastern Asia and South America and has land snails, particularly of the genus *Bradybaena*, grasshoppers of the genus *Conocephalus* or tree crickets (*Oecanthus*) as intermediate hosts.

Parasites of the circulatory system

Schistosomes

Schistosomes are flukes found in the circulatory system. The sexes are separate, the small adult female lying permanently in a longitudinal groove, the gynaecophoric canal, in the body of the male (see Fig. 1.109). The genus has been divided into four groups – *haematobium*, *indicum*, *mansoni* and *japonicum* – but the genus as currently defined is paraphyletic, so revisions are likely.

Indicum group

Schistosoma spindale

Schistosoma spindale (Phylum: Platyhelminthes; Class: Trematoda; Order: Strigeidida; Family: Schistosomatidae), commonly known as the Blood fluke, causes a disease called bilharziosis and is localised in the mesenteric veins of cattle, horses, pigs and occasionally dogs. This parasite is found in parts of Asia and the Far East and has snails (genera *Planorbis*, *Indoplanorbis*, *Galba*) as intermediate hosts.

Japonicum group

Schistosoma japonicum

Schistosoma japonicum (Phylum: Platyhelminthes; Class: Trematoda; Order: Strigeidida; Family: Schistosomatidae), commonly known as the Blood fluke, causes a disease called bilharziosis and is localised in the portal and mesenteric veins of cattle, horses, sheep, goats, dogs, cats, rabbits, pigs and humans. This parasite is present in Southeast Asia and has snails belonging to the genus *Oncomelania* as intermediate hosts.

Other schistosomes

For more general details of *Schistosoma* species see Chapter 8.

Trypanosomes

See Chapter 2 (Family Trypanosomatidae) for general description and Chapter 8 for detailed descriptions of individual species of trypanosomes and their control.

Trypanosoma brucei brucei

Trypanosoma brucei brucei (Phylum: Euglenozoa; Class: Kinetoplastea; Order: Trypanosomatida; Family: Trypanosomatidae) causes a disease commonly known as Nagana, and is localised in the blood but also extravascularly in, for example, the myocardium, central nervous system (CNS) and reproductive tract of cattle, horses, donkeys, zebu, sheep, goats, camels, pigs, dogs, cats and wild game species. This parasite is found in sub-Saharan Africa.

Treatment: The two drugs in common use in cattle are isometamidium and diminazene aceturate and both should be suitable for use in pigs. These are usually successful except where trypanosomes have developed resistance to the drug or in some very chronic cases. Treatment should be followed by surveillance, since reinfection, followed by clinical signs and parasitaemia, may occur within a week or two. Alternatively, the animal may relapse after chemotherapy due to a persisting focus of infection in the tissues or because the trypanosomes are drug resistant.

Trypanosoma congolense

Trypanosoma congolense (Phylum: Euglenozoa; Class: Kinetoplastea; Order: Trypanosomatida; Family: Trypanosomatidae) causes a disease commonly known as Nagana, Paranagana, Gambia fever, Ghindi or Gobial, and is localised in the blood of pigs and also horses, cattle, goats, sheep and dogs. It is distributed in sub-Saharan Africa.

Treatment: In infected cattle, the two drugs in common use are diminazene aceturate (Berenil®) and homidium salts (Ethidium® and Novidium®) and are appropriate for use in pigs infected with *T. congolense*. As with *T. brucei*, these drugs are usually successful except where trypanosomes have developed resistance to the drug or in some very chronic cases.

Trypanosoma simiae

Trypanosoma simiae, synonyms *Trypanosoma congolense simiae*, *Trypanosoma rodhaini* and *Trypanosoma porci* (Phylum: Euglenozoa; Class: Kinetoplastea; Order: Trypanosomatida; Family: Trypanosomatidae), is localised in the blood of pigs, camels, sheep and goats and is found in Central Africa.

Epidemiology: *Trypanosoma simiae* is mainly a parasite of warthogs transmitted by tsetse flies, in which the parasites develop in the midgut and proboscis. Tsetse flies also transmit the parasite to pigs, but transmission between pigs is usually mechanical.

Treatment: In pigs, *T. simiae* is the most important trypanosome pathogen and the rapid onset of death gives little chance of treatment. Isometamidium chloride at increased dose rates of 12.5–35 mg/kg i.m. or a combination of quinapyramine (7.5 mg/kg s.c.) and diminazene aceturate (5 mg/kg i.m.) can be used. A suramin–quinapyramine complex (4 ml per 5 kg) has shown some success in prophylaxis in young piglets for a period of three months, and in adults for five months.

Babesiosis

Two species of *Babesia* are found in pigs: *Babesia perroncitoi* is a small babesia; *Babesia trautmanni* is a large babesia. Infection is transmitted to pigs via tick vectors. The rapidly dividing parasites in the red cells produce destruction of the erythrocytes with accompanying haemoglobinaemia, haemoglobinuria and fever.

Pathology: The spleen is enlarged and there is pulmonary, renal and gastrointestinal hyperaemia and oedema. Subepicardial and subendocardial haemorrhages are present with petechiation present on the serous membranes.

Diagnosis: The history and clinical signs of fever, anaemia, jaundice and haemoglobinuria in pigs located in enzootic areas where ticks occur are usually sufficient to justify a diagnosis of babesiosis. For confirmation, examination of blood smears, stained with Giemsa, will reveal the parasites in the red cells.

Control and treatment: Tick control measures can be considered for controlling disease. Topical application of acaricides may provide some level of protection but may be difficult in pigs, be expensive and may have a negative cost–benefit. Under certain conditions, it may be more beneficial to attain endemic stability by allowing early infection and development of immunity. Diminazene aceturate at 3.5 mg/kg i.m. is effective.

Babesia perroncitoi

Babesia perroncitoi (Phylum: Apicomplexa; Class: Aconoidasida; Order: Piroplasmida; Family: Babesiidae) is localised in blood of pigs and distributed in southern Europe, West and Central Africa and Vietnam.

Epidemiology: Wild pigs may act as reservoirs of infection and the tick vectors include *Rhipicephalus* (*R. appendiculatus, R. sanguineus*) and *Dermacentor* (*D. reticulatus*).

Clinical signs: Clinical signs include fever, anaemia, haemoglobinuria, jaundice, oedema and incoordination. Abortion may occur in pregnant sows.

Babesia trautmanni

Babesia trautmanni (Phylum: Apicomplexa; Class: Aconoidasida; Order: Piroplasmida; Family: Babesiidae) is localised in blood of pigs and is distributed in southern Europe, Africa and parts of Asia.

Epidemiology: Infection and disease are seasonal according to the activity of the tick vector. Wild boar and warthogs may act as reservoirs of infection and the tick vectors include *Rhipicephalus* (*R. appendiculatus, R. sanguineus*), *Dermacentor* (*D. reticulatus*) and *Rhipicephalus* (*Boophilus*) *decoloratus*. Transovarian transmission has been reported in *R. sanguineus*.

Clinical signs: Clinical signs include fever, anaemia, haemoglobinuria, jaundice, oedema and incoordination. Abortion may occur in pregnant sows. Mortality may reach 50% and pigs of all ages are affected.

Mycoplasma suis

Mycoplasma suis, synonym *Eperythrozoon suis* (Phylum: Firmicutes; Classe: Mollicutes; Order: Mycoplasmatales; Family: Mycoplasmataceae), is a bacterium distributed worldwide and localised in the blood of pigs.

Epidemiology: Transmission is seasonal, being more common in summer and autumn when biting flies are active. The pig louse (*Haemotopinus suis*) has also been incriminated in transmission.

Pathogenesis: Of the *Mycoplasma* species, *M. suis* is the most pathogenic, and infection may be very severe and fatal. Pigs are first depressed and inappetent, have high fever and go on to develop anaemia, becoming weaker and constipated, then jaundiced. Infection in sows produces both acute and chronic syndromes.

Acute infections often occur *post partum* and affected animals are pyrexic and anorexic and may show agalactia and mammary and vulvular oedema. Chronic infections are usually subclinical and often difficult to diagnose. Affected animals are generally in poor condition, pale and jaundiced.

Clinical signs and pathology: Jaundice and anaemia in very young pigs. The main pathological changes occur in the liver and spleen. In the liver there is fatty degeneration and atrophy, and necrosis of central hepatic cells with widespread lymphatic infiltration. Reticuloendothelial cells in liver, spleen and lymph nodes are hypertrophied and filled with haemosiderin deposits.

Diagnosis: Identification from staining artefacts requires good blood smears and filtered Giemsa stain. The organisms appear as cocci or short rods on the surface of the erythrocytes, often completely surrounding the margin of the red cell. However, *Mycoplasma* organisms are relatively loosely attached to the red cell surface and are often found free in the plasma.

Control and treatment: Control of ectoparasite infections and possibly addition of arsenicals or tetracyclines to the diet have been advocated in countries where the disease is endemic. Tetracyclines and the arsenical roxarsone are reported to be effective.

Notes: The taxonomy of this species is subject to much debate and it is now considered to be in the bacterial genus *Mycoplasma* (class Mollicutes) based on 16S rRNA gene sequences and phylogenetic analysis.

Parasites of the nervous system

Toxoplasma gondii

For more details see Parasites of the locomotory system.

Parasites of the reproductive/urogenital system

Stephanurus dentatus

Stephanurus dentatus (Phylum: Nematoda; Class: Chromadorea; Order: Rhabditida; Family: Syngamidae), commonly known as the Pig kidney worm, is localised in the kidney, perirenal fat and occasionally the axial musculature and the spinal canal of pigs, wild boar and rarely cattle. This parasite is distributed mainly in warm and tropical regions of all continents and does not occur in Western Europe.

Epidemiology: Although the adult worms are never numerous, they are very fecund and an infected pig may pass a million eggs per day. The L_3 is susceptible to desiccation, so that stephanurosis is mainly associated with damp ground. Since it infects readily by skin penetration, the pigs' habit of lying around the feeding area when kept outside presents a risk, as does damp unhygienic accommodation for housed animals. Such conditions, coupled with prenatal infection and the longevity of the worm, ensure continuity of infection through many generations of pigs. All ages of pigs are susceptible to infection. Piglets can be infected *in utero*.

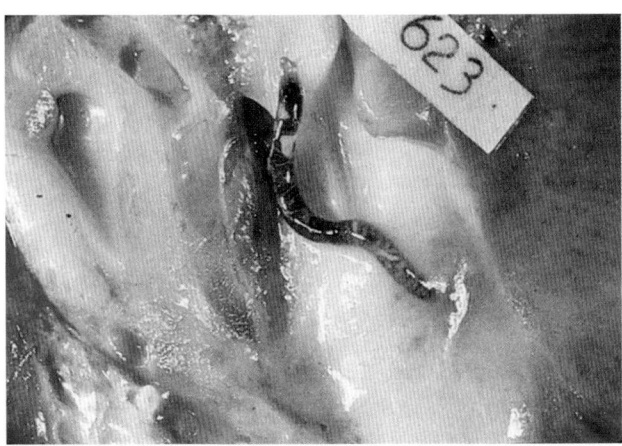

Fig. 11.7 *Stephanurus dentatus* worms in a kidney.

Pathogenesis: Although the favoured site is the perirenal fat, some worms occur in the kidney itself, in the calyces and pelvis (Fig. 11.7). Erratic migration is common in *Stephanurus* infection, and larvae have been found in most organs, including the lungs, spleen and spinal cord, and in muscle. In these sites they are trapped by encapsulation and never reach the perirenal area. Prenatal infection has been reported. The main pathogenic effect is due to the larvae, which by the late L_4 stage have heavily sclerotised buccal capsules capable of tearing tissue, and they cause much damage to the liver and occasionally other organs in their wanderings. In heavy infections there may be severe cirrhosis, thrombosis of hepatic vessels and ascites and, in rare cases, liver failure and death. In most infections, however, the effects are seen only after slaughter as patchy cirrhosis, and the main importance of the worm is economic, from liver condemnation. In general, the adult worms are not pathogenic. Usually the adult worms, soon after arrival at the perirenal site, are encapsulated in cysts, which may contain greenish pus. In rare cases the ureters may be thickened and stenosed, with consequent hydronephrosis.

Clinical signs and pathology: In most infections the only sign is failure to gain weight or, in more severe cases, weight loss. Where there is more extensive liver damage, there may be ascites, but it is only when there is massive invasion, comparable to acute fasciolosis in sheep, that death occurs. Percutaneous infection leads to the formation of nodules in the skin, with oedema and enlargement of the superficial lymph nodes. Migrating larvae produce acute inflammatory lesions, especially in the liver. Inflammation may lead to abscess formation and extensive liver cirrhosis. The adult parasite is not markedly pathogenic and is found in cysts 0.5–4 cm in diameter, each cyst containing a pair of worms. Cysts in the kidney may cause thickening of the ureter, which in chronic cases may be almost occluded.

Diagnosis: The clinical signs are likely to be few, and since most of the damage occurs during the prepatent phase, eggs may not be found in the urine. However, in endemic areas, where pigs are failing to thrive and where local abattoirs record appreciable numbers of cirrhotic livers, a presumptive diagnosis can be made. Worms can be identified at necropsy.

Control and treatment: One approach to control is based on the susceptibility of the L_3 to desiccation and on the fact that a major route of infection is percutaneous. It follows that the provision of impervious surfaces around the feeding areas for outdoor reared pigs, and simple hygiene, ensuring clean dry flooring in pig houses, will help to limit infection. This approach may be supplemented by segregating young pigs from those of more than nine months of age, which will be excreting eggs.

The 'gilt only' scheme, which was advocated by workers in the USA, consists essentially of using only gilts for breeding. The gilts are reared on land which is dry and exposed to the sun. A single litter is taken from them and as soon as the piglets can be weaned, the gilts are marketed. The scheme takes advantage of the extremely long prepatent period, which allows a single breeding cycle by the gilts to be completed before egg laying begins and so progressively eliminates infection. The boars used in the scheme are housed on concrete.

Regimens incorporating anthelmintic control recommend treatment of sows and gilts 1–2 weeks before putting to the boar, and again 1–2 weeks before farrowing. It should be remembered in designing a control system that the earthworm transport hosts present a continuous reservoir of infection. Levamisole, the modern benzimidazoles and ivermectin are effective.

Parasites of the locomotory system

Taenia solium

Taenia solium, synonyms *Cysticercus cellulosae* and *Cysticercus solium* (Phylum: Platyhelminthes; Class: Cestoda; Order: Cyclophyllidea; Family: Taeniidae), commonly known as the Human pork tapeworm, is localised in the small intestine of humans (final hosts) and in the muscle of pigs, wild boar, rarely dogs and humans (intermediate hosts). Note that humans can act as an intermediate as well as a definitive host. This cestode is most prevalent in South and Central America, India, Africa and parts of the Far East, apart from areas where there are religious sanctions on the eating of pork. It is now uncommon in many developed countries.

Epidemiology: In developing countries, this depends primarily on the close association of rural pigs with humans, and in particular their often unrestricted access to human faeces. Indifferent standards of meat inspection and illicit trading in uninspected pork are also major factors in the spread of the infection. Pigs may acquire massive infections because the gravid segments are not active and may remain in faeces. Humans normally become infected when they consume raw or undercooked pork. As noted above, humans may become infected with cysticerci and this may occur from the ingestion of eggs on vegetables or other foodstuffs contaminated with human faeces or handled by an infected person.

Pathogenesis: Clinical signs are inapparent in pigs naturally infected with cysticerci and generally insignificant in humans with adult tapeworms. However, when humans are infected with cysticerci, various clinical signs may occur depending on the location of the cysts in the organs, muscles or subcutaneous tissue. Cysticerci may be found in every organ of the body in humans but are most common in the subcutaneous tissue, eye and brain. Larvae that reach the brain develop in the ventricles and frequently become racemose in character. Most seriously, cysticerci that develop in the CNS produce mental disturbances or clinical signs of epilepsy or increased intracranial pressure. They may also develop in the eye with consequent loss of vision. In Latin America alone, it is estimated that almost 0.5 million people are affected, by either the nervous or ocular forms of cysticercosis.

Clinical signs and pathology: Infected pigs are usually asymptomatic. Infection is generally insignificant in humans, although adult tapeworms can occasionally cause abdominal discomfort and diarrhoea. However, when humans, acting as the intermediate host, are infected with cysticerci, various clinical signs may occur, depending on the location and number of cysts in the organs, muscles or subcutaneous tissue. CNS signs include mental disturbances or clinical signs of epilepsy and may be fatal. Loss of vision may occur when the eye is involved. Cysticerci, comprising a single large cyst and inverted scolex, measure 1–2 cm and are easily visible between muscle fibres. The cysticerci are rapidly ensheathed in connective tissue and create a crescentic zone of degenerative lysis around them, thereby allowing room to grow. Pigs are usually slaughtered at an age when all cysticerci are generally still viable.

Diagnosis: For all practical purposes, diagnosis in pigs depends on meat inspection procedures but this lacks sensitivity for low infection levels. Individual countries have different regulations regarding the inspection of carcasses, but invariably the masseter muscle, tongue and heart are incised and examined, and the intercostal muscles and diaphragm inspected. Proglottids can sometimes be seen in faeces. Cysticerci of *T. solium* are larger and more numerous than those of *T. saginata* (see Chapter 8). In humans, the diagnosis of cerebral cysticercosis depends primarily on the detection of cysticerci by computed tomography (CT) and on the finding of antibodies to cysticerci in the cerebrospinal fluid.

Control and treatment: Control depends ultimately on the enforcement of meat inspection regulations and deep-freezing procedures. Freezing pork at –10 to –8 °C continuously for four days kills the cysticerci but chilling the meat at 0 °C is not sufficient and cysts may remain viable in chilled meat for 70 days. The exclusion of pigs from contact with human faeces, the thorough cooking of pork and proper standards of personal hygiene will reduce the prevalence of infection. No effective drugs are available to kill cysticerci in the pig, although in humans praziquantel and albendazole are considered to be of some value as possible alternatives to surgery.

Notes: A third form of *Taenia* ('Asian *Taenia*') has been reported throughout eastern Asia and also from parts of East Africa and Poland. The 'Asian *Taenia*' appears to be closely related to *T. saginata* but its molecular profile indicates that it is genetically different. The cysticerci of this tapeworm are located in the liver of pigs and wild boar and occasionally in cattle, goats and monkeys. The 'Asian *Taenia*' is considered not to be an important cause of human cysticercosis.

Trichinella spiralis

For more details see section on Small intestine.

Toxoplasma gondii

Toxoplasma gondii (Phylum: Apicomplexa; Class: Conoidasida; Order: Eucoccidiorida; Family: Sarcocystidae) is a parasite distributed worldwide and localised in muscle, lung, liver, reproductive system and CNS of cats and other felids. This protozoan has any mammal, including humans, or birds as intermediate hosts. The final host, the cat, may also be an intermediate host and harbour extraintestinal stages of this parasite.

Epidemiology: The cat plays a central role in the epidemiology of toxoplasmosis, and infection in pigs may occur through ingestion of feed contaminated with cat faeces or through ingestion of bradyzoites and tachyzoites in the flesh of another intermediate host, such as rats.

Pathogenesis: Most *Toxoplasma* infections in animals are light and consequently asymptomatic. Toxoplasmosis has been occasionally reported in young pigs and may cause severe fetal losses in pregnant sows, but more usually is mild and unnoticed.

Pathology: In heavy infections, the multiplying tachyzoites may produce areas of necrosis in vital organs such as the myocardium, lungs, liver and brain. Examination of the brain may reveal focal microgliosis. The lesions often have a small central focus of necrosis that might be mineralised. Focal leucomalacia in cerebral white matter, due to anoxia arising from placental pathology, is often present.

Diagnosis: Tachyzoites of *T. gondii* are often difficult to find in tissue sections but are more likely to be present in sections of brain and placenta. Identification can be confirmed by immunohistochemistry, while the polymerase chain reaction may be used to identify parasite DNA in tissues. A number of serological tests have been developed, of which the dye test is the longest established serological method, and in many ways represents the gold standard. Its reliability for use in pigs is not known.

Control and treatment: On farms, control is difficult but where possible, animal feedstuffs should be covered to exclude access by cats and insects. Control of rats and regulation of feeding of swill to pigs are measures that will limit exposure to infection. Treatment is not indicated.

Sarcocystiosis

Sarcocystis is one of the most prevalent parasites of livestock and three species are reported in pigs (Table 11.3). Most cases of *Sarcocystis* infection are only revealed at meat inspection when the grossly visible sarcocysts in the muscle are discovered. Little is known of the epidemiology but from the high prevalence of symptomless infections observed in abattoirs, it is clear that where dogs and cats are kept in close association with farm animals or their feed, then transmission is likely.

Table 11.3 *Sarcocystis* species found in the muscles of pigs.

Species	Synonym	Definite host	Pathogenicity	Final host
Sarcocystis suicanis	*Sarcocystis porcicanis* *Sarcocystis miescheriana*	Dogs, wolves, foxes	+++	0
Sarcocystis porcifelis	*Sarcocystis suifelis*	Cats	0	0
Sarcocystis suihominis	*Isospora hominis*	Humans	+++	+++

0, non-pathogenic; +, mildly pathogenic; +++, severe pathogenicity.

The only control measures possible are those of simple hygiene. Farm dogs and cats should not be housed in, or allowed access to, fodder stores nor should they be allowed to defecate in pens where livestock are housed. It is also important that they are not fed uncooked meat.

Sarcocystis suicanis

Sarcocystis suicanis, synonyms *Sarcocystis porcicanis*, *Sarcocystis miescheriana* (Phylum: Apicomplexa; Class: Conoidasida; Order: Eucoccidiorida; Family: Sarcocystidae), is a parasite distributed worldwide and localised in the muscle of pigs and has dogs as final hosts.

Pathogenesis: *Sarcocystis suicanis* is pathogenic to the pig and is known to produce signs of enteritis, myositis and lameness. More generally, clinical signs are rarely observed and the most significant effect is the presence of cysts in the muscles of food animals, resulting in downgrading or condemnation of carcasses.

Clinical signs and pathology: In heavy infections of the intermediate hosts, there may be anorexia, fever, anaemia, loss of weight, a disinclination to move and sometimes recumbency. In pigs, meronts present in endothelial cells of capillaries in various organs lead to endothelial cell destruction. As the organisms enter muscle, a wide range of change may be encountered. Microscopic inspection of *Sarcocystis*-infected muscle often reveals occasional degenerate parasitic cysts surrounded by variable numbers of inflammatory cells (very few of which are eosinophils) or, at a later stage, macrophages and granulation tissue. Usually there is no muscle fibre degeneration, but there may be thin linear collections of lymphocytes between fibres in the region. The extent of muscle change bears little relationship to the numbers of developing cysts, but generally very low numbers of *Sarcocystis* produce no reaction. As cysts mature, the cyst capsule within the enlarged muscle fibre becomes thicker and more clearly differentiated from the muscle sarcoplasm.

Sarcocystis porcifelis

Sarcocystis porcifelis, synonym *Sarcocystis suifelis* (Phylum: Apicomplexa; Class: Conoidasida; Order: Eucoccidiorida; Family: Sarcocystidae), is localised in the muscle of pigs and has cats as final hosts. The geographical distribution of this parasite is unknown.

Clinical signs and pathology: The infection is usually asymptomatic. Cysts are found in oesophageal muscles, but their detailed pathology has not been described.

Sarcocystis suihominis

Sarcocystis suihominis, synonym *Isospora hominis* (Phylum: Apicomplexa; Class: Conoidasida; Order: Eucoccidiorida; Family: Sarcocystidae), is localised in the muscle of pigs and has humans and primates as final hosts. The geographical distribution of this parasite is unknown.

Pathogenesis: Infection is not pathogenic for non-human primates but is extremely pathogenic for humans and the pig intermediate host. In the pig, the principal pathogenic effect is attributable to the merogony stages in the vascular endothelium of the liver.

Clinical signs: Acute sarcocystiosis in pigs shows a biphasic fever between 5–9 and 11–15 days post infection. During the second phase, there is apathy, dyspnoea, anaemia and cyanosis of the skin, muscle spasms and hyperexcitability and prostration. Abortion may occur in pregnant sows.

Control: Contamination of animal feed and grazing land with human faeces should be avoided. Human infection can be prevented through adequate cooking or freezing of meat.

Notes: In humans, the ingestion of infected pork containing *S. suihominis* produces clinical signs of bloat, nausea, loss of appetite, stomach ache, vomiting, diarrhoea, difficulty breathing and rapid pulse within 6–42 hours. *Sarcocystis* may be responsible for several idiopathic diseases in humans, including cardiac diseases such as cardiomyopathy and myocarditis and rheumatic diseases. It has also been suggested that *Sarcocystis* may be associated with muscle aches and fatigue as part of chronic fatigue syndrome.

Parasites of the integument

Suifilaria suis

Suifilaria suis (Phylum: Nematoda; Class: Chromadorea; Order: Spirurida; Family: Filariidae) is localised in the subcutaneous and connective tissue of pigs and is distributed in southern Africa. The intermediate host of this parasite is not known.

Pathogenesis: The worms induce small, hard, whitish nodules in the subcutaneous and intermuscular connective tissues. Infection is generally considered to be non-pathogenic, although erupted skin vesicles may become secondarily infected, forming abscesses.

Clinical signs and pathology: Infection is usually asymptomatic, causing no effect on productivity. Vesicular nodules may form in the cutaneous and intermuscular connective tissue.

Diagnosis: This is normally based on clinical signs of small whitish nodules, which eventually burst. Vesicular eruptions contain the eggs.

Control and treatment: As the intermediate host is unknown, control is not feasible or usually required. Treatment is seldom required as infection is of little veterinary relevance.

ECTOPARASITES

LICE

Haematopinus suis

Haematopinus suis (Phylum: Arthropoda; Class: Insecta; Order: Psocodea; Suborder: Anoplura; Family: Haematopinidae), commonly known as the Hog louse, is found on the skin, most commonly around the skinfolds of the neck and jowl, the flanks and the insides of the legs on thin-coated animals. It occurs worldwide.

Epidemiology: Infection is primarily by physical contact between pigs, particularly in closely confined fattening animals and in suckling sows penned with their piglets. However, lice may also be acquired when animals are put into recently vacated dirty accommodation.

Pathogenesis: Infested animals show a reduction in weight gain and are more susceptible to other diseases. In severe infestations, piglets may die of anaemia. *Haematopinus suis* is believed to be a vector of the African swine fever, *Eperythrozoon suis*, and the virus of the swine pox.

Clinical signs and pathology: This louse is very common, and at low intensities is usually tolerated without any signs, apart from occasional mild irritation. It usually occurs in the folds of the neck and jowl, around the ears and on the flanks and backs (Fig. 11.8). The majority of nymphs occur on the head region. However, irritation is caused by the small but frequent blood meals, each of which is taken via a different puncture wound. In heavy infestations, pigs are restless and fail to thrive. Economically, the most important feature of pediculosis in pigs is probably skin damage from scratching, with reduction in hide value. In the most severe cases, pigs may rub most of the hair off their bodies and, if acquired by piglets, *H. suis* infestation may retard growth. Transfer is usually by contact but *H. suis* may survive for up to three days off its host. Hence, transfer can also occur when animals are put into recently vacated dirty accommodation. Both epidermis and corium may be affected by inflammatory lesions at the bite puncture sites. Initially, neutrophil infiltration with necrosis of epithelial cells prevails. This is followed by capillary proliferation with angioblast and fibroblast multiplication and straggled lymphoid infiltration.

Diagnosis: *Haematopinus suis* is the only louse found on pigs. Adults are easily seen on the skin and can be removed and identified under a light microscope.

Control and treatment: Generally, control is based on the application of insecticides or use of a macrocyclic lactone. For herd prophylaxis, gilts and sows should be treated before farrowing to prevent spread of infection to their piglets, and boars treated twice annually. Avermectins given parenterally or the organophosphate phosmet administered as a pour-on have both proved highly effective as a single treatment. Amitraz and deltamethrin are also effective. Once lice have been diagnosed, it is essential to treat the entire herd.

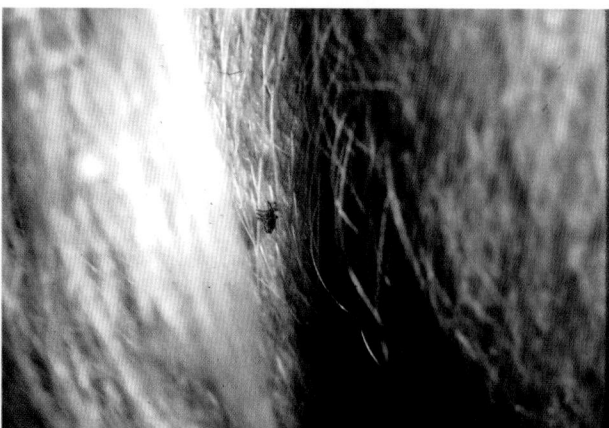

Fig. 11.8 Louse infestation.

FLEAS

Pulex irritans

Pulex irritans (Phylum: Arthropoda; Class: Insecta; Order: Siphonaptera; Family: Pulicidae), sometimes called the human flea, may infest humans and pigs but may also occasionally occur on dogs, cats, rats and badgers.

Epidemiology: Although described as the human flea, *P. irritans* can infest cats, dogs and many other domestic animals, although it is probably most common on pigs. It breeds profusely in pigsties and is usually the most important species in farm areas. People working with infested pigs can also easily become infested and start infestations in their homes.

Pathogenesis: The bites of *Pulex* can cause dermatitis and it may on occasion act as a vector of the plague pathogen *Yersinia pestis*.

Tunga penetrans

Tunga penetrans (Phylum: Arthropoda; Class: Insecta; Order: Siphonaptera; Family: Tungidae), commonly known as the Chigger, Jigger, Chigoe, bicho do pé or Sand flea, is an important parasite of humans in the Neotropical and Afro-tropical regions, but will also infest primates and pigs. In addition, reservoir hosts include cattle, sheep, horses, mules, rats, mice, dogs and other wild animals.

Epidemiology: The main habitat is warm dry soil and sand of beaches, stables and stock farms. On contact, the fleas invade unprotected skin. The most common site of involvement is the feet (interdigital skin and subungual area). The flea has limited jumping ability.

Pathogenesis: Once *T. penetrans* becomes engorged with blood, its presence causes great pain and may produce inflammation and localised ulcers. Tetanus and gangrene may result from secondary infections. Intense local irritation and pruritus are also symptomatic of more minor infestations. *Tunga penetrans* may also pose significant problems in dogs, particularly in the interdigital spaces, under the pads and the scrotum, but infestation tends to be highly localised. The presence of a number of adult *T. penetrans* in the paws can be crippling. The damage to the skin can facilitate the entry of other pathogens, leading to secondary infection and ulceration.

Clinical signs: The presence of the female flea can cause extreme itching, pain and inflammation, and secondary infections may occur. This flea occurs mainly on the feet of humans, causing severe irritation. In pigs, the main sites of attachment are the feet and scrotum, but these animals tolerate the infection with no signs of distress.

Diagnosis: The swelling produced by the female is easily visible and often surrounded by eggs. The nodule (usually on the foot in humans) slowly enlarges over a few weeks in a patient who has recently been in an endemic area. The nodule can range from 4 to 10 mm in diameter. Sometimes, a serosanguineous exudate oozes from the central opening.

Control and treatment: Tungiosis can be controlled by treating infested areas with pesticides (malathion and methoprene have been used successfully) and treating infected reservoir hosts.

Reported topical treatments in humans include cryotherapy or electrodesiccation of the nodules. Application of formaldehyde, chloroform or dichlorodiphenyltrichloroethane (DDT) to the infested skin has been used. Occlusive petroleum suffocates the organism. These treatments do not remove the flea from the skin, and they do not result in quick relief from painful lesions. The flea may also be gently removed with a needle or forceps. Surgical removal of the fleas is the recommended treatment.

A number of surgical treatment methods are available. The flea can be removed from its cavity with sterile instruments but this is more difficult when the flea is engorged. The orifice needs to be enlarged, and the entire nodule should be excised. An antibiotic ointment may be applied, along with systemic antibiotic therapy when indicated. Aggressive treatment of secondary infection and tetanus prophylaxis are important. In dogs, footbathing with 0.2% trichlorphon or metriphonate has been shown to be effective, as has subcutaneous injection of ivermectin (0.2 mg/kg body weight).

MITES

Sarcoptes scabiei

Sarcoptes scabiei (Phylum: Arthropoda; Class: Arachnida; Subclass: Acari; Order: Sarcoptiformes (Astigmata); Family: Sarcoptidae), commonly known as the Scabies mite, is found worldwide infesting all domestic mammals and humans.

Epidemiology: New hosts are infected by contact with infected individuals, presumably by the transfer of larvae, which are commonly present more superficially on the skin surface. Transmission occurs between mature animals and also from mother to offspring at birth. Transfer of different host-adapted populations of *S. scabiei* between different host species often results in only temporary infestations. Infestation may also occur by indirect transfer, since the mites have been shown to be capable of surviving off the host for short periods. The length of time that *S. scabiei* can survive off the host depends on environmental conditions but may be between two and three weeks. Consequently, animal bedding may become contaminated and is a possible source of infestation.

Pathogenesis: Host reactions occur primarily in response to the feeding and burrowing activity of the mites and their faecal deposits. This commonly occurs progressively three weeks into the initial infection. Lesions can occur anywhere on the body, but are usually found on the head where the hair is relatively thin. The infestation spreads quickly from the initial lesions to cause more generalised mange. In pigs, the ears are the most common site of infestation, and are usually the primary focus from which the mite population spreads to other areas of the body, especially the back, flanks and abdomen. Many pigs harbour inapparent infections throughout their lives, and the main mode of transmission appears to be between carrier sows and their piglets during suckling. Signs may appear on the face and ears within three weeks of birth, later extending to other areas. Transmission may also occur during service, especially from an infected boar to gilts.

Clinical signs and pathology: Affected pigs scratch continuously and may lose condition. Common signs are papular eruptions with erythema, pruritus and hair loss. As the infestation progresses, the skin becomes thickened, crusted with exudates and secondarily infected due to damage caused by the host scratching (Fig. 11.9).

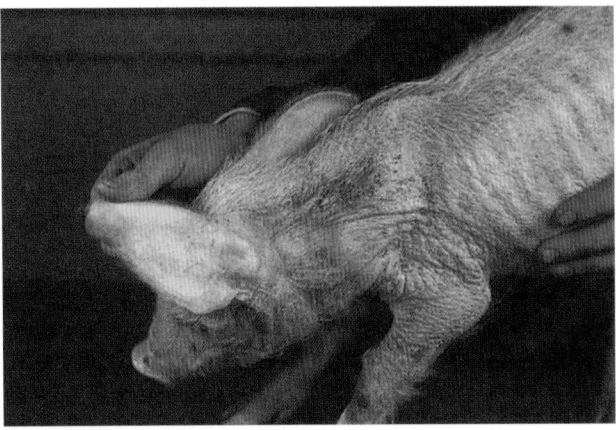
Fig. 11.9 Sarcoptic mange in a pig.

Scaly areas around the edge of lesions indicate the spread of mites. Severe cases exhibit loss of appetite and weight, impaired hearing, blindness and exhaustion. The first lesions appear as small red papules or weals and general erythema about the eyes, around the snout, on the concave surface of the external ears, in the axillae and on the front of the hocks where the skin is thin. Scratching results in excoriation of these affected areas and the formation of brownish scabs on the damaged skin. Subsequently, the skin becomes wrinkled, covered with crusty lesions and thickened.

Diagnosis: Useful diagnostic features of porcine sarcoptic mange include the following.

- The edges of the ears are often first affected and on rubbing, a scratch reflex is readily elicited.
- There is always intense itching, so in cases of dermatitis where there is no itch, sarcoptic mange can be eliminated as a possibility.
- It is a highly contagious condition, and single cases are rarely seen in groups of animals kept in close contact.

Confirmatory diagnosis is by examination of skin scrapings for the presence of mites. However, since these are sometimes difficult to demonstrate, a negative finding should not preclude a tentative diagnosis of mange and initiation of treatment. For confirmatory diagnosis in pigs, a reliable source of material for examination is wax from the ear.

Control and treatment: In pigs, a common control approach is to treat the sow (the main reservoir of infection) before she goes into the farrowing crate or pen. This procedure will be more successful than having to treat partly grown pigs. The offspring of treated sows show better growth rates and shorter finishing periods than those of untreated sows. It is most important that boars are routinely treated at six-monthly intervals, and any newly introduced boar is treated and quarantined as they can readily infect sows at service. In the treatment of affected pigs, acaricide may be applied weekly, by wash or spray, until the signs have regressed. It is recommended that phosmet is applied to the back of the sow 3–7 days before farrowing, pouring a small part of the dose into the ears. As an alternative, systemic macrocyclic lactones may be given. In pigs, effective preparations that have been used include amitraz, trichlorphon and bromocyclen. Newer and more convenient products with a better residual effect include the systemic organophosphate pour-on phosmet and the macrocyclic lactones.

Demodex phylloides

Demodex phylloides (Phylum: Arthropoda; Class: Arachnida; Subclass: Acari; Order: Trombidiformes (Prostigmata); Family: Demodicidae) is found in the hair follicles and sebaceous glands, particularly the eyelids, of pigs worldwide.

Epidemiology: Probably because of its location deep in the dermis, it is difficult to transmit *Demodex* between animals unless there is prolonged contact. Such contact occurs most commonly at suckling. This mange is rare in pigs, although sporadic incidences of up to 5% have been noted in Eastern European countries.

Pathogenesis: Infestation is usually confined to the head, where there is erythema, papules and thickened skin. If there is secondary bacterial infection or follicular rupture, pustules and nodules may be observed.

Clinical signs and pathology: Erythema, papules and thickened skin on the head. Lesions typically involve the ventral abdomen, ventral neck, eyelids and snout. They commence as small red macules, developing into cutaneous nodules, covered by surface scale. Excision of the nodules releases thick white caseous debris.

Diagnosis: For confirmatory diagnosis, deep scrapings are necessary to reach the mites deep in the follicles and glands. This is best achieved by taking a fold of skin, applying a drop of liquid paraffin, and scraping until capillary blood appears.

Control and treatment: Control is rarely applied. In many cases, demodicosis spontaneously resolves and treatment is unnecessary. The organophosphates (e.g. malathion, coumaphos, diazinon, fenchlorvos, chlorfenvinphos, phosmet or trichlorphon) and systemic macrocyclic lactones may be effective.

Notes: Species of the genus *Demodex* are highly specialised mites that live in the hair follicles and sebaceous glands of a wide range of wild and domestic animals, including humans. They are believed to form a group of closely related sibling species that are highly specific to particular hosts: *Demodex phylloides* (pig), *Demodex canis* (dog), *Demodex bovis* (cattle), *Demodex equi* (horse), *Demodex musculi* (mouse), *Demodex ratti* (rat), *Demodex caviae* (guinea pig), *Demodex cati* (cat) and *Demodex folliculorum* and *Demodex brevis* on humans. Various morphological variations may be seen on a host; these are sometimes, probably incorrectly, ascribed separate species status. A number of non-host-specific ectoparasites are found on pigs and are listed in the host–parasite checklist at the end of this chapter. More detailed descriptions of these parasites can be found in Chapter 3.

TICKS

Ornithodoros hermsi

Ornithodoros hermsi (Phylum: Arthropoda; Class: Arachnida; Order: Ixodida; Family: Argasidae), commonly known as the Sand tampan, is a parasite of small mammals, particularly rodents, and is found in North America (Rocky Mountains and Pacific coast).

Epidemiology: *Ornithodoros hermsi* is found in rural areas that are usually mountainous and forested. They live in dark cool places where rodents nest, such as woodpiles outside buildings, under houses, between walls or beneath floorboards inside cabins. They are most active during the summer months.

Pathogenesis: This species transmits *Borrelia hermsi*, the agent of tick-borne relapsing fever in America, and may also act as a vector for African swine fever virus. Rodents, including deer mice, squirrels and chipmunks, are the primary reservoir hosts for *B. hermsi*.

Ornithodoros moubata porcinus

Ornithodoros moubata porcinus (Phylum: Arthropoda; Class: Arachnida; Order: Ixodida; Family: Argasidae), commonly known as the Eyeless tampan or Hut tampan, feeds on warthogs, bushpigs, porcupines and domestic pigs in Africa, Madagascar and southern Europe.

Epidemiology: This tick spends the day sheltered in the burrows of its natural hosts (warthogs), or the cracks and crevices of pig housing, emerging to feed at night.

Pathogenesis: An important reservoir and vector of African swine fever virus and other viruses of suidae.

HOST–PARASITE CHECKLISTS

In the following checklists, the codes listed below apply.

Helminths

N, nematode; T, trematode; C, cestode; A, acanthocephalan.

Arthropods

F, fly; L, louse; S, flea; M, mite; Mx, maxillopod; Ti, tick.

Protozoa

Co, coccidia; Bs, blood sporozoa; Am, amoeba; Fl, flagellate; Ci, ciliate.

Miscellaneous 'protozoal organisms'

B, blastocyst; Mi, microsporidian; My, *Mycoplasma*; P, Pneumocystidomycete; R, *Rickettsia*.

Pig parasite checklist.

Section/host system	Helminths		Arthropods		Protozoa	
	Parasite	(Super)family	Parasite	Family	Parasite	Family
Digestive						
Mouth					Entamoeba suigingivalis	Entamoebidae (Am)
Oesophagus	Gongylonema pulchrum	Spiruroidea (N)				
Stomach	Hyostrongylus rubidus	Trichostrongyloidea (N)				
	Ollulanus tricuspis	Trichostrongyloidea (N)				
	Ascarops strongylina	Spiruroidea (N)				
	Ascarops dentata	Spiruroidea (N)				
	Gnathostoma hispidum	Spiruroidea (N)				
	Gnathostoma doloresi	Spiruroidea (N)				
	Physocephalus sexalatus	Spiruroidea (N)				
	Simondsia paradoxa	Spiruroidea (N)				
	Trichostrongylus axei	Trichostrongyloidea (N)				
Small intestine	Globocephalus urosubulatus	Ancylostomatoidea (N)			Cystoisospora suis	Sarcocystidae (Co)
	Ascaris suum	Ascaridoidea (N)			Eimeria debliecki	Eimeriidae (Co)
	Strongyloides ransomi	Strongyloidoidea (N)			Eimeria polita	Eimeriidae (Co)
	Trichinella spiralis	Trichinelloidea (N)			Eimeria scabra	Eimeriidae (Co)
	Macracanthorhynchus hirudinaceus	Oligacanthorhynchidae (A)			Eimeria spinosa	Eimeriidae (Co)
	Fasciolopsis buski	Fasciolidae (T)			Eimeria porci	Eimeriidae (Co)
	Postharmostomum suis	Brachylaemidae (T)			Eimeria neodeblicki	Eimeriidae (Co)
					Eimeria perminuta	Eimeriidae (Co)
					Eimeria suis	Eimeriidae (Co)
					Cryptosporidium parvum	Cryptosporidiidae (Co)
					Cryptosporidium suis	Cryptosporidiidae (Co)
					Giardia intestinalis	Giardiidae (Fl)
Caecum, colon	Oesophagostomum dentatum	Strongyloidea (N)			Tritrichomonas suis	Trichomonadidae (Fl)
	Oesophagostomum quadrispinulatum	Strongyloidea (N)			Tetratrichomonas buttreyi	Trichomonadidae (Fl)
	Oesophagostomum brevicaudum	Strongyloidea (N)			Trichomitus rotunda	Trichomonadidae (Fl)
	Oesophagostomum longicaudatum	Strongyloidea (N)			Entamoeba suis	Entamoebidae (Am)
	Oesophagostomum georgianum	Strongyloidea (N)			Iodamoeba buetschlii	Entamoebidae (Am)
	Oesophagostomum granatensis	Strongyloidea (N)			Endolimax nana	Entamoebidae (Am)
	Trichuris suis	Trichuroidea (N)			Chilomastix mesnili	Retortamonadidae (Fl)
	Gastrodiscus aegyptiacus	Gastrodiscidae (T)			Balantioides coli	Balantidiidae (Ci)
	Gastrodiscus hominis	Gastrodiscidae (T)				
Respiratory						
Nose					Tritrichomonas suis	Trichomonadidae (Fl)
Trachea, bronchi						
Lung	Metastrongylus apri	Metastrongyloidea (N)				
	Metastrongylus pudendotectus	Metastrongyloidea (N)				
	Metastrongylus salmi	Metastrongyloidea (N)				
	Echinococcus granulosus	Taeniidae (C)				
Liver						
	Ascaris suum	Ascaridoidea (N)				
	Toxocara canis	Ascaridoidea (N)				
	Fasciola hepatica	Fasciolidae (T)				
	Fasciola gigantica	Fasciolidae (T)				
	Echinococcus granulosus	Taeniidae (C)				
	Cysticercus tenuicollis (metacestode: Taenia hydatigena)	Taeniidae (C)				

(Continued)

Pig parasite checklist. *Continued*

Section/host system	Helminths		Arthropods		Protozoa	
	Parasite	(Super) family	Parasite	Family	Parasite	Family
Pancreas						
	Eurytrema pancreaticum	Dicrocoeliidae (C)				
Circulatory						
Blood	*Schistosoma suis*	Schistosomatidae (T)			*Trypanosoma brucei brucei*	Trypanosomatidae (Fl)
	Schistosoma spindale	Schistosomatidae (T)			*Trypanosoma congolense*	Trypanosomatidae (Fl)
	Schistosoma japonicum	Schistosomatidae (T)			*Trypanosoma suis*	Trypanosomatidae (Fl)
					Trypanosoma simiae	Trypanosomatidae ((Fl)
					Babesia perroncitoi	Babesiidae (Bs)
					Babesia trautmanni	Babesiidae (Bs)
Blood vessels						
Nervous						
CNS					*Toxoplasma gondii*	Sarcocystidae (Co)
Eye						
Reproductive/urogenital						
	Stephanurus dentatus	Strongyloidea (N)				
Kidneys	*Stephanurus dentatus*	Strongyloidea (N)				
Locomotory						
Muscle	*Cysticercus cellulosae* (metacestode: *Taenia solium*)	Taeniidae (C)			*Toxoplasma gondii*	Sarcocystidae (Co)
	Trichinella spirialis	Trichinelloidea (N)			*Sarcocystis suicanis*	Sarcocystidae (Co)
					Sarcocystis porcifelis	Sarcocystidae (Co)
					Sarcocystis suihominis	Sarcocystidae (Co)
Connective tissue						
Subcutaneous			*Cordylobia anthropophaga*	Calliphoridae (F)		
			Cochliomyia hominivorax	Calliphoridae (F)		
			Cochliomyia macellaria	Calliphoridae (F)		
			Chrysomya bezziana	Calliphoridae (F)		
			Chrysomya megacephala	Sarcophagidae (F)		
			Wohlfahrtia magnifica	Sarcophagidae (F)		
			Wohlfahrtia meigeni	Sarcophagidae (F)		
			Wohlfahrtia vigil	Oestridae (F)		
			Dermatobia hominis	Tungidae (S)		
			Tunga penetrans			
Integument						
Skin	*Suifilaria suis*	Filarioidea (N)	*Haematopinus suis*	Haematopinidae (L)		
			Sarcoptes scabiei	Sarcoptidae (M)		
			Demodex phylloides	Demodicidae (M)		
			Pulex irritans	Pulicidae (S)		

The following species of flies and ticks are found on pigs. More detailed descriptions can be found in Chapter 3.

Flies of veterinary importance on pigs.

Group	Genus	Species	Family
Blackflies Buffalo gnats	*Simulium*	spp.	Simuliidae (F)
Bot flies	*Dermatobia*	*hominis*	Oestridae (F)
Flesh flies	*Sarcophaga*	*fusicausa haemorrhoidalis*	Sarcophagidae (F)
	Wohlfahrtia	*magnifica meigeni vigil*	
Midges	*Culicoides*	spp.	Ceratopogonidae (F)
Mosquitoes	*Aedes* *Anopheles* *Culex*	spp. spp. spp.	Culicidae (F)
Muscids	*Hydrotaea*	*irritans*	Muscidae (F)
	Musca	*autumnalis domestica*	
	Stomoxys	*calcitrans*	
sand flies	*Phlebotomus*	spp.	Psychodidae (F)
Screwworms and blowflies	*Chrysomya*	*albiceps bezziana megacephala*	Calliphoridae (F)
	Cochliomyia	*hominivorax macellaria*	
	Cordylobia	*anthropophaga*	
Tabanids	*Chrysops*	spp.	Tabanidae (F)
	Haematopota	spp.	
	Tabanus	spp.	
Tsetse flies	*Glossina*	*fusca morsitans palpalis*	Glossinidae (F)

Tick species found on pigs.

Genus	Species	Common name	Family
Ornithodoros	*moubata*	Eyeless or hut tampan	Argasidae (Ti)
	savignyi	Eyed or sand tampan	
	hermsi	Sand tampan	
Dermacentor	*reticulatus*	Marsh tick	Ixodidae (Ti)
Hyalomma	*detritum*	Mediterranean *Hyalomma*	Ixodidae (Ti)
	marginatum	Mediterranean tick	
	truncatum	Bont-legged tick	
Ixodes	*ricinus*	Castor bean or European sheep tick	Ixodidae (Ti)
	holocyclus	Paralysis tick	
	rubicundus	Karoo paralysis tick	
	scapularis	Shoulder tick	
Rhipicephalus	*evertsi*	Red or red-legged tick	Ixodidae (Ti)
	sanguineus	Brown dog or kennel tick	

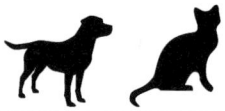
ENDOPARASITES

Parasites of the digestive system

MOUTH

Tetratrichomonas canistomae

Tetratrichomonas canistomae, synonym *Trichomonas canistomae* (Phylum: Metamonada; Class: Trichomonadea; Order: Trichomonadida; Family: Trichomonadidae), is a non-pathogenic parasite localised in the mouth of dogs, transmitted by ingestion of trophozoites from saliva during licking and groomimg. The diagnosis is made by morphological identification of the organisms from fresh and stained mouth swab preparations. The organisms can also be cultured in a range of media used for trichomonads. This parasite does not require treatment.

Notes: *Tetratrichomonas felistomae* is a parasite localised in the mouth of cats synonymized as *T. canistomae.*

OESOPHAGUS

Spirocerca lupi

Spirocerca lupi, synonym *Spirocerca sanguinolenta* (Phylum: Nematoda; Class: Chromadorea; Order: Spirurida; Family: Spirocercidae), commonly known as Oesophageal worm, is localised in the oesophagus, stomach and aorta of dogs, foxes, wild canids and occasionally cats and wild felids. This parasite occurs in tropical and subtropical areas and has coprophagous beetles as intermediate hosts (i.e. *Scarabeus sacer*, *Akis* spp., *Atenchus* spp., *Gymnopleurus* spp., *Cauthon* spp.), and many vertebrates such as rodents, birds, chickens, insectivores and reptiles can act as paratenic hosts.

Epidemiology: In endemic areas, the incidence of infection in dogs is often extremely high, sometimes approaching 100%. Probably this is associated with the many opportunities of acquiring infection from the variety of paratenic hosts.

Pathogenesis: The migrating larvae produce haemorrhages, scarring and/or the formation of fibrotic nodules on the internal wall of the aorta which, if particularly severe, may cause stenosis or even rupture. The oesophageal granulomas, up to 4 cm in size, associated with the adult worms may be responsible for a variety of clinical signs including dysphagia and vomiting arising from oesophageal obstruction and inflammation.

Two further complications are, first, the development of oesophageal osteosarcoma in a small proportion of infected dogs. These may be highly invasive and produce metastases in the lung and other tissues. Second, also relatively rare, is the occurrence of spondylosis of the thoracic vertebrae or of hypertrophic pulmonary osteoarthropathy of the long bones. The aetiology of these lesions is unknown. Occasionally *S. lupi* infection can induce a pyaemic nephritis.

Clinical signs: Despite the potential pathogenicity of this parasite, many infected dogs do not exhibit clinical signs even when extensive aortic lesions and large, often purulent, oesophageal granulomas are present. In some dogs, infection will induce persistent vomiting with worms passed in the vomit. In less serious cases, there may be difficulty in swallowing or interference with the action of the stomach. Aortic infection is not usually observed until sudden death is caused by rupture.

Pathology: The migrating larvae produce characteristic lesions in the wall of the aorta (Fig. 12.1) while the adults are found embedded in granulomatous lesions in the wall of the oesophagus and occasionally the stomach. Aortic lesions include haemorrhage and necrosis with eosinophilic inflammation, intimal roughening with thrombosis, aneurysm with rare aortic rupture, and subintimal and medial mineralisation and heterotopic bone deposition. Spondylosis of the ventral aspects of thoracic vertebrae occurs in some cases with exostoses of the vertebral bodies. Granulomas in the oesophagus contain pleomorphic fibroblasts. In some animals, mesenchymal neoplasms develop in the wall of the oesophageal

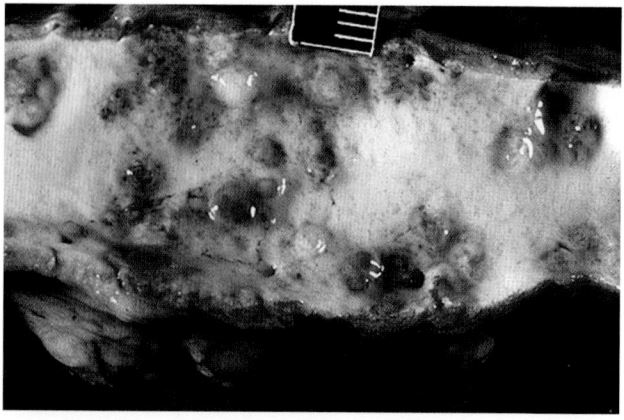

Fig. 12.1 Fibrotic nodules on the internal wall of the aorta from a dog infected with *Spirocerca lupi*.

Veterinary Parasitology, Fifth Edition. Domenico Otranto and Richard Wall.
© 2024 John Wiley & Sons Ltd. Published 2024 by John Wiley & Sons Ltd.

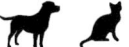

granuloma, with lesions showing cytological characteristics typical of fibrosarcoma and osteosarcoma, with local tissue invasion and, in many cases, pulmonary metastasis.

Diagnosis: The location and appearance of the granulomatous lesions, up to golf ball size, are usually sufficient for identification. Numerous pinkish-red, stout, spirally coiled worms may be seen on section of the granulomas, but these are difficult to extricate intact since they are coiled and up to 8 cm long. Eggs may be found in the faeces or vomit if there are fistulae in the oesophageal granulomas. However, the eggs are similar in appearance to those of other spirurids. Otherwise, diagnosis may depend on endoscopy or radiography.

Control and treatment: Control is difficult because of the ubiquity of the intermediate and paratenic hosts. Dogs should not be fed uncooked viscera from wild birds or from free-range domestic chickens. Treatment is rarely practical, but levamisole and albendazole have been reported to be of value. Levamisole is given at 5–10 mg/kg as a single dose. Doramectin, administered at intervals over 4–6 weeks followed by monthly treatment, has been successful at resolving the lesions in the oesophagus. Diethylcarbamazine at oral doses of 10 mg/kg twice daily for 10 days may kill adult worms but not larvae.

STOMACH

Ollulanus tricuspis

Ollulanus tricuspis (Phylum: Nematoda; Class: Chromadorea; Order: Rhabditida; Family: Molineidae) is a parasite localised in the stomach of cats and wild felids. It is occasionally found in pigs, foxes and domestic dogs and is distributed mainly in Europe, North and South America, Australasia and the Middle East.

Epidemiology: The parasite is common in some parts of the world, particularly in cat colonies and cats that roam. The parasite can replicate in the stomach without any need for external egg or larval phases and can spread via vomit. The disease spreads mainly among starving stray cats and sometimes stray dogs.

Pathogenesis: The parasite is considered non-pathogenic in cats. Heavy infections may induce a severe catarrhal gastritis and vomiting. Untreated cats may become emaciated. Little is known of its pathogenicity in other hosts, although a chronic gastritis has been reported in the pig.

Clinical signs and pathology: This infection could occasionally cause vomiting and emaciation. The worms lie beneath the mucus on the surface of the stomach, or partly in the gastric glands, and their presence may lead to mucosal lymphoid hyperplasia and elevated numbers of globule leucocytes in the gastric epithelium. Heavy infections cause hyperplasia of the gastric glands, causing the stomach mucosa to become convoluted and thrown into folds.

Diagnosis: Diagnosis of ollulanosis is seldom made because of their small size and lack of eggs and larvae in the faeces. Examination of vomit, following an emetic, for the presence of worms is a useful approach. At necropsy, recovery and identification of the very small worms from the gastric mucosa should lead to a diagnosis.

Control and treatment: Control of this infection is mainly achieved through the implementation of good hygiene procedures. Treatment with levamisole, ivermectin or repeated doses of oxfendazole 10 mg/kg twice daily for five days is effective.

Spirocerca lupi

See section entitled Oesophagus.

Gnathostoma spinigerum

Gnathostoma spinigerum (Phylum: Nematoda; Class: Chromadorea; Order: Spirurida; Family: Gnathostomatidae) is a parasite localised in the stomach of cats, dogs, humans, mink, polecats and several wild carnivores, and occurs in Thailand, Japan, Southeast Asia, China and Mexico. This parasite has many species of freshwater crustaceans and copepods as first intermediate hosts and small vertebrates including mammals, birds, reptiles, fish and amphibians as second intermediate hosts.

Epidemiology: Dogs, cats and several species of wild mammals are reservoirs of the parasite. These final hosts become infected primarily through eating infected fish or other animals that serve as paratenic hosts. In humans, the ingestion of raw or inadequately cooked fish is the major source of infection. Human infections are also reported from eating raw or poorly cooked catfish, eels, frogs, chickens, ducks and snakes.

Pathogenesis: *Gnathostoma spinigerum* is the most pathogenic *Gnathostoma* species, which in cats may cause fatal gastric perforation and peritonitis. In some cases, a number of larvae will migrate from the stomach to other organs, most commonly the liver, in which they burrow, leaving necrotic tracks in the parenchyma.

Clinical signs and pathology: This infection in the cat may cause acute abdominal signs. As in many spiruroid infections, the most obvious effect of gnathostomosis is the presence of fibrous growths on the stomach wall. These growths are of variable size, the largest being 3–4 cm in diameter, and are cavitated, amounting to thick-walled cysts containing worms and fluid. Ulceration and necrosis of the stomach wall are often present.

Diagnosis: The infection in the living animal can only be diagnosed by the finding of the greenish oval eggs, which have a thin cap at one pole, in the faeces. Often, however, eggs are not present in faeces.

Control and treatment: With the ubiquity of the first and second intermediate hosts, complete control cannot be achieved. Ensuring only well-cooked fish, eels or other intermediate hosts, such as snakes, frogs and poultry, are eaten can prevent infections. Potentially copepod-infested water should be boiled or treated. Treatment has not been fully investigated.

Notes: Like most spiruroids, *Gnathostoma* inhabits the upper alimentary tract, occurring in nodules in the stomach wall of omnivores and carnivores. It is exceptional in requiring two intermediate hosts in most species.

When visceral *larva migrans* due to *Gnathostoma* occurs in humans, *G. spinigerum* is the species usually involved, and the most common source of infection is inadequately cooked domestic poultry and fish

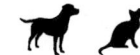

acting as second intermediate hosts. Infection is particularly common in Southeast Asia, Japan and China but occurs in many other countries. The worms never become fully adult, and the immature forms are most commonly found in subcutaneous tissues and other organs in nodules that appear and disappear irregularly as the parasites wander in various parts of the body. In humans, cutaneous gnathostomosis can result in pruritic swellings and eosinophilia with occasional abscess formation. Ocular gnathostomosis is characterised by haemorrhage, uveitis and perforation of the iris. A severe form of infection is central nervous system (CNS) gnathostomosis, leading to haemorrhage and intracranial necrotic tracks that can be fatal.

Physaloptera praeputialis

Physaloptera praeputialis (Phylum: Nematoda; Class: Chromadorea; Order: Spirurida; Family: Physalopteridae) is a parasite localised in the stomach and occasionally anterior duodenum by the gastric valve of cats, wild felids and occasionally dogs. This parasite has beetles, cockroaches, and crickets as intermediate hosts and lizards are paratenic hosts. It is distributed throughout China, Africa, North and South America.

Epidemiology: The epidemiology depends on the presence and abundance of the intermediate beetle hosts. Infection is more prevalent in outdoor cats that have access to intermediate hosts or paratenic hosts.

Pathogenesis: The adult worms have small teeth on their large triangular lips and attach strongly to the gastric mucosa, leaving small ulcers when they move to fresh sites. These feeding sites may continue to bleed. They may cause catarrhal gastritis, with emesis, and in heavy infections blood may appear in the faeces.

Clinical signs and pathology: In heavy infections there may be vomiting and some degree of anorexia. The faeces may appear dark in colour. Severely affected animals may lose weight. The presence of the adult worms may cause gastric ulceration and haemorrhage.

Diagnosis: Diagnosis is based on clinical signs and by the finding of the elongate eggs, thickened at either pole, in the faeces or vomit.

Control and treatment: The ubiquity of the insect intermediate hosts means that control is not usually feasible. Treatment with benzimidazoles over a five-day period has been reported to be effective. Pyrantel, praziquantel and febantel are also effective but elevated or repeated doses may be required.

Physaloptera rara

Physaloptera rara (Phylum: Nematoda; Class: Chromadorea; Order: Spirurida; Family: Physalopteridae) is a parasite localised in the stomach of cats and dogs, in North America.

Details of the life cycle, pathogenesis, treatment and control are essentially similar to those of *P. praeputialis*.

Spirura rinypleurites

Spirura ritypleurites (Phylum: Nematoda; Class: Chromadorea; Order: Spirurida; Family: Spiruridae) is a parasite localised in the stomach and occasionally the oesophagus of cats, foxes and rarely dogs and is endemic in parts of southern Europe, Africa and Asia. This parasite

has coprophagous beetles as intermediate hosts in which the eggs develop into larvae. Larvae may then be ingested by paratenic hosts, such as rodents and lizards, in which they become encapsulated.

Epidemiology: The epidemiology depends on the presence and abundance of the intermediate beetle hosts. Infection is more prevalent in outdoor cats that have access to intermediate hosts or paratenic hosts.

Clinical signs and pathology: Symptoms of nausea, vomiting and digestive upsets have been reported with no associated pathology.

Diagnosis: As for *Physaloptera* spp.

Control and treatment: Prevention is difficult because of the large number of intermediate and paratenic hosts. Treatment is not usually indicated but the use of benzimidazole over an extended period is likely to be effective.

Capillaria putorii

Capillaria putorii, synonym *Aonchotheca putorii* (Phylum: Nematoda; Class: Enoplea; Order: Enoplida; Family: Capillariidae), is a parasite localised in the stomach and small intestine of cats, dogs, mustelids, hedgehogs, bears, raccoons and bobcats and is distributed in Europe, New Zealand and Russia.

Epidemiology: Cats are thought to become infected by eating infective eggs from soil contaminated by hedgehog faeces.

Clinical signs and pathology: There are few reports on the clinical signs of infection in cats. Infected cats may present anorexia and intermittent bloody vomit. There is reported chronic hyperplastic pyloric gastritis and ulceration around the pylorus associated with the presence of worms, with eggs present in the pyloric mucus and the lumen of the pyloric glands.

Diagnosis: Identification of the characteristic eggs in faeces.

Control and treatment: The use of levamisole, given as two doses of 7.5 mg/kg at two-week intervals, and ivermectin 300 µg/kg has been reported to be effective.

SMALL INTESTINE

Toxocara canis

Toxocara canis (Phylum: Nematoda; Class: Chromadorea; Order: Ascaridida; Family: Ascarididae) is a parasite distributed worldwide localised in the small intestine of dogs and foxes.

Epidemiology: Surveys of *T. canis* prevalence in dogs have been carried out in most countries and have shown a wide range of infection rates, from 5% to over 80%. The highest rates of prevalence have been recorded in dogs of less than six months of age, with the fewest worms in adult animals. Infection induces immunity that results in loss of adult worms.

The widespread distribution and high intensity of infection with *T. canis* depend essentially on three factors. First, the females are extremely fecund, one worm being able to contribute about 700 eggs per gram of faeces (epg) per day, and egg counts of 15 000 epg are not uncommon in pups. Second, the eggs are highly resistant to climatic extremes, and can survive for years on the ground. Third,

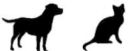

there is a constant reservoir of infection in the somatic tissues of the bitch, and larvae in these sites are not susceptible to most anthelmintics.

Pathogenesis: In moderate infections, the larval migratory phase is accomplished without any apparent damage to the tissues, and the adult worms provoke little reaction in the intestine. In heavy infections, the pulmonary phase of larval migration is associated with pneumonia, which is sometimes accompanied by pulmonary oedema; the adult worms cause mucoid enteritis, there may be partial or complete occlusion of the gut and, in rare cases, perforation with peritonitis or in some instances blockage of the bile ducts of the liver.

Clinical signs and pathology: In mild to moderate infections, there are no clinical signs during the pulmonary phase of larval migration. The adults in the intestine may cause tucked-up abdomen or potbelly, with failure to thrive, and occasional vomiting and diarrhoea. Entire worms are sometimes vomited or passed in the faeces. The signs in heavy infections during larval migration result from pulmonary damage and include coughing, increased respiratory rate and a frothy nasal discharge. Most fatalities from *T. canis* infection occur during the pulmonary phase, and pups which have been heavily infected transplacentally may die within a few days of birth. Nervous convulsions have been attributed by some clinicians to toxocarosis, but there is still some disagreement on whether the parasite can be implicated as a cause of these signs.

On *post mortem*, the animal appears poorly grown, potbellied and cachectic. Large numbers of maturing worms are present in the intestines and sometimes the stomach. Focal haemorrhages may be found in the lungs of puppies with migrating *T. canis* larvae. Inflammatory foci are often observed in the kidneys as white elevated spots 1–2 mm in diameter in the cortex beneath the capsule. In section, they are composed of a small focus of macrophages, lymphocytes, plasma cells and a few eosinophils, possibly containing larvae. Occasionally, granulomas may be found in the eye.

Diagnosis: Only a tentative diagnosis is possible during the pulmonary phase of heavy infections when the larvae are migrating, and is based on the simultaneous appearance of pneumonic signs in a litter, often within two weeks of birth. The eggs in faeces, subglobular and brown with thick pitted shells, are species diagnostic. The egg production of the worms is so high that there is no need to use flotation methods, and they are readily found in simple faecal smears to which a drop of water has been added.

Toxocara canis in the dog can be confused only with *Toxascaris leonina*, which is slightly smaller. Differentiation of these two species is difficult, as the only useful character, visible with a hand lens, is the presence of a small finger-like process on the tail of the male *T. canis*.

Control and treatment: The main aim is to prevent transmammary and intrauterine transmission of infection using the anthelmintic treatment regimens described. Hygienic disposal of dog faeces should be encouraged. Where practical, access of rodents to kennels should be prevented. The adult worms are easily removed by anthelmintic treatment. The most popular drug used has been piperazine, although this is being superseded by the benzimidazoles (fenbendazole and mebendazole) and by nitroscanate. Pyrantel and the avermectin selamectin are also effective. Although several anthelmintics have activity against larval stages and juvenile worms, none are fully effective at their removal.

A simple and frequently recommended regimen for control of toxocarosis in young dogs is as follows. All pups should be dosed at two weeks of age, and again 2–3 weeks later, to eliminate prenatally acquired infection. It is also recommended that the bitch should be treated at the same time as the pups. A further dose should be given to the pups at two months old to eliminate any infection acquired from the milk of the dam or from any increase in faecal egg output by the dam in the weeks following whelping. Newly purchased pups should be dosed twice at an interval of 14 days.

Since there are likely to be a few worms present, even in adult dogs and despite the diversion of the majority of larvae to the somatic tissues, it is recommended that adult dogs should be treated every 3–6 months throughout their lives.

It has been shown that daily administration of high doses of fenbendazole to the bitch from three weeks *pre partum* to two days *post partum* has largely eliminated transmammary and prenatal infection of the pups, although residual infection in the tissues of the bitch may persist. This regimen may be useful in breeding kennels.

Notes: Apart from its veterinary importance, this species is responsible for the most widely recognised form of visceral *larva migrans* in humans. Though this term was originally applied to invasion of the visceral tissues of an animal by parasites whose natural hosts were other animals, it has now, in common usage, come to represent this type of invasion in humans alone and, in particular, by the larvae of *T. canis*, although the larval stages of *T. mystax*, *T. leonina* and *T. vitulorum* (see Chapter 8) can be implicated. Its complementary term is cutaneous *larva migrans* (CLM) for infections by 'foreign' larvae that are limited to the skin.

The global condition occurs most commonly in children, often under five years of age, who have had close contact with household pets or who have frequented areas such as public parks where there is contamination of the ground by infective dog faeces. Surveys of such areas in many countries have almost invariably shown the presence of viable eggs of *T. canis* in around 10% of soil samples. Despite this high risk of exposure to infection, the reported incidence of clinical cases is small. For example, in 1979 a French survey of the world literature reported that only 430 cases of ocular and 350 cases of visceral *larva migrans* had been recorded. However, it has been suggested that 50–60 clinical cases occur in Britain each year, since many are not recorded.

In many cases, larval invasion is limited to the liver and may give rise to hepatomegaly and eosinophilia, but on some occasions a larva escapes into the general circulation and arrives in another organ, the most frequently noted being the eye. Here, a granuloma forms around the larva on the retina, often resembling a retinoblastoma. Only in rare cases does the granuloma involve the optic disc, with total loss of vision, and most reports are of partial impairment of vision, with endophthalmitis or granulomatous retinitis. Such cases are currently treated using laser therapy. In a few cases of epilepsy, *T. canis* infection has been identified serologically but the significance of the association has yet to be established.

Control of visceral *larva migrans* is based on the anthelmintic regimen described previously, on the safe disposal of dog faeces in houses and gardens, and on the limitation of access by dogs to areas where children play such as public parks and recreation grounds.

Other hosts apart from humans, such as sheep and pigs, can also suffer from migration of *T. canis* and *T. mystax* larvae through their tissues. In pigs, the larval migration can cause white-spot disease in the liver.

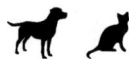

Toxocara mystax

Toxocara mystax, synonym *Toxocara cati* (Phylum: Nematoda; Class: Chromadorea; Order: Ascaridida; Family: Ascarididae), is a parasite distributed worldwide localised in the small intestine of cats.

Epidemiology: The epidemiology of *T. mystax* depends largely on a reservoir of larvae in the tissues of the dam, which are mobilised late in pregnancy and excreted in the milk throughout lactation. The paratenic host (e.g. rodents) is also of considerable significance because of the strong hunting instinct in cats. Exposure to the latter route of infection does not occur until kittens begin to hunt for themselves or to share the prey of their dams.

Pathogenesis: Because the majority of infections are acquired either in the milk of the dam or by ingestion of paratenic hosts, there is no migratory phase so any changes are usually confined to the intestine, showing as potbelly, diarrhoea, poor coat and failure to thrive.

Clinical signs and pathology: Unthriftiness, potbelly, diarrhoea. The larvae developing in the mucosa of the stomach may provoke a mild granulomatous reaction comprising lymphocytes and a few macrophages around the coiled larvae.

Diagnosis: The subglobular eggs, with thick pitted shells, are easily recognised in faeces.

Control and treatment: Since infection is first acquired during suckling, complete control would be based on removal of kittens from the dam and artificial rearing. Good hygiene is essential in catteries. Young kittens should be wormed regularly with an anthelmintic from 4–6 weeks of age at three-week intervals until four months of age and thereafter at regular intervals. Fenbendazole, mebendazole, piperazine and pyrantel are all effective against adult nematodes. The benzimidazole anthelmintics are more effective against larval ascarids.

Notes: *Toxocara mystax* has been reported as a rare cause of visceral *larva migrans* in humans.

Toxocara malayiensis

Toxocara malayiensis (Phylum: Nematoda; Class: Chromadorea; Order: Ascaridida; Family: Ascarididae) is a parasite localised in the small intestine of cats and is distributed in Malaysia. The epidemiology of this disease has not yet been described. The diagnosis is made by identification of the eggs in faeces, similar to those of *T. canis*. Details of the pathogenesis, pathology and clinical signs have not been reported. Control and treatment are presumed similar to *T. mystax*.

Toxascaris leonina

Toxascaris leonina, synonym *Toxascaris limbata* (Phylum: Nematoda; Class: Chromadorea; Order: Ascaridida; Family: Ascarididae), is a parasite distributed worldwide, particularly in the cooler regions, localised in the small intestine of dogs, cats and foxes.

Epidemiology: Infection normally occurs through the ingestion of the larvated eggs. Larvae of *T. leonina* may occur in mice with the encysted third-stage larvae distributed in many tissues. If a dog or cat ingests an infected mouse, the larvae are released and develop to maturity in the wall and lumen of the intestine of the final host.

Pathogenesis: Infection with *Toxascaris* is unlikely to occur in isolation and is more usually accompanied by a *Toxocara* infection. In puppies and young dogs less than two months of age, the infection is usually absent as there is no prenatal or lactogenic transmission. Damage is caused predominantly by the adult worms and is determined by the number of worms present in the intestine.

Clinical signs and pathology: Unthriftiness, potbelly, diarrhoea. The pathological effects due to *T. leonina* are rarely seen. Heavy infections may cause occlusion of the intestinal lumen and are usually associated with the mixed presence of *Toxocara* spp.

Diagnosis: *Toxascaris* is almost indistinguishable grossly from *T. canis*, the only point of difference being the presence of a finger-like process at the tip of the male tail of the latter. In the cat, differentiation from *T. mystax* is based on the shape of the cervical alae, which are lanceolate in *Toxascaris* but arrowhead shaped in *T. mystax*. The characteristic ovoid smooth-shelled eggs are easily recognised in the faeces.

Control and treatment: Ascarid infections in the domestic carnivores invariably include *Toxocara*, such that the measures recommended for control of the latter will also have an effect on *Toxascaris*. Since the two main reservoirs of infection are larvae in the prey and eggs on the ground, control has to be based on treatment of worm infection in the host animals, and on adequate hygiene to limit the possibility of acquisition of infection by ingestion of eggs. Fenbendazole, mebendazole, piperazine and pyrantel are all effective against adult nematodes. The benzimidazole anthelmintics are more effective against larval ascarids.

Notes: This genus occurs in domestic carnivores and, though common, is of less significance than *Toxocara* because its parasitic phase is non-migratory.

Ancylostoma caninum

Ancylostoma caninum (Phylum: Nematoda; Class: Chromadorea; Order: Rhabditida; Family: Ancylostomatidae), commonly known as the Canine hookworm, is a parasite distributed worldwide, mainly in the tropics and warm temperate areas. In other countries it is sometimes seen in dogs imported from endemic regions. This hookworm is localised in the small intestine of dogs, foxes and occasionally humans.

Epidemiology: In endemic areas the disease is most common in dogs under one year old. In older animals, the gradual development of age resistance makes clinical disease less likely, particularly in dogs reared in endemic areas, whose age resistance is reinforced by acquired immunity. The epidemiology is primarily associated with the two main sources of infection: transmammary in suckled pups and percutaneous or oral from the environment. An important aspect of transmammary infection is that disease may occur in suckled pups reared in a clean environment and nursed by a bitch which may have been recently treated with an anthelmintic and has a negative faecal egg count. Contamination of the environment is most likely when dogs are exercised on grass or earth runs that retain moisture and also protect larvae from sunlight. On such surfaces, larvae may survive for some weeks. In contrast, dry

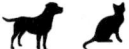

impervious surfaces, particularly if exposed to sunlight, are lethal to larvae within a day or so. Housing is also important and failure to remove soiled bedding, especially if the kennels are damp or have porous or cracked floors, can lead to a massive build-up of infection.

Pathogenesis: This is essentially that of an acute or chronic haemorrhagic anaemia. The disease is most commonly seen in dogs under one year old, and young pups, infected by the transmammary route, are particularly susceptible due to their low iron reserves. Transmammary infection is often responsible for severe anaemia in litters of young pups in their second or third week of life. Infection of the bitch on a single occasion has been shown to produce transmammary infections in at least three consecutive litters.

Following infection, blood loss starts about the eighth day of infection when the immature adult has developed the toothed buccal capsule, which enables it to grasp plugs of mucosa containing arterioles. Each worm removes about 0.1 ml of blood daily and in heavy infections of several hundred worms, pups quickly become profoundly anaemic. In lighter infections, common in older dogs, the anaemia is not so severe, as the marrow response is able to compensate for a variable period. The nutritional state of the individual will influence the progression of the anaemia. Ultimately, however, the dog may become iron deficient and develop a microcytic hypochromic anaemia. In previously sensitised dogs, skin reactions such as moist eczema and ulceration at the sites of percutaneous infection occur, especially affecting the interdigital skin.

It appears that dormant L_3 in the muscles of both bitches and dogs can recommence migration months or years later to mature in the host's intestine. Stress, severe illness or repeated large doses of corticosteroids can all precipitate these apparently new infections in dogs, which may perhaps now be resident in a hookworm-free environment. Experimentally, L_3 of some strains of *A. caninum* exposed to chilling before oral administration have been shown to remain in arrested development in the intestinal mucosa for weeks or months. The significance of this observation is still unknown, but it is thought that such larvae may resume development if the adult hookworm population is removed by an anthelmintic or at times of stress, such as lactation.

Clinical signs and pathology: In acute infections, associated with the sudden exposure of susceptible animals to large numbers of infective larvae, there is anaemia and lassitude and occasionally respiratory embarrassment. In suckled pups, the anaemia is often severe and is accompanied by diarrhoea, which may contain blood and mucus. Respiratory signs may be due to larval damage in the lungs or to the anoxic effects of anaemia. In more chronic infections, the animal is usually underweight, the coat is poor and there is loss of appetite and perhaps pica. Inconsistently, there are signs of respiratory embarrassment, skin lesions and lameness. The adverse effects of infection on the coat can have an economic impact where foxes are reared for their fur. Animals dying of ancylostomosis are extremely pale and there is often oedema of subcutaneous tissues and mesenteries, and serous effusion into the body cavities attributable to hypoproteinaemia. In chronic infections, cachexia may be evident. If recent exposure to heavy percutaneous infection has occurred, there may be dermatitis and numerous focal haemorrhages in the lung parenchyma. The liver is pale and the intestinal contents are mucoid and red in colour. Worms may be seen attached to the mucosa and pinpoint haemorrhagic sites may be scattered over the intestinal surface.

Diagnosis: This depends on the clinical signs and history supplemented by haematological and faecal examination. High faecal worm egg counts are valuable confirmation of diagnosis, but it should be noted that suckled pups may show severe clinical signs before eggs are detected in the faeces. The presence of a few hookworm eggs in the faeces, although giving confirmatory evidence of infection, does not necessarily indicate that an ailing dog is suffering from hookworm disease.

Control and treatment: A system of regular anthelmintic therapy and hygiene should be adopted. Weaned pups and adult dogs should be treated every three months. Pregnant bitches should be dosed at least once during pregnancy with an anthelmintic that has high efficacy against somatic larvae, so as to reduce transmammary infection, and the nursing litters dosed at least twice, at 1–2 weeks of age and again two weeks later, with a drug specifically recommended for use in pups. This will also help to control ascarid infections. The perinatal transfer of both *Ancylostoma* and *Toxocara* larvae may be reduced by the oral administration of fenbendazole daily from three weeks before to two days after whelping.

Kennel floors should be dry and free of crevices, and the bedding should be disposed of daily. Runs should preferably be of tarmac or concrete and kept as clean and dry as possible; faeces should be removed with a shovel before hosing. Paved surfaces can be sprayed with a 1% solution of sodium hypochlorite after first being cleaned. If an outbreak has occurred, earth runs may be treated with sodium borate, which is lethal to hookworm larvae, but this also kills grass. A second possibility, which is often used in fox farms, is the provision of wire-mesh flooring in the runs.

Affected dogs should be treated with an anthelmintic, such as mebendazole, fenbendazole, pyrantel or nitroscanate, all of which will kill both adult and developing intestinal stages; several of the macrocyclic lactones have similar activity. If the disease is severe, it is advisable to give parenteral iron and possibly vitamin B_{12} and to ensure that the dog has a protein-rich diet. Young pups may require a blood transfusion. Arrested fourth-stage larvae are often refractory to anthelmintic treatment and further treatment may be required after these larvae mature.

Notes: *Ancylostoma caninum* is more pathogenic for dogs than either *Ancylostoma braziliense* or *Uncinaria stenocephala* due to the greater level of blood loss. *Ancylostoma caninum* can occasionally use humans as a final host. Although infections do not reach full maturity, they may induce an eosinophilic enteritis.

Ancylostoma braziliense

Ancylostoma braziliense (Phylum: Nematoda; Class: Chromadorea; Order: Rhabditida; Family: Ancylostomatidae), commonly known as the Hookworm, is localised in the small intestine of dogs, foxes and cats, in tropical and subtropical regions. Details of the epidemiology, control and treatment are as for *A. caninum*.

Pathogenesis: While it may cause a degree of hypoalbuminaemia through intestinal leak of plasma, it is not a bloodsucker and consequently is of little pathogenic significance, causing only mild digestive upsets and occasional diarrhoea. The main importance of *A. braziliense* is that it is regarded as the primary cause of CLM or 'creeping eruption' in humans. CLM is characterised by tortuous erythematous inflammatory tracts within the dermis and by severe pruritus, and is caused by infective larvae penetrating the skin and

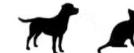

wandering in the dermis. These larvae do not develop but the skin lesions usually persist for weeks. The severity of the skin lesions is related to the degree of exposure to infective larvae.

Clinical signs and pathology: Mild digestive upset and diarrhoea in affected animals. In humans, there may be skin erythema and pruritus. Infected animals may show oedema of subcutaneous tissues and mesenteries, and serous effusion into the body cavities attributable to hypoproteinaemia. If recent exposure to heavy percutaneous infection has occurred, there may be dermatitis.

Diagnosis: Worms that have been heat-fixed bend markedly at the position of the vulva. This differs from *A. ceylanicum*.

Notes: Humans exposed to *A. braziliense* larvae can develop an erythematous and intensely pruritic eruption of the skin associated with migration of larvae (human CLM).

Ancylostoma tubaeforme

Ancylostoma tubaeforme, synonym *Strongylus tubaeforme* (Phylum: Nematoda; Class: Chromadorea; Order: Rhabditida; Family: Ancylostomatidae), commonly known as the Feline hookworm, is a parasite distributed worldwide and localised in the small intestine of cats. This infection is generally considered to be of low pathogenicity, although heavy infections may lead to a poor coat, anaemia and reduced growth. A strong immunity often develops to infection.

Ancylostoma ceylanicum

Ancylostoma ceylanicum (Phylum: Nematoda; Class: Chromadorea; Order: Rhabditida; Family: Ancylostomatidae), commonly known as Hookworm, is localised in the small intestine of dogs, cats, wild felids and humans and is found in Asia (Malaysia, Sri Lanka). The infections of this parasite are usually subclinical but heavy infections can induce anaemia and diarrhoea. The parasite can complete its life cycle in humans and may cause anaemia and abdominal pain, and skin penetration by infective larvae may induce cutaneous lesions. In the parasitological diagnosis, the heat-fixed female worms are not bent as occurs with *A. braziliense*.

All other details of these two species are in most respects similar to *A. caninum*.

Uncinaria stenocephala

Uncinaria stenocephala (Phylum: Nematoda; Class: Chromadorea; Order: Rhabditida; Family: Ancylostomatidae), commonly known as Northern hookworm, is localised in the small intestine of dogs, cats, foxes and other canids and felids. This hookworm occurs in temperate and sub-arctic areas, North America and northern Europe. Various mammals can act as paratenic hosts.

Epidemiology: Evidence suggests that in temperate climates like the UK, the seasonal pattern of infective larvae on paddocks used for greyhounds follows that described for gastrointestinal trichostrongyloids in ruminants, with a sharp rise in July and a peak in September, suggesting that development to the L_3 is heavily dependent on temperature.

Pathogenesis: The infection is not uncommon in groups of sporting and working dogs. The adult worms attach to the mucosa. They are not voracious bloodsuckers like *A. caninum*, but hypoalbuminaemia and low-grade anaemia, accompanied by diarrhoea, anorexia and lethargy, have been recorded in heavily infected pups. Probably the most common lesion in dogs made hypersensitive by previous exposure is pedal dermatitis, affecting particularly the interdigital skin.

Clinical signs and pathology: Anaemia, diarrhoea, anorexia, lethargy and interdigital dermatitis. Severe hookworm infections cause villous fusion and atrophy in the small intestine and an inflammatory response in the lamina propria.

Diagnosis: In areas where *A. caninum* is absent, the clinical signs of the patent infection, together with the demonstration of strongyle eggs in the faeces, are indicative of uncinariosis. Where *Ancylostoma* is also endemic, differential diagnosis may require larval culture, although the treatment is similar.

Control and treatment: Regular anthelmintic treatment and good hygiene as outlined for *Ancylostoma* will control *Uncinaria* infection. The combination of ivermectin and pyrantel pamoate or a formulation of chewable ivermectin can give high efficacy. The pedal dermatitis responds poorly to symptomatic treatment, but regresses gradually in the absence of reinfection. Fenbendazole, mebendazole, nitroscanate, piperazine, pyrantel and milbemycin oxime are active against the northern hookworm.

Strongyloides stercoralis

Strongyloides stercoralis, synonyms *Strongyloides canis*, *Strongyloides intestinalis*, *Anguillula stercoralis* (Phylum: Nematoda; Class: Chromadorea; Order: Rhabditida; Family Strongyloididae), commonly known as Threadworm, is localised in the small intestine of dogs, foxes, cats and humans. It is a parasite distributed worldwide, mainly in warmer climates of Europe (Portugal, France, Poland, Ukraine, Romania and Hungary).

Epidemiology: The dog may act as a natural host for this species. Transmission is either by the oral or percutaneous route or by autoinfection. The latter route can lead to cases of persistent strongyloidosis occurring without external reinfection. Unweaned puppies are infected orally via larvae adhering to the teats and larvae ingested with colostrum. Infection is most commonly seen in the summer when the weather is hot and humid and is frequently a kennel problem. A strain of *S. stercoralis* has become adapted to humans and usually occurs in warm climates.

Pathogenesis: Severe infections can occur in dogs, especially puppies. Mature parasites are found in the duodenum and proximal jejunum and, if present in large numbers, may cause inflammation with oedema and erosion of the epithelium. This results in a catarrhal enteritis with impairment of digestion and absorption. Migrating larvae can cause bronchopneumonia.

Clinical signs and pathology: Bloody diarrhoea, dehydration, sometimes death. Lesions consist of catarrhal inflammation of the small intestine while in severe infections there may be necrosis and sloughing of the mucosa. Adult worms establish in tunnels in the epithelium at the base of the villi in the small intestine. In young puppies, heavy invasion of the lungs by migrating larvae may result in petechial and ecchymotic haemorrhages.

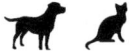

Table 12.1 *Strongyloides* species reported in cats.

Species	Description	Pathogenicity
Strongyloides planiceps	Parasitic females are 2.4–3.3 mm long (mean 2.8 mm). The tail of the parasitic female narrows abruptly to a blunt tip and the ovaries have a spiral appearance	Non-pathogenic
Strongyloides felis (syn. *Strongyloides cati*)	Similar to *S. planiceps*. Parasitic females of *S. felis* have a long tail narrowing slowly to the tip. Ovaries are straight	Non-pathogenic
Strongyloides tumefaciens	Parasitic female is about 5 mm long	Found in tumours in the mucosa of the large intestine

Diagnosis: The clinical signs in very young animals, usually within the first few weeks of life, together with the finding of large numbers of the characteristic eggs or larvae in the faeces are suggestive of strongyloidosis.

Control and treatment: Disinfection or replacement of kennels and bedding eliminates the sources of infection. Treatment in dogs with oral fenbendazole 10–20 mg/kg daily for three days is effective. Ivermectin is effective against adult worms.

Three other species of *Strongyloides* are found in cats (Table 12.1). Details of the life cycle, diagnosis, treatment and control of these species are as for *S. stercoralis*.

Trichinella spiralis

For more details see Chapter 11.

Alaria alata

Alaria alata (Phylum: Platyhelminthes; Class: Trematoda; Order: Strigeidida; Family: Diplostomatidae), commonly known as the Intestinal carnivore fluke, is localised in the small intestine of dogs, cats, foxes, mink, wild carnivores and rarely humans and is found in Eastern Europe. Freshwater snails (*Planorbis* spp.) can act as a first intermediate host. Frogs and toads can act as a second intermediate host.

Epidemiology: Infection is maintained in endemic areas where intermediate hosts are abundant. Transmammary infection has been reported with some species in cats and rodents.

Pathogenesis: Adult flukes attach to the mucous membrane of the small intestine (Fig. 12.2) but cause little harm. However, the migratory mesocercariae may cause clinical symptoms. Heavy infections may cause a severe duodenitis and pulmonary damage in dogs and cats. A fatal case has been recorded in humans through eating inadequately cooked frogs' legs; the principal lesions were in the lungs.

Clinical signs and pathology: Infection is not usually associated with clinical signs. The effects are generally limited to the attachment of flukes to the intestinal mucosa and may include local irritation, erosion and ulceration and the production of excessive intestinal mucus and, rarely, haemorrhagic enteritis.

Diagnosis: Diagnosis is by identifying the presence of eggs in the faeces.

Control and treatment: Dogs and cats should be prevented from catching or consuming paratenic hosts such as frogs, rodents and snakes. Treatment with praziquantel or niclosamide is recommended.

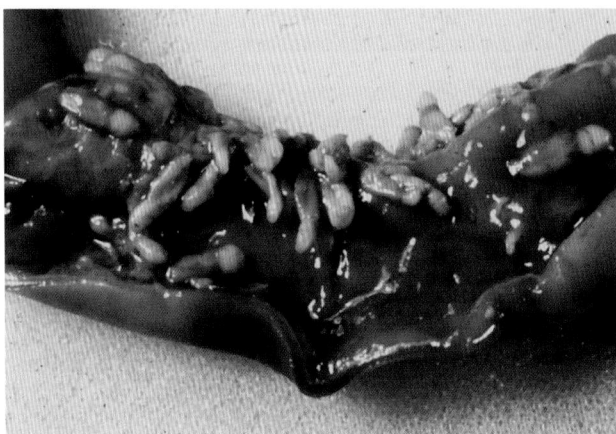

Fig. 12.2 *Alaria* spp. attached to the mucosa of the small intestine.

Other species of *Alaria* found in canids and felids are given in Table 12.2.

Table 12.2 Intestinal flukes of dogs and cats.

Species	Final hosts	Intermediate hosts	Distribution
Family Diplostomatidae			
Alaria alata	Dogs, cats, foxes, mink, wild carnivores, humans	1: Snails 2: Frogs and toads	Eastern Europe
Alaria americana	Dogs, foxes and other canids	1: Snails 2: Frogs and toads	North America
Alaria minnesotae	Cats, skunks	1: Snails 2: Frogs and toads	North America
Alaria canis	Dogs, foxes	1: Snails 2: Frogs and toads	North America
Alaria michiganensis	Dogs, foxes	1: Snails 2: Frogs and toads	North America
Alaria marcianae	Cats	1: Snails 2: Frogs and toads	North America
Family Nanophyetidae			
Nanophyetus salmincola	Dogs, cats, raccoons, mink, bears, lynx, fish-eating mammals, rarely humans	1: Snails 2: Fishes	North America, eastern Russia
Family Heterophyidae			
Heterophyes heterophyes	Dogs	1: Snails 2: Fishes	Egypt, Asia
Heterophyes nocens	Dogs	1: Snails 2: Fishes	Egypt, Asia
Metagonimus yokogawai	Dogs	1: Snails 2: Fishes	Asia, Balkans
Family Opisthorchiidae			
Cryptocotyle lingua	Gulls, foxes	1: Shellfish 2: Fishes	Europe (Germany, Denmark, UK)
Apophallus muehlingi	Gulls	1: Unknown 2: Fishes	Europe
Apophallus (Rossicotrema) donicus	Cats, dogs	1: Unknown 2: Fishes	Europe, North America
Family Echinostomatidae			
Echinochasmus perfoliatus	Dogs	1: Snails 2: Fishes	Europe, Asia
Euparyphium melis	Cats	1: Snails 2: Tadpoles	Europe
Euparyphium ilocanum	Dogs	1: Snails 2: Freshwater molluscs	Europe

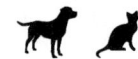

Nanophyetus salmincola

Nanophyetus salmincola, synonym *Troglotrema salmincola* (Phylum: Platyhelminthes; Class: Trematoda; Order: Plagiorchiida; Family: Nanophyetidae), is localised in the small intestine of dogs, foxes, coyotes, cats, raccoons, mink, bears, lynx, other fish-eating mammals and rarely humans and is distributed in North America (northwest Pacific) and eastern Russia. Snails (*Oxytrema silicula*, *Goniobasis*, *Semisulcospira* spp.) can act as first intermediate host. Various salmonid fish can act as second intermediate hosts.

Epidemiology: Infection is maintained in endemic areas where intermediate hosts are abundant.

Pathogenesis: The trematodes penetrate deeply into the mucosa of the duodenum or attach to the mucosa of other parts of the small or large intestine. In large numbers, they produce a superficial enteritis which may lead to haemorrhagic enteritis. The real importance of *N. salmincola* is its ability to transmit *Neorickettsia helminthoeca*, the agent of 'salmon poisoning', which frequently produces severe and fatal infections in dogs, foxes and other animals.

Clinical signs and pathology: The presence of large numbers of flukes may cause diarrhoea. With complicated infections involving *N. helminthoeca*, there is sudden onset of fever and complete loss of appetite. Within a few days there is purulent discharge from the eyes, vomiting and profuse diarrhoea, which may be haemorrhagic. Lymph nodes may be enlarged. Mortality varies from 50% to 90% of infected animals. In large numbers, superficial enteritis leading to haemorrhagic enteritis may occur.

Diagnosis: Diagnosis is by identifying the presence of eggs in the faeces.

Control and treatment: Dogs and cats should not be fed raw fish and should be kept away from salmon rivers and streams. Since the rickettsial organisms cause the main pathogenic effects, tetracycline therapy is indicated. High doses of albendazole or fenbendazole over a prolonged period can be effective in treating the fluke infection. Praziquantel given intramuscularly or subcutaneously is also effective.

Notes: *Nanophyetus* can occasionally infect humans, where it penetrates between the villi and causes inflamation and necrosis of the mucosa.

Several other trematodes parasitise the small intestine of dogs and cats and other definitive hosts, including birds and humans, but they are usually of minor veterinary significance and are briefly summarised in Table 12.2. More detailed descriptions are given in Chapter 1.

Diphyllobothrium latum

Diphyllobothrium latum, synonym *Dibothriocephalus latus* (Phylum: Platyhelminthes; Class: Cestoda; Order: Diphyllobothriidea; Family: Diphyllobothriidae), commonly known as the Broad tapeworm, is localised in the small intestine of humans and fish-eating mammals, such as dogs, foxes, cats, pigs, mink, seals and bears. This parasite is distributed in parts of Scandinavia, Russia, Japan and North America. Copepods of the genus *Diaptomus* can act as first

intermediate host. Freshwater fish (pike, trout, perch, minnow) can act as second intermediate host.

Epidemiology: *Diphyllobothrium latum* is essentially a parasite of humans since in other hosts the cestode produces few fertile eggs. The epidemiology is therefore largely centred around two factors: the access of human sewage to freshwater lakes and the ingestion of uncooked fish. Domestic animals, such as dogs or pigs, become infected by eating raw fish or fish offal.

Pathogenesis: In humans, infections are often asymptomatic but there can be fatigue, dyspepsia, vomiting and transient diarrhoea. Infection is usually asymptomatic in animals, although occasionally vitamin B_{12} deficiency can occur.

Clinical signs and pathology: In humans, infections are often asymptomatic but there can be fatigue, dyspepsia, vomiting and transient diarrhoea. The parasite does not induce damage to the intestine.

Diagnosis: This depends on detection of the characteristic eggs in the faeces.

Control and treatment: In areas where infection is common, domestic animals should not be fed fish products unless these have been thoroughly cooked or deep-frozen. Praziquantel and niclosamide are effective against the adult tapeworm.

Notes: *Diphyllobothrium latum* is an important cestode parasite of the small intestine of humans in northern climates; it may also infect other fish-eating mammals.

Dipylidium caninum

Dipylidium caninum (Phylum: Platyhelminthes; Class: Cestoda; Order: Cyclophyllidea; Family: Dipylidiidae), commonly known as the Double-pored or Cucumber seed tapeworm, is a parasite distributed worldwide and localised in the small intestine of dogs, foxes and cats and rarely humans. This parasite has fleas (*Ctenocephalides* spp., *Pulex irritans*) and biting lice (*Trichodectes canis*) as intermediate hosts and it is the most common tapeworm genus of domestic dogs and cats.

Epidemiology: *Dipylidium* infection is very common and, being dependent on the continuous presence of ectoparasites for its local endemicity, it is more prevalent in neglected animals, though infestations are also seen in well-kept dogs and cats.

Pathogenesis: The adult is non-pathogenic and several hundreds can be tolerated without clinical effect. They shed segments which, as they crawl actively from the anus, may cause some discomfort, and a useful sign of infection is excessive grooming of the perineum. It has been suggested that infected dogs form the habit of rubbing the anus along the floor, but impacted anal glands are a more common cause of this behaviour.

Clinical signs and pathology: The clinical signs are anal discomfort and itching. Adult tapeworms are of little pathogenic significance.

Diagnosis: Often the first indication of infection is the presence of a segment on the coat around the perineum. If the segment is freshly passed, preliminary identification may be made on the elongate shape and the double genital organs, which may be seen with a hand lens. If it is dried and distorted, it will be necessary to

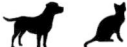

break it up with mounted needles in water, where the egg packets are easily seen under the microscope, thus differentiating the segment from that of *Taenia* spp. which contains only numerous single oncospheres.

Control and treatment: In *Dipylidium* infection, control and treatment must be instituted together, for it is clearly of no value to eliminate the adult tapeworm while leaving a reservoir in the animal's ectoparasites. Hence, administration of anthelmintics, such as nitroscanate and praziquantel, should be accompanied by the use of insecticides. It is also imperative that the animal's bedding and customary resting places should receive attention with insecticides to eliminate the immature stages of the flea, which are many times more numerous than the adult parasites feeding on the dog or cat.

Echinococcus

The taxonomy of *Echinococcus* has suffered from uncertainty regarding the taxonomic status of described species and subspecies. This has resulted in confusion regarding the nomenclature of intraspecific variants and impacted on the understanding of the epidemiology of echinococcosis, particularly the nature of transmission patterns. Recent application of molecular tools has led to the recognition of a series of largely host-adapted species that are maintained in distinct cycles of transmission.

Echinococcus granulosus possesses a high degree of genetic divergence and various strains (G1–G10) have been described which show differences in morphology, host range and pathogenicity and geographical distribution. Two former strains are now recognised as individual species: *Echinococcus equinus* (the former horse strain) and *Echinococcus orteleppi* (the former cattle strain). More strains or species of the *E. granulosus* complex undoubtedly exist.

Echinococcus multilocularis is primarily a parasite of foxes but is an important zoonosis also affecting dogs and cats. Two further species of *Echinococcus* occur in dogs: *Echinococcus oligarthrus* and *Echinococcus vogeli*. These are briefly summarised in the following sections. The metacestode stages can establish and develop in humans. Intermediate hosts include rodents such as the paca (*Cuniculus paca*), spiny rat (*Proechimys guyannensis*) and agouti (*Dasyprocta* spp.).

Echinococcus granulosus, Echinococcus equinus (G4), Echinococcus orteleppi (G5)

Echinococcus granulosus, *E. equinus* (G4), *E. orteleppi* (G5) (Phylum: Platyhelminthes; Class: Cestoda; Order: Cyclophyllidea; Family: Taeniidae), commonly known as the Dwarf dog tapeworm, causes a disease named hydatidosis and is distributed according to the species. *Echinococcus granulosus* is distributed worldwide and localised in the anterior small intestine of dogs and many wild canids such as coyotes, dingoes and wolves (final hosts). The parasite is localised in the liver and lungs of the intermediate hosts. Domestic and wild ruminants, humans and primates, pigs and lagomorphs act as intermediate hosts (horses and donkeys are resistant). *Echinococcus equinus* is distributed mainly in Europe and is localised in the anterior small intestine of dogs and red foxes. Horses, mules and donkeys act as the intermediate hosts. *Echinococcus orteleppi* is a parasite of dogs and cattle act as the intermediate hosts.

Epidemiology:
- *Echinococcus granulosus.* Only a few countries, notably Iceland and Eire, are free from *E. granulosus*. It is customary to consider the epidemiology as being based on two cycles: pastoral and sylvatic. In the pastoral cycle, the dog is always involved, being infected by the feeding of ruminant offal containing hydatid cysts. The domestic intermediate host will vary according to local husbandry but the most important is the sheep, which appears to be the natural intermediate host, scolices from these animals being the most highly infective for dogs. In parts of the Middle East, the camel is the main reservoir of hydatids, while in northern Europe and northern Russia it is the reindeer. The pastoral cycle is the primary source of hydatidosis in humans, infection being by accidental ingestion of oncospheres from the coats of dogs, or from vegetables and other foodstuffs contaminated by dog faeces. The sylvatic cycle occurs in wild canids and ruminants and is based on predation or carrion feeding. It is less important as a source of human infection, except in hunting communities where the infection may be introduced to domestic dogs by the feeding of viscera of wild ruminants.
- *Echinococcus equinus* (G4). Equine hydatidosis is most common in Europe, and in other parts of the world most cases have been recorded in imported European horses. The strain is highly specific for the horse and the eggs do not develop in the sheep. The domestic dog and red fox are the final hosts, and the cycle in countries of high prevalence depends on access by dogs to infected equine viscera. On mainland Europe, the most likely source is offal from horse abattoirs and in Britain the viscera of hunting horses, which are fed to foxhounds. The horse strain does not appear to be infective to humans.

Pathogenesis: The adult tapeworm is not pathogenic, and thousands may be present in the small intestine of a dog without clinical signs. In domestic animals, the hydatid in the liver or lungs is usually tolerated without any clinical signs, and the majority of infections are only revealed at the abattoir. Where oncospheres have been carried in the circulation to other sites, such as the kidney, pancreas, CNS or marrow cavity of long bones, pressure by the growing cyst may cause a variety of clinical signs.

In contrast, when humans are involved as an intermediate host, the hydatid in its pulmonary or hepatic site is often of pathogenic significance. One or both lungs may be affected, causing respiratory symptoms, and if several hydatids are present in the liver, there may be gross abdominal distension. If a cyst should rupture, there is a risk of death from anaphylaxis; alternatively, if the person survives, released daughter cysts may resume development in other regions of the body.

Clinical signs and pathology: Asymptomatic in the dog and infection in cattle, sheep and horses is also generally not associated with clinical signs. Human infection can result in respiratory distress or abdominal enlargement, depending on whether the lungs or liver are infected. There is no reported pathology in the final hosts.

Diagnosis: Diagnosis of infection in dogs with adult tapeworms is difficult, because the segments are small and are only shed sparsely. When found, identification is based on their size (2–3 mm), ovoid shape and single genital pore.

In some countries control regimens have involved the administration of purgative anthelmintics, such as arecoline hydrochloride,

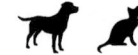

so that the whole tapeworm is expelled in mucus and can be searched for in the faeces. If a necropsy is available, the small intestine should be opened and immersed in shallow water, when the attached tapeworms will be seen as small slender papillae. Immunodiagnostic tests have been developed based on the detection of faecal antigen by the antibody sandwich enzyme-linked immunosorbent assay (ELISA) technique.

Control and treatment: This is based on the regular treatment of dogs to eliminate the adult tapeworms and on the prevention of infection in dogs by exclusion from their diet of animal material containing hydatids. This is achieved by denying dogs access to abattoirs and, where possible, by proper disposal of sheep carcasses on farms. In some countries these measures have been supported by legislation, with penalties when they are disregarded. In countries where no specific measures for hydatid control exist, it has been found that an incidental benefit from the euthanasia of stray dogs for rabies control has been a great reduction in the incidence of hydatid infection in humans.

A recombinant DNA vaccine has been developed for *E. granulosus* but it requires further refinement for practical application and is currently not available commercially. *Echinococcus* tapeworms are more difficult to remove than *Taenia* but several drugs, notably praziquantel, are now available which are highly effective. After treatment, it is advisable to confine dogs for 48 hours to facilitate the collection and disposal of infected faeces. In humans, hydatid cysts may be excised surgically, although mebendazole, albendazole and praziquantel therapies have been reported to be effective.

Echinococcus multilocularis

Echinococcus multilocularis (Phylum: Platyhelminthes; Class: Cestoda; Order: Cyclophyllidea; Family: Taeniidae), commonly known as the Dwarf fox tapeworm, causes a disease named alveolar echinococcosis, and is localised at the lower small intestine of wild canids (primarily foxes but in some areas coyotes, wolves and raccoon dogs may be involved), domestic dogs and cats, although cats are less suitable hosts than canids. This cestode is distributed in the northern hemisphere, including North America, Greenland, Scandinavia, Central Europe, Russia, Middle East and also India, China and Japan. This parasite is localised at the lungs, brain, muscles and lymph nodes of the intermediate hosts (i.e. mainly microtine rodents, such as voles, muskrats and lemmings, and insectivores). Some of the larger mammals, including humans, are also susceptible and may act as intermediate host.

Epidemiology: Though *E. multilocularis* has a wide distribution in the northern hemisphere, it is essentially a parasite of tundra regions, with its greatest prevalence being in the sub-arctic regions of Canada, Alaska and Russia. Its basic epidemiological cycle in these regions is in the arctic fox and wolf, and their prey, small rodents and insectivores. In North America, its range is extending south from Canada into the USA where the red fox and coyote act as final hosts. The cycle is therefore sylvatic, and most cases in humans occur in trappers and their families following contact with the contaminated fur of foxes and wolves. However, eating vegetables or fruit contaminated by infected foxes seeking garden voles may occasionally infect suburban humans.

In recent years, the population of red foxes has expanded in Europe and foxes have also extended their distribution into urban and periurban areas. The demonstration of an urban wildlife cycle of *E. multilocularis* in foxes has implications for human health in areas where this parasite is endemic. In addition, expansion of the synanthropic cycle, involving domestic dogs that prey on metacestode-infected rodents, may lead to an increase in the prevalence of human alveolar echinococcosis. *Echinococcus multilocularis* egg contamination has been predicted to be maximal where the urban and rural habitats overlap.

Pathogenesis: The larval metacestode stage develops primarily in the liver as the so-called multilocular or alveolar cyst, a diffuse growth with many compartments containing a gelatinous matrix into which the protoscolices are budded off. Growth of the intermediate stage is invasive, extending locally and capable of systemic metastases to other sites such as lungs, brain, muscles and lymph nodes. These hydatids are the causative agent of alveococcosis or alveolar echinococcosis.

Clinical signs and pathology: Usually asymptomatic in the definitive host. In the intermediate host, clinical signs are dependent on the level of infection and the location of the metacestode stages. Infection in humans often presents with few signs until the infection has markedly progressed. The slow infiltration of organs may cause symptoms resembling those of a slow-growing carcinoma. The adult tapeworm causes little damage in the intestine of the definitive host. In the liver, invasion by the metacestode stage can result in atrophy of the parenchyma and cause cirrhosis. Expansion of alveolar *Echinococcus* in the liver produces aggregates of small gelatinous cysts that appear similar to malignant neoplasia.

Diagnosis: The sedimentation and counting technique at necropsy is the well-established method for detection of intestinal *E. multilocularis* in the definitive host, although the intestinal scraping technique is also useful. More recent research techniques include the detection of copro-DNA by polymerase chain reaction (PCR) and of *E. multilocularis*-specific coproantigen in an ELISA-based assay. Serological and PCR-based tests are available for the early detection of infection in humans.

Control and treatment: Because of the large sylvatic reservoir, control of *E. multilocularis* is unlikely ever to be achieved. Precautionary measures include:

- the wearing of protective rubber gloves when handling fresh skins/furs of foxes, wolves, etc.
- thorough washing of forest fruits and berries prior to consumption in regions where infection is endemic
- treatment of dogs and cats with an effective cestocidal anthelmintic.

Dogs and cats can be treated with praziquantel or epsiprantel. Treatment of domestic intermediate hosts is not advised. The invasive growth in humans simulates malignant neoplasia, and because of its infiltrative spread in tissues and its readiness to develop metastatically, surgery is not advisable; instead treatment with mebendazole or praziquantel is recommended.

Echinococcus vogeli

Echinococcus vogeli (Phylum: Platyhelminthes; Class: Cestoda; Order: Cyclophyllidea; Family: Taeniidae) is localised at the small intestine of bush dogs (*Speothos venaticus*) and occasionally

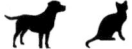

domestic dogs, and is distributed in Central and South America. Humans can be accidental hosts. This parasite is also localised at the liver, lung and other visceral organs of the intermediate hosts.

Notes: *Echinococcus shiquicus* is found in Tibet and cycles between a fox, *Vulpes ferrilata*, and the plateau pika.

Echinococcus oligarthrus
Echinococcus oligarthrus (Phylum: Platyhelminthes; Class: Cestoda; Order: Cyclophyllidea; Family: Taeniidae) is localised at the small intestine of cougars, jaguars, ocelots and other felids (humans can be an accidental hosts) and is distributed in Central and South America. This parasite is localised at the viscera, musculature and skin of the intermediate hosts. Other details for these species are similar to those for *E. multilocularis*.

Notes: Other details are similar in most respects to *D. latum*. Occasionally, humans may become infected with plerocercoids, either through drinking water containing procercoid-infected crustacea or from eating a plerocercoid-infected host such as a pig. This zoonosis, known as sparganosis (*Sparganum* was the old name for these plerocercoids), is characterised by the presence of larvae up to 35 mm long in the muscles and subcutaneous tissues, particularly the periorbital area, causing oedema and inflammation. Occasionally, the spargana disintegrate into several pieces (proliferating disease), which develop separately, and this can be fatal.

Other species of *Spirometra* found in dogs and cats are detailed in Table 12.3. Descriptive details of taeniid tapeworms of dogs are listed in Table 12.4.

Spirometra mansoni

Spirometra mansoni (Phylum: Platyhelminthes; Class: Cestoda; Order: Diphyllobothriidea; Family: Diphyllobothriidae), commonly known as the Tapeworm, is localised in the small intestine of dogs, cats, wild carnivores and occasionally humans and is distributed in South America and Asia. Copepods (host 1), amphibia, reptiles, birds and mammals (host 2) can act as intermediate hosts. The tapeworm is usually asymptomatic in animals, causing little effect in the intestine of dogs and cats.

Taenia hydatigena

Taenia hydatigena, synonyms *Taenia marginata*, *Cysticercus tenuicollis* (Phylum: Platyhelminthes; Class: Cestoda; Order: Cyclophyllidea; Family: Taeniidae), commonly known as the Thin-necked bladder worm, is a parasite distributed worldwide localised in the small intestine of dogs, foxes, weasels, stoats, polecats, wolves and hyenas. This parasite is localised in the abdominal cavity and liver of sheep, goats, cattle, deer, pigs and horses (intermediate hosts).

Table 12.3 Tapeworms of dogs and cats.

Genus	Species	Hosts	Intermediate hosts	Metacestode stages	Site
Echinococcus	*granulosus*	Dogs (wolves, foxes, jackals, dingoes, hyenas)	Livestock, humans	Hydatidosis, hydatid cyst	Liver, lungs, etc.
	equinus	Dogs	Horses		
	orteleppi	Dogs	Cattle		
Echinococcus	*multilocularis*	Foxes, dogs, cats	Rodents, humans, pigs, horses	Alveolar echinococcosis	Liver, lungs, etc.
Echinococcus	*vogeli*	Bush dogs, dogs, rarely humans	Rodents	Hydatid	Liver, lung and other visceral organs
Echinococcus	*oligarthus*	Cougars, jaguars, ocelots and other felids	Rodents	Hydatid	Viscera, musculature and skin
Taenia	*pisiformis*	Dogs, foxes	Rabbits	*Cysticercus pisiformis*	Abdominal cavity, liver
Taenia	*hydatigena*	Dogs, foxes	Livestock	*Cysticercus tenuicollis*	Abdominal cavity, liver
Taenia (syn. *Multiceps*)	*multiceps*	Dogs	Sheep, cattle, humans	*Coenurus cerebralis*	Brain, spinal cord
	skrjabini	Dogs, foxes	Sheep	*Coenurus skrjabini*	Muscle, subcutis
	gaigeri	Dogs, foxes	Goats	*Coenurus gaigeri*	Muscle, subcutis
Taenia	*ovis*	Dogs, foxes	Sheep, goats	*Cysticercus ovis*	Muscle
Taenia	*crassiceps*	Foxes, dogs	Small rodents	*Cysticercus longicollis*	Abdominal cavity
Taenia (syn. *Hydatigera*)	*taeniaeformis*	Cats	Small rodents	*Strobilocercus fasciolaris* (syn. *Crassicollis*)	Liver
Taenia (syn. *Multiceps*)	*serialis*	Dogs	Rabbits	*Coenurus serialis*	Connective tissue
Dipylidium	*caninum*	Dogs, cats, foxes	Fleas, lice	Cysticercoid	Abdominal cavity
Mesocestoides	*lineatus*	Dogs, foxes, cats	1: Oribatid mites 2: Mammals, reptiles, frogs, birds	Tetrathyridium	Abdominal cavity, liver
Diphyllobothrium	*latum*	Humans, dogs, pigs, cats	1: Copepods 2: Fishes	Plerocercoid	Abdominal cavity, muscle
Spirometra	*mansoni*	Dogs, cats, wild carnivores, and occasionally humans	1: Copepods 2: Amphibians, reptiles, birds	Plerocercoid	Muscles, subcutaneous tissues
Spirometra	*mansonoides*	Cats, bobcats and occasionally dogs	1: Crustacea 2: Rats, mice, snakes	Plerocercoid	Muscles, subcutaneous tissues
Spirometra	*erinacei*	Cats, foxes	1: Crustacea 2: Frogs	Plerocercoid	Muscles, subcutaneous tissues

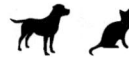

Table 12.4 Taeniid tapeworms of dogs.

Parasite species	Scolex size (mm)[a]	No. of hooks[a]	Length of hooks (μm) Large hooks[a]	Small hooks[a]	No. of testes (layers)	Genital pores	No. of uterine branches	Notes
Taenia hydatigena	206 (170–220)	28–36 (26–44)	191–218 (170–235)	118–143 (110–168)	600–700 (1)	5–10 prominent	6–10 that redivide	Lobes of ovary unequal in size. No vaginal sphincter. Testes extend to vitellarium, but not confluent behind
Taenia ovis (syn. *Taenia cervi*, *Taenia krabbei*, *Taenia hyaenae*)	180 (156–188)	30–34 (24–38)	170–191 (131–202)	111–127 (89–157)	350–750 (1)	15–30	11–20 that redivide	Lobes of ovary unequal in size. Well-developed vaginal sphincter. Testes extend to posterior edge of ovary
Taenia multiceps (syn. *Multiceps multiceps*) *Taenia skrjabini*, *Taenia* (*Multiceps*) *gaigeri*	160 (150–170)	22–30 (20–34)	157–177 (120–190)	98–136 (73–160)	284–388 (2)		14–20 that redivide	Lobes of ovary equal in size. Pad of muscle on anterior wall of vagina. Testes extend to vitellarium, but not confluent behind
Taenia serialis (syn. *Multiceps serialis*)	160 (135–175)	26–32	137–175	78–120			20–25	
Taenia pisiformis	250 (225–294)	34–48	225–294	132–177			5–15 Barely visible	

[a] Values in parentheses indicate ranges.

Notes: The correct nomenclature for the intermediate host stage is 'metacestode stage of *Taenia hydatigena*' rather than '*Cysticercus tenuicollis*'.

Clinical signs and pathology: Adult tapeworms in dogs are usually asymptomatic and, if untreated, they survive from several months to a year or more. In heavy infections there may be gastrointestinal disturbances such as diarrhoea, abdominal pain and anal pruritus that result from migration of proglottids from the perianal area. The infection usually causes little damage to the intestine although there have been occasional reports of obstruction when several worms are present.

Diagnosis: Often the first sign of tapeworm infection in dogs is the presence of proglottids in the faeces or more frequently the perianal area as a result of the active migration of the segments. These segments may cause itching and grooming of the perianal area.

Control and treatment: This is similar to that of other taeniids and involves control of infection in the final host and burial or disposal of ruminant carcasses and offal. Tapeworms can be removed from

dogs through the administration of an effective cestocidal anthelmintic, such as niclosamide, praziquantel, nitroscanate or multiple doses of mebendazole or fenbendazole (Table 12.5). No practical treatment is available for the intermediate host.

Taenia ovis

Taenia ovis, synonyms *Taenia cervi*, *Taenia krabbei*, *Taenia hyaenae*, *Cysticercus ovis*, *Cysticercus cervi*, *Cysticercus tarandi*, *Cysticercus dromedarii*, *Cysticercus cameli* (Phylum: Platyhelminthes; Class: Cestoda; Order: Cyclophyllidea; Family: Taeniidae), causes a disease commonly known as Cysticercosis, 'Sheep measles'. It is known as the sheep bladder worm, is a parasite distributed worldwide and localised in the small intestine of dogs, foxes and wild carnivores. This parasite is localised in the muscle, liver and other organs of the intermediate hosts such as sheep, goats (*Cysticercus ovis*), deer (*Cysticercus cervi*), reindeer (*Cysticercus tarandi*) and camels (*Cysticercus dromedarii*, *Cysticercus cameli*).

Table 12.5 Tapeworm treatments for dogs and cats.

Anthelmintic	Dose rate (mg/kg)	*Taenia* spp.	*Echinococcus* spp.	*Dipylidium*	Comments
Praziquantel	5 (oral)	+	+	+	Good activity against *E. multilocularis*
	8 (spot-on)	+	+	+	
	3.5–7.5 (injection)	+	+	+	
Dichlorophen	200	+			
Nitroscanate	50	+	(+)	+	Active against *E. granulosus*. Use in dogs only
Niclosamide	125	+		(+)	
Fenbendazole	100 single dose 50 for 3 days	+			
Mebendazole	Variable (3.5–50) Given for 2–5 days	(+)	(+)		Activity against tapeworms variable. Some activity against *E. granulosus*
Epsiprantel	5.5	+		+	Combined with pyrantel pamoate
Bunamidine		+	+	+	No longer available in many countries

+, active; (+), variable activity.

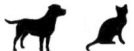

Notes: The correct nomenclature for the intermediate host stage is 'metacestode stage of *Taenia ovis*' rather than '*Cysticercus ovis*', etc.

Epidemiology: Adult tapeworms shed three segments each containing 78 000–95 000 eggs. Dogs can be infected by more than one adult tapeworm. The thick-shelled eggs can survive 90–150 days at 16 °C but survive for shorter periods at higher temperatures. Ruminants are infected by grazing pasture and forages contaminated with dog or fox faeces harbouring eggs of *T. ovis*.

Pathogenesis and clinical signs: Heavy infections in young dogs can sometimes cause diarrhoea and ill-thrift.

Diagnosis: Tapeworm infection in dogs is often recognised through the presence of shed proglottids and/or tapeworm segments in fresh faeces.

Control and treatment: Regular treatment of dogs with an effective anthelmintic will reduce contamination of the environment. Dogs should be denied access to raw sheep and goat meat and carcasses. A highly protective recombinant vaccine is available in some countries. The treatment is as for other taeniid species.

Taenia multiceps

Taenia multiceps, synonyms *Multiceps multiceps*, *Coenurus cerebralis*, *Taenia skrjabini*, *Coenurus skrjabini*, *Taenia (Multiceps) gaigeri*, *Coenurus gaigeri* (Phylum: Platyhelminthes; Class: Cestoda; Order: Cyclophyllidea; Family: Taeniidae), causes a disease commonly known as Gid, Sturdy or Staggers and is distributed worldwide, but absent from the USA and New Zealand. This parasite is localised in the small intestine of dogs, foxes, coyotes, jackals and wolves (final host) and in the brain and spinal cord of intermediate hosts (i.e. sheep, goats, cattle, deer, pigs, horses and humans).

Epidemiology: This is largely influenced by whether sheepdogs and stray dogs have access to the heads or spinal cords of infected intermediate hosts. Foxes are in general less efficient than dogs in contaminating pastures.

Clinical signs and pathology: Usually asymptomatic. There is no associated pathology. The diagnosis is as for *T. hydatigena*.

Control and treatment: This can be achieved through ensuring that dogs, in particular sheepdogs, do not have access to the heads of slaughtered or dead sheep or goats. It is essential that all sheep carcasses are buried as soon as possible. In areas where coenurosis is endemic, the regular deworming of dogs with an effective anthelmintic every 6–8 weeks will reduce contamination into the environment and, by breaking the sheep–dog cycle, may lead to eradication of the disease. Foxes are not thought to be an important final host for *T. multiceps*. The treatment is as for other taeniid species.

Taenia pisiformis

Taenia pisiformis, synonym *Cysticercus pisiformis* (Phylum: Platyhelminthes; Class: Cestoda; Order: Cyclophyllidea; Family: Taeniidae), is a parasite distributed worldwide localised in the small intestine of dogs, mainly hunting dogs, and foxes. This parasite is localised in the peritoneum and liver of the intermediate hosts such as rabbits and hares.

Notes: The correct nomenclature for the intermediate host stage is 'metacestode stage of *Taenia pisiformis*' rather than '*Cysticercus pisiformis*'.

Clinical signs and pathology: Infection is usually asymptomatic in both the final and the intermediate host. However, in heavy infections liver damage can occur in the intermediate host as a result of migration of juvenile worms through the liver parenchyma. This can lead to hepatitis and cirrhosis. In heavy infections the intermediate hosts may show emaciation and jaundice with pea-like cysts present on the peritoneum, wall of the mesentery and omentum.

Diagnosis: Infection of the intermediate host is detected through the presence of a single cyst or a cluster of several cysts in the abdominal cavity.

Control and treatment: Hunting dogs should be wormed regularly with an effective anthelmintic and should not be fed raw carcasses or offal from rabbits and hares. The treatment is as for other taeniid species.

Taenia serialis

Taenia serialis, synonyms *Multiceps serialis*, *Coenurus serialis* (Phylum: Platyhelminthes; Class: Cestoda; Order: Cyclophyllidea; Family: Taeniidae), is a parasite distributed worldwide and localised in the small intestine of dogs, mainly hunting dogs, foxes and other canids. This parasite is localised in the intramuscular and subcutaneous connective tissues of the intermediate hosts such as rabbits, hares and rarely rodents and humans.

Notes: The correct nomenclature for the intermediate host stage is 'metacestode stage of *Taenia serialis*' rather than '*Coenurus serialis*'. Another species, *Taenia brauni*, is very similar to *T. serialis* and is found in parts of Africa. The adult tapeworm occurs in the dog and other wild canids and the metacestode in rodents.

Clinical signs and pathology: Infection is usually asymptomatic in both the definitive and intermediate host. Pea-like cysts are present in subcutaneous or intramuscular connective tissue.

Diagnosis: Infection of the intermediate host is detected through the presence of cysts in subcutaneous or intramuscular connective tissue.

Control and treatment: Hunting dogs should be wormed regularly with an effective anthelmintic and should not be fed raw carcasses or offal from rabbits and hares. The treatment is as for other taeniid species.

Taenia taeniaeformis

Taenia taeniaeformis, synonyms *Hydatigera taeniaeformis*, *Taenia crassicollis*, *Cysticercus fasciolaris*, *Strobilocercus fasciolaris* (Phylum: Platyhelminthes; Class: Cestoda; Order: Cyclophyllidea; Family: Taeniidae), is a cosmopolitan parasite localised in the small intestine of cats, lynx, stoats and foxes. This parasite is localised in the liver of the intermediate hosts such as mice, rats, rabbits and squirrels.

Epidemiology: Rodents are infected by grazing pasture and forages contaminated with cat faeces harbouring eggs of *T. taeniaeformis*.

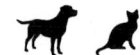

Two cycles can occur: an urban cycle, that involves the domestic cat and house and field rodents, and a sylvatic cycle that in North America uses bobcats and wild rodents.

Pathogenesis: Adult tapeworms are of minor pathogenic significance and infections are usually subclinical.

Diagnosis: Diagnosis depends on the demonstration of segments or individual taeniid eggs in the faeces. Specific identification of the adult tapeworm is a specialised task.

Control and treatment: Control depends on dietary methods that exclude access to the larval stage in the intermediate host. Where practical, cats should be prevented from eating rodents. Cats should be treated regularly with an effective cestocidal anthelmintic. For adult tapeworms a number of effective drugs are available, including praziquantel, mebendazole, fenbendazole and dichlorophen.

Mesocestoides lineatus

Mesocestoides lineatus, synonyms *Dithrydium variable*, *Tetrathyridium bailetti*, *Tetrathyridium elongatum* (Phylum: Platyhelminthes; Class: Cestoda; Order: Cyclophyllidea; Family: Mesocestoididae), is localised in the small intestine of dogs, cats, foxes, mink and wild carnivores in Europe, Asia and Africa. This parasite has oribatid mites (host 1) and birds, amphibians, reptiles and small mammals (host 2) as intermediate hosts. Adult tapeworms are of minor pathogenic significance and infections are usually subclinical with no reported clinical signs.

Notes: A related tapeworm, *Mesocestoides corti*, reproduces asexually in the intestine of the dog.

Macracanthorhynchus hirudinaceus

Macracanthorhynchus hirudinaceus (Phylum: Acanthocephala; Class: Archiacanthocephala; Order: Oligacanthorhynchida; Family: Oligacanthorhynchidae), commonly known as the Thorny-headed worm, is a parasite distributed worldwide but absent from certain

areas, for example parts of Western Europe, localised in the duodenum and proximal small intestine of pigs, wild boar, occasionally dogs, cats, wild carnivores and humans. This parasite has dung beetles and water beetles as intermediate hosts.

For more details see Chapter 11.

Coccidiosis

Dogs and cats are infected with coccidian parasites belonging to the genus *Cystoisospora*. In dogs, the common species are *Cystoisospora canis* and *Cystoisospora ohioensis*. In cats, the common species are *Cystoisospora felis* and *Cystoisospora rivolta*. At one time it was thought that species of the genus *Cystoisospora* were freely transmissible between dogs and cats, but it is now established that this is not the case.

Epidemiology: Crowding and lack of good sanitation promote spread of coccidiosis. Breeding establishments, kennels and rescue centres are potential sources of infection. Older dogs and cats are generally immune from disease, but may seed the environment with oocysts, leading to infection in young puppies and kittens that have no previous exposure.

Pathogenesis: There is no real evidence that these species are pathogenic on their own, but infection may be exacerbated by intercurrent viral disease or other immunosuppressive agents.

Clinical signs and pathology: Diarrhoea in young puppies or kittens. Coccidial stages are found in the epithelial cells lining the villi of the small intestine. In heavy infections there is villous stunting and reduction in the absorptive area of the lower small intestine leading to diarrhoea.

Diagnosis: Coccidiosis may be diagnosed on *post mortem* by finding coccidial stages in the intestines. Affected animals with diarrhoea or dysentery may be shedding oocysts in the faeces. The presence of oocysts is not in itself sufficient for diagnosis but should be considered with presenting signs of sudden onset of enteritis. Oocysts may need to be differentiated from the oocysts of other coccidial genera found in dogs (Table 12.6) and cats (Table 12.7 and Fig. 12.3).

Table 12.6 Coccidian parasites in the faeces of dogs.

Coccidian species	Alternative name	Intermediate hosts	Oocyst condition[a]	Oocyst size (μm)	Sporocyst size (μm)
Sarcocystis bovicanis	*Sarcocystis cruzi* *Sarcocystis fusiformis*	Cattle	S	19–21 × 15–18	16.3 × 10.8[b]
Sarcocystis ovicanis	*Sarcocystis tenella*	Sheep	S		14.8 × 9.9[b]
Sarcocystis suicanis	*Sarcocystis porcicanis* *Sarcocystis mieschiriana*	Pigs	S		12.7 × 10.1[b]
Sarcocystis equicanis	*Sarcocystis bertrami*	Horses	S		15.2 × 10[b]
Sarcocystis fayeri		Horses	S		12.0 × 7.9[b]
Sarcocystis capracanis		Goats	S		12–15 × 8–10[b]
Sarcocystis hircicanis		Goats	S		
Sarcocystis cameli		Camels	S		12 × 9[b]
Sarcocystis hovarthi	*Sarcocystis gallinarum*	Chickens	S		10–13 × 7–9[b]
Hammondia heydorni	*Toxoplasma heydorni*		U	13 × 11	
Cystoisospora canis	—		U	38 × 30	2 × 16
Cystoisospora ohioensis			U	23 × 19	14.5 × 10

[a] Sporulated (S) or unsporulated (U) oocysts in faeces.
[b] Sporocysts generally found free in faeces.

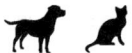

Table 12.7 Coccidian parasites in the faeces of cats.

Coccidian species	Alternative name	Intermediate hosts	Oocyst condition[a]	Oocyst size (μm)	Sporocyst size (μm)
Sarcocystis bovifelis	*Sarcocystis hirsuta*	Cattle	S	12–18 × 11–14	12.5 × 7.8[b]
Sarcocystis ovifelis	*Sarcocystis tenella*	Sheep	S		12.4 × 8.1[b]
Sarcocystis hircifelis	*Sarcocystis moulei*	Goats	S		12.4 × 9.1[b]
Sarcocystis porcifelis		Pigs	S		13.5 × 8[b]
Sarcocystis cuniculi	*Sarcocystis cuniculorum*	Rabbits	S		13 × 10[b]
Sarcocystis muris		Mice	S		10.3 × 8.5[b]
Besnoitia besnoiti	*Sarcocystis besnoiti*	Ruminants	U	14–16 × 12–14	
Toxoplasma gondii			U	13 × 12	9 × 6.5
Hammondia hammondi	*Toxoplasma hammondi* *Cystoisospora hammondi*	Rodents	U	13.2 × 10.6	9.8 × 6.5
Cystoisospora felis	*Cystoisospora felis*	—	U	41.6 × 30.5	22.6 × 18.4
Cystoisospora rivolta	*Cystoisospora rivolta*	—	U	25 × 21.1	15.2 × 11.6

[a] Sporulated (S) or unsporulated (U) oocysts in faeces.
[b] Sporocysts generally found free in faeces.

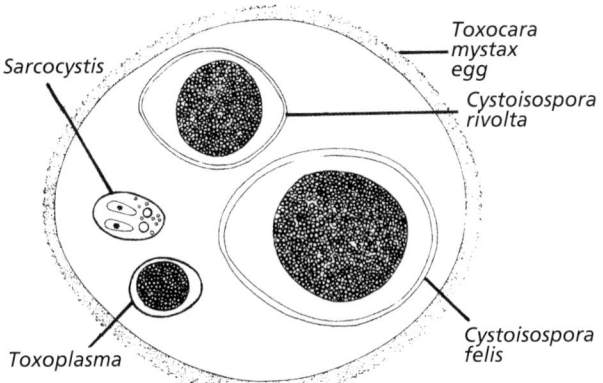

Fig. 12.3 Diagram of cat oocysts relative to ascarid eggs of *Toxocara mystax.*

Control and treatment: Good sanitation and isolation are effective measures in preventing coccidiosis. In kennels or rescue centres, animal accommodation should be cleaned daily. Standard disinfectants are ineffective against coccidial oocysts but ammonia-based products are effective. Information on treatment in the dog and cat is scanty, although by analogy with other host species, the use of sulfonamides, such as sulfadimidine, should be tried.

Cystoisospora canis

Cystoisospora canis, synonym *Isospora canis* (Phylum: Apicomplexa; Class: Conoidasida; Order: Eucoccidiorida; Family: Sarcocystidae), is a parasite localised in the small intestine of dogs. Three merogony generations occur in the subepithelium of the lamina propria of the small intestine. Gamonts appear within the epithelial cells about seven days post infection. The prepatent period is 9–11 days and infections can remain patent for about four weeks.

Cystoisospora ohioensis

Cystoisospora ohioensis, synonym *Isospora ohioensis* (Phylum: Apicomplexa; Class: Conoidasida; Order: Eucoccidiorida; Family: Sarcocystidae), is a parasite localised in the small intestine of dogs. All stages of the life cycle occur in the epithelium of the small

intestine; gamonts can also be found in the caecum and large intestine from 4–5 days post infection. The prepatent period is 4–5 days and patency is 3–5 weeks.

Cystoisospora felis

Cystoisospora felis, synonym *Isospora felis* (Phylum: Apicomplexa; Class: Conoidasida; Order: Eucoccidiorida; Family: Sarcocystidae), is a parasite localised in the small intestine of cats. In the life cycle of this parasite, all stages are found above the host cell nuclei in the epithelium of the lower small intestine. Gamonts appear from six days after infection. The prepatent period is 7–10 days. Infections can remain patent for about 1–3 weeks.

Cystoisospora rivolta

Cystoisospora rivolta, synonym *Isospora rivolta* (Phylum: Apicomplexa; Class: Conoidasida; Order: Eucoccidiorida; Family: Sarcocystidae), is a parasite distributed worldwide and localised in the small intestine of cats. In the life cycle of this parasite, meront stages are found in the epithelial cells and crypt cells of the lower small intestine, caecum and colon. Gamonts appear 3–4 days post infection. The prepatent period is 4–7 days and patency can persist for up to nine weeks.

Epidemiology: Rodents may ingest sporulated oocysts and become infected with asexual stages, thereby acting as reservoirs of infection. A number of rodent species can act as transport hosts. The life cycle is normally direct, although there is some evidence that a predator–prey relationship may be involved and that dogs and cats can acquire infection from the tissues of rodents.

Pathogenesis: The pathogenicity of *C. rivolta* is generally thought to be low, although severe diarrhoea in young kittens has been associated with high oocyst counts.

Sarcocystiosis

The previously complex nomenclature for the large number of *Sarcocystis* spp. has largely been discarded by many workers in favour of a new system based on their biology. The new names generally incorporate those of the intermediate and final hosts in that order.

At present the most important species recognised with the dog as a final host are:
- *Sarcocystis bovicanis* (*Sarcocystis cruzi*)
- *Sarcocystis ovicanis* (*Sarcocystis tenella*)
- *Sarcocystis capracanis*
- *Sarcocystis hircicanis*
- *Sarcocystis suicanis* (*Sarcocystis porcicanis, Sarcocystis miescheriana*)
- *Sarcocystis equicanis* (*Sarcocystis bertrami*)
- *Sarcocystis fayeri*
- *Sarcocystis hovarthi*
- *Sarcocystis cameli*.

The most important species recognised with the cat as a final host are:
- *Sarcocystis bovifelis* (*Sarcocystis hirsuta*)
- *Sarcocystis ovifelis* (*Sarcocystis tenella, Sarcocystis medusiformis*)
- *Sarcocystis porcifelis* (*Sarcocystis suifelis*).

Epidemiology: Little is known of the epidemiology, but from the high prevalence of symptomless infections observed in abattoirs, it is clear that where dogs and cats are kept in close association with farm animals or their feed, then transmission is likely. Sheepdogs and farm cats are known to play an important part in the transmission of *Sarcocystis* and care should be exercised that only cooked meat is fed to dogs and cats. Acute outbreaks of *Sarcocystis* in livestock are probably most likely when livestock which have been reared without contact with farm dogs in particular are subsequently exposed to large numbers of the sporocysts from dog faeces. The longevity of the sporocysts shed in the faeces is not known.

Clinical signs and pathology: Infection in the dog and cat is normally non-pathogenic although mild diarrhoea has occasionally been reported with some infections. Oocysts may be seen in the lamina propria and within the epithelium at the tips of the villi.

Diagnosis: Identification of oocysts in dog or cat faeces and differentiation from other coccidial species of dogs and cats (see Tables 12.6 and 12.7).

Control and treatment: The only control measures possible are those of simple hygiene. Farm dogs and cats should not be housed in, or allowed access to, fodder stores, nor should they be allowed to defecate in pens where livestock are housed. It is also important that they are not fed uncooked meat. There is no effective treatment for infection in dogs or cats.

Sarcocystis bovicanis

Sarcocystis bovicanis, synonyms *Sarcocystis cruzi, Sarcocystis fusiformis* (Phylum: Apicomplexa; Class: Conoidasida; Order: Eucoccidiorida; Family: Sarcocystidae), is a parasite distributed worldwide and localised in the small intestine of dogs, foxes, wolves and coyotes. This parasite has cattle as intermediate hosts.

Sarcocystis ovicanis

Sarcocystis ovicanis, synonyms *Sarcocystis tenella, Isospora bigemina* (Phylum: Apicomplexa; Class: Conoidasida; Order: Eucoccidiorida; Family: Sarcocystidae), is a parasite distributed worldwide and localised in the small intestine of dogs. This parasite has sheep as intermediate hosts.

Sarcocystis capracanis

Sarcocystis capracanis (Phylum: Apicomplexa; Class: Conoidasida; Order: Eucoccidiorida; Family: Sarcocystidae) is a parasite distributed worldwide and localised in the small intestine of dogs. This parasite has goats as intermediate hosts.

Sarcocystis hircicanis

Sarcocystis hircicanis (Phylum: Apicomplexa; Class: Conoidasida; Order: Eucoccidiorida; Family: Sarcocystidae) is a parasite distributed worldwide and localised in the small intestine of dogs. This parasite has goats as intermediate hosts.

Sarcocystis suicanis

Sarcocystis suicanis, synonyms *Sarcocystis porcicanis, Sarcocystis miescheriana* (Phylum: Apicomplexa; Class: Conoidasida; Order: Eucoccidiorida; Family: Sarcocystidae) is a parasite distributed worldwide and localised in the small intestine of dogs. This parasite has pigs as intermediate hosts.

Sarcocystis equicanis

Sarcocystis equicanis, synonym *Sarcocystis bertrami* (Phylum: Apicomplexa; Class: Conoidasida; Order: Eucoccidiorida; Family: Sarcocystidae), is a parasite distributed worldwide and localised in the small intestine of dogs. This parasite has horses as intermediate hosts.

Sarcocystis fayeri

Sarcocystis fayeri, synonym *Sarcocystis bertrami* (Phylum: Apicomplexa; Class: Conoidasida; Order: Eucoccidiorida; Family: Sarcocystidae), is a parasite distributed worldwide and localised in the small intestine of dogs. This parasite has horses as intermediate hosts.

Sarcocystis hovarthi

Sarcocystis hovarthi, synonym *Sarcocystis gallinarum* (Phylum: Apicomplexa; Class: Conoidasida; Order: Eucoccidiorida; Family: Sarcocystidae), is a parasite distributed worldwide and localised in the small intestine of dogs. This parasite has chickens as intermediate hosts.

Sarcocystis cameli

Sarcocystis cameli (Phylum: Apicomplexa; Class: Conoidasida; Order: Eucoccidiorida; Family: Sarcocystidae) is localised in the small intestine of dogs and occurs in North Africa (Egypt, Morocco, Sudan). This parasite has camels (bactrian and dromedary) as intermediate hosts.

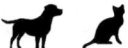

Sarcocystis bovifelis

Sarcocystis bovifelis, synonyms *Sarcocystis hirsuta, Sarcocystis fusiformis* (Phylum: Apicomplexa; Class: Conoidasida; Order: Eucoccidiorida; Family: Sarcocystidae), is a parasite distributed worldwide and localised in the small intestine of cats. This parasite has cattle as intermediate hosts.

Sarcocystis ovifelis

Sarcocystis ovifelis, synonyms *Sarcocystis tenella, Sarcocystis gigantea, Sarcocystis medusiformis, Isospora bigemina* (Phylum: Apicomplexa; Class: Conoidasida; Order: Eucoccidiorida; Family: Sarcocystidae), is a parasite distributed worldwide and localised in the small intestine of cats. This parasite has sheep as intermediate hosts.

Sarcocystis porcifelis

Sarcocystis porcifelis, synonym *Sarcocystis suifelis* (Phylum: Apicomplexa; Class: Conoidasida; Order: Eucoccidiorida; Family: Sarcocystidae), is a parasite distributed worldwide and localised in the small intestine of cats. This parasite has pigs as intermediate hosts.

Hammondia heydorni

Hammondia heydorni, synonyms *Cystoisospora hammondi, Toxoplasma hammondi* (Phylum: Apicomplexa; Class: Conoidasida; Order: Eucoccidiorida; Family: Sarcocystidae), is presumed to be a parasite distributed worldwide and localised in the small intestine of dogs. This parasite has cattle, sheep, goats, rodents and guinea pigs as intermediate hosts. The dog is infected following the consumption of zoite-containing tissues of the intermediate host. Direct dog-to-dog transmission does not occur.

Clinical signs and pathology: The pathology is not reported but the infection may cause diarrhoea in young puppies.

Diagnosis: Identification of oocysts in dog faeces and differentiation from other coccidial species of dogs (see Table 12.6).

Control and treatment: The only control measures possible are those of simple hygiene. Dogs should also not be fed raw or uncooked meat. Treatment is not indicated.

Hammondia hammondi

Hammondia hammondi, synonyms *Isospora hammondi, Toxoplasma hammondi* (Phylum: Apicomplexa; Class: Conoidasida; Order: Eucoccidiorida; Family: Sarcocystidae), is presumed to be a parasite distributed worldwide and localised in the small intestine of cats. This parasite has rodents (mice, rats and guinea pigs) as intermediate hosts. The cat is infected following the consumption of zoite-containing tissues of the intermediate host. Direct cat-to-cat transmission does not occur.

Pathogenesis: Non-pathogenic to either host, but it is important to recognise that the oocysts of *Hammondia* closely resemble those of *Toxoplasma* and that their differentiation in cat faeces is a specialist task.

Clinical signs and pathology: There are no associated clinical signs. Pathology is not reported.

Diagnosis: Identification of oocysts in cat faeces and differentiation from other coccidial species of cats (see Table 12.7).

Control and treatment: The only control measures possible are those of simple hygiene. Cats should not be fed raw or uncooked meat. Treatment is not indicated

Besnoitia besnoiti

Besnoitia besnoiti, synonyms *Sarcocystis besnoiti, Globidium besnoiti* (Phylum: Apicomplexa; Class: Conoidasida; Order: Eucoccidiorida; Family: Sarcocystidae), is presumed to be a parasite distributed worldwide (although important in tropical and subtropical countries, especially in Africa), and localised in the small intestine of cats and wild cats (lions, cheetahs and leopards). This parasite has cattle, goats and wild ruminants (wildebeest, impala and kudu) as intermediate hosts. In the life cycle, the ruminant intermediate hosts are infected by the ingestion of oocysts shed into the environment by infected cats. Cats are infected following ingestion of cysts present in the subcutaneous tissues of infected intermediate hosts. Therefore, the natural mode of transmission is by ingestion of pseudocysts present in the skin of animal carcasses. *Besnoitia besnoiti* is non-pathogenic in the cat final host.

Diagnosis: Identification of oocysts in cat faeces and differentiation from other coccidial species of cats (see Table 12.7).

Control and treatment: As for *Sarcocystis* species. There is no effective treatment for infection in cats.

Cryptosporidiosis

Recent molecular characterisations have shown that there is extensive host adaptation in *Cryptosporidium* evolution, and many mammals or groups of mammals have host-adapted *Cryptosporidium* genotypes that differ from each other in both DNA sequences and infectivity. These genotypes are now delineated as distinct species and include *Cryptosporidium hominis* (previously termed human genotype or genotype 1), *C. parvum* (also termed bovine genotype or genotype 2) and *C. canis* (dog genotype). Other genotypes have been associated with mice, pigs, bears, deer, marsupials, monkeys, muskrats, skunks, cattle and ferrets. Most of these organisms probably represent individual *Cryptosporidium* species.

Epidemiology: A variety of mammals act as hosts to *C. parvum* but *C. canis* appears to be adapted to dogs and *C. felis* to cats. Transmission appears to be mainly by the faecal–oral route.

Pathogenesis: Chronic diarrhoea may occur in dogs that are immunosuppressed because of concurrent illness or toxicity. Puppies with distemper virus, for example, have developed persistent diarrhoea and persistently excreted *Cryptosporidium* oocysts. Infection with *C. felis* in cats is not considered pathogenic.

Clinical signs and pathology: Infection with *Cryptosporidium* is generally asymptomatic but may cause acute diarrhoea in neonatal animals or more chronic diarrhoea in young immunosuppressed

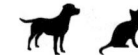

animals or in animals with intercurrent and debilitating diseases such as distemper in dogs or feline leukaemia virus (FeLV)/feline immunodeficiency virus (FIV) in cats. The meronts and gamonts develop in a parasitophorous envelope apparently derived from the microvilli and so the cell disruption seen with other coccidia does not apparently occur. However, mucosal changes are obvious in the ileum where there is stunting, swelling and eventually fusion of the villi. This has a marked effect on the activity of some of the membrane-bound enzymes.

Diagnosis: Oocysts may be demonstrated using Ziehl–Neelsen stained faecal smears in which the sporozoites appear as bright red granules. Speciation of *Cryptosporidium* is difficult, if not impossible, using conventional techniques. A range of molecular and immunological techniques has been developed that includes immunofluorescence or ELISA. More recently, DNA-based techniques have been used for molecular characterisation of *Cryptosporidium* species.

Control and treatment: Good hygiene and management are important in preventing disease from cryptosporidiosis. There is no known treatment. Supportive treatment and therapy of any concurrent illness may be required.

Cryptosporidium parvum

Cryptosporidium parvum (Phylum: Apicomplexa; Class: Conoidasida; Order: Cryptogregarinorida; Family: Cryptosporidiidae) is a parasite distributed worldwide and localised in the small intestine of cattle, sheep, goats, horses, deer, dogs, cats and humans.

Cryptosporidium canis

Cryptosporidium canis (Phylum: Apicomplexa; Class: Conoidasida; Order: Cryptogregarinorida; Family: Cryptosporidiidae) is a parasite distributed worldwide and localised in the small intestine of dogs, foxes and humans.

Cryptosporidium felis

Cryptosporidium felis (Phylum: Apicomplexa; Class: Conoidasida; Order: Cryptogregarinorida; Family: Cryptosporidiidae) is a parasite distributed worldwide and localised in the small intestine of cats, cattle and humans.

Other protozoa

Giardia is important because of water-borne outbreaks that have occurred in human populations. There is still some controversy over the classification of *Giardia* spp. The main species is *G. intestinalis*, although phylogenetic data suggest that *G. intestinalis* is a species complex composed of several species that are host specific. The current molecular classification places isolates into eight distinct assemblages. Some authors give separate specific names to *Giardia* organisms isolated from dogs and cats, for example *G. duodenalis* (Assemblage A), *Giardia enterica* (Assemblage B), *Giardia canis* (Assemblage C, D) and *Giardia cati* (Assemblage F), although species specificity of many isolates is unknown.

Giardia intestinalis

Giardia intestinalis, synonyms *Giardia duodenalis*, *Giardia lamblia*, *Lamblia lamblia* (Phylum: Metamonada; Class: Trepomonadea; Order: Diplomonadida; Family: Giardiidae), is a parasite distributed worldwide and localised in the small intestine of humans, cattle, sheep, goats, pigs, alpaca, dogs, cats, guinea pigs and chinchillas.

Epidemiology: Molecular studies have revealed a substantial level of genetic diversity in *G. intestinalis* isolates. Human isolates fall into two major groups (Assemblage A and B), with a wide host range in other mammals, and it may prove to be the case that some separate species names may be applicable. Other assemblages may also represent distinct species. Limited epidemiological studies suggest that in animal isolates, direct animal-to-animal contact and faecal soiling are the most likely methods of transmission, although water contamination can also be considered as a possible route. Zoonotic transmission has been reported from dogs.

Pathogenesis: While *Giardia* cysts are commonly excreted in the faeces of dogs and cats, there is no consistent relationship with diarrhoea or other signs of gastrointestinal problems, although they could act as reservoirs of infection for humans.

Clinical signs and pathology: When disease does occur, the signs often include chronic pasty diarrhoea, weight loss, lethargy and failure to thrive. There may be villous atrophy, crypt hypertrophy and an increased number of intraepithelial lymphocytes. Trophozoites may be seen between villi, attached by their concave surface to the brush border of epithelial cells.

Diagnosis: *Giardia* cysts can be detected in faeces by a number of methods. Traditional methods of identification involve direct examination of faecal smears, or faecal concentration by formalin-ethyl acetate or zinc sulfate methods and subsequent microscopic examination. It is generally recommended that three consecutive samples be examined as cysts are excreted intermittently.

Control and treatment: As infection is transmitted by the faecal–oral route, good hygiene and prevention of faecal contamination of feed and water are essential. A vaccine based on disrupted axenically cultured trophozoites is available commercially (GiardiaVax®) for use in dogs and cats. Several benzimidazole anthelmintics (e.g. albendazole, fenbendazole) and nitroimidazoles (metronidazole, tinidazole) are effective and may be of benefit in the treatment of *Giardia* infections in animals.

LARGE INTESTINE

Trichuris vulpis

Trichuris vulpis, synonym *Trichocephalus vulpis* (Phylum: Nematoda; Class: Enoplea; Order: Enoplida; Family: Trichuridae), commonly known as the Whipworm, is a parasite distributed in many parts of the world and localised in the large intestine of dogs, foxes and cats. Two other species, *Trichuris serrata* and *Trichuris campanula*, are occasionally found in the cats, mainly in North and South America and the Caribbean. Details on the life cycle, pathogenesis, treatment and control are essentially similar to those for *T. vulpis*. The adults are usually found in the caecum but are only occasionally present in sufficient numbers to be clinically significant.

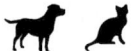

Epidemiology: The most important feature is the longevity of the eggs. Older dogs tend to have higher whipworm burdens than young dogs.

Pathogenesis: Most infections are light and asymptomatic. Occasionally, when large numbers of worms are present, they cause a haemorrhagic colitis and/or a diphtheritic inflammation of the caecal mucosa. This results from the subepithelial location and continuous movement of the anterior end of the whipworm as it searches for blood and fluid.

Clinical signs and pathology: Sporadic disease due to heavy infection is more common in dogs and is associated with an acute or chronic inflammation of the caecal mucosa with watery diarrhoea that often contains blood. Anaemia may be present and animals can lose weight. In severe cases, the mucosa of the large intestine is inflamed and haemorrhagic, with ulceration and formation of diphtheritic membranes.

Diagnosis: Since the clinical signs are not pathognomonic, diagnosis may depend on finding numbers of lemon-shaped *Trichuris* eggs in the faeces. Egg output is often low in *Trichuris* infections. However, since clinical signs may occur during the prepatent period, diagnosis may depend on necropsy or a favourable response to anthelmintic treatment. Occasionally, expelled adult worms may be present in faeces.

Control and treatment: Prophylaxis is rarely necessary. Attention should be paid to areas where eggs might continue to survive for long periods. Such areas should be thoroughly cleaned and disinfected or sterilised by wet or dry heat. For treatment, the pro-benzimidazoles and benzimidazoles, administered over several days, are effective against adult *Trichuris* but less so against the larval stage. Milbemycins are effective.

Entamoeba histolytica

Entamoeba histolytica, synonyms *Entamoeba dysenteriae*, *Endamoeba histolytica* (Phylum: Amoebozoa; Class: Archamoeba; Order: Entamoebida; Family: Entamoebidae), is a parasite distributed worldwide and localised in the large intestine and liver of humans, apes, monkeys, dogs, cats, pigs and rats. It is primarily a parasite of primates; humans are the reservoir for animals. Infection in dogs has only been reported sporadically and often through human contacts.

Pathogenesis: Two forms of the parasite exist. Non-pathogenic forms normally live in the lumen of the large intestine. Pathogenic forms invade the mucosa, causing ulceration and dysentery. From there, they may be carried via the portal system to the liver and other organs where large abscesses may form. The amoeba-like trophozoites secrete proteolytic enzymes and produce characteristic flask-shaped ulcers in the mucosa of the large intestine. Their erosion may allow the parasites to enter the bloodstream when the most common sequela is the formation of amoebic abscesses in the liver. The veterinary significance of amoebosis is that natural infections, usually without clinical signs, can occur occasionally in dogs from the human reservoir of active or carrier infections. Kittens are also susceptible to experimental infection, although they do not produce cysts. Monkeys have their own strains of *E. histolytica* and these can be infective to humans.

Clinical signs and pathology: Infection causes diarrhoea or dysentery. Pathogenic strains of amoebae penetrate the mucosa of the large intestine and multiply to form small colonies that extend into the submucosa and muscularis. In the absence of bacterial infection, there is little reaction but in complicated infections, there is hyperaemia and inflammation with predominant neutrophils. Amoebae may pass into the lymphatic system and mediastinal lymph nodes and from there migrate in the portal system to the liver where they may cause abscessation. Abscesses may also form in other organs including the lungs and brain.

Diagnosis: Motile organisms and cysts of *E. histolytica* may be detected in smears from faeces. Trophozoites and cysts can be stained with iodine, Trichrome or iron haematoxylin. The organisms can also be cultured in a number of media including Boeck and Drbohlav's, Dobell and Laidlaw's, TYI-S-33 and Robinson's. Isoenzyme markers can be used to differentiate the two forms seen, but there is some debate as to whether the two types represent different species or if they can change from one type to another under certain circumstances.

A number of serological tests have been evaluated for the diagnosis of *E. histolytica* infections. These include ELISA, latex agglutination, complement fixation and indirect haemagglutination. A number of PCR methods have also been used to detect *E. histolytica* in clinical samples. These are based on the amplification of specific DNA sequences that correlate to the pathogenic/non-pathogenic isoenzyme categorisation and appear to be very sensitive and specific.

Control and treatment: Dogs are not a significant reservoir of infection for humans so that prophylaxis ultimately depends on personal and sanitary hygiene in the human population. Treatment, if required, relies on the combined use of metronidazole and di-iodohydroxyquin.

Pentatrichomonas hominis

Pentatrichomonas hominis, synonyms *Pentatrichomonas felis*, *Cercomonas hominis*, *Monocercomonas hominis*, *Trichomonas felis*, *Trichomonas intestinalis* (Phylum: Metamonada; Class: Trichomonadea; Order: Trichomonadida; Family: Trichomonadidae), is a parasite distributed worldwide and localised in the large intestine of humans, monkeys, dogs, cats, rats, mice, hamsters and guinea pigs. This parasite is considered non-pathogenic and the diagnosis is through morphological identification of the organisms from fresh and stained faecal preparations. The organism can also be cultured in trichomonads culture medium. Treatment and control are not required.

Tritrichomonas foetus

Tritrichomonas foetus (Phylum: Metamonada; Class: Trichomonadea; Order: Trichomonadida; Family: Trichomonadidae) is localised in the ileum, caecum and colon of cats and cattle and diffused in USA and parts of Europe (Germany, Austria, France and UK) and possibly worldwide.

Notes: *Tritrichomonas foetus* has been found worldwide and is an important cause of infertility, abortion and endometritis in cattle, although the organism has been eradicated from many cattle

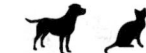

populations through the use of artificial insemination. A morphologically identical organism (*T. suis*) has been identified in pigs, in which it commonly causes asymptomatic infection of the nasal cavity, stomach and intestine. This organism is now considered synonymous with *T. foetus*. Reports of trichomonad-associated large bowel diarrhoea started to emerge in cats in the USA in 2000, which were subsequently confirmed to be *T. foetus*.

Epidemiology: In cats, transmission is probably via the faecal–oral route. Infection is most commonly seen in colonies of cats and multicat households. In these situations, the organism is presumably spread between cats by close contact.

Pathogenesis: The organisms are mainly localised to the epithelial surface, occasionally in the crypts of the colon, and cause an accompanying lymphocytic and neutrophilic inflammatory response. In some cases, the organisms have been seen to invade the lamina propria of the colon, resulting in a more severe inflammatory response. The organism has also been found in the uterus of a cat with pyometra, suggesting a possible link to reproductive tract disease in cats.

Clinical signs: Infection causes colitis with increased frequency of defecation; faeces are semi-formed to liquid, sometimes with fresh blood or mucus. With severe diarrhoea, the anus may become inflamed and painful, and the cat may become faecally incontinent. Although cats of all ages can be affected, *T. foetus*-associated diarrhoea is most commonly seen in young cats and kittens.

Diagnosis: There are three routine diagnostic methods: direct microscopy, culture of the organism and PCR analysis of faeces. In some countries, a liquid culture system is available (InPouch® TFFeline). The pouch can be inoculated with a small amount of faeces obtained within 1–2 hours of collection, and ideally incubated at 37 °C for between 18 and 24 hours and then at room temperature. The pouch can be examined microscopically (via an in-built viewing chamber) for the motile organisms every two days for 12 days. This test is considerably more sensitive than direct examination of faeces, and helpful in detecting infections when direct smears are negative.

Control and treatment: Dietary changes may improve faecal consistency and diarrhoea. Diarrhoea will usually resolve spontaneously in untreated cats although this may take several months. For treatment, the use of a number of antibiotics has been reported to improve clinical symptoms, possibly through reduction in resident bacterial microflora on which the organisms feed. Ronidazole has been shown to have a direct effect on the organisms, leading to a reduction in diarrhoea, although its use is cautioned because of possible neurotoxic side-effects in cats at higher doses.

Parasites of the respiratory system

Two species of the genus *Mammomonogamus*, which is closely related to *Syngamus*, are parasitic in the nasal cavities of cats. Infections are usually asymptomatic but affected animals may sneeze and have a nasal discharge due to irritation of the nasal mucosa. Adult worms are red in colour, 1–2 cm long and permanently joined *in copula*. Diagnosis is based on clinical signs and the finding of eggs in the faeces or adult worms on *post mortem*. Details of the life cycle are unknown and there is no known effective treatment.

Mammomonogamus ierei

Mammomonogamus ierei, synonym *Syngamus ierei* (Phylum: Nematoda; Class: Chromadorea; Order: Rhabtidida; Family: Syngamidae), is localised in the nasal cavities of cats and diffused in the Caribbean.

Eucoleus aerophila

Eucoleus aerophila, synonym *Capillaria aerophila* (Phylum: Nematoda; Class: Enoplea; Order: Enoplida; Family: Capillariidae), commonly known as the Tracheal worm, is a parasite distributed worldwide and localised in the trachea, bronchi, occasionally nasal passages and frontal sinuses of foxes, particularly those reared on fur farms, and mustelids; occasionally dogs, cats and humans. This parasite has earthworms as intermediate hosts.

Epidemiology: Although infection can be acquired through the consumption of infective earthworms, the major route of transmission is usually via the ingestion of embryonated infective eggs. *Eucoleus aerophila* is particularly a problem in farmed animals reared for their fur. Disease is usually seen in foxes of less than 18 months of age.

Pathogenesis: The nematode causes irritation to the respiratory mucosa with a resultant increase in secretion. There may be some constriction of the lumen of the air passages and some areas may show emphysema. Heavy infections can induce bronchopneumonia with occasional abscess formation in the lung tissue. Secondary bacterial infection can sometimes occur and this is often fatal in younger animals.

Clinical signs and pathology: Light infections are usually asymptomatic. The clinical signs of moderate to severe infection are those of rhinotracheitis and/or bronchitis and in this respect are similar to those caused by *Oslerus* or *Crenosoma* infection. In such cases, there may be a nasal discharge, a wheezing cough and/or sneezing. Dyspnoea can be observed in heavy infections. The effects depend on the number of worms present. Mild infections cause a mild catarrhal inflammation while heavy infections cause more severe irritation and obstruction to the lumen of the airways.

Diagnosis: The presence of eggs in faeces or sputum and a nasal discharge are indicative of infection. Note that the eggs are morphologically similar to those of *Capillaria plica* (see Parasites of the reproductive/urogenital system).

Control and treatment: On fox-rearing farms, care should be taken to ensure that runs are created in areas where the soil is dry and free-draining. Alternatively, the animals should be housed in cages raised above the soil. Breeding pens need to be cleaned thoroughly to reduce the accumulation of infective eggs. Periodic treatment with anthelmintic is essential.

Treatment with modern benzimidazoles or ivermection is effective. Levamisole 7.5 mg/kg on two consecutive days and repeated 14 days later is also effective.

Eucoleus boehmi

Eucoleus boehmi, synonym *Capillaria boehmi* (Phylum: Nematoda; Class: Enoplea; Order: Enoplida; Family: Capillariidae), commonly

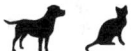

known as the Sinus worm, is a parasite localised in the frontal sinuses of foxes and, very rarely, dogs.

Notes: The taxonomy and systematics of these parasites have been changed many times because of a difficulty in designation of particular species' features and there are many synonyms in this group. Some species of *Capillaria* are now listed under the generic name *Eucoleus*, although they may universally still be referred to as *Capillaria*.

Crenosoma vulpis

Crenosoma vulpis (Phylum: Nematoda; Class: Chromadorea; Order: Rhabditida; Family: Crenosomatidae), commonly known as the Fox lungworm, is a parasite distributed worldwide and localised in the trachea, bronchi and bronchioles of dogs, foxes, wolves and raccoons. This parasite has slugs and snails (*Helix*, *Cepea*, *Arianta*, *Agrioli-max*, *Arion*) as intermediate hosts.

Epidemiology: *Crenosoma vulpis* is more common in the fox than in the dog, and can be a problem in farmed foxes. The infection has a seasonality corresponding to fluctuations in population of its snail vectors so that although cubs may begin to acquire L_3 in early summer, the highest incidence of clinical crenosomosis is seen in autumn.

Clinical signs and pathology: The spiny cuticular folds abrade the mucosa of the air passages with resulting bronchopneumonia and occlusion of the smaller bronchi and bronchioles. Therefore, symptoms are those of a chronic respiratory infection, with coughing, sneezing and nasal discharge associated with tachypnoea. Farmed foxes may become emaciated, with fur of poor quality. In the infrequent acute infections there may be high mortality. The gross lesions usually observed in dogs are greyish consolidations in dorsal regions of the caudal lobes. Histologically, the lesions are catarrhal eosinophilic bronchitis and bronchiolitis.

Diagnosis: Examination of faeces by smear, flotation or Baermann technique will reveal the L_1 with a straight tail, which differentiates it in fresh canine faeces from those of *Oslerus*, *Filaroides* and *Angiostrongylus*. The L_1 somewhat resembles that of *Strongyloides* spp. Infection should be differentiated from that caused by *Eucoleus aerophila* as the two disease entities are similar.

Control and treatment: The snail vectors may be eliminated by spraying fox runs with molluscicide and painting woodwork with creosote up to 20 cm from the ground. Faeces should be disposed of in a manner that will avoid access by molluscs. Treatment with diethylcarbamazine has been reported to be effective but is no longer widely available. Levamisole has reported activity at 8 mg/kg and ivermectin is likely to be active. Fenbendazole (50 mg/kg for 3–5 days) has had some success in removing *C. vulpis* in dogs.

Oslerus osleri

Oslerus osleri, synonym *Filaroides osleri* (Phylum: Nematoda; Class: Chromadorea; Order: Rhabditida; Family: Filaroididae), commonly known as the Dog lungworm, is a parasite distributed worldwide and localised in the bronchi and trachea of dogs and other wild canids such as dingoes.

Notes: Until recently, this genus was part of the larger genus *Filaroides*, but it has now been separated on morphological grounds from the other members. Though distinction has been made on morphology, it is also useful from the veterinary standpoint as it separates the single harmful species, *O. osleri* living in the upper air passages, from the relatively harmless species which are retained in the genus *Filaroides* and which live in the lung parenchyma.

Epidemiology: Transmission occurs when an infected bitch licks the pups and transfers the newly hatched L_1 present in the sputum. Though *Oslerus* has been recorded from many countries, there are few data on its local prevalence. In the UK, one survey has given a figure of 6% for all types of dogs. In further surveys in the same area, greyhounds have shown a prevalence rate of 18%, but there is no evidence of breed susceptibility. In general, the focus of infection appears to be the nursing bitch. Infection rates may be high in kennel-housed dogs.

Pathogenesis: The worms are embedded in fibrous nodules (2–20 mm) in the trachea at the region of the bifurcation and in the adjacent bronchi (Fig. 12.4). Rarely found deeper in the lungs. The nodules in which the worms live first appear at about two months after infection. They are pinkish-grey granulomas, and the small worms may be seen partly protruding from their surfaces. These nodules are fibrous in character and are very firmly applied to the mucosa; they may be up to 2 cm in diameter. Although the majority of worms occur near the tracheal bifurcation, a few may be found several centimetres from this area. Infection can cause chronic tracheobronchitis.

Clinical signs and pathology: Many infections are clinically inapparent, and the characteristic nodules are only discovered incidentally at necropsy. The major signs of *Oslerus* infection are respiratory distress and a dry rasping persistent cough, especially after exercise. The most severe cases have usually been seen in dogs of 6–12 months old, and obviously the infection is of greater importance in working dogs. Heavy chronic infections can impair appetite and lead to emaciation. In household pets, whose exercise

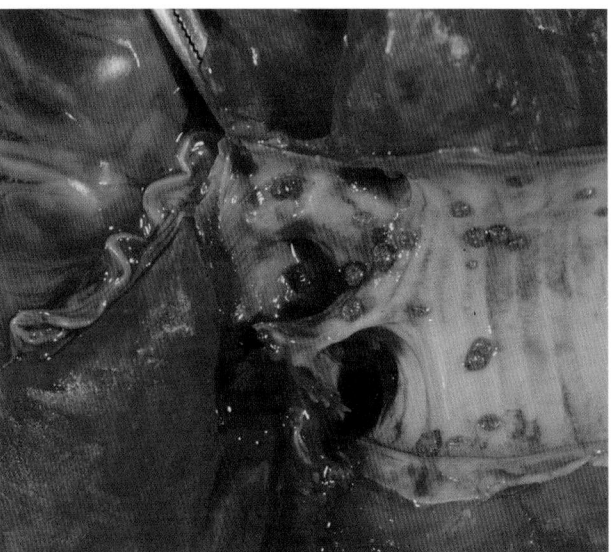

Fig. 12.4 Fibrous nodules in the bronchus caused by infection with *Oslerus osleri*.

is limited, the presence of the tracheal nodules is well tolerated and animals show little respiratory distress. Typical lesions are protruding submucosal nodules, greyish-white in colour, in the region of the tracheal bifurcation. Lesions vary in size from barely visible to larger nodules or protruding plaques that project over 1 cm into the lumen of the trachea. Smaller nodules contain immature worms and the larger ones a mass of tightly coiled adults. The worms lie in tissue spaces between the cartilage rings of the trachea and large bronchi. Live worms provoke formation of a thin capsule and lymphocytic infiltration locally. Superficially the nodules are covered by intact epithelium, except for small pores through which the female worms protrude their tails to lay eggs. Dead worms provoke a foreign body reaction with neutrophils and a few giant cells.

Diagnosis: Swabs of pharyngeal mucus give variable results and repeated sampling may be necessary. However, in paroxysmal coughing, large amounts of bronchial mucus are often expelled, containing large numbers of larvae. Less rewarding techniques are those based on faecal examination, by either flotation or the Baermann method. Although requiring general anaesthesia, bronchoscopy is the most reliable method, as it will not only indicate the presence, size and location of many of the nodules, but will also allow the collection of tracheal mucus for confirmatory examination for eggs and larvae; the latter are invariably coiled, sluggish and have an S-shaped tail. Large nodules may be detected by lateral thoracic radiography.

Control and treatment: Control is difficult unless infected bitches can be identified and treated before whelping and during lactation. In the past, the only certain method of control was the removal of pups from infected dams at birth, and hand rearing or fostering on uninfected bitches. There are reports of amelioration of clinical signs, apparently due to a reduction in the size of the nodules, after prolonged treatment with some benzimidazoles. Fenbendazole and albendazole at increased dosage rates are licensed for the treatment of *Oslerus* infection in dogs. The signs of infection have been reportedly cleared with ivermectin or doramectin.

Oslerus rostratus

Oslerus rostratus, synonyms *Anafilaroides rostratus*, *Filaroides rostratus* (Phylum: Nematoda; Class: Chromadorea; Order: Rhabditida; Family: Filaroididae), is localised in the lungs of cats and rodents and occurs in North America, Sri Lanka, Pacific Islands, southern Europe and the Middle East.

Filaroides hirthi

Filaroides hirthi (Phylum: Nematoda; Class: Chromadorea; Order: Rhabditida; Family: Filaroididae), commonly known as the Dog lungworm, is localised in the lungs of dogs and wild carnivores, in North America, Europe and Japan.

Epidemiology: Little is known of the epidemiology. *Filaroides hirthi* was first observed in a breeding colony of experimental beagles, and it would be fair to suggest, in view of its mode of transmission, that a high prevalence could be expected in dogs from breeding kennels.

Clinical signs and pathology: Infection is almost invariably asymptomatic, and is discovered only at *post mortem* examination.

However, in the rare heavy infection, hyperpnoea may occur. The chief lesions are the small, soft, greyish miliary nodules that are associated with the presence of worms and which are distributed subpleurally and throughout the lung parenchyma; in heavy infections, sometimes observed in experimental dogs subjected to immunosuppressive drugs, the nodules may coalesce into greyish masses.

Diagnosis: A squeeze preparation from a cut surface of the lung will show worm fragments, eggs and larvae and this, with the host and site, is sufficient for generic diagnosis. *Filaroides hirthi* has only been diagnosed in the live animal and this was in experimental dogs. The L_1, present in the faeces and sputum is coiled and the tail has a notch, followed by a constriction, and a terminal lance-like point. Zinc sulfate is an effective flotation solution for the detection of larvae.

Control and treatment: Control is unlikely to be required. Treatment with albendazole (orally at a dose rate of 25 mg/kg twice daily over five days) has been reported to be highly effective although treatment is rarely called for. Ivermectin has also shown efficacy.

Aelurostrongylus abstrusus

Aelurostrongylus abstrusus (Phylum: Nematoda; Class: Chromadorea; Order: Rhabditida; Family: Angiostrongylidae), commonly known as the Cat lungworm, is presumed to be a parasite distributed worldwide and localised in the lung parenchyma and small bronchioles of cats. This parasite has many terrestrial molluscs, such as snails and slugs, as intermediate hosts. The paratenic hosts include rodents, birds, amphibians and reptiles.

Notes: Other nematodes can invade the lungs of cats and other felines, such as the bobcat, ocelot and mountain lion, but generally they are considered to be of low pathogenicity unless present in high numbers.

Epidemiology: *Aelurostrongylus* infection is widespread, partly because it is almost indiscriminate in its ability to develop in slugs and snails, and partly because of its wide range of paratenic hosts. So far, all surveys have shown prevalences greater than 5%.

Pathogenesis: The worm generally has a low pathogenicity and the majority of infections are discovered only incidentally at *post mortem* examination as multiple small greyish foci or bigger consolidated granulomas in the lungs.

Clinical signs and pathology: The clinical effects are slight and in the resting cat are limited to a chronic mild cough. Following exercise or handling, there may be coughing, sneezing and nasal discharge with slight dyspnoea and production of mucoid sputum. In heavy experimental infections, the most severe signs have appeared at 6–12 weeks after infection, when egg laying is maximal. Heavy infections may be accompanied by dyspnoea, diarrhoea, anorexia and weight loss. In most cases, the lungs show only multiple small raised subpleural foci with greyish centres containing the worms and tissue debris, but in the rare severe infections, larger nodules are present, up to 1 cm in diameter with caseous centres, projecting from the lung surface; these nodules may coalesce to form areas of consolidation. Microscopically, the alveoli may be blocked with worms, eggs, larvae and cellular aggregations, which may progress to granuloma formation.

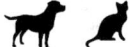

A characteristic change is muscular hypertrophy and hyperplasia, which affects not only the bronchioles and alveolar ducts but also the media of the pulmonary arteries. In these heavy infections, the pleural cavity can be filled with a whitish fluid and occasionally fatalities have been reported.

With the exception of the muscular changes, which appear to be irreversible, resolution is rapid and the lungs appear almost completely normal within six months of experimental infection, though a few worms may still be present.

Diagnosis: Repeated faecal examination by smear, flotation or Baermann technique may be necessary to find the characteristic L_1, which bears a subterminal spine on its S-shaped tail. Examination of pharyngeal swabs may be a useful additional procedure. At necropsy, a squeeze preparation from a cut surface of the lung will often show the worm material, including the characteristic L_1. Radiography has revealed the increased vascular and focal parenchymal densities which would be expected from the changes described above.

Control and treatment: In household pets, and especially those of a nomadic disposition or living in rural locations, access to the intermediate and paratenic hosts is difficult to prevent and control is not often easy or practical. Treatment with fenbendazole 50 mg/kg daily for three days has proved effective.

Troglostrongylus brevior

Troglostrongylus brevior (Phylum: Nematoda; Class: Chromadorea; Order: Rhabditida; Family: Crenosomatidae) is localised in the respiratory system of wild and domestic cats worldwide. In comparison to the better known *A. abstrusus*, *T. brevior* is larger in size and infects the bronchi and bronchioles of cats, mainly kittens, being also transmitted via the transmammary route.

Epidemiology: Since L_1 of *T. brevior* in faeces of infested cats are morphologically similar to those of *A. abstrusus*, very careful examination is needed to differentiate the two species. Thus, molecular analysis of faecal samples from parasitised cats is the way to differentiate the parasites and identify possible co-infestation. In recent years, several cases of *T. brevior* infestation have been reported in cats through Europe; the main risk factors of exposure are similar to those of *A. abstrusus* since the two species share the same biology and paratenic hosts. However, *T. brevior* is more frequent in young animals and kittens due to the fact that they are transmitted via the transmammary route.

Clinical signs and pathology: Due to localisation in the upper airways (i.e. bronchi, large bronchi or trachea) of infected animals, *T. brevior* has a more pathogenic potential compared to *A. abstrusus*. Infected animals may show mild respiratory symptoms to severe respiratory distress, with fatal outcomes mainly in kittens, in which other concomitant respiratory infections (e.g. feline calicivirus or feline herpes virus) might play a major role.

Diagnosis: As for *A. abstrusus*.

Treatment: Some of the macrocyclic lactones used against *A. abstrusus* infestation in cats have also been found to be safe and effective towards *T. brevior*.

Paragonimus westermani

Paragonimus westermani (Phylum: Platyhelminthes; Class: Trematoda; Order: Plagiorchiida; Family: Paragonimidae), commonly known as Oriental lung fluke, is localised in the lung of dogs, cats, pigs, goats, cattle, foxes, other carnivores, humans and primates, in Asia and North America. Snails (*Melania*, *Ampullaria*, *Pomatiopsis*) can act as first intermediate hosts. Crabs and crayfish can act as second intermediate hosts. There are over 10 species of *Paragonimus* which infect humans.

Epidemiology: Infection is maintained in endemic areas where intermediate hosts are abundant.

Pathogenesis: Parasites in the lungs are not usually of great importance, but some may lodge in the brain or other organs, causing more severe damage. Pulmonary signs are comparatively rare in cats or dogs and the veterinary interest is in the potential reservoir of infection for humans. Extrapulmonary infections may produce CLM and abscess formation in the skin and viscera. Brain and spinal cord involvement may lead to seizures, paraplegia and occasional deaths.

Clinical signs and pathology: In lung infections there may be a cough and eggs may be found in the sputum in large numbers. In the lungs, the parasitic cyst is surrounded by diffuse connective tissue and the cyst wall becomes infiltrated by leucocytes and giant cells. The cyst usually contains two parasites surrounded by a purulent fluid mixed with blood and eggs. Pleural adhesions sometimes occur and there is usually hyperplasia of the bronchial epithelium and focal areas of inflammation in the lung parenchyma.

Diagnosis: Diagnosis is by identifying the presence of eggs in the sputum or faeces.

Control and treatment: The complex life cycle makes control in endemic areas impossible. Treatment with high doses of albendazole, fenbendazole or niclofolan over a prolonged period can be effective. Praziquantel administered three times per day over three days can also remove flukes from the lungs.

Paragonimus kellicotti

Paragonimus kellicotti (Phylum: Platyhelminthes; Class: Trematoda; Order: Plagiorchiida; Family: Paragonimidae), commonly known as the Lung fluke, is localised in the lung of cats, pigs and dogs, in North America and South Africa. The intermediate host and pathogenesis of this parasite are the same as for *P. westermani*.

Pneumonyssoides caninum

Pneumonyssoides caninum, synonym *Pneumonyssus caninum* (Phylum: Arthropoda; Class: Arachnida; Subclass: Acari; Family: Halarachnidae), commonly known as the Nasal mite, is localised in the nasal cavity and sinuses of dogs and found worldwide; it is particularly prevalent in Scandanavia.

Epidemiology: The infection is probably transmitted by direct nose-to-nose contact between animals. This species appears to be particularly common in Scandinavia; a prevalence of 24% in pet dogs at necropsy has been reported in Sweden.

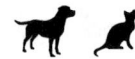

Pathogenesis: *Pneumonyssoides caninum* has been associated with head shaking and 'inverted' sneezing, as well as with chronic rhinitis, sinusitis and tonsillitis, although the majority of infections seem to be subclinical. In working and hunting dogs, the most obvious result of nasal mite infection is a markedly impaired sense of smell. There is evidence that *P. caninum* can penetrate host tissues and move beyond the respiratory system to cause lesions in the liver and kidney.

Clinical signs: The presence of mites causes excessive nasal secretion and hyperaemia of the nasal mucosa. Extreme infestations may result in listlessness, loss of appetite, irritation and scratching at the eyes, chronic sneezing, bronchial cough and rhinitis or sinusitis.

Diagnosis: The mites can be seen crawling over the tissue surface of the nasal sinuses. Specific diagnosis may be achieved through microscopic examination.

Control and treatment: Treatment with ivermectin has proved effective.

Linguatula serrata

Linguatula serrata (Phylum: Arthropoda; Class: Crustacea; Family: Linguatulidae), commonly known as the Tongue worm, is localised in the nasal cavity, sinuses and mesenteric lymph nodes of dogs, cats and foxes, the adult occurring in the nasal passages and sinuses. It is distributed in North America, Europe and Australia.

Pathogenesis and clinical signs: Infrequently, heavy infections in dogs may cause sneezing, coughing and a nasal discharge. The parasites live for about 15 months in the host, after which the animal usually recovers.

Diagnosis: Eggs may be found in the faeces or the nasal discharge. Encysted nymphs may be visible in cut surfaces of mesenteric glands.

Control and treatment: There is no specific treatment recommended, although systemic insecticides should be considered. It is possible to remove the parasites surgically. Infection can be avoided by preventing animals from eating potentially infected material.

Notes: Other species are parasites of tropical reptiles, such as snakes and crocodiles.

Pneumocystis carinii

Pneumocystis carinii, synonym *Pneumocystis jiroveci* (Kingdom: Fungi; Phylum: Ascomycota; Class: Pneumocystidomycetes; Family: Pneumocystidaceae), causes a disease commonly known as Pneumocystosis. It is localised in the lung and may infect humans, cattle, rats, ferrets, mice, dogs, horses, pigs and rabbits worldwide.

Epidemiology: Two major forms of *P. carinii* have been consistently identified from histological and ultrastructural analysis of organisms found in human and rat lung. These are a trophic form and a larger cyst stage containing eight intracystic stages.

The organism is apparently quite widely distributed in latent form in healthy individuals and in the dog, as well as a wide variety of other domestic and wild animals. The organism is thought to be transmitted by aerosol, although the natural habitats and modes of transmission of infections in humans are current areas of research. *Pneumocystis* DNA has been detected in air and water, suggesting that the free forms of the organism may survive in the environment long enough to infect a susceptible host. However, little information on the means of transmission exists currently. In humans, infections appear to spread between immunosuppressed patients colonised with *Pneumocystis* and immunocompetent individuals transiently parasitised with the organism. Human and non-human *Pneumocystis* species have been shown to be different and host specific, suggesting that zoonotic transmission does not occur.

Pathogenesis: *Pneumocystis* is one of the major causes of opportunistic mycoses in the immunocompromised, including those with congenital immunodeficiencies, retrovirus infections such as AIDS, and cases receiving immunosuppressive therapy.

Clinical signs and pathology: Not reported in dogs. The lesion is characterised by a massive plasma cell or histiocyte infiltration of the alveoli in which the organisms may be detected by a silver staining procedure. A foamy eosinophilic material is observed in the lungs during infection. This material is composed of masses of the organism, alveolar macrophages, desquamated epithelial alveolar cells, polymorphonuclear leucocytes and other host cells.

Diagnosis: Gomori's methenamine silver (GMS) and Giemsa stains may be used for microscopic visualisation of *Pneumocystis*. Toluidine blue (TBO) is the most effective for cyst stages while Giemsa stains are used to show trophozoites. Axenic culture methods have been described; however, *in vitro* cultivation, especially from clinical samples, is not always successful. Fluorescence antibody staining techniques can be used to detect both cyst and trophozoite stages of *P. carinii*. A number of PCR methods have been reported which amplify specific regions of DNA from *P. carinii* and are approximately 100 times more sensitive than conventional staining techniques.

Trimethoprim-sulfamethoxazole is the drug of choice for treatment and prophylaxis of *Pneumocystis* infections. Pentamidine and atovaquone are the alternative therapeutic agents in humans.

Control and treatment: Control is difficult given that the routes of transmission are unknown. Infection is generally asymptomatic in animals and is only likely to be detected in immunocompromised individuals.

Notes: Initially reported as a morphological form of *Trypanosoma cruzi*, this microorganism later proved to be a separate genus and was named *P. carinii* and classified as a protozoan until the late 1980s. Following further taxonomic revision, *Pneumocystis* is now classified as a fungus, not a protozoan. The taxonomy is still complicated in that *Pneumocystis* from humans and other animals are quite different and there appear to be multiple species in this genus. Genetic variations and DNA sequence polymorphisms are often observed, suggesting the existence of numerous strains even within a single species of *Pneumocystis*.

Parasites of the liver

Fasciola hepatica

For more details see Chapter 9.

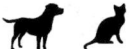

Capillaria hepatica

Capillaria hepatica, synonyms *Callodium hepatica*, *Hepaticola hepatica* (Phylum: Nematoda; Class: Enoplea; Order: Enoplida; Family: Capillariidae), is a parasite distributed worldwide and localised in the liver of rats, mice, squirrels, rabbits and farmed mustelids. Only occasionally reported in dogs, cats and humans.

Epidemiology: Although the prevalence of *C. hepatica* is high in the liver of rodents, it lacks host specificity and occurs in a variety of mammals. Human infection is acquired through ingestion of soil containing embryonated eggs or by consuming contaminated food or water.

Pathogenesis: Adult worms are found in the parenchyma of the liver where they provoke traumatic hepatitis. Eggs are laid in groups in the liver parenchyma from which there is no natural access to the exterior. Granulomas develop around the eggs, accompanied by fibrosis. Heavy infections can cause hepatitis and/or cirrhosis and ascites. The liver may be enlarged and severe infections can be fatal. Heavy infections in humans induce similar hepatic lesions to those seen in other mammalian hosts and hepatic capillariosis is usually fatal.

Clinical signs and pathology: Mild infections are usually asymptomatic. At necropsy, the liver may have yellowish-white streaks on the surface. The eggs, which are deposited in clusters, provoke the development of localised granulomas, which are visible through the capsule as yellowish streaks or patches.

Diagnosis: Most infections are discovered at routine necropsy. Granulomatous tissue in the liver parenchyma can be examined for the presence of eggs or worm fragments after squashing between microscope slides.

Control and treatment: Elimination of rodents will assist in control. Treatment with oral administration of a modern benzimidazole over several days can be effective at preventing egg deposition in the liver tissues. Once egg deposition has occurred, treatment may not be effective.

Clonorchis sinensis

Clonorchis sinensis, synonym *Opisthorchis sinensis* (Phylum: Platyhelminthes; Class: Trematoda; Order: Plagiorchiida; Family: Opisthorchiidae), commonly known as the Chinese or Oriental liver fluke, is localised in the bile ducts, pancreatic ducts and occasionally small intestine of humans, dogs, cats, pigs, mink and badgers. This fluke is prevalent in China, Taiwan, Korea, Vietnam, Japan, India and parts of the former Soviet Union. In the life cycle, two intermediate hosts are required. The operculated snails (*Parafossalurus*, *Bulimus*, *Bithynia*, *Melania* and *Vivipara*) can act as first intermediate hosts. Fish belonging to several genera of the family Cyprinidae (more than 40 have been reported naturally infected) can act as second intermediate hosts.

Notes: Opisthorchiids may be mistaken for dicrocoeliids as they are similar in size and location. However, in the former the ovary is anterior to the testes, whereas in the latter it is posterior to the testes.

Epidemiology: Carnivores or humans usually acquire infection by eating raw fish. In some fish, the metacercariae are found only under the scales and animals that are fed with the scales and offal of such fish become infected, while humans who eat the rest of the fish do not. Infection is usually aggregated in a small number of individuals.

Pathogenesis: The worms live in the narrow proximal parts of the bile ducts. The young flukes particularly, with their cuticular spines, cause cholangitis, pericholangitis and cholecystitis with desquamation of the epithelium, and may in rare cases bring about bile stasis by blocking up the passages, resulting in jaundice.

Clinical signs and pathology: Symptoms are not generally seen except in heavy infections. The symptoms in humans include anaemia, emaciation, ascites, jaundice and diarrhoea. Light infestations may cause little pathology but in heavier infections, there is fibrosis of the smaller bile ducts and cholangiohepatitis and severe biliary fibrosis may develop. Papillomatous or even adenomatous proliferation of the epithelium of the bile ducts occurs, together with cirrhosis of the liver, and this frequently leads to the formation of cysts enclosing eggs and flukes.

Diagnosis: Diagnosis is based on identification of the characteristic eggs in faecal samples, which have to be differentiated from the eggs of other trematodes such as *Heterophyes*, *Metagonimus* and other *Opisthorchis* species. Several serological tests have been developed, but most are non-specific. A reported ELISA may be of value.

Control and treatment: Cats and dogs act as reservoirs for human infection. Prevention relies on not feeding or eating raw, undercooked or improperly pickled, salted, smoked or dried fish. Freezing fish for a week at −10 °C may be beneficial, but even frozen fish has been incriminated with outbreaks of infection in non-endemic areas. In endemic areas, treatment of all infected persons and improved sanitation would help control infection. In those areas where fish are raised in ponds, human and animal faeces should be composted or sterilised before being applied as fertiliser to ponds. Treatment with praziquantel 25 mg/kg on three consecutive days has been reported to be effective.

Opisthorchis felineus

Opisthorchis felineus, synonyms *Opisthorchis tenuicollis*, *Opisthorchis viverrini* (Phylum: Platyhelminthes; Class: Trematoda; Order: Plagiorchiida; Family: Opisthorchiidae), commonly known as the Cat liver fluke, is localised in the bile ducts, pancreatic ducts and occasionally small intestine of cats, dogs, foxes, pigs, humans and cetaceans (seals, porpoises). This fluke is prevalent in southern Asia, Europe, Russia and Canada. In the life cycle, two intermediate hosts are required. Operculated snails (*Bithynia*) can act as first intermediate hosts. Freshwater fish belonging to several genera (*Leuciscus*, *Blicca*, *Tinca*, *Barbus*) can act as second intermediate hosts. In Europe, metacercariae are common in freshwater fish such as orfe, bream, tench and barbel. Most infections are asymptomatic, depending on the level and duration of infection. Adult flukes in the bile ducts, gallbladder and occasionally pancreatic duct cause thickening of the ducts, predisposing to cholangiocarcinoma and hepatocellular carcinoma. Light infestations may cause little pathology but in heavier infections, there is fibrosis of the smaller bile ducts, and cholangiohepatitis and severe biliary fibrosis may develop in advanced cases. Adenocarcinoma of the liver or pancreas has been reported in cats and humans.

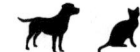

Notes: There is some uncertainty regarding the proper classification of opisthorchiid flukes and many texts suggest the reported species of *Opisthorchis* are synonymous.

Metorchis albidus

Metorchis albidus, synonyms *Distoma albicum, Opisthorchis albidus* (Phylum: Platyhelminthes; Class: Trematoda; Order: Plagiorchiida; Family: Opisthorchiidae), commonly known as the Liver fluke, is localised in the bile ducts and gallbladder of dogs, cats, foxes, seals, occasionally poultry and humans. It occurs in Europe, Asia and North America. In the life cycle, two intermediate hosts are required: freshwater snails (first intermediate host) and fish (*Blicca bjorkna*) (second intermediate host).

Metorchis conjunctus

Metorchis conjunctus (Phylum: Platyhelminthes; Class: Trematoda; Order: Plagiorchiida; Family: Opisthorchiidae), commonly known as the Liver fluke, is localised in the bile ducts and gallbladder of dogs, cats, foxes, mink and raccoons, in North America. In the life cycle, two intermediate hosts are required. Freshwater snails (*Amnicola*) can act as first intermediate hosts. Fish (*Catostomus*) can act as second intermediate hosts.

Platynosomum fastosum

Platynosomum fastosum, synonym *Eurytrema fastosum* (Phylum: Platyhelminthes; Class: Trematoda; Order: Plagiorchiida; Family: Dicrocoeliidae), commonly known as the Cat liver fluke, is localised in the bile and pancreatic ducts of cats. It is distributed in South America, the Caribbean, southern USA, Hawaii, West Africa, Malaysia and the Pacific Islands. This parasite has land snails (*Sublima*) and wood lice as intermediate hosts. Lizards are obligate paratenic hosts and the infection is maintained in endemic areas where intermediate hosts and lizards are abundant.

Pathogenesis: Most infections are well tolerated by the cat, causing only a mild inappetence, but in heavy infestations, so-called 'lizard

poisoning', cirrhosis and jaundice have been reported with diarrhoea and vomiting in terminal cases.

Clinical signs and pathology: In mild cases, vague chronic signs of unthriftiness may be observed. Severe infections cause anorexia, vomiting, diarrhoea and jaundice leading to death. Liver cirrhosis and cholangitis have been reported and the bile ducts are often markedly distended.

Diagnosis: Based on faecal examination for eggs and necropsy examination of the bile and pancreatic ducts for the presence of flukes.

Control and treatment: Preventing cats from hunting lizards can control infection. Treatment with praziquantel (20 mg/kg) and nitroscanate (100 mg/kg) is reported to be effective.

Eurytrema procyonis

Eurytrema procyonis (Phylum: Platyhelminthes; Class: Trematoda; Order: Plagiorchiida; Family: Dicrocoeliidae) is localised in the bile and pancreatic ducts of cats, foxes and racoons, in North America. This is a common parasite of the pancreatic ducts of the raccoon. Cats presumably become infected by ingestion of the intermediate host.

Pathogenesis: Infection is usually well tolerated and causes no apparent ill health. Infection in the cat has been reported to cause weight loss and vomiting due to pancreatic fibrosis and atrophy.

Clinical signs and pathology: Mild infections are usually asymptomatic. Periductal fibrosis may produce cord-like ducts and there may be atrophy of glandular acini.

Diagnosis: Based on faecal examination for eggs and necropsy examination of the bile and pancreatic ducts for the presence of flukes.

Control and treatment: This is difficult because of the longevity of the eggs, the wide distribution of the intermediate hosts and the number of reservoir hosts. Treatment with praziquantel may be effective against these flukes.

Several other species of liver flukes of the family Opisthorchiidae are found in dogs and cats and are summarised in Table 12.8. Details are essentially similar to those of other opisthorchiid flukes.

Table 12.8 Liver flukes of dogs and cats.

Species	Hosts	Intermediate hosts	Distribution
Opisthorchis sinensis	Humans, dogs, cats, pigs, mink, badgers	1: Freshwater snails (*Parafossalurus, Bulimus* spp., *Bithynia, Melania* and *Vivipara*) 2: Fishes (Cyprinidae)	China, Taiwan, Korea, Vietnam, Japan, India and parts of the former Soviet Union
Opisthorchis felineus	Cats, dogs, foxes, pigs, humans, cetaceans (seals, porpoises)	1: Freshwater snails (*Bithynia*) 2: Fishes (*Leuciscus, Blicca, Tinca, Barbus*)	Southern Asia, Europe, Russia, Canada
Metorchis albidus	Dogs, cats, foxes, seals	1: Freshwater snails (*Amnicola limosa porosa*) 2: Fishes (*Blicca bjorkna*)	Europe, Asia, North America
Metorchis conjunctus	Dogs, cats, foxes, mink, raccoons	1: Freshwater snails (*Amnicola limosa porosa*) 2: Fishes (common sucker, *Catostomus commersoni*)	North America
Platynosomum fastosum	Cats	Land snails (*Sublima*)	South America, the Caribbean, southern USA, West Africa, Malaysia and the Pacific Islands
Platynosomum concinnum	Cats	Crustacean (wood louse)	
Platynosomum illiciens	Cats	Lizard (paratenic)	
Parametorchis complexus	Cats, dogs	Not known but probably similar to other liver flukes	North America
Eurytrema procyonis	Cats, foxes, raccoons	Unknown, thought to be snail (*Mesodon*)	North America
Pseudamphistomum truncatum	Dogs, cats, foxes, rarely humans	1: Snails, unknown 2: Fishes (*Leuciscus, Sardinius, Blicca, Abramis*)	Europe, India

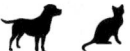

Leishmania infantum

Leishmania infantum, included in the *Leishmania donovani* complex (Phylum: Euglenozoa; Class: Kinetoplastea; Order: Trypanosomatida; Family: Trypanosomatidae), causes a disease commonly kown as Visceral leishmaniosis, Kala-azar, Infantile or Mediterranean leishmaniosis (*L. infantum*). The protozoan is transmitted by phlebotominae sand flies and localises in the skin, liver and spleen of humans, dogs, foxes (*Vulpes vulpes*), black rats (*Rattus rattus*), raccoons (*Nyctereutes procyonoides*), jackals (*Canis aureus*), wolves and fennic foxes (*Fennecus zerda*) and bush dogs (*Lycalopex vetulus*). It has a worldwide distribution including countries of the Mediterranean basin (Europe and Africa), Iran, Middle East, central and southern America (from Mexico to northern Argentina). In particular, *L. infantum* localises in the dermal, splenic, medullary and lymph node macrophages of dogs and wild canids, which act as main reservoirs. The domestic cat is an occasional host as well as black rats. In recent years canine leishmaniosis has expanded its range from the Mediterranean basin (Spain, France, Italy, Croatia, former Yugoslavia, Albania, Greece) to central European countries (e.g. Switzerland and Germany).

Epidemiology: Dogs are commonly infected and transmission is by sand flies of the genus *Phlebotomus* (*P. ariasi*, *P. neglectus*, *P. perfiliewi*, *P. perniciosus*, *P. longcuspis*, *P. chinensis*, *P. mongolensis* and *P. caucasius*) in the Mediterranean area and the genus *Lutzomyia* (*L. ongipalpis*, *L. evansi*, etc.) in Central and South America. The dog is the principal urban reservoir, with infection rates as high as 20% in some countries, and the most important source of human infection. It is probable that most dogs in endemic areas are exposed to disease and will either develop clinical or subclinical infection or become immune and resistant to infection. leishmaniosis is diagnosed in dogs in countries where sand fly vectors do not occur, suggesting a currently unknown mechanism of transmission. Vertical transmission from dam to offspring has been reported and transmission by infected blood transfusion has been described. However, this transmission route is less relevant than the vectorial one.

Pathogenesis: In dogs, *L. donovani infantum* may cause either visceral or cutaneous lesions, the latter being more common (Fig. 12.5). It may take months or even years for infected dogs to develop clinical signs, so that the disease may only become apparent long after dogs have left endemic areas. The disease is usually chronic with low mortality, although it can manifest as an acute, rapidly fatal form. Recovery depends on the proper expression of cell-mediated immunity; if this does not occur, the active lesion persists, leading to chronic enlargement of the spleen, liver and lymph nodes and persistent cutaneous lesions. Upon stimulation of Th2 lymphocyte lines, an immune, non-protective, antibody-mediated response may occur resulting in hypergammaglobulinaemia and formation of immune complexes. The deposition of immune complexes in numerous organs (i.e. liver, kidney, lymph nodes) and capillaries represents the basis of pathology and clinical alterations.

Clinical signs and pathology: In the cutaneous form in the dog, lesions are confined to shallow skin ulcers often on the lip or eyelid, from which recovery is often spontaneous. In the visceral form, dogs initially develop 'spectacles' due to depilation of hair around the eyes and this is followed by generalised loss of body hair and eczema, leishmanial organisms being present in large numbers in the infected skin. Intermittent fever, anaemia, cachexia and generalised lymphadenopathy are also typical signs, as well as mucosal and skin ulcers as a

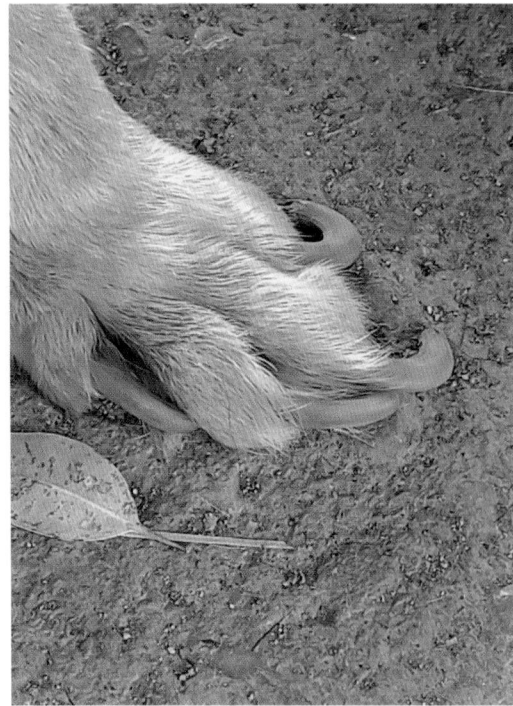

Fig. 12.5 Forelimbs of dog with cutaneous lesions of *Leishmania infantum*. (Courtesy of Andrea Zatelli).

result of the deposition of immune complexes and vasculites. Additional findings (due to the excessive antibody-mediated response) may include epistaxis and arthropathy, as well as diarrhoea (due to decreased albumins and renal failure). The serum protein electrophoretic profile is altered with a decreased albumin/globulins ratio. Long periods of remission followed by the reappearance of clinical signs are not uncommon. Visceral leishmaniosis is essentially a reticuloendotheliosis. Reticuloendothelial cells are increased in number and invaded by the parasites. The enormously enlarged spleen is congested with prominent Malpighian corpuscles. The liver is enlarged with fatty infiltration of Kupffer cells. Macrophages, myelocytes and neutrophils of the bone marrow are filled with parasites. Lymph nodes are usually enlarged and the intestinal mucosa is infiltrated with macrophages filled with parasites.

Diagnosis: This depends on demonstration of the amastigote parasites in smears or scrapings from affected skin or from lymph node or marrow biopsies. Confirmation in an individual case may be difficult, particularly if signs are non-specific. Intracellular or extracellular amastigotes can be identified in Giemsa, Romanowsky or Leishman's stained aspirates, impression or biopsy samples from lymph node, bone marrow, spleen or skin lesions. PCR and immunocytochemistry methods have been developed for use on these samples and offer greater sensitivity. Serological assays using the indirect fluorescent antibody test (IFAT), ELISA and Western blot have also been developed. Specialist laboratories can carry out culture and species identification using isoenzyme analysis and several methods of PCR amplifications.

Control and treatment: From a public health perspective, control of the population of stray dogs is crucial, whereas the euthanasia of infected dogs, other than being ethically unacceptable, has not proved to be relevant where it was used as control strategy

Table 12.9 Drugs used in the treatment of leishmaniosis in dogs.

Drug	Drug group	Dose rate	Notes
Meglumine antimoniate	Pentavalent antimonial	100 mg/kg s.c. for 3–4 weeks	Nephrotoxic. May cause pain and muscle fibrosis at injection site
Allopurinol	Pyrimidine derivative	20 mg/kg orally daily 20 mg/kg orally daily combined with meglumine antimoniate (100 mg/kg daily s.c. for 20 days), then continue with 20 mg/kg allopurinol indefinitely	
Amphotericin B	Polyene macrolide	0.5–0.8 mg/kg i.v. or s.c. 2–3 times weekly	Nephrotoxic. Administer until cumulative dose of 15 mg/kg is reached
		1–2.5 mg/kg i.v. in lipid emulsion twice weekly	Administer until cumulative dose of 10 mg/kg is reached
		3 mg/kg/day i.v. in liposamalised formulation	Administer until cumulative dose of 15 mg/kg is reached
Miltefosine	Alkylphosphocholine	2 mg/kg orally daily for 28 days	

(e.g. India, Brazil), partly because of the presence of other reservoirs. In some areas, the population of sand flies has been reduced as a result of mosquito control for malaria and as a result, the incidence of leishmaniosis has decreased. Generally, though, chemical control of sand fly vectors has had very limited success. A deltamethrin-impregnated collar offers some protection of dogs from sand fly bites and appears to decrease the rate of infection in dogs and people in endemic areas. Several drugs are used for treating canine leishmaniosis (Table 12.9). These include the pentavalent antimonials, of which meglumine antimoniate is the main drug, used either alone or in combination with other drugs, particularly allopurinol. Allopurinol can also be given alone following initial therapy with meglumine antimoniate. Other drugs that have been used include amphotericin B, pentamidine, allopurinol and ketoconazole. Other drugs, such as domperidone, are effective immunostimulants and can be considered either in combination with first-choice molecules or as monotherapy in cases of asymptomatic infections. Finally, considering the concern raised by selection of drug-resistant parasites, dogs should not be treated with molecules used for the treatment of human leishmaniosis.

A subunit vaccine has been developed in South America for the control of visceral leishmaniosis in dogs. This vaccine is based on a surface fucose–mannose–ligand antigen complex. A parasite lyophilisate vaccine (CaniLeish®), which contains excretory/secretory proteins of *L. infantum*, is commercially available in Europe for the immunisation of dogs.

Notes: *Leishmania donovani* is a highly fatal infection of humans and causes visceral leishmaniosis. In humans, the incubation period may be several months with spasmodic fever. Hepatomegaly and splenomegaly follow with mortality of 75–95%.

Hepatozoon canis

Hepatozoon canis, synonym *Leucocytozoon canis* (Phylum: Apicomplexa; Class: Conoidasida; Order: Eucoccidiorida; Family: Hepatozoidae), causes a disease commonly known as Canine hepatozoonosis and is localised in the blood, liver and kidney of dogs. This protozoan is distributed in southern Europe, Middle East, Africa, Southeast Asia and South America.

Notes: The closely related *Hepatozoon americanum* was initially reported to be a strain of *H. canis* but is now considered a separate species, based on clinical disease manifestations, pathology, and morphological and genetic differences.

Epidemiology: The main vector of *H. canis* is the brown dog tick, *Rhipicephalus sanguineus*, which is found in warm and temperate regions all over the world. Infection is transmitted trans-stadially from nymph to adult stages of the tick vectors. Infection appears to be mainly from ingestion of infected ticks. Vertical transmission has been reported.

Pathogenesis: Most dogs infected with *H. canis* appear to undergo a mild infection associated with a limited degree of inflammatory reaction. However, infection may vary from asymptomatic in dogs with a low parasitaemia to life-threatening in animals that present with a high parasitaemia. Symptoms may be exacerbated by the presence of concurrent infections with parvovirus, *Ehrlichia canis*, *Anaplasma platys*, *Toxoplasma gondii*, *Leishmania donovani infantum* or immunosuppression in the young neonate or those with primary or induced immunodeficiency. High parasitaemias can cause direct injury to the affected tissues and affect the immune system, leading to extreme loss of weight and cachexia, although infected dogs may maintain a good appetite.

Clinical signs and pathology: Infection with *H. canis* may be subclinical in some animals but produce severe and fatal disease in others. Mild disease is common and is usually associated with low-level *H. canis* parasitaemia (1–5%), frequently in association with a concurrent disease. A more severe disease, characterised by lethargy, fever and severe weight loss, is found in dogs with high parasitaemia often approaching 100% of circulating neutrophils. Dogs presenting with both leucocytosis and high parasitaemia may have a massive number of circulating gamonts (>50 000/μl blood). Infection may be found as an incidental finding in histopathological specimens in dogs from endemic areas. In dogs with low parasitaemias, few lesions are usually observed. In dogs with high parasitaemias, there may be hepatitis, pneumonia and glomerulonephritis associated with numerous meronts. Meronts and developing gamonts are also found in lymph nodes, spleen and bone marrow.

Diagnosis: Diagnosis is usually made on the identification of gamonts in the cytoplasm of neutrophils (more rarely monocytes) in Giemsa or Wright's stained blood smears. Between 0.5% and 5% of neutrophils are commonly infected, although this may reach as high as 100% in severe infections. IFAT and Western blot have been developed using gamont antigens. Dogs with a high parasitaemia frequently have neutrophilia and a normocytic, normochromic non-regenerative anaemia.

Control and treatment: Prophylaxis depends on regular tick control using an effective acaricide and close examination of animals for the presence of ticks. In areas where the disease is endemic, dogs should be prevented from scavenging or eating raw meat or organs from wildlife. The infection is treated with imidocarb dipropionate 5–6 mg/kg every 14 days until gamonts are no longer present in blood smears. Oral doxycycline 10 mg/kg daily for 21 days

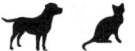

in combination with imidocarb may also be used. Treatment may take up to eight weeks to eliminate gamonts from peripheral blood and require regular haematological evaluation. Treatment of all infected dogs is recommended as parasitaemia may increase over time and develop into a severe infection. The prognosis for dogs with a low parasitaemia is generally good, but less favourable for those with a high parasitaemia.

Parasites of the circulatory system

Angiostrongylus vasorum

Angiostrongylus vasorum, synonym *Haemostrongylus vasorum* (Phylum: Nematoda; Class: Chromadorea; Order: Rhabditida; Family: Angiostrongylidae), commonly known as the French heartworm, is a parasite distributed worldwide, except in the Americas, apart from the Atlantic coastal provinces of Canada. It is prevalent in Western Europe and is localised in the right ventricle and pulmonary artery of dogs, foxes and other canids. The terrestrial molluscs, mainly snails and slugs, act as intermediate hosts.

Epidemiology: Though worldwide in general distribution, *A. vasorum* is only prevalent in certain localities, and these are invariably rural. In Europe, endemic foci have been recognised in Italy, France, Spain, Eire and England.

Pathogenesis: Canine angiostrongylosis is usually a chronic condition, extending over months or even years. Much of the pathogenic effect is attributable to the presence of the adult worms in the larger vessels and eggs and larvae in the pulmonary arterioles and capillaries. Blockage of these vessels results in circulatory impediment, which may eventually lead to congestive cardiac failure.

Clinical signs and pathology: In recently established infections the resting dog usually shows no clinical signs, but if a substantial number of worms is present, the active animal will often show tachycardia, tachypnoea and a heavy productive cough, the sputum sometimes showing blood. In longer established severe infections, signs are present even in the resting dog. There may be recurrent syncope. As a consequence of reduced blood-clotting capacity, slowly developing painless swellings may appear in dependent areas, such as the lower abdomen and intermandibular space, and on the limbs where bruising has occurred. Chronic infections may be accompanied by reduced appetite and anaemia, and ascites and deaths can occur. The rare acute infection, normally seen in young animals, manifests as dyspnoea and violent coughing, with whitish-yellow, occasionally bloody sputum. The cut surface of the lung is mottled and reddish-purple. One reported systemic effect, unusual in helminth infections, is interference with the blood-clotting mechanism, so that subcutaneous haematomas may be present. In the larger blood vessels, there is endarteritis and periarteritis which progress to fibrosis and at necropsy the vessels have a pipe-stem feel on palpation. The vascular change may extend to the right ventricle, with endocarditis involving the tricuspid valve.

Diagnosis: The L_1, which may be present in faeces and sputum, has a small cephalic button and a wavy tail with a subterminal notch, and its presence in association with respiratory and circulatory signs is accepted as confirmatory.

Control and treatment: Control is impractical in most cases, due to the ubiquity of the molluscan intermediate hosts. Treatment with mebendazole and fenbendazole (at increased dose rates), levamisole and ivermectin has proved effective.

Dirofilaria immitis

Dirofilaria immitis, synonym *Nochtiella immitis* (Phylum: Nematoda; Class: Chromadorea; Order: Spirurida; Family: Onchocercidae), commonly known as the Canine heartworm, is localised in the cardiovascular system: adults are found in the right ventricle, right atrium, pulmonary artery and posterior vena cava of dogs, foxes and wild canids. Occasionally cats and other wild felids and rarely humans may be infected. This parasite has mosquitoes of the genera *Aedes*, *Anopheles* and *Culex* as intermediate hosts and it is distributed in warm-temperate and tropical zones throughout the world, including North and South America, southern Europe, India, China, Japan and Australia.

Epidemiology: Host species vary in their susceptibility to infection, the dog being the most susceptible natural host. Infection commonly occurs in dogs older than one year. Intrauterine infection of puppies can also occur. The important factors in the spread of heartworm disease can be divided into those affecting the host and those affecting the vector.

Host factors include a high density of dogs in areas where the vectors exist, the lengthy patent period of up to five years during which time circulating microfilariae are present, and the lack of an effective immune response against established parasites. Also, diurnal periodicity of microfilaraemia ensures that high numbers of microfilariae are circulating in the peripheral blood during the period of mosquito activity.

Vector factors include the ubiquity of the mosquito intermediate hosts, their capacity for rapid population increase and the short development period from microfilariae to L_3 at optimal temperatures. At one point it was considered that the worms do not occur in areas where the temperature falls below 16 °C but more recently, spread has occurred to colder zones in Canada and the USA.

Pathogenesis: Pathogenic effects are associated with the adult parasites (Fig. 12.6). Many dogs infected with low numbers of *D. immitis* show no apparent ill effects and it is only in heavy chronic infections that circulatory distress occurs, primarily due to obstruction of normal blood flow, leading to chronic congestive right-sided heart failure. The presence of a mass of active worms can cause an

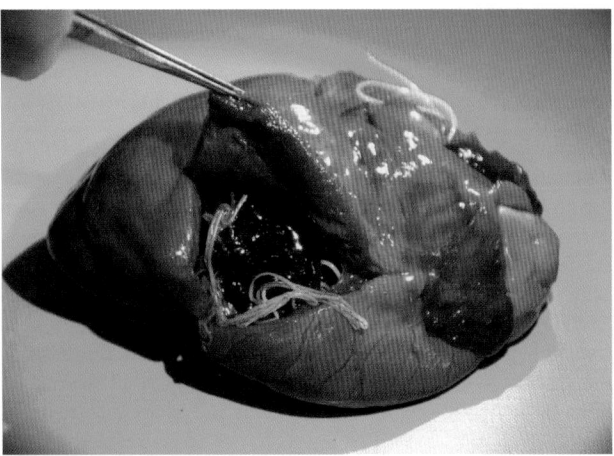

Fig. 12.6 *Dirofilaria immitis* in a section of an infected heart. (Courtesy of Riccardo Paolo Lia).

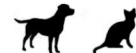

endocarditis in the heart valves and a proliferative pulmonary endarteritis, possibly due to a response to parasite excretory products. In addition, dead or dying worms may cause pulmonary embolism. After a period of about nine months the effect of the developing pulmonary hypertension is compensated for by right ventricular hypertrophy, which may lead to congestive heart failure with the usual accompanying signs of oedema and ascites. At this stage the dog is listless and weak.

A mass of worms may lodge in the posterior vena cava and the resulting obstruction leads to an acute, sometimes fatal syndrome known as the vena caval syndrome. This is characterised by haemolysis, haemoglobinuria, bilirubinaemia, icterus, dyspnoea, anorexia and collapse. Death may occur within 2–3 days. Very occasionally, there is blockage of the renal capillaries by microfilariae leading to a glomerulonephritis, possibly related to the deposition of immune complexes.

In cats, pulmonary hypertension, right-sided heart failure and caval syndrome are less common, and more commonly the presence of the parasites in the distal pulmonary arteries may induce a diffuse pulmonary pneumonia. Ectopic infections are more commonly seen in cats, with parasites reported in the eye, CNS and subcutaneous tissues.

Clinical signs and pathology: Heavily infected dogs are often listless and there is a gradual loss of condition and exercise intolerance. They have a chronic soft cough with haemoptysis, and in the later stages of the disease become dyspnoeic and may develop oedema and ascites. The acute vena caval syndrome described above is characterised by haemoglobinuria, icterus and collapse. Lighter infections in working dogs may be responsible for poor performance during periods of sustained exercise. Infected cats may show coughing; tachypnoea and dyspnoea and heavy infections can be fatal.

Heartworm disease is primarily a pulmonary vascular disease characterised by endarteritis with infiltration of leucocytes, mainly eosinophils, followed by myointimal proliferations which produce irregular rugose to villous projections that enmesh the worms. Thrombosis may be associated with either dead or live worms, and thromboembolism and pulmonary infarction following adulticide therapy. Pulmonary changes include haemosiderosis, diffuse interalveolar fibrosis and proliferation of alveolar epithelium. Dead worms commonly result in pulmonary granuloma formation. Additional lesions of heartworm disease include those of right heart failure, such as chronic congestion of the liver and occasionally ascites. Glomerulonephropathy occurs primarily due to glomerular deposition of immune complexes, leading to a mild to moderate proteinuria. Venal caval syndrome causes severe hepatic congestion leading to cavernous enlargement of hepatic venules with phlebosclerosis and thrombosis in the caudal vena cava and hepatic veins.

Diagnosis: This is based on the clinical signs of cardiovascular dysfunction and demonstration of the appropriate microfilariae in the blood. However, non-microfilaraemic dogs may still harbour adult parasites. Affected dogs are seldom less than one year old and most are over two years. In suspected cases in which the microfilariae cannot be demonstrated, thoracic radiography may show the thickening of the pulmonary artery, its tortuous course and right ventricular hypertrophy. Angiography may also be used to demonstrate the vascular changes more clearly. At necropsy, adult worms are often present in the right heart chambers and adjacent large blood vessels.

Immunodiagnostic tests are also available commercially to identify cases that do not have a detectable microfilaraemia. For example, there are a number of ELISA test kits for the detection of circulating heartworm antigens or specific antibodies, that will identify most mature infections and which are highly specific.

Identification of the microfilariae in the blood (samples ideally taken in the early evening) is aided by concentrating the parasites following lysis, filtration and then staining with methylene blue or May–Grunwald Giemsa. Commercial kits are available for this technique. Alternatively, one part of blood and nine parts of formalin are centrifuged and the sediment mixed with a blue stain and examined as a microscopic smear. The microfilariae have to be differentiated from those of *Acanthocheilonema reconditum*, a filarial parasite commonly found in the subcutis in dogs. Those of *D. immitis* are more than 300 μm in length and have a tapered head and a straight tail; those of *A. reconditum* are less than 300 μm in length and have a blunt head and a hooked posterior end. More precise differentiation may be achieved by using histochemical stains for acid phosphatase activity. *Dirofilaria immitis* shows distinct red acid phosphate-positive spots at the excretory pore and anus, while *A. reconditum* stains pink overall. Differential diagnosis may be achieved through the application of PCR-based recombinant DNA technology.

Heartworm infection in cats can be difficult to diagnose as a result of low parasite populations and a tendency to remain amicrofilaraemic.

Control and treatment: Mosquito control is difficult and therefore prophylaxis is based almost entirely on medication (Table 12.10). The drug widely used for this has been diethylcarbamazine, which in endemic areas is given orally to pups daily at 2–3 months of age. This kills developing larvae and so pre-empts the problems of treating patent infections and microfilaraemia. In tropical areas, the drug is given all year round but in more temperate zones, where the mosquito has a limited season, treatment commences one month prior to the mosquito season and ceases two months after it ends. Where prophylaxis is introduced in older dogs or after treatment of an infected dog, care must be taken to ensure that the dog is free from microfilarial infection as anaphylactoid reactions may occur in infected dogs after diethylcarbamazine treatment. Once prophylaxis is introduced, regular checks for microfilariae should be made every six months.

Drug treatment is complex, as the adult heartworms and microfilariae differ in their susceptibility to anthelmintics. Treatment should not be undertaken without a physical examination of the dog and an assessment of heart, lung, liver and kidney function.

Table 12.10 Drugs available for heartworm prevention.

Drug	Host	Recommended dosing interval	Route of administration
Ivermectin	Dogs, cats	Monthly	Oral tablet
Ivermectin (+ pyrantel)	Dogs	Monthly	Oral tablet
Ivermectin (+ imidacloprid)	Dogs	Monthly	Spot-on
Milbemycin oxime	Dogs	Monthly	Oral tablet
Milbemycin oxime (+ lufenuron)	Dogs	Monthly	Oral tablet
Moxidectin	Dogs	Monthly	Oral
Moxidectin microspheres	Dogs	Six-monthly	Injectable
Selamectin	Dogs, cats	Monthly	Spot-on
Diethylcarbamazine citrate (DEC) (oxibendazole)	Dogs	Daily	Oral

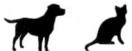

Table 12.11 Adulticides for dirofilariosis.

Chemical	Trade name	Dose rate	Comments
Thiacetarsamide sodium	Caparsolate	2.2 mg/kg twice daily for two days	Intravenous injection. No longer available
Melarsomine dihydrochloride	Immiticide	2.5 mg/kg i.m. repeated after 24 hours	In severely affected dogs, single injection given followed one month later by two injections 24 hours apart to reduce postadulticide complications

Where these functions are grossly abnormal, it may be necessary to give prior treatment for cardiac insufficiency. The usual recommendation is that infected dogs are first treated intravenously with thiacetarsamide twice daily over a two-day period or intramuscularly with melarsamide over two days to remove the adult worms; toxic reactions are not uncommon following this treatment due to the dying and disintegrating heartworms and resultant embolism; activity of the dog should be restricted for a period of 2–6 weeks. This drug should be used with extreme care (Table 12.11).

A further treatment with a different drug is then given six weeks later to remove the microfilariae that are not susceptible to thiacetarsamide or melarsamide. Several drugs are now available for this purpose; the traditional one was dithiazanine iodide, administered over seven days, and either this or levamisole given orally over a 10–14-day period has proved effective. The avermectins are also highly efficient against microfilariae, as is milbemycin at the heartworm prophylactic dose of 500 μg/kg. These induce rapid clearance of microfilariae but are not licensed for this purpose because of occasional toxic or microfilaricidal side-effects. Veterinarians who choose to use either drug as a microfilaricide should realise that this is an 'extra-label' application and that they take responsibility for administration of the correct dose and provide appropriate monitoring and aftercare.

With all these drugs, there is a risk of adverse reactions to dying microfilariae. In some severe cases, heartworms have been removed surgically rather than risk adverse reactions following drug therapy. Following treatment, it is usual to place dogs on a prophylactic programme and this is considered in the next section on control.

There are currently no licensed anthelmintics for treatment of cats.

The most up-to-date methods of preventing heartworm infection involve monthly administration, throughout the mosquito season, of ivermectin or milbemycin especially formulated for this use in dogs.

Notes: Of the two species occurring in domestic carnivores, *D. immitis* is by far the more important. The adults, which are found in the right side of the heart and adjacent blood vessels of dogs, are responsible for a debilitating condition known as canine heartworm disease. Although primarily a problem of warm countries where the mosquito intermediate host abounds, the disease has become much more widespread in the past decade and the problem in North America is now so extensive that special heartworm clinics have been created.

With regard to dirofilariosis in humans, *D. immitis* and *D. repens* can cause aberrant infections. *Dirofilaria immitis* induces pulmonary coin lesions that are normally of little pathological significance. *Dirofilaria repens* (see Parasites of the integument) more commonly occurs in subcutaneous nodules, particularly in the ocular area.

Schistosomes

Schistosomes are flukes found in the circulatory system. The sexes are separate, the small adult female lying permanently in a longitudinal groove, the gynaecophoric canal, in the body of the male. The genus has been divided into four groups – *haematobium*, *indicum*, *mansoni* and *japonicum* – but the genus as currently defined is paraphyletic so revisions are likely.

Indicum group

Schistosoma spindale

Schistosoma spindale (Phylum: Platyhelminthes, Class: Trematoda; Order: Strigeidida; Family: Schistosomatidae), commonly known as the Blood fluke, causes a disease named bilharziosis and is localised in the mesenteric veins of cattle, horses, pigs and occasionally dogs. This fluke has snails (*Planorbis*, *Indoplanorbis* spp., *Galba* spp.) as intermediate hosts and is found in parts of Asia and the Far East.

Japonicum group

Schistosoma japonicum

Schistosoma japonicum (Phylum: Platyhelminthes, Class: Trematoda; Order: Strigeidida; Family: Schistosomatidae), commonly known as the Blood fluke, causes a disease named bilharziosis and is localised in the portal and mesenteric veins of cattle, horses, sheep, goats, dogs, cats, rabbits, pigs and humans. This parasite has snails belonging to the genus *Oncomelania* as intermediate hosts and is found in parts of Asia and the Far East.

Trypanosomes

Members of the genus *Trypanosoma* are haemoflagellates of overwhelming importance in cattle in sub-Saharan Africa but also occur in many other hosts, including dogs and cats. See Chapter 2 (Trypanosomatidae) for a general description and Chapter 8 for detailed descriptions of individual species of trypanosomes and their control.

Trypanosoma brucei brucei

Trypanosoma brucei brucei (Phylum: Euglenozoa; Class: Kinetoplastea; Order: Trypanosomatida; Family: Trypanosomatidae) causes a disease commonly known as Nagana, is localised in the blood and also found extravascularly in, for example, the myocardium, CNS and reproductive tract of cattle, horses, donkeys, zebus, sheep, goats, camels, pigs, dogs, cats and wild game species. This protozoon is distributed in sub-Saharan Africa. The dog and cat are susceptible to *T. brucei brucei*. The disease is usually acute, and apart from signs of fever, anaemia and myocarditis, corneal opacity is often a feature. There may also be neurological changes resulting in aggressive signs, ataxia or convulsions. Dogs can be treated with either isometamidium or quinapyramine. Recommended doses are as follows: isometamidium 0.25–1 mg/kg i.m.; quinapyramine dimethylsulfate 5 mg/kg s.c.

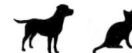

Trypanosoma brucei evansi

Trypanosoma brucei evansi, synonyms *Trypanosoma evansi*, *Trypanosoma equinum* (Phylum: Euglenozoa; Class: Kinetoplastea; Order: Trypanosomatida; Family: Trypanosomatidae), causes a disease commonly known as Surra, El debab, Mbori, Murrina, Mal de caderas, Doukane, Dioufar or Thaga and is localised in the blood of horses, donkeys, camels, cattle, zebus, goats, pigs, dogs, water buffalo, elephants, capybaras, tapirs, mongooses, ocelots, deer and other wild animals. This protozoon is endemic in North Africa, Central and South America, central and southern Russia, and parts of Asia (India, Myanmar, Malaysia, southern China, Indonesia, Philippines). Many laboratory and wild animals can be infected experimentally. Transmission is by biting flies and no cyclical development occurs in the vector, the trypanosomes remaining in the proboscis.

Epidemiology: This species, although closely related to the salivarian trypanosome *T. brucei brucei*, is mechanically transmitted by biting insects; the usual vectors are horse flies (*Tabanus*) but *Stomoxys*, *Haematopota* and *Lyperosia* can also transmit the infection. In Central and South America, the vampire bat is a vector and can transmit the disease (murrina).

Pathogenesis: Depending on the virulence of the strain and the susceptibility of the individual host, the disease may be acute in horses, camels and dogs. The syndrome is similar to that caused by the tsetse-transmitted trypanosomes. Anaemia is caused mainly by extravascular haemolysis through erythrophagocytosis in the mononuclear phagocytic systems of the spleen, liver and lungs, but as the disease becomes chronic there may be decreased haemoglobin synthesis. Leucopenia and thrombocytopenia are caused by mechanisms that predispose leucocytes and platelets to phagocytosis. Immunological mechanisms in the pathogenesis lead to extensive proliferation of activated macrophages, which engulf or destroy erythrocytes, leucocytes, platelets and haematopoietic cells.

Clinical signs and pathology: All domestic animals are susceptible but the disease is only fatal in horses, camels and dogs. The disease is manifested by pyrexia, progressive anaemia, loss of condition and depression. Recurrent episodes of fever occur during the course of disease. Oedematous swellings ranging from cutaneous plaques to frank oedema of the ventral abdomen and genitalia and petechial haemorrhages of the serous membranes are often observed. Nervous signs may occur and include circling, incoordination, staggering, head pressing, paraplegia, paralysis and prostration.

The carcass is often pale and emaciated and there may be oedematous swellings in the lower part of the abdomen and genital organs with serous atrophy of fat. The liver, lymph nodes and spleen are enlarged and the viscera are congested. Petechiae may appear on lymph nodes, pericardium and intestinal mucosa. The liver is hypertrophic and congested with degeneration and necrosis of the hepatocytes, dilation of blood vessels and parenchymal infiltration of mononuclear cells. A non-suppurative myocarditis, sometimes associated with hydropericarditis, has been reported, accompanied by degeneration and necrosis of the myocardial tissue. Other lesions can include glomerulonephritis, renal tubular necrosis, non-suppurative meningoencephalomyelitis, focal poliomalacia, keratitis, ophthalmitis, orchitis, interstitial pneumonia and bone marrow atrophy. Splenic and lymph node hypertrophy occur during the acute phase but the lymphoid tissues are usually exhausted and fibrotic in the chronic stage.

Diagnosis: The clinical signs of the disease, although indicative, are not pathognomonic. Confirmation of clinical diagnosis depends on the demonstration of trypanosomes in the blood. Occasionally, when the parasitaemia is massive, it is possible to detect motile trypanosomes in fresh smears of blood. More usually, both thick and thin smears of blood are air-dried and examined later. Thick smears, dehaemoglobinised before staining with Giemsa or Leishman's stain, offer a better chance of finding trypanosomes while the stained thin smears are used for differentiation of the trypanosome species.

More sensitive techniques utilise centrifugation in a microhaematocrit tube followed by microscopic examination of the interface between the buffy coat and the plasma; alternatively, the tube may be snapped, the buffy coat expressed on to a slide, and the contents examined under dark-ground or phase-contrast microscopy for motile trypanosomes. With these techniques, the packed red cell volume is also obtained, which is of indirect value in diagnosis if one can eliminate other causes of anaemia, especially helminthosis.

A number of serological tests have been described, including IFAT and ELISA, and have been partially validated but require further evaluation and standardisation.

Treatment: Dogs can be treated with quinapyramine.

Notes: The original distribution of this parasite coincided with that of the camel, and is often associated with arid deserts and semi-arid steppes.

Trypanosoma congolense

Trypanosoma congolense (Phylum: Euglenozoa; Class: Kinetoplastea; Order: Trypanosomatida; Family: Trypanosomatidae) causes a disease commonly known as Nagana, Paranagana, Gambia fever, Ghindi or Gobial and is localised in the blood of cattle, sheep, goats, horses, camels, dogs and pigs. It is distributed in sub-Saharan Africa. Reservoir hosts include antelopes, giraffes, zebras, elephants and warthogs. Dogs and cats are susceptible to *T. congolense*. The disease is usually acute, and apart from signs of fever, anaemia and myocarditis, corneal opacity is often a feature. There may also be neurological changes resulting in aggressive signs, ataxia or convulsions. Dogs can be treated with quinapyramine.

Trypanosoma cruzi

Trypanosoma cruzi, synonyms *Schizotrypanum cruzi*, *Trypanosoma lesourdi*, *Trypanosoma rhesii*, *Trypanosoma prowazeki*, *Trypanosoma vickersae* (Phylum: Euglenozoa; Class: Kinetoplastea; Order: Trypanosomatida; Family: Trypanosomatidae), causes a condition commonly known as Chagas disease and is localised in the blood, heart and muscle of humans, dogs, cats, primates and wild animals. This parasite is prevalent in South America.

Epidemiology: Reduviid bugs commonly defecate after feeding, and animals become infected when they lick the insect bites or eat the infected bugs. Transmission also occurs by ingestion of infected animals, via infected maternal milk, by fly contamination or contamination by urine or saliva of heavily infected animals.

Pathogenesis and clinical signs: Trypomastigote forms are found in blood, and amastigote forms are found in pseudocysts in skeletal

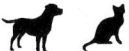

and cardiac muscle, the reticuloenthothelial system and other tissues. Infection causes generalised oedema, anaemia, hepatosplenomegaly and lymphadenitis. Depression, anorexia and weight loss can occur.

Diagnosis: In acute stages of the disease, trypomastigotes can be found in thick blood smears stained with Giemsa. The size and morphology make it relatively easy to distinguish from other trypanosomes found in primates. Complement fixation or ELISA serological tests are available for humans and may be helpful in screening.

Control and treatment: Control is based on eliminating the insect vector. Because the disease is zoonotic, owners should take precautions to avoid exposure or contamination of mucous membranes or skin with infective secretions. There is no effective treatment.

Babesia canis

Babesia canis, subspecies *Babesia canis canis*, *Babesia canis rossi*, *Babesia canis vogeli* (Phylum: Apicomplexa; Class: Aconoidasida; Order: Piroplasmida; Family: Babesiidae), causes a disease commonly known as Canine piroplasmosis, is localised in the blood of dogs and is distributed in southern Europe, Africa, Asia, USA, Central and South America. However, the three subspecies are nowadays considered as three different species transmitted by different tick species: *Babesia canis* by *Dermacentor reticulatus*, *B. rossi* by *Haemaphysalis leachi* and *B. vogeli* by *Rhipicephalus sanguineus* sensu lato (Table 12.12).

Pathogenesis: The severity of infection is determined by the strain of parasite as well as other factors, such as age, immune status and presence of concurrent infections. Haemolytic anaemia is the principal pathogenic mechanism caused by the parasite but other factors, such as immune-mediated destruction of erythrocytes, may occur. Infection may be classified as uncomplicated or complicated. The former is usually associated with mild to moderate anaemia, lethargy, weakness and hepatosplenomegaly. Complicated babesiosis refers to manifestations that cannot be explained by the haemolytic crisis alone and is characterised by severe anaemia and organic dysfunction. Mortality in complicated babesiosis often exceeds 80%.

Clinical signs and pathology: The more severe forms of the disease in adult dogs are associated with virulent infections (*B. rossi*, *B. canis*), while pups are more severely affected irrespective of the species of *Babesia*. Peracute infections are a feature of *B. rossi* and are characterised by rapid-onset collapse, with findings typical of hypotensive shock: pale (sometimes cyanotic) mucous membranes, tachycardia, weak pulse, weakness and depression. Severe intravascular haemolysis produces haemoglobinuria and there may be widespread organ dysfunction associated with hypotension and hypoxaemia leading to coma and death.

In acute cases the first sign is fever, followed by marked anaemia, jaundice, inappetence, marked thirst, weakness, prostration and often death. Petechial and ecchymotic haemorrhages may be observed on the gums or ventral abdomen of some dogs. In chronic cases the fever is not high and there is little jaundice. Anaemia is severe and affected animals are listless and become very weak and emaciated.

The disease may take on many different clinical forms. Involvement of the circulatory system may produce oedema, purpura and ascites, and there may be stomatitis and gastritis; involvement of the respiratory system may cause catarrh and dyspnoea. CNS involvement causes locomotor disturbances, paresis or epileptiform fits. Cerebral babesiosis may be confused with rabies.

The spleen is enlarged, with dark red soft pulp and prominent splenic corpuscles. The liver is enlarged and jaundiced, with pathological changes ranging from congestion to centrilobular necrosis. The heart, kidneys and muscles are icteric. There may be variable amounts of fluid in the pleural, pericardial and peritoneal cavities. Small haemorrhages are sometimes present on the heart, pleura, bronchi and intestines.

Diagnosis: Examination of blood smears, stained with Romanowsky stains such as Giemsa, will reveal the parasites in the red cells. Species identification between large and small *Babesia* is essential with regard to choice of therapeutic drugs.

A range of serological tests has been developed, with IFAT being the most reliable. Titres exceeding 1:80 are considered to be indicative of infection. Cross-reactivity occurs between species, and there may also be cross-reactivity with *Neospora* and *Toxoplasma*.

Control and treatment: Prophylaxis depends on regular treatment of dogs with a suitable acaricide, and since *R. sanguineus* s.l. may live in kennels, these should also be frequently treated with a suitable acaricide. For dogs visiting tick-endemic regions, tick prevention should be practised (e.g. fipronil application). In addition, surveillance of dogs exposed to infection is advisable so that treatment can be administered as early as possible. A vaccine has recently been launched in Europe for use against *B. canis*. The vaccine contains surface proteins expressed by cultures of *B. canis* and *B. rossi* and provides protection for up to six months.

For treatment, in every case, chemotherapy with imidocarb, phenamidine, diminazene acetate or trypan blue is advisable immediately after clinical diagnosis, since death may occur rapidly (Table 12.13). Diminazene has a low therapeutic index and toxicity appears to be dose related, although idiosyncratic reactions

Table 12.13 Babesicides for use in dogs against *B. canis*.

Drug	Recommended dose	Frequency	Comments
Imidocarb dipropionate	5 mg/kg s.c. or i.m.	Two at 14-day interval	Pain at injection site
Diminazene (di)aceturate	3.5 mg/kg i.m.	Single	Low therapeutic index
Phenamidine isethionate	15 mg/kg s.c.	Single or repeat 24 hours	Vomiting and CNS signs are common side-effects
Trypan blue	10 mg/kg i.v.		1% solution, tissue irritant

Table 12.12 Species of *Babesia* of dogs and their distribution.

Species	Distribution	Vector	Virulence
Babesia canis	Southern and central Europe	*Dermacentor reticulatus*	Moderate to severe
Babesia rossi	Southern Africa	*Haemaphysalis leachi*	Severe
Babesia vogeli	Africa, Asia, North and South America, Australia, Europe	*Rhipicephalus sanguineus*	Mild to moderate

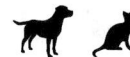

may occur. In addition to antibabesial treatment, supportive care should be provided. In dogs with severe anaemia, blood transfusion should be considered.

Babesia gibsoni

Babesia gibsoni (Phylum: Apicomplexa; Class: Aconoidasida; Order: Piroplasmida; Family: Babesiidae) causes a disease commonly known as Canine piroplasmosis, is localised in the blood of dogs and is distributed in Asia, North Africa and occasionally North America.

Epidemiology: Tick vectors are *Haemaphysalis bispinosa* and *Rhipicephalus sanguineus* sensu lato. For both species of *Babesia*, increasing numbers of cases are reported in parts of the world, such as northern Europe, where the disease did not previously exist and may be linked to establishment of ticks in previously non-enzootic regions, and with increasing international pet travel and trade.

Pathogenesis: Highly pathogenic in dogs, causing marked anaemia, remittent fever, haemoglobinuria, constipation, marked splenomegaly and hepatomegaly. The disease is usually chronic with remissions and relapses of fever. Death may not occur for many months.

Clinical signs and pathology: Similar to *B. canis*. In acute cases, the first sign is fever, followed by marked anaemia, jaundice, inappetence, marked thirst, weakness, prostration and often death. The pathology is as for *B. canis*.

Diagnosis: As for *B. canis*.

Control and treatment: Control is the same as for *B. canis*. No vaccine is available for this species. Diminazene is the drug of choice for the treatment of *B. gibsoni* since imidocarb is less effective against small babesial species (Table 12.14).

Notes: Phylogenetic analysis of DNA sequences has identified two strains of *Babesia gibsoni*: 'Asia' and 'California'. More recently, *Babesia vulpes* has been identified and appears to be endemic in Galacia, Spain, and transmitted by the tick *Ixodes hexagonus* (see below).

Babesia felis

Babesia felis, synonyms *Nuttallia felis*, *Babesia cati* (Phylum: Apicomplexa; Class: Aconoidasida; Order: Piroplasmida; Family: Babesiidae), is localised in the blood of cats and diffused in Africa.

Epidemiology: Natural hosts are wild cats such as lion and leopard. The highest prevalence is in young adult cats (<3 years old) during

the spring and summer in endemic regions. The vectors are unknown, although *Haemaphysalis leachi* has been incriminated in South Africa.

Pathogenesis: Infection usually manifests as an afebrile, chronic, low-grade disease.

Clinical signs and pathology: Affected animals show anorexia, depression, anaemia, emaciation, constipation and jaundice. There is splenomegaly and jaundice, and complications are wide-ranging and include hepatopathy, renal failure, pulmonary oedema and immune-mediated haemolytic anaemia often associated with feline immunodeficiency disease, FeLV or feline infectious anaemia (*Mycoplasma*).

Diagnosis: Examination of blood smears, stained with Romanowsky stains such as Giemsa, will reveal the parasites in the red cells. Species identification between large and small *Babesia* is essential with regard to choice of therapeutic drugs. Concurrent infection with other haemoparasites such as *Mycoplasma* (*Haemobartonella*) can be common in endemic areas and complicates the diagnosis.

Control and treatment: Reducing tick exposure is the best way to prevent infection, although this is rarely achievable in endemic areas. Care must be taken in cats with the use of acaricides due to their increased susceptibility to many compounds. The antimalarial drug primaquine phosphate 0.5 mg/kg orally is the drug of choice for treating *B. felis* infections. Although it reduces the parasitaemia, it does not sterilise the infection. Accurate dosing is required in cats to avoid toxicity, although vomiting is a common side-effect at this dose rate.

Babesia vulpes

Babesia vulpes, synonyms *Theileria annae*, *Babesia annae* (Phylum: Apicomplexa; Class: Aconoidasida; Order: Piroplasmida; Family: Theileriidae), is localised in the blood of dogs and foxes and diffused in parts of Europe (Spain). Reported infections of this parasite cause anaemia.

Cytauxzoon felis

Cytauxzoon felis, synonym *Theileria felis* (Phylum: Apicomplexa; Class: Aconoidasida; Order: Piroplasmida; Family: Theileriidae), is localised in the blood of cats and bobcats (*Lynx rufus*), and is distributed in USA.

Epidemiology: This species has been found in the erythrocytes and tissues of domestic cats in the USA. It is suspected that *Dermacentor variabilis* is the principal vector. The natural hosts are the North American wild cat species, such as the bobcat, and it is thought that transmission to domestic cats represents inadvertent infection of a dead-end host. The highest incidence of infection occurs during early summer through to autumn when ticks are most active.

Pathogenesis: Infection of domestic cats with the merogenous stage typically results in a rapidly progressive systemic disease with a high mortality rate. In natural infections with *C. felis*, there is an apparent variation in pathogenicity that may be associated with geographical location. During the merogenous phase, there is mechanical obstruction to blood flow through various organs,

Table 12.14 Babesicides for use in dogs against *B. gibsoni*.

Drug	Recommended dose	Frequency	Comments
Diminazene (di)aceturate	3.5 mg/kg i.m.	Single	Low therapeutic index
Phenamidine isethionate	15 mg/kg s.c.	Single or repeat 24 hours	Vomiting and CNS signs are common side-effects
Parvaquone	20 mg/kg s.c.	Single	
Clindamycin	25 mg/kg	Twice daily	

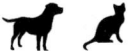

notably the lungs, resulting in a shock-like state. Intravascular and extravascular haemolysis occurs because of erythrocyte invasion by merozoites.

Clinical signs and pathology: Soon after infection, affected cats develop non-specific signs, such as anorexia, lymphadenopathy, fever and lethargy, but the course of the disease is usually rapid, with the onset of a severe clinical syndrome characterised by dehydration, pallor, dyspnoea, icterus, recumbency and death. Usually, by the time the cat is presented, it is severely ill. Most cats die within 9–15 days following infection by virulent strains, regardless of treatment. Affected animals are markedly dehydrated, with generalised pallor, jaundice and numerous petechiae and ecchymoses of the epicardium and serosal membranes of the abdominal organs, as well as the visceral pleura of the lungs and mucosa of the urinary bladder. Pulmonary vessels are enlarged and tortuous as a result of vascular occlusion by the tissue stages. The lymph nodes are enlarged, congested or haemorrhagic and oedematous and the spleen is markedly enlarged. Extraerythrocytic forms are found within phagocytes in the spleen, lymph nodes, lungs, liver, kidneys and sometimes veins of the heart, urinary bladder and bone marrow and contain hundreds of merozoites or indistinct Koch bodies.

Diagnosis: Diagnosis is made by the identification of erythrocytic piroplasms in blood smears stained with Wright's stain or Giemsa. Parasitaemias are typically low (1–4%) although in some acute infections as many as 25% of the red cells may be infected. *C. felis* is a small piroplasm that must be differentiated from *Babesia felis*, which is very similar in size and appearance under light microscopy but differs in geographical location. Dark-staining 'dot' forms may be mistaken for a more common and widespread parasite of cats, *Mycoplasma* (*Haemobartonella*) spp., the cause of feline infectious anaemia. Tissue meronts can be demonstrated in impression smears from bone marrow, spleen or lymph nodes, where they are typically numerous. There is currently no commercially available serological assay.

Control and treatment: Reducing tick exposure is the best way to prevent infection although this is rarely achievable in endemic areas. Care must be taken in cats with the use of acaricides due to their increased susceptibility to many compounds. Once diagnosed, the prognosis is poor and treatment often unsuccessful. Treatment with diminazene aceturate or imidocarb dipropionate, both at 2 mg/kg i.m., may be used but may result in transient worsening of the condition. Supportive fluid therapy or blood transfusion may also be beneficial.

Anaplasma phagocytophilum

Anaplasma phagocytophilum, synonyms *Anaplasma phagocytophila*, *Ehrlichia phagocytophila*, *Cytoecetes phagocytophila* (Phylum: Proteobacteria; Class: Alphaproteobacteria; Order: Rickettsiales; Family: Anaplasmataceae), causes a disease commonly known as Tick-borne fever, Pasture fever, Canine granulocytic ehrlichiosis, Human granulocytic ehrlichiosis, Equine granulocytic ehrlichiosis or Canine infectious thrombocytopenia and is localised in the blood of sheep, cattle, dog, horses, deer, rodents and humans. This protozoon is transmitted by ticks and has a cosmopolitan distribution (i.e. Europe, USA, South America, Australia).

Table 12.15 Tick-borne *Rickettsiales* of dogs.

Disease agent	Disease	Primary tick vectors	Distribution
Ehrlichia canis	Canine monocytic ehrlichiosis	*Rhipicephalus sanguineus*	Worldwide; tropical/temperate
Ehrlichia chaffeensis		*Amblyomma americanum*	Worldwide
Ehrlichia ewingii	Canine granulocytic ehrlichiosis	*Amblyomma americanum*	Southeastern and south central USA
Anaplasma phagocytophilum (including *A. platys*)		*Ixodes* spp. *Rhipicephalus sanguineus*	Worldwide
Rickettsia rickettsii	Rocky Mountain spotted fever	*Dermacentor varabilis* *Dermacentor andersoni*	North and South America
Rickettsia conorii	Boutonneuse fever Mediterranean fever Indian tick typhus East African tick typhus	*Rhipicephalus* spp. *Amblyomma* spp. *Hyalomma* spp.	Europe Asia, Africa

Epidemiology: Rodents as well as domestic and wild ruminants (sheep and deer) have been reported as reservoir hosts of *A. phagocytophilum* in Europe. The predominant reservoir host varies depending on the local natural and agricultural landscape. The vector of *A. phagocytophilum* in Europe is the common sheep tick *Ixodes ricinus* (Table 12.15). The organisms spend part of their normal life cycle within the tick and are transmitted trans-stadially. As the tick vector feeds on a wide range of vertebrate animals, transmission of the infectious agent to multiple host species may take place.

Pathogenesis: Organisms enter the dermis via a tick bite and are then spread via the blood and/or lymph and localise in mature granulocytes, mainly in neutrophils but also in eosinophils, of the peripheral blood. In dogs, severe pulmonary inflammation, alveolar damage and vasculitis of the extremities in the absence of bacterial organisms suggest an immunopathological course of events, such as cytokine-mediated stimulation of host macrophages and non-specific mononuclear phagocyte activity. The infection may also induce an overactive inflammatory response, such as a septic shock-like syndrome, or diffuse alveolar damage leading to respiratory distress syndrome. Phagocytic dysfunction of infected neutrophils may result in defective host defence and subsequent secondary infections have been reported.

Both animals and humans can be co-infected with various *Anaplasma*, *Ehrlichia*, *Borrelia*, *Bartonella*, *Rickettsia*, *Babesia* and arboviral species. Infection with any of these organisms causes a wide range of clinical and pathological abnormalities, ranging in severity from asymptomatic infection to death. The risk of acquiring one or more tick-borne infections may be dependent on the prevalence of multi-infected vectors. For example, *A. phagocytophilum* and *Borrelia burgdorferi* share both reservoir hosts and vectors, and in geographical areas where tick-borne fever is endemic, borreliosis is also prevalent.

Clinical signs and pathology: In dogs, the spectrum of clinical manifestations caused by *A. phagocytophilum* is wide but it most commonly presents as an acute febrile syndrome. The incubation period may vary from four to 14 days, depending on the immune

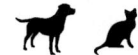

status of the infected individual and the bacterial strain involved. Infected dogs usually present with a history of lethargy and anorexia. Clinical examination commonly reveals fever, reluctance to move and occasionally splenomegaly. Less commonly, animals may show lameness, diarrhoea or nervous signs such as seizures. Systemic manifestations may include haemorrhage, shock and multiorgan failure. The disease is characterised by haematological changes typified by thrombocytopenia and leucopenia. The leucopenia is a result of early lymphopenia later accompanied by neutropenia. Thrombocytopenia is one of the most consistent haematological abnormalities in infected dogs. It may be moderate to severe and persists for a few days before returning to normal. Biochemical abnormalities may include mildly elevated serum alkaline phosphatase and alanine aminotransferase activities.

Diagnosis: *Anaplasma phagocytophilum* should be considered when an animal presents with an acute febrile illness in an endemic geographic area. Stained blood smears should be examined and with Wright's stain morulae typically appear as dark blue, irregularly stained densities in the cytoplasm of neutrophils. The colour of the morulae is usually darker than that of the cell nucleus. Morulae are often sparse and difficult to detect and a negative blood smear cannot rule out *A. phagocytophilum* infection. Specific diagnostic tests include IFAT, immunoblot analyses, ELISA and PCR analyses. The most widely accepted diagnostic criterion is a fourfold change in titre by IFAT. However, cross-reactivity may occur with other members of the genera *Anaplasma* and *Ehrlichia*. Thrombocytopenia can be a haematological finding although leucopenia has also been reported in rare cases.

Control and treatment: In dogs and cats, infections can be prevented to some extent by avoiding tick-infested areas. Careful daily inspection for, and removal of, ticks is recommended in combination with the application of residual acaricidal products. Spray, spot-on liquid or collar formulations are available with residual efficacy of one month or more, depending on the product. Doxycycline 5–10 mg/kg for three weeks appears to be the most effective regimen for treating infections in dogs and cats. Severe disease may require treatment for longer periods. The most common side-effects of doxycycline treatment are nausea and vomiting, which are avoided by administering the drug with food.

Notes: The newly reclassified *Anaplasma phagocytophilum* combo nov. (formerly known as three separate ehrlichiae: *E. phagocytophila*, *E. equi* and *Anaplasma platys* [formerly known as *E. platys*]) causes canine, equine and human granulocytic ehrlichiosis.

Ehrlichia canis

Ehrlichia canis (Phylum: Proteobacteria; Class: Alphaproteobacteria; Order: Rickettsiales; Family: Anaplasmataceae) causes a disease commonly known as Canine monocytic ehrlichiosis or Tropical canine pancytopenia, is localised in the blood of dogs and is distributed in Asia, Europe, Africa, Australia and America.

Epidemiology: *Ehrlichia canis* is transmitted by the brown dog tick, *Rhipicephalus sanguineus* sensu lato. Transmission has also been shown to occur experimentally with the American dog tick, *Dermacentor variabilis*. Transmission in the tick occurs transstadially but not transovarially. Larvae and nymphs become infected while feeding on rickettsaemic dogs and transmit the infection to the host after moulting to nymphs and adults, respectively. Adult

ticks have been shown to transmit infection 155 days after becoming infected. This phenomenon allows ticks to overwinter and infect hosts in the following spring. The occurrence and geographical distribution of *E. canis* are related to the distribution and biology of its tick vector. *Rhipicephalus sanguineus* s.l. ticks are abundant during the warm season, and disease in dogs is seen most commonly during the summer months. Dogs living in endemic regions and those travelling to endemic areas should be considered at risk of infection.

Pathogenesis: Following infection, ehrlichiae organisms enter the bloodstream and lymphatics and localise in macrophages, mainly in the spleen and liver, where they replicate by binary fission. From there, infected macrophages disseminate the infection to other organ systems. The incubation period is 8–20 days and is followed consecutively by an acute, a subclinical and a chronic phase. The acute phase may last 2–4 weeks and if not treated, may enter the subclinical phase. Dogs in this phase may remain persistent carriers of *E. canis* for months or years. The spleen plays a major role in the pathogenesis of the disease and persistence of infection appears to be within splenic macrophages. Some persistently infected dogs may recover spontaneously, but others subsequently develop the chronic severe form of the disease. Not all dogs develop the chronic phase, and factors leading to the development of this phase remain unclear. The prognosis at this stage is grave, and death may occur as a consequence of haemorrhage and/or secondary infection.

Immunological mechanisms appear to be involved in the pathogenesis of the disease, through the production of antibodies that bind to erythrocyte membranes and of platelet-bound antibodies which appear to play a role in the pathogenesis of thrombocytopenia. Other mechanisms involved in the development of the thrombocytopenia include increased platelet destruction and shortened platelet half-life during the acute phase and decreased production in the chronic phase. Meningitis and meningoencephalitis are associated with extensive lymphoplasmacytic and monocytic infiltration, perivascular cuffing and gliosis. On rare occasions morulae may be detected in the cerebrospinal fluid of dogs with neurological signs. The finding of circulating immune complexes in sera of naturally infected dogs suggests that some of the pathological and clinical manifestations are mediated by immune complexes.

Clinical signs: *Ehrlichia canis* infects all breeds of dogs; however, the German shepherd appears to be more susceptible to clinical disease and more severely affected than other breeds, with a higher mortality rate. There is no age predilection and both sexes are equally affected. The disease is manifested by a wide variety of clinical signs. During the acute phase, clinical signs range from mild and non-specific to severe and life-threatening. Common non-specific signs in this phase include depression, lethargy, anorexia, pyrexia, tachypnoea and weight loss. Specific signs include lymphadenomegaly, splenomegaly, petechiation and ecchymoses of the skin and mucous membranes, and occasional epistaxis. Less commonly, there is vomiting, and serous or purulent oculonasal discharge and dyspnoea. In the chronic severe form of the disease, clinical signs may be similar to those seen in the acute disease but more severe. There may be pallor of the mucous membranes and emaciation, and peripheral oedema, especially of the hindlimbs and scrotum, may also be seen. Entire bitches may show prolonged bleeding during oestrus, infertility, abortion and neonatal death. Secondary bacterial and protozoal infections may cause interstitial pneumonia and renal failure.

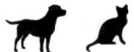

Ocular signs have been reported to occur during the acute and chronic phases and may manifest as conjunctivitis, petechiae and ecchymoses of the conjunctiva and iris, corneal oedema and panuveitis. Subretinal haemorrhage and retinal detachment resulting in blindness may occur due to a monoclonal gammopathy and hyperviscosity. Neurological signs include ataxia, seizures, paresis, hyperaesthesia and cranial nerve dysfunction, and may be attributed to meningitis or meningoencephalitis, which are more commonly seen during the acute phase.

Systemic manifestations may include haemorrhage, shock and multiorgan failure.

Pathology: Once present in tissues, *E. canis* organisms continue to invade, persist and replicate in cells. Circulating infected cells may induce vasculitis and subsequent intravascular coagulation which, in combination with an altered cell-mediated immunity, result in the destruction of platelets. Similar destruction of leucocytes and erythrocytes in combination with decreased erythrocyte production may cause clinical leucopenia and anaemia, respectively. During the subclinical phase, thrombocytopenia, leucopenia and anaemia may continue. Hyperglobulinaemia may be observed in the chronic stages, which is unrelated to serum antibody levels. Bone marrow may be impaired during the chronic phase, although the mechanisms for suppression are not completely understood.

Diagnosis: Diagnosis of *E. canis* infection is based on history, clinical presentation and clinical pathological findings supported by serology. Residence in or travel to known endemic areas and a history of tick infestation should increase the suspicion of infection.

In general, *Ehrlichia* can be distinguished by the type of cell they invade. As the name of the disease it causes implies, *E. canis* invades mononuclear cells. Intracytoplasmic *E. canis* morulae may be visualised in monocytes during the acute phase of the disease in some cases. Examination of the buffy coat enhances the chance of visualising morulae in smears. During the acute phase, there is an increase in the mean platelet volume, mild leucopenia and anaemia, and megaplatelets appear in the blood smear reflecting active thrombopoiesis. Monocytosis and reactive monocytes and large granular lymphocytes are also seen. During the subclinical phase, a mild thrombocytopenia is commonly found, with severe pancytopenia as a result of a suppressed hypocellular bone marrow.

On blood biochemistry, there is hypoalbuminaemia and hyperglobulinaemia, the latter mainly due to hypergammaglobulinaemia, which is usually polyclonal, as determined by serum protein electrophoresis. On rare occasions, monoclonal gammopathy may be noticed and may result in a hyperviscosity syndrome. Pancytopenic dogs manifest significantly lower concentrations of total protein, total globulin and γ-globulin concentrations compared with non-pancytopenic dogs. Mild transient increase in serum alanine aminotransferase and alkaline phosphatase may also be present. Antiplatelet antibody test as well as Coombs' test may be positive in infected dogs.

IFAT is the most widely used serological assay for the diagnosis of canine ehrlichiosis, and titres at a dilution equal to or greater than 1:40 are considered evidence of exposure. Two consecutive tests are recommended, 1–2 weeks apart, with a fourfold increase in antibody titre indicative of active infection. In areas endemic for other *Ehrlichia* species, serological cross-reactivity may complicate the diagnosis. ELISAs for *E. canis* antibodies have been developed and several commercial dot-ELISA antibody tests have been developed for rapid in-clinic use. PCR assays using specific primers for *E. canis* have also been developed. Concurrent infections with other tick-borne pathogens, such as *Babesia* spp. and *Hepatozoon canis*, are common in endemic areas and it is therefore important to examine blood smears of infected dogs microscopically and to consider multiple serological or PCR screening for co-infecting organisms.

Control: No effective anti-*E. canis* vaccine has been developed and tick control remains the most effective preventive measure against infection. Breaking the life cycle of the tick vector at the level of the canine host will eliminate the source of numerous pathogenic agents, in addition to ehrlichiae, that infect dogs and may decrease the risk of transmission to humans for those tick vectors with broad host ranges. Common acaracides such as amitraz, fipronil and pyrethrins, when used according to the manufacturer's instructions, are effective. By targeting the vector, the life cycle and consequently transmission of ehrlichiae will be interrupted. In endemic areas, low-dose oxytetracycline treatment (6.6 mg/kg) once daily has been suggested as an additional prophylactic measure.

Treatment: Doxycycline 10 mg/kg once daily by mouth (or 5 mg/kg twice daily), for a minimum of three weeks, is the treatment of choice for acute infections, and most acute cases respond and show clinical improvement within 24–72 hours. Dogs in the subclinical phase may need prolonged treatment, while those suffering from the chronic severe form of the disease are usually unresponsive to treatment. Other drugs with known efficacy against *E. canis* include tetracycline hydrochloride (22 mg/kg), oxytetracycline (25 mg/kg) and chloramphenicol (50 mg/kg) all given at eight-hourly intervals. Despite treatment, antibody titres may persist for months and even years. Their persistence may represent an aberrant immune response, or treatment failure, but progressive decrease in γ-globulin concentrations is associated with elimination of the rickettsia. *Ehrlichia canis* antibodies do not provide protection against rechallenge, and seropositive dogs remain susceptible.

Ehrlichia chaffeensis

Ehrlichia chaffeensis (Phylum: Proteobacteria; Class: Alphaproteobacteria; Order: Rickettsiales; Family: Anaplasmataceae) causes a disease commonly known as Canine monocytic ehrlichiosis, is localised in the blood of dogs, humans and deer, and occurs in states of the southern USA. *Ehrlichia chaffeensis* is transmitted by *Amblyomma americanum* (Lone Star tick) and to a lesser extent by *Dermacentor variabilis*. Persistently infected white-tailed deer (*Odocoileus virginianus*), and possibly canids, serve as reservoirs.

Pathogenesis and clinical signs: Experimental infections in dogs have shown fever only. The clinical significance of natural canine infection has yet to be determined.

Diagnosis: The IFAT detects exposure to the rickettsia, but it cannot differentiate between antibodies to other canine ehrlichiae. Species identification is by Western immunoblot analysis and by PCR using species-specific primers.

Control and treatment: As for *E. canis*, although treatment is not usually required.

Ehrlichia ewingii

Ehrlichia ewingii (Phylum: Proteobacteria; Class: Alphaproteobacteria; Order: Rickettsiales; Family: Anaplasmataceae) causes a disease commonly known as Canine granulocytic ehrlichiosis, is localised in the

blood of dogs, and is found in southeast and south central USA. The main tick vector is *Amblyomma americanum* but the organism has been identified in a number of other tick species, including *Rhipicephalus sanguineus* sensu lato, *Dermacentor variabilis*, *Ixodes scapularis* and *I. pacificus*.

Epidemiology: Ehrlichiosis caused by *E. ewingii* has been diagnosed in the USA only. It occurs mainly in the spring and early summer.

Pathogenesis: Following infection, ehrlichiae enter the bloodstream and lymphatics and localise in neutrophils. The pathogenesis of polyarthritis, observed more often with infection by granulocytic ehrlichiae, arises from haemarthrosis and immune complex deposition into the joints.

Clinical signs and pathology: The condition is usually an acute mild disease that may lead to polyarthritis in chronically infected dogs. Lameness, joint swelling, stiff gait and fever are common clinical signs. Haematological changes are mild and include thrombocytopenia and anaemia. After entering the canine host through the bite of the tick vector, ehrlichial organisms travel through the circulation, invade cells and disseminate to various tissues. Once in tissues, they continue to invade, persist and replicate in cells. Polyarthritis may arise from haemarthrosis and immune complex deposition into the joints and is often accompanied by neutrophilic inflammation.

Diagnosis: Diagnosis of *E. ewingii* infection is based on history, clinical presentation and clinical pathological findings supported by serology. Residing in, or travel to, known endemic areas and a history of tick infestation should increase the suspicion of infection. Visualisation of morulae in the respective cell types provides a definitive diagnosis and allows differentiation between the monocytic and granulocytic ehrlichiae. Intracytoplasmic *E. ewingii* morulae may be seen within neutrophils.

The IFAT is the serological assay most widely used for the diagnosis of canine ehrlichiosis. However, as *E. ewingii* has not yet been cultured *in vitro*, antigen is not readily available for IFAT. In areas endemic for other *Ehrlichia* species, serological cross-reactivity with the monocytic *Ehrlichia* spp. may complicate diagnosis. Anti-*E. ewingii* antibodies strongly cross-react with *E. canis* and *E. chaffeensis*, and do not (or weakly) react with *A. phagocytophilum*. Western immunoblot and species-specific PCR assays should be used to confirm the ehrlichial species. Species determination is important, as *A. phagocytophilum* is also associated with intraneutrophilic morula formation and similar clinical signs in dogs.

Control and treatment: Tick control is the most effective preventive measure against infection. By targeting the vector, the life cycle and consequently transmission of ehrlichiae will be interrupted. Common acaracides such as amitraz, fipronil and pyrethrins, when used according to the manufacturer's instructions, are effective in controlling ticks. Treatment with tetracyclines, especially doxycycline, elicits rapid clinical improvement.

Notes: *Ehrlichia ewingii* and the newly reclassified *Anaplasma phagocytophilum* combo nov. cause canine and human granulocytic ehrlichiosis. *Ehrlichia ewingii* has been implicated as the cause of human infections in the USA, particularly in immunocompromised people. The role of the dog as a zoonotic reservoir for *E. ewingii* infection is unknown.

Rickettsia rickettsii

Rickettsia rickettsii (Phylum: Proteobacteria; Class: Alphaproteobacteria; Order: Rickettsiales; Family: Rickettsiaceae) causes a disease commonly known as Rocky Mountain spotted fever, is localised in the blood vessels of dogs and humans, and occurs in USA, Canada and Central America.

Epidemiology: Two tick species, *Dermacentor andersoni* (wood tick) and *D. variabilis* (dog tick), both three-host ticks, appear to be mainly involved in the transmission of *R. rickettsii*. Only a small proportion of ticks may be infected in the overall population of a given area. In addition to the low prevalence of infection, infected ticks are not immediately infectious but become so following tick attachment and blood feeding for periods of 5–20 hours. Dogs usually develop illness during the warmer months of the year when questing ticks are active. This seasonality is less noticeable at lower latitudes.

Pathogenesis: Following infection, the organisms enter the bloodstream and infect endothelial cells, causing widespread vasculitis leading to activation of the coagulation and fibrinolytic pathways. Thrombocytopenia occurs through coagulatory and immune-mediated mechanisms. In chronic untreated cases, organs such as the skin, brain, heart and kidneys may develop multiple foci of necrosis and vascular injury leads to leakage of intravascular fluids and oedema. Fluid accumulation in tissues such as the CNS can cause significant brain oedema, resulting in progressive mental and cardiorespiratory depression.

Clinical signs and pathology: Infected dogs usually develop fever within several days after tick exposure. This is usually accompanied by signs of lethargy, mental dullness, inappetence, arthralgia and myalgia, manifest as difficulty in rising and eventual reluctance to walk. Lymphadenomegaly of all peripheral lymph nodes is apparent, and subcutaneous oedema and dermal necrosis may develop in severely affected animals. Petechial haemorrhages may occur rarely on the mucous membranes, and more commonly in the ocular fundus. Neurological signs may appear due to meningitis and can include hyperaesthesia, seizures, vestibular dysfunction and a variety of manifestations depending on the lesion localisation. Recovery is rapid and complete in those animals receiving treatment early, before the onset of organ damage or neurological complications. Once the neurological signs have developed, recovery is delayed or signs may become permanent. On *post mortem*, there are usually widespread petechial and ecchymotic haemorrhages, lymphadenomegaly and splenomegaly. Microscopically, there is a widespread necrotising vasculitis in many organs.

Diagnosis: Clinical laboratory findings are non-specific for a generalised acute-phase inflammatory reaction. There is usually a leucopenia in the acute stages followed by a moderate leucocytosis. A left shift and toxic granulation of neutrophils may be observed in animals with the most severe tissue necrosis. Thrombocytopenia is one of the most consistent laboratory findings. Serum biochemical abnormalities include hypoalbuminaemia, elevated serum alkaline phosphatase activity and variable hyponatraemia and hyperbilirubinaemia. Conduction disturbances related to myocarditis may be seen on electrocardiography and a diffuse increase in pulmonary interstitial density on radiography. A micro-immunofluorescence (Micro-IF) test is used to determine specific antibodies. Titres above 1:1024 generally indicate recent exposure. PCR-specific primers have been used to identify organisms in blood or tissue

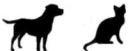

specimens. Rickettsial isolation involves risk and can only be done in secure biocontainment facilities.

Control and treatment: Prevention can be achieved by tick control and periodic treatment with systemic or topically applied acaricides. If left untreated, the disease is highly fatal and treatment should be instituted whenever the disease is suspected. Tetracyclines are the antibiotics of choice and should be administered for at least seven days, but are only effective if they are given prior to the onset of tissue necrosis or organ failure. Recovery is usually associated with protective immunity.

Notes: Rocky Mountain spotted fever is an important zoonotic disease because of its high prevalence and potentially fatal outcome if diagnosis is delayed or missed. Early signs in humans may be vague and misdiagnosis can occur until a rash develops later in the course of disease.

Rickettsia conorii

Rickettsia conorii (Phylum: Proteobacteria; Class: Alphaproteobacteria; Order: Rickettsiales; Family: Rickettsiaceae) causes a disease commonly known as Boutonneuse fever, Mediterranean spotted fever, Indian tick typhus and East African tick typhus, and is localised in the blood of rodents, dogs, cattle, sheep, goats and humans. The vector of the pathogen that causes Mediterranean boutonneuse fever is *Rhipicephalus sanguineus* s.l. Apart from dogs, sheep and cattle, other small free-living mammals, such as rats, mice and shrews, are believed to play an important role in the cycle of infection within tick vectors. Infections appear to be non-pathogenic.

Diagnosis: The rickettsiae can be demonstrated by staining blood or organ smears with Giemsa or may be detected serologically.

Control and treatment: Not usually required although if infection is suspected, tetracyclines are usually effective.

Rickettsia felis

Rickettsia felis (Phylum: Proteobacteria; Class: Alphaproteobacteria; Order: Rickettsiales; Family: Rickettsiaceae) is localised in the blood vessels of cats, humans and dogs, and is diffused in North and South America and Europe. In endemic areas of the USA, opossums are major reservoirs for *R. felis*. Infection of dogs and cats is transmitted by the cat flea, *Ctenocephalides felis*. Cats infected with *R. felis* through exposure to infected fleas develop a subclinical infection. Prevention can be achieved by flea control and periodic treatment with systemic or topically applied insecticides. Treatment with tetracyclines is likely to be effective but seldom indicated.

Notes: *Rickettsia felis* causes flea-transmitted human typhus along with *Rickettsia typhus*; the latter is transmitted by rodent fleas.

Mycoplasma haemofelis

Mycoplasma haemofelis, synonyms *Haemobartonella felis*, *Candidatus Mycoplasma turicensis*, *Mycoplasma haemominutum* (Phylum: Firmicutes; Class: Mollicutes; Order: Mycoplasmatales; Family: Mycoplasmataceae), is localised in the blood of cats, in northern and southern Europe.

Epidemiology: Transmission of the disease probably depends on arthropods including lice, fleas, ticks and biting flies and, at least in the case of *M. felis*, by ingestion of blood during fighting. Infection is most common in young cats.

Pathogenesis: Haemoplasmas induce anaemia by haemolysis and sequestration. The disease may be acute or chronic with periodic recrudescence of clinical signs. Recovered cats may remain carriers. Infection with *Candidatus M. haemominutum* does not often result in clinical signs but a fall in packed cell volume does occur.

Clinical signs and pathology: In the acute form, there is intermittent fever with a progressive anaemia. There are no specific or pathognomonic pathological findings, although cats with concurrent FeLV infection develop more pronounced lesions. Tissues are usually pale and on occasions jaundiced. The liver is often pale and jaundiced. Splenomegaly and lymph node enlargement have been reported. Histology of the liver includes centrilobular congestion and degeneration, and in cats with concurrent FeLV there may be haemosiderosis. In the spleen, there is congestion, extramedullary haemopoiesis, follicular hyperplasia, erythrophagocytosis and haemosiderosis.

Diagnosis: The organisms can be detected in blood smears stained with Romanowsky stain.

Control and treatment: Control blood-sucking arthropods with insecticides and instigate prompt treatment following cat fights. Treatment with tetracyclines is effective.

Notes: The taxonomy of this species is subject to much debate and there is a proposal to reclassify it into the bacterial genus *Mycoplasma* (class Mollicutes) based on 16S rRNA gene sequences and phylogenetic analysis. DNA studies have additionally demonstrated the existence of two distinct species of *M. felis*: *Mycoplasma haemofelis* (large species) and *Candidatus Mycoplasma haemominutum* (small species). A third species, *Candidatus Mycoplasma turicensis*, has also been reported.

Parasites of the nervous system

EYES

Thelazia callipaeda

Thelazia callipaeda (Phylum: Nematoda; Class: Chromadorea; Order: Spirurida; Family: Thelaziidae), commonly known as the Oriental eyeworm, is localised in the eye, conjunctival sac and lacrimal duct of dogs, cats, foxes, wolves, beech martens, bears, rabbits and humans. This parasite has lachryphagus drosophilids of the subfamily Steganinae of the genera *Amiota* and *Phortica* as intermediate hosts.

Epidemiology: *Thelazia* infections occur seasonally and are linked to periods of maximum activity of *Phortica* spp. flies. Although considered present in dogs and humans only from Russia and the Middle East (i.e. Indonesia, Thailand, China, Korea, Myanmar, India and Japan), *T. callipaeda* has been reported in Europe (Italy, France, Portugal, Spain, Switzerland, Germany, Balkans) in dogs, cats, foxes, wolves and humans, and recently in the USA. All cases of human thelaziosis were associated with the close proximity of

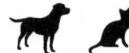

infested dogs in a certain area and the age of patients (i.e. higher incidence in children and elderly people).

Pathogenesis: Lesions are caused by the serrated cuticle of the worm and most damage results from movement by the active young adults, causing lacrimation followed by conjunctivitis. As a result of the discomfort caused by the presence of the nematodes, patients often rub their eyes, thus inducing secondary bacterial infection (e.g. *Pasteurella* spp., *Chlamydia* spp., *Staphylococcus* spp). Although most nematodes localise in the conjunctival sac and the lateral and medial canthi of the eyes, they can also occur in the anterior chamber or the vitreous body. The severity of thelaziosis depends mainly on the number of nematodes in the eye, their specific localisation, the host's immune response and secondary bacterial infections.

Clinical signs and pathology: This infection can cause conjunctivitis and excessive lacrimation. The invasion of the lacrimal gland and ducts may cause inflammation leading to occlusion and reduced tear production. Mechanical irritation of the conjunctiva produces inflammation, while damage to the cornea leads to opacity, keratitis, corneal ulceration and photophobia.

Diagnosis: This is based on observation of the parasites (which appear as cream-coloured filaments) in the conjunctival sac or on the conjunctiva following local anaesthesia, or finding larvae in the lacrimal secretion by microscopy (Fig. 12.7). The clinical diagnosis of human thelaziosis may be difficult if only a small number of nematodes or immature stages are present in the conjunctival sac. The infection could be characterised by symptoms similar to an allergic or bacterial conjunctivitis.

Control and treatment: Prevention is difficult because of the ubiquitous nature of the fly vectors. Treatment is surgical removal with forceps following the application of an ocular local anaesthetic (e.g. lidocaine 1%). In particular, parasites are mechanically removed by irrigating the conjunctival sac with sterile saline or using ophthalmological forceps. Spot-on formulation of imidacloprid 10% and moxidectin 2.5% has proven successful in the control of canine thelaziosis and also made it possible to overcome problems derived from mechanical removal of the parasites or the animals' reluctance to accept local instillation of drugs into the eyes. Milbemicin is equally effective. Again, the

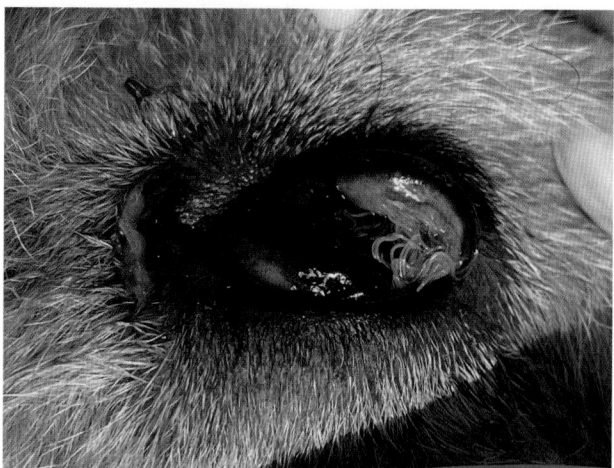

Fig. 12.7 *Thelazia* in the eye of an infected dog.

administration of products containing moxidectin has been shown to protect dogs during an entire season in endemic areas. This chemoprophylactic approach is useful in reducing the prevalence of canine thelaziosis and the risk of human infection. In cases of secondary bacterial infection, the use of antibiotic eye preparations may be indicated.

Thelazia californiensis

Thelazia californiensis (Phylum: Nematoda; Class: Chromadorea; Order: Spirurida; Family: Thelaziidae), commonly known as the Eyeworm, is localised in the eye, conjunctival sac and lacrimal duct of dogs and cats, but also humans. This nematode occurs in North America and has muscid flies as intermediate hosts.

CENTRAL NERVOUS SYSTEM

Taenia solium

Taenia solium, synonym *Cysticercus cellulosae* (Phylum: Platyhelminthes; Class: Cestoda; Order: Cyclophyllidea; Family: Taeniidae), commonly known as the Human pork tapeworm, is localised in the CNS of humans. This parasite has pigs, wild boar, rarely dogs and humans as intermediate hosts. Dogs that become infected with the metacestode stage can also show signs of cerebral cysticercosis with convulsions.

Encephalitozoon cuniculi

Encephalitozoon cuniculi, synonym *Nosema cuniculi* (Phylum: Microsporidia; Class: Microsporea; Order: Microsporida; Family: Unikaryonidae), is distributed worldwide and is localised in the blood of rabbits, dogs, foxes, cats, mice, rats and humans.

Epidemiology: Not reported in dogs, although in other hosts transmission via urine from infected animals has been described.

Pathogenesis: The parasite develops within parasitophorous vacuoles in macrophages and other cells, especially vascular endothelial cells.

Clinical signs and pathology: Infection in dogs is usually asymptomatic, but there may be loss of condition, posterior weakness, incoordination, apathy and epileptiform seizures. In the dog, non-suppurative nephritis, encephalitis and vasculitis have been reported.

Diagnosis: Diagnosis in the live animal is difficult and is usually based on identifying the lesions on histopathology and observation of the organisms in Giemsa, Gram or Goodpasture-carbol fuchsin stains. A serum ELISA test is available.

Notes: Three strains of *Encephalitozoon* have been identified: strain I ('rabbit strain'); strain II ('rodent strain'); strain III ('dog strain'). Each of the three strains has been reported in humans and infections in dogs may therefore pose a potential zoonotic risk.

Toxoplasma gondii

For more details see Parasites of the locomotory system.

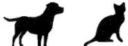

Neospora caninum

Neospora caninum, synonym *Histoplasma gondii* (Phylum: Apicomplexa; Class: Conoidasida; Order: Eucoccidiorida; Family: Sarcocystidae), is a parasite distributed worldwide and localised in the blood of dogs, coyotes, wolves and dingoes. This parasite has cattle, sheep, goats, deer, horses, dogs, foxes, chicken and wild birds as intermediate hosts.

Epidemiology: The dog and other canids are the final hosts, and can also act as intermediate hosts in prenatal infections. In naturally infected dogs, the main route of transmission is thought to be transplacental, with chronically infected bitches developing a parasitaemia during gestation that leads to successive litters becoming infected. Infected pups may either show clinical signs or carry infection subclinically, leading to disease later in life following immunosuppressive illness or administration of immunosuppressive drugs.

Pathogenesis: Neosporosis occurs most severely in transplacentally infected puppies and is characterised by a progressive ascending paralysis, particularly of the hindlimbs. Polymyositis and hepatitis may also occur. Clinical signs are first noticed at 1–6 months of age but can be seen in adults and older dogs. Sudden death due to myocarditis has been reported.

Clinical signs and pathology: Fatal, ascending hindleg paralysis. Lesions are most commonly seen in the brain, spinal cord, nerve roots and skeletal muscles but any organ may be involved, including the skin. In the brain, the grey matter is most severely affected, while the submeningeal white matter tends to be most severely affected in the spinal cord. Tachyzoite proliferation is associated with focal malacia, suppuration and granulatomous reaction. Chronic lesions are characterised by lymphoplasmacytic perivascular infiltrations and gliosis. A marked fibrosis may develop, particularly in submeningeal areas of the cerebral and cerebellar cortex. Parasitised muscle fibres undergo rapid necrosis, and there are massive infiltrations of macrophages, lymphocytes and plasma cells. Tissue cysts are scarce and usually found only in the CNS.

Diagnosis: History of neurological signs, muscle weakness with a progressive ascending paralysis. An IFAT is available; titres of 1:50 or greater are considered positive. A cerebrospinal fluid PCR can be used in diagnosing active CNS infection.

Control and treatment: Dogs should not be allowed to eat aborted fetuses or fetal membranes, and their faeces should be prevented from contaminating bovine feedstuffs. If canine neosporosis is diagnosed early, treatment with trimethoprim, sulfadiazine, pyrimethamine and clindamycin might be useful. Decoquinate has been shown to kill *N. caninum* tachyzoites in cultures.

Onchocerca lupi

Onchocerca lupi (Phylum: Nematoda; Class: Chromadorea; Order: Spirurida; Family: Onchocercidae) is a vector-borne nematode localised in the eyes of dogs, cats and humans. This filarioid is responsible for severe nodular eye lesions in the hosts. The biological cycle, in particular the identity of the insect vector, and spread of *O. lupi* in dog populations are to date unknown.

Epidemiology: The infestation is endemic in canine populations in several European countries (e.g. Austria, Greece, Portugal,

Romania, Spain) and in the Middle East (Israel, Iran), as well as in dogs and cats from the United States. In dogs, the infestation occurs exclusively in adult individuals (probably due to the long prepatent period) and, in particular, in animals aged between one and 15 years (mean 5.3 years). The suspected susceptibility of male dogs and the German shepherd breed is probably related to an increased use of these individuals as guard dogs and, consequently, to a greater exposure to the vector. As for humans, the zoonotic potential of *O. lupi* has been demonstrated in patients from Iran, Tunisia, Turkey, the United States and Europe. Data about the biology and arthropod vector of this onchocercid are still missing.

Pathogenesis, clinical signs and pathology: The pathogenesis of canine onchocercosis has not yet been clarified. For example, regarding the granulomatous formations, it is not known whether these are caused by the filarioid itself, rather than as a result of the host immune response. In most cases, canine onchocercosis occurs in an acute clinical form, characterised by lacrimation, conjunctivitis and exophthalmos. In addition, as demonstrated by histological examinations, adults contained in the granuloma may cause a modest fibrosis and infiltration of monocytic cells, while microfilariae may determine acute inflammation, with an eosinophilic or lymphocytic dermatitis. In chronic cases, inflammation of the visual apparatus is a common finding, combined with the presence of nodules with thickened portions due to the clustering and entanglement of adult filaroids, which may deepen into the periocular connective tissue and reach up to 2 cm in diameter. In humans, the symptomatic picture is characterised by the presence of a non-painful conjunctival/subconjunctival mass, associated with inflammation, oedema and discomfort. However, human infection may be severe due to the localisation of the parasite in the spinal canal of the patient.

Diagnosis: As for *Cercopitiphilaria* spp., *O. lupi* is diagnosed through the identification of microfilariae at the skin level, by sampling small dermal fragments with a sterile scalpel or skin punch biopsy of the interscapular area. The specimens, immersed in saline solution, are incubated at room temperature (20 °C) for about 12 hours and then used for morphological evaluation. No serological test is commercially available. In addition, the lack of circulating microfilariae and clear ocular lesions in the host makes diagnosis more difficult. In cases of overt onchocercosis (acute or chronic), ocular lesions should be differentiated from retrobulbar abscesses, tumours and prolapse of the nictitating gland.

Treatment: *Onchocerca lupi* infestations are currently treated by surgical excision of the parasites within the nodule and, in some cases, the entire eyeball. This intervention must be supported by proper instrumental examinations (e.g. computed axial tomography or ultrasonography) to precisely define the location of nodules at the ocular level. Although no molecule is registered for the treatment of *O. lupi* infestations, macrocyclic lactones and oxfendazole are potential candidates against microfilariae and adults, respectively.

Parasites of the reproductive/urogenital system

Capillaria plica

Capillaria plica, synonym *Pearsonema plica* (Phylum: Nematoda; Class: Enoplea; Order: Enoplida; Family: Capillariidae), commonly

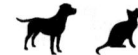

known as the Bladder hairworm, is a parasite distributed in many parts of the world, localised in the urinary bladder of foxes, dogs, wolves and more rarely cats. This parasite has earthworms as intermediate hosts and transmission occurs via ingestion of infective larvae present in earthworms.

Pathogenesis: It is rarely of pathogenic significance, but can occasionally induce cystitis where secondary bacterial infection occurs.

Clinical signs and pathology: Infections are usually asymptomatic. Cystitis and difficulty in urinating have been observed. Most infections are harmless; the anterior end of the worm embedded in the surface epithelium provokes a light cellular reaction in the lamina propria.

Diagnosis: Diagnosis is based on finding the typical *Capillaria* eggs in urine.

Control and treatment: Care should be taken to ensure that runs are clean, dry and free-draining. Successful treatment with fenbendazole 50 mg/kg orally daily for three days has been reported.

Capillaria feliscati

Capillaria feliscati, synonym *Pearsonema feliscati* (Phylum: Nematoda; Class: Enoplea; Order: Enoplida; Family: Capillariidae), commonly known as the Bladder hairworm, is a parasite distributed in many parts of the world, localised in the urinary bladder of cats. This parasite has earthworms as intermediate hosts. *Capillaria feliscati* lie free on the surface of the bladder mucosa.

Dioctophyma renale

Dioctophyma renale, synonyms *Dictophyme renale*, *Eustrongylus gigas* (Phylum: Nematoda; Class: Enoplea; Order: Enoplida; Family: Dioctophymatidae), commonly known as the Giant kidney worm, is localised in the kidney parenchyma and abdominal cavity of dogs, foxes, mink, ferrets, otters, pine martens and polecats; it is sporadically reported in cats, pigs, horses, cattle and humans. This parasite is distributed in temperate and sub-arctic areas, in North and South America, and Asia. Its main endemic area is the northern part of North America, chiefly Canada. It occurs sporadically in Europe. This parasite has aquatic oligochaete annelids (e.g. *Lumbriculus variegatus*) as intermediate hosts.

Epidemiology: As in many of the parasitic infections of domestic carnivores, there is a large reservoir in wild animals from which the intermediate and paratenic hosts are infected. Ranch mink probably acquire infection from their fish diet, and domestic dogs by casual ingestion of infected annelids, frogs or fish.

Pathogenesis: The final effect of infection is destruction of the kidney. Usually only one kidney is affected, the right being more often involved than the left. The parenchyma is destroyed, leaving only the capsule as a distended sac containing the worms; though there may be three or four worms in a kidney, occasionally there is only one. Rarely, the worms may occur in the abdominal cavity, either free or encapsulated, and in the subcutaneous connective tissue.

Clinical signs and pathology: The main signs are dysuria with some haematuria, especially at the end of micturition; in a few cases there is lumbar pain. However, most cases are completely asymptomatic, even when one kidney has been completely destroyed.

Worms in the abdominal cavity can cause a chronic peritonitis. Adult worms in the renal pelvis are very destructive, initially causing haemorrhagic pyelitis which becomes suppurative, and the parenchyma is eventually destroyed until only the tunic contains the worm and exudate. In the abdominal cavity, the worm often entwines a lobe of the liver and may cause erosion of the hepatic capsule, leading to haemorrhage or infarction and rupture.

Diagnosis: The eggs are quite characteristic, being ovoid and yellowish-brown with pitted shells, and their occurrence in the urine, singly or in clumps or chains, is diagnostic.

Control and treatment: Elimination of raw fish from the diet. Treatment is rarely called for, although surgery may be attempted in confirmed cases.

Notes: *Dioctophyma* (red scourge) infection in humans has been mainly recorded in North America, but other cases have occurred throughout the world. Annelid intermediate hosts in the drinking water are infective and uncooked frogs and fish act as paratenic hosts. The adult worms are found in a thick-walled cyst in the kidney (usually the right) and may cause loin pain and haematuria.

Parasites of the locomotory system

Trichinella spiralis

For more details see Chapter 11.

Toxoplasma gondii

Toxoplasma gondii (Phylum: Apicomplexa; Class: Conoidasida; Order: Eucoccidiorida; Family: Sarcocystidae) is distributed worldwide and localised in the muscles, lungs, liver, reproductive system and CNS of cats and other felids. This parasite has any mammal, including humans, or bird as intermediate hosts. Treatment is not indicated. Note that the final host, the cat, may also be an intermediate host and harbour extraintestinal stages.

Epidemiology: Most cats become infected by ingesting *Toxoplasma*-infected animals, usually rodents, whose tissues contain tachyzoites or bradyzoites. Direct transmission of oocysts between cats can also occur. The ingestion of mature bradyzoites is the most important route and results in the shedding of higher numbers of oocysts than when infection is acquired from other stages. Following infection, the cyst wall is digested in the cat's stomach, and in the intestinal epithelium the liberated bradyzoites initiate a cycle of merogonous and gametogonous development culminating in the production of oocysts in 3–10 days. Oocysts are shed for only 1–2 weeks. During this cycle in the intestinal mucosa, the organisms may invade the extraintestinal organs where the development of tachyzoites and bradyzoites proceeds as in intermediate hosts.

Dogs are infected by the ingestion of undercooked meat containing *Toxoplasma* cysts.

The cat plays a central role in the epidemiology of toxoplasmosis and the disease is virtually absent from areas where cats do not occur. Epidemiological investigations in the USA and elsewhere indicate that 60% of cats are serologically positive to *Toxoplasma* antigen, the majority acquiring infection by predation. As might be expected, infections are more prevalent in stray cats. Congenital

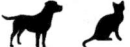

infection is rare. Following infection, cats shed oocysts for only 1–2 weeks, after which they are resistant to reinfection. However, a proportion remain as carriers, perhaps due to the persistence of some meronts, and reactivation of infection with shedding of oocysts may occur in association with intercurrent disease, during the periparturient period in queens or following corticosteroid therapy. However, the oocysts appear to be very resistant and this compensates for the comparatively short period of oocyst excretion.

Pathogenesis: Most *Toxoplasma* infections in animals are light and consequently asymptomatic.

Clinical signs and pathology:

- Cats: Despite the fact that cats are frequently infected, clinical disease is rare, although enteritis, enlarged mesenteric lymph nodes, pneumonia, degenerative changes in the CNS and encephalitis have been recorded in experimental infections. Congenital transmission, although uncommon, has occurred following activation of bradyzoite cysts during pregnancy.
- Dogs: The onset of illness is marked by fever with lassitude, anorexia and diarrhoea. Pneumonia and neurological manifestations are common. Infection may occur in conjunction with distemper and has also been incriminated in distemper vaccination breakdowns. At necropsy, bradyzoite cysts can be demonstrated in cells in the brain and respiratory tract; the associated lymph nodes are enlarged.

Diagnosis: Diagnosis is usually based on serological testing by latex agglutination test or ELISA.

Hepatozoon americanum

Hepatozoon americanum (Phylum: Apicomplexa; Class: Conoidasida; Order: Eucoccidiorida; Family: Hepatozoidae) causes a disease commonly known as Canine hepatozoonosis and is localised in the blood and muscle of dogs in southeast USA.

Epidemiology: The main vector of *H. americanum* is the Gulf Coast tick, *Amblyomma maculatum*, which is found in southern North America, Central America and the northern parts of South America. Infection is transmitted trans-stadially from nymph to adult stages of the tick vectors. Larval *A. maculatum* can also become infected and transmit *H. americanum* as newly moulted nymphs or adults. Infection appears to be mainly from ingestion of infected ticks. Vertical transmission has been reported.

Pathogenesis: The earliest lesions occur in skeletal muscle with the formation of characteristic 'onion skin' cysts comprising meronts and mucopolysaccharide lamellar membranes laid down by the host cells. Clinical signs in infected dogs result from the pyogranulomatous inflammatory response that occurs after the encysted mature meront ruptures, releasing merozoites into the surrounding tissue. Some cysts undergo merogony very rapidly while others appear to enter dormancy. Prolonged infection may occur from a single infecting episode perpetuated by repeated merogonic cycles. Infected dogs commonly develop osteoproliferative lesions, most frequently on the diaphysis of long bones. Pain results from both the pyogranulomatous inflammation in skeletal muscle and the osteoproliferative lesions. Prolonged infection may persist, perpetuated by prolonged merogony cycles. Muscle atrophy becomes apparent with chronic disease and can result in secondary weakness.

Clinical signs and pathology: Dogs infected with *H. americanum* are often presented with fever, generalised pain or hyperaesthesia, muscle atrophy, weakness, depression, reluctance to rise and mucopurulent ocular discharge. Muscle atrophy becomes apparent with chronic disease and can result in secondary weakness. Most dogs maintain a relatively normal appetite, but weight loss is common due to muscle atrophy and chronic cachexia. Mucopurulent ocular discharge is common and is sometimes associated with decreased tear production. Less frequently, clinical signs include polyuria and polydipsia, abnormal lung sounds or cough, pale mucous membranes and lymphadenomegaly. On *post mortem*, chronically infected dogs show cachexia and muscle atrophy, and osteoproliferative lesions may be apparent on bone surfaces. Grossly, pyogranulomas may appear as multiple foci, 1–2 mm in diameter, diffusely scattered predominantly in skeletal and cardiac muscle; they may also be found sporadically in other tissues including adipose tissue, lymph node, intestinal smooth muscle, spleen, skin, kidney, salivary gland, liver, pancreas and lung. Vascular changes in various organs include fibrinoid degeneration of vessel walls, mineralisation and proliferation of vascular intima, and pyogranulomatous vasculitis. Renal lesions are frequently present and include focal pyogranulomatous inflammation with mild glomerulonephritis, lymphoplasmacytic interstitial nephritis, mesangioproliferative glomerulonephritis and occasionally amyloidosis. Amyloid deposits may also be found in spleen, lymph nodes, small intestine and liver. Occasional findings include pulmonary congestion, splenic coagulative necrosis, lymphadenopathy and congestion of the gastric mucosa.

Diagnosis: Diagnosis is based on the identification of gamonts in blood smears is unreliable because of the low numbers present in circulating blood. Blood samples should be examined rapidly using buffy coat smears. Muscle biopsy of the biceps or epaxial muscles is the most consistent method of identification of the characteristic cysts with pyogranuloma formation and the presence of parasites. An ELISA for *H. americanum* has been reported. Infected dogs have a marked neutrophilia, a mild to moderate normocytic normochromic non-regenerative anaemia and thrombocytosis.

Control and treatment: The control is the same as for *H. canis*. There is no effective treatment capable of eliminating all stages. Clinical remission can be obtained rapidly using a combination of trimethoprim-sulfadiazine (15 mg/kg twice daily), clindamycin (10 mg/kg three times daily) and pyrimethamine (0.25 mg/kg daily) over a period of 14 days. Palliative therapy with non-steroidal anti-inflammatory drugs (NSAIDs) may also be required to reduce fever and pain.

Parasites of the integument

Rhabditis strongyloides

Rhabditis strongyloides, synonym *Pelodera strongyloides* (Phylum: Nematoda, Class: Chromadorea, Order: Rhabditida; Family: Rhabditidae), is presumed to be a parasite distributed worldwide and localised in the subcutaneous tissue and skin of dogs, cattle and horses.

Epidemiology: These worms are saprophytic, living in warm moist soil rich in organic matter, and significant infections probably require the host's skin to be continually moist and dirty. Cases have

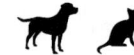

been most frequently reported in dogs housed in kennels with damp hay or straw bedding.

Pathogenesis: Worms invade the hair follicles, causing an intense pruritus. Lesions, usually confined to areas of the body in contact with the ground, show hair loss, erythema and pustule formation if infected with bacteria. The intense itching is probably induced by an allergic reaction to the parasite.

Clinical signs and pathology: Pruritus, erythema and pustule formation. The worms invade the follicles, attracting large numbers of eosinophils. An acute dermatitis develops, commonly with suppurative folliculitis due to secondary bacterial infection.

Diagnosis: The very small worms, 1–2.8 mm in length with a rhabditiform oesophagus, may be recovered from skin scrapings.

Control and treatment: The condition can be prevented by housing animals on clean dry bedding. The treatment is symptomatic.

Acanthocheilonema reconditum

Acanthocheilonema reconditum, synonym *Dipetalonema reconditum* (Phylum: Nematoda; Class: Chromadorea; Order: Spirurida; Family: Onchocercidae), is localised in the subcutaneous tissues, kidney and body cavity of dogs and various canids. It is found in Africa, the USA and Europe. This parasite has fleas (*Ctenocephalides canis*, *C. felis*, *Pulex irritans*) and lice (*Heterodoxus spiniger*, *Linognathus setosus*) as intermediate hosts.

Epidemiology: Infection is presumably common in areas where the parasite and intermediate hosts co-exist.

Clinical signs and pathology: The worms are not usually considered pathogenic. The presence of adult worms may occasionally cause subcutaneous abscessation and ulceration.

Diagnosis: *Acantocheilonema reconditum* often occurs in the same endemic area as *Dirofilaria immitis* and the presence of its microfilariae may lead to misdiagnosis on blood examination. Identification of the microfilariae in the blood (samples ideally taken in the early evening) is aided by concentrating the parasites following lysis and filtration and then staining with methylene blue or May–Grunwald Giemsa. Commercial kits are available for this technique. Alternatively, one part of blood and nine parts of formalin are centrifuged and the sediment mixed with a blue stain and examined as a microscopic smear. The microfilariae have to be differentiated from those of *D. immitis*, which are more than 300 μm in length and have a tapered head and a straight tail; those of *A. reconditum* are less than 300 μm in length and have a blunt head and a hooked posterior end. More precise differentiation may be achieved by using histochemical stains for acid phosphatase activity. *Dirofilaria immitis* shows distinct red acid phosphate-positive spots at the excretory pore and anus, while *A. reconditum* stains pink overall. Differential diagnosis may be achieved through the application of PCR-based recombinant DNA technology.

Control and treatment: Preventive measures include control of the intermediate hosts. Drug therapy is not usually indicated.

Cercopithifilaria grassii

Cercopithifilaria grassii, synonyms *Dipetalonema grassi*, *Acanthocheilonema grassi* (Phylum: Nematoda; Class: Chromadorea;

Order: Spirurida; Family: Onchocercidae), causes a disease commonly known as Subcutaneous filarioidosis and is localised in the subcutaneous tissue of dogs in southern Europe and Africa. This parasite has ticks and fleas as intermediate hosts and treatment is not required.

Epidemiology: Infection is presumably common in areas where the parasite and intermediate hosts co-exist.

Pathogenesis: *Cercopithifilaria grassii* inhabits the thoracic cavity and subcutaneous tissues. It is considered to be of low pathogenicity.

Clinical signs and pathology: Infection with this parasite is usually asymptomatic. No pathology is associated with the infection.

Diagnosis: Identification of the microfilariae in the blood (samples ideally taken in the early evening) is aided by concentrating the parasites following lysis and filtration and then staining with methylene blue or May–Grunwald Giemsa. Alternatively, one part of blood and nine parts of formalin are centrifuged and the sediment mixed with a blue stain and examined as a microscopic smear. The microfilariae are large with a hook-shaped tail.

Cercopithifilaria bainae

Cercopithifilaria bainae (Phylum: Nematoda; Class: Chromadorea; Order: Spirurida; Family: Onchocercidae) is localised in the subcutaneous tissue of dogs and diffused in the Mediterranean basin. This parasite has *Rhipicephalus sanguineus* sensu lato as intermediate host.

Epidemiology: The prevalence of infestation is up to 45.4% in dog populations of the Mediterranean basin. The presence of *C. bainae* within the arthropod vector follows a seasonal dynamic in the Mediterranean. In Italy, although animals are exposed to the infestation throughout the entire year, the proportion of ticks infected increases between April and July, with peaks at the beginning of the summer.

Pathogenesis, clinical signs and pathological findings: Although the pathogenetic role of *C. bainae* is still poorly investigated and in the majority of cases the infestation appears asymptomatic, the presence of microfilariae in the host can cause erythematous papules and dermatitis, with onset of perivascular and interstitial dermatitis, presence of neutrophils, eosinophils and lymphocytes.

Diagnosis: *Cercopithiifilaria bainae* infestations are diagnosed by searching for microfilariae in the skin. This procedure is based on the sampling of small skin fragments (3 mm in diameter) using a sterile scalpel or skin punch biopsy at the interscapular area or the neck, which are then immersed in a physiological saline solution. Following incubation at 37 °C for one hour or at room temperature for about 12 hours, the microfilariae migrate from the dermis into the solution and therefore can be found in the sediment and identified at the morphological and molecular level. In the former case, only a few microlitres of sample are required for the visualisation of microfilariae by light microscopy, facilitated by the addition of a few drops of methylene blue (1%) in the sediment. In the second case, following DNA extraction, specific target genes are amplified.

Control and treatment: Although no molecules with filaricidal activity are registered for *C. bainae* infestations, macrocyclic

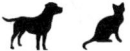

lactones are effective against microfilariae. Moreover, the prevention of infestation is possible by using repellents or acaricides towards the arthropod vector, directly on the dog or in the environment.

Notes: In recent years, the examination of skin fragments has revealed the presence of *Cercopithifilaria* sp. II sensu Otranto et al., 2012 in dogs from Greece, Italy (Basilicata and Sicily regions), Portugal and Spain. However, although the morphology of the microfilariae is clear and distinctive (i.e. about 280 μm in length with characteristic cuticle expansions called wings), the adults of this species have not yet been described, so their taxonomic position is still not determined.

Acanthocheilonema dracunculoides

Acanthocheilonema dracunculoides, synonym *Dipetalonema dracunculoides* (Phylum: Nematoda; Class: Chromadorea; Order: Spirurida; Family: Onchocercidae), is localised in the peritoneum of dogs and hyenas and is found in Africa (Kenya) and parts of India. This parasite has ticks and fleas as intermediate hosts.

Pathogenesis and clinical signs: Not considered pathogenic.

Notes: All other details are essentially as for *D. reconditum*.

Dirofilaria repens

Dirofilaria repens, synonym *Nochtiella repens* (Phylum: Nematoda; Class: Chromadorea; Order: Spirurida; Family: Onchocercidae), is localised in the subcutaneous and intermuscular tissues of dogs, cats, foxes, bears and occasionally humans. This parasite has mosquitoes of the genera *Aedes, Mansonia, Anopheles* and *Culex* as intermediate hosts. It is distributed in the Mediterranean basin (Italy, Spain, Greece, France, former Yugoslavia), Middle East, sub-Saharan Africa and Asia. Recently, it has been reported in USA.

Epidemiology: Infection is by biting mosquitoes and transmission is generally confined to warmer months when mosquitoes are active.

Pathogenesis: The adults are found in nodules in subcutaneous and intermuscular tissues and the microfilariae in the blood and lymph. *Dirofilaria repens* is responsible for cutaneous dirofilariosis, causing mild skin lesions and localised itching. It is of little pathogenic significance in dogs.

In humans, infection is usually asymptomatic. Subcutaneous nodules are found in the breasts, arms, legs, scrotum, eyelid, conjunctivae, penis and testes.

Clinical signs and pathology: Itching, mild skin lesions and subcutaneous nodules. The presence of the adult parasites causes a local inflammatory reaction with accumulations of eosinophils and mononuclear cells.

Diagnosis: As the microfilariae of *D. repens* and *D. immitis* are morphologically similar, techniques such as isoenzyme characterisation and recombinant DNA application are required to distinguish these species.

Control and treatment: Mosquito control is difficult and therefore prophylaxis is based almost entirely on preventive medication with avermectins or milbemycins as used for *D. immitis*. Treatment is achieved by the surgical removal of the parasites from skin lesions.

Dracunculus medinensis

Dracunculus medinensis (Phylum: Nematoda; Class: Chromadorea; Order: Spirurida; Family: Dracunculidae), commonly known as the Guinea worm and Medina worm, is localised in the subcutaneous connective tissue of humans and occasionally cattle, horses, dogs, cats and other mammals. This parasite has copepod crustaceans (*Cyclops* spp.) as intermediate hosts and is found in Africa, the Middle East and parts of Asia.

Pathogenesis: Following initial infection, there are virtually no signs of disease until the gravid adult female emerges in the subcutaneous tissues of the extremities. Pathogenesis is associated with cutaneous ulcer formation.

Clinical signs: The migration of the worm to the surface of the skin may induce pruritus and urticaria and a blister on an extremity.

Diagnosis: Symptoms of dracunculosis are pathognomonic.

Pathology: Secondary bacterial infection of the ulcer lesion or degeneration of worms can cause marked abscessation.

Control and treatment: This is best achieved through the provision of clean drinking water or water that has been adequately sieved to remove any copepods. For treatment, the worm may be gradually removed through the lesion by winding it round a small stick at a rate of about 2 cm each day; alternatively, it may be surgically excised. Treatment with thiabendazole or niridazole, administered over several days, might be effective. Ivermectin or albendazole may be useful but efficacy data are lacking.

Dracunculus insignis

Dracunculus insignis (Phylum: Nematoda; Class: Chromadorea; Order: Spirurida; Family: Dracunculidae), commonly known as the North American guinea worm, is localised in the subcutaneous connective tissue of raccoons and other carnivores, including dogs and cats, and diffused in North America. This parasite has copepod cructaceans (*Cyclops* spp.) as intermediate hosts.

Notes: Other aspects are essentially similar to *D. medinensis*.

Cutaneous leishmaniosis

Several species of *Leishmania* are responsible for cutaneous leishmaniosis, characterised by a moist ulcerative lesion at the site of insect bites that may become large and granulomatous.

Leishmania infantum

For more details see Parasites of the liver.

Leishmania tropica

Leishmania tropica, synonym *Leishmania tropica* complex (Phylum: Euglenozoa; Class: Kinetoplastea; Order: Trypanosomatida; Family:

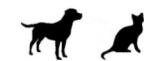

Trypanosomatidae), causes a disease commonly known as Cutaneous leishmaniosis, 'dry' Oriental sore or Jericho boil and is localised in the skin of rock hyraxes (*Procavia capensis*) but also humans and dogs. It is distributed in central and southwest Asia and equatorial and southern Africa, Kenya and Namibia.

Epidemiology: The disease is urban in distribution and dogs are commonly infected. Transmission is by sand flies of the genus *Phlebotomus* (*P. sergenti*, *P. guggisbergi*), particularly in cities and rocky areas in semi-arid regions.

Pathogenesis: *Leishmania tropica* causes cutaneous leishmaniosis or 'Oriental sore', the lesions developing at the site of the insect bite. Gradually the lesion enlarges, remaining red but without heat or pain. Resolution involves immigration of leucocytes, which isolate the infected area leading to necrosis and granuloma formation. Macrophages infected with *Leishmania* organisms are eventually destroyed, and the animal recovers and is immune to reinfection.

Clinical signs and pathology: It may take many months or even years for infected dogs to develop clinical signs, so that the disease may only become apparent long after dogs have left endemic areas. Lesions are confined to shallow skin ulcers often on the lip or eyelid, from which recovery is often spontaneous. The basic lesions are foci of activated proliferating macrophages infected with *Leishmania* organisms. In some cases, these are ultimately surrounded by plasma cells and lymphocytes leading to necrosis and granuloma formation.

Diagnosis: See *Leishmania infantum*

Control and treatment: See *Leishmania infantum*.

Notes: Other *Leishmania* species reported in dogs include:

- *Leishmania aethiopica* found in the highlands of Ethopia and Kenya
- *Leishmania major* in North Africa, Israel, southwest Asia (Algeria to Saudi Arabia), central Asia (Iran to Uzbekistan) and West Africa
- *Leishmania peruviana* found on the mountain slopes of the western Andes in Peru and Bolivia.

ECTOPARASITES

FLEAS

Ctenocephalides felis

Ctenocephalides felis (Phylum: Arthropoda; Class: Insecta; Order: Siphonaptera; Family: Pulicidae), commonly known as the Cat flea, is a blood-sucking ectoparasite that feeds on cats, but will also readily infest dogs and a range of other mammals. There are four subspecies: *C. felis felis* is widespread, *C. f. strongylus* occurs in Africa, *C. f. damarensis* in southwestern Africa and *C. f. orientalis* in India, Sri Lanka and Southeast Asia.

Epidemiology: The cat flea, *C. f. felis*, is the most common species of flea found on domestic cats and dogs throughout North America and northern Europe. Significantly more cats are usually infested with fleas than dogs, however, perhaps because of their tendency to roam, increasing their contact with other cats. Fleas may be found on pets throughout the year but, in the northern hemisphere, numbers tend to increase around late spring and early autumn when ambient conditions are favourable for larval development. Since

C. felis are able to survive for long periods off the host, they do not require direct contact for transmission.

Pathogenesis: The response to a flea bite is a raised, slightly inflamed wheal on the skin, associated with mild pruritus, but though the animal will scratch intermittently there is little distress. However, after repeated flea bites over a period of several months, a proportion of dogs and cats develop flea-bite allergy, which is often associated with profound clinical signs.

Since each female *C. f. felis* can ingest as much as 13.6 μl of blood per day, severe infestations may lead to iron deficiency anaemia. Anaemia caused by *C. f. felis* is particularly prevalent in young animals and has been reported in cats and dogs and, very rarely, goats, cattle and sheep.

Flea-bite allergy is a hypersensitive reaction to components of the flea saliva released into the skin during feeding. The allergy shows a seasonality in temperate areas, appearing in summer when flea activity is highest, though in centrally heated homes exposure may be continuous. In warmer regions, such as the western states of the USA, the problem occurs throughout the year. As would be expected, the most commonly affected areas in both dogs and cats are the preferential biting sites of the fleas, namely the back, the ventral abdomen and the inner thighs. In the dog the primary lesions are discrete crusted papules which cause intense pruritus. The most important damage, however, is subsequently inflicted by the animals themselves, in scratching and biting the affected areas, to produce areas of alopecia or moist dermatitis ('wet eczema'). In older dogs which have been exposed for many years, the skin may become thickened, folded and hairless, and in these animals the pruritus is much less intense. In the cat, flea-bite allergy produces the condition commonly known as Miliary dermatitis or Eczema, readily detectable on palpation, in which the skin is covered with innumerable small, brown, crusty papules that cause marked pruritus. In cats, there are two distinct clinical manifestations associated with flea allergy: miliary dermatitis and feline symmetrical alopecia.

Flea allergy dermatitis is one of the most common causes of dermatological disease of dogs and cats. Dermatitis associated with allergy to flea bites is characterised by intense pruritus and reddening of the skin, with itching persisting up to five days after the bite. The resultant licking, chewing and scratching can lead to hair loss, self-induced trauma and secondary infection. Other symptoms include restlessness, irritability and weight loss, though the intensity of irritation varies greatly with the individual attacked.

All cats and dogs can become allergic to fleas, though atopic hosts are predisposed to developing reactivity. One bite may be sufficient to cause an allergic reaction. Intermittent flea exposure encourages development of a flea allergy, while continual exposure appears to protect against it, as does contact with fleas at an early age. Though little is known about the allergens responsible for evoking the allergic response, recent findings suggest that multiple proteins are important in flea-bite hypersensitivity. In studies which have attempted to determine how flea antigens react with IgG or IgE, at least 15 different flea components have been found to bind IgE. No pattern of reactivity or differences in antibody structure have been observed which distinguish hosts with flea allergy from those without, suggesting that there is little association between particular antibody responses and allergic reactivity to fleas. Both immediate and delayed hypersensitivity can be observed, and individuals will vary in the strength and proportion of each type of sensitivity they express. Hosts chronically infested with *C. f. felis* rarely develop a state of natural tolerance resulting in a loss of clinical signs.

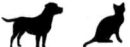

Cats kept in a flea-infested environment groom at twice the rate of cats in a flea-free environment. In normal grooming, a cat may ingest almost 50% of its resident flea population within a few days and cats fitted with Elizabethan collars, which prevent grooming, harbour much greater populations of fleas than cats free to groom. The removal of fleas during grooming reduces the chance of finding them during a skin and coat examination. This is a particular diagnostic problem in cats with a low flea burden but marked flea-bite hypersensitivity. In such cases, since many of the groomed fleas are ingested, examination of the mouth may reveal fleas caught in the spines of the cat's tongue.

Fleas are vectors of a range of viruses and bacteria, and pathogen transmission is enhanced by their promiscuous feeding habits. Most species of flea are host preferential rather than host specific and will try to feed on any available animal. For example, *C. felis* has been found on over 50 different host species. Other factors which contribute to the potential of *C. felis* as a vector include transovarial transmission of some pathogens (*Rickettsia* species) and the transmission of pathogens such as *Bartonella henselae* through adult flea faeces.

Fleas act as intermediate hosts for the common tapeworm of dogs and cats, *Dipylidium caninum*. Tapeworm eggs, along with general organic debris, are ingested by flea larvae. The tapeworm eggs hatch in the midgut of the flea larva and the worm larvae penetrate the gut wall, passing into the haemocoel. The tapeworm larvae develop within the flea body cavity throughout larval, pupal and adult flea development, eventually encapsulating as an infective cysticercoid. After ingestion of the adult flea by the host, cysticercoids are liberated and develop into tapeworms in the digestive tract.

Ctenocephalides felis felis also acts as an intermediate host of the non-pathogenic subcutaneous filarioid nematode of dogs, *Acanthocheilonema reconditum*, which adults may ingest during blood feeding.

Clinical signs: Host animals scratch and bite at the affected area and the bite may produce a small raised wheal on the skin.

Diagnosis: When the signs are indicative of flea infestation but no parasites can be found, the host should be sprayed with an insecticide, placed on a large sheet of plastic or paper, and vigorously combed or groomed. The combings and debris should be examined for fleas or flea faeces, which show as dark brown-black crescentic particles. Consisting almost entirely of blood, these will produce a spreading reddish stain when placed on moist tissue.

Another technique is the use of a vacuum cleaner with fine gauze inserted behind the nozzle; the latter is applied to the host or its habitat and the fleas are retained on the gauze.

Control and treatment: For optimal control, the adults already infesting the host animal should be killed immediately and reinfestation from the environment prevented. A wide range of products is available. Many of the new chemicals with excellent long-acting flea adulticidal activity also have contact ovicidal and/or larvicidal activity. In addition, combination with insect growth regulators (chitin synthesis inhibitors, juvenile hormone analogues) applied directly to the animal not only increases ovicidal and/or larvicidal activity but also delivers it effectively to the sleeping areas most likely to be infested without unnecessarily contaminating the environment. Insect growth regulators do not kill adult fleas and are not suitable by themselves for flea control, unless used in a completely closed environment. For flea infestations of domestic

animals, frequent vacuuming can help to reduce environmental infestation and pet bedding should be washed at high temperatures.

In flea-bite allergy, where there is much distress, corticosteroids may be used topically or systemically as palliative treatment. Since in-contact animals may also harbour fleas without developing allergy, these should also be treated.

For specific treatment, insecticides are available, mainly in the form of powders, sprays, shampoos or spot-on preparations. These historically have generally been organophosphate compounds, pyrethrum and its derivatives, or carbamates. The insect growth regulator lufenuron, a benzoylurea derivative, is given orally for use against fleas in dogs. When ingested by fleas during feeding, the compound is transferred to the eggs and blocks the formation of chitin, thereby inhibiting the development of flea larvae.

Of the newer generation of ectoparasiticides, fipronil is given either by spray or spot-on for the control of fleas and ticks in both dogs and cats, giving protection for 2–3 months. Imidacloprid is a systemic neurotoxic insecticide that is chemically related to the tobacco toxin nicotine. It is highly effective at killing adult fleas for up to one month after application. Fleas are not required to bite the animal to receive a lethal dose, which can be absorbed through the cuticle.

Newer and recently introduced flea compounds include indoxacarb, which is a pro-insecticide that requires activation in the target insect to an active metabolite that causes paralysis and death. Afoxolaner and fluralaner belong to a new class of insecticide, the isoxazoles, which act as non-competitive γ-aminobutyric acid (GABA) receptor agonists, binding to chloride channels in nerve and muscle cells of the target parasites. Given orally, they protect against fleas and ticks for up to three months.

Ctenocephalides canis

Ctenocephalides canis (Phylum: Arthropoda; Class: Insecta, Order: Siphonaptera, Family: Pulicidae), commonly known as the Dog flea, has pathogenesis and treatment similar to that of *C. f. felis*.

Epidemiology: The behavioural differences between dog and cat fleas seem largely to involve the range of environmental conditions which their larvae are capable of tolerating. While household dogs in northern Europe and North America are more likely to be infested by the cat flea, working dogs in kennels and dogs in rural areas or at higher altitudes are more likely to be infested by *C. canis*.

Archaeopsylla erinacei

Archaeopsylla erinacei (Phylum: Arthropoda; Class: Insecta; Order: Siphonaptera; Family: Pulicidae), commonly known as the Hedgehog flea, occurs on hedgehogs and may be transferred to dogs and cats following contact.

Dogs and cats may also be infested by rabbit fleas and a range of bird fleas (see Chapter 3).

LICE

Heavy louse infestation is known as pediculosis. Blood-sucking lice have been implicated in the transmission of disease such as anaplasmosis. However, lice are predominantly of importance in dogs and

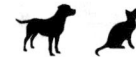

cats because of the direct damage they cause, either by blood feeding or chewing the skin or hair. Clinical importance is therefore usually a function of their density. Transmission of lice is usually by direct physical contact.

Clinical signs and pathology: The most notable sign of louse infestation is a scruffy, dry hair or coat. Restlessness, rubbing and damage to the coat suggest that lice are present, and when the hair is parted the parasites will be found. Heavy infestations cause intense pruritus, associated with papulocrustous dermatitis or with patchy alopecia.

Diagnosis: The lice and their eggs may be seen within the hair and on the skin when the coat is parted. The lice may be removed and identified under a light microscope.

Control and treatment: Since lice spend their entire life on the host animal, control is readily achieved through the use of topical insecticides on all in-contact animals. Lice can be spread on dirty, shared grooming equipment so appropriate hygiene is essential.

Lice are killed by most organophosphates (e.g. chlorpyrifos, malathion or diazinon), amitraz, pyrethroids (e.g. permethrin) and carbamates (e.g. carbaryl). Organophosphates and permethrin should not be used in cats; amitraz should be used only with care at half the dose applied to dogs. The more recent products imidacloprid, fipronil and the macrocyclic lactone selamectin may also be particularly effective with high safety margins. However, since the eggs are relatively resistant to most insecticides, repeat treatments 14 days apart may be recommended for some products in order to kill newly hatched lice.

Felicola subrostratus

Felicola subrostratus, synonym *Felicola subrostrata* (Phylum: Arthropoda; Class: Insecta; Order: Psocodea; Suborder: Ischnocera; Family: Trichodectidae), is a chewing louse, commonly known as the Cat biting louse. It is found on the skin of cats, most commonly on the face, pinnae or dorsum, and occurs worldwide.

Epidemiology: Generally, infestation occurs via close bodily contact. This species of louse is highly host specific. Infestations may be common in catteries, where asymptomatic carriers may act as reservoirs. Kittens may be particularly susceptible to infestation.

Pathogenesis: This is a chewing louse and is the only species of louse that commonly occurs on cats. Pediculosis is now rare and generally is seen only in elderly or chronically ill animals. It is more problematic in long-haired breeds and pathogenic populations may develop under thickly matted or neglected fur. Infestations most commonly occur on the face, back and pinnae, causing a dull ruffled coat, scaling, crusts and alopecia.

Heterodoxus spiniger

Heterodoxus spiniger (Phylum: Arthropoda; Class: Insecta; Order: Psocodea; Suborder: Amblycera; Family: Boopidae) is a large chewing louse louse found on the skin of dogs and other carnivores, largely in tropical and subtropical regions between latitudes 40° N and 40° S.

Epidemiology: Infection occurs after direct contact with an infested host animal. Cross-contamination between different host species is possible if the animals have physical contact.

Pathogenesis: Lice infestations often accompany manifestations of poor health such as internal parasitism, infectious disease, malnutrition and poor sanitation. This species may transmit the tapeworm *Dipylidium caninum* when lice are ingested during grooming.

Notes: It is thought that *H. spiniger* evolved in Australasia as a louse of marsupials that subsequently switched to dingo hosts, and now parasitises a number of canids and other carnivores. *Heterodoxus spiniger* can be found anywhere on the body of the host.

Linognathus setosus

Linognathus setosus (Phylum: Arthropoda; Class: Insecta; Order: Psocodea; Suborder: Anoplura; Family: Linognathidae), commonly known as the Dog sucking louse, is a sucking louse found on the skin of dogs, particularly on the head and neck areas, and occurs worldwide.

Epidemiology: Generally, for the transfer of louse infestation, close bodily contact is necessary. Lice dropped or pulled from the host die in a few days, but eggs that have fallen from the host may continue to hatch over 2–3 weeks in warm weather. Therefore, bedding used by infested hosts should be disinfected.

Pathogenesis: *Linognathus setosus* is a common and widespread parasite of dogs, particularly the long ears of breeds such as the spaniel, basset and Afghan hounds. It may cause anaemia and is usually of greater pathogenic significance in younger animals. *Linognathus setosus* is primarily found in the head and neck areas and is especially common under the collar.

Linognathus setosus has been shown to harbour immature stages of the filarial nematode *Acanthocheilonema reconditum*, which parasitises dogs. However, it is unknown whether the lice act as efficient vectors of these parasites.

Trichodectes canis

Trichodectes canis (Phylum: Arthropoda; Class: Insecta; Order: Pscoptera; Suborder: Ischnocera; Family: Trichodectidae), commonly known as the Dog biting louse, is a chewing louse found on the skin of dogs and wild canids, most commonly in the head, neck and tail regions. It occurs worldwide.

Pathogenesis: *Trichodectes canis* can be a harmful ectoparasite of dogs, particularly in puppies and old or debilitated dogs. It is most commonly found on the head, neck and tail attached to the base of hairs. It feeds on tissue debris. It is a highly active species and infestation produces intense irritation around predilection sites. Lice often congregate around body orifices or wounds seeking moisture. Intense pruritus, scratching, biting, sleeplessness, nervousness and a matted coat are all typical of *T. canis* infestation. Skin damage caused by scratching results in inflammation, excoriation, alopecia and secondary bacterial involvement.

Trichodectes canis is important as a vector of the tapeworm *Dipylidium caninum*. Lice become infected when they ingest

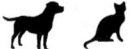

D. caninum eggs from dried host faeces. The tapeworm develops into a cysticercoid stage within the louse, where it remains quiescent until the louse is ingested by a dog during grooming. In the gut of the dog, the cystercoid is liberated and develops into an adult tapeworm.

FLIES

Psychodidae

Phlebotomus/Lutzomyia spp. (Phylum: Arthropoda; Class: Insecta; Order: Diptera; Sub-class: Nematocera; Family: Psychodidae), commonly known as Phlebotomine sand flies, are blood-feeding flies that feed on a wide range of mammals, reptiles, birds and humans. These insects bite areas of exposed skin such as the ears, eyelids, nose, feet and tail. The genus *Phlebotomus* is of veterinary importance in the Old World and *Lutzomyia* is of importance in the New World. They are widely distributed in the tropics, subtropics and the Mediterranean area. Most species prefer semi-arid and savannah regions to forests.

Epidemiology: In common with many other small biting flies, only the females suck blood. They prefer to feed at night, resting in shaded areas during the day. Since they are capable of only limited flight, nuisance due to biting may be confined to certain areas near the breeding sites. There is some seasonality in activity, the numbers of flies increasing during the rainy season in the tropics, whereas they are only present during the summer months in temperate zones. Adults often accumulate in the burrows of rodents or in other shelters, such as caves, where the microclimate is suitable.

Pathogenesis: These flies inflict a painful bite, causing irritation and blood loss, which may lead to a reduction in weight gain. Apart from their biting nuisance in localised areas, phlebotomine sand flies are important as vectors of various pathogens. Of particular importance is leishmaniosis in humans and dogs, caused by the protozoan *Leishmania* spp. The diseases caused in humans are commonly classified as either visceral (kala-azar) or cutaneous infections. Dogs, cats, rodents and other wild animals act as reservoirs of infection. Dogs affected with cutaneous leishmaniosis have a non-pruritic exfoliative dermatitis with alopecia and peripheral lymphadenopathy. Systemic leishmaniosis leads to splenomegaly, hepatomegaly, generalised lymphadenopathy, lameness, anorexia, weight loss and death. The disease has also been reported in cats. In North America, sand flies may also act as vectors of vesicular stomatitis of cattle and horses, which is caused by a rhabdovirus.

Clinical signs: The bites of these flies are painful and irritating to the host, giving rise to wheals in soft-skinned animals. Sand flies particularly bite areas of exposed skin such as the ears, eyelids, nose, feet and tail.

Diagnosis: Sand flies may be visible on the host during the night. During the day, sand flies can most often be collected in the field and are not usually seen on animals.

Control and treatment: There have been few large-scale attempts to control phlebotomine sand flies, probably due to the fact that leishmaniosis has merited insufficient attention as a disease, and also because little is known in detail of the biology and ecology of the developing stages of these flies. The adults are, however, susceptible to most insecticides, and where there have been spraying campaigns to control the mosquito vectors of malaria, these have effectively controlled *Phlebotomus*. Removal of dense vegetation may reduce the suitability of the environment for the breeding of these flies.

The most effective method to prevent fly bites and transmission of infection is to ensure that animals avoid areas of high fly density and are kept indoors when fly activity is highest. Flies spend limited time on their hosts and are difficult to control using insecticides unless these have rapid killing or repellent activity. Permethrin and deltamethrin are the only insecticides with sufficient repellent activity and rapidity of action to make them suitable for the control of sand fly biting in dogs. Neither drug is suitable for cats.

Notes: The large family Psychodidae, subfamily Phlebotominae contains a single genus of veterinary importance in the Old World, *Phlebotomus*, and a single genus of veterinary importance in the New World, *Lutzomyia*. In some areas of the world, the term 'sand flies' includes some biting midges and blackflies, so phlebotomines should be distinguished by referring to them as 'phlebotomine sand flies'.

CULICIDAE

Culicidae (Phylum: Arthropoda; Class: Insecta; Order: Diptera; Sub-Order: Nematocera; Family: Culicidae) are a diverse group of over 3000 species. They occur worldwide from the tropics to the Arctic. There are three genera of medical and veterinary importance: *Anopheles*, *Aedes* and *Culex*.

Pathogenesis: Mosquitoes may cause considerable annoyance by biting. Mosquito populations can reach large sizes, especially in parts of the southern USA. Several species of *Aedes*, *Culex* and *Anopheles* can be vectors of the dog heartworm, *Dirofilaria immitis*, although this occurs mainly in tropical and subtropical regions. *Aedes sierrensis* is one of the main carriers of *D. immitis* and will attack mammals of all sizes.

See Chapters 3 and 8 for further details.

Cordylobia anthropophaga

Cordylobia anthropophaga (Phylum: Arthropoda; Class: Insecta; Order: Diptera; Family: Calliphoridae), commonly known as the Tumbu, Mango or Putzi fly, is an agent of subcutaneous myiasis found in sub-Saharan Africa where the domestic dog is an important host.

Pathogenesis: The larvae develop under the skin and produce a painful swelling, 10 mm in diameter, with a small central opening. The swelling is initially pruritic, becoming more painful as the larva grows. Serous fluid may exude from the lesion.

BUGS

Triatoma and Rhodnius

Rhodnius, *Triatoma* and *Panstrongylus* (Phylum: Arthropoda; Class: Insecta; Order: Hemiptera; Family: Reduviidae), also commonly kown as Triatome, Cone-nose, Kissing or Assassin bugs, are

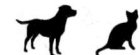

blood feeders on a wide range of wild and domestic animals, including dogs, cats, cattle, sheep, goats and humans. Over 100 species are found in South and Central America and the southern and midwestern USA, predominantly in tropical regions. Important species include *Triatoma infestans* and *Rhodnius prolixus*. However, five species of *Linshcosteus* are found in India and seven species of *Triatoma* are found in Southeast Asia and one in Africa.

Epidemiology: Some species of triatomine bug, including *Triatoma infestans*, live in and near human dwellings and poultry houses where they hide in cracks and crevices in the structure. During the night, they emerge to search for warm-blooded hosts. The interval between feeding and defecation is critical in determining the effectiveness of disease transmission. Infected dogs provide a reservoir of infection for the vector and thus human infection.

Pathogenesis: Triatomines are important vectors of the protozoan *Trypanosoma cruzi*. This causes Chagas disease in humans and a disease of similar pathology in dogs. Although cats are susceptible to infection, there are no reports of clinical disease. As it feeds, the bug defecates and the parasite is transmitted in the faeces which is rubbed into the feeding wound or into the eyes or the mouth. Infection may also be transmitted by the ingestion of infected bugs or infected prey.

Clinical signs: The bite causes irritation and swelling. Heavy infestations in poultry houses may result in chronic blood loss and mortality in young birds.

Pathology: The lesions produced at the feeding site may vary considerably between individual hosts. The wounds created are usually seen as erythematous papules or wheals surrounding the central puncture site. The wheals may persist for several weeks. Pruritis may be intense, resulting in secondary traumatic lesions.

Control and treatment: Long-term control of bugs in the domestic environment or animal house can be achieved by spraying dwellings with formulations of pyrethroid insecticide. This is often enough to eliminate existing populations of the bugs within a house, although reintroductions are possible. Dogs may be treated with pour-on formulations of pyrethroid insecticide to repel or kill host-seeking bugs.

MITES

Infestation by mites is called acariasis and can result in severe dermatitis, known as mange, which may cause significant welfare problems and economic losses.

All mites are small, usually less than 1 mm in length. The body shows no segmentation, although it can have various sutures and grooves. Adult and nymphal mites have four pairs of legs; larvae have only three pairs. The body is usually soft but may carry a number of hardened plates. Eyes are usually absent and hence most mites are blind. Hairs, or setae, many of which are sensory in function, cover the body of many species of mite. The mouthparts are highly specialised, consisting of a pair of chelicerae, which may be used for tearing, grasping or piercing.

Cheyletiella blakei

Cheyletiella blakei (Phylum: Arthropoda; Class: Arachnida; Subclass: Acari; Order: Trombidiformes (Prostigmata); Family: Cheyletidae) is found on the skin of cats, usually on the face, but may spread all over the body. It is found worldwide.

Epidemiology: This highly contagious, though mild, mange can spread rapidly through catteries and kennels. Transmission is usually by direct contact with infested animals, but the adult parasite can survive for over 10 days off the host and therefore bedding and furniture can act as a source of infestation. *Cheyletiella* mites may be phoretic on cat and dog fleas (*Ctenocephalides* spp.) and may be transmitted by these ectoparasites.

Pathogenesis: The mite is not usually highly pathogenic and is more often found in young animals in good physical condition. Long-haired cats tend to be more commonly infested than short-haired cats. This parasite is readily transferred to humans even on short contact, where it causes severe irritation and intense pruritus. A positive diagnosis on a pet may be associated with a history of persistent skin rash in the owner's family. Human cases will resolve spontaneously when the animal source has been treated.

Clinical signs and pathology: *Cheyletiella blakei* most commonly infests the facial area of cats, causing mild eczema-like skin conditions and associated pruritus. It is a characteristic of the dermatitis caused by *Cheyletiella* that many skin scales are shed into the fur, giving it a powdery or mealy appearance, and the presence of moving mites among this debris has given it the common name of 'walking dandruff'. The pathology of *Cheyletiella* infestation is poorly understood. In many cases, there is very little skin reaction or pruritus. In the rare severe case, heavy infestations can result in the formation of small, crusty, erythematous papules involving much of the body surface; crusts are formed, but often there is only slight hair loss.

Diagnosis: In any case of excessive scurf or dandruff in the cat, *Cheyletiella* should be considered in the differential diagnosis. On parting the coat along the back, and especially over the sacrum, scurf will be seen, and if this is combed out onto dark paper, the movement of mites will be detected among the debris. Scraping is not necessary as the mites are always on the skin surface or in the coat.

Control and treatment: The cats, all in-contact animals and their surroundings should be treated to control infestation rates. This is particularly important in catteries, which often serve as a source of mite infestation.

Cats can be treated with a number of topical acaricidal shampoos, such as carbamates (e.g. carbaryl) and fipronil. Selenium sulfide shampoos have also been recommended for cats. Some products with low residual activity may require three successive weekly treatments.

Cheyletiella yasguri

Cheyletiella yasguri (Phylum: Arthropoda; Class: Arachnida; Subclass: Acari; Order: Trombidiformes (Prostigmata); Family: Cheyletidae) is found on the skin of dogs, usually on the dorsum and head but may spread all over the body. It is found worldwide.

Clinical signs and pathology: The mite is not highly pathogenic and is often found in young animals in good physical condition. *Cheyletiella* may be more common on short-haired breeds of dog and many individuals act as asymptomatic carriers. It is a

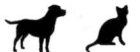

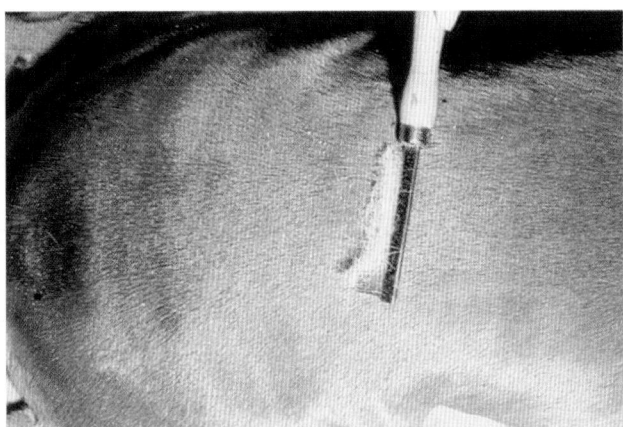

Fig. 12.8 Marked 'dandruff' associated with *Cheyletiella* infection.

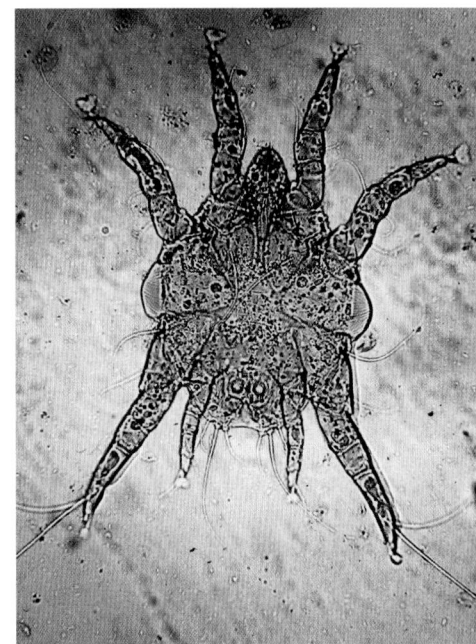

Fig. 12.9 Male *Otodectes cynotis*.

characteristic of the dermatitis caused by *Cheyletiella* that many skin scales are shed into the hair or fur, giving it a powdery or mealy appearance (Fig. 12.8). There is very little skin reaction or pruritus. In the rare severe case, involving much of the body surface, crusts are formed but there is only slight hair loss. This parasite is readily transferred to humans even on short contact, where it causes severe irritation and intense pruritus. Cases will resolve spontaneously when the animal source has been treated.

Diagnosis: A positive diagnosis on a pet may be associated with a history of persistent skin rash in the owner's family.

Control and treatment: Dogs can be treated with a number of topical acaricidal shampoos, such as carbamates (e.g. carbaryl), organophosphates (e.g. phosmet, chlorpyrifos, malathion or diazinon), permethrin, amitraz and fipronil. Oral milbemycin may be effective. Some of the older products with low residual activity may require three successive weekly treatments.

All other details are as for *C. blakei*.

Otodectes cynotis

Otodectes cynotis (Phylum: Arthropoda; Class: Arachnida; Subclass: Acari; Order: Sarcoptiformes (Astigmata); Family: Psoroptidae), commonly known as the Ear mite, is localised in the external ear canal of dogs and cats and a number of other small mammals, including the ferret and red fox (Fig. 12.9). The mite may secondarily infest other parts of the body including the head, back, tip of tail and feet. It is found worldwide.

Epidemiology: Transfer may occur through direct contact or from infested female hosts to their pups or kittens.

Pathogenesis: Most animals harbour this mite and in adult animals it has almost a commensal association with the host, signs of irritation appearing only sporadically with the transient activity of the mites. The development of clinical signs reflects the development of allergic hypersensitivity by the host to antigenic substances produced by the mites while they are feeding. This can result in responses ranging from asymptomatic to severe otitis and convulsive seizures in different individual hosts. Young animals probably acquire the mites from their mothers during suckling.

Early in infections, there is a brownish waxy exudate in the ear canal, which becomes crusty (Fig. 12.10). The mites live deep in the crust, next to the skin. Secondary bacterial infection may result. Scratching may cause excoriation of the posterior surface of the ear pinna. The resultant violent head shaking and ear scratching are a common cause of aural haematomas. In long-standing cases a severe purulent otitis may result.

Clinical signs and pathology: In general, the ear canals become inflamed and excessively moistened with accumulations of brown-black exudates in cats and grey deposits. This is accompanied by pruritus and intense itching that causes the host to scratch the ears, shake the head or hold it to one side and turn in circles. Signs of severe untreated cases include emaciation, spasms, self-induced trauma and convulsions, including epileptiform fits. Perforation of the tympanic membrane can result. The clinical signs may be seen in dogs at an earlier stage than in cats and foxes, which do not appear to be affected until the infestation has reached high numbers

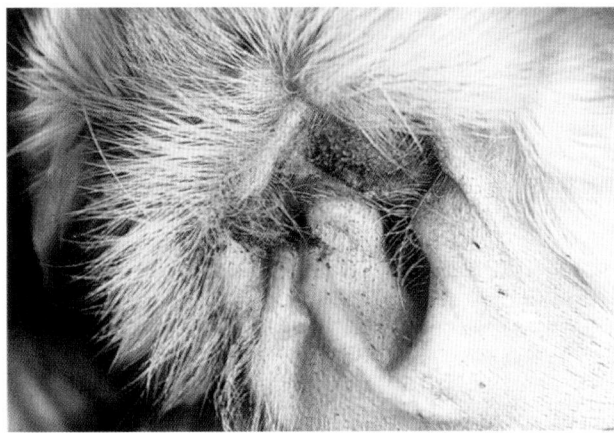

Fig. 12.10 Dark waxy exudate caused by *Otodectes* infection in the dog.

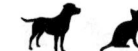

and the disease is advanced. The canal becomes full of cerumen, blood and mite faeces, giving rise to a characteristic otitis externa. Mechanical irritation may account for some of the pruritus but, in addition, the presence of IgE-like antibodies suggests that hypersensitivity also contributes to the pruritus.

Diagnosis: Tentative diagnosis is based on the behaviour of the animal and the presence of dark waxy deposits and exudate in the ear canal. Confirmation depends on observing the mites either within the ear or by removing some of the deposit and exudate and placing it on a dark surface where the mites will be seen by a hand lens as whitish moving specks.

Control and treatment: Any bedding should be replaced or thoroughly disinfected. In view of the ubiquity and high infectivity of the mite, all dogs or cats in the same household, or those in close contact in kennels and catteries, should be treated at the same time as clinically affected animals. In heavy infestations, concurrent whole-body treatment may also be required to kill any mites that have moved out of the ear canal.

Topical application of systemic selamectin and imidacloprid has been found to give good control in both dogs and cats. There are also many effective preparations available commercially as eardrops, including, for dogs, permethrin, thiabendazole and monosulfiram. With these preparations, treatment should be repeated to kill any newly hatched mites. In cats, treatments with milbemycin and ivermectin may be used, and in both cats and dogs fipronil eardrops may be effective. When eardrops are used, the ear canal should first be thoroughly cleaned; after the eardrops have been instilled, the base of the ear should be massaged to disperse the oily preparation.

Sarcoptes scabiei

Sarcoptes scabiei (Phylum: Arthropoda; Class: Arachnida; Subclass: Acari; Order: Sarcoptiformes (Astigmata); Family: Sarcoptidae), commonly known as the Scabies mite, is a burrowing mite found on all domestic mammals and humans worldwide.

Pathogenesis:

- Dogs. The predilection sites for the mites are thinly haired areas such as the ears (Fig. 12.11), muzzle, face and elbows but, as in other manges, severe infestations may extend over the whole body. Visually, the condition begins as erythema, with papule formation, and this is followed by scale and crust formation and alopecia (Fig. 12.12). It is a characteristic of this form of mange that there is intense pruritus, which often leads to self-inflicted trauma. After a primary infection, dogs begin to scratch within a week, often before lesions are visible. In cases that are neglected for a number of months, the whole skin surface may be involved, dogs becoming progressively weak and emaciated. A strong sour odour is a notable feature of this form of mange.
- Cats. Sarcoptic mange is rare in cats. In the few recorded cases, the changes have been similar to those in *Notoedres* infection, with progressive hair loss from the ears, face and neck, extending to the abdomen.

Clinical signs and pathology: Dogs with chronic generalised disease develop seborrhoea, severe thickening of the skin, crust build-up, peripheral lymphadenopathy and emaciation. However,

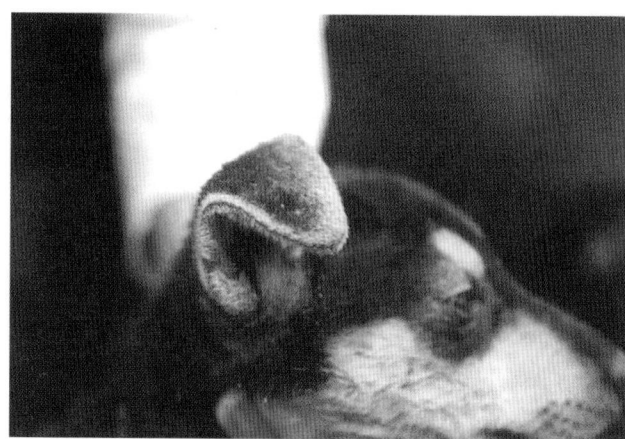

Fig. 12.11 Thickened ear edge characteristic of sarcoptic mange.

the lesions associated with canine sarcoptic mange are very nonspecific. Usually there is dramatic epidermal hyperplasia and a subtle, diffuse and uniform eosinophilic perivascular dermatitis. However, cases may present with no eosinophilic infiltrate and sacroptic mange should be a differential diagnosis for any hyperplastic pruritic dermatitis.

Control and treatment: Based on the protected location of the parasites, the duration of the life cycle and the necessity of killing all mites, dogs should be bathed weekly with an acaricidal preparation for four weeks, or longer if necessary, until lesions have disappeared. Because this is a highly contagious mange, affected dogs should be isolated and it should be explained to owners that rapid cure cannot be expected. To ensure that an outbreak is contained, all dogs on the premises should be treated if possible. In severely distressed dogs, oral or parenteral corticosteroids are valuable in reducing the pruritus and so preventing further excoriation.

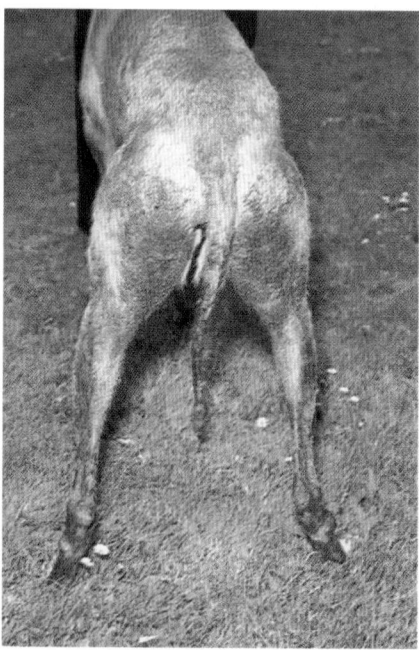

Fig. 12.12 Severe sarcoptic mange in a dog.

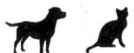

Treatment can be either topical or systemic. For topical treatment in dogs, effective acaricides include the organochlorines γ-hexachlorocyclohexane and bromocyclen, and organophosphates such as phosmet and amitraz, but the availability of some of these compounds is limited or non-existent in some countries. Lime-sulfur is highly effective and safe for use in young animals; several dips five days apart are recommended. Many preparations are combined with a surfactant, which aids contact with the mites by removing skin scales and softening crusts and other debris. Selamectin spot-on is effective. Other macrocyclic lactones, such as moxidectin and ivermectin, are not registered for the treatment of sarcoptic mange in dogs but have been reported to be effective, depending on the dosage and route of administration. Hair can be clipped, the crusts and dirt removed by soaking with a good antiseborrhoeic shampoo, and an acaricidal dip applied. In cats, lime-sulfur dips at 10-day intervals have been used. Selamectin spot-on may give good control, although this is not an approved application.

Control: For more detailed descriptions see Chapter 11.

Notoedres cati

Notoedres cati (Phylum: Arthropoda; Class: Arachnida; Subclass: Acari; Order: Sarcoptiformes (Astigmata); Family: Sarcoptidae), commonly known as the Notoedric cat mite, is found on the ears of domestic cats, but it may occasionally infest dogs or rabbits, also wild cats, foxes, canids and civets. It occurs worldwide.

Epidemiology: Notoedric mange is highly contagious and transmission from host to host is by the spread of larvae or nymphs. It occurs in local, limited outbreaks but usually the prevalence is very low. It is rarely seen in northern Europe, for example, but is more common in eastern Europe. Where it is present, it is more commonly encountered in neglected or feral animals and where cats are housed in groups.

Pathogenesis: *Notoedres cati* typically burrows in the stratum corneum and the stratum germinativum, occasionally invading hair follicles and sebaceous glands, causing hyperkeratosis and thickening of the epidermis. The infection appears as dry, encrusted, scaly lesions on the edges of the ears and on the face, the skin being thickened and somewhat leathery. Advanced lesions can give cats a wrinkled thickened skin with hyperkeratinisation and hyperpigmentation, causing an 'old age' appearance. The associated pruritus is often intense, and there may be severe excoriation of the head and neck from scratching. In typical cases the lesions appear first on the medial edge of the ear pinna and then spread rapidly over the ears, face, eyelids and neck. It may be spread to the feet and tail by contact when the cat grooms and sleeps.

Clinical signs and pathology: Intense pruritus, erythema, skin scaling, greyish-yellow crusts and loss of hair. Scratching, to alleviate itching, leads to excoriation of the skin, inflammation and secondary bacterial infections. If untreated, the affected animal can become severely debilitated and notoedric mange may be fatal in 4–6 months. Infestation is associated with erythematous dermatosis, marked epidermal hyperplasia, dermal inflammation consisting principally of mononuclear cells and regional lymphadenopathy.

Diagnosis: *Notoedres cati* occur in clumps in the skin, and are usually initially found around the head and ears causing an ear canker.

Transient dermatitis can occur in humans. Diagnosis may initially be based on the intense pruritus, the location of lesions and the rapid spread to involve all kittens in a litter. Confirmation is achieved by finding the mites in skin scrapings.

Control and treatment: All in-contact animals should be treated and bedding replaced. Skin crusts should first be softened with liquid paraffin or soap solution before applying an acaricide. Lime-sulfur dips at 10-day intervals may be used. A 1% solution of selenium sulfide is also recommended for use in cats; treatment should be given at weekly intervals for 4–6 weeks, the prognosis being good. Although not licensed for the treatment of cats, selamectin and ivermectin may prove effective against *Notoedres*, although sudden death in kittens has been reported with the use of ivermectin.

Notes: This genus has somewhat similar behaviour and pathogenesis to *Sarcoptes*, but has a more restricted host range.

Demodex canis

Demodex canis (Phylum: Arthropoda; Class: Arachnida; Subclass: Acari; Order: Trombidiformes (Prostigmata); Family: Demodicidae) is a parasite of dogs, localised in the hair follicles and sebaceous glands. It is found worldwide.

Epidemiology: Probably because of its location deep in the dermis, it is very difficult to transmit *Demodex* between animals unless there is prolonged contact. It is thought that most infections are acquired in the early weeks of life during suckling. This view is supported by the fact that lesions first appear on the muzzle, face, periorbital region and forelimbs.

Pathogenesis: For the most part, *Demodex* mites are non-pathogenic and form a normal part of the skin fauna. Occasionally they can cause significant clinical disease, particularly in dogs, where they cause demodectic mange or demodicosis.

Early in infection, there is a slight loss of hair on the face and forelimbs, followed by thickening of the skin (Fig. 12.13). The mange may progress no further than the in-contact areas; many of these localised mild infections resolve spontaneously without treatment. On the other hand, lesions may spread over the entire body, and this generalised demodicosis may take one of two forms.

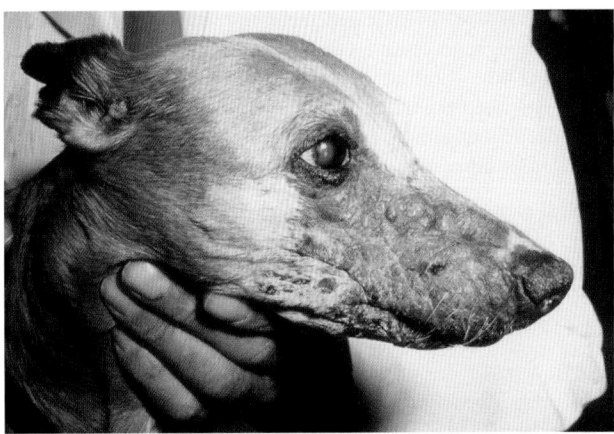

Fig. 12.13 Demodectic mange on the muzzle of a dog.

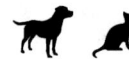

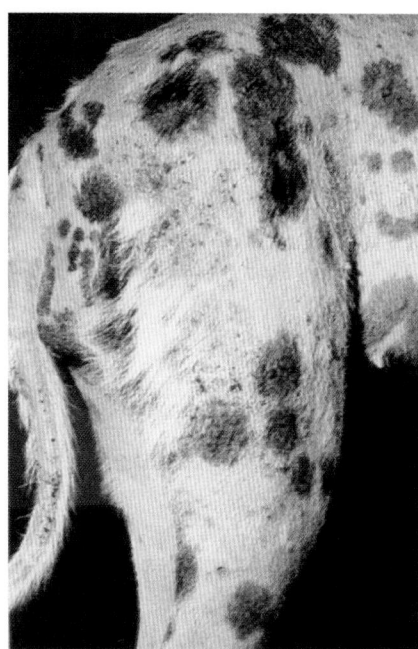

Fig. 12.14 Pustular demodectic mange.

- Squamous demodicosis is the less serious. It is a dry reaction, with little erythema but widespread alopecia, desquamation and thickening of the skin. In some cases of this type, only the face and paws are involved.
- Pustular or follicular demodicosis is the severe form, and follows bacterial invasion of the lesions, often by staphylococci. The skin becomes wrinkled and thickened, with many small pustules from which serum, pus and blood ooze, giving this form its common name of 'red mange' (Fig. 12.14). Affected dogs have an offensive odour. Prolonged treatment is necessary and survivors may be severely disfigured, so early euthanasia is sometimes requested by owners and by pedigree breeders.

The pathogenesis of *Demodex* is more complex than that of other mange mites because immune factors appear to play a large part in its occurrence and severity. It is thought that certain bitches carry a genetically controlled factor that results in immunodeficiency in their offspring, making them more susceptible to mite invasion. It has been observed that littermates from such a bitch often develop the generalised form of demodectic mange simultaneously, even though they have been reared separately. In addition, *Demodex* itself is thought to cause a cell-mediated immunodeficiency that suppresses the normal T-lymphocyte response. This defect disappears when the mites have been eradicated from the animal. Demodectic mange may erupt when dogs are given immunosuppressants for other conditions.

Clinical signs and pathology: In early infection, there is a slight loss of hair on the face and forelimbs, followed by thickening of the skin. Infection may resolve spontaneously or spread over the entire body. A common notable feature of all types of demodectic mange is the absence of pruritus, but this is not universal.

In squamous demodicosis, there is little erythema but widespread alopecia, desquamation and thickening of the skin. In severe pustular or follicular demodicosis, the lesions observed are variable and may include comedones, follicular papules and casts. More severely affected patients have deep folliculitis and furunculosis with severe haemorrhagic exudation and thick crusting. Demarcation between affected areas and normal skin is abrupt. Lymphadenopathy is common. There is bacterial invasion of the lesions, often by staphylococci. Dogs with chronic generalised demodicosis have depressed cell-mediated immune responsiveness, associated with the secondary bacterial infections. In some dogs only pododemodicosis is present. Pain and pedal oedema are especially prominent in large dogs.

Diagnosis: For confirmatory diagnosis, deep scrapings are necessary to reach the mites deep in the follicles and glands. This is best achieved by taking a fold of skin, applying a drop of liquid paraffin and scraping until capillary blood appears. Even in normal dogs, a few commensal mites may be found in the material but the presence of a high proportion of larvae and nymphs will indicate a rapidly increasing population and hence an active infection. Skin biopsy, to detect mites in the follicles, has been used in severely affected dogs but is rarely necessary.

Control and treatment: In controlling the endemicity of demodicosis, it should be noted that since certain bitches are more prone than others to have susceptible offspring, it may be advisable to discard these from breeding establishments.

Of the available acaricides, the most widely used is amitraz although the organophosphate cythioate may also be applied. With their deep location in the dermis, the mites are not readily accessible to most topically applied acaricides, so repeated treatment is necessary and rapid results should not be expected. In localised squamous mange, recovery may be expected in 1–2 months but in the generalised pustular form, the prognosis should indicate that recovery will take at least three months, and should, even so, be guarded.

Treatment with oral or injectable ivermectin 250–300 μg/kg, milbemycin 2 mg/kg and moxidectin 400 μg/kg have all been used successfully for generalised canine demodicosis. Ivermectin and moxidectin should be initiated at lower doses and patients monitored for possible adverse effects during therapy. Where pyoderma is severe, antibiotic therapy may be necessary.

Notes: Species of the genus *Demodex* are believed to form a group of closely related sibling species, which are highly specific to particular hosts: *Demodex phylloides* (pigs), *Demodex canis* (dogs), *Demodex bovis* (cattle), *Demodex equi* (horses), *Demodex musculi* (mice), *Demodex ratti* (rats), *Demodex caviae* (guinea pigs), *Demodex cati* (cats) and *Demodex folliculorum* and *Demodex brevis* (humans). Various morphological variations may be seen on a host, which are sometimes given separate species status.

Demodex cati

Demodex cati (Phylum: Arthropoda; Class: Arachnida; Subclass: Acari; Order: Trombidiformes (Prostigmata); Family: Demodicidae) is a parasite of cats, localised in the hair follicles and sebaceous glands. It is found worldwide.

Pathogenesis: Demodicosis is rare in cats. It manifests as a localised self-limiting form confined to the eyelids and periocular region and is of the mild squamous type, with some alopecia. Feline demodicosis is usually associated with underlying debilitating disease such as diabetes mellitus, FeLV infection and systemic lupus erythematosus.

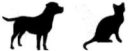

Clinical signs: Erythema, papules and thickened skin crusts, alopecia. Generalised demodicosis is very rare but has been reported with variable pruritus, alopecia, scaling, crusting and hyperpigmentation on the head, neck, legs and trunk.

Diagnosis: For confirmatory diagnosis, deep scrapings are necessary to reach the mites deep in the follicles and glands. This is best achieved by taking a fold of skin, applying a drop of liquid paraffin and scraping until capillary blood appears.

Control and treatment: Control is rarely applied. In cats, 2% lime-sulfur dips may be effective when given every 5–7 days for six dips; amitraz rinses at 0.0125–0.025% have also been used successfully. In many cases demodicosis in cats resolves spontaneously and treatment is unnecessary.

A number of non-specific ectoparasites, particularly fleas and ticks, are also found on dogs and cats and are listed in the host–parasite checklists at the end of this chapter.

Neotrombicula autumnalis

Neotrombicula autumnalis (Phylum: Arthropoda; Class: Arachnida; Subclass: Acari; Order: Trombidiformes (Prostigmata); Family: Trombiculidae), commonly known as the Harvest mite, is commonly found in clusters on the foot and up the legs of dogs, on the genital area and eyelids of cats, on the face of cattle and horses and on the heads of birds, having been picked up from the grass. This species is widespread within Europe.

Epidemiology: In Europe the activity of *N. autumnalis* is most pronounced in late summer and autumn, and larvae are most active on dry sunny days. They parasitise almost all domestic mammals, including humans, and some ground-nesting birds. *Neotrombicula autumnalis* may be particularly abundant in closely cropped chalk grassland but may also be found in wooded areas and scrub.

Clinical signs: Infestation can result in pruritus, erythema, wheals, papules and excoriation leading to hair loss.

Diagnosis: Small clusters of orange larval mites may be seen on the skin surface. Microscopic examination may then be used to identify individual species.

Control and treatment: Area-wide control is usually impractical, unnecessary and can result in environmental impacts; problems should be managed by avoidance of sites of known mite risk. In most cases, the dermatitis should resolve a few days after the larvae have left the skin, although acaridial treatment may be necessary. Topical acaricides, such as organophosphates (e.g. phosmet, chlorpyriphos, malathion or diazinon), fipronil or lime-sulfur can be used, depending on the host infested.

Eutrombicula alfreddugesi

Eutrombicula alfreddugesi (Phylum: Arthropoda; Class: Arachnida; Subclass: Acari; Order: Trombidiformes (Prostigmata); Family: Trombiculidae), commonly known as Chigger mites, are blood-feeding mites that infest a range of hosts including dogs, cats, cattle, horses, rabbits and birds. This species is the most important and widespread of the trombiculid mites of veterinary interest in the

New World. It is common from eastern Canada through to South America.

Epidemiology: *Eutrombicula alfreddugesi* is particularly common at the margins of woodland, scrub and grassland, but is not highly habitat specific. In the northern parts of its range, it may be most active between July and September whereas in more southern habitats, it may be active all year round. *Eutrombicula alfreddugesi* parasitises a wide range of mammals and birds.

Eutrombicula splendens

Eutrombicula splendens (Phylum: Arthropoda; Class: Arachnida; Subclass: Acari; Order: Trombidiformes (Prostigmata); Family: Trombiculidae), commonly known as the Chigger mite, is morphologically similar and frequently sympatric with *E. alfreddugesi* in North America. It is generally confined to the east of North America, from Ontario in Canada to the Gulf States, although it may also be abundant in Florida and parts of Georgia.

Lynxacarus radovskyi

Lynxacarus radovskyi (Phylum: Arthropoda; Class: Arachnida; Subclass: Acari; Order: Sarcoptiformes (Astigmata); Family: Epidermoptidae), commonly known as the Cat fur mite, is found on cats in tropical environments throughout North and South America and Australia.

Epidemiology: Transmission appears to occur by direct contact. The isolation of infested animals is therefore important to prevent further transmission to other animals in the household.

Pathogenesis: Common clinical signs are a dry, dull coat. Vomiting, constipation and hairballs may be caused by excess grooming induced by the infestation.

Diagnosis: The large eggs can be found attached to the hair of the cat. The mites can be found on the skin, particularly on the tail head, tail tip and perineal areas.

Treatment: Ivermectin 300 µg/kg administered subcutaneously is reported to be highly effective.

TICKS

Ixodes canisuga

Ixodes canisuga (Phylum: Arthropoda; Class: Arachnida; Order: Ixodida; Family: Ixodidae), commonly known as the Dog tick, is found on a range of mammals, particularly dogs but also foxes, sheep, horses and mules throughout Europe, as far east as Russia.

Epidemiology: This species, sometimes called the British dog tick, has been found in a variety of hosts. It is particularly recognised as a problem in kennels, where the tick is capable of survival in crevices and cracks in the floors and walls.

Pathogenesis: Infestation may cause dermatitis, pruritus, alopecia and anaemia, but it is not an important vector of disease. It may be a particular problem in packs of dogs in kennels.

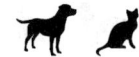

Treatment: In companion animals, topical acaricidal compounds such as fipronil (phenylpyrazole), imidacloprid (chloronicotinyl), selamectin (macrocyclic lactone), amitraz (formamidine), afoxolaner and fluralaner (isoxazolines) and the organophosphates (e.g. malathion, ronnel, chlorpyrifos, fenthion, dichlorvos, cythoate, diazinon, propetamphos, phosmet) and carbamates can be used to kill ticks on the host. Pyrethroids (e.g. permethrin, deltamethrin) should not be used on cats.

Ixodes ricinus

See Chapter 9.

Ixodes hexagonus

Ixodes hexagonus (Phylum: Arthropoda; Class: Arachnida; Order: Ixodida; Family: Ixodidae), commonly known as the Hedgehog tick, is found in Europe and northwest Africa on hedgehogs but also other mammals, particularly cats, but also dogs, foxes, sheep and horses.

Epidemiology: The main host is the European hedgehog, and the movement of this host to urbanised areas may increase the risk of both people and their animals being exposed to infectious diseases carried by *I. hexagonus*. The ticks may be active from early spring to late autumn, but are probably most active during April and May. This species inhabits sheltered habitats such as burrows and kennels and may infest pets in large numbers when they are exposed.

Pathogenesis: On dogs and cats, adult females usually attach themselves behind the ears, on the jaws, neck and groin, causing localised dermatitis and the risk of wound infection. These ticks are often found to be responsible when dogs become repeatedly infested with ticks, particularly around the head area. It may also become a more significant pest in places where *I. ricinus* is absent. *Ixodes hexagonus* is a biological vector of *Borrelia* spp. and the pathogens that cause tick-borne encephalitis.

Treatment: see *Ixodes canisuga*.

Dermacentor variabilis

Dermacentor variabilis (Phylum: Arthropoda; Class: Arachnida; Order: Ixodida; Family: Ixodidae), commonly known as the American dog tick or Wood tick, will feed on a wide range of domestic and wild mammal species, particularly on dogs, horses, cattle and humans, and is found in North America, to the east of the Rocky Mountains.

Epidemiology: The larval and nymphal stages feed on wild rodents, particularly the short-tailed meadow mouse (*Microtus* spp.), while the preferred hosts of adults are larger mammals, particularly wild and domestic carnivores.

Pathogenesis: *Dermacentor variabilis* is an important parasite of wild and domestic carnivores. The feeding activity of *D. variabilis* may cause tick paralysis in dogs. In cattle, it may transmit bovine anaplasmosis. It is also an important vector of *Rickettsia rickettsii* (Rocky Mountain spotted fever) in the USA and is able to transmit the bacteria which causes tularaemia (hunter's disease). It also transmits St Louis encephalitis virus and several studies have shown that it may carry the Lyme disease bacterium *Borrelia burgdorferi*.

Rhipicephalus sanguineus

Rhipicephalus sanguineus (Phylum: Arthropoda; Class: Arachnida; Order: Ixodida; Family: Ixodidae), commonly known as the Brown dog tick or Kennel tick, occurs worldwide, largely on dogs. It is often found in the ears and between the toes. This species is believed to have originated in Africa but is now considered to be the most widely distributed tick species in the world (see Chapter 3).

Pathogenesis: *Rhipicephalus sanguineus* is primarily parasitic on dogs and is responsible for the transmission of *Babesia canis* and *Ehrlichia canis* and can also cause tick paralysis in the dog. There seems little doubt that it can also transmit many protozoal, viral and rickettsial infections of animals and humans. These include *Theileria equi* and *B. caballi* of equines, *Anaplasma marginale* in North America, *Hepatozoon canis* of dogs, *Coxiella burnetii*, *Rickettsia conorii*, *R. canis*, *R. rickettsii*, *Pasteurella tularensis*, *Borrelia hispanica* and the viruses that cause Nairobi sheep disease and other viral diseases of sheep in Africa. *Rhipicephalus sanguineus* is also a vector for East Coast fever (*Theileria parva*) among cattle, *Babesia perroncitoi* and *B. trautmanni* among pigs, and also transmits Rocky Mountain spotted fever in some areas of the USA and Mexico.

Hyalomma marginatum

The adult form of *Hyalomma marginatum* (Phylum: Arthropoda; Class: Arachnida; Order: Ixodida; Family: Ixodidae) parasitises wild herbivores and livestock (particularly equines and ruminants). Immature stages primarily parasitise small wild mammals, lizards and birds. They are found throughout Africa, Asia Minor and southern Europe.

Pathogenesis: The salivary secretions of this species may produce tick paralysis. *Hyalomma marginatum* subspecies are important vectors of disease: in dogs they transmit *Babesia canis*; in cattle *Babesia ovis*, *Rickettsia aeschlimanii* and Crimean–Congo haemorrhagic fever; and in horses *Babesia caballi* and *Theileria equi*.

Another species of *Haemaphysalis* of veterinary importance in dogs and cats is shown in Table 12.16.

Table 12.16 *Haemaphysalis* sp. of veterinary importance in dogs and cats.

Species	Distribution	Hosts	Pathogenesis
Haemaphysalis leachi	Africa, Australia and Asia	Primarily dogs and wild carnivores but also occasionally cattle	*Babesia canis* in dogs, tick-bite fever *Rickettsia conorii* and *Coxiella burnetii* in cattle

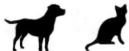

HOST–PARASITE CHECKLISTS

In the following checklists, the codes listed below apply.

Helminths

N, nematode; T, trematode; C, cestode; A, acanthocephalan.

Arthropods

F, fly; L, louse; S, flea; M, mite; Ti, tick; Pn, pentostomid.

Protozoa

Co, coccidia; Bs, blood sporozoa; Am, amoeba; Fl, flagellate; Ci, ciliate.

Miscellaneous 'protozoal organisms'

B, blastocyst; Mi, microsporidian; My, *Mycoplasma*; P, Pneumocystidomycete; R, *Rickettsia*.

Dog parasite checklist.

Section/host system	Helminths		Arthropods		Protozoa	
	Parasite	(Super) family	Parasite	Family	Parasite	Family
Digestive						
Mouth					*Tetratrichomonas canistomae*	Trichomonadidae (Fl)
Oesophagus	*Spirocerca lupi*	Spiruroidea (N)				
Stomach	*Ollulanus tricuspis*	Trichostrongyloidea (N)				
	Capillaria putorii	Trichuroidea (N)				
	Gnathostoma spinigerum	Spiruroidea (N)				
	Physaloptera praeputialis	Physalopteroidea (N)				
	Physaloptera rara	Physalopteroidea (N)				
	Spirura ritypleurites	Spiruroidea (N)				
	Spirocerca lupi	Spiruroidea (N)				
Small intestine	*Toxocara canis*	Ascaridoidea (N)			*Cystoisospora canis*	Sarcocystidae (Co)
	Toxocara leonina	Ascaridoidea (N)			*Cystoisospora ohioensis*	Sarcocystidae (Co)
	Ancylostoma caninum	Ancylostomatoidea (N)			*Hammondia hedorni*	Sarcocystidae (Co)
	Ancylostoma braziliense	Ancylostomatoidea (N)			*Sarcocystis bovicanis*	Sarcocystidae (Co)
	Ancylostoma ceylanicum	Ancylostomatoidea (N)			*Sarcoystis ovicanis*	Sarcocystidae (Co)
	Uncinaria stenocephala	Ancylostomatoidea (N)			*Sarcoystis suicanis*	Sarcocystidae (Co)
	Strongyloides stercoralis	Strongyloidoidea (N)			*Sarcoystis capracanis*	Sarcocystidae (Co)
	Diphyllobothrium latum	Diphyllobothriidae (C)			*Sarcoystis hircicanis*	Sarcocystidae (Co)
	Dipylidium caninum	Dilepididae (C)			*Sarcoystis equicanis*	Sarcocystidae (Co)
	Echinococcus granulosus	Taeniidae (C)			*Sarcoystis fayeri*	Sarcocystidae (Co)
	Echinococcus equinus	Taeniidae (C)			*Sarcoystis hovarthi*	Sarcocystidae (Co)
	Echinococcus orteleppi	Taeniidae (C)			*Sarcoystis cameli*	Sarcocystidae (Co)
	Echinococcus multilocularis	Taeniidae (C)			*Cryptosporidium parvum*	Cryptosporidiidae (Co)
	Echinococcus vogeli	Taeniidae (C)			*Cryptosporidium canis*	Cryptosporidiidae (Co)
	Spirometra mansoni	Diphyllobothriidae (C)			*Giardia intestinalis*	Giardiidae (Fl)
	Spirometra mansonoides	Diphyllobothriidae (C)				
	Taenia hydatigena	Taeniidae (C)				
	Taenia multiceps	Taeniidae (C)				
	Taenia ovis	Taeniidae (C)				
	Taenia pisiformis	Taeniidae (C)				
	Taenia serialis	Taeniidae (C)				
	Taenia crassiceps	Taeniidae (C)				
	Mesocestoides lineatus	Mesocestoididae (C)				
	Alaria alata	Diplostomatidae (T)				
	Alaria americana	Diplostomatidae (T)				
	Alaria canis	Diplostomatidae (T)				
	Alaria michiganensis	Diplostomatidae (T)				
	Heterophyes heterophyes	Heterophyidae (T)				
	Heterophyes nocens	Heterophyidae (T)				
	Metagonimus yokagawai	Heterophyidae (T)				
	Apophallus donicum	Opisthorchiidae				
	Apophallus muhlingi	Opisthorchiidae				
	Cryptocotyle lingua	Opisthorchiidae				
	Echinochasmus perfoliatus	Echinostomatidae (T)				
	Euparyphium ilocanum	Echinostomatidae (T)				
	Nanophyetus salmincola	Nanophyetidae (T)				
	Macracanthorhynchus hirudinaceus	Oligacanthorhynchidae				
	Macracanthorhynchus catalinum	Oligacanthorhynchidae				
	Oncicola canis	Oligacanthorhynchidae				
	Trichinella spiralis	Trichinelloidea (N)				
Caecum, colon	*Trichuris vulpis*	Trichuroidea (N)			*Entamoeba histolytica*	Entamoebidae (Am)
					Trichomonas intestinalis	Trichomonadidae (Fl)
					Pentatrichomonas hominis	Trichomonadidae (Fl)

Respiratory

Location	Parasite	Higher taxon
Nose	Eucoleus boehmi	Trichuroidea (N)
	Pneumonyssoides caninum	Halarachnidae (M)
	Linguatula serrata	Linguatulidae (Pn)
Trachea, bronchi	Oslerus (Filaroides) osleri	Metastrongyloidea (N)
Lung	Capillaria aerophila	Trichuroidea (N)
	Crenosoma vulpis	Metastrongyloidea (N)
	Filaroides hirthi	Metastrongyloidea (N)
	Filaroides milksi	Metastrongyloidea (N)
	Paragonimus westermani	Paragonimidae (T)
	Paragonimus kellicotti	Paragonimidae (T)
	Pneumocystis carinii	Pneumocystidaceae (P)

Liver

Parasite	Higher taxon
Fasciola hepatica	Fasciolidae (T)
Capillaria hepatica	Trichuroidea (N)
Clonorchis sinensis	Opisthorchiidae (T)
Opisthorchis felineus	Opisthorchiidae (T)
Metorchis albidus	Opisthorchiidae (T)
Metorchis conjunctus	Opisthorchiidae (T)
Parametorchis complexus	Opisthorchiidae (T)
Leishmania donovani complex	Trypanoscmatidae (Fl)
Hepatozoon canis	Hepatozoidae (Bs)

Pancreas

Parasite	Higher taxon
Pseudamphistomum truncatum	Opisthorchiidae (T)

Circulatory

Location	Parasite	Higher taxon
Blood	Angiostrongylus vasorum	Metastrongyloidea (N)
	Dirofilaria immitis	Filarioidea (N)
	Trypanosoma brucei brucei	Trypanosomatidae (Fl)
	Trypanosoma congolense	Trypanosomatidae (Fl)
	Trypanosoma evansi	Trypanosomatidae (Fl)
	Trypanosoma cruzi	Trypanosomatidae (Fl)
	Babesia canis canis	Babesiidae (Bs)
	Babesia canis rossi	Babesiidae (Bs)
	Babesia canis vogeli	Babesiidae (Bs)
	Babesia gibsoni	Babesiidae (Bs)
	Babesia vulpes	Theileriidae (Bs)
	Anaplasma phagocytophilum (platys)	Anaplasmataceae (R)
	Ehrlichia canis	Anaplasmataceae (R)
	Ehrlichia chaffeensis	Anaplasmataceae (R)
	Ehrlichia ewingii	Anaplasmataceae (R)
Blood vessels	Schistosoma japonicum	Schistosomatidae (T)
	Schistosoma spindale	Schistosomatidae (T)
	Schistosoma incognitum	Schistosomatidae (T)
	Heterobilharzia americana	Schistosomatidae (T)
	Rickettsia rickettsii	Rickettsiaceae (R)
	Rickettsia conorii	Rickettsiaceae (R)
	Rickettsia felis	Rickettsiaceae (R)
Lymphatics	Brugia pahangi	Filarioidea (N)
	Brugia malayi	Filarioidea (N)

Nervous

Location	Parasite	Higher taxon
CNS	Taenia solium	Taeniidae (C)
	Encephalitozoon cuniculi	Unikaryonidae (Mi)
	Toxoplasma gondii	Sarcocystidae (Co)
	Neospora caninum	Sarcocystidae (Co)
Eye	Thelazia callipaeda	Spiruroidea (N)
	Thelazia californiensis	Spiruroidea (N)

(Continued)

Dog parasite checklist. *Continued*

Section/host system	Helminths		Arthropods		Protozoa	
	Parasite	(Super) family	Parasite	Family	Parasite	Family
Reproductive/urogenital						
Kidneys	*Capillaria plica*	Trichuroidea (N)				
	Dioctophyma renale	Dioctophymatoidea (N)				
Locomotory						
Muscle	*Toxocara canis*	Ascaridoidea (N)			*Toxoplasma gondii*	Sarcocystidae (Co)
	Trichinella spiralis	Trichinelloidea (N)			*Hepatozoon americanum*	Hepatozoidae (Co)
					Trypanosoma cruzi	Trypanosomatidae (Fl)
Connective tissue						
Subcutaneous	*Acanthocheilonema reconditum*	Filarioidea (N)	*Cordylobia anthropophaga*	Calliphoridae (F)		
	Acanthocheilonema grassi	Filarioidea (N)	*Cochliomyia hominivorax*	Calliphoridae (F)		
	Acanthocheilonema dracunculoides	Filarioidea (N)	*Cochliomyia macellaria*	Calliphoridae (F)		
	Dirofilaria repens	Filarioidea (N)	*Chrysomya bezziana*	Calliphoridae (F)		
	Dracunculus medinensis	Dracunculoidea (N)	*Chrysomya megacephala*	Sarcophagidae (F)		
	Dracunculus insignis	Dracunculoidea (N)	*Wohlfahrtia magnifica*	Sarcophagidae (F)		
	Rhabditis strongyloides (Pelodera)	Rhabditoidea (N)	*Wohlfahrtia meigeni*	Sarcophagidae (F)		
			Wohlfahrtia vigil	Oestridae (F)		
			Dermatobia hominis			
Integument						
Skin			*Heterodoxus spiniger*	Boopidae (M)	*Leishmania donovani* complex	Trypanosomatidae (Fl)
			Linognathus setosus	Linognathidae (L)	*Leishmania tropica*	Trypanosomatidae (Fl)
			Trichodectes canis	Trichodectidae (L)	*Leishmania aethiopica*	Trypanosomatidae (Fl)
			Cheyletiella yasguri	Cheyletidae (M)	*Leishmania major*	Trypanosomatidae (Fl)
			Otodectes cyanoti	Psoroptidae (M)	*Leishmania peruviana*	Trypanosomatidae (Fl)
			Sarcoptes scabiei	Sarcoptidae (M)		
			Notoedres cati	Sarcoptidae (M)		
			Demodex canis	Demodicidae (M)		
			Dermanyssus gallinae	Dermanyssidae (M)		
			Neotrombicula autumnalis	Trombiculidae (M)		
			Ceratophyllus gallinae	Ceratophyllidae (S)		
			Ctenocephalides canis	Pulicidae (S)		
			Ctenocephalides felis	Pulicidae (S)		
			Pulex irritans	Pulicidae (S)		
			Archaeopsylla erinacei	Pulicidae (S)		
			Spilopsyllus cuniculi	Pulicidae (S)		
			Echidnophaga gallinacea	Pulicidae (S)		

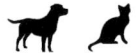

The following species of flies and ticks are found on dogs. More detailed descriptions can be found in Chapter 3.

Flies of veterinary importance on dogs.

Group	Genus	Species	Family
Blackflies Buffalo gnats	Simulium	spp.	Simuliidae (F)
Bot flies	Dermatobia	hominis	Oestridae (F)
Midges	Culicoides	spp.	Ceratopogonidae (F)
Mosquitoes	Aedes	spp.	Culicidae (F)
	Anopheles	spp.	
	Culex	spp.	
Muscids	Musca	domestica	Muscidae (F)
	Stomoxys	calcitrans	
Sand flies	Phlebotomus	spp.	Psychodidae (F)
Screwworms and blowflies	Chrysomya	albiceps bezziana megacephala	Calliphoridae (F)
	Cochliomyia	hominivorax macellaria	
	Cordylobia	anthropophaga	
Tabanids	Chrysops	spp.	Tabanidae (F)
	Haematopota	spp.	
	Tabanus	spp.	

Tick species found on dogs.

Genus	Species	Common name	Family
Otobius	megnini	Spinose ear tick	Argasidae (Ti)
Ornithodoros	moubata	Eyed tampan	Argasidae (Ti)
	porcinus		
Amblyomma	americanum	Lone Star tick	Ixodidae (Ti)
	cajennense	Cayenne tick	
	hebraeum	South African bont tick	
	maculatum	Gulf Coast tick	
	variegatum	Tropical bont tick	
Dermacentor	andersoni	Rocky Mountain wood tick	Ixodidae (Ti)
	pictus		
	eticulatus	Marsh tick	
	variabilis	American dog tick	
	venustus		
Haemaphysalis	bispinosa	New Zealand cattle or bush tick	Ixodidae (Ti)
	concinna		
	leachi	Yellow dog tick	
	punctata		
Hyalomma	marginatum	Bont-legged tick	Ixodidae (Ti)
	dromedarii	Camel Hyalomma	
	aegypticum	Tortoise Hyalomma	
Ixodes	canisuga	British dog tick	Ixodidae (Ti)
	hexagonus	Hedgehog tick	
	ricinus	Castor bean or European sheep tick	
	holocyclus	Australian paralysis tick	
	pacificus	Western black-legged tick	
	persulcatus	Taiga tick	
	rubicundus	South African paralysis tick	
	scapularis	Shoulder or black-legged tick	
Rhipicephalus	appendiculatus	Brown ear tick	Ixodidae (Ti)
	bursa		
	capensis	Cape brown tick	
	evertsi	Red-legged tick	
	sanguineus	Brown dog or kennel tick	
	simus		
Rhipicephalus (Boophilus)	annulatus	Texas cattle fever tick	Ixodidae (Ti)
	mircoplus	Pantropical cattle tick	

Cat parasite checklist.

Section/host system	Helminths		Arthropods		Protozoa	
	Parasite	(Super) family	Parasite	Family	Parasite	Family
Digestive						
Mouth					Tetratrichomonas felistomae	Trichomonadidae (Fl)
Oesophagus	Spirocerca lupi	Spiruroidea (N)				
Stomach	Ollulanus tricuspis	Trichostrongyloidea (N)				
	Gnathostoma spinigerum	Spiruroidea (N)				
	Physaloptera praeputialis	Physalopteroidea (N)				
	Physaloptera rara	Physalopteroidea (N)				
	Spirura ritypleurites	Spiruroidea (N)				
	Capillaria putorii	Trichuroidea (N)				
Small intestine	Toxascaris leonina	Ascaridoidea (N)			Cystoisospora felis	Sarcocystidae (Co)
	Toxocara mystax	Ascaridoidea (N)			Cystoisospora rivolta	Sarcocystidae (Co)
	Toxocara malayiensis	Ascaridoidea (N)			Hammondia hammondi	Sarcocystidae (Co)
	Ancylostoma braziliense	Ancylostomatoidea (N)			Sarcocystis bovifelis	Sarcocystidae (Co)
	Ancylostoma ceylanicum	Ancylostomatoidea (N)			Sarcocystis ovifelis	Sarcocystidae (Co)
	Ancylostoma tubaeforme	Ancylostomatoidea (N)			Sarcocystis porcifelis	Sarcocystidae (Co)
	Uncinaria stenocephala	Ancylostomatoidea (N)			Sarcocystis hircifelis	Sarcocystidae (Co)
	Strongyloides stercoralis	Strongyloidoidea (N)			Sarcocystis cuniculi	Sarcocystidae (Co)
	Strongyloides planiceps	Strongyloidoidea (N)			Sarcocystis muris	Sarcocystidae (Co)
	Strongyloides felis	Strongyloidoidea (N)			Besnoitia besnoiti	Sarcocystidae (Co)
	Strongyloides tumefaciens	Strongyloidoidea (N)			Cryptosporidium parvum	Cryptosporidiidae (Co)
	Diphyllobothrium latum	Diphyllobothriidae (C)			Cryptosporidium felis	Cryptosporidiidae (Co)
	Dipylidium caninum	Dilepididae (C)			Giardia intestinalis	Giardiidae (Fl)
	Echinococcus multilocularis	Taeniidae (C)				
	Echinococcus oligarthrus	Taeniidae (C)				
	Taenia taeniaeformis	Taeniidae (C)				
	Spirometra mansoni	Diphyllobothriidae (C)				
	Spirometra mansonoides	Diphyllobothriidae (C)				
	Spirometra erinacei	Diphyllobothriidae (C)				
	Mesocestoides lineatus	Mesocesoididae (C)				
	Alaria alata	Diplostomatidae (T)				
	Alaria minnesotae	Diplostomatidae (T)				
	Alaria marcianae	Diplostomatidae (T)				
	Heterophyes heterophyes	Heterophyidae (T)				
	Metagonimus yokagawai	Heterophyidae (T)				
	Heterophyes nocens	Heterophyidae (T)				
	Apophallus donicum	Opisthorchiidae				
	Apophallus muhlingi	Opisthorchiidae				
	Cryptocotyle lingua	Opisthorchiidae				
	Echinochasmus perfoliatus	Echinostomatidae (T				
	Euparyphium melis	Echinostomatidae (T)				
	Nanophyetus salmincola	Nanophyetidae (T)				
	Macracanthorhynchus hirudinaceus	Oligacanthorynchidae (A)				
	Macracanthorhynchus catalinum	Oligacanthorynchidae (A)				
	Oncicola campanulatus	Oligacanthorynchidae (A)				
Caecum, colon	Trichuris vulpis	Trichuroidea (N)			Entamoeba histolytica	Entamoebidae (Am)
	Trichuris serrata	Trichuroidea (N)			Pentatrichomonas hominis	Trichomonadidae (Fl)
	Trichuris campanula	Trichuroidea (N)			Tritrichomonas foetus	Trichomonadidae (Fl)

Location	Parasite	Taxon	Parasite	Taxon
Respiratory				
Nose			*Linguatula serrata*	Linguatulidae (Pn)
Trachea, bronchi				
Lung	*Capillaria aerophila*	Trichuroidea (N)		
	Aelurostrongylus abstrusus	Metastrongyloidea (N)		
	Troglostrongylus brevior	Metastrongyloidea (N)		
	Oslerus rostratus	Metastrongyloidea (N)		
	Metathelazia californica	Metastrongyloidea (N)		
	Mammomonogamus ierei	Strongyloidea (N)		
	Mammomonogamus mcgaughei	Strongyloidea (N)		
	Paragonimus westermani	Paragonimidae (T)		
	Paragonimus kellicotti	Paragonimidae (T)		
Liver	*Capillaria hepatica*	Trichuroidea (N)	*Leishmania donovani* complex	Trypanosomatidae (Fl)
	Fasciola hepatica	Fasciolidae (T)		
	Clonorchis sinensis	Opisthorchiidae (T)		
	Opisthorchis felineus	Opisthorchiidae (T)		
	Opisthorchis viverrini	Opisthorchiidae (T)		
	Metorchis albidus	Opisthorchiidae (T)		
	Metorchis conjunctus	Opisthorchiidae (T)		
	Parametorchis complexus	Opisthorchiidae (T)		
	Pseudamphistomum truncatum	Opisthorchiidae (T)		
	Eurytrema procyonis	Dicrocoeliidae (T)		
	Platynostomum fastosum	Dicrocoeliidae (T)		
Pancreas	*Eurytrema procyonis*	Dicrocoeliidae (T)		
	Platynosomum fastosum	Dicrocoeliidae (T)		
	Pseudamphistomum truncatum	Opisthorchiidae (T)		
Circulatory				
Blood	*Schistosoma japonicum*	Schistosomatidae (T)	*Trypanosoma brucei brucei*	Trypanosomatidae (Fl)
			Trypanosoma cruzi	Trypanosomatidae (Fl)
			Babesia felis	Babesiidae (Bs)
			Cytauxzoon felis	Theileriidae (Bs)
Blood vessels	*Dirofilaria immitis*	Filarioidea (N)	Hepatozoon spp.	Hepatozoidae (Bs)
Lymphatics	*Schistosoma rodhaini*	Schistosomatidae (T)	*Rickettsia felis*	Rickettsiaceae (R)
	Brugia pahangi	Filarioidea (N)	*Mycoplasma haemofelis*	Mycoplasmataceae (My)
	Brugia malayi	Filarioidea (N)	(syn. *Haemobartonella felis*)	

(Continued)

Cat parasite checklist. *Continued*

Section/host system	Helminths Parasite	(Super) family	Arthropods Parasite	Family	Protozoa Parasite	Family
Nervous						
CNS					*Encephalitozoon cuniculi*	Unikaryonidae (Mi)
					Toxoplasma gondii	Sarcocystidae (Co)
Eye	*Thelazia californiensis*	Spiruroidea (N)				
	Thelazia callipaeda	Spiruroidea (N)				
	Onchocerca lupi	Filarioidea (N)				
Reproductive/urogenital						
Kidneys	*Capillaria plica*	Trichuroidea (N)				
	Capillaria feliscati	Trichuroidea (N)				
	Dioctophyma renale	Dioctophymatoidea (N)				
Locomotory						
Muscle	*Toxocara mystax*	Ascaridoidea (N)			*Toxoplasma gondii*	Sarcocystidae (Co)
	Trichinella spiralis	Trichuroidea (N)			*Trypanosoma cruzi*	Trypanosomatidae (Fl)
Connective tissue						
Subcutaneous	*Dirofilaria repens*	Filarioidea (N)	*Cordylobia anthropophaga*	Calliphoridae (F)		
	Dracunculus medinensis	Dracunculoidea (N)	*Cochliomyia hominivorax*	Calliphoridae (F)		
	Dracunculus insignis	Dracunculoidea (N)	*Cochliomyia macellaria*	Calliphoridae (F)		
			Chrysomya bezziana	Calliphoridae (F)		
			Chrysomya megacephala	Calliphoridae (F)		
			Wohlfahrtia magnifica	Sarcophagidae (F)		
			Wohlfahrtia meigeni	Sarcophagidae (F)		
			Wohlfahrtia vigil	Sarcophagidae (F)		
			Dermatobia hominis	Oestridae (F)		
Integument						
Skin	*Cercopithifilaria bainae*	Spiruroidea (N)	*Felicola subrostratus*	Trichodectidae (L)	*Leishmania donovani* complex	Trypanosomatidae (Fl)
	Cercopithifilaria grassii	Spiruroidea (N)	*Demodex cati*	Demodicidae (M)		
			Otodectes cynotis	Psoroptidae (M)		
			Noteodres cati	Sarcoptidae (M)		
			Sarcoptes scabiei	Sarcoptidae (M)		
			Cheyletiella blakei	Cheyletidae (M)		
			Lynxacarus radovskyi	Epidermoptidae (M)		
			Cheyletiella parasitovorax	Cheyletidae (M)		
			Neotrombicula autumnalis	Trombiculidae (M)		
			Dermanyssus gallinae	Dermanyssidae (M)		
			Ceratophyllus gallinae	Ceratophyllidae (S)		
			Ctenocephalides canis	Pulicidae (S)		
			Ctenocephalides felis	Pulicidae (S)		
			Pulex irritans	Pulicidae (S)		
			Spilopsyllus cuniculi	Pulicidae (S)		
			Archaeopsylla erinacei	Pulicidae (S)		
			Echidnophaga gallinacea	Pulicidae (S)		

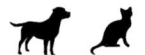

The following species of flies and ticks are found on cats. More detailed descriptions can be found in Chapter 3.

Flies of veterinary importance on cats.

Group	Genus	Species	Family
	Simulium	spp.	Simuliidae (F)
Bot flies	*Dermatobia*	*hominis*	Oestridae (F)
Midges	*Culicoides*	spp.	Ceratopogonidae (F)
Mosquitoes	*Aedes*	spp.	Culicidae (F)
	Anopheles	spp.	
	Culex	spp.	
Muscids	*Musca*	*domestica*	Muscidae (F)
	Stomoxys	*calcitrans*	
Sand flies	*Phlebotomus*	spp.	Psychodidae (F)
Screwworms and blowflies	*Chrysomya*	*albiceps* *bezziana* *megacephala*	Calliphoridae (F)
	Cochliomyia	*hominivorax* *macellaria*	
	Cordylobia	*anthropophaga*	
Tabanids	*Chrysops*	spp.	Tabanidae (F)
	Haematopota	spp.	
	Tabanus	spp.	

Tick species found on cats.

Genus	Species	Common name	Family
Otobius	*megnini*	Spinose ear tick	Argasidae (Ti)
Ornithodoros	*moubata*	Eyed tampan	Argasidae (Ti)
	porcinus		
Amblyomma	*americanum*	Lone Star tick	Ixodidae (Ti)
	cajennense	Cayenne tick	
	hebraeum	South African bont tick	
	maculatum	Gulf Coast tick	
	variegatum	Tropical bont tick	
Dermacentor	*andersoni*	Rocky Mountain wood tick	Ixodidae (Ti)
	pictus		
	reticulatus	Marsh tick	
	variabilis	American dog tick	
	venustus		
Haemaphysalis	*bispinosa*	Yellow dog tick	Ixodidae (Ti)
	concinna		
	leachi		
	punctata		
Ixodes	*dammini*		Ixodidae (Ti)
	hexagonus	Hedgehog tick	
	ricinus	Castor bean or European sheep tick	
	holocyclus	Australia paralysis tick	
	pacificus	Western black-legged tick	
	persulcatus	Taiga tick	
	pilosus	Russet, sour veld or bush tick	
	scapularis	Shoulder or black-legged tick	
Rhipicephalus	*evertsi*	Red or red-legged tick	Ixodidae (Ti)
	sanguineus	Brown dog or kennel tick	
	simus		

ENDOPARASITES

Parasites of the digestive system

OESOPHAGUS

Eucoleus annulata

Eucoleus annulata, synonym *Capillaria annulata* (Phylum: Nematoda; Class: Enoplea; Order: Enoplida; Family: Capillariidae), commonly known as Hairworms or Threadworms, occur worldwide in the oesophagus of chickens, turkeys, ducks and wild birds. This parasite has earthworms as intermediate hosts.

Epidemiology: Young birds are most susceptible to *Eucoleus* infections while adults may serve as carriers. The epidemiology is largely based on the ubiquity of the earthworm intermediate host.

Clinical signs and pathology: Like *Trichuris*, the anterior ends of the parasite are buried in the mucosa and even light infections can produce a catarrhal inflammation and thickening of the oesophagus and crop wall. Light infections of less than 100 worms may cause poor weight gain and lowered egg production. Heavy infections often induce inappetence and emaciation, diphtheritic inflammation and marked thickening of the wall; in such cases mortality may be high.

Diagnosis: Because of the non-specific nature of the clinical signs and the fact that, in heavy infections, these may appear before *Eucoleus* eggs are present in the faeces, diagnosis depends on necropsy and careful examination of the oesophagus and crop for the presence of the worms. This may be carried out by microscopic examination of mucosal scrapings squeezed between two glass slides; alternatively, the contents should be gently washed through a fine sieve and the retained material resuspended in water and examined against a black background.

Control and treatment: Control depends on regular anthelmintic treatment accompanied, if possible, by moving the birds to fresh ground. Scrubbing and heat treatment of affected surfaces are essential, as is the provision of fresh litter in chicken houses. Levamisole in the drinking water is highly effective, as are several benzimidazoles given in the feed. Elevated oral doses of these anthelmintics, administered over several days, also give high efficacy.

Notes: The taxonomy and systematics of these parasites have been changed many times because of a difficulty in designation of particular species' features and there are many synonyms in this group. Therefore, some species of *Capillaria* are now listed under the generic name *Eucoleus*, although they may still be universally referred to as *Capillaria*.

Eucoleus contorta

For details see section entitled Crop.

Gongylonema ingluvicola

For details see section entitled Crop.

Dispharynx nasuta

For details see section entitled Proventriculus.

Echinuria uncinata

For details see section entitled Proventriculus.

Trichomonas gallinae

Trichomonas gallinae, synonyms *Cercomonas gallinae*, *Trichomonas columbae* (Phylum: Metamonada; Class: Trichomonadea; Order: Trichomonadida; Family: Trichomonadidae), causes a disease commonly known as Canker, Frounce or Roup. It occurs worldwide in the oesophagus, crop and proventriculus of different species, such as pigeons, turkeys, chickens and raptors (e.g. hawks, falcons and eagles).

Epidemiology: Turkeys and chickens are infected through drinking contaminated water, the source of contamination being feral pigeons and other wild birds that also use the water source. Trichomonads enter the water from the mouths, not the faeces, of the wild birds. *Trichomonas gallinae* has no cysts and is very sensitive to drying, so direct contamination is necessary.

Clinical signs and pathology: In turkeys and chickens, lesions most commonly occur in the crop, oesophagus and pharynx and are uncommon in the mouth. Severely affected birds lose weight, stand huddled with ruffled feathers, and may fall over when forced to move. Yellow necrotic lesions are present in the oesophagus and

Veterinary Parasitology, Fifth Edition. Domenico Otranto and Richard Wall.
© 2024 John Wiley & Sons Ltd. Published 2024 by John Wiley & Sons Ltd.

crop and a greenish fluid containing large numbers of trichomonads may be found in the mouth. The early lesions in the pharynx, oesophagus and crop are small, whitish to yellowish caseous nodules. These may grow and remain circumscribed and separate, or may coalesce to form thick, caseous, necrotic masses that may occlude the lumen. The circumscribed disc-shaped lesions are often described as 'yellow buttons'. The lesions in the liver, lungs and other organs are solid, yellowish, caseous nodules up to 1 cm or more in diameter.

Diagnosis: The clinical signs are pathognomonic and can be confirmed by identifying the characteristic motile trichomonads from samples taken from lesions in the mouth or from fluid.

Control and treatment: Control in chickens and turkeys depends on preventing access of wild pigeons to drinking water. Nitroimidazole compounds, such as dimetridazole and metronidazole, are effective but their availability has declined in many countries through legislative changes and toxicity concerns.

CROP

Gongylonema ingluvicola

Gongylonema ingluvicola (Phylum: Nematoda; Class: Chromadorea; Order: Spirurida; Family: Gongylonematidae), commonly known as the Gullet worm, is a parasite localised in the crop of chickens, turkeys, partridges, pheasants and quails in North America, Asia, Africa, Australia and Europe. This nematode has cockroaches (*Blatella germanica*) and beetles of the species *Copris minutus* as intermediate hosts.

Pathogenesis: The adult parasites are moderately pathogenic, depending on the number of worms embedded in the epithelium.

Clinical signs and pathology: Light infections are often asymptomatic. Heavier infections may produce regurgitation and can induce hypertrophy and cornification of the epithelium of the crop in fowls.

Diagnosis: Usually an incidental finding on *post mortem*.

Trichomonas gallinae

For details see section entitled Oesophagus.

Eucoleus contorta

Eucoleus contorta, synonym *Capillaria contorta* (Phylum: Nematoda; Class: Enoplea; Order: Enoplida; Family: Capillariidae), is distributed worldwide and found in the oesophagus and crop of chickens, turkeys, pheasants, partridges, ducks and wild birds. This parasite has earthworms as intermediate hosts.

Epidemiology: Young birds are most susceptible to *Eucoleus* infections while adults may serve as carriers. *Eucoleus contorta* is important since, having a direct life cycle, it occurs indoors in birds kept on deep litter and outdoors in free-range systems, allowing large numbers of infective eggs to accumulate.

Clinical signs and pathology: Low infections are frequently asymptomatic, possibly causing some reduction in growth and lower egg production. Severely infected birds often become anaemic, weak and emaciated. Large numbers of worms produce an inflammation varying from catarrhal to diphtheritic.

Control: Control depends on regular anthelmintic treatment accompanied, if possible, by moving the birds to fresh ground. Scrubbing and heat treatment of affected surfaces are essential, as is the provision of fresh litter in chicken houses.

Details of the pathogenesis, diagnosis and treatment are as for *E. annulata*.

Eucoleus annulata

For details see section entitled Oesophagus.

PROVENTRICULUS

Several spiruroid worms are found in the oesophagus, crop and proventriculus of poultry. The life cycles of these parasites are indirect, involving a range of invertebrate hosts. Infections with these parasites are more common in free-ranging birds. Attempts to control the poultry spiruroids are unlikely to be successful because of the ready availability of the intermediate hosts.

Tetrameres americana

Tetrameres americana, synonym *Tropisurus americana* (Phylum: Nematoda; Class: Chromadorea; Order: Spirurida; Family: Tetrameridae), commonly known as the Globular roundworm, is a parasite of the proventriculus of chickens, turkeys, ducks, geese, grouse, quails and pigeons that commonly occurs in Africa and North America. Infection is more common in free-ranging birds. This parasite has cockroaches, grasshoppers and beetles as intermediate hosts.

Pathogenesis: The females in the glands of the proventriculus are blood suckers and can cause anaemia as well as local erosion. Heavy infections may be fatal in chicks, but this genus is usually present only in moderate numbers and is well tolerated. The migration of juvenile stages into the wall of the proventriculus can cause inflammation and thickening.

Clinical signs and pathology: Infected fowl may become anaemic and lose condition. Heavy infections, particularly in young chickens, can induce thickening of the proventriculus with oedema and, in some instances, this can lead to partial blockage of the lumen. Heavy infections can be fatal. The wall of the proventriculus may be thickened to an extent that the lumen is almost obliterated.

Diagnosis: At necropsy, the female *Tetrameres* appear as dark red spots when viewed from the serosal surface of the proventriculus.

Tetrameres fissispina

Tetrameres fissispina, synonym *Tropisurus fissispina* (Phylum: Nematoda; Class: Chromadorea; Order: Spirurida; Family: Tetrameridae), is a parasite of the proventriculus of ducks, geese, chickens, turkeys, pigeons and wild aquatic birds. It is distributed

Table 13.1 Species of *Tetrameres* found in poultry.

Species	Hosts	Intermediate hosts	Geographical distribution
Tetrameres americana	Chickens, turkeys, ducks, geese, grouse, quails, pigeons	Cockroaches, grasshoppers and beetles	Africa and North America
Tetrameres fissispina	Ducks, geese, chickens, turkeys, pigeons and wild aquatic birds	Aquatic crustaceans, grasshoppers, earthworms	Most parts of the world
Tetrameres crami	Domestic and wild ducks	Amphipods	North America
Tetrameres confusa	Chickens	?	Brazil
Tetrameres mohtedai	Chickens	?	India
Tetrameres pattersoni	Quails	?	?

in most parts of the world and has aquatic crustaceans such as *Daphnia* and *Gammarus*, grasshoppers and earthworms as intermediate hosts. Details of the life cycle, pathogenesis, clinical signs, diagnosis and pathology are as for *T. americana*.

Species of *Tetrameres* found in poultry are listed in Table 13.1. Details on pathogenicity in the host species are essentially similar to those for *T. americana*.

Dispharynx nasuta

Dispharynx nasuta, synonyms *Dispharynx spiralis*, *Acuaria spiralis*, *Acuaria nascuta* (Phylum: Nematoda; Class: Chromadorea; Order: Spirurida; Family: Acuaridae), commonly known as the Spiral stomach worm, is a parasite of the oesophagus and proventriculus of chickens, turkeys, pigeons, guinea fowl, grouse, pheasants and other birds. This parasite is distributed in Asia, Africa and the Americas, and has various isopods, such as sowbugs (*Porcellio scaber*) and pillbugs (*Armadillidium vulgare*), as intermediate hosts.

Pathogenesis: Mild infections usually provoke only a slight nodular inflammatory reaction in the mucosa with excessive mucus production.

Clinical signs and pathology: Most mild infections with *Dispharynx* are inapparent. Heavily infected young birds can rapidly lose weight, become emaciated and anaemic. Death rates can be high. In severe infections, deep ulcers and hypertrophy can occur in the mucosa of the proventriculus in which the anterior ends of the worms are embedded.

Diagnosis: A tentative diagnosis is based on the presence of spiruroid eggs, which are difficult to differentiate. Species identification is usually based on morphological identification of adult worms on *post mortem*.

Echinuria uncinata

Echinuria uncinata, synonym *Acuaria uncinata* (Phylum: Nematoda; Class: Chromadorea; Order: Spirurida; Family: Acuaridae), occurs worldwide and is localised in the oesophagus, proventriculus and

gizzard of ducks, geese, swans and various aquatic birds. This nematode has *Daphnia* and *Gammarus* as intermediate hosts.

Pathogenesis: The worms can cause an inflammation of the alimentary tract and the formation of caseous nodules. These nodules can be very large in the gizzard and proventriculus and interfere with the passage of food.

Clinical signs: Infected birds may become weak and emaciated and deaths have been reported.

Hystrichis tricolor

Hystrichis tricolor (Phylum: Nematoda; Class: Enoplea; Order: Enoplida; Family: Dioctophymatidae) is a parasite of the proventriculus and oesophagus of domestic and wild ducks and anatid birds. It has oligochaetes (annelids) as intermediate hosts. The extent of distribution is not known but it occurs occasionally in Europe.

Pathogenesis: The parasite induces nodule formation (pea-sized tumours) on the wall of the proventriculus and oesophagus. Sometimes these can perforate to the pleural cavity.

Clinical signs: Low infections are usually asymptomatic but heavy burdens can induce emaciation.

Eustrongyloides tubifex

Eustrongyloides tubifex, synonyms *Strongylus tubifex*, *Eustrongylus tubifex*, *Hystrichis tubifex* (Phylum: Nematoda; Class: Enoplea; Order: Enoplida; Family: Dioctophymatidae), is a parasite of the oesophagus and proventriculus of waterfowl. It has aquatic oligochaetes as intermediate hosts and fish as paratenic hosts. This parasite is distributed in many parts of the world.

Pathogenesis: Generally considered to be of low pathogenicity and of little veterinary significance, although the parasites can induce the formation of nodules in the wall of the anterior digestive tract.

Trichomonas gallinae

For details see section entitled Oesophagus. For treatment and control, see section entitled Gizzard.

GIZZARD

Several species of gizzard worms are found in ducks and geese. The following applies to all species. The infective L_3 require adequate moisture, such as pond margins, to survive as they are very susceptible to desiccation.

Pathogenesis: Adult birds may not show clinical symptoms but act as carriers. These parasites are found in the upper alimentary tract, particularly the gizzard, and may cause heavy mortality in goslings, ducklings and other young aquatic fowl. Young goslings and ducklings are particularly susceptible. The worms burrow into the mucosa of the gizzard, cause irritation and ingest blood.

Clinical signs and pathology: Young fowl may become inappetent, and show diarrhoea and anaemia. Over time, the birds become emaciated and weak and, when heavily infected, fatalities can occur. Often older fowls show few clinical signs but act as reservoirs of infection. Severe infections induce haemorrhages on the gizzard mucosa, and this may be accompanied by catarrhal inflammation. Heavy infections can cause necrosis of the horny lining of the gizzard, forming reddish-brown loose folds containing many embedded worms.

Diagnosis: At necropsy, worms may be recovered from the mucosa of the gizzard following incubation in warm saline for 1–2 hours. *Amidostomum* spp., which possess a buccal capsule, are the main trichostrongyloids of the gizzard.

Control and treatment: Gizzard worm infection may be prevented by ensuring that birds do not run on the same ground each year. It is important to restrict access of wild aquatic fowl to areas where geese are raised. Treatment with one of the modern benzimidazoles or levamisole, often administered in feed or drinking water, is effective.

Amidostomum anseris

Amidostomum anseris, synonym *Amidostomum nodulosum* (Phylum: Nematoda; Class: Chromadorea; Order: Rhabditida; Family: Amidostomidae), commonly known as the Gizzard worm, is distributed worldwide and localised in the gizzard, occasionally proventriculus and oesophagus of domestic and wild geese, ducks and other aquatic fowl.

Cheilospirura hamulosa

Cheilospirura hamulosa, synonym *Acuaria hamulosa* (Phylum: Nematoda; Class: Chromadorea; Order: Spirurida; Family: Acuariidae), occurs worldwide, particularly in Europe, Africa, Asia and the Americas. It is a nematode of the gizzard of chickens and turkeys which has grasshoppers (*Melanoplus*), weevils and beetles as intermediate hosts.

Pathogenesis: Generally, mild to moderate infections are of low pathogenicity. In heavy infections, many adult worms penetrate under the keratinised layer of the gizzard where they are found embedded in soft orange-coloured nodules. The keratinised layer of the gizzard may become necrotic, and rupture of the gizzard can occur.

Clinical signs and pathology: Mild infections are usually asymptomatic, whereas severe infections can lead to emaciation, weakness and anaemia. In mild infections, the worms are noticed only if the horny lining of the gizzard is removed and are found in soft yellowish-red nodules. In severe cases, the horny lining may be partly destroyed, with the worms found below the necrotic material within the altered musculature of the gizzard.

Diagnosis: This is best achieved through necropsy of an affected chicken, as the eggs of several species of *Cheilospirura* appear very similar.

Other species of spiruroid worms found in the gizzard are of minor significance.

Echinuria uncinata

For details see section entitled Proventriculus.

SMALL INTESTINE

Ascaridia galli

Ascaridia galli, synonyms *Ascaridia lineata*, *Ascaridia perspicillum* (Phylum: Nematoda; Class: Chromadorea; Order: Ascaridida; Family: Ascaridiidae), is a parasite occurring worldwide in the small intestine of chickens, turkeys, geese, ducks, guinea fowl and several wild galliform birds.

Epidemiology: Adult birds are symptomless carriers, and the reservoir of infection is on the ground, either as free eggs or in earthworm transport hosts. Infection is heaviest in young chicks.

Pathogenesis: *Ascaridia* is not a highly pathogenic worm, and any effects are usually seen in young birds of around 1–2 months of age, adults appearing relatively unaffected. The main effect is seen during the prepatent phase, when the larvae are in the duodenal/intestinal mucosa. There they cause enteritis, which is usually catarrhal, but in very heavy infections may be haemorrhagic. In moderate infections the adult worms are tolerated without clinical signs, but when considerable numbers are present, the large size of these worms may cause intestinal occlusion and death. Nutritional deficiency may predispose birds to the establishment of infection.

Clinical signs and pathology: Heavily infected birds may become anaemic and show intermittent diarrhoea and anorexia, later becoming unthrifty and emaciated. This can lead to a decrease in egg production. Enteritis or haemorrhagic enteritis may be seen when large numbers of young parasites penetrate the duodenal or jejunal mucosa. The embedded larvae cause haemorrhage and extensive destruction of the glandular epithelium, and proliferation of mucous secretory cells may result in adhesion of the mucosal villi. Damage to the epithelia may not only be caused by the larvae, but also by the adult worms in the form of pressure atrophy of the villi with occasional necrosis of the mucosal layer. In chronic infections, a loss of muscle tone may be seen, and the intestinal wall may assume a flabby appearance. During the histotropic phase, there is loss of blood and reduced blood sugar and the ureters frequently become distended with urates.

Diagnosis: In infections with adult worms, the eggs will be found in faeces, but since it is often difficult to distinguish these from the slightly smaller eggs of *Heterakis*, confirmation must be made by *post mortem* examination of a casualty when the large white worms will be found. In the prepatent period, larvae will be found in the intestinal contents and in scrapings of the mucosa.

Control and treatment: When birds are reared on a free-range system and ascaridiosis is a problem, the young birds should, if possible, be segregated and reared on ground previously unused by poultry. Rotation of poultry runs is advisable. Since the nematode may also be a problem in deep-litter houses, feeding and watering systems which limit the contamination of food and water by faeces should be used. Treatment with piperazine salts, levamisole or a benzimidazole, such as flubendazole, mebendazole or fenbendazole, can be administered in the feed (30 ppm over seven days; 60 ppm over seven days; 60 ppm over three days, respectively). Levamisole is effective at 30 mg/kg given orally, or 300 ppm in the feed.

Ascaridia dissimilis

Ascaridia dissimilis (Phylum: Nematoda; Class: Chromadorea; Order: Ascaridida; Family: Ascaridiidae) is a parasite of the small intestine of turkeys, presumably distributed worldwide. This parasite is considered non-pathogenic.

Epidemiology and pathogenesis: Adult birds are symptomless carriers, and the reservoir of infection is on the ground, either as free eggs or in earthworm transport hosts.

Clinical signs and pathology: Moderate infections are frequently inapparent. They are not associated with any pathology.

Diagnosis: Adult worms may be found in the intestine on *post mortem* or the characteristic ascarid eggs may be seen in faeces.

Control and treatment: For control, strict hygiene and feeding and watering systems that limit the contamination of food and water by faeces should be used. Treatment is not usually required, although treatment with piperazine salts, levamisole or a benzimidazole, such as fenbendazole, is effective.

Capillaria caudinflata

Capillaria caudinflata, synonym *Aonchotheca caudinflata* (Phylum: Nematoda; Class: Enoplea; Order: Enoplida; Family: Capillariidae), occurs worldwide in the small intestine of chickens, turkeys, geese, pigeons and wild birds. This nematode has earthworms as intermediate hosts.

Pathogenesis: The anterior ends of the worms are embedded in the mucosa. Light infections can produce a catarrhal inflammation; heavy infections may cause a haemorrhagic enteritis with bloody diarrhoea.

Clinical signs: Heavy infections often induce anaemia and the birds become weak and emaciated.

Capillaria obsignata

Capillaria obsignata, synonyms *Baruscapillaria obsignata*, *Capillaria columbae* (Phylum: Nematoda; Class: Enoplea; Order: Enoplida; Family: Capillariidae), is distributed worldwide and localised in the small intestine of pigeons, chickens, turkeys, pheasants and wild birds.

Epidemiology: Young birds are most susceptible to *Capillaria* infections while adults may serve as carriers. *Capillaria obsignata* is important since, having a direct life cycle, it occurs indoors in birds kept on deep litter and outdoors in free-range systems, allowing large numbers of infective eggs to accumulate.

Pathogenesis: *Capillaria obsignata* can be highly pathogenic in chickens and pigeons, leading to fatalities. Birds become listless, emaciated and diarrhoeic. Details of the dianosis, epidemiology, treatment and control for these species are as for *E. annulata*.

Hartertia gallinarum

Hartertia gallinarum (Phylum: Nematoda; Class: Chromadorea; Order: Spirurida; Family: Hartertiidae) is a parasite of the small intestine and gizzard of chickens and bustards. This nematode has termites as intermediate host. It is widespread in Europe, Africa and Asia but has not been found in the New World.

Pathogenesis and clinical signs: Infections are rarely fatal but when large numbers of worms are present, there may be inflammation of the intestine. Diarrhoea and emaciation may occur, often accompanied by a decrease in egg production.

Diagnosis: Differentiation of eggs in faeces is difficult as they are morphologically similar to those of other poultry spiruroids. Diagnosis is usually confirmed at necropsy.

Control and treatment: Where feasible, removal of termite nests from areas adjacent to runs used for poultry will be beneficial. No treatment has been reported.

Tapeworms

Tapeworms are a feature of poultry reared on pasture, infection being acquired through ingestion of infected intermediate hosts, such as beetles, earthworms, ants, grasshoppers or flies. Infection is uncommon in intensive indoor systems as suitable intermediate hosts are usually absent.

The most important and pathogenic species is *Davainea proglottina*, which penetrates the duodenal mucosa, and in young birds can induce a necrotic haemorrhagic enteritis that can be fatal. *Raillietina echinobothrida* is also pathogenic, inducing a hyperplastic enteritis and multiple caseous nodules where the scolex attaches to the wall of the intestine. Many other tapeworm species produce only mild symptoms, unless infections are heavy when loss of productivity may be seen. Effective treatment of avian tapeworms is achieved with praziquantel, flubendazole, mebendazole, febantel or niclosamide. The dose rate and duration of administration vary between species of poultry. Control depends on the treatment of infected birds with a suitable anthelmintic and the destruction or removal of intermediate hosts where possible.

Davainea proglottina

Davainea proglottina (Phylum: Platyhelminthes; Class: Cestoda; Order: Cyclophyllidea; Family: Davaineidae) is a parasite distributed in most parts of the world, colonising the small intestine, in particular the duodenum of chickens, turkeys, pigeons and other gallinaceous birds. It has gastropod molluscs of the genera *Agriolimax*, *Arion*, *Cepaea* and *Limax* as intermediate hosts.

Epidemiology: Infection can be common in free-range fowl as suitable intermediate hosts are often available. Young birds tend to be more severely affected than older fowl.

Pathogenesis: This is the most pathogenic of the poultry cestodes, the doubly armed scolex penetrating deeply between the duodenal villi. Heavy infections may cause haemorrhagic enteritis while light infections cause retarded growth and weakness.

Clinical signs and pathology: Moderate infections can lead to reduced weight gain, inappetence and lowered egg production. Large numbers of parasites may induce emaciation and dyspnoea and even be fatal. The mucosal membranes are thickened and haemorrhagic with localised patches of necrosis. Fetid mucus may be present.

Diagnosis: This is best achieved at necropsy through microscopic examination of mucosal scrapings from the duodenum and anterior small intestine. The tapeworm can easily be overlooked due to its minute size.

Raillietina cesticillus

Raillietina cesticillus, synonym *Skrjabinia cesticillus* (Phylum: Platyhelminthes; Class: Cestoda; Order: Cyclophyllidea; Family: Davaineidae), occurs worldwide in the small intestine of chickens, turkeys and guinea fowl. It has various genera of beetles, including the families Carabidae, Scarabaeidae and Tenebrionidae, and the meal beetles *Tribolium* spp., as intermediate hosts.

Epidemiology: Young birds are usually more susceptible to infection than adults. Infection rates depend on the availability of the intermediate hosts. Beetles are numerous for free-range fowl but some beetles may also breed in litter bedding. Eggs are reasonably resistant to environmental conditions and will survive for several months.

Clinical signs and pathology: Infections may cause reduction in growth rate. Heavy infection can lead to emaciation and weakness. In heavy infections, the embedded scolices of this parasite can produce caseous nodules in the wall of the small intestine and catarrhal enteritis.

Diagnosis: This is best achieved at necropsy through microscopic examination of mucosal scrapings from the small intestine.

Raillietina echinobothrida

Raillietina echinobothrida (Phylum: Platyhelminthes; Class: Cestoda; Order: Cyclophyllidea; Family: Davaineidae) commonly causes Nodular tapeworm disease. It occurs worldwide and is localised in the small intestine of chickens, turkeys and other fowl. It has ants of the genera *Pheidole* and *Tetramorium* as intermediate hosts.

Pathology: *Raillietina echinobothrida* is more pathogenic than either *R. cesticillus* or *R. tetragona*. In heavy infections, the embedded scolices of this parasite produce large caseous nodules in the subserous and muscular layers of the wall of the posterior small intestine. Hyperplastic enteritis may occur at the site of attachment. The lesions in the intestine are similar to those associated with avian tuberculosis.

Raillietina tetragona

Raillietina tetragona (Phylum: Platyhelminthes; Class: Cestoda; Order: Cyclophyllidea; Family: Davaineidae) occurs worldwide in the posterior half of small intestine of chickens, guinea fowl and pigeons. It has ants of the genera *Pheidole*, *Onthophagus* and *Tetramorium*, and house flies as intermediate hosts (Fig. 13.1).

Pathogenesis: In heavy infections, the embedded scolices of this parasite produce large caseous nodules in the wall of the small intestine.

Pathology: *Raillietina tetragona* is usually less pathogenic than either *R. echinobothrida* or *R. cesticillus*.

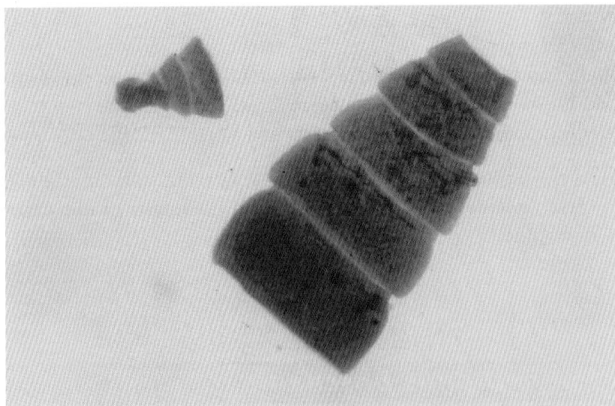

Fig. 13.1 *Raillietina tetragona*: scolex and proglottids.

Hymenolepis carioca

Hymenolepis carioca, synonym *Echinolepis carioca* (Phylum: Platyhelminthes; Class: Cestoda; Order: Cyclophyllidea; Family: Hymenolepididae), is a parasite of the small intestine of chickens, turkeys and other fowl, having dung and flour beetles, and sometimes *Stomoxys* spp., as intermediate hosts. It is distributed in most parts of the world but is common in the USA. It is usually considered to be of low pathogenicity although large numbers of tapeworms may cause diarrhoea.

Hymenolepis lanceolata

Hymenolepis lanceolata, synonym *Drepanidotaenia lanceolatum* (Phylum: Platyhelminthes; Class: Cestoda; Order: Cyclophyllidea; Family: Hymenolepididae), is a cosmopolitan parasite of the small intestine of ducks and geese, having aquatic copepod crustaceans as intermediate hosts.

Clinical signs and pathology: Large numbers of tapeworms may cause diarrhoea while moderate to heavy infections can induce a catarrhal enteritis and necrosis of the mucosa. Heavy infections can be fatal.

Intestinal flukes

Intestinal flukes are found in both the small and large intestines. The majority of avian intestinal trematodes parasitise aquatic fowl and birds, and are of importance where birds forage in habitats that support the snail intermediate hosts. Large numbers of flukes can irritate the intestinal mucosa, inducing a catarrhal haemorrhagic enteritis and diarrhoea. Young birds are particularly susceptible to infection, showing progressive emaciation, and fatalities can be high. Various anthelmintics are available for treatment. Praziquantel or flubendazole, administered over several days, are effective in aquatic fowl. Niclosamide (not for geese) and fenbendazole are effective against Echinostomatidae.

Echinoparyphium recurvatum

Echinoparyphium recurvatum (Phylum: Platyhelminthes; Class: Trematoda; Order: Plagiorchiida; Family: Echinostomatidae) is a parasite of the small intestine, particularly of the duodenum of ducks, geese, chickens and pigeons, having snails (e.g. *Galba* spp. and *Planorbis* spp.) as first intermediate hosts, and frogs, tadpoles, snails (e.g. *Valvata piscinalis* and *Planorbis albus*), freshwater clams and mussels as second intermediate hosts. This parasite is distributed worldwide, particularly in Asia and North Africa.

Heavy infections may induce weakness, anaemia and emaciation. A catarrhal enteritis is often present, and the intestinal mucosa is oedematous.

Thorny-headed worms

Polymorphus boschadis

Polymorphus boschadis, synonyms *Polymorphus minutus*, *Echinorhynchus polymorphus* (Phylum: Acanthocephala; Class: Archiacanthocephala; Order: Oligacanthorhynchida; Family: Polymorphidae), commonly known as the Thorny-headed worm, occurs worldwide in the small intestine of ducks, geese, chickens, swans and various wild aquatic birds. This parasite has crustaceans such as the freshwater shrimp *Gammarus pulex*, and sometimes the crayfish *Potamobius astacus*, as intermediate hosts.

Pathogenesis and pathology: The worm causes inflammation of the intestinal mucosa and localised haemorrhage, which in heavy infection can induce anaemia. Worms use their armed proboscis to penetrate deep into the mucosa of the intestine and nodules frequently form at the point of attachment. Heavy infections can be fatal.

Diagnosis: Characteristic eggs are detectable in faeces or the adult worms may be seen at necropsy.

Filicollis anatis

Filicollis anatis (Phylum: Acanthocephala; Class: Archiacanthocephala; Order: Oligacanthorhynchida; Family: Polymorphidae), commonly known as the Thorny-headed worm, occurs worldwide in the small intestine of ducks, geese, swans and wild aquatic birds. This parasite has crustaceans, in particular isopods such as *Asellus aquaticus*, as intermediate hosts.

Clinical signs and pathology: Clinical signs are characterised by loss of weight, emaciation and, in heavy infections, death. Male worms penetrate the mucosa of the intestine and nodules may occur at the point of attachment. The female penetrates deep into the wall of the intestine and often its proboscis is situated directly under the peritoneum, leading to rupture in severe cases. The worm produces inflammation of the intestinal mucosa and localised haemorrhage.

Diagnosis: Characteristic eggs are detectable in faeces or the adult worms may be seen at necropsy.

Treatment and control: Details of treatment and control are as for *P. boschadis*.

Coccidiosis in chickens

Seven species of *Eimeria* are found in domestic chickens (Table 13.2); identification is based on location in the intestine and associated pathology. Specific identification is based on the nature and location of the lesions in the intestine together with careful

Table 13.2 Predilection sites and prepatent periods of *Eimeria* species in chickens.

Species	Predilection site	Prepatent period (hours)
Eimeria acervulina	Duodenum	89
Eimeria brunetti	Lower small intestine, caeca, rectum	120
Eimeria maxima	Mid-small intestine	120
Eimeria mitis	Small intestine, caeca, rectum	91
Eimeria necatrix	Small intestine	138
Eimeria praecox	Small intestine	84
Eimeria tenella	Caeca	132

examination of fresh smears for developmental stages of the parasite.

Epidemiology: The appearance and development of coccidiosis in poultry houses are dependent on a complex interplay of many factors. In fresh litter, few coccidia are present and there may be only a few oocysts scattered around. From the moment a few chicks are infected, rapid multiplication commences and a week later, new oocysts are excreted in large quantities. The infection usually begins to spread at full rate around the third or fourth week after housing. As exposure and immunity increase, the chicks will then gradually recover and withstand the infection.

Rearing of thousands of birds on litter-covered floors in enormous houses may result in a tremendous and dangerous build-up of the oocyst population. Whether or not infection leads to the occurrence of disease outbreaks is to a great extent determined by the numbers of oocysts to which birds are exposed. However, serious outbreaks of clinical coccidiosis with acute mortality are highly exceptional in modern broiler farms because of the stringent monitoring and control measures employed. Where outbreaks do occur, clinical signs can be ascribed to one, or a combination of two, or rarely three, coccidial species. Management-related factors, such as stocking density, size of the farm, period of vacancy, quality of the litter, inadequate cleaning, ventilation system, presence of animals of different ages and anticoccidials used, will play an important part in influencing the numbers of oocysts that birds will be exposed to, and whether and to what extent coccidiosis will develop. The occurrence and incidence of disease are also, to a great extent, affected by the type of chicks reared, breed sensitivities to infection, their initial health, acquired immunity and the interference of other diseases. The damaging nature and the location of the coccidia in the intestine will differ to such an extent that ultimately a complex and unique picture will develop on individual poultry farms. A change from litter-covered floors to wire-floored pens greatly reduces the exposure to coccidia. Outbreaks of coccidiosis rarely occur in laying hens maintained in cages. In general, the prophylactic use of anticoccidial drugs is not required if the cages are kept clean and the faeces do not contaminate watering and feeding systems.

Oocysts are disseminated via the faeces and the litter, with dust within the poultry buildings, inside and outside the house by invertebrates and vermin, while mechanical ventilation systems serve to scatter the oocysts outside the house. Faecal contamination of vehicles and personnel can spread the infection to other farms. Measures such as thorough cleaning and disinfecting with oocidal agents, batch depopulation between grow-outs, and admitting as few visitors as possible are essential to maintain proper hygiene standards. Today most poultry enterprises rely on floor-rearing methods for broiler production or breeder flocks and use continuous medication programmes. Poultry producers also attempt to control coccidiosis by employing good sanitary programmes. Litters should be kept dry so that oocysts cannot sporulate. Wet litter must be cleaned out and replaced with dry litter. When broiler houses are emptied for a new batch of chickens, the litter should be piled up for about 24 hours so that the heat generated can destroy the majority of oocysts. Disinfection is usually impractical since oocysts are resistant to disinfectants used against bacteria, viruses or fungi.

Diagnosis: Diagnosis is best based on *post mortem* examination of a few affected birds. This can be made at microscopic level, either by examining the faeces for the presence of oocysts or by examination of scrapings or histological sections of affected tissues. Although oocysts may be detected on faecal examination, it would be wrong to diagnose solely on such evidence for two reasons. First, the major pathogenic effect usually occurs prior to oocyst production and, second, depending on the species involved, the presence of large numbers of oocysts is not necessarily correlated with severe pathological changes in the gut. At necropsy, the location and type of lesions present provide a good guide to the species, and this can be confirmed by examination of the oocysts in the faeces and the meronts and oocysts present in scrapings of the gut. A reliable species diagnosis based on oocyst morphology is not possible as the dimensions and other features overlap between species (see Table 4.12). Species diagnosis is based on a combination of characteristics, including site of development in the intestinal tract, type of macroscopic lesions and size of meronts in mucosal smears. The mature meronts may be identified histologically by their location, size and the number of merozoites they contain.

Control: Prevention of avian coccidiosis is based on a combination of good management and the use of anticoccidial compounds in the feed or water. Thus, litter should always be kept dry and special attention given to litter near water fonts or feeding troughs. Fonts that prevent water reaching the litter should always be used and they should be placed on drip trays or over the droppings pit. Feeding and watering utensils should be of such a type and height that droppings cannot contaminate them. Good ventilation will also reduce the humidity in the house and help to keep litter dry. Preferably, clean litter should always be provided between batches of birds. If this is not possible, the litter should be heaped and left for 24 hours after it has reached a temperature of 50 °C; it should then be forked over again and the process repeated to ensure that all the oocysts in the litter have been destroyed.

The use of anticoccidial agents depends on the type of management concerned. Broiler chicks are on lifetime-medicated feed and the anticoccidials used are maintained at a level sufficient to prevent merogony. The drugs available for use singly or in various combinations are amprolium, clopidol, diclazuril, ethopabate, halofuginone, lasalocid, maduramicin, monensin, narasin, nicarbazin, robenidine, salinomycin and sulfaquinoxaline. It is recommended that drugs are switched between batches of broilers, the so-called 'rotation programme', or within the lifespan of each batch, the 'shuttle programme'. Most drugs have a minimum period for which they must be withdrawn before the birds can be slaughtered for human consumption. This is usually 5–7 days.

Where replacement laying birds spend their whole life on wire floors, no medication is necessary; if they are reared on litter, for eventual production on wire, then a full level of coccidiostat is given as for broilers. If they are reared on litter, for production on litter, then a programme of anticoccidials designed to stimulate immunity is used. Preparations frequently used either singly or in combination

are amprolium, ethopabate, lasalocid, monensin and sulfaquinoxaline. The procedure is to administer these drugs in a decreasing level over the first 16 or 18 weeks of life. This may be done as a two-stage reduction, i.e. between 0 and 8 weeks and 8 and 16 weeks, or, alternatively, as a three-stage reduction, from 0–6 weeks, 6–12 weeks and 12–18 weeks. Using this technique, complete protection against coccidial challenge is maintained in the very young birds and the reduced drug rate in older birds allows limited exposure to developing coccidia so that acquired immunity can develop.

When in-feed coccidiostats are used, there are two further factors to consider. First, outbreaks of coccidiosis may occur in birds on medicated feed either because the level of coccidiostat used is too low or because conditions in the house have changed to allow a massive sporulation of oocysts which, on ingestion, the level of drug can no longer control. Second, the influence of intercurrent infections in affecting appetite, and therefore uptake of coccidiostat, should also be considered.

Several commercial vaccines have been developed for the control of coccidiosis in chickens. Live vaccines containing oocysts of wild-type strains of four, or eight, species of coccidia are available in the USA. Young chicks are given the vaccine either in a spray cabinet or orally on the feed. Successful immunisation has also been achieved with oocysts attenuated by irradiation or by selection of selected 'precocious' strains of each of the pathogenic species of coccidia that affect poultry. These strains show rapid development *in vivo* with minimal damage to the intestine but stimulate an effective immunity. For success, both techniques depend on subsequent exposure to oocysts to boost immunity and this may not occur unless litter is sufficiently moist to allow sporulation. There is considerable interest in developing more efficient vaccines, in view of the increasing problem of drug resistance in coccidiosis. A subunit transmission-blocking vaccine which targets the sexual macrogametocyte stages and thus reduces oocyst output has been developed. The vaccine comprises affinity-purified antigens from the gametocyte stages of *Eimeria maxima*. It provides a good level of protection across three species of *Eimeria* (*E. maxima*, *E. tenella* and *E. acervulina*) and is administered to laying hens where protection is passed, via the yolk, to their broiler offspring. Unfortunately, it is an expensive vaccine to manufacture, and work is ongoing to test whether recombinant forms of the gametocyte proteins are as effective at producing antigenicity as the natural proteins.

Treatment: This should be introduced as early as possible after a diagnosis has been made. Sulfonamide drugs have been the most widely used and it is recommended that these be given for two periods of three days in the drinking water, with an interval of two days between treatments. Where resistance has occurred to sulfonamides, mixtures of amprolium and ethopabate have given good results. Toltrazuril has been introduced for the treatment of outbreaks of coccidiosis and its use is restricted to those cases where other treatments have been ineffective. In the successful treatment of an outbreak of coccidiosis, the aim is to treat birds already affected and at the same time allow sufficient merogonous development in the clinically unaffected birds to stimulate their resistance.

Intestinal coccidiosis

This form of the disease tends to be chronic and may be associated with several species of *Eimeria*. Mortality may not be heavy but morbidity may retard growth significantly. Usually more than one species is present. Specific identification is based on the nature and location of the lesions in the intestine together with careful examination of fresh smears for developmental stages of the parasite.

Eimeria acervulina

Eimeria acervulina (Phylum: Apicomplexa; Class: Conoidasida; Order: Eucoccidiorida; Family: Eimeriidae) occurs worldwide in the duodenum of chickens (Fig. 13.2). The sporocysts emerge from the oocysts in the gizzard and the sporozoites are activated and emerge in the small intestine. Most enter the duodenum. The meronts are found in the epithelial cells of the villi of the anterior small intestine where they lie above the host nucleus. There are four merogony generations. The first-generation meronts lie at the base of the glands of the crypts of the duodenum. Second-generation meronts are found at the neck of the glands, third-generation meronts lie at the base of the villi and fourth-generation meronts lie on the sides and tips of the villi. The sexual stages are found above the host cell nuclei, in the epithelial cells of the villi and to a lesser extent in the gland cells, and are seen four days after infection. They take 40 hours to mature. The prepatent period is 89 hours. The sporulation time is 24 hours (Table 13.3).

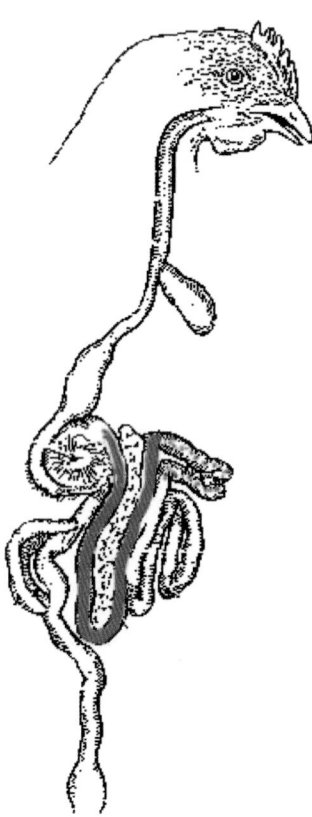

Fig. 13.2 Predilection site of *Eimeria acervulina*.

Table 13.3 *Eimeria acervulina*.

Lesions: whitish ladder-like streaks to coalescent plaques affecting mainly duodenum (Fig. 13.3)
Mean oocyst size (µm): 18 × 14
Shape and length/width index: ovoid, 1.25
Prepatent period (hours): 89
Sporulation time (hours): 24

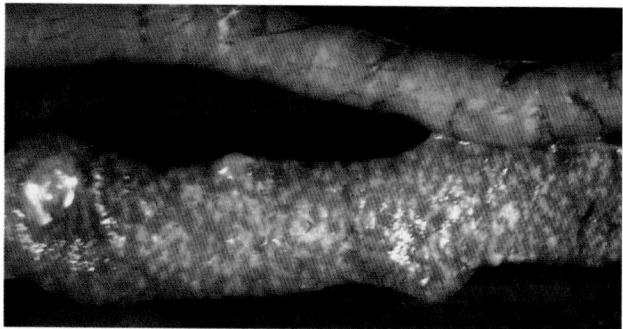

Fig. 13.3 Duodenal lesions of *Eimeria acervulina*.

Pathogenesis: The disease is usually chronic, with birds showing poor weight gains but little mortality. Clinical disease occurs about three days following the ingestion of large numbers of oocysts.

Clinical signs and pathology: *Eimeria acervulina* is generally considered to be moderately pathogenic, but heavy infections can cause severe signs and death. Symptoms include diarrhoea, dejection, ruffled feathers and drooping wings, inappetence, weight loss and depressed weight gain. The lesions in light infections consist of white transverse streaks in the duodenum and upper small intestine (Fig. 13.3). In heavier infections the lesions coalesce and the intestinal wall becomes thickened and congested with marked whitish mucoid exudate. Very large numbers of gamonts and oocysts can be seen in smears from the duodenum and on histopathology (Fig. 13.4).

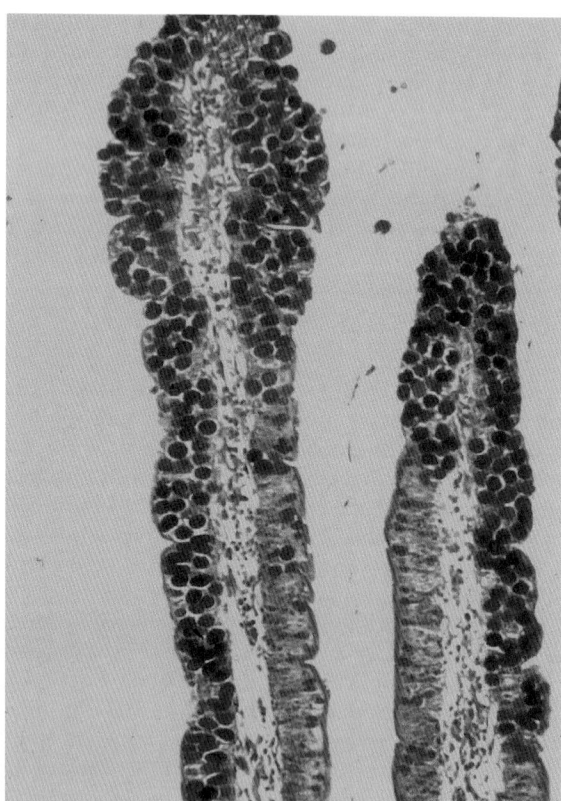

Fig. 13.4 Gamonts of *Eimeria acervulina* within enterocytes of small intestinal villi.

Lesions are scored +1 to +4 as follows.

1 Scattered white plaque-like lesions containing developing oocysts confined to the duodenum. These lesions are elongated with the longer axis transversely oriented on the thickened intestinal walls like the rungs of a ladder. They may be seen from either the serosal or mucosal intestinal surfaces. The birds would not be clinically affected and weight gains would not be affected.

2 Lesions are much closer together but not coalescent and may extend below the duodenum in young birds. The intestinal walls are not thickened and the gut contents are normal. The birds would show a depression in weight gain.

3 The lesions are clearly recognisable from the mucosal and serosal surfaces, are more numerous and beginning to coalesce. The intestinal wall is thickened, and the intestinal contents are watery due to excessive mucus secretion. The birds have diarrhoea and their weight gains are decreased.

4 The mucosal wall is greyish with colonies completely coalesced. In extremely heavy infections the entire mucosa may be bright red in colour. Individual lesions may be indistinguishable in the upper intestine. Typical ladder-like lesions appear in the middle part of the intestine. The intestinal wall is very much thickened and the intestine is filled with a creamy exudate, which may contain numbers of oocysts. The birds show diarrhoea, severe weight loss, poor feed conversion and skin depigmentation.

Eimeria brunetti

Eimeria brunetti (Phylum: Apicomplexa; Class: Conoidasida; Order: Eucoccidiorida; Family: Eimeriidae) occurs worldwide in the small and large intestine of chickens (Fig. 13.5). The first-generation

Table 13.4 *Eimeria brunetti.*

Lesions: coagulation, necrosis and bloody enteritis in lower intestine (Fig. 13.6)
Mean oocyst size (μm): 26 × 22
Shape and length/width index: ovoid, 1.31
Prepatent period (hours): 120
Sporulation time (hours): 24–48

meronts are found in the epithelial cells in the base of the villi in the mid-intestine. There are at least three merogony generations. Second-generation meronts are found subepithelially at the tips of the villi in the lower small intestine three days post infection. Third-generation meronts are first seen at 84 hours, mature by four days after infection and are located in the lower small intestine and large intestine. Gamonts are seen from day 5 at the tips and sides of the villi in the lower small intestine and large intestine, either above the host cell nuclei or on the basement membrane. The prepatent period is 120 hours. The sporulation time is 24–48 hours (Table 13.4).

Pathogenesis: The pathogenicity of this species is high, but mortality is variable. Lesions are most pronounced in the posterior small intestine.

Clinical signs: *Eimeria brunetti* is markedly pathogenic, but its effects depend on the degree of infection. Light infections may be asymptomatic. Heavier infections reduce weight gain or cause weight loss. The birds develop fluid droppings containing blood-tinged mucus and mucous casts. They become depressed and deaths may occur. The symptoms continue for five days before recovery.

Pathology: The gut wall becomes thickened and a pink or blood-tinged catarrhal exudate appears 4–5 days after experimental inoculation. In early or light infections, haemorrhagic ladder-like streaks are present on the mucosa of the lower small intestine and rectum. In heavy infections, a characteristic necrotic enteritis appears that may involve the entire intestinal tract, but which is more usually found in the lower small intestine, colon and tubular part of the caeca (Fig. 13.6). A patchy or continuous dry caseous necrotic membrane may line the intestine, and the intestine may be filled with sloughed necrotic material. Circumscribed white patches may be visible through the serosa and there may be intestinal perforation with resultant peritonitis.

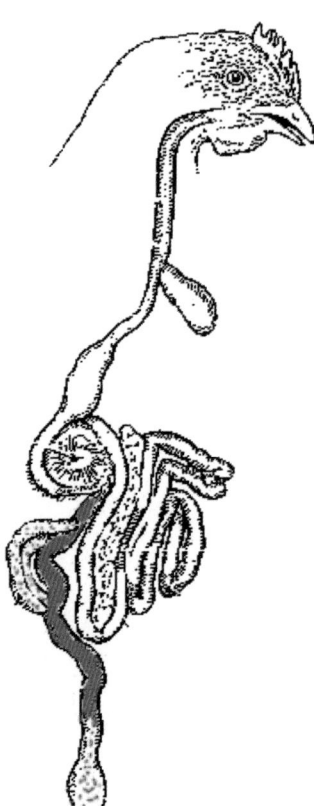

Fig. 13.5 Predilection site of *Eimeria brunetti*.

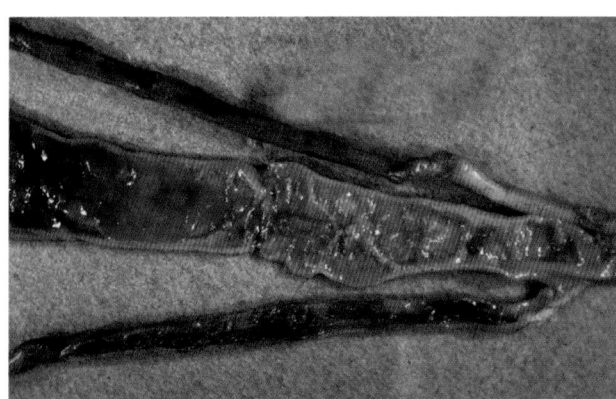

Fig. 13.6 Lesions of *Eimeria brunetti* in lower small intestine.

Lesions are scored +1 to +4 as follows.

1 Gross lesions are very distinct with some greying and reddening of the mucosal surfaces with a few petechiae visible from the serosal surface, appearing as pits on the mucosal surface.

2 Intestinal walls may appear grey in colour, and the lower portion may be thickened with flecks of pinkish material sloughed from the intestine. More petechiae are present, with the greatest number appearing on day 5 after infection. They may appear as early as day 3.5 and occur from the yolk stalk posteriorly. Mild mucosal roughening can be detected by feel.

3 Intestinal walls are thickened and a blood-tinged exudate is present. Transverse streaks may be present in the lower rectum with lesions in the caecal tonsils. Weight gains and feed conversion are reduced.

4 Severe coagulative necrosis of the lower intestine can result in erosion of the entire mucosa. This is apparent as a thickening of the intestine wall, and in some birds a dry necrotic membrane may line the intestine (pseudomembranous necrosis) and caseous cores may plug the caeca. Lesions may extend into the middle or upper intestine, and the necrosis may be severe enough to cause intestinal obstruction and death of the bird.

Eimeria maxima

Eimeria maxima (Phylum: Apicomplexa; Class: Conoidasida; Order: Eucoccidiorida; Family: Eimeriidae) occurs worldwide in the small intestine of chickens (Fig. 13.7). The meronts are located above the host cell nuclei (or occasionally beside them) in the epithelial cells of the tips of the villi of the duodenum and

Table 13.5 *Eimeria maxima*.

Lesions: thickened mid-intestine with petechial haemorrhage and blood-tinged exudate (Fig. 13.8)
Mean oocyst size (μm): 30 × 20
Shape and length/width index: ovoid, 1.47
Prepatent period (hours): 120
Sporulation time (hours): 30–48

upper ileum. There are three asexual generations. The first-generation meronts lie deep in the epithelial cells of the deep glands of the duodenum. They appear 48 hours after inoculation and contain 25–50 loosely packed merozoites. The second-generation meronts are in the epithelial cells of the small intestine villi near the openings of the crypts and appear on the third day after infection and produce about 12 merozoites. Third-generation meronts are in the epithelial cells along the sides of the superficial villi and sometimes near the tips, appearing during the fourth day after infection and producing about 12 merozoites. Gamonts are located below the host cell nuclei and, as they enlarge the host cells, are displaced towards the centre of the villi and come to lie in their interior. After fertilisation, an oocyst wall is laid down and the oocysts break out of the villi and are passed in the faeces. The prepatent period is 120 hours. Sporulation time is 30–48 hours (Table 13.5).

Pathogenesis: Strains of *Eimeria maxima* differ in their pathogenicity, which can be very variable, but some strains can be responsible for high morbidity and mortality may approach 25%. Lesions occur most frequently in the mid small intestine, although the whole of the small intestine may be involved. Clinical disease occurs about three days following the ingestion of large numbers of oocysts. Asexual stages cause relatively little damage, with the most serious effects being due to the sexual stages.

Clinical signs and pathology: Symptoms include diarrhoea, depression, ruffled feathers, decreased growth rate or weight loss and, in some cases, death. Birds that recover soon return to normal. The principal lesions are haemorrhages in the mid small intestine. The intestinal muscles lose their tone, and the intestine becomes flaccid and dilated with a somewhat thickened wall. There is catarrhal enteritis; the intestinal contents are viscid and mucoid and are grey-brown or pink-orange in colour (Fig. 13.8). Occasionally there are blood flecks in the intestinal contents, but in

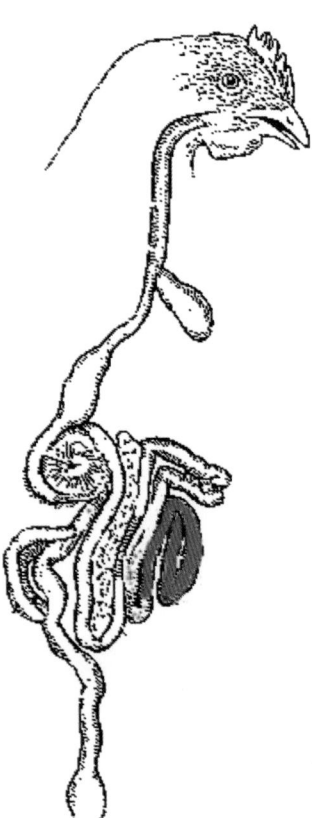

Fig. 13.7 Predilection site of *Eimeria maxima*.

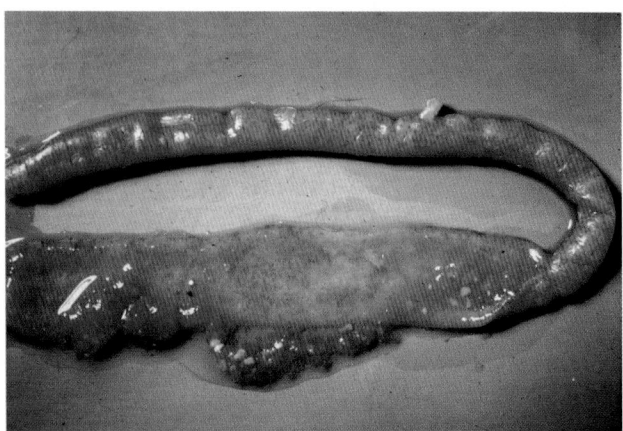

Fig. 13.8 Lesions of *Eimeria maxima*: mid small intestine.

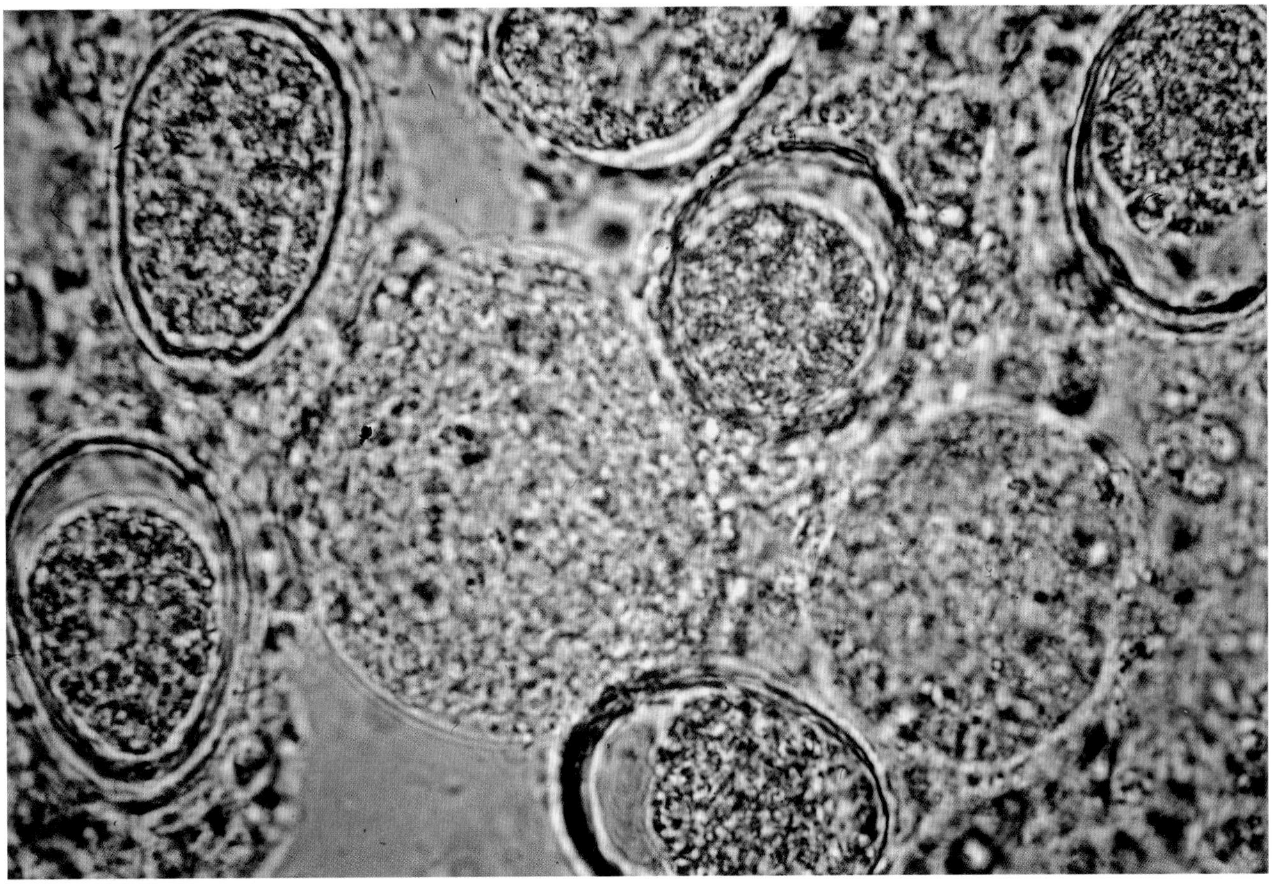

Fig. 13.9 Oocysts and gamonts of *Eimeria maxima* in mucosal smear of the mid small intestine.

heavy infections haemorrhage may be pronounced and blood may pass into the caeca. Gametocytes or characteristic large yellowish oocysts may be seen in smears from the intestinal mucosa (Fig. 13.9).

Lesions are scored +1 to +4 as follows.

1 Small red petechiae may appear on the serosal side of the midintestine surface on days 6 and 7 of infection. There is no thickening of the intestine, although small amounts of orange mucus may be present. Birds show some weight loss and skin depigmentation.

2 The serosal surface may be speckled with numerous red petechiae. The intestine may be filled with orange mucus, with little or no thickening of the intestine.

3 The intestinal wall is ballooned and thickened. The mucosal surface is roughened, and intestinal contents filled with pinpoint blood clots and mucus.

4 The intestinal wall may be ballooned for most of its length and greatly thickened and contains numerous blood clots and digested red blood cells, giving a characteristic colour and putrid odour.

Eimeria mitis

Eimeria mitis (Phylum: Apicomplexa; Class: Conoidasida; Order: Eucoccidiorida; Family: Eimeriidae) occurs worldwide in the small and large intestine of chickens (Fig. 13.10). No discrete lesions are

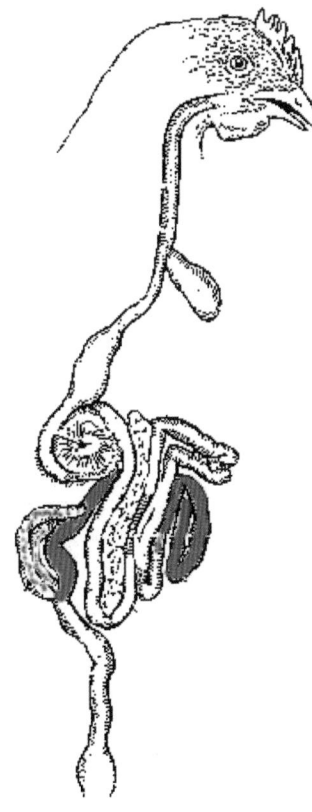

Fig. 13.10 Predilection site of *Eimeria mitis*.

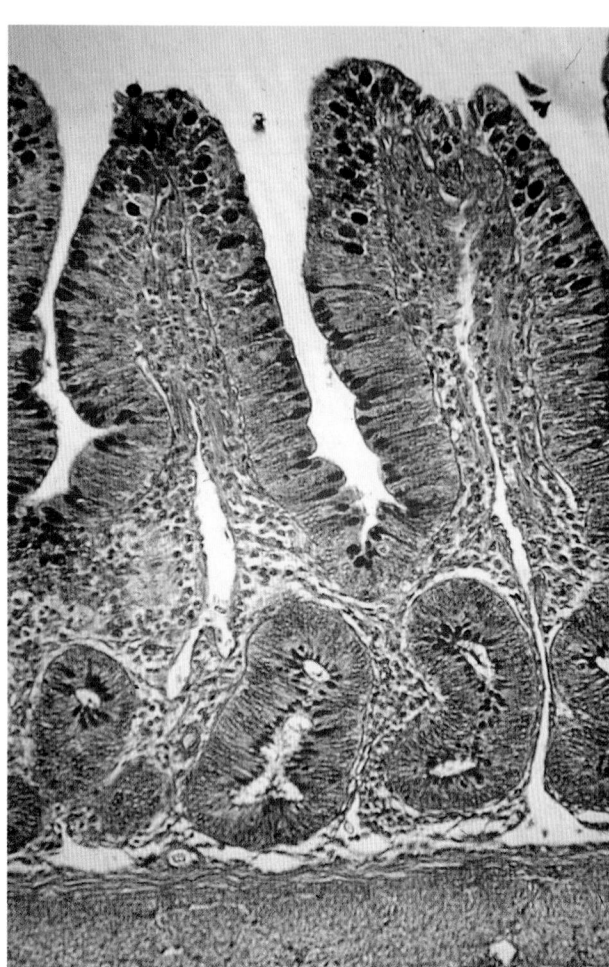

Fig. 13.11 Endogenous stages of *Eimeria mitis* in the villi of the small intestine.

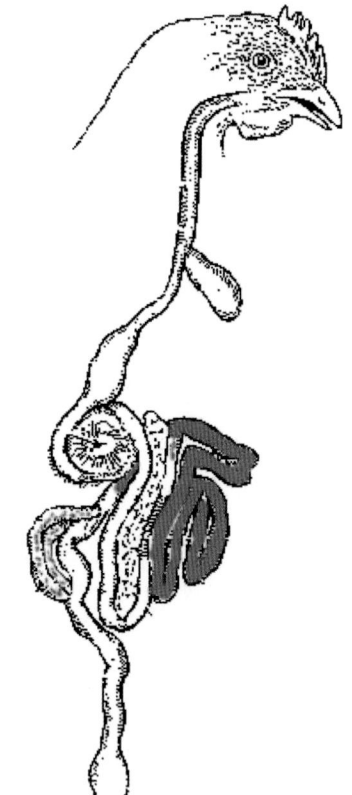

Fig. 13.12 Predilection site of *Eimeria necatrix*.

produced with this species, but infection can cause a decrease in body weight gain. The endogenous stages are in the epithelial cells of the villi and occasionally in the crypts of the small intestine (Fig. 13.11), also the caeca and rectum. The number of meront generations is unknown. Asexual and sexual stages occur together. The prepatent period is 91 hours. The sporulation time is 18–24 hours (Table 13.6).

Clinical signs and pathology: Generally, older chickens are affected by the species found in the small intestine, and clinical signs are similar to those of caecal coccidiosis. Subclinical infections are more common than overt disease and may be suspected when pullets have poor rates of growth and feed conversion, and the onset of egg-laying is delayed. Infection produces little pathology, although there may be small petechiae in the lower small intestine and mucoid exudates in the lumen.

Table 13.6 *Eimeria mitis.*

Lesions: no discrete lesions, mucoid exudate and areas of small petechiation
Mean oocyst size (μm): 16 × 15
Shape and length/width index: subspherical, 1.09
Prepatent period (hours): 91
Sporulation time (hours): 18–24

Eimeria necatrix

Eimeria necatrix (Phylum: Apicomplexa; Class: Conoidasida; Order: Eucoccidiorida; Family: Eimeriidae) occurs worldwide in the small intestine of chickens (Fig. 13.12). It is one of the most pathogenic species of coccidia affecting these birds. Following ingestion of sporulated oocysts and excystation, sporozoites enter the epithelial cells of the small intestine, pass through the epithelium into the lamina propria at the centre of the villi, and migrate towards the muscularis mucosae. Many sporozoites are engulfed by macrophages during this passage and are transported to the epithelial cells of the fundus. The macrophages invade these cells and appear to disintegrate, leaving the sporozoites unharmed. The sporozoites round up to form first-generation meronts, found above the host cell nuclei in the epithelial cells of the crypts of the small intestine. Second-generation meronts develop deep in the mucosa (Fig. 13.13). The prepatent period is 138 hours and the patent period about 12 days. Sporulation time is 18–24 hours (Table 13.7).

Clinical signs: Symptoms seen include diarrhoea (mucoid and sometimes bloody), dejection, ruffled feathers and drooping wings, inappetence, weight loss and depressed weight gain. Death usually occurs 5–7 days after infection, often before oocysts are passed in the faeces. Birds that recover often remain unthrifty and emaciated.

Pathology: The principal lesions are in the small intestine, especially the middle third. Small white opaque foci are seen by the fourth day after infection. These are the second-generation meronts

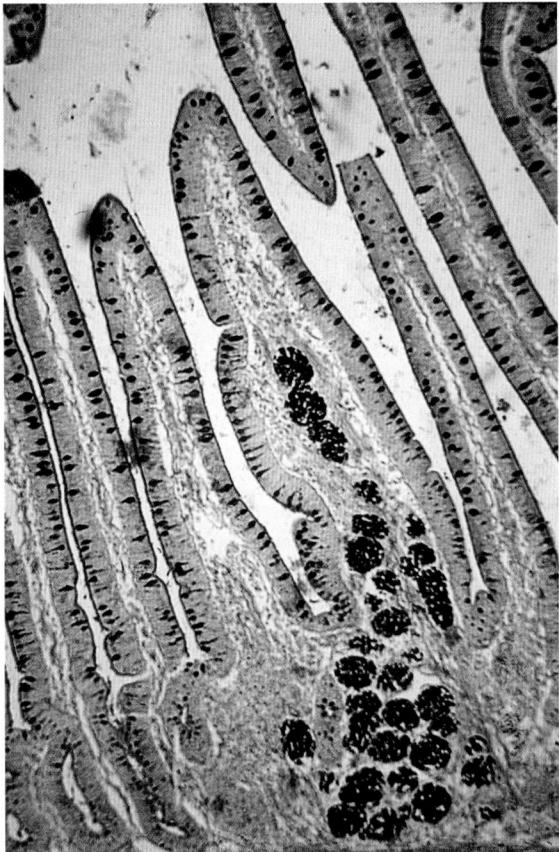

Fig. 13.13 Histological section showing second-generation meronts of *Eimeria necatrix* deep in the mucosa.

Table 13.7 *Eimeria necatrix.*

Lesions: ballooning intestine with white spots (meronts), petechiation and blood-filled exudate (Fig. 13.15)
Mean oocyst size (µm): 20 × 17
Shape and length/width index: subspherical, 1.19
Prepatent period (hours): 138
Sporulation time (hours): 18–24

(Fig. 13.14), and they are often so deep in the mucosa that they are most visible from the serosal surface. Severe haemorrhage may occur by day 5 or 6 and the small intestine may be markedly swollen and filled with clotted or unclotted blood. The wall is thickened and dull red and petechiae are present in the white foci as a result of release of the second-generation merozoites (Fig. 13.15). The gut wall may lose its contractility, become friable, and the epithelium may slough and be replaced by a network of fibrin-containing mononuclear cells. This network is replaced by connective tissue resulting in permanent scarring, which interferes with intestinal absorption.

Lesions are scored +1 to +4 as follows.

1 The presence of small scattered petechiae and white spots visible from the serosal surface.
2 Numerous petechiae on the serosal surface and some slight ballooning of the intestine.
3 Extensive haemorrhage into the lumen and the presence of red or brown mucus, extensive petechiae on the serosal surface, marked ballooning of the intestine and absence of normal intestinal contents.
4 Ballooning may be extensive, and haemorrhage may give an intensive dark colour to the intestinal contents.

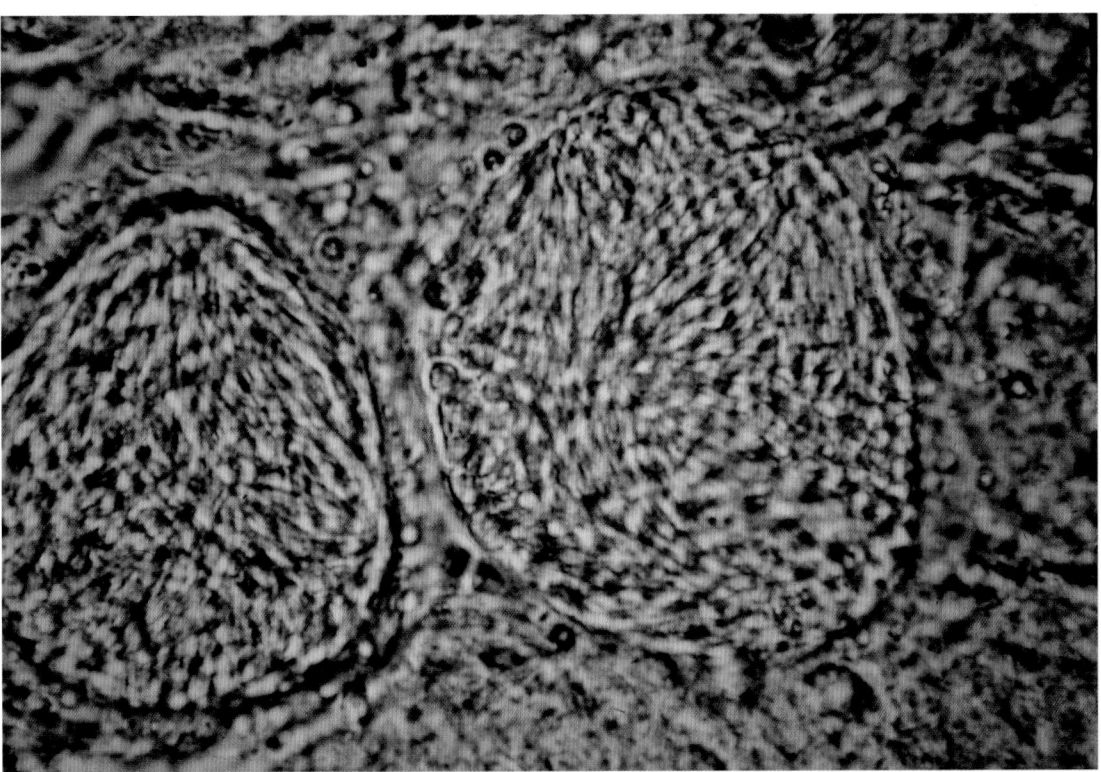

Fig. 13.14 Second-generation meronts of *Eimeria necatrix* in mucosal smear of mid small intestine.

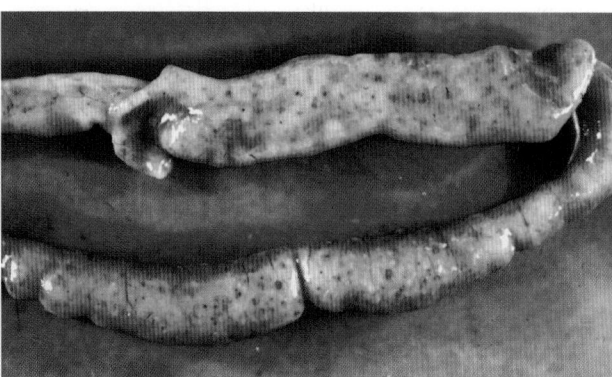

Fig. 13.15 Lesions of *Eimeria necatrix*: mid small intestine.

Eimeria praecox

Eimeria praecox (Phylum: Apicomplexa; Class: Conoidasida; Order: Eucoccidiorida; Family: Eimeriidae) occurs worldwide in the small intestine of chickens and is generally considered non-pathogenic (Fig. 13.16). The endogenous stages occur in the epithelial cells of the villi, usually along the sides of the villi, and lie below the host cell nucleus. There are at least three, and possibly four, generations of merogony. The second meront generation is seen as early as 36 hours after infection. Later development is irregular, and both asexual and sexual generations are seen together. The prepatent period is 84 hours and the patent period approximately four days. The sporulation time is 48 hours (Table 13.8).

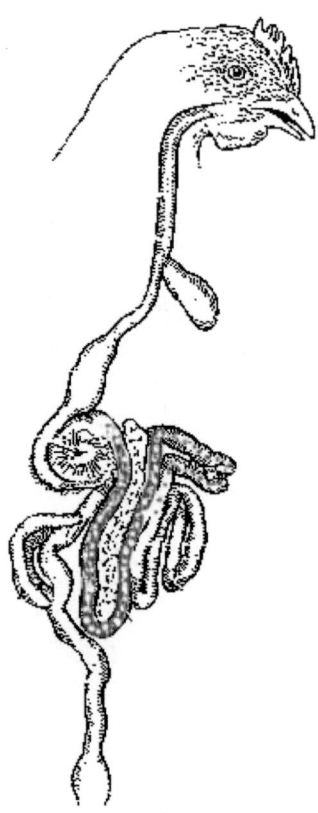

Fig. 13.16 Predilection site of *Eimeria praecox*.

Table 13.8 *Eimeria praecox.*

Lesions: no lesions, mucoid exudate
Mean oocyst size (µm): 21 × 17
Shape and length/width index: ovoid, 1.24
Prepatent period (hours): 84
Sporulation time (hours): 48

Clinical signs and pathology: There are no associated clinical signs. A mucoid exudate is the only lesion seen. Endogenous stages can be detected in the wall of the small intestine by histopathology.

Coccidiosis in turkeys

Seven species of *Eimeria* have been identified in turkeys; identification is based on location in the intestine and associated pathology (Table 13.9). Specific identification is based on the nature and location of the lesions in the intestine together with careful examination of fresh smears for the developmental stages of the parasite.

Epidemiology: The appearance and development of coccidiosis are similar to those described for chickens. Acute infections with pathogenic species occur in young turkey poults 2–10 weeks of age, causing enteritis with variable mortality. Deep-litter houses offer optimal conditions of temperature and humidity for oocyst sporulation, and with overcrowding the risk of heavy infection is further increased.

Diagnosis: Diagnosis is best based on *post mortem* examination of a few affected birds. The oocysts may be identified according to shape and size. At necropsy, the location and type of lesions present provide a good guide to the species, which can be confirmed by examination of the oocysts in the faeces, and the meronts and oocysts present in scrapings of the gut.

Control: Prevention of turkey coccidiosis is based on a combination of good management and the use of anticoccidial compounds in the feed or water. Thus, litter should always be kept dry and special attention given to litter near water fonts or feeding troughs. Drinkers that prevent water reaching the litter should always be used and they should be placed on drip trays or over the droppings pit. Feeding and watering utensils should be of such a type and height that droppings cannot contaminate them. Good ventilation will also reduce the humidity in the house and help to keep litter dry. Preferably, clean litter should always be provided between batches of birds. If this is not possible, the litter should be heaped and left for 24 hours after it has reached a temperature of 50 °C; it should then be forked over again and the process repeated to ensure that all the oocysts in the litter have been destroyed.

Table 13.9 Predilection sites and prepatent periods of *Eimeria* species in turkeys.

Species	Predilection site	Prepatent period (hours)
Eimeria adenoides	Lower small intestine, caeca	104–132
Eimeria dispersa	Duodenum, upper small intestine	120–144
Eimeria meleagridis	Ceaca	144
Eimeria meleagrimitis	Duodenum	144
Eimeria gallopavonis	Ileum, rectum, caeca	144
Eimeria innocua	Small intestine	120
Eimeria subrotunda	Small intestine	96

When in-feed coccidiostats are used, there are two further factors to consider. First, outbreaks of coccidiosis may occur in birds on medicated feed either because the level of coccidiostat used is too low or because conditions in the house have changed to allow a massive sporulation of oocysts which, on ingestion, the level of drug can no longer control. Second, the influence of intercurrent infections in affecting appetite, and therefore uptake of coccidiostat, should also be considered.

Treatment: Anticoccidial drugs, such as lasolocid, monensin, robenidine, amprolium, ethopabate and clopidol/methylbenzoquate, can be used for prophylaxis by incorporation in the feed for the first 12–16 weeks of life. Low doses of anticoccidial drugs can be used to allow immunity to develop, particularly in breeding birds. Monensin should be used under veterinary guidance because of its greater toxicity for turkeys than for chickens.

Intestinal coccidiosis

As with coccidiosis in chickens, more than one species is usually present in outbreaks of disease. Specific identification is based on the nature and location of the lesions in the intestine together with careful examination of fresh smears for the developmental stages of the parasite.

Eimeria adenoides

Eimeria adenoides (Phylum: Apicomplexa; Class: Conoidasida; Order: Eucoccidiorida; Family: Eimeriidae) occurs worldwide in the in the lower small intestine, caeca and rectum of turkeys and has two generations of meronts. First-generation meronts can be seen in the epithelial cells as early as six hours after inoculation. Second-generation meronts mature 96–108 hours after inoculation. Sexual stages can be detected as early as 120 hours post infection. The prepatent period is 104–132 hours and the patent period 7–20 days. Sporulation time is 24 hours.

Pathogenesis: *Eimeria adenoides* is one of the most pathogenic species of coccidia in turkeys. Clinical signs first appear four days after infection, coincident with the rupture of the second-stage meronts. Initially the intestines appear grossly normal until this point; thereafter, the walls of the lower third of the small intestine, caeca and rectum become swollen and oedematous, with petechial haemorrhages visible from the mucosal surface only. The lower intestine becomes filled with mucus. The infected epithelial cells break away, leaving the villi denuded. The blood vessels become engorged and cellular infiltration of the submucosa and epithelium increases progressively. In birds that recover from the disease, and in those that received a low infection dose, resolution is rapid. Vascularity is greatly reduced and the deep glands are almost free of parasites by day 7. The intestine is almost normal by day 9 or 10 post infection.

Clinical signs and pathology: The affected poults are dull, listless and anorexic, stand with ruffled feathers and have their heads tucked under their wings. Their droppings are white and mucoid and may contain blood. Heavy infections can result in mortality. Most of the terminal intestine is congested and contains large numbers of merozoites and long streaks of blood. Caseous material, composed of cellular debris, gametes and a few immature oocysts, accumulates. With time, the caseous exudate is composed largely of oocysts. The faeces in severe cases are relatively fluid and may be blood-tinged and contain mucous casts 2.5–5 cm long. Caseous plugs may be present in the caeca. The terminal intestine may contain creamy white mucus and petechiae may be present in the mucosa. As recovery proceeds, the intestinal contents appear normal but still contain large numbers of oocysts.

Eimeria dispersa

Eimeria dispersa (Phylum: Apicomplexa; Class: Conoidasida; Order: Eucoccidiorida; Family: Eimeriidae) occurs worldwide in the duodenum and upper small intestine of turkeys. First-, second-, third- and fourth-generation meronts are present 30, 48, 72 and 96 hours after infection, respectively. Sporozoites and first-generation meronts lie close above the epithelial cell nuclei; second-, third- and fourth-generation meronts are also above the host cell nucleus, but lie near the brush border of the host cell. The mature macrogamonts and microgamonts can be found in the small intestine villous epithelial cells 96 hours after infection. The prepatent period is 120–144 hours. Oocyst sporulation time is 48 hours.

Clinical signs and pathology: This is a mildly pathogenic species that produces creamy mucoid exudates in the small intestine of young turkeys and depressed weight gains. Symptoms are characterised by diarrhoea, weight loss, ruffled feathers, droopiness and growth retardation. With pathogenic strains, the most severe lesions occur 5–6 days after infection. The entire small intestine is markedly dilated, and the duodenum and anterior jejunum are creamy white when seen through the serosal surface. The anterior half of the small intestine is filled with creamy, yellowish, sticky, mucoid material. The wall of the anterior intestine is oedematous but there is little epithelial sloughing. Recovery is rapid and the intestine appears virtually normal eight days post infection.

Eimeria gallopavonis

Eimeria gallopavonis (Phylum: Apicomplexa; Class: Conoidasida; Order: Eucoccidiorida; Family: Eimeriidae) is a moderately pathogenic parasite distributed worldwide and localised in the small and large intestine of turkeys. Endogenous stages occur in the epithelial cells at the tips of the villi and lie above the host cell nucleus. The first-generation meronts occur in the ileum and rectum. There appear to be two sizes of second-generation meronts, with smaller ones occurring in the rectum and ileum, more rarely the caeca, and larger ones only in the rectum. A few third-generation meronts are found in the rectum producing 10–12 merozoites. These and second-generation meronts develop into gamonts found primarily in the rectum and occasionally the ileum and caeca. The prepatent period is 144 hours. Oocyst sporulation time is 24 hours.

Clinical signs and pathology: Symptoms are characterised by watery or mucoid diarrhoea, depression, ruffled feathers and anorexia. This species is found in the ileum, rectum and less commonly the caeca. The intestine is inflamed and oedematous with soft white caseous material in the lumen.

Eimeria meleagrimitis

Eimeria meleagrimitis (Phylum: Apicomplexa; Class: Conoidasida; Order: Eucoccidiorida; Family: Eimeriidae) occurs worldwide in the duodenum of turkeys. The sporocysts emerge from the oocysts in the gizzard and the sporozoites are activated and emerge from the sporocysts in the small intestine. The sporozoites invade the tips of the villi and migrate down the villi in the lamina propria until they reach the glands. First-generation meronts can be found in the gland epithelial cells as early as 12 hours after infection and are mature by 48 hours. The first-generation merozoites invade the adjacent epithelial cells, forming colonies of second-generation meronts that mature at about 66 hours after infection. Third-generation meronts may appear as early as 72 hours after inoculation and are mature by 96 hours. Macrogametes and microgamonts appear 114 hours after infection. The prepatent period is 144 hours. Oocyst sporulation time is 24–72 hours.

Pathogenesis: *Eimeria meleagrimitis* is moderately to markedly pathogenic and has three generations of merogony, with disease occurring after the rupture of the third-stage meronts, at about four days after infection. It is usually located in the small intestine anterior to the yolk stalk but may extend throughout the intestine.

Clinical signs: Disease is seen in turkey poults 2–10 weeks of age and rarely in older birds because of acquired immunity. The affected poults are dull and listless, stand with ruffled feathers and have their heads tucked under their wings. Feed consumption drops following infection and affected birds are huddled together with closed eyes, drooping wings and ruffled feathers. Their droppings are white and mucoid and, at the peak of the disease, intestinal cores may be passed and the faeces may contain a few flecks of blood. Death occurs 5–7 days after infection, particularly in young poults under six weeks old.

Pathology: Lesions are seen from the end of the fourth day after infection. The jejunum is slightly thickened and dilated and contains an excessive amount of clear colourless fluid, or mucus containing merozoites, small amounts of blood and other cells. By days 5–6 after infection, the duodenum is enlarged and its blood vessels are engorged. It contains a reddish-brown necrotic core that is firmly adherent to the mucosa and extends a little way into the upper small intestine. The remainder of the intestine is congested, and petechial haemorrhages may be present in the mucosa of most of the small intestine. The mucosa begins to regenerate on day 6 or 7 after infection. A few petechiae are present in the duodenum and jejunum. There are small streaks of haemorrhage and spotty congestion in the ileum. The posterior part of the jejunum and ileum may contain greenish mucoid casts, 5–10 cm long and 3–6 mm in diameter. Necrotic material may be found in the ileum or faeces.

Coccidiosis in ducks and geese

Eimeria anseris

Eimeria anseris (Phylum: Apicomplexa; Class: Conoidasida; Order: Eucoccidiorida; Family: Eimeriidae) is a parasite of the small and large intestine of domestic geese, blue geese (*Anser caerulescens*) and Richardson's Canada geese (*Branta canadensis hutchinsi*). It is distributed in Europe, occurring in young birds, and is associated with birds kept under intensive conditions. The life cycle is typically coccidian, although precise details are lacking. There appears to be only one merogony generation. Endogenous stages occur in compact clumps under the intestinal epithelium near the muscularis mucosae, in the epithelial cells of the villi of the small intestine and, in heavy infections, also in the caeca and rectum. The gamonts are mostly in the subepithelial tissues but invade the epithelium in heavy infections. The prepatent period is 6–7 days and patent period 2–8 days.

Pathogenesis: There is comparatively little information on coccidiosis of ducks and geese. *Eimeria anseris* has been reported as causing acute intestinal coccidiosis with haemorrhage in goslings.

Clinical signs and pathology: The infection causes diarrhoea with mucus and haemorrhage. There may be intestinal hyperaemia and mucus production with flecks of coagulated blood within the gut lumen. Oocysts are found in small discrete papilliform lesions.

Diagnosis: Diagnosis is best based on *post mortem* examination of a few affected birds. At necropsy, the location and type of lesions present provide a good guide to the species, which can be confirmed by examination of the oocysts in the faeces, and the meronts and oocysts present in scrapings of the gut.

Control and treatment: Prevention is based on good management, avoidance of overcrowding and stress, and attention to hygiene. Contact with wild geese should be avoided wherever possible. Little is known about treatment but, by analogy with other hosts, one of the sulfonamide drugs should be tried.

Eimeria nocens

Eimeria nocens (Phylum: Apicomplexa; Class: Conoidasida; Order: Eucoccidiorida; Family: Eimeriidae) is a parasite of the small intestine of domestic geese and blue geese (*Anser caerulescens*). It is distributed in Europe and North America. Specific details of the life cycle are lacking. Developmental stages occur in the epithelial cells of the tips of villi at the posterior part of the small intestine but may also occur beneath the epithelium. The younger developmental stages lie near the host cell nuclei, and as they grow they displace the nuclei and eventually destroy the cell and come to lie free and partly beneath the epithelium. The prepatent period is 4–9 days.

Epidemiology: *Eimeria nocens* occurs in young birds and is associated with birds kept under intensive conditions, which offer optimal conditions of temperature and humidity for oocyst sporulation. Overcrowding further exacerbates infection levels and risks from disease.

Clinical signs and pathology: *Eimeria nocens* has been reported as causing acute intestinal coccidiosis in goslings with diarrhoea with mucus and flecks of blood. There may be intestinal hyperaemia and mucus production with small flecks of coagulated blood within the gut lumen.

Diagnosis, control and treatment: As for *E. anseris*.

Tyzzeria perniciosa

Tyzzeria perniciosa (Phylum: Apicomplexa; Class: Conoidasida; Order: Eucoccidiorida; Family: Eimeriidae) is a parasite of the small intestine of domestic ducks, pintail ducks and diving ducks

(*Aythya erythropus*). It is presumably distributed worldwide, and is highly pathogenic for ducklings.

Clinical signs and pathology: Infected birds stop eating, lose weight and become weak; there can be a high mortality. Clinical signs are characterised by anorexia, diarrhoea with mucus and haemorrhage. On *post mortem*, inflammation and haemorrhagic areas are seen throughout the small intestine, and especially in the upper part of the intestine. The intestinal wall is thickened and round white spots are visible through the serosal surface. In severe cases, the lumen is filled with blood and often cheesy exudates. The intestinal epithelium sloughs off in long pieces, often forming a lifting 'tube'.

Diagnosis: Diagnosis is best based on *post mortem* examination and by examination of the oocysts in the faeces. Masses of very small, rounded oocysts are present in smears and scrapings of the gut.

Control and treatment: As for *E. anseris*.

Coccidiosis in gamebirds

Pheasants

The development of intensive management systems by pheasant-rearing farms has led to an increase in coccidiosis. The significance of coccidiosis in wild pheasants is difficult to assess because natural predators and scavengers deal promptly with weak or dead birds. Treatment with clopidol, lasalocid, amprolium or potentiated sulfonamides (sulfaquinolaxaline or sulfadimidine) is generally effective, although specific efficacy data are lacking. Apart from the usual measures of isolation and rigorous hygiene, the use of preventive medication in intensively reared pheasants provides a means of controlling the disease where outbreaks occur.

Eimeria colchici

Eimeria colchici (Phylum: Apicomplexa; Class: Conoidasida; Order: Eucoccidiorida; Family: Eimeriidae) is a parasite localised in the caeca of phaesants. It is distributed in the USA and Europe (e.g. UK, Bulgaria, Czech Republic, Slovakia). The life cycle is typically coccidian. First-generation meronts are found deep in the glands of the mucosal lining of the mid small intestine; second-generation meronts appear in colonies in the lamina propria at the base of the villi; small third-generation meronts develop in the glands of the caeca. The gametocytes develop in the epithelial cells lining the caecal mucosa. The prepatent period is six days. Sporulation time is two days.

Pathogenesis: *Eimeria colchici* is the most pathogenic species of coccidia in pheasants, producing weight loss and mortality in infected birds.

Clinical signs and pathology: The infection causes diarrhoea and white soiling around the vent. There is hyperaemia and mucoid enteritis in the small intestine caused by the second-generation meronts. Dead birds have soft white cores in the caeca and lower small intestine. In the caeca, there is extensive invasion of the mucosa by gametocytes, with the entire epithelium and subepithelial cells of the lamina propria infected. The cores are composed of oocysts, necrotic debris and food material.

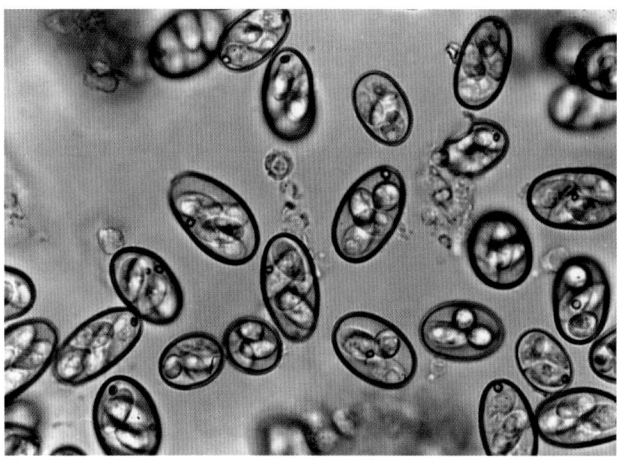

Fig. 13.17 Sporulated oocysts of *Eimeria colchici* isolated from faeces.

Diagnosis: *Post mortem* examination of affected birds reveals the characteristic white cores, and examination of scrapings or histological sections of affected tissues shows large numbers of gametocytes in the caeca. On faecal examination, there are large numbers of oocysts in a white caseous exudate, and these are readily identifiable after sporulation (Fig. 13.17).

Eimeria duodenalis

Eimeria duodenalis (Phylum: Apicomplexa; Class: Conoidasida; Order: Eucoccidiorida; Family: Eimeriidae) is a protozoon of the small intestine of pheasants, distributed in Europe (e.g. UK, France, Lithuania, Kazakhstan) and the USA. First-generation meronts appear in the epithelial cells towards the tips of the duodenal villi. Second- and third-generation meronts follow on quickly in the same site but extending further along the intestinal tract. Gametocytes and third-generation meronts are present together and the infection may extend throughout the entire small intestine, with the villi heavily parasitised and multiple infections of individual epithelial cells occurring frequently. The prepatent period is five days. Sporulation time is 1–2 days.

Epidemiology: Coccidiosis in pheasants occurs most frequently in young birds reared under intensive conditions. Disease surveys carried out in the UK have shown that *E. duodenalis* accounted for 10–15% of the coccidiosis cases where species identification was possible.

Clinical signs and pathology: As the specific name implies, this parasite develops in the duodenum and upper small intestine where it can cause a mucoid enteritis. Light infections are generally asymptomatic but heavier infections may cause mucoid diarrhoea. The intestines of the birds that die are congested and contain a pinkish mucoid exudate, while the caeca may be distended with a foamy yellow fluid. Scrapings from the small intestine show masses of small subspherical oocysts.

Diagnosis: *Post mortem* examination of affected birds reveals a mucoid enteritis in the duodenum and upper small intestine, and examination of scrapings or histological sections of affected tissues shows large numbers of small subspherical oocysts in the small intestine.

Eimeria megalostoma

Eimeria megalostoma (Phylum: Apicomplexa; Class: Conoidasida; Order: Eucoccidiorida; Family: Eimeriidae) is a protozoon of pheasants, distributed in North America, the UK and Kazakhstan. The significance of coccidiosis in wild pheasants is difficult to assess because natural predators and scavengers deal promptly with weak or dead birds. No information is available about the pathogenesis. The infection occurs only rarely in small numbers and has not been associated with outbreaks of disease.

Diagnosis: Diagnosis is based on oocyst morphology from faecal samples. Where possible, *post mortem* examination of affected birds and examination of scrapings or histological sections of affected tissues should be undertaken.

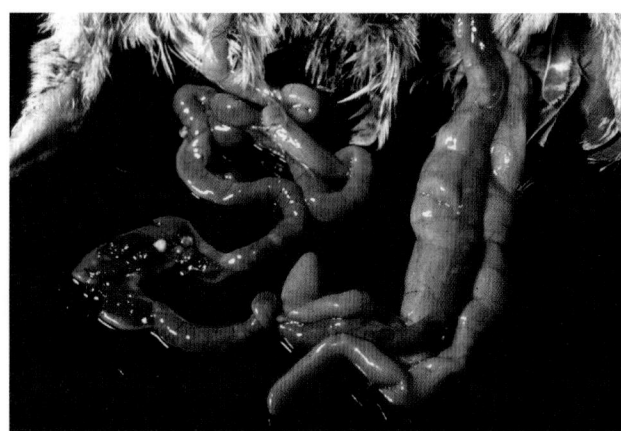

Fig. 13.18 Caecal lesions of *Eimeria phasiani.*

Eimeria phasiani

Eimeria phasiani (Phylum: Apicomplexa; Class: Conoidasida; Order: Eucoccidiorida; Family: Eimeriidae) is a parasite of the small and large intestine of pheasants. It is distributed in Europe (e.g. UK, France, Germany, Czech Republic, Slovakia, Lithuania, Kazakhstan) and the USA. Development of the endogenous stages occurs in the small intestine and there is a gradual spread down the gut as the infection proceeds. First-generation meronts develop in the epithelial cells lining the glands of the ascending duodenum and upper small intestine. Second-generation meronts are most numerous towards the tips of the villi in the upper small intestine. Third-generation meronts and gametocytes are found throughout the small intestine and also in the proximal part of the caeca, being most numerous towards the tips of the villi. The prepatent period is five days. Sporulation time is two days.

Epidemiology: Coccidiosis in pheasants occurs most frequently in young birds reared under intensive conditions. Disease surveys carried out in the UK have shown that *E. phasiani* accounted for approximately 15% of the coccidiosis cases where species identification was possible. In studies conducted in the Czech Republic/Slovakia, *E. phasiani* occurred less frequently than *E. colchici* in wild pheasants but was most prevalent during the winter and spring, when it was identified in 18–41% of the samples examined. Mortality can reach 50% in 2–3-week-old pheasants.

Clinical signs and pathology: Infection can result in anorexia, depression and a reduction in weight gain, and in heavy infections causes liquid faeces with mucus and a little blood. The main lesions consist of mucoid enteritis in the small intestine. The intestines of heavily infected birds are hyperaemic and show petechial haemorrhages, while the lumen may be filled with blood-streaked mucus (Fig. 13.18). The developmental stages of *E. phasiani* occur below the nucleus of the host cell, causing ballooning of the infected cell with enlargement of the nucleus. Oocysts occur throughout the small intestine and in the proximal part of the caeca.

Diagnosis: *Post mortem* examination of affected birds reveals a mucoid enteritis, and examination of scrapings or histological sections of affected tissues shows large numbers of gametocytes in the small intestine and proximal part of the caeca.

Partridges

Several species of coccidia have been described in partridges, based mainly on oocyst morphology. Details on life cycle, pathogenesis, treatment and control are lacking. Prevention, as with other hosts, should be based on good management, avoidance of overcrowding and stress, and attention to hygiene.

Eimeria legionensis

Eimeria legionensis (Phylum: Apicomplexa; Class: Conoidasida; Order: Eucoccidiorida; Family: Eimeriidae) is a parasite of the small intestine of red-legged partridges (*Alectoris rufa*) and rock partridges (*Alectoris graeca*). Its distribution is still unknown, but it has been reported in the UK and Bulgaria.

Pathology: Dead birds have soft white cores in the caeca and lower small intestine. In the caeca there is extensive invasion of the mucosa by gametocytes, with the entire epithelium and subepithelial cells of the lamina propria infected. The cores are composed of oocysts, necrotic debris and food material.

Diagnosis: *Post mortem* examination of affected birds reveals the characteristic white cores, and examination of scrapings or histological sections of affected tissues shows large numbers of gametocytes in the caeca. On faecal examination there are large numbers of oocysts in a white caseous exudate.

Quails

Several species of coccidia have been described in these species (see checklist table), based mainly on oocyst morphology. Details on life cycle, pathogenesis, treatment and control are lacking.

Guinea fowl

Eimeria grenieri

Eimeria grenieri (Phylum: Apicomplexa; Class: Conoidasida; Order: Eucoccidiorida; Family: Eimeriidae) is a parasite of the small intestine of guinea fowl. It is distributed in Europe and

Africa. *Eimeria grenieri* has been reported to cause disease in guinea fowl, inducing diarrhoea and weight loss. The life cycle is typically coccidian and there appear to be three merogony generations. First-generation meronts are in the epithelial cells of the crypts below the host cell nucleus near the muscularis mucosae of the duodenum. Second-generation meronts are in the crypts of the lower part of the villi of the upper and middle small intestine. Third-generation meronts are in the middle to tips of the villi of the middle to lower small intestine. The gamonts are in the caecal epithelium. The prepatent period is 4–5 days and the patent period three days.

Other protozoa

Cryptosporidium baileyi

For more details see section on Large intestine.

Cryptosporidium meleagridis

Cryptosporidium meleagridis (Phylum: Apicomplexa; Class: Conoidasida; Order: Cryptogregarinorida; Family: Cryptosporidiidae) is a presumably worldwide distributed parasite of the small intestine of turkeys, chickens, ducks and parrots. Transmission occurs mainly via the faecal–oral route.

Pathogenesis: Infection with this parasite has been associated with diarrhoea and a low death rate in 10–14-day-old turkey poults. *Cryptosporidium meleagridis* also infects other avian hosts (e.g. parrots) and is also the third most common *Cryptosporidium* parasite in humans.

Clinical signs and pathology: Diarrhoea. Following ingestion, the sporozoites invade the microvillous brush border of the proventriculus, intestines and lungs and the trophozoites rapidly differentiate to form meronts with 4–8 merozoites. Only a single merogony generation has been reported. There is villous atrophy and crypt hyperplasia in the ileum of affected turkeys and humans.

Diagnosis: Oocysts may be demonstrated using Ziehl–Neelsen stained faecal smears in which the sporozoites appear as bright red granules. Speciation of *Cryptosporidium* is difficult, if not impossible, using conventional techniques. A range of molecular and immunological techniques has been developed that includes immunofluorescence and enzyme-linked immunosorbent assay (ELISA). More recently, DNA-based techniques have been used for the molecular characterisations of *Cryptosporidium* species.

Control and treatment: Good hygiene and management are important in preventing disease from cryptosporidiosis. Thus, litter should always be kept dry and special attention given to litter near water fonts or feeding troughs. Fonts that prevent water reaching the litter should always be used and they should be placed on drip trays or over the droppings pit. Feeding and watering utensils should be of such a type and height that droppings cannot contaminate them. Batch rearing of birds, depopulation and adequate disinfection procedures should help limit levels of infection. Antibiotics to control secondary bacterial infections of the respiratory form may be required but there is no reported effective treatment. Good ventilation in poultry houses is also essential.

Spironucleus meleagridis

Spironucleus meleagridis, synonym *Hexamita meleagridis* (Phylum: Metamonada; Class: Trepomonadea; Order: Diplomonadida; Family: Spironucleidae), is the aetiological agent of infectious catarrhal enteritis, also known as hexamitosis or spironucleosis. It occurs worldwide in the small intestine and caeca of turkeys, ducks and gamebirds (e.g. pheasants, quails and partridges).

Epidemiology: Infection is transmitted through contaminated feed and water. Carrier adult birds are the most important sources of infection for young poults. Wild gamebirds may be a source of infection to birds reared outdoors in natural pens. Hot weather and overcrowding predispose to infection and the severity of a disease outbreak.

Pathogenesis: Spironucleosis is a disease of young birds with adults as symptomless carriers. The mortality in a flock varies and can be as high as 80%, reaching a peak in the flock at 7–10 days after the first bird dies, but heavy losses seldom occur in birds over 10 weeks old. The incubation period is 4–7 days. Affected birds are ruffled, have a foamy watery diarrhoea, lose weight rapidly and may become weak and die.

Diagnosis: Infection can be diagnosed by finding the characteristic motile protozoa in fresh scrapings from the small intestine. The organism can be differentiated from other flagellates in the gut by its small size, absence of an undulating membrane and characteristic motion. The organism can also be demonstrated in Giemsa-stained smears from the small intestine (Fig. 13.19).

Control and treatment: Control depends on good management and hygiene. Young birds should be raised in batches away from other birds of different age groups. Separate utensils should be used for different groups of birds and they should be kept raised or on wire mesh floors. Outdoor natural pens should be moved periodically and contact with pheasants, quails or partridges prevented. Dimetridazole 125–200 g/tons in feed or 12 g/l in drinking water for up to 15 days can be used in prevention. Dimetridazole 27 g per 100 l of drinking water for 12 days, or 54 g per 100 l for 3–5 days then 27 g per 100 l for 12 days are effective treatments. However, in many countries products containing dimetridazole (and other nitroimidazole compounds) are becoming unavailable for legislative reasons.

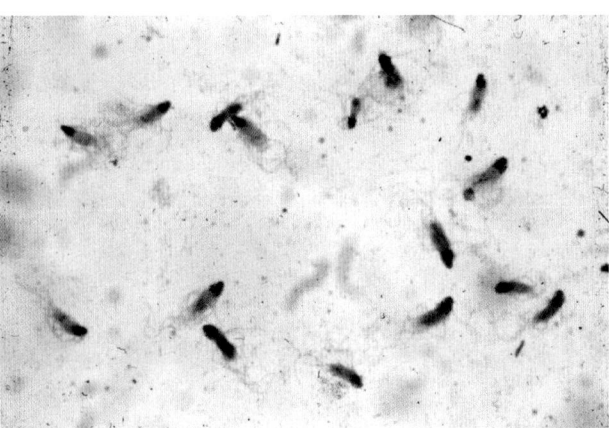
Fig. 13.19 Motile protozoa of *Spironucleus meleagridis* in the mucosal scrapings of small intestine.

LARGE INTESTINE

Several species of *Heterakis* are found in poultry.

Heterakis gallinarum

Heterakis gallinarum, synonyms *Heterakis papillosa*, *Heterakis gallinae*, *Heterakis vesicularis* (Phylum: Nematoda; Class: Chromadorea; Order: Ascaridida; Family: Heterakiidae), commonly known as the Poultry caecal worm, occurs worldwide in the caeca and rarely in the small and large intestine of chickens, turkeys, pigeons, pheasants, partridges, grouse, quails, guinea fowl, ducks, geese and a number of wild galliform birds.

Epidemiology: *Heterakis gallinarum* is widespread in most poultry flocks and is of little pathogenic significance in itself, but is of great importance in the epidemiology of *Histomonas*. Larvated eggs can remain viable in soil for about one year and can be a source of infection in free-range birds. Additionally, paratenic hosts such as earthworms can transmit infection.

Pathogenesis: *Heterakis gallinarum* is the most common nematode parasite of poultry and is usually regarded as being non-pathogenic, although heavy infections can induce thickening of the caecal mucosa. Its chief pathogenic importance is as a vector of the protozoan *Histomonas meleagridis*, the causal agent of 'blackhead' (enterohepatitis) in turkeys. The organism can be transmitted from fowl to fowl in the egg of *Heterakis* and in earthworms containing hatched larvae of the worm.

Clinical signs and pathology: Frequently, *H. gallinarum* alone produces an asymptomatic infection. The caeca may show marked inflammation and thickening of the mucosa with petechial haemorrhages.

Diagnosis: *Heterakis gallinarum* infection is usually only diagnosed accidentally, by the finding of eggs in faeces or the presence of worms at necropsy. Differentiation between the three species of *Heterakis* is based on the shape of the oesophagus and the length and shape of the spicules.

Control and treatment: Control of *H. gallinarum* is only necessary when histomonosis is a problem in turkeys. It is largely based on hygiene and in backyard flocks, the two most important factors are the segregation of turkeys from other domestic poultry and the removal and disposal of litter from poultry houses. Where the problem is serious and continuous, it may be advisable to administer either piperazine or levamisole intermittently in the feed or water in addition to continuous *Histomonas* chemoprophylaxis. Treatment with piperazine salts, levamisole or a benzimidazole is effective. Flubendazole, mebendazole or fenbendazole can be administered in the feed (30 ppm over seven days; 60 ppm over seven days; 60 ppm over three days; respectively). Levamisole is effective at 30 mg/kg orally or 300 ppm in the feed.

Heterakis isolonche

Heterakis isolonche (Phylum: Nematoda; Class: Chromadorea; Order: Ascaridida; Family: Heterakiidae), commonly known as the Caecal worm, is distributed worldwide in the caeca and rarely in the large and small intestine of pheasants, grouse, quails, ducks and chickens.

Epidemiology: Infection is common in birds raised in permanent grass pens. Larvated eggs can remain viable in soil for about one year. Additionally, paratenic hosts such as earthworms can transmit infection.

Pathogenesis: *Heterakis isolonche* of gamebirds is in itself pathogenic, causing a severe inflammation of the caeca with nodules projecting from both peritoneal and mucosal surfaces. These can cause ulceration of the mucosa and diarrhoea with progressive emaciation and there may be high mortality in heavily infected flocks.

Clinical signs and pathology: Infections with *H. isolonche* may produce nodular typhlitis, diarrhoea, emaciation and death. In *H. isolonche* infection, the hatched larvae enter the caecal mucosa and develop to maturity in nodules. Each nodule has an opening into the gut through which the eggs reach the lumen. The caeca may show marked inflammation and thickening of the mucosa with nodule formation and petechial haemorrhages.

Diagnosis: *Heterakis isolonche* infection is diagnosed at necropsy by the finding of caecal nodules containing adult worms and, if necessary, confirmed microscopically by examination of the spicules.

Control and treatment: Where *H. isolonche* infection is endemic in pheasantries, the runs should be abandoned and pheasant chicks reared on fresh ground. The treatment is the same as for *H. gallinarum*.

Trichostrongylus tenuis

Trichostrongylus tenuis (Phylum: Nematoda; Class: Chromadorea; Order: Rhabditida; Family: Trichostrongylidae) is a parasite of the small intestine and caeca of gamebirds (e.g. grouse, partridges, pheasants), chickens, ducks, geese, turkeys and emus. It is distributed in North America, Asia and Europe.

Epidemiology: High stocking densities can lead to build-up of large numbers of infective larvae with associated high morbidity and mortality, particularly in grouse.

Pathogenesis: *Trichostrongylus tenuis* has been implicated in outbreaks of severe enteritis in gamebirds. Moderate to severe infections cause diarrhoea, which is often fatal. Lighter infections result in a chronic syndrome characterised by anaemia and emaciation.

Clinical signs and pathology: Reduced appetite, anaemia and general emaciation. Light infections produce few pathological effects, but heavy infections can induce an acute haemorrhagic typhlitis.

Diagnosis: Adult worms are recovered on *post mortem*.

Control and treatment: Where gamebirds are farmed, the pens should be moved regularly to prevent the accumulation of larvae and, if possible, the runs should not be placed in the same areas in successive years. On game farms, therapy with levamisole in the drinking water has proved useful. Formulations of fenbendazole and flubendazole are available for incorporation into feed or grit.

Capillaria anatis

Capillaria anatis, synonyms *Capillaria brevicollis*, *Capillaria collaris*, *Capillaria mergi*, *Thornix anatis* (Phylum: Nematoda; Class: Enoplea; Order: Enoplida; Family: Capillariidae), occurs worldwide

Table 13.10 Species of *Eucoleus/Capillaria* found in gamebirds.

Species	Hosts	Location
Eucoleus (Capillaria) contorta	Chickens, turkeys, ducks, pheasants and wild birds	Oesophagus, crop
Eucoleus (Capillaria) annulata	Chickens, turkeys, ducks and wild birds	Oesophagus, crop
Eucoleus (Capillaria) perforans	Pheasants, guinea fowl	Oesophagus, crop
Capillaria uropapillata	Pheasants	Oesophagus, crop
Capillaria phasianina	Pheasants, grey partridges	Small intestine, caeca
Capillaria anatis	Chickens, turkeys, gallinaceous birds (e.g. pheasants, partridges), pigeons, ducks, geese	Caeca

in the caeca of chickens, turkeys, gallinaceous birds (e.g. pheasants and partridges), pigeons, ducks and geese.

Pathogenesis: The anterior ends of the worms are embedded in the mucosa. Heavy infection can induce haemorrhagic enteritis with bloody diarrhoea. The caecal wall is often thickened.

Clinical signs and pathology: Infected birds may become weak and emaciated and can be anaemic. Chronically infected birds have thickened intestinal walls covered with a catarrhal exudate.

Control and treatment: As for other *Capillaria* species (Table 13.10).

Strongyloides avium

Strongyloides avium (Phylum: Nematoda; Class: Chromadorea; Order: Rhabditida; Family: Strongyloididae), commonly known as the Threadworm, occurs worldwide in the caeca and small intestine of chickens, turkeys, geese, quails and wild birds. *Strongyloides* can be a serious pathogen in young floor-reared birds.

Epidemiology: *Strongyloides* spp. infective larvae are not ensheathed and are susceptible to extreme climatic conditions. However, warmth and moisture favour development and allow the accumulation of large numbers of infective stages.

Clinical signs and pathology: Acute heavy infections cause weakness, emaciation and bloody slimy diarrhoea. Mature parasites in the caeca, if present in large numbers, may cause inflammation with oedema and erosion of the epithelium.

Diagnosis: Small embryonated eggs may be found in the faeces. Adult parasites can be demonstrated in mucosal scrapings from the caecal mucosa on *post mortem*.

Control and treatment: No information is available.

Caecal flukes

See general comments in the section on intestinal flukes. See also Table 13.11.

Chicken caecal coccidiosis

Two species of coccidia are found in chickens, of which *Eimeria tenella* is the most important throughout the world.

Eimeria tenella

Eimeria tenella (Phylum: Apicomplexa; Class: Conoidasida; Order: Eucoccidiorida; Family: Eimeriidae) occurs worldwide in the caeca of chickens (Fig. 13.20). Following ingestion, the oocyst wall breaks in the gizzard, releasing the sporocysts. The sporozoites are activated by bile or trypsin when the sporocysts reach the small intestine, and they escape from the sporocysts. The sporozoites enter the epithelial cells either directly or following ingestion by a macrophage. The sporozoite rounds up to form a first-generation meront, each containing about 900 merozoites, which are approximately 2–4 µm long. These emerge into the caeca about 2.5–3 days after infection and invade new host cells. Second-generation meronts are formed, and these lie above the host cell nucleus producing 200–350 merozoites, which are approximately 16 µm long and are found five days after inoculation. They invade new host cells to form either the third-generation meronts (which lie beneath the host cell nucleus and produce 4–30 third-generation merozoites which are about 7 µm long and which invade new cells to form gamonts) or the gamonts directly. The macrogametes and microgamonts lie below the host cell nuclei. The microgamonts form many biflagellate microgametes, which fertilise the macrogametes. The resulting oocysts lay down a resistant wall, break out of the cells into the gut lumen and are then passed in the faeces. The prepatent period is 132 hours. Sporulation time is 18–48 hours (Table 13.12).

Epidemiology: *Eimeria tenella* is the species primarily responsible for caecal coccidiosis, which mainly occurs in chickens of 3–7 weeks of age.

Table 13.11 Caecal flukes found in poultry.

Parasite	Family	Size (mm)	Predilection site	Final host	Intermediate hosts	Geographical location
Notocotylus attenuatus	Notocotylidae	3–5 × 1	Caeca and rectum	Chickens, ducks, geese, wild aquatic birds	Various snails	Many parts of the world
Catatropis verrucosa	Notocotylidae	2–6 × 1–2	Caeca	Chickens, ducks, geese, wild aquatic birds	Various snails	Worldwide
Brachylaemus commutatus	Brachylaemidae	4–7 × 1–2	Caeca	Chickens, turkeys, other fowl, pigeons and pheasants	Land snails	Southern Europe, Africa, parts of Asia
Postharmostomum commutatum (syn. P. gallinarum)	Brachylaemidae		Caeca	Chickens, turkeys, guinea fowl, pheasants, pigeons	Various snails	North Africa, North America, southern Europe, parts of Southeast Asia
Echinostoma revolutum	Echinostomatidae	1–1.5	Caeca and rectum	Ducks, geese, pigeons, various fowl, aquatic birds	1: Aquatic snails 2: Various aquatic snails and tadpoles	Worldwide
Echinostoma paraulum (syn. Echinoparyphium paraulum)	Echinostomatidae	1–1.5	Caeca and rectum	Ducks, pigeons	1: Aquatic snails 2: Fish	Worldwide

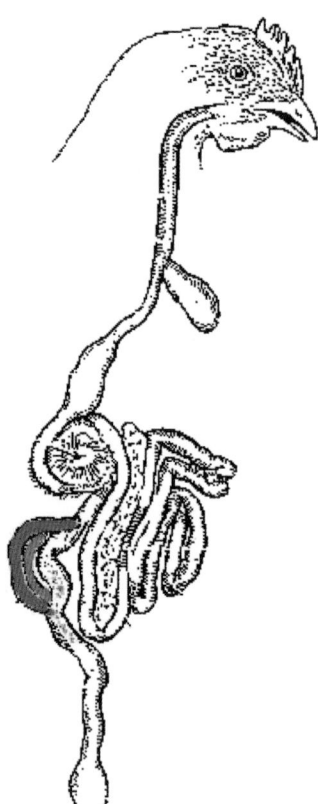

Fig. 13.20 Predilection site of *Eimeria tenella*.

Table 13.12 *Eimeria tenella*.

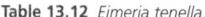

Lesions: haemorrhage in caecal lumen followed by thickening of mucosa and formation of caecal cores with clotted blood (Fig. 13.21)
Mean oocyst size (μm): 25 × 19
Shape and length/width index: ovoid, 1.16
Prepatent period (hours): 132
Sporulation time (hours): 18–48

The prevalence of disease due to this species, and caecal coccidiosis, has declined since many of the anticoccidial drugs in general use were developed specifically to control this pathogenic species.

Pathogenesis: The first-stage meronts of this species develop deep in the glands. The second-stage meronts are also unusual in that the epithelial cells in which they develop leave the mucosa and migrate into the lamina propria and submucosa. When these meronts mature and rupture, about 72 hours after ingestion of oocysts, haemorrhage occurs, the mucosal surface is largely detached and clinical signs become apparent.

Clinical signs and pathology: Clinical disease occurs when large numbers of oocysts are ingested over a short period and is characterised by the presence of soft faeces often containing blood. The chicks are dull and listless, with drooping feathers. In subclinical infections, there are poor weight gains and food conversion rates. At *post mortem*, the caeca are often found to be dilated and contain a mixture of clotted and unclotted blood (Fig. 13.21). In longer-standing infections, the caecal contents become caseous and adherent to the mucosa. As regeneration of the mucosa occurs,

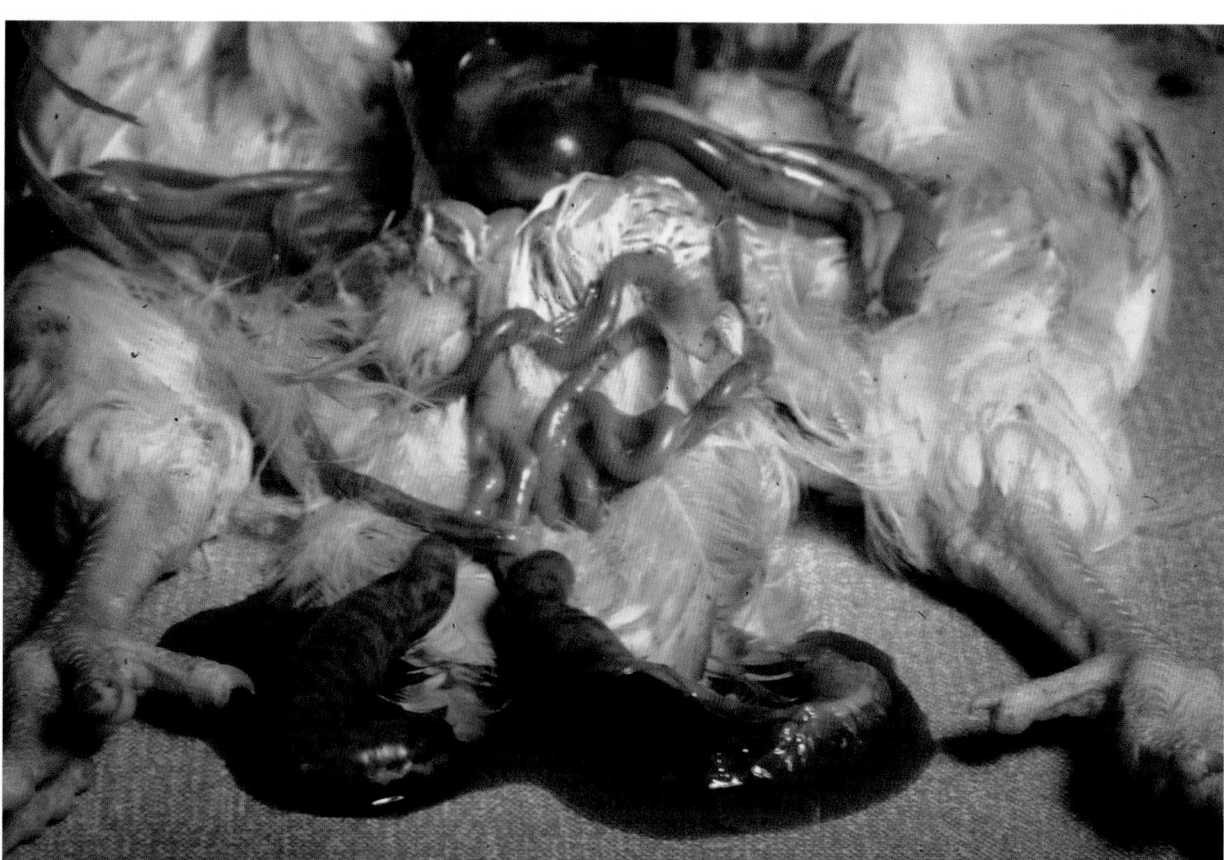

Fig. 13.21 Lesions of *Eimeria tenella* in caeca.

these caecal plugs are detached and caseous material is shed in the faeces.

Lesions are scored +1 to +4 as follows.
1 Very few small scattered petechiae on the caecal wall with no thickening of the caecal walls and normal caecal contents.
2 Lesions more numerous with noticeable blood in the caecal contents. The caecal wall is somewhat thickened with normal caecal contents.
3 Large amounts of blood and caecal cores present. The caecal walls are greatly thickened with little, if any, faecal contents in the caeca.
4 Caecal walls are greatly distended with blood or large caseous cores.

Wenyonella gallinae

Wenyonella gallinae (Phylum: Apicomplexa; Class: Conoidasida; Order: Eucoccidiorida; Family: Eimeriidae) is a parasite of caeca and rectum of chickens in India.

Clinical signs and pathology: This protozoon may cause diarrhoea with blackish green, semi-solid excreta. The terminal part of the intestine is thickened and congested, with pinpoint haemorrhages in the mucosa.

Diagnosis: Diagnosis is based on *post mortem* examination, by examining the faeces for the presence of oocysts or by examination of scrapings or histological sections of affected tissues. At necropsy, the location and type of lesions present provide a good guide to the species, and this can be confirmed by examination of the sporulated oocysts, which contain four sporocysts each with four sporozoites.

Control and treatment: Prevention of infection is based on good management. Chicken-rearing areas should always be kept dry and special attention given to litter near water drinkers and feeders. Anticoccidial compounds used for control of *Eimeria* species in chickens should be equally effective.

Turkey caecal coccidiosis

Eimeria adenoides

For more details see section on Small intestine.

Eimeria gallopavonis

For more details see section on Small intestine.

Eimeria meleagridis

Eimeria meleagridis (Phylum: Apicomplexa; Class: Conoidasida; Order: Eucoccidiorida; Family: Eimeriidae) occurs worldwide in the caeca of turkeys. It is a relatively non-pathogenic species, producing masses of ovoid oocysts in a white discharge from the caeca and lower small intestine. Infection is not associated with clinical signs and the endogenous stages can be seen on histopathology in the caeca. There are two to three merogony stages. The first-generation meronts appear in the middle small intestine 2–5 days after infection; second-generation meronts appear 60 hours after infection in the caeca and are mature by 70 hours. There

may be a third asexual generation, but most of the second-generation merozoites develop into sexual stages. Gamonts appear in the caeca, rectum and to a small extent the ileum. The prepatent period is 144 hours. The sporulation time is 15–72 hours.

Cryptosporidium baileyi

Cryptosporidium baileyi (Phylum: Apicomplexa; Class: Conoidasida; Order: Cryptogregarinorida; Family: Cryptosporidiidae) occurs worldwide in the small and large intestine, cloaca, bursa of Fabricius, nasopharynx, sinuses, trachea and conjunctiva of chickens, turkeys, ducks, cockatiels, quails and ostriches. Oocysts, each with four sporozoites, are liberated in the faeces. Following ingestion, the sporozoites invade the microvillous brush border of the proventriculus, intestines and lungs and the trophozoites rapidly differentiate to form meronts with 4–8 merozoites. There appear to be three merogony generations and both thin- and thick-walled oocysts have been observed. The prepatent period is three days and patent period 10–20 days.

Epidemiology: Transmission appears to be mainly by the faecal–oral route, although in the respiratory form infection may be spread by coughing and sneezing.

Pathogenesis: *Cryptosporidium baileyi* cryptosporidiosis is a disease of the epithelial lining of the bursa of Fabricius and cloaca of chickens, although the trachea and conjunctiva are lesser sites of infection. The presence of developmental stages in the microvillous region of enterocytes of the ileum and large intestines is not usually associated with clinical signs. Similarly, heavy infection of the bursa of Fabricius and cloaca does not appear to result in clinical illness (Figs 13.22–13.24). In the respiratory form of infection, up to 50% of a broiler flock may show clinical signs, and mortalities may reach 10%. Conjunctivitis has been reported in several species of birds.

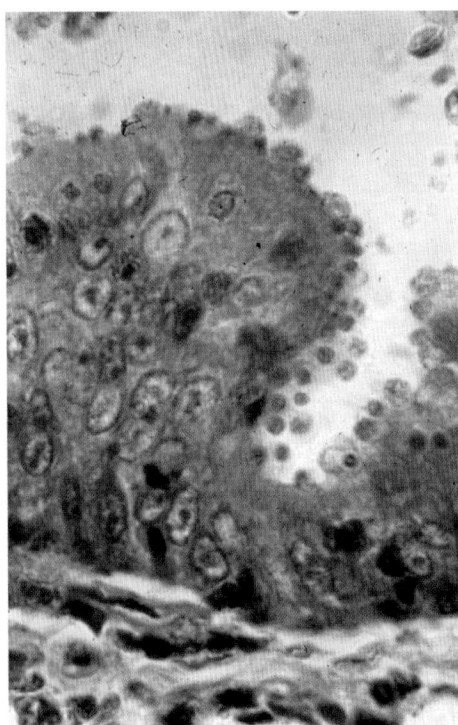

Fig. 13.22 *Cryptosporidium baileyi*: cloacal bursa.

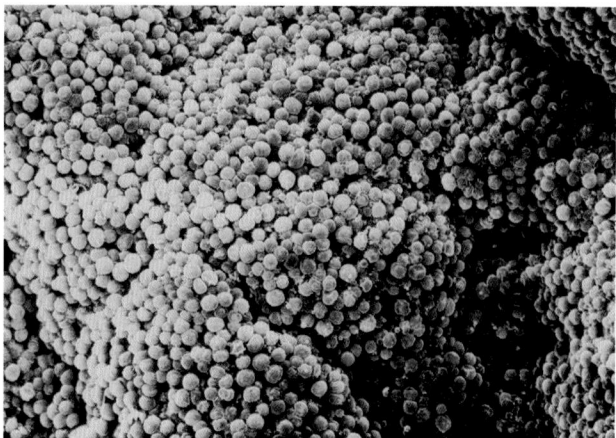

Fig. 13.23 Scanning electron micrograph of cloacal bursa showing numerous stages of *Cryptosporidium baileyi*.

Clinical signs and pathology: Enteric infections are not associated with clinical signs. In the respiratory form, initially disease is accompanied by sneezing and coughing, followed by head extension to facilitate breathing. Severe signs of respiratory disease last up to four weeks after infection. Villous atrophy, shortening of microvilli and enterocyte detachment are the major pathological changes associated with intestinal cryptosporidiosis. In respiratory cryptosporidiosis, gross lesions consist of excess mucus in the trachea, nasal mucosal congestion and atrophic bursa of Fabricius. Cryptosporidia are found in the nasopharynges, trachea, bronchi and bursa, but are not seen in the small intestine. With the respiratory form of cryptosporidiosis, there is epithelial cell deciliation and hyperplasia, mucosal thickening and discharge of mucocellular exudate into the airways in young broilers. Bronchopneumonia may be present in severely infected birds.

Diagnosis, control, and treatment: As for *C. mealeagridis*.

Histomonas meleagridis

For details see Parasites of the liver.

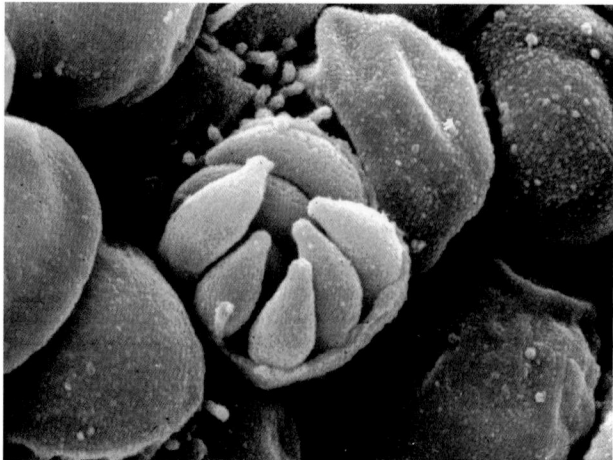

Fig. 13.24 Scanning electron micrograph of meront of *Cryptosporidium baileyi*.

Parasites of the respiratory system

Syngamus trachea

Syngamus trachea, synonyms *Syngamus parvis*, *Syngamus gracilis* (Phylum: Nematoda; Class: Chromadorea; Order: Rhabditida; Family: Syngamidae), is commonly known as the Gapeworm. It occurs worldwide in the trachea or lungs of chickens, turkeys, gamebirds (e.g. pheasants, partridges and guinea fowl), pigeons and various wild birds.

Epidemiology: Gapeworm infection primarily affects young domestic chickens of less than 2–3 months of age but turkeys of all ages are susceptible, the adults often acting as carriers. All ages of other passeriform and galliform species are susceptible to infection. Infrequently, *S. trachea* can infect anseriform birds. Eggs may survive for up to nine months in soil and L$_3$ for years within the earthworm or other transport hosts. Disease is seen most frequently in breeding and rearing establishments where outdoor pens, such as those used for breeding pheasants, are in use. Eggs, passed by wild birds such as rooks and blackbirds, may initiate infection; these may also infect earthworms. Infection is usually highest during the summer when earthworms are active. Infected chicks normally develop an age resistance by 2–3 months of age and markedly reduce their worm burdens. Partial immunity to reinfection is established.

Pathogenesis: The effects of *S. trachea* are most severe in young birds, especially game chicks and turkey poults. In these, migration through the lungs in heavy infections may cause emphysema and oedema and result in pneumonia and death. In less severe infections, the adult worms cause a haemorrhagic tracheitis with excess mucus production, which may lead to partial occlusion of the airways and difficulty in breathing. In turkeys, the male worms can be substantially embedded in the mucosa of the trachea, inducing the formation of nodules.

Clinical signs and pathology: These are most commonly seen in young chicks and poults. Pneumonia during the prepatent phase may cause signs of dyspnoea and depression, whereas the presence of adult worms and excess mucus in the trachea lead to signs of respiratory distress, asphyxia or suffocation, with the bird gasping for air; often there is a great deal of head shaking and coughing as it tries to rid itself of the obstruction. The clinical picture of 'gapes' may thus range from gasping, dyspnoea and death to, in less severely affected animals, weakness, anaemia and emaciation. The carcasses of infected birds are emaciated and anaemic and worms are found in the posterior part of the trachea, attached to the mucosa and surrounded by mucus, which may be streaked with blood. In turkeys, male worms become deeply embedded in the wall of the trachea, causing the development of nodules.

Diagnosis: This is based on clinical signs and the finding of eggs in the faeces. Disease is probably best confirmed by *post mortem* examination of selected cases when reddish worms will be found attached to the tracheal mucosa. The infected trachea often contains an increased amount of mucus.

Control and treatment: Young birds should not be reared with adults, especially turkeys, and to prevent infection becoming established, runs or yards should be kept dry and contact with wild birds prevented. The continuous rearing of birds on the same ground should also be avoided. Drug prophylaxis may be practised over the period when outbreaks are normally expected. It is not usually feasible to eliminate the paratenic hosts. In-feed modern benzimidazoles are effective, administered usually over a period of several days. Birds need to be monitored, as severely affected ones may not ingest adequate anthelmintic. Nitroxynil and levamisole are also very efficacious when given in the water.

Cyathostoma bronchialis

Cyathostoma bronchialis, synonym *Syngamus bronchialis* (Phylum: Nematoda; Class: Chromadorea; Order: Rhabditida; Family: Syngamidae), commonly known as the Gapeworm, is a parasite occurring worldwide in the trachea and bronchi of geese, ducks and swans.

Epidemiology: Severe infections are often associated with the ingestion of transport hosts such as earthworms, slugs, snails and invertebrates. Larvae may encyst and survive for years within invertebrate hosts. Infections often occur seasonally when, for instance, large numbers of earthworms occur on the surface after heavy rain.

Pathogenesis and clinical signs: Young birds are most susceptible to disease and heavy infections can be pathogenic, leading to emaciation and death. In heavy infections, these may include depression of food intake, asphyxia and dyspnoea.

Typhlocoelum cymbium

Typhlocoelum cymbium, synonym *Tracheophilus sisowi* (Phylum: Platyhelminthes; Class: Trematoda; Order: Plagiorchiida; Family: Cyclocoelidae), is a parasite of the trachea and bronchi of ducks, having snails of the genera *Helisoma* and *Planorbis* as intermediate host. Its distribution is described in Europe, Asia and Central America. The parasites cause obstruction of the trachea and affected birds may die of asphyxia. There is no reported treatment and control is impractical.

Cytodites nudus

Cytodites nudus (Phylum: Arthropoda; Class: Arachnida; Subclass: Acari; Order: Astigmata (Sarcoptiformes); Family: Cytoditidae), commonly known as the Air sac mite, is localised in the lungs and found in a range of birds, particularly poultry and canaries. It is distributed worldwide. Infestation may be spread by the host through coughing.

Pathogenesis: Small infestations may have no obvious effect; large infestations may cause accumulation of mucus in the trachea and bronchi, leading to coughing and respiratory difficulties, air sacculitis and weight loss. Balance may be affected in infested birds. Weakness, emaciation and death have been described with heavy infections.

Clinical signs and pathology: Coughing, respiratory difficulties, pulmonary oedema, weight loss, loss of balance or coordination. Death is usually associated with peritonitis, enteritis, emaciation and respiratory complications.

Diagnosis: Positive diagnosis is only possible at *post mortem*, when necropsy reveals white spots on the surface of air sacs.

Control and treatment: It is important to treat all the birds in an aviary when commencing a preventive programme. Treatment with topical moxidectin every three weeks as necessary may be effective.

Parasites of the liver

Histomonas meleagridis

Histomonas meleagridis (Phylum: Metamonada; Class: Trichomonadea; Order: Trichomonadida; Family: Dientamoebidae) causes a disease commonly known as 'Blackhead' or Infectious enterohepatitis. It occurs worldwide in the caeca and liver of turkeys, gamebirds (e.g. pheasants, partridges) and occasionally chickens.

Epidemiology: Although showing no signs of *Histomonas* infection, domestic chickens are commonly infected with *Heterakis gallinarum*, whose eggs, if fed to turkeys, will regularly produce histomonosis. Typically, histomonosis occurs when turkey poults are reared on ground shared with, or recently vacated by, domestic chickens. However, since the organism may survive in embryonated *Heterakis* eggs in soil or as larvae in earthworms for over two years, outbreaks may arise on apparently clean ground. Young turkeys may also become infected when reared by broody hens which are carriers.

Pathogenesis: The disease is essentially one of young turkeys up to 14 weeks old and is characterised by necrotic lesions in the caeca and liver. The earliest lesions are small ulcers in the caeca, but these quickly enlarge and coalesce so that the entire mucosa becomes necrotic and detaches, forming, with the caecal contents, a caseous plug. The liver lesions are circular and up to 1 cm in diameter with yellow depressed centres; they are found both on the surface and in the substance of the liver. Mortality in poults may reach 100% and in birds which recover, the caecum and liver may be permanently scarred.

Clinical signs and pathology: Infection is often mild and asymptomatic in chickens. Turkey poults become dull, the feathers are ruffled and the faeces become sulfur-yellow in colour eight days or more after infection. Unless treated, the birds usually die within 1–2 weeks. In older turkeys, the disease is more usually a chronic wasting syndrome followed by recovery and subsequent immunity. The name 'blackhead' was first coined to describe the disease when cyanosis of the head and wattles was thought to be a characteristic feature. However, this sign is not necessarily present and anyway is not confined to histomonosis.

The principal lesions of histomonosis appear in the caecum and liver. One or both caeca may be affected with small raised pinpoint ulcers, which subsequently enlarge and may affect the whole mucosa, occasionally ulcerating and perforating the caecal wall, causing peritonitis. The mucosa becomes thickened and necrotic and may be covered with a characteristic foul-smelling yellowish exudate that can eventually form hard dry caecal cores adhering to the caecal wall. The caeca are markedly inflamed and often enlarged. Liver lesions are pathognomonic and consist of circular, depressed, yellowish areas of necrosis and tissue degeneration, varying in size up to 1 cm or more and extending deeply into the liver (Fig. 13.25). In older birds, the lesions may be confluent and other organs such

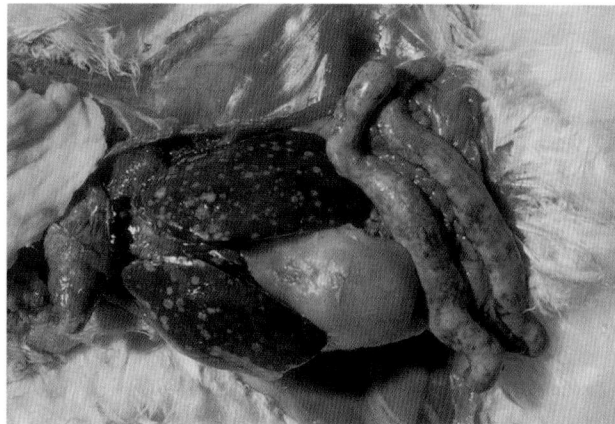

Fig. 13.25 Liver lesions due to *Histomonas meleagridis.*

as the kidney and lung may occasionally be involved. The parasites can be readily found on histopathological examination. Affected lesions are hyperaemic, haemorrhagic and necrotic with lymphocytic and macrophage infiltration and the presence of giant cells.

Control and treatment: Histomonosis can be prevented through good management. Turkeys should be reared on ground not used by domestic chickens for at least two years, or on fresh litter or wire floors raised above the ground. In gamebird-rearing facilities (pheasant, partridge), young birds should be cared for in raised pens and their droppings removed regularly. When poults are old enough to be moved to rearing pens, they should be placed on clean ground where birds have not been previously kept for at least two years, as *Heterakis* eggs may remain viable in soil or earthworms for some time, depending on the climate and soil type. The use of anthelmintics for the control of *Heterakis* worms can be an effective measure in limiting infection and spread. A number of drugs are effective, particularly the nitroimidazole compounds such as dimetridazole. These have been withdrawn in many countries because of concerns over human toxicity and carcinogenicity, and therefore few, if any, effective treatments are available.

Diagnosis: This is based on history, clinical signs and necropsy findings. Although rarely necessary, histological sections of liver or caecum may be prepared for specialist examination.

Parasites of the circulatory system

Bilharziella polonica

Bilharziella polonica (Phylum: Platyhelminthes; Class: Trematoda; Order: Strigeidida; Family: Schistosomatidae) is a parasite of the mesenteric and pelvic veins of ducks. It has snails of the genus *Planorbis* as intermediate hosts and is distributed in Europe and North America.

Pathogenesis and clinical signs: Generally considered to be non-pathogenic. Eggs in the wall of the intestine may produce inflammation. Parasites have been found in the pancreas, spleen and kidneys, but in these organs they eventually die.

Control and treatment: Not required.

Leucocytozoon caulleryi

Leucocytozoon caulleryi (Phylum: Apicomplexa; Class: Aconoidasida; Order: Haemosporida; Family: Plasmodiidae) is a blood parasite of chickens and guinea fowl, distributed in Asia. Some strains of *L. caulleryi* are non-pathogenic and others are highly pathogenic, killing a high percentage of chickens in a flock.

Epidemiology: The incidence of disease is linked to the presence and relative abundance of the midge vectors, *Culicoides* spp. In Japan, outbreaks occur frequently in June when the rice paddy fields are ready for planting and offer ideal conditions for midges to breed.

Clinical signs and pathology: Affected chickens are listless, diarrhoeic and anaemic with pallid combs and wattles. There is marked haemorrhage in the lungs, liver and kidneys and there may be gross haemorrhage from the kidney lesions into the peritoneal cavity due to the presence of megalomeronts, which cause haemorrhage on rupture.

Diagnosis: Gamonts can be seen in Giemsa-stained blood smears, the gamont being rounded in *L. caulleryi*. There are no pigment granules. On *post mortem* there are haemorrhages, splenomegaly and hepatomegaly and many organs have grossly visible white dots due to the presence of the meronts.

Control and treatment: Control requires elimination of the arthropod vector from the environment of the host. Insecticidal sprays and repellents sprayed within houses may be used to reduce the insect populations. Treatment is not usually effective, although pyrimethamine (1 ppm), sulfadimethoxine (10 ppm) or clopidol (125 ppm) in feed may prevent but not cure infections of *L. caulleryi*.

Leucocytozoon sabrazesi

Leucocytozoon sabrazesi, synonyms *Leucocytozoon schueffneri*, *Leucocytozoon macleani* (Phylum: Apicomplexa; Class: Aconoidasida; Order: Haemosporida; Family: Plasmodiidae), is a blood parasite of chickens and guinea fowl, distributed in Southeast Asia and Indonesia.

Epidemiology: The incidence of disease is linked to the presence and relative abundance of the midge vectors, *Culicoides* spp.

Clinical signs and pathology: It occurs uncommonly but can cause significant losses in flocks. Clinical signs include pyrexia, diarrhoea, leg paralysis, discharge from the mouth and anaemia. Pathology is as for *L. caulleryi*.

Diagnosis: Gamonts can be seen in Giemsa-stained blood smears, the gamont being elongate in *L. sabrazesi*. On *post mortem* there are haemorrhages, splenomegaly and hepatomegaly, and many organs have grossly visible white dots due to the presence of the meronts.

Treatment: Treatment is not usually effective.

Leucocytozoon smithi

Leucocytozoon smithi, synonyms *Leucocytozoon schueffneri*, *Leucocytozoon macleani* (Phylum: Apicomplexa; Class: Aconoidasida; Order: Haemosporida; Family: Plasmodiidae), is a blood parasite of turkeys distributed in Europe and North America.

Epidemiology: The vectors of *L. smithi* are blackflies of the genus *Simulium* and disease occurs in domestic and wild turkeys in North America and Europe, in mountainous or hilly areas where suitable blackfly breeding habitats occur.

Pathogenesis: *Leucocytozoon smithi* is markedly pathogenic for turkeys, and extremely heavy losses have been reported. Adult birds are less seriously affected than poults, and the disease runs a slower course, but they may even die. Recovered birds continue to carry parasites in their blood. Some birds recover completely but in other birds, persistent infection may lead to lethargy, lack of libido in male birds and persistent coughing. Sudden stress in these birds may lead to death.

Clinical signs and pathology: Affected poults are anorexic and lethargic and have difficulty in moving; in the later stages there may be incoordination, and the birds may suddenly collapse, become comatose and die. Birds surviving for 2–3 days after signs of disease appear tend to recover. Affected birds are anaemic and emaciated. The spleen and liver are enlarged and there is enteritis involving the duodenum, sometimes extending throughout the small intestine.

Diagnosis: Diagnosis is based on finding and identifying the gamonts in Giemsa-stained blood smears, or the meronts in tissue sections.

Control and treatment: Prevention depends on blackfly control. Ideally, turkeys should not be raised in areas where blackflies occur in significant numbers, or they should be raised under conditions that prevent them from being bitten by blackflies by rearing in screened quarters using 32–36 mesh screening. No effective treatment has been reported.

Leucocytozoon simondi

Leucocytozoon simondi (Phylum: Apicomplexa; Class: Aconoidasida; Order: Haemosporida; Family: Plasmodiidae) is a blood parasite of ducks and geese. It is distributed in northern USA, Canada, Europe and Vietnam.

Epidemiology: The vectors of *L. simondi* are various species of blackflies (*Simulium* and other simuliids) and disease occurs commonly in domestic ducks and geese in mountainous or hilly areas where cold rapid streams act as suitable blackfly breeding habitats.

Pathogenesis: *Leucocytozoon simondi* is markedly pathogenic for ducks and geese. The heaviest losses occur among young birds with very rapid onset. Adult birds are more chronically affected and the disease develops more slowly in them. Mortality is low but if it does occur, is seldom less than four days after the appearance of signs. Death usually occurs as the peripheral parasitism approaches its peak, 10–12 days after infection. Ducklings that recover often fail to grow normally, and recovered birds remain carriers.

Clinical signs and pathology: Acutely affected ducklings are listless and inappetent, with rapid laboured breathing due to obstruction of the lung capillaries with meronts. They may go through a short period of nervous excitement just before death. Adult birds are thin and listless. Main lesions are splenomegaly with liver hypertrophy and degeneration. Anaemia and leucocytosis are present, and the blood clots poorly.

Diagnosis: Diagnosis is based on finding and identifying the gamonts in Giemsa-stained blood smears, or the meronts in tissue sections.

Control and treatment: Prevention depends on blackfly control. Ideally, ducks and geese should not be raised in areas where blackflies occur in significant numbers, or they should be raised under conditions that prevent them from being bitten by blackflies by rearing in screened quarters using 32–36 mesh screening. Since wild ducks and geese are reservoirs of infection for domestic birds, the latter should not be raised close to places where wild birds congregate. No effective treatment has been reported.

Plasmodium gallinaceum

Plasmodium gallinaceum, synonym *Plasmodium metataticum* (Phylum: Apicomplexa; Class: Aconoidasida; Order: Haemosporida; Family: Plasmodiidae), is a blood parasite causing avian malaria in chickens and guinea fowl. It is distributed in Southeast Asia, Indonesia, Malaysia, Borneo, India and Sri Lanka. The distribution in domestic chickens coincides with the natural host, the jungle fowl.

Epidemiology: In Sri Lanka the mosquito vector is *Mansonia crassipes*. In other areas of its geographical range, the vectors are unknown and detailed epidemiological studies have not been conducted. A range of anopheline species of the genera *Anopheles*, *Armigeres*, *Culex*, *Culiseta* and *Mansonia* have been shown experimentally to be capable of transmitting infection.

Pathogenesis: *Plasmodium gallinaceum* can be highly pathogenic in domestic chickens, particularly when European breeds are introduced into endemic areas where the cycle is maintained in wild red jungle fowl. Anaemia is caused by destruction of circulating erythrocytes by developing meronts (Fig. 13.26). Neurological complications are caused by obstruction of capillaries in the brain by extraerythrocytic meronts.

Clinical signs and pathology: Birds with acute infection may be lethargic, anaemic with pale combs, diarrhoeic and show partial or total paralysis. There may be pallor of the carcass due to anaemia, brown-tinged skin and mucous membranes due to pigment deposition, splenomegaly and darkening of the viscera, especially liver, spleen, lungs and brain due to accumulation of pigment. Microscopic lesions are most evident in the blood. In the kidneys there may be accumulation of pigment in macrophages, fatty degeneration of the parenchyma and possibly immune complex glomerulonephritis. In the lungs there may be accumulation of

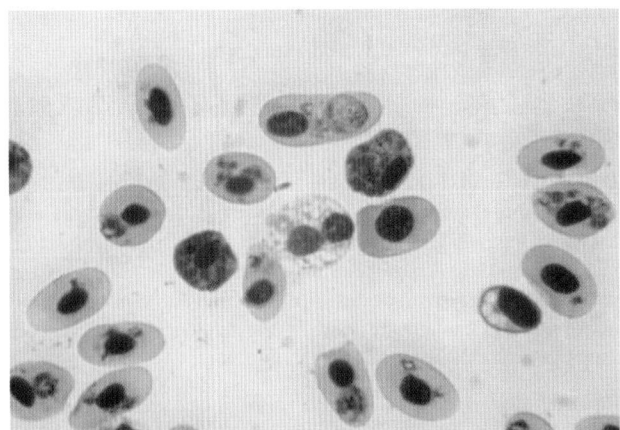

Fig. 13.26 Intraerythrocytic stages of *Plasmodium gallinaceum*.

pigment in macrophages in the capillaries, obstruction of the blood vessels and lymphatics and pulmonary oedema.

Diagnosis: Parasites can be seen in Giemsa-stained blood smears. The presence of meronts with numerous merozoites and round gametocytes that displace the host cell nucleus is distinctive for *P. gallinaceum*.

Control and treatment: Mosquito control can potentially reduce transmission of this parasite, but detailed control methods have not been studied. More potentially effective measures include keeping poultry in mosquito-proof buildings or keeping domestic chickens in areas away from the wild reservoir hosts. Sulfonamide drugs (sulfachloropyrazine and sulfamonomethoxine) and halofuginone have been shown to be effective in the laboratory.

Plasmodium juxtanucleare

Plasmodium juxtanucleare, synonym *Plasmodium japonicum* (Phylum: Apicomplexa; Class: Aconoidasida; Order: Haemosporida; Family: Plasmodiidae), is a blood parasite causing avian malaria in chickens, red jungle fowl (*Gallus gallus*) in Sri Lanka, grey wing francolins (*Francolinus africanus*) in South Africa and bamboo partridges (*Bambusicola thoracica*) in Taiwan. It is distributed in South and Central America (e.g. Mexico, Brazil, Uruguay), Asia (e.g. Sri Lanka, Philippines, Taiwan, Japan, Malaysia), East Africa (Tanzania) and South Africa.

Epidemiology: *Plasmodium juxtanucleare* is a parasite of wild birds that infects domestic chickens when wild reservoir birds and mosquito vectors are present. Infection is spread by culicine mosquitoes of the genus *Culex* (e.g. *C. sitiens*, *C. annulus*, *C. gelidus* and *C. tritaeniorhynchus* in Malaysia; *C. saltanensis* in Brazil). Natural vectors in other parts of its range are unknown and detailed epidemiological studies have not been undertaken.

Pathogenesis: This species is highly pathogenic, causing severe anaemia through erythrocyte destruction and organ damage due to massive numbers of exoerythrocytic forms. Central nervous system (CNS) signs are associated with exoerythrocytic forms, causing damage to endothelial cells of the brain capillaries.

Clinical signs and pathology: Affected birds are lethargic, depressed, progressively emaciated and anaemic. Severely affected birds have a protruding abdomen caused by splenic and hepatic enlargement and ocular haemorrhage may occur. Affected birds may show paralysis or CNS signs. Coma and death occur in heavy infections after a short period of time. The liver and spleen are enlarged and dark brown-black in colour. Exoerythrocytic stages can be seen in the endothelial cells and reticuloendothelial cells of the liver, spleen and brain.

Diagnosis: Giemsa-stained blood smears usually reveal numerous meronts and gamonts in the erythrocytes and infected cells also have dark pigment granules (digested haemoglobin). As blood samples cool, motile microgametes may be seen in the plasma in wet smears. This species can be distinguished from *P. gallinaceum* by its more elongate gametocytes and by the tendency of the meront stages to cling closely to the host cell nucleus.

Control and treatment: Since mosquitoes spread malaria, prevention depends on mosquito control. Residual spraying of poultry houses with insecticides may be effective. Birds can also be raised in screened quarters in areas where mosquitoes are particularly prevalent. Affected birds or flocks may be treated with primaquine 100 mg/kg orally or sulfonamide-trimethoprim combinations may be tried. Sulfonamide drugs (i.e. sulfachloropyrazine, sulfamonomethoxine) and halofuginone, which are effective against other *Plasmodium* species in birds, may also be effective.

Notes: Closely related species that occur in cage birds, pigeons, waterfowl, guinea fowl, pheasants, quails and turkeys include *P. vaughani*, *P. rouxi*, *P. nucleophilum*, *P. kempi*, *P. leanucleus* and *P. dissanaikei*.

Plasmodium durae

Plasmodium durae, synonym *Plasmodium japonicum* (Phylum: Apicomplexa; Class: Aconoidasida; Order: Haemosporida; Family: Plasmodiidae), is a blood parasite causing avian malaria in turkeys and francolins (*Francolinus leucoscepus*, *F. levaillantii levaillantii*). It is distributed in sub-Saharan Africa (e.g. Kenya, Nigeria, Zimbabwe, South Africa) and the vectors involved in transmission are not fully known.

Pathogenesis: *Plasmodium durae* is highly pathogenic in domestic turkeys and, depending on strain and geographic location, causes death in up to 90% of young turkey poults. Adult birds often develop right pulmonary hypertension as a consequence of hypoxic pulmonary arterial hypertension. Developing exoerythrocytic meronts may block cerebral capillaries such that infected birds can exhibit neurological signs and paralysis before death.

Clinical signs and pathology: Young poults show few clinical signs until immediately prior to death, when severe convulsions may occur. Adult birds are lethargic and anorexic and may develop oedematous legs and gangrene of the wattles. Pathology is as for *P. juxtanucleare*.

Diagnosis: The parasites can be identified in Giemsa-stained thin blood smears. Meronts are small and rounded and the gametocytes are elongate and do not curve around the host erythrocyte nucleus.

Control and treatment: Control is as for other avian malaria species. Sulfonamide drugs (i.e. sulfachloropyrazine, sulfamonomethoxine) and halofuginone may be effective in treatment. Sulfamonomethoxine does not provide full protection from mortality when given after the appearance of circulating parasites and sulfachloropyrazine, while reducing mortality, has no effect on the parasitaemia, suggesting activity against exoerythrocytic meronts.

Notes: Closely related species of the subgenus *Giovannolaia* reported in ducks, geese, turkeys, francolins, guinea fowl, quails, partridges and pigeons include *P. fallax*, *P. circumflexum*, *P. polare*, *P. lophurae*, *P. gabaldoni*, *P. pinotti*, *P. pediocetti*, *P. formosanum*, *P. anasum* and *P. hegneri*.

Aegyptianella moshkovskii

Aegyptianella moshkovskii (Phylum: Proteobacteria; Class: Alphaproteobacteria; Order: Rickettsiales; Family: Anaplasmataceae) is a blood pathogen of chickens, turkeys, pheasants and wild birds. It is distributed in Africa, India, Southeast Asia, Egypt, Russia and parts of the eastern CIS states.

Epidemiology: Infection is transmitted by the soft tick, *Argas persicus*. Indigenous poultry rarely suffer the acute disease, but freshly introduced stock are especially susceptible and may die within a few days. Recovered birds are frequently carriers.

Pathogenesis: Both species of *Aegyptianella* are pathogenic. The following descriptions apply to both species. The intraerythrocytic parasites cause severe anaemia, jaundice and frequent death. The incubation period is 12–15 days.

Clinical signs and pathology: Affected animals show ruffled feathers, anorexia, droopiness and diarrhoea and hyperthermia may be found. The clinical condition is often complicated by fowl spirochaetosis, which is also transmitted by *A. persicus*. Anaemia, jaundice, enlargement of the liver and the spleen, yellow-green kidneys and petechial haemorrhage of the serosa may be seen at necropsy.

Diagnosis: Diagnosis is based on the demonstration of organisms in Giemsa-stained blood smears. Intraerythrocytic forms (marginal bodies) and extraerythrocytic forms may be seen in leucocytes, lymphocytes, monocytes and in the plasma.

Control and treatment: Tick control and treatment of premises where adults and nymphal ticks may hide in cracks and crevices. After cleaning, premises should be treated with an acaricide, such as carbaryl, coumaphos or malathion. Tetracycline compounds (e.g. oxytetracycline, chlortetracycline, 15–30 mg/kg orally) are effective and usually recommended for treatment.

Parasites of the nervous system

Oxyspirura mansoni

Oxyspirura mansoni, synonym *Oxyspirura parvorum* (Phylum: Nematoda; Class: Chromadorea; Order: Spirurida; Family: Thelaziidae), commonly known as the Eye worm, is a parasite of the eye of chickens, turkeys, guinea fowl and peafowl. It is distributed in many areas of the world, particularly the tropical and subtropical regions, and is not present in Europe. The genus *Oxyspirura* in birds is the equivalent of *Thelazia* in mammals. This parasite has cockroaches (*Pycnoscelus surinamensis*) and mayflies as intermediate hosts.

Pathogenesis: It occurs on the conjunctiva, under the nictitating membrane, or in the nasal/lacrimal ducts or conjunctival sacs. Although not a highly pathogenic genus, moderate infections can induce inflammation of the eye, with the nictitating membrane becoming oedematous. Heavy infections may cause blindness or occlusion of the nasal passages.

Clinical signs and pathology: Birds may be observed scratching the eyes if they become irritated. Affected birds develop ophthalmitis, the eye becoming inflamed and watery. Untreated heavy infections can cause ophthalmia with erosion of the eyeball.

Diagnosis: A definitive diagnosis is made by finding the parasite in the conjunctival sac. It may be necessary to instil local anaesthetic into the eye to allow removal. Examination of lacrimal secretions may reveal eggs or first-stage larvae.

Control and treatment: Attempts to control the poultry spiruroids are unlikely to be fully successful because of the ready availability of the intermediate hosts. Reduction and restriction of cockroaches will be beneficial. Oral or topical levamisole or tetramisole and ivermectin have been used successfully to treat infections. Removal with fine forceps after instillation of local anaesthetic has been reported.

Philophthalmus gralli

Philophthalmus gralli (Phylum: Platyhelminthes; Class: Trematoda; Order: Plagiorchiida; Family: Philophthalmidae), commonly known as the Oriental avian eye fluke, is a parasite of conjunctival sac of ostriches, chickens, wild birds and humans. It has freshwater snails as intermediate hosts and is distributed in the USA, Indo-China, parts of Europe and Africa.

Pathogenesis: Infection may cause congestion and erosion of the conjunctivae, and conjunctivitis with persistent lacrimation.

Clinical signs: The flukes can cause lacrimation and conjunctivitis and can be a localised problem in captive farmed ostriches where they have access to standing water.

Parasites of the reproductive/urogenital system

Prosthogonimus pellucidus

Prosthogonimus pellucidus, synonyms *Prosthogonimus intercalandus*, *Prosthogonimus cuneatus* (Phylum: Platyhelminthes; Class: Trematoda; Order: Plagiorchiida; Family: Prosthogonimidae), commonly known as the Oviduct fluke, occurs worldwide in the cloaca, oviduct and bursa of Fabricius of chickens, turkeys, other fowl, geese and ducks. This parasite has two different intermediate hosts: the first is an aquatic snail such as *Bithynia tentaculata* and the second is a nymphal stage of various dragonflies.

Epidemiology: Occurrence is seasonal, with the main peak of infection in the spring and summer in temperate regions.

Pathogenesis: *Prosthogonimus* is considered to be the most pathogenic of the trematodes that infect poultry and ducks in America and Europe. Usually, chickens are mainly affected. Even moderate infections can inflame the oviduct, resulting in the formation of eggs with a soft shell or lacking a shell. Large numbers of flukes can be fatal.

Clinical signs and pathology: Infected birds may have an enlarged flaccid abdomen, become listless, show discharge of a limey secretion from the cloaca and may lay abnormally formed eggs. The feathers around the cloaca become soiled. Sometimes there is complete cessation of egg laying. The oviduct is often severely inflamed with a thick yellow-white secretion in the lumen. Irritation in the oviduct can cause a reversal of peristalsis, resulting in egg, bacteria and parasite material entering the abdominal cavity and causing peritonitis. The comb and wattles can become cyanotic in chronically infected birds. Sometimes there is a whitish milky discharge from the cloaca.

Diagnosis: Fluke eggs can be identified in secretions from the cloaca or found in the abdominal cavity at necropsy.

Control and treatment: Reduction of snails and their habitats will limit infection in the final hosts and, where possible, flocks should be denied access to the margins of ponds and lakes. Albendazole, fenbendazole, flubendazole 5 mg/kg or praziquantel 5–10 mg/kg can be used for treatment.

Eimeria truncata

Eimeria truncata (Phylum: Apicomplexa; Class: Conoidasida; Order: Eucoccidiorida; Family: Eimeriidae) occurs worldwide in the kidneys of domestic geese, greylag geese (*Anser anser*), Canada geese (*Branta canadensis*), Ross' geese (*Anser rossi*) and ducks. Complete details on the life cycle are lacking. Meronts and gamonts occur in the epithelial cells of the kidney tubules. The prepatent period is 5–14 days. Sporulation time is 1–5 days.

Epidemiology: *Eimeria truncata* occurs as a sporadic parasite in domestic geese and is most likely to occur when geese are kept in crowded unsanitary conditions. Contact with wild geese may introduce the infection.

Pathogenesis: *Eimeria truncata*, found in the kidneys of geese, can cause an acute nephritis especially where domestic geese are reared intensively. It is highly pathogenic for young goslings and can cause up to 100% mortality within a few days of onset of clinical symptoms. Outbreaks have also been recorded in geese in wildfowl sanctuaries.

Clinical signs and pathology: Symptoms are characterised by marked weakness, emaciation, polydipsia, muscular incoordination and death. The kidneys are markedly enlarged, light in colour and show numerous small white nodules, streaks and lines on the surface and throughout the cortex and medulla. Infected cells are eventually destroyed and the adjacent cells show pressure atrophy and destruction. Affected tubules are packed with urates and oocysts and gamonts in various stages of development (Fig. 13.27) and may be enlarged up to 5–10 times the diameter of normal tubules.

Diagnosis: Infection is diagnosed by identification of oocysts in urates or by the characteristic kidney lesions on *post mortem* or histopathology.

Control and treatment: Prevention is based on good management, avoidance of overcrowding and stress, and attention to hygiene. Contact with wild geese should be avoided wherever possible. Little is known about treatment but, by analogy with other hosts, one of the sulfonamide drugs should be tried.

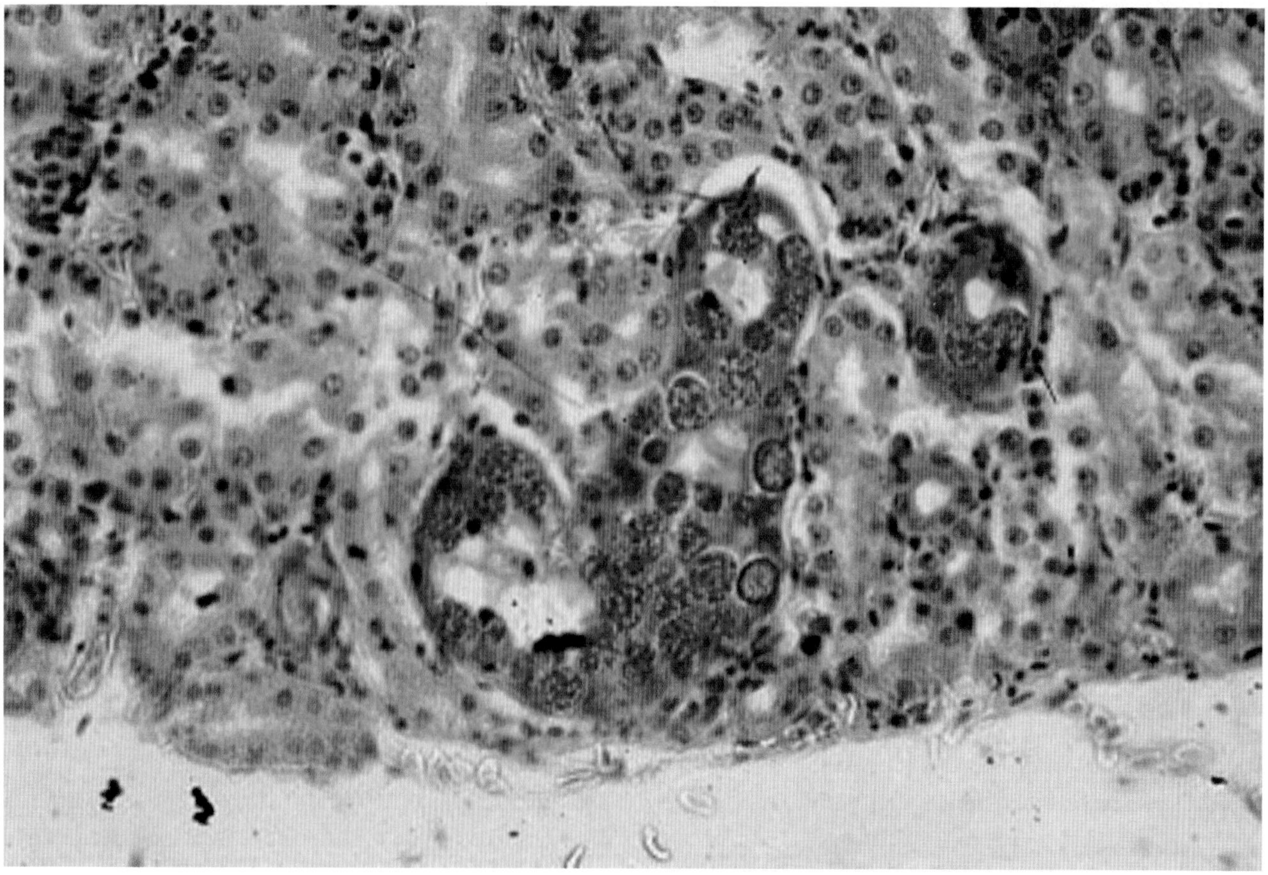

Fig. 13.27 Gamonts of *Eimeria truncata* in kidney epithelial cells.

Parasites of the locomotory system

Sarcocystis hovarthi

Sarcocystis hovarthi, synonym *Sarcocystis gallinarum* (Phylum: Apicomplexa; Class: Conoidasida; Order: Eucoccidiorida; Family: Sarcocystidae), is a parasite of dogs, presumably distributed worldwide, which has chickens as intermediate hosts.

Epidemiology: Little is known of the epidemiology, but where dogs are kept in close association with chickens or their feed then transmission is likely.

Pathogenesis: Infections in chickens are generally inapparent but have been reported to cause severe myositis or muscular dystrophy with muscle weakness and inability to stand.

Diagnosis: *Ante mortem* diagnosis is difficult and most cases of *Sarcocystis* infection are only revealed at *post mortem* when grossly visible sarcocysts in the muscle are discovered or detected by microscopic examination.

Control and treatment: The only control measures possible are those of simple hygiene. Farm dogs should not be housed in, or allowed access to, fodder stores nor should they be allowed to defecate in pens where chickens are housed. It is also important that dogs are not fed raw or uncooked chicken. Treatment is not indicated.

Toxoplasma gondii

Toxoplasma gondii (Phylum: Apicomplexa; Class: Conoidasida; Order: Eucoccidiorida; Family: Sarcocystidae) occurs worldwide in the muscle, lung, liver, reproductive system and central nervous system of cats and other felids. This parasite has all warm-blooded mammals and birds as intermediate hosts.

Epidemiology: The cat plays a central role in the epidemiology of toxoplasmosis and infection in poultry may occur through ingestion of feed contaminated with cat faeces or through ingestion of bradyzoites and tachyzoites in the flesh of another intermediate host, such as rats.

Pathogenesis and clinical signs: Most *Toxoplasma* infections in animals are light and consequently asymptomatic. Toxoplasmosis has been occasionally reported in poultry and is usually mild and unnoticed.

Diagnosis: Tachyzoites of *T. gondii* are often difficult to find in tissue sections but are more likely to be present in sections of brain and placenta. Identification can be confirmed by immunohistochemistry, while the polymerase chain reaction may be used to identify parasite DNA in tissues.

Control and treatment: As for *Sarcocystis hovarthi*.

Parasites of the integument

Avioserpens taiwana

Avioserpens taiwana, synonyms *Filaria taiwana*, *Oshimaia taiwana*, *Avioserpens denticulophasma*, *Petroviprocta vigissi* (Phylum: Nematoda; Class: Chromadorea; Order: Spirurida; Family:

Dracunculidae), is a parasite of the subcutaneous tissue of ducks. This parasite has copepods (*Cyclops*) as intermediate hosts and is distributed in China and Taiwan.

Epidemiology: Found in domesticated ducks in China, mainly in the dry season (January to April), and in Taiwan, where disease may also occur in September to October. It affects ducks aged three weeks to two months.

Pathogenesis: The worms cause the formation of swellings under the mandible, which are at first soft and movable and after about one month become hard and painful and may reach the size of a large nut. They interfere with swallowing and respiration and may cause death from inanition or asphyxia. Occasionally the swellings occur on the shoulders and legs and interfere with the bird's movements. Numerous microfilariae are found in the blood. The adult worms eventually rupture and disintegrate, and healing occurs, although if the worms die in the swellings, abscesses may form. The disease lasts about 11 months.

Clinical signs and pathology: Hard painful swellings located under the mandible, and occasionally on the shoulders and legs. Surviving birds have poor growth rates. For pathology, no lesions are described.

Diagnosis: Identification of the adult worms within subcutaneous swellings.

Control and treatment: Ducklings should be provided with water free from *Cyclops* and should not be allowed access to marshland. Removal of the worms through an incision into the most prominent part of the swelling and antiseptic treatment of the swelling are effective.

Collyriclum faba

Collyriclum faba, synonym *Monostoma faba* (Phylum: Platyhelminthes; Class: Trematoda; Order: Plagiorchiida; Family: Collyriclidae), commonly known as the Skin or Cystic fluke, is a parasite of chickens, turkeys and wild birds, having snails and dragonfly nymphs as intermediate hosts. It is distributed in Europe, Asia, North and South America.

Epidemiology: Only birds with access to marshy areas where the intermediate hosts occur are likely to become infected.

Pathogenesis: Commonly found in tissue around the cloaca but in heavy infections flukes may also be present along the thorax, abdomen, beak and neck. Such infections produce anaemia and loss of body condition and can be fatal.

Clinical signs and pathology: Young birds may show difficulty in moving, inappetence, anaemia, emaciation and even death. The presence of cysts can lead to disfigurement of the skin. The flukes are located in hard whitish-grey subcutaneous cysts that measure around 3–10 mm in diameter. These cysts have a central pore and contain a pair of flukes and are usually filled with dark fluid and eggs.

Diagnosis: Typical cysts are found around the cloacal opening and along the thorax and abdomen. Each cyst has a central opening and a pair of flukes.

Control and treatment: Birds should be restricted from entering marshy areas. Surgical removal is the only effective treatment.

Laminosioptes cysticola

Laminosioptes cisticola (Phylum: Arthropoda; Class: Arachnida; Subclass: Acari; Order: Astigmata (Sarcoptiformes); Family: Laminosioptidae), commonly known as the Subcutaneous mite or Fowl cyst mite, is localised in the subcutaneous tissues, lung or peritoneum of chickens, turkeys, pigeons and, occasionally, wild birds. It is particularly common in Europe and is also found in the USA, South America and Australia.

Epidemiology: It is estimated that around 1% of free-living urban pigeons harbour *L. cysticola*. The mode of transmission of this mite is unknown.

Pathogenesis: *Laminosioptes* is not usually associated with clinical signs and is only discovered at meat inspection, when infected carcasses are condemned partly on aesthetic grounds and partly because the infection appears somewhat similar to avian tuberculosis.

Clinical signs and pathology: The parasites are not usually regarded as pathogenic, although occasionally neurological signs including circling, loss of balance, wing droop and death have been reported. Aggregations of these small oval mites are found in yellow nodules, several millimetres in diameter, in the subcutaneous muscle fascia and in deeper tissues in the lungs, peritoneum, muscle and abdominal viscera. The subcutaneous nodules are often calcified, but these only contain dead mites as the calcareous deposits are produced around the mites after they have died. Active mites occur in the deep tissues. The nodules created by the mites reduce the value of meat intended for human consumption.

Diagnosis: The nodules may be seen in living birds by parting the breast feathers and sliding the skin back and forth with the fingertips. Examination of the nodules under a dissection microscope usually allows identification of the mite species.

Control and treatment: Destroying or quarantining infected birds reduces infestations within the flock. Ivermectin may be effective, but euthanasia may be required for rapid elimination of infected birds.

Notes: It has been reported that the fowl cyst mite may cause a granulomatous pneumonia in dogs.

ECTOPARASITES

HEMIPTERA

Cimex

Cimex (Phylum: Arthropoda; Class: Insecta; Order: Hemiptera; Family: Cimicidae), commonly known as the Bed bug, is a blood-feeding temporary ectoparasite of birds and mammals, including humans. Two species are of particular importance: *Cimex lectularius* is a cosmopolitan species of temperate and subtropical regions feeding on humans, chickens and other domestic animals, and also bats; *C. hemipterus* is tropical and subtropical, and feeds on humans and chickens. In terms of veterinary parasitology, infestations within poultry houses can be highly problematic.

Epidemiology: Twenty-one species of *Cimex* are mainly parasites of bats, with one species associated with birds. *Cimex lectularius* and *C. hemipterus* feed principally on humans. While *C. lectularius* is a cosmopolitan species of temperate and subtropical regions, *C. hemipterus* is present in tropical and subtropical areas.

Pathogenesis: Although bed bugs have been suspected in the transmission of many disease organisms, in most cases conclusive evidence is lacking, or experimental data have demonstrated that bed bugs are incompetent vectors. Scratching of the bite site can lead to secondary bacterial infection. The primary concern is the disturbance caused by nuisance biting which, with heavy infestations, may be significant.

Clinical signs and pathology: The bite causes irritation and swelling. Heavy infestations in poultry houses may result in chronic blood loss and mortality in young birds. Bed bugs are obligate blood feeders and will seek out hosts to acquire a blood meal, but they do not live on humans or burrow into their skin. They are nocturnal and their activity peaks before dawn. They are negatively phototactic which, combined with positive thigmotaxis, ensures that they hide away in cracks and crevices during the day, including under and within the seams of mattresses, bed frames and other furniture, floorboards, paintings and carpets, behind skirting boards, in various cracks and crevices of walls and behind loose wallpaper. Bed bugs are attracted by body heat and carbon dioxide (and perhaps skin odours) of a host, mainly coming out at night to bite the sleeping victim; temperature receptors are probably located on the basal segments of the antennae.

Control and treatment: Bed bugs, once rife all over the world, had been made rare in many countries by the domestic (and commercial) use of chlorinated hydrocarbon pesticides such as DDT from the 1950s. However, more recently, populations of bed bugs are becoming increasingly widespread and problematic once again. As bed bugs are cryptic in their habits and insecticides do not kill the eggs, complete control is usually not possible with an initial treatment. A postcontrol treatment evaluation and retreatment, approximately 10–12 days (dependent on ambient temperatures) following the initial treatment, is essential and, in some cases, more than two evaluations and treatments may be necessary.

LICE

Heavy louse infestation is known as pediculosis and is particularly common in poultry. All species on birds are chewing lice and are therefore of importance because of the direct damage they cause by chewing the skin or feathers, although some blood feeding may occur when the bases of feathers are damaged. Clinical importance is therefore usually a function of the density of the lice present. Transmission is usually by direct physical contact.

Epidemiology: Eggs ('nits') are glued to the feathers where they may be seen with the naked eye. The lice normally feed on fragments of skin or feather. Adult lice may live for several weeks on the host but can remain alive only for about one week off the host. Infection occurs after direct contact with an infested host animal. Cross-contamination between different host species is possible if the animals have physical contact.

Pathogenesis: Although there are differences in pathogenicity between the species of louse found on poultry, the effects of avian pediculosis are broadly similar, varying only in degree. Heavy infestations decrease reproductive potential in males, egg production in females and weight gain in growing chickens. The skin lesions are also sites for secondary bacterial infections. While most lice are not highly pathogenic to mature birds in low numbers, they may be fatal to chicks. As in the other pediculoses, the condition in domestic birds is often itself a symptom of ill health from other causes, such as other infections, malnutrition or inadequate, overcrowded and unhygienic housing. Chewing lice may occasionally cause severe anaemia by puncturing small feathers and feeding on the blood that oozes out.

Clinical signs and pathology: Restlessness, feather damage, emaciation and markedly reduced performance are all symptoms of severe pediculosis. Infected birds are unable to rest, cease feeding and may injure themselves by scratching and feather plucking, with results often more serious than any immediate damage by the lice. The pathology of louse infestation is highly variable. In heavy infestations the skin becomes inflamed, erythematous and eventually covered by scabs and blood clots, involving much of the body surface.

Diagnosis: Adult lice and eggs can be seen on the skin and feathers and removed for microscopic examination and identification.

Control and treatment: Topical insecticidal compounds, such as permethrin, carbaryl, malathion, cypermethrin or rotenone, can be used to kill lice. However, as the insecticides are unable to kill the eggs, two applications are necessary at an interval of 10–14 days. Deep-litter or free-range birds may be more easily treated by scattering carbaryl, coumaphos, malathion or stirophos dust on the litter. Regular checking and spraying of birds will enable infestation rates to be controlled. In addition, cross-contamination should be avoided. This is achieved by treating any birds in the environment of the chickens and restricting contact between wild birds and poultry. The housing and nesting should be thoroughly cleaned to eliminate sources of reinfestation such as egg-laden feathers. Although methods such as dusting the nesting material or providing insecticide-treated laying boxes can be used to avoid undue handling of birds, the results obtained from treating individual birds are undoubtedly better.

As would be expected, the practice of debeaking allows an increase in infestations by preventing birds from preening and grooming but is increasingly considered unacceptable on welfare grounds.

Cuclotogaster heterographus

Cuclotogaster heterographus (Phylum: Arthropoda; Class: Insecta; Order: Psocodea; Suborder: Ischnocera; Family: Philopteridae), commonly known as the Head louse, is found on poultry worldwide.

Pathogenesis: As the common name, chicken head louse, suggests, *C. heterographus* occurs mainly on the skin and feathers of the head, although it occurs occasionally on the neck and elsewhere. *Cuclotogaster heterographus* feeds on tissue debris, skin scales and scabs and can digest keratin from feathers and down. Infestation with *C. heterographus* is particularly important in young birds. Infestations of young birds and chicks may be pathogenic and sometimes fatal; the birds become weak and droopy and may die within a month. When birds become fairly well feathered, head lice infestation decreases, but can increase again when the birds reach maturity.

Goniocotes gallinae

Goniocotes gallinae (Phylum: Arthropoda; Class: Insecta; Order: Psocodea; Suborder: Ischnocera; Family: Philopteridae), commonly known as the Fluff louse, occurs on poultry worldwide.

Pathogenesis: *Goniocotes gallinae* may occur on the down feathers anywhere on the body but are often found in the fluff at the bases of feathers, the preferred sites being the back and the rump. These lice generally occur in low densities and so have little effect on the host. However, cases of severe *Goniocotes* infestation can cause restlessness, damaged plumage, anaemia and markedly reduced performance.

Goniodes dissimilis

Goniodes dissimilis (Phylum: Arthropoda; Class: Insecta; Order: Psocodea; Suborder: Ischnocera; Family: Philopteridae), commonly known as the Brown chicken louse, is found on the skin and feathers of chickens worldwide.

Pathogenesis: *Goniodes dissimilis* is more abundant in temperate habitats. Birds are unable to rest, cease feeding and may injure themselves by scratching and feather plucking. In general, young birds suffer more severely, with loss of body weight, debility and perhaps death.

Goniodes gigas

Goniodes gigas (Phylum: Arthropoda; Class: Insecta; Order: Psocodea; Suborder: Ischnocera; Family: Philopteridae), commonly known as the Large chicken louse, is found on the skin and feathers of chickens worldwide, but is more abundant in tropical areas.

Goniodes meleagridis

Goniodes meleagridis (Phylum: Arthropoda; Class: Insecta; Order: Psocodea; Suborder: Ischnocera; Family: Philopteridae), commonly known as the Large turkey louse, is found on the skin and feathers of turkeys worldwide.

Epidemiology: Infection occurs after direct contact with an infested host animal. Cross-contamination between different host species is possible if the animals have physical contact.

Pathogenesis: Birds are unable to rest, cease feeding and may injure themselves by scratching and feather plucking, with results often more serious than any immediate damage by the lice. This species of louse is most common in adult birds, but young birds that do become infested suffer more severely, with loss of body weight, debility and perhaps death. These lice can digest keratin; they bite off pieces of feather, breaking these up with comb-like structures in their crops and digesting them with secretions aided by bacterial action. They will ingest not only the sheaths of growing feathers but also down and skin scabs.

Clinical signs: In general, young birds suffer more severely, with loss of body weight, debility and perhaps death. In adult laying birds the effect on body weight is slight, and the main loss is in depression of egg production.

Lipeurus caponis

Lipeurus caponis (Phylum: Arthropoda; Class: Insecta; Order: Psocodea; Suborder: Ischnocera; Family: Philopteridae), commonly known as the Wing house is found on the skin and/or wing and tail feathers of chickens worldwide.

Pathogenesis: *Lipeurus caponis* is common on the underside of the wing and tail feathers of chicken and other fowl throughout the world. Pathogenic effects are usually slight in healthy animals and include restlessness, irritation and general unthriftiness. Young birds may be susceptible to heavy infestation, especially where underlying disease or malnutrition is debilitating.

Menacanthus stramineus

Menacanthus stramineus (Phylum: Arthropoda; Class: Insecta; Order: Psocodea; Suborder: Amblycera; Family: Menoponidae), commonly known as the Yellow body or Chicken body louse, is found worldwide, infesting chickens, turkeys, guinea fowl, peafowl, pheasants, quail and cage birds (canaries).

Epidemiology: This species is the most common and destructive louse of domestic chickens. It is widespread and often reaches pest proportions. It is most common on the breast, thighs and around the vent. In heavy infestations, the lice may also be found under the wings and on other parts of the body, including the head. After introduction into a flock, *M. stramineus* spreads from bird to bird by contact. Cross-contamination between different host species is possible if the animals have physical contact. Large populations are particularly common on caged layers.

Pathogenesis: *Menacanthus stramineus* is the most pathogenic louse of adult birds, and may lead to fatalities in chicks. It is an extremely active species which lays its eggs in clusters mainly in the anal region. Infestation can result in severe irritation, causing skin inflammation and localised scabs and blood clots, especially in the region of the vent and, in young birds, on the head and throat. Birds become restless and do not digest their food properly. Ultimately, infestation may result in decreased hen weight, decreased clutch size and death in young birds and chicks. Populations may reach as many as 35000 lice per bird. Lice infestations often accompany manifestations of poor health such as internal parasitism, infectious disease, malnutrition and poor sanitation. Although found naturally infected with the virus of eastern encephalomyelitis, it is not considered an important vector.

Menopon gallinae

Menopon gallinae (Phylum: Arthropoda; Class: Insecta; Order: Psocodea; Suborder: Amblycera; Family: Menoponidae), commonly known as the Shaft louse, is found worldwide on the skin and feathers of chickens, turkeys and ducks.

Pathogenesis: This louse feeds only on feathers and, although common, is rarely a serious parasite in adult birds. The shaft louse does not usually infest young birds until they are well feathered, but heavy infestations in young birds may prove fatal. *Menopon gallinae* rests on the body feather shafts of chickens and feeds on parts of the feathers. The louse occurs largely on the thighs and breast. It may also infest turkeys and ducks, particularly if kept in close association with chickens.

Menopon leucoxanthum

Menopon leucoxanthum (Phylum: Arthropoda; Class: Insecta; Order: Psocodea; Suborder: Amblycera; Family: Menoponidae), commonly known as the Shaft louse, is a small, rapidly moving louse found worldwide that especially favours the preen gland, inhibiting production of the oily secretion and causing 'wet feather'.

Epidemiology: Infection occurs after direct contact with an infested host animal. Cross-contamination between different host species is possible if the animals have physical contact.

Pathogenesis: Partly due to irritation, birds preen continuously but without the oily secretion, the feathers cannot be waterproofed. Unable to repel water and injured by constant preening, the plumage becomes tattered and dirty, with broken feathers. Water can penetrate to the skin, and when much of the body is affected, the birds are soaked and may die of pneumonia following chilling. Although the damaged plumage may be replaced at the annual moult, it soon degenerates, as a result of the excessive preening, into its former sodden condition.

Clinical signs: Wet damaged plumage.

Large numbers of closely related species of lice may be found on ducks, geese and other waterfowl (Table 13.13). Of epidemiological significance is that these species are among the least specific of all lice. The lice can be found on the skin and feathers in all areas of the body. In ducks, infection with lice can damage feathers, affecting water resistance and insulation so that the birds may die from cold. Treatment and control are as for *Menopon leucoxanthum*. Similarly, a number of closely related species of lice are found on gamebirds (Table 13.14). Host specificity is unknown.

Table 13.13 Other lice of ducks, geese and other waterfowl.

Family	Genus	Key representative species
Philopteridae	Anaticola	Anaticola anseris, Anaticola crassicornis, Anaticola tadornae, Anaticola thoracicus
Philopteridae	Acidoproctus	Acidoproctus rostratus
Philopteridae	Anatoecus	Anatoecus dentatus, Anatoecus brunneiceps, Anatoecus cygni, Anatoecus icterodes
Philopteridae	Ornithobius	Ornithobius cygni, Ornithobius mathisi, Ornithobius waterstoni
Menoponidae	Holomenopon	Holomenopon leucoxanthum
Menoponidae	Ciconiphilus	Ciconiphilus decimfasciatus, Ciconiphilus parvus, Ciconiphilus pectiniventris, Ciconiphilus cygni, Ciconiphilus quadripustulatus
Menoponidae	Trinoton	Trinoton anserium, Trinoton squalidurn, Trinoton querquedula

Table 13.14 Lice of gamebirds.

Family	Genus	Key representative species
Philopteridae	Goniocotes	Goniocotes chryocephalus, Goniocotes obscurus, Goniocotes microthorax
Philopteridae	Goniodes	Goniodes colchici, Goniodes dispar
Philopteridae	Lipeurus	Liperus maculosus
Philopteridae	Cuclotogaster	Cuclotogaster heterogrammicus, Cuclotogaster obsuricor
Philopteridae	Lagopoecus	Lagopoecus colchicus
Menoponidae	Amyrsidea	Amyrsidea perdicis
Menoponidae	Menacanthus	Menacanthus stramineus, Menacanthus layali
Menoponidae	Menopon	Menopon pallens

FLEAS

Echidnophaga gallinacea

Echidnophaga gallinacea (Phylum: Arthropoda; Class: Insecta; Order: Siphonaptera; Family: Pulicidae), commonly known as the Sticktight flea, is a burrowing flea important mainly in domestic poultry but may also infest cats, dogs, rabbits and humans. These fleas are most common in tropical areas throughout the world, but may also be found in many subtropical and temperate habitats.

Epidemiology: These fleas are not host specific and may attack any available mammal or bird for a blood meal. As they are able to survive off the host, transmission can occur from bedding and housing. Primarily important as a parasite of birds, the adult sticktight flea is an especially serious pest of chickens. However, it may also be found on humans, rats, cats, dogs, horses and larger insectivores. Infestations on dogs may be persistent if they are continually exposed to a source of infestation, and fleas are found on the poorly haired areas of the ventrum, scrotum, interdigital and periorbital skin and around the pinnae of the ears.

Pathogenesis: The burrowing of adults and subsequent emergence of larvae through the skin tissue can result in areas of ulceration, leading to secondary bacterial infection. Sticktight fleas can occur at densities of over 100 individuals per bird, all concentrated on the head. As a result, infestation of poultry may reduce growth and egg production. Severe infestation can lead to anaemia. Ocular ulceration, caused by self-trauma, may result in blindness and starvation. The skin over the nodules often becomes ulcerated, and young birds may be killed by heavy infections. Sticktight fleas may become abundant in poultry yards and adjacent buildings. They are potentially able to transmit the plague and murine typhus but since the females spend most of their lives attached to a single host, they are not considered to be significant vectors of disease.

Clinical signs: Signs include restlessness and scratching of affected areas. The bites may be visible on the skin. Allergic dermatitis may be seen but should be differentiated from other similar conditions such as sarcoptic mange.

Diagnosis: Diagnosis is not easy as adults may leave the host, and eggs and larvae are difficult to find. Poultry sometimes have clusters of these fleas around the eyes, comb, wattles and other bare spots. These dark brown fleas have their heads embedded in the host's flesh and cannot be brushed off.

Control and treatment: Sticktight fleas can be removed with tweezers by grasping and pulling firmly. An antibiotic ointment should be applied to the area to prevent infection. If fleas are too numerous to remove individually, a flea product registered for on-animal use should be applied according to label instructions. Several organophosphate-, carbamate- and pyrethrin-based insecticides are effective when applied as a solution. Should sticktight fleas become established in a poultry house, drastic measures may have to be adopted to get rid of them. All litter should be removed and burnt, and the poultry house sprayed with an insecticide.

Ceratophyllus gallinae

Ceratophyllus gallinae (Phylum: Arthropoda; Class: Insecta; Order: Siphonaptera; Family: Ceratophyllidae), commonly known as the European chicken flea, Infests poultry, Wild birds, Dogs, Cats and occasionally Humans. It is found predominantly in the Old World but has been introduced into southeastern Canada and northeastern USA.

Epidemiology: *Ceratophyllus gallinae* is the most common flea of domestic poultry. It is not host specific and may attack any available mammal or bird for a blood meal. As it is able to survive off the host, transmission can occur from bedding and housing. This flea is highly mobile on the host and can be especially common in host nesting material. It will feed readily on humans and domestic pets, and is often acquired in the handling of poultry and from injured wild birds brought into houses. It has also been known to migrate into rooms from nests under adjacent eaves. When such nests are removed, they should be incinerated, otherwise the hungry fleas may parasitise domestic pets and humans. In wild birds, flea reproduction and feeding activity are synchronised with the breeding season of the birds; in domestic chickens, flea activity may continue all year round.

Pathogenesis: *Ceratophyllus gallinae* is not considered to be an important vector of disease. Feeding activity may cause irritation, restlessness and, with heavy infestations, anaemia.

Clinical signs: Symptoms include restlessness and scratching of affected areas. The bites may be visible on the skin. Allergic dermatitis may be seen but should be differentiated from other similar conditions such as sarcoptic mange.

Diagnosis: Diagnosis is not easy as adults may leave the host and eggs and larvae are difficult to find.

Notes: The European chicken flea, *Ceratophyllus gallinae*, is a very common flea of poultry and also infests more than 75 species of wild bird and some mammals. In Europe, the vast majority of its hosts are hole-nesting tits, particularly great tits and blue tits. This species originated in Europe and has spread with poultry operations round the world. It is difficult to eradicate, as it is able to feed on many different species and is highly adaptable.

MITES

Infestation by mites can result in severe dermatitis, which may cause significant welfare problems and economic losses.

Clinical signs and pathology: Mites cause feeding lesions most commonly seen on the breast or legs of the bird. The feeding nymphs and adults cause irritation, restlessness and debility, and in heavy infections there may be severe, and occasionally fatal, anaemia. Newly hatched chicks may die rapidly as a result of mite activity. Egg production may decrease significantly. The effects of mites are highly variable but may include hyperkeratosis, acanthosis, epidermitis, dermatitis, poor feather growth and loss of feathers.

Diagnosis: The mites may be found in poultry housing during the day, particularly in cracks or where roost poles touch supports, or on birds at night. The mites can be observed in these locations with the naked eye, particularly after feeding when they appear red. Masses of mites may be found in the nasopharyngeal system of dead birds.

Dermanyssus gallinae

Dermanyssus gallinae (Phylum: Arthropoda; Class: Arachnida; Subclass: Acari; Order: Mesostigmata; Family: Dermanyssidae), commonly known as the Poultry red mite or Roost mite, is found worldwide on domestic poultry and wild birds; it may occasionally be parasitic on mammals, including humans.

Epidemiology: The red mite or chicken mite, *Dermanyssus gallinae*, is one of the most common mites of poultry. It is a mesostigmatid mite that feeds off the blood of fowl, pigeons, caged birds and many other wild birds. It occasionally bites mammals, including humans, if the usual hosts are unavailable. Populations generally increase during the winter months and decrease in the summer months, and infestation intensity increases during the host breeding period. The presence of nestlings may stimulate rapid reproduction and an exponential increase in mite numbers, so that at the time of fledging there is a significantly higher proportion of nymphs in the nest than adults. Mites are transmitted by mite dispersion between farms (via transport of crates, egg flats or even on humans themselves) or by direct contact between birds. *Dermanyssus gallinae* may be an important pest of poultry flocks maintained on the floor in barn or deep-litter systems, but is less important in caged production facilities. Since *Dermanyssus* can survive for long periods in the absence of a host, a poultry house may remain infested several months after birds are removed. Infestation of pigeons is common. Cats and dogs may become infested as a result of contact with poultry, and human carriers are also important.

Pathogenesis: In Australia, *D. gallinae* is a vector of *Borrelia anserina*, the cause of avian spirochaetosis. However, in general, *D. gallinae* is not considered an important vector of disease.

Clinical signs: The mite is a particular threat to fowl housed in old buildings. It causes feeding lesions, which are most likely to be seen on the breast or legs of the bird. The mites can directly cause irritation and anaemia, and can lower egg production and weight gain. Newly hatched chicks may rapidly die as a result of mite activity.

Control and treatment: Buildings and equipment should be cleaned, scalded with boiling water and treated with an acaricide such as carbaryl or synergised pyrethroids. Dimethoate and fenthion may be used as residual house sprays when poultry are not present. Where the mites have invaded dwelling houses, their ability to survive in nests, without feeding for several months, makes these important as reservoir sites, and all nests should be removed from eaves once the fledglings have departed. Buying in mite-free birds and using good sanitation practices are important to prevent a build-up of mite populations. Treatment of birds is only palliative, and attention should be paid to the mite habitats in buildings. Individual birds may be treated by spraying or dusting the birds with an acaricide such as a pyrethroid or carbaryl, coumaphos, malathion or stirofos. Systemic control by repeated treatment with ivermectin (1.8–5.4 mg/kg) or moxidectin (8 mg/kg) is effective for short periods.

Notes: *Dermanyssus* readily infects other animals and can cause erythema and intense pruritus in cats that occupy old wooden poultry houses. Humans may develop skin lesions when mites enter rooms from wild birds' nests in the eaves of houses.

Ornithonyssus sylviarum

Ornithonyssus sylviarum, synonyms *Liponyssus sylviarum*, *Macronyssus silviarum* (Phylum: Arthropoda; Class: Arachnida; Subclass: Acari; Order: Mesostigmata; Family: Macronyssidae), commonly known as the Northern fowl mite, is distributed worldwide in temperate areas and found on poultry and wild birds.

Epidemiology: As *O. sylviarum* is almost a permanent parasite, infection occurs via contact or by placing birds in accommodation recently vacated by infected stock.

Pathogenesis: *Ornithonyssus sylviarum* is a blood-sucking ectoparasite. It occasionally bites mammals, including humans, if the usual hosts are unavailable. This mite is capable of transmitting fowlpox, St Louis encephalitis, Newcastle disease, chlamydiosis and western equine encephalomyelitis. The viruses that cause western equine encephalitis and St Louis encephalitis have both been detected in *O. sylviarum* from nests of wild birds in North America and it is likely that this mite acts as a vector for their transmission among avian hosts. They may bite humans, causing pruritus.

Clinical signs and pathology: White or off-white eggs can be seen in the vent area on feather shafts. Feathers may become matted and severe scabbing may develop, particularly around the vent. Infested chickens show a grey-black discolouration of the feathers due to the large number of mites present. In heavy infections, birds are restless and lose weight from irritation, egg production may be reduced and there may be severe anaemia. Common signs, apart from debility, are thickened crusty skin and soiled feathers around the vent. Feeding activity of the mite causes pruritus, feather damage, weakness, anaemia and death. Scratching of the bites may result in secondary bacterial infection.

Diagnosis: The mites are found on the birds or in their nests and housing. Although similar in superficial morphology to the common chicken mite *Dermanyssus gallinae*, *Ornithonyssus sylviarum* can be distinguished behaviourally by the fact that it is present on birds in large numbers during the day.

Control and treatment: As for *D. gallinae*.

Ornithonyssus bursa

Ornithonyssus bursa, synonym *Liponyssus bursa* (Phylum: Arthropoda; Class: Arachnida; Subclass: Acari; Order: Mesostigmata; Family: Macronyssidae), commonly known as the Tropical fowl mite, is a parasite found on poultry and wild birds in tropical habitats: southern Africa, India, China, Australia, Colombia, Panama and USA.

Epidemiology: In warmer climates *O. bursa* is thought to replace the northern fowl mite, *O. sylviarum*.

For further details see *O. sylviarum*.

Knemidocoptes gallinae

Knemidocoptes gallinae, synonyms *Knemidokoptes laevis gallinae*, *Cnemidocoptes gallinae*, *Neocnemidocoptes gallinae* (Phylum: Arthropoda; Class: Arachnida; Subclass: Acari; Order: Astigmata (Sarcoptiformes); Family: Knemidocoptidae), is commonly known as the Depluming itch mite. It is found worldwide on chickens, turkeys, pheasants and geese.

Epidemiology: Infestation is especially prevalent in spring and summer and may disappear in autumn. New hosts are infected by contact. Infection may remain latent for a long time with a small static mite population until stress, such as chill or movement to a strange cage, occurs and then the population increases.

Pathogenesis: The parts of the body most commonly infected are the head, neck, back, abdomen and upper legs. Severe cases can result in emaciation and death.

Clinical signs and pathology: *Knemidocoptes gallinae* burrows into the feather shafts and the intense pain and irritation cause the bird to pull out body feathers. This is known as 'depluming itch'. The condition is characterised by intense scratching and feather loss over extended areas of the body. Feathers fall out, break off or are pulled out by the bird. Mites may be found embedded in the tissue at the base of feather quills, causing scaling, papules and thickening of the skin. The burrowing activity of the mites causes hyperkeratosis, thickening and wrinkling of the skin, and sloughing of the keratinous layers. Proliferative skin lesions may be observed on the legs, with digit necrosis observed in some birds.

Diagnosis: The progressive feather loss and scratching indicate the presence of the parasite. Identification of the mite species can be achieved through examination of mites found on feather shafts or skin scrapings taken from the edge of lesions.

Control and treatment: Repeated treatments of acaricides will prevent reinfestations. All housing should be thoroughly disinfected. Acaricidal dusts may be applied. Birds may also be treated with ivermectin; two to three treatments at 10-day intervals may be required to completely eliminate the mites. The ivermectin may be applied on the skin behind the neck, orally or injected. For individual birds, repeated topical application of paraffin may also be effective, if time-consuming.

Knemidocoptes mutans

Knemidocoptes mutans, synonym *Cnemidocoptes mutans* (Phylum: Arthropoda; Class: Arachnida; Subclass: Acari; Order: Astigmata (Sarcoptiformes); Family: Knemidocoptidae), commonly known as the Scaly leg mite, is found worldwide on chickens and turkeys beneath the scales of the feet and legs.

Epidemiology: Infection may remain latent for a long time with a small static mite population until stress, such as chill or movement to a new environment, occurs and then the population increases. The condition is more common in birds allowed access to the ground and therefore tends to be more prevalent in barnyard and deep-litter systems than in caged production facilities. The mites are highly contagious.

Pathogenesis: In poultry, *K. mutans* affects the skin beneath the leg scales, causing the scales to loosen and rise, and giving a ragged appearance to the usually smooth limbs and toes (Fig. 13.28). Lameness and distortion of the feet and claws may be evident. The mites crawl onto the feet of the birds from the ground, and the lesions develop from the toes upwards.

Clinical signs and pathology: Raised scales on the feet and legs. The infestation may result in lameness and malformation of the feet. Occasionally the neck and comb may be affected. As the disease progresses over the course of several months, birds stop feeding and eventually die. The parasites pierce the skin underneath the scale, causing an inflammation with exudate that hardens on the surface and displaces the scales.

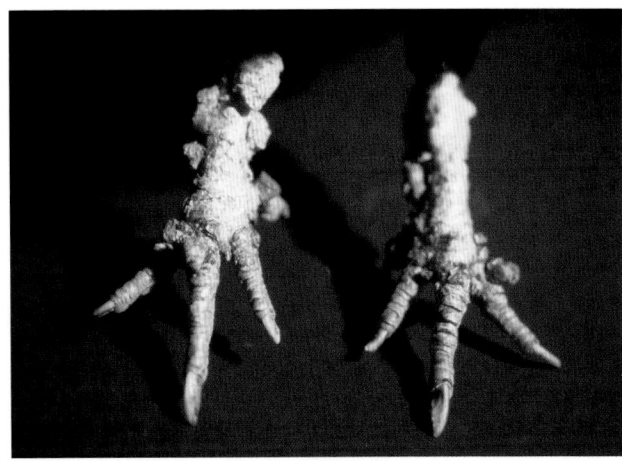

Fig. 13.28 Damage to the scales of the legs and feet caused by burrowing of the mite *Knemidocoptes mutans*.

Diagnosis: The raised scales on the legs and feet indicate the presence of the parasite. Confirmation is achieved by finding the mites in skin scrapings taken from lesions. Mature adult mites are often found beneath the crusts.

Control and treatment: The poultry house should be thoroughly cleaned and the perches and nesting boxes sprayed with acaricide. For 'scaly leg', the legs should be dipped into an acaricide solution. The treatment should be repeated several times at 10-day intervals. Birds can be treated by dipping the legs in a bath containing hexachlorocyclohexane (0.1%), sulfur solution (10%) or sodium fluoride (0.5%). Oral or topical ivermectin may also be effective.

Megninia ginglymura

Megninia ginglymura (Phylum: Arthropoda; Class: Arachnida; Subclass: Acari; Order: Astigmata (Sarcoptiformes); Family: Analgidae), commonly known as the Feather mite, occurs worldwide, infesting a wide range of birds including chickens, turkeys, pigeons and passeriformes and is found usually at the base of the feathers on the body and wings. Some species in this genus may also occur beneath the skin.

Epidemiology: More than 25 species of the superfamily Analgoidea, including *Megninia cubitalis*, are found on domestic poultry throughout the world. *Megninia columbae* may be found on pigeons.

Clinical signs and pathology: *Megninia ginglymura* may cause feather-pulling activity in pullets. Birds may become weak and irritated with damaged feathers. The infestation may lead to dermatitis with secretion. Records of economic damage by these mites are rare, but up to 20% decrease in egg production has been reported with heavy infestation.

Treatment: The application of acaricides such as pyrethrum, trichlorphon, dichlorvos or oral or topical ivermectin or selamectin may be effective. There are a large number of closely related species of feather, follicle and quill mites that may be found on a wide range of birds (Table 13.15). Quill mites may be found within the shaft of living feathers whereas feather mites are located externally, usually at the base of the feather. Feather follicle mites are found in the feather follicles of the skin. The mites cause restlessness and feather plucking.

Table 13.15 Feather and quill mites of domestic and wild birds.

Family	Genus	Key representative species
Analgidae	Megninia	Megninia cubitalis, Megninia ortari
Dermoglyphidae	Dermoglyphus	Dermoglyphus elongatus, Dermoglyphus passerinus
Freyanidae	Freyana	Freyana largifolia, Freyana anatina, Freyana canayi
Epidermoptidae	Epidermoptes	Epidermoptes bilobatus
Epidermoptidae	Rivoltasia	Rivoltasia bifurcata
Epidermoptidae	Microlichus	Microlichus avus
Epidermoptidae	Promyialges	Promyialges macdonaldi, Promyialges pari, Promyialges uncus
Pterolichidae	Pterolichus	Pterolichus bolus, Pterolichus obtusus
Pterolichidae	Sideroferus	Sideroferus lunula
Hypoderidae	Hypodectes	Hypodectes propus
Trombiculidae	Neoschongastia	Neoschongastia americana, Neoschongastia kallipygos
Syringophilidae	Syringophilus	Syringophilus bipectinatus

Treatment and control may be achieved through the application of acaricides such as pyrethrum, trichlorphon and dichlorvos; oral or topical ivermectin or selamectin may also be effective.

TICKS

Argas persicus

Argas persicus (Phylum: Arthropoda; Class: Arachnida; Order: Ixodida; Family: Argasidae), commonly known as the Fowl tick, Chicken tick, Adobe tick or Blue bug, is an important parasite of chickens, turkeys and wild birds found worldwide, but especially in the tropics.

Pathogenesis: Although common pests of chickens and turkeys, they are not usually a significant veterinary problem, except in small housed flocks. They will bite humans, particularly if living in proximity to an infested flock. Infestation may cause irritation, sleeplessness, loss of egg productivity and anaemia, which can prove fatal. Each tick requires a considerable quantity of blood for engorgement, and therefore heavy infestations can take enough blood to bring about the death of their host. Most species are nocturnal and are parasites of birds, bats, reptiles or, occasionally, small insectivorous mammals, and seldom attack humans. These ticks may transmit *Borrelia anserina*, the cause of fowl spirochaetosis, and *Aegyptianella pullorum*, a rickettsial infection. The spirochaetes may be passed from one generation of ticks to the next through the egg, and transmitted to the host by biting or by faecal contamination.

Clinical signs and pathology: The adult ticks, particularly the engorged females, are easily seen on the skin, commonly beneath the wings. Egg laying decreases and may stop altogether as a result of the infestation. However, the ticks only feed for a limited period. Inflammation and raised areas will be present from tick bites. Small granulomatous reactions may form at the site of tick bites, consisting of a mixed inflammatory cell response with fibrosis.

Diagnosis: The parasites may be found on the host or in cracks of the woodwork and walls around the animal housing. Microscopic examination may then be used to identify individual species.

Control and treatment: Control of argasid ticks can be assisted by elimination of cracks in walls and perches, which provide shelter to the free-living stages. Treatment should be repeated at monthly intervals. In poultry houses, all new birds should be treated prior to introduction into an existing flock.

Argas reflexus

Argas reflexus (Phylum: Arthropoda; Class: Arachnida; Order: Ixodida; Family: Argasidae), commonly known as the Pigeon tick, is a parasite of pigeons which is abundant in the Middle and Near East, from where it has spread into Europe and most of Asia.

Epidemiology: This species lives in close association with its host, *Columba livia*.

Pathogenesis: Heavy infestations may cause death from anaemia. This tick may also transmit fowl spirochaetosis. It occasionally bites humans, causing allergy. Its northern distribution through Europe is limited by the temperature requirement of its eggs and oviposition in summer months, since *A. reflexus* eggs show low levels of cold tolerance. Typical winter temperatures of 3 °C lead to approximately 50% mortality in *A. reflexus* eggs.

Argas walkerae

Argas walkerae (Phylum: Arthropoda; Class: Arachnida; Order: Ixodida; Family: Argasidae), commonly known as the Chicken tick, is a parasite of chickens found in southern Africa.

Pathogenesis: It causes considerable economic losses, especially where it transmits *Aegyptianella pullorum* and *Borrelia anserina*. In addition, it may secrete a neurotoxin during feeding, frequently resulting in fatal paralysis.

HOST–PARASITE CHECKLISTS

In the following checklists, the codes listed below apply.

Helminths

N, nematode; T, trematode; C, cestode; A, acanthocephalan.

Arthropods

F, fly; L, louse; S, flea; M, mite; Mx, maxillopod; Ti, tick; B, bug.

Protozoa

Co, coccidia; Bs, blood sporozoa; Am, amoeba; Fl, flagellate; Ci, ciliate.

Miscellaneous 'protozoal organisms'

B, blastocyst; Mi, microsporidian; My, *Mycoplasma*; P, Pneumocystidomycete; R, *Rickettsia*.

Chicken parasite checklist.

Section/host system	Helminths		Arthropods		Protozoa	
	Parasite	(Super) family	Parasite	Family	Parasite	Family
Digestive						
Pharynx					Trichomonas gallinae	Trichomonadidae (Fl)
Oesophagus	Gongylonema ingluvicola	Spiruroidea (N)			Trichomonas gallinae	Trichomonadidae (Fl)
	Dispharynx nasuta	Acuarioidea (N)				
	Eucoleus (Capillaria) annulata	Trichuroidea (N)				
	Eucoleus (Capillaria) contorta	Trichuroidea (N)				
Crop	Gongylonema ingluvicola	Spiruroidea (N)			Trichomonas gallinae	Trichomonadidae (Fl)
	Eucoleus (Capillaria) annulata	Trichuroidea (N)				
	Eucoleus (Capillaria) contorta	Trichuroidea (N)				
Proventriculus	Gongylonema ingluvicola	Spiruroidea (N)			Trichomonas gallinae	Trichomonadidae (Fl)
	Dispharynx nasuta	Acuarioidea (N)				
	Tetrameres americana	Spiruroidea (N)				
	Tetrameres fissispina	Spiruroidea (N)				
	Tetrameres confusa	Spiruroidea (N)				
	Tetrameres mohtedai	Spiruroidea (N)				
Gizzard	Cheilospirura hamulosa	Acuarioidea (N)				
	Histiocephalus laticaudatus	Spiruroidea (N)				
	Streptocara crassicauda	Acuarioidea (N)				
Small intestine	Capillaria caudinflata	Trichuroidea (N)			Eimeria acervulina	Eimeriidae (Co)
	Capillaria bursata	Trichuroidea (N)			Eimeria brunetti	Eimeriidae (Co)
	Capillaria obsignata	Trichuroidea (N)			Eimeria maxima	Eimeriidae (Co)
	Ascaridia galli	Ascaridoidea (N)			Eimeria mitis	Eimeriidae (Co)
	Hartertia gallinarum	Spiruroidea (N)			Eimeria necatrix	Eimeriidae (Co)
	Raillietina echinobothrida	Davaineidae (C)			Eimeria praecox	Eimeriidae (Co)
	Raillietina tetragona	Davaineidae (C)			Cryptosporidium meleagridis	Cryptosporidiidae (Co)
	Raillietina cesticillus	Davaineidae (C)				
	Davainea proglottina	Davaineidae (C)				
	Cotugnia digonopora	Davaineidae (C)				
	Amoebotaenia sphenoides	Dilepididae (C)				
	Choanotaenia infundibulum	Dilepididae (C)				
	Metroliasthes lucida	Paruterinidae (C)				
	Fimbriaria fasciolaris	Hymenolepididae (C)				
	Hymenolepis carioca	Hymenolepididae (C)				
	Hymenolepis cantaniana	Hymenolepididae (C)				
	Echinoparyphium recurvatum	Echinostomatidae (T)				
	Hypoderaeum conoideum	Echinostomatidae (T)				
	Polymorphus boschadis	Polymorphidae (A)				
Caeca	Capillaria anatis	Trichuroidea (N)			Eimeria tenella	Eimeriidae (Co)
	Heterakis gallinarum	Ascaridoidea (N)			Wenyonella gallinae	Eimeriidae (Co)
	Heterakis isolonche	Ascaridoidea (N)			Histomonas meleagridis	Dientamoebidae (Fl)
	Heterakis dispar	Ascaridoidea (N)			Tetratrichomonas gallinarum	Trichomonadidae (Fl)
	Heterakis brevispeculum	Ascaridoidea (N)			Tritrichomonas eberthi	Trichomonadidae (Fl)
	Trichostrongylus tenuis	Trichostrongyloidea (N)			Pentatrichomonas gallinarum	Trichomonadidae (Fl)
	Subulura suctoria	Subuluroidea (N)			Chilomastix gallinarum	Retortamonadoididae (Fl)
	Strongyloides avium	Strongyloidoidea (N)			Entamoeba gallinarum	Entamoebidae (Am)
	Echinostoma revolutum	Echinostomatidae (T)				
	Catatropis verrucosa	Notocotylidae (T)				
	Brachylaemus commutatus	Brachylaemidae (T)				
	Postharmostomum commutatum	Brachylaemidae (T)				
	Notocotylus attenuatus	Notocotylidae (T)				

(Continued)

Chicken parasite checklist. *Continued*

Section/host system	Helminths		Arthropods		Protozoa	
	Parasite	(Super) family	Parasite	Family	Parasite	Family
Rectum	*Notocotylus attenuatus*	Notocotylidae (T)			*Cryptosporidium baileyi*	Cryptosporidiidae (Co)
	Echinostoma revolutum	Echinostomatidae (T)				
Cloacal bursa	*Prosthogonimus pellucidus*	Prosthogonimidae (T)			*Cryptosporidium baileyi*	Cryptosporidiidae (Co)
	Prosthogonimus macrorchis	Prosthogonimidae (T)				
	Prosthogonimus ovatus	Prosthogonimidae (T)				
	Plagiorchis arcuatus	Plagiorchiidae (T)				
Respiratory						
Nares						
Trachea, bronchi	*Syngamus trachea*	Strongyloidea (N)	*Cytodites nudus*	Cytoditidae (A)		
Lung						
Air sacs						
Liver					*Histomonas meleagridis*	Dientamoebidae (Fl)
Pancreas						
Circulatory						
Blood					*Leucocytozoon caulleryi*	Plasmodiidae (Bs)
					Leucocytozoon sabrazesi	Plasmodiidae (Bs)
					Plasmodium gallinaceum	Plasmodiidae (Bs)
					Plasmodium juxtanucleare	Plasmodiidae (Bs)
					Trypanosoma avium	Trypanosomatidae (Fl)
					Trypanosoma gallinarum	Trypanosomatidae (Fl)
					Aegyptianella pullorum	Anaplasmataceae (R)
					Aegyptianella moshkovskii	Anaplasmataceae (R)
Blood vessels						
Nervous						
CNS						
Eye	*Oxyspirura mansoni*	Spiruroidea (N)				
	Philophthalmus gralli	Philophthalmidae (T)				
Reproductive/urogenital						
Oviduct	*Plagiorchis arcuatus*	Plagiorchiidae (T)				
	Prosthogonimus pellucidus	Prosthogonimidae (T)				
	Prosthogonimus macrorchis	Prosthogonimidae (T)				
	Prosthogonimus ovatus	Prosthogonimidae (T)				
Kidneys						
Locomotory						
Muscle					*Sarcocystis hovarthi*	Sarcocystidae (Co)
					Toxoplasma gondii	Sarcocystidae (Co)

Connective tissue				
Subcutaneous	Collyriclum faba	Collyriclidae (T)	Laminosioptes cysticola	Laminosioptidae (M)
	Dithydium variable	Mesocestoididae (C)	Wohlfahrtia magnifica	Sarcophagidae (F)
	(metacestode stage of Mesocestoides lineatus)		Cochliomyia hominivorax	Calliphoridae (F)

Integument				
Skin	Collyriclum faba	Collyriclidae (T)	Dermanyssus gallinae	Dermanyssidae (M)
			Ornithonyssus bursa	Macronyssidae (M)
			Ornithonyssus sylviarum	Macronyssidae (M)
			Knemidocoptes mutans	Knemidocoptidae (M)
			Knemidocoptes gallinae	Knemidocoptidae (M)
			Epidermoptes bilobatus	Epidermoptidae (M)
			Rivoltasia bifurcata	Epidermoptidae (M)
			Megninia cubitalis	Analgidae (M)
			Megninia ginglymura	Analgidae (M)
			Megninia ortari	Analgidae (M)
			Pterolichus obtusus	Pterolichidae (M)
			Neotrombicula autumnalis	Trombiculidae (M)
			Neoschongastia americana	Trombiculidae (M)
			Androlaelaps casalis	Laelapidae (M)
			Syringophilus bipectinatus	Syringophilidae (M)
			Dermoglyphus elongatus	Dermoglyphidae (M)
			Cuclotogaster heterographus	Philopteridae (L)
			Goniocotes gallinae	Philopteridae (L)
			Goniodes gigas	Philopteridae (L)
			Goniodes dissimilis	Philopteridae (L)
			Lipeurus caponis	Philopteridae (L)
			Numidilipeurus tropicalis	Philopteridae (L)
			Menacanthus stramineus	Menoponidae (L)
			Menopon gallinae	Menoponidae (L)
			Echidnophaga gallinacea	Pulicidae (S)
			Ctenocephalides felis	Pulicidae (S)
			Ceratophyllus gallinae	Ceratophyllidae (S)
			Ceratophyllus columbae	Ceratophyllidae (S)
			Cimex lectularis	Cimicidae (B)

The following species of flies and ticks are found on poultry. More detailed descriptions can be found in Chapter 17.

Flies of veterinary importance on chickens.

Group	Genus	Species	Family
Blackflies Buffalo gnats	*Simulium*	spp.	Simuliidae (F)
Midges	*Culicoides*	spp.	Ceratopogonidae (F)
Mosquitoes	*Aedes*	spp.	Culicidae (F)
	Anopheles	spp.	
	Culex	spp.	
Muscids	*Musca*	domestica	Muscidae (F)
	Stomoxys	calcitrans	
Sand flies	*Phlebotomus*	spp.	Psychodidae (F)
Screwworms and blowflies	*Chrysomya*	albiceps bezziana megacephala	Calliphoridae (F)
	Cochliomyia	hominivorax macellaria	
	Cordylobia	anthropophaga	
	Wohlfahrtia	magnifica	Sarcophagidae (Fl)

Tick species found on chickens.

Genus	Species	Common name	Family
Argas	*persicus*	Fowl tick	Argasidae
	walkerae		
	reflexus		
Ornithodoros	*moubata*	Eyeless tampan	Argasidae
	savignyi	Eyed tampan	
Haemaphysalis	*cinnabarina*		Ixodidae
	leporispalustris		
Amblyomma	*hebraeum*		Ixodidae
	americanum		
Ixodes	*ricinus*	European sheep, castor bean tick	Ixodidae
	holocyclus		

Turkey parasite checklist.

Section/host system	Helminths		Arthropods		Protozoa	
	Parasite	(Super) family	Parasite	Family	Parasite	Family
Digestive						
Pharynx						
Oesophagus	Eucoleus (Capillaria) annulata	Trichuroidea (N)			Trichomonas gallinae	Trichomonadidae (Fl)
	Eucoleus (Capillaria) contorta	Trichuroidea (N)				
	Gongylonema ingluvicola	Spiruroidea (N)				
	Dispharynx nasuta	Acuarioidea (N)				
Crop	Eucoleus (Capillaria) annulata	Trichuroidea (N)			Trichomonas gallinae	Trichomonadidae (Fl)
	Eucoleus (Capillaria) contorta	Trichuroidea (N)				
	Gongylonema ingluvicola	Spiruroidea (N)				
Proventriculus	Gongylonema ingluvicola	Spiruroidea (N)			Trichomonas gallinae	Trichomonadidae (Fl)
	Dispharynx nasuta	Acuarioidea (N)				
	Tetrameres americana	Spiruroidea (N)				
	Tetrameres fissispina	Spiruroidea (N)				
Gizzard	Cheilospirura hamulosa	Acuarioidea (N)				
	Streptocara crassicauda	Acuarioidea (N)				
Small intestine	Capillaria obsignata	Trichuroidea (N)			Eimeria adenoides	Eimeriidae (Co)
	Capillaria caudinflata	Trichuroidea (N)			Eimeria dispersa	Eimeriidae (Co)
	Capillaria bursata	Trichuroidea (N)			Eimeria gallopavonis	Eimeriidae (Co)
	Ascaridia galli	Ascaridoidea (N)			Eimeria innocua	Eimeriidae (Co)
	Ascaridia dissimilis	Ascaridoidea (N)			Eimeria meleagrimitis	Eimeriidae (Co)
	Raillietina cesticillus	Davaineidae (C)			Eimeria subrotunda	Eimeriidae (Co)
	Raillietina echinobothrida	Davaineidae (C)			Cryptosporidium meleagridis	Cryptosporididae (Co)
	Davainea proglottina	Davaineidae (C)			Spironucleus meleagridis	Hexamitidae (Fl)
	Choanotaenia infundibulum	Dilepididae (C)				
	Metroliasthes lucida	Paruterinidae (C)				
	Hymenolepis carioca	Hymenolepidae (C)				
	Hymenolepis cantaniana	Hymenolepidae (C)				
	Hypoderaeum conoideum	Echinostomatidae (C)				
Caeca	Capillaria anatis	Trichuroidea (N)			Eimeria adenoides	Eimeriidae (Co)
	Heterakis gallinarum	Ascaridoidea (N)			Eimeria gallopavonis	Eimeriidae (Co)
	Trichostrongylus tenuis	Trichostrongyloidea (N)			Histomonas meleagridis	Dientamoebidae (Fl)
	Subulura suctoria	Subuluroidea (N)			Tetratrichomonas gallinarum	Trichomonadidae (Fl)
	Strongyloides avium	Strongyloidoidea (N)			Tritrichomonas eberthi	Trichomonadidae (Fl)
	Brachylaemus commutatus	Brachylaemidae (T)			Pentatrichomonas gallinarum	Trichomonadidae (Fl)
	Postharmostomum commutatum	Brachylaemidae (T)			Chilomastix gallinarum	Trichomonadidae (Fl)
					Spironucleus meleagridis	Hexamitidae (Fl)
					Entamoeba gallinarum	Entamoebidae (Am)
Cloacal bursa	Prosthogonimus pellucidus	Prosthogonimidae (T)			Cryptosporidium baileyi	Cryptosporididae ((Co)
	Prosthogonimus macrorchis	Prosthogonimidae (T)				
	Prosthogonimus ovatus	Prosthogonimidae (T)				
	Plagiorchis arcuatus	Plagiorchidae (T)				
Respiratory						
Nares			Cytodites nudus	Cytodites nudus		
Trachea	Syngamus trachea	Strongyloidea (N)				
Liver						Histomonas meleagridis	Dientamoebidae (Fl)

(Continued)

Turkey parasite checklist. *Continued*

	Helminths		Arthropods		Protozoa	
Section/host system	Parasite	(Super) family	Parasite	Family	Parasite	Family
Pancreas						
Circulatory						
Blood					*Haemoproteus meleagridis*	Plasmodiidae (Bs)
					Leucocytozoon smithi	Plasmodiidae (Bs)
					Plasmodium durae	Plasmodiidae (Bs)
Blood vessels					*Aegyptianella pullorum*	Anaplasmataceae (R)
					Aegyptianella moshkovskii	Anaplasmataceae (R)
Nervous						
CNS						
Eye	*Oxyspirura mansoni*	Spiruroidea (N)				
Reproductive/urogenital						
Oviduct	*Prosthogonimus pellucidus*	Prosthogonimidae (T)				
	Prosthogonimus macrorchis	Prosthogonimidae (T)				
	Prosthogonimus ovatus	Prosthogonimidae (T)				
	Plagiorchis arcuatus	Plagiorchidae (T)				
	Notocotylus attenuatus	Notocotylidae (T)				
Kidneys						
Locomotory						
Connective tissue						
Subcutaneous	*Collyriclum faba*	Collyriclidae (T)	*Laminosioptes cysticola*	Laminosioptidae (M)	*Toxoplasma gondii*	Sarcocystidae (Co)
	Dithridium variable (metacestode stage of *Mesocestoides lineatus*)	Mesocestoididae (C)	*Cochliomyia hominivorax*	Calliphoridae (F)		
			Wohlfahrtia magnifica	Sarcophagidae (S)		
Integument						
Skin	*Collyriclum faba*	Collyriclidae (T)	*Dermanyssus gallinae*	Dermanyssidae (M)		
			Ornithonyssus bursa	Macronyssidae (M)		
			Ornithonyssus sylviarum	Macronyssidae (M)		
			Knemidocoptes gallinae	Knemidokoptidae (M)		
			Knemidocoptes mutans	Knemidokoptidae (M)		
			Megninia ginglymura	Analgidae (M)		
			Androlaelaps casalis	Laelapidae (M)		
			Freyana chanayi	Freyanidae (M)		
			Pterolichus obtusus	Pterolichidae (M)		
			Neotrombicula autumnalis	Trombiculidae (M)		
			Neoschongastia americana	Trombiculidae (M)		
			Syringophilus bipectinatus	Syringophilidae (M)		
			Goniodes meleagridis	Philopteridae (L)		
			Menacanthus stramineus	Menoponidae (L)		
			Menopon gallinae	Menoponidae (L)		
			Cuclotogaster heterographus	Philopteridae (L)		
			Echidnophaga gallinacea	Pulicidae (S)		
			Ceratophyllus gallinae	Ceratophyllidae (S)		

Flies of veterinary importance on turkeys.

Group	Genus	Species	Family
Blackflies Buffalo gnats	*Simulium*	spp.	Simuliidae (F)
Midges	*Culicoides*	spp.	Ceratopogonidae (F)
Mosquitoes	*Aedes*	spp.	Culicidae (F)
	Anopheles	spp.	
	Culex	spp.	
Muscids	*Musca*	*domestica*	Muscidae (F)
	Stomoxys	*calcitrans*	
Sand flies	*Phlebotomus*	spp.	Psychodidae (F)
Screwworms and blowflies	*Chrysomya*	*albiceps bezziana megacephala*	Calliphoridae (F)
	Cochliomyia	*hominivorax macellaria*	
	Cordylobia	*anthropophaga*	
	Wohlfahrtia	*magnifica*	Sarcophagidae (Fl)

Tick species found on turkeys.

Genus	Species	Common name	Family
Argas	*persicus*	Fowl tick	Argasidae
	walkerae		
	reflexus		
Ornithodoros	*moubata*	Eyeless tampan	Argasidae
	savignyi	Eyed tampan	
Haemaphysalis	*cinnabarina*		Ixodidae
	leporispalustris		
Amblyomma	*hebraeum*		Ixodidae
	americanum		
Ixodes	*ricinus*	European sheep, castor bean tick	Ixodidae
	holocyclus		

Duck parasite checklist.

Section/host system	Helminths		Arthropods		Protozoa	
	Parasite	(Super) family	Parasite	Family	Parasite	Family
Digestive						
Pharynx						
Oesophagus	Eucoleus (Capillaria) annulata	Trichuroidea (N)				
	Eucoleus (Capillaria) contorta	Trichuroidea (N)				
	Echinuria uncinata	Acuarioidea (N)				
	Typhlocoelum cucumerinum	Cyclocoelidae (T)				
	Hystrichis tricolor	Dioctophymatoidea (N)				
	Eustrongyloides papillosus	Dioctophymatoidea (N)				
Crop	Eucoleus (Capillaria) contorta	Trichuroidea (N)				—
Proventriculus	Echinuria uncinata	Acuarioidea (N)				
	Tetrameres americana	Spiruroidea (N)				
	Tetrameres crami	Spiruroidea (N)				
	Tetrameres fissispina	Spiruroidea (N)				
	Hystrichis tricolor	Dioctophymatoidea (N)				
	Eustrongyloides papillosus	Dioctophymatoidea (N)				
Gizzard	Amidostomum anseris	Trichostrongyloidea (N)				
	Amidostomum acutum	Trichostrongyloidea (N)				
	Epomidiostomum uncinatum	Trichostrongyloidea (N)				
	Epomidiostomum orispinum	Trichostrongyloidea (N)				
	Histiocephalus laticaudatus	Spiruroidea (N)				
	Echinuria uncinata	Acuarioidea (N)				
	Steptocara craussicauda	Acuarioidea (N)				
Small intestine	Ascaridia galli	Ascaridoidea (N)			Eimeria anatis	Eimeriidae (Co)
	Porrocaecum crassum	Ascaridoidea (N)			Tyzzeria perniciosa	Eimeriidae (Co)
	Contracaecum spiculigerum	Ascaridoidea (N)			Spironucleus meleagridis	Hexamitidae (Fl)
	Capillaria bursata	Trichuroidea (N)			Cryptosporidium meleagridis	Cryptosporidiidae (Co)
	Polymorphus boschadis	Polymorphidae (A)				
	Filicollis anatis	Polymorphidae (A)				
	Echinoparyphium recurvatum	Echinostomatidae (T)				
	Hypoderaeum conoideum	Echinostomatidae (T)				
	Apatemon gracilis	Strigeidae (T)				
	Parastrigea robusta	Strigeidae (T)				
	Cotylurus cornutus	Strigeidae (T)				
	Hymenolepis lanceolata	Hymenolepididae (C)				
	Fimbriaria fasciolaris	Hymenolepididae (C)				
Caeca	Heterakis dispar	Ascaridoidea (N)			Tetratrichomonas anatis	Trichomonadidae (Fl)
	Heterakis isolonche	Ascaridoidea (N)			Cochlosoma anatis	Trichomonadidae (Fl)
	Heterakis gallinarum	Ascaridoidea (N)			Entamoeba anatis	Entamoebidae (Am)
	Heterakis brevispeculum	Ascaridoidea (N)			Entamoeba gallinarum	Entamoebidae (Am)
	Trichostrongylus tenuis	Trichostrongyloidea (N)				
	Capillaria anatis	Trichuroidea (N)				
	Subulura suctoria	Subuluroidea (N)				
	Echinostoma revolutum	Echinostomatidae (T)				
	Echinostoma paraulum	Echinostomatidae (T)				
	Notocotylus attenuatus	Notocotylidae (T)				
	Catatropis verrucosa	Notocotylidae (T)				
Cloaca, cloacal bursa, rectum	Prosthogonimus pellucidus	Prosthogonimidae (T)			Cryptosporidium baileyi	Cryptosporidiidae (Co)
	Prosthogonimus macrorchis	Prosthogonimidae (T)				
	Prosthogonimus ovatus	Prosthogonimidae (T)				
	Notocotylus attenuatus	Notocotylidae (T)				

Respiratory		
Nares	*Hyptiasmus tumidus*	Cyclocoelidae (T)
Trachea, bronchi	*Cyathostoma bronchialis*	Strongyloidea (N)
	Typhlocoelum cymbium	Cyclocoelidae (T)
	Typhlocoelum cucumerinum	Cyclocoelidae (T)
Lung		
Air sacs	*Typhlocoelum cucumerinum*	Cyclocoelidae (T)
Liver		
Pancreas		
Circulatory		
Blood	*Leucocytozoon simondi*	Plasmodiidae (Bs)
	Haemoproteus nettionis	Plasmodiidae (Bs)
	Aegyptianella pullorum	Anaplasmataceae (R)
Blood vessels	*Bilharziella polonica*	Schistosomatidae (T)
Nervous		
CNS		
Eye		
Reproductive/urogenital		
Oviduct	*Prosthogonimus pellucidus*	Prosthogonimidae (T)
	Prosthogonimus macrorchis	Prosthogonimidae (T)
	Prosthogonimus ovatus	Prosthogonimidae (T)
Kidneys	*Eimeria truncata*	Eimeriidae (Co)
Locomotory		
Connective tissue		
	Toxoplasma gondii	Sarcocystidae (Co)
Subcutaneous	*Avioserpens taiwana*	Dracunculoidea (N)
	Collyriclum faba	Collyriclidae (T)
	Splendidofilaria fallisensis	Filarioidea (N)

(Continued)

713

Duck parasite checklist. *Continued*

| Section/host system | Helminths | | Arthropods | | Protozoa | |
	Parasite	(Super) family	Parasite	Family	Parasite	Family
Integument						
Skin	Collyriclum faba	Collyriclidae (T)	Anaticola anseris	Philopteridae (L)		
			Anaticola crassicornis	Philopteridae (L)		
			Anaticola tadornae	Philopteridae (L)		
			Anaticola thoracicus	Philopteridae (L)		
			Acidoproctus rostratus	Philopteridae (L)		
			Anatoecus dentatus	Philopteridae (L)		
			Anatoecus brunneiceps	Philopteridae (L)		
			Anatoecus cygni	Philopteridae (L)		
			Anatoecus icterodes	Philopteridae (L)		
			Ornithobius cygni	Philopteridae (L)		
			Ornithobius mathisi	Philopteridae (L)		
			Ornithobius waterstoni	Philopteridae (L)		
			Menopon gallinae	Menoponidae (L)		
			Menopon leucoxanthum	Menoponidae (L)		
			Holomenopon leucoxanthum	Menoponidae (L)		
			Ciconiphilus decimfasciatus	Menoponidae (L)		
			Ciconiphilus parvus	Menoponidae (L)		
			Ciconiphilus pectiniventris	Menoponidae (L)		
			Ciconiphilus cygni	Menoponidae (L)		
			Ciconiphilus quadripustulatus	Menoponidae (L)		
			Trinoton anserium	Menoponidae (L)		
			Trinoton squalidum	Menoponidae (L)		
			Trinoton querquedula	Menoponidae (L)		

Goose parasite checklist.

	Helminths		Arthropods		Protozoa	
Section/host system	**Parasite**	**(Super) family**	**Parasite**	**Family**	**Parasite**	**Family**
Digestive						
Pharynx						
Oesophagus	*Echinuria uncinata*	Acuarioidea (N)				
	Eustrongyloides papillosus	Dioctophymatoidea (N)				
Crop						
Proventriculus	*Echinuria uncinata*	Acuarioidea (N)				
	Tetrameres americana	Spiruroidea (N)				
	Tetrameres fissispina	Spiruroidea (N)				
	Eustrongyloides papillosus	Dioctophymatoidea (N)				
Gizzard	*Amidostomum anseris*	Trichostrongyloidea (N)				
	Epomidiostomum uncinatum	Trichostrongyloidea (N)				
	Epomidiostomum orispinum	Trichostrongyloidea (N)				
	Epomidiostomum skrjabini	Trichostrongyloidea (N)				
	Echinuria uncinata	Acuarioidea (N)				
	Steptocara craussicauda	Acuarioidea (N)				
Small intestine	*Ascaridia galli*	Ascaridoidea (N)			*Eimeria anseris*	Eimeriidae (Co)
	Contracaecum spiculigerum	Ascaridoidea (N)			*Eimeria nocens*	Eimeriidae (Co)
	Capillaria caudinflata	Trichuroidea (N)			*Tyzzeria anseris*	Eimeriidae (Co)
	Polymorphus boschadis	Polymorphidae (A)				
	Filicollis anatis	Polymorphidae (A)				
	Hypoderaeum conoideum	Echinostomatidae (T)				
	Echinoparyphium recurvatum	Echinostomatidae (T)				
	Hymenolepis lanceolata	Hymenolepididae (C)				
	Fimbriaria fasciolaris	Hymenolepididae (C)				
Caeca	*Heterakis gallinarum*	Ascaridoidea (N)			*Tetratrichomonas anseris*	Trichomonadidae (Fl)
	Heterakis dispar	Ascaridoidea (N)			*Entamoeba gallinarum*	Entamoebidae (Am)
	Heterakis brevispeculum	Ascaridoidea (N)				
	Capillaria anatis	Trichuroidea (N)				
	Trichostrongylus tenuis	Trichostrongyloidea (N)				
	Strongyloides avium	Strongyloidoidea (N)				
	Echinostoma revolutum	Echinostomatidae (T)				
	Notocotylus attenuatus	Notocotylidae (T)				
	Catatropis verrucosa	Notocotylidae (T)				
Cloacal bursa, rectum	*Prosthogonimus ovatus*	Prosthogonimidae (T)				
	Notocotylus attenuatus	Notocotylidae (T)				
Respiratory						
Nares	*Hyptiasmus tumidus*	Cyclocoelidae (T)				
Trachea, bronchi	*Cyathostoma bronchialis*	Strongyloidea (N)				
Lung						
Air sacs						

(Continued)

Goose parasite checklist. *Continued*

Section/host system	Helminths		Arthropods		Protozoa	
	Parasite	(Super) family	Parasite	Family	Parasite	Family
Liver						
Pancreas						
Circulatory						
Blood					*Leucocytozoon simondi*	Plasmodiidae (Bs)
					Haemoproteus nettionis	Plasmodiidae (Bs)
					Aegyptianella pullorum	Anaplasmataceae (R)
Blood vessels						
Nervous						
CNS						
Eye						
Reproductive/urogenital						
Oviduct	*Prosthogonimus pellucidus*	Prosthogonimidae (T)				
	Prosthogonimus ovatus	Prosthogonimidae (T)				
Kidneys					*Eimeria truncata*	Eimeriidae (Co)
Locomotory						
Connective tissue					*Toxoplasma gondii*	Sarcocystidae (Co)
Subcutaneous	*Collyriclum faba*	Collyriclidae (T)				
	Splendidofilaria fallisensis	Filarioidea (N)				
Integument						
Skin	*Collyriclum faba*	Collyriclidae (T)	*Anaticola anseris*	Philopteridae (L)		
			Anaticola crassicornis	Philopteridae (L)		
			Anaticola tadornae	Philopteridae (L)		
			Anaticola thoracicus	Philopteridae (L)		
			Acidoproctus rostratus	Philopteridae (L)		
			Anatoecus dentatus	Philopteridae (L)		
			Anatoecus brunneiceps	Philopteridae (L)		
			Anatoecus cygni	Philopteridae (L)		
			Anatoecus icterodes	Philopteridae (L)		
			Ornithobius cygni	Philopteridae (L)		
			Ornithobius mathisi	Philopteridae (L)		
			Ornithobius waterstoni	Philopteridae (L)		
			Holomenopon leucoxanthum	Menoponidae (L)		
			Ciconiphilus decimfasciatus	Menoponidae (L)		
			Ciconiphilus parvus	Menoponidae (L)		
			Ciconiphilus pectinventris	Menoponidae (L)		
			Ciconiphilus cygni	Menoponidae (L)		
			Ciconiphilus quadripustulatus	Menoponidae (L)		
			Trinoton anserium	Menoponidae (L)		
			Trinoton squalidum	Menoponidae (L)		
			Trinoton querquedula	Menoponidae (L)		
			Knemidocoptes gallinae	Knemidocoptidae (M)		

Pheasant parasite checklist.

Section/host system	Helminths		Arthropods		Protozoa	
	Parasite	(Super) family	Parasite	Family	Parasite	Family
Digestive						
Pharynx						
Oesophagus	Eucoleus (Capillaria) perforans	Trichuroidea (N)				
	Eucoleus (Capillaria) annulata	Trichuroidea (N)				
	Eucoleus (Capillaria) contorta	Trichuroidea (N)				
	Capillaria uropapillata	Trichuroidea (N)				
	Dispharynx nasuta	Acuarioidea (N)				
	Gongylonema ingluvicola	Spiruroidea (N)				
Crop	Eucoleus (Capillaria) perforans	Trichuroidea (N)				
	Eucoleus (Capillaria) annulata	Trichuroidea (N)				
	Eucoleus (Capillaria) contorta	Trichuroidea (N)				
	Capillaria uropapillata	Trichuroidea (N)				
	Gongylonema ingluvicola	Spiruroidea (N)				
Proventriculus	Dispharynx nasuta	Acuarioidea (N)				
	Gongylonema ingluvicola	Spiruroidea (N)				
Gizzard						
Small intestine	Ascaridia galli	Ascaridoidea (N)			Eimeria colchici	Eimeriidae (Co)
	Capillaria caudinflata	Trichuroidea (N)			Eimeria duodenalis	Eimeriidae (Co)
	Capillaria obsignata	Trichuroidea (N)			Eimeria megalostoma	Eimeriidae (Co)
	Capillaria phasianina	Trichuroidea (N)			Eimeria pacifica	Eimeriidae (Co)
	Capillaria bursata	Trichuroidea (N)			Eimeria phasiani	Eimeriidae (Co)
	Hymenolepis cantaniana	Hymenolepididae (C)			Spironucleus meleagridis	Hexamitidae (Fl)
Caeca	Heterakis gallinarum	Ascaridoidea (N)			Tetratrichomonas gallinarum	Trichomonadidae (Fl)
	Heterakis isolonche	Ascaridoidea (N)			Spironucleus meleagridis	Hexamitidae (Fl)
	Capillaria phasianina	Trichuroidea (N)			Histomonas meleagridis	Dientamoebidae (Fl)
	Capillaria anatis	Trichuroidea (N)				
	Trichostrongylus tenuis	Trichostrongyloidea (N)				
	Postharmostomum commutatum	Brachylaemidae (T)				
	Brachylaemus commutatus	Brachylaemidae (T)				
	Subulura suctoria	Subuluroidea (N)				
Cloacal bursa, rectum						
Respiratory						
Nares						
Trachea, bronchi	Syngamus trachea	Strongyloidea (N)				
Lung						
Air sacs						
Liver					Histomonas meleagridis	Dientamoebidae (Fl)

(Continued)

Pheasant parasite checklist. *Continued*

Section/host system	Helminths		Arthropods		Protozoa	
	Parasite	(Super) family	Parasite	Family	Parasite	Family
Pancreas						
Circulatory						
Blood					*Aegyptianella moshkovskii*	Anaplasmataceae (R)
Blood vessels						
Nervous						
CNS						
Eye						
Reproductive/urogenital						
Oviduct						
Kidneys						
Locomotory						
Muscle					*Toxoplasma gondii*	Sarcocystidae (Co)
Connective tissue						
Subcutaneous						
Integument						
Skin	*Dithyridium variable*	Mesocestoididae (C)	*Dermanyssus gallinae*	Dermanyssidae (M)		
			Menacanthus stramineus	Menoponidae (L)		
			Amyrsidea perdicis	Menoponidae (L)		
			Goniocotes chryocephalus	Philopteridae (L)		
			Gonoides colchici	Philopteridae (L)		
			Liperus maculosus	Philopteridae (L)		
			Lagopoecus colchicus	Degeeriellidae (L)		
			Knemidocoptes gallinae	Knemidocoptidae (M)		

Partridge parasite checklist (R, red-legged partridge; G, grey partridge; Ro, rock partridge; C, chukar partridge).

Section/host system	Helminths		Arthropods		Protozoa	
	Parasite	(Super) family	Parasite	Family	Parasite	Family
Digestive						
Pharynx						
Oesophagus	Eucoleus (Capillaria) perforans	Trichuroidea (N)				
	Eucoleus (Capillaria) annulata	Trichuroidea (N)				
	Eucoleus (Capillaria) contorta	Trichuroidea (N)				
	Capillaria uropapillata	Trichuroidea (N)				
	Dispharynx nasuta	Acuarioidea (N)				
	Gongylonema ingluvicola	Spiruroidea (N)				
Crop	Eucoleus (Capillaria) perforans	Trichuroidea (N)				
	Eucoleus (Capillaria) annulata	Trichuroidea (N)				
	Eucoleus (Capillaria) contorta	Trichuroidea (N)				
	Capillaria uropapillata	Trichuroidea (N)				
	Gongylonema ingluvicola	Spiruroidea (N)				
Proventriculus	Dispharynx nasuta	Acuarioidea (N)				
	Gongylonema ingluvicola	Spiruroidea (N)				
Gizzard						
Small intestine	Ascaridia galli	Ascaridoidea (N)			Eimeria caucasica (Ro)	Eimeriidae (Co)
	Capillaria caudinflata	Trichuroidea (N)			Eimeria procera (G)	Eimeriidae (Co)
	Capillaria obsignata	Trichuroidea (N)			Eimeria koifoidi (G, Ro, C)	Eimeriidae (Co)
	Capillaria phasianina	Trichuroidea (N)			Eimeria legionensis (R, Ro)	Eimeriidae (Co)
					Spironucleus meleagridis	Hexamitidae (Fl)
Caeca	Heterakis gallinarum	Ascaridoidea (N)			Tetratrichomonas gallinarum	Trichomonadidae (Fl)
	Capillaria anatis	Trichuroidea (N)				
	Capillaria phasianina	Trichuroidea (N)				
	Trichostrongylus tenuis	Trichostrongyloidea (N)				
	Subulura suctoria	Subuluroidea (N)				
Cloacal bursa, rectum						
Respiratory						
Nares						
Trachea, bronchi	Syngamus trachea	Strongyloidea (N)				
Lung						
Air sacs						
Liver					Histomonas meleagridis	Dientamoebidae (Fl)

(Continued)

Partridge parasite checklist (R, red-legged partridge; G, grey partridge; Ro, rock partridge; C, chukar partridge). *Continued*

Section/host system	Helminths		Arthropods		Protozoa	
	Parasite	(Super) family	Parasite	Family	Parasite	Family
Pancreas						
Circulatory						
Blood						
Blood vessels						
Nervous						
CNS						
Eye						
Reproductive/urogenital						
Oviduct						
Kidneys						
Locomotory						
Muscle					*Toxoplasma gondii*	Sarcocystidae (Co)
Connective tissue						
Subcutaneous						
Integument						
Skin	*Dithyridium variable*	Mesocestoididae (C)	*Dermanyssus gallinae*	Dermanyssidae (M)		
			Goniocotes microthorax (G)	Philopteridae (L)		
			Goniocotes obscurus (R)	Philopteridae (L)		
			Goniodes dispar	Philopteridae (L)		
			Amyrsidea perdicis	Menoponidae (L)		
			Menacanthus layali (R)	Menoponidae (L)		
			Menacanthus stramineus	Menoponidae (L)		
			Menopon pallens	Menoponidae (L)		
			Lipeurus maculosus (G)	Philopteridae (L)		
			Cuclotogaster heterogrammicus (G)	Philopteridae (L)		
			Cuclotogaster obsuricor (R)	Philopteridae (L)		
			Lagopoecus colchicus	Degeeriellidae (L)		

Quail parasite checklist.

Section/host system	Helminths		Arthropods		Protozoa	
	Parasite	(Super) family	Parasite	Family	Parasite	Family
Digestive						
Pharynx						
Oesophagus	Eucoleus (Capillaria) annulata	Trichuroidea (N)				
	Eucoleus (Capillaria) contorta	Trichuroidea (N)				
	Gongylonema ingluvicola	Spiruroidea (N)				
Crop	Eucoleus (Capillaria) annulata	Trichuroidea (N)				
	Eucoleus (Capillaria) contorta	Trichuroidea (N)				
	Gongylonema ingluvicola	Spiruroidea (N)				
Proventriculus	Dispharynx nasuta	Acuarioidea (N)				
	Tetrameres americana	Spiruroidea (N)				
	Tetrameres pattersoni	Spiruroidea (N)				
	Gongylonema ingluvicola	Spiruroidea (N)				
Gizzard						
Small intestine	Ascaridia galli	Ascaridoidea (N)			Eimeria bateri	Eimeriidae (Co)
	Hymenolepis cantaniana	Hymenolepididae (C)			Eimeria coturnicus	Eimeriidae (Co)
	Strongyloides avium	Strongyloidoidea (N)			Eimeria taldykurganica	Eimeriidae (Co)
					Eimeria tsunodai	Eimeriidae (Co)
					Eimeria uzura	Eimeriidae (Co)
					Spironucleus meleagridis	Spironucleidae (Fl)
Caeca	Heterakis gallinarum	Ascaridoidea (N)			Tetratrichomonas gallinarum	Trichomonadidae (Fl)
	Heterakis isolonche	Ascaridoidea (N)				
	Capillaria anatis	Trichuroidea (N)				
	Subulura suctoria	Subuluroidea (N)				
	Strongyloides avium	Strongyloidoidea (N)				
Large intestine, cloacal bursa, rectum					Cryptosporidium baileyi	Cryptosporidiidae (Co)
Respiratory						
Nares						
Trachea, bronchi						
Lung						
Air sacs						

(Continued)

Quail parasite checklist. *Continued*

Section/host system	Helminths		Arthropods		Protozoa	
	Parasite	(Super) family	Parasite	Family	Parasite	Family
Liver						
Pancreas						
Circulatory						
Blood						
Blood vessels						
Nervous						
CNS						
Eye						
Reproductive/urogenital						
Oviduct						
Kidneys						
Locomotory						
Connective tissue					Toxoplasma gondii	Sarcocystidae (Co)
Subcutaneous						
Integument						
Skin			Menacanthus stramineus	Menoponidae (L)		

Guinea fowl parasite checklist.

Section/host system	Helminths Parasite	Helminths (Super) family	Arthropods Parasite	Arthropods Family	Protozoa Parasite	Protozoa Family
Digestive						
Pharynx						
Oesophagus	Eucoleus (Capillaria) perforans	Trichuroidea (N)				
Crop	Eucoleus (Capillaria) perforans	Trichuroidea (N)				
Proventriculus	Dispharynx nasuta	Acuarioidea (N)				
Gizzard						
Small intestine	Ascaridia galli	Ascaridoidea (N)			Eimeria grenieri	Eimeriidae (Co)
	Railietina tetragona	Davaineidae (C)			Eimeria numidae	Eimeriidae (Co)
	Railietina cesticillus	Davaineidae (C)				
Caeca	Heterakis gallinarum	Ascaridoidea (N)			Tetratrichomonas gallinarum	Trichomonadidae (M)
	Heterakis brevispeculum	Ascaridoidea (N)			Pentatrichomonas gallinarum	Trichomonadidae (Fl)
	Subulura suctoria	Subuluroidea (N)			Entamoeba gallinarum	Entamoebidae (Am)
	Postharmostomum commutatum	Brachylaemidae (T)				
Cloacal bursa, rectum						
Respiratory						
Nares						
Trachea, bronchi	Syngamus trachea	Strongyloidea (N)				
Lung						
Air sacs						
Liver						
Pancreas						
Circulatory						
Blood					Leucocytozoon caulleryi	Plasmodiidae (Bs)
					Leucocytozoon sabrazesi	Plasmodiidae (Bs)
					Plasmodium gallinaceum	Plasmodiidae (Bs)
Blood vessels						
Nervous						
CNS						
Eye	Oxyspirura mansoni	Spiruroidea (N)				
Reproductive/urogenital						
Oviduct						
Kidneys						
Locomotory						
Muscle					Toxoplasma gondii	Sarcocystidae (Co)
Connective tissue						
Subcutaneous						
Integument						
Skin			Menacanthus stramineus	Menoponidae (L)		
			Lipeurus maculosus	Philopteridae (L)		

CHAPTER 14
Parasites of ungulates

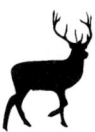

DEER

ENDOPARASITES

Parasites of the digestive system

Oesophagus

Gongylonema pulchrum

Gongylonema pulchrum, synonym *Gongylonema scutatum* (Phylum: Nematoda; Class: Chromadorea; Order: Spirurida; Family: Gongylonematidae), commonly known as the Gullet worm, is a parasite distributed worldwide and is localised in the oesophagus and rumen of sheep, goats, cattle, buffalo, deer, horses and camels, and the oesophagus of donkeys, pigs, humans and primates (for more details see Chapter 9). This parasite has coprophagous beetles and cockroaches as intermediate hosts.

Rumen and reticulum

Gongylonema verrucosum

Gongylonema verrucosum (Phylum: Nematoda; Class: Chromadorea; Order: Spirurida; Family: Gongylonematidae), commonly known as the Rumen gullet worm, is localised in the rumen, reticulum and omasum of cattle, sheep, goats and deer. This parasite has coprophagous beetles and cockroaches as intermediate hosts.

Paramphistomum and other rumen flukes

Several species of rumen fluke belonging to genera in the families Paramphistomatidae and Gastrothylacidae are found in deer and are summarised in Table 14.1. The taxonomy of the paramphistomes is complex and unresolved and many of the species described may be synonymous, being differentiated mainly on size and shape of the suckers. For more details on these rumen fluke species refer to Chapters 1, 8 and 9.

Abomasum

A number of ostertagian parasites are found in the abomasa of various deer hosts (Table 14.2). Species descriptions are provided in Chapter 1 (Family Trichostrongylidae). There have been few specific studies on the pathogenesis of abomasal parasites in deer.

Ostertagia ostertagi

Ostertagia ostertagi, synonyms *Ostertagia lyrata*, *Skrjabinagia lyrata* (Phylum: Nematoda; Class: Chromadorea; Order: Rhabditida; Family: Trichostrongylidae), commonly known as the Brown stomach worm, is a parasite distributed worldwide and is localised in the abomasum of cattle, deer and, very occasionally, goats.

Ostertagia leptospicularis

Ostertagia leptospicularis, synonym *Ostertagia crimensis* (Phylum: Nematoda; Class: Chromadorea; Order: Rhabditida; Family: Trichostrongylidae), commonly known as the Brown stomach worm, is a parasite distributed worldwide and is localised in the abomasum of fallow deer, roe deer, red deer, sika deer, moose, reindeer, cattle, sheep, goats and camels. It is considered a polymorphic species with two male morphs, *Ostertagia leptospicularis* and *Skrjabinagia kolchida* (for more details see Chapter 1).

Spiculopteragia bohmi

Spiculopteragia bohmi, synonyms *Apteragia bohmi*, *Rinadia bohmi* and morph species *Spiculopteragia mathevossiani*, *Rinadia mathevossiani* (Phylum: Nematoda; Class: Chromadorea; Order: Rhabditida; Family: Trichostrongylidae), is localised in the abomasum of red deer, roe deer, sika deer, fallow deer, moose and reindeer.

Pathogenesis: Worm burdens in deer are generally light, with lesions in the abomasum resembling those of ostertagiosis in cattle. Clinical disease is uncommon in free-ranging deer and occurs uncommonly in captive animals.

Veterinary Parasitology, Fifth Edition. Domenico Otranto and Richard Wall.
© 2024 John Wiley & Sons Ltd. Published 2024 by John Wiley & Sons Ltd.

Table 14.1 Rumen flukes of deer.

Species	Hosts	Site	Intermediate hosts
Paramphistomatidae			
Paramphistomum cervi (syn. *Paramphistomum explanatum*)	Cattle, sheep, goats, deer, buffalo, antelope	Rumen	Freshwater snails (*Bulinus* spp., *Planorbis* spp.)
Paramphistomum microbothrium	Cattle, sheep, goats, deer, buffalo, antelope	Rumen	Freshwater snails (*Fossaria* spp., *Bulinus* spp.)
Paramphistomum streptocoelium (syn. *Ceylonocotyle streptocoelium*, *Orthocoelium streptocoelium*)	Cattle, sheep, goats and wild ruminants	Rumen	Freshwater snails (*Glyptanisus* spp.)
Cotylophoron cotylophorum (syn. *Paramphistomum cotylophorum*)	Sheep, goats, cattle and wild ruminants	Rumen, reticulum	Freshwater snails (*Bulinus* spp.)
Calicophoron calicophorum (syn. *Paramphistomum calicophorum*)	Cattle, sheep, other ruminants	Rumen, reticulum	Water snails
Gastrothylacidae			
Gastrothylax crumenifer	Cattle, buffalo, zebu, sheep and other ruminants	Rumen, reticulum	Freshwater snails
Fischoederius elongatus	Cattle, buffalo, zebu, sheep and other ruminants; rarely humans	Rumen, duodenum	Freshwater snails
Fischoederius cobboldi	Cattle, buffalo, zebu, sheep and other ruminants	Rumen, duodenum	Freshwater snails

Table 14.2 Ostertagian parasites of deer.

Species	Host
Ostertagia ostertagi *Ostertagia* (syn. *Skrjabinagia*) *lyrata*	Cattle, deer and occasionally goats
Ostertagia leptospicularis (syn. *Ostertagia crimensis*) Morph species: *Skrjabinagia* (*Ostertagia*) *kolchida* (syn. *Grosspiculagia podjapolskyi*)	Deer, cattle, sheep and goats
Spiculopteragia spiculoptera	Deer (red deer, fallow deer, roe deer), cattle, sheep, goats
Spiculopteragia asymmetrica	Deer (roe deer, sika deer, fallow deer)
Apteragia quadrispiculata	Deer (roe deer, sika deer, fallow deer)
Spiculopteragia (*Apteragia*) *bohmi* Morph species: *Spiculopteragia* (*Rinadia*) *mathevossiani*	Mouflon, deer (fallow deer, roe deer)

Table 14.3 Cattle and sheep nematodes found in the abomasum of deer.

Species	Superfamily	Hosts	Geographical distribution
Ostertagia ostertagi *Ostertagia lyrata*	Trichostrongyloidea	Cattle, deer and occasionally goats	Worldwide
Teladorsagia circumcincta	Trichostrongyloidea	Sheep, goats, deer, camels, llamas	Worldwide
Haemonchus contortus	Trichostrongyloidea	Sheep, goats, cattle, deer, camels, llamas	Worldwide
Trichostrongylus axei	Trichostrongyloidea	Cattle, sheep, goats, deer, horses, donkeys, pigs and occasionally humans	Worldwide
Parabronema skrjabini	Spiruroidea	Sheep, goats, cattle, camels	Central and East Africa, Asia and some Mediterranean countries, notably Cyprus

Control and treatment: Both benzimidazoles and macrocyclic lactones have been shown to be effective against gastrointestinal nematodes in deer. For most anthelmintics, the dose rate in deer is that recommended for cattle or higher.

Deer can be infected with other species of abomasal nematodes found in cattle and sheep (Table 14.3). Detailed descriptions of these nematode species can be found in Chapter 1.

Intestines

A number of intestinal species have been reported in deer (Table 14.4) but are generally of little clinical significance. The majority of these are parasites of cattle or sheep and are described in more detail in Chapters 8 and 9 for these hosts.

A range of protozoa similar to those present in domesticated ruminants is found in the intestine of deer. Similarly, several species of *Eimeria* have been reported in various species of deer but their significance is not known (Table 14.5). Reported species of *Eimeria* may be synonymous and host specificity between species is unknown due to lack of cross-transmission studies.

Parasites of the respiratory system

Cephenemyia trompe

Cephenemyia trompe (Phylum: Arthropoda; Class: Insecta; Family: Oestridae), commonly known as the Reindeer throat bot or Deer nose bot, is a larval parasite found in reindeer/caribou, deer and moose throughout the northern Holarctic region including Europe and North America.

Epidemiology: *Cephenemyia trompe* is considered a serious problem in domestic reindeer management in Scandinavia. It is estimated that in Sweden, the losses due to *C. trompe* and the warble fly *Oedemagena tarandi* equate to approximately 15% of the income from reindeer production.

Pathogenesis: Although the larvae occasionally cause death from suffocation, their general effect is loss of condition. The adult flies cause disturbance and avoidance responses, which reduce feeding and result in loss of condition. In summer, keratitis and blindness may occur in reindeer if larvae are deposited in the eye.

Table 14.4 Intestinal parasites in deer.

Species	(Super)family	Hosts	Geographical distribution
Small intestine			
Trichostrongylus vitrinus	Trichostrongyloidea	Sheep, goats, deer and occasionally pigs and humans	Mainly temperate regions of the world
Trichostrongylus longispicularis	Trichostrongyloidea	Cattle, sheep, goats, deer, camels, llamas	Ruminants in Australia and cattle in America and parts of Europe
Nematodirus spathiger	Trichostrongyloidea	Sheep, goats, occasionally cattle and other ruminants	Cosmopolitan, but more prevalent in temperate zones
Nematodirus filicollis	Trichostrongyloidea	Sheep, goats, occasionally cattle and deer	Cosmopolitan, but more prevalent in temperate zones
Cooperia curticei	Trichostrongyloidea	Sheep, goats, deer	Worldwide
Cooperia onchophora	Trichostrongyloidea	Cattle, sheep, goats, deer	Worldwide
Cooperia punctate	Trichostrongyloidea	Cattle, deer	Worldwide
Cooperia pectinata	Trichostrongyloidea	Cattle, deer	Worldwide
Bunostomum trigonocephalum	Ancylostomatoidea	Sheep, goats, camels, deer	Worldwide
Capillaria bovis (syn. C. brevipes)	Trichuroidea	Cattle, sheep, goats, deer	Worldwide
Moniezia benedeni	Anoplocephalidae	Cattle, red deer, roe deer, camels Intermediate hosts: forage mites	Worldwide
Large intestine			
Oesophagostomum venulosum	Strongyloidea	Sheep, goats, deer, camels	Worldwide
Oesophagostomum columbianum	Strongyloidea	Sheep, goats, deer, camels	Worldwide; more important in tropical and subtropical areas
Chabertia ovina	Strongyloidea	Sheep, goats, occasionally deer, cattle and other ruminants	Worldwide but more prevalent in temperate regions
Trichuris ovis	Trichuroidea	Sheep, goats, occasionally cattle and other ruminants	Worldwide
Trichuris globulosa	Trichuroidea	Cattle, occasionally sheep, goats, camelss and other ruminants	Worldwide
Trichuris capreoli	Trichuroidea	Deer	?
Skrjabinema parva	Oxyuroidea	Deer (white-tailed)	North America

Table 14.5 *Eimeria* spp. of deer.

Roe deer	Red deer/wapiti	Reindeer
Eimeria capreoli	Eimeria asymmetrica	Eimeria arctica
Eimeria catubrina	Eimeria austriaca	Eimeria mayeri
Eimeria panda	Eimeria cervi	Eimeria tarandi
Eimeria patavina	Eimeria elaphi	
Eimeria ponderosa	Eimeria robusta	
Eimeria rotunda	Eimeria sordida	
Eimeria superba	Eimeria wapiti	

Table 14.6 Other species of bot flies (Family Oestridae) in deer.

Genus	Species	Host(s)	Region
Pharyngomyia	picta	Red deer, sika deer, fallow deer, roe deer	Europe, Central Asia
Cephenemyia	auribarbis	Red deer, fallow deer, mule deer, white-tailed deer	Europe, North America
	phobifer	Mule deer	North America
	jellisoni	Moose, elks	North America
	stimulator	Roe deer	Eurasia

Clinical signs and pathology: There are few external signs of the presence of deer nose bots, although there may be some nasal discharge. Occasionally, heavy infections may cause death by suffocation. Behaviour such as snorting and lowering or shaking of the head may indicate the migration of mature larvae within the nasal passages or oviposition activity of the adult fly. The retropharyngeal pouch may be enlarged and its epithelium may be pitted or eroded and become partly detached, necrotic and oedematous in infected deer.

Diagnosis: Occasionally a larva may be found on the ground after a severe sneezing attack, but often a positive diagnosis can only be made at necropsy.

Control and treatment: Nose bots are generally well tolerated in wild hosts and treatment is not usually required and control is impractical.

Other species of bot flies in deer are listed in Table 14.6.

Dictyocaulus viviparus

Dictyocaulus viviparus (Phylum: Nematoda; Class: Chromadorea; Order: Rhabditida; Family: Dictyocaulidae), commonly known as the Gullet worm, is distributed worldwide, but is especially important in temperate climates with a high rainfall. It is localised in the bronchi and trachea of cattle, buffalo, red deer and camels.

Epidemiology: Clinical disease is more prevalent in autumn in deer calves kept under intensive conditions. The prepatent period in red deer is 20–24 days and larvae are excreted for approximately 25 days.

Pathogenesis: Larval migration produces only a mild inflammatory response in the lungs. Thus, larger numbers of immature worms reach the pulmonary bronchi and heavy burdens of mature worms are well tolerated.

Clinical signs and pathology: In contrast with *D. viviparus* infection in cattle, coughing is not a common sign of affected red deer. Clinical signs commonly associated with lungworm infection are loss of condition, dull coat as well as inappetence, reduced weight gain, fever, tachycardia, tachypnoea, dyspnoea and death in severe cases. Gross pathological changes in lungs include consolidation of the dorsal portion of the diaphragmatic lobes, excess mucus and lungworms in the trachea, bronchi and bronchioles, and enlarged bronchial lymph nodes. Death results from asphyxiation due to obstruction of the trachea and bronchi with adult lungworms and mucus.

Diagnosis: Presumptive diagnosis of infection can be made on clinical signs if young susceptible deer develop respiratory problems or inappetence. On *post mortem* examination, the diagnosis is confirmed by finding large numbers of lungworms and mucus in pulmonary airways and pneumonic changes in the lungs. Mature *D. viviparus* infection can be detected by recovery of first-stage larvae from faecal samples by the Baermann technique (see Chapter 4).

Control and treatment: The importance and widespread occurrence of *D. viviparus* infection in farmed red deer have prompted a number of recommendations for its control. Clinical disease is exacerbated by stressors such as malnutrition and transport and is often associated with high stocking densities. These conditions can be reduced by not allowing deer to graze pasture previously grazed by cattle. Any introduced deer should be treated on arrival and then three and six weeks later. Live lungworm vaccine has been used as a preventive. Benzimidazole anthelmintics and macrocyclic lactones are generally effective at increased dose rates.

Dictyocaulus eckerti

Dictyocaulus eckerti, synonym *Dictyocaulus noerneri* (Phylum: Nematoda; Class: Chromadorea; Order: Rhabditida; Family: Dictyocaulidae), is a parasite distributed worldwide, but is especially important in temperate climates with a high rainfall. It is localised in the bronchi and trachea of roe deer, fallow deer and various other deer.

Dictyocaulus capreolus

Dictyocaulus capreolus (Phylum: Nematoda; Class: Chromadorea; Order: Rhabditida; Family: Dictyocaulidae) is localised in the bronchi and trachea of roe deer, and moose, and is found in Europe.

Varestrongylus sagittatus

Varestrongylus sagittatus, synonym *Bicaulus sagittatus* (Phylum: Nematoda; Class: Chromadorea; Order: Rhabditida; Family: Protostrongylidae), commonly known as the Small lungworm, is localised in the lungs of red deer and fallow deer, and is distributed throughout Europe. This parasite has slugs and snails as intermediate hosts.

Pathogenesis and clinical signs: Infection can cause pulmonary oedema, emphysema and inflammation of the lungs. Secondary bacterial infection can lead to pneumonia, emaciation and death.

Diagnosis: *Varestrongylus* first-stage larvae have a dorsal, posteriorly directed spine.

Treatment: Treatment with fenbendazole or mebendazole given over 3–5 days has been reported to be effective.

The following metastrongylid parasites have also been reported in the lungs of various deer hosts. Control is impractical and rarely, if ever, indicated.

Protostrongylus rufescens

Protostrongylus rufences (Phylum: Nematoda; Class: Chromadorea; Order: Rhabditida; Family: Protostrongylidae) is localised on small bronchioles of sheep, goats, deer and wild small ruminants. This parasite has snails (e.g. *Helicella*, *Theba*, *Abida*, *Zebrina*, *Arianta*) as intermediate hosts.

Muellerius capillaris

Muellerius capillaris (Phylum: Nematoda; Class: Chromadorea; Order: Rhabditida; Family: Protostrongylidae), commonly known as the Nodular lungworm, is localised in the lungs of sheep, goats, deer and wild small ruminants. This parasite has snails (e.g. *Helix*, *Succinea*) and slugs (e.g. *Limax*, *Agriolimax*, *Arion*) as intermediate hosts.

Cystocaulus ocreatus

Cystocaulus ocreatus (Phylum: Nematoda; Class: Chromadorea; Order: Rhabditida; Family: Protostrongylidae), commonly known as the Small lungworm, is distributed worldwide and is localised in the lungs of sheep, goats, deer and wild small ruminants. This parasite has snails (e.g. *Helicella*, *Helix*, *Theba*, *Cepaea*, *Monacha*) as intermediate hosts.

Echinococcus granulosus

For more details see Parasites of the liver.

Parasites of the liver

Fascioloides magna

Fascioloides magna (Phylum: Platyhelminthes; Class: Trematoda; Order: Plagiorchiida; Family: Fasciolidae), commonly known as the Large American liver fluke, is localised in the liver and bile ducts of white-tailed deer, elks, Red deer and moose, but also of cattle, sheep, goats, pigs, horses and llamas. This fluke is distributed in North America, central, eastern and southwestern Europe, South Africa and Mexico. A variety of freshwater snails (e.g. *Fossaria*, *Galba*, *Stagnicola*) are intermediate hosts.

Epidemiology: The various snail intermediate hosts tend to occur in stagnant semi-permanent water that contains large amounts of dead or dying vegetation, swamp areas, or pools and streams. *Fascioloides magna* is indigenous to North America and is common in Canada and the Great Lake areas where the white-tailed deer and elks are commonly infected.

Pathogenesis: In deer (and cattle), the flukes are frequently encapsulated in thin-walled fibrous cysts in the liver parenchyma and this restricted migration results in low pathogenicity.

Clinical signs and pathology: In deer and cattle the parasites can cause hepatic damage on reaching the liver but the flukes rapidly become encapsulated by the host reaction and clinical signs are minimal. In deer, encapsulated thin-walled fibrous cysts are found in the liver parenchyma.

Diagnosis: This is based primarily on clinical signs. Cysts and the large flukes are usually seen on *post mortem* examination. Faecal examination for the presence of fluke eggs is a useful aid to diagnosis.

Control and treatment: Elimination of the snail intermediate hosts is difficult due to their varied habitats. For cattle and sheep, the commonly used flukicides such as triclabendazole, closantel, clorsulon and albendazole are effective. Mature *F. magna* are susceptible to oxyclosanide.

Fasciola hepatica

Fasciola hepatica (Phylum: Platyhelminthes; Class: Trematoda; Order: Plagiorchiida; Family: Fasciolidae), commonly known as the Liver fluke, is a parasite distributed worldwide and is localised in the liver of sheep, cattle, goats, horses, deer, humans and other mammals. The parasite has snails of the genus *Galba* as intermediate host. The most common, *Galba truncatula*, is an amphibious snail with a wide distribution throughout the world.

Fasciola gigantica

Fasciola gigantica (Phylum: Platyhelminthes; Class: Trematoda; Order: Plagiorchiida; Family: Fasciolidae), commonly known as the Tropical large liver fluke, is localised in the liver of cattle, buffalo, sheep, goats, pigs, camels, deer and humans. This fluke is distributed in Africa, Asia, Europe and the USA. The intermediate hosts are snails of the genus *Galba*; in southern Europe it is *Galba auricularia*, which is also the important species in the southern USA, the Middle East and the Pacific Islands.

Dicrocoelium dendriticum

Dicrocoelium dendriticum (Phylum: Platyhelminthes; Class: Trematoda; Order: Plagiorchiida; Family: Dicrocoeliidae), known as the small lanceolate fluke, is localised in the liver of sheep, goats, cattle, deer and rabbits, occasionally horses and pigs. It is distributed worldwide except for South Africa and Australia. In Europe, the prevalence is high but in the British Isles prevalence is low, being confined to small foci throughout the country. Two intermediate hosts are required: the first host is land snails of many genera, principally *Cionella lubrica* in North America and *Zebrina detrita* in

Europe (some 29 other species have been reported to serve as first intermediate hosts of the genera *Abida*, *Theba*, *Helicella* and *Xerophila*). Brown ants of the genus *Formica*, frequently *Formica fusca*, represent the second intermediate host.

Stilesia hepatica

Stilesia hepatica (Phylum: Platyhelminthes; Class: Cestoda; Order: Cyclophyllidea; Family: Anoplocephalidae) is distributed in Africa and Asia and is localised in the bile ducts of sheep, deer and other ruminants. The intermediate host is probably an oribatid mite.

For more details of these species see Chapters 8 and 9.

Taenia hydatigena

Taenia hydatigena, synonyms *Taenia marginata*, *Cysticercus tenuicollis* (Phylum: Platyhelminthes; Class: Cestoda; Order: Cyclophyllidea; Family: Taeniidae), is localised in the abdominal cavity and liver of the intermediate hosts (sheep, cattle, deer, pigs and horses) and in the small intestine of the definitive hosts (dogs, foxes, weasels, stoats, polecats, wolves and hyenas).

Echinococcus granulosus

Echinococcus granulosus (Phylum: Platyhelminthes; Class: Cestoda; Order: Cyclophyllidea; Family: Taeniidae), commonly known as the Dwarf dog tapeworm, is the causative agent of hydatidosis. This parasite is distributed worldwide and is localised mainly in the liver and lungs in the intermediate hosts (domestic and wild ruminants, deer, humans, primates, pigs and lagomorphs; horses and donkeys are resistant) and small intestine in the definitive host (dogs and many wild canids).

For more details of these species see Chapter 9.

Parasites of the circulatory system

Babesia bovis

Babesia bovis, synonym *Babesia argentina* (Phylum: Apicomplexa; Class: Aconoidasida; Order: Piroplasmida; Family: Babesiidae), is localised in the blood of cattle, buffalo and deer (roe deer, red deer), and is distributed throughout Australia, Africa, Central and South America, Asia and southern Europe.

For more details see Chapter 8.

Anaplasma marginale

Anaplasma marginale (Phylum: Proteobacteria; Class: Alphaproteobacteria; Order: Rickettsiales; Family: Anaplasmataceae) is localised in the blood of cattle and wild ruminants, and is distributed throughout Africa, southern Europe, Australia, South America, Asia, former Soviet States and in the USA.

Anaplasma centrale

Anaplasma centrale (Phylum: Proteobacteria; Class: Alphaproteobacteria; Order: Rickettsiales; Family: Anaplasmataceae) is localised in the blood of cattle, deer and wild ruminants, and is found distributed throughout Africa, southern Europe, Australia, South America, Asia, former Soviet States and in the USA.

For more details of these species see Chapter 8.

Parasites of the nervous system

Elaphostrongylus cervi

Elaphostrongylus cervi, synonym *Elaphostrongylus crangiferi* (Phylum: Nematoda; Class: Chromadorea; Order: Rhabditida; Family: Protostrongylidae), is localised in the connective tissue and central nervous system (CNS) of red deer, roe deer and sika deer from most countries of northern and central Europe, Commonwealth of Independent States (CIS), and is also present in New Zealand. Various land and freshwater snails and slugs are intermediate hosts. This parasite affects a number of deer species and the prevalence of infection is generally high in both wild and farmed deer.

Pathogenesis: The severity of clinical disease is very much influenced by the level of infection and location in the body. Light infections are usually subclinical. Three clinical syndromes are described:

- acute disease characterised by hindlimb paralysis and perhaps blindness resulting from damage to the CNS
- chronic ill-thrift, resulting from connective tissue damage
- verminous pneumonia, resulting from larval migration.

Additionally, there may be economic losses through trimming, downgrading or condemnation of carcass.

Clinical signs and pathology: Most infections are inapparent. Clinical signs include exercise intolerance, hindlimb incoordination and nervous disorders. Connective tissue lesions are most likely to be found in the muscles of the neck, shoulders, flanks and loins. These consist of green discoloration of fascial sheets and chronic granulomas with encapsulated degenerated worms. Similar lesions may be seen in regional lymph nodes. Worms associated with CNS lesions are most likely to be seen in the subdural and subarachnoid spaces. Pulmonary lesions consist of a diffuse interstitial pneumonia with focal emphysema and consolidation.

Diagnosis: Diagnosis is based on finding the infective larvae in faeces using the Baermann method. The first-stage larvae have a characteristic dorsal spine on their tails and look very like the protostrongylid larvae of *Muellerius* spp. that infest sheep.

Control and treatment: Control is difficult given the ubiquitous nature of the intermediate hosts. Fenbendazole given on three consecutive days has been reported to be effective.

Parelaphostrongylus tenuis

Parelaphostrongylus tenuis, synonyms *Odocoileostrongylus tenuis*, *Elaphostrongylus tenuis* (Phylum: Nematoda; Class: Chromadorea; Order: Rhabditida; Family: Protostrongylidae), causes a condition commonly known as Cerebrospinal nematodosis, Meningeal worm, Moose sickness or Moose disease and is found in the veins and venous sinuses of cranial meninges, CNS of white-tailed deer, moose, wapiti, other deer species, llamas, guanacos, alpacas and camels. It has been reported rarely in sheep and goats from North America. The parasite has snails and slugs as intermediate hosts. *Parelaphostrongylus tenuis* is a common parasite of white-tailed deer in North America. Infection occurs in moose that share the same range as white-tailed deer.

Pathogenesis: In the white-tailed deer, the parasite causes little clinical effect but in other cervids and camelids (and in sheep and goats) it can cause debilitating neurological signs and in North America is the causative agent of 'moose sickness'. Llamas and their relatives are susceptible to *P. tenuis*.

Clinical signs: Signs of infection are rare in white-tailed deer. Infected moose may show swaying, paraparesis, torticollis, circling, blindness, ataxia, paresis, difficulty in standing, weight loss and death. In red deer (wapiti), there is progressive neurological disease and death.

Diagnosis: Based on finding adult worms in the CNS. *P. tenuis* does not normally mature in the abnormal hosts and larvae will not be present in faeces.

Control and treatment: Not practical. Strict management of national and international deer translocations should be practised wherever possible.

Parasites of the reproductive/urogenital system

No parasites of veterinary significance reported.

Parasites of the locomotory system

Taenia ovis

Taenia ovis, synonyms *Taenia cervi*, *Taenia krabbei*, *Taenia hyenae*, *Cysticercus ovis*, *Cysticercus cervi*, *Cysticercus tarandi*, *Cysticercus dromedarii*, *Cysticercus cameli* (Phylum: Platyhelminthes; Class: Cestoda; Order: Cyclophyllidea; Family: Taeniidae), is a parasite distributed worldwide and is localised in the small intestine of the definitive hosts (e.g. dogs, foxes, wild carnivores) and on muscle of the intermediate hosts (sheep, goats, deer, reindeer and camels). Wild canids are infested by consuming the cysticercus in the intermediate host. The intermediate host is infected through the ingestion of tapeworm eggs that hatch in the intestine. Deer are infected by grazing pasture and forages contaminated with carnivore faeces harbouring taenid eggs.

Pathogenesis: Cysticerci may cause economic loss through condemnation at meat inspection.

Clinical signs and pathology: Infected intermediate hosts do not usually show clinical signs of disease. The mature, ovoid, white cysticerci are grossly visible in the muscle, heart, lung, liver and brain.

Diagnosis: Through the identification of cysts at *post mortem* inspection.

Treatment and control: Control is not practical.

Notes: The correct nomenclature for the intermediate host stage is 'metacestode stage of *Taenia ovis*' rather than '*Cysticercus ovis*'. It is now thought that *Taenia cervi*, which is found mainly in red deer and roe deer, and *Taenia krabbei*, found mainly in reindeer, are synonymous with *T. ovis*, and that they are one and the same species present in different hosts.

Sarcocystiosis

Several species of *Sarcocystis* have been reported in deer (Table 14.7). Specific descriptions are outwith the scope of this book. As with cattle and sheep, infections are only diagnosed at *post mortem* or on histology when the sarcocysts in muscle are discovered (Fig. 14.1).

Table 14.7 *Sarcocystis* species found in deer.

Species	Deer host(s)	Final hosts	Distribution
Sarcocystis cervicanis	Red deer	Dogs	Europe
Sarcocystis grueneri	Red deer, reindeer	Dogs, foxes, coyotes	Eurasia
Sarcocystis wapiti	Red deer, roe deer	Dogs, coyotes	North America
Sarcocystis sybillensis	Red deer, roe deer	Dogs	North America
Sarcocystis capreolicanis	Roe deer	Dogs, foxes	Europe
Sarcocystis gracilis	Roe deer	Dogs, foxes	Eurasia
Sarcocystis rangi	*Sarcocystis rangi*	Dogs	Europe
Sarcocystis tarandivulpis	Reindeer	Dogs, foxes, raccoon dogs	Europe
Sarcocystis tarandi	Reindeer	Unknown	Europe
Sarcocystis rangiferi	Reindeer	Unknown	Europe
Sarcocystis alceslatranis	Moose	Dogs, coyotes	North America, Europe
Sarcocystis jorrini	Fallow deer		Europe

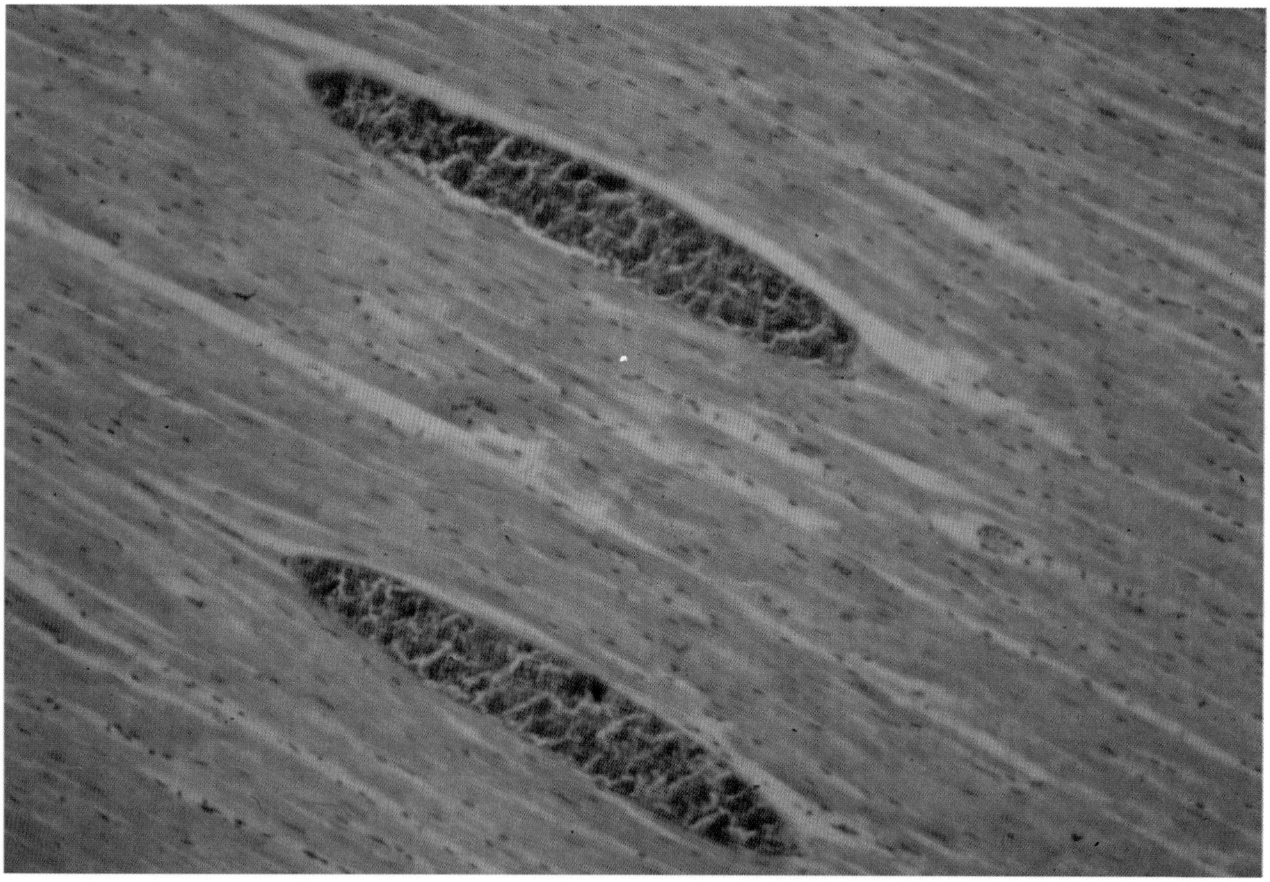

Fig. 14.1 Sarcocysts in the heart muscle of a red deer (*Cervus elaphus*).

Parasites of the connective tissue

Elaeophora schneideri

Elaeophora schneideri (Phylum: Nematoda; Class: Chromadorea; Order: Spirurida; Family: Onchocercidae) causes a disease commonly known as Filarial dermatosis or 'Sore head' and is localised in the blood vessels of sheep, goats and deer (elks, moose, mule deer) of western and southern USA. This parasite has tabanid flies as intermediate host.

Pathogenesis: It is thought that the natural hosts of *E. schneideri* are deer, in which the infection is asymptomatic.

For more details see Chapter 9.

Hypoderma diana

Hypoderma diana (Phylum: Arthropoda; Class: Insecta; Family: Oestridae), commonly known as the Deer warble fly, is a larval parasite of deer and occasionally horses and sheep. It is found throughout the northern hemisphere.

Epidemiology: *Hypoderma diana* is present in a great variety of habitats, overlapping the territory of its hosts. It is spread throughout Europe and Asia, from 30° to 60°N, living in several different ecological zones, such as mixed, deciduous and coniferous forests, wooded steppes and wetlands. The adult fly is most active in May and June, particularly on warm sunny days. The main factors influencing the flight and oviposition of female flies are ambient air temperature and light, as a result of which they are most active at midday. As in other species, the extent of parasitism and prevalence is higher in younger animals, possibly due to a measure of resistance in adults built up through repeated contact with the parasite. The degree of parasitism in male deer is usually higher than in females and castrated animals.

Pathogenesis: The deer warble fly is most active in May and June, but it is not recognised as a cause of 'gadding' in deer. The mature larvae occur subcutaneously along the back and hide damage occurs with linear perforations.

Clinical signs and pathology: Except for poor growth in severe cases, the hosts show no symptoms until the larvae appear along the back, when the swellings can be seen and felt. The larval migration is not usually noticed clinically, but heavy infestations may reduce growth. Occasionally the pressure of larvae on the spinal cord can cause paralysis. When the larvae reach the skin on the animal's back, large, soft, painful swellings of up to 3 mm in diameter develop. The larvae lie in cysts containing yellow purulent fluid. Deer warble larvae induce a pronounced tissue inflammation. The cellular reaction is predominantly eosinophilic and lymphocytic. The presence of the larvae also induces the production of a thickened connective tissue-lined cavity surrounding the larva, filled with inflammatory cells, particularly eosinophils.

Diagnosis: The presence of the larvae under the skin of the back of deer allows diagnosis of warble flies. The eggs may also be found on the hairs of the animals in the summer.

Treatment and control: Like other species, *H. diana* is highly susceptible to systemically active organophosphate insecticides and the macrocyclic lactones ivermectin, doramectin, eprinomectin and moxidectin. For farm-raised deer a control programme may be implemented, with regular treatment timed in relation to the local population dynamics of *Hypoderma*. Animals may be given some protection by being herded into corrals, shelters or shaded areas to reduce the risk of infestation when adult flies are active. It is more difficult to develop effective control measures for diseases in wild and semi-wild deer. Here it is important that any attempted parasite controls do not have an effect on the environment in which the animals live. For free-range deer that cannot be captured, food may be supplemented with oral forms of antiparasitic preparations. However, care must be taken in selecting a suitable food medium for the antiparasitic agent, since it cannot be freely distributed around the environment because it may be eaten by other animals; neither can the volume ingested be controlled.

Notes: With the success of control measures against warbles in cattle, it is important to realise that *H. diana*, although capable of infecting many species of deer, will not infect cattle. As a consequence of this, even in areas where (as is commonly the case) almost all the deer carry the parasitic larvae, cattle are not at risk.

Hypoderma tarandi

Hypoderma tarandi, synonym *Oedemagena tarandi* (Phylum: Arthropoda; Class: Insecta Family: Oestridae), commonly known as the Reindeer warble, occurs in the subcutaneous connective tissue of reindeer/caribou and musk ox in the circum-arctic and subarctic regions of Europe, Asiatic Russia and America

Epidemiology: Fawns and yearlings are most affected by this parasite, which produces large oedematous swellings. These swellings may suppurate and attract blowflies, which then oviposit in the wound.

Pathogenesis: The adult flies cause gadding, and the newly hatched larvae may cause dermatitis with local oedema when they penetrate the skin. However, the main importance of this genus is economic, from damage to hides by the L_3. In Sweden this loss can amount to one-fifth of the total income from reindeer herds. Up to 200 holes may be found in typically infested reindeer skins in Russia.

Clinical signs and pathology: Except for poor growth in severe cases, the hosts show no symptoms until the larvae appear along the back, when the swellings can be seen and felt. The larval migration is not usually noticed clinically, but heavy infestations may reduce growth. Occasionally, the pressure of larvae on the spinal cord can cause paralysis. When the larvae reach the skin on the animal's back, large, soft, painful swellings may be observed. The larvae lie in cysts containing yellow purulent fluid. Attacks by reindeer warble flies laying eggs can cause irritation to reindeer. Host animals may injure themselves as a result. Reindeer warble larvae induce a pronounced tissue inflammation. The cellular reaction is predominantly eosinophilic and lymphocytic. The presence of the larvae also induces the production of a thickened connective tissue-lined cavity surrounding the larva, filled with inflammatory cells, particularly eosinophils.

Diagnosis: The presence of the larvae under the skin of the back allows diagnosis of reindeer warble flies. The eggs may also be found on the hairs of the animals in the summer.

Treatment and control: Injectable ivermectin, doramectin, eprinomectin or moxidectin administered between November and January is extremely effective in eliminating these parasites. In control schemes, a single annual treatment in autumn is usually recommended before the larvae have reached the back and perforated the hide.

Notes: Limited geographical distribution but of local veterinary importance.

ECTOPARASITES

Flies

Lipoptena spp.

Lipoptena spp. (Phylum: Arthropoda; Class: Insecta; Order: Diptera; Family: Hippoboscidae), commonly known as Deer keds, are blood-feeding flies found on deer and elk. *Lipoptena depressa* is found in North America and *Lipoptena cervi* in Europe and Asia (but it has also been introduced into North America).

Pathogenesis: These species are primarily a nuisance and a cause of disturbance.

Lice

Lice infestations are frequently encountered in deer. It is beyond the scope of this book to provide detailed descriptions of all the species of lice that may be encountered on deer throughout the world. Some of the more common species that may be encountered are provided in Table 14.8.

Treatments with insecticides, such as carbaryl, cypermethrin, deltamethrin, diazinon, lindane and malathion, are usually effective in controlling lice on deer. Insecticidal dust bags or 'back rubbers' can be used as self-dosing rubbing stations for deer and other ungulates. Because louse populations on most temperate ungulates increase during the cooler months, insecticides should ideally be administered to them in the autumn/winter. Avermectins are generally less effective against chewing lice but may be effective against sucking lice. Animals destined to be introduced into established herds should be quarantined and where necessary treated.

Ticks

Ixodes scapularis

Ixodes scapularis, synonym *Ixodes dammin* (Phylum: Arthropoda; Class: Arachnida; Order: Ixodida; Family: Ixodidae), commonly known as the Shoulder tick or Black-legged tick, may be commonly found on deer but may also occur on a range of other mammals and birds throughout North America, particularly in and around wooded areas east of the Rocky Mountains.

Epidemiology: *Ixodes scapularis* requires a high relative humidity to survive, and its patterns of feeding activity reflect this requirement. With feeding restricted to times of year when conditions of temperature and humidity are appropriate, distinct restricted seasonal periods of activity result, usually in spring and autumn. As a result of its requirement for high humidity, in general it is associated with areas of deciduous woodland containing small mammals and deer.

Pathogenesis: *Ixodes scapularis* inflicts a very painful bite. Nymphal and adult stages of this tick are the most common vector for Lyme disease in North America. They are also implicated in the transmission of *Francisella tularensis*. These ticks are major vectors for the transmission of human babesiosis and human granulocytic ehrlichiosis and are responsible for the transmission of anaplasmosis and piroplasmosis.

Dermacentor albipictus

Dermacentor albipictus (Phylum: Arthropoda; Class: Arachnida; Order: Ixodida, Family: Ixodidae), commonly known as the Winter tick or Moose tick, feed particularly on moose but will also feed on a wide variety of domestic and wild mammals, including horses, cattle and humans. The species is found throughout the northern USA and Canada, particularly in upland and mountainous areas.

Epidemiology: This is a one-host species of tick. The larva, nymph and adult all attach to, and develop on, a single host. This species feeds only in winter, usually between October and March/April, on horses, deer and related large mammals. Under normal conditions this tick species produces one generation per year.

Table 14.8 Lice on deer.

Lice	Family	Host(s)	Region
Solenopotes tarandi	Linognathidae	Reindeer/caribou	Eurasia, North America
Solenopotes binipilosus	Linognathidae	White-tailed deer, black-tailed deer, mule deer	North, Central and South America
Solenopotes burmeisteri	Linognathidae	Elk, Red deer, sika deer	Eurasia
Solenopotes capreoli	Linognathidae	Roe deer	Eurasia
Solenopotes ferrisi	Linognathidae	Black-tailed deer	North America
Solenopotes muntiacus	Linognathidae	Muntjac	South Asia
Bovicola forficula	Bovicolidae	Muntjac	Asia
Bovicola longicornis	Bovicolidae	Red deer	Europe
Bovicola maai	Bovicolidae	Sika deer	Eurasia
Bovicola meyeri	Bovicolidae	Roe deer	Eurasia
Bovicola tibialis	Bovicolidae	Fallow deer	Europe
Tricholipeurus indicus	Philopteridae	Muntjac	Asia

Pathogenesis: *Dermacentor albipictus* may cause tick paralysis and is a vector of anaplasmosis and possibly Rocky Mountain spotted fever. Heavy infestations with *D. albipictus* cause hair loss and a condition known as 'ghost moose' in northern parts of the USA. Heavy infection can occur in the long winter coats of mammals such as horses, deer, elks and moose, causing debilitation and anaemia, particularly when there are food shortages.

Mites

Sarcoptes scabiei

Sarcoptes scabiei (Phylum: Arthropoda; Class: Arachnida; Subclass: Acari; Order: Astigmata (Sarcoptiformes); Family: Sarcoptidae) is a burrowing mite found in the skin of red deer, roe deer, moose and reindeer.

For more details see Chapters 3 and 11.

A number of non-obligate ectoparasites are found on deer and these are listed in the host–parasite checklists at the end of this chapter.

CAMELS

ENDOPARASITES

Parasites of the digestive system

Gongylonema pulchrum

Gongylonema pulchrum (Phylum: Nematoda; Class: Chromadorea; Order: Spirurida; Family: Gongylonematidae), commonly known as the Gullet worm, is a parasite distributed worldwide and is localised in the oesophagus and rumen of sheep, goats, cattle, buffalo, deer, horses and camels, and the oesophagus of donkeys pigs, humans and primates (for more details see Chapter 9). This parasite has coprophagous beetles and cockroaches as intermediate hosts.

Gongylonema verrucosum

Gongylonema verrucosum (Phylum: Nematoda; Class: Chromadorea; Order: Spirurida; Family: Gongylonematidae), commonly known as the Rumen gullet worm, is localised in the rumen, reticulum and omasum of cattle, sheep, goats, deer and camels. This parasite has coprophagous beetles and cockroaches as intermediate hosts. For more details see Chapter 9.

Studies on the helminth parasites of camels are few, and published information consists mainly of case reports and lists of reported helminths. Many of the species reported are accidental infections with parasite species of domestic ruminants and their significance and pathogenicity are generally not known. The most important species, against which treatment is targeted, is the camel stomach worm *Haemonchus longistipes*. This nematode, either alone or in mixed infections with *Trichostrongylus* spp., may cause a debilitating and sometimes fatal condition.

Limited information is available on the efficacy of anthelmintics against gastrointestinal nematodes in camels. Benzimidazoles and ivermectin given at cattle dose rates have reported efficacy against a number of gastrointestinal nematode species found in camels. Ivermectin has been reported as less effective against *Nematodirus* spp. and *Trichuris* spp.

Monthly treatments of young animals during the rainy season can help reduce parasitic burdens. Removal of faeces around watering points and keeping these areas dry can also reduce numbers of infective larvae.

Abomasum

Haemonchus longistipes

Haemonchus longistipes (Phylum: Nematoda; Class: Chromadorea; Order: Rhabditida; Family: Trichostrongylidae), commonly known as the Camel stomach worm, is localised in the abomasum of camels and sheep from Africa and Middle East.

Epidemiology: The epidemiology is similar to that reported with haemonchosis in domestic ruminants. The prevalence of this parasite varies from region to region and from season to season in the same region. Higher prevalence rates have been reported during the rainy season with a drop in prevalence during the dry season.

Clinical signs and pathogenesis: *Haemonchus longistipes* is a voracious blood sucker, producing symptoms similar to those of *Haemonchus contortus* in domestic ruminants. Infection has been reported to cause anaemia, oedema, emaciation and death.

Camelostrongylus mentulatus

Camelostrongylus mentulatus (Phylum: Nematoda; Class: Chromadorea; Order: Rhabditida; Family: Trichostrongylidae) is localised in the abomasum and small intestine of camels, llamas, sheep and goats of the Middle East, Australia and South America. It is generally of low pathogenicity and considered of little importance, though heavy infections can produce gastric hyperplasia and increase in abomasal pH, similar to that seen in *Ostertagia* spp. infection.

Physocephalus sexalatus

Physocephalus sexalatus, synonym *Physocephalus cristatus* (Phylum: Nematoda; Class: Chromadorea; Order: Spirurida; Family: Spirocercidae), is a parasite of pigs, camels and occasionally rabbits and hares. It has been reported in dromedary camels in Iran. The parasite has coprophagous beetles as intermediary hosts.

Other parasites of cattle or sheep and wild ruminants have been reported in the abomasum of camels (Table 14.9).

Small intestine

Species of nematodes and cestodes reported in the small intestines of camels are generally of little clinical significance and only brief

Table 14.9 Cattle and sheep parasites found in the abomasum of camels.

Species	(Super)family	Hosts	Geographical distribution
Teladorsagia circumcincta	Trichostrongyloidea	Cattle, sheep, goats, deer, camels, llamas	Worldwide
Ostertagia leptospicularis	Trichostrongyloidea	Deer (roe deer), cattle, sheep, goats, camels	Many parts of the world, particularly Europe and New Zealand
Haemonchus contortus	Trichostrongyloidea	Sheep, goats, cattle, deer, camels, llamas	Worldwide
Marshallagia marshalli	Trichostrongyloidea	Sheep, goats and wild small ruminants	Tropics and subtropics including southern Europe, USA, South America, India and Russia
Trichostrongylus axei	Trichostrongyloidea	Cattle, sheep, goats, deer, horses, donkeys, pigs and occasionally humans	Worldwide
Parabronema skrjabini	Spiruroidea	Sheep, goats, cattle, camels	Central and East Africa, Asia and some Mediterranean countries, notably Cyprus

Table 14.10 Cattle and sheep parasites found in the small intestines of camels.

Species	(Super)family	Hosts	Geographical distribution
Nematodes			
Trichostrongylus longispicularis	Trichostrongyloidea	Cattle, sheep, goats, deer, camels, llamas	Ruminants in Australia and cattle in America and parts of Europe
Trichostrongylus vitrinus	Trichostrongyloidea	Sheep, goats, deer, camels, occasionally pigs and humans	Mainly temperate regions of the world
Trichostrongylus colubriformis	Trichostrongyloidea	Sheep, goats, cattle, camels and occasionally pigs and humans	Worldwide
Trichostrongylus probolorus	Trichostrongyloidea	Sheep, camels, humans	?
Nematodirus spathiger	Trichostrongyloidea	Sheep, goats, occasionally cattle and other ruminants	Cosmopolitan, but more prevalent in temperate zones
Nematodirus helvetianus	Trichostrongyloidea	Cattle, occasionally sheep, goats and other ruminants	?
Nematodirus abnormalis	Trichostrongyloidea	Sheep, goats, camels	Europe, Asia, North America, Australia and Russia
Cooperia oncophora	Trichostrongyloidea	Cattle, sheep, goats, deer	Worldwide
Cooperia surnabada (syn. Cooperia mcmasteri)	Trichostrongyloidea	Cattle, sheep, camels	Parts of Europe, North America and Australia
Bunostomum trigonocephalum	Ancylostomatoidea	Sheep, goats, camels	Worldwide
Strongyloides papillosus	Strongyloidoidea	Sheep, cattle, other ruminants and rabbits	Worldwide
Cestodes			
Moniezia benedeni	Anoplocephalidae	Cattle, red deer, roe deer, camels Intermediate hosts: forage mites	Worldwide
Moniezia expansa	Anoplocephalidae	Sheep, goats, occasionally cattle Intermediate hosts: forage mites	Worldwide
Thysaniezia ovilla (syn. Thysaniezia giardia)	Anoplocephalidae	Cattle, sheep, goats, camels and wild ruminants Intermediate hosts: oribatid mites and psocid lice	Southern Africa
Avitellina centripunctata (syn. Avitellina woodlandi)	Anoplocephalidae	Sheep and other ruminants Intermediate hosts: oribatid mites or psocid lice	Europe, Africa and Asia. Widespread in camels in Asia and Africa
Stilesia globipunctata	Anoplocephalidae	Sheep, cattle and other ruminants Intermediate hosts: oribatid mites or psocid lice	Southern Europe, Africa and Asia

Table 14.11 Cattle and sheep parasites found in the large intestine of camels.

Species	(Super)family	Hosts	Geographical distribution
Oesophagostomum venulosum (syn. Oesophagostomum virginimembrum)	Strongyloidea	Sheep, goats, deer, camels	Worldwide
Oesophagostomum columbianum	Strongyloidea	Sheep, goats, deer, camels	Worldwide; more important in tropical and subtropical areas
Chabertia ovina	Strongyloidea	Sheep, goats, occasionally deer, cattle and other ruminants	Worldwide but more prevalent in temperate regions
Trichuris ovis	Trichuroidea	Sheep, goats, occasionally cattle and other ruminants	Worldwide
Trichuris globulosa	Trichuroidea	Cattle, occasionally sheep, goats, camels and other ruminants	Worldwide

details are listed below. Cattle or sheep parasites found in the small intestine are listed in Table 14.10 and those of the large intestine are given in Table 14.11. Further details of these parasites can be found in Chapters 8 and 9. A more detailed list of helminth species found in camels is provided in the parasite checklist at the end of the chapter.

Nematodirella dromedarii

Nematodirella dromedarii (Phylum: Nematoda; Class: Chromadorea; Order: Rhabditida; Family: Molineidae) is localised in the small intestine of dromedary camels, and presumably distributed throughout the host range of Asia and North Africa.

Nematodirella cameli

Nematodirella cameli (Phylum: Nematoda; Class: Chromadorea; Order: Rhabditida; Family: Molineidae) is localised in the small intestine of Bactrian camels, reindeer and elks from Russia and CIS countries.

Coccidia

Eimeria bactriani

Eimeria bactriani, synonym *Eimeria nolleri* (Phylum: Apicomplexa; Class: Conoidasida; Order: Eucoccidiorida; Family: Eimeriidae), is localised in the small intestine of camels (Bactrian, dromedary) from Germany, Russia and former Soviet states. The epidemiology, pathogenesis and clinical signs of this parasite are not reported. The life cycle is typically coccidian with endogenous stages found in the small intestine, although the number of merogony stages is unknown. Sporulation time is 9–15 days.

Diagnosis: Based on clinical signs and the demonstration of oocysts in diarrhoeic faeces.

Control and treatment: Little is known about treatment but, by analogy with other hosts, one of the sulfonamide drugs should be tried if disease is suspected. Prevention is based on good management, avoidance of overcrowding and stress, and attention to hygiene, particularly watering areas, which should be protected from faecal contamination.

Notes: There is controversy regarding the specific name of this organism. In some texts it is referred to as *Eimeria nolleri.*

Eimeria cameli

Eimeria cameli (Phylum: Apicomplexa; Class: Conoidasida; Order: Eucoccidiorida; Family: Eimeriidae) is distributed worldwide and is localised in the small and large intestine of camels (Bactrian, dromedary). This is the most frequently encountered *Eimeria* species in camels in North Africa. Giant meronts are found in the small intestine and gamonts are found in the ileum and occasionally the caecum. Sporulation time is 9–15 days.

Epidemiology: Young camels are much more susceptible to infection.

Pathogenesis and clinical signs: Infections can produce severe enteritis leading to progressive weight loss and emaciation. Watery diarrhoea, sometimes containing blood, has been found in heavy infections. Diarrhoea and secondary bacterial infections may aggravate the condition, leading to death in young camels.

Pathology: Presence of the parasite may cause inflammatory lesions in the small intestine and giant meronts may be visible with the naked eye. Cystic structures containing oocysts may be seen in the mucosa on histopathology.

Control and treatment: As for *E. bactriani.*

Eimeria dromedarii

Eimeria dromedarii (Phylum: Apicomplexa; Class: Conoidasida; Order: Eucoccidiorida; Family: Eimeriidae) is distributed worldwide and is localised in the small intestine of camels (Bactrian, dromedary). This species is found frequently, often together with *E. cameli.* Giant meronts are found in the small intestine and gamonts are found in the ileum and occasionally the caecum. Sporulation time is 15–17 days.

Cystoisospora orlovi

Cystoisospora orlovi, synonym *Isospora orlovi* (Phylum: Apicomplexa; Class: Conoidasida; Order: Eucoccidiorida; Family: Sarcocystidae), is a parasite of camels, found in Russia and former Soviet states. Another species, *Isospora cameli,* has been reported in India. It is not clear if these species are valid.

Cryptosporidium parvum

For more details, see Chapter 8.

Parasites of the respiratory system

Cephalopina titillator

Cephalopina titillator, synonym *Cephalopsis titillator* (Phylum: Arthropoda; Class: Insecta; Order: Diptera; Family: Oestridae), commonly known as the Camel nasal bot fly, is a larval parasite found in the nasal cavities of camels over the entire range of both species: sub-Saharan Africa, Middle East, Australia and Asia.

Epidemiology: Infestation of up to 90% of camel herds has been recorded.

Pathogenesis: The larvae irritate and damage the mucosa. Camels snort, sneeze and are restless, and may even stop feeding, especially during the emergence of mature larvae from the nostrils. When large numbers of larvae are present, the animals' breathing and working capacity may be severely impaired. Unlike many oestrids, adult *Cephalopina* do not panic the animals, and large numbers are often seen resting on the head and around the nostrils.

Clinical signs and pathology: Snorting, sneezing, increased grooming, nasal discharge, bleeding from the nostrils, coughing and reduced milk production and body weight. The larval phase usually occupies about 11 months and is associated with inflammation, sometimes purulent, of the nasopharyngeal mucosa.

Diagnosis: The adult flies may be visible and recognisable on the host. The eggs are also easily identifiable on the host. Larvae present in the pharynx may be seen on direct inspection.

Treatment and control: Macrocyclic lactones, rafoxanide, trichlorphon and nitroxynil have all been reported to be effective against the larvae of *C. titillator*. The most effective means of control of this parasite is to remove the eggs from the host's coat. This requires, where possible, daily examination of the animal, paying particular attention to the area around the nostrils.

Oestrus ovis

Oestrus ovis (Phylum: Arthropoda; Class: Insecta; Order: Diptera; Family: Oestridae), commonly known as the Sheep nasal bot, is a larval parasite found in the nasal passages primarily of sheep and goats but also ibex, camels and humans.

For more details, see Chapter 9.

Dictyocaulus filaria

Dictyocaulus filaria (Phylum: Nematoda; Class: Chromadorea; Order: Rhabditida; Family: Dictyocaulidae) is distributed worldwide and is localised in the lungs of sheep, goats, camels and a few wild ruminants. *Dictyocaulus filaria* is found in the respiratory tract of camels in Africa. Severe infections cause depression, coughing, dyspnoea and loss of condition.

For more details see Chapter 9.

Dictyocaulus viviparus

Dictyocaulus viviparus, synonym *Dictyocaulus cameli* (Phylum: Nematoda; Class: Chromadorea; Order: Rhabditida; Family: Dictyocaulidae), is a parasite distributed worldwide and localised in the lungs of cattle, deer and camels.

Pathogenesis and clinical signs: As for *D. filaria*.

For more details see Chapter 8.

Echinococcus granulosus

For more details see Parasites of the liver.

Parasites of the liver

Fasciola hepatica

Fasciola hepatica (Phylum: Platyhelminthes; Class: Trematoda; Order: Plagiorchiida; Family: Fasciolidae), commonly known as the Liver fluke, is distributed worldwide, and is localised in the liver of sheep, cattle, goats, horses, deer, humans and other mammals.

For more details see Chapter 9.

Fasciola gigantica

Fasciola gigantica (Phylum: Platyhelminthes; Class: Trematoda; Order: Plagiorchiida; Family: Fasciolidae), commonly known as the Tropical large liver fluke, is localised in the liver of cattle, buffalo, sheep, goats, pigs, camels, deer and humans.

For more details see Chapter 8.

Echinococcus granulosus

Echinococcus granulosus (Phylum: Platyhelminthes; Class: Cestoda; Order: Cyclophyllidea; Family: Taeniidae) is localised in the liver and lungs of the intermediate host (domestic and wild ruminants, humans and primates, pigs and lagomorphs) and small intestine of the definitive host (dogs and many wild canids).

For more details see Chapter 9.

Parasites of the pancreas

Eurytrema pancreaticum

Eurytrema pancreaticum, synonyms *Distoma pancreaticum*, *Eurytrema ovis* (Phylum: Platyhelminthes; Class: Trematoda; Order: Plagiorchiida; Family: Dicrocoeliidae), commonly known as the Pancreatic fluke, is localised in the pancreatic ducts of cattle, buffalo, sheep, goats, pigs, camels and humans from South America, Asia and Europe. Two intermediate hosts are required for the parasite: host 1 is land snails, particularly of the genus *Bradybaena*, and host 2 is grasshoppers of the genus *Conocephalus* or tree crickets (*Oecanthus*).

Parasites of the circulatory system

Elaeophora schneideri

For more details see Chapter 9.

Dipetalonema evansi

Dipetalonema evansi, synonym *Deraiophoronema evansi* (Phylum: Nematoda; Class: Chromadorea; Order: Spirurida; Family: Onchocercidae), commonly known as Subcutaneous filaroidosis, is localised in the heart, arteries and veins, pulmonary arteries, spermatic arteries and lymph nodes of camels from North Africa, Asia, eastern Russia and Australia. This parasite has mosquitoes of the genus *Aedes* as intermediate hosts.

Epidemiology: Infection is presumably common in areas where the parasite and intermediate hosts co-exist. In the eastern former Soviet states, infection may occur in up to 80% of camels.

Clinical signs and pathology: Light infections are inapparent. Heavy infections can cause emaciation, arteriosclerosis and heart insufficiency and parasitic orchitis in the spermatic vessels. The presence of the parasites in an artery or vein leads to inflammation of the vessel wall and thrombosis may occur. Fibrosis leads to a granulomatous arteritis or phlebitis, and possible occlusion of the vessel lumen. Aneurysms may occur in the spermatic vessels.

Diagnosis: Filarial nematodes within arteries cannot be detected clinically. Identification of the microfilariae in the blood (samples ideally taken in the early evening) is aided by concentrating the parasites following lysis, filtration and then staining with methylene blue or May–Grunwald Giemsa. Alternatively, one part of blood and nine parts of formalin are centrifuged and the sediment mixed with a blue stain and examined as a microscopic smear.

Control and treatment: Mosquito control methods, such as the use of insect repellents, may limit exposure. Stibophen used prophylactically may help limit infection. Ivermectin 200 µg/kg can be used to eliminate microfilariae. Stibophen 0.5 mg/kg i.v. is effective both therapeutically and prophylactically during the periods of mosquito activity.

Schistosomes

Schistosomes are flukes found in the circulatory system. The sexes are separate, the small adult female lying permanently in a longitudinal groove, the gynaecophoric canal, in the body of the male. The genus has been divided into four groups – *haematobium*, *indicum*, *mansoni* and *japonicum* – but the genus as currently defined is paraphyletic so revisions are likely.

Haematobium group

Schistosoma bovis

Schistosoma bovis (Phylum: Platyhelminthes; Class: Trematoda; Order: Strigeidida; Family: Schistosomatidae), commonly known as the Blood fluke, causes a disease commonly known as Bilharziosis, is localised on the portal and mesenteric veins and urogenital veins of cattle, sheep, goats and camels (dromedary) and is distributed throughout Africa, Middle East, southern Asia and southern Europe. The parasite has snails as intermediate hosts (*Bulinus contortus*, *B. truncates*, *Physopsis africana*, *P. nasuta*).

Other schistosomes

Schistosoma turkestanica

Schistosoma turkestanica, synonym *Orientobilharzia turkestanicum* (Phylum: Platyhelminthes; Class: Trematoda; Order: Strigeidida; Family: Schistosomatidae), is localised in the mesenteric veins and small veins of the pancreas and liver of cattle, buffalo, sheep, goats, camels, horses, donkeys, mules and cats from Asia, Middle East and parts of Europe. This parasite has snails (*G. euphratica*) as intermediate host.

Trypanosomes

Trypanosoma brucei brucei

Trypanosoma brucei brucei (Phylum: Euglenozoa; Class: Kinetoplastea; Order: Trypanosomatida; Family: Trypanosomatidae) causes a disease commonly known as Nagana and is localised in the blood and also in extravascular sites (for example, the myocardium, CNS and reproductive tract) of cattle, horses, donkeys, zebus, sheep, goats, camels, pigs, dogs, cats and wild game species, particularly antelope, and is distributed over approximately 10 million km² of sub-Saharan Africa between latitudes 14°N and 29°S. Antelopes are the natural host species and are reservoirs of infection for domestic animals. Horses, mules and donkeys are very susceptible, and the disease is very severe in sheep, goats, camels and dogs (see respective hosts).

Treatment: The two drugs in common use in camels are diminazene aceturate and suramin. Treatment should be followed by surveillance since reinfection, followed by clinical signs and parasitaemia, may occur within a week or two.

For more details see Chapter 8.

Trypanosoma brucei evansi

Trypanosoma brucei evansi, synonyms *Trypanosoma evansi*, *Trypanosoma equinum* (Phylum: Euglenozoa; Class: Kinetoplastea; Order: Trypanosomatida; Family: Trypanosomatidae), causes a disease commonly known as El debab, Surra, Mbori, Murrina, Mal de caderas, Doukane, Dioufar or Thaga and is localised in the blood of horses, donkeys, camels, cattle, zebus, goats, pigs, dogs, water buffalo, elephants, capybaras, tapirs, mongooses, ocelots, deer and other wild animals. Many laboratory and wild animals can be infected experimentally. The parasite is distributed in North Africa, Central and South America, central and southern Russia and parts of Asia (India, Myanmar, Malaysia, southern China, Indonesia, Philippines). The original distribution of this parasite coincided with that of the camels, and is often associated with arid deserts and semi-arid steppes.

Control and treatment: Suramin or quinapyramine (Trypacide®) are the drugs of choice for treatment and also confer a short period of prophylaxis. For more prolonged protection, a modified quinapyramine known as Trypacide Pro-Salt is also available. Unfortunately, drug resistance, at least to suramin, is not uncommon. Currently in camels, isometamidium is administered intravenously because of local tissue reactions.

For more details see Chapter 10.

Trypanosoma congolense

Trypanosoma congolense (Phylum: Euglenozoa; Class: Kinetoplastea; Order: Trypanosomatida; Family: Trypanosomatidae) causes a disease commonly known as Nagana, Paranagana, Gambia fever, Ghindi or Gobial and is localised in the blood of cattle, sheep, goats, horses, camels, dogs and pigs. Reservoir hosts include antelopes, giraffes, zebras, elephants and warthogs and the parasite is widely distributed in tropical Africa between latitudes 15°N and 25°S.

Pathogenesis: With *T. congolense*, there are many strains that differ markedly in virulence. The signs caused by this species are similar to those caused by other trypanosomes, but the CNS is not affected.

Control and treatment: Isometamidium is the drug of choice but is administered intravenously because of local tissue reactions. Diminazene is contraindicated in the camels.

For more details see Chapter 8.

Trypanosoma vivax

Trypanosoma vivax (Phylum: Euglenozoa; Class: Kinetoplastea; Order: Trypanosomatida; Family: Trypanosomatidae) causes a disease commonly known as Nagana or Souma and is localised in the blood of cattle, sheep, goats, camels, horses, antelopes and giraffes. It is distributed throughout Central Africa, West Indies, Central and South America (Brazil, Venezuela, Bolivia, Colombia, Guyana, French Guiana) and Mauritius.

For more details see Chapter 8.

Rickettsiosis

Although *Rickettsia* are now considered to be in the kingdom Bacteria, for historical reasons they are included within parasitological texts and for this reason mention is made of some genera and species of importance.

Anaplasma marginale

Anaplasma marginale (Phylum: Proteobacteria; Class: Alphaproteobacteria; Order: Rickettsiales; Family: Anaplasmataceae) is localised in the blood of cattle, sheep, goats, camels and wild ruminants and is found throughout Africa, southern Europe, Australia, South America, Asia, former Soviet states and the USA.

For more details see Chapter 8.

Anaplasma centrale

Anaplasma centrale (Phylum: Proteobacteria; Class: Alphaproteobacteria; Order: Rickettsiales; Family: Anaplasmataceae) is localised in the blood of cattle and wild ruminants, and sheep may perhaps act as reservoirs of infection. It is distributed throughout Africa, southern Europe, Australia, South America, Asia, former Soviet states and the USA.

For more details see Chapter 8.

Parasites of the eye

Thelazia rhodesi

Thelazia rhodesi (Phylum: Nematoda; Class: Chromadorea; Order: Spirurida; Family: Thelaziidae), commonly known as the Cattle eyeworm, is localised in the eye, conjunctival sac and lacrimal duct of cattle, buffalo, occasionally sheep, goats and camels. The parasite has muscid flies as intermediate hosts, particularly *Fannia* spp.

For more details see Chapter 8.

Thelazia leesi

Thelazia leesi (Phylum: Nematoda; Class: Chromadorea; Order: Spirurida; Family: Thelaziidae), commonly known as the Eyeworm, is localised in the conjunctival sac of camels and is distributed throughout Africa, Asia and Russia. The parasite has muscid flies as intermediate hosts. Heavy infections may cause irritation and keratitis with epiphora.

Parasites of the nervous system

Taenia multiceps

The metacestoid form of *Taenia multiceps* (Phylum: Platyhelminthes; Class: Cestoda; Order: Cyclophyllidea; Family: Taeniidae) is *Multiceps multiceps*, synonym *Coenurus cerebralis*, which causes a disease commonly known as Gid, Sturdy, Staggers or Coenurosis. It is a parasite distributed worldwide and is localised in the brain and spinal cord of the intermediate hosts (sheep, cattle, deer, pigs, horses, camels, humans) and in the small intestine of the definitive hosts (dogs, foxes, coyotes, jackals).

For more details see Chapter 9.

Parasites of the locomotory system

Taenia ovis

Taenia ovis, synonyms *Taenia cervi*, *Taenia krabbei*, *Taenia hyenae* (Phylum: Platyhelminthes; Class: Cestoda; Order: Cyclophyllidea; Family: Taeniidae), is the adult form of the metacestoid *Cysticercus cervi* (*C. tarandi*, *C. dromedarii*, *C. camelsi*). This parasite is distributed worldwide and is localised in the small intestine of the definitive host (dogs, foxes, wild carnivores e.g. hyenas), and in the muscle of the intermediate hosts (sheep, goats, deer, reindeer and camels). Infection is usually asymptomatic.

Sarcocystis

Several species of *Sarcocystis* have been reported in camels. Further general details on nomenclature, diagnosis and epidemiology are given in Chapter 2.

Sarcocystis cameli

Sarcocystis cameli (Phylum: Apicomplexa; Class: Conoidasida; Order: Eucoccidiorida; Family: Sarcocystidae) is localised in the muscle of the intermediate hosts (camels – Bactrian and dromedary) and in the small intestine of the definitive host (dogs) and is present in North Africa (Egypt, Morocco, Sudan) and Asia.

Epidemiology: Little is known of the epidemiology but from the high prevalence of symptomless infections observed in abattoirs, it is clear that where dogs are kept in close association with camels or their feed, then transmission is likely. The parasite is widespread within its endemic range, with a high percentage of camels found to be infected at slaughter.

Clinical signs and pathology: The tissue cysts may be visible to the naked eye but are more likely to be detected on histopathology. Myocardial lesions and emaciation have both been attributed to infection.

Diagnosis: *Ante mortem* diagnosis is difficult and most cases of *Sarcocystis* infection are only revealed at *post mortem* when the grossly visible sarcocysts in the muscle are discovered.

Control and treatment: The only control measures possible are those of simple hygiene. Dogs should not be fed raw or uncooked camel meat. Treatment is not usually indicated.

Toxoplasma gondii

For more details see Chapter 11.

Parasites of the connective tissue

In camels, three species of filarial worms have been reported to cause skin nodules, 0.5–4 cm in diameter, on various parts of the body. The intermediate hosts are various species of biting flies.

ECTOPARASITES

Flies

Wohlfahrtia nuba

Wohlfahrtia nuba (Phylum: Arthropoda; Class: Insecta; Order: Diptera; Family: Sarcophagidae), commonly known as the Flesh fly, is an obligate agent of myiasis that primarily infests camels. It is found in North Africa and the Near East.

Epidemiology: *Wohlfahrtia nuba* may be an occasional secondary facultative invader of wounds, particularly of camels, in North Africa and the Middle East.

Pathogenesis: When present in an infected wound or as a secondary invader at an existing myiasis, larvae extend and deepen the lesion. The irritation and distress caused by the lesion are extremely debilitating and the host animal can rapidly lose condition. If untreated, repeated infestation may quickly lead to the death of the host within 1–2 weeks.

Clinical signs: Animals infested by flesh fly larvae may appear dull, lethargic and separate from the herd or flock. They may cease feeding and show weight loss. Wounds with foul-smelling odour will be observed on inspection.

Diagnosis: Flesh fly larvae are diagnosed by removal of the larvae and identification under a dissecting microscope.

Treatment and control: The larvae should be removed and identified and the wound thoroughly cleaned and disinfected. Organophosphate and pyrethroid insecticides are effective against newly hatched larvae, immature forms and adult flies. Larvae inside wounds must be treated with a suitable larvicide. Spraying or dipping animals with an approved insecticide and treating infested wounds can protect against new infestations for 7–10 days.

Hippobosca camelina

Hippobosca camelina (Phylum: Arthropoda; Class: Insecta; Order: Diptera; Family: Hippoboscidae), commonly known as the Camel fly, is a blood-sucking fly found on the skin of camels in sub-Saharan Africa.

Epidemiology: The adult flies are most abundant on the host during the summer months.

Pathogenesis: This species is primarily a nuisance and a cause of disturbance. There is no evidence that it plays any role in the transmission of camel trypanosomosis.

Clinical signs: The adult flies are clearly visible when feeding on the host animal. Irritation at the feeding sites may be observed.

Diagnosis: Observation of adult flies on the host animal.

Treatment and control: This is best achieved by topical application of insecticides, preferably those with some repellent and residual effect, such as the synthetic pyrethroids permethrin and deltamethrin.

Lice

Microthoracius cameli

Microthoracius cameli (Phylum: Arthropoda; Class: Insecta; Order: Psocodea; Family: Microthoraciidae), commonly known as the Camel sucking louse, is a spindle-shaped parasite (**Fig. 14.2**) found on the skin of camels worldwide, in association with its host

Epidemiology: Infection occurs after direct contact with an infested host animal. Cross-contamination between different host species is possible if the animals have physical contact.

Pathogenesis: These lice are blood feeders and heavy infestations can significantly reduce weight gain and milk production.

Clinical signs and pathology: The signs of infestation are variable. Light infestation may have no obvious effects but pruritus, dermatitis and hair loss are usually evident at heavier parasite intensities.

Diagnosis: The lice and their eggs can be seen on the skin of the host animal when the hair is parted.

Treatment and control: Macrocyclic lactones, such as moxidectin, in a repeated treatment programme of 7–10 days may be effective.

Notes: Microthoraciidae contains four species in the genus *Microthoracius*; three species parasitise llamas. The fourth species, *M. cameli*, is parasitic on camels. The closely related *M. mazzai* is an economically important parasite of alpacas (see host section in this chapter).

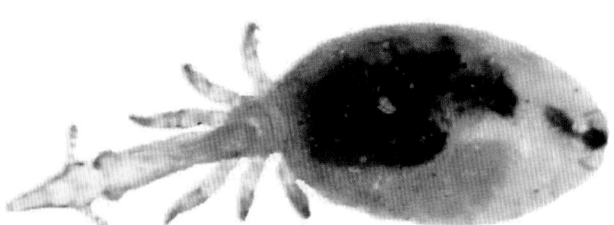

Fig. 14.2 *Microthoracius* spp.

Ticks

Ornithodoros savignyi

Ornithodoros savignyi (Phylum: Arthropoda; Class: Arachnida; Order: Ixodida; Family: Argasidae), commonly known as the Sand tampan, will feed on most mammals but particularly on camels and poultry. It is found throughout Africa, India and the Middle East.

Pathogenesis: Toxicosis may occur in response to the tick saliva, characterised by cutaneous oedema, haemorrhage, rapidly progressing weakness and prostration. Toxicosis can suppress the host's immune system, allowing the reactivation of chronic infections. Such toxicosis with *O. savignyi* occurs in young calves and lambs, especially when there are large tick populations and multiple bites.

Hyalomma dromedarii

Hyalomma dromedarii (Phylum: Arthropoda; Class: Arachnida; Order: Ixodida; Family: Ixodidae), commonly known as the Camel tick, is of veterinary significance primarily in camels, but may also be of importance in ruminants and horses. It is found from India to Africa.

Epidemiology: This is predominantly a two-host species of tick.

Pathogenesis: Tick bites may cause damage at the site of attachment, which may predispose to secondary bacterial infection. This genus is mainly responsible for tick toxicosis in parts of Africa and the Indian subcontinent. The 'toxin' produced by the adult tick causes a sweating sickness in ruminants and pigs characterised by widespread hyperaemia of the mucous membranes and a profuse moist eczema.

Clinical signs and pathology: There are no obvious signs of tick infestation other than the presence of the parasites and the local skin reactions to their bites. Small granulomatous reactions may form at the site of tick bites, consisting of a mixed inflammatory cell response with fibrosis.

Diagnosis: The adult ticks, particularly the engorged females, are easily seen on the skin. The main predilection sites are the face, ears, axilla and inguinal region.

Notes: In some circumstances, a variable life cycle has been reported for *H. dromedarii*, with a three-host life cycle observed on sheep or cattle. It appears that the type of host, rearing conditions, density and age of the larvae may influence the life cycle adopted by this species.

Mites

Sarcoptes scabiei

Sarcoptes scabiei subspecies *cameli* (Phylum: Arthropoda; Class: Arachnida; Subclass: Acari; Order: Astigmata (Sarcoptiformes); Family: Sarcoptidae) is a burrowing mite that causes mange in camels in Africa and Asia.

Epidemiology: New hosts are infected by contact with infected individuals, presumably by the transfer of larvae, which are commonly present more superficially on the skin surface. Transmission occurs between mature animals and also from mother to offspring at birth.

Pathogenesis and clinical signs: Host reaction starts on the head, neck, mammary glands, prepuce and flanks. The first lesions appear as erythema and papules and cause intense pruritus with hair loss, which becomes reddened and moist. The lesions may become generalised with hyperkeratosis on the neck and legs, with intense pruritus leading to loss of appetite, weight loss and emaciation.

Treatment and control: Spray treatments of lindane or organophosphates repeated after 1–2 weeks and ivermectin given twice at two-week intervals have been reported to be effective. It is important to treat the whole herd and new introductions.

Notes: Sarcoptic mange is one of the most important diseases of camels and can also be transmitted to humans.

Chorioptes bovis

Chorioptes bovis, synonyms *Chorioptes ovis*, *Chorioptes equi*, *Chorioptes caprae*, *Chorioptes cuniculi* (Phylum: Arthropoda; Class: Arachnida; Subclass: Acari; Order: Astigmata (Sarcoptiformes); Family: Psoroptidae), is a non-burrowing mite found on the skin, particularly the legs, feet, base of tail and upper rear surface of the udder of cattle, sheep, horses, goats, camels, llamas and rabbits. It has been reported in dromedary camels in zoos.

For more details see Chapter 8.

LLAMAS, ALPACAS, GUANACOS, VICUÑAS

Several species of parasites are unique to camelids, for example coccidia and lice. However, there are a number of parasites for which camelids are an alternative or aberrant host. Parasites unique to these hosts are covered in detail in this chapter; others which are parasites of cattle or sheep will be mentioned or briefly described, and are covered in greater detail under their respective host chapters.

ENDOPARASITES

Parasites of the digestive system

Gongylonema pulchrum

Gongylonema pulchrum (Phylum: Nematoda; Class: Chromadorea; Order: Spirurida; Family: Gongylonematidae), commonly known as the Gullet worm, is distributed worldwide and is localised in the oesophagus and rumen of sheep, goats, cattle, buffalo, deer and camels, and the oesophagus of donkeys, pigs, horses, humans and primates. This parasite has coprophagous beetles and cockroaches as intermediate hosts.

For more details see section on Deer, and Chapter 9.

Abomasum

The following nematode species have been reported in the abomasum of camelids in their country of origin, Peru. Their pathogenicities are unknown.

Camelostrongylus mentulatus

Camelostrongylus mentulatus (Phylum: Nematoda; Class: Chromadorea; Order: Rhabditida; Family: Trichostrongylidae) is localised in the abomasum and small intestine of camels, llamas, sheep and goats, and is distributed in the Middle East, Australia and South America. Generally of low pathogenicity, it is considered of little importance. Heavy infections can produce gastric hyperplasia and increase in abomasal pH, similar to that seen in *Ostertagia* spp. infection.

Additionally, several cattle and sheep nematode species have been reported in farmed camelids (Table 14.12).

Small intestine

Intestinal species reported in camelids are generally of little clinical significance. Many of the species listed are parasites of cattle or sheep and are described in more detail under the chapters for these hosts.

Lamanema chavezi

Lamanema chavezi (Phylum: Nematoda; Class: Chromadorea; Order: Rhabditida; Family: Molineidae) is localised in the small intestine, with immature stages in the liver and lungs of alpacas and vicuñas in South America.

Clinical signs and pathology: Large infections can cause respiratory and hepatic failure. The penetration and migration of larvae through the wall of the intestine can cause catarrhal haemorrhagic enteritis with localised necrosis. Areas of congestion may be present in the lungs with petechial haemorrhages and necrosis in the hepatic tissue. These liver lesions can calcify following remigration of larvae to the intestine.

Nematodirus lamae

Nematodirus lamae (Phylum: Nematoda; Class: Chromadorea; Order: Rhabditida; Family: Molineidae) is localised in the small intestine of alpacas, llamas and vicuñas in South America.

Table 14.13 lists parasites of cattle or sheep which have been reported in the small intestine of camelids.

Cryptosporidium parvum

For more details see Chapter 8.

Giardia intestinalis

Giardia intestinalis, synonyms *Giardia duodenalis*, *Giardia lamblia*, *Lamblia lamblia* (Phylum: Metamonada; Class: Trepomonadea; Order: Diplomonadida; Family: Giardiidae), is distributed worldwide and is localised in the small intestine of humans, cattle, sheep, goats, pigs, horses, alpacas, dogs, cats, guinea pigs and chinchillas.

Table 14.12 Cattle and sheep parasites found in the abomasa of camelids.

Species	(Super)family	Hosts	Geographical distribution
Teladorsagia circumcincta	Trichostrongyloidea	Cattle, sheep, goats, deer, camels, llamas	Worldwide
Ostertagia leptospicularis	Trichostrongyloidea	Deer (roe deer), cattle, sheep, goats, camels	Many parts of the world, particularly Europe and New Zealand
Haemonchus contortus	Trichostrongyloidea	Sheep, goats, cattle, deer, camels, llamas	Worldwide
Marshallagia marshalli	Trichostrongyloidea	Sheep, goats and wild small ruminants	Tropics and subtropics including southern Europe, USA, South America, India and Russia
Trichostrongylus axei	Trichostrongyloidea	Cattle, sheep, goats, deer, horses, donkeys, pigs and occasionally humans	Worldwide

Table 14.13 Cattle and sheep parasites found in the small intestine of camelids.

Species	(Super)family	Hosts	Geographical distribution
Nematodes			
Trichostrongylus vitrinus	Trichostrongyloidea	Sheep, goats, deer, llamas and occasionally pigs and humans	Worldwide
Trichostrongylus colubriformis	Trichostrongyloidea	Sheep, goats, deer, llamas and occasionally pigs and humans	Worldwide
Trichostrongylus longispicularus	Trichostrongyloidea	Cattle, sheep, goats, deer, camels, llamas	Australia, America and parts of Europe
Nematodirus helvetianus	Trichostrongyloidea	Cattle, occasionally sheep, goats and other ruminants	Worldwide
Nematodirus battus	Trichostrongyloidea	Sheep, goats, camelids, occasionally cattle	UK, Norway, Sweden, Netherlands, Canada
Cooperia surnabada (syn. *Cooperia mcmasteri*)	Trichostrongyloidea	Cattle, sheep, camels	Parts of Europe, North America and Australia
Bunostomum trigonocephalum	Ancylostomatoidea	Sheep, goats, camels	Worldwide
Strongyloides papillosus	Strongyloidoidea	Sheep, cattle, other ruminants and rabbits	Worldwide
Cestodes			
Moniezia expansa	Anoplocephalidae	Sheep, goats, occasionally cattleIntermediate hosts: forage mites	Worldwide

Table 14.14 Cattle and sheep parasites found in the large intestine of camelids.

Species	(Super)family	Hosts	Geographical distribution
Oesophagostomum venulosum	Strongyloidea	Sheep, goats, deer, camels	Worldwide
Oesophagostomum columbianum	Strongyloidea	Sheep, goats, deer, camels	Worldwide; more important in tropical and subtropical areas
Chabertia ovina	Strongyloidea	Sheep, goats occasionally deer, cattle and other ruminants	Worldwide but more prevalent in temperate regions
Trichuris ovis	Trichuroidea	Sheep, goats, occasionally cattle and other ruminants	Worldwide
Skrjabinema ovis	Oxyuroidea	Sheep, goats, guanacos	Worldwide

Clinical signs and pathogenesis: Infections in alpacas are considered non-pathogenic.

For more details see Chapter 8.

Large intestine

See Table 14.14 for cattle and sheep parasites found in the large intestine of camelids.

Parasites of the respiratory system

Cephenemyia spp.

Cephenemyia spp. (Phylum: Arthropoda; Class: Insecta; Order: Diptera; Family: Oestridae), commonly known as Deer nasopharyngeal bots or Throat bots, are larval parasites found in the nasopharynx of llamas.

Clinical signs: As the llama is an aberrant host, the signs of infection can be more marked and a granulomatous swelling may occur in the nasal cavity and nasopharynx, with coughing and sneezing. Breathing can become impaired.

For more details see section on Deer.

Dictyocaulus filaria

Dictyocaulus filaria (Phylum: Nematoda; Class: Chromadorea; Order: Rhabditida; Family: Dictyocaulidae) is distributed worldwide and is localised in lungs of sheep, goats, camelids and a few wild ruminants. *Dictyocaulus filaria* is found in the respiratory tract of camelids in many areas of the world. Severe infections cause depression, coughing, dyspnoea and loss of condition. Benzimidazoles, levamisole and avermectins are all reported to be effective against this species in camels.

For more details of these species see Chapter 9.

Dictyocaulus viviparus

Dictyocaulus viviparus, synonym *Dictyocaulus cameli* (Phylum: Nematoda; Class: Chromadorea; Order: Rhabditida; Family: Dictyocaulidae), is distributed worldwide and is localised in the lungs of cattle, deer, camels or camelids. It is similar to *D. filaria*.

For more details see Chapter 8.

Parasites of the liver

Fasciola hepatica

Fasciola hepatica (Phylum: Platyhelminthes; Class: Trematoda; Order: Plagiorchiida; Family: Fasciolidae) is commonly known as the Liver fluke and is localised in the liver of sheep, cattle, goats, horses, deer, humans and other mammals.

For more details see Chapter 9.

Fasciola gigantica

Fasciola gigantica (Phylum: Platyhelminthes; Class: Trematoda; Order: Plagiorchiida; Family: Fasciolidae) is commonly known as the Tropical large liver fluke and is localised in the liver of cattle, buffalo, sheep, goats, pigs, camels, deer and humans.

For more details see Chapter 8.

Dicrocoelium dendriticum

Dicrocoelium dentriticum, synonym *Dicrocoelium lanceolatum* (Phylum: Platyhelminthes; Class: Trematoda; Order: Plagiorchiida; Family: Dicrocoeliidae), is distributed worldwide (except for South Africa and Australia) and is localised in the liver of sheep, goats, cattle, deer, llamas and rabbits, and occasionally horses and pigs.

For more details see Chapter 9.

Echinococcus granulosus

Echinococcus granulosus (Phylum: Platyhelminthes; Class: Cestoda; Order: Cyclophyllidea; Family: Taeniidae), commonly known as the Dwarf dog tapeworm, is the causative agent of hydatidosis. It is distributed worldwide and is localised mainly in the liver and lungs in the intermediate hosts (domestic and wild ruminants, deer, humans, primates, pigs and lagomorphs; horses and donkeys are resistant) and small intestine in the definitive host (dogs and many wild canids).

For more details see Chapter 9.

Parasites of the nervous system

Parelaphostrongylus tenuis

Parelaphostrongylus tenuis, synonym *Odocoileostrongylus tenuis*, *Elaphostrongylus tenuis* (Phylum: Nematoda; Class: Chromadorea;

Order: Rhabditida; Family: Protostrongylidae) causes a disease commonly known as Cerebrospinal nematodosis, Meningeal worm, Moose sickness or Moose disease, and is localised in the veins and venous sinuses of cranial meninges and CNS of white-tailed deer, moose, wapitis, other deer species, llamas, guanacos, alpacas and camels. It has been reported rarely in sheep and goats from North America. The parasite has snails and slugs are intermediate hosts.

Clinical signs and pathogenesis: Clinical signs include ataxia, circling, lameness, paraplegia, hypermetria and blindness. The parasite is well adapted to its normal definitive host but in an aberrant host such as the llama, migration of the larvae in the spinal cord can cause neurological symptoms which relate to their exact location.

Control: Management procedures such as fencing to protect farmed camelids from white-tailed deer can be effective. Where applicable, a molluscicide may be used to reduce the numbers of snails and slugs.

For more details see section on Deer.

Parasites of the reproductive/ urogenital system

No parasites of veterinary significance reported.

Parasites of the locomotory system

Toxoplasma gondii

See section on Camels.

Sarcocystiosis

Several species of *Sarcocystis* have been reported in camelids (Table 14.15). Specific descriptions are outwith the scope of this book. Further general details on nomenclature, diagnosis and epidemiology are given in Chapter 2.

ECTOPARASITES

Microthoracius mazzai

Microthoracius mazzi (Phylum: Arthropoda; Class: Insecta; Order: Psocodea; Family: Microthoraciidae) commonly known as the

llama louse, is a spindle-shaped parasite found on the skin of alpacas and llamas worldwide, in association with its host.

Epidemiology: Infection usually occurs after direct contact with an infested host animal. Cross-contamination between different host species is possible if the animals have physical contact. Transfer may occur from a contaminated environment or grooming equipment as the lice can survive for short periods off the host.

Pathogenesis: These lice are blood feeders and heavy infestations can significantly reduce weightgain and milk production.

Clinical signs: The signs of infestation are variable. Light infestation may have no obvious effects but pruritus, dermatitis and hair loss are usually evident at heavier parasite loads. Anaemia may be seen in young animals with heavy infestations.

Diagnosis: The lice can be seen in the hair of the host animal when the hair is parted. The eggs (nits) may be seen glued to hair shafts.

Treatment and control: Dips, dusts and sprays containing coumaphos, malathion or permethrin may be effective, particularly if applied after shearing. Macrocyclic lactones, such as ivermectin, doramectin and moxidectin, given in a repeated treatment programme of 7–10 days may also be highly effective.

Psoroptes ovis

Psoroptes ovis, synonyms *Psoroptes communis* var. *ovis*, *Psoroptes cuniculi*, *Psoroptes cervinus*, *Psoroptes bovis*, *Psoroptes equi*, *Psoroptes aucheniae* (Phylum: Arthropoda; Class: Arachnida; Subclass: Acari; Order: Astigmata (Sarcoptiformes); Family: Psoroptidae), are non-burrowing mange mites found on the skin of sheep, cattle, goat, horses, rabbits and camelids. They are found worldwide, particularly in Europe and South America

For more details see Chapter 9.

Chorioptes bovis

Chorioptes bovis, synonyms *Chorioptes ovis*, *Chorioptes equi*, *Chorioptes caprae*, *Chorioptes cuniculi* (Phylum: Arthropoda; Class: Arachnida; Subclass: Acari; Order: Astigmata (Sarcoptiformes); Family: Psoroptidae), is a non-burrowing mite found on the skin, particularly on the legs, feet, base of tail and upper rear surface of the udder of cattle, sheep, horses, goats, camels, llamas and rabbits.

For more details see Chapter 8.

Sarcoptes scabiei

Sarcoptes scabiei (Phylum: Arthropoda; Class: Arachnida; Subclass: Acari; Order: Astigmata (Sarcoptiformes); Family: Sarcoptidae) is a burrowing mite found on the skin of llamas, guanacos, alpacas, and vicuñas.

For more details see Chapters 3 and 11.

A number of non-obligate ectoparasites are found on camelids and these are listed in the host–parasite checklists at the end of this chapter.

Table 14.15 *Sarcocystis* species found in camelids.

Species	Camelid host(s)	Final host	Distribution
Sarcocystis aucheniae (syn. *Sarcocystis tiopodi*, *Sarcocystis guanicocanis*)	Llamas, guanacos, alpacas	Dogs	South America
Sarcocystis lamacenis	Llamas	Unknown	South America

Table 14.16 Rumen flukes found in buffalo.

Species	Hosts	Site	Intermediate hosts
Paramphistomatidae			
Paramphistomum cervi (syn. Paramphistomum explanatum)	Cattle, sheep, goats, deer, buffalo, antelopes	Rumen	Freshwater snails (Bulinus spp., Planorbis spp.)
Paramphistomum microbothrium	Cattle, sheep, goats, deer, buffalo, antelopes	Rumen	Freshwater snails (Fossaria spp., Bulinus spp.)
Cotylophoron cotylophorum (syn. Paramphistomum cotylophorum)	Sheep, goats, cattle and wild ruminants	Rumen, reticulum	Freshwater snails (Bulinus spp.)
Calicophoron calicophorum (syn. Paramphistomum calicophorum)	Cattle, sheep, other ruminants	Rumen, reticulum	Water snails
Carmyerius gregarious	Cattle, buffaloes	Rumen	Water snails
Gastrothylacidae			
Gastrothylax crumenifer	Cattle, buffalo, zebu, sheep and other ruminants	Rumen, reticulum	Freshwater snails
Fischoederius elongates	Cattle, buffalo, zebu, sheep and other ruminants; rarely humans	Rumen, duodenum	Freshwater snails
Fischoederius cobboldi	Cattle, buffalo, zebu, sheep and other ruminants	Rumen, duodenum	Freshwater snails

WATER BUFFALO

The water buffalo, or domestic Asian water buffalo (*Bubalus bubalis*), is a large buffalo found on the Indian subcontinent. Buffalo breeds and populations have been established in countries throughout Europe, the Middle East, Asia, North and South America, China and Australia.

ENDOPARASITES

Parasites of the digestive system

Gongylonema pulchrum

Gongylonema pulchrum, synonym *Gongylonema scutatum* (Phylum: Nematoda; Class: Chromadorea; Order: Rhabditida; Family: Gongylonematidae), commonly known as the Gullet worm, is distributed worldwide and is localised in the oesophagus and rumen of sheep, goats, cattle, buffalo, deer, horses and camels, and the oesophagus of donkeys pigs, humans and primates. This parasite has coprophagous beetles and cockroaches as intermediate hosts.

For more details, see section on Deer, and Chapter 9.

Rumen and reticulum

Several species of rumen fluke belonging to genera of the families Paramphistomatidae and Gastrothylacidae are found in buffalo and are summarised in Table 14.16. For more details on these rumen fluke species refer to Chapters 1, 8 and 9.

Abomasum

Mecistocirrus digitatus

Mecistocirrus digitatus (Phylum: Nematoda; Class: Chromadorea; Order: Rhabditida; Family: Trichostrongylidae) is localised in the

Table 14.17 Cattle parasites found in the abomasum of water buffalo.

Species	(Super)family	Hosts	Geographical distribution
Ostertagia ostertagi	Trichostrongyloidea	Cattle, deer and occasionally goats	Worldwide
Haemonchus contortus	Trichostrongyloidea	Sheep, goats, cattle, deer, camels, llamas	Worldwide
Trichostrongylus axei	Trichostrongyloidea	Cattle, sheep, goats, deer, horses, donkeys, pigs and occasionally humans	Worldwide

abomasum of cattle, buffalo, zebus, sheep and goats, occasionally the stomach of pigs and rarely humans. The parasite is distributed in tropical and subtropical regions, particularly Central America and parts of Asia.

The nematode species listed in Table 14.17 have been reported in the abomasum of water buffalo in various countries in which they are found. Their pathogenicities are unknown.

Intestines

Toxocara vitulorum

Toxocara vitulorum, synonym *Neoascaris vitulorum* (Phylum: Nematoda; Class: Chromadorea; Order: Ascaridida; Family: Ascarididae), is localised in the small intestine of cattle, buffalo and zebus, rarely sheep and goats, and is distributed in Africa, India and Asia.

Epidemiology: Infection is highly prevalent in water buffalo calves between two weeks and three months of age and can be responsible for high morbidity and mortality rates in calves, resulting in serious economic losses. Infection can be transmitted by the transplacental and transmammary routes. Peak egg output occurs between 30 and 45 days post infection. Following peak infection around four months of age, the onset of immunity results in a rapid decline in faecal egg output.

Table 14.18 Cattle parasites found in the intestines of water buffalo.

Species	(Super)family	Hosts	Geographical distribution
Small intestine			
Trichostrongylus longispicularis	Trichostrongyloidea	Cattle, sheep, goats, deer, camels, llamas	Ruminants in Australia, cattle in America and parts of Europe
Nematodirus helvetianus	Trichostrongyloidea	Cattle, occasionally sheep, goats and other ruminants	Worldwide
Cooperia oncophora	Trichostrongyloidea	Cattle, sheep, goats, deer	Worldwide
Bunostomum phlebotomum	Ancylostomatoidea		Worldwide
Agriostomum vryburgi	Strongyloidea	Cattle, buffalo, oxen and zebu	
Strongyloides papillosus	Strongyloidoidea	Sheep, cattle, other ruminants, rabbits	Worldwide
Capillaria bovis	Trichuroidea	Cattle, sheep, goats	Worldwide
Moniezia benedeni	Anoplocephalidae	Cattle, buffalo	Worldwide
Avitellina centripunctata	Anoplocephalidae	Sheep and other ruminants	Europe, Africa and Asia
Large intestine			
Oesophagostomum radiatum	Strongyloidea	Cattle, buffalo	Worldwide
Trichuris discolor	Trichuroidea	Cattle, buffalo, occasionally sheep, goats	Europe, Asia, USA

Table 14.19 Cattle coccidia reported in the intestines of water buffalo.

Species	Site	Distribution
Eimeria alabamensis	Small and large intestine	Presumed worldwide, mainly Europe
Eimeria auburnensis	Small intestine	Worldwide
Eimeria bovis	Small and large intestine	Worldwide
Eimeria brasiliensis	Unknown	Worldwide
Eimeria bukidnonensis	Small and large intestine	Worldwide
Eimeria canadensis	Unknown	Worldwide
Eimeria cylindrical	Unknown	Worldwide
Eimeria ellipsoidalis	Small intestine	Worldwide
Eimeria subspherica	Unknown	Worldwide
Eimeria wyomingensis	Unknown	Worldwide
Eimeria zuernii	Small and large intestine	Worldwide

Clinical signs: The presence of adult worms in the small intestine of young calves results in growth reduction and diarrhoea.

Control and treatment: Adult worms are sensitive to a wide range of anthelmintics and young calves should be treated at 3–6 weeks of age.

A number of intestinal helminths of cattle have been reported in water buffaloes (Table 14.18). These parasites are described in more detail in Chapter 8.

Several species of *Eimeria* have been described and appear specific to water buffalo. In addition, species found in cattle have also been reported in water buffalo but their significance is not known (Table 14.19).

Cryptosporidium parvum

Cryptosporidium parvum (Phylum: Apicomplexa; Class: Conoidasida; Order: Cryptogregarinorida; Family: Cryptosporidiidae) is distributed worldwide and is localised in the small intestine of cattle, sheep, goats, horses, deer and humans. *Cryptosporidium* oocysts have been found in buffalo faeces from all countries where they are bred.

Parasites of the respiratory system

Mammomonogamus laryngeus

Mammomonogamus laryngeus, synonym *Syngamus laryngeus* (Phylum: Nematoda; Class: Chromadorea; Order: Rhabditida; Family: Syngamidae), commonly known as the Gapeworm, is localised in the larynx of cattle, buffalo, goats, sheep, deer and rarely humans. It is distributed in Asia, Central Africa, South America and Caribbean islands. Infections are usually asymptomatic.

Dictyocaulus viviparus

Dictyocaulus viviparus (Phylum: Nematoda; Class: Chromadorea; Order: Rhabditida; Family: Dictyocaulidae) is distributed worldwide, but is especially important in temperate climates with a high rainfall. This parasite is localised in the bronchi and trachea of cattle, buffalo, deer (red deer) and camels.

Parasites of the liver

Fasciola gigantica

Fasciola gigantica (Phylum: Platyhelminthes; Class: Trematoda; Order: Plagiorchiida; Family: Fasciolidae), commonly known as the Tropical large liver fluke, is localised in the liver of cattle, buffalo, sheep, goats, pigs, camels, deer and humans, and distributed in Africa, Asia, Europe and the USA. The intermediate hosts are snails of the genus *Galba*; in southern Europe it is *Galba auricularia*, which is also the important species in the southern USA, the Middle East and the Pacific Islands.

Epidemiology: Infection can have a huge economic impact as water buffalo are the main beasts of labour in rice fields in some countries, and important for meat and milk production. In India and Pakistan, young calves acquire infection during early winter and suffer an acute condition leading to death.

Clinical signs: Fluke infections in buffalo are usually chronic, leading to weight loss and poor performance.

Diagnosis: Diagnosis is based on clinical signs or the presence of eggs in faeces.

Fasciola hepatica

Fasciola hepatica (Phylum: Platyhelminthes; Class: Trematoda; Order: Plagiorchiida; Family: Fasciolidae), commonly known as the Liver fluke, is distributed worldwide and is localised in the liver of sheep, cattle, goats, horses, deer, humans and other mammals. The parasite has snails of the genus *Galba* as intermediate hosts.

Gigantocotyle explanatum

Gigantocotyle explanatum, synonyms *Explanatum explanatum*, *Paramphistomum explanatum* (Phylum: Platyhelminthes; Class: Trematoda; Order: Plagiorchiida; Family: Paramphistomatidae), is localised in the liver, intrahepatic ductules, bile ducts, gallbladder and duodenum of cattle, buffalo and other ruminants and is distributed in the Indian subcontinent, Southeast Asia, tropical and subtropical regions of the Middle East and Africa. The parasite has snails as intermediate hosts.

Clinical signs and pathology: Infection may cause general wasting of body condition, diarrhoea and loss of weight. Large numbers of immature flukes can cause amphistomosis with enteritis which in some cases, particularly in young buffalo, can be fatal to the host. The flukes can cause connective tissue proliferation and haemorrhages at the site of attachment. There is extensive fibrosis and hyperplasia of the bile ducts and multifocal granulomatous nodules occur over their luminal surface.

Echinococcus granulosus

Echinococcus granulosus (Phylum: Platyhelminthes; Class: Cestoda; Order: Cyclophyllidea; Family: Taeniidae), commonly known as the Dwarf dog tapeworm, the causative agent of hydatidosis, is distributed worldwide and is localised mainly in the liver and lungs in the intermediate hosts (domestic and wild ruminants, deer, humans and primates, pigs and lagomorphs; horses and donkeys are resistant) and small intestine in the definitive hosts (dogs and many wild canids).

Parasites of the pancreas

Eurytrema pancreaticum

Eurytrema pancreaticum, synonyms *Distoma pancreaticum*, *Eurytrema ovis* (Phylum: Platyhelminthes; Class: Trematoda; Order: Plagiorchiida; Family: Dicrocoeliidae), commonly known as the Pancreatic fluke, is localised in the pancreatic ducts of cattle, buffalo, sheep, goats, pigs, camels and humans from South America, Asia and Europe. Two intermediate hosts are required for the parasite, a land snail (host 1), particularly of the genus *Bradybaena*, and grasshoppers (host 2) of the genus *Conocephalus*, or tree crickets

(*Oecanthus*). Buffalo are commonly infected with pancreatic fluke in Southeast Asia and Brazil. Infections cause little effect on the host although general weight loss may occur in heavy infections.

Parasites of the circulatory system

Elaeophora poeli

Elaeophora poeli (Phylum: Nematoda; Class: Chromadorea; Order: Spirurida; Family: Onchocercidae) causes a disease commonly known as Large aortic filariasis, is localised in the blood vessels of cattle, buffalo, zebus and is distributed in parts of Africa, Asia and the Far East. It is possible that tabanid flies represent the intermediate host.

Schistosomes

Indicum group

Schistosoma nasale

Schistosoma nasale, synonym *Schistosoma nasalis* (Phylum: Platyhelminthes; Class: Trematoda; Order: Strigeidida; Family: Schistosomatidae), is localised in the veins of nasal mucosa of cattle, goats, sheep, buffalo and horses. This parasite is distributed in India, Pakistan and Southeast Asia. It has snails (*Galba luteola*, *G. acuminata*, *Indoplanorbis exustus*) as intermediate hosts.

For other *Schistosoma* spp. of the *Indicum* group, see Chapter 8.

Other schistosomes

Schistosoma turkestanica

Schistosoma turkestanica, synonym *Orientobilharzia turkestanicum* (Phylum: Platyhelminthes; Class: Trematoda; Order: Strigeidida; Family: Schistosomatidae), is localised in the mesenteric veins and small veins of the pancreas and liver of cattle, buffalo, sheep, goats, camels, horses, donkeys, mules and cats. This parasite is distributed in Asia, Middle East and parts of Europe. The parasite has snails (*Galba euphratica*) as intermediate hosts.

Description: Small species, the male measuring around 4.2–8 mm and the female 3.4–8 mm in length. The spirally coiled ovary is positioned in the anterior part of the body. In the male there are around 70–80 testes. The female uterus is short and contains only one egg at a time, which measures 72–77 by 16–26 μm with a terminal spine and a short appendage at the opposite end.

Trypanosomes

Trypanosoma evansi

Trypanosoma evansi, synonym *Trypanosoma equinum* (Phylum: Euglenozoa; Class: Kinetoplastea; Order: Trypanosomatida; Family: Trypanosomatidae), causes a disease commonly known as El debab,

Surra, Mbori, Murrina, Mal de caderas, Doukane, Dioufar or Thaga, and is localised in the blood of horses, donkeys, camels, cattle, zebus, goats, pigs, dogs, water buffalo, elephants, capybaras, tapirs, mongooses, ocelots, deer and other wild animals. Many laboratory and wild animals can be infected experimentally. The parasite is distributed in North Africa, Central and South America, central and southern Russia, and parts of Asia (e.g. India, Myanmar, Malaysia, southern China, Indonesia, Philippines).

Epidemiology: Surra is widely prevalent on the Indian subcontinent and parts of Southeast Asia. Buffalo can be considered reservoir hosts, although clinical signs may manifest if animals are stressed or through the presence of intercurrent diseases. Infection is also widespread in North Africa and South America.

Pathogenesis: Surra is a chronic infection in water buffalo, characterised by weight loss, infertility and abortion. There is also enlargement of the lymph nodes, mucous discharge from the eyes, emaciation, hindlimb weakness and recumbency.

Control and treatment: The drug of choice in buffalo is 10% quinapyrimine sulfate 5 mg/kg subcutaneously.

For more details see Chapter 10.

Trypanosoma theileri

Trypanosoma theileri (Phylum: Euglenozoa; Class: Kinetoplastea; Order: Trypanosomatida; Family: Trypanosomatidae) is distributed worldwide and is localised in the blood of cattle and buffalo. The parasite has tabanid flies as intermediate host. Infections are usually asymptomatic.

Babesiosis

Babesia bovis

Babesia bovis, synonym *Babesia argentina* (Phylum: Apicomplexa; Class: Aconoidasida; Order: Piroplasmida; Family: Babesiidae), is localised in the blood of cattle, buffalo and deer (roe deer, red deer) and is distributed in Australia, Africa, Central and South America, Asia and southern Europe.

Babesia bigemina

Babesia bigemina (Phylum: Apicomplexa; Class: Aconoidasida; Order: Piroplasmida; Family: Babesiidae) causes a disease commonly known as Texas fever and is localised in the blood of cattle and buffalo. It is endemic in Australia, Africa, North, Central and South America, Asia and southern Europe.

For more details on these species see Chapter 8.

Babesia orientalis

Babesia orientalis (Phylum: Apicomplexa; Class: Aconoidasida; Order: Piroplasmida; Family: Babesiidae) causes a disease commonly known as Buffalo babesiosis and is localised in the blood of buffalo, typically in China. The parasite is found in water buffalo

only, and is transmitted by *Rhipicephalus haemaphysaloides* ticks. Infection is characterised by fever, icterus, haemoglobinuria and high mortality.

Theileriosis

Theileria parva

Theileria parva (Phylum: Apicomplexa; Class: Aconoidasida; Order: Piroplasmida; Family: Theileriidae) causes a disease commonly known as East Coast fever or Corridor fever. It is localised in the blood and lymphatics of cattle and buffalo, distributed in East and Central Africa.

Epidemiology: Occurs in some regions of Africa where cattle and buffalo share the same pasture. Infection is transmitted by the tick *Rhipicephalus appendiculatus*. *Theileria parva lawrencei* is transmitted from the African buffalo and becomes indistinguishable in its behaviour from *Theileria parva parva* following several passages in cattle.

Theileria annulata

Theileria annulata (Phylum: Apicomplexa; Class: Aconoidasida; Order: Piroplasmida; Family: Theileriidae) causes a disease commonly known as Mediterranean theileriosis or Mediterranean Coast fever. The protozon is localised in the blood and lymphatics of cattle and domestic buffalo and is distributed in Mediterranean countries (Portugal and Spain, Balkans), the Middle East, Indian subcontinent and China.

Theileria orientalis complex

Theileria orientalis complex, synonyms *Theileria mutans*, *Theileria buffeli*, *Theileria sergenti* (Phylum: Apicomplexa; Class: Aconoidasida; Order: Piroplasmida; Family: Theileriidae), causes a disease commonly known as Benign theileriosis. The protozon is localised in the blood of cattle and buffalo and is distributed in southern Europe, Middle East, Asia and Australia.

For more details on *Theileria* species see Chapter 8.

Ehrlichia ruminantium

Ehrlichia ruminantium, synonym *Cowdria ruminantium* (Phylum: Proteobacteria; Class: Alphaproteobacteria; Order: Rickettsiales; Family: Anaplasmataceae), is localised in the blood of cattle, sheep, goats, buffalo and wild ruminants and is distributed throughout Africa south of the Sahara and the Caribbean (Guadeloupe, Marie-Galante and Antigua).

Parasites of the nervous system

Thelazia rhodesi

For more details see Chapter 8.

Parasites of the reproductive/urogenital system

No parasites of veterinary significance reported.

Parasites of the locomotory system

There is uncertainty as to the number of distinct *Sarcocystis* species that occur in water buffalo because studies have shown that some species are capable of developing in more than one intermediate host. Morphological similarities have been reported for *Sarcocystis sinensis* found in buffalo and *S. hominis* in cattle, and it appears that cattle and water buffalo can each serve as a competent intermediate host for each species.

Parasites of the connective tissue

Parafilaria bovicola

Parafilaria bovicola (Phylum: Nematoda; Class: Chromadorea; Order: Spirurida; Family: Filariidae) is transmitted by muscid flies (*Musca autumnalis* in Europe), which are the intermediate hosts. Infection by this nematode causes the formation of verminous nodules localised in the subcutaneous and intermuscular connective tissue of cattle and buffalo and is distributed in Africa, Asia, southern Europe and Sweden.

Setaria labiato-papillosa

Setaria labiato-papillosa, synonym *Setaria cervi* (Phylum: Nematoda; Class: Chromadorea; Order: Spirurida; Family: Onchocercidae), commonly known as Bovine abdominal filariasis, is distributed worldwide and is localised in the peritoneum and pleural cavity of cattle, buffalo, bisons, yaks and various deer and antelopes, and rarely sheep. The parasite has mosquitoes (*Aedes, Culex*) as intermediate hosts.

ECTOPARASITES

Haematopinus tuberculatus

Haematopinus tuberculatus (Phylum: Arthropoda; Class: Insecta; Order: Psocodea; Suborder: Anoplura; Family: Haematopinidae), commonly known as the Buffalo louse, is found on the skin. It is originally a parasite of buffalo but now infests cattle in Africa.

Pathogenesis: Populations build up during the winter when the animal's coat is longer and thicker but it is not generally considered of any great clinical importance.

Sarcoptes scabiei

Sarcoptes scabiei (Phylum: Arthropoda; Class: Arachnida; Subclass: Acari; Order: Astigmata (Sarcoptiformes); Family: Sarcoptidae) is a burrowing mite distributed worldwide that causes mange in buffalo.

HOST–PARASITE CHECKLISTS P803

In the following checklists, the codes listed below apply.

Helminths

N, nematode; T, trematode; C, cestode; A, acanthocephalan.

Arthropods

F, fly; L, louse; S, flea; M, mite; Mx, maxillopod; Ti, tick.

Protozoa

Co, coccidia; Bs, blood sporozoa; Am, amoeba; Fl, flagellate; Ci, ciliate.

Miscellaneous 'protozoal organisms'

B, blastocyst; Mi, microsporidian; My, *Mycoplasma*; P, Pneumocystidomycete; R, *Rickettsia*.

Deer parasite checklist.

	Helminths		Arthropods		Protozoa	
Section/host system	**Parasite**	**(Super) family**	**Parasite**	**Family**	**Parasite**	
Digestive						
Oesophagus	*Gongylonema pulchrum*	Spiruroidea (N)				
Rumen/reticulum	*Gongylonema verrucosum*	Spiruroidea (N)				
	Paramphistomum cervi	Paramphistomatidae (T)				
	Paramphistomum microbothrium	Paramphistomatidae (T)				
	Paramphistomum streptocoelium	Paramphistomatidae (T)				
	Cotylophoron cotylophorum	Paramphistomatidae (T)				
	Calicophoron calicophorum	Paramphistomatidae (T)				
	Gastrothylax crumenifer	Gastrothylacidae (T)				
	Fischoederius elongatus	Gastrothylacidae (T)				
	Fischoederius cobboldi	Gastrothylacidae (T)				
Abomasum	*Spiculopteragia spiculoptera*	Trichostrongyloidea (N)				
	Spiculopteragia asymmetrica	Trichostrongyloidea (N)				
	Apteragia quadrispiculata	Trichostrongyloidea (N)				
	Spiculopteragia bohmi	Trichostrongyloidea (N)				
	Ostertagia leptospicularis	Trichostrongyloidea (N)				
	Ostertagia ostertagi	Trichostrongyloidea (N)				
	Teladorsagia circumcincta	Trichostrongyloidea (N)				
	Haemonchus contortus	Trichostrongyloidea (N)				
	Trichostrongylus axei	Trichostrongyloidea (N)				
	Parabronema skrjabini	Spiruroidea (N)				
Small intestine	*Trichostrongylus vitrinus*	Trichostrongyloidea (N)			*Eimeria capreoli*	Eimeriidae (Co)
	Trichostrongylus longispicularis	Trichostrongyloidea (N)			*Eimeria catubrina*	Eimeriidae (Co)
	Nematodirus spathiger	Trichostrongyloidea (N)			*Eimeria panda*	Eimeriidae (Co)
	Nematodirus filicollis	Trichostrongyloidea (N)			*Eimeria patavina*	Eimeriidae (Co)
	Cooperia oncophora	Trichostrongyloidea (N)			*Eimeria ponderosa*	Eimeriidae (Co)
	Cooperia curticei	Trichostrongyloidea (N)			*Eimeria rotunda*	Eimeriidae (Co)
	Cooperia pectinata	Trichostrongyloidea (N)			*Eimeria superba*	Eimeriidae (Co)
	Cooperia punctata	Trichostrongyloidea (N)			*Eimeria asymmetrica*	Eimeriidae (Co)
	Bunostomum trigonocephalum	Ancylostomatoidea (N)			*Eimeria austriaca*	Eimeriidae (Co)
	Capillaria bovis	Trichuroidea (N)			*Eimeria cervi*	Eimeriidae (Co)
	Moniezia benedeni	Anoplocephalidae (C)			*Eimeria elaphi*	Eimeriidae (Co)
					Eimeria robusta	Eimeriidae (Co)
					Eimeria sordida	Eimeriidae (Co)
					Eimeria wapiti	Eimeriidae (Co)
					Eimeria arctica	Eimeriidae (Co)
					Eimeria mayeri	Eimeriidae (Co)
					Eimeria tarandi	Eimeriidae (Co)
					Cryptosporidium parvum	Cryptosporidiidae (Co)
					Cryptosporidium ubiquitum	Cryptosporidiidae (Co)
Caecum, colon	*Chabertia ovina*	Strongyloidea (N)				
	Oesophagostomum columbianum	Strongyloidea (N)				
	Oesophagostomum venulosum	Strongyloidea (N)				
	Skrjabinaema parva	Strongyloidea (N)				
	Trichuris ovis	Trichuroidea (N)				
	Trichuris globulosa	Trichuroidea (N)				
	Trichuris capreoli	Trichuroidea (N)				

(Continued)

Deer parasite checklist. *Continued*

Section/host system	Helminths		Arthropods		Protozoa	
	Parasite	(Super)family	Parasite	Family	Parasite	Family
Respiratory						
Trachea, bronchi			*Cephenemyia trompe*	Oestridae (F)		
			Cephenemyia auribarbis	Oestridae (F)		
			Cephenemyia jellisoni	Oestridae (F)		
			Cephenemyia phobifer	Oestridae (F)		
			Cephenemyia stimulator	Oestridae (F)		
			Pharyngomyia picta	Oestridae (F)		
Lung	*Dictyocaulus viviparous*	Trichostrongyloidea (N)				
	Dictyocaulus eckerti	Trichostrongyloidea (N)				
	Dictyocaulus capreolus	Trichostrongyloidea (N)				
	Protostrongylus rufescens	Metastrongyloidea (N)				
	Muellerius capillaris	Metastrongyloidea (N)				
	Cystocaulus ocreatus	Metastrongyloidea (N)				
	Varestrongylus sagittatus	Metastrongyloidea (N)				
	Varestrongylus capreoli	Metastrongyloidea (N)				
	Echinococcus granulosus	Taeniidae (C)				
Liver	*Fasciola hepatica*	Fasciolidae (T)				
	Fasciola gigantica	Fasciolidae (T)				
	Fascioloides magna	Fasciolidae (T)				
	Dicrocoelium dendriticum	Dicrocoeliidae (T)				
	Dicrocoelium hospes	Dicrocoeliidae (T)				
	Stilesia hepatica	Anoplocephalidae (C)				
	Echinococcus granulosus	Taeniidae (C)				
	Cysticercus tenuicollis	Taeniidae (C)				
	(metacestode: *Taenia hydatigena*)					
Pancreas						
Circulatory						
Blood					*Babesia bovis*	Babesiidae (Bs)
					Theileria cervi	Theileriidae (Bs)
					Anaplasma marginale	Anaplasmataceae (R)
					Anaplasma centrale	Anaplasmataceae (R)
Blood vessels						
Nervous						
CNS	*Elaphostrongylus cervi*	Metastrongyloidea (N)				
	Parelaphostrongylus tenuis	Metastrongyloidea (N)				
Eye						

Reproductive/urogenital

Locomotory

Location	Parasite	Family
Muscle	Cysticercus ovis (metacestode: Taenia ovis)	Taeniidae (C)
	Toxoplasma gondii	Sarcocystidae (Co)
	Sarcocystis cervicanis	Sarcocystidae (Co)
	Sarcocystis grueneri	Sarcocystidae (Co)
	Sarcocystis wapiti	Sarcocystidae (Co)
	Sarcocystis sybillensis	Sarcocystidae (Co)
	Sarcocystis capreolicanis	Sarcocystidae (Co)
	Sarcocystis gracilis	Sarcocystidae (Co)
	Sarcocystis rangi	Sarcocystidae (Co)
	Sarcocystis tarandivulpis	Sarcocystidae (Co)
	Sarcocystis tarandi	Sarcocystidae (Co)
	Sarcocystis rangiferi	Sarcocystidae (Co)
	Sarcocystis alceslatranis	Sarcocystidae (Co)
	Sarcocystis jorrini	Sarcocystidae (Co)

Connective tissue

Location	Parasite	Family
	Elaeophora schneideri	Filarioidea (N)
Subcutaneous	Hypoderma diana	Oestridae (F)
	Hypoderma tarandi	Oestridae (F)
	Lucilia spp.	Calliphoridae (F)
	Cordylobia anthropophaga	Calliphoridae (F)
	Cochliomyia hominivorax	Calliphoridae (F)
	Chrysomya bezziana	Calliphoridae (F)
	Chrysomya megacephala	Calliphoridae (F)
	Wohlfahrtia magnifica	Sarcophagidae (F)
	Wohlfahrtia nuba	Sarcophagidae (F)
	Sarcophaga dux	Sarcophagidae (F)
	Dermatobia hominis	Oestridae (F)

Integument

Location	Parasite	Family
Skin	Besnoitia tarandi	Sarcocystidae (Co)
	Bovicola longicornis	Bovicolidae (L)
	Bovicola tibialis	Bovicolidae (L)
	Bovicola meyeri	Bovicolidae (L)
	Bovicola maai	Bovicolidae (L)
	Bovicola forficula	Bovicolidae (L)
	Tricholipeurus indicus	Philopteridae (L)
	Solenopotes burmeisteri	Linognathidae (L)
	Solenopotes capreoli	Linognathidae (L)
	Solenopotes ferrisi	Linognathidae (L)
	Solenopotes muntiacus	Linognathidae (L)
	Solenopotes tarandi	Linognathidae (L)
	Solenopotes biniplosus	Linognathidae (L)
	Sarcoptes scabiei	Sarcoptidae (M)

The following species of flies and ticks are found on deer. More detailed descriptions can be found in Chapter 3.

Flies of veterinary importance on deer.

Group	Genus	Species	Family
Blackflies Buffalo gnats	*Simulium*	spp.	Simuliidae (F)
Bot flies	*Cephenemyia*	*trompe*	Oestridae (F)
	Dermatobia	*hominis*	
Flesh flies	*Sarcophaga*	*dux*	Sarcophagidae (F)
	Wohlfahrtia	*magnifica nuba*	
Hippoboscids	*Lipoptena*	*depressa cervi*	Hippoboscidae (F)
Midges	*Culicoides*	spp.	Ceratopogonidae (F)
Mosquitoes	*Aedes*	spp.	Culicidae (F)
	Anopheles	spp.	
	Culex	spp.	
Muscids	*Musca*	spp.	Muscidae (F)
	Stomoxys	*calcitrans*	
Sand flies	*Phlebotomus*	spp.	Psychodidae (F)
Screwworms and blowflies	*Chrysomya*	*bezziana megacephala rufifaces albiceps*	Calliphoridae (F)
	Cochliomyia	*hominivorax macellaria*	
	Cordylobia	*anthropophaga*	
	Calliphora	spp.	
	Lucilia	spp.	
Tabanids	*Chrysops*	spp.	Tabanidae (I)
	Haematopota	spp.	
	Tabanus	spp.	

Tick species found on deer.

Genus	Species	Common name	Family
Ornithodoros	*hermsi*	Sand tampan	Argasidae (Ti)
	savignyi	Eyed or sand tampan	
	turicata		
Otobius	*megnini*	Spinose ear tick	Argasidae (Ti)
Amblyomma	*americanum*	Lone Star tick	Ixodidae (Ti)
	cajennense	Cayenne tick	
	maculatum	Gulf Coast tick	
Dermacentor	*andersoni*	Rocky Mountain wood tick	Ixodidae (Ti)
	variablilis	American dog tick	
	albipictus	Moose tick	
	marginatus	Sheep tick	
	nitens	Tropical horse tick	
	reticulatus	Marsh tick	
	silvarum		
	occidentalis	Pacific Coast tick	
Haemaphysalis	*punctata*	Bush tick	Ixodidae (Ti)
	longicornis	Bush tick	
	bispinosa	Bush tick	
	concinna	Bush tick	
Hyalomma	*anatolicum*	Bush tick	Ixodidae (Ti)
	excavatum	Brown ear tick	
	marginatum	Mediterranean *Hyalomma*	
	scupense		
Ixodes	*ricinus*	Castor bean or European sheep tick	Ixodidae (Ti)
	holocyclus		
	persulcatus	Taiga tick	
	pacificus	Western black-legged tick	
	rubicundus	Karoo paralysis tick	
	scapularis		
Rhipicephalus	*bursa*		Ixodidae (Ti)
	capensis	Cape brown tick	
	sanguineus	Brown dog or kennel tick	
Rhipicephalus (*Boophilus*)	*annulatus*	Texas cattle fever tick	Ixodidae (Ti)
	microplus	Pantropical or southern cattle tick	

Camel parasite checklist.

Section/host system	Helminths		Arthropods		Protozoa	
	Parasite	(Super)family	Parasite	Family	Parasite	Family
Digestive						
Oesophagus	Gongylonema pulchrum	Spiruroidea (N)				
Rumen/reticulum	Gongylonema pulchrum	Spiruroidea (N)				
	Gongylonema verrucosum	Spiruroidea (N)				
Abomasum	Haemonchus longistipes	Trichostrongyloidea (N)				
	Haemonchus contortus	Trichostrongyloidea (N)				
	Teladorsagia circumcincta	Trichostrongyloidea (N)				
	Ostertagia leptospicularis	Trichostrongyloidea (N)				
	Camelostrongylus mentulatus	Trichostrongyloidea (N)				
	Marshallagia marshalli	Trichostrongyloidea (N)				
	Trichostrongylus axei	Trichostrongyloidea (N)				
	Impalaia nudicollis	Trichostrongyloidea (N)				
	Impalaia tuberculata	Trichostrongyloidea (N)				
	Parabronema skrjabini	Spiruroidea (N)				
	Physocephalus sexalatus	Spiruroidea (N)				
Small intestine	Nematodirus abnormalis	Trichostrongyloidea (N)			Eimeria bactriani	Eimeriidae (Co)
	Nematodirus helvetianus	Trichostrongyloidea (N)			Eimeria cameli	Eimeriidae (Co)
	Nematodirus mauritanicus	Trichostrongyloidea (N)			Eimeria dromedarii	Eimeriidae (Co)
	Nematodirus spathiger	Trichostrongyloidea (N)			Eimeria pellerdyi	Eimeriidae (Co)
	Nematodirella dromedarii	Trichostrongyloidea (N)			Eimeria rajasthani	Eimeriidae (Co)
	Nematodirella camesi	Trichostrongyloidea (N)			Cystoisospora orlovi	Sarcocystidae (Co)
	Cooperia oncophora	Trichostrongyloidea (N)			Cryptosporidium parvum	Cryptosporidiidae (Co)
	Cooperia sumabada	Trichostrongyloidea (N)				
	Trichostrongylus colubriformis	Trichostrongyloidea (N)				
	Trichostrongylus longispicularis	Trichostrongyloidea (N)				
	Trichostrongylus probolorus	Trichostrongyloidea (N)				
	Trichostrongylus vitrinus	Trichostrongyloidea (N)				
	Bunostomum trigonocephalum	Ancylostomatoidea (N)				
	Strongyloides papillosus	Strongyloidoidea (N)				
	Moniezia benedeni	Anoplocephalidae (C)				
	Moniezia expansa	Anoplocephalidae (C)				
	Avitellina centripunctata	Anoplocephalidae (C)				
	Avitellina woodlandi	Anoplocephalidae (C)				
	Stilesia globipunctata	Anoplocephalidae (C)				
	Stilesia vittata	Anoplocephalidae (C)				
	Thysaniezia ovilla	Anoplocephalidae (C)				
Caecum, colon	Chabertia ovina	Strongyloidea (N)			Balantidium coli	Balantiidae (Ci)
	Oesophagostomum columbianum	Strongyloidea (N)			Buxtonella sulcata	Pycnotrichidae (Ci)
	Oesophagostomum venulosum	Strongyloidea (N)			Entamoeba wenyoni	Entmaoebidae (Am)
	Trichuris ovis	Trichuroidea (N)				
	Trichuris globulosa	Trichuroidea (N)				
	Trichuris camelsi	Trichuroidea (N)				
Respiratory						
Nasal cavities			Cephalopina titillator	Oestridae (F)		
			Oestrus ovis	Oestridae (F)		
Trachea, bronchi	Dictyocaulus viviparus	Trichostrongyloidea (N)				
	Dictyocaulus filaria	Trichostrongyloidea (N)				
Lung	Echinococcus granulosus	Taeniidae (C)				

Camel parasite checklist. *Continued*

Section/host system	Helminths		Arthropods		Protozoa	
	Parasite	(Super)family	Parasite	Family	Parasite	Family
Liver						
	Fasciola hepatica	Fasciolidae (T)				
	Fasciola gigantica	Fasciolidae (T)				
	Dicrocoelium dendriticum	Dicrocoeliidae (T)				
	Echinococcus granulosus	Taeniidae (C)				
Pancreas						
	Eurytrema pancreaticum	Dicrocoeliidae (T)				
Circulatory						
Blood	*Schistosoma bovis*	Schistosomatidae (T)			*Trypanosoma brucei*	Trypanosomatidae (Fl)
	Schistosoma mattheei	Schistosomatidae (T)			*Trypanosoma congolense*	Trypanosomatidae (Fl)
	Schistosoma indicum	Schistosomatidae (T)			*Trypanosoma vivax*	Trypanosomatidae (Fl)
	Schistosoma turkestanica	Schistosomatidae (T)			*Trypanosoma evansi*	Trypanosomatidae (Fl)
					Theileria camelensis	Theileriidae (Bs)
					Theileria dromedari	Theileriidae (Bs)
					Anaplasma centrale	Anaplasmataceae (R)
					Anaplasma marginale	Anaplasmataceae (R)
Blood vessels	*Elaeophora schneideri*	Filarioidea (N)				
	Dipetalonema evansi	Filarioidea (N)				
	Onchocerca armillata	Filarioidea (N)				
Nervous						
CNS	*Coenurus cerebralis* (metacestode: *Taenia multiceps*)	Taeniidae (C)				
Eye	*Thelazia rhodesi*	Spiruroidea (N)				
	Thelazia leesi	Spiruroidea (N)				
Reproductive/urogenital						
Locomotory						
Muscle	*Cysticercus ovis* (metacestode: *Taenia ovis*)	Taeniidae (C)			*Sarcocystis cameli*	Sarcocystidae (Co)
					Sarcocystis ippeni	Sarcocystidae (Co)
					Toxoplasma gondii	Sarcocystidae (Co)
Connective tissue						
	Onchocerca fasciata	Filarioidea (N)				
	Onchocerca gutturosa	Filarioidea (N)				
Subcutaneous	*Onchocerca fasciata*	Filarioidea (N)	*Lucilia cuprina*	Calliphoridae (F)		
	Onchocerca gibsoni	Filarioidea (N)	*Cordylobia anthropophaga*	Calliphoridae (F)		
	Onchocerca gutturosa	Filarioidea (N)	*Cochliomyia hominivorax*	Calliphoridae (F)		
			Chrysomya bezziana	Calliphoridae (F)		
			Chrysomya megacephala	Calliphoridae (F)		
			Wohlfahrtia magnifica	Sarcophagidae (F)		
			Wohlfahrtia nuba	Sarcophagidae (F)		
			Sarcophaga dux	Sarcophagidae (F)		
			Dermatobia hominis	Oestridae (F)		
Integument						
Skin			*Hippobosca camelina*	Hippoboscidae (F)		
			Sarcoptes scabiei	Sarcoptidae (M)		
			Chorioptes bovis	Psoroptidae (M)		
			Microthoracius cameli	Microthoracidae (L)		

The following species of flies and ticks are found on camels. More detailed descriptions can be found in Chapter 3.

Flies of veterinary importance on camels.

Group	Genus	Species	Family
Blackflies Buffalo gnats	*Simulium*	spp.	Simuliidae (F)
Bot flies	*Cephalopina*	*titillator*	Oestridae (F)
Flesh flies	*Sarcophaga*	*dux*	Sarcophagidae (F)
	Wohlfahrtia	*magnifica nuba*	
Hippoboscids	*Hippobosca*	*camelsina maculate*	Hippoboscidae (F)
Midges	*Culicoides*	spp.	Ceratopogonidae (F)
Mosquitoes	*Aedes*	spp.	Culicidae (F)
	Anopheles	spp.	
	Culex	spp.	
Muscids	*Haematobia*	*irritans*	Muscidae (F)
	Musca	*autumnalis domestica*	
	Stomoxys	*calcitrans*	
Sand flies	*Phlebotomus*	spp.	Psychodidae (F)
Screwworms and blowflies	*Chrysomya*	*bezziana*	Calliphoridae (F)
	Cochliomyia	*hominivorax*	
	Cordylobia	*anthropophaga*	
	Calliphora	spp.	
	Lucilia	spp.	
Tabanids	*Chrysops*	spp.	Tabanidae (F)
	Haematopota	spp.	
	Tabanus	spp.	
Tsetse flies	*Glossina*	*fusca morsitans palpalis*	Glossinidae (F)

Tick species found on camels.

Genus	Species	Common name	Family
Ornithodoros	*savignyi*	Eyed or sand tampan	Argasidae (Ti)
Otobius	*megnini*	Spinose ear tick	Argasidae (Ti)
Amblyomma	*lepidum*		Ixodidae (Ti)
	gemma		
	variegatum	Variegated or tropical bont tick	
Dermacentor	*marginatus*	Ornate sheep tick	Ixodidae (Ti)
	reticulatus	Marsh tick	
	silvarum		
Haemaphysalis	*punctata*	Bush tick	Ixodidae (Ti)
Hyalomma	*anatolicum*	Bont-legged tick	Ixodidae (Ti)
	dromedarii	Camel tick	
	detritum	Bont-legged tick	
	impressum		
	marginatum	Mediterranean tick	
Ixodes	*ricinus*	Castor bean or European sheep tick	Ixodidae (Ti)
	holocyclus	Paralysis tick	
	rubicundus	Karoo paralysis tick	
Rhipicephalus	*evertsi*	Red-legged tick	Ixodidae (Ti)
	bursa		
	pulchellus	Zebra tick	
	sanguineus	Brown dog or kennel tick	
Rhipicehalus (Boophilus)	*decoloratus*	Blue tick	Ixodidae (Ti)

Camelids (llamas, alpacas, guanacos, vicuñas) parasite checklist.

| Section/host system | Helminths | | Arthropods | | Protozoa | |
	Parasite	(Super)family	Parasite	Family	Parasite	Family
Digestive						
Oesophagus	Gongylonema pulchrum	Spiruroidea (N)				
Rumen/reticulum	Gongylonema pulchrum	Spiruroidea (N)				
Stomach	Graphinema aucheniae	Trichostrongyloidea (N)				
	Spiculopteragia peruvianus	Trichostrongyloidea (N)				
	Camelostrongylus mentulatus	Trichostrongyloidea (N)				
	Teladorsagia circumcincta	Trichostrongyloidea (N)				
	Marshallagia marshalli	Trichostrongyloidea (N)				
	Haemonchus contortus	Trichostrongyloidea (N)				
	Trichostrongylus axei	Trichostrongyloidea (N)				
	Ostertagia leptospicularis	Trichostrongyloidea (N)				
Small intestine	Lamanema chavezi	Trichostrongyloidea (N)			Eimeria lamae	Eimeriidae (Co)
	Nematodirus lamae	Trichostrongyloidea (N)			Eimeria alpacae	Eimeriidae (Co)
	Nematodirus helvetianus	Trichostrongyloidea (N)			Eimeria punoensis	Eimeriidae (Co)
	Nematodirus battus	Trichostrongyloidea (N)			Eimeria macusaniensis	Eimeriidae (Co)
	Trichostrongylus vitrinus	Trichostrongyloidea (N)			Cryptosporidium parvum	Cryptosporidiidae (Co)
	Trichostrongylus colubriformis	Trichostrongyloidea (N)			Giardia intestinalis	Giardiidae (Fl)
	Trichostrongylus longispicularis	Trichostrongyloidea (N)				
	Cooperia surnabada	Trichostrongyloidea (N)				
	Bunostomum trigonocephalum	Ancylostomatoidea (N)				
	Strongyloides papillosus	Strongyloidoidea (N)				
	Moniezia expansa	Anoplocephalidae (C)				
Caecum, colon	Oesophagostomum venulosum	Strongyloidea (N)				
	Oesophagostomum columbianum	Strongyloidea (N)				
	Chabertia ovina	Strongyloidea (N)				
	Trichuris ovis	Trichuroidea (N)				
	Skrjabinema ovis	Oxyuroidea (N)				
Respiratory						
Nose			Cephenemyia spp.	Oestridae (F)		
Trachea, bronchi	Dictyocaulus viviparus	Trichostrongyloidea (N)				
	Dictyocaulus filaria	Trichostrongyloidea (N)				
Lung						
Liver						
	Fasciola hepatica	Fasciolidae (T)				
	Fasciola gigantica	Fasciolidae (T)				
	Fascioloides magna	Fasciolidae (T)				
	Dicrocoelium dendriticum	Dicrocoeliidae (T)				
	Echinococcus granulosus	Taeniidae (C)				

Site	Species	Taxonomic group
Pancreas		
Circulatory		
Blood		
Blood vessels		
Nervous		
CNS	Parelaphostrongylus tenuis	Metastrongyloidea (N)
Eye	Thelazia rhodesi	Spiruroidea (N)
Reproductive/urogenital		
Locomotory		
Muscle	Toxoplasma gondii	Sarcocystidae (Co)
	Sarcocystis aucheniae	Sarcocystidae (Co)
	Sarcocystis lamacenis	Sarcocystidae (Co)
Connective tissue		
Subcutaneous	Cochliomyia hominivorax	Calliphoridae (F)
Integument		
Skin	Microthoracius mazzai	Microthoraciidae (L)
	Bovicola breviceps	Bovicolidae (L)
	Sarcoptes scabiei	Sarcoptidae (M)
	Psoroptes ovis	Psoroptidae (M)
	Chorioptes bovis	Psoroptidae (M)

Tick species found on camelids.

Genus	Species	Common name	Family
Otobius	*megnini*	Spinose ear tick	Argasidae (Ti)
Amblyomma	*americanum*	Lone Star tick	Ixodidae (Ti)
	cajennense	Cayenne tick	
	hebraeum	South African bont tick	
	maculatum	Gulf Coast tick	
	variegatum		
Dermacentor	*andersoni*	Rocky Mountain wood tick	Ixodidae (Ti)
	marginatus	Sheep tick	
	reticulatus	Marsh tick	
	occidentalis	Pacific Coast tick	
	variabilis	American dog tick	
Haemaphysalis	*punctata*		Ixodidae (Ti)
	concinna	Bush tick	
	bispinosa	Bush tick	
	longicornis		
Hyalomma	*dromedarii*	Camel *Hyalomma*	Ixodidae (Ti)
	marginatum	Mediterranean *Hyalomma*	
Ixodes	*ricinus*	Castor bean or European sheep tick	Ixodidae (Ti)
	holocyclus		
	rubicundus	Karoo paralysis tick	
	scapularis		
Rhipicephalus	*evertsi*	Red or red-legged tick	Ixodidae (Ti)
	sanguineus	Brown dog or kennel tick	
	simus	Glossy tick	
Rhipicehalus (Boophilus)	*annulatus*	Texas cattle fever tick	Ixodidae (Ti)
	decoloratus	Blue tick	
	microplus	Tropical cattle tick	

Buffalo parasite checklist.

Section/host system	Helminths			Arthropods		Protozoa	
	Parasite	(Super)family	Family	Parasite	Family	Parasite	Family
Digestive							
Oesophagus	Gongylonema pulchrum	Spiruroidea (N)					
Rumen/reticulum	Gongylonema pulchrum	Spiruroidea (N)					
	Paramphistomum cervi	Paramphistomatidae (T)					
	Paramphistomum microbothrium	Paramphistomatidae (T)					
	Cotylophoron cotylophoron	Paramphistomatidae (T)					
	Calicophoron calicophorum	Paramphistomatidae (T)					
	Carmyerius gregarius	Gastrothylacidae (T)					
	Gastrothylax cruminifer	Gastrothylacidae (T)					
	Fischoederius elongatus	Gastrothylacidae (T)					
	Fischoederius cobboldi	Gastrothylacidae (T)					
Stomach	Mecistocirrus digitatus	Trichostrongyloidea (N)					
	Ostertagia ostertagi	Trichostrongyloidea (N)					
	Haemonchus contortus	Trichostrongyloidea (N)					
	Trichostrongylus axei	Trichostrongyloidea (N)					
Small intestine	Toxocara vitulorum	Ascaridoidea (N)				Eimeria ankarensis	Eimeriidae (Co)
	Nematodirus helvetianus	Trichostrongyloidea (N)				Eimeria bareillyi	Eimeriidae (Co)
	Cooperia onchophora	Trichostrongyloidea (N)				Eimeria gokaki	Eimeriidae (Co)
	Trichostrongylus longispicularis	Trichostrongyloidea (N)				Eimeria ovoidalis	Eimeriidae (Co)
	Bunostomum phlebotomum	Ancylostomatoidea (N)				Eimeria thianethi	Eimeriidae (Co)
	Agriostomum vryburgi	Ancylostomatoidea (N)				Eimeria alabamensis	Eimeriidae (Co)
	Strongyloides papillosus	Strongyloidoidea (N)				Eimeria aubernensis	Eimeriidae (Co)
	Capillaria bovis	Trichuroidea (N)				Eimeria bovis	Eimeriidae (Co)
	Moniezia benedeni	Anoplocephalidae (C)				Eimeria brasiliensis	Eimeriidae (Co)
	Avitellina centripunctata	Anoplocephalidae (C)				Eimeria bukidnonensis	Eimeriidae (Co)
						Eimeria canadensis	Eimeriidae (Co)
						Eimeria cylindrica	Eimeriidae (Co)
						Eimeria ellipsoidalis	Eimeriidae (Co)
						Eimeria subspherica	Eimeriidae (Co)
						Eimeria wyomingensis	Eimeriidae (Co)
						Eimeria zuernii	Eimeriidae (Co)
						Cryptosporidium parvum	Cryptosporidiidae (Co)
Caecum, colon	Oesophagostomum radiatum	Strongyloidea (N)				Eimeria bovis	Eimeriidae (Co)
	Trichuris discolor	Trichuroidea (N)				Eimeria zuernii	Eimeriidae (Co)
	Homalogaster paloniae	Gastrodiscidae (T)					
Respiratory							
Larynx	Mammomonogamus laryngeus	Strongyloidea (N)					
Trachea, bronchi	Dictyocaulus viviparus	Trichostrongyloidea (N)					
Lung							
Liver							
	Fasciola gigantica	Fasciolidae (T)					
	Fasciola hepatica	Fasciolidae (T)					
	Gigantocotyle explanatum	Paramphistomatidae (T)					
	Echinococcus granulosus	Taeniidae (C)					
Pancreas							
	Eurytrema pancreaticum	Dicrocoeliidae (T)					

Buffalo parasite checklist. *Continued*

Section/host system	Helminths		Arthropods		Protozoa	
	Parasite	(Super)family	Parasite	Family	Parasite	Family
Circulatory						
Blood					Trypanosoma brucei evansi	Trypansomatidae (Fl)
					Trypanosoma theileri	Trypansomatidae (Fl)
					Babesia bovis	Babesiidae (Bs)
					Babesia bigemina	Babesiidae (Bs)
					Babesia orientalis	Babesiidae (Bs)
					Theileria parva	Theileriidae (Bs)
					Theileria annulata	Theileriidae (Bs)
					Theileria orientalis complex	Theileriidae (Bs)
					Ehrlichia ruminantium	Anaplasmataceae (R)
Blood vessels	Elaeophora poeli	Filarioidea (N)				
	Schistosoma indicum	Schistosomatidae (T)				
	Schistosoma nasale	Schistosomatidae (T)				
	Schistosoma spindale	Schistosomatidae (T)				
	Schistosoma turkestanica	Schistosomatidae (T)				
Nervous						
CNS						
Eye	Thelazia rhodesi	Spiruroidea (N)				
Reproductive/urogenital						
Locomotory						
Muscle					Sarcocystis sinensis	Sarcocystidae (Co)
Connective tissue						
Subcutaneous	Parafilaria bovicola	Filarioidea (N)				
	Setaria labiato-papillosa	Filarioidea (N)				
	Setaria digitatus	Filarioidea (N)				
Integument						
Skin	Stephanofilaria zaheeri	Filarioidea (N)	Haematopinus tuberculatus	Haematopinidae (L)		
			Sarcoptes scabiei	Sarcoptidae (M)		
			Psoroptes natalensis	Psoroptidae (M)		

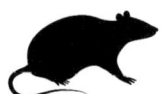
RABBITS

ENDOPARASITES

Parasites of the digestive system

Helminth infections are rarely seen in domestic rabbits unless they are kept in conditions that expose them to the infective stages resulting from contact with wild rabbits. The following species, with the exception of *Passalurus*, are therefore generally only found in wild rabbits, and treatment of domesticated rabbits for many of these parasites is therefore rarely indicated. When treatment is required, fenbendazole and mebendazole are effective. In-feed medication with flubendazole can also be given over 10 days.

A more detailed list of helminth species found in both domesticated and wild rabbits is provided in the parasite checklist at the end of the chapter.

Graphidium strigosum

Graphidium strigosum (Phylum: Nematoda; Class: Chromadorea; Order: Rhabditida; Family: Trichostrongylidae), commonly known as the Rabbit strongyle, is localised in the stomach and small intestine of rabbits and hares and is distributed in Europe.

Clinical signs and pathology: Infections may range from few effects to destruction of the gastric mucosa according to parasitic load. The most common clinical signs are diarrhoea, anaemia, emaciation and sometimes death if untreated.

Diagnosis: This is based on identification of the eggs in faeces or adult worms in the stomach on *post mortem*.

Obeliscoides cuniculi

Obeliscoides cuniculi (Phylum: Nematoda; Class: Chromadorea; Order: Rhabditida; Family: Trichostrongylidae) is localised in the stomach of rabbits, hares and occasionally white-tailed deer. It is distributed throughout the USA. The parasite can occasionally undergo hypobiosis.

Trichostrongylus retortaeformis

Trichostrongylus retortaeformis (Phylum: Nematoda; Class: Chromadorea; Order: Rhabditida; Family: Trichostrongylidae) is distributed worldwide and is localised in the small intestine of rabbits and hares.

Pathogenesis: The parasites penetrate the mucosa, causing desquamation and, in heavy infections, inflammation of the intestine with excess mucous exudate.

Diagnosis: This is based on clinical signs, seasonal occurrence of disease and, if possible, lesions at *post mortem* examination. Faecal egg counts are a useful aid to diagnosis, although faecal cultures are necessary for generic identification of larvae.

Nematodirus leporis

Nematodirus leporis (Phylum: Nematoda; Class: Chromadorea; Order: Rhabditida; Family: Trichostrongylidae) is localised in the small intestine of rabbits and hares.

Pathogenesis: Clinical signs become noticeable with severe infestations, leading to diarrhoea and loss of weight. Necropsy shows that the large numbers of worms form clumps resembling cottonwool and are usually intertwined around the intestinal villi, causing atrophy, degeneration and necrosis of the surface enterocytes.

Tapeworms

Tapeworms of the genus *Cittotaenia* are up to 80 cm long and 1 cm wide with proglottids broader than long, each containing two sets of genital organs. Eggs are about 64 µm in diameter and have a pyriform apparatus. Forage mites, mainly of the family Oribatidae, represent the intermediate hosts and the infection occurs in domesticated rabbits grazing contaminated grass. Heavy infections may cause digestive disturbances, emaciation and occasionally death. Diagnosis is based largely on the presence of mature proglottids in the faeces. For information on the main species, see the checklist table.

Oxyurid worms

Passalurus ambiguus

Passalurus ambiguus (Phylum: Nematoda; Class: Chromadorea; Order: Oxyurida; Family: Oxyuridae), commonly known as the Rabbit pinworm, is distributed worldwide and localised in the caecum and colon of rabbits and hares.

Veterinary Parasitology, Fifth Edition. Domenico Otranto and Richard Wall.
© 2024 John Wiley & Sons Ltd. Published 2024 by John Wiley & Sons Ltd.

Pathogenesis: Rabbits can harbour large numbers of oxyurid worms with no clinical signs. These worms can present a problem in rabbit colonies.

Control and treatment: Single treatments are not very effective because of the direct life cycle and rapidity of reinfection. Fenbendazole 50 mg/kg in feed for five days is effective.

Coccidiosis

There are more than 30 species of coccidia described from lagomorphs. The more common species from domestic rabbits are given in Table 15.1. The intestinal species *Eimeria flavescens* and *Eimeria intestinalis* are the most pathogenic, causing destruction of crypts in the intestine and resulting in diarrhoea and emaciation, with disease most common around weaning. Coccidial infections are seen commonly on commercial rabbit farms.

Diagnosis: As in other hosts, diagnosis is best made by a *post mortem* examination. Species identification is based on pathological lesions and location within the intestine. Identification is possible with oocysts recovered from faeces following sporulation. In practice, the demonstration of many oocysts in the faeces is often used as an indication that rabbits require treatment.

Treatment and control: A number of coccidiostats are available for prophylactic use, including robenidine and clopidol. Sulfonamides (sulfadimidine or sulfaquinoxaline) are used for treatment, usually given as two seven-day courses in drinking water, one week apart to allow for the possibility of reinfection. Control of rabbit coccidiosis involves the daily cleaning of cages, hutches or pens and the provision of clean feeding troughs. In many large units, control is achieved by rearing animals on wire floors; alternatively, coccidiostats such as amprolium, clopidol or robenidine are incorporated in the feed.

Eimeria flavescens

Eimeria flavescens (Phylum: Apicomplexa; Class: Conoidasida; Order: Eucoccidiorida; Family: Eimeriidae) is distributed worldwide and localised in the small and large intestines (Fig. 15.1) of hosts. There are five merogony stages. The first-generation meronts are in the glands of the lower small intestine, the second- to fifth-generation meronts in the caecum and colon. The second-, third- and fourth-generation meronts are in the superficial epithelium

Table 15.1 Common *Eimeria* species in rabbits.

Species	Predilection site	Prepatent period (days)
Eimeria flavescens	Small and large intestine	9
Eimeria intestinalis	Small intestine	9–10
Eimeria exigua	Small intestine	7
Eimeria perforans	Small intestine	5
Eimeria irresidua	Small intestine	9
Eimeria media	Small intestine	5–6
Eimeria vejdovskyi	Small intestine	10
Eimeria coecicola	Large intestine	9
Eimeria magna	Small intestine	7
Eimeria pyriformis	Colon	9
Eimeria stiedae	Liver, bile ducts	18

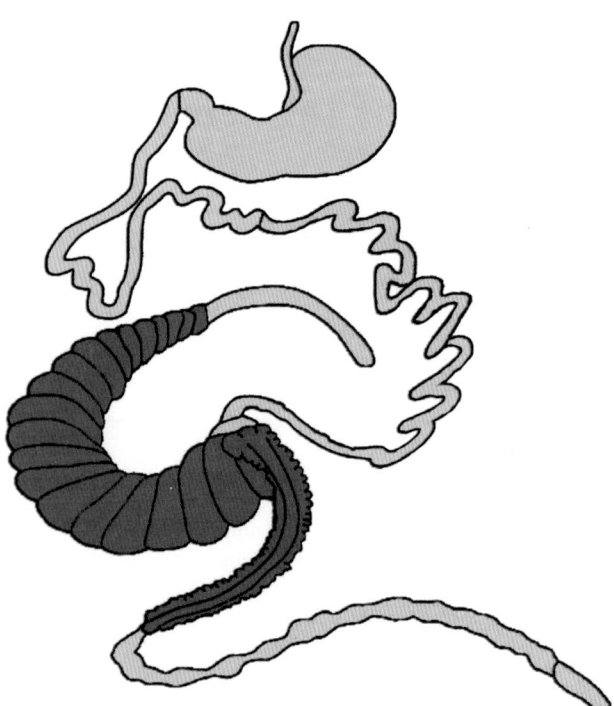

Fig. 15.1 Predilection site of *Eimeria flavescens.*

and the fifth-generation meronts and the gamonts are in the crypts (Figs 15.2 and 15.3). Gamonts and gametes appear about seven days after infection, and oocysts appear in the faeces about nine days after infection. Sporulation time is four days.

Pathogenesis: *Eimeria flavescens* is highly pathogenic for young rabbits, causing high morbidity and mortality, and is a major problem on commercial rabbit farms.

Clinical signs and pathology: There is thickening of the intestinal wall of the caecum and colon with petechial haemorrhages and loss of epithelium in the caecum and colon (Fig. 15.4).

Eimeria intestinalis

Eimeria intestinalis (Phylum: Apicomplexa; Class: Conoidasida; Order: Eucoccidiorida; Family: Eimeriidae) is distributed worldwide, and localised in the small intestine of lagomorphs (Fig. 15.5). There are three merogony stages. First-generation meronts are at the base of the villi in the lower ileum. There appear to be two types of second-generation meronts in the distal part of the villi, followed by third-generation meronts in the same location on the villi. Gamonts begin developing eight days post infection, and are located above the host cell nucleus in the epithelial cells of the villi (Fig. 15.6). The prepatent period is 9–10 days and the patent period 6–10 days. Sporulation time is three days.

Pathogenesis, clinical signs and pathology: *Eimeria intestinalis* is highly pathogenic. This species causes diarrhoea and emaciation. There is oedema of the intestinal wall with destruction of the crypts in the ileum and lower jejunum. Greyish-white foci may coalesce to form a sticky purulent layer in the small intestine (Fig. 15.7).

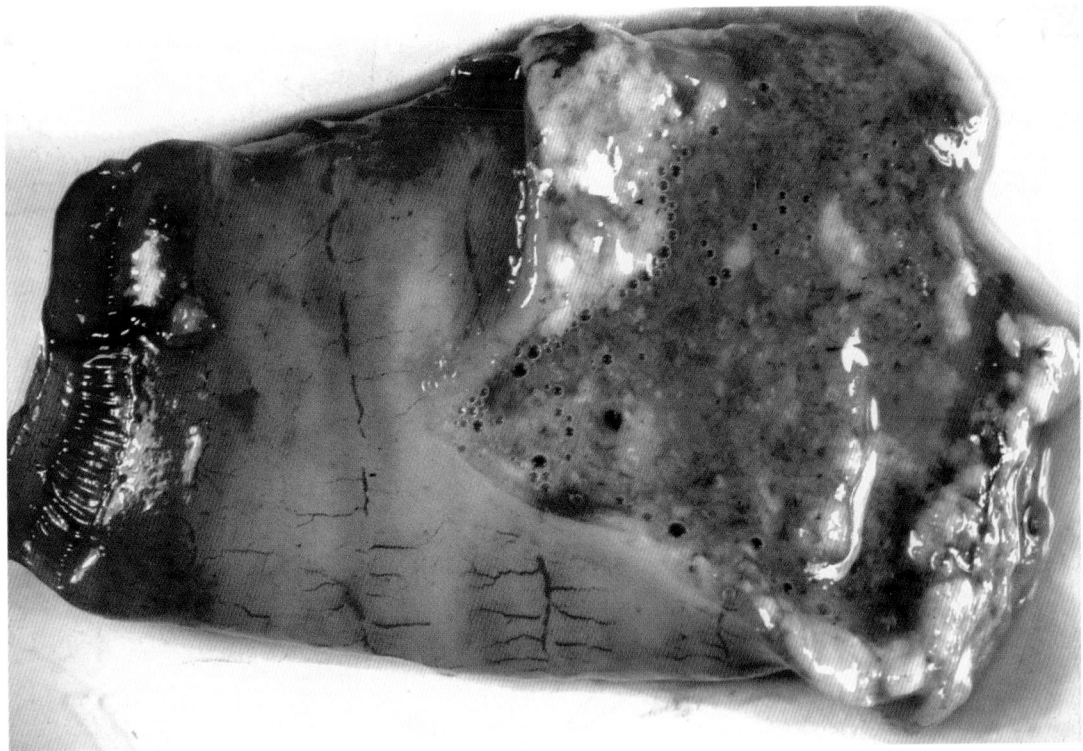

Fig. 15.2 Thickened and inflamed intestine due to the presence of *Eimeria flavescens*.

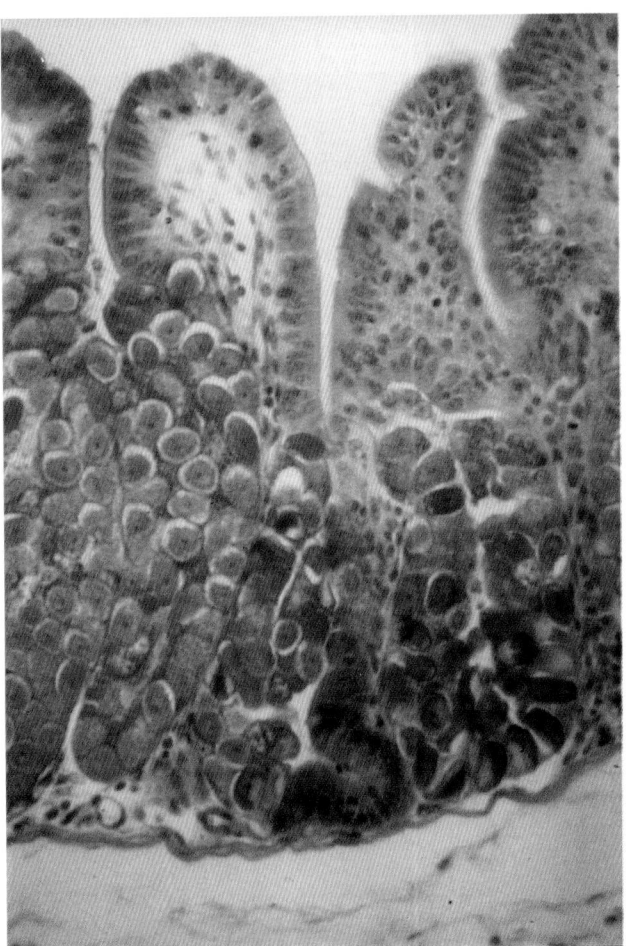

Fig. 15.3 Meronts of *Eimeria* within crypt epithelial cells of the caecum.

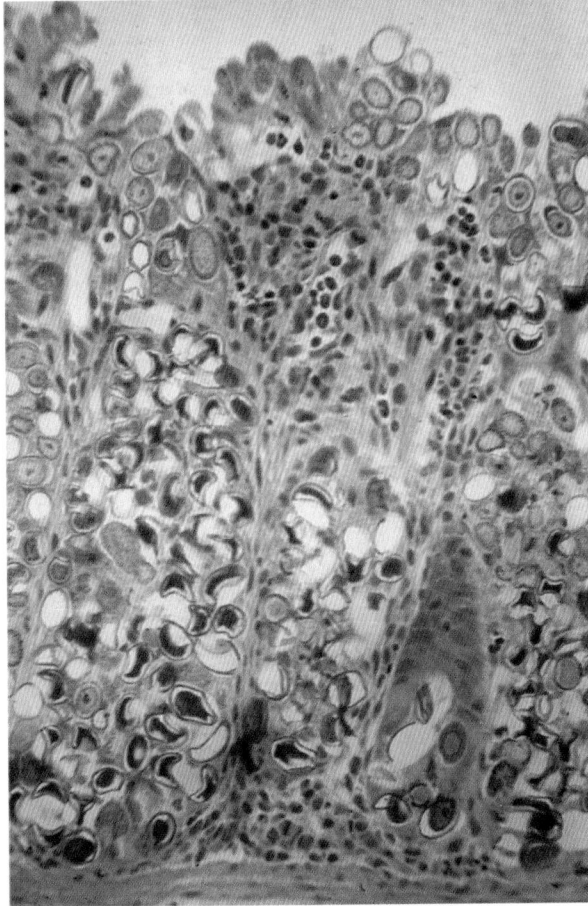

Fig. 15.4 Gamonts and oocysts of *Eimeria flavescens* in the mucosa of the large intestine.

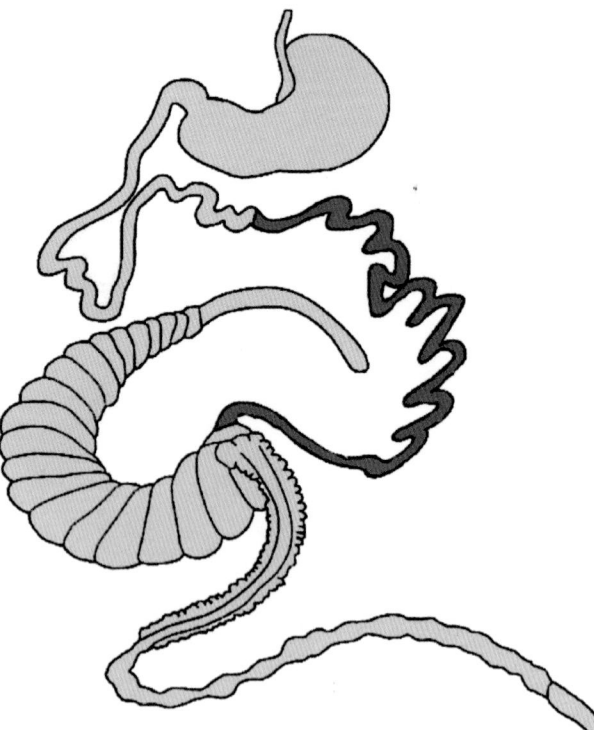

Fig. 15.5 Predilection site of *Eimeria intestinalis*.

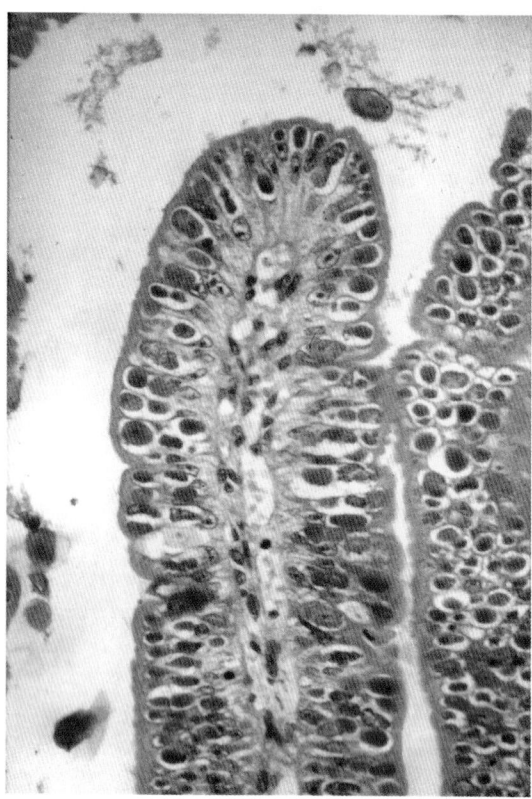

Fig. 15.6 Gamonts of *Eimeria intestinalis* within epithelial cells of the villi of the small intestine.

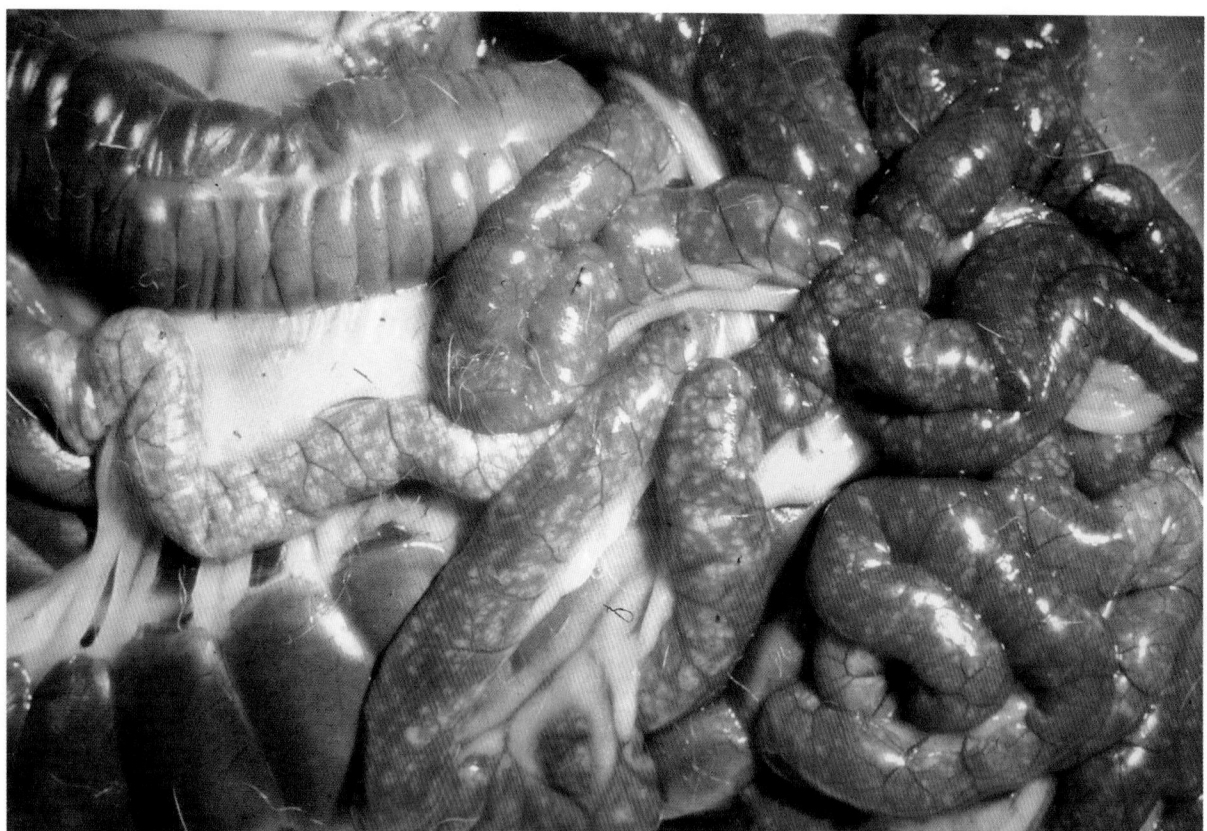

Fig. 15.7 Focal lesions associated with *Eimeria intestinalis* infection in the small intestine.

Eimeria perforans

Eimeria perforans (Phylum: Apicomplexa; Class: Conoidasida; Order: Eucoccidiorida; Family: Eimeriidae) is distributed worldwide, and localised in the small intestine of rabbits (Fig. 15.8). The endogenous stages are found in the epithelial cells of the villi and crypts of the small intestine, especially the middle section. There are two asexual generations, followed by gametogony. The prepatent period is five days and the patent period is 12–32 days. Sporulation time is 1.5–2 days.

Pathogenesis, clinical signs and pathology: *Eimeria perforans* is one of the less pathogenic intestinal coccidia of rabbits. It may cause mild to moderate signs in a heavy infection. Symptoms are usually mild but in heavy infections, there may be anorexia, diarrhoea, weakness, weight loss and growth retardation. The duodenum may be enlarged and oedematous, and may appear a chalky white colour. The jejunum and ileum may contain white spots and streaks and petechiae have been observed in the caecum.

Eimeria irresidua

Eimeria irresidua (Phylum: Apicomplexa; Class: Conoidasida; Order: Eucoccidiorida; Family: Eimeriidae) is distributed worldwide and localised in the small intestine of hosts (Fig. 15.9). There are four merogony stages. First-generation meronts are in the crypts, second-generation meronts are in the lamina propria and third- and fourth-generation meronts and gamonts are in the villous epithelium in the jejunum and to a lesser extent the ileum. The prepatent period is nine days. Sporulation time is four days.

Pathogenesis: Mildly pathogenic, causing a depression in weight gain and in some cases diarrhoea. During this time, there is a reduction in food and water consumption as well as faecal excretion. Occasionally causes mortality depending on the level of infection.

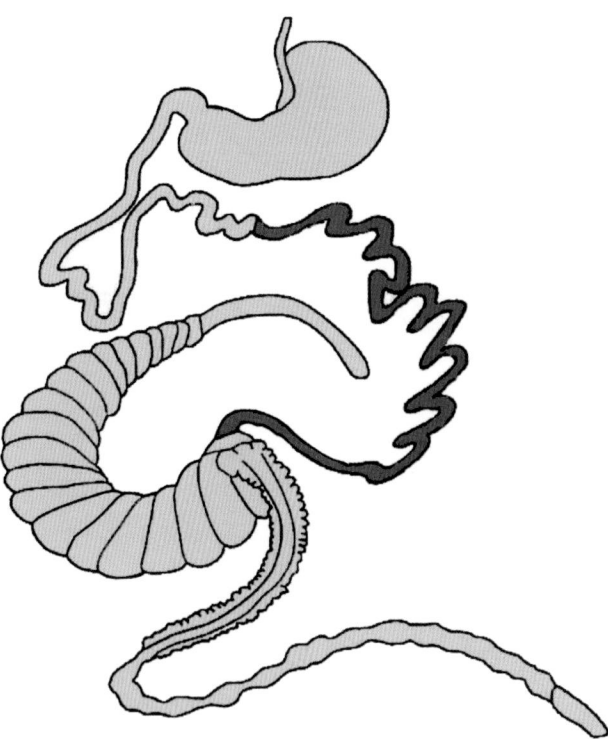

Fig. 15.9 Predilection site of *Eimeria irresidua*.

Clinical signs and pathology: Catarrhal inflammation of the small intestine, particularly the jejunum, may be seen. On *post mortem*, there may be enteritis, with gross thickening of the intestine. Large numbers of meronts and gamonts may be found in mucosal scrapings (Fig. 15.10). Histopathological examination shows a congested and thickened mucosa with villous atrophy, villous fusion and crypt hyperplasia with numerous parasite stages present within the mucosa (Fig. 15.10).

Eimeria media

Eimeria media (Phylum: Apicomplexa; Class: Conoidasida; Order: Eucoccidiorida; Family: Eimeriidae) is distributed worldwide, and localised in the small intestine of hosts (Fig. 15.11). There are two

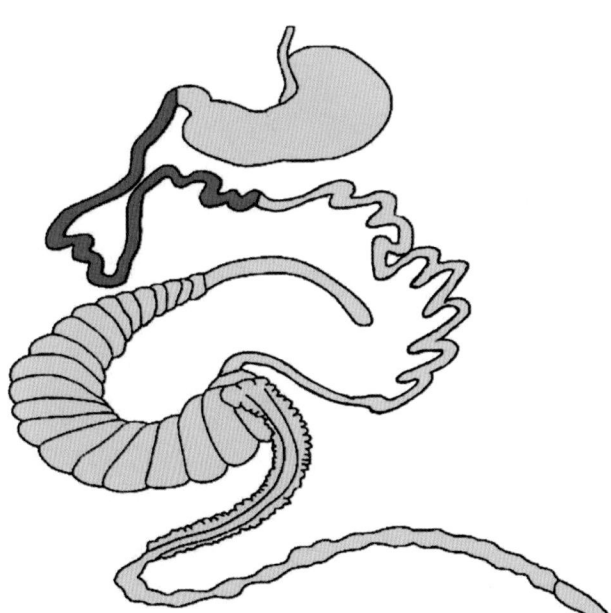

Fig. 15.8 Predilection site of *Eimeria perforans*.

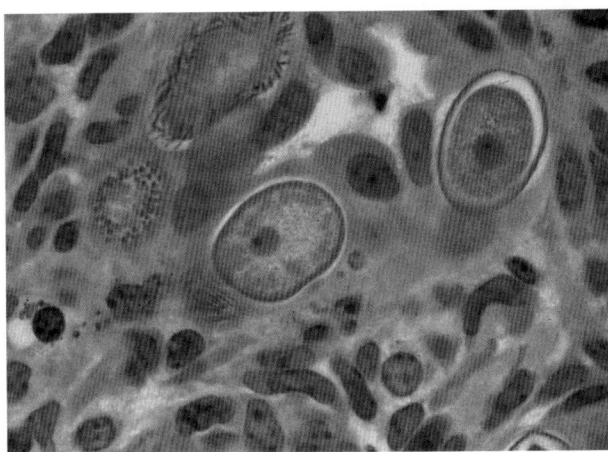

Fig. 15.10 Gamonts of *Eimeria irresidua*.

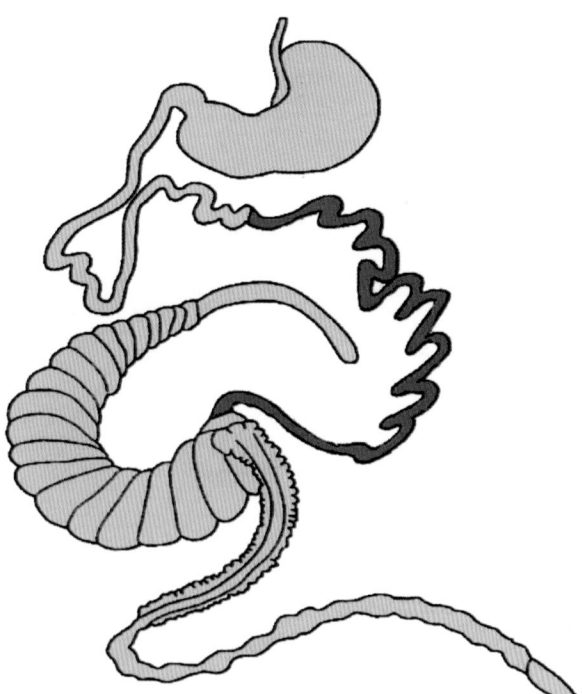

Fig. 15.11 Predilection site of *Eimeria media*.

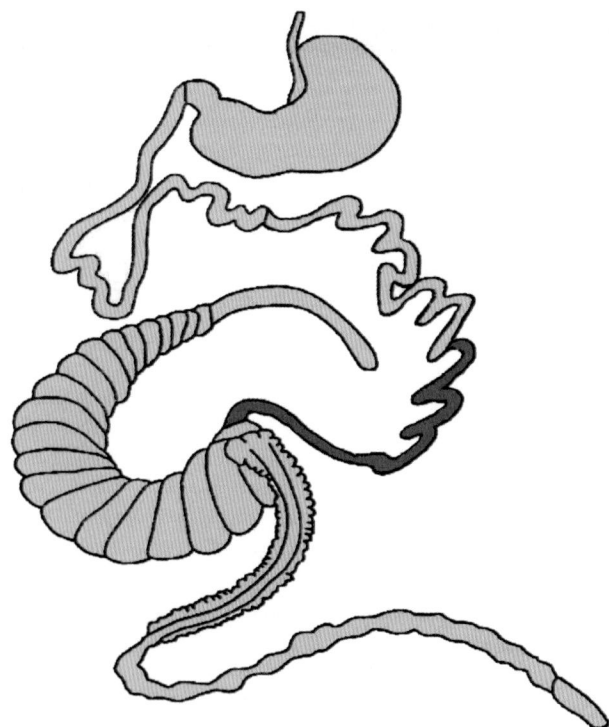

Fig. 15.12 Predilection site of *Eimeria vejdovskyi*.

merogony stages. The endogenous stages are found above or below the host cell nuclei of the epithelial cells and submucosa of the villi of the small intestine, mainly jejunum and ileum. The prepatent period is 5–6 days and the patent period is 15–18 days. Sporulation time is two days.

Pathogenesis: *Eimeria media* is slightly to moderately pathogenic, leading to a depression in weight gain and, in some cases, diarrhoea.

Clinical signs and pathology: During the infection, there is a reduction in food and water consumption as well as faecal excretion. The affected parts of the intestine, mainly the duodenum, are oedematous with greyish foci. In heavy infections, the lesions may extend into the large intestine.

Eimeria vejdovskyi

Eimeria vejdovskyi (Phylum: Apicomplexa; Class: Conoidasida; Order: Eucoccidiorida; Family: Eimeriidae) is localised in the small intestine of hosts (Fig. 15.12), and has an unknown distribution but probably worldwide. This species is considered only slightly pathogenic. Development takes place in the ileum and lower jejunum but details of the life cycle are unknown. The prepatent period is 10 days. The sporulation time is two days.

Clinical signs and pathology: Infections are usually asymptomatic but heavy infections may cause slight depression of growth. Lesions occur only in the ileum and distal jejunum following heavy infection.

Eimeria coecicola

Eimeria coecicola (Phylum: Apicomplexa; Class: Conoidasida; Order: Eucoccidiorida; Family: Eimeriidae) is distributed worldwide and localised in the large intestine of hosts (Fig. 15.13). The number of

generations is unknown. The meronts are in the epithelial cells of the ileum and the gamonts in the epithelial cells of the vermiform process of the caecum. The gamonts are usually sited beneath the host cell nucleus. The prepatent period is 9–11 days and the patent period 7–9 days. Sporulation time is four days.

Clinical signs and pathology: This species is not considered pathogenic. The infection is not associated with clinical signs. In heavy infections, lesions may be seen in the crypts of the vermiform appendix.

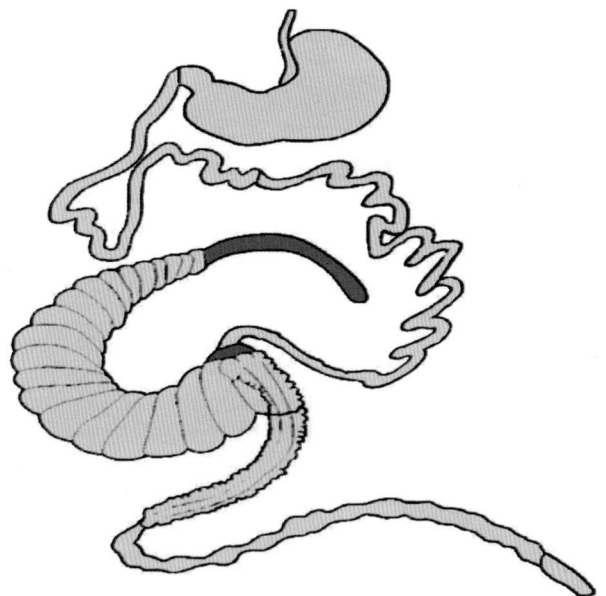

Fig. 15.13 Predilection site of *Eimeria coecicola*.

Eimeria magna

Eimeria magna (Phylum: Apicomplexa; Class: Conoidasida; Order: Eucoccidiorida; Family: Eimeriidae) is distributed worldwide, and localised in the small intestine of hosts (Fig. 15.14). There are two or three merogony stages. The meronts develop in the villous epithelial cells from the middle of the jejunum to the posterior end of the ileum. They lie either above or below the host cell nucleus. The prepatent period is seven days and the patent period is 12–21 days. Sporulation time is 2–3 days.

Clinical signs and pathology: *Eimeria magna* is mildly to moderately pathogenic. The infection causes a depression in weight gain and in some cases diarrhoea. During this time, there is a reduction in food and water consumption as well as faecal excretion. A large amount of mucus may be passed in the faeces. Death may occur, depending on the level of infection. The intestinal mucosa is hyperaemic and inflamed. Epithelial sloughing may occur. Large numbers of meronts and gamonts may be found in mucosal scrapings. Histopathological examination shows a congested and thickened mucosa with villous atrophy, villous fusion and crypt hyperplasia.

Eimeria pyriformis

Eimeria pyriformis (Phylum: Apicomplexa; Class: Conoidasida; Order: Eucoccidiorida; Family: Eimeriidae) is distributed worldwide, and localised in the colon of hosts (Fig. 15.15). There are three generations of meronts found in the proximal and distal colon. The prepatent period is nine days and the patent period is 5–10 days. Sporulation time is four days.

Clinical signs and pathology: *Eimeria pyriformis* is mildly to moderately pathogenic. Infection causes anorexia, diarrhoea, weakness,

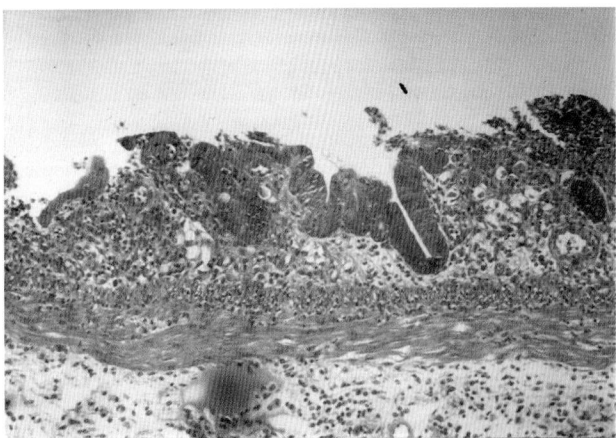

Fig. 15.15 Mucosa of the colon infected with *Eimeria pyriformis*.

weight loss and growth retardation, and in heavy infections can result in death. The wall of the large intestine is thickened and inflamed with large numbers of endogenous parasite stages found within crypt epithelial cells on histopathology (Fig. 15.16).

Parasites of the respiratory system

Several protostrongylid nematodes are found in the lungs of wild rabbits. These are listed in the parasite checklist at the end of the chapter.

Echinococcus granulosus

For more details see Chapter 9.

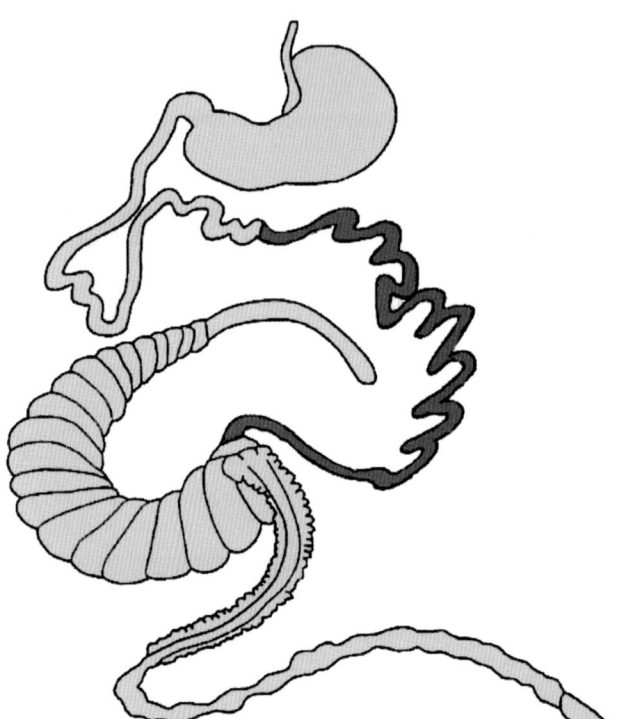

Fig. 15.14 Predilection site of *Eimeria magna*.

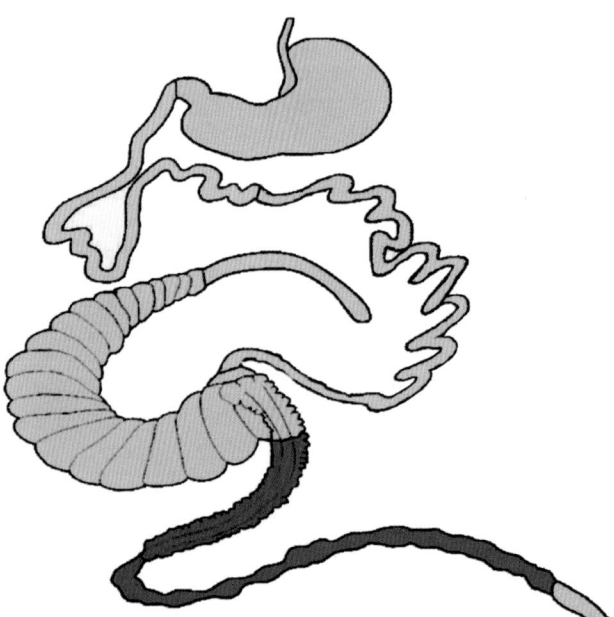

Fig. 15.16 Predilection site of *Eimeria pyriformis*.

Parasites of the liver

Capillaria hepatica

Capillaria hepatica, synonyms *Callodium hepatica*, *Hepaticola hepatica* (Phylum: Nematoda; Class: Enoplea; Order: Enoplida; Family: Capillariidae), is localised in the liver of rats, mice, squirrels, rabbits and farmed mustelids. Occasionally it infects dogs, cats and humans. For more information see section on Rats and mice.

Fasciola hepatica

Fasciola hepatica (Phylum: Platyhelminthes; Class: Trematoda; Order: Plagiorchiida ; Family: Fasciolidae), commonly known as the Liver fluke, is distributed worldwide and localised in the liver of sheep, cattle, goats, horses, deer, humans and other mammals. This parasite has snails of the genus *Galba* as intermediate hosts, in which the most common is *Galba truncatula*, an amphibious snail with a wide distribution throughout the world. For more details, see Chapter 9.

Taenia serialis

Taenia serialis, synonym *Coenurus serialis* (Phylum: Platyhelminthes; Class: Cestoda; Order: Cyclophyllidea; Family: Taeniidae), is distributed worldwide and localised in the intramuscular and subcutaneous connective tissue of intermediate hosts and the small intestine in he definitive hosts. Dogs, foxes and other canids are considered final hosts, while rabbits, hares, rarely rodents, human and primates are intermediate hosts. For more information see Chapter 12.

Eimeria stiedai

Eimeria stiedai (Phylum: Apicomplexa; Class: Conoidasida; Order: Eucoccidiorida; Family: Eimeriidae) has a worldwide distribution and is localised in the liver and bile ducts of hosts (Fig. 15.17). The sporozoites emerge from the sporocysts in the small intestine and migrate to the liver via the lymph vessels. Merogony occurs above the host cell nucleus in the epithelial cells of the bile ducts. The number of asexual generations is uncertain but there appear to be at least six. In due course, some merozoites form macrogametes and others form microgamonts. The latter produce large numbers of comma-shaped biflagellate microgametes. These fertilise the macrogametes which lay down an oocyst wall, break out of the host cell and pass into the intestine with the bile, and then out in the faeces. The prepatent period is 18 days and the patent period is 21–30 days. The sporulation time is 2–3 days.

Pathogenesis: This species, which occurs in the bile ducts, reaches the liver via the portal vein and then locates in the epithelium of the bile ducts where it results in a severe cholangitis.

Clinical signs and pathology: Grossly, the liver is enlarged and studded with white nodules (Fig. 15.18). Some of the symptoms seen are due to interference with liver function. Mild cases may be asymptomatic. In more severe infections, the animals become inappetent and lose weight. There may be diarrhoea, jaundice, ascites

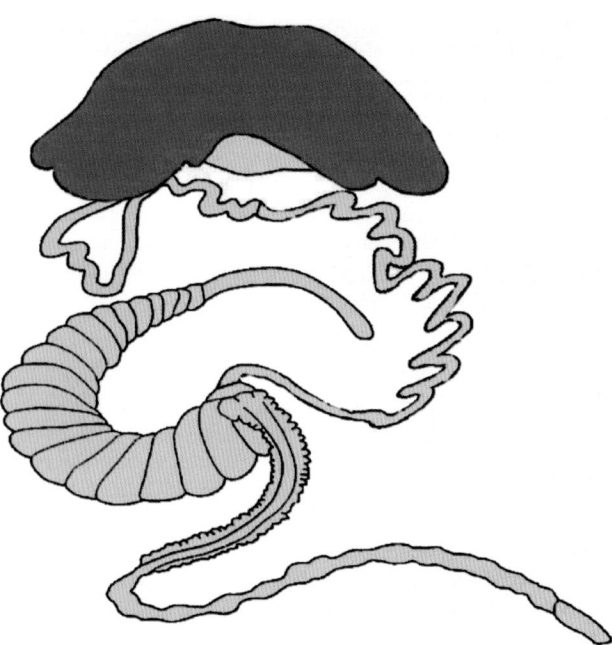

Fig. 15.17 Predilection site of *Eimeria stiedai*.

and polyuria. The symptoms may become chronic or death may occur in 21–30 days. The liver may become markedly enlarged, and white circular nodules or elongated cords may be visible. These nodules are initially sharply circumscribed but later coalesce. The bile ducts are grossly enlarged and filled with developing parasites. There is pronounced hyperplasia of the bile duct epithelial cells and the epithelium is thrown into folds. Each cell contains one or more parasites (Figs 15.19 and 15.20).

Other parasites found in the liver of wild rabbits are listed in the parasite checklist at the end of the chapter.

Parasites of the circulatory system

Rickettsia conorii

Rickettsia conorii (Kingdom: Bacteria; Phylum: Proteobacteria; Class: Alphaproteobacteria; Order: Rickettsiales; Family: Rickettsiaceae) causes a disease commonly known as Boutonneuse fever, Mediterranean spotted fever, Indian tick typhus and East African tick typhus, and is distributed in southern Europe, Africa, India and the Oriental region. The bacterium is localised in the blood of rodents, dogs, cattle, sheep, goats and humans. For a more detailed description see Chapter 12.

Hepatozoon cuniculi

Hepatozoon cuniculi (Phylum: Apicomplexa; Class: Conoidasida; Order: Eucoccidiorida; Family: Hepatozoidae) is localised in the spleen of rabbits and is distributed in Italy. The pathological effect of this protozoon is unknown.

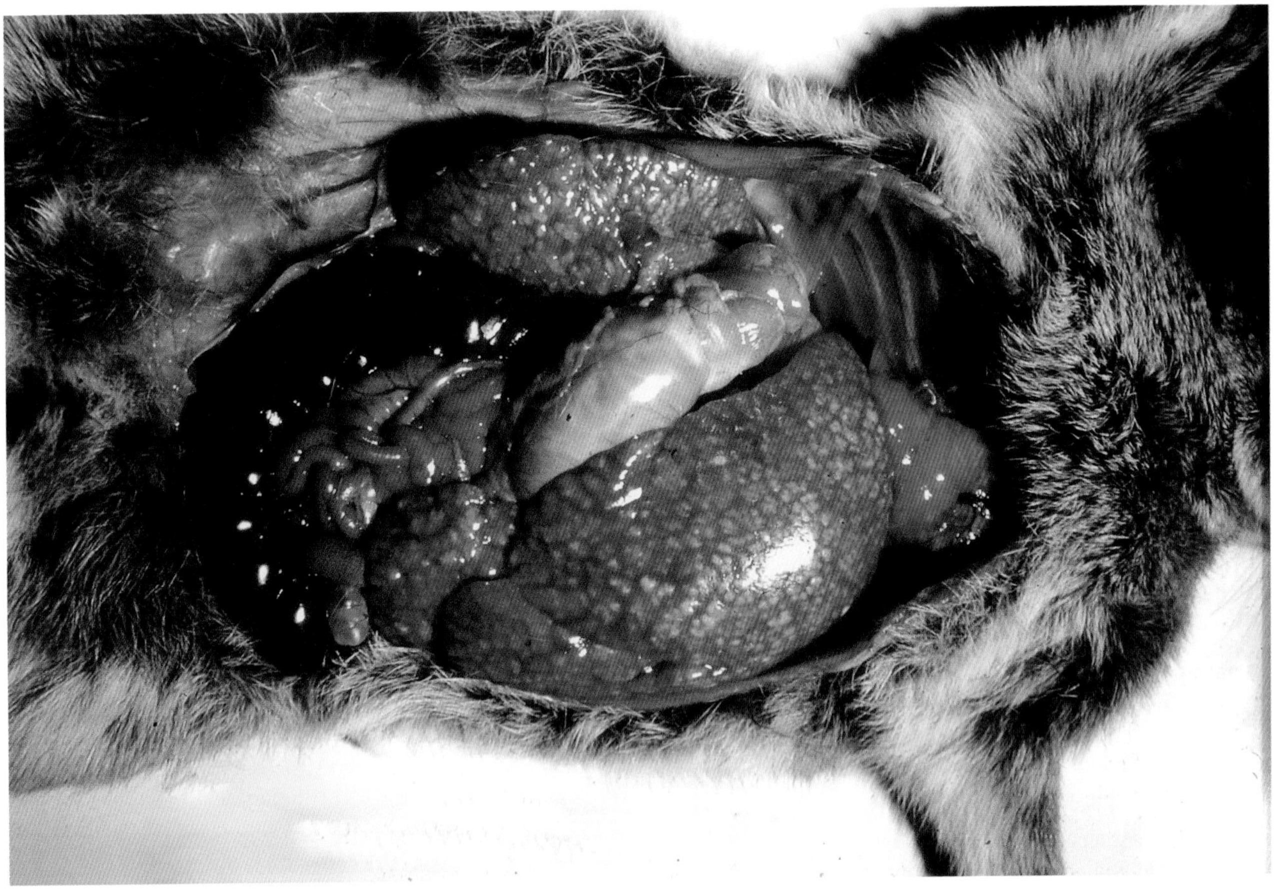

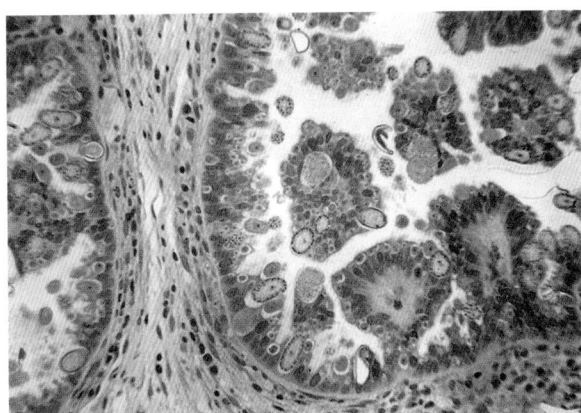

Fig. 15.18 Rabbit liver infected with *Eimeria stiedai*.

Parasites of the nervous system

Encephalitozoon cuniculi

Encephalitozoon cuniculi, synonym *Nosema cuniculi* (Phylum: Microsporidia; Class: Microsporea; Order: Microsporida; Family: Unikaryonidae), is localised in the blood of rabbits, dogs, red foxes (*Vulpes vulpes*), blue foxes (*Alopex lagopus*), silver foxes, cats, mice, rats, humans and monkeys. It has a cosmopolitan distribution.

Epidemiology: Transplacental infection occurs in rabbits and rodents but is probably rare, with most infections in these animals acquired by ingestion of spores. Evidence suggests that infection in rabbits is common in many countries.

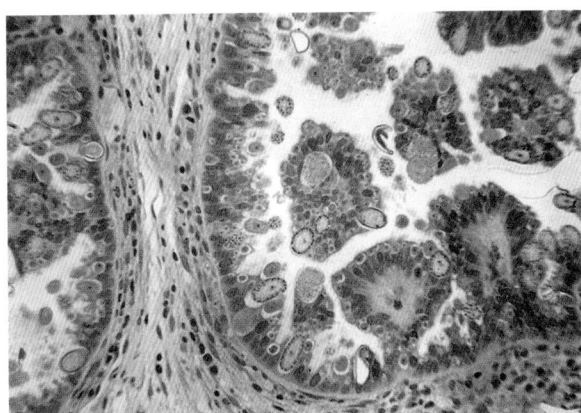

Fig. 15.19 Hyperplastic bile duct epithelium with endogenous stages of *Eimeria stiedai*.

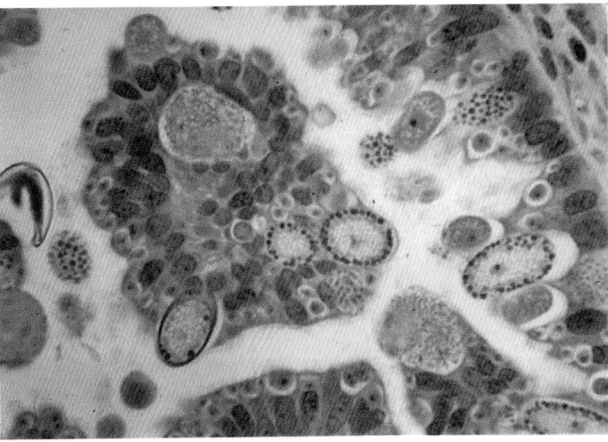

Fig. 15.20 Gamonts of *Eimeria stiedai*.

Pathogenesis: In rabbits, infection is very common, causing granuloma formation in the kidneys, liver and brain. Infection in the brain causes convulsions, tremors, torticollis, ataxia, urinary incontinence, coma and death.

Clinical signs and pathology: Many infected rabbits are asymptomatic, although clinical signs such as head tilt, urinary incontinence, posterior paresis and anterior uveitis have been reported. In the rabbit, microscopic lesions consist of focal granulomas and pseudocysts in the brain and kidneys, with occasional severe focal interstitial nephritis.

Diagnosis: Diagnosis in the live animal is difficult and is usually based on identifying the lesions on histopathology and observation of the organisms in Giemsa, Gram or Goodpasture-carbol fuchsin stains. A serum enzyme-linked immunosorbent assay (ELISA) is available.

Control and treatment: Control in rabbits depends on testing individuals, isolation and treatment. The primary source of infection is urinary excretion and ingestion of spores. Strict hygiene should therefore be followed, with raised food dishes and use of water bottles rather than bowls. Rabbits should not be housed in tiered hutches where urine contamination of cages below is common. Treatment with benzimidazoles (fenbendazole, oxfendazole and albendazole) has been reported in rabbits. Fenbendazole 20 mg/kg for 28 days, or albendazole 10–15 mg/kg for three months, can be given. Corticosteroids may suppress granuloma formation but should be used with caution.

Notes: There are reports of *E. cuniculi* acting as a zoonosis, particularly in immunocompromised individuals. Three strains of *Encephalitozoon* have been identified: strain I ('rabbit strain'), strain II ('rodent strain') and strain III ('dog strain'). Each of the three strains has been reported in humans and infections in rabbits may therefore pose a potential zoonotic risk.

Parasites of the reproductive/ urogenital system

No parasites of veterinary significance reported.

Parasites of the locomotory system

Toxoplasma gondii

Toxoplasma gondii (Phylum: Apicomplexa; Class: Conoidasida; Order: Eucoccidiorida; Family: Sarcocystidae) has as intermediate hosts any mammal, including humans, or birds, and as final hosts cats and other felids. This species is localised in the muscle, lung, liver, reproductive system and central nervous system of hosts. For more details see Chapter 9.

Sarcocystis cuniculi

Sarcocystis cuniculi (Phylum: Apicomplexa; Class: Conoidasida; Order: Eucoccidiorida; Family: Sarcocystidae) is distributed worldwide, and localised in the muscle of cats (final host) or rabbits (intermediate host) with no pathogenic effects.

Epidemiology: Little is known of the epidemiology but it is clear that where cats are able to hunt or catch rabbits then transmission is likely. The longevity of the sporocysts shed in the faeces is not known.

Diagnosis: Diagnosis is made by microscopic identification of the characteristic cysts. They may sometimes be visible macroscopically.

Pelecitus scapiceps

Pelecitus scapiceps, synonyms *Dirofilaria scapiceps*, *Loaina scapiceps* (Phylum: Nematoda; Class: Chromadorea; Order: Spirurida; Family: Onchocercidae), is distributed in North America and elsewhere, and is localised in the synovial sheaths of the feet of rabbits and hares. This nematode has several species of mosquitoes as intermediate hosts. This filarioid is usually non-pathogenic. Swelling and tenosynovitis can occur in affected tissues. Control and treatment are usually not necessary.

Diagnosis: At necropsy, adult worms may be seen in the connective tissue surrounding the tendons of the hock and occasionally in the intermuscular fascia near the knee joint. Microfilariae may be seen in blood smears if the host has a patent infection.

ECTOPARASITES

Mites

Psoroptes cuniculi

Psoroptes cuniculi, synonyms *Psoroptes ovis*, *Psoroptes cervinus*, *Psoroptes bovis*, *Psoroptes equi* (Phylum: Arthropoda; Class: Arachnida; Subclass: Acari; Order: Sarcoptiformes (Astigmata); Family: Psoroptidae), commonly known as the Ear canker mite, is a non-burrowing mite localised in the ears of rabbits (particularly in farmed or laboratory animals), goats, sheep and horses. It is found worldwide.

Epidemiology: When in its preclinical phase deep in the ear, transmission between animals is uncommon. In many cases the infestation remains localised within the ear, particularly if the host is healthy and in good condition. However, if the infestation spreads out of the ear, transmission is more likely, primarily through physical contact but also via the environment. The classification of *Psoroptes* mites is complex and *P. cuniculi* shows minimal genetic or morphological differentiation from *P. ovis*. Species designation is based on the site of infestation, and whether *P. cuniculi* is a genuine species requires further investigation.

Pathogenesis: Mites described as *P. cuniculi* occur in the ears, where the mites may be found at relatively low intensities but occasionally proliferate, causing severe mange in which the auditory canal may be completely blocked with greyish debris. If untreated, the infection may extend over the rest of the body with scabs, loss of hair and excoriation from scratching. The initial preclinical stages may last for several months, during which the infestation is difficult to spot and causes few obvious problems to the infested rabbit. Mites are non-burrowing and therefore are found only in exudate, not in tissue.

Clinical signs and pathology: In the initial stages of the infection, small skin scales appear deep in the ear canal. These yellow-grey scales can be relatively thick; they contain large numbers of parasites, mite eggs, skin cells and blood. If untreated, the scales begin to crust and may eventually grow to a thickness of 10 mm and fill the ear in severe cases. Scratching behaviour and shaking of the head may occur, and scabs and loss of hair may be observed in the ears. At low population densities, little pathology may be evident. In a rapidly expanding population, however, there may be chronic erosive and proliferative eosinophilic dermatitis. Eventually, the mites may spread out of the ear and over the rest of the body. However, once on the body, they would be indistinguishable from *P. ovis*.

Diagnosis: A sample of scab should be taken from the infected area. When placed in a glass jar or beaker, the highly mobile mites will leave the scab and start to migrate up the sides of the jar. They can then be collected and examined under a microscope for key features: oval outline, all legs projecting beyond the body margin, three-jointed pretarsus.

Control and treatment: All in-contact animals should be treated. The housing must be disinfected to prevent reinfection. The off-host survival time is probably the same as for *P. ovis* at around 18 days. Regular inspection of the animal, paying particular attention to the ears, should help to control the parasite and reduce the effects of subsequent infestations. Treatment is as for otodectic mange of cats and dogs. Insecticidal preparations, such as diazinon applied daily for four days and repeated in 10 days, have been found to be effective. Treatment with injected ivermectin is highly successful. The infected bedding should be burnt and the housing thoroughly disinfected. The crust will resolve itself, without the need to clean the ears, falling off approximately 10 days after the first treatment.

Cheyletiella parasitivorax

Cheyletiella parasitivorax (Phylum: Arthropoda; Class: Arachnida; Subclass: Acari; Order: Trombidiformes (Prostigmata); Family: Cheyletidae), commonly known as the Rabbit fur mite (Fig. 15.21), is most frequently found in the fur of rabbits on the dorsum, above the tail and on the neck but may occur all over the body. It occurs worldwide but particularly in North America, Europe, Asia, Australia and New Zealand.

Epidemiology: *Cheyletiella parasitivorax* is a common fur mite of rabbits. It is highly contagious and can spread rapidly through rabbit colonies. Transmission is usually by direct contact with infested animals, although the parasite can survive for over 10 days off the host and therefore bedding and housing can act as a source of infestation.

Pathogenesis: *Cheyletiella* is relatively common in rabbits but the mite is not highly pathogenic at low densities and is often found in young animals in good physical condition. It is a characteristic of the dermatitis caused by *Cheyletiella* that many skin scales are shed into the fur, giving it a powdery or mealy appearance, and the presence of moving mites among this debris has given it the common name of 'walking dandruff'. There is usually very little skin reaction or pruritus. In the rare severe case, involving much of the body surface, crusts are formed. *Cheyletiella parasitivorax* is capable of transmitting the myxomatosis virus among European rabbits.

Clinical signs and pathology: Infestation can result in eczema-like skin conditions and associated pruritus and hair loss. Severe cases may show serous exudate and extensive alopecia. The pathology of *Cheyletiella* infestation is poorly understood. In many cases there is very little skin reaction or pruritus. However, in severe cases rabbits may show alopecia with red scaly skin and dermatitis with hyperkeratosis.

Diagnosis: In any case of excessive scurf or dandruff, *Cheyletiella* should be considered in the differential diagnosis. On parting the coat along the back, and especially over the sacrum, scurf will be seen, and if this is combed out on to dark paper, the movement of mites will be detected among the debris. Skin scraping is not necessary as the mites are always on the skin surface or in the coat.

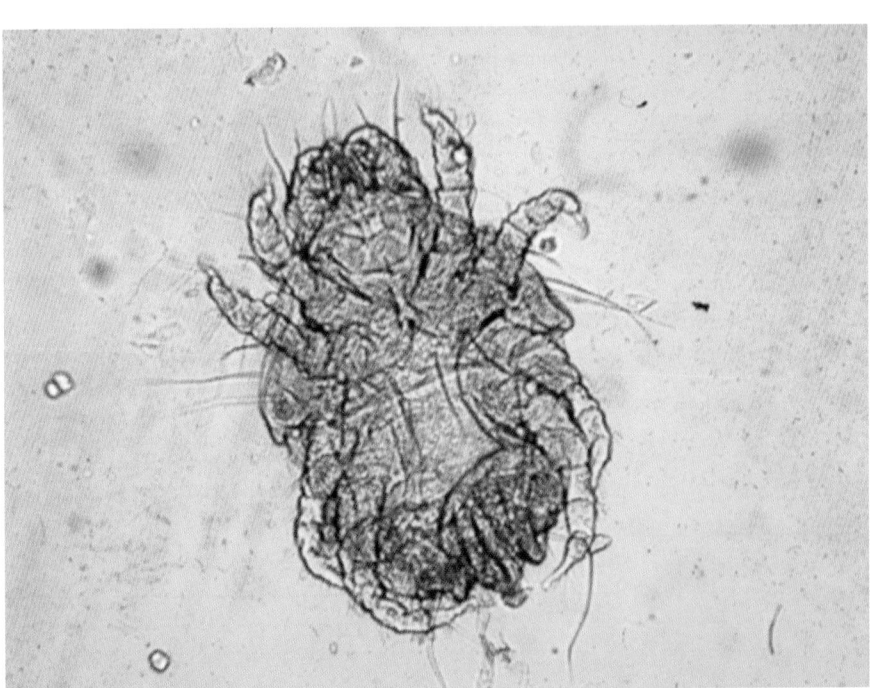

Fig. 15.21 *Cheyletiella parasitivorax.*

Control and treatment: All in-contact animals should be treated, bedding replaced and housing disinfected. Topical acaricides, such as pyrethrin and dichlorvos-containing sprays, are effective against *Cheyletiella*. Systemic treatment with ivermectin on three occasions, seven days apart, is effective. Selamectin spot-on has also been used effectively. Fipronil should only be used with great caution because it has been associated with deaths in some cases.

Notes: Of all the mite infestations of domestic animals, this is one of the most readily transferable to humans. The mites can penetrate clothing and are easily transferred, even on short periods of contact. It is often found that when a positive diagnosis has been made on a pet, there is a history of persistent skin rash in the owner's family. In contrast to the condition in its natural hosts, the infestation in humans causes severe irritation and intense pruritus. The early sign is an erythema, which may progress to a vesicular and pustular eruption. Cases in humans invariably resolve spontaneously when the animal source has been treated.

Leporacarus gibbus

Leporacarus gibbus, synonyms *Listrophorus gibbus*, *Listracarus gibbus* (Phylum: Arthropoda; Subclass: Acari; Class: Arachnida; Order: Sarcoptiformes (Astigmata); Family: Listrophoridae), commonly known as the Rabbit fur mite, is a non-burrowing mite occasionally present at low to moderate densities on domestic rabbits. It occurs worldwide. Treatment and control are as for *C. parasitivorax*.

Pathogenesis and clinical signs: *Leporacarus gibbus* may co-occur with *C. parasitivorax*. This mite is generally considered to be non-pathogenic and is found primarily on the back and abdomen.

Diagnosis: Hair plucks can be examined under a dissecting microscope or with a hand lens for the characteristic brown mite or its eggs.

For occasional mite parasites of rabbits, see Table 15.2.

Fleas

Spilopsyllus cuniculi

Spilopsyllus cuniculi (Phylum: Arthropoda; Class: Insecta; Order: Siphonaptera; Family: Pulicidae), commonly known as the Rabbit flea or European rabbit flea (Fig. 15.22), is most frequently found on the ears of rabbits and hares but may also infest dogs and cats. It occurs worldwide.

Epidemiology: The fleas can survive for up to nine months at low temperatures without feeding. The main method of transmission is from the mother to her young.

Table 15.2 Occasional mite parasites of rabbits.

Notoedres cati (see Chapter 12)
Chorioptes bovis (see Chapter 8)
Sarcoptes scabiei (see Chapter 11)
Neotrombicula autumnalis (see Chapter 17)
Dermanyssus gallinae (see Chapter 13)

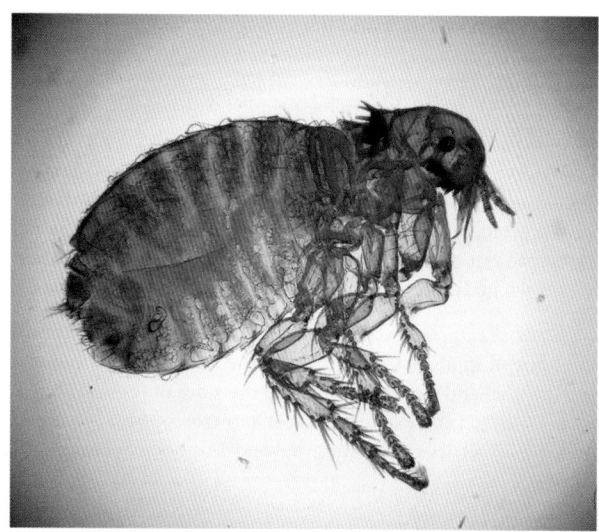

Fig. 15.22 *Spilopsyllus cuniculi.*

Pathogenesis: When rabbits are not breeding, the distribution of *S. cuniculi* is related to skin temperature, with fleas usually congregating on the ears. Because they assemble here in large numbers, the intensity of bites may cause considerable irritation and tissue damage. The rabbit flea may also be found on cats and dogs which hunt or frequent rabbit habitats. On these hosts, they are commonly found on the face and attached to the margin of the pinna. *Spilopsyllus cuniculi* is the main vector of myxomatosis and also transmits the non-pathogenic *Trypanosoma nabiasi*.

Clinical signs and pathology: These fleas may cause a great deal of irritation and tissue damage at the congregation sites on the ears.

Diagnosis: The fleas may be seen on the skin of the host animal, particularly around the ears. They have a more sedentary habit than most fleas, and will remain on the ear even when it is handled.

Control and treatment: Control is not usually considered necessary. In cases of repeated infestation, the source should be identified and contact prevented; all in-contact animals should be treated; bedding should be replaced and housing disinfected. Imidacloprid may be used in rabbits to kill adult fleas on contact. Fipronil should only be used with extreme care in rabbits due to its potential toxicity.

Table 15.3 lists species of fleas which have also been found on rabbits. For more details see also Chapter 3.

Flies

Lucilia sericata

Lucilia sericata, synonym *Phaenicia sericata* (Phylum: Arthropoda; Class: Insecta; Order: Diptera; Family: Calliphoridae), is commonly known as the Greenbottle or Sheep blowfly. The larvae cause myiasis

Table 15.3 Occasional flea parasites of rabbits.

Ctenocephalides felis (see Chapter 12)
Ctenocephalides canis (see Chapter 12)
Echidnophaga gallinacae (see Chapter 13)

in rabbits and may be found worldwide, particularly in temperate areas.

Epidemiology: Seasonal risk is associated with the presence of flies; hence it is predominantly a summer problem in temperate areas but may occur all year round in warmer areas.

Pathogenesis: Blowfly strike of domestic rabbits and occasionally other domestic mammals and birds may be very common, particularly if dirty, debilitated by clinical disease or wounded. Strike is a very serious condition in rabbits and death may result within a few days.

Clinical signs and pathology: Infested animals show extensive skin ulceration, shock, weakness, depression, lethargy and anorexia. Struck animals have a rapid increase in body temperature and respiratory rate. They show extensive tissue damage, become anaemic and suffer severe toxaemia. Infestation is most common around the anus, and may be associated with wet faecally soiled fur, often when rabbits are fed an inappropriate diet or are unable to groom themselves.

Diagnosis: This is based on the clinical signs and recognition of maggots in the lesion.

Control and treatment: Once the problem is diagnosed, the area surrounding the lesion should be clipped. Where possible, larvae should be removed. The use of a hair-drier, at a low heat setting, to direct dry air towards the maggots has been reported as an effective way to cause them to drop off the host. However, in advanced infestations the rabbit may require sedation, intravenous fluid therapy and analgesia. Ivermectin may be used to kill any remaining feeding larvae. Unless caught in its early stages, the prognosis must be guarded, since myiasis can be extremely damaging to rabbits relatively quickly. To prevent fly strike, formulations of pour-on cyromazine are available specifically for rabbits, offering prevention for up to 8–10 weeks. Longer-term steps should be taken to prevent diarrhoea and faecal contamination of the hair, either through worm control or diet as required.

Note: Several other species of blowfly or fleshfly may also strike rabbits in various parts of the world. The treatment is as described above for *L. sericata*.

Wohlfahrtia vigil

Wohlfahrtia vigil (Phylum: Arthropoda; Class: Insecta; Order: Diptera; Family: Sarcophagidae), commonly known as the Grey flesh fly, is an obligate agent of myiasis that primarily infests mink, foxes, rabbits and other wild mammals. Dogs and cats may also occasionally be attacked. It is found throughout North, Central and South America.

Pathogenesis: *Wohlfahrtia vigil* can cause rapid and severe myiasis in most animals. The myiasis caused is furuncular rather than cutaneous. Furuncles similar to those of *Dermatobia* are produced, although those of *W. vigil* can contain up to five larvae with a small pore opening to the outside.

Cuterebra

For details see section on Rats and mice.

GUINEA PIGS

ENDOPARASITES

Parasites of the digestive system

Small intestine

Hymenolepis diminuta

For details see section on Rats and mice.

Hymenolepis nana

For details see section on Rats and mice.

Eimeria caviae

Eimeria caviae (Phylum: Apicomplexa; Class: Conoidasida; Order: Eucoccidiorida; Family: Eimeriidae) is distributed worldwide, and is localised in the large intestine of guinea pigs. Following ingestion of oocysts, sporozoites enter the intestinal epithelium to become first-generation meronts. Following a further three merogony generations, gamonts appear in epithelial cells of the large intestine, leading to the excretion of oocysts in the faeces. The prepatent period is about seven days and the patent period approximately 4–5 days.

Epidemiology: Crowding and lack of good sanitation promote the spread of coccidiosis. Breeding establishments and rescue centres are potential sources of infection. Older guinea pigs are generally immune from disease but may seed the environment with oocysts, leading to infection in young animals that have no previous exposure.

Pathogenesis: *Eimeria caviae* is usually non-pathogenic but may occasionally cause diarrhoea and mortality.

Clinical signs and pathology: Clinical signs include unthriftiness and poor weight gain in young animals; droppings are slimy and contain blood. Lesions seen at *post mortem* occur in the mucosa of the colon and consist of small white or pale yellow plaques and petechial haemorrhages. In severe infections, the whole mucosa may be destroyed. There have also been reports of hepatomegaly with focal necrosis containing oocysts.

Diagnosis: Diagnosis is based on identification of oocysts in the faeces in association with clinical and pathological findings.

Control and treatment: Good sanitation and isolation are effective measures in preventing coccidiosis. If possible, guinea pigs should be housed on wire floor cages to reduce the incidence of infection. Standard disinfectants are ineffective against coccidial oocysts but ammonia-based products are effective. Information on treatment in the guinea pig is scanty, although by analogy with other host species, the use of sulfonamides, such as sulfamezathine, should be tried.

Cryptosporidium wrairi

Cryptosporidium wrairi (Phylum: Apicomplexa; Class: Conoidasida; Order: Cryptogregarinorida; Family: Cryptosporidiidae) has an unknown distribution, and is localised in the small intestine of guinea pigs.

Epidemiology: The primary route of infection is mainly direct animal-to-animal transmission via the faecal–oral route.

Pathogenesis: The infection has only been reported in small guinea pigs (weighing 200–300 g) and is not associated with diarrhoea or overt signs of disease.

Clinical signs and pathology: Clinical signs are usually inapparent. There may be chronic enteritis depending on the severity of infection. Lesions are usually focal when only limited areas of the intestine are affected. The organisms are more numerous in the posterior ileum and are distributed over the entire surface of the intestinal villi but are more numerous towards the tips and absent in the crypts. Control and treatment are not required.

Diagnosis: Oocysts may be detected using Ziehl–Neelsen stained faecal smears in which the sporozoites appear as bright red granules. Speciation of *Cryptosporidium* is difficult, if not impossible, using conventional techniques. A range of molecular and immunological techniques has been developed that includes immunofluorescence and ELISA. More recently, DNA-based techniques have been used for the molecular characterisation of *Cryptosporidium* species.

Giardia intestinalis

For more details see Chapter 12.

Large intestine

Paraspidodera uncinata

Paraspidodera uncinata (Phylum: Nematoda; Class: Chromadorea; Order: Ascaridida; Family: Aspidoderidae) is distributed worldwide, and is localised in the large intestine of guinea pigs and agoutis.

Epidemiology: This caecal worm occurs naturally in the caecum and colon of the wild guinea pig in South America and in laboratory guinea pigs around the world. Infection is usually associated with guinea pigs housed in outdoor runs. It is generally considered non-pathogenic.

Clinical signs and pathology: Heavy infections may cause weight loss, debility and diarrhoea.

Diagnosis: Diagnosis is based on the identification of eggs in the faeces or adult worms in the large intestine.

Control and treatment: Control is based on good hygiene and management. To treat, piperazine 3 g/l in the drinking water for seven days is effective. Ivermectin 200–500 µg/kg body weight given subcutaneously is also likely to be effective.

A number of protozoa are found in the caecum of the guinea pig. All are considered non-pathogenic. *Entamoeba caviae* and *Tritrichomonas caviae* are common in the caeca of laboratory guinea pigs (see checklist table).

Parasites of the respiratory system

No parasites of veterinary significance reported.

Parasites of the liver

No parasites of veterinary significance reported.

Parasites of the circulatory system

No parasites of veterinary significance reported.

Parasites of the nervous system

No parasites of veterinary significance reported.

Parasites of the reproductive/urogenital system

Klossiella cobayae

Klossiella cobayae (Phylum: Apicomplexa; Class: Conoidasida; Order: Eucoccidiorida; Family: Klossiellidae) is distributed worldwide, and is localised in the kidney of guinea pigs. The mature zygote is 30–40 µm in diameter and produces 30 or more sporocysts each containing about 30 sporozoites. Control and treatment are not required.

Epidemiology: Sporocysts are passed in the urine and infection takes place by the ingestion of sporulated sporocysts.

Clinical signs and pathology: It is usually considered non-pathogenic. A chronic to subacute nephritis with degenerative lesions has been described. Only heavily parasitised kidneys have gross lesions, which appear as tiny grey foci on the cortical surface. Microscopically, these foci are areas of necrosis, with perivascular infiltration of inflammatory cells, especially lymphocytes, with an increase in interstitial fibroblasts.

Diagnosis: Sporocysts may be detected in urine sediments or trophozoite stages may be found on *post mortem* in the kidney. The site and location are pathognomonic.

Parasites of the locomotory system

Toxoplasma gondii

For more details see section on Rabbits (Parasites of the locomotory system).

Parasites of the integument

No parasites reported.

ECTOPARASITES

Lice

Gyropus ovalis

Gyropus ovalis (Phylum: Arthropoda; Class: Insecta; Order: Psocodea; Suborder: Amblycera; Family: Gyropidae) is commonly known as the Guinea pig louse and is found on the skin of guinea pigs and rodents. It occurs worldwide (see Fig. 3.63).

Epidemiology: Infection occurs after direct contact with an infested host animal. Cross-contamination between different host species is possible if the animals have physical contact.

Pathogenesis: This species tears pieces of skin until blood pools and then feeds from these pools. Underlying skin may be dry or oily and thickened or crusty. Severely infected animals may show secondary bacterial infection and stress, including weight loss. Infestation often accompanies manifestations of poor health, such as internal parasitism, infectious disease, malnutrition and poor sanitation.

Clinical signs and pathology: The signs of infestation are variable. Light infestation may have no obvious effects but pruritus, dermatitis, scratching and hair loss are usually evident with heavier parasite loads.

Diagnosis: The lice and their eggs can be seen on the skin of the host animal when the hair is parted.

Control and treatment: Prevention of infestation includes the use of clean bedding, which should be changed regularly. The cage and other areas where guinea pigs roam should be cleaned and rinsed thoroughly with a diluted bleach solution. Since lice spend their entire life on the host animal, control is readily achieved through the use of topical insecticides. Treatment of *G. ovalis* involves dusting of the guinea pig and bedding with carbaryl 5% powder lightly once per week, dipping in 2.5% lime-sulfur solution once per weeks for 4–6 weeks, or treatment with ivermectin. However, since the eggs are quite resistant to most insecticides, repeat treatments 14 days apart are recommended to kill newly hatched nymphs. Imidacloprid is a very safe and effective treatment for guinea pig lice and can be used on pregnant females and newly weaned young. One application lasts for 30 days.

Notes: Closely related to the very similar *Gliricola porcelli*.

Gliricola porcelli

Gliricola porcelli (Phylum: Arthropoda; Class: Insecta; Order: Psocodea; Suborder: Amblycera; Family: Gyropidae), commonly known as the Guinea pig louse, is a very similar species to *G. ovalis* and is found in the body fur of guinea pigs worldwide. For pathogenesis, treatment and control, see *G. ovalis*.

Trimenopon hispidium

Trimenopon hispidium (Phylum: Arthropoda; Class: Insecta; Order: Psocodea; Suborder: Amblycera; Family: Trimenoponidae), commonly known as the Guinea pig louse, occurs in the hair of guinea pigs worldwide.

Pathogenesis: Lice of this genus are very rare and light infestations are easily overlooked. Occasional heavy infestations may cause excessive scratching leading to alopecia and a roughened coat. For treatment and control see *G. ovalis*.

Mites

Chirodiscoides caviae

Chirodiscoides caviae, synonym *Campylochirus caviae* (Phylum: Arthropoda; Class: Arachnida; Subclass: Acari; Order: Sarcoptiformes (Astigmata); Family: Atopomelidae), commonly known as the Guinea pig fur mite, is found on the skin of guinea pigs worldwide (see Fig. 3.102). New hosts are infected by contact with infested individuals.

Pathogenesis: *Chirodiscoides caviae* is commonly found on Guinea pigs. Light infestations probably have little effect and are easily overlooked. The mites may cause inflammation, scaling, crusting and pruritic dermatitis, leading to scratching and alopecia.

Clinical signs: Subclinical cases may be asymptomatic; clinical cases show pruritus and alopecia usually along the posterior trunk of the body.

Diagnosis: For confirmatory diagnosis, coat brushings must be examined; *C. caviae* is found only in the fur.

Control and treatment: Systemic treatment with ivermectin on three occasions, seven days apart, may be effective. All in-contact animals should be treated and the cage or housing should be cleaned.

Trixacarus caviae

Trixacarus caviae (Phylum: Arthropoda; Class: Arachnida; Subclass: Acari; Order: Sarcoptiformes (Astigmata); Family: Sarcoptidae), commonly known as the Guinea pig mite (Fig. 15.23), is found on the skin of guinea pigs; it originated in South America but has now spread worldwide.

Epidemiology: *Trixacarus caviae* superficially resembles *Sarcoptes scabiei*. New hosts are infected by contact with infected individuals.

Table 15.4 shows the differentiation among adult female *Trixacarus caviae*, *Sarcoptes scabiei* and *Notoedres cati*.

Pathogenesis: These are burrowing mites, and the burrowing activity results in irritation, inflammation and pruritus, causing biting, scratching and rubbing of the infested areas and leading to alopecia. The infestation spreads quickly from the initial lesions to cause more generalised mange. Death may occur within 3–4 months of infestation. Transmission is by close physical contact and from mother to offspring.

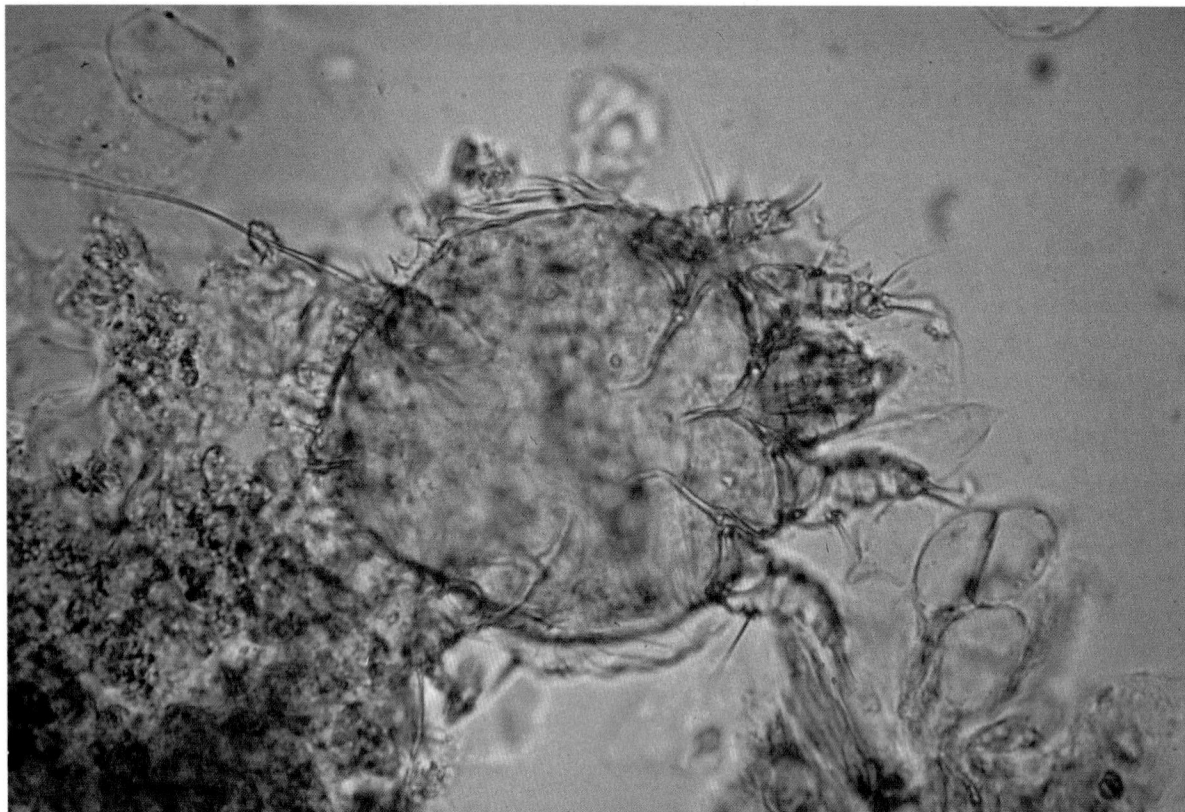

Fig. 15.23 *Trixacarus caviae.*

Clinical signs and pathology: Infestation causes irritation, biting, scratching, rubbing and general restlessness. Affected areas display marked acanthosis and hyperkeratosis and may become secondarily infected with bacteria.

Diagnosis: Confirmatory diagnosis is by examination of skin scrapings for the presence of mites. However, since these are sometimes difficult to demonstrate, a negative finding should not preclude a tentative diagnosis of mange and initiation of treatment.

Control and treatment: All bedding must be replaced, and housing and the guinea pig's local environment thoroughly cleaned. Ivermectin may be administered twice at intervals of 7–10 days.

For further details about *Sarcoptes* mites, see Chapter 3.

Demodex caviae

Demodex caviae (Phylum: Arthrpoda; Class: Arachnida; Subclass: Acari; Order: Trombidiformes (Prostigmata); Family: Demodicidae)

Table 15.4 Differentiation between adult female *Trixacarus caviae*, *Sarcoptes scabiei* and *Notoedres cati*.

	Trixacarus caviae	*Sarcoptes scabiei*	*Notoedres cati*
Length (µm)	230–240	400–430	225–250
Anus position	Dorsal	Terminal	Dorsal
Dorsal setae	All dorsal setae simple (not spine-like)	Some stout dorsal spines	All dorsal setae simple (not spine-like)
Dorsal scales	Many, pointed	Many, pointed	Few, rounded

is localised in the hair follicles and sebaceous glands of guinea pigs, found worldwide.

Psoroptes cuniculi

Psoroptes cuniculi, synonyms *Psoroptes ovis*, *Psoroptes cervinus*, *Psoroptes bovis*, *Psoroptes equi*, *Psoroptes aucheniae* (Phylum: Arthropoda; Class: Arachnida; Subclass: Acari; Order: Astigmata (Sarcoptiformes); Family: Psoroptidae), commonly known as the Ear canker mite, is localised in the ear canals of guinea pigs and is found worldwide. For details, see section on Rabbits.

RATS AND MICE

ENDOPARASITES

Parasites of the digestive system

Small intestine

Nippostrongylus brasiliensis

Nippostrongylus brasiliensis, synonyms *Nippostrongylus muris*, *Heligmosomum muris* (Phylum: Nematoda; Class: Chromadorea; Order: Rhabditida; Family: Helligmoneillidae), is distributed worldwide and is localised in the small intestine of rats, mice, hamsters, gerbils, rabbits and chinchillas.

Epidemiology: This parasite is common in wild rats but can become problematic in animal colonies where management and sanitation are poor.

Pathogenesis: Initial light infections cause inflammation of the skin, lungs and intestines. Severe infections cause verminous pneumonia and death.

Diagnosis: Diagnosis depends on the identification of the eggs in faeces or adult worms in the intestine on *post mortem*.

Control and treatment: In laboratory colonies of rodents, eradication depends on strict hygiene and good management. Piperazine 5 g/l in the drinking water and ivermectin by injection are effective.

Nematospiroides dubius

Nematospiroides dubius, synonym *Heligmosomoides polygyrus* (Phylum: Nematoda; Class: Chromadorea; Order: Rhabditida; Family: Helligmoneillidae), is distributed in North America and Europe, and is localised in the small intestine of rats and mice.

Epidemiology: Internal autoinfection occurs in humans but infection in rodents usually involves an intermediate host.

Pathogenesis: Infections are usually asymptomatic but may produce small cysts in the intestinal wall. Diagnosis is made by the identification of the eggs in faeces or the adult worms in the small intestine. Control and treatment are as for *N. brasiliensis*.

Notes: *Nematospiroides dubius* is widely used as a laboratory model for nematode infection studies.

Hymenolepis nana

Hymenolepis nana, synonyms *Rodentolepis nana*, *Hymenolepis fraterna*, *Vampirolepis nana* (Phylum: Platyhelminthes; Class: Cestoda; Order: Cyclophyllidea; Family: Hymenolepididae), commonly known as the Dwarf tapeworm, is distributed worldwide but most frequently found in Asia, Africa, South America and parts of southern Europe. This species is localised in the small intestine of rats, mice, birds, humans and primates, and has flour beetles (*Tenebrio*) and fleas as intermediary hosts.

Epidemiology: Internal autoinfection occurs in humans but infection in rodents usually involves an intermediate host. Under conditions of poor hygiene, infected rodents will contaminate food with their faeces, leading to human infection. In addition, such an environment will support the intermediate hosts. Human prevalence is highest in children.

Pathogenesis: Infections in laboratory rodents are relatively uncommon and usually asymptomatic.

Clinical signs and pathology: Heavy infestations can cause weight loss, vomiting and occasionally obstruction of the intestine. In humans, heavy infections, may cause enteritis, anorexia and anal pruritus.

Diagnosis: Identification of the eggs in faeces or the adult worms in the small intestine.

Control and treatment: In laboratory colonies of rodents, eradication depends on strict hygiene and elimination of potential intermediate hosts. The treatment is not usually indicated. Niclosamide

mixed in powdered feed at 10 mg per 100 mg body weight for two seven-day periods, one week apart, has been reported to be effective; alternatively, praziquantel 5–10 mg/kg repeated in 10 days may be used.

Notes: *Hymenolepis nana* is of peripheral veterinary importance in that it is a common tapeworm of humans and of laboratory and wild rodents. This is the only species of tapeworm for which an intermediate host is not necessary since the parasite can also be transmitted by direct ingestion of eggs.

Hymenolepis diminuta

Hymenolepis diminuta, synonym *Rodentolepis diminuta* (Phylum: Platyhelminthes; Class: Cestoda; Order: Cyclophyllidea; Family: Hymenolepididae), commonly known as the Rat tapeworm, is localised in the small intestine of rats, mice and occasionally dogs and humans. The intermediate hosts are larvae, nymphs and adults of various species of moths, cockroaches, fleas, flour beetles and millipedes.

All other details are as for *H. nana*, except that *H. diminuta* requires an intermediate host whereas *H. nana* can complete its full life cycle within the intestinal tract of the definitive host. Because *H. diminuta* infection is dependent on ingestion of an infected insect, infection of humans is less likely to occur.

Coccidia

Eimeria nieschulzi

Eimeria nieschulzi, synonym *Eimeria halli* (Phylum: Apicomplexa; Class: Conoidasida; Order: Eucoccidiorida; Family: Eimeriidae), is distributed worldwide and localised in the small intestine of rats (*Rattus norvegicus* and *R. rattus*). Crowding and lack of good sanitation promote the spread of coccidiosis. Infection is by ingestion of sporulated oocysts. First-generation meronts occur after 36 hours followed by three further merogony generations and gametogony within the epithelial cells of the small intestine. The prepatent period is seven days and patency 4–5 days. Sporulation time is approximately 72 hours.

Pathogenesis and clinical signs: *Eimeria nieschulzi* primarily affects young animals. Those that recover are immune but disease may occur in adults under periods of stress. Infected animals may display weakness, diarrhoea and emaciation.

Diagnosis: Diagnosis is based on identification of oocysts in the faeces in association with clinical and pathological findings.

Control and treatment: Infection is usually self-limiting in the individual and colony. Good sanitation and isolation are effective measures in preventing coccidiosis. Wherever possible, rats should be housed on wire floor cages to reduce the incidence of infection. Standard disinfectants are ineffective against coccidial oocysts but ammonia-based products are effective. As treatment, none of the available anticoccidials have been reported as effective in the rat.

Eimeria falciformis

Eimeria falciformis (Phylum: Apicomplexa; Class: Conoidasida; Order: Eucoccidiorida; Family: Eimeriidae) is distributed worldwide, and is localised in the small and large intestine of mice (*Mus musculus*). Infection is by ingestion of sporulated oocysts. The number of merogony stages has not been determined. The prepatent period is four days.

Epidemiology: Crowding and lack of good sanitation promote spread of coccidiosis. Breeding establishments and laboratory mice are potential sources of infection. In one study, eight out of 10 conventional laboratory mouse colonies were found to be infected.

Clinical signs and pathology: Mild infections have little effect but severe ones cause anorexia, diarrhoea and sometimes death. Catarrhal enteritis, haemorrhage and epithelial sloughing have been reported.

Diagnosis: Diagnosis is based on identification of oocysts in the faeces in association with clinical and pathological findings.

Control and treatment: Control depends on good hygiene and isolation as effective measures in preventing coccidiosis. Wherever possible, laboratory mice should be housed on wire floor cages to reduce the incidence of infection. Standard disinfectants are ineffective against coccidial oocysts but ammonia-based products are effective. Deriving a new colony by Caesarean section can eliminate infection. As treatment, none of the available anticoccidials have been reported as effective in the mouse. Several other species of coccidia are found in rats and mice worldwide but are generally considered non-pathogenic and control measures are not usually required.

Cryptosporidium muris

Cryptosporidium muris (Phylum: Apicomplexa; Class: Conoidasida; Order: Cryptogregarinorida; Family: Cryptosporidiidae) is distributed worldwide, and is localised in the small intestine of rats, mice, hamsters, squirrels, Siberian chipmunks, wood mice (*Apodemus sylvaticus*), bank voles (*Clethrionomys glareolus*), Patagonian mara (*Dolichotis patagonum*), rock hyraxes, Bactrian camels, mountain goats, humans and cynomolgus monkeys. Transmission occurs mainly via the faecal–oral route. Infections in rodents appear to cause few pathogenic effects.

Clinical signs and pathology: Infections are usually asymptomatic, and in heavy infections there may be large numbers of parasites within the gastric glands of the stomach (pars glandularis), with meronts and gamonts extending from the isthmus down to the base of each gland (Fig. 15.24). Infection results in thickening of the glandular mucosa, with some glands becoming dilated and hypertrophied, and parasitised glands lined with undifferentiated cells.

Diagnosis: Oocysts may be demonstrated using Ziehl–Neelsen-stained faecal smears in which the sporozoites appear as bright red granules. Speciation of *Cryptosporidium* is difficult, if not impossible, using conventional techniques. A range of molecular and immunological techniques has been developed that includes ELISA. More recently, DNA-based techniques have been used for the molecular characterisation of *Cryptosporidium* species. Control and treatment are not required.

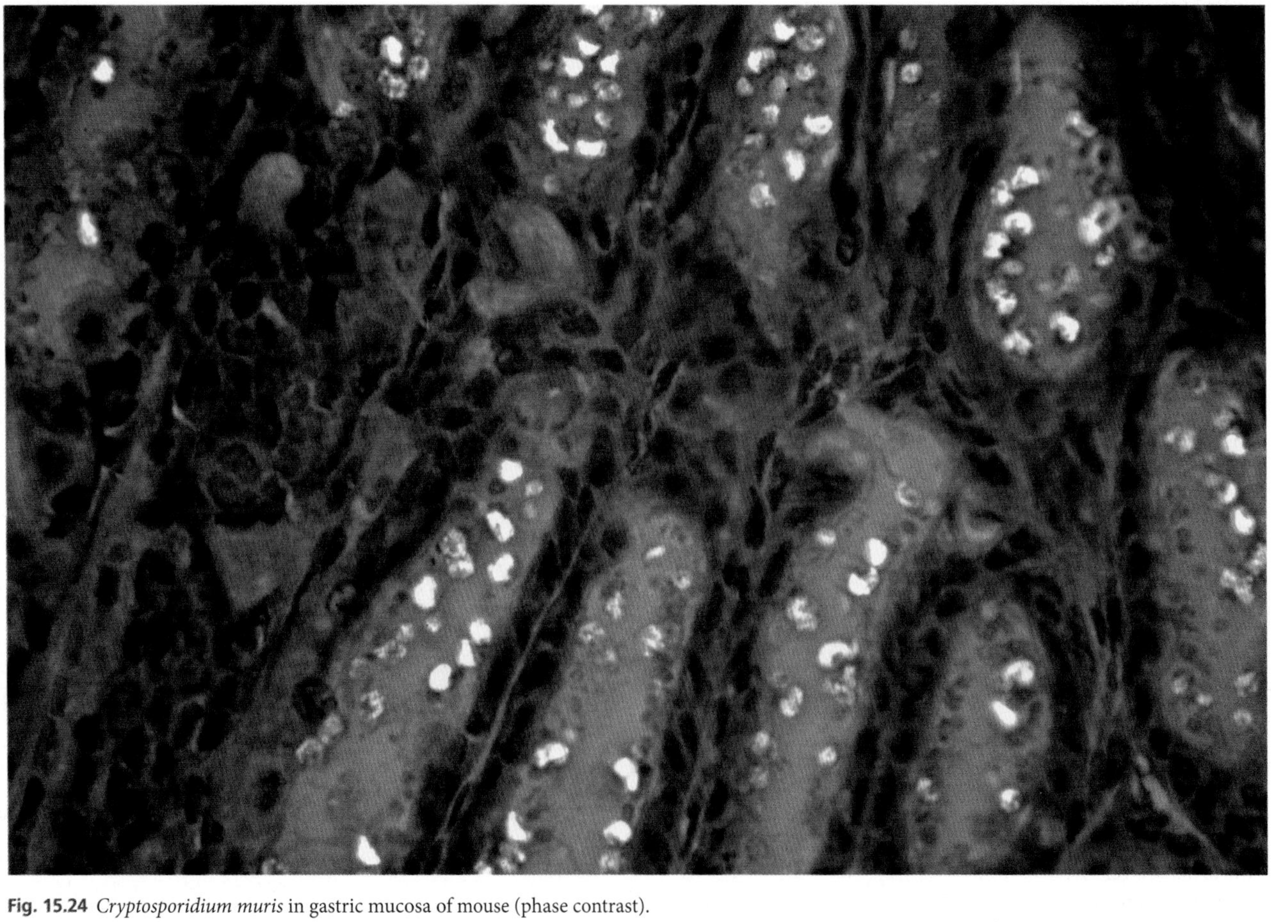

Fig. 15.24 *Cryptosporidium muris* in gastric mucosa of mouse (phase contrast).

Giardia muris

Giardia muris (Phylum: Metamonada; Class: Trepomonadea; Order: Diplomonadida; Family: Giardiidae) is distributed worldwide, and is localised in the small intestine of rodents, such as mice, rats and hamsters.

Epidemiology: Limited epidemiological studies suggest that direct animal-to-animal contact and faecal contamination are the most likely methods of transmission, although water contamination can also be considered as a possible route. Infections are generally asymptomatic.

Clinical signs and pathology: Can cause chronic enteritis in young mice. The pathology has not been described. There may be villous atrophy, crypt hypertrophy and an increased number of intraepithelial lymphocytes. Trophozoites may be seen between villi, attached by their concave surface to the brush border of epithelial cells.

Diagnosis: *Giardia* cysts can be detected in faeces by a number of methods. Traditional methods of identification involve direct examination of faecal smears, or faecal concentration by formaline-thyl acetate or zinc sulfate methods and subsequent microscopic examination. It is generally recommended that three consecutive samples be examined as cysts are excreted intermittently.

Control and treatment: As infection is transmitted by the faecal–oral route, good hygiene and prevention of faecal contamination of feed and water are essential. Metronidazole 0.5% in the drinking water for 10 days is reported to be effective.

Spironucleus muris

Spironucleus muris, synonyms *Hexamita muris*, *Octomitus muris*, *Syndyomita muris* (Phylum: Metamonada; Class: Trepamonadea; Order: Diplomonadida; Family: Spironucleidae), is localised on the small intestine and caecum of mice, rats and hamsters. Incidence of infection is occasional.

Epidemiology: Infection is common in some rodent colonies. Transmission presumably occurs by ingestion of trophozoites or cysts from faeces or by faecal contamination.

Pathogenesis, clinical signs and pathology: Infection causes enteritis and diarrhoea in laboratory rodents. With chronic infections, there is weight loss and listlessness and diarrhoea is uncommon. Lesions are generally confined to the anterior small intestine with inflammation of the duodenum, and the duodenal crypts are cystic and filled with trophozoites of *S. muris*.

Diagnosis: Identification of characteristic trophozoites in mucosal smears or on histopathology. Cysts may be seen in fresh faecal smears or in smears stained with Giemsa.

Control and treatment: Control relies mainly on good hygiene and management in rodent colonies and culling of animals with symptoms of diarrhoea unresponsive to treatment or those showing chronic weight loss.

Large intestine

Pinworms

Pinworms are relatively common but non-pathogenic parasites in the large intestine of laboratory rodents. Crowding and lack of good sanitation promote spread of infection. Diagnosis is based on identification of oocysts in the faeces. Suggested treatment is piperazine 4–7 g/ml given as three separate seven-day courses in drinking water; ivermectin 0.4 mg/kg by injection or orally twice five days apart; or fenbendazole 0.1% in feed for 3–4 weeks. However, eradication is extremely difficult and repeat anthelmintic treatment may be required. Human infections have been reported with *Syphacia* spp. in laboratory workers.

Endolimax nana

Endolimax nana, synonyms *Amoeba limax*, *Entamoeba nana*, *Entamoeba intestinalis*, *Entamoeba suis*, *Entamoeba ratti* (Phylum: Amoebozoa; Class: Archamoebea; Order: Entamoebida; Family: Entamoebidae), is distributed worldwide, is localised in the large intestine of humans, apes, monkeys, pigs and rats and is non-pathogenic protozoa.

Notes: *Endolimax nana* is common in humans, primates and pigs.

Enteromonas hominis

Enteromonas hominis, synonyms *Octomitus hominis*, *Tricercomonas intestinalis*, *E. bengalensis* (Phylum: Metamonada; Class: Trepomonadea; Order: Diplomonadida; Family: Enteromonadidae), is localised on the caecum of rats, hamsters, humans and primates (chimpanzees, macaques) with a worldwide distribution.

Parasites of the respiratory system

Angiostrongylus cantonensis

Angiostrongylus cantonensis, synonym *Parastrongylus cantonensis* (Phylum: Nematoda; Class: Chromadorea; Order: Rhabditida; Family: Angiostrongylidae), is commonly known as the Rat lungworm. This parasite is distributed in Asia and Pacific islands, Australia, India, Africa, Caribbean, parts of the USA and recently in Europe (Canary and Balearic Islands). This species is localised in the pulmonary veins of rats and humans, and has molluscs, such as land snails of the genera *Agrolimax*, *Limax* and *Deroceras*, as intermediate hosts. Crustaceans, such as prawns and crabs, and amphibians can act as paratenic hosts.

Epidemiology: Rate of infection in rats and in the intermediate hosts is usually highest during the rainy seasons.

Pathogenesis: Light infections are usually asymptomatic. Heavy infestations can lead to uncoordinated movement and weakness.

Clinical signs and pathology: There may be blood-stained fluid from the eyes and a bloody nasal discharge. The presence of parasites in the lung can cause coughing and sneezing. In humans, signs may include a stiff neck, headache, paraesthesiae, nausea, vomiting and fever. The migration of larvae is accompanied by an eosinophilic reaction. In the lung, there may be intra-alveolar haemorrhages and, in the brain, granulomatous reactions, haemorrhage and abscesses. The lung parenchyma may become consolidated.

Diagnosis: Presence of larvae in faeces. An ELISA has been developed for detection of infection in humans.

Control and treatment: Control in humans is through education and cooking of the snail hosts and thorough washing of raw vegetables and salad greens. As treatment, mebendazole and albendazole have been used. Anthelmintic treatment is not usually recommended for treatment of infection in humans.

Notes: Humans can be a paratenic host following the ingestion of infective intermediate hosts. *A. cantonensis* can cause meningitis and meningoencephalitis with mild to moderate symptoms, often of sudden onset, with intense headaches, vomiting, moderate intermittent fever and, in about 50% of cases, coughing, anorexia, malaise, constipation and somnolence, and in severe cases coma and death.

Parasites of the liver

Capillaria hepatica

Capillaria hepatica, synonyms *Callodium hepatica*, *Hepaticola hepatica* (Phylum: Nematoda; Class: Enoplea ; Order: Enoplida; Family: Capillariidae), is localised in the liver of rats, mice, squirrels, rabbits and farmed mustelids, being occasionally found in dogs, cats, humans and primates.

Epidemiology: Although the prevalence of *C. hepatica* is high in the liver of rodents, it lacks host specificity and occurs in a variety of mammals.

Pathogenesis: Adult worms are found in the parenchyma of the liver where they provoke traumatic hepatitis. Eggs are laid in groups in the liver parenchyma from which there is no natural access to the exterior. Granulomas develop around the eggs, accompanied by fibrosis. Heavy infections can cause hepatitis and/or cirrhosis and ascites. The liver may be enlarged and severe infections can be fatal.

Clinical signs and pathology: Mild infections are usually asymptomatic. At necropsy, the liver may have yellowish-white streaks on the surface. The eggs, which are deposited in clusters, provoke the development of localised granulomas, which are visible through the capsule as yellowish streaks or patches.

Diagnosis: Most infections are discovered at routine necropsy. Granulomatous tissue in the liver parenchyma can be examined for the presence of eggs or worm fragments after squashing between microscope slides.

Taenia taeniaeformis

Taenia taeniaeformis, synonyms *Hydatigera taeniaeformis*, *Taenia crassicollis*, *Cysticercus fasciolaris*, *Strobilocercus fasciolaris* (Phylum: Platyhelminthes; Class: Cestoda; Order: Cyclophyllidea; Family: Taeniidae), has a cosmopolitan distribution and is localised in the small intestine in definitive hosts (cats, lynx, stoats, foxes), and in the liver of intermediate hosts (mice, rats, rabbits, squirrels).

Epidemiology: Rodents are infected by grazing pasture and forages contaminated with cat faeces harbouring eggs of *T. taeniaeformis*. Two cycles can occur: an urban cycle that involves the domestic cat and house and field rodents, and a sylvatic cycle that occurs in North America and which involves bobcats and wild rodents.

Pathology: Each strobilocercus is found within a pea-sized nodule partially embedded in the liver parenchyma.

Notes: The correct nomenclature for the intermediate host stage is 'metacestode stage of *T. taeniaeformis*' rather than '*C. fasciolaris*'.

Hepatozoon muris

Hepatozoon muris, synonyms *Hepatozoon perniciosum*, *Leucocytozoon muris*, *Leucocytozoon ratti* (Phylum: Apicomplexa; Class: Conoidasida; Order: Eucoccidiorida; Family: Hepatozoidae), is distributed in France, Israel, India and South Africa, and is localised in the liver and blood (lymphocytes) of rats. The vector is the spiny rat mite *Echinolaelaps echidninusi* and control of the mites will prevent transmission of the parasite. Diagnosis is based on the detection of gamonts in blood smears. No effective treatment has been reported.

Clinical signs and pathology: It is a non-pathogenic protozoon. Anaemia, emaciation, splenomegaly and hepatic degeneration have been reported in rats with severe infections but these changes may have been caused by a concurrent heavy infection with the mite vector.

Parasites of the circulatory system

Angiostrongylus costaricensis

Angiostrongylus costaricensis (Phylum: Nematoda; Class: Chromadorea; Order: Rhabditida; Family: Angiostrongylidae) is mainly distributed in Central and South America, in particular Costa Rica, occasionally being reported in other parts of the world. This parasite is localised in the mesenteric arteries and arterioles of rodents (common in the cotton rat) but can also infect humans. Terrestrial molluscs, such as slugs and snails, are considered the intermediate hosts, and the slug *Vaginulus plebeius* is the main vector responsible for the infection in cotton rats and humans.

Epidemiology: The cotton rat (*Sigmodon hispidus*) is the most common definitive host in the Americas. Infection of humans in endemic areas is probably through accidental ingestion of infected slugs on vegetables or salads or via infected mucous trails on green vegetation.

Pathogenesis: Heavy infections with adult worms in rats can cause obstruction and necrosis of the gut wall and the mesentery and may sometimes be fatal.

Clinical signs and pathology: In humans, infection causes anorexia, vomiting, diarrhoea and fever. Large infections can induce local haemorrhages in the arterioles. In cases where large numbers of eggs have been shed into the mesenteric capillaries, the serosal surface can have a yellowish coloration. In humans, the adult parasites are frequently present in the ileocaecocolic arteries where they induce thickening of the intestinal wall and a granulomatous eosinophilic inflammatory response. The syndrome is termed abdominal angiostrongylosis.

Diagnosis: The L1 may be detected in faeces. At necropsy, adult worms can often be seen in the mesenteric vessels.

Control and treatment: Control is not practical in rodents. Control of slugs and rodents and greater public awareness of the zoonotic disease should reduce infection in humans. Thorough washing of vegetables and salad greens is important. Anthelmintic treatment is not advised in humans.

Notes: Other *Angiostrongylus* species are found in wild rodents, such as *Angiostrongylus mackerrasae* (rats in Australia) and *Angiostrongylus schimidti* (rice rat in the USA).

Parasites of the nervous system

No parasites of veterinary significance reported.

Parasites of the reproductive/urogenital system

Trichosomoides crassicauda

Trichosomoides crassicauda (Phylum: Nematoda; Class: Enoplea; Order: Enoplida; Family: Trichuridae), commonly known as the Bladder threadworm, is distributed worldwide and localised in the bladder of rats. Transmission in laboratory animals occurs from parents to offspring. Laboratory rats have been treated successfully with either orally or subcutaneously administered ivermectin.

Clinical signs and pathology: The parasite is generally considered non-pathogenic. However, urinary calculi and bladder tumours associated with infection have been reported. The female worms either occur free in the urinary bladder or are embedded in the bladder wall. The presence of the worms can cause granulomatous lesions in the lungs and white nodules in the bladder wall.

Klossiella muris

Klossiella muris (Phylum: Apicomplexa; Class: Conoidasida; Order: Eucoccidiorida; Family: Klossiellidae) is distributed worldwide and localised in the kidney of mice. Infections in mice appear to cause few pathogenic effects and are usually asymptomatic. Control and treatment are not required.

Epidemiology: Sporocysts are passed in the urine and infection takes place by the ingestion of the sporulated sporocysts.

Clinical signs and pathology: Only heavily parasitised kidneys have gross lesions, which appear as tiny grey foci on the cortical surface. Microscopically these foci are areas of necrosis, with perivascular infiltration of inflammatory cells, especially lymphocytes, with an increase in interstitial fibroblasts.

Diagnosis: Sporocysts may be detected in urine sediments or trophozoite stages may be found on *post mortem* in the kidney. The site and location are pathognomonic.

Parasites of the locomotory system

Toxoplasma gondii

For more details see section on Rabbits (Parasites of the locomotory system).

ECTOPARASITES

Lice

Polyplax spinulosa

Polyplax spinulosa (Phylum: Arthropoda; Class: Insecta; Order: Psocodea; Suborder: Anoplura; Family: Polyplacidae) infests the fur of mice and rats and is found worldwide. Adult lice, nymphs or eggs may be found on the fur and can cause pruritus, restlessness, debilitation and anaemia.

Pathogenesis: These blood-sucking lice are commonly encountered in wild rats and mice but rarely seen in laboratory rodents. They cause irritation, restlessness and constant scratching, particularly behind the ears. Anaemia, unthrifty appearance and debilitation occur in heavy infestations.

Control and treatment: Lice may be killed by most organophosphates (e.g. diazinon, malathion methoxychlor) and pyrethroids (e.g. permethrin). Topical application of fipronil or imidacloprid or systemic ivermectin may also be highly effective but care must be taken because adverse responses to ivermectin have been reported in some strains of mice.

Polyplax serrata

Polyplax serrata (Phylum: Arthropoda; Class: Insecta; Order: Psocodea; Suborder: Anoplura; Family: Polyplacidae), commonly known as the Spined rat louse, is found in the fur of mice. It may be a vector for murine eperythrozoonosis. For control and treatment see *P. spinulosa*.

Mites

Ornithonyssus bacoti

Ornithonyssus bacoti, synonyms *Liponyssus bacoti*, *Macronyssus bacoti* (Phylum: Arthropoda; Class: Arachnida; Order: Mesostigmata; Family: Macronyssidae), commonly known as the Tropical rat mite, is found on the skin of rats, mice, hamsters and a wide variety of mammals and birds and occurs worldwide.

Epidemiology: A common parasite worldwide, despite its name. It is particularly common in laboratory rodent colonies. Being an almost permanent parasite, infection is by contact or contamination from accommodation recently vacated by infected stock.

Pathogenesis: Bites are painful and in heavy infections hosts are restless and lose weight from irritation and there may be severe anaemia.

Clinical signs and pathology: Skin irritation and dermatitis. Feeding results in severely pruritic papular dermatitis, thickened crusty skin and soiled fur.

Diagnosis: White or off-white eggs can be seen in the hair. Mites should be collected and identified under a dissecting microscope.

Control and treatment: Treatment includes the application of topical acaricides such as pyrethrin or systemic ivermectin given orally or topically. Repeat treatments will be required to kill newly hatched nymphs.

Myocoptes musculinus

Myocoptes musculinus (Phylum: Arthropoda; Class: Arachnida; Order: Sarcoptiformes (Astigmata); Family: Myocoptidae) infests the fur of mice but will also infest guinea pigs, and is found worldwide. New hosts are infected by contact with infected individuals.

Pathogenesis: This mite causes myocoptic mange in wild and laboratory mice. It is extremely widespread but usually of little pathogenic significance. Problems may occur, however, in crowded laboratory colonies or in animals in poor condition. Lesions are often found along the head and neck and between the shoulder blades. With heavy infestation, mice may scratch constantly, leading to self-induced skin trauma and alopecia.

Clinical signs and pathology: Infestations may be asymptomatic but the mite may cause erythema, inflammation, scaling, crusting and pruritic dermatitis with secondary alopecia. Chronic cases may develop secondary bacterial infection.

Diagnosis: For confirmatory diagnosis, skin scrapings or coat brushings must be examined for eggs and mites.

Control and treatment: All in-contact animals should be treated, and the cage or housing should be cleaned. Application of pyrethrin dusts, or oral or systemic ivermectin on three occasions seven days apart, may be effective. Adverse reactions to ivermectin have been reported in some strains of mice.

Leptotrombidium deliense

Leptotrombidium deliense (Phylum: Arthropoda; Class: Arachnida; Order: Trombidiformes (Prostigmata); Family: Trombiculidae), commonly known as the Scrub typhus mite or Chigger, infests the fur of ground-dwelling rodents and can be found in Southeast Asia and Japan

Pathogenesis: Only the larvae blood feed. Infestation causes pruritus, erythema and scratching, though there may be considerable

individual variation in response. The larvae of this species are vectors of scrub typhus caused by *Rickettsia tsutsugamushi*.

Notes: There are several closely related species in the genus *Leptotrombidium*. For further details see Chapter 3.

Myobia musculi

Myobia musculi (Phylum: Arthropoda; Class: Arachnida; Order: Sarcoptiformes (Astigmata); Family: Mobidae) infests the fur of mice and is found worldwide. For control and treatment see *M. musculinus*.

Pathogenesis and clinical signs: Light infestations are asymptomatic and hence often go unnoticed. Larger mite populations result in alopecia, dermatitis, pruritus and a harsh coat. The preferred site of infestation is the head and underside of the neck. *M. musculi* has a worldwide distribution.

A large number of other closely related species of mites may also occasionally be found on rats and mice (Table 15.5); treatment and control are as for *M. musculinus*. Distinguishing between individual genera and species is beyond the scope of this text.

Notes: *Radfordia ensifera* and *Radfordia affinis* are closely related species of Myobidae, normally found on rats and mice, respectively. They are morphologically similar to *M. musculi* but can be distinguished by the presence of two tarsal claws as opposed to just one (see Fig. 3.108). *Radfordia ensifera* produces intense itching, leading to scabs most frequently seen on the shoulders, neck and face.

Fleas

Nosopsyllus fasciatus

Nosopsyllus fasciatus (Phylum: Arthropoda; Class: Insecta; Order: Siphonaptera; Family: Ceratophyllidae), commonly known as the Northern rat flea, infests the fur and skin of rats and mice but may

Table 15.5 Other species of mites found on rats and mice.

Species	Family	Details
Psorobia simplex (syn. Psorergates simplex)	Psorergatidae	A follicular mite that causes small white intradermal nodules. Closely related to the more pathogenically important Psorobia ovis (see Chapter 9)
Demodex musculi, Demodex ratticola	Demodicidae	Largely non-pathogenic but may occasionally cause follicular dermatitis (see Demodex, Chapter 12)
Notoedres muris	Sarcoptidae	An ear mite of rats. It is relatively rare. It burrows into skin and may result in yellowish crusty-looking warts on edges of ears and nose (see Notoedres cati, Chapter 12)
Ornithonyssus sylviarum	Macronyssidae	See Chapter 13
Dermanyssus gallinae	Dermanyssidae	See Chapter 13
Liponyssoides sanguineus	Dermanyssidae	House mouse mite. A blood-feeding mite of mice and rats found worldwide. It readily bites humans and may act as a vector of rickettsial pox caused by infection with Rickettsia akari. Distinguished from D. gallinae by more pointed posterior of dermal shield
Laelaps nuttalli Hirstionyssus isabellinus Eulaelaps stabularis	Laelapidae	Adults have a single dorsal shield and the sternal plates are wider than long. Though capable of biting, they more commonly feed on skin debris and serous exudate, infesting already abraded areas of skin
Laelaps echidninus		The spiny rat mite. A known vector of a number of disease agents such as Francisella tularensis and Hepatozoon muris
Androlaelaps casalis		Common on a wide variety of rodents; there are several species within this genus (e.g. A. rotundus, A. frontalis and A. sinuosa). Androlaelaps casalis may also cause dermatitis of humans
Haemogamasus pontiger	Haemogamasidae	Identified by the deeply concave posterior margin of the sternal shield. A widespread predatory mite, usually free-living in straw and nests but may be found on rodents and other small mammals.

also bite humans. Although originally European in distribution, this species has now been transported to temperate habitats worldwide.

Epidemiology: *Nosopsyllus fasciatus* fleas are not host specific and may attack any available mammal or bird for a blood meal. As they are able to survive off the host, transmission can occur from the bedding and housing. This flea is highly mobile on the host and can be especially common in host nesting material.

Pathogenesis: Its main hosts are rodents, particularly the Norway rat, *Rattus norvegicus*. However, it has also been found on house mice, gophers and many other hosts. The northern rat flea will attack and feed on humans, although it is not thought to be an important vector of plague. It is known to be a vector of *Hymenolepis diminuta* in parts of Europe, Australia and South America.

Clinical signs and pathology: Symptoms include restlessness and scratching of affected areas. The bites may be visible on the skin. Allergic dermatitis may be seen but should be differentiated from other similar conditions such as sarcoptic mange.

Diagnosis: Diagnosis is not easy as adults may leave the host and eggs and larvae are difficult to find. The bites of these fleas are similar to those of mosquitoes, lice and mites, with inflammation and itchiness.

Control and treatment: Should this species become established in pet rats or mice, the animal should be treated, all litter and bedding should be removed and burnt, and the cage sprayed with an insecticide. If there is invasion of other domestic hosts or humans from wild animals, the source must be eradicated. Several organophosphate, carbamate and pyrethrin-based insecticides are effective. Imidacloprid and fipronil may be highly effective and kill adult fleas on contact.

Xenopsylla cheopis

Xenopsylla cheopis (Phylum: Arthropoda; Class: Insecta; Order: Siphonaptera; Family: Pulicidae), commonly known as the Oriental or Black rat flea, can be found on the skin of rats. This species may also infest mice, cottontail rabbits and ground squirrels and will also bite humans. Its distribution largely follows that of its primary host the black rat (*R. rattus*) worldwide. It is one of the most abundant fleas in the southern states of the USA. It is particularly common in urban areas. Diagnosis can be achieved by identifying the flea species on the host.

Epidemiology: The fleas are able to survive off the host for long periods, making infection possible from the environment. They are uncommon in laboratory or pet rats and mice so their presence may indicate that there is contamination by wild rodents.

Pathogenesis: The bites of the flea may prove irritating to the host animal, causing it to scratch and rub itself. *Xenopsylla cheopis* is also an intermediate host of helminths, such as *H. diminuta* and *H. nana*. This parasite is the main vector of *Yersinia pestis*, the cause of bubonic plague in humans. *Xenopsylla cheopis* acquires *Y. pestis* when feeding on its usual hosts. When the bacilli multiply in its gut, the proventriculus becomes blocked so that blood cannot be ingested; the hungry flea moves from host to host in attempts to feed, and in its wanderings the infection may be transferred from its endemic base in rodents to the human population. Bacteria secreted

in faeces may also enter a host through abrasions. Though now rare in humans, plague still exists in wild rodents ('sylvatic plague') in parts of Africa, Asia, South America and the western states of the USA. *Xenopsylla cheopis* is also a vector of murine typhus (*Rickettsia typhi*). In the case of typhus, the disease is only transmitted by rickettsia in faeces. However, the pathogen can invade the ovary, leading to its transovarial transmission via eggs.

Clinical signs and pathology: The adult fleas may be seen on the skin and coat of the host animal. Other signs are the host scratching affected areas. Flea feeding does not appear to produce histopathology at flea feeding sites nor does the elevated blood basophilic response of infested rats affect subsequent feeding or longevity of the fleas.

Control and treatment: For optimal control, nesting material must be removed and replaced, the housing treated and reinfestation from the environment or introduced animals prevented. A wide range of products is available to treat infested hosts. Imidacloprid and fipronil may be used in rats to kill adult fleas on contact. Growth regulators such as methoprene or pyriproxyfen are another effective longer-term alternative.

Leptopsylla segnis

Leptopsylla segnis (Phylum: Arthropoda; Class: Insecta; Order: Siphonaptera; Family: Leptopsyllidae), commonly known as the Mouse flea, can be found on mice and rats in Europe and the east and west coasts of the USA. For control and treatment see *X. cheopis*.

Epidemiology: Found largely in temperate areas and does not survive hot dry conditions.

Pathogenesis: Bites cause irritation, causing the host to scratch and rub, and may provoke allergic responses. This species of flea has been infected experimentally with plague and murine typhus but generally it is considered a poor disease vector.

Flies

Cuterebra

Cuterebra (Phylum: Arthropoda; Class: Insecta; Family: Oestridae; Subfamily: Cuterebrinae), commonly known as the New World skin bot fly, causes subdermal myiasis (warbles) in rodents but may also occasionally infest dogs and cats in the New World.

Epidemiology: Twenty-six species are known to occur in the USA and Canada. They are also found in Mexico and the neotropical regions but the taxonomy of this genus is not yet clearly defined. In most regions there is only a single generation per year; adults are active in spring and summer and overwinter as pupae in the ground.

Pathogenesis: The larvae cause subdermal nodules. They are not commonly seen in laboratory colonies but may be found in animals maintained outdoors.

Clinical signs and pathology: Symptoms include the swellings and lesions made by the larvae. In the warble formed around each larva, a thin layer of necrotic tissue develops, and the larva feeds off the tissue debris and exudate. In general, the cuterebrid species are of little economic veterinary importance. However, occasional fatal cases of infestation have been recorded in cats and dogs.

Diagnosis: The presence of one or more superficially situated swellings with central openings indicates myiasis. Specific diagnosis can only be made after extraction and identification of the larvae.

Control and treatment: Area-wide control is impractical; for long-term management, areas of known fly activity should be avoided. Surgical removal of larvae can be performed relatively easily if required for infected captive animals. The cyst opening should be enlarged by incision and the parasite excised. The wound should then be rinsed with an antiseptic solution and a topical antibiotic administered.

PRIMATES

Numerous parasites have been described from all the major non-human primate groups. Some of these are considered to be non-pathogenic, or at least their detrimental effects on the host have yet to be elucidated. However, a large number are pathogenic and can create opportunities for secondary infections that may be fatal, especially following immunosuppression and stress. Because of their close relationship with humans, a number of human diseases have been reported in species of monkeys used for experimental purposes.

Non-human primates are classified according to the currently most widely accepted taxonomy. Prosimians include the lemurs and lorises; New World monkeys include species in the families Cebidae, Pitheciidae and Atelidae; Old World monkeys are classified within the superfamily Cercopithecoidea, which has two subfamilies, Cercopithecinae and Colobinae; and the apes include species in the families Hylobatidae (lower apes) and Pongidae (great apes). While extensive checklists of parasites exist for specific species of non-human primates, it is outside the scope of this section to cover all primate parasites in detail, and reference will be made mainly to the more common parasites encountered in laboratory primates and those more commonly seen in zoological collections.

ENDOPARASITES

Parasites of the digestive system

Mouth

Gongylonema macrogubernaculum

Gongylonema macrogubernaculum (Phylum: Nematoda; Class: Chromadorea; Order: Spirurida ; Family: Gongylonematidae) is localised on the oesophagus, tongue and buccal cavity of monkeys from the Old World and New World. This parasite has coprophagous beetles and cockroaches as intermediate hosts.

Epidemiology: Infection is very much dependent on the presence and abundance of the intermediate hosts, dung beetles and cockroaches.

Clinical signs and pathology: Usually asymptomatic. Adult worms bury in tunnels in the squamous epithelium of the oesophagus, lips and buccal cavity.

Diagnosis: Scrapings of the tongue or oral mucosa and identification of the eggs.

Control and treatment: Control is not practical nor necessary. Ivermectin, benzimidazole anthelmintics (mebendazole, thiabendazole) and levamisole all have reported activity.

Trichomonas tenax

Trichomonas tenax, synonyms *Tetratrichomonas buccalis*, *Trichomonas buccalis* (Phylum: Metamonada; Class: Trichomonadea; Order: Trichomonadida; Family: Trichomonadidae), is distributed worldwide and localised in the mouth of macaques (rhesus, crab-eating), baboons, chimpanzees and humans. The body is ovoid, ellipsoidal or pyriform, 4–16 by 2–15 μm, with four anterior flagella and a short undulating membrane with no free anterior flagella. The costa is slender and an accessory filament is present. The capitulum of the axostyle is enlarged and spatulate and the axostyle itself is slender and extends some way beyond the body.

Notes: A number of flagellate protozoa are found throughout the gastrointestinal tract of primates and, with the exception of one or two species, are generally considered to be non-pathogenic. Some of the enteric trichomonads that infect non-human primates are also known to infect humans but are probably non-pathogenic to humans.

Entamoeba gingivalis

Entamoeba gingivalis, synonyms *Amoeba gingivalis*, *Amoeba buccalis*, *Amoeba dentalis*, *Endamoeba buccalis*, *Entamoeba maxillaris*, *Entamoeba canibuccalis* (Phylum: Amoebozoa; Class: Archamoebea; Order: Entamoebida; Family: Entamoebidae), is distributed worldwide and is localised in the mouth of humans, chimpanzees, macaques and baboons.

Notes: This species occurs commonly in the human mouth as a harmless commensal feeding on epithelial cells and bacteria.

Stomach

Several species of nematodes have been reported from the stomach and upper gastrointestinal tract of monkeys and apes (Table 15.6).

Entamoeba histolytica

For details see section on Large intestine.

Small intestine

Helminths

A large number of helminth parasites have been reported from the intestine of non-human primates but only some are peculiar to these hosts. Primates can, under certain circumstances, become infected with common helminths affecting humans and may be used as experimental models for some major helminth diseases affecting humans.

Table 15.6 Species of stomach/oesophageal worms in primates.

Species	Hosts	Site	Distribution
Superfamily Trichostrongyloidea			
Nochtia nochti	Old World monkeys	Stomach	Africa, Asia
Superfamily Gongylonematidae			
Gongylonema pulchrum	Sheep, goats, cattle, pigs, zebu, buffalo, horses, donkeys, deer, camels, humans, primates	Oesophagus, stomach	Worldwide
Gongylonema macrogubernaculum	Old World and New World monkeys	Oesophagus, stomach	Unknown
Superfamily Spiruroidea			
Streptopharagus armatus	Rhesus, cynomolgus monkeys, Japanese macaques, guenons, baboons, gibbons	Stomach	Africa, Asia
Streptopharagus pigmentatus	Rhesus, cynomolgus monkeys, Japanese macaques, guenons, baboons, gibbons	Stomach	Africa, Asia
Protospirura muricola	New World and Old World monkeys	Stomach	Africa, Asia, Central and South America
Physaloptera tumefasciens	Macaques	Stomach	Asia
Physaloptera dilatata	New World monkeys, marmosets	Stomach	Central and South America
Physaloptera caucasica (syn. Abbreviata caucasica)	Rhesus macaques, baboons, orangutans	Oesophagus, stomach, small intestine	Africa, Asia
Physaloptera poicilometra (syn. Abbreviata poicilometra)	Mangabeys, guenons	Stomach	Africa
Superfamily Subuluroidea			
Subulura distans	Old World monkeys (baboons, mangabeys, macaques)	Stomach	Africa, Asia

Ancylostoma duodenale

Ancylostoma duodenale (Phylum: Nematoda; Class: Chromadorea; Order: Rhabditida; Family: Ancylostomatidae), commonly known as the Old World hookworm, is distributed in southern Europe, northern Africa, India, China, Southeast Asia, parts of the USA and Caribbean islands. This parasite is localised in the small intestine of humans and primates such as mandrills, baboons, gibbons, chimpanzees, gorillas and other species of monkeys.

Pathogenesis: Light infections cause abdominal pain and loss of appetite. Heavy infections cause iron deficiency anaemia, oedema and 'pot belly', dyspnoea on exercise and debilitation.

Diagnosis: Diagnosis is based on finding eggs (see Fig. 1.55) in the faeces or adult worms in the intestine on *post mortem*.

Control and treatment: Strict sanitation is required, and routine screening and treatment should be maintained in primate colonies to ensure adequate control. Ivermectin and mebendazole are reportedly effective.

Necator americanus

Necator americanus (Phylum: Nematoda; Class: Chromadorea; Order: Rhabditida; Family: Ancylostomatidae), commonly known as the New World hookworm, is distributed in the USA, Brazil, Africa, China, India, Southeast Asia and Pacific islands. This parasite is localised in the small intestine of humans, primates, pigs and dogs.

Strongyloides stercoralis

Strongyloides stercoralis, synonyms *Strongyloides canis*, *Strongyloides intestinalis*, *Anguillula stercoralis* (Phylum: Nematoda; Class: Chromadorea; Order: Rhabditida; Family: Strongyloididae),

commonly known as the Threadworm, is distributed worldwide in warmer climates and in Europe (Portugal, France, Poland, Ukraine, Romania, Hungary). This parasite is localised in the small intestine of dogs, foxes, cats, humans, apes and monkeys.

Epidemiology: Transmission is via the faecal–oral route or via skin penetration by the infective larvae. A strain of *S. stercoralis* has become adapted to humans and usually occurs in warm climates. Infection in primates should be considered a potential zoonotic risk.

Pathogenesis: Severe infections have been reported in chimpanzees, gibbons, orangutans, patas monkeys and woolly monkeys. Histologically, there is a multifocal erosive and ulcerative enteritis. The mucosa contains numerous parasites within epithelial tunnels or lumina of the intestinal crypts. The intestinal villi are shortened, blunted and fused. In cases of autoinfection, there may be a severe and acute granulomatous or necrotising enterocolitis associated with varying degrees of lymphatic obstruction with submucosal and serosal oedema.

Clinical signs and pathology: Bloody diarrhoea, dehydration, sometimes death. Other clinical signs include dermatitis, urticaria, anorexia, depression, listlessness, debilitation, vomiting and emaciation. Lesions consist of catarrhal to haemorrhagic or necrotising enterocolitis, and multifocal and diffuse haemorrhage in the lungs with granulomas on the pleural surface. Filariform larvae are also seen in many tissues throughout the body, most commonly in the liver and lymph nodes.

Diagnosis: The clinical signs, particularly in young animals, together with the finding of large numbers of the characteristic eggs or larvae in the faeces, are suggestive of strongyloidosis.

Control and treatment: Strict hygiene, daily removal of faeces and keeping water and food free of contamination are important control measures. It is important to keep enclosures and bedding dry to reduce levels of infective larvae. Newly acquired primates should be checked on arrival and treated if infected. Ivermectin 200 µg/kg and moxidectin 0.5 mg/kg are effective in primates. Benzimidazoles such as thiabendazole, albendazole and mebendazole are also reported to be effective.

Notes: *Strongyloides stercoralis* can cause several forms of disease in humans.

1 Penetration and subcutaneous migration of filariform larvae (*larva migrans*) can cause an itching dermatitis that often resolves spontaneously.
2 Migration in the mucosa of the intestinal tract can cause a chronic intestinal syndrome. Symptoms include sporadic diarrhoea, epigastric abdominal pain, heartburn, bloating and weight loss.
3 A mild transient pulmonary form can occasionally occur that induces mild coughing.
4 Occasionally, disseminated infection can induce neurological manifestations, such as Gram-negative polymicrobial meningitis. Less frequently, *S. stercoralis* has been associated with cerebral and cerebellar abscesses.

Several other species of *Strongyloides* have been reported from primates and are summarised in Table 15.7. Some of these species may be synonymous.

Ascaris lumbricoides

Ascaris lumbricoides (Phylum: Nematoda; Class: Chromadorea; Order: Ascaridida; Family: Ascarididae) is localised in the small intestine of humans and some primates, worldwide.

Pathogenesis: Generally of little clinical significance, although fatal cases have been reported in monkeys and apes due to intestinal blockage when large numbers of worms are present.

Diagnosis: The typical ascarid eggs can be detected in faeces (see Fig. 1.64).

Control and treatment: Strict hygiene and treatment with anthelmintics. Piperazine, mebendazole and pyrantel are reported to be effective.

Notes: *Ascaris lumbricoides* is the ascarid species found in humans. Ascarid worms isolated from primates are morphologically identical to *A. lumbricoides* and therefore pose a potential zoonotic threat.

Other small intestinal nematode species of primates are listed in Table 15.8.

Intestinal trematodes

Intestinal flukes are found in both the small and large intestines of primates but natural transmission is unlikely to occur in laboratory

Table 15.7 Other *Strongyloides* species reported in non-human primates.

Species	Hosts	Site
Strongyloides fulleborni	Old World monkeys (rhesus, cynomolgus monkeys, baboons, etc.), apes (chimpanzees)	Small intestine
Strongyloides cebus	New World monkeys (cebus, woolly, spider, squirrel monkeys, marmosets)	Small intestine

Table 15.8 Other small intestinal nematode species of primates.

Species	Superfamily	Hosts
Globocephalus simiae	Ancylostomatoidea	Old World monkeys
Angiostrongylus costaricensis	Metastrongyloidea	Rats, human, marmosets
Pterygodermatities nycticebi	Spiruroidea	Loris, tamarins, marmosets, gibbons
Molineus elegans	Trichostrongyloidea	Squirrel monkeys
Molineus torulosus	Trichostrongyloidea	Cebus, squirrel and owl monkeys
Molineus vexillarius	Trichostrongyloidea	Marmosets
Nematodirus weinbergi	Trichostrongyloidea	Apes
Tupaiostrongylus liei	Trichostrongyloidea	Prosimians (tree shrews)
Tupaiostrongylus major	Trichostrongyloidea	Prosimians (tree shrews)
Tupaiostrongylus minor	Trichostrongyloidea	Prosimians (tree shrews)

or captive primates due to the absence of intermediate hosts. Fluke species that may be encountered in wild-caught individuals are listed in Table 15.9.

Cestodes

A range of tapeworm species has been described in primates. Tapeworm genera and species are shown in Table 15.10. Similar to the situation with intestinal flukes, most reported species of tapeworms are mainly seen in wild-caught primate species as they require an intermediate host to complete the life cycle.

Hymenolepis nana

Hymenolepis nana, synonyms *Rodentolepis nana*, *Hymenolepis fraternal*, *Vampirolepis nana* (Phylum: Platyhelminthes; Class: Cestoda; Order: Cyclophyllidea; Family: Hymenolepididae), commonly known as the Dwarf tapeworm, is distributed worldwide but most frequently found in Asia, Africa, South America and parts of southern Europe. This species is localised in the small intestine of rats, mice, birds, humans and primates (final hosts) and has flour beetles (*Tenebrio*) or fleas as intermediate hosts. Diagnosis is based on the identification of the eggs in faeces or the adult worms in the small intestine.

Clinical signs and pathology: Infections in laboratory primates are usually asymptomatic, although heavy infections can cause catarrhal enteritis and abscessation of the mesenteric lymph nodes.

Control and treatment: Control is difficult because infection can be transmitted in a number of ways. Eradication depends on strict hygiene, elimination of potential intermediate hosts, screening of newly arrived individuals and treatment. Effective drugs include niclosamide and praziquantel.

Notes: *Hymenolepis nana* is of some veterinary importance in that it is a common tapeworm of humans and laboratory animals. This is the only species of tapeworm for which an intermediate host is not necessary since the parasite can also be transmitted by direct ingestion of eggs.

Table 15.9 Intestinal flukes in primates.

	Prosimians	New World monkeys	Old World monkeys	Apes
Family Lecithodendriidae	*Novetrema nycticebi*	*Phaneropsolus orbicularis*	*Phaneropsolus simiae*	*Phaneropsolus longipenis*
	Odeningotrema apidon		*Phaneropsolus aspinosus*	
	Odeningotrema bivesicularis		*Phaneropsolus oviforme*	
	Phaneropsolus bonnie		*Primatotrema macacae*	
	Phaneropsolus lakdivensis		*Primatotrema kellogi*	
	Phaneropsolus longipenis			
	Phaneropsolus perodictici			
	Phaneropsolus oviforme			
Family Paramphistomatidae			*Watsonius watsoni*	
			Watsonius deschieni	
			Watsonius macaci	
			Gastrodiscoides hominis	
			Chiorchis noci	
Family Diplostomidae	*Neodiplostomum tamarini*			
Family Heterophyidae			*Haplorchis pumelo*	
			Haplorchis yokogawi	
			Metagonimus yokogawi	
			Pygidiopsis summa	
Family Echinostomatidae			*Echinostoma aphylactum*	
			Echinostoma ilocanum	
Family Notocotylidae		*Ogmocotyle ailuri*		
		Ogmocotyle indica		
Family Plagiorchiidae		*Plagiorchis multiglandularis*		

Table 15.10 Intestinal tapeworms in primates.

	Prosimians	New World monkeys	Old World monkeys	Apes
Family Anoplocephalidae	*Tupaitaenia guentini*	*Bertiella mucronata*	*Bertiella studeri*	*Bertiella studeri*
	Atriotaenia megastoma	*Bertiella fallax*	*Bertiella satyri*	*Bertiella mucronata*
		Bertiella satyri	*Bertiella okabei*	
		Moniezia rugosa	*Matheovataenia cruzsilvai*	
		Atriotaenia megastoma		
		Matheovataenia brasiliensis		
		Paratriotaenia oedipomidatus		
Family Davaineidae	*Raillietina rothlisbergeri*	*Raillietina alouattae*		
		Raillietina demerariensis		
Family Dilepididae		*Choanotaenia infundibulum*		
Family Hymenolepidae	*Hymenolepis diminuta*	*Hymenolepis nana*	*Hymenolepis nana*	*Hymenolepis nana*
		Hymenolepis cebidarum	*Hymenolepis diminuta*	

Acanthocephalans

Acanthocephalan species reported in primates belong to the genera *Moniliformis* or *Prosthenorchis*. *Prosthenorchis* spp. are distributed throughout Central and South America and have been reported in a variety of New World monkeys. *Prosthenorchis elegans* occurs in the caecum and colon and *Prosthenorchis spirula* in the terminal ileum. The life cycle is indirect, with beetles and cockroaches acting as intermediate hosts. Clinical signs vary in severity and can include diarrhoea, anorexia, debilitation, dehydration and death.

Protozoa

Coccidian infections are generally considered to be of little importance in monkeys, with few reports of associated diseases. Several species of *Eimeria* and *Isospora* (*Cystoisospora*) have been reported in species of monkeys but their significance is not known (Table 15.11). Reported species of *Eimeria* may be synonymous and host specificity between species is unknown due to lack of cross-transmission studies.

Cryptosporidium parvum

Cryptosporidium parvum (Phylum: Apicomplexa; Class: Conoidasida; Order: Cryptogregarinorida; Family: Cryptosporidiidae) is distributed worldwide, and is localised in the small intestine of cattle, sheep, goats, horses, deer, humans and primates (macaques, monkeys).

Epidemiology: A variety of mammals act as hosts to *C. parvum* but little is known of the importance of their involvement in

Table 15.11 Coccidia species from primates.

Prosimians	New World monkeys	Old World monkeys	Apes
Eimeria galago	Cystoisospora aectopitheci	Cystoisospora papionis	Cystoisospora spp.
Eimeri ferruginea	Cystoisospora callimico		
Eimeria lemuris			
Eimeria modesta			
Eimeria otolicni			
Eimeria pachylepyron			
Eimeria tupaiae			

transmitting or maintaining infection. In many instances where *Cryptosporidium* is diagnosed in animals, it appears that infections usually originate from the same host species. The primary route of infection is mainly direct animal to animal via the faecal–oral route and infected monkeys should be considered to have a high potential for zoonotic transmission.

Pathogenesis: *Cryptosporidium* has been reported in several species of macaques, monkeys and lemurs. In rhesus monkeys, it has been associated with acquired immune deficiency syndrome. In these animals, the organisms may be identified in multiple sites including the intestine, stomach, bile and pancreatic ducts.

Clinical signs and pathology: Clinical disease was associated with depression, dehydration, weight loss and intractable diarrhoea. Lesions in the small intestine consist of stunting and fusion of the villi, hyperplasia of the surface epithelium, with focal areas of necrosis and crypt regeneration and adherent trophozoites on the enterocysts of the villi and within the crypts.

Diagnosis: Oocysts may be demonstrated using Ziehl–Neelsen-stained faecal smears in which the sporozoites appear as bright red granules (see Fig. 2.81) or by fluorescence staining with auramine O. Speciation of *Cryptosporidium* is difficult, if not impossible, using conventional techniques. A range of molecular and immunological techniques has been developed that includes immunofluorescence and ELISA. More recently, DNA-based techniques have been used for the molecular characterisation of *Cryptosporidium* species.

Control and treatment: Good hygiene and management are important in preventing disease from cryptosporidiosis. Care should be taken in handling neonatal monkeys; in addition to wearing protective clothing, handlers should follow strict personal hygiene practices. There is no known treatment, although spiramycin may be of some value, and the infection is difficult to control since the oocysts are highly resistant to most disinfectants except formol-saline and ammonia. Symptomatic treatment may be given in the form of anti-diarrhoeals and fluid and electrolyte replacement therapy.

Giardia intestinalis

Giardia intestinalis, synonyms *Giardia duodenalis*, *Giardia lamblia*, *Lamblia lamblia* (Phylum: Metamonada; Class: Trepomonadea; Order: Diplomonadida; Family: Giardiidae), is localised in the small intestine of humans, primates, cattle, sheep, goats, pigs, horses, alpacas, dogs, cats, guinea pigs and chinchillas, worldwide.

Epidemiology: *Giardia* is commonly seen in rhesus and cynomolgus monkeys, chimpanzees and other non-human primates. Molecular studies have revealed a substantial level of genetic diversity in *G. intestinalis* isolates. Human isolates fall into two major groups (assemblage A and B) with a wide host range in other mammals and some separate species names may be applicable. Other assemblages may also represent distinct species. Limited epidemiological studies suggest that in animal isolates, direct animal-to-animal contact and faecal soiling are the most likely methods of transmission, although water contamination may also be a possible route.

Clinical signs and pathology: When disease does occur, the signs often include chronic pasty diarrhoea, weight loss, lethargy and failure to thrive. The diarrhoea may be continuous or intermittent. There may be villous atrophy, crypt hypertrophy and an increased number of intraepithelial lymphocytes. Trophozoites may be seen between villi, attached by their concave surface to the brush border of epithelial cells.

Diagnosis: *Giardia* cysts can be detected in faeces by a number of methods. Traditional methods of identification involve direct examination of faecal smears, or faecal concentration by formalin-ethyl acetate or zinc sulfate methods and subsequent microscopic examination. It is generally recommended that three consecutive samples be examined as cysts are excreted intermittently.

Control and treatment: As infection is transmitted by the faecal–oral route, good hygiene and prevention of faecal contamination of feed and water are essential. Treatment with quinacrine and metronidazole has been reported to be effective. Quinacrine is not well tolerated in some species such as squirrel monkeys.

Cyclospora cayatenensis

Cyclospora cayatenensis (Phylum: Apicomplexa; Class: Conoidasida; Order: Eucoccidiorida; Family: Eimeriidae) is localised in the small intestine of humans, monkeys and reptiles. It is distributed in developing tropical or subtropical regions. Oocysts are small, 8–10 μm in diameter, and when sporulated contain two sporocysts, each with two sporozoites.

Pathogenesis: The clinical significance in monkeys is unknown. The organism has been reported from chimpanzees and baboons but may well occur in other species of monkeys. Infection in humans can cause severe watery diarrhoea.

Treatment: Trimethoprim-sulfamethoxazole results in rapid improvement in humans and should be equally effective in primates.

Large intestine

Enterobius vermicularis

Enterobius vermicularis (Phylum: Nematoda; Class: Chromadorea; Order: Oxyurida; Family: Oxyuridae), commonly known as the Pinworm, is distributed worldwide and is localised in the caecum and colon of humans and apes (chimpanzees).

Pathogenesis: Infections are usually innocuous, although fatal cases in chimpanzees may be characterised by ulcerative colitis, and peritonitis has been reported.

Clinical signs and pathology: Anal pruritus and irritation, which may lead to self-mutilation and restlessness.

Diagnosis: Pinworm infection can be diagnosed either by observing adult worms emerging from the anus or by use of sticky tape on the anus and microscopic identification of the characteristic ellipsoidal asymmetrical eggs.

Control and treatment: Control is based on strict hygiene procedures and treatment of infected animals. Pyrantel pamoate and benzimidazole anthelmintics are effective. Other species of pinworms found in primates are listed in Table 15.12.

Oesophagostomum spp.

Oesophagostomum spp. (Phylum: Nematoda; Class: Chromadorea; Order: Rhabditida; Family: Strongylidae), commonly known as the Nodular worm, is widespread on Asia and Africa, and is localised in the caecum and colon of primates, such as macaques, mangabeys, guenons, chimpanzees and gorillas.

Pathogenesis: The presence of larvae causes the formation of smooth elevated nodules, 2–4 mm in diameter, in the mucosa of the large intestine, and these may be blackish in colour if associated with haemorrhages. Older nodules become caseous and contain mineralised deposits. Histopathologically, the nodules are surrounded by a fibrous capsule and contain inflammatory cells, mainly neutrophils, macrophages, eosinophils, lymphocytes and plasma cells, and with foreign body giant cells also present.

Clinical signs and pathology: Infections are usually asymptomatic but severely infected animals may show general unthriftiness and debilitation, characterised by weight loss and diarrhoea.

Diagnosis: Eggs present in the faeces must be differentiated from other strongyle eggs and faecal culture may be required to identify the larvae. *Post mortem* diagnosis is based on the presence of typical nodular lesions.

Control and treatment: Good hygiene practices and treatment of infected animals are required to control nodular worm infections. Benzimidazole anthelmintics and levamisole are reportedly effective.

Notes: At least 11 species have been described, the main species being *Oesophagostomum apiostomum*, *Oeshophagostomum bifurcatum*, *Oesophagostomum aculeatum* and *Oesophagostomum stephanostomum*.

Trichuris trichiura

Trichuris trichiura (Phylum: Nematoda; Class: Enoplea; Order: Enoplida; Family: Trichuridae), commonly known as the Whipworm, is localised in the large intestine of humans and primates.

Pathogenesis: Light infections do not usually cause any significant problems. Heavy infections have been reported to result in anorexia, grey mucoid diarrhoea and sometimes death in primates.

Diagnosis: Identification of eggs, with characteristics polar plugs, in the faeces (Fig. 15.25).

Control and treatment: Strict personal hygiene is required for all animal care personnel because of the risk of zoonotic transmission. Mebendazole, flubendazole and levamisole are reportedly effective.

Ternidens deminutus

Ternidens deminutus (Phylum: Nematoda; Class: Chromadorea; Order: Rhabditida; Family: Rhabditidae) is distributed in Africa and Asia and is localised in the caecum and colum of Old World monkeys (macaques, guenons, baboons), apes (chimpanzees, gorillas) and humans. Adult worms are 8–16 mm long and have a large globose buccal capsule with three forked teeth at the base.

Entamoeba histolytica

Entamoeba histolytica, synonyms *Entamoeba dysenteriae*, *Amoeba coli*, *Entamoeba pitheci* (Phylum: Amoebozoa; Class: Archamoebea; Order: Entamoebida; Family: Entamoebidae), is localised in the large intestine, liver, lungs, rarely brain, spleen and stomach of humans, apes, monkeys, dogs, cats, pigs and rats. This aemoeba has a worldwide distribution.

Table 15.12 Other species of pinworms.

	Prosimians	New World monkeys	Old World monkeys	Apes
Superfamily Oxyuroidea	Enterobius lemoris	Trypanoxyuris trypanuris	Enterobius brevicauda	Enterobius anthropopitheci
	Primasubulura otolicini	Trypanoxyuris atelis	Enterobius bipapillata	Enterobius buckleyi
		Trypanoxyuris duplicideus	Enterobius pitheci	Enterobius lerouxi
		Trypanoxyuris lagothricis	Enterobius parallela	Probstmayria gombensis
		Trypanoxyuris clementinae	Enterobius zakari	Probstmayria gorillae
		Trypanoxyuris minutus	Enterobius chabaudi	Probstmayria simiae
		Trypanoxyuris satanus	Enterobius inglisi	
		Trypanoxyuris scleratus	Enterobius pesteri	
		Trypanoxyuris brachylelesi	Enterobius macaci	
		Trypanoxyuris callithricis	Enterobius presbytis	
		Trypanoxyuris callicebi	Probstmayria natalensis	
		Trypanoxyuris oedepi		
		Trypanoxyuris goedeli		
		Oxyuronema atelophorum		
		Primasubulura jacchi		

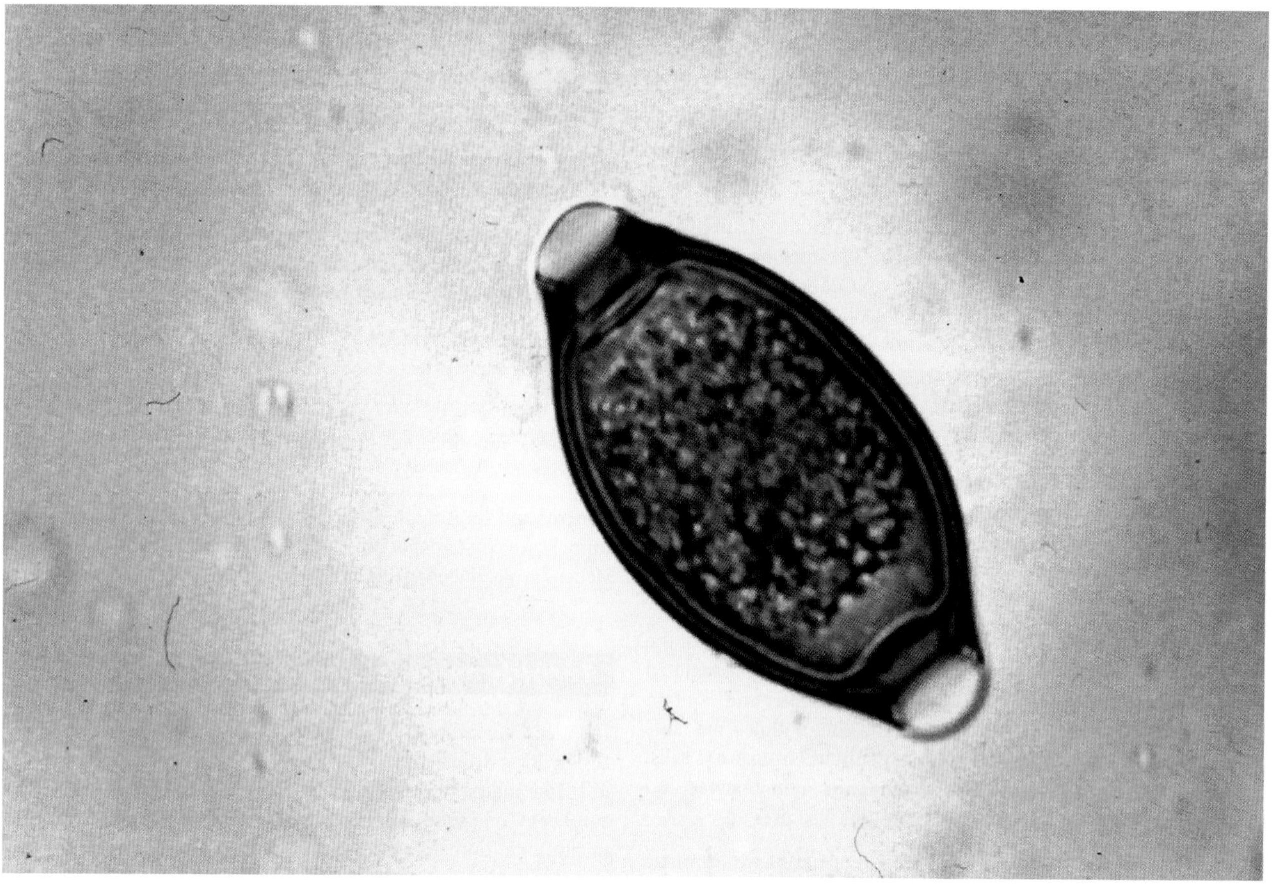

Fig. 15.25 *Trichuris* egg.

Epidemiology: *Entamoeba histolytica* is primarily a parasite of primates and humans that are reservoirs for other animal species.

Pathogenesis: Non-pathogenic forms of the organism normally live in the lumen of the large intestine. Pathogenic forms invade the mucosa, causing ulceration and dysentery. From there, they may be carried via the portal system to the liver and other organs where large abscesses may form. The amoeba-like trophozoites secrete proteolytic enzymes and produce characteristic flask-shaped ulcers in the mucosa of the large intestine. Their erosion may allow the parasites to enter the bloodstream, when the most common sequela is the formation of amoebic abscesses in the liver. Infections with *E. histolytica* can cause considerable problems in colonies of chimpanzees. Infection has also been found in many species of monkeys throughout the world. Spider monkeys are particularly susceptible, often developing liver infections. Gastric amoebosis has been reported in proboscis monkeys, colobus monkeys, silver leaf monkeys and langurs.

Clinical signs and pathology: Infections may be asymptomatic or produce mild to severe clinical signs, with invasion of the mucosa causing diarrhoea or dysentery. Clinically affected animals may show apathy, lethargy, weakness, dehydration, weight loss, anorexia, vomiting and severe haemorrhagic or catarrhal diarrhoea. Pathogenic strains of amoebae penetrate the mucosa of the large intestine and multiply to form small colonies that extend into the submucosa and muscularis. In the absence of bacterial infection, there is little reaction but in complicated infections there is

hyperaemia and inflammation with predominantly neutrophils. Amoebae may pass into the lymphatic system and mediastinal lymph nodes and from there migrate in the portal system to the liver where they may cause abscessation. Abscesses may also form in other organs including the lungs and brain.

Diagnosis: Diagnosis is based on identification of the causative agent in faeces or associated with typical lesions. These organisms are common non-pathogenic commensals in the digestive tract of non-human primates and their presence in the faeces of animals is not necessarily a definitive diagnosis. Motile organisms and cysts of *E. histolytica* may be detected in smears from faeces. Trophozoites and cysts can be stained with iodine, trichrome or iron haematoxylin. The organisms can also be cultured in a number of media, including Boeck and Drbohlav's, Dobell and Laidlaw's, TYI-S-33 and Robinson's. Isoenzyme markers can be used to differentiate the two forms seen but there is some debate as to whether the two types represent different species or if they can change from one type to another under certain circumstances.

A number of serological tests have been evaluated for the diagnosis of *E. histolytica* infections, including ELISA, latex agglutination, complement fixation and indirect haemagglutination. A number of polymerase chain reaction (PCR) methods have also been used to detect *E. histolytica* in clinical samples. These are based on the amplification of specific DNA sequences that correlate to the pathogenic/non-pathogenic isoenzyme categorisation and appear to be very sensitive and specific.

Control and treatment: Strict sanitation is important in the prevention of amoebiasis. Trophozoites are killed by common disinfectants but cysts are more resistant and steam cleaning may be required. Infected humans are a potential source of infection for monkeys, so routine screening of handlers or laboratory technicians is required. Insects, such as flies and cockroaches, act as mechanical vectors and should be controlled. Treatment, if required, relies on the combined use of metronidazole and di-iodohydroxyquin.

Entamoeba hartmanni

Entamoeba hartmanni (Phylum: Amoebozoa; Class: Archamoebea; Order: Entamoebida; Family: Entamoebidae) is distributed worldwide and localised in the large intestine of humans, apes and monkeys. *Entamoeba hartmanni* resembles the small form of *E. histolytica*, being slightly smaller with rounded trophozoites measuring 3–10.5 µm and a nucleus 1.5–2.5 µm in size. The peripheral chromatin is usually more variable and consists of widely separated discrete granules. Cysts are also smaller, measuring 3.8–8.0 µm in size.

Notes: True incidence is not known as this species has often been considered synonymous with *E. histolytica*.

A number of other species of amoebae are found in monkeys and apes but are generally considered to be non-pathogenic commensals.

Entamoeba coli

Entamoeba coli, synonyms *Amoeba coli*, *Endamoeba hominis*, *E. cynocephalusae* (Phylum: Amoebozoa; Class: Archamoebea; Order: Entamoebida; Family: Entamoebidae), is a non-pathogenic amoeba distributed worldwide and localised in the large intestine of humans, apes, monkeys, pigs and white-tailed deer. Trophozoites are 15–50 µm in diameter. The nucleus is large and eccentric and has a ring of coarse peripheral granules with scattered chromatin granules. The cysts are 10–33 µm and have eight nuclei and contain splinter-like chromatin granules.

Notes: This is the most common species of amoeba in humans.

Entamoeba chattoni

Entamoeba chattoni, synonym *Entamoeba polecki* (Phylum: Amoebozoa; Class: Archamoebea; Order: Entamoebida; Family: Entamoebidae), is localised in the large intestine of macaques, other species of monkeys and rarely humans. The geographical distribution of this parasite is unknown. *Entamoeba chattoni* trophozoites are 9–25 µm long. The nucleus has a small central endosome with a row of fine peripheral granules. Cysts are 6–18 µm in size and usually uninucleate.

Iodamoeba buetschlii

Iodamoeba buetschlii, synonyms *Iodamoeba wenyonii*, *Iodamoeba suis*, *Entamoeba williamsi*, *Endolimax williamsi* (Phylum: Amoebozoa; Class: Archamoebea; Order: Entamoebida; Family: Entamoebidae), is non-pathogenic, distributed worldwide and localised in the large intestine of pigs, humans, apes (chimpanzees, gorillas) and monkeys.

Endolimax nana

Endolimax nana, synonyms *Amoeba limax*, *Entamoeba nana*, *Entamoeba intestinalis*, *Entamoeba suis*, *E. ratti* (Phylum: Amoebozoa; Class: Archamoebea; Order: Entamoebida; Family: Entamoebidae), is a non-pathogenic amoeba localised in the large intestine of humans, apes, monkeys, pigs and rats. It has a worldwide distribution.

Notes: *Endolimax nana* is common in humans, primates and pigs.

Pentatrichomonas hominis

Pentatrichomonas hominis, synonyms *Pentatrichomonas felis*, *Cercomonas hominis*, *Monocercomonas hominis*, *Trichomonas felis*, *Trichomonas intestinalis* (Phylum: Metamonada; Class: Trichomonadea; Order: Trichomonadida; Family: Trichomonadidae), is a non-pathogenic protozoon localised in the large intestine of humans, monkeys, dogs, cats, rats, mice, hamsters and guinea pigs. It has a worldwide distribution.

Diagnosis: Morphological identification of the organisms from fresh and stained faecal preparations. The organism can also be cultured in trichomonad culture medium. Control and treatment are not required.

Dientamoeba fragilis

Dientamoeba fragilis (Phylum: Metamonada; Class: Trichomonadea; Order: Trichomonadida; Family: Dientamoebidae) is localised in the caecum and colon of humans and monkeys worldwide.

Pathogenesis: Generally considered to be non-pathogenic but can cause diarrhoea in humans, with mild to moderate abdominal pain.

Enteromonas hominis

Enteromonas hominis, synonyms *Octomitus hominis*, *Tricercomonas intestinalis*, *Enteromonas bengalensis* (Phylum: Metamonada; Class: Trepamondea; Order: Diplomonadida; Family: Enteromonadidae), is localised in the caecum of rats, hamsters, humans and primates (chimpanzees, macaques).

Retortamonas intestinalis

Retortamonas intestinalis, synonyms *Embadomonas intestinalis*, *Waskia intestinalis* (Phylum: Metamonada; Class: Trepomonadea; Order: Retortamonadida; Family: Retortamonadidae), is localised in the large intestine of humans, chimpanzees and monkeys.

Tritrichomonas mobilensis

Tritrichomonas mobilensis (Phylum: Metamonada; Class: Trichomonadea; Order: Trichomonadida; Family: Trichomonadidae) is localised in the large intestine of squirrel monkeys. Treatment with metronidazole has been reported to be effective. Trophozoites are lanceolate shaped, 7–10.5 μm long, and there are three anterior flagella with a well-developed undulating membrane that extends the length of the body and has a long trailing posterior flagellum. The nucleus is ovoid and situated anteriorly.

Pathogenesis: The clinical significance of this species is uncertain. Invasive infection has been reported in squirrel monkeys leading to focal epithelial necrosis and associated inflammatory response.

Chilomastix mesnili

Chilomastix mesnili, synonyms *Chilomastix suis*, *C. hominis*, *Macrostoma mesnili* (Phylum: Metamonada; Class: Trepomonadea; Order: Retortamonadida; Family: Retortamonadidae), is a non-pathogenic protozoon distributed worldwide and localised in the caecum and colon of humans, apes (chimpanzees, orangutans), monkeys (macaques) and pigs. The diagnosis is based on identification of trophozoites or cysts in large intestinal contents or faeces and control and treatment are not required.

Balantioides coli

Balantioides coli, synonym *Balantidium coli* (Phylum: Ciliophora; Class: Litostomatea; Order: Vestibuliferida; Family: Balantidiidae), is localised in the large intestine of pigs, humans, camels, apes, monkeys, dogs (rarely) and rats. It has a worldwide distribution.

Epidemiology: *Balantioides coli* exists as a common commensal in the large intestine of most monkeys. Humans and apes may occasionally become clinically affected through faecal contamination of foodstuffs or hands. Transmission occurs by ingestion of cysts or trophozoites. The cysts are resistant to environmental conditions and can survive for weeks in faeces.

Clinical signs and pathology: Generally, it is non-pathogenic and is a common inhabitant of the caecum of non-human primates. However, infection can cause severe ulcerative enterocolitis in great apes. Signs in clinically affected apes include weight loss, anorexia, muscle weakness, lethargy, watery diarrhoea, tenesmus and rectal prolapse. The organisms are found in enormous numbers in the lumen of the large intestine with normal caecal mucosa. However, the organism may be found within mucosal ulcers initiated by other infections. It produces hyaluronidase, which might help to enlarge the lesions by attacking the intercellular ground substance.

Diagnosis: *Balantioides* is easily recognised by microscopic examination of intestinal contents or by histological examination of intestinal lesions (see Figs 2.97, 2.98 and 2.99).

Control and treatment: Strict sanitation to prevent ingestion of cysts or faeces should prevent infection in non-human primate colonies. Tetracyclines, metronidazole and di-iodohydroxyquin are effective.

Peritoneum

A variety of filarial worms (Filarioidea) commonly parasitise primates, being found in the subcutaneous tissues and the abdominal and thoracic cavities (Table 15.13). Worms in the abdominal cavity may cause fibrinopurulent peritonitis with associated fibrinous adhesions. Transmission of these parasites within primate colonies is unlikely and no special control measures are required other than control of possible arthropod vectors.

The larval forms of several species of pentastomids are also found in the peritoneum and peritoneal cavity of primates, which act as intermediate hosts to the adult stages which are found in either dogs or snakes depending on the genus.

Linguatula serrata is a parasite of dogs and nymph stages have been reported in the viscera of Old World and New World monkeys. Species of *Armillifer* and *Porocephalus* are parasites of snakes with nymph stages reported in prosimians, Old World and New World monkeys and apes throughout Africa, Asia and South America.

Parasites of the respiratory system

Anatrichosoma cynomolgi

Anatrichosoma cynomolgi, synonyms *Anatrichosoma cutaneum*, *Anatrichosoma rhina*, *Anatrichosoma nacepobi* (Phylum: Nematoda; Class: Enoplea; Order: Enoplida; Family: Trichuridae), is localised in the nasal mucosa, nares and skin of Old World primates (macaques, mangabeys, langurs, baboons), New World primates (marmosets), apes (orangutans, gibbons) and humans. It is distributed in Asia and Africa.

Pathogenesis: Female worms migrate through the stratified layers of the squamous epithelium, forming tunnels and pustules around the nares.

Diagnosis: Nasal or skin scrapings reveal the characteristic eggs. Nasal mites (genus *Rhinophaga*) are also found in the nasal cavity and upper respiratory tract of Old World monkeys and apes (Table 15.14). Their presence can cause inflammation and nasal polyp formation.

Table 15.13 Filarial worms of the peritoneal cavity.

	Prosimians	New World monkeys	Old World monkeys	Apes
Family Onchocercidae		Mansonella barbascalensis	Mansonella digitatum	Mansonella vanhoofi
		Mansonella zakii		
		Mansonella nicollei		
		Dipetalonema gracile		
		Dipetalonema caudispina		
		Dipetalonema graciliformis		
		Dipetalonema robini		
		Dipetalonema tenue		

Table 15.14 Nasal mites of primates.

Species	Hosts	Site
Rhinophaga papinois	Baboon	Maxillary sinuses
Rhinophaga elongate	Baboon	Nasal cavities
Rhinophaga dinolti	Rhesus monkey	Nasal cavities, lung
Rhinophaga cercopitheci	Guenon	Frontal sinuses, lungs
Rhinophaga pongicola	Orangutan	Maxillary sinuses

Filaroides spp.

Filaroides spp. (Phylum: Nematoda; Class: Chromadorea; Order: Rhabditida; Family: Filaroididae) are localised in the lungs of New World monkeys (marmosets, squirrels, cebus and howlers). Infections are usually asymptomatic and the worms usually produce varying numbers of small subpleural nodules.

Notes: Reported species include *Filaroides barretoi*, *Filaroides gordius* and *Filaroides cebus*. A related species, *Filariopsis arator*, also occurs in New World primates.

Paragonimus westermani

Paragonimus westermani (Phylum: Platyhelminthes; Class: Trematoda; Order: Plagiorchiida; Family: Paragonimidae), commonly known as the Oriental lung fluke, is distributed in Asia and North America. This trematode is localised in the lungs of dogs, cats, pigs, goats, cattle, foxes, other carnivores, humans and primates (cynomolgus monkeys).

Epidemiology: Infections in cynomolgus monkeys are associated with the ingestion of crabs or crayfish.

Pathogenesis: Infection causes focal emphysema and the formation of cysts (2–3 cm in size) that may cause pleural adhesions.

Clinical signs and pathology: In lung infections there may be a cough, and eggs may be found in the sputum in large numbers. Parasites in the lungs are not usually of great importance but some may lodge in the brain or other organs, causing more severe damage. Pulmonary signs are comparatively rare in cats or dogs and veterinary interest is in the potential reservoir of infection for humans. Extrapulmonary infections may produce cutaneous *larva migrans* and abscess formation in the skin and viscera. Brain and spinal cord involvement may lead to seizures, paraplegia and occasional deaths.

Diagnosis: Diagnosis is by identifying the presence of eggs in the sputum or faeces (see Fig. 1.102).

Pneumonyssus simicola

Pneumonyssus simicola (Phylum: Arthropoda; Class: Arachnida; Subclass: Acari; Family: Halarachnidae), commonly known as Lung mites, are localised in the lungs of Old World monkeys (rhesus, cynomolgus, patas, colobus, proboscis, celebes apes, mangabeys, baboons, langurs) and apes (chimpanzees, gorillas, orangutans) in Africa and Asia. *Pneumonyssus simicola* is very common in imported rhesus monkeys.

Pathogenesis: Infections result in pale spots throughout the lung parenchyma and pleural adhesions may be present. The lesions are soft and pale and contain 1–20 mites. They are surrounded by a brown to black pigment and are characterised by localised bronchiolitis, focal pneumonitis, alveolar consolidation and occasional bronchiolectasis. The inflammatory cell exudate comprises neutrophils, eosinophils and macrophages containing pigment and refractile crystals.

Clinical signs: Infections are usually asymptomatic and clinical signs are uncommon. Death has been reported in rhesus monkeys with massive infestations.

Diagnosis: Diagnosis in the live animal is difficult. Tracheobronchial washings may demonstrate lung mite larvae but negative washings are not conclusive that infections do not exist. Gross lesions are characteristic but need to be differentiated from tuberculosis.

Control and treatment: There is no reported effective treatment and control can only be achieved through the establishment of mite-free colonies.

Other *Pneumonyssus* species in the respiratory tract of primates are listed in Table 15.15.

Parasites of the liver

Capillaria hepatica

Capillaria hepatica, synonyms *Callodium hepatica*, *Hepaticola hepatica* (Phylum: Nematoda; Class: Enoplea; Order: Enoplida; Family: Capillariidae), is localised in the liver of rats, mice, squirrels, rabbits and farmed mustelids. Occasionally it can infect dogs, cats, humans and primates including New World monkeys (*Cebus*, squirrel, spider), Old World monkeys (rhesus) and apes (chimpanzees).

Pathogenesis: Adult worms are found in the parenchyma of the liver where they provoke traumatic hepatitis. Eggs are laid in groups in the liver parenchyma from which there is no natural access to the exterior. Granulomas develop around the eggs, accompanied by fibrosis. Fatal hepatitis has been reported in primates.

Table 15.15 *Pneumonyssus* species in the respiratory tract of primates.

Species	Hosts	Site
Pneumonyssus duttoni	Old World monkeys	Lungs
Pneumonyssus longus	Old World monkeys, apes	Lungs, bronchi, trachea
Pneumonyssus oudemansi	Old World monkeys, apes	Lungs, bronchi, trachea
Pneumonyssus africanus	Old World monkeys	Bronchi
Pneumonyssus mossambicensis	Old World monkeys	Lungs
Pneumonyssus congoensis	Old World monkeys	Trachea, lungs
Pneumonyssus rodhaini	Old World monkeys	Lungs, nasal fossae
Pneumonyssus vitzthumi	Old World monkeys	Lung, maxillary sinuses, nasal fossae
Pneumonyssus vocalis	Old World monkeys	Larynx, vocal pouches

Clinical signs and pathology: Mild infections are usually asymptomatic. At necropsy, the liver may have yellowish-white streaks on the surface. The eggs, which are deposited in clusters, provoke the development of localised granulomas, which are visible through the capsule as yellowish streaks or patches.

Diagnosis: Most infections are discovered at routine *post mortem*. Granulomatous tissue in the liver parenchyma can be examined for the presence of eggs or worm fragments after squashing between microscope slides.

Notes: Although the parasite can infect humans, the zoonotic risk is low.

Echinococcus granulosus

Echinococcus granulosus (Phylum: Platyhelminthes; Class: Cestoda; Order: Cyclophyllidea; Family: Taeniidae), commonly known as the Dwarf dog tapeworm, causes hydatidosis. It is distributed worldwide and localised mainly in the liver and lungs of intermediate hosts and the small intestine of definitive hosts. The final hosts are dogs and many wild canids, while domestic and wild ruminants, humans and primates, pigs and lagomorphs act as intermediate hosts. Horses and donkeys are resistant to the infection.

Pathogenesis: Hydatid cysts have been described from a number of Old World monkeys (guenons, colobus, mangabeys, mandrill, macaques, celebes ape, baboons), New World monkeys (marmosets), apes (chimpanzees, gorillas, orangutans) and prosimians (lemurs). Cysts may be located in the abdomen, thoracic cavity, liver, lungs or subcutis.

Clinical signs and pathology: Infections are usually asymptomatic but may cause abdominal distension or localised swellings depending on the size and location of the cysts.

Diagnosis: The diagnosis of hydatidosis is not usually made until the cysts reach a large size and symptoms may be mistaken for a tumour. Ultrasound and radiography have been used in diagnosis in apes. Serological tests developed for use in humans have also proven useful.

Notes: Considerable phenotypic and genetic variability has been observed within the species *E. granulosus* and several strains have been identified based on molecular genotyping. New data demonstrate that '*E. granulosus*' is an assembly of several rather diverse strains and genotypes (designated G1–G10) that show fundamental differences not only in their epidemiology but also in their pathogenicity to humans.

Two other species, *Echinococcus multilocularis* in lemurs, macaques, gorillas, gibbons and orangutans and *Echinococcus vogeli* in great apes (gorillas, orangutans and chimpanzees), have also been reported.

Flukes

A number of species of flukes have been reported in primates (Table 15.16). Reported fluke species are invariably seen in wild-caught primates as they require an intermediate host to complete their life cycles.

Entamoeba histolytica

For more details see section on Large intestine.

Parasites of the pancreas
Eurytrema pancreaticum

Eurytrema pancreaticum, synonyms *Distoma pancreaticum*, *Eurytrema ovis* (Phylum: Platyhelminthes; Class: Trematoda; Order: Plagiorchiida; Family: Dicrocoeliidae), commonly known as the Pancreatic fluke, is distributed in South America, Asia and Europe. This parasite is localised in the pancreatic ducts, and rarely the bile ducts, of cattle, buffalo, sheep, goats, pigs, camels, humans and primates. Two intermediate hosts are required: land snails, particularly of the genus *Bradybaena*, as host 1 and grasshoppers of the genus *Conocephalus* or tree crickets (*Oecanthus*) as host 2.

Parasites of the circulatory system

Schistosomes

Schistosomes are flukes found in the circulatory system. The sexes are separate, the small adult female lying permanently in a longitudinal groove, the gynaecophoric canal, in the body of the male. The genus has been divided into four groups – *haematobium*, *indicum*, *mansoni* and *japonicum* – but the genus as currently defined is paraphyletic so revisions are likely.

Several species of *Schistosoma* have been reported to infect non-human primates but are generally of little consequence in captive animals and are usually only observed as incidental findings on *post mortem*. Infected primates are not of direct public health

Table 15.16 Fluke species from primates.

	Prosimians	New World monkeys	Old World monkeys	Apes
Family Dicrocoelidae		*Athesmia heterolecithodes*	*Brodenia lacinata*	*Eurytrema brumpti*
		Controrchis biliophilus	*Dicrocoelium colobusciola*	*Dicrocoelium lanceolatum*
			Dicrocoelium lanceolatum	*Dicrocoelium macaci*
			Dicrocoelium macaci	*Eurytrema satoi*
			Euparadistomum cercopitheci	
			Eurytrema satoi	

significance because of the need for an obligate intermediate molluscan host.

Haematobium group

Schistosoma haematobium

Schistosoma haematobium (Phylum: Platyhelminthes; Class: Trematoda; Order: Strigeidida; Family: Schistosomatidae) is distributed in Africa and Middle East and localised in the bladder veins and urethra of humans and primates (mangabeys, patas monkeys, guenons, baboons). This parasite has snails (*Bulinus*) as intermediate hosts.

Schistosoma mattheei

Schistosoma mattheei (Phylum: Platyhelminthes; Class: Trematoda; Order: Strigeidida; Family: Schistosomatidae) is distributed in South and Central Africa and Middle East and localised in the portal and mesenteric and bladder veins of cattle, sheep, goats, camels, rodents, humans and primates (baboons). This parasite has snails (*Bulinus*) as intermediate hosts.

Mansoni group

Schistosoma mansoni

Schistosoma mansoni (Phylum: Platyhelminthes; Class: Trematoda; Order: Strigeidida; Family: Schistosomatidae) is localised in the mesenteric veins of hosts. It is distributed in South America, the Caribbean, Africa and Middle East.

Brugia spp.

The lymphatic filarial worms (*Brugia* spp.) are carried by many species of mosquito and occur in Southeast Asia, notably Malaysia, causing elephantiasis in humans (Table 15.17). The most important human species, *Brugia malayi*, is also infective for monkeys and domestic and wild carnivores. Adult parasites inhabit lymph nodes and afferent lymphatic vessels.

Trypanosoma cruzi

Trypanosoma cruzi, synonyms *Schizotrypanum cruzi*, *Trypanosoma lesourdi*, *Trypanosoma rhesii*, *Trypanosoma prowazekii*, *Trypanosoma vickersae* (Phylum: Euglenozoa; Class: Kinetoplastea; Order: Trypanosomatida; Family: Trypanosomatidae), which causes Chagas disease, is distributed in South America and localised in the blood, heart and muscles of humans, dogs, cats, New World primates and wild animals. This parasite has reduviid bugs (assassin or kissing bugs) as intermediate hosts.

Epidemiology: Reduviid bugs commonly defecate after feeding, and animals become infected when they lick the insect bites or eat the infected bugs. Transmission also occurs by ingesting infected animals, via infected maternal milk, by fly contamination or contamination by urine or saliva of heavily infected animals.

Pathogenesis: Trypomastigote forms are found in blood, and amastigote forms are found in pseudocysts in skeletal and cardiac muscle, the reticuloenthothelial system and other tissues. Infection causes generalised oedema, anaemia, hepatosplenomegaly and lymphadenitis.

Clinical signs and pathology: Depression, anorexia and weight loss can occur. Myocarditis is commonly seen in non-human primates, leading to destruction of myocardial fibres caused by the parasite pseudocysts.

Diagnosis: In acute stages of the disease, trypomastigotes can be found in thick blood smears stained with Giemsa. The size and morphology make it relatively easy to distinguish from other trypanosomes found in primates. Complement fixation or ELISA serological tests are available for humans and may be helpful in screening monkeys.

Control and treatment: Control is based on eliminating the insect vector. Because the disease is zoonotic, handlers should take precautions to avoid exposure or contamination of mucous membranes or skin to infective secretions. There is no effective treatment.

Plasmodium

Plasmodium spp. cause malaria in both humans and animals. Malaria is one of the most common haemoprotozoal parasitic diseases of primates in tropical and subtropical regions. Malaria parasites that infect the apes are different from those affecting monkeys and are homologous to human malaria parasites and morphologically indistinguishable. The parasites are classified on the basis of the host infected, the parasite morphology and the type of cyclic fever produced (quotidian, 24 hours; tertian, 48 hours; quartan, 72 hours). Reported species are summarised in Table 2.45.

Pathogenesis: Malaria infections in most primates are generally not fatal. However, they may cause debilitation and disease which can be precipitated by stress, concurrent disease or immunosuppression. Infection causes hepatosplenomegaly and lymphoid hyperplasia in the spleen, liver and bone marrow. Myeloid hyperplasia of the bone marrow leads to erythropoiesis and malarial pigmentation (hemozoin) in the Kupffer cells of the liver, in bone marrow macrophages and in the red pulp of the spleen. Splenic rupture, nephron necrosis in the kidney and haemorrhages in the brain have been reported in infected animals.

Table 15.17 Lymphatic filarial worms in primates.

	Prosimians	New World monkeys	Old World monkeys	Apes
Family Onchocercidae	*Brugia tupaiae*		*Brugia malayi*	
			Brugia pahangi	

Diagnosis: Diagnosis depends on the morphological identification of the organisms in the erythrocytes in blood smears stained with Giemsa. Fluorescent antibody tests have been developed for non-human primates to determine current, or previous, malaria infections.

Treatment: Malaria in primates can be treated with chloroquine given intramuscularly, followed by primaquine given orally. These drugs should be given separately because of the increased risk of toxicity when given together.

Control: Effective mosquito control is essential to prevent malaria transmission in primate colonies. Infected primates are also a source of infection to humans, if the mosquito vectors are present, and appropriate steps should be taken to minimise risk of zoonotic transmission.

Malaria parasites of prosimians

Plasmodium hylobati

Plasmodium hylobati, synonyms *Plasmodium eylesi*, *Plasmodium jefferyi* and *Plasmodium youngi* (Phylum: Apicomplexa; Class: Aconoidasida; Order: Haemosporida; Family: Plasmodiidae), is localised in the blood of gibbons and is distributed in Southeast Asia.

Pathogenesis: *Plasmodium hylobati*, *P. eylesi* and *P. youngi* produce a quartan malaria in gibbons and are reported to be pathogenic, producing a fever associated with the parasitaemia.

Malaria parasites of Old World monkeys

Plasmodium knowlesi

Plasmodium knowlesi (Phylum: Apicomplexa; Class: Aconoidasida; Order: Haemosporida; Family: Plasmodiidae) is localised in the blood of cynomolgus monkeys, leaf monkeys, pig-tailed macaques, rhesus monkeys and humans. It is distributed in Southeast Asia.

Pathogenesis: This quotidian malaria parasite produces a virulent infection in rhesus monkeys that is almost always fatal and resembles acute *Plasmodium falciparum* infection in humans.

Plasmodium cynomolgi

Plasmodium cynomolgi (Phylum: Apicomplexa; Class: Aconoidasida; Order: Haemosporida; Family: Plasmodiidae) is localised in the blood of toque monkeys, pig-tailed macaques, bonnet macaques, leaf monkeys, rhesus monkeys and humans. It is distributed in Southeast Asia, East Indies and Philippines.

Pathogenesis: A tertian malaria parasite of low pathogenicity that causes a low-grade parasitaemia resembling *Plasmodium ovale* infection in humans.

Plasmodium gonderi

Plasmodium gonderi (Phylum: Apicomplexa; Class: Aconoidasida; Order: Haemosporida; Family: Plasmodiidae) is distributed in West and Central Africa and localised in the blood of mangabeys and drills.

Pathogenesis: A tertian malaria parasite that produces a high, chronic parasitaemia in rhesus monkeys, and which can also infect baboons, guenons and humans.

Plasmodium fieldi

Plasmodium fieldi (Phylum: Apicomplexa; Class: Aconoidasida; Order: Haemosporida; Family: Plasmodiidae) is distributed in the Malay Peninsula and localised in the blood of cynomolgus monkeys and pig-tailed macaques.

Pathogenesis: A tertian malaria parasite that can cause severe disease in rhesus monkeys that is often fatal.

Plasmodium fragile

Plasmodium fragile (Phylum: Apicomplexa; Class: Aconoidasida; Order: Haemosporida; Family: Plasmodiidae) is localised in the blood of toque monkeys and bonnet macaques. It is distributed in southern India and Sri Lanka.

Pathogenesis: A tertian malaria parasite that causes severe disease and death in rhesus monkeys.

Plasmodium siminovale

Plasmodium siminovale (Phylum: Apicomplexa; Class: Aconoidasida; Order: Haemosporida; Family: Plasmodiidae) is localised in the blood of toque monkeys in Sri Lanka.

Pathogenesis: A tertian malaria parasite of low pathogenicity but which can cause severe anaemia and is similar to *P. ovale* infection in humans.

Plasmodium coatneyi

Plasmodium coatneyi (Phylum: Apicomplexa; Class: Aconoidasida; Order: Haemosporida; Family: Plasmodiidae) is localised in the blood of cynomolgus monkeys in the Malay Peninsula and Philippines.

Pathogenesis: A tertian malaria parasite similar to *P. knowlsei* that causes severe anaemia in rhesus monkeys.

Plasmodium inui

Plasmodium inui (Phylum: Apicomplexa; Class: Aconoidasida; Order: Haemosporida; Family: Plasmodiidae) is localised in the blood of cynomolgus monkeys, pig-tailed macaques, Celebes black apes and humans, in southeast Asia extending from India to the Philippines.

Pathogenesis: A quartan malaria parasite of low pathogenicity that causes a mild to moderate non-fatal illness resembling *Plasmodium malariae* infection in humans.

Malaria parasites of New World monkeys

Plasmodium simium

Plasmodium simium (Phylum: Apicomplexa; Class: Aconoidasida; Order: Haemosporida; Family: Plasmodiidae) is localised in the blood of howler monkeys, spider monkeys, capuchins, woolly monkeys, squirrel monkeys and humans in the south of Brazil. This causes a tertian malaria resembling *P. vivax* infection in humans.

Plasmodium brazilianum

Plasmodium brazilianum (Phylum: Apicomplexa; Class: Aconoidasida; Order: Haemosporida; Family: Plasmodiidae) is localised in the blood of howler monkeys, spider monkeys, capuchins, woolly monkeys, squirrel monkeys and humans. It is distributed in Mexico, Central America and South America.

Pathogenesis: A quartan malaria parasite that causes severe symptoms and is considered to be the same as *P. malariae* infection in humans.

Plasmodium rodhaini

Plasmodium rodhaini (Phylum: Apicomplexa; Class: Aconoidasida; Order: Haemosporida; Family: Plasmodiidae) is localised in the blood of chimpanzees, gorillas and humans. It is distributed in West and Central Africa. It causes a quartan malaria that is considered synonymous with *P. malariae* infection in humans.

Malaria parasites of apes

Plasmodium reichenowi

Plasmodium reichenowi (Phylum: Apicomplexa; Class: Aconoidasida; Order: Haemosporida; Family: Plasmodiidae) is localised in the blood of chimpanzees, gorillas and humans in West, Central and East Africa. It causes a mildly pathogenic quartan malaria similar to *P. falciparum* infection in humans.

Plasmodium schwetzi

Plasmodium schwetzi (Phylum: Apicomplexa; Class: Aconoidasida; Order: Haemosporida; Family: Plasmodiidae) is localised in the blood of chimpanzees, gorillas and humans in West Africa. It causes a mildly pathogenic tertian malaria similar to *P. vivax* infection in humans, often in subclinical forms.

Hepatocystis kochi

Hepatocystis kochi (Phylum: Apicomplexa; Class: Aconoidasida; Order: Haemosporida; Family: Plasmodiidae) is localised in the blood of Old World monkeys and apes (gibbons, orangutans). It is distributed in the Indian subcontinent and sub-Saharan Africa with a high incidence in primates within endemic areas.

Clinical signs and pathology: Infected primates have numerous scattered greyish-white foci on the surface of the liver due to the presence of mature merocysts. Histologically, the cysts are surrounded by neutrophils. Following rupture of the cyst, a granulomatous inflammatory reaction occurs with infiltration of lymphocytes and macrophages. Because of this location, clinical disease, cyclical fever and blood parasitaemia do not usually occur in infected animals.

Diagnosis: Diagnosis is based on demonstration and identification of the parasite in blood smears or finding the typical hepatic lesions on *post mortem*.

Control and treatment: An effective vector control programme prevents spread within primate colonies. Treatment is not usually required.

Other *Hepatocystis* species in monkeys are listed in Table 15.18.

Babesia pitheci

Babesia pitheci (Phylum: Apicomplexa; Class: Aconoidasida; Order: Piroplasmida; Family: Babesiidae) is localised in the blood of Old World monkeys (mangabeys, guenons, macaques, baboons) and New World monkeys (marmosets). This parasite is considered to be only slightly pathogenic.

Parasites of the nervous system

Taenia multiceps

Taenia multiceps, synonyms *Multiceps multiceps*, *Coenurus cerebralis* (Phylum: Platyhelminthes; Class: Cestoda; Order: Cyclophyllidea; Family: Taeniidae), causes a disease commonly known as Gid and Coenurosis, is distributed worldwide and localised in the CNS, subcutaneous tissues, liver and other organs (intermediate hosts) and small intestine (final hosts). Final hosts are dogs, foxes, coyotes and jackals. Sheep, cattle, deer, pigs, horses, camels, humans and primates (macaques, vervets, baboons) are considered intermediate hosts.

Pathogenesis: The coenurus takes about eight months to mature in the CNS and as it develops, it causes damage to the brain tissue resulting in neurological disturbances. These cysts can cause pressure atrophy, which may lead to perforation of the skull. When cysts locate in the spinal cord, the resulting pressure can lead to paresis of the hindlimbs. Although an acute form of coenurosis can occur, chronic disease is more frequently identified. The migration of large numbers of larval stages through the brain can rapidly lead to neurological dysfunction and death.

Table 15.18 Other *Hepatocystis* species.

Species	Hosts	Vectors
Hepatocystis semnopitheci	Monkeys	Midges (*Culicoides*)
Hepatocystis taiwanensis	Monkeys	Midges (*Culicoides*)
Hepatocystis bouillezi	Monkeys	Midges (*Culicoides*)
Hepatocystis cercopitheci	Monkeys	Midges (*Culicoides*)
Hepatocystis foleyi	Monkeys	Midges (*Culicoides*)

Clinical signs and pathology: Clinical signs depend on the number of cysts present and their location. When the CNS is involved, neurological symptoms may occur. The cyst or cysts are mainly located in one cerebral hemisphere and occur less frequently in the cerebellum and spinal cord (see Fig. 9.27). The growth of the cysts within the brain or skull causes pressure atrophy of adjacent cerebral tissue. The migration of large numbers of immature stages in the brain of lambs can lead to acute meningoencephalitis. In acute cases of coenurosis, pale yellow tracts are frequently present on the surface of the brain. They comprise necrotic tissue with marked cellular infiltration. In chronic coenurosis there may be compression of brain tissue by the developing cyst and the increased intracranial pressure can result in local softening of the bones of the skull, either above the cyst or in other areas.

Diagnosis: Diagnosis can be made by radiography or the finding of masses in the subcutaneous tissues. Identification is based on the morphology of the scolices.

Thelazia callipaeda

Thelazia callipaeda (Phylum: Nematoda; Class: Chromadorea; Order: Spirurida; Family: Thelaziidae), commonly known as the Eye worm, is localised in the eye, conjunctival sac and lacrimal duct of dogs, cats, humans and primates, and is distributed in Asia, Europe and the USA. This parasite has drosophilid flies of the genera *Amiota* and *Phortica* as intermediate hosts. For more details see Chapter 12.

Acanthamoeba spp.

Acanthamoeba spp. (Phylum: Amoebozoa; Class: Discosea; Order: Centramoebida; Family: Acanthamoebidae) have a presumed worldwide distribution and are localised in the brain and lung of Old World monkeys and humans. *Acanthamoeba* are opportunistic pathogens that have reportedly caused meningoencephalitis and keratitis in humans. Relatively small amoebae with a vesicular nucleus and a large endosome but without well-developed cytoplasm. Cysts have a single nucleus.

Naegleria fowleri

Naegleria fowleri (Phylum: Percolozoa; Class: Heterolobosea; Order: Schizopyrenida; Family: Vahlkampfidae) has a presumed worldwide distribution and is localised in the CNS and nasal mucosa of Old World monkeys and humans. *Naegleria* are opportunistic pathogens found in water, faeces and sewage, and cause amoebic meningoencephalitis in humans. The trophozoites are characterised by a nucleus and surrounding halo. They travel by pseudopodia, temporary round processes which fill with granular cytoplasm. The pseudopodia form at different points along the cell, thus allowing the trophozoite to change direction. There is no effective treatment.

Encephalitozoon cuniculi

Encephalitozoon cuniculi, synonym *Nosema cuniculi* (Phylum: Microsporidia; Class: Microsporea; Order: Microsporida; Family: Unikaryonidae), is distributed worldwide, and localised in the brain, kidney, heart and lungs of rabbits, dogs, red foxes (*Vulpes vulpes*), blue foxes (*Alopex lagopus*), silver foxes, cats, mice, rats, humans and monkeys.

Parasites of the reproductive/ urogenital system

Schistosoma haematobium

For more details see Parasites of the circulatory system.

Klossiella spp.

An unknown species of *Klossiella* has been reported from the kidneys of marmosets. In other hosts, where these parasites are more commonly found, infections are not considered significant.

Parasites of the locomotory system

Infections with *Sarcocystis* have been described in the skeletal muscle, and occasionally in the heart and smooth muscle, of a number of primate species. The two main species reports in rhesus monkeys involve *Sarcocystis kortei* and *Sarcocystis nesbitti*. Other unnamed species have been reported from both Old World and New World monkeys. Their life cycles and definitive hosts are also unknown.

Parasites of the integument

Subcutaneous filarial worms

A variety of filarial worms (Filarioidea) commonly parasitise primates, being found in the subcutaneous tissues and the abdominal and thoracic cavities (Table 15.19). Subcutaneous worms cause little if any inflammatory response, whereas those in the serous cavities may cause a fibrinopurulent peritonitis or pleuritis with associated fibrinous adhesions. Transmission of these parasites within primate colonies is unlikely and no special control measures are required other than control of possible arthropod vectors.

Sarcocystis spp.

Sarcocystis spp. (Phylum: Apicomplexa; Class: Conoidasida; Order: Eucoccidiorida; Family: Sarcocystidae) are localised in the muscle of hosts. Reported species include *S. kortei* and *S. nesbitti* from Old World monkeys.

Clinical signs and pathology: Lesions associated with naturally occurring infections are rare. Infection causes inflammation characterised by infiltrates of lymphocytes, plasma cells and eosinophils associated with degeneration of cysts within the muscle fibres.

Diagnosis: Sarcocystiosis is usually an incidental finding, and diagnosis is based on the identification of the characteristic intramuscular cysts.

Table 15.19 Filarial worms of the subcutis in primates.

	Prosimians	New World monkeys	Old World monkeys	Apes
Family Onchocercidae	Dipetalonema petteri	Mansonella atelenis	Dirofilaria corynoides	Dirofilaria immitis (pongoi)
		Mansonella parvum	Dirofilaria immitis	Mansonella rohdani
		Mansonella panamensis	Dirofilaria repens	Mansonella streptocerca
		Mansonella saimiri	Dirofilaria magnilarvatum	Mansonella leopoldi
		Mansonella columbiensis	Cercopithifilaria papionis	Mansonella gorrillae
		Dipetalonema tenue	Cercopithifilaria degraffi	Mansonella lopeensis
			Cercopithifilaria verveti	Loa loa
			Cercopithifilaria narokensis	
			Cercopithifilaria eberhardi	
			Loa papionis	

Toxoplasma gondii

For details see section on Rabbits (Parasites of the locomotory system).

Trypanosoma cruzi

For details see Parasites of the circulatory system.

ECTOPARASITES

Lice

Chewing lice (Suborders Ambylocera and Ischnocera) are rare on primates and of little significance (Table 15.20). In contrast, numerous species of sucking lice (Suborder Anoplura) have been reported from a wide variety of primates (Table 15.21). Many species of sucking lice are considered interchangeable between apes, humans and New World monkeys and thus some of the species' names used may be synonymous or no longer valid. For further details of the lice genera see Chapter 3 (Order Psocodea).

Mites

Sarcoptes scabiei

Sarcoptes scabiei (Phylum: Arthropoda; Class: Arachnida; Subclass: Acari; Order: Sarcoptiformes (Astigmata); Family: Sarcoptidae), commonly known as a Scabies mite, is a burrowing mite that causes mange in all domestic mammals, including humans and primates (cynomolgus monkeys, drills, chimpanzees, gorillas, orangutans, gibbons) worldwide.

Epidemiology: Infestations on primates are transmissible to humans by direct contact and infected animals should be handled with caution.

Table 15.20 Chewing lice of primates.

	Prosimians	New World monkeys	Old World monkeys	Apes
Family Trichodectidae	Trichodectes mjoebergi	Trichodectes armatus	Trichodectes colobi	
		Trichodectes semiarmatus	Eutrichophilus setosus	
		Cebidicola armatus		
		Cebidicola semiarmatus		
Family Philopteridae	Trichophilopterus ferresti			
Family Gyropidae		Aotiella aotophilus		

Table 15.21 Sucking lice of primates.

	Prosimians	New World monkeys	Old World monkeys	Apes
Family Pedicinidae			Pedicinus eurigaster	Pedicinus schaeffi
			Pedicinus obtusus	
			Pedicinus patas	
			Pedicinus pictus	
			Pedicinus hamadryas	
			Pedicinus mjobergi	
			Pedicinus schaeffi	
Family Pediculidae		Pediculus humanus		Pediculus humanus
		Pediculus mjöbergi		Pediculus schaeffi
Family Pthiridae				Pthirus pubis

Table 15.22 Other mite species found on primates.

	Prosimians	New World monkeys	Old World monkeys	Apes
Family Sarcoptidae			*Sarcoptes pitheci*	
			Prosarcoptes pitheci	
			Pithesarcoptes talapoini	
Family Psoroptidae			*Paracoroptes gordoni*	
Family Psorergatidae			*Psorergates cercopitheci*	
Family Atopomelidae		*Listrocarpus hapeli*		
		Listrocarpus saimirii		
		Listrocarpus lagothrix		

Pathogenesis: Host reactions occur primarily in response to the feeding and burrowing activity of the mites and their faecal deposits.

Clinical signs: Signs include intense pruritus, anorexia, emaciation and self-mutilation with bleeding and secondary bacterial dermatitis. There may be thickening of the skin and hair loss.

Diagnosis: Confirmatory diagnosis is by examination of skin scrapings for the presence of mites. However, since these are sometimes difficult to demonstrate, a negative finding should not preclude a tentative diagnosis of mange and initiation of treatment.

Control and treatment: Infected animals should be treated with an acaricide and successful treatment has been reported with ivermectin.

Other mite species found on primates are listed in Table 15.22.

Fleas

There is little information on flea infestations in primates. Most recorded species are opportunistic species that are natural parasites of other animals. Flea species are covered in more detail in Chapter 3.

Flies

The larval bots of several species of flies in the families Cuterebrinae and Calliphoridae are reported to infect primates. Further details are provided in the checklist at the end of this chapter and in Chapter 3.

Ticks

A number of species of ixodid ticks have been reported from numerous species of primates throughout the areas of the world where wild primates are found. Ticks are important as vectors of

disease, many of which are zoonotic, and their importance in primates is very much dependent on tick abundance and species distribution. In captive primates, ticks are less of a problem because when engorged they drop off, and under conditions of captivity the hosts are unlikely to become reinfested.

Where they do occur, tick infestations are generally asymptomatic but with heavy parasite loads irritation and anaemia may manifest. Because ticks can be vectors of zoonotic diseases, newly acquired primates should be quarantined, examined and treated if infested.

HOST–PARASITE CHECKLISTS

In the following checklists, the codes listed below apply.

Helminths

N, nematode; T, trematode; C, cestode; A, acanthocephalan.

Arthropods

F, fly; L, louse; S, flea; M, mite; Mx, maxillopod; Ti, tick; Pn, pentastomid.

Protozoa

Co, coccidia; Bs, blood sporozoa; Am, amoeba; Fl, flagellate; Ci, ciliate.

Miscellaneous 'protozoal organisms'

B, blastocyst; Mi, microsporidian; My, *Mycoplasma*; P, Pneumocystidomycete; R, *Rickettsia*.

Rabbit parasite checklist.

Section/host system	Helminths		Arthropods		Protozoa	
	Parasite	(Super) family	Parasite	Family	Parasite	Family
Digestive						
Oesophagus						
Stomach	Graphidium strigosum	Trichostrongyloidea (N)				
	Obeliscoides cuniculi	Trichostrongyloidea (N)				
Small intestine	Trichostrongylus retortaeformis	Trichostrongyloidea (N)			Eimeria flavescens	Eimeriidae (Co)
	Trichostrongylus colubriformis	Trichostrongyloidea (N)			Eimeria exigua	Eimeriidae (Co)
	Trichostrongylus vitrinus	Trichostrongyloidea (N)			Eimeria intestinalis	Eimeriidae (Co)
	Trichostrongylus calcaratus	Trichostrongyloidea (N)			Eimeria irresidua	Eimeriidae (Co)
	Nematodirus leporis	Trichostrongyloidea (N)			Eimeria magna	Eimeriidae (Co)
	Strongyloides papillosus	Strongyloidoidea (N)			Eimeria media	Eimeriidae (Co)
	Cittotaenia ctenoides	Anoplocephalidae (C)			Eimeria perforans	Eimeriidae (Co)
	Cittotaenia denticulata	Anoplocephalidae (C)			Eimeria vejdovskyi	Eimeriidae (Co)
	Cittotaenia pectinata	Anoplocephalidae (C)				
	Paranoplocephala cuniculi	Anoplocephalidae (C)				
Caecum, colon	Passalurus ambiguus	Oxyuroidea (N)			Eimeria pyriformis	Eimeriidae (Co)
	Passalurus nonannulatus	Oxyuroidea (N)			Eimeria coecicola	Eimeriidae (Co)
	Dermatoxys veligera	Oxyuroidea (N)			Eimeria flavescens	Eimeriidae (Co)
	Trichuris leporis	Trichuroidea (N)			Entamoeba cuniculi	Entamoebidae (Fl)
					Retortamonas cuniculi	Retortamonadorididae (Fl)
Respiratory						
Nose						
Trachea, bronchi						
Lung	Protostrongylus tauricus	Metastrongyloidea (N)				
	Protostrongylus pulmonaris	Metastrongyloidea (N)				
	Protostrongylus oryctolagi	Metastrongyloidea (N)				
	Echinococcus granulosus	Taeniidae (C)				
Liver						
	Capillaria hepatica	Trichuroidea (N)			Eimeria stiedai	Eimeriidae (Co)
	Fasciola hepatica	Fasciolidae (T)				
	Echinococcus granulosus	Taeniidae (C)				
	Cysticercus serialis	Taeniidae (C)				
	(metacestode: Taenia serialis)					
Pancreas						
Peritoneum	Cysticercus serialis	Taeniidae (C)				
	(metacestode: Taenia serialis)					
Circulatory						
Blood						
Blood vessels					Rickettsia conorii	Rickettsiaceae (R)
					Hepatozoon cuniculi	Hepatozoidae (Co)
Spleen						

(Continued)

Rabbit parasite checklist. *Continued*

Section/host system	Helminths		Arthropods		Protozoa	
	Parasite	(Super) family	Parasite	Family	Parasite	Family
Nervous						
CNS					*Encephalitozoon cuniculi*	Unikaryonidae (Mi)
Eye						
Ear			*Psoroptes cuniculi*	Psoroptidae (A)		
Reproductive/urogenital						
Kidneys						
Locomotory						
Muscle					*Sarcocystis cuniculi* *Toxoplasma gondii*	Sarcocystidae (Co) Sarcocystidae (Co)
Connective tissue	*Pelecitus scapiceps* *Coenurus serialis* (metacestode: *Taenia serialis*)	Filarioidea (N) Taeniidae (C)				
Subcutaneous			*Cordylobia anthropophaga* *Cordylobia rhodaini* *Dermatobia hominis*	Calliphoridae (F) Calliphoridae (F) Oestridae (F)		
Integument						
Skin			*Leporacarus gibbus* *Notoedres cati* *Sarcoptes scabiei* *Chorioptes bovis* *Cheyletiella parasitivorax* *Neotrombicula autumnalis* *Dermanyssus gallinae* *Spilopsyllus cuniculi* *Ctenocephalides felis* *Ctenocephalides canis* *Echidnophaga gallinacea* *Lucilia sericata* *Wohlfahrtia vigil*	Listrophoridae (L) Sarcoptidae (M) Sarcoptidae (M) Psoroptidae (M) Cheyletidae (M) Trombiculidae (M) Dermanyssidae (M) Pulicidae (S) Pulicidae (S) Pulicidae (S) Pulicidae (S) Calliphoridae (F) Sarcophagidae (F)		

Guinea pig parasite checklist.

Section/host system	Helminths		Arthropods		Protozoa	
	Parasite	(Super) family	Parasite	Family	Parasite	Family
Digestive						
Oesophagus						
Stomach						
Small intestine	Hymenolepis diminuta	Hymenolepididae (C)			Eimeria caviae	Eimeriidae (Co)
	Hymenolepis nana	Hymenolepididae (C)			Cryptosporidium wrairi	Cryptosporidiidae (Co)
					Giardia intestinalis	Giardiidae (Fl)
Caecum, colon	Paraspidodera uncinata	Ascaridoidea (N)			Entamoeba caviae	Entamobidae (Am)
					Tritrichomonas caviae	Trichomonadidae (Fl)
					Caviomonas mobilis	Caviomonadidae (Fl)
					Enteromonas caviae	Enteromonadidae (Fl)
					Monocercomonoides caviae	Polymastigidae (Fl)
					Monocercomonoides quadrifunilis	Polymastigidae (Fl)
					Monocercomonoides wenrichi	Polymastigidae (Fl)
					Monocercomonoides exilis	Polymastigidae (Fl)
					Protomonas brevifilia	Proteromonadidae (Fl)
					Hexamastix caviae	Hexamastigidae (Fl)
					Hexamastix robustus	Hexarrastigidae (Fl)
					Chilomitus caviae	Monocercomonadidae (Fl)
					Chilomitus conexus	Monocercomonadidae (Fl)
					Retortamonas caviae	Retortamonadidae (Fl)
					Tritrichomonas caviae	Trichomonadidae (Fl)
Respiratory						
Nose						
Trachea, bronchi						
Lung						
Liver						
Pancreas						
Circulatory						
Blood						
Blood vessels						
Nervous						
CNS						
Eye						
Reproductive/urogenital						
Kidneys					Klossiella cobayae	Klossiellidae (Co)
Locomotory						
Muscle					Toxoplasma gondii	Sarcocystidae (Co)
Connective tissue						
Subcutaneous			Cuterebra spp.	Oestridae (F)		
Integument						
Skin			Trixacarus caviae	Sarcoptidae (M)		
			Psoroptes cuniculi	Psoroptidae (M)		
			Demodex caviae	Demodicidae (M)		
			Chirodiscoides caviae	Atopomelidae (M)		
			Gliricola porcelli	Gyropidae (L)		
			Gyropus ovalis	Gyropidae (L)		
			Trimenopon hispidium	Trimenoponidae (L)		
			Ctenocephalides felis	Pulicidae (S)		

803

Rat parasite checklist.

Section/host system	Helminths		Arthropods		Protozoa	
	Parasite	(Super) family	Parasite	Family	Parasite	Family
Digestive						
Oesophagus						
Stomach						
Small intestine	Nematospiroides dubius	Trichostrongyloidea (N)			Eimeria nieschulzi	Eimeriidae (Co)
	Nippostrongylus brasiliensis	Trichostrongyloidea (N)			Eimeria hasei	Eimeriidae (Co)
	Hymenolepis diminuta	Hymenolepididae (C)			Eimeria nochti	Eimeriidae (Co)
	Hymenolepis nana	Hymenolepididae (C)			Eimeria ratti	Eimeriidae (Co)
					Cryptosporidium muris	Cryptosporidiidae (Co)
					Giardia muris	Giardiidae (Fl)
					Spironucleus muris	Spironucleidae (Fl)
Caecum, colon	Aspiculuris tetraptera	Oxyuroidea (N)			Eimeria separata	Eimeriidae (Co)
	Syphacia muris	Oxyuroidea (N)			Tetratrichomonas microti	Trichomonadidae (Fl)
	Syphacia obvelata	Oxyuroidea (N)			Tritrichomonas muris	Trichomonadidae (Fl)
	Trichuris muris	Trichuroidea (N)			Tritrichomonas minuta	Trichomonadidae (Fl)
					Tritrichomonas wenyoni	Trichomonadidae (Fl)
					Spironucleus muris	Spironucleidae (Fl)
					Enteromonas hominis	Enteromonadidae (Fl)
					Entamoeba muris	Entamobidae (Am)
					Endolimax nana	Entamobidae (Am)
Respiratory						
Nose						
Trachea, bronchi						
Lung	Angiostrongylus cantonensis	Metastrongyloidea (N)				
Liver	Capillaria hepatica	Trichuroidea (N)				
	Cysticercus fasciolaris (metacestode: Taenia taeniaeformis)	Taeniidae (C)				
Pancreas						
Circulatory						
Blood	Angiostrongylus costaricensis	Metastrongyloidea (N)			Hepatozoon muris	Hepatozoidae (Co)
Blood vessels						
Nervous						
CNS						
Eye						

Reproductive/urogenital			
Kidneys	Trichosomoides crassicauda		Trichuroidea (N)
Locomotory			
Muscle		Toxoplasma gondii	Sarcocystidae (Co)
Connective tissue			
Subcutaneous	Cuterebra spp.	Oestridae (F)	
Integument			
Skin	Notoedres muris	Sarcoptidae (M)	
	Demodex ratticola	Demodecidae (M)	
	Radfordia ensifera	Myobidae (M)	
	Leptotrombidium deliense	Trombiculidae (M)	
	Dermanyssus gallinae	Dermanyssidae (M)	
	Liponyssoides sanguineus	Dermanyssidae (M)	
	Haemogamasus pontiger	Haemogamasidae (M)	
	Androlaelaps casalis	Laelapidae (M)	
	Hirstionyssus isabellinus	Laelapidae (M)	
	Laelaps echidnina	Laelapidae (M)	
	Laelaps nuttali	Laelapidae (M)	
	Eulaelaps stabularis	Laelapidae (M)	
	Ornithonyssus sylviarum	Macronyssidae (M)	
	Ornithonyssus bacoti	Macronyssidae (M)	
	Psorobia simplex	Psorergatidae (M)	
	Trimenopon jenningsi	Trimenoponidae (M)	
	Polyplax spinulosa	Polyplacidae (L)	
	Xenopsylla cheopis	Pulicidae (S)	
	Nosopsyllus fasciatus	Ceratopyllidae (S)	
	Leptopsylla segnis	Leptopsyllidae (S)	

Mouse parasite checklist.

Section/host system	Helminths		Arthropods		Protozoa	
	Parasite	(Super) family	Parasite	Family	Parasite	Family
Digestive						
Oesophagus						
Stomach						
Small intestine	Nematospiroides dubius	Trichostrongyloidea (N)			Cryptosporidium muris	Cryptosporididae (Co)
	Nippostrongylus brasiliensis	Trichostrongyloidea (N)			Giardia muris	Giardiidae (Fl)
	Hymenolepis diminuta	Hymenolepididae (C)			Spironucleus muris	Hexamitidae (Fl)
	Hymenolepis nana	Hymenolepididae (C)			Eimeria falciformis	Eimeriidae (Co)
					Eimeria musculi	Eimeriidae (Co)
					Eimeria scheuffneri	Eimeriidae (Co)
					Eimeria krijgsmanni	Eimeriidae (Co)
					Eimeria keilini	Eimeriidae (Co)
					Eimeria hindlei	Eimeriidae (Co)
Caecum, colon	Aspiculuris tetraptera	Oxyuroidea (N)			Tetratrichomonas microti	Trichomonadidae (Fl)
	Syphacia muris	Oxyuroidea (N)			Tritrichomonas muris	Trichomonadidae (Fl)
	Syphacia obvelata	Oxyuroidea (N)			Tritrichomonas minuta	Trichomonadidae (Fl)
	Trichuris muris	Trichuroidea (N)			Tritrichomonas wenyoni	Trichomonadidae (Fl)
					Spironucleus muris	Hexamitidae (Fl)
					Entamoeba muris	Entamobidae (Am)
Respiratory						
Nose						
Trachea, bronchi						
Lung						
Liver	Capillaria hepatica	Trichuroidea (N)				
	Cysticercus fasciolaris (metacestode: Taenia taeniaeformis)	Taeniidae (C)				
	Echinococcus granulosus	Taeniidae (C)				
Pancreas						
Circulatory						
Blood						
Blood vessels						
Nervous						
CNS						
Eye						

Reproductive/urogenital			
Kidneys	*Klossiella muris*		Klossiellidae (Co)
Locomotory			
Muscle	*Toxoplasma gondii*		Sarcocystidae (Co)
	Sarcocystis muris		Sarcocystidae (Co)
Connective tissue			
Subcutaneous	*Cuterebra* spp.	Oestridae (Fl)	
Integument			
Skin	*Myobia musculi*	Myobiidae (M)	
	Myocoptes musculinus	Myocoptidae (M)	
	Radfordia affinis	Myobiidae (M)	
	Demodex musculi	Demodicidae (M)	
	Psorogates simplex	Psorogatidae (M)	
	Ornithonyssus bacoti	Macronyssidae (M)	
	Trichoecius romboutsi	Myocoptidae (M)	
	Liponyssoides sanguineus	Dermanyssidae (M)	
	Haemogamasus pontiger	Haemogamasidae (M)	
	Hirstionyssus isabellinus	Laelapidae (M)	
	Laelaps echidninus	Laelapidae (M)	
	Laelaps nuttali	Laelapidae (M)	
	Eulaelaps stabularis	Laelapidae (M)	
	Leptotrombidium deliense	Trombiculidae (M)	
	Polyplax serrata	Polyplacidae (L)	
	Polyplax spinulosa	Polyplacidae (L)	
	Xenopsylla cheopis	Pulicidae (S)	
	Nosopsyllus fasciatus	Ceratopyllidae (S)	
	Leptopsylla segnis	Leptopsyllidae (S)	

807

Primate parasite checklist.

	Helminths		Arthropods		Protozoa	
Section/host system	Parasite	(Super) family	Parasite	Family	Parasite	Family
Digestive						
Mouth	Gongylonema macrogubernaculum	Spiruroidea (N)			Trichomonas tenax	Trichomonadidae (Fl) E
Oesophagus	Gongylonema macrogubernaculum	Spiruroidea (N)			Entameoba gingivalis	Entamoebidae (Am)
Stomach	Nochtia nochti	Trichostrongyloidea (N)			Entamoeba histolytica	Entamoebidae (Am)
	Gongylonema pulchrum	Spiruroidea (N)				
	Gongylonema macrogubernaculum	Spiruroidea (N)				
	Streptopharagus armatus	Spiruroidea (N)				
	Streptopharagus pigmentatus	Spiruroidea (N)				
	Protospirura muricola	Spiruroidea (N)				
	Physaloptera tumefasciens	Physalopteroidea (N)				
	Physaloptera dilatata	Physalopteroidea (N)				
	Physaloptera caucasica	Physalopteroidea (N)				
	Physaloptera poicilometra	Physalopteroidea (N)				
	Subulura distans	Subuluroidea (N)				
Small intestine	Ancylostoma duodenale	Ancylostomatoidea (N)			Eimeria galago	Eimeriidae (Co)
	Necator americanus	Ancylostomatoidea (N)			Eimeria ferruginea	Eimeriidae (Co)
	Strongyloides stercoralis	Strongyloidoidea (N)			Eimeria lemuris	Eimeriidae (Co)
	Strongyloides fulleborni	Strongyloidoidea (N)			Eimeria modesta	Eimeriidae (Co)
	Strongyloides cebus	Strongyloidoidea (N)			Eimeria otolicni	Eimeriidae (Co)
	Ascaris lumbricoides	Ascaridoidea (N)			Eimeria pachylepyron	Eimeriidae (Co)
	Globocephalus simiae	Ancylostomatoidea (N)			Eimeria tupaiae	Eimeriidae (Co)
	Angiostrongylus costaricensis	Metastrongyloidea (N)			Isospora aectopitheci	Eimeriidae (Co)
	Pterygodermatities alphi	Spiruroidea (N)			Isospora callimico	Eimeriidae (Co)
	Pterygodermatities nycticebi	Spiruroidea (N)			Isospora papionis	Eimeriidae (Co)
	Molineus elegans	Trichostrongyloidea (N)			Isospora spp.	Eimeriidae (Co)
	Molineus torulosus	Trichostrongyloidea (N)			Cyclospora cayetenensis	Eimeriidae (Co)
	Molineus vexillarius	Trichostrongyloidea (N)			Cryptosporidium parvum	Cryptosporidiidae (Co)
	Nematodirus weinbergi	Trichostrongyloidea (N)			Giardia intestinalis	Giardiidae (Fl)
	Tupaiostrongylus liei	Trichostrongyloidea (N)			Tritrichomonas mobilensis	Trichomonadidae (Fl)
	Tupaiostrongylus major	Trichostrongyloidea (N)			Spironucleus pitheci	Spironucleidae (Fl)
	Tupaiostrongylus minor	Trichostrongyloidea (N)			Balantidium coli	Balantididae (Ci)
	Novetrema nycticeba	Lecithodendriidae (T)				
	Odeningotrema apidon	Lecithodendriidae (T)				
	Odeningotrema bivesicularis	Lecithodendriidae (T)				
	Phaneropsolus bonnie	Lecithodendriidae (T)				
	Phaneropsolus lakdivensis	Lecithodendriidae (T)				
	Phaneropsolus longipenis	Lecithodendriidae (T)				
	Phaneropsolus perodictici	Lecithodendriidae (T)				
	Phaneropsolus orbicularis	Lecithodendriidae (T)				
	Phaneropsolus simiae	Lecithodendriidae (T)				
	Phaneropsolus aspinosus	Lecithodendriidae (T)				
	Phaneropsolus oviforme	Lecithodendriidae (T)				
	Primatotrema macacae	Lecithodendriidae (T)				
	Primatotrema kellogi	Lecithodendriidae (T)				

Location	Species	Family
	Watsonius watsoni	Paramphistomatidae (T)
	Watsonius deschieni	Paramphistomatidae (T)
	Watsonius macaci	Paramphistomatidae (T)
	Gastrodiscoides hominis	Gastrodiscidae (T)
	Chiorchis noci	Heterophyidae (T)
	Neodiplostomum tamarini	Diplostomidae (T)
	Haplorchis pumilo	Heterophyidae (T)
	Haplorchis yokogawi	Heterophyidae (T)
	Metagonimus yokogawai	Heterophyidae (T)
	Pygidiopsis summa	Heterophyidae (T)
	Echinostoma aphylactum	Echinostomatidae (T)
	Echinostoma ilocanum	Echinostomatidae (T)
	Ogmcotyle ailuri	Notocotylidae (T)
	Ogmcotyle indica	Notocotylidae (T)
	Plagiorchis multiglandularis	Plagiorchidae (T)
	Bertiella mucronata	Anoplocephalidae (C)
	Bertiella fallax	Anoplocephalidae (C)
	Bertiella satyri	Anoplocephalidae (C)
	Bertiella studeri	Anoplocephalidae (C)
	Bertiella okabei	Anoplocephalidae (C)
	Moniezia rugosa	Anoplocephalidae (C)
	Tupaitaenia guentini	Anoplocephalidae (C)
	Atriotaenia megastoma	Anoplocephalidae (C)
	Matheovataenia brasiliensis	Anoplocephalidae (C)
	Matheovataenia cruzsilvai	Anoplocephalidae (C)
	Paratriotaenia oedipomidatus	Anoplocephalidae (C)
	Raillietina rothlsbergeri	Davaineidae (C)
	Raillietina alouattae	Davaineidae (C)
	Raillietina demerariensis	Davaineidae (C)
	Choanotaenia infundibulum	Dilepididae (C)
	Hymenolepis nana Hymenolepis diminuta	Hymenolepidae (C)
	Hymenolepis cebidarum	Hymenolepidae (C)
	Prosthenorchis spirula	Oligacanthorhynchidae (A)
Caecum, colon	*Oesophagostomum apiostomum*	Strongyloidea (N)
	Oesophagostomum bifurcatum	Strongyloidea (N)
	Oesophagostomum aculeatum	Strongyloidea (N)
	Oesophagostomum stephanostomum	Strongyloidea (N)
	Ternidens deminutus	Trichuroidea (N)
	Trichuris trichiura	Oligacanthorhynchidae (A)
	Prosthenorchis elegans	Oxyuroidea (N)
	Enterobius vermicularis	Oxyuroidea (N)
	Enterobius lemoris	Oxyuroidea (N)
	Enterobius brevicauda	
	Entamoeba histolytica	Entamoebidae (Am)
	Entamoeba hartmanni	Entamoebidae (Am)
	Entamoeba coli	Entamoebidae (Am)
	Entamoeba chattoni	Entamoebidae (Am)
	Iodamoeba buetschlii	Entamoebidae (Am)
	Endolomax nana	Entamoebidae (Am)
	Pentatrichomonas hominis	Trichomonadidae (Fl)
	Tritritrichomonas wenyoni	Trichomonadidae (Fl)
	Tritrichomonas mobilensis	Trichomonadidae (Fl)
	Dientamoeba fragilis	Monocercomonadidae (Fl)

(Continued)

809

Primate parasite checklist. *Continued*

Section/host system	Helminths		Arthropods		Protozoa	
	Parasite	(Super) family	Parasite	Family	Parasite	Family
	Enterobius bipapillata	Oxyuroidea (N)			*Enteromonas hominis*	Enteromonadidae (Fl)
	Enterobius pitheci	Oxyuroidea (N)			*Retortamonas intestinalis*	Retortamonadorididae (Fl)
	Enterobius parallela	Oxyuroidea (N)			*Chilomastix mesnili*	Retortamonadorididae (Fl)
	Enterobius zakari	Oxyuroidea (N)			*Spironucleus pitheci*	Spironucleidae (Fl)
	Enterobius chabaudi	Oxyuroidea (N)			*Balantidium coli*	Balantidiidae (Ci)
	Enterobius inglisi	Oxyuroidea (N)				
	Enterobius pesteri	Oxyuroidea (N)				
	Enterobius macaci	Oxyuroidea (N)				
	Enterobius presbytis	Oxyuroidea (N)				
	Enterobius anthropopitheci	Oxyuroidea (N)				
	Enterobius buckleyi	Oxyuroidea (N)				
	Enterobius lerouxi	Oxyuroidea (N)				
	Trypanoxyuris	Oxyuroidea (N)				
	Trypanoxyuris trypanuris	Oxyuroidea (N)				
	Trypanoxyuris atelis	Oxyuroidea (N)				
	Trypanoxyuris duplicideus	Oxyuroidea (N)				
	Trypanoxyuris lagothricis	Oxyuroidea (N)				
	Trypanoxyuris clementinae	Oxyuroidea (N)				
	Trypanoxyuris minutus	Oxyuroidea (N)				
	Trypanoxyuris satanus	Oxyuroidea (N)				
	Trypanoxyuris sceratus	Oxyuroidea (N)				
	Trypanoxyuris brachylelesi	Oxyuroidea (N)				
	Trypanoxyuris callithricis	Oxyuroidea (N)				
	Trypanoxyuris callicebi	Oxyuroidea (N)				
	Trypanoxyuris oedepi	Oxyuroidea (N)				
	Trypanoxyuris goedeli	Oxyuroidea (N)				
	Oxyuronema atelophorum	Oxyuroidea (N)				
	Primasubulura otolicni	Subuluroidea (N)				
	Primasubulura jacchi	Subuluroidea (N)				
	Probstmayria natalensis	Oxyuroidea (N)				
	Probstmayria gombensis	Oxyuroidea (N)				
	Probstmayria gorillae	Oxyuroidea (N)				
	Probstmayria simiae	Oxyuroidea (N)				
Respiratory						
Nose	*Anatrichosoma cynmologi*	Trichuroidea (N)	*Rhinophaga papinois*	Halarachnidae (M)		
			Rhinophaga elongata	Halarachnidae (M)		
			Rhinophaga dinolti	Halarachnidae (M)		
			Rhinophaga cercopitheci	Halarachnidae (M)		
			Rhinophaga pongicola	Halarachnidae (M)		
Larynx			*Pneumonyssus vocalis*	Halarachnidae (M)		
Trachea, bronchi			*Pneumonyssus congoensis*	Halarachnidae (M)		
			Pneumonyssus longus	Halarachnidae (M)		
			Pneumonyssus oudemansi	Halarachnidae (M)		
			Pneumonyssus africanus	Halarachnidae (M)		
Lung	*Filaroides barretoi*	Metastrongyloidea (M)	*Pneumonyssus simicola*	Halarachnidae (M)	*Pneumocystis carinii*	Pneumocystidaceae (P)
	Filaroides gordius	Metastrongyloidea (M)	*Pneumonyssus duttoni*	Halarachnidae (M)		
	Filaroides cebus	Metastrongyloidea (M)	*Pneumonyssus longus*	Halarachnidae (M)		
	Filariopsis arator	Metastrongyloidea (M)	*Pneumonyssus oudemansi*	Halarachnidae (M)		
	Paragonimus westermani	Paragonimidae (T)	*Pneumonyssus mossambicensis*	Halarachnidae (M)		
			Pneumonyssus congoensis	Halarachnidae (M)		
			Pneumonyssus rodhaini	Halarachnidae (M)		
			Pneumonyssus vitzthumi	Halarachnidae (M)		

Organ system	Species	Family
Liver		
	Capillaria hepatica	Trichuroidea (N)
	Echinococcus granulosus	Taeniidae (C)
	Athesmia heterolecithodes	Dicrocoeliidae (T)
	Controrchis biliophilus	Dicrocoeliidae (T)
	Brodenia lacinata	Dicrocoeliidae (T)
	Dicrocoelium colobusciola	Dicrocoeliidae (T)
	Dicrocoelium lanceolatum	Dicrocoeliidae (T)
	Dicrocoelium macaci	Dicrocoeliidae (T)
	Euparadistomum cercopitheci	Dicrocoeliidae (T)
	Eurytrema satoi	Dicrocoeliidae (T)
	Eurytrema brumpti	Dicrocoeliidae (T)
	Entamoeba histolytica	Entamoebidae (Am)
Pancreas		
	Eurytrema pancreaticum	Dicrocoeliidae (T)
Circulatory		
Blood	*Trypanosoma cruzi*	Trypanosomatidae (Fl)
	Spironucleus eylesi	Spironucleidae (Fl)
	Plasmodium hylobati	Plasmodiidae (Bs)
	Plasmodium jefferyi	Plasmodiidae (Bs)
	Plasmodium youngi	Plasmodiidae (Bs)
	Plasmodium knowlesi	Plasmodiidae (Bs)
	Plasmodium cynomolgi	Plasmodiidae (Bs)
	Plasmodium gonderi	Plasmodiidae (Bs)
	Plasmodium fieldi	Plasmodiidae (Bs)
	Plasmodium fragile	Plasmodiidae (Bs)
	Plasmodium siminovale	Plasmodiidae (Bs)
	Plasmodium coatneyi	Plasmodiidae (Bs)
	Plasmodium inui	Plasmodiidae (Bs)
	Plasmodium shorti	Plasmodiidae (Bs)
	Plasmodium simium	Plasmodiidae (Bs)
	Plasmodium brazilianum	Plasmodiidae (Bs)
	Plasmodium rodhaini	Plasmodiidae (Bs)
	Plasmodium pitheci	Plasmodiidae (Bs)
	Plasmodium silvaticum	Plasmodiidae (Bs)
	Plasmodium reichenowi	Plasmodiidae (Bs)
	Plasmodium schwetzi	Plasmodiidae (Bs)
	Hepatocystis kochi	Hepatozoidae (Bs)
	Hepatocystis semnopitheci	Hepatozoidae (Bs)
	Hepatocystis taiwanensis	Hepatozoidae (Bs)
	Hepatocystis bouillezi	Hepatozoidae (Bs)
	Hepatocystis cercopitheci	Hepatozoidae (Bs)
	Hepatocystis foleyi	Hepatozoidae (Bs)
	Babesia pitheci	Babesiidae (Bs)
Blood vessels	*Schistosoma haematobium*	Schistosomatidae (T)
	Schistosoma mattheei	Schistosomatidae (T)
	Schistosoma mansoni	Schistosomatidae (T)
Lymphatics	*Brugia malayi*	Filarioidea (N)
	Brugia pahangi	Filarioidea (N)
	Brugia tupaiae	Filarioidea (N)

(Continued)

Primate parasite checklist. *Continued*

Section/host system	Helminths		Arthropods		Protozoa	
	Parasite	(Super) family	Parasite	Family	Parasite	Family
Nervous						
CNS	Coenurus cerebralis (metacestode: Taenia multiceps)	Taeniidae (C)			Naegleria fowleri	Vahlkampfidae (Am)
					Encephalitozoon cuniculi	Unikaryonidae (Mi)
Eye	Thelazia callipaeda	Spiruroidea (N)			Acanthamoeba spp.	Acanthamoebidae (Am)
Reproductive/urogenital						
	Schistosoma haematobium	Schistosomatidae (T)				
Kidneys					Klossiella spp.	Klossiellidae (Co)
Locomotory						
Muscle			Linguatula sericata	Linguatulidae (Pn)	Trypanosoma cruzi	Trypanosomatidae (Fl)
					Sarcocystis kortei	Sarcocystidae (Co)
					Sarcocystis nesbitti	Sarcocystidae (Co)
					Toxoplasma gondii	Sarcocystidae (Co)
Connective tissue						
Peritoneum	Mansonella barbascalensis	Filarioidea (N)				
	Mansonella zakii	Filarioidea (N)				
	Mansonella nicollei	Filarioidea (N)				
	Mansonella digitatum	Filarioidea (N)				
	Mansonella vanhoofi	Filarioidea (N)				
	Dipetalonema gracile	Filarioidea (N)				
	Dipetalonema caudispina	Filarioidea (N)				
	Dipetalonema graciliformis	Filarioidea (N)				
	Dipetalonema robini	Filarioidea (N)				
	Dipetalonema tenue	Filarioidea (N)				
Subcutaneous	Dirofilaria corynodes	Filarioidea (N)			Trypanosoma cruzi	Trypanosomatidae (Fl)
	Dirofilaria immitis (pongoi)	Filarioidea (N)				
	Dirofilaria repens	Filarioidea (N)				
	Dirofilaria magnilarvatum	Filarioidea (N)				
	Mansonella atelensis	Filarioidea (N)				
	Mansonella parvum	Filarioidea (N)				
	Mansonella panamensis	Filarioidea (N)				
	Mansonella saimiri	Filarioidea (N)				
	Mansonella columbiensis	Filarioidea (N)				
	Mansonella rohdani	Filarioidea (N)				
	Mansonella streptocera	Filarioidea (N)				
	Mansonella leopoldi	Filarioidea (N)				
	Mansonella gorillae	Filarioidea (N)				
	Mansonella lopeensis	Filarioidea (N)				
	Cercopithifilaria papionis	Filarioidea (N)				
	Cercopithifilaria degraffi	Filarioidea (N)				
	Cercopithifilaria verveti	Filarioidea (N)				
	Cercopithifilaria narokensis	Filarioidea (N)				
	Cercopithifilaria eberhardi	Filarioidea (N)				
	Dipetalonema petteri	Filarioidea (N)				
	Dipetalonema tenue	Filarioidea (N)				
	Loa papionis	Filarioidea (N)				
	Loa loa	Filarioidea (N)				

Integument		
Skin	Trichodectes armatus	Trichodectidae (L)
	Trichodectes semiarmatus	Trichodectidae (L)
	Trichodectes colobi	Trichodectidae (L)
	Trichodectes mjoebergi	Trichodectidae (L)
	Eutrichophilus setosus	Trichodectidae (L)
	Cebidicola armatus	Trichodectidae (L)
	Cebidicola semiarmatus	Trichodectidae (L)
	Trichophilopterus ferresti	Philptertidae (L)
	Aotiella aotophilus	Gyropidae (L)
	Pedicinus eurigaster	Pedicinidae (L)
	Pedicinus obtusus	Pedicinidae (L)
	Pedicinus patas	Pedicinidae (L)
	Pedicinus pictus	Pedicinidae (L)
	Pedicinus hamadryas	Pedicinidae (L)
	Pedicinus mjobergi	Pedicinidae (L)
	Pedicinus schaeffi	Pedicinidae (L)
	Pediculus humanus	Pediculidae (L)
	Pthirus pubis	Pthiridae (L)
	Sarcoptes scabiei	Sarcoptidae (M)
	Sarcoptes pitheci	Sarcoptidae (M)
	Prosarcoptes pitheci	Sarcoptidae (M)
	Pithesarcoptes talapoini	Sarcoptidae (M)
	Paracoroptes gordoni	Psoroptidae (M)
	Psorergates cercopitheci	Psorergatidae (M)
	Listrocarpus hapeli	Atopomelidae (M)
	Listrocarpus saimirii	Atopomelidae (M)
	Listrocarpus lagothrix	Atopomelidae (M)

Tick species reported on primates.

Genus	Species	Hosts	Family
Argas	*reflexus*		Argasidae (Ti)
Ornithodoros	*talaje*		Argasidae (Ti)
Amblyomma	*hebraeum*	Prosimians, Old World monkeys	Ixodidae (Ti)
	variegatum	Prosimians	
Dermacentor	*auratus*	Old World monkeys	Ixodidae (Ti)
Haemaphysalis	*aculeate*	Old World monkeys	Ixodidae (Ti)
	bispinosa	Old World monkeys	
	cuspidate	Old World monkeys	
	hylobatis	Apes	
	koningsbergeri	Prosimians	
	kysanurensis	Old World monkeys	
	leachi	Prosimians	
	lemuris	Prosimians	
	parmata	Old World monkeys	
	spinigera	Old World monkeys	
	turturis	Old World monkeys	
Hyalomma	*truncatum*	Old World monkeys	Ixodidae (Ti)
Ixodes	*cavipalpus*	Old World monkeys	Ixodidae (Ti)
	ceylonensis	Old World monkeys	
	lemuris	Prosimians	
	loricatus	New World and Old World monkeys	
	petauristae	Old World monkeys	
	rasus	Old World monkeys	
	schillingsi	Old World monkeys	
Rhipicephalus	*appendiculatus*	Old World monkeys	Ixodidae (Ti)
	evertsi	Old World monkeys	
	haemaphysaloides	Old World monkeys	
	pulchellus	Old World monkeys	
	sanguineus	Old World monkeys	
	simus	Old World monkeys	
Rhipicephalus (Boophilus)	*annulatus*	Old World monkeys	Ixodidae (Ti)

CHAPTER 16

Parasites of exotics

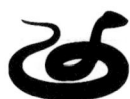

PIGEONS

ENDOPARASITES

Parasites of the digestive system

Dispharynx nasuta

For details see section on Crop and proventriculus.

Crop and proventriculus

Trichomonas gallinae

Trichomonas gallinae, synonyms *Cercomonas gallinae*, *Trichomonas columbae* (Phylum: Metamonada; Class: Trichomonadea; Order: Trichomonadida; Family: Trichomonadidae), causes a disease commonly known as Canker, Frounce or Roup. The infection is distributed worldwide and localised in the pharynx, oesophagus, crop and proventriculus of pigeons, turkeys, chickens and raptors (e.g. hawks, falcons, eagles).

Epidemiology: In pigeons and doves, trichomonosis is transmitted from the adults to the squabs in the 'pigeon milk' which is produced in the crop. The squabs become infected within minutes of hatching. Hawks and wild raptors become infected by eating infected birds.

Pathogenesis: The domestic pigeon is the primary host but the parasite has been found in birds of prey that feed on pigeons, and it has been experimentally established in a wide range of other birds. *Trichomonas gallinae* is extremely common in domestic pigeons and often causes serious losses. Previous infection leads to a varying degree of immunity, and adult pigeons that have survived infection as squabs are asymptomatic carriers. Infection with a relatively harmless strain produces immunity against virulent strains. Injection of plasma from infected pigeons also confers immunity. In pigeons, trichomonosis is essentially a disease of young birds; 80–90% of adults are infected but show no signs of disease. Trichomonosis varies from a mild condition to a rapidly fatal one with death 4–18 days after infection (there are strain differences in virulence). *Trichomonas gallinae* parasitises the mouth, sinuses, orbital region, pharynx, oesophagus, crop and even proventriculus but is not found beyond the proventriculus. It often occurs in the liver and, to a lesser extent, in other organs including the lungs, air sacs, heart, pancreas and, more rarely, spleen, kidneys, trachea and bone marrow.

Clinical signs and pathology: Severely affected birds lose weight, stand huddled with ruffled feathers and may fall over when forced to move. Yellow necrotic lesions are present in the mouth, oesophagus and crop of pigeon squabs and a greenish fluid containing large numbers of trichomonads may be found in the mouth. The early lesions in the pharynx, oesophagus and crop are small, whitish to yellowish caseous nodules. These grow in size and may remain circumscribed and separate or may coalesce to form thick, caseous, necrotic masses that may occlude the lumen. The circumscribed disc-shaped lesions are often described as 'yellow buttons'. The lesions in the liver, lungs and other organs are solid, yellowish, caseous nodules up to 1 cm or more in diameter.

Diagnosis: The clinical signs are pathognomonic and can be confirmed by identifying the characteristic motile trichomonads from samples taken from lesions in the mouth or from fluid.

Control and treatment: Control of trichomonosis in pigeons depends on elimination of the infection from the adult birds by drug therapy. Carnidazole is used for the treatment and prophylaxis of trichomonosis in pigeons at a dose rate of 10 mg for adult birds and 5 mg for squabs. Other nitroimidazole compounds, such as dimetridazole and metronidazole, are also effective but their availability has declined in many countries through legislative changes and toxicity concerns.

Ornithostrongylus quadriradiatus

Ornithostrongylus quadriradiatus (Phylum: Nematoda; Class: Chromadorea; Order: Rhabditida; Family: Ornithostrongylidae) is localised in the crop, proventriculus and small intestine of pigeons and doves, and occurs in North America, South Africa, Australia and Europe.

Epidemiology: The parasite may be responsible for heavy losses in breeding establishments.

Pathogenesis: The worms are voracious blood feeders which burrow into the mucosa and in severe infections cause a catarrhal enteritis.

Clinical signs and pathology: The infection causes an enteritis and anaemia, and high parasitic loads may result in severe mortality in domestic pigeons. Haemorrhagic enteritis with ulceration and necrosis may occur in severe infections.

Diagnosis: Identification of the worms on *post mortem* or eggs in the faeces.

Veterinary Parasitology, Fifth Edition. Domenico Otranto and Richard Wall.
© 2024 John Wiley & Sons Ltd. Published 2024 by John Wiley & Sons Ltd.

Control and treatment: Facilities where pigeons or doves are kept should be cleaned regularly to avoid build-up of eggs and infective larvae. Oral benzimidazoles used for other nematode species should be effective.

Spiruroid nematodes

Several species of spiruroid worms belonging to the genera *Tetrameres* and *Dyspharynx* are found in the proventriculus of pigeons. These species have been described in detail in Chapter 13.

Tetrameres americana

Tetrameres americana, synonym *Tropisurus americana* (Phylum: Nematoda; Class: Chromadorea; Order: Spirurida; Family: Tetrameridae), is localised in the proventriculus of chickens, turkeys, ducks, geese, grouse, quails and pigeons, and occurs in Africa and North America. This parasite has cockroaches, grasshoppers and beetles as intermediate hosts.

Dispharynx nasuta

Dispharynx nasuta, synonyms *Dispharynx spiralis*, *Acuaria spiralis*, *Acuaria nasuta* (Phylum: Nematoda; Class: Chromadorea; Order: Spirurida; Family: Acuaridae), commonly known as the Spiral stomach worm, is localised in the oesophagus and proventriculus of chickens, turkeys, pigeons, guinea fowl, grouse, pheasants and other birds, and is distributed in Asia, Africa and the Americas. This parasite has various isopods such as sowbugs (*Porcellio scaber*) and pillbugs (*Armadillidium vulgare*) as intermediate hosts.

Small intestine

Ascaridia columbae

Ascaridia columbae, synonym *Ascaridia maculosa* (Phylum: Nematoda; Class: Chromadorea; Order: Ascaridida; Family: Ascaridiidae), is presumably distributed worldwide and is localised in the small intestine of pigeons. This parasite is considered non-pathogenic.

Epidemiology: Adult birds are asymptomatic carriers, and the reservoir of infection is on the ground, either as free eggs or in earthworm transport hosts. Infection is heaviest in young squabs.

Diagnosis: Adult worms may be found in the intestine on *post mortem* or the characteristic ascarid eggs may be seen in faeces.

Control and treatment: Strict hygiene and feeding and watering systems, which will limit the contamination of food and water by faeces, should be used for control.

The following helminths have been reported in the intestines of pigeons and have been described in detail in Chapter 13. Treatment is not usually required although the use of piperazine salts, levamisole or a benzimidazole such as fenbendazole is effective. Capsules containing fenbendazole or cambendazole are effective and can be given by mouth to pigeons.

Capillaria caudinflata

Capillaria caudinflata, synonym *Aonchotheca caudinflata* (Phylum: Nematoda; Class: Enoplea; Order: Enoplida; Family: Capillariidae), is distributed worldwide and localised in the small intestine of chickens, turkeys, geese, pigeons and wild birds. This parasite has earthworms as intermediate hosts.

Control and treatment: Oral capsules containing fenbendazole or cambendazole are effective.

Davainea proglottina

Davainea proglottina (Phylum: Platyhelminthes; Class: Cestoda; Order: Cyclophyllidea; Family: Davaineidae) is a parasite distributed in most parts of the world, and localised in the small intestine, particularly the duodenum, of chickens, turkeys, pigeons and other gallinaceous birds. This parasite has gastropod molluscs such as *Agriolimax*, *Arion*, *Cepaea* and *Limax* and land snails as intermediate hosts.

Raillietina tetragona

Raillietina tetragona (Phylum: Platyhelminthes; Class: Cestoda; Order: Cyclophyllidea; Family: Davaineidae) is distributed worldwide and localised in the posterior half of the small intestine of chickens, guinea fowl and pigeons. This parasite has ants of the genera *Pheidole* and *Tetramorium* and house flies as intermediate hosts.

Echinoparyphium recurvatum

Echinoparyphium recurvatum (Phylum: Platyhelminthes; Class: Trematoda; Order: Plagiorchiida; Family: Echinostomatidae) is distributed worldwide (mainly in Asia and North Africa) and localised in the small intestine, particularly the duodenum, of ducks, geese, chickens, pigeons and humans. This parasite has two intermediate hosts during its life cycle: host 1: snails such as *Galba* spp. and *Planorbis* spp; host 2: frogs, tadpoles and snails, such as *Valvata piscinalis* and *Planorbis albus*, and shellfish.

Eimeria labbeana

Eimeria labbeana, synonyms *Eimeria peifferi*, *Eimeria columbarum* (Phylum: Apicomplexa; Class: Conoidasida; Order: Eucoccidiorida; Family: Eimeriidae), is distributed worldwide and localised in the small intestine of pigeons (*Columba domestica*), rock doves (*Columba livia*) and collared doves (*Streptopelia decaoto*). After the sporulated oocysts are ingested, the sporozoites are released and invade the epithelial cells of the intestine. First-generation meronts are present 20–48 hours after infection in the epithelial cells of the anterior ileum. Mature second-generation meronts are present 96 hours and mature third-generation meronts 144 hours after infection. The macrogametes are in the epithelial cells of the ileum. The prepatent period is about five days. The sporulation time is four days or less.

Epidemiology: Transmission is via the faecal–oral route and is more common in young birds. Sources of infection include dirty contaminated baskets, eating or drinking contaminated food or water, or drinking from contaminated water in roosts such as roof guttering.

Pathogenesis: *Eimeria labbeana* is slightly to markedly pathogenic, depending on the strain of parasite and age of the birds. Adults are fairly resistant, although fatal infections have been seen. The birds become weak and emaciated, eat little but drink a great deal and have a greenish diarrhoea. The heaviest losses occur among squabs in the nest. A high percentage of the squabs may die, and those that recover are often somewhat stunted.

Clinical signs and pathology: Light infections are usually asymptomatic. In heavier infections, birds are listless, have a puffed-up appearance and show weakness, emaciation and diarrhoea. In severe infections there is inflammation of the intestinal mucosa with the lumen filled with a haemorrhagic exudate.

Diagnosis: Diagnosis is based on identification of oocysts in the faeces in association with any clinical and pathological findings.

Control and treatment: Prevention is based on good management, avoidance of overcrowding and stress, and attention to hygiene. Sulfonamides administered in the drinking water (e.g. sulfamethoxine 120 g per 2000 ml) are effective in treating infection. Clazuril 2.5 mg given as an oral tablet per pigeon, regardless of weight, is also effective. All birds in the same loft are usually treated simultaneously to prevent reinfection of untreated birds.

Caeca/large intestine

Heterakis gallinarum

Heterakis gallinarum, synonyms *Heterakis papillosa*, *Heterakis gallinae*, *Heterakis vesicularis* (Phylum: Nematoda; Class: Chromadorea; Order: Ascaridida; Family: Heterakiidae), commonly known as the Poultry caecal worm, is distributed worldwide and localised in the caeca, and rarely large and small intestine, of chickens, turkeys, pigeons, pheasants, partridges, grouse, quails, guinea fowl, ducks, geese and a number of wild galliform birds.

Echinostoma revolutum

Echinostoma revolutum (Phylum: Platyhelminthes; Class: Trematoda; Order: Plagiorchiida; Family: Echinostomatidae) is distributed worldwide and localised in the caeca and rectum of ducks, geese, pigeons, various fowls and aquatic birds.

Notes: *Echinostoma revolutum* can also infect humans. *E. paraulum* occurs in the small intestine of ducks and pigeons and can cause weakness, inappetence and diarrhoea in the latter.

Parasites of the respiratory system

Syngamus trachea

Syngamus trachea, synonyms *Syngamus parvis*, *Syngamus gracilis* (Phylum: Nematoda; Class: Chromadorea; Order: Rhabditida; Family: Syngamidae), commonly known as the Gapeworm, is distributed worldwide and localised in the trachea or lungs of chickens, turkeys, gamebirds (pheasant, partridge, guinea fowl), pigeons and various wild birds.

For more details see Chapter 13.

Cytodites nudus

Cytodites nudus (Phylum: Arthropoda; Class: Arachnida; Subclass: Acari; Order: Sarcoptiformes (Astigmata); Family: Cytoditidae), commonly known as the Air sac mite, is localised in the lung or air sac of birds, particularly poultries and canaries, and is found worldwide. Infestation may be spread through coughing.

Pathogenesis: Small infestations may have no obvious effect; large infestations may cause accumulation of mucus in the trachea and bronchi, leading to coughing and respiratory difficulties, air sacculitis and weight loss. Balance may be affected in infested birds. Weakness, emaciation and death have been described with heavy infections.

Clinical signs and pathology: Coughing, respiratory difficulties, pulmonary oedema, weight loss, loss of balance or coordination. Death is usually associated with peritonitis, enteritis, emaciation and respiratory complications.

Diagnosis: Positive diagnosis is only possible at *post mortem*, when necropsy reveals white spots on the surface of air sacs.

Control and treatment: It is important to treat all the birds in an aviary when commencing a preventive programme. Treatment with topical moxidectin every three weeks as necessary may be effective.

Parasites of the circulatory system

Leucocytozoon marchouxi

Leucocytozoon marchouxi, synonym *Leucocytozoon turtur* (Phylum: Apicomplexa; Class: Aconoidasida; Order: Haemosporida; Family: Plasmodiidae), is distributed worldwide and localised in the blood of pigeons and doves. Vectors are members of the genus *Simulium* (blackflies).

Pathogenesis: Until recently, this species was considered non-pathogenic in pigeons and doves but the parasite has been shown to be pathogenic to pink pigeons (*Columba mayeri*).

Diagnosis: Demonstration of gametocytes in blood smears (Figs 16.1 and 16.2).

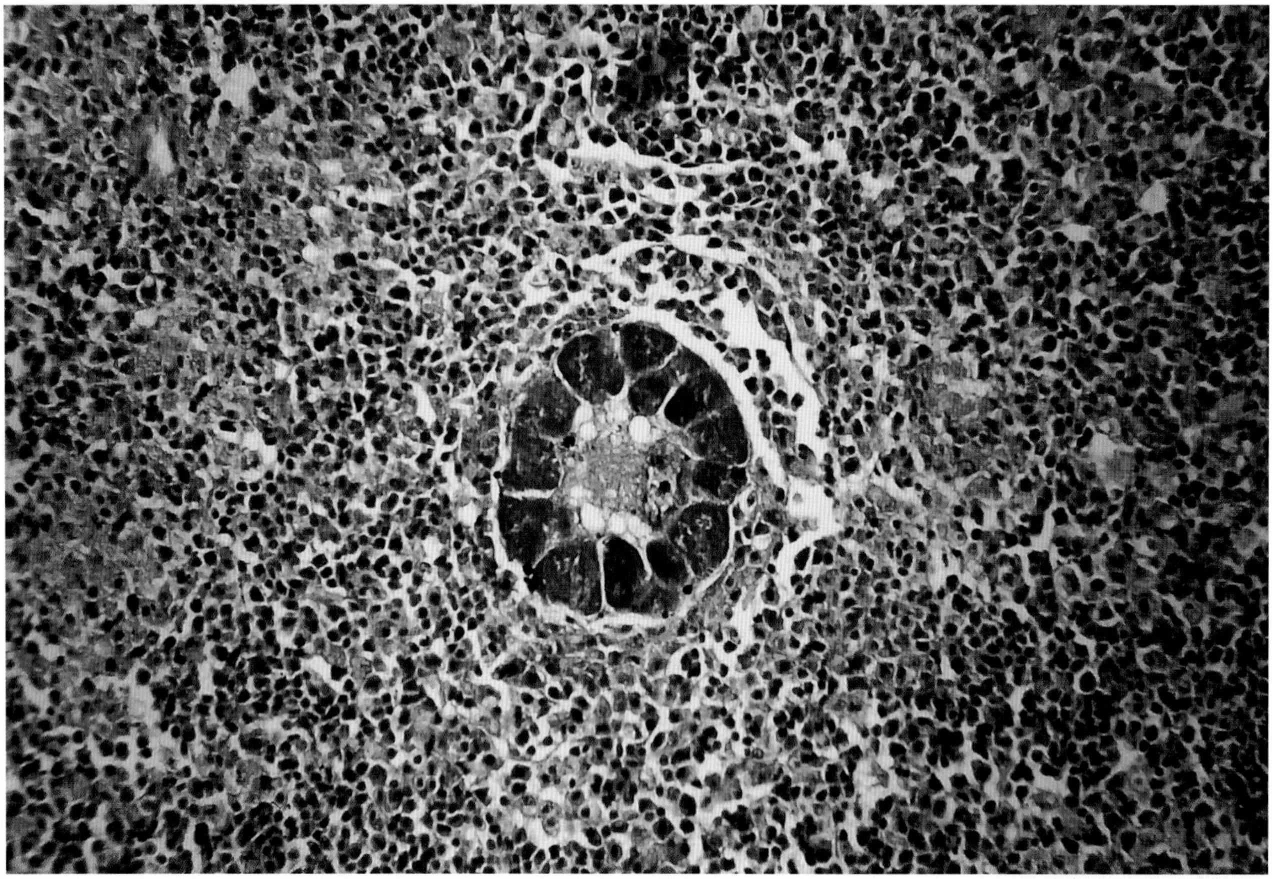

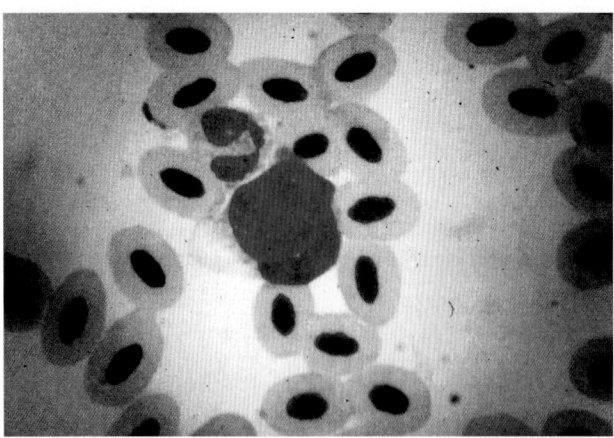

Fig. 16.1 Macrogamont of *Leucocytozoon marchouxi*.

Control and treatment: Not usually required although general insect control or preventive measures may limit infection.

Haemoproteus columbae

Haemoproteus columbae (Phylum: Apicomplexa; Class: Aconoidasida; Order: Haemosporida; Family: Plasmodiidae) is distributed worldwide and localised in the blood of domestic and wild pigeons, doves and other wild birds. Vectors are hippoboscid flies in the genus *Pseudolynchia*.

Fig. 16.2 Megalomeront of *Leucocytozoon marchouxi* in the spleen.

Pathogenesis: Generally considered to be of low pathogenicity in adult birds but an acute form of infection has been reported in squabs. The clinical presentation is characterised by anorexia and anaemia.

Diagnosis: Demonstration of gametocytes in blood smears.

Control and treatment: Not usually required although general insect control or preventive measures may limit infection.

Parasites of the nervous system

No parasites of veterinary significance.

Parasites of the reproductive/ urogenital system

No parasites of veterinary significance.

Parasites of the integument

Laminosioptes cysticola

Laminosioptes cysticola (Phylum: Arthropoda; Class: Arachnida; Subclass: Acari; Order: Sarcoptiformes (Astigmata); Family: Laminosioptidae), commonly known as the Subcutaneous mite or Fowl cyst mite, is localised in the subcutaneous tissues, lung or peritoneum of chickens, turkeys and pigeons, and occasionally in wild birds. It is particularly abundant in Europe and is also found in the USA, South America and Australia.

Epidemiology: It is estimated that around 1% of free-living urban pigeons harbour *L. cysticola*. The mode of transmission of this mite is unknown.

Pathogenesis: The mites are found in the subcutaneous muscle fascia and in deeper tissues in the lungs, peritoneum, muscle and abdominal viscera. *Laminosioptes* is not usually associated with clinical signs and is only discovered in pigeons at *post mortem*. Active mites occur in the deep tissues. The nodules created by the mites reduce the value of meat intended for human consumption.

Clinical signs and pathology: The parasites are not usually regarded as pathogenic. Aggregations of these small oval mites are found in yellow nodules, several millimetres in diameter, in the subcutaneous muscle fascia and in deeper tissues in the lungs, peritoneum, muscle and abdominal viscera. The subcutaneous nodules are often calcified but these only contain dead mites as the calcareous deposits are produced around the mites after they have died.

Diagnosis: The nodules may be seen in living birds by parting the breast feathers and sliding the skin back and forth with the fingertips. Examination of the nodules under a dissection microscope usually allows identification of the mite species.

Control and treatment: Destroying or quarantining the infected birds may be required to achieve long-term reduction in infestations within a flock. Macrocyclic lactones may be effective.

Pelecitus clavus

Pelecitus clavus, synonym *Eulimdana clava* (Phylum: Nematoda; Class: Chromadorea; Order: Spirurida; Family: Onchocercidae), is distributed worldwide and localised in the subcutaneous and connective tissues of pigeons and many other wild birds.

Epidemiology: *Pelecitus* spp. can be of zoonotic significance in some areas of the world, infecting the eyes and periorbital region of humans.

Pathogenesis: These parasites are considered to be of low pathogenicity in birds.

Notes: Another species, *Pelecitus mazzanti*, is also found in pigeons.

ECTOPARASITES

Other species of mites found in pigeons are listed in Table 16.1.

Columbicola columbae

Columbicola columbae (Phylum: Arthropoda; Class: Insecta; Order: Psocodea; Suborder: Ischnocera; Family: Philopteridae), commonly known as the Slender pigeon louse, is found on the wings or anterior part of the body of pigeons and doves worldwide.

Epidemiology: Infection occurs after direct contact with an infested host animal. Cross-contamination between different host species is possible if the animals have physical contact.

Pathogenesis: Infection may cause a mild pruritus, and in common with most pediculosis, heavy infestations are usually seen only in diseased and debilitated birds, causing feather damage and irritation.

Clinical signs and pathology: Lice are rarely linked to significant pathology associated with feather damage and irritation.

Diagnosis: Adult lice (Fig. 16.3) may be seen moving around the plumage or eggs may be seen attached to feathers.

Control and treatment: Although methods such as dusting the litter or providing insecticide-treated laying boxes are used to avoid undue handling of birds, the results obtained from treating individual birds are undoubtedly better. Regular checking and spraying of

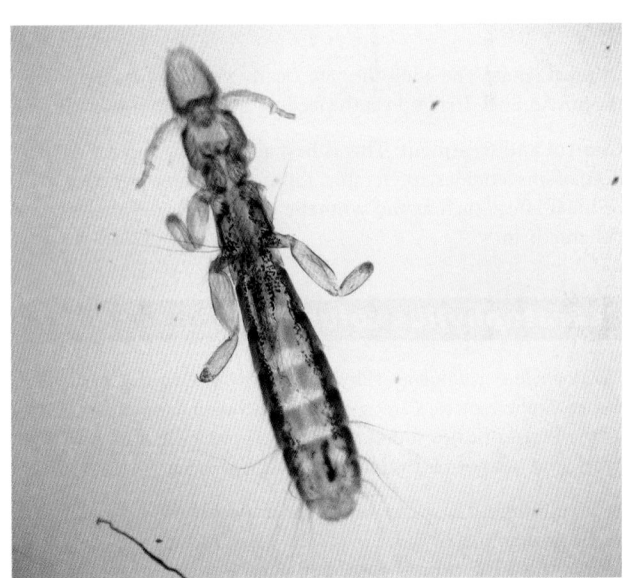

Fig. 16.3 *Columbicola columbae.*

Table 16.1 Mites of pigeons (see also Chapter 3).

Species	Common name	Host	Clinical signs
Hypodectes propus (Family Hypoderidae)		Pigeons and doves	Presence of the parasite in the subcutaneous tissue causes itching, feather loss and restlessness
Dermanyssus gallinae (Family Dermanyssidae)	Poultry red mite	Domestic poultry and wild birds; occasionally parasitic on mammals, including humans	Mites feed on birds at night, spending the day within the structure of the poultry house or nest
Ornithonyssus sylviarum Synonym: *Liponyssus sylviarum* (Family Macronyssidae)	Northern fowl mite	Poultry and wild birds	Presence of mites at the base of the feathers, particularly the vent area, causes irritation
Ornithonyssus bursa Synonym: *Liponyssus bursa* (Family Macronyssidae)	Tropical fowl mite	Poultry and wild birds	

birds will enable infestation rates to be controlled. In addition, cross-contamination should be avoided. This is achieved by treating any birds in the environment of the pigeons and restricting contact between wild birds and pigeons. The housing and nesting should be thoroughly cleaned to eliminate sources of reinfestation such as egg-laden feathers.

Topical insecticidal compounds, such as permethrin, carbaryl, malathion and cypermethrin, can be used to kill lice. However, as the insecticides are unable to kill the eggs, two applications are necessary at an interval of 10 days.

Pseudolynchia canariensis

Pseudolynchia canariensis (Phylum: Arthropoda; Class: Insecta; Order: Diptera; Family: Hippoboscidae), commonly known as the Pigeon louse fly, occurs worldwide on the skin of pigeons but other domestic birds may also be infested. The adult flies are found on the host animal.

Epidemiology: The adult flies are most abundant on the host during the summer months.

Pathogenesis: The adult flies bite and blood feed, resulting in nuisance and disturbance. Heavily infested birds may be restless and emaciated and become susceptible to secondary infections. The flies may act as vectors of *Haemoproteus columbae* and *H. sacharovi*.

Clinical signs: The adult flies are clearly visible when feeding on the host animal. Irritation at the feeding sites may be observed.

Control and treatment: This is best achieved by topical application of insecticides, preferably those with some repellent and residual effect such as the synthetic pyrethroids permethrin and deltamethrin.

Ceratophyllus columbae

Ceratophyllus columbae (Phylum: Arthropoda; Class: Insecta; Order: Siphonaptera; Family: Ceratophyllidae), commonly known as the Pigeon flea, is found on pigeons predominantly in the Old World but has been introduced into the Americas.

Epidemiology: These fleas are not host specific and may attack any available mammal or bird for a blood meal. As they are able to survive off the host, transmission can occur from bedding and housing. This flea is highly mobile on the host and can be especially common in host nesting material. *Ceratophyllus columbae* feeds readily on humans and domestic pets, and is often acquired in the handling of pigeons and wild birds. It has also been known to migrate into rooms from nests under adjacent eaves. When such nests are removed, they should be incinerated; otherwise the underfed fleas may parasitise domestic pets and humans.

Pathogenesis: Feeding activity may cause irritation, restlessness and, with heavy infestations, anaemia. In wild birds, flea reproduction and feeding activity are synchronised with the breeding season. Adult *C. columbae* may also feed on humans and domestic pets.

Clinical signs: Symptoms include restlessness and scratching of affected areas. The bites may be visible on the skin. Allergic dermatitis may be seen.

Diagnosis: Diagnosis is not easy as adults may leave the host and eggs and larvae are difficult to find. The bites of these fleas are similar to those of mosquitoes, lice and mites, with inflammation and itchiness.

Control and treatment: Should fleas become established, drastic measures may have to be adopted to get rid of them. All litter and nest material should be removed and burnt, and the housing sprayed with an insecticide. Topical treatment of affected birds with insecticidal products such as permethrin, carbaryl, malathion and rotenone is effective.

Argas reflexus

Argas reflexus (Phylum: Arthropoda; Class: Arachnida; Subclass: Acari; Order: Ixodida; Family: Argasidae), commonly known as the Pigeon tick, is found on birds, most commonly pigeons, in Europe, Russia, Asia, North and West Africa.

Epidemiology: *Argas reflexus* eggs show limited levels of cold tolerance; winter temperatures of 3 °C cause approximately 50% mortality. This limits its northern distribution through Europe.

Pathogenesis: Infestation may cause irritation, sleeplessness, loss of egg productivity and anaemia, which can prove fatal. Heavy infestations can remove enough blood to bring about the death of their host. This species transmits *Borrelia anserina*, the cause of fowl spirochaetosis, and *Aegyptianella pullorum*, a rickettsial infection. It may also be a vector of West Nile and Chenuda viruses and the Quaranfil virus group.

Clinical signs and pathology: Inflammation and raised areas will be present from tick bites. Larvae may be found living in the feathers. These ticks can cause sleeplessness, loss of productivity and anaemia, which can prove fatal. Small granulomatous reactions may form at the site of tick bites, consisting of a mixed inflammatory cell response with fibrosis.

Diagnosis: The adult ticks, particularly the engorged larvae, may be seen on the skin. Nymphs and adult ticks may be found in cracks in the woodwork. Red spots may be seen on the skin where the ticks have fed.

Control and treatment: Argasid ticks, which exist in lofts and enclosures, can be controlled by application of an acaricide to their environment coupled with treatment of the population on the host. Environmental treatment of roosts and lofts may be performed using acaricidal sprays or emulsions containing organophosphates or pyrethroids. All niches and crevices in affected buildings should be sprayed, and nesting boxes and perches should also be painted with acaricides. At the same time as premises are treated, birds should be dusted with a suitable acaricide or, in the case of larger animals, sprayed or dipped. Treatment should be repeated at monthly intervals. All new animals should be treated prior to introduction into an existing flock.

RATITES (OSTRICH, RHEA, EMU)

Ostriches (*Struthio camelus*) in the wild are mainly confined to the drier parts of Africa but have been imported into many countries for intensive farming. Emus (*Dromaius novaehollandiae*) occur naturally throughout most regions of Australia. The subspecies of greater rhea (*Rhea americana*) and lesser rhea (*Pterocnemia pennata*) inhabit the open plains of central and southern regions of South America. Captive ratites may be infected with their own specific parasites but may also be carrying parasites from other birds or mammals.

ENDOPARASITES

Parasites of the digestive system

Proventriculus and gizzard

Libyostrongylus douglassi

Libyostrongylus douglassi (Phylum: Nematoda; Class: Chromadorea; Order: Rhabditida; Family: Trichostrongylidae), commonly known as the Wireworm, is localised in the proventriculus and gizzard of ostriches and is distributed in Africa, North and South America and Europe.

Epidemiology: Eggs and first-stage larvae can survive desiccation for around 30 months in hot arid environments.

Pathogenesis: The young worms penetrate deeply into the mucosa of the glands of the proventriculus. Adults live on the surface of the epithelium (Fig. 16.4) where they feed on blood, causing a severe inflammatory reaction and anaemia. In severe infections there may be impaction of the proventriculus.

Clinical signs and pathology: Chicks are most susceptible to infection and become anaemic, weak and emaciated with heavy mortality in untreated cases. There may be lower egg production and constipation. Sometimes chicks are unable to support their head and develop a 'hockey-stick' appearance of the neck as a result of muscular weakness. Pathological findings often include hypertrophy and erythema of the glandular mucosa of the proventriculus. There may also be muscle atrophy and cachexia.

Diagnosis: Diagnosis is based on finding eggs in the faeces or identifying the worms in the proventriculus and gizzard on *post*

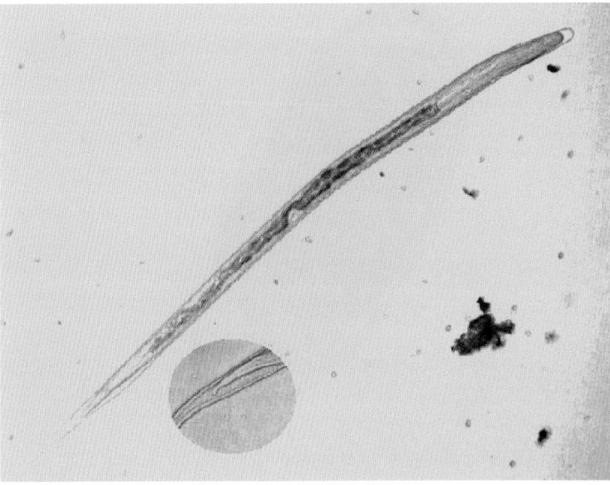

Fig. 16.5 *Libyostrongylus douglassi* L$_3$. Inset shows magnified larval tail tip within the third cuticle.

mortem. Larval culture is frequently used to differentiate eggs from the usually non-pathogenic species *Codiostomum struthionis*, which is often also present in ostriches (Fig. 16.5).

Control: Appropriate hygiene and husbandry measures, including removal of faeces aimed at limiting pasture contamination, which will avoid the exposure to dangerous levels of infective larvae. Rotation of pasture is useful where practicable. The exposure of young susceptible birds to infection can be reduced by penning the juveniles separately from the adults. It is important to isolate and treat all new birds to prevent introduction of infection on ostrich farms.

Treatment: Levamisole (30 mg/kg), fenbendazole (15 mg/kg), ivermectin orally (200 mg/kg) and ivermectin as a subcutaneous injection (300 mg/kg) are effective in the treatment of wireworm infection in young ostriches.

Spiruroid nematodes

Several species of spiruroid worms belonging to the genera *Spirura* and *Odontospirura* are found in the proventriculus of rheas. These species are essentially similar to spiruroid worm species found in the proventriculus of poultries (see Chapter 13). Diagnosis is based on the presence of spiruroid eggs in the faeces or the presence of the worms in the proventriculus on *post mortem*.

Small intestine

Deletrocephalus dimidiatus

Deletrocephalus dimidiatus (Phylum: Nematoda; Class: Chromadorea; Order: Rhabditida; Family: Deletrocephalidae) is localised in the small intestine of greater rheas (*Rhea americana*) and lesser rheas (*Pterocnemia pennata*) and is distributed in South America, North America and Europe. The life cycle is thought to be direct, with birds ingesting infective larvae while foraging. There are limited reports on the distribution and pathogenicity of this parasite in rheas.

Clinical signs: Heavy infections cause diarrhoea in chicks.

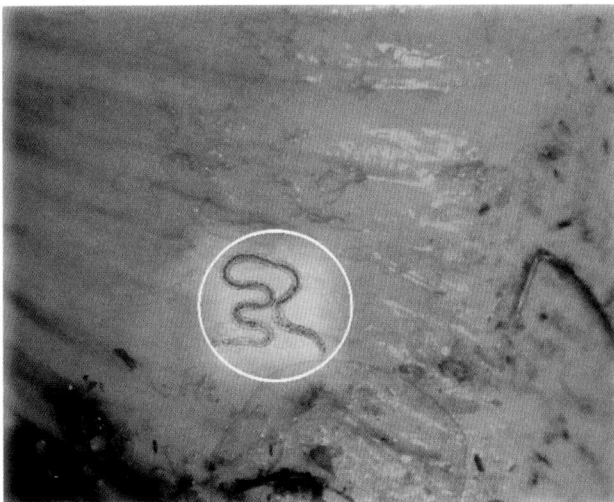

Fig. 16.4 *Libyostrongylus douglassi*: mucosal surface of proventriculus. Inset shows magnified worm.

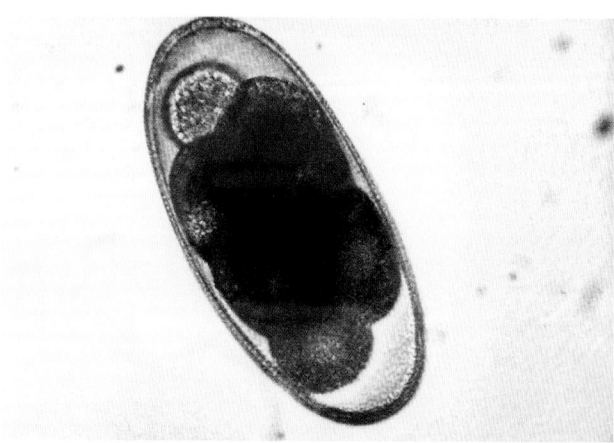

Fig. 16.6 *Deletrocephalus dimidiatus* egg.

Diagnosis: Diagnosis is based on finding eggs in the faeces (Fig. 16.6) or by identifying the worms in the intestine on *post mortem*.

Control and treatment: Rearing of chicks away from adult birds and regular cleaning of pens may help limit infection. There is little information on the treatment of this parasite in rheas. Benzimidazoles and ivermectin have been used in the treatment of nematodes in ostrich, and therefore may be of benefit.

Houttuynia struthionis

Houttuynia struthionis (Phylum: Platyhelminthes; Class: Cestoda; Order: Cyclophyllidea; Family: Davaineidae) is localised in the small intestine of ostriches and rheas, distributed in Africa and South America, and reported in imported ostriches in the USA and Europe. The tapeworm is seen especially in ostrich chicks but has also been reported in rheas, causing unthriftiness, loss of appetite, emaciation and diarrhoea. Affected chicks lose their appetite and may die.

Diagnosis: Diagnosis is based on finding tapeworm segments or eggs in the faeces or identifying the worms in the proventriculus and gizzard on *post mortem*.

Control and treatment: As the intermediate host is not known, specific control measures are not possible. Rearing of chicks away from adult birds, regular cleaning of pens and insect control would seem expedient. Praziquantel (7.5 mg/kg orally) or niclosamide (100 mg/kg orally) is effective; also fenbendazole (25 mg/kg) or oxfendazole (5 mg/kg orally).

Large intestine

Codiostomum struthionis

Codiostomum struthionis (Phylum: Nematoda; Class: Chromadorea; Order: Rhabditida; Family: Strongylidae) is localised in the large intestine and caecum of ostriches and rheas and is distributed in Africa and South America.

Pathogenesis: Infection is reported to impair water absorption in the gut.

Clinical signs and pathology: Small worm burdens are generally considered to be non-pathogenic but heavy infections can cause anaemia and poor growth rates. The intestinal mucosa may be thickened and contain nodules. Some areas can be haemorrhagic and contain small ulcers.

Diagnosis: The eggs are identical to those of *L. douglassi* and diagnosis is based on identification of adult worms in the caeca and colon or on the morphology of the L_3 following larval culture.

Control and treatment: As for *Libyostrongylus*.

Parasites of the respiratory system

Syngamus trachea

Syngamus trachea (Phylum: Nematoda; Class: Chromadorea; Order: Rhabditida; Family: Syngamidae), commonly known as the Gapeworm, is distributed worldwide and localised in the trachea of chickens, turkeys, gamebirds (pheasants, partridges, guinea fowl), pigeons, ostriches, emus, rheas and various wild birds.

For more details see Chapter 13.

Cyathostoma variegatum

Cyathostoma variegatum (Phylum: Nematoda; Class: Chromadorea; Order: Rhabditida; Family: Syngamidae), commonly known as the Gapeworm, is localised in the trachea and bronchi of ducks and emus and occurs in Australia. Paratenic hosts may be involved in transmission. It has been reported to cause severe respiratory distress in young emus.

Control and treatment: Ivermectin is likely to be effective.

Parasites of the circulatory system

Leucocytozoon struthionis

Leucocytozoon struthionis (Phylum: Apicomplexa; Class: Aconoidasida; Order: Haemosporida; Family: Plasmodiidae) is localised in the blood of ostriches and is distributed in Africa. This parasite has blackflies (*Simulium*) as intermediate hosts.

Pathogenesis: Although it is considered of low pathogenicity, it has been found in association with myocarditis in young ostrich chicks. During early parasitaemia it may cause anaemia.

Diagnosis: Identification of either gamonts in blood or megalomeronts in tissue.

Parasites of the nervous system

Philophthalmus gralli

Philophthalmus gralli (Phylum: Platyhelminthes; Class: Trematoda; Order: Plagiorchiida; Family: Philophthalmidae), commonly known as the Oriental avian eye fluke, is localised in the conjunctival sac of ostriches, chickens, wild birds and humans, and is distributed in the

USA, Indo-China, parts of Europe and Africa. This parasite has freshwater snails as intermediate hosts, and can be a problem in captive farmed ostriches where they have access to standing water.

Pathogenesis and clinical signs: Infection may cause congestion and erosion of the conjunctivae, and conjunctivitis with persistent lacrimation.

Bayliascaris procyonis

Bayliascaris procyonis (Phylum: Nematoda; Class: Chromadorea; Order: Ascaridida; Family: Ascarididae) is localised in the brain and spinal cord of intermediate hosts such as ostriches, emus, dogs, cats, rodents and lagomorphs, and is distributed in North America, Europe and Japan. This parasite has raccoons as definitive hosts.

Epidemiology: *Bayliascaris procyonis* is found abundantly in its definitive host, the raccoon. The parasite can infect a wide range of wild and domestic animals. Many animals act as intermediate hosts and infection results in penetration of the gut wall by the larvae and subsequent invasion of tissue, resulting in severe disease. The raccoon plays an important role in the life cycle of the disease. Raccoons are solitary but will frequently defecate in communal latrines, which are an abundant source of *B. procyonis* eggs. The eggs can remain viable for years.

Pathogenesis: Can cause damage to the central nervous system in ostriches and emus.

Clinical signs: Infected birds show behavioural changes as a result of the visceral larval migration. Ataxia, muscle weakness and recumbency may occur.

Diagnosis: Diagnosis is usually based on the presence of the larvae in tissues at necropsy.

Notes: Visceral *larva migrans* resulting from infection with *Bayliascaris* species occurs in a range of hosts including various poultries, rabbits and small mammals. The larvae invade the central nervous system of the intermediate host and increase in size as they migrate, causing them to be highly pathogenic. *Bayliascaris* spp. can also infect humans and provoke severe brain damage.

ECTOPARASITES

Lice

Struthiolipeurus struthionis

Struthiolipeurus struthionis (Phylum: Arthropoda; Class: Insecta; Order: Psocodea; Suborder: Ischnocera; Family: Philopteridae), commonly known as the Ostrich louse or Feather louse, is found on the skin or feathers of ostriches.

Pathogenesis and clinical signs: This is a chewing louse that damages the feathers, reducing the value of especially white plumes. The damage causes the feathers to have a moth-eaten appearance.

Diagnosis: Lice and eggs may be found in the feathers close to the skin (Fig. 16.7).

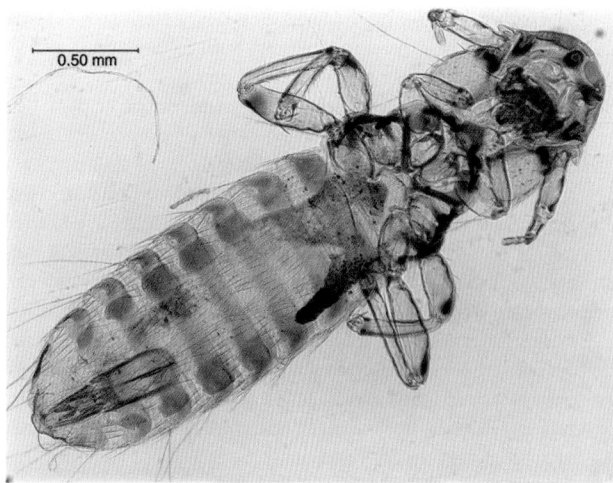

Fig. 16.7 *Struthiolipeurus struthionis.* (Courtesy of Dr Vince Smith).

Control and treatment: Treatment with pyrethroid is recommended; carbaryl dust (5%) may also be effective.

A variety of other lice may also be found on ostriches including *Struthiolipeurus nandu, S. stresemanni* and *S. rheae. Meinertzhageniella lata* and *M. schubarti* have been reported in rheas, and *Dahlemhornia asymmetrica* in emus.

Mites

Gabucinia spp.

Gabucinia spp. (Phylum: Arthropoda; Class: Arachnida; Subclass: Acari; Order: Sarcoptiformes (Astigmata); Family: Gabuciniidae), commonly known as Shaft or Quill mites, are found in the ventral groove of the feather shaft of ostriches and feed on blood and contents of the feather sheath.

Pathogenesis and clinical signs: Quill mites are very common but occasionally become a problem in ostriches kept under intensive conditions. Large numbers of mites cause severe feather damage, leading to scarring of the skin and a reduction in the economic value of the infested animal.

Diagnosis: Mites may be observed at the base of the feathers as small dust-like elongated particles.

Control and treatment: Treatment with ivermectin (0.2 mg/kg) at 30-day intervals has been reported to be effective.

Notes: There are several species in this genus, which infest a range of wild birds, but *Gabucinia sculpturata* and *Gabucinia (Pterolichus) bicaudatus* are the most common and well described in ostriches.

Numerous species of ticks have also been reported to infest ostriches in their native ranges. These are summarised in the parasite checklist at the end of this chapter.

REPTILES

Reptiles are represented by four orders of animals comprising approximately 5500 species. Species of reptiles belonging to the Testudinata (tortoises, terrapins, turtles) and Squamata, divided into the suborders Sauria (lizards) and Serpentes (snakes), are increasingly kept and bred in captivity, both in zoological and in private collections, and kept as individual pets.

Reptiles in the wild are infected with a wide range of parasites, especially given the extremely varied range of prey animals and their potential to act as intermediate/paratenic hosts for many species of parasites. Generally, however, if well fed and non-stressed, parasitised animals can remain comparatively healthy even when carrying burdens of several species of parasites. Parasites with heteroxenous life cycles, requiring two or more hosts, are only likely to be encountered in wild-caught animals.

Parasitic infections are frequently encountered in captive-bred reptiles and this section concentrates only on these infections, rather than those found in wild-caught specimens. Given the range of reptile species kept in captivity, it is beyond the scope of this book to provide detailed descriptions of all the species of parasites that may be encountered. As such, only a general overview is provided, with more detailed descriptions of those parasite species considered to be of importance.

It is not uncommon to encounter 'pseudoparasites', namely parasites of the prey host (e.g. the oxyurid parasite *Syphacia* of rodents, seen in snake faeces) or normal commensals of the gut flora in herbivorous animals (e.g. the ciliate *Nyctotherus* in iguanas and tortoises). For this reason, it is important to know both the taxonomic identification and the diet of captive reptiles prior to attempted parasite identification and instigation of potentially unnecessary treatment.

ENDOPARASITES

Parasites of the digestive system

Helminths

While cestode, trematode and acanthocephalan parasites are commonly found in wild-caught reptiles, their complex life cycles, which may involve one or more intermediate hosts, mean that they are rarely found in captive reptiles and as a consequence these parasite classes are not discussed further.

Nematodes

Reptile digestive tracts can be infected with a wide range of trichostrongylid, strongylid, ascarid and other nematode superfamilies. Both strongyles and trichostrongyles can be found in the alimentary tracts of reptiles, especially snakes.

Kalicephalus spp.

Kalicephalus spp. (Phylum: Nematoda; Class: Chromadorea; Order: Rhabditida; Family: Diaphanocephalidae) is localised in the small intestine of snakes.

Epidemiology: Infection is by ingestion of contaminated food or water or percutaneously. There is low host specificity and many species of snake can be infected, which is important where several species are kept together.

Clinical signs and pathology: *Kalicephalus* causes a wide range of signs, including lethargy, regurgitation, diarrhoea, anorexia and debility. The larvae may undergo visceral *larva migrans* and can cause respiratory problems. Adult worms embedded in the oesophageal, gastric and intestinal mucosa cause ulceration, usually with a secondary bacterial infection. Build-up of necrotic debris may cause occlusion of the oesophagus.

Diagnosis: The embryonated eggs or larvae may be found in faecal smears or on microscopy of oral and oesophageal mucus, or tracheal washings.

Control and treatment: Good husbandry is very important in controlling and preventing infection. Treatment is often unsuccessful, although fenbendazole (50–100 mg/kg) or oxfendazole (60 mg/kg) may be tried. Ivermectin 200 mg/kg by subcutaneous injection has also been reported to be effective but should be used with caution in some species of reptiles. Recovery can be very protracted.

Within the Ascaridoidea, certain genera and species of worms parasitise particular host groups: *Ophidascaris* and *Polydelphus* are found only in snakes; *Angusticaecum* and *Sulcascaris* are found in chelonia. The pathogenic effects of ascarid nematodes depend on parasite numbers, food availability and an infected animal's overall condition. Clinical signs, such as regurgitation and obstipation, may be seen. The presence of worms in the gastrointestinal tract may cause gastritis, ulceration and perforation of the stomach wall, and in the intestines, intestinal obstruction, intussusception and necrotic enteritis leading to coelomitis and death. Such sequelae may be seen following treatment with anthelminitics in reptiles with heavy worm burdens.

Diagnosis of these infections is based on microscopic examination of eggs found in the faeces. Ascarid eggs are round with thick heavily pitted walls (Fig. 16.8). Control of ascarid nematodes depends on routine parasitological screening of all new arrivals and treatment of all infected animals with anthelmintics. Fenbendazole 50–100 mg/kg by mouth or stomach tube is generally reported to be effective.

Oxyurid parasites belonging to the superfamily Oxyuridoidea are commonly found in reptiles and at least 12 different genera have been described in snakes, lizards and testudines. These small nematodes ('pinworms') may be present in large numbers in the large intestine, colon and rectum, causing discomfort. Some

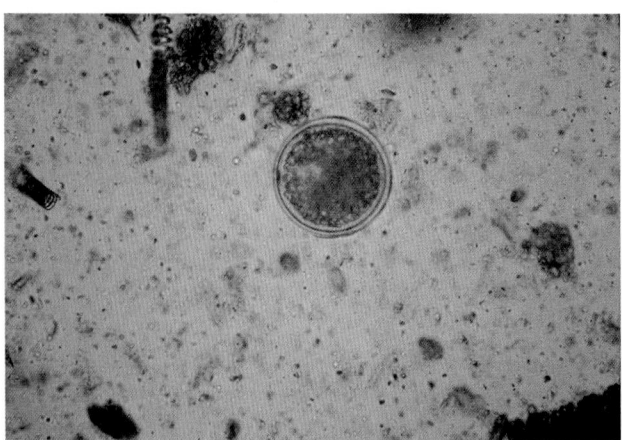

Fig. 16.8 Ascarid (*Angusticaecum* spp.) egg from a Hermann's tortoise (*Testudo hermanni*).

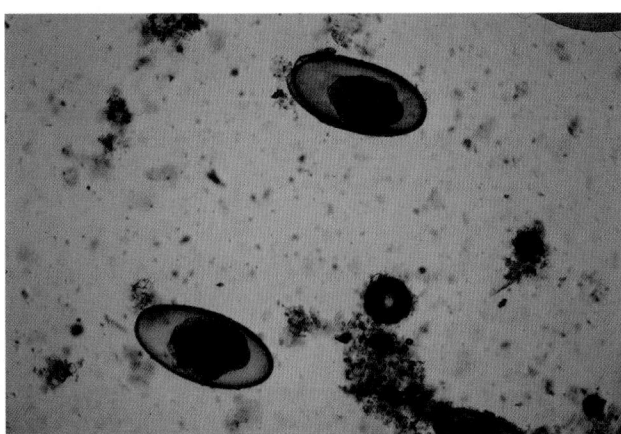

Fig. 16.9 Oxyurid egg (*Tachygonetria* spp.) from a Hermann's tortoise (*Testudo hermanni*).

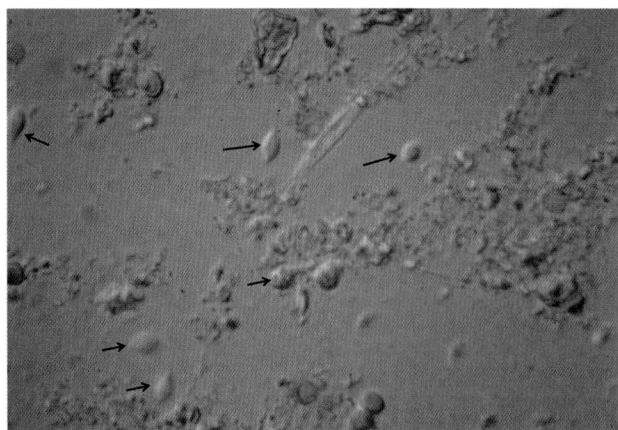

Fig. 16.11 Flagellate protozoa (arrows) in snake faeces (wet mount ×400).

species are viviparous but the majority are oviparous or ovoviviparous and a common feature of their eggs is an asymmetrical flattening on one side. Diagnosis of oxyurid infections is based on identification of the eggs in faeces (Figs 16.9 and 16.10), or the adults from faeces or *post mortem* specimens. Treatment is as for ascarid infections.

Strongyloides and *Rhabdias* spp., belonging to the superfamily Rhabditoidea, are slender hair-like worms. Only females are parasitic and these produce larvated, oval and thin-shelled eggs. After hatching, larvae may develop through four larval stages into free-living adult male and female worms and this can be followed by a succession of free-living generations. In *Strongyloides* infection, there is anorexia, weight loss, diarrhoea, dehydration and death. *Rhabdias* are primarily respiratory parasites but can be associated with enteritis. Treatment with fenbendazole, as for other worm species, is usually effective.

Several species of *Capillaria* (Trichuroidea) have been reported in reptiles. These are very fine filamentous worms found mainly in the gastrointestinal tract but may also infest other organs such as the liver and reproductive organs. Transmission is direct from one infected reptile to another via the larvated egg, which is barrel-shaped with bipolar plugs.

Protozoa

Flagellate protozoa are commonly seen in the faeces of reptiles (Fig. 16.11). *Spironucleus* (*Hexamita*) has been reported to cause fatal renal disease in aquatic chelonia (terrapins). A number of other flagellates have been reported in reptiles. These include *Chilomastix*, *Enteromonas*, *Trichomonas* and *Pentatrichomonas*. *Monocercomonas* has been recorded in both Old World and New World lizards and snakes of several different genera and species. Definitive diagnosis is made by identifying the organisms by their characteristic flagella, nuclear complement and other morphological characteristics. Most of these organisms are sensitive to oral metronidazole (100–275 mg/kg).

Several other types of protozoa can often be present in clinically normal reptiles and may become pathogenic only if and when the host is stressed or becomes immunologically incompetent for one reason or another. *Nyctotherus* (Fig. 16.12) and other protozoa, such as *Balantioides* and *Paramecium*, are thought to serve as beneficial commensals required for the processing of dietary cellulose and complex carbohydrate constituents. Correct identification is essential otherwise they become the objects of unnecessary (and possibly harmful) treatment. Neonatal common iguanas, for example, acquire their intestinal microflora by actively seeking out and ingesting the fresh stools of older lizards. When the normal microflora is substantially disturbed or destroyed, the gut must be reinoculated with a culture or other source of bacterial and protozoan organisms from a healthy animal as close to the genus and species of the sick reptile as possible.

Entamoeba invadens

Entamoeba invadens (Phylum: Amoebozoa; Class: Archamoebea; Order: Entamoebida; Family: Entamoebidae) is localised in the large intestine of reptiles.

Epidemiology: There does not appear to be any particular host susceptibility or resistance, although it is seen more commonly in captive boas and pythons. Cysts can survive for 7–14 days in the environment.

Pathogenesis: *Entamoeba invadens* usually lives as a commensal symbiont in turtles, some tortoises and crocodilians that serve as

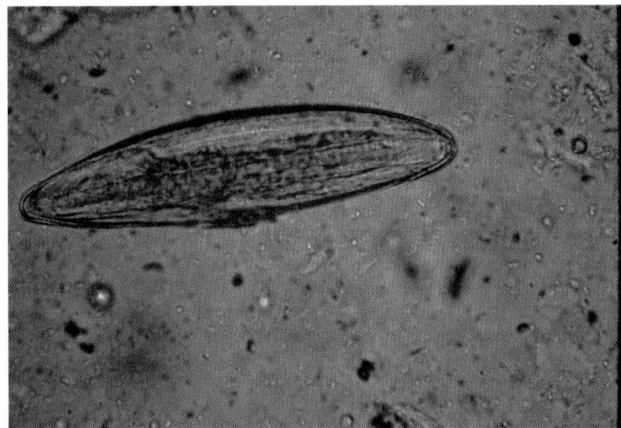

Fig. 16.10 Oxyurid egg from a snake.

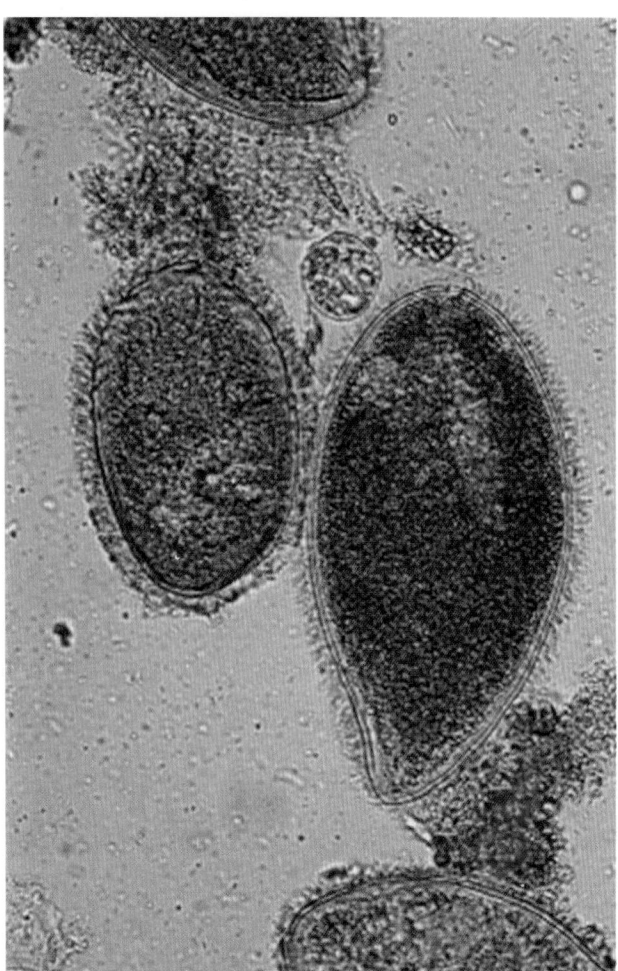

Fig. 16.12 Ciliate (*Nyctotherus*) from an iguana.

healthy reservoirs of the organism. Contamination of the water supply of snakes and lizards with *Entamoeba* can sometimes lead to enteritis, hepatitis and, occasionally, nephritis. It has been reported in cases of human and animal amoebic meningoencephalitis.

Clinical signs and pathology: There are few specific or pathognomonic signs attributable to amoebiasis in reptiles. The clinical signs of infection are usually related to regurgitation of undigested food, weight loss, dehydration, lethargy and severe diarrhoea, sometimes accompanied with blood- or bile-tinged green mucus and/or tags of intestinal mucosa. Rupture of hollow viscus organs has been reported in some cases. Occasionally, rectal or cloacal prolapse occurs. Microscopically, the characteristic lesions produced by *E. invadens* are severe intestinal erosion, inflammation and, often, ulceration. The affected gut wall is thickened, ulcerated and focally necrotic, and often a fibrinonecrotic pseudomembrane is found in the intestinal lumen overlying the foci of inflammation. Typically, the ileum and colon are the most severely affected intestinal segments. The liver shows focal areas of necrosis and evidence of fatty degeneration. Pulmonary abscessation has also been associated with more chronic infections.

Diagnosis: Positive diagnosis of amoebiasis depends on finding elongated uninucleate trophozoites and/or cysts containing four nuclei in the faeces. Cysts are more easily detected if stained with Lugol's iodine.

Control and treatment: Strict hygiene and quarantine are important in preventing transmission of *E. invadens* cysts. All cages and water containers should be cleaned routinely with disinfectant. Metronidazole 275 mg/kg as a single oral treatment has been reported to be effective. An alternative treatment is 160 mg/kg orally for three days. Supportive medical care, consisting of fluid and multivitamin complex therapy and increased ambient environmental temperature, should also be provided.

Reptiles and amphibians may serve as natural hosts to other amoebae. *Acanthamoeba* has elongate filiform pseudopodia and a large nuclear karyosome. Amoeboid forms of the genus *Naegleria* have broad pseudopodia but may also exist as flagellate forms with two flagella and a large central nuclear karyosome. It is thought that the flagellate form is infective for both vertebrates and invertebrates. Many of these organisms appear to share a commensal relationship with their hosts but some infections have been associated with gastric, intestinal, hepatic, brain and renal lesions. Because of the potential for human infection, care must be taken when working with reptiles harbouring these organisms.

Several genera of coccidia (Eimeriidae) have been reported from reptiles. These include *Eimeria*, *Isospora*, *Caryospora*, *Cyclospora*, *Hoarella*, *Octosporella*, *Pythonella*, *Wenyonella*, *Dorisiella* and *Tyzzeria*. *Eimeria*, *Isospora* and *Caryospora* are the most frequently observed genera in reptiles, particularly lizards and snakes. *Isospora* has also been reported in crocodilians. Only *Eimeria* have been found in testudines. *Wenyonella* has only been reported in snakes. Determining the number of sporocysts and sporozoites present within the sporulated oocysts is used for differentiating the genera (see Table 2.16).

However, it is important to be aware that in some species of carnivorous snakes and lizards, some of the *Isospora* recorded may in fact be *Toxoplasma* and *Sarcocystis*. *Eimeria* species recorded in snakes may similarly be parasites of the prey host.

Parasites of the genus *Cryptosporidium* are of increasing importance in reptiles. Two species have been reported: *C. serpentis* and *C. saurophilum* in snakes and lizards.

Cryptosporidium serpentis

Cryptosporidium serpentis (Phylum: Apicomplexa; Class: Conoidasida; Order: Cryptogregarinorida; Family: Cryptosporidiidae) is presumably distributed worldwide and localised in the stomach of snakes and lizards. Transmission appears to be mainly by the faecal–oral route.

Pathogenesis: Infection has been reported in snakes belonging to a number of species and genera, with infected animals showing a severe chronic hypertrophic gastritis. Signs include postprandial regurgitation and firm mid-body swelling. Infection usually occurs in mature snakes, the clinical course is usually protracted, and once infected most snakes remain infected. *C. serpentis* apparently also infects lizards and has been found in savannah monitors.

Clinical signs and pathology: Postprandial regurgitation, mid-body swelling and chronic weight loss. Oedema and thickening of gastric mucosa with exaggeration of normal longitudinal rugae with copious mucus adhesion. Histologically, there is mucosal petechiation, ecchymotic haemorrhages and focal necrosis. There is hypertrophy of mucous neck cells with excess mucus in the gastric pits and adherent to the surface epithelium. The lamina propria is oedematous with lymphocyte and scattered heterophil infiltration. Trophozoites can be seen on the brush border of surface and glandular epithelial cells. In some animals there may be replacement of glandular cells by cuboidal or columnar epithelial cells, epithelial hyperplasia and mucosal necrosis with abscess formation and oedema.

Diagnosis: Oocysts may be demonstrated using Ziehl–Neelsen-stained faecal smears in which the sporozoites appear as bright red granules. Speciation of *Cryptosporidium* is difficult, if not impossible, using conventional techniques. A range of molecular and immunological techniques has been developed that includes immunofluorescence and enzyme-linked immunosorbent assay (ELISA). More recently, DNA-based techniques have been used for the molecular characterisation of *Cryptosporidium* species.

Control and treatment: Strict hygiene and quarantine of imported or captive reptiles is required. Chronically infected animals showing weight loss, emaciation and gastric enlargement should be culled. There is no effective treatment.

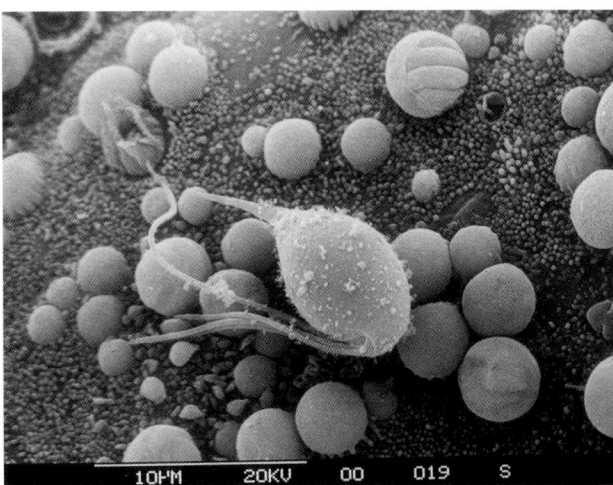

Fig. 16.14 Scanning electron micrograph of lizard intestine showing several stages of *Cryptosporidium saurophilum* and flagellated trichomonad (foreground).

Cryptosporidium saurophilum

Cryptosporidium saurophilum (Phylum: Apicomplexa; Class: Conoidasida; Order: Cryptogregarinorida; Family: Cryptosporidiidae) is presumably distributed worldwide and localised in the intestine and cloaca of lizards and snakes. Transmission appears to be mainly by the faecal–oral route.

Pathogenesis: No pathological changes have been found in the intestine and cloaca of infected adult lizards but weight loss, abdominal swelling and mortality have occurred in some colonies of juvenile geckos (*Eublepharis macularius*).

Clinical signs and pathology: Weight loss and abdominal swelling have been reported. Cryptosporidia are found on the mucosal surfaces of the lower intestine and cloaca of lizards and are associated with mucosal thickening and hyperplastic and hypertrophic epithelia (Figs 16.13 and 16.14). *C. saurophilum* infection in snakes is not totally restricted to the intestine and may also affect the stomach.

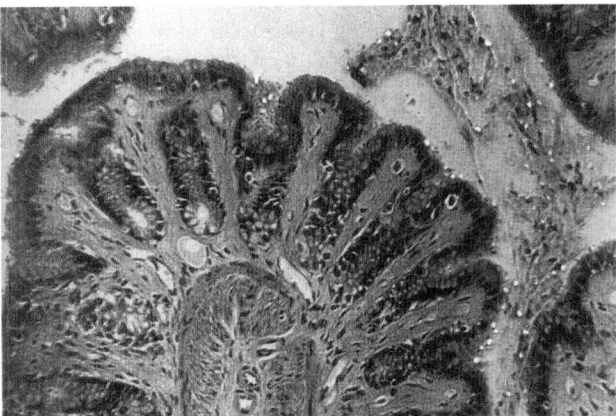

Fig. 16.13 *Cryptosporidium saurophilum* in lizard intestine (phase contrast).

Diagnosis: As for *C. serpentis*.

Control and treatment: As for *C. serpentis*.

Parasites of the respiratory system

Rhabdias spp.

Rhabdias spp. (Phylum: Nematoda; Class: Chromadorea; Order: Rhabditida; Family: Rhabdiasidae) is localised in the lungs of snakes and squamate reptiles.

Pathogenesis and clinical signs: Infection often causes minimal damage but may result in inflammation, hypoxia and pneumonia and secondary bacterial infection of the oral/respiratory mucosa with production of mucous exudate. Percutaneous infections may cause skin lesions.

Diagnosis: The larvae may be found in faecal smears or on microscopy of tracheal washings.

Control and treatment: Levamisole 10 mg/kg into the coelomic cavity and repeated after two weeks is effective. Ivermectin 200 µg/kg by subcutaneous injection has also been reported to be effective.

Parasites of the circulatory system

A wide range of haemoprotozoan parasites can be found in the blood of reptiles. The major genera found include *Haemoproteus*, *Leucocytozoon*, *Plasmodium*, *Trypanosoma*, *Hepatozoon* and *Haemogregarina*. As these parasites are transmitted by arthropod vectors, they are unlikely to be found in captive reptiles unless recently caught from the wild.

Parasites of the reproductive/ urogenital system

Klossiella boae

Klossiella boae (Phylum: Apicomplexa; Class: Conoidasida; Order: Eucoccidiorida; Family: Klossiellidae) is a parasite of unknown distribution localised in the kidneys of *Boa constrictor*.

Epidemiology: Sporocysts are passed in the urine and infection takes place by ingestion of the sporulated sporocysts.

Pathology: Vegetative forms develop in renal tubular epithelial cells.

Diagnosis: Sporocysts may be detected in urine sediments or trophozoite stages may be found on *post mortem* in the kidney. The site and location are pathognomonic.

Control and treatment: Not required, although some of the sulfonamide antibiotics, such as sulfaquinoxaline or sulfamethoxazole-trimethoprim, should be effective.

Sarcocystis, Besnoitia and *Toxoplasma* are occasionally found in reptiles in histological sections of *post mortem* material. Occasionally, oocysts of *Sarcocystis* are seen in the faeces of a predator reptile. The intermediate host is often a higher vertebrate such as a rodent but can include other reptile species.

ECTOPARASITES

Reptiles can be affected by a wide range of ectoparasites in the wild. Both ticks and mites are frequently encountered in wild-caught specimens but are generally less of a problem in captive-bred reptiles with a few exceptions.

Mites

Mesostigmata

One of the most commonly encountered mites is the snake mite, *Ophionyssus natricis*, which is described in detail in the following text. Other species of mesostigmatid mites found on snakes and occasionally lizards include *Ophionyssus lacertinus*, *O. mabuya* and *Neoliponyssus saurarum*.

    Entonyssus, *Entophionyssus* and *Mabuyonyssus* mites belonging to the family Entonyssidae are parasites of the trachea and lungs of snakes.

Ophionyssus natricis

Ophionyssus natricis, synonyms *Ophionyssus serpentium*, *Serpenticola serpentium* (Phylum: Arthropoda; Class: Arachnida; Subclass: Acari; Order: Mesostigmata; Family: Macronyssidae), commonly known as the Snake mite (Fig. 16.15), is usually localised on the skin beneath the scales of snakes and lizards. It is found worldwide.

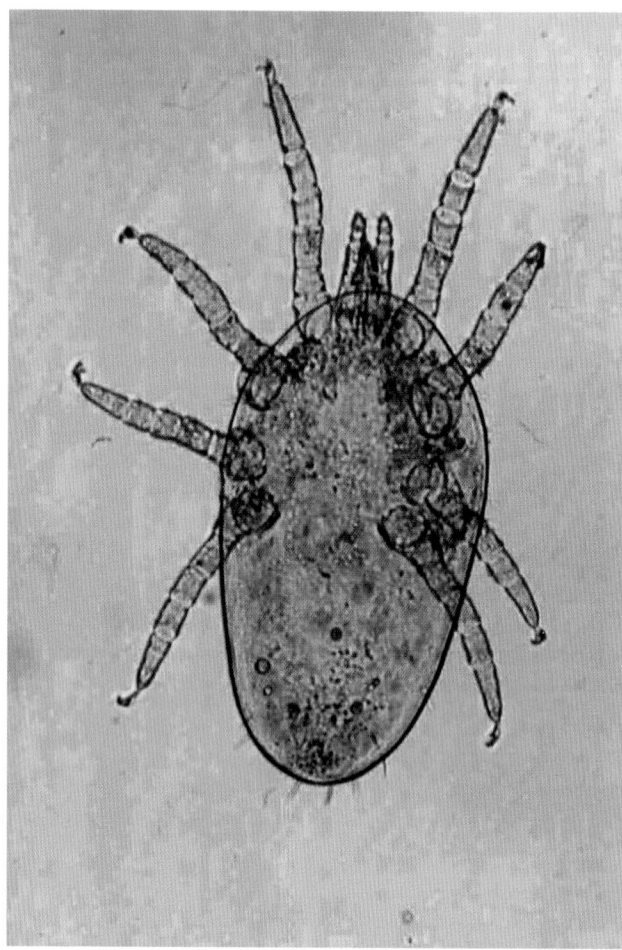

Fig. 16.15 *Ophionyssus natricis.*

Epidemiology: This mite is the most serious ectoparasite of captive snakes and lizards. The source of infection is other snakes or contaminated equipment or cages.

Pathogenesis and clinical signs: The number of mites on captive snakes is frequently large. The mites feed on blood and are found at several locations, usually on the rim of the eye or beneath scales anterior to the neck. Heavy infestations are characterised by irritation, listlessness, debilitation, anaemia and death.

Diagnosis: Mite infestations are often diagnosed by direct observation of the mites or mite faeces on the snake.

Control and treatment: Newly acquired snakes should be quarantined, inspected and placed in clean sterilised cages. If cages or cage contents become infested, thorough cleaning and treatment with acaricides or steam sterilisation are necessary. Infected animals may be treated with insecticides applied sparingly to skin by wiping with a cloth sprayed with an insecticidal flea spray preparation used on small animals (e.g. containing permethrin). Injectable ivermectin 200 µg/kg has also been reported to be effective. Isoxazoline drugs have been successfully used for the oral treatment of captive ball pythons (fluralaner), in Burmese pythons (afoxolaner 2.0 mg/kg) and in eastern rat snake and Sumatran short-tailed python (afoxolaner 2.5 mg/kg).

Prostigmata

Trombiculid mites (Family Trombiculidae), during their larval stages only, feed on reptiles for 2–10 days before dropping off, moulting to protonymphs and then to deutonymphs, which feed on insects and spiders. The adult mites feed on detritus in the environment.

The family Pterygosomatidae are specialised parasitic mites of lizards, parasitising only certain species that include the agamids (Agamidae), geckoes (Gekonidae), iguanas (Iguanidae) and zonures (Zonuridae). *Geckobiella* and *Pimeliaphilus* infest primarily geckoes; *Hirstiella* infests iguanas and geckoes; *Ixodiderma* infests zonures; *Scapothrix* and *Zonurobia* infest zonures, with some infections causing severe dermatitis.

Cloacarus (family Cloacaridae) are found in the cloacal mucosa of aquatic terrapins; members of the family Ophioptidae are found beneath the scales of snakes.

Ticks

At least seven genera of ticks have been found on reptiles and include *Amblyomma*, *Aponomma*, *Hyalomma*, *Haemaphysalis*, *Ixodes*, *Argas* and *Ornithodoros*. These tick genera are covered in more detail in Chapter 3.

Hyalomma aegyptium was seen frequently in northern Europe on tortoises imported from southern Europe for the pet trade. This practice has now ceased and there is no evidence of establishment outside its natural range. The relapsing fever tick, *Ornithodoros turicata*, native to the USA and Mexico, has been reported on box turtles (*Terrepene* spp.).

Hyalomma aegyptium

Hyalomma aegyptium (Phylum: Arthropoda; Class: Arachnida; Order: Ixodida; Family: Ixodidae), commonly known as the Tortoise tick, feeds on tortoises (*Testudo* spp.) and lizards but may also feed on dogs and horses. It is found throughout southern Europe and southwest Asia. The tick has a role in the cryptic cycle of Crimean–Congo haemorrhagic fever (CCHF), which is a widespread disease caused by a tick-borne virus (*Nairovirus*) of the Bunyaviridae family. CCHF virus causes a severe haemorrhagic fever in humans, with a fatality rate of 10–40%.

Epidemiology: This species is a two-host tick. *Hyalomma aegyptium* is found mainly in arid areas, sheltering in burrows of its tortoise host.

Treatment and control: Individual ticks can be removed carefully with forceps.

Other *Amblyomma* species of ticks affecting reptiles are listed in Table 16.2.

Insects

Several fly species are known to attack reptilian hosts and may be responsible for transmission of diseases in the wild. Phlebotomine sand flies are known to transmit *Leishmania* to reptiles, and mosquitoes transmit a range of haemoparasites, filarial worms and arboviruses to reptiles.

Myiasis has been reported in tortoises, with blowfly larvae causing lesions especially around the cloaca, following diarrhoea or trauma to the cloaca. Treatment is by cleaning and debriding the lesion, followed by disinfection and application of a topical insecticide.

HOST–PARASITE CHECKLISTS

In the following checklists, the codes listed below apply.

Helminths

N, nematode; T, trematode; C, cestode; A, acanthocephalan.

Arthropods

F, fly; L, louse; S, flea; M, mite; Mx, maxillopod; Ti, tick.

Protozoa

Co, coccidia; Bs, blood sporozoa; Am, amoeba; Fl, flagellate; Ci, ciliate.

Miscellaneous 'protozoal organisms'

B, blastocyst; Mi, microsporidian; My, *Mycoplasma*; P, Pneumocysti-domycete; R, *Rickettsia*.

Table 16.2 Other *Amblyomma* tick species in reptiles.

Species	Hosts	Geographical distribution	Pathogenesis
Amblyomma sparsum	Reptiles, tortoises	Sub-Saharan Africa	These species are of particular importance because they are vectors of the rickettsia *Ehrlichia ruminantium*, the causal agent of heartwater in cattle, sheep, goats, deer and buffalo. Infected ticks may be present on imported reptiles, facilitating the transmission of disease into new areas such as the USA
Amblyomma marmorium	Tortoises	Sub-Saharan Africa	

Pigeon parasite checklist.

Section/host system	Helminths Parasite	(Super)family	Arthropods Parasite	Family	Protozoa Parasite	Family
Digestive						
Pharynx					Trichomonas gallinae	Trichomonadidae (Fl)
Oesophagus	Dispharynx nasuta	Acuarioidea (N)			Trichomonas gallinae	Trichomonadidae (Fl)
Crop	Ornithostrongylus quadriradiatus	Trichostrongyloidea (N)			Trichomonas gallinae	Trichomonadidae (Fl)
	Capillaria contorta	Trichuroidea (N)				
Proventriculus	Ornithostrongylus quadriradiatus	Trichostrongyloidea (N)			Trichomonas gallinae	Trichomonadidae (Fl)
	Tetrameres americana	Spiruroidea (N)				
	Tetrameres fissispina	Spiruroidea (N)				
	Dispharynx nasuta	Acuarioidea (N)				
Gizzard						
Small intestine	Ornithostrongylus quadriradiatus	Trichostrongyloidea (N)			Eimeria labbeana	Eimeriidae (Co)
	Ascaridia columbae	Ascaridoidea (N)			Wenyonella columbae	Eimeriidae (Co)
	Capillaria caudinflata	Trichuroidea (N)			Spironucleus columbae	Spironucleidae (Fl)
	Capillaria obsignata	Trichuroidea (N)				
	Davainea proglottina	Davaineidae (C)				
	Raillietina tetragona	Davaineidae (C)				
	Echinoparyphium recurvatum	Echinostomatidae (T)				
	Hypoderaeum conoideum	Echinostomatidae (T)				
Large intestine, caeca	Heterakis gallinarum	Ascaridoidea (N)				
	Capillaria anatis	Trichuroidea (N)				
	Echinostoma revolutum	Echinostomatidae (T)				
	Brachylaemus commutatus	Brachylaemidae (T)				
Respiratory						
Nares						
Trachea, bronchi	Syngamus trachea	Strongyloidea (N)				
Lung			Laminosioptes cysticola	Laminosioptidae (M)		
Air sacs			Cytodites nudus	Cytoditidae (M)		
Liver						
Pancreas						
Circulatory						
Blood					Leucocytozoon marchouxi	Plasmodiidae (Bs)
					Haemoproteus columbae	Plasmodiidae (Bs)
					Haemoproteus sacharovi	Plasmodiidae (Bs)
Blood vessels						
Nervous						
CNS						
Eye						

Organ system	Species	Family / group
Reproductive/urogenital		
Oviduct		
Kidneys		
Locomotory		
Muscle	*Toxoplasma gondii*	Sarcocystidae (Co)
Connective tissue		
Subcutaneous	*Pelecitus clavus*	Filarioidea (N)
	Laminosioptes cysticola	Laminosioptidae (M)
	Hypodectes propus	Hypoderatidae (M)
Integument		
Skin	*Dermanyssus gallinae*	Dermanyssidae (M)
	Ornithonyssus sylviarum	Macronyssidae (M)
	Ornithonyssus bursa	Macronyssidae (M)
	Pseudolynchia canariensis	Hippoboscidae (F)
	Columbicola columbae	Philopteridae (L)
	Ceratophyllus columbae	Ceratophyllidae (S)

Tick species found on pigeons.

Genus	Species	Common name	Family
Argas	*Persicus*	Fowl tick	Argasidae (A)
Argas	*Reflexus*	Pigeon tick	Argasidae (A)

Ratite parasite checklist: ostrich (O), emu (E) and rhea (R).

Section/host system	Helminths		Arthropods		Protozoa	
	Parasite	(Super) family	Parasite	Family	Parasite	Family
Digestive						
Pharynx						
Oesophagus						
Crop						
Proventriculus	Libyostrongylus douglassi (O)	Trichostrongyloidea (N)				
	Libyostrongylus dentatus (O)	Strongyloidea (N)				
	Spirura uncinipenis (R)	Spiruroidea (N)				
	Spirura zschokkei (R)	Spiruroidea (N)				
	Odontospirura cetiopenis (R)	Spiruroidea (N)				
Gizzard	Odontospirura cetiopenis (R)	Spiruroidea (N)				
	Libyostrongylus douglassi (O)	Trichostrongyloidea (N)				
	Libyostrongylus dentatus (O)	Trichostrongyloidea (N)				
Small intestine	Deletrocephalus dimidiatus (R)	Strongyloidea (N)			Eimeria spp. (O, R)	Eimeriidae (Co)
	Paradeletrocephalus minor (R)	Strongyloidea (N)			Spironucleus meleagridis	Spironucleidae (Fl)
	Trichostrongylus tenuis (E)	Trichostrongyloidea (N)			Cryptosporidium baileyi (O)	Cryptosporidiidae (Co)
	Houttuynia struthionis (O, R)	Davaineidae (C)			Retortamonas spp.	Retortamonadidae (Fl)
Caeca	Trichostrongylus tenuis (E)	Trichostrongyloidea (N)			Blastocystis galli (O)	Blastocystidae (B)
Large intestine	Codiostomum struthionis (O, R)	Strongyloidea (N)			Histomonas meleagridis (O, R)	Dientamoebidae (Fl)
Cloacal bursa					Trichomonas spp.	Trichomonadidae (Fl)
Rectum					Balantioides coli (O)	Balantiidae (Ci)
					Balantioides struthionis (O)	Balantiidae (Ci)
					Blastocystis galli (O)	Blastocystidae (B)
Respiratory						
Nares						
Trachea, bronchi	Syngamus trachea (O, R, E)	Strongyloidea (N)				
	Cyathostoma variegatum (E)	Strongyloidea (N)				
Lung	Paronchocerca struthionis (O, R)	Filarioidea (N)				
Air sacs						
Liver						
Pancreas						
Circulatory						
Blood					Plasmodium struthionis (O)	Plasmodiidae (Bs)
					Plasmodium spp. (O, R)	Plasmodiidae (Bs)
					Leucocytozoon struthionis (O)	Plasmodiidae (Bs)
Blood vessels	Paronchocerca struthionis (O, R)	Filarioidea (N)			Aegyptianella pullorum (O)	Anaplasmataceae (R)

(Continued)

Ratite parasite checklist: ostrich (O), emu (E) and rhea (R). *Continued*

Section/host system	Helminths		Arthropods		Protozoa	
	Parasite	(Super) family	Parasite	Family	Parasite	Family
Nervous						
CNS	Baylliascaris procyonis (O, E)	Ascaridoidea (N)				
	Chandlerella quiscali (E)	Filarioidea (N)				
Eye	Philophthalmus gralli (O)	Philophthalmidae (T)				
Reproductive/urogenital						
Oviduct						
Kidneys						
Locomotory						
Muscle						
Connective tissue	Dicheilonema spicularia (O)	Filarioidea (N)				
	Dicheilonema rhea (R)	Filarioidea (N)				
Subcutaneous						
Integument						
Skin			Gabucinia sculpturata	Gabuciniidae (L)		
			Gabucinia bicaudatus	Gabuciniidae (L)		
			Struthiolipeurus struthionis	Philopteridae (L)		
			Struthiolipeurus nandu	Philopteridae (L)		
			Struthiolipeurus stresemanni	Philopteridae (L)		
			Struthiolipeurus rheae	Philopteridae (L)		
			Meinertzhageniella lata	Philopteridae (L)		
			Meinertzhageniella schubarti	Philopteridae (L)		
			Dahlemhornia asymmetrica	Philopteridae (L)		

Tick species found on ostriches.

Genus	Species	Common name	Family
Argas	persicus	Fowl tick	Argasidae (A)
	walkerae	Chicken tick	
Otobius	megnini	Spinose ear tick	Argasidae (A)
Amblyomma	hebraeum	South African bont tick	Ixodidae (A)
	gemma		
	lepidum		
	variegatum		
Haemaphysalis	punctata		Ixodidae (A)
Hyalomma	dromedarii	Camel tick	Ixodidae (A)
	impeltatum		
	marinatum		
	rufipes		
	truncatum		
Rhipicephalus	sanguineus	Brown dog or kennel tick	Ixodidae (A)
	turanicus		

Reptiles parasites checklist.

Section/host system	Helminths		Arthropods		Protozoa	
	Parasite	(Super) family	Parasite	Family	Parasite	Family
Digestive						
Stomach					Cryptosporidium serpentis	Cryptosporidiidae (Co)
Small intestine	Kalicephalus spp.	Diaphanocephaloidea (N)				
Large intestine, cloaca					Entamoeba invadens	Entamoebidae (Am)
					Cryptosporidium saurophilum	Cryptosporidiidae (Co)
Respiratory						
Lung	Rhabdias spp.	Rhabditoidea (N)				
Kidney					Klossiella boae	Klossiellidae (Co)
Skin			Ophionyssus natricis	Macronyssidae (M)		
			Hyalomma aegyptium	Ixodidae (Ti)		

Glossary

A

Acanthocephala: Gr. ákantha: 'hook' and kephalé: 'head' (= hooked head). Helminth phylum characterised by the cephalic end being covered in spines.

Acarid: Gr. akarés: 'small'. Arthropods belonging to the class Arachnida, subclass Acari. In general usage, the term 'mites' refers to the Acarina, causative agents of mange of humans and animals.

Amastigote: Gr. a-: privative and mástix, -igos: 'whip'. Intracellular stage lacking an external flagellum (e.g. *Leishmania* spp.).

Amblyomma spp.: Gr. amblýs: 'blunt' and omma: 'eye'. Genus of ornate ticks belonging to the family Ixodidae presenting eyes and festoons at the margin of the dorsal scutum.

Anaplasma spp.: Gr. aná: 'sopra' and plasma: 'shape', 'shaped object'. Genus of Protozoa of the order Rickettsiales and family Anaplasmataceae.

Ancylostomatidae: Gr. ánkylos: 'curved' and stoma, -tos: 'mouth'. Family of haematophagous nematodes belonging to the order Strongylida featuring a curved cephalic end, hook-shaped, presenting teeth or cutting plates.

Anisakis spp.: Gr. anisakis: 'different'. Genus of nematodes belonging to the order Ascaridida and family Anisakidae that infect humans and use fish as paratenic hosts.

Anoplura: Gr. ánoplos: 'without arms' and ourá: 'tail'. Suborder of lice featuring an elongated head and biting buccal apparatus.

Apicomplexa: Lat. apex: 'tip'. Phylum of Protozoa characterised by the presence of an apical complex, visible via electron microscopy, that participates in the mechanism of penetration of the host cell by the parasite.

Apterous: Gr. a-: privative 'without' and pterón: 'wing' (= 'without wings'). Suffix that usually indicates orders of wingless insects (e.g. Siphonaptera).

Arachnida: Gr. aráchne: 'spider'. Class of the phylum Arthropoda.

Argasidae: Gr. argós: 'incomplete', 'inactive'. Family of ticks belonging to the suborder Metastigmata, lacking a dorsal scutum and also known as 'soft ticks'.

Arthropoda: Gr. arthron: 'joint' and pous, podós: 'foot'. Phylum of invertebrates with limbs featuring joints.

Ascaridida: Gr. askarízein: 'jumping'. Order of nematodes that localise to the intestine without anchoring themselves to the intestinal wall, but floating against the direction of movement of the digesta in order to survive intestinal peristalsis.

Astigmata: Gr. a- privative: 'without' and stígma, -tos: 'sign'. Suborder of sarcoptiform acarids lacking respiratory plates.

B

Babesiidae: Family of Protozoa belonging to the order Piroplasmida named after the Romanian veterinarian Victor Babes (1854–1926).

Blasto-: Gr. blastós: 'embryo' and 'embryonation'. In composite words, indicates a 'seed' or 'embryo' or 'cell'.

Boophilus spp.: Gr. bous, boós: 'bovine' and 'associate'. Formerly considered as a genus of one-host and species-specific ticks of the family Ixodidae, often infecting cattle, now subsumed within the genus *Rhipicephalus*.

Botridia: Gr. bóthros: 'cavity'. Adhesive organs located on the scolex of Pseudophyllidea.

Brachycera: Gr. brachýs: 'short' and kéras: 'horn', 'antenna' (= 'with short antennae'). Together with Nematocera and Cyclorrhapha, the Brachicera represent a suborder of the class Insecta and order Diptera.

Bradyzoite: Gr. bradýs: 'slow' and zóon: 'animal'. Slowly replicating developmental stage of *Toxoplasma*. Bradyzoites are enclosed in the terminal cysts.

C

Calliphoridae: Gr. kállos: 'beauty' and phérein: 'carrying'. Family belonging to the order Diptera, often featuring bright iridescent colours. Of veterinary interest are species whose larvae cause cutaneous and wound myiases.

Capillaria spp.: Lat. capillus: 'hair'. Genus of nematodes of the family Trichuridae, characterised by a hair-thin body.

Cercaria: Gr. kérkos: 'tail'. Larval form of helminth of the class Digenea, featuring a tail that allows free movement to seek suitable intermediate hosts.

Cestoda: Gr. kestós: 'belt'. Class of the phylum Platyhelminthes including helminths characterised by segmented, flattened bodies, featuring a scolex (cephalic end), neck (growth region) and strobila (made of a chain of proglottids).

Chelicerae: Gr. chelé: 'claw' and kéras: 'horn'. Appendices on the head of arachnids that penetrate and anchor the parasite to the skin of the host during feeding.

Cimicidae: Lat. cimex: 'bed bug'. Family belonging to the class Insecta and order Hemiptera, including haematophagous species.

Coenurus spp.: Gr. koinós: 'common' and ourá: 'tail'. Vesicle, which may become rather large (cyst), containing significant amounts of fluids and with several scolexes originating from the internal wall (e.g. *Coenurus cerebralis* larval form of *Multiceps multiceps*).

Cryptosporidiidae: Gr. kryptós: 'hidden' and spóros: 'seed'. Refers to Protozoa of the phylum Apicomplexa, class Sporozoasida, characterised by sporulated oocysts containing free sporozoites that are not contained within sporocysts.

Ctenocephalides spp.: Gr. ktéis, ktenós: 'comb' and kephalé 'head'. Insects belonging to the order Siphonaptera featuring 'combs' localised to the head.

Cyclophyllidea: Gr. kýklos: 'circle', phýllon: 'leaf' and èidos: 'shape'. Order belonging to the class Cestoda whose scolex features four rounded structures (suckers) that adhere to host tissues. See also Pseudophyllidea.

Cyclorrhapha: Gr. kýklos: 'circle' and raphé: 'seam'. Previously considered as a suborder of the class Insecta, order Diptera, now subsumed within the Brachycera, characterised by a circular opening of the puparium.

Cysticercus: Gr. kýstis: 'vesicle' and kérkos: 'tail'. Non-replicating larval form of some Taeniidae (e.g. *Taenia solium*, *T. saginata*, *T. hydatigena*), made of a vesicle containing more or less abundant fluids with an invaginated scolex.

D

Dermacentor spp.: Gr. dérma: 'skin' and kentéin: 'stinging'. Genus of ticks belonging to the family Ixodidae. Refers to the biting of animal skin.

Dermanyssidae: Gr. dérma: 'skin' and nýssein: 'biting'. Family of acarids of the order Parasitiformes, suborder Gamasida.

Veterinary Parasitology, Fifth Edition. Domenico Otranto and Richard Wall.
© 2024 John Wiley & Sons Ltd. Published 2024 by John Wiley & Sons Ltd.

Digenea: Gr. di-: 'twice', 'double' and ghénos: 'generation'. Subclass of parasites belonging to the phylum Platyhelminthes.

***Dipetalonema* spp.:** Gr. di-: 'double', pétalon: 'petal' and nema: 'thread'. Genus of nematodes belonging to the order Spirurida, family Filariidae with flattened extremities.

Diphyllobothriidae: Gr. di-: 'double', phýllon: 'leaf' and bothríon: 'cavity'. Family of parasites belonging to the class Cestoda featuring two cavities on the scolex.

***Dipylidium* spp.:** Gr. dípylos: 'with two doors'. Genus belonging to the class Cestoda, order Cyclophyllidea with two genital openings for each proglottid.

***Dirofilaria* spp.:** Lat. dirus: 'vicious' and filum: 'thread'. Genus of nematodes belonging to the order Spirurida, family Filariidae.

E

***Echinococcus* spp.:** Gr. echínos: 'spiky' and kókkos: 'grain'. Cestode belonging to the family Taeniidae, with rounded armed scolex.

Eimeriidae: Family of Coccidia belonging to the order Eucoccidiida, named after the German scientist Theodor Eimer (1843–1898).

Eucoccidiida: Gr. kókkos: 'grain' (= 'grain-like protozoa with rounded shape'). Refers to Protozoa of the phylum Apicomplexa, class Sporozoasida, that replicate in the intestine.

Eyespot: Lat. ocellus, dim. of oculus: 'eye'. Organelle for vision made of pigmented, photosensitive cells, typical of several invertebrate organisms.

F

Filariidae: Lat. filum: 'thread'. Family of nematodes of the order Spirurida.

G

Gamasida: Lat. scien. gamasus. Suborder of Acarids (known also as Mesostigmata); species that infect animals are haematophagous.

***Gasterophilus* spp.:** Gr. gastér, gastrós: 'stomach' and phílos: 'associate'. Genus of Diptera of the suborder Cyclorrhapha, family Oestridae, named after the localisation of the larvae in the gastrointestinal tract of infected hosts.

***Giardia* spp.:** Genus of Protozoa belonging to the order Diplomonadida, family Diplomonadidae, named after the French zoologist Alfred Giard (1846–1908).

Glossinidae: Gr. glóssa: 'tongue'. Family of Diptera, including the single genus *Glossina* spp., that includes species of biting flies commonly known as 'tsetse'.

H

***Habronema* spp.:** Gr. habrós: 'delicate' and néma: 'thread'. Nematodes belonging to the family Spiruridae, ~10 mm long and characterised by a thin, thread-like body.

***Haemaphysalis* spp.:** Gr. háima, -tos: 'blood' and physallís: 'vesicle'. Genus of ticks belonging to the family Ixodidae.

***Haematobia* spp.:** Gr. háima, -tos: 'blood' and bía: 'strength', 'violence'. Blood-feeding fly (Diptera) belonging to the suborder Brachycera (Cyclorrhapha), featuring a biting buccal apparatus.

Haematophagous: Gr. háima, -tos: 'blood' and phaghéin: 'to feed'. Organisms that feed on blood.

Haematopinidae: Gr. háima, -tos: 'blood' and pínein: 'to drink'. Haematophagous lice, obligate ectoparasites belonging to the order Psocodea (Phthiraptera), suborder Anoplura.

Haemosporida: Gr. háima: 'blood' and spóros: 'seed'. Order of Protozoa of the class Aconoidasida, whose schizogony is completed within red or white blood cells or reticuloendothelial cells of vertebrate hosts.

Helminth: Gr. hélmins: 'worm'. Generally refers to parasites belonging to the classes Nematoda, Cestoda and Trematoda.

Hemiptera: Gr. hemi-: 'half' and pterón: 'wing'. Order of insects whose anterior pair of wings is partially sclerotised, thus appearing like a half wing (families Cimicidae and Reduviidae).

Heteroptera: Gr. hetero- 'hetero-' and pterón: 'wing'. Suborder of insects within the order Hemiptera, whose anterior pair of wings is partially sclerotised, thus appearing like a half wing.

Hexacanth: Gr. hexa-: 'six' and ákantha: 'spine'. Organism featuring six spines (refers to cestode embryos of the family Taeniidae).

Hippoboscidae: Gr. híppos: 'horse' and boské: 'pasture', 'meal'. Family of Diptera of the suborder Brachycera (Cyclorrhapha) that feed on equids as well as small and large ruminants.

***Histomonas* spp.:** Gr. histós: 'tissue' and monás: 'unit'. Genus of Protozoa that infects primarily birds.

***Hyalomma* spp.:** Gr. hýalos: 'glass' and ómma: 'eye'. Genus of ticks of the family Ixodidae, featuring eyes and ornate scutum.

Hydatid or hydatid cyst: Gr. hýdor, -atos: 'water'. Embryonic vesicle, also large in size, containing significant amount of fluids and containing several daughter and granddaughter cysts with several scolexes originating from the germinal membrane. The hydatid or hydatid cyst localises to the parenchyma of organs of intermediate hosts.

I

Insecta: Lat. in -séctor: 'in parts'. Class of invertebrates belonging to the phylum Arthropoda, characterised by three body segments, i.e. head, thorax and abdomen.

Ixodes ricinus: Gr. ixódes: 'tenacious' and Lat. ricinus: 'castor'. Tick species belonging to the family Ixodidae, whose superficial appearance resembles a castor bean.

Ixodidae: Gr. ixódes: 'tenacious'. Family of ticks of the suborder Ixodida, featuring a chitinous dorsal scutum, also known as 'hard ticks'.

K

Kinetoplastida: Gr. kinetós: 'motile' and plastós: 'shaped'. Order of Protozoa belonging to the phylum Sarcomastigophora characterised by the presence of a kinetoplast and a flagellum.

Kinetoplast: Gr. kinetós: 'motile' and plastós: 'shaped'. Cylindrical or stick-like organelle made of mitochondrial DNA (self-replicating), located in the cytoplasm of Kinetoplastida near the basal body of the flagellum, which allows movement of the latter.

L

***Leishmania* spp.:** Genus of Protozoa of the order Kinetoplastida, family Trypanosomatidae, named after the English explorer William B. Leishman (1865–1926).

***Linognathus* spp.:** Gr. láinos: 'made of stone' and gnáthos: 'jaw'. Genus of sucking louse of the suborder Anoplura, family Linognathidae. The term derives from the consistency of the buccal apparatus.

M

Malaria: mal'aria, Italian popular slang that attributed the onset of disease to swampy environments lacking sanitation. The term then became widespread worldwide.

Mallophaga: Gr. mallós: 'fleece' and phaghéin: 'to feed'. A paraphyletic grouping of lice belonging to the order Psocodea (Phthiraptera). They are chewing lice that feed on skin debris and sloughing cells.

Mange: Lat. volg. ronea (aranea): 'scabies'; 'rust' (similar to the colour of the skin infected by mange). Cutaneous disease of domestic and wild animals, and of humans, caused by acarids.

Mastigophora: Gr. mástix, -igos: 'whip' and phérein: 'to carry' (= 'carrying a whip'). Subphylum of Protozoa belonging to the phylum Sarcomastigophora.

Merogony: Gr. méros: 'part', 'division' and theme -gon (from ghennáo): 'reproducing'. Synonym of schizogony. Asexual reproductive process typical of Protozoa of the class Sporozoasida that leads to the formation of merozoites (synonym schizozoites).

Merozoite: Gr. méros: 'part', 'division', and zóon: 'living organism', 'animal'. Synonym of schistozoites. Developmental stage of some protozoa of the class Sporozoasida originated by merogony (synonym schizogony).

Mesostigmata: Gr. mésos: 'median' and stígma, -tos: 'sign'. Order of acarids featuring a pair of stigma localised to the basis of the II, III or IV pair of legs. Also known as Gamasida.

Metacercariae: Gr. metá: 'after' and kérkos: 'tail'. Larval form of helminths belonging to the class Digenea, developing from the cercaria.

Metastigmata: Gr. metá: 'after' and stígma, -tos: 'stigma, sign'. Suborder of acarids featuring a pair of stigma localised to the middle-posterior part of the body. Also known as Ixodida.

Microsporida: Gr. mikrós: 'small' and spóros: 'seed'. Order of Protozoa.

Miracidium: Gr. meirákion: 'young'. Juvenile larva of digeneans.

Monogenea: Gr. mónos: 'sole', 'unique' and ghénos: 'generation'. Order of parasites of the phylum Platyhelminthes, class Trematoda, whose life cycle includes one phase of sexual reproduction.

N

Nemathelminthes: Gr. néma, -tos: 'thread', hélmins, -inthos: 'worm'. Phylum of endoparasites with an elongated, cylindrical body (worm-like).

Nematocera: Gr. néma, -tos: 'thread' and kéras, -tos: 'horn', 'antenna'. Suborder of insects of the order Diptera that, unlike the Brachycera, feature long, multi-annulated antennae.

Nematoda: Gr. néma, -tos: 'thread' and -oeidés: 'similar to' (= 'thread-shaped'). Class of roundworms.

O

Onchocerca spp.: Gr. ónkos: 'mass', 'tumour' and kérkos: 'tail'. Genus of nematodes belonging to the order Spirurida, family Filariidae. Parasites of ligaments, intramuscular and subcutaneous connective tissue of mammals, that cause cutaneous, tumour-like masses.

Oocyst: Gr. oón: 'egg' and kýstis: 'vesicle'.

Ornithodoros spp.: Gr. órnis, -ithos: 'bird' and dóron: 'present'. Genus of ticks of the family Argasidae that mainly infests birds.

P

Paramphistomatidae: Gr. pará: 'near', amphís: 'at the two poles' and stoma: 'mouth'. Family of flatworms characterised by the presence of two polar opposite suckers.

Parasite: Gr. parásitos: 'commensal'.

Pediculidae: Lat. pedículus: 'louse'. Family of lice of the suborder Anoplura.

Phlebotomus spp.: Gr. phleps, -phlebós: 'vein' and témnein: 'to cut' (= 'that cuts veins'). Genus of haematophagous insects of the order Diptera, suborder Nematocera, family Psychodidae. Known vectors of *Leishmania* spp.

Phthiraptera: Gr. phthir 'lice' and aptera 'wingless'. Formerly considered as an order containing the parasitic lice, now subsumed into the order Psocodea.

Phylum: Gr. phýlon: 'lineage'. Indicates a taxonomic group hierarchically underneath kingdom but above class.

Piroplasmida: See Piroplasmosis. Order of Protozoa of the phylum Apicomplexa.

Piroplasmosis: Lat. pirum: 'pear' and plasma: 'shaped' (= 'pear-shaped'). Refers to the classic shape that Protozoa of the genus *Babesia* display within infected red blood cells.

Plasmodium spp.: Lat. scient. Plasmodium (from plasma): 'group of parts held together'. Genus of Protozoa belonging to the order Haemosporida, family Plasmodiidae, including the causative agents of malaria.

Platyhelminthes: Gr. platýs: 'flat' and helmins, -inthòs: 'worm'. Phylum of dorsoventrally flattened endoparasites.

Proglottid: Lat. scient. proglottis (F. Dujardin in 1843), from Gr. pro-: 'in front' and glótta: 'tongue'. Refers to individual segments that follow the neck of cestodes and that together form the strobila (chain).

Promastigote: Gr. pro-: 'in front' and mástix, -igos: 'whip'. Protozoa whose flagellum originates from a kinetoplast located in front of the nucleus, near the basal body, and that allows parasite movement (e.g. infective metacyclic form of *Leishmania* spp.).

Prostigmata: Gr. pro-: 'in front' and stígma, -tos: 'stigma, sign'. Suborder of trombidiform acarids featuring respiratory spiracles localised anteriorly to the basis of the chelicerae.

Protozoa: Gr. prótos: 'first' and zóon: 'animal'. Subkingdom of unicellular eukaryotic organisms.

Pseudophyllidea: Gr. pséudo-, with pseudés: 'false' and phýllon: 'leaf'. Order of the class Cestoda whose unarmed scolex features two adhesive, lateral organs known as botrids. Also see Cyclophyllidea.

Psychodidae: Gr. psyché: 'soul'. Family of Diptera of the suborder Nematocera, termed after their silent flight that makes them unperceivable. Also known as 'papataci' (= 'feeding in silence').

Pterygota: Gr. pterugōtós, 'winged'; includes all orders of winged insects and the orders that are secondarily wingless.

R

Rhipicephalus spp.: Gr. rhipís: 'fan' and kephalé: 'head'. Genus of ticks of the family Ixodidae.

S

Sarcocystis spp.: Gr. sarx, sarcós: 'flesh' and kýstis: 'vesicle'. Genus of Protozoa of the phylum Apicomplexa, class Sporozoasida, order Eucoccidida, family Sarcocystidae, that parasitise the muscles of mammals, humans included, and birds, forming muscular cysts.

Sarcomastigophora: Gr. sarx, sarcós: 'flesh', mástix, -igos: 'whip' and phérein: 'to carry'. Phylum of Protozoa with a flagellum.

Sarcophagidae: Gr. sarx, sarcós: 'flesh' and phaghéin: 'to feed'. Family of Diptera of the suborder Brachycera (Cyclorrhapha), superfamily Muscoidea. Species of veterinary interest have larvae that feed on wounds or skin of animals.

Schistosomatidae: Gr. schistós: 'divided', and sóma, -tos: 'body'. Family of the phylum Platyhelminthes, named after the morphology of the adult male, characterised by the presence of a gynaecophorous canal that accommodates the female during mating.

Schizogony: Gr. schízein: 'to separate' and -gon from ghígnomai: 'to generate', 'to reproduce'. Form of asexual reproduction typical of some Sarcodina and Apicomplexa, whose daughter cells are generated by binary fission of the parasite nucleus, followed by segmentation of the cytoplasm (schizonts) and that result in the formation of separate bodies with small nuclei (schizo- or merozoites).

Scolex: Gr. skólex, -kos: 'worm'; the anterior end of cestodes (head).

Simuliidae: Lat. simulus: 'to simulate'. Family of Diptera of the suborder Nematocera characterised by a humped, oval thorax.

Siphonaptera: Gr. síphon, and apteros: 'wingless'. Order of blood-feeding, wingless insects, known as fleas, with buccal apparatus similar to a tube.

Spiracle: Lat. spiraculum, from spirare: 'to breathe'. External opening of the respiratory system of insects.

Spirocerca spp.: Gr. spéira: 'spiral' and kérkos: 'tail'. Genus of nematodes of the order Spirurida, family Spiruridae. The tail of the male is spiral shaped.

Spirurida: Gr. spéira: 'spiral' and ourá: 'tail'. Order of nematodes that includes species with varying localisation (gastrointestinal and respiratory tract and, more frequently, orbital cavities).

Sporoblast: Gr. sporá: 'to seed', 'seed' and blastós: 'germination'. Protoplasmatic mass contained within the sporocysts of coccidia.

Sporocyst: Gr. sporá: 'to seed', 'seed' and kýstis: 'vesicle', 'cyst'. Cyst containing spores or gametes. Refers to reproducing forms of coccidia and digeneans.

Sporogony: Gr. sporá: 'to seed', 'seed' and -gon from ghígnomai: 'to generate'. In protozoa, replication by multiple fission of a sporont leading to the formation of sporocysts and sporozoites.

Sporont: Gr. sporá: 'to seed', 'seed'. Evolutionary form of the zygote of coccidia enclosed within a oocyst that, following sporogony, produces sporoblasts that develop into sporocysts containing sporozoites.

Sporozoite: Gr. sporá: 'to seed', 'seed' and zóon: 'living organism'. Reproductive cell of several animals able to generate a new individual.

Stigma: Gr. stigma: 'sign'. External opening of the respiratory system of ticks and mites.

Stomoxynae: Gr. stóma: 'mouth' and oxýs: 'acute', 'pointy' (= 'with a pointy mouth'). Diptera of the family Muscidae with a biting, long and hard buccal apparatus. Includes the genera *Stomoxys* spp., *Haematobia* spp. and *Lyperosia* spp.

Strobila: Gr. stróbilos: 'spinning wheel', 'pine cone'. Series of proglottids that, together, form the body of cestodes.

Strobilocercus: Gr. stróbilos: 'spinning wheel' and kérkos: 'tail'. Larval form of cestodes made of a poorly developed vesicle followed by a short, evaginated strobila. Typical of *Taenia taeniaeformis* and found in the liver of the intermediate host (rodent).

T

Tachyzoite: Gr. tachýs: 'fast', and zóon: 'animal'. Fast-replicating developmental stage of *Toxoplasma*. Tachyzoites can be found inside the pseudocysts.

Taeniidae: Gr. tainía, Lat. taenia: 'tape'. Family of cestodes of the order Cyclophyllidea, including the genera *Taenia* spp., *Multiceps* spp. and *Echinococcus* spp.

Tetraphyllidea: Gr. tetra-: 'four', phýllon: 'leaf'. Order of cestodes characterised by a scolex with four suckers of varying shape.

***Theileria* spp.:** Genus of Protozoa of the order Piroplasmida, family Theileriidae, named after the South African veterinarian Arnold Theiler (1867–1936).

Thelaziidae: Gr. thelázein: 'to suck'. Spirurids that feed on ocular secretions.

Tick: from German Zecke: 'tick' (stechen: 'to bite'). Haematophagous arthropod.

***Toxoplasma* spp.:** Gr. tóxon: 'arc' and plásma: 'shape' (= 'curved'). Genus of Protozoa of the phylum Apicomplexa, family Sarcocystidae, named after the half-moon shape of tachyzoites inside the pseudocysts.

Trematoda: Gr. trematódes: 'provided with intestinal opening' (tréma: 'opening'). Class of parasites of the phylum Platyhelminthes with a dorsoventrally flattened, non-segmented body and suckers that adhere to the site of localisation.

Trichocephalida: Gr. thríx, trichós: 'hair' and kephalé: 'head'. Order of nematodes characterised by a very thin body. Includes the genera *Trichuris*, *Capillaria* and *Trichinella*.

Trichomonadida: Gr. thríx, trichós: 'hair' and monás: 'unit'. Order of Protozoa of the phylum Sarcomastigophora, subphylum Mastigophora, class Zoomastigophorasida, characterised by the presence of 3–4 flagellae.

Trichostrongylidae: Gr. thríx, trichós: 'hair' and strongýlos: 'rounded'. Family of nematodes belonging to the order Strongylida, very small, mainly infecting the gastrointestinal tract of ruminants.

Trichuridae: Gr. thríx, trichós: 'hair' and ourá: 'tail'. Family of nematodes of the order Orichocephalida, including the genera *Trichuris* spp., *Capillaria* spp. and *Trichinella* spp. Particularly the males are characterised by a spiral-shaped tail and a very thin anterior end.

Trombiculidae: Gr. thrómbos: 'blood clot', referring to the colour. Family of trombidiform acarids of the suborder Prostigmata.

Trophozoite: Gr. trophé: 'nutrient' and zóon: 'living organism', 'animal'. Motile stage of endocellular protozoans able to feed.

Trypanosomatidae: Gr. trýpanon: 'perforating' and sóma: 'body'. Family of Protozoa of the phylum Sarcomastigophora, characterised by an undulating membrane that supports a long flagellum.

Tsetse: From Tswana, local language of South Africa, tsetse: 'fly'. Commonly referring to flies (Diptera: Glossinidae) of the genus *Glossina* spp.

U

***Uncinaria* spp.:** Lat. uncinus: 'hook'. Genus of nematodes of the family Ancylostomatidae with a buccal capsule featuring cutting plates and two teeth.

W

***Wuchereria* spp.:** Genus of nematodes of the family Filariidae, named after the scientist Otto Wucherer (1820–1874).

X

***Xenopsylla*:** Gr. xénos: 'stranger' and psýlla: 'flea'. Genus of the order Siphonaptera, family Pulicidae.

Z

Zoonosis: Gr. zóon: 'animal' and nósos: 'illness' (= 'disease transmitted from animals to humans').

References and further reading

Abbott, K.A., Taylor, M.A. & Stubbings, L.A. (2012) *Sustainable Worm Control Strategies for Sheep. A Technical Manual for Veterinary Surgeons and Advisors*, 4th edn. SCOPS (Sustainable Control of Parasites). www.scops.org.uk/content/SCOPS-Technical-manual-4th-Edition-June-2012.pdf

Adler, P.H., Cheke, R.A. & Post, R.J. (2010) Evolution, epidemiology, and population genetics of black flies (Diptera: Simuliidae). *Infection Genetics and Evolution*, **10**, 846–865.

Alban, L., Pozio, E., Boes, J. *et al.* (2011) Towards a standardised surveillance for *Trichinella* in the European Union. *Preventive Veterinary Medicine*, **99**, 148–160.

Angulo-Valadez, C.E., Ascencio, F., Jacquiet, P., Dorchies, P. & Cepeda-Palacios, R. (2011) Sheep and goat immune responses to nose bot infestation: a review. *Medical and Veterinary Entomology*, **25**, 117–125.

Arias-Robledo, G., Wall, R., Szpila, K. *et al.* (2019) Ecological and geographical speciation in *Lucilia bufonivora*: the evolution of amphibian obligate parasitism. *International Journal for Parasitology*: *Parasites and Wildlife*, **10**, 218–230.

Arlian, L.G. (2002) Arthropod allergens and human health. *Annual Review of Entomology*, **47**, 395–433.

Arthur, D.R. (1962) *Ticks and Disease*. International Series of Monographs on Pure and Applied Biology, Vol. 9. Pergamon Press, London.

Arthur, D.R. (1963) *British Ticks*. Butterworths, London.

Axtell, R.C. & Arends, J.J. (1990) Ecology and management of arthropod pests of poultry. *Annual Review of Entomology*, **35**, 101–126.

Baker, A.S. (1999) *Mites and Ticks of Domestic Animals. An Identification Guide and Information Source*. Natural History Museum, London.

Baker, E.W., Evans, T.M., Gould, D.J. *et al.* (1956) *A Manual of Parasitic Mites of Medical or Economic Importance*. National Pest Control Association, New York.

Baker, E.W., Camin, J.H., Cunliffe, F. *et al.* (1958) *Guide to the Families of Mites*. Contribution No. 3, Institute of Acarology, University of Maryland.

Baneth, G. (2011) Perspectives on canine and feline hepatozoonosis. *Veterinary Parasitology*, **181**, 3–11.

Baylis, M., Parkin, H., Kreppel, K., Carpenter, S., Mellor, P.S. & Mcintyre, K.M. (2010) Evaluation of housing as a means to protect cattle from *Culicoides* biting midges, the vectors of bluetongue virus. *Medical and Veterinary Entomology*, **24**, 38–45.

Black, W.C. & Piesman, J. (1994) Phylogeny of hard- and soft-tick taxa (Acari: Ixodida) based on mitochondrial 16S rDNA sequences. *Proceedings of the National Academy of Sciences USA*, **91**, 10034–10038.

Bezerra-Santos, M.A., Mendoza-Roldan, J.A., Lia, R.P. *et al.* (2022) Description of *Joyeuxiella pasqualei* (Cestoda: Dipylidiidae) from an Italian domestic dog, with a call for further research on its first intermediate host. *Parasitology*, **149**, 1769–1774.

Bezerra-Santos, M.A., Dantas-Torres, F., Mendoza-Roldan, J.A., Thompson, R.A., Modry, D. & Otranto, D. (2023) Invasive mammalian wildlife and the risk of zoonotic parasites. *Trends in Parasitology*, **39**, 786–798.

Boatin, B., Molyneux, D.H., Hougard, J.M. *et al.* (1997) Patterns of epidemiology and control of onchocercosis in West Africa. *Journal of Helminthology*, **71**, 91–101.

Burgess, I. (1994) *Sarcoptes scabiei* and scabies. *Advances in Parasitology*, **33**, 235–293.

Calvete, C., Estrada, R., Miranda, M.A., Borras, D., Calvo, J.H. & Lucientes, J. (2009) Ecological correlates of bluetongue vírus in Spain: predicted spatial occurrence and its relationship with the observed abundance of the potential *Culicoides* spp. vector. *Veterinary Journal*, **182**, 235–243.

Calvete, C., Estrada, R., Miranda, M.A. *et al.* (2010) Protection of livestock against bluetongue virus vector *Culicoides imicola* using insecticide-treated netting in open areas. *Medical and Veterinary Entomology*, **24**, 169–175.

Campbell, W.C. & Rew, R.S. (eds) (1986) *Chemotherapy of Parasitic Diseases*. Plenum Press, New York.

Carpenter, S., Mellor, P.S. & Torr, S.J. (2008) Control techniques for *Culicoides* biting midges and their application in the U.K. and north-western Palaearctic. *Medical and Veterinary Entomology*, **22**, 175–187.

Carpenter, S., Wilson, A. & Mellor, P.S. (2009) *Culicoides* and the emergence of bluetongue virus in northern Europe. *Trends in Microbiology*, **17**, 172–178.

Castellani, A. & Chalmers, A.J. (1910) *Manual of Tropical Medicine*. Baillière, Tindall & Cox, London.

Chapman, R.F. (1971) *The Insects: Structure and Function*. English Universities Press, London.

Clutton-Brock, J. (1987) *A Natural History of Domesticated Mammals*. Cambridge University Press, Cambridge.

Colebrook, E. & Wall, R. (2004) Ectoparasites of livestock in Europe and the Mediterranean region. *Veterinary Parasitology*, **120**, 251–274.

Colwell, D.D., Hall, M.J.R. & Scholl, P.J. (2006) *Oestrid Flies: Biology, Host–Parasite Relationships, Impact and Management*. CABI Publishing, Wallingford.

Conboy, G. (2009) Helminth parasites of the canine and feline respiratory tract. *Veterinary Clinics of North America Small Animal Practice*, **39**, 1109–1126.

Crawford, S., James, P.J. & Maddocks, S. (2001) Survival away from sheep and alternative methods of transmission of sheep lice (*Bovicola ovis*). *Veterinary Parasitology*, **94**, 205–216.

Cringoli, G., Maurelli, M.P., Levecke, B. *et al.* (2017) The Mini-FLOTAC technique for the diagnosis of helminth and protozoan infections in humans and animals. *Nature Protocols*, **12**, 1723–1732.

Dantas-Torres, F. (2008) The brown dog tick, *Rhipicephalus sanguineus* (Latreille, 1806) (Acari: Ixodidae): from taxonomy to control. *Veterinary Parasitology*, **152**, 173–185.

Dantas-Torres, F., Chomel, B.B. & Otranto, D. (2012) Ticks and tick-borne diseases: a One Health perspective. *Trends in Parasitology*, **28**, 437–446.

Dantas-Torres, F., Miró, G., Baneth, G. *et al.* (2019) Canine leishmaniosis control in the context of One Health. *Emerging Infectious Diseases*, **25**, 1.

Davies, J.B. (1994) Sixty years of onchocercosis vector control: a chronological summary with comments on eradication, reinvasion, and insecticide resistance. *Annual Review of Entomology*, **39**, 23–45.

Veterinary Parasitology, Fifth Edition. Domenico Otranto and Richard Wall.
© 2024 John Wiley & Sons Ltd. Published 2024 by John Wiley & Sons Ltd.

Deplazes, P., Eckert, J., Mathis, A., Von Samson-Himmelstjerna, G. & Zahner, H. (2016) *Parasitology in Veterinary Medicine*. Wageningen Academic Publishers, Wageningen.

De Waal, D.T. (1992) Equine piroplasmosis: a review. *British Veterinary Journal*, **148**, 6–13.

Dryden, M.W. & Rust, M.K. (1994) The cat flea: biology, ecology and control. *Veterinary Parasitology*, **52**, 1–19.

Dumler, J.S., Barbet, A.F., Bekker, C.P. *et al.* (2001) Reorganization of genera in the families Rickettsiaceae and Anaplasmataceae in the order *Rickettsiales*: unification of some species of *Ehrlichia* with *Anaplasma*, *Cowdria* with *Ehrlichia*, and *Ehrlichia* with *Neorickettsia*, descriptions of five new species combinations and designation of *Ehrlichia equi* and 'HGE agent' as subjective synonyms of *Ehrlichia phagocytophila*. *International Journal of Systematic and Evolutionary Microbiology*, **51**, 2145–2165.

Edwards, F.W., Oldroyd, H. & Smart, J. (1939) *British Blood-Sucking Flies*. British Museum, London.

Edwards, K., Jepson, R.P. & Wood, K.F. (1960) Value of plasma pepsinogen estimation. *British Medical Journal*, **1**, 30.

Eidmann, H. & Kuhlhorn. F. (1970) *A Text-Book of Entomology*. Paul Parey, Hamburg.

Estrada-Pena, A., Venzal, J.M. & Sanchez Acedo, C. (2006). The tick *Ixodes ricinus*: distribution and climate preferences in the western Palaearctic. *Medical and Veterinary Entomology*, **20**, 189–197.

Estrada-Peña, A., Mihalca, A.D. & Petney, T.N. (2017) *Ticks of Europe and North Africa: A Guide to Species Identification*. Springer, New York.

Ewald, P.W. (1993) The evolution of virulence. *Scientific American*, **268**, 56–62.

Fain, A. (1994) Adaptation, specificity and host–parasite coevolution in mites (Acari). *International Journal for Parasitology*, **24**, 1273–1283.

Fassi Fehri, M.M. (1987) Diseases of camels. *Scientific and Technical Review. Office International des Epizooties Paris*, **6**, 337–354.

Figueiredo, R. & Gil-Azevedo, L.H. (2010). The role of Neotropical blackflies (Diptera: Simuliidae) as vector of the onchocercosis: a short review of the ecology behind the disease. *Oecologia Australis*, **14**, 745–755.

Georgi, J.R. & Georgi, M.E. (1990) *Parasitology for Veterinarians*. W.B. Saunders, Philadelphia.

Grimaldi, D. & Engel, M.S. (2004) *Evolution of the Insects*. Cambridge University Press, Cambridge.

Gullan, P.J. & Cranston P.S. (1994) *The Insects: An Outline of Entomology*. Chapman & Hall., London.

Hall, M.J.R. & Smith, K.G.V. (1993) Diptera causing myiasis in man. In: *Medical Insects and Arachnids* (eds R.P. Lane & R.W. Crosskey), pp. 429–469. Springer, Dordrecht.

Hall, M.J.R. & Wall, R. (1994) Myiasis of humans and domestic animals. *Advances in Parasitology*, **35**, 258–334.

Harwood, R.F. & James, M.T. (1979) *Entomology in Human and Animal Health*. Macmillan, New York.

Hassan, M.U., Khan, M.N., Abubakar, M., Waheed, H.M., Iqbal, Z. & Hussain, M. (2010) Bovine hypodermosis: a global aspect. *Tropical Animal Health and Production*, **42**, 1615–1625.

Hinkle, N.C., Rust, M.K. & Reierson, D.A. (1997) Biorational approaches to flea (Siphonaptera: Pulicidae) suppression: present and future. *Journal of Agricultural Entomology*, **14**, 309–321.

Hodda, M. (2022). Phylum Nematoda: a classification, catalogue and index of valid genera, with a census of valid species. *Zootaxa*, **5114**, 1–289.

Hoogstraal, H. (1985) Argasid and nuttalliellid ticks as parasites and vectors. *Advances in Parasitology*, **24**, 135–238.

Hprak, I.G. (1971) Paramphistomiasis of domestic ruminants. *Advances in Parasitology*, **9**, 33–72.

Jacobs, D.E. (1986) *A Colour Atlas of Equine Parasites*. Baillière Tindall, London.

Jorgensen, R. (1975) Isolation of infective *Dictyocaulus* larvae from herbage. *Veterinary Parasitology*, **1**, 61–67.

Kassai, T. (1999) *Veterinary Helminthology*. Butterworth-Heinemann, Oxford.

Kaufmann, J. (1996) *Parasitic Infections of Domestic Animals: A Diagnostic Manual*. Birkhausse Verlag, Basel.

Keirans, J.E. & Robbins, R.G. (1999) A world checklist of genera, subgenera, and species of ticks (Acari: Ixodida) published from 1973–1997. *Journal of Vector Ecology*, **24**, 115–129.

Kettle, D.S. (1984) *Medical and Veterinary Entomology*. Croom Helm, London.

Kim, K.C. & Merritt, R.W. (eds) (1987) *Black Flies. Ecology, Population Management and Annotated World List*. Pennsylvania State University, University Park, PA.

Klomper, J.S.H., Black, W.C., Keirans, J.E. & Oliver, J.H. Jr (1996) Evolution of ticks. *Annual Review of Entomology*, **41**, 141–162.

Klowden, M.J. (2007) *Physiological Systems in Insects*, 2nd edn. Academic Press, Burlington, MD.

Krinsky, W.L. (1976) Animal disease agents transmitted by horse flies and deer flies. *Journal of Medical Entomology*, **13**, 225–275.

Lane, R.P. & Croskey, R.W. (eds) (1993) *Medical Insects and Arachnids*. Chapman & Hall, London.

Levine, N.D. (1985) *Veterinary Protozoology*. Iowa State University Press, Ames, IA.

Lewis, R.E. (1998) Resumé of the Siphonaptera of the world. *Journal of Medical Entomology*, **35**, 377–389.

Lichtenfels, J.R., Kharchenko, V.A. & Dvojnos, G.M. (2008) Illustrated identification keys to strongylid parasites (Strongylidae: Nematoda) of horses, zebras and asses (Equidae). *Veterinary Parasitology*, **156**, 4–161.

Long, P.L. (ed.) (1990) *Coccidiosis of Man and Domestic Animals*. CRC Press, Boca Raton, FL.

Lusat, J., Bornstein, S. & Wall, R. (2011) *Chorioptes* mites: a re-evaluation of species integrity. *Medical and Veterinary Entomology*, **25**, 370–376.

Mendoza Roldan, J.A. & Otranto, D. (2023) Zoonotic parasites associated with predation by dogs and cats. *Parasites and Vectors*, **16**, 55.

Mendoza-Roldan, J.A., Modry, D. & Otranto, D. (2020) Zoonotic parasites of reptiles: a crawling threat. *Trends in Parasitology*, **36**, 677–687.

Miró, G. & López-Vélez, R. (2018) Clinical management of canine leishmaniosis versus human leishmaniosis due to *Leishmania infantum*: Putting "One Health" principles into practice. *Veterinary Parasitology*, **254**, 151–159.

Mulen, G. & Durden, L. (2002) *Medical and Veterinary Entomology*. Academic Press, Amsterdam.

Navarro, E., Serrano-Heras, G., Casteano, M.J. & Solera, J. (2015) Real-time PCR detection chemistry. *Clinica Chimica Acta*, **429**, 231–250.

Otranto, D. (2001). The immunology of myiasis: parasite survival and host defense strategies. *Trends in Parasitology*, **17**, 176–182.

Otranto, D. & Deplazes, P. (2019) Zoonotic nematodes of wild carnivores. *International Journal for Parasitology: Parasites and Wildlife*, **9**, 370–383.

Otranto, D., Dantas-Torres, F., Brianti, E. *et al.* (2013) Vector-borne helminths of dogs and humans in Europe. *Parasites and Vectors*, **6**, 1–14.

Pegler, K.R., Evans, L., Stevens, J.R. & Wall, R. (2005) Morphological and molecular comparison of host-derived populations of parasitic *Psoroptes* mites. *Medical and Veterinary Entomology*, **19**, 392–403.

Piesman, J. & Eisen, L. (2008) Prevention of tick-borne diseases. *Annual Review of Entomology*, **53**, 323–343.

Pozio, E. & Murrell, K.D. (2006) Systematics and epidemiology of *Trichinella*. *Advances in Parasitology*, **63**, 367–439.

Reinecke, R.K. (1983) *Veterinary Helminthology*. Butterworth, Durban, Pretoria.

Rogers, D.J. & Randolph, S.E. (2006) Climate change and vector-borne diseases. *Advances in Parasitology*, **62**, 345–381.

Rinaldi, L., Krücken, J., Martinez-Valladares, M. *et al.* (2022) Advances in diagnosis of gastrointestinal nematodes in livestock and companion animals. *Advances in Parasitology*, **118**, 85–176.

Rothschild, M. (1965) Fleas. *Scientific American*, **213**, 44–53.

Ruggiero, M.A., Gordon, D.P., Orrell, T.M. *et al.* (2015) A higher level classification of all living organisms. *PloS One*, **10**, e0119248.

Russell, R.C., Otranto, D. & Wall, R.L. (2013) *Encyclopedia of Medical & Veterinary Entomology*. CAB International, Wallingford.

Sanders, A., Froggatt, P., Wall, R. & Smith K.E. (2000) Life-cycle stage morphology of *Psoroptes* mange mites. *Medical and Veterinary Entomology*, **14**, 131–141.

Shtakelbergh, A.A. (1956) *Diptera Associated with Man from the Russian Fauna*. Moscow.

Smart, J.A. (1943) *Handbook for the Identification of Insects of Medical Importance*. British Museum (Natural History), London.

Smith, K.G.V. (1989) An introduction to the immature stages of British flies: Diptera larvae, with notes on eggs, puparia and pupae. *Handbooks for the Identification of British Insects*, **10** (14), 1–280.

Snodgrass, R.E. (1935) *Principles of Insect Morphology*. McGraw-Hill, New York.

Soe, A.K. & Pomroy, W.E. (1992) New species of *Eimeria* (Apicomplexa: Eimeriidae) from the domesticated goat *Capra hircus* in New Zealand. *Systematic Parasitology*, **23**, 195–202.

Sonenshine, D.E. (1991) *Biology of Ticks*, Vol. 1. Oxford University Press, New York.

Soulsby, E.J.L. (1968) *Helminths, Arthropods and Protozoa of Domesticated Animals*, 6th edn. Baillière Tindall, London.

Soulsby, E.J.L. (1982) *Helminths, Arthropods and Protozoa of Domesticated Animals*, 7th edn. Baillière Tindall, London.

Stevens, J.R., Wallman, J.F., Otranto, D., Wall, R. & Pape, T. (2006) The evolution of myiasis in humans and other animals in the Old and New Worlds (part II): biological and life-history studies. *Trends in Parasitology*, **22**, 181–188.

Taylor, M.A. (1992) Anthelmintic resistance in helminth parasites of domestic animals. *Agricultural Zoology Reviews*, **5**, 1–50.

Thompson, R.C.A. & Monis, P. (2012) *Giardia*: from genome to proteome. *Advances in Parasitology*, **78**, 57–95.

Thompson, R.C.A., Olsen, M.E., Zhu, G., Enomota, S., Abramamson, M.S. & Hijawi, N.S. (2005) *Cryptosporidium* and cryptosporidiosis. *Advances in Parasitology*, **59**, 78–162.

Toft, J.D. & Eberhard, M.L. (1998) Parasitic diseases. In: *Nonhuman Primates in Biomedical Research* (eds B.T. Bennett, C.R. Abee & R. Henricksen), pp. 111–205. Academic Press, San Diego, CA.

Urech, R., Bright, R.L., Green, P.E. *et al.* (2012) Temporal and spatial trends in adult nuisance fly populations at Australian cattle feedlots. *Australian Journal of Entomology*, **51**, 88–96.

Varcasia, A., Tamponi, C., Tosciri, G. *et al.* (2015) Is the red fox (*Vulpes vulpes*) a competent definitive host for *Taenia multiceps*? *Parasites and Vectors*, **8**, 1–6.

Vercruysse, J. & Rew, R.S. (2002) *Macrocyclic Lactones in Antiparasitic Therapy*. CABI Publishing, Wallingford.

Walker, A. (1994) *Arthropods of Humans and Domestic Animals*. Chapman & Hall, London.

Wall, R. (2007) Psoroptic mange: rising prevalence in UK sheep flocks and prospects for its control. In: *Emerging Pests and Vector-Borne Diseases in Europe* (eds W. Takken & B.G.J. Knols). Ecology and Control of Vector-Borne Diseases Series, Vol. 1, pp. 227–239. Wageningen Academic Publishers, Wageningen.

Wall, R. & Beynon, S. (2011) Area wide impacts of macrocyclic-lactone parasiticides in cattle dung. *Medical & Veterinary Entomology*, **26**, 1–8.

Wall, R. & Ellse, L. (2011) Climate change and livestock disease: integrated management of blowfly strike in a warmer environment. *Global Change Biology*, **17**, 1770–1777.

Wigglesworth, V.B. (1972) *The Principles of Insect Physiology*. Chapman & Hall, London.

Williams, J.C., Knox, J.W., Sheehan, D. & Fuselier, R.H. (1977) Efficacy of albendazole against inhibited early 4th stage larvae of *Ostertagia ostertagi*. *Veterinary Record*, **101**, 484.

Wilson, A.J. & Mellor, P.S. (2009) Bluetongue in Europe: past, present and future. *Philosophical Transactions of the Royal Society of London Series B Biological Sciences*, **364**, 2669–2681.

Woldehiwet, Z. & Ristic, M. (1993) *Rickettsial and Chlamydial Diseases of Domestic Animals*. Pergamon Press, Oxford.

Zajac, A. M., Conboy, G.A., Little, S.E. & Reichard, M.V. (2012) *Veterinary Clinical Parasitology*. Wiley Blackwell, Oxford.

Zumpt, F. (1965) *Myiasis in Man and Animals in the Old World*. Butterworth, London.

Index

Page references to *Figures* will contain the letter '*f*' following the number, while references to *Tables* will contain the letter '*t*'.

Veterinary Parasitology, Fifth Edition. Domenico Otranto and Richard Wall.
© 2024 John Wiley & Sons Ltd. Published 2024 by John Wiley & Sons Ltd.

amitraz 391, 394, 476
  cattle 476, 478
  dogs and cats 637, 638, 648, 651, 653, 654, 655, 656
  horses 571
  pigs 594, 595
  sheep and goats 532, 536
  see also formamidines
Amoeba buccalis see Entamoeba gingivalis
Amoeba coli see Entamoeba histolytica
Amoeba dentalis see Entamoeba gingivalis
Amoeba gingivalis see Entamoeba gingivalis
Amoebotaenia 130
Amoebotaenia cuneata see Amoebotaenia sphenoides
Amoebotaenia sphenoides 130, 132
Amoebozoa 139
Amphotericin B, 389
Amprolium 387, 397
Ampullaria 105
anaemia 142, 204, 215, 257, 262, 269, 301, 383, 396, 400, 403, 405, 413, 420
  camelids 743
  cattle 420, 427, 428, 433, 439, 440, 444, 446, 447, 449, 450, 451, 452, 453, 454, 455, 456, 458, 463, 472, 474, 478, 480, 481
  deer 733
  dogs and cats 605, 606, 619, 625, 627, 628, 629, 631, 632, 633, 634, 635, 637, 638, 639, 655
  horses 553, 554, 555, 556, 558, 560, 561, 562, 563, 565, 566, 570
  pigeons 815, 818
  pigs 577, 579, 586, 589, 590, 593, 594
  poultry and gamebirds 667, 668, 669, 670, 672, 686, 690, 692, 693, 694, 695, 697, 699, 701, 702, 704
  primates 785, 796, 800
  rabbits 761
  ratites 821, 822
  rats and mice 781
  reptiles 828
  sheep and goats 488, 493, 498, 499, 505, 510, 514, 515, 516, 518, 523, 524, 528, 529, 532, 533, 537
Anaerononadea 159
Anafilaroides rostratus see Oslerus rostratus
anal groove, mites 302
anal shield, mites 279
Analgidae 289–90
Anaplasma spp. 212–13, 235, 389
Anaplasma centrale 213, 456, 729, 738
Anaplasma marginale 213, 314
  camels 738
  cattle 455–6, 480
  deer 728
  dogs and cats 656
  sheep and goats 537
Anaplasma phagocytophilum 212–13
  cattle 456
  dogs 635–6
  horses 564
  sheep and goats 523–4
  small ruminants 457
Anaplasmataceae 212–14
anaplasmosis 355, 356
Anaticola 264
Anatoecus 264
Anatrichosoma spp. 84, 87
Anatrichosoma cutaneum see Anatrichosoma cynomolgi

Anatrichosoma cynomolgi 792
Anatrichosoma nacepobi see Anatrichosoma cynomolgi
Anatrichosoma rhina see Anatrichosoma cynomolgi
Ancylostoma (hookworms) 6, 41, 328*f*, 381, 785
Ancylostoma braziliense 43, 605–6
Ancylostoma caninum 41–2, 43, 44, 604–5
Ancylostoma ceylanicum 43, 606
Ancylostoma duodenale 43–4
Ancylostoma tubaeforme 43, 606
Ancylostomatidae 41–5
Ancylostomatoidea 41
Androlaelaps 300
Androlaelaps casalis (poultry litter mite) 300
Angiostrongylidae 50–2
Angiostrongylus spp. 46, 50
Angiostrongylus cantonensis 50, 779–80
Angiostrongylus costaricensis 50–1, 780–1
Angiostrongylus vasorum 50, 333*f*, 629
Angostrongylidae 46
Anguillula stercoralis see Strongyloides stercoralis
Angusticaecum (Chelonia) 55, 63, 330*f*
Anisakidae 55
Anisakis 55, 63
Anopheles 79, 226, 227
Anoplocephala spp. 126, 279, 327*f*, 380
Anoplocephala magna 126, 552
Anoplocephala perfoliata 126, 551–2
Anoplocephalidae 117, 126–30
Anoplocephaloides mamillana see Paranoplocephala mamillana
Anoplura (sucking lice) 256, 257–61, 257*f*
anteaters 277
anterior station development, trypanosomes 141
anthelmintics
  administration methods 384–5
  camels 733
  cats 631
  cattle 380, 381, 382
    resistance 395
    treatment of whole herd 396
  chemical groups/mode of action 379–83
  combination products 384
  deer 725, 727
  groups 379*t*
  herbal/plant 408
  horses 380, 382
    resistance 395–6
  impact on host immunity 401
  lambs 492
  multiple active products 384–5
  poultry and gamebirds 666, 667, 670, 671, 691, 692
  primates 784, 786, 789
  properties 383–4
  prophylactic use
    cattle 384, 424
    horses 384
    rumen-dwelling boluses 384
    sheep and goats 491–2, 517
  rats and mice 779, 780, 781
  reptiles 824
  resistance
    cattle nematodes 395, 425
    DNA-based diagnostics 346
    horse nematodes 395–6
    management strategies 396
    multiple active agents 384, 385
    non-chemical control 407

  sheep 346, 395, 396
    small ruminants 395
  sheep and goats 396, 490–2, 517
  therapeutic use 384
    targeted selective treatment 380
    treatment of whole herd/flock 396
  water buffalo 745
antibacterials 388–9
  see also antibiotics
antibiotics
  aminoglycoside 389
  for *Cryptosporidium meleagridis* 685
  for *Dictyocaulus viviparus* 436
  ionophore 397
  lincosamide 389
  macrolide 389
  for *Rickettsia rickettsii* 638
  sulfonamide 828
  tetracycline 389
anticholinesterase 386
anticoccidial drugs 387, 388, 389, 396
  antiprotozoal resistance 396
  cattle 431, 454
  chemical 397
  compounds 389, 396, 397, 680, 689
  poultry 672, 673, 680, 681, 688, 689
  rats and mice 777, 778
  resistance 397
  sheep and goats 502
antifolate drugs 386
antigens
  excretory/secretory 404–5
  hidden 405–6
  natural 404
  surface and somatic 404
  see also vaccines
antimonials 385
antiparasitics 379–98
antiprotozoals 379
  administration methods 389, 390*t*
  chemical groups/mode of action 385–9
  resistance 396–7
  use of 389
antitrypanosomal drugs 386
Aonchotheca caudinflata see Capillaria caudinflata
Aonchotheca putorii see Capillaria putorii
Aotiella 263
Apatemon 115, 116
Apatemon gracilis 116
apes 786, 789
  intestinal protozoa 586, 587
  lice 799
  malaria parasites 797
  pinworm 788
  subcutaneous filarial worms 799*t*
Aphodius 132
Apicomplexa 139, 159–95
apodemes, arthropods 217
Aponomma see Amblyomma (Aponomma)
Apophallus spp. 108, 112
Apophallus donicum 108
Apophallus muhlingi 108
apotele, mites 279
appendicular ovipositor, flies 220
aprinocid 387
Apteragia bohmi see Spiculopteragia bohmi
Apteragia quadrispiculata 17
Apteragia spiculoptera see Spiculopteragia spiculoptera

Paramphistomatidae 93, 96*f*, 98–9
Paramphistomum spp. 98, 98*t*, 99*f*, 326*f*
  cattle 419–20
  deer 724
  egg identification 331
  sheep and goats 488
Paramphistomum cervi 98–9, 420, 488
Paramphistomum cotylophoron see Cotylophoron cotylophorum
Paramphistomum explanatum see Gigantocotyle explanatum; Paramphistomum cervi
Paramphistomum fraturnum see Gigantocotyle explanatum
Paramphistomum ichikawa 420
Paramphistomum microbothrium 420
Paramphistomum streptocoelium 420
Paranoplocephala spp. 126
Paranoplocephala cunniculi 126
Paranoplocephala mamillana 126–7, 552
Parascaris spp. 55, 60, 382
Parascaris equorum 60, 327*f*, 383, 395, 550–1
parasitic bronchitis 436
  in adult cattle 438
  postpatent 437
  preventing 438
  reinfection syndrome 438
  see also Dictyocaulus viviparus
parasitic disease, epidemiology 411–18
  acquired immunity, absence of 415–16
  age immunity, absence of 416
  biotic potential 411
  breeds 416
  diapause 412
  effluent, role of 417
  environmental contamination 416–17
  genetic factors, influence of 416
  host species 416
  hypobiosis 412
  immune status of host 411–12
  increased numbers of infective stages 411–12
  infected vectors, role of 417
  livestock 417–18
  mechanical fragmentation 418
  new stock, introduction of 416–17
  nutrition, impact on parasite infections 413–14
  populations of parasite 416
  risk-based and targeted selective treatment 417
  seasonal development 413
  sex 416
  spatial scale 418
  stock management 411, 413
  timing of treatment application 417
  see also infective stages
parasitic gastroenteritis (PGE) 490
Parasitiformes 275
Paraspidodera spp. 55, 64
Paraspidodera uncinata 64, 774
Parastrigea 115, 116
Parastrigea robusta 116
parbendazole 379
Parelaphostrongylus spp. 46, 49
Parelaphostrongylus tenuis 49, 729, 742–3
paromomycin 389
Paronchocerca spp. 77, 84
Paronchocerca ciconarum 84
Paronchocerca struthionis 84
partridges
  antiprotozoals 388

coccidiosis 684
  Eimeria oocysts 179*t*
  parasite checklist 719–20*t*
  see also gamebirds
Paruterinidae 117, 132
parvaquone 386
Passalurus spp. 64, 65
Passalurus ambiguus 65–6, 329*f*, 761–2
pasture(s)
  bioactive forages or nutraceuticals 409
  butterfly route 340
  control 424
  counts of nematode larvae 340
  management
    bovine ostertagiosiis 424
    treatment of whole flock/herd 396
  safe, move to 424
peanut agglutinin-fluorescein isothiocyanate 339, 377
Pearsonema feliscati see Capillaria feliscati
Pearsonema plica see Capillaria plica
Pedicinidae 261
Pediculidae 258, 261
pediculosis 257, 411
  avian 698, 699
  bovine 474, 475*f*
  cattle 474
  dogs and cats 647, 648
  equine 569, 570
  pigeons 815
  pigs 594
  sheep and goats 532
  see also lice
Pediculus spp. 214, 257, 261
Pediculus humanus capitis 261
Pediculus humanus humanus 261
Pelecitus spp. 77, 82
Pelecitus clavus 82, 819
Pelecitus scapiceps 82, 770
Pelodera strongyloides see Rhabditis strongyloides
pentamidine 385, 386
Pentastomida 216, 322
Pentatrichomastix caviae see Hexamastix caviae
Pentatrichomastix robustus see Hexamastix caviae; Hexamastix muris
Pentatrichomonas spp 147, 153
Pentatrichomonas felis see Pentatrichomonas hominis
Pentatrichomonas gallinarum 153
Pentatrichomonas hominis 153, 619, 791
pepper ticks 306
pepsin/hydrochloric acid (HCl) 377
Percolozoa 141
peripylaria 147
peritremes, mites 280
permethrin 390, 391, 394
Peromyscus leucopus (white-footed mice) 307
Persicargas 319
Petroviprocta vigissi see Avioserpens taiwana
Phaneropsolus 108
Pharyngodonidae 66
pheasants
  coccidiosis 387, 683–4
  Eimeria oocysts 178*t*
  parasite checklist 717–18*t*
  see also gamebirds
phenamidine 385
phenathridiums 387–8
phenidium chloride 387
phenol derivatives 381

phenothiazine 383
phenylpyrazoles 391
phenylurea 386
Philophthalmidae 102
Philophthalmus spp. 102
Philophthalmus gralli 102, 695, 822–3
Philopteridae 264–6, 365
Phlebotominae *see* phlebotomine sandflies (Phlebotominae)
phlebotomine sandflies (Phlebotominae) 649
  adult morphology 224–5
  identification 358
  Leishmania transmission 224, 829
  see also Psychodidae (*Phlebotomus*)
Phlebotomus 147, 224–5
  identification 358, 360*f*
Phlebotomus papatasi 224*f*, 358, 360*f*
Phormia spp. 238, 238*f*, 245, 364
Phormia regina 245, 361, 363*f*
Phortica variegata 71
phosmet 390
phospate buffered saline (PBS) 339, 377
phosphoglyceromutase 383
phospholipase C 385
Phthiraptera *see* Psocodea
phylum 1
Physaloptera spp. 66, 75, 76*f*
Physaloptera praeputialis 75–6, 602
Physaloptera rara 75, 76, 602
Physalopteridae 75
Physalopteroidea 75
Physocephalus spp. 66, 67, 68
Physocephalus cristatus see Physocephalus sexalatus
Physocephalus sexalatus 68, 327*f*, 578, 733
pigeon tick *see Argas reflexus* (pigeon tick)
pigeons
  anthelmintics 382
  antiprotozoals 388
  circulatory system parasites 817–18
  coccidiosis 388
  ectoparasites 819–20
  Eimeria oocysts 179*t*
  endoparasites 815–19
  mites 819*t*
  parasite checklist 830–1*t*
  respiratory system parasites 817
  ticks 832*t*
pigs
  anthelmintics 382
  antiprotozoals 387
  circulatory system parasites 589–90
  coccidiosis 388
  connective tissue parasites 592, 593
  digestive system parasites 577–87
  ectoparasites 593–6
  Eimeria oocysts 171*t*, 352*f*, 353*t*
  endoparasites 577–93
  fleas 594–5
  Helminth eggs 327*f*
  integumentary parasites 593
  lice 593–4
  liver parasites 588
  locomotory system parasites 591–6
  metastrongyloidea 46
  pancreas parasites 588
  parasite checklist 597–8*t*
  reproductive/urogenital system parasites 590–1
  respiratory system parasites 587–8